Principles of

Neuropsychopharmacology

Principles of
Neuropsychopharmacology

Robert S. Feldman
University of Massachusetts

Jerrold S. Meyer
University of Massachusetts

Linda F. Quenzer
University of Hartford

Sinauer Associates, Inc., Publishers
Sunderland, Massachusetts

ABOUT THE COVER

The plasma membrane norepinephrine (NE) transporter is responsible for the synaptic reuptake of NE and is a target of several psychoactive drugs, including tricyclic antidepressants
and cocaine. The cover image is an in vitro autoradiogram for which [^{3}H]nisoxetine was
used to localize NE transporter sites in a horizontal section through a 25-day-old rat brain.
Areas showing relatively high transporter densities (red and yellow) include the anteroven-
tral, paraventricular, and lateral geniculate nuclei of the thalamus, the septal nuclei, and the
periaqueductal gray. Note the virtual absence of the transporter in the striatum (blue).
(Autoradiogram by Alison McReynolds and Jerrold S. Meyer, University of Massachusetts.)

Principles of Neuropsychopharmacology

Library of Congress Cataloging-in-Publication Data
Feldman, Robert S. (Robert Simion), 1918–
    Principles of neuropsychopharmacology / Robert S. Feldman, Jerrold S. Meyer,
Linda F. Quenzer.
    p. cm.
ISBN 0-87893-175-9 (hardcover)
1. Neuropsychopharmacology. I. Meyer, Jerrold S., 1947–
II. Quenzer, Linda F. III. Title.
    [DNLM: 1. Psychotropic Drugs—pharmacology. 2. Central Nervous System—
drug effects. 3. Mental Disorders—drug therapy. QV 77.2
F312p 1996]
RM315.F434 1996
615'.78—dc20
DNLM/DLC
for Library of Congress   96-33066
                                                   CIP

Manufactured in the United States of America

10 9 8 7 6 5 4

Brief Contents

Contents

Preface

In 1984, two of us (R.S.F. and L.F.Q.) published *Fundamentals of Neuropsychopharmacology,* which presented in a single volume the basic principles of the study of drugs that influence neural systems and induce changes in behavior. This book is a successor to *Fundamentals,* but it cannot properly be called a second edition because it differs from the previous book in profound ways that reflect the revolutionary changes in the field of neuropsychopharmacology over the last 12 years.

Our goal in writing this new text is to acknowledge and document the tremendous technical advances that have taken place in neuropsychopharmacology without losing sight of the continuing important role played by more traditional neurochemical, pharmacological, and behavioral methods. To accomplish this larger goal, a colleague (J.S.M.) with a deep knowledge of neurochemistry and extensive teaching experience joined us as a third author.

Two major revolutions have occurred in the field since 1984, both driven by the development of new technologies. One is the rise of molecular neuropharmacology: students must now be conversant with an array of methodologies that were unimaginable to earlier generations of pharmacologists. Stunning new techniques in molecular biology have enabled modern researchers to discover novel neurotransmitter receptors, to elucidate the primary structures of receptors without having to purify the receptor protein, to characterize receptor signal transduction mechanisms, to determine how various drug treatments alter receptor gene expression, and to observe how animals respond behaviorally in the absence of a specific receptor or other gene product. The second revolution stems from the growth and refinement of brain imaging techniques, especially positron-emission tomography (PET) and functional magnetic resonance imaging (fMRI), which have permitted, in human subjects, the noninvasive localization of specific brain areas involved in various neuropathological disorders and in the responses to numerous psychotropic drugs.

In a sense, the present book is also revolutionary in its attempt to incorporate these new techniques while addressing all levels of psychotropic drug assessment, from molecular and biochemical characterization, to behavioral effects in animal test paradigms, and finally to clinical applications. Also, because we believe that students should appreciate that science is an evolutionary process in which the great discoveries of today are built upon the brilliant and ground-breaking work of our scientific forebears, most topics are introduced with a historical account of early research in that area.

The breadth of this approach (and, as those familiar with *Fundamentals* will note, the increased length it required) led to our decision to change the book's title to *Principles of Neuropsychopharmacology,* which we feel more accurately captures its wide scope. *Principles of Neuropsychopharmacology* expands on the contents of *Fundamentals* with extensive and up-to-date coverage of all major neurotransmitter systems, as well as completely new chapters on cocaine and amphetamine, nicotine and caffeine, alcohol, mind-altering drugs, and Parkinson's disease and Alzheimer's disease.

First and foremost, *Principles of Neuropsychopharmacology* is intended as a text for courses in psycho- or neuropharmacology at the advanced undergraduate or beginning graduate level, and in schools of medicine or nursing. To make the book accessible to students with less background in chemistry or the life sciences, discussion of each topic progresses logically from simpler to more difficult concepts, and the difficult concepts are carefully explained when introduced. While we believe that our broad approach is a unique and valuable feature, we also recognize that some instructors may not wish to cover all topics we present or may simply not have the necessary time, particularly in a one-semester course. Hence, many chapters are subdivided into relatively self-contained parts, which should facilitate focusing on either molecular–biochemical or behavioral aspects of those chapters. We have chosen to provide extensive citations to both the primary literature and recent review articles, and the book should serve as a handy reference source. Because students, researchers, and practitioners will undoubtedly come to the book from a variety of specialized fields, we have also presented pertinent reviews of basic pharmacology, methods in experimental psychology, neurocytology, neuroanatomy, and some topics in biochemistry.

Throughout each chapter, we have provided the chemical structures of important drugs when they are first mentioned. These structures should serve as a useful reference source for students and researchers alike. Even though we do not discuss structure–activity relationships for every drug depicted, the inclusion of chemical structures is meant to encourage students to compare similarly acting compounds and to relate drug effects to drug chemistry.

The book is organized into four main parts: Part I covers the foundations of the field in chapters on basic principles of pharmacology, pharmacological methods, neuroanatomy, neurocytology, and neurophysiology; Part II deals with the biochemistry of the neurotransmitter systems most pertinent to psychopharmacology; Part III discusses a number of important licit and illicit drugs; Part IV describes several mental illnesses and neurological disorders that are commonly treated with psychotropic drugs.

Achieving the goals we set forth for this volume was most challenging, but we hope that we have succeeded in conveying the excitement we feel about how much has been learned and how much still remains to be understood about how drugs act on the nervous system. We would appreciate any comments you wish to offer about *Principles of Neuropsychopharmacology.* We can be reached by mail at the Department of Psychology, Tobin Hall, University of Massachusetts, Amherst, MA 01003, or by e-mail at pon@sinauer.com.

ROBERT S. FELDMAN

JERROLD S. MEYER

LINDA F. QUENZER

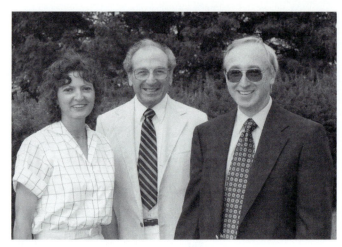

Linda F. Quenzer, Robert S. Feldman, and Jerrold S. Meyer

ACKNOWLEDGMENTS

A book of this kind ultimately represents the efforts of many individuals. We would like to acknowledge the expertise and professionalism of our copy editors, Norma Roche and Elaine Brown. We also wish to thank the staff at Sinauer Associates, particularly our project editor Kerry Falvey, electronic production specialist Janice Holabird, and production manager Christopher Small for their hard work and dedication. Most of all we owe tremendous gratitude to Peter Farley, our editor, for his patience and perseverance despite our many missed deadlines, and for his vision in wanting to make this book the best of its kind. Finally, we would like to thank the following reviewers, whose comments and suggestions contributed importantly to the book:

Rita Balice-Gordon *University of Pennsylvania School of Medicine*

Neil S. Buckholtz *National Institute on Aging*

Marilyn E. Carroll *University of Minnesota*

Steven R. Childers *Bowman Gray School of Medicine*

Adrian J. Dunn *Louisiana State University Medical Center*

Ray W. Fuller Late, *Lilly Research Laboratories*

Monique Garbarg *Centre Paul Broca de l'INSERM, Paris*

Stephen A. George *Amherst College*

John Hannigan *Wayne State University*

Bertha Madras *Harvard Medical School*

James I. Nagy *University of Manitoba*

John W. Olney *Washington University School of Medicine*

Elaine Sanders-Bush *Vanderbilt University School of Medicine*

Ratna Sircar *Albert Einstein College of Medicine*

J. Michael Walker *Brown University*

Michael J. Zigmond *University of Pittsburgh*

Basic Concepts

Chapter 1

Principles of Pharmacology

Pharmacology is the scientific study of the actions of drugs and their effects on living organisms. Neuropharmacology and psychopharmacology are concerned with drug-induced modification of nervous system function and behavior, respectively.

When we speak of **drug action**, we are referring to the specific molecular changes produced by a drug. These molecular changes lead to more widespread alterations in physiological or psychological functions, which we consider **drug effects**. Drugs are incapable of creating new cellular functions; they can only modify existing biological systems by increasing or decreasing their cellular activity. For instance, drugs can increase or decrease heart rate, attenuate anxiety, or reduce pain. Lacking total specificity, drugs almost always have several effects. Amphetamine, for example, increases motor activity, increases heart rate, and decreases appetite.

The distinction between drug action and drug effect is a real one. Some examples will demonstrate that the site of drug action is not necessarily the site of drug effect. Lysergic acid diethylamine (LSD) has an inhibitory action on clusters of nerve cells in the pons and medulla of the brain stem. The effects of this drug action are widespread, including increased heart rate and blood pressure, sweating and chills, sometimes nausea and vomiting, and optical distortions and an exaggerated imagination.

A second example demonstrates that similar drug effects can be initiated by quite different drug actions. Both carbachol and morphine reduce the size of the pupil of the eye. The site of action of carbachol is the nerve endings in the iris. Direct external application of the drug to the eye causes a decrease in pupil size—an effect frequently desired in acute cases of glaucoma. In contrast, application of morphine to the eye has no effect, although morphine administered by injection significantly decreases pupil size (frequently referred to as "pinpoint pupils"). Morphine is known to act on areas of the brain that modify the pupillary response to light. Although both drugs decrease pupil size, the sites of their neurochemical actions are quite different.

Determinants of Drug Action

One goal of neuropsychopharmacology is to find or develop chemical substances that act upon the nervous system in such a way as to alter behavior that has been compromised by injury, disease, or environmental stress. Additionally, neuropharmacologists are interested in identifying the neural substrates of behavior by utilizing chemical agents as probes. These goals can be reached by studying the neurochemical actions of drugs that yield specific behavioral effects. Ultimately, as we shall see, it is the chemical nature of a substance that determines its action. But first, this chapter will describe the variables that determine the characteristics of drug action in general: where a drug acts, how quickly it acts, and for how long it acts.

In the interval between the administration of a drug and a measurable change in nervous system activity and behavior, many intervening processes occur. The drug must be absorbed into the blood and transported to its sites of action, or **target sites**, where it initiates chemical reactions that ultimately may bring about changes in mood, behavior, or thinking. These processes are similar for any pharmacological agent, whether it acts on the brain, the heart, or other organs, and they influence drug action and drug effects. Figure 1.1 diagrams the multiple events that begin with the administration of a drug. The principal processes are listed below, then described in detail later in the chapter.

1. *Routes of administration.* How and where a drug is administered will determine how quickly and how completely the drug is absorbed into the blood.
2. *Absorption and distribution.* Because a drug rarely acts where it initially contacts the body, it must pass through a variety of cell membranes and enter the blood plasma, which transports the drug to virtually all the cells in the body.
3. *Binding.* Once transport has occurred, the drug binds primarily to those cells having particular chemical receptors, which, when combined with the drug, modify the biological activity of the cells. These cells are the drug's target sites. Here the drug may increase or decrease enzyme activ-

ity or alter membrane properties. If these events occur in the nervous system, behavioral changes can result. A drug may also bind to plasma proteins (which usually prevents the drug from leaving the bloodstream), or it may be stored temporarily in bone or fat.

4. *Inactivation.* Drug inactivation occurs primarily as a result of metabolic processes in the liver. The amount of drug in the body at any one time is dependent on the dynamic balance between absorption and inactivation. Therefore, inactivation influences both the intensity and duration of drug effects.
5. *Excretion.* The liver metabolites are excreted with the urine or feces. Some drugs, such as phenobarbital, which is metabolized slowly, are excreted in an unaltered form by the kidneys.

Most of the phenomena discussed in this chapter are not limited to psychoactive drugs, but describe the essentials of drug action in general. Where possible, examples involving behavior-modifying agents will be used. Much more detail regarding these drugs follows in later chapters.

Routes of Administration

The route of administration of a drug determines how much drug reaches its site of action and how quickly the

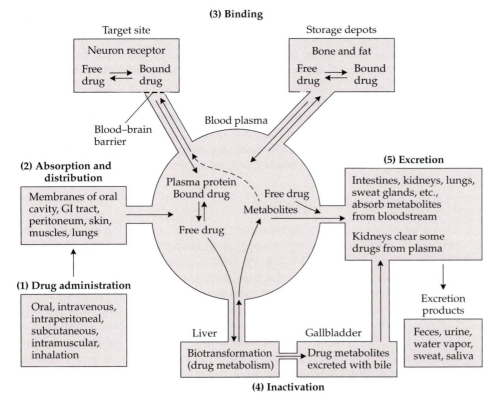

(3) Binding

Target site
Neuron receptor
Free drug ⇄ Bound drug

Storage depots
Bone and fat
Free drug ⇄ Bound drug

Blood–brain barrier

Blood plasma

(2) Absorption and distribution
Membranes of oral cavity, GI tract, peritoneum, skin, muscles, lungs

Plasma protein Bound drug
Free drug
Free drug
Metabolites

(5) Excretion
Intestines, kidneys, lungs, sweat glands, etc., absorb metabolites from bloodstream

Kidneys clear some drugs from plasma

(1) Drug administration
Oral, intravenous, intraperitoneal, subcutaneous, intramuscular, inhalation

Liver
Biotransformation (drug metabolism)

Gallbladder
Drug metabolites excreted with bile

Excretion products
Feces, urine, water vapor, sweat, saliva

(4) Inactivation

1.1 ADMINISTRATION, DISTRIBUTION, AND FATE OF PSYCHOTROPIC DRUGS. After injection into the bloodstream or absorption at the site of administration, the drug molecules are distributed in blood plasma throughout the whole body. Some drugs bind to plasma proteins, maintaining an equilibrium between bound and free drug in the bloodstream. An equilibrium is also maintained between plasma levels of the drug and that stored in bone and fat. Free drug that can pass the blood–brain barrier forms complexes with neuronal receptor sites to initiate drug action. The drug that is circulated in the liver may be metabolized and the metabolites collected into the gallbladder, emptied into the intestines with bile, and excreted with feces. Liver metabolites may also return to the bloodstream to be absorbed by the kidneys, lungs, and sweat glands and excreted, or they may themselves be active agents that stimulate neuronal receptors. The kidneys, as well as the lungs and glands, may clear some drugs directly from the blood plasma.

drug effect occurs. **Intravenous injection (i.v.)** is the most rapid method of drug administration because the agent is placed directly into the blood to be carried to the sites of action. By delivering the drug directly into the blood, the time of passage through cell membranes such as the gastric wall is eliminated. In addition, the amount of drug in the blood is readily controlled, unlike the variable amount resulting from absorption from the gastrointestinal (GI) tract following oral administration. Intravenous administration is used if a rapid effect is required, if the drug would be altered in the GI tract, or if the drug would be irritating if injected into muscle or other tissue. In addition, the drug can be infused slowly over a long time by means of an infusion pump, which maintains a constant blood level of drug over a prolonged period of time. The quick onset of the drug effect is a potential hazard of the intravenous injection method. An overdose or a dangerous allergic reaction to the drug will leave little time for corrective measures, and the drug cannot be removed from the body as it can be, for example, from the stomach by pumping. Also, too rapid a rate of infusion produces a drug mass that may lead to cardiac arrhythmias or arrest, a precipitous drop in blood pressure, depressed respiration, or convulsions. Such catastrophic effects can occur even with chemically inert substances if they are injected rapidly enough. Development of aseptic techniques has reduced the rate of infection following intravenous drug administration in the clinic; however, self-administration of drugs by addicts is the cause of numerous infections such as hepatitis, acquired immune deficiency syndrome (AIDS), and endocarditis. Also, embolism may occur if a particulate suspension is injected or if a precipitate is formed when the drug is placed in the blood.

An alternative to the intravenous procedure is **intramuscular injection (i.m.)**, which has the advantage of slower and more even absorption over a period of time. Drugs that are administered intramuscularly are usually absorbed within 10–30 minutes. Absorption can be further slowed by combining the drug with a vasoconstrictor, such as ephedrine, because the rate of drug absorption is dependent upon the rate of blood flow to the muscle. To provide slow and even absorption and sustained action, the drug may be injected as a suspension in some kind of vegetable oil. Fairly large volumes of drug can be injected into muscle, but intramuscular injection is not appropriate with irritating substances.

In **subcutaneous administration (s.c.)**, the drug is injected just below the skin and is absorbed at a rate dependent on blood flow to the site. In laboratory animals such as rats or rabbits, the drug is injected into the scruff of the neck. Absorption is fairly slow and steady with this method, although considerable variation in absorption occurs even within the same individual. Injection of a drug in a nonaqueous solution (such as peanut oil) or implantation of a drug pellet further slows the rate of absorption. Subcutaneous implantation of drug-containing pellets is most often used to administer hormones. Such pellets release their contents at a rate dependent upon the surface area of the pellet, its rate of erosion, and the solubility of the drug in body fluids. A variation of this method widely used for chronic administration of gonadal steroids to laboratory animals is the implantation of hormone-filled capsules made of silicone rubber tubing, which allows absorption of the hormone over several months. Because this method provides even, sustained delivery of a drug over time without frequent administration, it is also employed to develop tolerance to and dependence on morphine and other drugs in laboratory animals.

The most common method of drug administration to animals is by the **intraperitoneal (i.p.)** route. Intraperitoneal injection deposits the drug in the peritoneum (body cavity), from which it is absorbed into blood capillaries. The absorption of the drug is quite rapid because of the rich vascularization of the peritoneum and the organs within it. Although this is the method most often used with research animals, a certain amount of experimental variability can be attributed to differences in drug absorption depending upon where within the peritoneum the drug is deposited. Intraperitoneal injections are rarely given to humans because of the danger of intraperitoneal infection.

Oral administration is the most popular route for clinical treatment because it is safe, self-administered, and economical. To be effective, the drug must be soluble in stomach fluids, resistant to acid degradation, and able to pass through the stomach wall to reach blood capillaries. In the stomach, low solubility of drug tablets as well as the presence of food will slow absorption. Drugs such as insulin that can be destroyed by gastric acid or by other digestive processes obviously cannot be administered orally. Many drugs are not fully absorbed until they reach the small intestine, whose absorptive characteristics differ from those of the stomach (see below). Food in the stomach slows gastric emptying and thus delays intestinal absorption. Because of these factors, plasma levels of orally administered drugs are often irregular and unpredictable.

Fatty or waxy coatings on orally administered drug tablets may be used to resist degradation in the stomach while allowing disintegration in the intestine. Such preparations are used to reduce stomach irritation, delay the onset of drug effect, or provide a high drug concentration locally in the intestine for optimal effect. Sustained-release preparations are usually multicoated in such a way as to allow the outer layer to dissolve in the stomach for rapid action followed by an inner tablet coated to dissolve at a later time in the intestine for delayed absorption. One danger of such sustained-release medication is that if the rate of release is greater than anticipated in a given individual—for example, due to an uncontrolled dietary factor—a toxic level of drug may occur. Similarly, if the release rate is unexpectedly low, insufficient drug availability may jeopardize treatment. The way the drug is prepared, including types of coatings, particle size, shape of the tablet, proportion of inert substances, and compression of the tablet, also has a significant effect on its ultimate bioavailability.

Several difficulties of absorption following oral administration can be avoided for some drugs by **sublingual administration** (under the tongue). This method provides more rapid, even, and complete absorption than from the GI tract because it uses richly vascularized tissues and avoids the destruction of the drug by gastric substances and liver enzymes. An example of such a drug is nitroglycerin. When a tablet of this substance is placed under the tongue, it is absorbed quickly and acts rapidly to relax the smooth muscles of the cardiovascular system. The muscle relaxation increases the blood supply to the heart muscles, and quickly relieves the pain of angina pectoris. Clearly, neither irritating nor bad-tasting drugs can be administered in this way.

Inhalation is a rapid means of administering gaseous and volatile drugs such as anesthetic gases. Absorption is rapid because the area of the absorbing surfaces, the alveolar sacs in the lung with their rich capillary supply and the mucous membranes of the respiratory tract, is very large. Inhalation is a very effective way of self-administering nicotine, which is released from the smoke of burning cigarette tobacco. Tetrahydrocannabinol (THC), an active ingredient of marijuana, also is rapidly absorbed from the lungs following inhalation of burning-induced smoke. Inhalation in the case of THC is the preferred method for self-administration because oral absorption is slow and little active drug actually reaches the brain through that route because of liver biotransformation. Cocaine is a third example of a self-administered drug frequently taken by inhalation. The smoking of freebase cocaine produces a very rapid rise in blood level and almost instant central nervous system (CNS) effects, which peak in about 5 minutes.

Topical application of drugs to mucous membranes such as the conjunctiva of the eye, nasopharynx, vagina, colon, and urethra generally provides local drug effects. However, some drugs can be readily absorbed into the general circulation from these membranes, leading to widespread systemic effects. Direct application of finely powdered cocaine to the nasal mucosae by sniffing leads to rapid absorption, producing profound effects on the CNS that peak in about 15–30 minutes. Cocaine addicts whose nasal mucosae have been damaged by chronic cocaine "snorting" may resort to applying the drug to the rectum, vagina, or inside the penis.

Although the skin provides an effective barrier to the diffusion of water-soluble drugs, certain lipid-soluble substances are capable of penetrating it slowly. Toxic effects can occur by accidental absorption through the skin of chemicals used in industrial or agricultural environments. Among these potentially hazardous compounds are carbon tetrachloride, tetraethyl lead, and organic phosphate insecticides (e.g., parathion, DFP, and malathion). The development of **transdermal drug delivery** (i.e., through the skin) by means of skin patches has provided a means of controlled and sustained delivery at a preprogrammed rate. The patches consist of either a microporous membrane fixed between the drug reservoir and the skin or a polymer matrix saturated with the drug in high concentration. Transdermal delivery has been used to treat angina pectoris with nitroglycerin, motion sickness with scopolamine, and cigarette craving with nicotine patches.

Special injection methods must be used for some drugs that act on nerve cells because the blood–brain barrier (discussed below) prevents or slows the passage of the drugs from the blood into neural tissue. One special method, spinal anesthesia, is used clinically during childbirth. Anesthetics are administered directly into the cerebrospinal fluid (CSF) surrounding the spinal cord of the mother. Depending on the precise locus of administration, spinal anesthesia may be either epidural, when it is injected into the outer lining of the spinal cord, or subarachnoid, when it is injected between the vertebrae. The extent of the area anesthetized depends upon the amount and strength of local anesthetic injected. In laboratory experiments, a stereotaxic apparatus and microsyringe or cannula are employed to facilitate precise drug injection into discrete areas of brain tissue (**intracranial administration**), into the cerebrospinal fluid–filled chambers, the ventricles (**intracerebroventricular administration [i.c.v.]**) or into the cisterns (**intracisternal administration [i.c.]**). In this way experimenters can study the electrophysiological, biochemical, or behavioral effects of drugs on particular nerve cell groups, especially those that lie in close proximity to the ventricles or the cisterns.

Because the route of administration significantly affects the rate of absorption, plasma levels of the same drug administered by different routes vary significantly. Figure 1.2 shows the rapid rise in plasma level of a drug given intravenously and the rate of decline, which reflects drug metabolism and elimination. A much lower level is achieved after subcutaneous administration of the same drug, but the drug remains in the blood for a longer time. Because absorption in this case is slow, metabolism of part of the active drug can occur before absorption is completed. Thus, no sharp peak occurs, and a lower plasma drug level is maintained over a longer period of time.

The principal goal of any drug regimen is to maintain the plasma concentration of the drug at a constant desired level for the time required. As plasma drug level at any given moment is the result of absorption and degradation (or elimination), one would expect an inconstant level over time. For instance, after oral adminis-

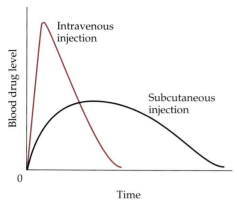

1.2 BLOOD DRUG LEVEL following single intravenous and subcutaneous injections.

tration, the plasma level of a drug that is readily absorbed increases rapidly. As Figure 1.3 shows, drug administration at time A produces a high drug level in the blood (peak 1). Almost immediately, however, the drug begins to disappear from the blood because of metabolism, excretion, or storage at inactive sites, as described below. By time B, the plasma drug level has fallen to one-half the peak 1 value. That rate is expressed in terms of **drug half-life** ($t_{\frac{1}{2}}$) (also known as *half-time*), that is, the time it takes for the plasma drug concentration to fall to half its peak level. During the second half-life the drug level falls to 25%, during the third half-life to 12.5%, and so on, until after 6 half-lives, 98.4% of the drug has been eliminated. For many drugs, the next dose should be administered before the plasma drug level has fallen significantly. For those drugs whose half-life is short, administration must be frequent.

Half-life also determines the time needed to reach steady state plasma levels. For any given daily dose of a drug, the **steady state plasma level** (Figure 1.3, time C) is achieved after a period of time equal to five half-lives. The steady state level is the concentration of the drug in the blood after equilibrium between its absorption/distribution phase and its metabolism/excretion phase is reached. The blood level achieved is directly related to the dose of the drug administered.

One method used to avoid peaks and troughs in drug blood level is continuous intravenous infusion, which is the only method capable of producing stable plasma drug levels. However, subcutaneous pellet implantation is a reasonable substitute and has become technically more sophisticated in recent years. In addition to the development of implantation materials (e.g., silicone rubber capsules) that can release drug at a constant rate for up to 13 months, other researchers have developed implantable infusion pumps that can deliver a constant drug dose to a specific target area intravenously, subcutaneously, or directly into the brain via a cannula and connecting tubing. The osmotic minipumps used frequently in animal research utilize the force generated by an osmotic gradient across a semipermeable diaphragm separating the target tissue from a chamber containing the drug. As water moves into it from the surrounding medium, the drug chamber swells and forces the infusion fluid, now containing drug, out through a delivery port. Of particular interest is the development of a pump that can be implanted under the skin of the scalp and connected with a brain ventricle, which contains CSF. This system has been used to treat meningitis with high concentrations of antibiotics, which normally would not reach the CSF through the blood–brain barrier. Pulsatile administration is possible with pumps that mimic the normal circadian rhythmicity of hormonal surges. For instance, diabetics can adjust the flow of insulin from an external pump to adapt to shifts in glucose levels. Techniques are being developed to provide feedback regulation of such pumps. A sensor element that monitors blood sugar level could regulate the infusion rate of insulin released by an implantable pump, thereby mimicking the body's normal homeostatic control of insulin. As more is learned about the neurochemical basis of neurological and psychiatric disorders, a drug delivery system that can administer drugs to specific and localized sites within the brain may have important potential.

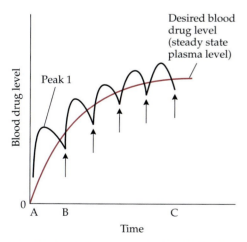

1.3 CHANGES IN BLOOD DRUG LEVEL during repeated administration and continuous infusion. The scalloped line represents the pattern of accumulation during repeated administration (at arrows) of a drug. The shape of the scallop is dependent upon both the rate of absorption and the rate of elimination. The smooth line represents drug accumulation in the blood during continuous intravenous infusion of the same drug.

Drug Absorption and Distribution

Once a drug has been administered, it is absorbed from the site of administration into the blood to be circulated throughout the body and ultimately to the brain, the primary target site for psychoactive drugs. We have already shown that the rate of absorption depends on several factors. Clearly, the route of administration affects absorption because it determines the area of the absorbing surface, the number of cell layers between the site of administration and the blood, the amount of drug destroyed by liver metabolism or extreme acidity (e.g., in the stomach), and the extent of binding to food or inert complexes. Absorption is also dependent on the solubility and ionization of the drug, on drug concentration, and on individual differences in age, sex, and body size.

Effects of Age, Sex, and Body Size

In a general way, the drug dosage required to achieve a desired effect is related to the size of the individual. In studies using laboratory animals, drug dose in milligrams (mg) is based on the number of kilograms (kg) of body weight. However, because drug effects are directly related to the amount of drug reaching the target site, the volume of body fluid is a significant determinant of drug action. For the most part, the larger the individual, the more the drug will be diluted in its larger fluid volume, and less of the drug will reach the target sites in a given unit of time. The sex of the individual also plays a part in determining plasma drug level because in females, the ratio of adipose tissue to body water is greater than in males. Thus, the total fluid volume is relatively smaller in women than in men, producing a higher drug concentration at the target site in women. In obese people as well, a larger fraction of the body weight is fat, so the total fluid volume is a smaller percentage of total body weight. However, the relatively larger adipose pool may sequester lipid-soluble drugs, thereby reducing their target site availability (see the section on silent receptors below). It should be obvious also that the smaller fluid volume of a child means that a standard dose of a drug will be more concentrated at the target site and will produce a greater pharmacological effect.

An important example of these general rules is provided by the action of ethyl alcohol (ethanol), a drug that affects the CNS. The effects of this drug on thinking and behavior (such as instability of gait, slurred speech, and delayed reaction time) are directly related to the plasma level of the drug. It should not be surprising that the effects of the same amount of ethanol will be much different for a 100-pound woman and her 200-pound husband, not only because the mg drug/kg body weight ratio is different, but because fluid/fat ratios also differ between the two. After ingesting 1.0 ounce of pure ethanol (in the form of 2 ounces of spirits or 2 cans of beer), the woman in our example may have a blood ethanol level of approximately 0.090 mg ethanol/100 ml blood. In contrast, under the same conditions, her husband, at 200 pounds, may have a blood ethanol level of 0.037 mg/100 ml. Clearly, these two individuals can expect quite different effects on behavior following the same dose.

Drug Transport across Membranes

Perhaps the single most important factor in achieving therapeutic plasma drug levels is the rate of passage of the drug through the various cell layers (and their respective membranes) between the site of administration and the blood.

Passive diffusion. Passive diffusion is characterized by the movement of a dissolved substance through a biological barrier (a membrane) in a direction from higher to lower concentration. The concentration gradient directs the movement, and no energy is required. An example of this process is the passage of ethanol from intestine to blood. As the ethanol moves from the intestine, it passes into the bloodstream, where its concentration is lower. From there it is circulated in the blood away from the intestine. Thus, the level of ethanol on the blood side of the barrier remains low, and passive diffusion continues at a constant rate. For many drugs, diffusion is that simple, and depends only on the concentration gradient and the blood flow to the absorbing area. However, the selective permeability of membranes prevents many molecules from passively penetrating the membrane barrier, regardless of the concentration gradients that exist. Therefore, passive diffusion also depends upon the drug's molecular shape and weight, its lipid solubility, and its degree of ionization (charge).

Lipid solubility. Membranes have a high lipid content. Lipids are molecules that have the characteristics of fats. Thus, it is reasonable to expect that drugs that are lipid soluble will more readily permeate a lipid membrane, just as oil of turpentine will readily mix with oil-base paint. Conversely, substances that are soluble in water, such as sugar, will not dissolve in oil.

The lipid solubility of a given substance can be estimated in the following way: A radiolabeled drug is mixed with water. The mixture is then added to the same volume of oil, such as olive oil, and again thoroughly mixed. After settling, the oil and water form two distinct layers. The oil floating on top can then be drawn off, and the radioactivity of the oil and the water can be measured separately. The amount of radioactivity in each solvent is directly related to the amount of drug dissolved in that solvent. The concentration of the drug in oil divided by its concentration in water is the oil/water **partition coefficient**. It is the relative affinity of the drug for either oil or water that determines how rapidly it leaves the water in the blood or stomach juices and enters the lipid layers of membranes. The partition coefficient also determines how readily a drug will pass lipid barriers to enter the brain. The abused narcotic drug heroin, for example, is a simple modification of the parent compound morphine. Heroin, or diacetylmorphine, is more soluble in lipids than is morphine and penetrates to brain tissue more readily, thus having a quicker onset of action and more potent reinforcing properties.

The ionization factor. Most drugs are not readily lipid soluble because they are weak acids or weak bases that can become ionized under certain conditions. To facilitate an understanding of the role of ionization in transmembrane diffusion, let us first briefly review some basic concepts in chemistry. We are all aware that some substances dissolve quickly and completely in water, whereas other substances do so slightly or not at all. Thus, water solubility, like lipid solubility, is a relative matter. Water solubility and ionization are associated phenomena because the molecules of soluble substances are formed by ionic bonding of atoms. For example, common table salt (sodium chloride, NaCl) is formed by combining an atom of sodium, which can readily give up one of its electrons (a negative charge), and an atom of chlorine, which can readily accept the negative charge. These bonds are relatively strong in the crystalline state but are weak in water solutions because the dissociated atoms of water (H^+ and OH^-) pull the NaCl molecules apart to form ions. The more soluble a substance, the more easily it can be pulled apart by the dissociated atoms of water. Thus, the sodium atom, having lost one of its electrons, has a net positive charge of 1 (Na^+, a cation), whereas the chlorine atom has, by addition of an electron, a net negative charge of 1 (Cl^-, an anion). Ions are defined as atoms or groups of atoms (molecules) that have gained an electric charge (+ or −) after dissociating from a stable configuration. The extent of ionization of a substance is an intrinsic property of the molecule and depends upon the electron attraction and repulsion of various atoms in the molecule.

Ionization also depends on the acidity or the alkalinity of the solvent, which is expressed as pH. pH is defined as the negative logarithm of the concentration of hydrogen ions (H^+) in solution. Distilled water has a hydrogen ion concentration of 10^{-7} M (0.0000001 moles/liter). This represents a pH level of 7, called neutral because this concentration of H^+ ions equals the concentration of OH^- ions. Acids have a lower pH, signifying a greater concentration of H^+; for example, vinegar has a pH of 2.2 ($10^{-2.2}$ M). Solutions having a greater concentration of OH^- than H^+ ions are called alkaline or basic and have pH values higher than 7. Thus, a saturated solution of magnesium hydroxide [$Mg(OH)_2$] has a pH of 10.5, indicating a relatively smaller concentration of H^+ ions in solution. (Magnesium hydroxide is commonly used as an antacid to neutralize stomach hyperacidity.)

Because transmembrane diffusion of a drug molecule depends upon ionization, which in turn is dependent upon the pH of the solvent, it is important to note that body compartments differ in their pH levels. For example, gastric juice is very acidic (pH 2.0–3.0), whereas the contents of the small intestine may vary in pH from 5.0 to 6.6. Blood is slightly basic (or alkaline) with a pH of 7.4; kidney urine is acidic, its pH varying from 4.5 to 7.0. As will be seen, the differences in pH that exist between these compartments play an important role in drug ionization and translocation from one compartment to another, for example, from the stomach to the bloodstream or from the bloodstream into the kidney urine.

Lipid solubility–ionization interactions. Drugs that are lipid soluble, and hence relatively insoluble in water, also have very little charge; that is, they are largely unionized. Consequently, they mix freely with lipid layers that are nonpolar, which means that they too have no electrostatic charges. In contrast, drugs that are ionized are bound to water molecules by the electrostatic attraction between the drug and water ions and do not readily move from the aqueous to the lipid components of membranes. Because many drugs are either weak acids or weak bases, they are capable of ionizing at a particular range of acidity or alkalinity (pH) of the solvent. The extent of ionization of a drug is expressed as the **pK_a** of the drug. The pK_a is the negative logarithm of the acid dissociation constant and is equal to the pH of the aqueous solution in which that drug would be 50% ionized and 50% un-ionized. Drugs that are weak acids ionize more readily in an alkaline environment and become less ionized in an acidic environment. The reverse is true of drugs that are weak bases. Since the lipid/water partition coefficients are quite different for the ionized and un-ionized forms of the same drug, rates of passage through the lipid membrane will be different for the two forms.

If we put the weak acid aspirin* (acetylsalicylic acid), which has a pK_a of 3.5, into the stomach, we would have the equilibrium

Un-ionized   Ionized

---

*The six-sided ring structure seen in the aspirin molecule is a common feature in many organic compounds found in biological systems as well as in drugs. It is a typical cyclic hydrocarbon because it consists of hydrogen and carbon atoms arranged in a ring. The alternating single and double bonds are not static, but are constantly interchanging. A carbon atom is present at every angle, and a hydrogen atom is attached to the carbon (unless another atom or group of atoms is indicated). There are hundreds of thousands of organic compounds consisting of combinations of these and other rings, some with fewer sides and angles, some with more. Many other atoms, either singly or in chains, can be attached to these rings at the angles.

Table 1.1   Percentage of Weak Acids and Bases Absorbed in One Hour from Rat Stomach at Different pH Levels

	pK_a	pH of Stomach 2–3	~8[a]
Acids			
Salicylic acid (weak)	3.0	61 ± 7	13 ± 1
Benzoic acid (weak)	4.2	55 ± 3	—
Thiopental (very weak)	7.6	46 ± 3	34 ± 2
Secobarbital (very weak)	7.9	30 ± 2	—
Bases			
Acetanilid (very weak)	0.3	36 ± 3	—
Caffeine (very weak)	0.8	24 ± 3	—
Aniline (weak)	4.6	6 ± 4	56 ± 3
Dextrorphan (weak)	9.2	0 ± 2	16 ± 1
Ephedrine (weak)	9.6	3 ± 3	—

[a]This pH level was obtained by treatment with $NaHCO_3$.
Source: After Pratt and Taylor, 1990.

From chemical principles we know that by increasing H^+ (from HCl in the stomach) we drive the reaction to the left, or increase the un-ionized form of the drug. The reduced charge increases the lipid solubility of the drug. Thus, aspirin readily passes through stomach membranes into the blood, which carries it to the target sites where it initiates an action that reduces pain. In the intestine, where the pH is about 5.0–6.6 and the H^+ concentration is lower, the reaction is driven to the right, toward dissociation. The ionization of aspirin in the intestine reduces its absorption through that membrane relative to the amount that is absorbed in the stomach.

Now it should be clear how the pH of the body compartment's fluid and the degree of ionization of the drug determines where relative distribution of the drug occurs. In our example, aspirin in the acidic gastric fluid is primarily in the un-ionized form, and thus passes through the stomach wall into the blood. In the blood (pH 7.4), however, aspirin becomes ionized, and so it is said to be "trapped" within the plasma compartment and does not return to the stomach. In contrast, drugs that are weak bases, such as strychnine, will be more ionized in the stomach, where the pH is low. They will therefore be "trapped" and will not readily pass the gastric wall.

Table 1.1 shows the rate of absorption of selected acids and bases from rat stomach in a 1-hour period. Weak acids, such as salicylic and benzoic, are absorbed well because they are almost completely un-ionized at the low gastric pH. Weak bases, such as aniline, dextrorphan, and ephedrine, tend to be absorbed less well. Note that salicylic absorption is significantly reduced by changing the stomach pH with the addition of sodium bicarbonate ($NaHCO_3$, pH 8), but the absorption of very weakly acidic drugs is not altered because they are almost completely un-ionized even at the more basic pH.

Conversely, the weak bases, which are poorly absorbed from the stomach, are more readily absorbed at pH 8.

Table 1.2 shows the rate of absorption of drugs from rat intestine at various pH levels in a one-hour period. For bases, intestinal absorption increases with pH, while acids show an inverse relationship, that is, less absorption at higher pH.

Recall that other factors also have an influence on drug absorption. For instance, we have shown that any drug meant to be absorbed from the intestine must be resistant to the low pH and the digestive processes in the stomach. Further, despite our earlier emphasis on the importance of ionization, the much greater surface area of the small intestine, as compared with the stomach, provides a much greater opportunity for absorption of weak bases or weak acids. In addition, the passage of orally ingested material through the intestine is much slower than through the stomach, further increasing total absorption time. Thus, the rate at which the stomach empties into the intestine very often is the significant rate-limiting factor. For this reason, medication is often prescribed to be ingested before meals and with sufficient fluid to move the agent through the stomach and into the intestine.

Once the drug has entered the blood, it is carried throughout the body and can act at any number of receptor sites. In general, those parts of the body that are well vascularized will have the highest concentration of drug. The amount of drug reaching each organ is determined by the blood flow through that organ and the rate of passage across the vascular endothelium (i.e., the blood vessel walls), through the interstitial fluid (the fluid filling the extracellular space), and through the cell walls of the organ. High concentrations of lipid-soluble drugs will be found in the heart, brain, kidneys, and liver. As the brain receives perhaps 20% of the blood that

Table 1.2 Percentage of Weak Acids and Bases Absorbed from Rat Intestine at Various pH Levels

		pH of intestinal solution			
	pK_a	3.6–4.3	4.7–5.0	7.2–7.1	8.0–7.8
Acids					
5-Nitrosalicylic acid	2.3	40 ± 0	27 ± 2	<2	<2
Salicylic acid	3	64 ± 4	35 ± 4	30 ± 4	10 ± 3
Benzoic acid	4.2	62 ± 4	36 ± 3	35 ± 4	5 ± 1
Bases					
Aniline	4.6	40 ± 7	48 ± 5	58 ± 5	61 ± 8
Aminopyrine	5	21 ± 1	35 ± 1	48 ± 2	52 ± 2
Quinine	8.4	9 ± 3	11 ± 2	41 ± 1	54 ± 5

Source: Modified from Pratt and Taylor, 1990.

leaves the heart, lipid-soluble drugs are readily distributed to brain tissue. However, because of the existence of the blood–brain barrier, passive diffusion of water-soluble or ionized molecules into the brain is low.

The blood–brain barrier. Because of our primary interest in the effects of drugs on neural tissue, it is important to understand the unique characteristics of drug transport to brain cells. Our first consideration is the special features of the external and internal fluid environments of the brain. There are three fluid compartments that affect the brain. The first is the blood plasma, which is supplied by a dense vascular network that permeates the whole brain so that no nerve cell is farther than 40–50 micrometers (μm, 1 millionth of a meter) from a capillary. This network supplies the major items of sustenance for the brain, such as oxygen, glucose and other sugars, and amino acids. It also carries away carbon dioxide and other waste products. Lipid-soluble or un-ionized substances, including some drugs, readily diffuse through the capillary walls and become part of the neuronal environment.

The second fluid compartment is the cerebrospinal fluid (CSF), which fills the subarachnoid space that surrounds the entire bulk of the brain and spinal cord and fills the cerebral ventricles, the cisternae, the spinal canal, and their interconnecting channels (aqueducts; Figure 1.4). The CSF is manufactured by cells in the choroid plexus, which lines the cerebral ventricles. The CSF is secreted at a constant rate by the epithelial cells of the choroid plexus. The entire volume of CSF is replaced six or seven times per day, while the excess volume is drained through capillaries and the cerebral veins in the subarachnoid space. The composition of the CSF differs significantly from that of the blood plasma in that it is almost devoid of protein. Also, the contents of the CSF remain quite stable, in contrast to the wide fluctuations that occur in the blood plasma. In addition, many substances that diffuse out of the blood and affect other organs in the body do not seem to enter the CSF. This barrier between the brain capillaries and the CSF constitutes the **blood–CSF barrier**.

The third compartment is the interstitial or extracellular fluid (ECF), which exists in the intercellular spaces or channels between the capillaries, glial cells, and neurons. ECF resembles CSF, although differences in chemical composition occur depending on the brain region. The channels containing ECF are open to the flow of the CSF, but there is a major barrier between brain capillaries and the ECF. This barrier is known as the **blood–brain barrier**.

The earliest investigators of the blood–brain barrier believed that its selective permeability was due to tight packing of glial feet around the brain capillaries and the absence of an intercellular space between the capillaries and the neurons. However, these conditions were later found to be due to tissue shrinkage during preparation for microscopic study. Figure 1.5 presents schematic diagrams of the relationships between capillaries, glia, and neurons. Notice that there are sufficient intercellular channels to allow the diffusion of substances directly from capillaries to neurons. Thus, in order to explain the blood–brain barrier, investigators have had to look at morphological features other than glial cells and intercellular spaces. It is now believed that the morphology of brain capillaries provides an adequate explanation for this barrier effect.

Figure 1.6 compares typical nonneural capillaries and capillaries that infiltrate neural tissue. The walls of capillaries are made up of endothelial cells one layer thick (about 1 μm) surrounded by an amorphous mucopolysaccharide matrix called the basement membrane. The latter layer is about 50 nm thick (nm = nanometer: 10^{-9} meter, or 10^{-6} millimeter) and it contributes to the permeability of the capillary. The endothelial layer of a nonneural capillary has small gaps (intercellular clefts) about 9 nm wide between adjacent cells or where the cells circle upon themselves. There are also fenestrae

(a)

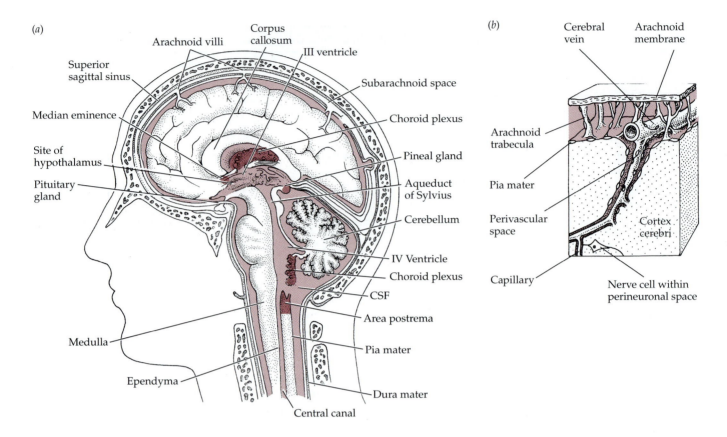

(b)

1.4 DISTRIBUTION OF CEREBROSPINAL FLUID and its relation to larger blood vessels and to structures surrounding the brain (a). CSF is drained into the venous system through the arachnoid villi (b).

(larger openings) about 9–15 nm wide in nonneural capillaries. Through these openings small molecules can pass. In addition, nonneural capillaries have **pinocytotic vesicles** that envelop larger molecules and transport them through the capillary wall. In brain capillaries, the intercellular clefts are closed because the adjoining edges are fused, forming **tight junctions**. Fenestrae are absent, and pinocytotic vesicles are rare. Surrounding brain capillaries are numerous **astrocytic processes**, or **glial feet**, as shown in Figures 1.5 and 1.6, covering about 85% of the basement membrane that fills the gap between the endothelial cells and the glial feet.

It is now apparent how molecules having a molecular weight (mol wt) as large as 20,000–40,000 can equilibrate between blood plasma and the ECF in nonneural tissue in half-lives of 10–30 seconds following an intravenous injection (that is, within 10–30 seconds, half of the molecules have left the blood plasma and entered the ECF). Larger molecules, such as albumin (60,000 mol wt), remain in the blood plasma much longer, with a half-life of several hours. In the brain, however, because of the absence of clefts and fenestrae, even water-soluble molecules with molecular weights as low as 2,000 cannot enter the brain ECF from capillaries.

The chemical composition of the internal fluid compartment of the brain—the CSF and the ECF—must be kept constant relative to the blood plasma in order to maintain the proper functioning of the nervous system. Concentrations of electrolytes and ionic sodium and potassium must be carefully balanced, and an appropriate pH must be maintained. Most organs of the body can function normally during small fluctuations in these factors, but the brain can be adversely affected by any changes that exceed narrow deviations from the norm.

Before we go on, we must emphasize that the blood–brain barrier is selectively permeable rather than impermeable. The barrier reduces diffusion of water-soluble or ionized molecules, but does not impede the passage of lipid-soluble or un-ionized molecules. In addition, water-soluble materials that are moved by specific transport processes (e.g., glucose and other sugars, amino acids) are not impeded by the barrier. (See the section on facilitated diffusion in Chapter 3.)

Finally, the blood–brain barrier is not "intact" along the entire capillary–brain ECF interface. There are places where fenestrae in the capillary endothelium permit proteins and small organic molecules to pass into brain ECF and thus, presumably, to interact with neurons. Examples of these areas (see Figure 1.4) are the **area postrema**, a highly vascularized strip of tissue found in the medulla along the lateral border of the caudal end of the fourth ventricle; the **median eminence** of the hypothalamus; the **choroid plexus**; and the **pineal gland**. The area

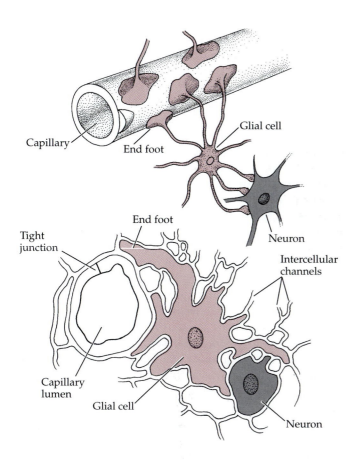

1.5. SPATIAL RELATIONSHIPS OF CAPILLARIES, GLIA, AND NEURONS. The intercellular channels between the cells provide a means for small molecules to pass between capillaries and neurons.

Capillary

End foot

Glial cell

End foot

Neuron

Tight junction

Intercellular channels

Capillary lumen

Glial cell

Neuron

leasing factors access to the hypothalamic/pituitary portal blood system. These peptides, such as corticotropin-releasing factor and growth hormone–releasing hormone, are formed in the hypothalamus and regulate hormone secretion by the anterior pituitary. They are not readily diffusible across endothelial membranes, but can pass through the fenestrae into the blood going to the pituitary (see Chapter 11).

The choroid plexi synthesize and secrete the CSF, which fills the cisternae, the lateral ventricles, and the third and fourth ventricles and surrounds the brain and spinal cord. The fluid substrate for the manufacture of CSF comes from the blood. Waste products from the brain pass into the CSF and then into the blood to be excreted (the so-called "sink" function of the CSF). Close association between the blood and the choroid plexi is critical to the maintenance of both vital functions. Finally, the pineal gland also maintains a close association with blood capillaries. Its role in seasonal changes in reproductive status in some mammalian species requires the release of pineal hormones into the blood. Its responsiveness to environmental changes may require that it also have a blood hormone–monitoring function.

The practical consequence of the limited permeability of the blood–brain barrier is that in order for a systemically administered psychotropic drug to be effective, it must remain un-ionized at plasma pH and must have a fairly high lipid/water partition coefficient. Dopamine and other amine neurotransmitters, for example, do not pass the blood–brain barrier when administered intravenously. However, since the amino acid precursor to

postrema is adjacent to the **chemical trigger zone**, otherwise known as the "vomiting center." Because some toxic substances in the blood are stimuli for vomiting, the freer passage of materials from blood to this area of the brain provides a more efficient coupling of a toxic stimulus and a vomiting response. In the case of the median eminence of the hypothalamus, one known role of the fenestrated capillaries is to allow hypothalamic re-

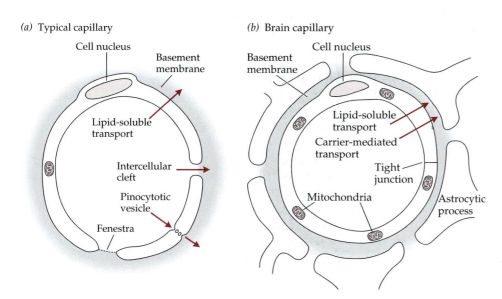

(a) Typical capillary

Cell nucleus

Basement membrane

Lipid-soluble transport

Intercellular cleft

Pinocytotic vesicle

Fenestra

(b) Brain capillary

Cell nucleus

Basement membrane

Lipid-soluble transport

Carrier-mediated transport

Tight junction

Mitochondria

Astrocytic process

1.6 TYPICAL (NONNEURAL) AND BRAIN (NEURAL) CAPILLARIES. In typical capillaries, small molecules can pass by diffusion from the blood through the intercellular clefts to the extracellular fluid. Fenestrae are typically found in these capillaries, through which fluids pass in high volume, as in the kidney. Pinocytosis, though somewhat inefficient, is the mechanism for transporting large molecules. In brain capillaries, intercellular clefts are replaced with tight junctions that block the passage of water-soluble molecules, even of small size; fenestrae are absent and pinocytotic vesicles are rare. (After Oldendorf, 1975.)

dopamine, L-dihydroxyphenylalanine (L-DOPA), can move from the blood to the brain via a transporter mechanism, L-DOPA can be used effectively to treat Parkinson's disease. In other cases, minor differences in drug molecules are responsible for a relative selectivity of drug action. Physostigmine, a tertiary amine, readily crosses the blood–brain barrier and is useful for treating the intoxication caused by some anticholinergic pesticides by increasing the availability of the neurotransmitter acetylcholine. In contrast, the highly charged structure of neostigmine is excluded from the brain and increases acetylcholine only peripherally. Neostigmine is used to treat myasthenia gravis without significant CNS side effects (see Chapter 7).

The placental barrier.   A second barrier unique to mammalian females, called the **placental barrier**, occurs between the maternal vascular system and that of the fetus. The mature placenta contains a network of maternal blood sinuses (cavities) surrounding fingerlike processes (villi) that contain fetal capillaries. Exchange of nutrients, oxygen, and carbon dioxide, as well as various drugs, occurs between the maternal arterial supply to the intervillous spaces and the fetal capillaries in the villi. The membranes separating the two blood systems are similar to other cell membranes in terms of permeability: that is, lipid-soluble substances diffuse easily, water-soluble substances pass less easily depending on their molecular size, and large organic molecules are essentially excluded. The rate of transplacental transfer of many drugs is similar to that between blood and brain; however, the placental membranes are much more permeable to water-soluble molecules than are brain capillaries. Therefore, the potential for transfer of drug from mother to child must be recognized. It is well known that opiates such as heroin readily reach the fetal circulation, and newborn infants of heroin- or methadone-addicted mothers experience many of the signs of opiate withdrawal. Tranquilizers of the phenothiazine and reserpine class pass the placenta and produce characteristic depressant effects in the newborn. Gaseous anesthetics, ethyl alcohol, many barbiturates, and cocaine all readily pass into fetal circulation.

Drug Binding

Depot Binding

High concentrations of drug may be found in various organs that are well supplied with blood. In addition to these reservoirs, drug binding occurs at inactive binding sites where no measurable biological effect is initiated. Such sites, sometimes called **silent receptors**, include those in plasma protein, muscle, bone, and fat. Of the plasma binding sites, the protein albumin is responsible for a significant amount of total binding.

The binding of a drug to inactive sites (**depot binding**) in many cases has a significant effect upon drug distribution. Depot binding may slow the onset of drug action, prolong it, or prevent it from occurring. Depot binding effectively reduces the concentration of drug at its sites of action since only unbound drug can readily pass across membranes. Because bound and unbound drug are in equilibrium, as the unbound drug leaves the circulation, the inactive drug complex in the depot begins to dissociate (unbind) and makes more unbound drug available for diffusion. In the case of a drug that binds readily to silent receptors, the onset of the drug's action at its active sites may be delayed because the effective drug concentration is dependent upon its release from inactive sites. Variation in the amount of depot binding among individuals in part explains the differences in dose required to achieve a therapeutic effect. Some evidence of genetic differences among individuals in the extent of protein binding has been found. Furthermore, certain diseases, such as liver disease, renal failure, and protein-wasting diseases, including cancer, significantly alter the amount of albumin in the blood and consequently modify the amount of depot binding.

Serum albumin is a natural carrier of free fatty acids in plasma, but the same binding sites show varying affinity for many drugs. Since binding to albumin is rather nonselective, many drugs with similar physicochemical characteristics compete with one another and with endogenous substances for these sites. The competition may lead to much higher than expected free drug blood levels of one of the drugs. The elevated drug level may be responsible for increased therapeutic effects, increased toxicity, or an increased rate of biotransformation and excretion. Since many psychotropic drugs, including the antidepressant imipramine, the tranquilizer diazepam, and the antiepileptic drug phenytoin, show extensive plasma protein binding, the competition for silent receptors is an important consideration when evaluating potential drug interactions.

Depot binding also explains why small doses of some drugs initially produce very little effect. Once these sites have been filled, plasma drug levels and therapeutic effects more closely reflect the dose administered. An example of this occurs with the drug chloroquine, which is used to counteract the malaise associated with malaria. Since chloroquine readily binds to receptors in the liver, the liver sites must be saturated before a plasma drug level effective in treating malaria can be attained.

Because bound drug cannot be altered by liver enzymes, depot binding may also prolong drug action. As the unbound pool of drug is eliminated from the body, the equilibrium is maintained by increased dissociation of drug from the inactive sites to enter the circulation and replenish some of the drug that is lost by metabolism and excretion. In contrast, a drug may form inactive complexes so readily and be released into the blood so slowly that an effective plasma concentration is never achieved, preventing any drug action from occurring.

The depots may also be responsible for terminating a drug's action, as in the case of barbiturates, which are CNS depressant drugs. Thiopental, a barbiturate used for intravenous anesthesia, is highly lipid soluble and readily passes from the blood to various tissues. The rapid onset of the drug's effects after intravenous infusion is due to its rapid entry into the brain while the blood level is still very high. Its effect is of very short duration, however, because the blood level falls rapidly as a result of distribution of the drug to other tissues. As the blood level falls, thiopental moves from the brain to the blood to maintain equilibrium. High levels of thiopental can be found in the brain 30 seconds after intravenous infusion. However, within 5 minutes, brain levels of the drug drop to threshold anesthetic concentrations. Within 30 minutes of administration, the brain may give up as much as 90% of the initial peak concentration to various inactive binding sites such as muscle and fat (Harvey, 1985). In this way, thiopental induces sleep almost instantaneously, but is effective for only about 5 minutes, followed by rapid recovery.

These examples emphasize several of the pharmacological factors contributing to the final drug effect. Thus far, we have considered what happens to the drug between administration and binding to an active receptor at the target tissue. Of importance are (1) the route of administration, (2) factors that regulate the passage of drug across cell membranes and through various fluid compartments, and (3) binding of drug to inactive sites ("silent receptors"). In the next section we explore the relationship of the drug to its site of biological action.

Receptor Binding

A **receptor** is a molecule, usually a protein, that is present on the surface of or within a cell and which is the initial site of action of a biologically active agent. Modern biochemical and molecular biological techniques have made possible the purification and characterization of many of the receptors for psychoactive drugs. A discussion of receptor labeling techniques and kinetic analysis of binding is presented in Chapter 2.

While several types of receptors are now known, the ability to recognize specific endogenous chemical messengers is a characteristic of all of them. The often-used analogy of a lock and key suggests that only a limited group of neurochemicals or hormones can bind to a particular receptor protein to initiate or mediate a cellular response. Molecules that have the best chemical "fit" (i.e., have the highest affinity for the receptor) tend to produce the greatest response from the cell. The relationship between drug, receptor, and pharmacological effect can be inferred from analysis of the dose–response curve, as described in the following sections. A second common feature of receptors is that the binding of a specific ligand (molecule) to the receptor produces a physicochemical transformation of the receptor protein molecule that alters subsequent cellular events.

Of the various types of receptors, those found on the cell surface are most often studied by neuropharmacologists. Neuronal receptors embedded in the cell membrane bind neurotransmitters or drugs that mimic or block the actions of neurotransmitters. For example, pilocarpine mimics the action of acetylcholine on the receptors of the cells of the salivary glands and thereby causes salivation, whereas atropine blocks those receptors and causes a dry mouth. The majority of these chemical messengers are relatively polar compounds and cannot easily enter the cell. For this reason, receptors on the cell surface are responsible for transducing the message from outside the cell to bring about changes in intracellular enzymatic processes or ion permeability. Which of the many intracellular changes occurs depends upon whether the receptor is coupled to a specific ion channel or to a second messenger (see Chapter 5).

The second general type of receptor is found within the target cell, in the cytoplasm for some classes of receptors (e.g., for the glucocorticoids) or in the nucleus for other classes (e.g., for the sex steroids). Most of the hormones that act on the brain to influence neural events utilize this type of receptor. The hydrophobic characteristic of some hormones (e.g., sex steroids) allows them to cross the cell membranes readily. For other hormones, special transport mechanisms must be assumed. Hormonal binding to intracellular receptors alters cell function by triggering changes in the expression of the genetic material within the nucleus. Changes in gene expression produce differences in protein synthesis that mediate the hormone's cellular effects. Molecular biological research has begun to unravel how the hormone–receptor complex alters gene expression (see Pratt and Taylor, 1990). Sex hormones act in this way to facilitate mating behavior and other activities related to reproduction.

Law of Mass Action

Once a drug has reached a specific tissue receptor, in the simplest case, the response is proportional to the fraction of receptors occupied at any given moment. Binding usually is a dynamic state, with drug molecules constantly binding to and breaking away from receptor molecules; in other words, the binding is reversible. The classic **law of mass action** best sums up drug–receptor interaction:

$$D + R \rightleftharpoons DR^* \rightarrow \text{biological effect}$$

The law says that the drug (D) and free receptors (R) must combine to form an active complex (DR*), which leads to a cellular response in proportion to the fraction of receptors occupied. The active form (DR*) is in equilibrium with the inactive components (D, R); that is, the drug associates with the receptor and then dissociates. The reversibility of drug–receptor interactions indicates that covalent chemical bonds ordinarily are not formed between the two molecules. Rather, the binding may involve a complex product of several types of weaker, noncovalent interactions. These include **ionic** or **electrostatic** interactions in which bonds form between charged groups on the drug and the receptor; **hydrogen bonds**; and **hydrophobic interactions** mediated by van der Waals forces. Although a complete discussion of these molecular interactions is beyond the scope of this chapter, the interested reader will find pertinent information in any text on general chemistry.

Dose–Response Relationships

From the law of mass action (D + R $\rightleftharpoons$ DR*) and elementary chemistry, we know that, with receptor number (R) held constant, when we increase the concentration of drug (D), we drive the reaction to the right, forming greater amounts of drug–receptor complex (DR*) and attaining greater effect. A **dose–response curve**, which describes the amount of biological or behavioral effect (response) for a given drug concentration (dose), is shown in Figure 1.7. With increasing drug concentration (which, in turn, increases the amount of DR* complex) there is an increase in biological or behavioral effect until the maximum effect is achieved. This maximum is achieved when receptors are fully occupied, except when **spare receptors** are present.

If we were to graph the effects of a family of drugs with similar molecular structure, we would expect a relationship similar to the one shown in Figure 1.7. That figure shows the dose–response characteristics for hydromorphine, morphine, and codeine—all drugs from the opiate analgesic class that reduce pain. For each drug, increasing the dose produces greater analgesia (elevation in pain threshold) until the maximum response is achieved. The differences among the three drugs at any arbitrarily selected fixed dose indicate their potency. For example, at 10 mg (dotted line), the analgesic effect of hydromorphine is maximal. The same dose of morphine produces a much smaller elevation in the pain threshold, and a 10 mg dose of codeine produces no measurable analgesic effect. Even at ten times that dose (100 mg), codeine does not produce its maximal effect. Because of this difference, we would say that hydromorphine is more potent than morphine, and each is more potent than codeine. **Potency** is determined by the accessibility of the drug to the receptor and the affinity of the drug for the receptor, as well as the efficacy of the drug at the receptor. Efficacy refers to the percentage of maximal change elicited when the drug binds to the receptor. For a further discussion of affinity and efficacy, see the section on receptor binding in Chapter 2.

Despite the great differences in potency among the three opiate drugs in Figure 1.7, their maximum effectiveness is the same. A large amount of codeine will be

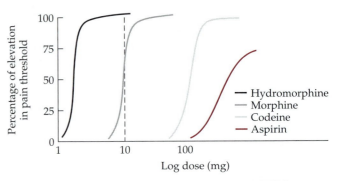

1.7 DOSE–RESPONSE CURVES FOR FOUR ANALGESIC AGENTS. Each curve represents the increase in the pain threshold (the magnitude of painful stimulus required to elicit pain) as a function of dose. (After Levine, 1983.)

as effective as either of the other drugs administered at a lower dose. The fact that the curves are identical in shape and approach the same maximum suggests that the drugs act at the same receptor. When we look at the dose–response curve for aspirin (see Figure 1.7), we see that it is not parallel to the other three and does not reach the same maximum regardless of how high a dose is administered. Although aspirin also reduces pain, it acts on a different receptor and works by a different mechanism.

Assuming that accessibility of the drug to the receptor and the structural specificity of the receptor determine the relative potency of a family of drugs, we can infer from the previous example that hydromorphine more readily reaches the opiate receptor and fits it more closely than does morphine. A minor molecular modification of morphine produces codeine, which shows less effectiveness in lowering pain. Chemists have synthesized a wide variety of morphinelike painkillers, hoping to produce a drug that is more effective than morphine.

Drugs are absorbed and distributed throughout the entire body, where multiple sites of action (receptors) mediate different biobehavioral effects. Furthermore, receptors for the same drug in different target tissues may not have identical characteristics. For this reason, there is a unique dose–response curve for each biobehavioral effect a drug produces. This multiplicity reflects the various receptors acted on by the drug. It should not be surprising that the order of potency for structurally similar drugs is not the same for every biobehavioral effect. Thus, we may see a distinct family of curves for each response we are measuring. Table 1.3 shows the multiple effects of several drugs in the xanthine class: caffeine, theophylline, and theobromine. Notice that the order of potency for the three drugs in stimulating the CNS is caffeine > theophylline > theobromine. In contrast, when cardiovascular stimulation is measured, theophylline (which is found in tea) is more potent than either of the other two, whereas caffeine (found in coffee) stimulates the cardiovascular system least.

Table 1.3 Relative Biological Activity of the Xanthines

Biological Effect	Caffeine	Theophylline	Theobromine
CNS and respiratory stimulation	1	2	3
Cardiac stimulation	3	1	2
Coronary dilation	3	1	2
Smooth muscle relaxation	3	1	2
Skeletal muscle stimulation	1	2	3
Diuresis	3	1	2

[a] 1 = most active; 3 = least active.
Source: After Ritchie, 1975.

Side Effects and the Therapeutic Index

Among the multiple responses to a drug, some are undesirable or even dangerous; these are known as **side effects**. The therapeutic usefulness of a drug must be balanced against the extent of its side effects. For instance, amphetamine-like agents may be prescribed for short-term weight reduction because they significantly reduce appetite, but because they also stimulate the CNS, a major side effect is sleeplessness. Under other conditions, for example, in the treatment of narcolepsy (an illness characterized by uncontrolled, sudden lapses into sleep), the stimulating properties of amphetamine are the desired therapeutic action, while loss of appetite in the treated individuals may be a serious side effect. A discussion of side effects reemphasizes the fact that drugs have neither a single site of action nor a single biobehavioral effect. Drugs that act on the CNS also have potent peripheral effects if the appropriate receptors are present. For instance, amphetamine acts on the CNS, causing alertness, hyperactivity, and appetite suppression, but in addition, it stimulates the sympathetic nervous system, causing cardiac arrhythmias and hypertension as well as dry mouth, diarrhea, and a host of other changes. Recall, however, that not all drugs that have peripheral effects act on the CNS because the blood–brain barrier effectively excludes many chemicals from neural tissue.

In a therapeutic situation, the extent of disagreeable or harmful side effects must be carefully considered. Figure 1.8 depicts the curves for two distinct pharmacological effects of drug A, which is prescribed to induce sleep. The solid curve shows the percentage of individuals who fall asleep at various doses of the drug. The colored curve shows the percentage of persons who suffer respiratory depression from various doses of the same drug. Comparing the dose at which 50% of the people fall asleep (**effective dose 50, or ED_{50}**) with the dose at which 50% show respiratory depression (**toxic dose 50 = TD_{50}**), it can be seen that for most individuals, the toxic dose is several times higher than the dose producing the desired effect. Therefore, pharmacologists would say that the drug has a relatively favorable **therapeutic index (TI)**, which is the ratio of the TD_{50} to the ED_{50} (TI = TD_{50}/ED_{50}). In other words, the drug in this case is fairly safe. In contrast, drug B has an unfavorable TI because the TD_{50} is not very different from the ED_{50}. Thus, there is a small margin of safety and a danger of serious side effects for many people who might use the drug.

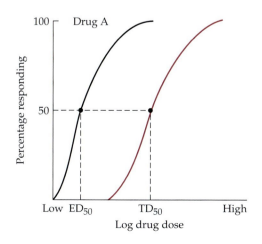
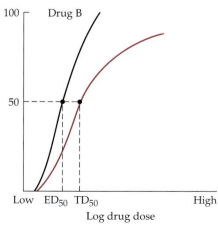

1.8 DRUGS WITH HIGH AND LOW THERAPEUTIC INDICES. Comparisons between the dose–response curves for an effective dose (sleep induction, black curve) and a toxic dose (respiratory depression, colored curve) for two drugs. For drug A, the difference in average dose for the two effects (ED_{50}, TD_{50}) is large enough for the drug to be considered fairly safe. This is not true of drug B.

Another way of assessing safety of a drug is to compare the ED_{50} with the **lethal dose 50 (LD_{50})**, the dose that will kill 50% of the animals tested (usually mice). In this case the TI would be LD_{50}/ED_{50}. To ensure the safety of drugs even more, some pharmacologists propose that the TI should be the ratio of the dose that kills 1% of the subjects (LD_1) to an ED_{99}. Using the formula LD_1/ED_{99}, a drug with a favorable TI would almost certainly be safe. An example of such a drug is aspirin, which is freely available without medical regulation. Even so, regardless of the TI, there are frequent poisonings and occasional deaths following overdoses of aspirin, especially among children.

In drug therapy, potential benefit must clearly outweigh potential hazard. For this reason, given a choice of drugs, the drug with the higher TI would be used. However, in a case in which there is no alternative to a drug, one must ask whether the disorder being treated is sufficiently severe or life threatening to warrant the risk of medication with possible toxicity. This question is especially relevant for psychotropic drugs because chemotherapy for some psychiatric illnesses is often accompanied by disabling side effects (see Chapter 18).

Receptor Antagonists

Thus far, the picture of drug–receptor interaction presented here has been quite simple. However, few drugs follow these simple rules. Some drugs bind to receptors but fail to initiate an intracellular effect. These drugs are called **antagonists** because, although they have no effect per se, they can effectively block the action of a neurotransmitter or an **agonist**, a drug that binds to the same receptors as the neurotransmitter and *does* initiate intracellular changes. Thus, we might modify the law of mass action to include a role for antagonists, such that:

for agonists: $D + R \rightleftharpoons DR^* \rightarrow$ biological effect

for antagonists: $A + R \rightleftharpoons AR \rightarrow$ no biological effect

While most antagonists follow the principle of reversible binding described previously for agonists, other antagonists may have a very great affinity for the receptor and form almost inseparable bonds. These **irreversible antagonists** leave receptors inoperative for a long time, or even permanently. In the case of those antagonists considered irreversible, recovery of function is possible only after the cells synthesize new receptors to take the place of the ones that have been inactivated. An irreversible antagonist may be used therapeutically when a long-lasting blocking effect is desired.

An important distinction between antagonists can be made based on their specificity for the receptor. **Competitive antagonists** bind to the same receptor as the neurotransmitter or active drug and can be displaced from those sites by an excess of the agonist. In this case the potency of the agonist is largely dependent upon the concentrations of each agent. Recall that this follows the law of mass action, such that

$$D + A + R \rightleftharpoons DR^* + AR$$

The effect of the competition between the two agents for a fixed quantity of receptor is to reduce the rate of formation of the active drug–receptor unit. The ratio of drug–receptor interaction (DR^*) to the total possible number of molecule–receptor interactions ($DR^* + AR$) is directly proportional to the ratio of the amount of drug (D) to the total amount of free drug plus free antagonist (D + A).

$$\frac{D}{D+A} \; \alpha \; \frac{DR^*}{DR^* + AR}$$

Figure 1.9a illustrates the effect of a competitive antagonist (naloxone). The black line shows a typical dose–response curve for the analgesic effect of morphine on rats as measured by the hotplate test. This test measures the latency of response to the application of a thermal stimulus to the feet (see Chapter 2). When the rats were pretreated with an intraperitoneal dose of 10 mg of naloxone per kg of body weight, the dose–response curve shifted to the right, demonstrating that for any given dose of morphine, the naloxone-pretreated rats showed less analgesia. The addition of naloxone diminished the potency of morphine. Figure 1.9a also shows that the inhibitory action of naloxone was overcome by increasing the amount of morphine administered; that is,

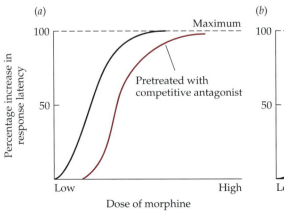

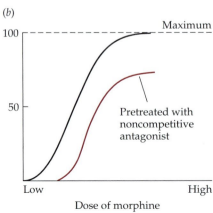

1.9 COMPETITIVE AND NONCOMPETITIVE DRUG ANTAGONISM. (*a*) The effect of a competitive antagonist (naloxone) on the analgesic effect of morphine. Pretreatment with naloxone decreases the potency of morphine, as shown by the shift of the dose–response curve to the right. The maximum effect of the drug can still be achieved by increasing the dose of morphine. (*b*) Pretreatment with a noncompetitive antagonist not only decreases the potency of the drug, but the antagonism cannot be entirely overcome by increasing drug dosage.

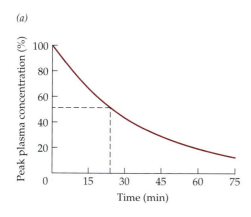

(a)

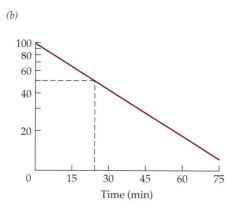

(b)

1.10 DRUG CLEARANCE CURVES. Exponential clearance of intravenously administered penicillin from the bloodstream of a dog. (*a*) The half-life (dashed line), which represents the time required for clearance of 50% of the peak drug concentration, is 25 minutes. (*b*) The drug clearance curve can be linearized by plotting on a semilogarithmic scale.

the same maximum effect (analgesia) was achieved, but more morphine was required. Because the competitive antagonist binds to the same receptors as the active drug, it is assumed that a higher concentration of active drug can compete more effectively for the fixed number of receptors.

A **noncompetitive antagonist** cannot be overcome by increasing the amount of agonist (Figure 1.9*b*). In this case, not only is the dose–response curve shifted to the right, but the maximum effect achieved is also reduced. The reduction of the maximum response occurs because no amount of agonist can fully restore function in the presence of the antagonist. A noncompetitive antagonist may act on a cell in such a way as to prevent agonist–receptor coupling. Alternatively, the antagonist may bind to the same receptor as the active drug, but at a different site on the molecule. An example of this has been discovered for the NMDA receptor, which is one type of receptor used by excitatory amino acid neurotransmitters such as glutamic acid (see Chapter 10). NMDA receptor functions are stimulated when glutamic acid or a related agonist molecule binds to the receptor. These functions are antagonized in the presence of phencyclidine (PCP), an abused dissociative anesthetic drug, despite the fact that PCP does not appear to interact with the agonist binding site. This finding suggests that PCP and related drugs bind to a separate site on the NMDA receptor to block its activity. In addition, a noncompetitive antagonist may act at an entirely different site along the neural pathways mediating the final response so that the agonist is simply incapable of displacing the antagonist. Noncompetitive antagonists may be reversible; that is, removal of the antagonist restores the system to normal. In other cases, they can be irreversible, in which case synthesis of new receptors is required before full functioning can occur.

Drugs may also be mixed agonist–antagonists. These agents possess some of the same pharmacological effects as an agonist, but when administered together with that agonist, reduce the agonist's potency. One such drug is nalorphine, which has some analgesic action and produces certain autonomic effects resembling those produced by morphine. However, it is not constipating,

and tends to produce dysphoria (unpleasant feelings) rather than euphoria. If nalorphine is given with morphine, it reduces the analgesia as well as the morphine-induced autonomic effects (vomiting, pinpoint pupils, drowsiness, etc.). Further discussion of mixed agonist–antagonists and their relationship to drug receptors can be found in the chapter on opiates (Chapter 12).

Drug Inactivation and Elimination

Drug Clearance

Drugs are eliminated from the body by the concerted action of several mechanisms, beginning with metabolism of the drug and ending with excretion of the metabolites that have been formed. One of the most common methods of assessing the rate of elimination of a drug is to measure the clearance of the drug from the blood plasma once a peak drug level has been established. With repeated blood sampling, the decline in plasma drug concentration provides a direct index of the clearance rate. Drug clearance is usually exponential, which in practical terms means that a constant fraction of the drug is removed in each time interval.

To give an example, the half-life of intravenously injected penicillin in a dog is approximately 25 minutes. In other words, 25 minutes (1 half-life) after the peak plasma penicillin concentration has been reached, the drug concentration is reduced to about 50% of its initial value (Figure 1.10*a*). After 50 and 75 minutes (i.e., 2 and 3 half-lives) have elapsed, the concentration is reduced to 25% and 12.5%, respectively. The half-life of a drug can be estimated most accurately by linearizing the clearance data using a semilogarithmic plot (Figure 1.10*b*).

Drug Metabolism

Most drugs are chemically altered by the body before they are excreted. These chemical changes can occur in many tissues and organs, including the intestine, the plasma, the kidney, and the brain. However, the greatest number of the chemical changes that we call drug metabolism or biotransformation occur in the liver. Biotransformation of a drug usually produces one or more inactive metabolites that are excreted more readily than the parent drug. In some instances liver metabolism produces an active metabolite from an inactive drug. An example of this occurs with tremorine, which is converted to oxotremorine in the liver. When injected into mice, tremorine produces shaking and tremors of the whole body. However, if tremorine is administered along with a metabolism inhibitor, no tremors occur.

In some cases, a variety of metabolites are formed from the same compound. One such drug is diazepam (Valium)*. This commonly used tranquilizer is metabolized into a large number of compounds, some of which are active tranquilizers themselves and others that are inactive metabolites. In this case, the formation of active metabolites helps to explain the long duration of the drug's potent antianxiety effects.

The ability of an enzyme to alter a drug is dependent on the formation of an enzyme–drug complex, which may be described as

$$E + D \rightleftharpoons E \bullet D \rightarrow P + E$$

where E = enzyme; D = drug; E • D = enzyme–drug complex; and P = products of metabolism.

This formula is another example of the law of mass action and is very much like the drug–receptor interaction described earlier. In fact, one might consider an enzyme to be another type of receptor with a degradative effect. Many of the principles of enzyme–drug interaction are similar to those of receptor activity. In general, both are described by the law of mass action. In particular, enzymes and drugs combine in a reversible fashion, and the bonds formed are primarily ionic (electrostatic) bonds. Further, the drug–enzyme complex initiates a sequence of events that lead to an end product. Also, although enzymes usually show some specificity based on the conformation of "active sites," their specificity is not absolute. While an enzyme can act on drugs that are structurally similar to a naturally occurring substrate, some enzymes show very little specificity and can metabolize a wide variety of compounds. The lack of specificity of some enzymes is the basis for many instances of cross-tolerance among drugs (discussed in later sections). There are two principal ways in which a drug molecule can be modified: **synthetic reactions** and **nonsynthetic reactions**.

Synthetic reactions.   Synthetic reactions, also called **conjugations**, involve the chemical coupling of the drug with some molecule provided by the body. An enzyme acts as a catalyst for the coupling reaction. The catalytic activity of an enzyme is characterized by the fact that the enzyme is required for the reaction to occur, but no part of the enzyme molecule itself is incorporated into the new product. As the formula in the preceding section shows, the enzyme–substrate interaction produces products of metabolism plus unaltered enzyme, which can rebind to new unmodified drug.

The products of synthetic reactions are most often more water soluble and less lipid soluble than the parent drug, and therefore more likely to be excreted through the kidney. Usually the end product is pharmacologically inactive. The chemical groups on the drug that provide sites for conjugation are carboxyl (COOH), hydroxyl (OH), amino (NH$_2$), and sulfhydryl (SH). In order for conjugation to occur, one of these groups must be present. Drugs that have no site for conjugation may undergo a nonsynthetic reaction before undergoing a synthetic reaction. Drugs that have multiple sites for conjugation will produce a variety of metabolites, depending on the sites altered.

The most common synthetic reaction is conjugation with glucuronic acid, C$_6$H$_{10}$O$_7$, an acid derived from glucose. Aspirin (acetylsalicylic acid, Figure 1.11), for example, is first converted to salicylic acid by hydrolysis, a nonsynthetic reaction in which the molecule is cleaved by the addition of water (step 1). It can then undergo conjugation with glucuronic acid (step 2) at one of two sites, forming two different metabolites. Both of the glucuronide-modified molecules produced are highly water soluble and ionized and therefore are rapidly excreted by the kidneys. It should also be mentioned that salicylic acid can undergo a variety of other metabolizing reactions at the same sites—for example, conjugation with glycine—and form other metabolites.

It is important to recognize that salicylic acid is an active metabolite of aspirin. In fact, aspirin was derived from salicylic acid for systemic use because the latter is extremely irritating and can be used only externally. If the nonsynthetic metabolism of aspirin were inhibited, its painkilling effects would be greatly reduced. If the conjugation with glucuronic acid were inhibited, the analgesic effect of salicylic acid would be prolonged. Clearly, drug metabolism can produce active or inactive metabolites.

In other synthetic reactions, other chemical molecules are attached at the conjugation sites. Among the most common additions are two amino acids (glutamine and glycine) and sulfate. In addition, both acetylation and methylation are conjugation reactions, in which an

---

*A drug that is sold commercially, either by prescription or over the counter, has a chemical name that indicates its chemical composition, a generic name that is a much shortened form of the chemical name but still can be unique for it, and one of many trade names. For example, the popular antianxiety drug known by the trade name Valium (always capitalized) has a chemical name, 7-chloro-1,3-dihydro-1-methyl-5-phenyl-2H-1,4-benzodiazepin-2-one, and a generic name, diazepam. Sometimes a generic name is so widely recognized that it is also used as a trade name. Acetylsalicylic acid, for example, is known almost solely by its generic name, aspirin. In fact, almost all chemical compounds have a generic name, such as salt, lime, milk of magnesia, and penicillin.

acetyl group (O=C—CH$_3$) and a methyl group (—CH$_3$) are added, respectively.

Nonsynthetic reactions. Nonsynthetic reactions are those in which the parent drug is modified by oxidation, reduction, or hydrolysis. These reactions differ from conjugation in several respects. The products of these reactions are not necessarily inactive and, in fact, may be more active than the parent drug. In general, drugs that undergo nonsynthetic reactions are not eliminated from the body without undergoing a conjugation reaction in a second step. In the example of aspirin metabolism above (see Figure 1.11), the first step is a nonsynthetic hydrolysis. The product of that step, salicylic acid, is as active as the parent compound. Like conjugation reactions, nonsynthetic reactions are dependent on the presence of an appropriate chemical group, but the presence of the group does not guarantee that a particular nonsynthetic reaction will occur.

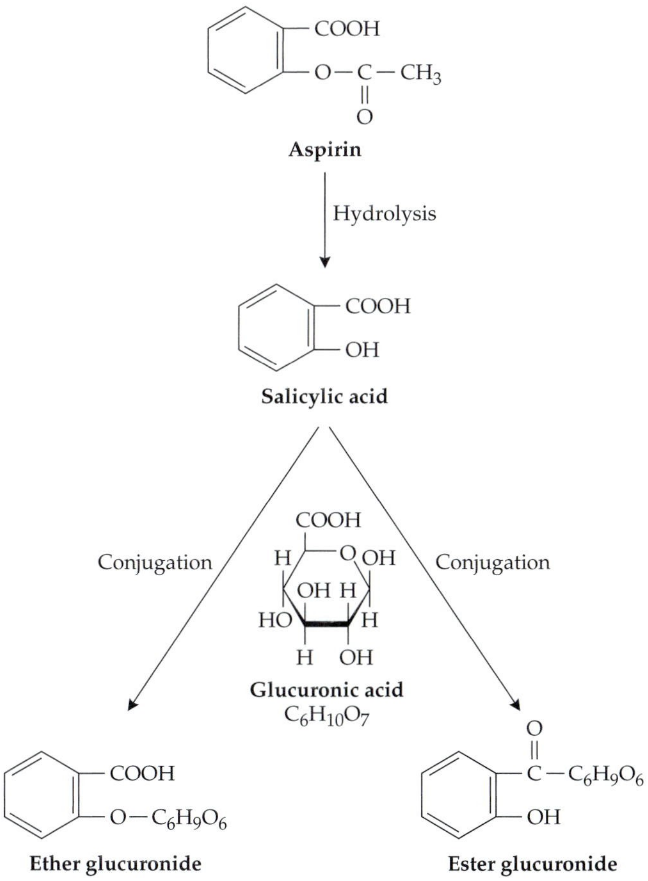

Aspirin

Hydrolysis

Salicylic acid

Conjugation

Conjugation

Glucuronic acid
C$_6$H$_{10}$O$_7$

Ether glucuronide

Ester glucuronide

1.11 METABOLISM OF ASPIRIN. Alternative routes of the two-step metabolism of acetylsalicylic acid (aspirin). Aspirin first undergoes nonsynthetic hydrolysis to form salicylic acid (an active metabolite). The second step is conjugation with glucuronic acid (a synthetic reaction) at either of two sites, which produces one of two highly water soluble metabolites that are readily excreted from the body. Conjugation with several other molecules may also occur, producing additional metabolites.

Liver microsomal enzymes. A large number of drug-metabolizing reactions are catalyzed by liver enzymes located on the **smooth endoplasmic reticulum**, a network of tubules within the liver cell cytoplasm. These enzymes catalyze many of the oxidation and reduction reactions and some of the hydrolysis reactions. They also catalyze one synthetic reaction: conjugation with glucuronic acid. They are often called **microsomal enzymes** because, when liver cells are homogenized and the cell constituents separated by sucrose gradient centrifugation (see Chapter 2), the enzymes are found in the microsomal fraction, which contains primarily smooth endoplasmic reticulum with some contamination by membrane fragments from other organelles. The microsomal enzymes lack a great deal of specificity and can metabolize a wide variety of compounds. However, they are limited to catalyzing reactions of compounds that are lipid soluble. Lipid solubility enhances the penetration of a drug into the endoplasmic reticulum and its binding with the enzyme system.

The metabolizing enzymes of the liver are of particular interest to psychopharmacologists because a large number of drugs that alter mood and behavior cause an increase in liver enzyme activity with repeated exposure to the drug. Various therapeutic agents, pesticides, herbicides, food additives, and carcinogenic compounds are known to increase the rate of their own biotransformation. For example, repeated use of barbiturates, which are used to elicit sedation and sleep, increases the capacity of the liver enzymes to metabolize the drugs into inactive compounds. Therefore, with chronic use, rapid metabolism reduces the plasma levels of these drugs and diminishes the pharmacological effect. Such changes in drug metabolism explain in part why some drugs lose their effectiveness with repeated use—a phenomenon known as tolerance (see below).

Renal Excretion

A final biological process affecting the amount of drug–receptor interaction at any one time is the rate of excretion. Drugs are eliminated from the body either unchanged or as metabolites. The most important organ of elimination is the kidney, although small amounts of some drugs are eliminated from the lungs, in the sweat, saliva, and feces, or in milk.

The human kidneys are paired organs each about the size of a fist. They are responsible for filtering products of metabolism from the blood and maintaining appropriate levels of various ions and other substances. The kidney excretes the end products of body metabolism (e.g., urea) as well as excess sodium, potassium, and chloride. However, the organ conserves water, sugar, and necessary amounts of sodium, potassium, and chloride.

The anatomy of the kidney facilitates maximum interaction between the internal and external environment. The functional unit of the kidney is the **nephron** (Figure

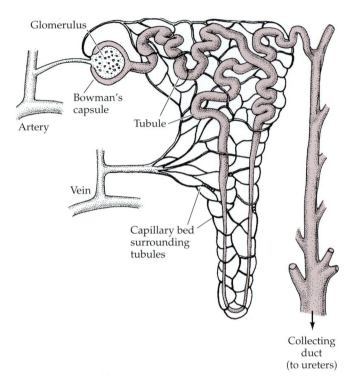

Glomerulus

Bowman's capsule

Artery

Tubule

Vein

Capillary bed surrounding tubules

Collecting duct (to ureters)

1.12   A SINGLE NEPHRON WITHIN A KIDNEY. This highly magnified view shows how the large surface area of the tubule and the close relationship of the blood vessel to the tubule enable maximum internal–external fluid exchange. (After Julien, 1985.)

1.12), which contains a long, unbranched tubule that begins in a capsulelike structure (**Bowman's capsule**) that encircles a network of capillaries called the **glomerulus**. There are approximately 1–3 million nephrons per human kidney, with a total of about 35 miles of tubules. With approximately 1,300 ml of blood passing through each kidney per minute, the pressure of the blood in the glomeruli causes the fluid constituents of the blood to leave the capillaries and flow into Bowman's capsules (as the glomerular filtrate) at the rate of 125 ml per minute. Because the capsules are continuous with the tubules, the filtrate passes into the tubules, from which 124 ml is reabsorbed into the blood via the capillary beds surrounding the tubules. Only 1 ml of fluid is left to be excreted as urine. Within the reabsorbed fraction is virtually all of the sodium, chloride, glucose, amino acids, proteins, and other substances necessary for the body. Left in the tubules are chemical substances (such as some drugs, end products of metabolism, urea, uric acid, and creatinine) that are of little or no use to the body, as well as substances that are exchanged for sodium (such as potassium, hydrogen, and ammonia). Hormones from the hypothalamus regulate the amount of water and sodium that is reabsorbed, determining the concentration of the urine that passes to the urinary bladder for excretion (see Chapter 11).

Most drugs are readily filtered by the kidney unless they are bound to plasma proteins or are of large molec-

ular size. However, the reabsorption of water from the tubules produces a drug concentration gradient so that the drug is more highly concentrated in the kidney tubules than in the blood plasma. Because of this gradient, and because many drugs are small molecules with little charge, they also are often reabsorbed into the bloodstream. For this reason, kidney clearance of unaltered drugs is rather ineffective.

In order to eliminate drugs from the body via the kidneys more readily, the reabsorption process must be reduced. The ionization of drugs reduces reabsorption (from kidney tubule to blood) because it makes the drug less lipid soluble. Most drug metabolism transforms an essentially nonionic drug molecule into a metabolite with a greater charge. This process of drug metabolism or biotransformation occurs primarily, but not entirely, in the liver.

Reabsorption from the tubules, like diffusion across other membranes, is pH-dependent. When tubular urine is made more alkaline, weak acids are excreted more rapidly because they become more ionized and are reabsorbed less well; that is, they are "trapped" in the tubular urine. If the urine is acidic, the drug will be less ionized and more easily reabsorbed; thus excretion will be less. The opposite is true for a weakly basic drug. This principle of altering urinary pH is frequently used in treatment of drug toxicity, when it is highly desirable to remove the offending drug from the body. In the case of phenobarbital poisoning, for example, kidney excretion of this weakly acidic substance is greatly enhanced by alkalinization of the urine with sodium bicarbonate. This treatment leads to ionization and trapping of the drug in the tubules, from whence it is readily excreted.

Tolerance and Sensitization

Tolerance is defined as a diminished response to the administration of a drug after repeated exposure to that drug. In other words, tolerance has developed when increasingly larger doses of a given drug must be administered to obtain the same magnitude of biological effect that occurred with the original dose. It is well known, for example, that the daily dose of morphine must be gradually increased in order to maintain a quantitatively similar degree of analgesia.

We should be aware that not all of the biobehavioral effects of a particular drug demonstrate tolerance equally. This can sometimes be beneficial, as in the case of the tranquilizer chlordiazepoxide (Librium). In animal studies, it has been shown that this drug initially has both sedative and antianxiety effects, but with repeated administration, tolerance develops for the sedative effect but not for the antianxiety effect. Therapeutically, this property is of significance for patients who need the reduction in anxiety but who must continue to function without sedation. The reduction in sedation occurs only with chronic use of the drug. As with most drugs, tolerance disappears after a period of abstinence. Thus, for an individual who uses the drug infrequently, the sedative effect will continue to be apparent, and the patient will require time to adapt (i.e., become tolerant) to the initial side effects.

Another example of the differential development of tolerance occurs with the use of the barbiturates. Although the sedative property of barbiturates undergoes tolerance, the depression of respiratory centers in the brain stem apparently does not show the same extent of tolerance. Consequently, after repeated administration of the barbiturate, the dose that effectively produces sedation and the lethal dose become more similar; hence, the probability of lethal overdose becomes significantly greater.

We should also keep in mind that for some drugs tolerance can appear at the second administration, whereas for others repeated doses over a period of many days are required. Furthermore, the appearance of tolerance is related to the amount of drug administered as well as to the temporal sequence of administration. Thus, a drug administered in large doses at short intervals will produce more tolerance than smaller doses of the same drug at longer intervals. Keep in mind that tolerance is reversible, reflecting the dynamics of the biological system upon which the drug acts. When drug administration is stopped, tolerance disappears gradually, at a rate depending on the particular drug involved.

Cross-Tolerance

The development of tolerance to one drug can diminish the pharmacological effectiveness of a second drug. This phenomenon is called **cross-tolerance** and is the basis for a number of drug interactions. It is known, for example, that the effective anticonvulsant dose of phenobarbital is significantly larger in a patient who has a history of chronic alcohol use than in a patient who has not developed tolerance to alcohol. Because tolerance to alcohol diminishes the effectiveness of the barbiturates, we say that cross-tolerance exists between alcohol and phenobarbital. Cross-tolerance also exists among several hallucinogenic drugs, for instance, LSD, psilocybin, and mescaline.

Drug Disposition Tolerance

Based on our previous discussion of the importance of the receptor in pharmacological activity, we will assume that the quantitative effect of a drug is determined by its concentration and chemical reaction at a specific receptor site.

Tolerance is defined as a diminished response to drug administration after repeated exposure. We can see from the law of mass action (above) that there are only a few ways in which an individual can become tolerant to a drug. Tolerance can be the consequence of (1) a decrease in the effective concentration of the agonist at the

site of action (bioavailability), (2) a reduction in the number of receptors or in their reactivity, or (3) a change in the response elicited (compensation) because of the activation of a homeostatic mechanism. In the first case, tolerance can develop if, with repeated drug administration, there is a reduction in the concentration of the drug at its receptor. **Drug disposition tolerance** (metabolic tolerance) occurs when a drug produces effects that reduce its own absorption, increase its binding to an inert complex, alter its rate of transfer across a biological membrane, or increase its own rate of elimination.

The only well-documented way of reducing the drug concentration at the receptor is by increasing the rate of drug metabolism. Drug disposition tolerance can be shown for drugs like the sedative pentobarbital, which increases its own rate of biotransformation through induction of liver microsomal enzymes. In one experiment, rabbits responded to pentobarbital treatment by falling asleep. Rabbits pretreated with pentobarbital for 3 days slept a much shorter time after an intravenous test dose than did drug-naive controls (Remmer, 1962). Because the blood drug levels were the same for each group at the moment of awakening, the reduced sleeping time can be attributed to increased metabolism without a change in the animals' sensitivity to a given drug concentration. The biological half-life of pentobarbital in the tolerant animals was 26 minutes as compared with 79 minutes for the drug-naive controls. Clearly, the metabolism of pentobarbital was much greater in the pretreated animals. The increased rate of metabolism was not due to more efficient enzyme activity, but to greater amounts of enzyme, as reflected in an increase in smooth endoplasmic reticulum, the structure associated with drug-metabolizing enzymes in the liver cells. Thus, treatment with certain drugs over a period of time can increase the amount of liver microsomal enzymes, which then reduce the blood drug level and thereby reduce the pharmacological effect.

Evidence suggests that high blood drug levels have to be maintained for some time to induce an increase in the amount of liver microsomal enzymes. This characteristic is demonstrated by the finding that mice and rabbits, which metabolize drugs very rapidly, have to be given a drug several times daily for several days in order to achieve the high blood levels of drug necessary to increase the rate of metabolism. Since dogs metabolize drugs much more slowly, they maintain higher levels of drug in the blood and develop tolerance at a faster rate.

One interesting aspect of drug disposition tolerance is that its appearance is also dependent upon the route of administration of the drug. Intravenous administration of a drug to a tolerant and a nontolerant animal should produce the same maximum (peak) effect because absorption is rapid, and the dose should produce the same drug concentration in both animals (Figure 1.13). Thus, a lethal dose of drug administered intravenously would be equally effective in the tolerant and nontolerant individuals. However, because the rate of metabolism of the drug in the tolerant animals is greater, the pharmacological effect (assuming it was nonlethal) would be terminated sooner. This same relationship would not be true if the drug were administered subcutaneously. The slow rate of absorption following subcutaneous administration is a balance between absorption rate and elimination rate. Tolerant animals that are metabolizing faster would have a lower effective drug concentration at any one time than would nontolerant animals. Hence, when a drug is given to a tolerant individual by a slow-absorption route, both the peak effect and duration of action will be reduced.

As mentioned earlier, some liver microsomal enzymes are not very specific for their substrate; that is, they metabolize a variety of drugs. Therefore, cross-tolerance between many drugs is possible. However, the occurrence of cross-tolerance is not solely related to rate of metabolism. For many drugs, pretreatment with one drug produces tolerance to a second drug even though the rate of drug metabolism is not altered.

Pharmacodynamic Tolerance

The most dramatic form of tolerance that develops to the actions of certain drugs on the CNS cannot be explained on the basis of altered metabolism or altered concentration of drug reaching the brain. Therefore, some change in receptors, either in the number of receptors, in their affinity for the drug, or coupling to second messengers, might be suspected. In some instances, no mechanism has yet been determined to explain the appearance of this **pharmacodynamic**, or **cellular**, **tolerance**, so we speak of adaptation of the cells to the presence of the drug. This type of tolerance occurs for the barbiturates (e.g., pentobarbital) and is manifested by a decrease in drug-induced sedation with repeated doses. Pharmacodynamic tolerance also occurs for ethanol, amphetamine, caffeine, and many other psychotropic drugs. Table 1.4 demonstrates that some drugs, but not others, undergo both types of tolerance.

Tolerance to the opiates (e.g., morphine, heroin) is characterized by a shorter duration of action, a reduced intensity of the analgesic, euphoric, and sedative effects, and a significant increase in the average lethal dose. Although some metabolic tolerance may occur, it has been shown that at equal brain drug levels, tolerant animals show much less analgesic and sedative effect than nontolerant animals. One possible biochemical basis for the reduced effectiveness of these drugs was suggested some years ago. By examining cells maintained in a cell culture medium, Sharma, Klee, and Nirenberg (1975) measured both an acute effect of morphine and a change in the effect after several days of exposure to the drug. They found that by binding to its receptor, morphine initially reduces the activity of adenylyl cyclase, an enzyme that directs cellular processes. After several days of treatment with morphine, however, the adenylyl cyclase was

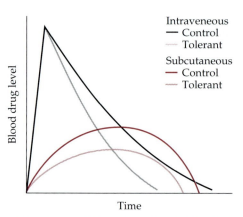

1.13 EFFECT OF TOLERANCE ON BLOOD DRUG LEVEL. The graphs show blood levels of a drug administered intravenously and subcutaneously to tolerant and nontolerant individuals. The difference in peak blood drug levels and the duration of drug concentration in the blood is related to both the method of administration and the metabolic rate in each individual.

no longer easily inhibited by the drug; much more morphine had to be added to the cells to produce inhibition. Apparently, adaptive changes in the receptor, the enzyme regulated by the receptor, or the mechanism by which they are coupled occurred after prolonged exposure to morphine. (For further discussion, see the section of Chapter 12 dealing with opiate dependence or Louie, Law, and Low, 1985).

Behavioral Tolerance

Many drugs with CNS effects, particularly those that are abused, develop tolerance of the cellular type. Although tolerance in some cases can be explained by changes in cell physiology and chemistry, a behavioral component has been demonstrated by several investigators. The Pavlovian conditioning theory proposed by Siegel (1985) suggests that this **behavioral tolerance** is at least in part due to the learning of an association between the effects of a given drug and the environmental cues that reliably precede the drug effects. The learned response is triggered by the environmental signals (conditioned stimuli) even before the drug (unconditioned stimulus) is administered. This "anticipatory" response by an animal is frequently compensatory in nature. For instance, in animals that have repeatedly experienced the hypoglycemic effects of injected insulin, the injection procedure alone (in the same environment) leads to elevated blood sugar. One could argue that the apparent decrease in effectiveness of insulin in these subjects over time is due to the animal's ability to compensate for the drug effect. Of course, it can also be argued that the neural changes that underlie behavioral tolerance are unspecified subtle alterations in physiology similar to cellular tolerance.

Similar results have been found for other tolerance-inducing drugs and physiological variables. Dafters and Anderson (1982), for example, found tolerance to the effects of ethyl alcohol on heart rate only in the environ-

Table 1.4	Types of Tolerance Exhibited by Several Drugs or Drug Classes	
Drug or drug class	Pharmacodynamic tolerance	Drug disposition tolerance
Barbiturates	+	+
Ethanol	+	+
Meprobamate	+	+
Morphine	+	+
Amphetamine	+	−
Cocaine	+	−
Caffeine	+	−
Nicotine	+	−
LSD	+	−

ment in which ethyl alcohol had been previously administered. Their finding of environment-specific tolerance could be explained in part as a conditioned compensatory slowing of heart rate. Experiments utilizing behavioral measures as the dependent variables are more difficult to interpret, but clearly suggest that conditioned drug effects can alter the pharmacological response to drugs. The role of conditioning in the development of tolerance, sensitization, and drug abuse should be a concern for both the research psychopharmacologist and the clinician. The role of Pavlovian conditioning in the development of tolerance to opiates is described in Chapter 12.

Tolerance to a psychotropic drug is often manifested in a task in which learning plays some part. For example, a psychotropic drug might initially disrupt the performance of a task (such as maze running for food reward), but repeated administrations may have less and less effect. The improved performance could be identified as a type of tolerance, but the apparent tolerance could be due to the learning of a new skill (the ability to run a maze in the drugged state), which we would expect to improve with practice. One example of this phenomenon is the alcoholic who learns to maneuver fairly efficiently while highly intoxicated to avoid detection, whereas a less experienced alcohol abuser with the same blood alcohol level may appear behaviorally to be quite intoxicated (see Krasnegor, 1978).

State-dependent learning. Tasks learned in the presence of a psychotropic drug may subsequently be performed better in the drugged state than in the nondrugged state. Conversely, learning acquired in the nondrugged state may be more available in the nondrugged state. This phenomenon has been called **state-dependent learning** and illustrates the difficulty in transferring learned performance from a drugged to a nondrugged condition. An example is the alcoholic who during a binge hides his supply of liquor for later consumption but is unable to find it while he is sober (in the nondrugged state). Once he has returned to the alcoholic state, he can readily locate his cache.

One explanation for state dependency is that the drug effect may become part of the environmental "set"; that is, it may assume the properties of a stimulus itself. A drugged subject learns to perform a particular task in relationship to all the internal and external cues in the environment, including, it is argued, drug-induced cues. Thus, in the absence of drug-induced cues, performance deteriorates in much the same way as if the test apparatus were altered. It has been shown in animal studies that the decrease in performance is very much related to the change in environmental cues and that a particular drugged state does provide readily discriminable stimuli (Overton, 1984). (Further discussion of the cueing properties of drugs follows in Chapter 2.)

The appearance of state-dependent learning probably has great importance in clinical pharmacology. It would not be surprising, for example, if a new behavior acquired during psychotherapy by a patient who was also receiving psychotropic medication did not transfer to the nondrugged state when the drug was discontinued.

Tolerance by Indirect Mechanisms

Looking once again at the law of mass action, we can see that tolerance might also occur at the final step in the drug–receptor interaction sequence—the response stage—as a consequence of the operation of homeostatic adjustment.

An example of this type of tolerance occurs when the drug does not produce all of its effects by direct action, but instead triggers the release of an endogenous, physiologically active substance from storage vesicles. If stores of the endogenous substance become depleted because the interval between doses of a drug that releases them is too short to allow reaccumulation, then tolerance to that drug will appear. Tolerance of this type develops to morphine-induced vasodilation. One effect of morphine is the release of stored histamine, which produces a dilation of cutaneous blood vessels, seen in humans as flushing in the face, neck, and upper thorax. If small doses of morphine are administered to an animal over several weeks, very little tolerance to peripheral vasodilation occurs because stores of histamine can be replenished. With larger doses, tolerance develops rapidly because stores of histamine become depleted; that is, histamine synthesis cannot keep up with demand. When tolerance of this type occurs very rapidly, it is called **tachyphylaxis**.

A second example of a physiological, homeostatic adjustment to a drug effect is the operation of the negative feedback mechanism, which can be seen in the response to treatment with thyroid hormone. Thyroid hormone produces an acute increase in cellular metabolism and a perception of increased energy and vigor. However, when administered to a healthy individual, some of the thyroid hormone circulates to the pituitary gland. The pituitary, in turn, signals the thyroid gland to stop releasing natural thyroid hormone. Although the administration of the hormone leads initially to high blood hormone levels, the thyroid gland very quickly responds by turning down the normal hormone release, thereby restoring the previous level of thyroid hormone in the blood. The restoration of normal hormone levels reduces the rate of cellular metabolism and may elicit a feeling of fatigue. Clearly, the effectiveness of the exogenous hormone has been diminished by the negative feedback mechanism.

Sensitization or Reverse Tolerance

Despite the fact that repeated drug administration produces tolerance for many drugs, reverse tolerance, or sensitization, has been described for some others, most notably CNS stimulants such as cocaine and amphetamine. **Sensitization** is the enhancement of particular drug effects following repeated administration of the same dose of drug. For instance, a single administration of cocaine to animals significantly increases the motor activity and stereotypy produced by subsequent stimulant administration. Chronic administration of high doses of cocaine has also been shown to produce an increased susceptibility to cocaine-induced catalepsy, hyperthermia, and convulsions (Post and Weiss, 1988). As was true for tolerance, the development of sensitization is dose dependent, and the interval between treatments is important. Further, cross-sensitization between cocaine and other psychomotor stimulants has been documented. The augmentation of response to drug challenge tends to persist over long periods of abstinence, indicating that long-term physiological changes occur as a result of stimulant administration.

No definitive explanation for the phenomenon of sensitization exists, although several factors have been considered as possible contributors. Post and Weiss (1988) have shown that conditioning plays a significant role in the appearance of sensitization. Pretreatment with cocaine and subsequent testing in a dissimilar environment yielded significantly less sensitization than that occurring in the identical environment. Others (Pettit et al., 1990) have demonstrated changes in the pharmacodynamics of the drug. They recorded an elevation in the concentration of cocaine in dopamine-rich brain areas following chronic cocaine administration.

Neurochemical explanations for sensitization to stimulants focus on dopamine cell activity because dopamine is the neurotransmitter believed to mediate the stimulant drug effects. Evidence has been found for in vivo increases in extracellular dopamine (Patrick et al., 1991), changes in pre- and postsynaptic dopamine receptors (Peris et al., 1990; Vezina and Stewart, 1989), and modifications of other neurochemical mechanisms (Segal and Kuczenski, 1992; Karler, Calder, and Turkanis, 1991). Furthermore, since protein synthesis inhibitors have been shown to block the induction of stimulant sensitization without altering the acute response to the drugs, it is possible that altered gene expression is involved in the phenomenon (Karler, Finnegan, and Calder, 1993; also see Chapter 13).

Placebo Effects

A **placebo** is a pharmacologically inert compound administered to an individual in place of an active drug. The act of administering a drug is an important part of the relationship between physician and patient or researcher and subject, and both parties have expectations regarding the outcome of treatment. Expectations, motivations, and enhanced suggestibility lead to effects that are unrelated to the drug's chemical activity. It is difficult to separate the pharmacological effects of drugs from the effects arising from psychic and emotional factors because these **placebo effects** are "real." Indeed, it is frequently difficult to distinguish between organic disease and the readily measurable symptoms generated by psychological processes. Likewise, the effects of a placebo are not necessarily limited to subjective perceptions of efficacy, but include physiological changes, such as altered gastric acid secretion, blood vessel dilation, and hormonal changes. It is not surprising that the mere act of administering a drug may provide striking therapeutic effects as well as various side effects. For example, when surgical patients suffering from steady, severe wound pain are injected subcutaneously with saline, three or four out of ten report satisfactory relief of pain (Lasagna et al., 1954). One might consider the total drug effect as a placebo effect overlaid by active drug effects. For instance, morphine's effectiveness can be seen as the sum of a placebo effect and its pharmacodynamic (drug–receptor interaction) effects. If 70% of a group tested for pain relief were satisfactorily improved by morphine, 30% to 40% of the total number experiencing pain relief would have to be subtracted as placebo responders in order to determine the true effectiveness of the drug.

Although the percentage of placebo responders varies from situation to situation, every therapeutic treatment must be assumed to elicit placebo effects. Even environmental conditions alter the response to drugs, particularly psychotropic drugs. To demonstrate this phenomenon, a group of normal human subjects was regulated on food and water intake and physical exercise. The response measured was the amount of urine output induced by the drinking of a large quantity of water (the drug) in a short period of time. For the 2 weeks of the study, water was administered and urine collected in the same manner in the same laboratory. After the 2 weeks, a very small dose (1 oz) of water (test dose) was administered. When administered in the same environment, the test dose resulted in urine output similar to that following the larger conditioning doses. In a very different experimental setting, urine output was directly proportional to water intake. Clearly the therapeutic environment influenced the subjects and modified the response of a regulatory mechanism (Levine, 1983).

In investigations of drug effects, the placebo is an essential part of the experimental design because it enables the separation of the effect of the drug from that of suggestion. In order to evaluate the contribution of placebo effects to the total drug effect, a control group is utilized that is identical to the experimental group in all ways except for the substitution of the inert substance for the test drug. Even in animal experimentation, all placebo subjects are exposed to the same environmental conditions as the experimental animals, including handling, injection with an inert substance (usually saline), or sham surgery. The placebo must be included in each individual experiment because there seems to be no simple, reliable way to eliminate those subjects in the group who will be placebo responders. Neither superficial observations nor classic measures of intelligence are correlated with the response. With more elaborate psychological testing, placebo responders have been found to be generally less mature, more anxious, and more emotionally labile. However, the number of placebo responders varies from experiment to experiment, and almost any individual will respond to a placebo under some circumstances.

Because of the large contribution of emotional factors to drug response and the high and variable incidence of placebo responders, a **double-blind experiment** is highly desirable. In these experiments, neither the patient nor the observer knows what treatment the patient has received. Such precautions ensure that the results of any given treatment will not be colored by overt or covert prejudices on the part of either the patient or the observer. Obviously, the ability to maintain blindness is reduced if the active drug has noticeable side effects. Occasionally a relatively benign drug that has some perceptible physiological effect is used in lieu of a totally inert placebo. Unfortunately, appropriate experimental design and controls are not often readily applicable in the clinical setting. Also, ethical concerns are raised if treatment is withheld for reasons of experimental design. Therefore, a new drug is usually compared with a known effective drug rather than a placebo.

Summary

Drugs are chemical substances that cause changes in physiological systems. This chapter attempts to show the mechanisms by which drugs are able to reach and affect organ function with reasonable efficacy and safety. The principles of drug administration, absorption and distribution, dose requirements, metabolism, excretion, and tolerance apply to all drug treatment and determine the amount of active drug reaching its principal site of action. The binding of a drug to its receptor is the critical event in drug action. Pharmacology studies the relationship between drug, receptor, and biobehavioral effect, as described by dose–response curve analysis.

Drugs do not cause behaviors outside of the species-typical repertoire. Rather, they can alter the probability of the occurrence of a particular behavior at a given time. The behaviors are complex because they are the consequence of highly varied experiences as well as variations in physiology both within and between species. Behavioral pharmacology systematically begins with standard procedures and measurements to establish a norm (baseline behavior) against which to compare behavioral drug effects. Techniques useful to behavioral pharmacologists are discussed in Chapter 2.

Chapter 2

Methods in Neuropsychopharmacology

The current explosion in neuroscience research is in no small part due to improvements in biochemical techniques. The research methods currently available are vastly more sensitive and more specific than ever before. Analytical techniques such as high-performance liquid chromatography and gas chromatography coupled with mass spectrometry are now being applied to problems in neuroscience in which minute quantities of biological substances must be identified. The ability to label compounds radioactively has prompted the refinement of enzyme assays using isotope tracers and receptor labeling techniques. Despite the tremendous improvement in methods of quantification and localization, most researchers in neuropharmacology anticipate even greater advances in the future.

In Chapter 1 we saw that pharmacological effects are dependent upon reversible physiochemical interactions between drugs and cellular molecules (receptors) that are coupled to intracellular biological events. The notion of the receptor may be the single most important concept in pharmacology. Certainly, the idea that biological effects can be initiated by the binding of specific biochemical substances to complementary receptor proteins is the essence of neuroscience today. In general terms, we might say that neuropharmacologists measure biological responses following the addition of a known pharmacological agent. In the past, dose–response curves mapped neuropharmacological changes in intact tissues (or whole animals) and were interpreted to define receptor properties. Refinements in techniques have given researchers more direct measures of receptor function. Such measures include the quantification of intracellular biochemical products whose formation is coupled to the receptor. The characteristics of the receptor can be defined by drug-induced changes in cell products such as cyclic AMP (see Chapter 6) without direct measurement of binding. These studies require the assumption that the drug binds to a specific recognition site and, via one or more steps, induces a measurable response. Since indirect measures of receptor occupancy involve tissue-specific responses, generalizations to similar, but not identical, systems must be conservative.

As is true of our knowledge of neuropharmacology in general, the conclusions drawn from such experiments clearly depend upon the specificity and the sensitivity of the methods used. The selection of a particular experimental method reflects the underlying assumptions made by the researcher regarding the advantages and disadvantages of the technique and the characteristics of the neuronal system under evaluation. Whether or not those assumptions stand the test of time dictates the ultimate value of the experimental results. As our techniques change, our understanding advances in incremental steps, which become accepted "knowledge" only when corroborated by several laboratories using various methods over a period of time.

Recent developments in biochemistry and technology have paved the way for more direct measures of cell function and more precise descriptions of neuronal membrane receptors. Our emphasis in the first part of this chapter will be on direct methods of measurement or visualization of neurotransmitters and their receptors, including receptor binding assays, histochemistry and immunocytochemistry, autoradiography, and high-pressure liquid chromatography, as well as brain metabolism and imaging methods such as tomography (CAT and PET) and magnetic resonance imaging (MRI).

The second half of the chapter is devoted to methods of evaluating drug effects on behavior. In general, the measurement of drug–receptor mediation of behavior is less precise than the measurement of receptor mediation of biochemical events because vertebrate behavior is rarely simple enough to be coupled to a receptor without many intervening events. Evaluation of the simplest behavioral responses, such as pharmacologically induced changes in spinal reflexes or in the latency of startle following acoustic stimuli (Davis et al., 1984), along with receptor localization, provides the most direct approach to examining the neurochemical basis of behavior. However, behavioral psychopharmacology can provide very important clinical information without any consideration of receptors per se. As is true of the methods of chemical analysis, recent advances in techniques of behavioral analysis are helping to refine the definition and evaluation of the neuropharmacology of behavior. Also, computerized collection and analysis of data further enhances the detailed investigation of behavior. Some of these techniques, including operant techniques and ethological methods, will be discussed in Part II.

Part I
Neurochemical Techniques

Neurotransmitter Measurement and Localization

Histofluorescent Techniques

In the early 1950s Eränkö discovered that treatment of adrenal glands with liquid formalin made it possible to induce fluorescence in the cells with ultraviolet light. Those experiments began a new era in histochemistry and initiated a surge of interest in the further development of the technique, which identifies and maps specific cell types based on their chemical constituents. Although it has broad applications in many biomedical fields, histochemistry (and its most recent offspring, immunocytochemistry) has a special role in neuroscience because it can localize a number of chemical substances that are known to have profound effects on nerve cells.

Eränkö's discovery and subsequent work led to the development of the **formaldehyde-induced fluorescence (FIF)** technique for visualizing the catecholamine neurotransmitters and hormones. Catecholamine molecules (dopamine, norepinephrine, and epinephrine) contain both a catechol group and single amine group (NH_2) (see Chapter 7), and are found within the central and peripheral nervous systems as well as in the adrenal glands. Hillarp and Falck and their colleagues (Falck et al., 1962) further modified the technique to visualize norepinephrine in nerve cells by exposure of dried tissue to formaldehyde vapor. Formaldehyde induces fluorescence via a condensation reaction with catecholamines to form green fluorescent products (3,4-dihydro-isoquinoline derivatives).

The specificity of the fluorescent techniques depends upon the presence of certain molecular groups that are necessary for the formation of fluorophores. For example, using a multistep procedure, catecholamines can be converted to strongly fluorescent compounds, while other compounds that do not have the required structure do not react and so are only weakly fluorescent or nonfluorescent. Histamine, which is a monoamine, does not develop sufficient fluorescence with FIF visualization, whereas a method using orthophthaldialdehyde instead of formaldehyde does induce histamine fluorescence. However, although histamine can be visualized in the gut, where it occurs in large concentrations, the method is not sensitive enough to identify histamine-containing nerve cells in the CNS.

In contrast to catecholamines and histamine, the indolamine serotonin, which is found in large concentrations in the gut as well as within nerve cells, can react with formaldehyde to produce yellow fluorescent products (β-carboline derivatives) that can be visualized by fluorescent microscopy (Dahlstrom and Fuxe, 1964). Fortunately, the monoamines fluoresce green while serotonin produces a yellowish color, which provides a basis for discrimination between the two. Also, different frequencies of ultraviolet and visible light can discriminate between amines.

A description of the FIF technique and the chemical reactions involved is given by Lindvall and Björklund (1987). Following perfusion with fixative to maintain tissue structural integrity, the tissue is frozen and freeze-dried to extract water vapor. The dried tissue is then treated with formaldehyde vapor and embedded (often in paraffin) before being sliced into thin sections for examination under a fluorescent microscope.

Many modifications of the FIF technique have been developed (Steinbusch, DeVente, and Schipper, 1986) to increase both its sensitivity and its specificity. These improvements mean that lower concentrations of monoamines can be more readily detected. Despite these improvements, distinguishing between cells containing different amines remains a problem, particularly when the concentration of one is very low compared with that of the second. In these cases, pharmacological manipulations such as prior selective depletion of one amine improve the probability of accurate evaluation. Unfortunately, the rapid fading of the fluorophore complicates the photographic procedure for permanent recording of the results. Despite these difficulties, few methods have had such an impact on neuroscience. The earliest and most detailed maps of amine-containing neuronal pathways in the brain were completed using this histochemical technique (see Chapter 7). The use of histofluorescence, along with the more recently developed method of immunohistochemistry, continues to offer new and exciting possibilities for examining the CNS.

Immunocytochemistry

Immunocytochemistry (ICC) is a method that identifies a tissue constituent by means of a specific antigen–antibody reaction labeled with a visible tag. This method is dependent upon the action of the immune system, which produces specific proteins (antibodies) that attack and neutralize foreign substances (antigens) in the body. In essence, the method binds antibodies to a protein (enzymes or receptors) in brain and then uses them to estimate the amount and location of the protein. The principal steps are (1) producing a specific antibody, (2) applying it to the brain tissue, where it will bind selectively to the antigenic substance it was derived from, and (3) attaching the bound antibody to a label suitable for light or electron microscopy. Recent advances in methods of protein purification have made it possible to raise antibodies against many cell constituents, including neurotransmitters (e.g., peptides, dopamine, and serotonin), neurotransmitter synthesizing enzymes, and most recently, neurotransmitter receptors. Thus, it is possible to map the distribution of the neuronal systems using immunocytochemistry (see Color Plate 2).

The first step, antibody production, uses standard methods in immunology. The substance to be mapped is the antigenic substance. The antigenic substance (a large enzyme or a small molecule coupled to a larger, more antigenic substance) is injected repeatedly at various intervals into a host (any one of a number of species, most often rabbit) along with other substances that boost the subsequent immune reaction (e.g., Freund's adjuvant). Blood samples are tested for the presence and concentration of antibody at various intervals. With this method, the host produces polyclonal antibodies; that is, a heterogeneous mixture of antibodies developed to many components of the antigen as well as to the whole antigen. In addition, since antibody production by the host is a continuous process, antibody sampled at any one time will be different from that taken at any other time. To avoid these difficulties, a monoclonal antibody may be produced.

Monoclonal antibodies. The production of **monoclonal antibodies** requires a cell culture technique such as that devised by Kohler and Milstein (1975). Cells from the spleen of a mouse that have been sensitized to a designated antigen are fused with tumor cells, which have the characteristics of rapid replication and immortality (Figure 2.1). When the spleen cells fuse with the tumor cells, they combine the specific antibody production of the spleen cells with the growth properties of the tumor cells. Each hybrid cell, called a hybridoma, produces antibodies with a unique structure, just as in the case of spleen cells in an intact host that contribute to the polyclonal antibodies described above. However, in this case, individual antibody-producing cells are isolated and cloned (i.e., large numbers of identical offspring of each cell are grown in culture). The clonal cell lines are then screened for their antibody characteristics, and only those clones that produce antibodies meeting predetermined criteria are maintained. If radioactively labeled amino acids are added to the culture medium at this point, the label will be incorporated into the antibody and can later be used to map the antibody using autoradiography (see below). Several reports provide details on methodology for the production of monoclonal antibodies to neuronal markers (MacMillan and Cuello, 1986), including the CNS peptide substance P (Cuello, Priestley, and Milstein,

2.1 MONOCLONAL ANTIBODY PRODUCTION. Important steps include (1) sensitization of a host and preparation of sensitized spleen cells, (2) cell fusion between spleen cells and tumor cells, (3) selection of desired hybrid cells (screening), and (4) growing of the selected cell lines in culture medium. (After Mudgett-Hunter, 1986.)

1982), the endogenous opiate peptide enkephalin (Cuello et al., 1984), and the neurotransmitter serotonin (Steinbusch, Verhofstad, and Joosten, 1978).

The monoclonal antibody technique has been a significant advance for neurobiology as well as for most biomedical fields (Mudgett-Hunter, 1986). This cell culture technique has several advantages over in vivo polyclonal antibody production. First, whereas polyclonal antibodies are in limited supply, monoclonal antibodies can be reproduced in unlimited quantity and for an indefinite period of time because cell lines can be frozen, stored, and reactivated after long intervals. Second, the cultured cells produce a single, identical antibody for as long as the cells are viable, while in vivo polyclonal antibody production changes throughout the life of the host. Third, the feasibility of selecting a monoclonal antibody that does not cross-react with other antigens is a powerful advantage of the cell culture technique: the more specific the antibody, the more precise the mapping. Also, since selection of antibody is possible, the antigen used to generate the antibody need not be purified. This advantage has been important in the case of those enzymes whose purification has not yet been accomplished.

Antibody binding and labeling.   The development of antibody (either poly- or monoclonal) is the first step in the ICC process. The next step, the preparation of brain tissue and its exposure to the antibody, can follow several different procedures depending on the antigen of interest, the anticipated labeling technique, and the method of visualization (light or electron microscopy or autoradiography). A summary of methods is given by Pickel and Teitelman (1987).

Because even the thinnest tissue sections do not permit the resolution necessary to visualize antibody molecules attached to antigen, it is necessary to mark the antibody with a label that allows its visualization by light or electron microscopy. A variety of labels are available, although many conventional labels are not intense enough to be detected in low concentrations. For light microscopy, highly fluorescent compounds such as fluorescein and certain enzymes such as intestinal alkaline phosphatase, which form visible reaction products, are most commonly used. Markers for electron microscopy depend on the electron density of heavy metals such as ferritin and colloidal gold.

More important than the marker per se is the manner of linkage of the label to the antibody. It is the linkage that determines assay sensitivity by specifying both labeling intensity and nonspecific background labeling. In a one-step procedure (direct mode), the label can be attached directly to the antibody before it is applied to the tissue section. The two-step method (indirect mode), involves applying unlabeled antibody in the form of rabbit antiserum to the tissue to localize the antigen. In the second step, the reaction is visualized by a labeled antibody (second antibody) that has been prepared to the immunoglobulin of the first antibody (for example, fluorescence-labeled goat-antirabbit immunoglobulin G). The relative merits of each method have been explored extensively elsewhere (Sternberger, 1986) and will not be discussed in this chapter.

Until recently, one of the most commonly used methods, developed by Sternberger, was the PAP method because it depends on the formation of a peroxidase–antiperoxidase complex. It was developed to increase specificity and decrease background labeling. This method entails the use of a second antibody with two combining sites, only one of which is allowed to react with the first antibody. The second combining site undergoes a second immunological reaction with antibody to horseradish peroxidase complexed with peroxidase, which, when developed, permits visualization by light or electron microscopy. By using this method along with electron microscopy, the ultrastructural localization of neuronal constituents, present even in very low concentrations, is possible. For example, vasoactive intestinal peptide (VIP) is a neurosecretory peptide found in the CNS and in nerve endings that innervate glands. Using PAP intensification of the immunocytochemical signal in combination with electron microscopy, Johannson and Lundberg (1982) found VIP in large, dense core vesicles in nerve endings in the cat submandibular gland. The terminals contained small, clear vesicles, believed to contain the neurotransmitter acetylcholine, and the large, dense core vesicles in a proportion of 9:1. Such evidence supports the idea that VIP coexists with acetylcholine and may act as a neuromodulator (see Chapter 11).

Both histofluorescence and ICC provide morphological information on the location, size, and shape of nerve cells. In addition, these methods can be used along with quantitative fluorometric techniques to measure concentrations of amines or antibodies in a given brain area (Berkenbosch et al., 1987; Schipper and Tilders, 1982). This technique involves impregnating samples of molded gelatin with known concentrations of test compound; that is, the substance to be quantified in the tissue. The gelatin must undergo the same preparation procedures of fixation, embedding, and staining as the experimental tissue. The amount of staining of the gelatin sections can be quantified and a linear relationship determined between the known amount of test compound added to each slice of gelatin and the intensity of immunostaining. The amount of the substance in the experimental samples can be determined by comparing the intensity of immunostaining with the standard curve.

The importance of the histofluorescence and ICC techniques to neurobiology is clear. Both methods have seen extensive use in the localization and measurement of neurochemicals. The application of these techniques to problems in developmental biology, psychopharmacology, and physiological psychology is limited only by the fluorescent nature of cellular components or the ability to raise antibodies. These methods can be used to visualize changes in the distribution of neurochemicals following in vitro manipulation of neurotransmitter release, uptake, or metabolism. Furthermore, disturbances in the neurotransmitter system induced by drugs in vivo or by disease can also be analyzed. Over time, each of these methods has become increasingly refined. The use of antibodies to selected neural components means that ICC can provide information on specific cellular chemicals regardless of their inherent ability to fluoresce. Therefore, ICC can provide information not only on fluorescent amines but also on neuropeptides and cellular enzymes. Additionally, ICC can quantify amines in brain areas too small for microdissection and can localize chemicals in subsets of neurons or within subcellular structures in a single neuron.

Autoradiography

One technique that can be used very effectively in conjunction with ICC is autoradiography. **Autoradiography** is the mapping of cellular components that have been radioactively labeled. A molecule (ligand) that is radioactively labeled (now a radioligand) is incorporated into a tissue either by in vitro incubation or by injecting the agent into an experimental animal in vivo. The tissue of interest is then thinly sliced and mounted on a slide. The slide is either dipped in liquid photographic emulsion, which is then allowed to harden (microautoradiography), or placed against photographic film (macroautoradiography) and stored, to allow the radioactive material to act on the film. After exposure, the film or emulsion is processed to develop the autoradiogram.

Autoradiograms are formed by the darkening of silver halide grains in the film by the charged particles that are emitted from the radioactive compound during its constant disintegration. Since the effect of the disintegration is additive, the extent of film darkening is directly, although not linearly, related to the amount of radioactive material concentrated at the site (see Figure 2.17). It is now common to enhance the readability of autoradiograms by digitally applying "false colors," which map a color spectrum onto the gray scale (see cover illustration, and Color Plates 1, 3, and 4).

Originally, a densitometer was used to measure the optical density of several parts of a structure of interest and the results were averaged. Newer computerized scanning methods map densities over the entire sample with high resolution and display the results as a picture. There are a variety of scanners available to produce these visualizations, and they vary in sensitivity, maximum capacity, accuracy (signal-to-noise ratio), scan time, resolution, and cost.

Once the relative densities are mapped, the autoradiogram can be examined for both the localization of radioactive tracer and quantitative analysis of the radioligand incorporated. Qualitative analysis of the tissue compares the optical density of a given structure with that of other structures. The amount of radioactivity responsible for a measured optical density can be calculated based on an estimate of the number of grains that would be expected to be developed by each nuclear disintegration. In this way, quantitative analysis determines the amount of radioactivity in the structure. Alternatively, the quantity can be calculated by the use of standard precalibrated amounts of radioactivity that are placed adjacent to the tissue specimen and treated identically. Direct comparison of the optical densities produced by these standards and the samples provides a reasonable method of quantification.

While macroautoradiography is most often used for quantitative studies of the distribution of radiolabeled tracer in the brain—for example, to map the uptake of radiolabeled neurotransmitter into cells—the resolution of microautoradiography is much greater because of the radionuclides (radioactive atomic nuclei) used to label tracers and film emulsions used. The radionuclides used for microautoradiography tend to have lower electron emission energies, which means that the electrons from radioactive decay travel a shorter distance in the emulsion and minimize the production of an image at a distance from their origin. For that reason, radioiodine (^{125}I) produces images with very high spatial resolution, as well as tritium (^{3}H), which is a commonly used beta emitter. Although sometimes used, radioactive carbon (^{14}C) produces much poorer resolution. The photographic emulsions consist of a dense suspension of crystals whose size is a second factor in determining resolution. Crystals of 0.5 mm are used for light microscope examination, while for electron microscopic autoradiography, crystals of 0.05 mm are used. Furthermore, for electron microscopic microautoradiography, the exposed photographic emulsions are processed so that each grain is not entirely developed, and the image consists of portions of grains near the image centers, further enhancing resolution. An excellent description of these techniques and the underlying physics and chemistry of the reactions is provided by Lear (1986).

In vivo autoradiography can be used not only to visualize labeled brain areas and the intracellular locations of tracers, but also can be used to trace dynamic processes such as blood flow, cell metabolism, cellular uptake, and biochemical reactions. In addition, the technique can be used to visualize labeled drug and neurotransmitter binding to receptor sites. These applications will be described briefly in later sections of this chapter.

In Situ Hybridization

In situ hybridization (ISH) is a histochemical technique that makes it possible to localize cells containing a specific nucleic acid sequence (DNA or RNA) in much the same manner in which ICC localizes cells containing a particular protein. This technique has been developed to provide highly specific detection of very small quantities of genetic material—even a few molecules per cell. It is used in biomedical fields to identify the nucleic acid sequence of a virus in infected tissue, to examine the genetically determined proteins regulating developmental processes, and to identify unique gene sequences in chromosomes as a preliminary step in gene assembly and cloning.

For neuropharmacology, in situ hybridization is immensely useful in detecting the specific messenger RNA molecules that are responsible for directing the manufacture of the wide variety of proteins essential to neuron function, such as enzymes, structural proteins, receptors, ion channels, and peptide neurotransmitters. (For an introduction to gene chemistry, see Chapter 3.) It is useful not only in detecting the locations of cells expressing specific mRNAs, but also in the quantitative measurement of drug-induced changes in regional mRNA levels (which reflect alterations in gene expression). Chronic cocaine use, for example, apparently alters the mRNA levels of opiate neuropeptides in discrete cell populations in the striatum of postmortem tissue (Hurd and Herkenham, 1993).

Because each protein has a unique amino acid sequence, the DNA and coinciding mRNA responsible for directing its synthesis by necessity have unique base pair sequences. In order to identify cells containing a unique protein in low concentration, in situ hybridization is used to locate those cells containing the mRNA responsible for directing the synthesis of that protein. The technique depends on the fact that the probes, labeled single-stranded fragments of DNA or RNA made up of base pair sequences complementary to those of the nucleic acid of interest, can be linked to the cellular RNA, forming stable hybrids.

The ISH method can use either tissue slices or cultured cells. After the tissue is fixed, it is frozen, sliced, and mounted on slides. The tissue is then covered with hybridization buffer, which contains a probe for the nucleic acid of interest. The probe is a specific DNA or RNA fragment that has been labeled with ^{32}P, ^{35}S, ^{3}H, ^{125}I, or a nonradioactive label. The targets for the probe are sequences of nucleic acids that are complementary to the chosen probe. Detection occurs following the binding of the complementary nucleotides to the probe. After incubation with the probe, the tissue is washed and dehydrated before being placed in contact with X-ray film for several days. After X-ray film exposure, the sections are developed, stained, and evaluated microscopically. Figure 2.2 outlines and describes the essential steps in this procedure.

ISH is both slow and labor-intensive, but it provides exceptional specificity and very high affinity. Although light microscopic examination is most usual, protocols have been developed to allow visualization at the electron microscopic level in order to study subcellular localization of the nucleic acids and the morphology of the cells expressing the nucleic acid (Soghomonian, 1990).

Further recent developments have provided opportunities for quantitative analysis of messenger RNA levels within single cells in histological sections using video-based computer image analysis (Smolen and Beaston-Wimmer, 1990).

Tissue preparation.   Tissue fixation and preparation is one variable that determines the sensitivity of ISH. Other methods of RNA detection, such as Northern blotting, utilize homogenized tissue from which RNA is extracted. ISH preserves cell integrity and morphology in order to localize nucleic acids within cells. For that reason, tissue preparation for ISH is concerned with preserving cell morphology while maximizing the accessibility of probe to target without loss of nucleic acids.

Probe characteristics.   A second critical consideration in the design of an ISH assay involves the characteristics of the probe, probe labeling, and the sensitivity of detection methods. There are three main types of probes: complementary DNA (cDNA), RNA (riboprobes), and oligonucleotide probes. Each has distinct advantages and disadvantages as listed in Table 2.1. A complete discussion of probe types and their methodological advantages will not be presented here, but can be found in several sources (Chesselet, 1990; Polak and McGee, 1990; Tecott et al., 1994).

Briefly, the RNA and DNA probes are produced by cloning procedures in which bits of the partially purified nucleic acid of interest are incorporated into cloning vehicles (vectors) such as plasmids or bacteriophages. When the vector is introduced into a suitable bacterial host (usually *E. coli*), all descendants of the affected bacteria will contain the recombinant nucleic acid. In order to increase the specificity of the probe, the cloned recombinant may be cloned into another vector (subcloning), which is grown in large quantity before it is used as a hybridization probe. In contrast, oligonucleotides of a defined sequence can be manufactured by automated DNA synthesizers and require no cloning procedures.

Double-stranded cDNA is easily labeled by a variety of methods, and radiolabeling produces probes with high **specific activity** (a large total amount of radioactivity per gram of material labeled). However, the double strand must be separated by denaturing before being used, and many of the strands may recombine (reanneal) rather than hybridizing with mRNA, the intended target. In such a case, only a small amount of probe may be available for hybridization. The denatured strands may also partially reassociate, thereby impairing probe penetration. The introduction of single-stranded cDNA probes has theoretically reduced the reannealing problem, thus potentially enhancing the strength of the signal. However, the preparation of single-stranded probe is technically more difficult and limited by low efficiency. In addition, a subcloning step is required.

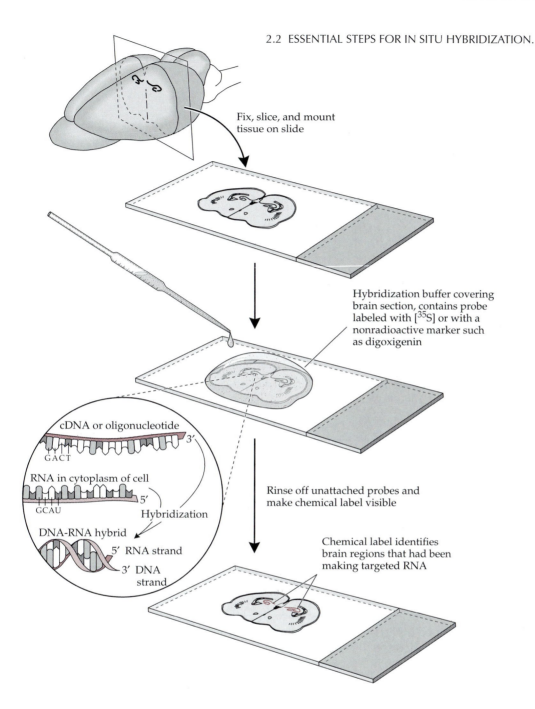

2.2 ESSENTIAL STEPS FOR IN SITU HYBRIDIZATION.

Fix, slice, and mount tissue on slide

Hybridization buffer covering brain section, contains probe labeled with [^{35}S] or with a nonradioactive marker such as digoxigenin

cDNA or oligonucleotide
3'
GACT

RNA in cytoplasm of cell
5'
GCAU
Hybridization

DNA-RNA hybrid
5' RNA strand
3' DNA strand

Rinse off unattached probes and make chemical label visible

Chemical label identifies brain regions that had been making targeted RNA

The single-stranded RNA probes have the potential for high specific activity and low potential for reannealing. Also, the probe–target hybrid (RNA–RNA) is more stable than the DNA–RNA hybrid, but RNA probes also tend to produce higher levels of nonspecific binding (i.e., binding to tissue components other than the target).

The third general type of probe is the synthetic oligonucleotide, which can be manufactured with the ideal sequence to enhance specificity and the ideal length to maximize penetration. However, because only short sequences are available, the amount of label carried per unit is smaller, making detection more difficult. Although preparation of the sequence requires a DNA synthesizer and known mRNA sequences, the process of manufacture by automated apparatus is quicker and easier than the more involved procedure of separation and cloning used to produce the other probes.

Although many probe labels are available, radioisotopes are the most common and can be used with any of the available probes. The selection of a radioisotope is dependent on considerations of (1) sensitivity, (2) anatomical resolution, and (3) speed of development. Tritium (^{3}H), for example, produces high resolution and low background labeling, but its low-energy emission requires long exposure times (weeks or months). ^{32}P-labeled probes have higher energy, so they require shorter

Table 2.1   Advantages and Disadvantages of Probes Used for In Situ Hybridization

Probe Type	Advantages	Disadvantages
DNA (double strand)	Easy to use Subcloning unnecessary Choice of labeling methods High specific activity Possibility of signal amplification (networking)	Reannealing during hybridization (decreased probe availability) Probe denaturation required, increasing probe length and decreasing tissue penetration Hybrids less stable than RNA probes
DNA (single strand)	No probe denaturation needed No reannealing during hybridization (single strand)	Technically complex Subcloning required Hybrids less stable than RNA probes
RNA	Stable hybrids (RNA–RNA) High specific activity No probe denaturation needed No reannealing Unhybridized probe enzymatically destroyed, sparing hybrid	Subcloning needed Less tissue penetration
Oligonucleotide	No cloning or molecular biology expertise required Stable Good tissue penetration (small size) Constructed according to recipe from amino acid data No self-hybridization	Limited labeling methods Lower specific activity, so less sensitive Dependent on published sequences Less stable hybrids Access to DNA synthesizer needed

(1–7 days) exposure, but resolution to the single-cell level is lost due to the long path of the energetic emissions. Probes labeled with ^{35}S are also used. These provide high specific activity and adequate cellular resolution, but in some cases a high level of nonspecific binding has been observed.

In general, nonradioactive labels are less sensitive and do not permit quantitative analysis. Furthermore, these labels cannot be used with all probes. Nevertheless, nonradioactive labeling is being developed because it reduces radiation hazards and avoids the inconvenience of specialized storage and limited half-life. Additionally, nonradioactive labeling significantly reduces assay time because the prolonged autoradiographic development step is eliminated. Resolution is often improved because the label is confined to the particular cell compartment containing the target nucleotide, whereas high-energy radioactive labels often produce more diffuse silver grain patterns. Nonradioactive labels for nucleotide probes include nonprotein antigens (e.g., biotin, digoxigenin), fluorescent compounds (e.g., fluorescein, ethidium), and enzymes (e.g., alkaline phosphatase, horseradish peroxidase, or firefly luciferase) similar to those used for immunoassays (see below; Bolch, 1990).

Hybridization conditions.   In addition to tissue preparation and probe variables, a third factor determining the specificity of ISH is hybridization reaction conditions. Among the critical factors are hybridization temperature and pH, probe concentration, time of reaction, and ionic characteristics of the hybridization buffer. Details of the techniques and evaluation for specific applications can be found in several sources (Diamandis, 1990; Chesselet, 1990; Eberwine, Valentino, and Barchas, 1994; Polak and McGee, 1990).

In situ hybridization is particularly useful in neuropharmacology for several reasons. First, the sensitivity of the technique permits the detection of the very small numbers of cells in the CNS that express a particular gene, which otherwise could not be detected. ISH theoretically permits the study of gene expression at the level of the single cell. Second, as more conventional tracing methods show, neuroactive substances are transported far from their site of synthesis. ISH can identify the population of cells actually manufacturing a particular protein. The method can be readily coupled with other neuropharmacological techniques, such as immunohistochemistry, neurotransmitter receptor labeling, or glucose utilization, to evaluate not only the gene but also the product expressed by the gene. Third, ISH can identify those cells whose activity has been altered by environmental events or drugs. Changes in gene expression may be temporary following a transitory stimulus, or may reflect more adaptive long-term changes, representing neuronal plasticity. Further, inherited neurological and neuropsychiatric disorders linked to abnormalities in gene expression can readily be evaluated using animal mutants and environmental manipulations that are linked to the expression of the disorder.

Immunoassay Techniques

Immunoassay is a well-established technique for detecting and quantifying physiologically important molecules at trace levels. Immunoassay is a modification of the competitive binding assay, which is based on the competition between labeled and unlabeled ligand for a limited number of binding sites. The principal difference is that in competitive binding assays, the binding sites are proteins that have a high specificity and affinity for the ligand, while immunoassays utilize an antibody to the ligand (antigen) of interest.

Briefly, the procedure involves the addition of a known concentration of antibody plus saturating concentrations of labeled antigen to each of several assay tubes. These pools of marker are then diluted with different known concentrations of unlabeled antigen. Competition between labeled and unlabeled antigen for the limited binding sites results in less labeled antigen being bound to the antibody: the higher the concentration of unlabeled competitor antigen, the lower the ratio of bound to total labeled antigen. When the percentage of bound labeled antigen to total labeled antigen is plotted as a function of the concentration of the unlabeled antigen, it produces a dose–response curve similar to the one shown in Figure 2.3a. This plot is used as a standard curve against which samples containing unknown amounts of antigen can be tested. By using the standard curve, the amount of labeled antigen found in each test sample can be translated into the amount of unlabeled antigen present in the sample. Plotting the dose–response curve on a semilogarithmic scale straightens the curve and makes it easier to use (Figure 2.3b).

In order to form the standard curve, it is necessary to known how much labeled ligand is bound to the antibody and how much is unbound (free). Some immunoassay techniques require physical separation of the labeled ligand bound to antibody and the free labeled ligand; such assays are called heterogeneous assays. Homogeneous assays do not require this physical separation because the signal of the label is changed when the ligand binds to the antibody, making it distinguishable from the unbound labeled ligand.

Radioimmunoassays.

Radioimmunoassays (RIAs) use radioisotopes as the ligand label and so are heterogeneous by necessity because the binding of antigen to antibody does not change the radioactive signal. The isotope most often used is ^{125}I because it has high specific activity and a reasonable half-life of 60 days. Separation of bound and free radioligand can be achieved in several ways, including solid-phase separation, which involves the adsorption of the free antigen onto charcoal, leaving the

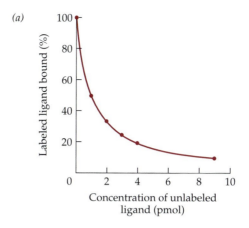

(a)

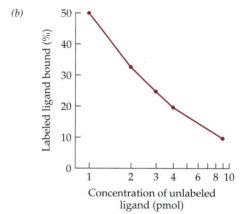

(b)

2.3 STANDARD CURVES FOR IMMUNOASSAYS. (a) The percentage of labeled ligand bound is plotted as a function of the concentration of unlabeled ligand to create the standard curve. As the concentration of unlabeled ligand increases, competition with labeled ligand for the limited binding sites favors the unlabeled ligand. The concentration of unlabeled ligand in experimental samples can be estimated by comparing the percentage of labeled ligand bound under the same conditions with the standard curve. (b) The same data plotted on a semilogarithmic scale to facilitate the evaluation of unknowns.

antigen–antibody complex in the supernatant after low-speed centrifugation. A second method is the double antibody technique, which utilizes a second antibody, or anti-antibody, prepared against the antibody that has combined with antigen. The second antibody is added in high concentration to precipitate all of the antibody–antigen complex, leaving the free antigen in the supernatant. A third method uses ammonium sulfate precipitation. In the ammonium sulfate method, saturated ammonium sulfate is added to each assay tube in sufficient concentration to precipitate the complex, but not the free antigen, which remains in the supernatant.

Since the original immunoassay method was developed, a number of modifications have been made that greatly enhance sensitivity and selectivity and reduce processing time. First, the substitution of monoclonal antibodies for antisera greatly improves specificity. Since monoclonal antibodies of known specificity can be obtained in virtually unlimited quantities (see above), the reliability of repeated assays is enhanced.

Second, new techniques have been developed using nonradioactive labels that equal or exceed the radionuclides in detectability. In addition, nonradioactive labels reduce radiation hazards and avoid technical problems related to short half-life. Some of the nonradioactive labeling–detection systems use fluorescent or chemiluminescent labels, electroactive metal ions, enzymes, or a combination of enzyme labeling and electrochemical detection of some component in the assay system. For example, enzymes may be used in electrochemical immunoassays as a label attached to either the antibody or the antigen. When the antigen–antibody complex is formed, the enzyme catalyzes the production of an electrochemically detectable product. The rate at which the product is formed reflects the concentration of analyte (i.e., that which is analyzed) in the sample. The reaction mixture may be separated and analyzed by liquid or high-pressure liquid chromatography using an amperometric or electrochemical detector (see below). Another example of a nonradioactive label is a releasable electroactive metal ion. Antibody–antigen binding releases the metal ion label, which can be measured by voltammetry (see the section on electrochemistry below).

Third, innovations such as the immobilization of antibody or antigen on a solid phase by passive adsorption or covalent bonding have increased reliability and allowed rapid processing of large numbers of samples. A very popular assay of this type is the enzyme-linked immunosorbent assay (ELISA), which involves the application of antibody to the walls of plastic cuvettes (sampling tubes) that can be prepared ahead and stored. Any antigen in the sample added to the tubes binds to sites on the fixed antibody (capture antibody). After the tubes are washed, an excess of the antibody labeled with enzyme is added, which also binds to the antigen, making a "sandwich." After washing, a substrate for the enzyme is added and the colored reaction product formed is measured by absorbance.

Additional design modifications have utilized nonradioactive labels and a homogenous protocol that avoids the separation step required by more conventional heterogenous RIAs. Homogeneous assays depend upon a change in the intensity of the label's signal when the labeled antigen binds to the antibody. For example, the antigen label may be an enzyme whose rate of function increases when it is bound to the antibody. The amount of bound and free antigen can be determined by the rate of enzymatic production of the product. In this case, the more antigen–antibody binding, the more product is formed. Such amplification of the antigen–antibody interaction increases the sensitivity of the assay. Numerous sources provide a more detailed discussion of immunoassay methodology (Diamandis, 1990; Heineman et al., 1987; Kaplan, Szabo, and Opheim, 1988).

Column Chromatography

Chromatography refers to any of several processes that are used to separate complex mixtures into individual compounds based on their physiochemical interactions with a stationary component of the system. The principal components of any chromatographic system include a mobile phase and a stationary phase. The mobile phase carries the complex sample to be separated through a column containing the stationary phase, which selectively retards the passage of the constituent components of the complex sample, leading to their separation. The final separation products may be extruded from the column at varying rates and collected in a specialized detector for identification and quantification. Alternatively, the materials retained in the column may be washed from the column by subsequent solvent elutions and the liquid collected in tubes for further analysis. The two principal methods of chromatography, gas chromatography and liquid chromatography, are classified according to the nature of the mobile phase. A variety of gas and liquid column chromatography methods, categorized by column type, method of separation, and type of detector used, are listed in Table 2.2.

Liquid chromatography. In liquid chromatography, the sample is introduced into a liquid mobile phase and is followed by the eluant. The rate of movement of the mobile phase through a packed vertical glass column is determined by gravity or by a low-pressure pump. In **high-performance liquid chromatography** (**HPLC**), the mobile phase is forced through a relatively short (10–20 cm), narrow-bore (2–4 mm) stainless steel column by a high-pressure pump developing pressures of 1,000–3,000 psi. Figure 2.4 is a schematic diagram of the basic components of a typical HPLC system. An important advantage of HPLC is rapid separation, which takes minutes rather than hours for each sample. Depending on the characteristics of the stationary phase, the sample will be separated according to molecular size and shape, polar functional groups, or magnitude and charge of ionic species.

Methods of separation. The methods of separation depend on the characteristics of the sample, such as polarity, size, and structure, and on characteristics of the solid phase. The four general classes of chromatographic separation are adsorption, partition, ion exchange, and steric exclusion. Steric exclusion (molecular sieve) is a type of liquid–solid chromatography that separates molecules by size and shape. ("Liquid–solid" refers to the form of the mobile phase and the form of the stationary phase, respectively.) The column is packed with porous material selected on the basis of pore size, depending on the size of the molecules being separated. As the sample, which is dissolved in the liquid mobile phase, passes down the column, the smallest molecules are momentar-

Table 2.2 Options Available with Liquid and Gas Chromatography Methods

| Method | Options | | |
	Column Type	Detectors	Separation
Liquid	Open column	Photometer	Liquid–liquid adsorption
	HPLC (closed column)	Fluorescence	Liquid–solid ion exchange
		Electrochemical	Liquid–solid steric exclusion
		Mass spectrometer	Liquid–liquid partition
Gas	Packed column	Flame photometer	Gas–solid adsorption
	Capillary wall coated column	Ionization	Gas–liquid partition
		Mass spectrometer	

ily trapped when they enter the pores (Figure 2.5). The largest molecules move quickly between the packing particles because they are excluded from the pores. Smaller molecules are partially restricted. Based on this relative retention, the molecules are eluted in order of size, beginning with the largest.

A second separation technique is ion exchange chromatography, which is used for separating molecules based on ionic charge. The stationary phase consists of resin beads to which charged molecular groups are covalently attached. In the case of cation (+) exchange, the tightly bound ions are negatively charged (e.g., SO_3^- in Figure 2.6a) and are associated with positive ions (Na^+) that are loosely attached by electrostatic charges. When positively charged molecules in the sample to be separated come into contact with the functional group, they displace the weakly attached cations (Na^+) and remain attached to the resin. The remainder of the mixture is washed through the column. By rinsing the column with a solution of hydrochloric or perchloric acid, the adsorbed cationic substance is released from the column and collected in the effluent. Anion exchange can be accomplished in the same way by substituting a positively charged covalently bound ion to attract the anions from solution (Figure 2.6b).

In liquid–liquid partition chromatography, the stationary phase support is coated with a monolayer of water or some other polar solvent. The mobile phase is a solvent immiscible in the stationary phase. The compounds in the eluate are distributed between the mobile phase and stationary phase depending on their relative solubility in each. If a material is soluble in the mobile phase, it will elute quickly. Affinity for the polar stationary phase will retain the compound on the column for a longer time. Separation is based on polarity: the least polar compounds are eluted first, and most polar are held longer in the polar liquid stationary phase. Gas–liquid chromatography also can separate materials by means of a partition mechanism. In this case the mobile phase is an inert carrier of the sample components, which are differentially distributed in the liquid-coated stationary phase based on polarity.

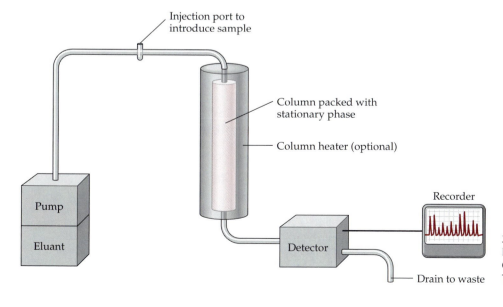

2.4 TYPICAL COMPONENTS OF A HIGH-PERFORMANCE LIQUID CHROMATOGRAPHY (HPLC) SYSTEM.

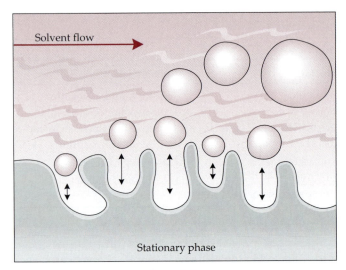

 ...

2.5 THE PRINCIPLE OF STERIC EXCLUSION CHROMATOGRA-PHY. The packed porous material making up the stationary phase is chosen based on pore size. As the sample, which is dissolved in the liquid mobile phase, is washed down the column by solvent, the smallest molecules are frequently trapped in pores along the column, thereby slowing their passage. Larger molecules are trapped less often because their size excludes them from more of the pores, and so the largest molecules reach the detector in a proportionately shorter time.

Adsorption chromatography is based on the interaction of the sample components with a three-dimensional binding site on the support matrix, which differentially retains materials based on their structure and polarity. The stationary phase is most often a polar silica or alumina gel, which retains components of the sample by both hydrogen bonding and dipole interactions. Strength of adsorption is determined by the number of attractive groups and the total surface area. Compounds are eluted from the column because of competition between the sample components and the eluant for the binding sites. By varying the solvent, specific compounds can be eluted. "Strong" solvents compete effectively for the chromatographic sites, thus producing rapid elution of sample components. "Weak" solvents compete less well and displace only those materials that are weakly adsorbed. Separation by adsorption can be used with either liquid or gas chromatography.

Methods of detection. Specialized detectors are often connected to the system to identify the separated components as they are eluted from the column. These detectors produce an electrical signal proportional to the concentration of each separated component. Photometers are among the most commonly used detectors. Light of specific wavelengths is directed through the elution sample toward a photodetector, which measures the absorbance of light by the sample. Because some materials have maximum absorption at very short wavelengths, lamps emitting ultraviolet light can be used. The use of ultraviolet light detection is common in the measurement of proteins, peptides, and many drugs. The absorbance of the eluate is plotted over time; changes in absorbance are directly related to the concentration of the compound present in the effluent. The changes produce a signal that is recorded as a chromatogram.

Another common HPLC detector measures the electrochemical characteristics of the eluate. Of the electrochemical detection methods, amperometric detection is the most often used. In an amperometric cell, the column effluent passes electrodes to which a voltage (usually between +1.3 and −1.2 V) is applied. As the potential becomes more positive, the surface becomes a better oxidant (electron sink), and the molecules in the column effluent tend to give up electrons (oxidation). Negatively charged electrodes encourage the effluent molecules to accept electrons (reduction). In either case, the movement of electrons causes a current to flow that is proportional to the instantaneous concentration of the molecules in the column effluent. Since the amount of voltage applied determines the amount of oxidation or reduction, the sensitivity of this method can be easily manipulated, and very low detection limits (1 pmol) can be achieved. Since only compounds electroactive at the selected potential are detected, coeluting compounds without the same electroactivity do not cause interference. A typical chromatogram resulting from electrochemical detection is seen in Figure 2.7. For neuropharmacologists, electrochemical detection is particularly useful to analyze biogenic amines, amino acids, and acetylcholine.

Gas chromatography. Gas chromatography, either gas–liquid or gas–solid, differs from liquid chromatogra-

(a)

Resin beads

$SO_3^- \cdot Na^+$
$SO_3^- \cdot Na^+$
$SO_3^- \cdot Na^+$

(b)

Resin beads

$CH_2 - CH_2 - N^+ \overset{H}{\underset{C_2H_5}{<}}\overset{C_2H_5}{\cdot} \quad Cl^-$

$CH_2 - CH_2 - N^+ \overset{H}{\underset{C_2H_5}{<}}\overset{C_2H_5}{\cdot} \quad Cl^-$

$CH_2 - CH_2 - N^+ \overset{H}{\underset{C_2H_5}{<}}\overset{C_2H_5}{\cdot} \quad Cl^-$

2.6 STATIONARY PHASE MATERIALS FOR ION EXCHANGE CHROMATOGRAPHY. (a) Typical cation (sulfonate) exchange resin with SO_3^- tightly bound to the resin beads and Na^+ loosely attached by electrostatic charges. (b) An anion (diethylaminoethyl$^+$) exchange resin with diethylaminoethyl$^+$ tightly bound to the resin and Cl^- loosely attached by electrostatic charges.

The detectors most often used are thermal conductivity or flame ionization detectors. Thermal conductivity detectors contain pairs of wires (filaments) that form a bridge and change electrical resistance with changes in temperature. The wires are heated electrically, and carrier gas alone flows steadily across one filament to cool it slightly. Carrier gas and separated compound flow across the other filament and usually increase the temperature and resistance of that wire. The difference in resistance produces an unbalanced bridge circuit, and the resulting electric charge is recorded as a peak. The electric charge is proportional to the concentration of the effluent.

Flame ionization detectors consist of a small chamber in which hydrogen gas and oxygen mix with the column effluent and are burned. As the sample burns, ions are formed and are attracted to an oppositely charged electrode. The current produced is proportional to the concentration of ions formed.

The most sophisticated detector, the mass spectrometer, provides unambiguous identification of the components of a mixture and is sensitive to picogram (10^{-12} g) quantities. It can be used in conjunction with either gas or liquid chromatography. Samples are bombarded by electrons to form charged molecular ions and fragments, which are filtered in terms of their mass-to-charge ratio (m/e) and are measured by electron multiplier. Identification is based on the unique and reproducible fragmentation pattern produced by the molecular ions. Because analysis is complex, mass spectrometers are connected to computer systems that collect the mass fragmentation data and search libraries of known compounds for comparison. High specificity and sensitivity make chromatography–mass spectrometry ideal for measuring the minute amounts of neurochemical compounds collected from discrete brain sites by microdialysis (see below). For further detail of procedures in chromatography and immunoassay, see Bishop, Duben-Engelkirk, and Fody (1996), or other texts in clinical chemistry.

In Vivo Microdialysis

The demonstration of calcium-dependent excitation-induced release of neurotransmitters and drug modification of that release is a significant focus of neuropharmacological research. In order to evaluate synaptic activity, it is important to be able to separate the neurochemical contents of the intracellular and extracellular spaces. In vitro studies of neurotransmitter release use nerve preparations, cultured cells, synaptosomes, or brain slices with or without preincubation in a radioactive tracer. The cells may be stimulated by electric current, ion-induced depolarization, or drug application. Stimulation is followed by collection of the extracellular fluids (ECF), which are presumed to contain materials released from the cells. The complex materials collected are then separated and analyzed by any one of several methods, including bioassay, RIA, and gas or liquid chromatogra-

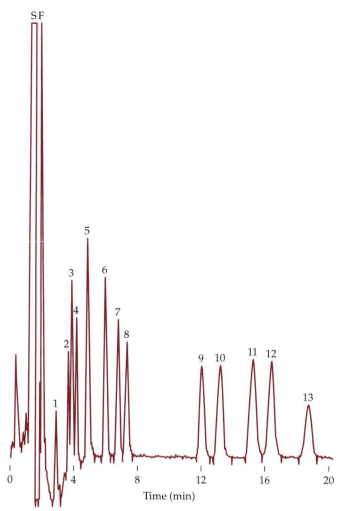

2.7 TYPICAL CHROMATOGRAM RESULTING FROM ELECTRO-CHEMICAL DETECTION. The peaks in the chromatogram are directly related to current flow, which is proportional to the concentration of molecules in the effluent over time. The chromatogram's 13 peaks correspond to various monoamines. (From Hadfield et al., 1985)

phy in that it is designed to separate and quantify volatile materials or those that can be made volatile in a heated (up to 400°C) column. The injection port is hot enough to flash-volatize the sample. The stationary phase is a nonvolatile liquid or solid, while the mobile phase is an inert gas (e.g., helium or nitrogen) that carries the volatile sample through the column. The effluent passes through a detector that produces an electrical signal proportional to the concentration of the volatile components. As with HPLC, the compounds can be identified by differences in retention time, and concentration can be calculated by estimating the area under the peak. Resolution (i.e., clear separation of sample components into discrete bands or peaks) has been improved by replacing the usual packed column with extremely thin quartz capillary tubing coated with a layer of the stationary phase on the inside.

phy, depending on the characteristics of the compound of interest and the sensitivity required.

While the in vivo demonstration of stimulus-induced release of neurotransmitter is relatively easy in the peripheral nervous system, it is a much more difficult task in the less accessible CNS. For peripheral synapses, afferent fibers can be stimulated while their terminals are in a bath that can be sampled and assayed. To perform similar release experiments in the CNS, in vivo assays use stereotaxic implantation of stimulation and collection equipment. One such device is the cortical cup, which collects the materials pooling at the brain surface following stimulation (Moroni and Pepeu, 1984). A second device, the push–pull cannula, involves a set of two concentric tubes that provide a means of perfusing specific areas of the CNS and collecting extracellular fluids following stimulation. The cannula has the advantage of being able to monitor deeper structures and localize the site of liberation to some extent. Implantation of the device allows measurements to be made in freely moving animals under relatively normal conditions, as shown in Figure 2.8 (Philippu, 1984).

The development of brain sampling techniques has been limited by the large amount of sample required for the identification and quantification of brain materials, which are normally found in low concentrations. The continuing improvement of highly sensitive analytic techniques (such as HPLC) has made it possible to measure minute amounts of endogenous chemicals and has subsequently paved the way for the development of microcollection techniques such as in vivo microdialysis (Benveniste and Huttemeier, 1990; Ungerstedt, 1984). **Microdialysis** is a technique that can both administer and collect substances at remote brain regions with a high degree of accuracy. The sampling can be done in a freely moving animal on an almost continuous basis, limited only by the amount of time needed to fill the sample loop of the HPLC injector. Such rapid sample collection is important for kinetic analysis. Further, since the tissue is not directly exposed to moving fluid, as in earlier collection methods, microdialysis may be more physiological in nature and minimizes cell damage.

Microdialysis is based on the principle of dialysis, in which a semipermeable membrane separating two solutions allows some diffusion to occur. The collection system consists of a double tubular membrane probe that is continuously flushed on one side with a solution devoid of the materials of interest, while the other side meets the interstitial fluid. Materials of interest diffuse from the interstitial fluid into the collecting tube. The solution in the collecting tube is constantly renewed so that a concentration gradient is maintained across the membrane. The movement of the fluid through the probe carries the substance of interest to the sampling site for analysis. If a substance is to be administered, it must be more concentrated in the perfusion fluid than in the extracellular space, which causes it to move out of the probe into the interstitial fluid.

One type of microdialysis probe, as shown schematically in Figure 2.9, contains a membrane connected with inlet and outlet tubes to apply solutions and collect samples, respectively. Configurations vary somewhat, but the outer diameter is usually as small as 300–800 μm, which minimizes tissue damage at the site of implantation. However, some limited damage does occur, and injury-induced release of substances into ECF occurs during the first hour of perfusion. In general, experiments are not begun until a stable baseline of sampled materials is achieved. The length of the probe depends on the brain region to be sampled, making essentially every part of the brain accessible. The membrane is sealed along its length except at the specific target site. Diffusion across this small portion of membrane takes place in a relatively narrow zone (less than a few hundred mi-

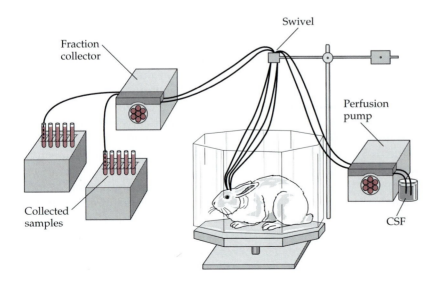

2.8 BRAIN SAMPLING TECHNIQUES USING IMPLANTED DEVICES such as the push–pull cannula or microdialysis probe allow the collection of samples in a freely moving animal under relatively normal conditions. The collected samples undergo further evaluation by any one of several analytic techniques, such as HPLC. (After Philippu, 1984).

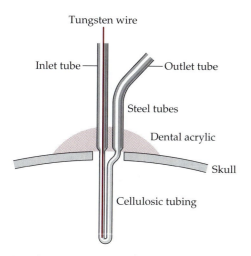

2.9 ONE TYPE OF MICRODIALYSIS PROBE, which uses flexible cellulosic tubing (outer diameter 0.25 mm) bent into a loop. The tungsten wire is used to straighten the tubing during implantation and is removed afterward. The nonimplanted ends of the tubing are inserted into steel tubes 0.64 mm in diameter, which are fastened to the skull with dental acrylic. (After Ungerstedt, 1984).

crometers in width) around the probe so that sampling can be localized to very small areas. The probe is implanted in an anesthetized animal by means of a micromanipulator attached to a stereotaxic frame. After implantation, the probe is fixed to the skull so that experiments can be carried out in awake and mobile animals, as shown previously in Figure 2.8.

Among the factors that affect recovery of the materials of interest are the physiochemical properties of the membrane, which determine the characteristics of the substances that can move freely through it. Also the size and design of the probe affect the surface-to-volume ratio. Since dialysis occurs at the interface between the ECF and the dialysis membrane, the total surface area of the membrane in relation to the volume of perfusate modifies collection of the sample. Further, the speed of perfusion determines the concentration gradient that develops and hence the rate of movement of materials across the membrane. The isotonicity of the perfusion solution is important because, ideally, the solution should differ from the ECF only in the solutes of interest. Technical difficulties may arise when the substance to be recovered is already contained in the perfusion medium and a substitution must be made that maintains the osmotic concentration.

The development and refinement of intracranial dialysis is important to neuropsychopharmacology because this method can be used effectively in several types of experiments combining biochemical and behavioral analyses. For example, research has evaluated the effects of repeated doses of amphetamine on extracellular concentrations of the neurotransmitter dopamine in dopamine-rich brain areas (Segal and Kuczenski, 1992). Since the sample collection was made in freely moving animals, correlated changes in behavior, such as behavioral sensitization, could be monitored simultaneously.

Further examples of the type of research that can be conducted with microdialysis include cerebral administration of drugs at discrete locations and recovery of neurotransmitter or metabolites in intact animals. The ability to monitor the concentration of free drug in the CNS following systemic administration contributes to pharmacokinetic analysis. Collection of extracellular materials at nerve terminals following discrete electrical stimulation of neural pathways is another valuable role. In addition, it is possible to collect endogenous compounds during ongoing behaviors such as sleep and waking, feeding, or operant tasks. Quite clearly, this technique provides an additional window into the functioning CNS.

Electrochemistry

In addition to in vivo microdialysis, a second method, electrochemical analysis, can be used in a complementary fashion to evaluate the relative activity of brain pathways in freely moving animals. Whereas microdialysis collects samples of ECF that are then separated and quantified, electrochemical analysis utilizes implanted microelectrodes to measure the concentration of electroactive compounds such as oxidizable monoamine neurotransmitters (e.g., norepinephrine, dopamine, serotonin) or their metabolites that have overflowed into the ECF. Because the microelectrodes are very small in diameter (1–1,000 μm), tissue damage is kept to a minimum and measurements can be made in very small, selected brain areas following activation of neural pathways. Modifications of the basic method provide the means not only for the measurement of slow concentration changes such as those following drug administration or behavioral stimulation, but also for continuous measurement of rapid concentration changes occurring within less than 1 second.

Several related electrochemical techniques (voltammetry, amperometry, and coulometry) that are available involve the measurement of electrical signals produced by chemical changes within an electrochemical cell. The cell consists of two electrodes (detector and reference) that provide an interface between a chemical system and an electrical system. The electrical system controls the voltage and current applied to a particular chemical system and measures the electrochemical current produced.

In vivo voltammetry is used to measure such things as the overflow of neurotransmitter (e.g., dopamine, norepinephrine, serotonin) into the extracellular space following exocytotic release or behaviorally induced changes in neuroactive substances, such as neurotransmitter metabolites. A small electric potential is applied to an electrode stereotaxically implanted in the extracellular space in the neural tissue to be studied. The applied electric potential produces electrolysis of electroactive compounds near the electrode surface, which results in a measurable electric current. Electrolysis occurs by reduction (a gain of one or more electrons) or by oxidation (a loss of one or more electrons). The substance to be measured can be identified by varying the electric potential applied (linear potential scanning) and obtaining information regarding the oxidation and re-reduction of the substance at the electrode. Slow linear potential scanning requires from one to a few minutes total recording time. Fast cyclic voltammetry uses much more rapid potential scanning and requires only 10–15 milliseconds to collect the required data, which makes it a powerful tool for in situ neural monitoring. To quantify the amount of substance released into ECF, the oxidation current curves occurring before and during activation-induced exocytosis are integrated and compared.

A second, related method of measurement requires that the electric potential of the detector electrode be set at a predetermined level at which oxidation occurs and is held steady at that level. The current that occurs under that condition is measured at a fixed time in the pulse (chronoamperometry) or integrated over a time interval in the pulse (chronocoulometry). The pulses last 20–100 milliseconds and are repeated every 50–100 milliseconds. Although somewhat slower than fast cyclic voltammetry, these methods also are capable of monitoring very rapid concentration changes in the ECF.

As with most analytical techniques, specificity and background interference pose potential problems for electrochemical measures (Adams, 1990). Many substances of interest to neuropharmacologists, such as the catecholamines dopamine and norepinephrine, and their metabolites, have closely spaced or overlapping oxidation potentials. Additionally, large quantities of oxidizable compounds of little interest are present in neural tissue. For example, ascorbic acid oxidizes at a potential similar to the catecholamines. Since it is present in concentrations 100 to 1,000 times greater than the catecholamines, it is capable of significant interference. Fortunately, recent developments in electrode selectivity have provided a means of accurately identifying many of the compounds of importance to neuroscientists, although electrochemical sensors for amino acids, peptides, and other neuroactive substances are not yet available.

Electrochemical analysis is still a rapidly developing technique, and careful verification of the identity of the substance measured is required (Marsden et al., 1988; Wightman et al., 1987). Adequate controls require the use of several standard neuropharmacological methods, such as injecting an exogenous sample of the proposed substance locally near the in vivo electrode to show that it oxidizes/reduces at the same voltage as the electrochemical peak. Alternatively, an enzyme known to specifically alter the substance to be verified can be injected into the vicinity of the electrode to produce a reduced electrochemical signal. Anatomical specificity can be demonstrated by lesioning or stimulating the pathway to eliminate or increase the electrochemical signal. Finally, it is common to compare values derived electrochemically with the values generated by other methods, such as in vivo microdialysis.

Voltammetric analysis has several advantages that make it an important tool in neuropsychopharmacology. First, it provides the opportunity to make repeated measures in the same animal without the use of radiolabeling or sacrificing the animal. Second, since the technique can be used with many different preparations, including brain slices, anesthetized animals, and active animals, it can be readily combined with electrophysiological or neuropharmacological methods. For example, combining voltammetry with electrophysiological recording can provide information on the relationship of extracellular electrical events and neurotransmitter release, or the relationship between ion fluxes in the ECF and release. Third, neuropharmacologists are excited by the opportunity to make on-line measurements of dynamic chemical changes associated with biogenic amine release. For example, real-time evaluation of neurotransmitter release was demonstrated by Wightman and colleagues (Wightman et al., 1988), who characterized with great detail and mathematically modeled dopamine overflow and uptake in the rat striatum following electrical stimulation of ascending neurons. Finally, the miniaturization of microelectrodes to tip diameters as fine as 1 μm has been achieved. Beveled carbon fiber electrodes can be used to impale large neurons, such as those of *Apylsia*, for monitoring instantaneous intracellular changes. The use of microcomputers with data capture devices that readily discriminate between signal and noise has further improved the sensitivity of electochemical detection and enhanced its value as a neurobiological tool. Voltammetric analysis has proved useful in research concerned with neurotransmitter turnover following intraperitoneal or intravenous drug treatment. It can also be used to monitor neurochemical changes internally generated by circadian rhythms, hormonal states, or stages of sleep and arousal. In both cases, behavioral changes can be simultaneously monitored. In addition to these relatively slow concentration changes, electrochemical analysis is capable of measuring rapid concentration changes that occur in less than 1 second after the initiation of stimulation and rapidly return to baseline within 60 seconds. Stimulation can be achieved by intracerebral injection of drugs or hormones, electrical stimulation of neuronal systems at cell bodies or terminals or along ascending pathways, or iontophoretic application of drugs. Clearly, electrochemical analysis is a significant tool for measuring the dynamic and fleeting neurochemical changes occurring with the CNS.

Receptor Measurement and Localization

Radioligand Binding

Although the concept of specific neurotransmitter and drug receptors was developed in the early 1900s by Langley (1906), the ability to measure neurotransmitter receptors in homogenized brain tissue was not achieved for another 60 years. The production of highly specific and tightly binding molecules that would have high radiolabeled specific activity was necessary before the receptor binding technique could be developed. Since then, radioligand binding of receptor proteins has exploded into the most prolific speciality within neuroscience.

The **radioligand binding** method is relatively simple. A ligand that is radioactively labeled (now the radioligand) is selected to bind to the receptor of interest. The radioligand is incubated with the tissue homogenate or tissue slice under conditions that optimize its binding. Unbound radioligand is removed either by washing and rapid filtration or by centrifugation, depending on the affinity of the ligand for the binding site. The amount of radioligand bound to the tissue is then measured with a scintillation (or gamma) counter.

The assay conditions in general are determined empirically; that is, in developing a binding assay, the optimum binding conditions, such as temperature, pH, and concentration of various salts such as Na^+, must be identified to maximize binding, and the appropriate radioligand must be selected. Ligands are labeled with either ^3H or ^{125}I. Tritium-labeled ligands have the advantage of a long half-life (12 years) compared with 60 days for ^{125}I. A second advantage is that the exchange of the ^3H for the H ion in the radiolabeling procedure is less likely to change the biological characteristics of the drug or neurotransmitter. In contrast, the "bulky" ^{125}I group may alter the biological properties of the ligand. Radioiodine labeling has certain other advantages, however, including a higher specific activity. Because very small amounts of bound radioligand can still be detected by the gamma counter, ^{125}I-labeled ligands can be used to assay receptors with low concentrations. Also, when radioligands with high specific activity are used, they can be added in smaller quantities, thus increasing the relative amount of radioactivity specifically bound to the receptor by minimizing binding to other cell components.

Regardless of the radioligand used, the stability of the radioligand under incubation and separation procedures must be determined to assure that the compound remains unaltered either by assay conditions or by metabolizing enzymes present in the tissue. The stability of the ligand–receptor complex must also be considered when choosing the method of separation of bound and free ligand. A discussion of separation techniques and modifications of the general procedure can be found in several sources (Bennett and Yamamura, 1985; Schwarz, 1986; Young, Frey, and Agranoff, 1986).

Interpretation of Ligand–Receptor Binding

Although the radioligand binding procedure is quite simple, interpretation of the results is more complex. Several criteria must be met before the results can be interpreted as radioligand binding to the specific biological receptors of interest, rather than binding to other sites by ionic attraction or experimental artifact. The criteria essential for concluding that receptor binding has occurred include (1) specificity, (2) saturability and high affinity, (3) reversibility, and (4) biological relevance.

Specificity. Specificity of binding means that the ligand is binding only to the receptor we are interested in and to nothing else. Specificity must be carefully determined because physiological membrane receptors are few in number, whereas the number of inert binding sites in the tissue and in adsorptive materials used in the assay procedure is assumed to be very large. Such nonspecific binding may include ionic attraction to glass incubation tubes, filters, or incubation medium additives, such as albumin. Nonspecific sites also may include functional structures such as metabolizing enzymes or other cellular constituents. The ultimate test for specificity is comparison with known properties (number of sites, affinity, reversibility, localization) of the biologically active receptor. Since those properties are often unknown preceding the binding study, researchers depend on empirical estimates of specific and nonspecific binding. Such estimates can be made by adding large amounts of unlabeled (nonradioactive) ligand to the assay materials to displace radioligand-bound receptors. Nonspecific binding is defined as that binding of the radioligand that is not displaced by the addition of the nonradioactive compound. Because the unlabeled compound is added in very high concentrations—as much as 10,000 times the concentration of the radioligand—it competes successfully and, in principle, completely with the radioligand for the specific receptor sites. Under these conditions, the labeled ligand has only a 1 in 10,000 chance of occupying a receptor. Since the unlabeled compound occupies practically all the receptors, any bound radioactivity is considered to be attached to nonspecific sites. There is no direct measure of specific binding. These experiments can only measure total binding and, when unlabeled ligand is added, estimate baseline or background levels of nonspecific binding. Specific binding is calculated by subtracting nonspecific binding from total binding. Figure 2.10 illustrates the relationship between total binding, nonspecific binding, and specific binding. Since many receptor agonists and antagonists are capable of

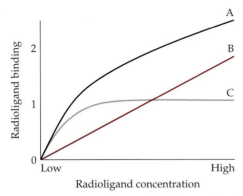

2.10 HYPOTHETICAL BINDING CURVES. When various amounts of radioligand are added to tissue samples, the total binding at each concentration can be plotted as a total binding curve (A). Nonspecific binding (B) is determined by introducing an excess of an unlabeled compound that will displace the radioligand bound to receptors. The radioligand binding that remains is nonspecific. The difference between these two curves represents binding that is specific for the receptors (C).

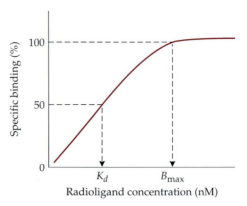

2.11 A HYPOTHETICAL SATURATION CURVE. As radioligand concentration increases, specific binding to the receptor also increases until all the sites are filled (B_{max}). The K_d is defined as the ligand concentration at which 50% of the receptors are occupied.

binding to the receptor of interest, the particular nonradioactive ligand used is an important variable in binding studies and can contribute to over- or underestimation of receptor binding.

Receptor sites may also show a steric specificity. In the case of ligands with an asymmetric carbon atom, the (–)-isomer (which is the prevalent configuration for naturally occurring agonists) is bound to specific receptor sites more readily than the (+)-isomer (which also tends to be biologically inactive). Since the two isomers are mirror images of each other, their adsorptive and ionic attractions for membranes or assay components should be the same, but their binding to a specific protein receptor will differ.

Saturability and high affinity.   Specific receptor binding is saturable; that is, as increasing amounts of radioligand are added to a fixed amount of tissue, binding steadily increases until all the receptors are occupied, at which time no further specific binding can occur. The concept of saturability indicates a finite and limited number of binding sites.

This concept is illustrated in Figure 2.11, a hypothetical saturation curve for a radioligand. Increasing the amount of radioligand produced increasing amounts of specific binding until a concentration was reached, beyond which specific binding became relatively constant. The asymptote indicates the **maximum concentration of available binding sites (B_{max})** in the tissue. The rate at which saturation is reached (the slope of the curve) reflects the affinity (K_d, or **dissociation constant**) of the ligand for the receptor. In this case, calculation of K_d would show that the ligand has a relatively high affinity well within the range expected for a biologically significant receptor, generally between 10^{-8} and 10^{-11} M.

In contrast, nonspecific binding tends to demonstrate relatively low affinity and nonsaturability. Nonsaturability means that with increasing concentrations of radioligand (over a typical range), an increasing amount of binding occurs (see Figure 2.10, curve B). Unfortunately, there are instances in which saturable nonspecific binding of certain ligands, such as peptide hormones, to particular kinds of filters and glass materials has been demonstrated. Also, since a radioligand may bind to more than one type of receptor, saturability is a necessary, but not a sufficient, criterion for specific binding.

Reversibility.   Not only the rate of association, but also the rate of dissociation of ligand and receptor is critical. Certainly, the dissociation rate should be consistent with the reversal of physiological effects of the labeled drug or neurotransmitter. The importance of dissociation rate in describing the kinetics (i.e., the temporal characteristics) of a binding reaction will be discussed more fully in the following section.

The ability of agents other than the principal ligand to inhibit its binding or displace it further describes the specificity and reversibility of binding. In **competition experiments**, the specificity of the binding is defined by measuring the displacement of the bound ligand by various compounds. Those drugs that mimic or antagonize the ligand's biological action should also be effective in displacing the radioligand from the receptor. Therefore, interpretation of data from displacement studies is limited by the known specificity of the competitors.

Biological relevance.   An important consideration in evaluating receptor binding is the relationship of the ligand–receptor interaction to a subsequent biological response. First, in the case of CNS receptor sites, binding experiments must demonstrate that binding is proportional to tissue concentration—that is, as the amount of receptor protein increases, maximum binding also increases. Second, the binding distribution in the brain and within the various cellular compartments must be consistent with the proposed neurochemical function of the ligand. Thus, those brain areas known to be activated by a particular neurotransmitter under study should possess appropriate neurotransmitter receptors. Similarly, ligands specific for receptor proteins serving synaptic transmission are expected to be associated with synaptic membrane portions of nerve cells, rather than binding to nuclear cell membranes or mitochondria. Third, a direct relationship between receptor binding and biological effect should exist. Under ideal conditions, receptor binding and biological response should be measured in the same, simple, intact system before disruptive procedures are performed on the cells. For example, the binding of labeled insulin to fat cells is saturable and of high affinity (K_d approximately 10^{-11} M), a value that correlates well with the known biological effects (initiating glucose uptake) of insulin in the same cells (Jacobs and Cuatrecasas, 1983).

The complexity of the structure and function of the CNS usually prohibits direct comparison of binding and function in the same cells. However, by using displacement studies, investigators can evaluate the ability of chemical derivatives to compete for binding in relation to their relative effectiveness as agonists in neurochemical or clinical tests. For example, inhibitors of the amino acid transmitter glycine are effective to varying extents in producing convulsive behavior in animals. Their order of potency in eliciting convulsions is similar to their order of effectiveness in displacing [³H]glycine from its receptor (Young, 1984). Results of such studies, however, show only a correlation between phenomena and cannot be considered evidence for a causal relationship. Also, experiments of this type rarely produce perfectly parallel results in binding affinity and functional potency. Particularly in the case of animal behavior, drug effects are dependent on many factors in addition to drug–receptor interaction. For instance, absorption

and biodistribution of the drug in the intact animal contributes to the disparity between predictions made based on in vitro binding results and in vivo behavioral measures. Furthermore, agonists initiate a chain of events that provide amplification or modification of the initial binding step. Therefore, the characteristics of binding may not directly reflect the effectiveness of the agonist at the measurable physiological endpoint. By necessity, neurochemical assays vary in assay conditions, such as ionic requirements and pH, that cannot be duplicated in binding assays, thus making direct comparisons between the two somewhat tenuous. Nevertheless, in many neuropharmacological studies, compelling relationships between receptor occupation and pharmacological effect have been uncovered. In some cases, as for the group of antianxiety drugs called the benzodiazepines, prediction of behavioral effects based on receptor binding results is possible (Creese, 1985).

Several typical displacement curves resulting from a competition experiment appear in Figure 2.12. In this type of experiment, the tissue is incubated with the same concentration of radioligand in all tubes. The competitor is added in various concentrations to pairs or triplicates of tubes. Radioligand binding is thus determined at each concentration of competitor. As the concentration of competitor increases, more of it will preferentially bind to the receptor, thus reducing the radioligand binding. A curve of this type can be prepared for each of several competitors. The most effective competitors are those that displace the radioligand at relatively low concentrations (Figure 2.12, curve A). Weaker competitors (Figure 2.12, curves B and C) require higher concentrations to effectively displace the radioligand. To compare their relative effectiveness in displacing the radioligand, an **inhibition concentration 50 (IC$_{50}$)** is calculated for each competitor. The IC$_{50}$ is the concentration of competitor that is required to inhibit or reduce radioligand binding to half its maximal value (50%). The lower the IC$_{50}$, the more effective the drug is in competing with the ligand for the receptor.

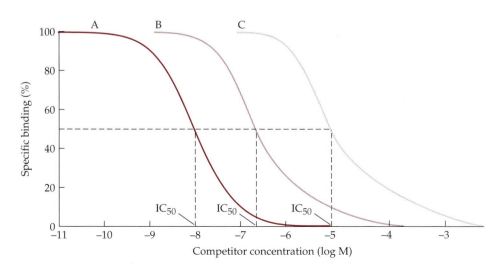

2.12 RESULTS OF A COMPETITION EXPERIMENT. Semilog plot of competition binding data using three competitors (A, B, and C). Tissue is incubated with a constant concentration of radioligand. The various amounts of competing drug added to the incubation tubes are plotted on the abscissa. The specific binding of the radioligand is plotted on the ordinate. Binding observed in the absence of competitor is designated as 100%. With increasing concentrations of competitor, specific binding of the radioligand decreases. The IC$_{50}$ is the concentration of competitor required to displace binding to half of the 100% value. The smaller the IC$_{50}$, the more effective the competitor.

Ligand–Receptor Kinetics

The pharmacological action of a drug is dependent on its interaction with specific receptors. Both the number of receptors acted upon and the affinity of the drug for the receptors are highly significant factors in determining drug effect. The simplest interaction between a drug (or neurotransmitter) and its receptor is the bimolecular reaction described by the law of mass action (see Chapter 1). The application of the law of mass action to the study of dose–response relationships is generally credited to the work of A. J. Clark during the 1920s (Clark, 1933). As shown in Equation 2.1, a ligand (L) interacts with a receptor (R) to produce a conformational change in the receptor, yielding an activated complex (RL*). Thus, the amount of RL* formed is proportional to both the concentration of the drug and the concentration of unoccupied receptor. The brackets in the equation denote "concentration."

$$\textbf{(2.1)} \qquad [R] + [L] \underset{k_{-1}}{\overset{k_1}{\rightleftharpoons}} [RL^*] \rightarrow \text{biobehavioral effect}$$

Receptor occupancy theory assumes that biological activity is directly proportional to the number of binding sites occupied; that is, the greater the occupancy of receptors (RL*), the greater the biological effect. It is important to notice the bidirectional nature of Equation 2.1, which represents the processes of association (formation of the RL* complex) and dissociation (separation of the RL* complex into its component parts, R = unoccupied receptor and L = uncoupled, or "free" ligand). Equilibrium is reached when the rate at which the receptor-ligand complex forms is equal to the rate at which it dissociates. Kinetic experiments are used to measure these rates. The rate of association is determined by incubating a radioligand with the receptor-containing tissue and measuring the amount of specific binding at various times. Figure 2.13 shows a typical association curve (solid-color line), which increases steeply at first and then more gradually until equilibrium is reached. The slope of the linear rising portion of the curve is defined as the association rate constant (k_1) for the specific ligand under the particular assay conditions. Equilibrium under usual assay conditions (25°–37°C) is reached in 30–90 minutes.

The rate of dissociation is determined by adding a large excess of unlabeled ligand to the incubation medium after equilibrium has been reached (Figure 2.13, time A). As the radioligand begins to dissociate from the receptor, the unlabeled ligand is more likely to bind because it is present in relatively large amounts. Specific binding is determined at various times following the addition of the unlabeled ligand (Figure 2.13, shaded-color line), and the slope of the straight line that best fits the data provides an estimate of the dissociation of radioligand and receptor (k_{-1}).

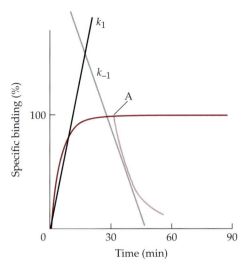

2.13 HYPOTHETICAL ASSOCIATION AND DISSOCIATION CURVES. The solid-color line represents the association of a radioligand with its receptors. After maximum binding has occurred (association and dissociation are in equilibrium), excess unlabeled ligand is added (at time A). The shaded-color line represents the dissociation of the radioligand from its receptors in the presence of large amounts of unlabeled ligand. The slopes of the straight lines that best fit the empirical data provide estimates of the rates of association (k_1) and dissociation (k_{-1}).

If we compare the rate of association (k_1) with the rate of dissociation (k_{-1}), we can learn something about the affinity of the ligand for the receptor. Those ligands demonstrating rapid binding and relatively slow dissociation are said to have greater affinity for the receptor. Since ligands with greater affinity would bind more receptors in a unit of time than ligands with relatively less affinity for the same receptors, we might expect a greater biological effect using higher affinity ligands.

Biochemical convention dictates that we describe this affinity numerically in an inverse way. The slope of a curve is difficult to measure, but mathematically manipulating the numbers by inverting them makes a curve linear, at least conceptually. The inversion allows some relatively simple mathematical operations that yield biologically important numbers representing affinity and also estimates of the number of receptors present. Hence we most frequently describe affinity in terms of the K_d, or dissociation constant: affinity is proportional to $1/K_d$, so affinity is said to be high if the concentration of a drug that results in 50% saturation of the receptors is low. The dissociation constant is expressed in moles per liter and is expected to be equivalent to the concentration of drug that produces a response that is 50% of the maximum (ED_{50}) attainable by that drug. Thus,

$$\textbf{(2.2)} \qquad K_d = \frac{k_{-1}}{k_1}$$

The more rapid the association relative to dissociation (i.e., when k_1 is greater than k_{-1}), the smaller the K_d, and the greater the affinity. Since we know from Equation 2.1 that k_1 describes the rate of formation of the complex RL^* while k_{-1} describes the rate of dissociation of the complex into its parts (R and L), we can combine Equations 2.1 and 2.2 so that

$$(2.3) \qquad K_d = \frac{k_{-1}}{k_1} = \frac{[R][L]}{[RL^*]}$$

We must assume that cells contain a finite number of receptors, represented by the value B_{max}, such that the total population of receptors is equal to the sum of those receptors associated with the ligand and those that are not associated with it.

$$[RL^*] + [R] = B_{max}$$

If we multiply both sides of this equation by [L], we find that

$$(2.4) \qquad [L][RL^*] + [L][R] = [L]B_{max}$$

Since from Equation 2.3 we already know that

$$[L][R] = [RL^*]K_d$$

we can substitute $[RL^*][K_d]$ for [L][R] in Equation 2.4, giving us

$$[L][RL^*] + [RL^*]K_d = [L]B_{max}$$

which can be simplified to

$$[RL^*]([L] + K_d) = [L]B_{max}$$

or solving for $[RL^*]$:

$$(2.5) \qquad [RL^*] = \frac{B_{max}[L]}{[L] + K_d}$$

Equation 2.5 expresses a relationship identical to the law of mass action (see Chapter 1) and the Michaelis–Menten equation, which is used to characterize the velocity of enzyme–substrate interactions. The relationship can be represented graphically by a simple rectangular hyperbola, for example, the saturation binding curve (see Figure 2.11) or its semilog transformation, which yields the classic sigmoidal curve (Figure 2.14) characteristic of dose–response relationships. The sigmoidal curve is the most commonly used because it provides the opportunity to see changes at low concentrations of ligand (or agonist) that would be too close together on an arithmetic scale. Additionally, the sigmoidal curve has the advantage of providing a center of symmetry at 50% of

the maximal response that can approximate a straight line, the slope of which describes its rate of change.

Using Figure 2.14 and Equation 2.5, you will find that when ligand concentration is zero, there is no binding (and therefore no effect). When ligand concentration equals K_d, binding is half-maximal. As [L] increases above K_d, B_{max} is approached by incrementally smaller approximations. By plugging the empirical values from saturation binding experiments into Equation 2.5 and calculating for K_d, we can determine the affinity of the ligand for the receptor.

In summary, this section on ligand–receptor kinetics has provided a mathematical description of the dynamic relationship between the concentration of receptors and that of ligands in relationship to total receptor population (B_{max}) and affinity (K_d) between ligand and receptor. Furthermore, we see that the K_d can be determined by two empirical methods: (1) comparison of the association and dissociation rates, and (2) analysis of the half-maximal binding of ligand saturation data.

The calculation of K_d using the method described is valid only when certain assumptions are met. We must assume: (1) that the response is proportional to the number of receptors occupied, (2) that each drug molecule binds to only one receptor, and that binding at one receptor has no effect on subsequent binding to other receptors, and (3) that only a small amount of available drug is bound at any time. Although these assumptions are sometimes true, often they are not. For this reason, receptor occupancy theory has been modified to deal with cases in which other relationships between receptor occupation and drug effect exist.

Efficacy. One such modification of occupancy theory was proposed to explain why different but chemically related drugs have quite different abilities to elicit a re-

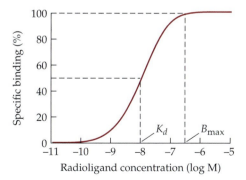

2.14 SEMILOG PLOT OF SATURATION CURVE DATA. Plotting saturation curve data on a log scale for radioligand concentration produces a sigmoidal dose–response curve. The ligand concentration that produces maximum (100%) binding (B_{max}) and the concentration that produces half the maximum (50%) binding (K_d) are readily determined.

sponse, with some even acting as antagonists. Since such variability cannot be explained solely in terms of the law of mass action, an additional factor, called **efficacy** (**E**) by Stephenson and intrinsic activity by Ariens, was defined. Efficacy refers to the properties of drugs that relate to the strength of the effect they elicit. Each drug acting on a specific receptor type has a different value for efficacy, which is expressed as a proportionality constant related to the drug's intrinsic ability to elicit a response once it has combined with the receptor. High efficacy means that each drug–receptor complex (RL*) produces a high level of physiological response, whereas low efficacy results in a lesser degree of response. The fewer the receptors that must be occupied to produce a response, the greater the efficacy of the agonist.

Efficacy is quite separate from affinity (K_d), and the two can vary independently within a series of related agonist agents. In other words, although two drugs may have identical rates of association and dissociation, one may be more effective in eliciting a response when it binds to a receptor. One reasonable explanation for differences in efficacy is that different agonists do not produce identical changes in receptor conformation (shape) when they bind and therefore do not produce identical intracellular events. As Figure 2.15 shows, changes in efficacy alone can shift the dose–response curve as well as the maximal response, even when affinity is held constant. Notice that as efficacy decreases, the dose–response curve shifts to the right, demonstrating the need for higher concentrations to achieve the same response. When efficacy falls below certain values, the maximum attainable response also decreases. Since we know that differences in drug concentration relative to affinity also produce shifts in dose–response curves, we must conclude that the dose–response curve reflects two factors: affinity and efficacy.

In Chapter 1 we introduced the concept of competitive drug antagonism. We explained that an antagonist binds to a receptor, usually with high affinity, but does not produce a biological effect. The absence of biological effect is due to the antagonist's low or zero efficacy, which means that although the drug readily binds, it does not change the conformation of the receptor to its activated state and hence is incapable of initiating the next step of the biological sequence. A pure agonist has both affinity and efficacy, while a mixed agonist–antagonist has affinity for the receptor but a low efficacy. Since agonists and competitive antagonists vie for the same receptors, an agonist in the presence of an antagonist must be present at a higher concentration in order to produce the same magnitude of response as the agonist alone. If enough agonist is administered, the maximum effect can be reached, as is demonstrated by the parallel shift in the dose–response curve (see Chapter 1).

Receptor occupancy theory has also been modified to account for receptors with multiple active sites or

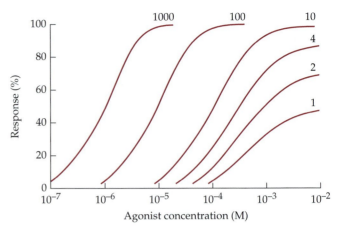

2.15 EFFECTS OF VARIATIONS IN EFFICACY. Hypothetical dose–response curves showing the effect of varying drug efficacy (E) while affinity (K_d) is held constant. Efficacy and affinity often vary independently in series of related agonists. The numbers on the curves are values of E.

cases in which binding by a single drug molecule either increases or decreases the ability of a second molecule to bind (cooperativity). To deal with cases in which the occupation of the receptor by the ligand may be less significant than the rate of occupation of the receptor, the "rate theory" of receptor binding was developed. Further modifications of receptor occupancy theory have been necessary to analyze results that indicate the existence of multiple receptor subtypes, a topic we will discuss in the following sections. Additional discussion of receptor occupancy theory is beyond the scope of this chapter, but in-depth discussions can be found in several excellent texts (Bentley, 1981; Limbird, 1986).

Mathematical Transformations and Data Plotting

There are three ways to evaluate receptor binding data. First, visual inspection of the experimental results can provide an initial appreciation of trends. Second, classic biochemical analyses using mathematical transformations of the data will frequently provide a linear representation of the results, which is easier to visualize graphically. Third, when results are complicated by the presence of multiple interacting binding sites or receptor subtypes, the use of computer analysis to describe the nonlinear results provides a powerful tool.

Among the many graphic approaches available to analyze binding data, the most commonly used is the **Scatchard plot** analysis. Using the data from a saturation binding experiment (see Figure 2.11), the values are replotted in the form of bound ligand/free ligand (B/F or [RL*]/[L]) on the y-axis versus bound ligand (B or [RL*]) on the x-axis (Figure 2.16). Free ligand (or ligand that is not bound) is often difficult to quantify. In most binding experiments the amount of ligand used is many times in excess of the available receptor, and free ligand is computed by subtracting bound from total. If a single class of receptors is present, the saturation curve is transformed into a straight line whose x-intercept indicates receptor concentration (B_{max}; that is, when B/F = 0). The dissociation constant is calculated from the slope of that straight line ($-1/K_d$). Analysis is more complex when the ligand binds to several independent or interacting binding sites and the plot becomes concave upward (Figure 2.16*b*). In that case, computer analysis provides the most effective means of fitting the data to a multireceptor model, producing two straight lines representing receptors with different affinities for the ligand. Further discussion of computer modeling can be found in several sources (Lundeen and Gordon, 1986; Motulsky and Insel, 1987).

Other mathematical transformation and plotting techniques are available to the researcher interested in radioligand binding. Some of these include the Hill plot, the Schild plot, and the Eadie–Hofstee plot. Each method available has unique benefits for evaluating complex data as well as certain drawbacks. All of the transformations are capable of distorting the data such that small

experimental errors are changed into larger deviations (Motulsky and Insel, 1987). Also, interpretations of results may be misleading unless the underlying assumptions for rigorous evaluation are met and appropriate ligand concentrations are used in the assay (Klotz, 1983).

The radioligand receptor binding method is currently the most popular technique for evaluating receptor density and affinity. Other techniques used to evaluate receptors include autoradiography, photoaffinity labeling, antireceptor antibodies, radionuclide scans and solubilization, purification, and reconstitution of receptors.

Receptor Autoradiography

In vitro receptor binding. Autoradiographic **in vitro receptor binding** applies the standard techniques of autoradiography described earlier to the study of ligand binding to receptor sites. This method uses frozen tissue sections that are mounted on glass slides. Following incubation with a radioligand (either labeled drug or neurotransmitter), the unbound radioactivity is washed away before autoradiographic processing. Many of the measurements made in homogenate binding studies (e.g., receptor number and affinity, results of competition experiments, association and dissociation rates) can also be made using the autoradiographic technique. The method is extremely useful in studying the effects of brain lesions on receptor binding because each lesioned animal can be evaluated independently by comparing the lesioned and nonlesioned sides of the brain. Additionally, since the anatomy of the brain is preserved, lesion size and placement can be evaluated. Further, the in vitro method can use different ligands in adjacent brain sections to evaluate multiple receptors. This method has been used quite effectively to study changes in pathological postmortem human brain.

Autoradiographic receptor mapping has been applied to questions about how various psychotropic drugs produce their behavioral effects. For instance, correlations between clinical effects and binding sites in brain have been found by mapping the binding of the drug [³H]strychnine (Kuhar, 1982). Such studies suggest that the increased acuity of perception that follows strychnine administration may be related to high concentrations of binding in various sensory areas. High spinal cord and brain stem binding may be related to the clinical effects of hyperreflexia and muscle spasm. Used in this manner, the technique is useful as an initial probe into the localization of brain function.

In vitro autoradiographic mapping of receptor binding can also be used in combination with immunohistochemistry. In one such study (Kito and Miyoshi, 1985), immunohistochemical labeling of glutamic acid decarboxylase (GAD, an enzyme that synthesizes the neurotransmitter GABA) and in vitro autoradiographic mapping of labeled flunitrazepam (a tranquilizer) were

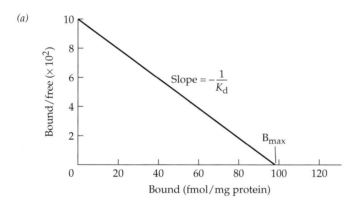

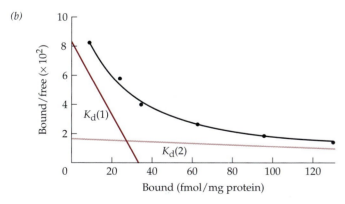

2.16 SCATCHARD PLOT. (*a*) Saturation curve data plotted with bound ligand on the abscissa and the ratio of bound to free ligand on the ordinate produces a straight line. The x-intercept indicates receptor concentration (B_{max}). The slope of the line is used to calculate the dissociation constant. (*b*) Scatchard plot analysis of ligand binding to multiple binding sites produces a curve that is concave upward. Computer analysis provides two straight lines that best fit the empirical data, representing two receptor types with different affinities for the ligand.

accomplished in the same slice. The results showed, in electron microscopic detail, that nerve endings in the striatum contained both GAD immunoreactivity and drug binding sites. Studies of this type can provide unique information about drug–brain–behavior interactions.

In vivo receptor binding.   The combination of **in vivo receptor binding** and autoradiography allows highly detailed mapping of ligand binding in the intact animal. This method involves systemically injecting radiolabeled ligand into a conscious animal. The ligand enters the general circulation, diffuses into the brain, and binds to receptors. The animal is then sacrificed, and the brain (or other body parts) is sliced and mounted on microscope slides for subsequent autoradiographic processing. In vivo binding and mapping by autoradiography provides the researcher with anatomical detail at the light microscope level that was not previously possible with the tissue dissection and homogenate binding techniques.

Despite the elegance of this technique, it is not without pitfalls. The analysis of results is far more complex than for the binding methods described previously. Because the initial labeling procedure occurs in the intact animal, factors such as blood levels of free ligand, biodistribution, diffusion through the blood–brain barrier, and metabolism of the tracer must be considered. In addition, as with in vitro assays, successful in vivo binding is dependent on ligand specific activity, receptor density, and binding affinity. These and other related factors are discussed in detail elsewhere (Young, Frey, and Agranoff, 1986).

Several neurotransmitter receptor types have been labeled successfully using in vivo techniques, including muscarinic cholinergic, enkephalinergic, and dopaminergic receptors. For instance, the feasibility of labeling dopamine receptors in vivo using radioactive spiperone was demonstrated a number of years ago (Kuhar et al., 1978). [^{3}H]Spiperone was injected into the tail veins of mice. Subsequent autoradiographic mapping of the brain showed binding sites that matched the known distribution of dopamine receptors. The drug binding showed pharmacological specificity (i.e., the radioligand could be displaced only by dopaminergic agents) and was distributed within the cell constituents in the manner expected for dopamine receptors. Careful verification of the identity of labeled proteins is a vital step in the development of this technique.

Although in vivo binding has been accomplished with a limited number of ligands, it provides a means of measuring synaptic transmitter levels or receptor occupancy at specific synapses under defined behavioral or pathological conditions. Furthermore, in vivo binding studies using PET visualization of human brain (see below) permit such measurements to be made in an intact, functioning subject. The availability of the technique has initiated a new area of clinical research. For those disorders (e.g., Parkinson's disease, Alzheimer's disease, Huntington's disease, schizophrenia, temporal lobe epilepsy) that have demonstrated postmortem receptor alterations in vitro, receptor labeling in vivo may show a correlation between receptor changes and progress of the disease as well as therapeutic responses (Young, Frey, and Agranoff, 1986).

Receptor Isolation and Labeling

Receptor solubilization.   In addition to localizing and quantifying drug and neurotransmitter receptors in the nervous system, neurobiologists are increasingly interested in understanding the molecular mechanisms of drug–receptor–effector interactions. One method currently available for studying these interactions is **receptor solubilization**. It is possible to biochemically dissect a receptor protein from the cell membrane (by solubilization) and characterize its general properties (e.g., affinity for ligand, temperature dependence) and physiochemical characteristics (e.g., size, molecular weight, amino acid sequence). In some cases, the isolated receptors can be reinserted into artificially prepared membranes whose characteristics are controlled. The reconstitution of receptor in a known membrane provides a well-controlled, functioning model of receptor–membrane interaction. A detailed discussion of receptor solubilization and reconstitution can be found in several sources (Newby, 1984; White, 1986). The reconstitution of the acetylcholine receptor in artificial membrane to measure ion conductances through the receptor-regulated channel is described in more detail in Chapter 6.

Photoaffinity labeling.   A useful adjunct to the solubilization technique is affinity or **photoaffinity labeling**. The affinity procedure is used to change a ligand that specifically and reversibly binds hydrostatically (ionically) to a receptor into a compound that binds covalently (essentially irreversibly) to that receptor. The method requires the attachment of a chemically labile group to the ligand. This group provides the covalent bond between ligand and receptor. The bound ligand can be detected by means of a marker that is radioactive or fluorescent.

Photoaffinity labeling uses this principle by adding to the ligand a photolabile group that is unreactive in the dark. When exposed to light, it is converted to an extremely reactive intermediate, which forms a covalent bond between the ligand and the binding site. In some cases, no photolabile group needs to be added: ultraviolet irradiation of certain ligands covalently links the ligand to the receptor. Among the ultraviolet-sensitive psychotropic drugs are the benzodiazepines (Möhler, Richards, and Wu, 1981), phencyclidine, and chlorpromazine (Oswald and Changeux, 1981).

The advantages of the photoaffinity method include the ability to bind the modified ligand to the receptor before photoactivation in order to confirm the specificity of binding. A second advantage is that an unreactive ligand can label components inside the cell before being activated, thereby avoiding external modification of the cell.

The photoaffinity labeling technique is useful for the isolation, localization, and characterization of receptors (Sokolovsky, 1984). The covalent binding of a labeled ligand to the receptor is important in the receptor solubilization procedure. When a membrane is disrupted and the receptor protein removed, the physiological functions of the receptor, including its ability to bind to the ligand, are often lost. Without measurable function, the receptor cannot be readily separated. However, with labels covalently bound to the receptor, its identification and separation are possible even if the protein is distorted or denatured.

Photoaffinity labeling is useful in other types of research as well. First, the use of photoaffinity labeling facilitates the identification and quantification of receptors, especially when receptor proteins constitute only a small proportion of total membrane protein, as, for example, in developing organisms. Second, covalent binding to a receptor produces prolonged stimulation or inactivation of the resulting molecular events, which can then be more easily studied biochemically or physiologically. For instance, affinity-labeled probes of the benzodiazepine receptor produced long-lasting anticonvulsant effects that were consistent with covalent attachment to the binding site (Williams et al., 1981).

Finally, photoaffinity labeling can be used to study the primary structure of receptor binding sites (Thomas and Tallman, 1984) and can aid in identifying the amino acid residues in the vicinity of the receptor. Also, the interconversion of high- and low-affinity binding sites that occurs for some receptors treated with metal ions, heat, or GTP can be observed (Gurwitz and Sokolovsky, 1980).

Brain Metabolism and Imaging Methods

Enzyme Kinetics

Enzymes are proteins that act as biological catalysts to speed up reaction rates, but are not used up in the process. Many different enzymes are found in every cell, and each has a role in a relatively specific reaction. Virtually every conversion of a reactant (substrate) to a product is catalyzed by a preferred enzyme. There are many enzymes of interest to neuropharmacologists, particularly those involved in the synthesis or metabolism of neurotransmitters, neuromodulators, or second messengers, as well as those responsible for general cell function. Assays that directly or indirectly measure enzymatic activity in the nervous system are among the most common tools in neuropsychopharmacology.

In general, the presence of a particular enzyme is of less significance than the rate of the reaction it catalyzes and the conditions that determine that rate. For example, neuropharmacologists are interested in identifying the conditions that regulate the rate of synthesis of the neurotransmitter, norepinephrine. Since the rate of formation of the final product (norepinephrine) is determined by the activity of the first enzyme in a multiple-step sequence, many efforts have been directed toward understanding the function of that rate-limiting enzyme, tyrosine hydroxylase.

Because enzymes play a vital role in neuronal activity, their function will be discussed in greater detail in subsequent chapters of this text. This section provides a brief outline of the general procedure for evaluating enzyme activity. The details of evaluating particular enzymes will be left for the individual to investigate using texts in biochemistry or enzymology.

The activity of an enzyme (E) depends upon its ability to combine reversibly with a substrate (S) to form an enzyme–substrate complex (ES), which then irreversibly decomposes to yield products (P) and the free enzyme in its original form. The substrate fits partially or entirely into the active site of the enzyme. The formation of the complex resembles the reversible drug–receptor binding described earlier, according to the law of mass action:

$$E + S \rightleftharpoons ES \rightarrow E + P$$

The binding of the substrate to the enzyme has a specificity determined by the enzyme's amino acid sequence, which is responsible for the three-dimensional configuration of the protein. Once the enzymatic reaction leads to a physical change in the substrate, the products do not remain bound, and the free enzyme is able to bind to another substrate molecule. Some enzymes require the presence of a coenzyme, such as pyridoxal (vitamin B_6) or thiamine phosphate (vitamin B_1). Enzymes may also require a cofactor, such as a specific ion, to induce the necessary configuration for attachment of the substrate. Among the most common cofactors are calcium, magnesium, zinc, manganese, copper, and iron.

The rate of an enzyme reaction as a function of time can be measured in vitro by incubating the enzyme preparation (e.g., tissue homogenate) with tagged reactant (substrate or cofactor) under specific reaction conditions. The rate of (1) use of substrate over time, (2) increase in the reaction product, or (3) increase or decrease of a required cofactor can then be determined. The assay is based on the assumption that if the substrate is available in saturating concentrations (i.e., enough substrate is available to saturate or occupy all the binding sites on the enzyme), the amount of product formed will depend on the activity of the enzyme and the duration of the reaction. Factors that affect the velocity of the enzymatic reaction include concentration of reactants, pH, temperature, ionic strength, presence of specific ions, and presence of inhibitors. Each factor can alter the configuration of the enzyme and thereby alter its activity. The optimum values of each factor that affect the velocity of the reaction are empirically determined for each enzyme.

The relationship between enzyme and substrate is reminiscent of the receptor–ligand interaction described earlier. In fact, by relabeling the y-axis "velocity" and the x-axis "substrate concentration," Figure 2.11 can be made to show that relationship graphically. The linear portion of Figure 2.11 shows that with a fixed amount of enzyme, the reaction rate (velocity) varies directly with the substrate concentration when the concentration is low. As more enzyme binding sites become occupied, the addition of further substrate produces a diminished increment of reaction velocity. When binding sites are saturated, reaction velocity is independent of substrate concentration. The relationship described, based on the law of mass action, is identical with the Michaelis–Menten equation discussed in Chapter 1 and in the section on ligand–receptor kinetics earlier in this chapter.

Autoradiography of Dynamic Cell Processes

One important application of autoradiography is the tracing of dynamic processes such as cerebral blood flow, cell metabolism and uptake, and biochemical processes. In order to measure the rate of any biological process, a tracer technique is required, because measuring steady state concentrations of reactants or products does not tell us about the speed of the process. Indeed, the amount of a known chemical may appear unchanged despite the fact that rates of its synthesis and breakdown are changing greatly, although perhaps in parallel.

The classic biochemical method of studying reaction rates is to label one reactant of a chemical reaction and measure in vitro the rate of formation of a labeled product or the rate of disappearance of the labeled reactant. In order to study rates, measurements are taken as a function of time, and inferences are made based on the collection of data. The development of quantitative autoradiography has provided a means to both quantify and localize a tagged reactant that has been administered in vivo. Thus, we are able to apply kinetic models (i.e., models describing the rate of a reaction) to examine the dynamic processes of the CNS in diverse neural systems of the same animal. The parallel development of PET scan techniques (see below) has made it possible to measure in vivo tracer changes in humans.

Macroautoradiography of the brain was developed in the late 1950s to trace blood flow in the brain of the rat (Freygang and Sokoloff, 1958). The technique has been modified (Sakurada et al., 1978) and successfully applied to the study of steady state oxygen consumption in the brain, local cerebral glucose utilization, and local rates of cerebral protein synthesis. Furthermore, the technique can be readily used to show labeled drug distribution in the brain (or in the whole body) as well as labeled ligand binding to neurotransmitter receptor sites (see above). It can also be used for immunologically locating specific cellular components.

2-Deoxyglucose autoradiography.   The study of brain utilization of glucose is extremely important because the brain is one of the most metabolically active organs in the body. Despite its relatively small size (approximately 2% of body weight), it accounts for 20% of the total oxygen consumption. Since neural stores of energy-rich substrates for metabolism are small, the brain is highly dependent on the continuous availability of glucose in the cerebral circulation.

The [^{14}C]2-deoxyglucose (2-DG) method developed by Sokoloff and colleagues (1977) measures and visualizes glucose utilization simultaneously in all brain areas following experimental manipulation. Since a direct relationship is assumed to exist between nerve function and glucose utilization, the pictures reveal a dynamic biochemical process that represents physiological function. It is possible to identify brain structures with altered neural activity during various conditions, such as sensory or motor stimulation, drug treatment, or disease (Sokoloff, 1986).

The technique is based on the ability of [^{14}C]2-DG to be transported into cells in the same manner as glucose. The amount of glucose incorporated into a cell is directly proportional to the metabolic activity of the cell. Once in the cell, [^{14}C]2-DG is converted (phosphorylated) by the enzyme hexokinase to form [^{14}C]2-deoxyglucose-6-phosphate. [^{14}C]2-deoxyglucose-6-phosphate cannot be further metabolized in the usual manner to fructose-6-phosphate. Since it does not readily pass the cell membrane, [^{14}C]2-deoxyglucose-6-phosphate accumulates in the cell. When the amount of radioactivity taken up into specific cells is quantified, using either quantitative autoradiography or positron emission tomography (PET) scans (see following sections), the regional metabolic rate for glucose utilization can be directly calculated. If the rate of glucose utilization is known, the extent of cell activity can be determined. The visualization of stimulus-evoked metabolic response is a very useful tool for studying functional neural pathways in the brain.

The 2-DG technique has been used extensively to map such things as the pathways of higher visual functions, metabolic changes during stages of sleep, and during psychotic episodes, and it has been used in a vast number of neuropharmacological investigations involving experimental modifications of neurochemistry (McCulloch, 1982; Sokoloff, 1986). For instance, McCulloch and coworkers (1982) have been able to create dose–response curves for the effects of drugs on glucose utilization in various dopamine-containing neural pathways. One such neural system projects from the retina to the superficial layer of the superior colliculus in the rat (Figure 2.17). They found that systemic injection of 1.5 mg/kg body weight apomorphine (a dopamine agonist) increased optical density (representing glucose utilization) bilaterally in the superior colliculus. However, following enucleation of one eye, apomorphine increased optical density bilaterally only in the deep layer of the superior colliculus. In the superficial layer, apomorphine increased optical density only on the ipsilateral side. This study and others of this type (Soncrant, 1986) demonstrate that quantitative surveys of the brain for sites of drug-induced neural activity allow comparisons of the relative potencies of drugs and provides information on structure–function relationships.

One great advantage of the 2-DG method is that the manipulations can be made on conscious animals, thereby avoiding the contamination of results by anesthetics. Additionally, the method provides an opportunity to evaluate behavior simultaneously. For example, Allen and coworkers (1981) have mapped glucose utilization in the female rat brain following vaginocervical stimulation, which also elicited lordosis (the crouching stance with raised hindquarters denoting sexual receptivity). The structures showing increased 2-DG uptake included the preoptic nucleus of the hypothalamus, mesencephalic reticular formation, and dorsal raphe nucleus, among others. Previous experiments using physi-

ological and pharmacological manipulation have shown the importance of these structures to sexual behavior in the female rat. However, vaginocervical stimulation also alters progesterone secretion, facilitates transport of sperm from vagina to cervix, and inhibits somatic reflexes, locomotion, and response to pain. The glucose mapping suggests the concurrent processing of this sensory stimulation by several neural areas, although no specific behavioral or physiological function can be ascribed to a particular brain area.

Critical evaluation of the 2-DG method has raised several empirical concerns and has led to several modifications of the original method (McCulloch, 1982; Duncan and Stumpf, 1991). First, since glucose utilization in brain structures varies with changes in physiological variables such as body temperature, blood pressure, and respiration, drug-induced changes in metabolism represent the average of all the drug's effects. A change in a single brain area cannot be assumed to be uniquely related to a specific response. Second, the close relationship between glucose utilization and cellular activity may be altered under conditions of low food consumption when ketone bodies contribute a greater proportion of energy than normal. Whether low food consumption is due to deprivation or induced anorexia, the condition violates an important underlying assumption in the 2-DG methodology. Finally, there is a twofold difference in cerebral glucose use during the normal circadian cycle. Neuropharmacological modifications of cell me-

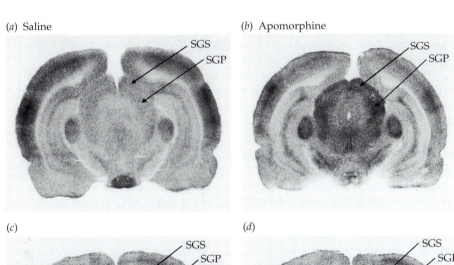

(a) Saline

(b) Apomorphine

(c)

(d)

Saline, right eye enucleated

Apomorphine, right eye enucleated

2.17 REPRESENTATIVE AUTORADIOGRAPHS FROM A 2-DG STUDY. These autoradiographs represent brain slices at the level of the superior colliculus from dark-adapted rats studied in the dark. SGS = stratum griseum superficiale; SGP = stratum griseum profundum. (a) Saline, intact visual system. (b) Apomorphine (1.5 mg/kg), intact visual system. (c) Saline, right eye enucleated. (d) Apomorphine (1.5 mg/kg), right eye enucleated. (From McCulloch et al., 1982; courtesy of James McCulloch.)

tabolism may therefore be somewhat dependent on the time of day of testing.

In summary, the [^{14}C]2-DG method provides a quantitative description of spatial and temporal patterns of neuronal activity in functional units of the CNS involved in physiological responses to sensory or pharmacological manipulation. Its major advantage is that investigations are not limited to a small preselected area of the brain, but rather, can evaluate global brain activity. However, recent research suggests that 2-DG studies alone do not provide a comprehensive evaluation of brain activity. Measurement of intercellular constituents (such as *c-fos* mRNA or fos protein) that reflect changes in the rate of protein synthesis in the cell following experimental manipulation can be measured using in situ hybridization or immunocytochemistry (see above). This type of data can provide complementary information on neural activation at a cellular level (Duncan and Stumpf, 1991).

In Vivo Imaging

The in vitro imaging techniques discussed so far have provided much information about the workings of the CNS. In addition to these methods, new techniques have been devised to examine brain function without injury to the subject. Among the most exciting of these new methods are computerized tomography (CT) scanning, positron emission tomography (PET) scanning, and magnetic resonance imaging (MRI). In each case, detailed examination of fine brain structures is possible while the individual is thinking, learning, or initiating movement. Because these methods are not invasive, they allow examination of CNS function in healthy as well as in diseased states. These methods not only provide neurobiologists with opportunities to localize brain function, but also allow them to identify the patterns of brain activity associated with different functional states.

Computerized tomography.   **Computerized tomography** (**CT**) is a technique developed by Hounsfield and Cormack, for which they received the Nobel Prize for Physiology and Medicine in 1979. CT resembles the conventional X-ray technique, but has been modified to greatly increase resolution of the image and to provide imaging in three dimensions. The conventional X-ray technique provides a static picture of the brain. That picture is dependent on differences in the absorption of X-rays by various brain areas as the rays are aimed through the tissue at a sensitive photographic plate. Since bone absorbs a great deal of radiation, it is clearly shown on the film as a light area, while air absorbs little radiation and appears dark on the film. Unfortunately, the difference in absorbance among different tissues is not large, so that even very different tissues, such as the gray and white matter of the brain, cannot be distinguished by conventional X-ray techniques.

In contrast, CT uses a series of narrow, parallel beams of radiation aimed through the tissue and toward a "film" of sensitive scintillation crystals (X-ray detectors). The X-ray source is rotated around the head while the detectors move on the opposite side in parallel. At each point of rotation, the source and detectors also move linearly. In this manner they make a series of radiation transmission readings. The radiation absorption of each brain region is calculated by a computer to yield a summation of all the readings passing through that region. Thus, each visually displaced brain "slice" is a summation of thousands of intersecting radiation transmission measurements. The measurements are translated into numbers and then into a visual display as relatively dark or light areas. For the first time, in situ resolution in brain tissue of less than 1 mm is possible, and such anatomic detail provides a much enhanced capacity for evaluation. Nevertheless, CT scans provide information only on the structure of the brain, not on its function.

Positron emission tomography.   A further advance in noninvasive visualization of brain tissue is the **positron emission tomography** (**PET scan**). Whereas CT scans provide a static view of brain slices, PET scans can be used to explore dynamic brain function. PET combines the CT technique with radioisotope imaging. CT measures transmission of X-rays through tissue, while PET measures the emission of inhaled or injected radiation after its distribution in the brain. To map the distribution of compounds of interest (e.g., drugs, glucose, water, neurotransmitters), an unstable, positron-emitting isotope must first be made and then bound to the compound before being introduced into the subject. The isotopes used for PET scans are listed in Table 2.3 along with their respective half-lives.

Positron-emitting isotopes that will be inhaled or injected into the subject are made in a cyclotron by forcing a proton at high speed into the nucleus of a stable isotope of the appropriate element. The addition of the extra proton makes the isotope unstable, forcing the proton to split into two parts: a neutron, which remains within the nucleus, and a positron, which is expelled from the nucleus. When the positron collides with an electron in the atomic orbit shells, two gamma rays are emitted at exactly 180° from one another. Crystal photomultipliers that surround the head are used to detect these gamma rays (Figure 2.18). The detectors record an event only when two essentially simultaneous detections are made. This allows calculation of the precise location of gamma emission and eliminates effects of stray radiation. Computer analysis of the gamma ray emissions translates the nuclear events into a visualization of the brain. The distance between the nucleus and the collision between positron and electron determines the resolution possible in PET scans. This distance varies for the commonly used isotopes; for instance, 2 mm for ^{18}F and 8 mm for ^{15}O. For this reason, ^{18}F scans can have greater resolution than those using other isotopes. However, because of the rela-

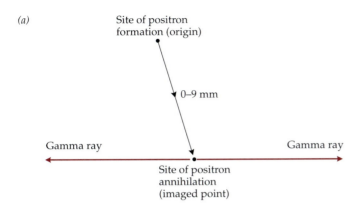

(a)

Site of positron
formation (origin)

0–9 mm

Gamma ray · Gamma ray

Site of positron
annihilation
(imaged point)

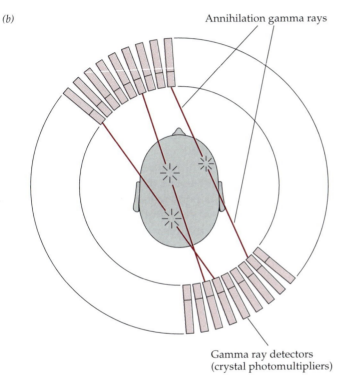

(b)

Annihilation gamma rays

Gamma ray detectors
(crystal photomultipliers)

2.18 THE PET SCANNING TECHNIQUE. The emission of positrons from labeled body structures is used for imaging. (*a*) The site of positron annihilation that is imaged may be several millimeters from the site of origin. The distance between sites of origin and annihilation varies for each isotope and determines the resolution of the scan. (*b*) Gamma rays that result from positron annihilation are detected by crystal photomultipliers that surround the head. The two gamma rays ultimately reach a pair of detectors that record an event only when two simultaneous detections are made. This method of coincident detection permits precise localization of the site of gamma ray emission. (After Oldendorf, 1980.)

vestigations using different stimulus modes and varying complexity of stimuli have demonstrated a direct relationship between intensity and complexity of tasks and metabolic activity (Greenberg et al., 1981; Mazziotta and Phelps, 1986; Reivich et al., 1986). Clearly PET is capable of mapping brain response to sensory input and provides researchers with opportunities to begin correlating structure with function in the living brain.

Glucose utilization mapping using PET can identify not only which brain areas become more active and which do not, but also which areas are interrelated. A correlational method developed recently makes it possible to identify which brain regions function together during a particular experimental manipulation. When two brain regions are functionally coupled, increased activity in one depends on increased activity in the other. A plot of the regional cerebral metabolic rate for glucose for one region against the second will demonstrate a statistically significant correlation coefficient. The size of the correlation coefficient is proportional to the strength of the coupling between the two areas. If two regions are not functionally related, the statistical manipulation will reveal a small correlation coefficient. Details of the use of the correlational matrix and implementation of the approach are described more fully by Horwitz, Soncrant, and Rapoport (1986).

Changes in glucose metabolism can also be mapped early in the course of certain neurological disorders that only later result in sufficient atrophy to be identified by CT scan. Among the disorders that can be identified by PET scanning of glucose utilization are various forms of dementia, convulsive states, and Huntington's disease.

tively long half-life of ^{18}F, the isotope is moderately toxic, while the other isotopes in Table 2.3 are considered lower in toxicity (Moseley, 1986). The relative benefits and dangers of the different isotopes are evaluated for each patient and experimental protocol.

2-DG with PET scans. The importance of mapping glucose utilization has already been described. It should be no surprise that such investigations have been undertaken with humans utilizing the PET scan technique and [^{18}F]2-DG. In one such study (Mazziotta and Phelps, 1985), glucose metabolism was measured in a normal individual during visual stimulation. The pattern of glucose use was traced while the eyes were closed, then open, then looking at a complex scene. With eyes open, glucose metabolism increased in the primary visual cortex. When the subject viewed the scene, primary visual cortex glucose utilization increased further, and the visual association cortex also became more active. Such in-

Table 2.3	Isotopes Used in PET Scans	
Isotope	Half-life (min)	Distance between nucleus and collision (mm)
[15]Oxygen	2.03	8.2
[13]Nitrogen	9.97	5.39
[11]Carbon	20.4	4.11
[68]Gallium	68.2	—
[18]Fluorine	109.8	2.39

In many cases, glucose uptake is impaired in proportion to the severity of clinical symptoms. For example, in senile dementia and presenile dementia of the Alzheimer's type, glucose metabolism in the brain is prematurely reduced, particularly in the parieto-temporal cortex and the frontal association cortex. Lateral asymmetry in cortical glucose metabolism can be correlated with language and visuospatial dysfunction in Alzheimer's patients. Indeed, PET scanning of glucose utilization is useful in determining the efficacy of therapy for dementia (Alavi and Reivich, 1986; Haxby et al., 1985; Kuhl, Metter, and Riege, 1985).

Mapping of CNS receptors.   PET has also been effectively used to map CNS neurotransmitters and receptors in vivo. This technique provides an opportunity to visualize synaptic events in various disease states as well as following drug administration. Not only can the distribution of receptors be visualized, but quantitative analysis of the number of receptors and their binding characteristics can also be accomplished (see Baron and Maziere, 1986). Furthermore, PET has proved useful in quantitative measures of receptor occupancy in relation to clinical drug treatment. Color Plate 5 shows a PET scan visualization of the binding of neuroleptic drugs (drugs used to treat schizophrenia) to two types of receptors in schizophrenic patients. The figure demonstrates the ability to image neurotransmitter receptors, as labeled by psychotropic drugs, in the living human brain using the PET technique.

The possibilities for PET scanning research seem quite limitless. However, the procedure for producing the short-lived positron-emitting isotopes needed is very costly due to the requirement of an on-site cyclotron. Relatively few research centers presently have such equipment. Thus, widespread use of PET scanning is unlikely in the near future.

Magnetic resonance imaging.   **Magnetic resonance imaging (MRI)**, or nuclear magnetic resonance (NMR), is a third technique for in vivo, noninvasive biochemical analysis. Since the physics of MRI is very complex, it will be discussed only in general terms. Several excellent sources of detailed information on MRI are available (Brant-Zawadzki, 1987; Oldendorf, 1985). MRI is based on the principle that certain atomic nuclei resonate and emit a radio frequency signal when placed in strong magnetic fields. The frequencies given off are distinct for different atoms as well as for the same atomic nucleus in different chemical or physical environments. In addition, relaxation times (the time it takes for a nucleus to return to its previous state after removal of the magnetic field) vary for different nuclei and local tissue conditions. Using computer techniques similar to those applied to CT and PET, one can translate the frequency characteristics of the signals coming from atomic nuclei

in the brain into images. This method, therefore, can distinguish different body tissues based on their individual chemical composition. It allows researchers to study anatomy, metabolism, and biochemistry in both normal and diseased nervous systems.

Hydrogen, for example, is a strong resonator that is found in high proportion in body tissue, since 75% of the body is water. Because different tissues contain different amounts of water, they can be distinguished by scanning the magnetic-induced resonance and relaxation time of hydrogen. The radio frequency signal can be manipulated so that the relaxation time of protons in water can be enhanced (i.e., exaggerated) to differentiate very clearly among tissue types, such as gray and white matter. Since cell death or disease frequently alters distribution of water, these local cell conditions can readily be discriminated from normal brain tissue. Because of the high resolution of the image, even small tumors, infarctions (scars), or plaques (patches of diseased neurons) of multiple sclerosis can be distinguished, thus providing a powerful tool for clinical diagnosis (Aichner and Willeit, 1986; Grucker et al., 1986).

MRI scanning techniques are being developed to measure the concentrations of sodium ions (Na^+) and various phosphorus-containing compounds. Sodium scans will provide a very rapid identification of cell death because in dying tissue Na^+ concentrations increase more rapidly than water increases.

Phosphorus imaging is of great interest because of the importance of phosphorus in the energy cycle. Even at this early stage of their development, these scans can display separately the phosphorus-containing compounds necessary for energy production, such as organic phosphates, phosphocreatine, and ATP. Finally, researchers have recently developed a **functional MRI (fMRI)** method based on the difference in magnetic susceptibility between oxyhemoglobin and deoxyhemoglobin. Neuronal activity leads to a greater increase in regional blood flow than in regional oxygen consumption. This results in enhanced oxygen content of venous blood, and hence, a stronger MRI signal (Cohen and Bookheimer, 1994).

Part I Summary

This portion of Chapter 2 has described some of the methods available to the neuropsychopharmacologist to study receptors and other components of the nervous system by labeling, quantifying, and visualizing. The list of topics discussed is far from complete, but the chapter describes those methods that are most commonly used and those whose further development in the future may provide a new direction for neuropsychopharmacology. Part II will introduce some of the most important methodologies available to evaluate pharmacological effects on behavior.

Part II
Techniques in Behavioral Pharmacology

Behavioral pharmacology is a relatively new area of study that examines the interaction between drug action and behavior. The need for such a discipline became apparent during the 1950s when several drugs from diverse classes were found to be clinically useful in modifying behavior. The methods of behavioral pharmacology provide the techniques with which scientists can objectively define and measure behavior, as well as the changes in behavior elicited by chemical agents. Behaviors are complex because they are the consequence of highly varied experiences, as well as variations in physiology both within and between species. Their measurement is complicated by the fact that drug-induced behavioral effects are modified by variables other than the drug itself. These variables include previous experience, current "mental set," and environmental factors, as well as route of drug administration, the dose-dependent nature of drug effects, and the interaction between dose and baseline rate of behavior. It must be appreciated that drugs do not create behavior per se; that is, drugs do not cause behaviors outside of the species-typical repertoire. Rather, they can alter the probability of the occurrence of a particular behavior at a given time. Behavioral pharmacology systematically begins with standard procedures and measurements to establish a dose and baseline rate of behavior.

The evaluation and quantification of behavior is important to neuropsychopharmacologists for at least three reasons. First, researchers can use drugs with a known mechanism of action to study the neurochemical or physiological basis of behavior. With these tools, they can also examine the action of other drugs whose mechanism of action is unknown. Second, behavior can be used to screen families of drugs to identify their relative potencies, their spectrum of behavioral effects, their structure–activity relationships, and so forth. In both cases, other tools, such as brain lesions or electrical stimulation of the brain, may be used along with drug administration. Third, behavioral pharmacologists can study drug-induced modifications of animal behavior, which provide models of pathological conditions in humans that cannot be studied directly in a patient population.

There is a close relationship in psychopharmacology between clinical research and laboratory studies with animals. Animal studies clearly have several advantages over clinical studies using patient populations. The most obvious advantage is that the use of animals allows rigorous and objective experimental controls. The living conditions (e.g., diet, exercise, room temperature) of animal subjects can be regulated far more precisely than those of humans. In addition, their past history, as well as their genetic background, is well known. Furthermore, drugs can be administered to animal subjects in ways not generally appropriate for humans. For example, drugs can be administered to animals over a long period of time to determine toxic effects or the potential for addiction. Finally, animals are the most appropriate subjects for the study of mechanisms of drug action because an understanding of the electrophysiological and neurochemical bases of drug effects often requires invasive techniques that are obviously unethical with human subjects.

The focus of Part II of this chapter is the measurement of drug-induced behavioral changes using animal subjects. It is not intended to be a complete compendium of behavioral techniques, but rather, an introduction to the variety of methods available to psychopharmacologists. As is true of the neuropharmacological methods described in Part I, techniques for measuring behavior are constantly being changed to improve their specificity, reliability, and validity.

Animal Care Guidelines

The Health Extension Act of 1985 provides strict guidelines for the care of animals to be used in biomedical and behavioral research. The goal of the legislation is humane animal maintenance and experimentation that limits both the use of animals and animal distress. Each research institution is required to form an Institutional Animal Care and Use Committee made up of a minimum of three members, including at least one individual who is not associated with the research institution and at least one who is a doctor of veterinary medicine. The committee reviews each research protocol that uses animals in the institution and evaluates the design and conduct of proposed experiments. Procedures involving animals must be designed and performed with due consideration of their relevance to human or animal health, the advancement of knowledge, or the good of society. For each protocol, alternative methods such as mathematical models, computer simulation, and in vitro biological systems must be considered. The procedures performed must avoid or minimize discomfort, distress, and pain when consistent with sound scientific practices. Procedures that may cause more than momentary pain should be performed with appropriate sedation, analgesia, or anesthesia. In every case, adequate presurgical and postsurgical veterinary medical and nursing practices must be applied. In any case in which animals would suffer severe or chronic pain or distress that cannot be relieved, they must be painlessly sacrificed at the end of the procedure.

In addition to the assessment of proposed research, the Public Health Service also requires periodic inspection of animal care facilities to ensure that the living conditions of the animals are appropriate for their species and contribute to their health and comfort. Included in the inspection is an evaluation of the size, temperature, ventilation, and lighting of the living space, as well as the general condition and cleanliness of the facility, the feeding and watering system, sanitation, and mode of transit. Medical care for animals must be available and provided by a qualified veterinarian.

New Drug Evaluation

Behavioral pharmacology is one part of the evaluation of new psychotropic drugs. The development of new drugs is a multistep procedure usually requiring many years of systematic evaluation and testing. The earliest psychotropic drugs had their origins in herbal or animal extract remedies that had been used for years for a variety of purposes. More recently, since the "receptor revolution," scientists have begun to design and synthesize new drug molecules that fit a particular receptor structure with the hope that the drug will produce more specific drug action with fewer undesirable side effects. In both cases, drug evaluation involves progressive screening for structural specificity, specific biobehavioral activity, toxicity, side effects, teratogenicity, and so forth.

Many preclinical screening procedures involve in vitro neuropharmacological methods, such as receptor binding, cell culture, and bioassays in which drugs are applied to cells or tissues in a laboratory dish. The pharmacokinetics of new compounds—that is, their rates of absorption, distribution, metabolism, and excretion—are, by necessity, evaluated in vivo. Furthermore, animal studies provide important information about the effective dose range as well as the toxic and lethal doses. Extensive behavioral testing provides both a screening method and a tool for further drug development. Following preclinical evaluation, a drug considered safe may be tested clinically on a limited basis, using healthy volunteers or patients. After its safety, side effects, and response variability have been assessed in this way, the drug may be approved for use in large clinical trials. If the results of these trials demonstrate effectiveness without inappropriate risk, the FDA can give the drug provisional approval for use by physicians, who are required to report therapeutic results and side effects on a regular basis.

Although our discussion in this chapter is limited to animal testing, keep in mind that drug testing on humans frequently uncovers subtle or unusual drug effects that animal tests are unable to reveal. It is very difficult, for example, to develop animal tests to screen drugs that alter a purely cognitive aspect of human activity. Many of the manifestations of psychiatric disorders, as well as drug actions related to these disorders, are described in typically human terms, such as facial expression, altered mood, or manner of speech. Nevertheless, psychopharmacology has evolved to the point at which distinct classes of drugs have been found to alter one or several measurable animal behaviors in a predictable fashion. In addition, imprecision in evaluating drug effects on human behavior occurs because of difficulty in matching control and experimental groups, in establishing diagnostic criteria, and because human subjects vary in the durations of illnesses, previous histories of medication and substance abuse (e.g., alcoholism), lifestyle, nutrition, age, sex, and placebo effects. The methods of behavioral pharmacology provide an important step between basic science and the treatment of psychological disabilities prevalent today.

Some animal tests used to evaluate drug effects on physiology closely approximate their human counterparts, particularly when the drug-induced changes can be recorded in physiological terms such as blood pressure, muscle tension, or body temperature. We would say that these measures have high **face validity** because they closely resemble the human conditions they are attempting to predict. For many drug effects, however, this is not the case, and the animal response does not resemble the human condition. In these instances, a correlated, quantifiable measure in an animal is substituted for a more cognitive human behavior. Should such a correlation be close, a drug that modifies rat behavior in a certain way can be expected to alter a particular human behavior, even though the two behaviors seem unrelated. For instance, if a new drug were to produce an abnormal posture in rats called catalepsy (see below), tests on humans might show it to be an antipsychotic. Tests such as these have low face validity. However, if the drug effects in the laboratory test closely parallel or predict the clinical effect, the measures may be said to demonstrate **construct validity** or **empirical validity**.

To be optimal, a behavioral test on animals should meet several criteria (Glick, 1976; Treit, 1985): (1) It should be specific for the class of drug being screened; that is, other types of drugs should not have the same effect. (2) It should be sensitive to all drugs having the desired pharmacological effect, in a dose-dependent fashion. (3) The rank order of potencies of drugs in the screening test should match their order of potency in therapeutic action. Unless these criteria are satisfactorily met, the results of the screening procedure must be evaluated cautiously. In addition, an optimal behavioral measure will have high **reliability**, meaning that under the defined conditions of testing, the results will be the same from one time to another and from one laboratory to another.

Keep in mind that a correlational model needs only to be predictive; no logical or functional connection is required between the measure used for screening and the target clinical response. However, more isomorphism between the model and the target behavior is needed if the model is to be useful as a tool for research into the mechanisms of drug action or into the neurochemical basis of the behavior. Unfortunately, it is often difficult to see overt similarities between human pathology and animal behavior. Measuring a behavior—for example, running—may tell us little about its underlying motivation, since animals run for many different reasons. A homologous model (Treit, 1985) is one that is based on apparent similarities between the processes that underlie the human condition and the animal response in the model. For instance, a researcher may make the assumption that aversive stimuli, either real or anticipated, cause anxiety in both humans and animals and that, therefore, the animal response to aversive stimuli is an appropriate model of human anxiety. In other words, the homologous model attempts to specify the underlying causes of the test response. These types of assumptions are necessary to probe the neurochemistry of behavior, but the development of such a model may depend on knowledge of the very processes that the model is designed to investigate.

Primary Evaluation

In general, preclinical drug evaluation proceeds in two distinct steps: primary evaluation and secondary testing. Primary evaluation usually begins with observation and simple behavioral measures that utilize untrained animals and a minimum of instrumentation, such as measures of motor activity. Among the observations made are measures of tremors, ptosis (drooping eyelids), salivation, defecation, catalepsy, hyper- or hyporeflexia, response to tail pinch, and changes in eating or drinking. The screening method varies for different species, depending on the usual behavior of each species. For example, the rotarod, a test that measures motor coordination (Watzman and Barry, 1968), is frequently used for rodents, but rarely used for larger animals such as dogs or monkeys. Animals are placed on a slowly rotating rod or drum, and the time it takes them to fall off is recorded. The difference between the pre- and postdrug scores gives a measure of ataxia, coordination, vestibular control, and muscular strength.

To further characterize behavior, measures of catalepsy can be made. **Catalepsy** is the abnormal maintenance of distorted postures, often called "waxy flexibility." Animals demonstrating catalepsy will remain in bizarre postures when positioned by the experimenter. The time it takes for the animal to return to normal posture gives an indication of the extent of catalepsy. The use of catalepsy as a test to identify drugs that can alleviate the symptoms of schizophrenia demonstrates the usefulness of screening tests that are unrelated to human behavior. The relative potency of some drugs in producing catalepsy in rats parallels their relative potency in clinical treatment of certain forms of mental illness.

Measures of Motor Activity

If CNS effects are seen during initial testing, primary evaluation is continued with measures of motor activity. In addition to identifying drugs that produce sleep or anesthesia (loss of consciousness from which one is not easily aroused), activity measures also reflect loss of coordination and sedation. Spontaneous locomotor activity is measured using a variety of tests that measure unrestrained movement within a prescribed area. A "jiggle cage," for example, is a box balanced on a single central pivot point; a switch closes and activates a counter whenever movement of the animal brings the cage edge in contact with the sensors located on the periphery. An alternative method employs infrared light beams (invisible to rodents) directed across the cage which, when broken, activate a counter that records one movement. A third method involves automated video tracking of movement in conjunction with computerized analysis. These automated counting procedures enable measurement of animal activity in a setting that is not disruptive to normal behavior; that is, it can be done in the dark and without the presence of the investigator. Also, more than one activity cage can be operated simultaneously so that the activity of more than one animal can be measured at the same time.

A less automated technique involves placing the animal subject in a prescribed area that is divided into squares. An investigator must be present to record the number of squares traversed in a unit of time. In general, we consider such observational methods less reliable than totally automated procedures because experimenter expectations may bias the results.

One distinct advantage of nonautomated techniques is that observation of animal behavior in an unstructured environment may provide important information about drug effects quite apart from general motor activity. The importance of nonautomated observation has been demonstrated in the case of the CNS stimulant amphetamine. Amphetamine at low doses significantly increases general motor activity in rats, whereas at higher doses, the activity score is much lower. This reduced activity, however, is not due to a cessation of all behavior. Rather, the animals spend much of their time performing sterotyped head movements and repetitive sniffing, licking, and gnawing with only infrequent bursts of locomotor activity. The repetitive actions are significant drug-induced behaviors, but in motor activity tests that are not sensitive to small movements of the head and neck, this behavior will go unrecorded. Therefore, direct observation is essential during primary evaluation of drug effects.

Regardless of the method of measurement chosen, it is necessary to consider the many factors that can alter motor activity in addition to the pharmacological manipulation under study. Motor activity is altered by curiosity and fear as well as by circadian rhythms, food and water deprivation, handling and rearing conditions, and the age, sex, and strain of the animals. In addition, environmental factors such as lighting, odor, novelty, temperature, and background noise interact with drug treatment to alter motor activity (Kelley, 1993). Despite the simplicity of measuring motor activity, adequate controls over extraneous variables are vital to the interpretation of data.

Interactions with Other Drugs

Much drug screening involves interactions with other drugs. In many cases, drugs administered alone may not produce characteristic behavioral effects in animals except at very high doses. For example, in general, antidepressant drugs do not have unique behavioral effects alone, but do interact with certain other drugs in unique ways. Antidepressant drugs alone have no effect on body temperature, but they potentiate (or accentuate) the increase in body temperature produced by treatment with amphetamine. The probable mechanism for this interaction will become clearer when the drug's effects on the chemical signals of the brain are discussed in Chapter 16.

A second significant drug interaction is that of antidepressants with reserpine. Used to treat hypertension, reserpine may cause depression in patients. In animals, low to moderate doses produce calming and sedation; higher doses eliminate all motor activity. The behavior-depressant action of reserpine is frequently used as a model of human depression. The classic antidepressant drugs antagonize the effects of reserpine on animal activity, but do not increase motor activity when given alone.

One of the most widely used initial screening tests for identifying antianxiety drugs (see Chapter 16) is the prevention of pentylenetetrazol-induced seizures in mice. In an unprotected animal, intravenous infusion of pentylenetetrazol produces an almost immediate onset of **clonic seizures** (alternating contraction of opposing muscles, causing limb shaking). Pretreatment with an effective antianxiety drug, such as diazepam, protects against the seizure. The relative potency of drugs in this animal test generally parallels their clinical pattern of anxiety reduction (see below).

Secondary Evaluation

The remainder of the procedures described in this chapter are considered techniques of secondary evaluation. Each of them is more complex than the simple observational methods described thus far. These methods of measuring behavior have their origins in ethological observations of animals in their natural environment. Natural behaviors have been developed into quantifiable measures that can be used in a more controlled environment. Of particular interest are feeding and drinking, social and reproductive behaviors, aggression, responses to pain and stress, and learning. We will briefly describe only those behavioral tests that are relevant to discussions in subsequent chapters or serve as models of clinical drug response.

Measures of Analgesia

Analgesia is the reduction of perceived pain without loss of consciousness. Pain is a motivational state arising from excessive stimulation of a number of sensory modalities and can be elicited by heat, extreme cold, electrical impulses, chemical irritation, and so forth. In general, pain is considered to have two distinct components: the physiological sensation and the emotional response to the physiological sensation. A separation of the two components is demonstrated by the athlete who sustains a serious injury during the heat of competition but is unaware of the pain until the arousal surrounding competition subsides. (For a more detailed discussion of the phenomenon of pain, see Chapter 12.)

Because of the dual nature of pain, the quantification of pain (and hence of analgesia) using human self-report techniques in the clinical setting, where anxiety and anticipation of pain influence a patient's response, is difficult. Analgesia testing with humans in the laboratory setting is also frequently misleading because the response to some types of experimentally induced pain is quite different from that to chronic or pathological pain. In other cases in which the induced pain is a very reliable model, it is understandably difficult to secure subjects.

An alternative method for measuring the analgesic properties of drugs is the use of animal models. We cannot know whether the animal "feels pain," but we can measure the animal's avoidance of a noxious stimulus, and we can call this avoidance a "pain reaction." The responses that the stimulus elicits might really measure a "sensation" threshold rather than a pain threshold. Of greatest value in analgesic testing would be a method to measure the modulation of severe and continuous pain, such as in carcinoma, a goal that cannot be met with animal testing. Nevertheless, animal testing does allow more controlled measures and eliminates some of the complications of the human emotional response.

Tail-flick test.   One of the simpler tests designed to measure drug-induced analgesia is the **tail-flick test**, which was developed by D'Amour and Smith (1941). In this test, a beam of light, the intensity of which is controlled by a rheostat, is focused on an ink-blackened portion of a rat's tail (Figure 2.19a). The latency between onset of the stimulus and the animal's removal of its tail from the beam of light is assumed to be correlated with pain intensity. The test was originally developed for use with human subjects, with whom the light was focused on a blackened spot on the forehead. The stimulus was repeated every 30 seconds at increasing intensities until an intensity was reached at which the subject just perceived pain. Using a similar threshold technique for animals eliminates the problems normally associated with subjective reports on pain by human subjects in the laboratory setting. However, an important consideration when using the tail-flick test is the age of the rats tested, because age-related increases in epidermal cornification raise pain thresholds and hence increase variability among animals.

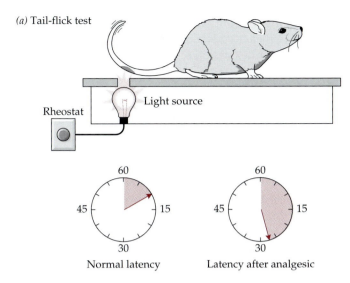

(a) Tail-flick test

Rheostat

Light source

Normal latency

Latency after analgesic

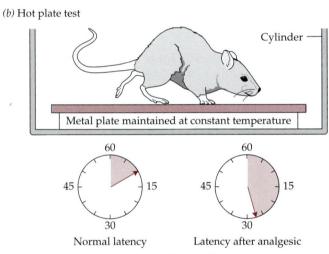

(b) Hot plate test

Cylinder

Metal plate maintained at constant temperature

Normal latency

Latency after analgesic

2.19 TESTS OF ANALGESIA. (a) The tail-flick test evaluates the response to a thermal stimulus by measuring the time between onset of the light beam and the movement of the tail. (b) The hot plate test measures the latency to kicking with the hind paws or attempting to escape the cylinder. (After Hamilton and Timmons, 1990.)

The tail-flick test is simple, rapid, and reproducible, and shows a relatively small individual variation. However it is not adequate for determining analgesic properties of compounds under conditions of severe, protracted, pathological pain. Nevertheless, there is a good relationship between the analgesic effect measured with the tail-flick test and the efficacy of various analgesic agents.

Hot plate test. Another method of measuring analgesic drug action using thermal stimuli is the **hot plate test** (Figure 2.19b) introduced by Woolfe and Macdonald (1944). The animal to be tested is placed in a cylinder on a metal plate maintained at a constant temperature, which can be varied between 55° and 70°C. Most often the animal's initial response is to sit on its hind legs and

lick its forepaws. Because that response can easily be confused with the common grooming response, drug evaluation is based on the second, more delayed, response of kicking with the hind paws or attempting to escape the cylinder. The sensitivity of this test is approximately equal to that of the tail-flick test. It seems to produce reliable and fairly stable pain thresholds with which to measure analgesic activity.

Flinch–jump procedure. The **flinch–jump procedure**, which was developed by Evans (1961), is based on the finding that an electric shock delivered to a rat's feet through the grid floor of a testing apparatus will elicit two distinguishable responses. At low shock intensities, the animal will be startled or "flinch" but show no signs of agitation. At higher intensities, the animal will remove two or more paws from the grid at the time of the shock onset (called a "jump"); the jump is often accompanied by vocalization, running, and other signs of a highly emotional reaction. As a rule, the animals are given a series of shocks (1 second in duration) varying from 0.1 to 3.4 mA in both ascending and descending order. The effect of various analgesic drugs can thus be readily determined over a range of shock intensities and with great sensitivity. One might assume that the flinch response reflects the first perception of pain by the animal and the jump response reflects an emotionally aroused reaction to the pain and, therefore, that the method provides information on the two factors believed to contribute to the human response to pain. Clearly, it is impossible to determine whether the flinch response indicates the first recognition of pain or just the perception of electric shock. Furthermore, although electric shock is easy to apply, it is quite difficult to control. Even when voltage is known, biological tissues offer impedance that cannot be controlled. Other tests that apply electric shock to the tooth pulp or the tail have been used, but in most cases these tests show considerable variability and therefore do not have the sensitivity of the flinch–jump test.

Tests of Learning and Memory

Psychopharmacologists have developed several types of tests to evaluate learning and memory in animals. There are a number of reasons for doing this. First, objective measures are necessary if we are to understand the behavioral and biological basis of memory and cognition. In turn, this information may lead to the development of new ways to manipulate the neurotransmitters involved in these functions. Second, these measures can be used to evaluate drugs that may be useful in overcoming deficits in human function due to normal aging or disease processes, such as Alzheimer's disease, or following neurological injuries. The strategies of such research require the study of drug effects on normal animals to determine whether a compound enhances the rate of learning or the ability to remember a new response. Additionally, this research must involve animals with "naturally" occurring cognitive defects, such as aged animals, poor learners, or those with genetic deficiencies, as well as animals with induced memory impairments following lesions, electrical stimulation of the brain, or drug-induced chemical changes.

Preclinical evaluation of drugs affecting memory in animals involves observing their behavior in experiments consisting of a presentation of information (the training stage) followed by a delay and the opportunity for performance (the test stage). Higher cognitive processes can be assessed by providing situations in which reorganization of the information presented is necessary before the appropriate response can be made. It is important to realize that these tests very often do not determine whether altered performance is due to drug-induced changes in attention, motivation, arousal, or to other factors that contribute to overall performance.

Passive avoidance.   **Passive avoidance**, or inhibitory avoidance, is one type of test commonly used with rodents. It is called "passive" because the correct response involves *not* performing a typical behavior in order to avoid an aversive consequence. In the training stage, the animal is punished, usually with a foot shock, for making a highly probable response, such as stepping off a platform onto the grid floor of the test chamber or entering a dark compartment. In the test stage, the animal is returned to the test apparatus after a fixed time interval (e.g., 24 hours). Memory is measured by the latency to make the response previously punished; the longer the latency, the better the memory. One major advantage of this technique is that it requires a minimal amount of training and is quick to perform. Also, the procedure is reasonably sensitive and provides a precise determination of the duration of memory retention. Unfortunately, the variability in latencies between subjects is quite high because animals differ in their tolerance to shock and because changes in arousal can alter latency, independent of drug effect (Heise, 1987). For these reasons, large numbers of subjects are usually necessary. (For details of the procedure see Sahgal, 1993.)

Some investigators (LeDoux, 1993; Tomaz et al., 1993) have argued that passive avoidance tests, as well as conditioned emotional response tests (see below), evaluate only a special category of memory that involves the learning and storage of information about the emotional significance of events. These tests are used in memory studies but are also considered models of anxiety. Recently a new test, the elevated plus-maze (see below), has been developed to measure drug effects on anxiety and memory simultaneously (Tomaz et al., 1993). Results from these investigators and others (see Izquierdo and Medina, 1991) suggest that the brain sys-

tems serving memory and anxiety overlap and that the function of the amygdala and its connections is critical to both. (Further discussion of measures of anxiety follows in later sections.)

Mazes.   The evolution of the maze as a tool for the measurement of learning shows a trend toward simplification. Early investigators used complex forms called **multiple T mazes**. A hungry animal was placed in the start box of an apparatus like the one in Figure 2.20*a*. The animal would explore the maze, which was made up of a series of two-direction choice points, until it reached the goal box, where it found a small piece of food. On subsequent trials, learning was evaluated based on the number of errors at choice points and the time taken to reach the goal box. Modifications of the multiple T maze include the Hebb–Williams maze, in which the route to the goal can be altered so that the animal must show some flexibility in learning each new pattern of responding.

Use of the multiple T maze declined as interest in a single choice point test, the **simple T maze**, increased. The simple T maze has a single stem or alley and one choice point, which leads to either available reinforcement (usually food) or an empty goal box depending on the choice made (Figure 2.20*b*). The use of this single choice point test provides information on the manner in

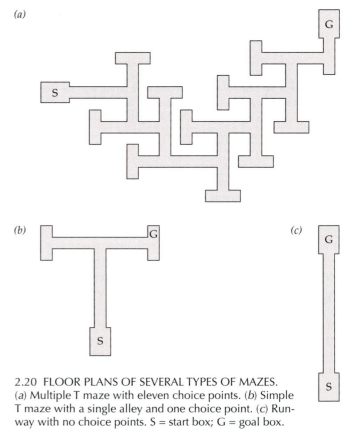

2.20 FLOOR PLANS OF SEVERAL TYPES OF MAZES. (*a*) Multiple T maze with eleven choice points. (*b*) Simple T maze with a single alley and one choice point. (*c*) Runway with no choice points. S = start box; G = goal box.

which a single discrimination, for example, left versus right or dark arm versus light arm, is learned. Interest in the simple T maze reflects the idea that it is beneficial to study the smallest possible unit of learning before examining the more complex problem of how the units are combined. The learning of a single discrimination can also be readily demonstrated using operant techniques, as described below. Such tasks involving choice measure both learning and motivation.

A final simplification of the maze is the **runway** (Figure 2.20*c*), which provides no opportunity for choice but measures response latency (time between placement in the start box and leaving the start box) and response duration (total time to goal box). Measures of latency and speed are in general assumed to reflect the motivation of the animal and so may be used along with other measures of learning.

Measures of Spatial Learning

Learning tasks that require the acquisition of spatial information are currently of great interest to neuropsychopharmacologists who are investigating the role of cholinergic neurons, hippocampal function, and memory deficits due to Alzheimer's disease. Among the spatial tasks utilized are the radial arm maze and the Morris water maze.

Radial arm maze. The **radial arm maze** developed by Olton and colleagues (Olton, Collison, and Werz, 1977) was designed to evaluate the ability to remember spatial information. The maze is made up of multiple arms radiating away from a central choice point (Figure 2.21). A small piece of food is placed at the end of each arm. When a hungry rat is placed in the central point, it explores the arms and eats the food. With very little experience, a normal rat learns to forage efficiently by visiting each arm only once on a given day, indicating effective spatial memory for that particular episode. The task can be made more complex by blocking some arms on the initial trial before the animal is returned to the central choice point. The animal is expected to remember which arms have been entered and move down only those that still contain food. The duration of memory can be measured by varying the time interval between the first exploration and the subsequent trials. In the radial arm maze, the animal acquires trial-unique information that has been presented within that day's session. Acquisition of trial-unique information assesses working memory rather than measuring learning that has accumulated over days of testing (reference memory).

Among the advantages of the radial arm maze are the ease with which animals learn the task and the flexibility it provides. For example, animals can be tested across a wide range of delays to evaluate duration of memory, and the number of arms can be increased or decreased to change memory load. Because each day's

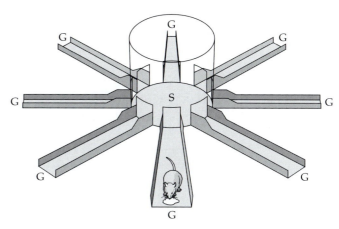

2.21 THE RADIAL ARM MAZE has a central start box (S) and a number of arms or alleys radiating from the center. Goal areas (G) containing food are at the end of each arm.

sequence is different, the experimenter can examine the behavioral effects of various pharmacological agents and a range of doses in a single subject. Rawlins and Deacon (1993) describe procedural details of the technique.

Morris water maze. A test of spatial learning developed by Morris (1984), the **Morris water maze**, uses a large circular pool of water that has been made opaque by the addition of milk or a dye. A platform that is hidden from view just below the surface of the water provides the means of escape (Figure 2.22). The subject demonstrates that it has acquired and retained the spatial location of the submerged platform by navigating from different starting positions to the platform. Since there are no local cues to direct the escape behavior, successful escape requires the learning of the spatial position of the platform relative to distal landmarks. When curtains surrounding the pool are drawn, performance falls to chance levels, demonstrating the importance of distal cues. The principal measure of performance is the latency to escape, although video tracking with a microcomputer link permits charting of the pathway taken, as well as measurement of path length and path directionality as a deviation from the correct path.

The water maze test has several advantages. No extensive pretraining is required, and normal animals learn where the platform is located very rapidly, so testing can be carried out over short periods of time. Escape from water motivates without the use of food or water deprivation or electric shock, which is advantageous for lesion and drug studies, although at the same time the experimenter loses the ability to vary motivational level or reinforcement magnitude. Also, water provides an intramaze environment that controls for olfactory cues. Among the disadvantages of the water maze is that the experiment must be run by hand rather than with automated equipment. Also, water immersion itself may

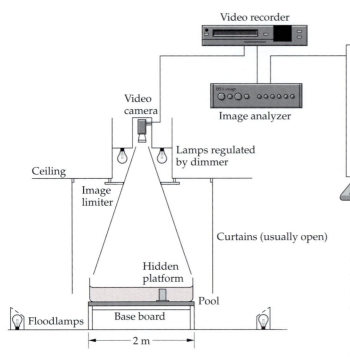

Video recorder

Video monitor

Video camera

Image analyzer

Lamps regulated by dimmer

Ceiling

Image limiter

Curtains (usually open)

Hidden platform

Pool

Floodlamps　Base board

← 2 m →

Computer

2.22　THE MORRIS WATER MAZE. (a) Schematic view of the water maze. The circular pool is filled with opaque water. The escape platform is approximately 9 cm in diameter and 1 cm below the water level. Curtains can be closed to eliminate some or all distal cues. A video camera is mounted above the pool and is connected to the video recorder and computer link. Software evaluates significant characteristics of the swim path. (After Stewart and Morris, 1993.)

cause endocrinological or other stress effects, which may interact with the manipulations (e.g., lesions or drugs) of interest.

Despite these few disadvantages, numerous recent studies have used the Morris water maze to examine the developmental and neural mechanisms of spatial learning. The importance of hippocampal function for place navigation acquisition and of discrete cortical areas for long-term storage of spatial memory have been demonstrated. Further, the significance of several neurotransmitter systems to spatial learning has been described and reviewed (McNamara and Skelton, 1993; Stewart and Morris, 1993).

Tests of Delayed Reaction

The **delayed matching test** assesses the type of memory often impaired by brain damage in humans and is similar to tasks on the Weschler Memory Scale, used to define amnesic syndrome. In this test the animal is asked to compare its short-term memory of a visual stimulus with an actual stimulus. The test has high face validity because many everyday experiences require this type of memory. It is currently of great interest because electrical stimulation and lesion studies have suggested a role for temporal lobe structures and acetylcholine neurons in this type of memory (Kovner and Stamm, 1972; Olton, 1985).

At the beginning of the trial, one or more stimuli are presented as the sample. After a short delay, during which the sample stimulus is removed, the animal is given a choice between two or more visual stimuli, one of which is the same as the sample (Figure 2.23a). If the

animal chooses the pattern that matches the sample, it is given a food reward (reinforcement); an incorrect response yields no reward. In order to make the correct choice after the interval, the animal must "remember" the initial stimulus. Of course, the test can be modified to evaluate the recognition of the novel stimulus in an analogous manner, in which case the animal is reinforced for selecting the stimulus different from that which was initially presented. The relative advantages and disadvantages of these two approaches have been discussed elsewhere (Aggleton, 1993). The test can be adapted to most animals by requiring a species-appropriate behavior: nonhuman primates most often have to touch the correct picture or push or pull a button; rodents may press a lever or run down the appropriate arm of a T maze; pigeons peck at a disk.

As early as 1913, Hunter, in a classic experiment, showed that a rat could learn a delayed response to a problem. In a modified maze, as shown in Figure 2.23b, a rat was placed in a start box from which it could see three light bulbs, one of which was lit to signal the presence of food in the corresponding arm of the maze. After the light was turned off, the rat was kept in the start box for a period of time and then released. In order to get the food, the rat had to "remember" which of the lights had been on. Hunter found that rats could perform the task successfully with a delay of up to 10 seconds; cats, 18 seconds; dogs, 3 minutes; a 2-year-old child, 50 seconds, and a 5-year-old child, 20 minutes or more.

The delayed matching test and other models that employ choice procedures are particularly useful in separating memory from performance. Stimulant drugs, for example, tend to increase responding in tests in which lever pressing is required (see below). When that measure is used alone, it is not clear whether the increased responding is due to generally increased motor behavior or enhanced learning. By using a delayed matching choice design such as a Y maze, one can see that stimulants tend to increase responding but have no effect on the accuracy of the choice behavior—that is, they have no memory-enhancing effects.

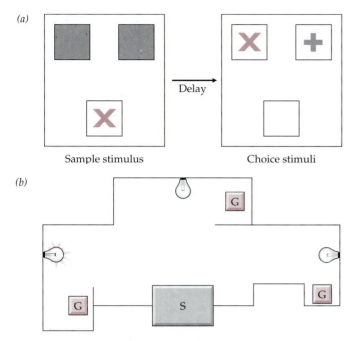

(a)

Sample stimulus   Choice stimuli

(b)

2.23 DELAYED REACTION TESTS. (*a*) In a delayed matching test, a sample stimulus is presented first. Following a delay during which the sample is removed, the choice stimuli are presented. A match to the sample is rewarded with food. (*b*) Floor plan of the delayed response experiment designed by Hunter. Only the goal box (G) indicated by the lighted bulb contains food. A transparent start box (S) holds the subject for varying periods of time after the stimulus light goes off.

Measures of Anxiety

There are many (20–30) biobehavioral measures available to identify novel anxiolytic (antianxiety) compounds and to predict their safety and efficacy. The tests employed vary in their complexity and their usefulness for studying the neural mechanisms of anxiolytic drug action and the biological basis of anxiety (Andrews and Broekkamp, 1993; Green, 1991; Treit, 1985). Many use simple or unconditioned animal reactions, such as exploratory or social behaviors, while others employ traditional animal learning paradigms. Most use induced fear as an analogy to human anxiety. Some depend on the memory of an aversive event to modify subsequent behavior (see "Passive avoidance" above) and so are frequently used as memory tests.

Measuring spontaneous behaviors. Among those tests that use spontaneous, unconditioned behaviors in a relatively uncontrolled environment are antagonism of pentylenetetrazol (PTZ)-induced seizures, the light–dark crossing task, the elevated plus-maze, and the social interaction paradigm. The ability of antianxiety drugs to antagonize PTZ-induced seizures was described earlier in this chapter as an example of a simple screening measure that relies on drug interactions rather than complex behaviors. Despite the low face validity, or isomorphism

between seizures in rodents and human anxiety, this test is very sensitive to a wide variety of agents, and the relative potency of drugs in blocking seizures is similar to their order of potency in relieving anxiety in humans. Furthermore, the test separates antiepileptic agents from antianxiety agents based on which component of the behavioral seizure (tonic or clonic) is inhibited. The simplicity, speed, and low cost of this test make it very popular as a screening tool, but it does not provide a real "model" of human anxiety.

The **light–dark crossing task** (Blumstein and Crawley, 1983) is a modification of simple spontaneous exploration that takes advantage of rodents' natural tendency to avoid brightly lighted areas. The simple testing apparatus consists of a two-compartment box with one side brightly lighted and the other side dark. The animal subject is placed in the bright side, and the number of crossings between the bright and dark sides is electronically recorded, along with the amount of time spent on each side and total motor activity. Anxiolytics produce a dose-dependent increase in the number of crossings and in overall motor activity, as well as increasing the amount of time spent in the light. The order of potency of drugs in increasing crossing behavior is in agreement with their order of potency in relieving clinical anxiety. The finding that drug-treated animals do not increase motor activity above that of saline-treated controls in a one-chamber, evenly lighted apparatus suggests that the activity of a nondrugged animal is suppressed by light and is "released" to normal by antianxiety agents. The release of behavior under aversive control enhances the analogy to human anxiety (Treit, 1985).

The **rat social interaction test**, which measures interactions between two male rats placed in a test chamber, is a second type of anxiety test that relies on spontaneous behaviors and rodents' tendency to avoid bright light and unfamiliar surroundings (File, 1980). The underlying assumption is that by using a novel test chamber or increasing the brightness of the chamber, anxiety is increased and social interaction decreases. Antianxiety drugs are expected to increase social behaviors under these test conditions, and chlordiazepoxide does so in a dose-dependent manner. Other anxiolytics tend to increase social interaction regardless of the test conditions and may do so in a nonspecific stimulatory manner. Differences in baseline social activity measures due to time of day, animal weight, and other factors may contribute to the variability reported in this test.

The **elevated plus-maze** (Pellow et al., 1985) is a cross-shaped maze that has two open arms and two arms enclosed by sides, but with an open roof. The entire maze is elevated 50 cm above the floor and depends on rodents' unconditioned aversion to heights and open spaces for its effectiveness as a test for anxiety. Saline-treated controls demonstrate a preference for the closed alleys by spending a significantly greater amount of time in them than in the open alleys. A greater amount of anxiety-related behavior (e.g., freezing, defecation) is observed in the open arms, and higher plasma corticosterone concentrations have been measured in rats confined to the open arms as compared to the closed arms. The test involves placing an animal in the center of the maze and observing the number of entries into the open, "fear-inducing" arms compared with the closed, "safe" arms, as well as the ratio of time spent in the open versus the closed arms. This quick and simple test shows a selective increase in open arm exploration following treatment with antianxiety drugs and a reduction following treatment with caffeine and amphetamine, drugs considered to be anxiogenic (increasing anxiety) in nature. Antischizophrenic drugs and antidepressants reduce exploratory behaviors in general. As is true of the other tasks described thus far, the elevated plus-maze depends on spontaneous behavior, so no lengthy training is necessary. In addition, no noxious stimuli are required, nor is manipulation of appetitive behaviors, for example, by food or water deprivation.

The three tests described above are based on spontaneous behavior in a relatively uncontrolled environment. For that reason, they are relatively quick and easy to perform. However, their results are not always consistent from laboratory to laboratory because of differences in animal age and baseline activity as well as differences in the apparatus, lighting, and defined dependent variables.

Measuring trained behaviors.   In contrast to the spontaneous behavior models described thus far, tests based on learned behaviors require a certain amount of training and hence are generally more costly and time-consuming. The **conditioned emotional response (CER)**, described more fully below, depends on a classically conditioned association between a signal and the onset of an unavoidable electric shock. When the signal is presented during ongoing behavior, the behavior is suppressed (i.e., "freezing" occurs). Although the CER resembles anxiety in humans, drug testing produces no consistent results; that is, results from different laboratories show that antianxiety drugs increase, decrease, or have no effect on behavior generated in this paradigm. In addition, drugs of other classes also decrease the CER or show no effect.

One variation on the CER that has demonstrated potential for screening antianxiety agents is the **potentiated startle paradigm** (Davis, 1979). Rats are first trained to associate a stimulus (e.g., a light) with the onset of foot shock. When this conditioned "fear" stimulus is presented with a sudden loud noise, the startle reflex that occurs naturally in response to the noise is potentiated. Anxiolytics selectively block this potentiation without affecting the unconditioned startle reflex that occurs when noise is presented alone. This test has been praised both for its isomorphism with human anxiety and its reliance on an elicited (as opposed to spontaneous) response in a relatively controlled environment, which may provide more consistent results because there are fewer opportunities for confounding variables (Green, 1991). However, the test has not yet been commonly used and requires greater empirical validation.

Other anxiolytic tests use operant conditioning, rather than classical conditioning, as their basis. One of the most common is the **Geller–Seifter conflict test** (Geller, 1962), which is described below. It is sufficient at this point to say that the Geller conflict test is a reasonably reliable predictor of anxiolytics and has been widely tested with many species including rats, pigs, cats, goldfish, pigeons, squirrel monkeys, and humans. It has the advantage of measuring drug effects on both appetitive behavior and conflict (approach–avoidance) behavior in the same animal on a given trial. Its usefulness as a screen for antianxiety agents is discussed more fully in Chapter 16.

Schedule-Controlled Behavior

Within the past few years, great interest has developed in the use of conditioned behaviors to study drug effects. This technique entails the selection of a small, clearly definable portion of a complex behavior pattern that can be modified by changing elements in the environment and by drug action. An example of such a behavior is lever pressing by a rat. Although lever pressing is not a normal component of a rat's behavioral repertoire, it can be readily quantified, and its use avoids an anthropomorphic interpretation of animal behavior.

The underlying principle of operant conditioning is that consequences control behavior. An animal performs because it is reinforced for doing so. Reinforcement can be positive (food or water for a hungry or thirsty animal) or negative (electric shock that can be avoided if the animal makes the correct response). Animals learn to respond to obtain rewards and avoid punishment.

The experiments are carried out in an operant chamber, or Skinner box, which is a soundproof box with a grid floor that can be electrified (for shock delivery), a food or water dispenser (for rewards), lights or loudspeaker (for stimulus cue presentation), and levers (one or more) that the animal can press (Figure 2.24). The equipment is almost always automatically controlled so that cues (if used) can be presented at specified times. The animal's lever pressing is converted to an electrical signal to enable automatic recording of responses and reinforcement delivery. The animal is conditioned to press the lever to obtain rewards or avoid punishment. Because the experiment must occur rapidly with precise timing and with many repetitions, accurate programming and recording of the experiments is important. Computerized stimulus presentation and data collection provide the opportunity to measure not only the total number of responses per unit time, but also response

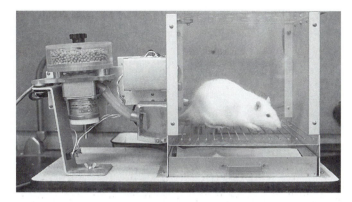

2.24 RAT IN A SKINNER BOX. A rat can be trained to press the lever (response), which activates a food delivery mechanism (reinforcement). An animal can also learn to press the lever to terminate or postpone shocks that can be delivered through the grid floor.

rates and interresponse times, which provide a stable and sensitive measure of continuous behavior.

In addition to the computerized tabulation of responses, a visual representation of the results can be generated by using a cumulative recorder, in which a sheet of paper moves over a roll at a set speed and a pen marks a step across the paper whenever a lever press is made. Delivery of reinforcement is also recorded (Figure 2.25).

Because the required behavior is not "natural" (that is, it does not appear in the animal's natural environment), it must be trained ("shaped"). When hungry, an animal in a Skinner box performs many behaviors in rapid succession, one of which may be pressing a lever. The animal must learn that pressing the lever produces a desirable result (e.g., delivery of food). The experimenter helps by presenting the reinforcer immediately after the correct response and before another behavior can occur. Because the response is trained, it can be similar for diverse species, both in its form and its consequences.

The arrangement of times or circumstances in which lever pressing produces reinforcement is called the **schedule of reinforcement**. Many different schedules of reinforcement can be used for studying behavior. Representing behavior as a temporal distribution of responses allows us to examine precisely the effect of a drug on the patterning of behavior. Also, drug–behavior interaction can be analyzed by determining how changes in the schedule modify the effect of the drug. Because there are a large number of possible reinforcement schedules, each eliciting a distinct pattern of behavior, the combinations of drug and schedule are very numerous and represent many volumes of research. This section describes only the most elementary and most commonly used operant behavior techniques, and uses examples of drug effects that are explained more thoroughly in later chapters.

Positive Reinforcement Schedules

Continuous reinforcement schedule. Perhaps the simplest schedule is **continuous reinforcement (CRF)**, which means that each lever press is reinforced by the delivery of a food pellet (or other reinforcer), regardless of how often the animal responds. CRF may be used initially during shaping in order to hasten the rate of training. However, animals working on CRF are not particularly resistant to extinction; that is, they stop responding soon after the reinforcer is eliminated.

Ratio schedules. A variation of the CRF schedule is the **fixed ratio (FR) schedule**, which requires a fixed number of responses before a reinforcer is delivered. Thus, an FR-3 schedule means that the animal must press the lever three times to receive one food pellet. Changing the fixed ratio—for example, from 3 to 20 or 45—will tell us how hard the animal is willing to work for the reinforcement. As a rule, animals respond at continuous, very high rates when working on an FR schedule. A typical cumulative recording of response rate under an FR schedule, as well as several of the other schedules described, is shown in Figure 2.26. Notice the steady rate of lever pressing and regular delivery of reinforcement under the FR schedule.

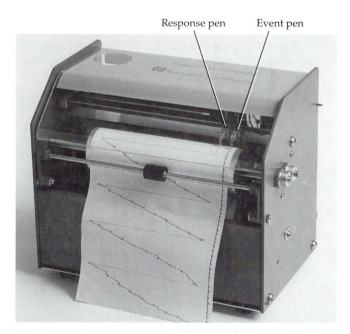

2.25 CUMULATIVE RECORDER. The paper unrolls under the two pens at a constant speed (5 mm/min). Each occurrence of a lever press moves the response pen a small increment to the left. Reinforcements are indicated by a short diagonal slash on the cumulative record or by a similar mark made by the event pen on the right. The event pen can also be used to indicate additional events during an experimental session, such as the onset of a discriminable stimulus (a light or a sound.) (Courtesy of Gerbrands Corporation, Arlington, Massachusetts.)

Variable ratio (VR) schedules differ from FR schedules only in that they are characterized by the average number of responses required before reinforcement is delivered. A VR-10 schedule means that on the average, reinforcement occurs after every 10 responses, but varies from trial to trial—for example, after 2, 11, 20, 8, and 9 responses. As is true for the FR schedule, response rate is high for the VR schedule, and responding is very persistent. A slot machine is programmed to deliver payoffs on a variable ratio schedule; a person cannot predict how many responses are required for the payoff.

The simple FR schedule has been used very effectively in identifying drugs that have abuse potential—that is, drugs that are capable of bringing about psychological dependence. We assume that if a drug maintains responding in the same way that food or water does, it must have reinforcing properties. The procedure requires that the reinforcement for lever pressing be an injection of the drug rather than food. The injection must be directly into the blood or into the brain so that the reinforcing effect can be perceived rapidly by the animal. This drug **self-administration method** is a very accurate indicator of abuse potential in humans. For instance, animals will readily self-administer morphine and amphetamine, which are certainly abused by humans, whereas drugs in the phenothiazine class are neither self-administered by animals nor abused by humans. More details on the self-administration method can be found in Chapter 12 and in a paper by Caine and coworkers (Caine, Lintz, and Koob, 1993). This method is used frequently and is an excellent example of the utility of animal testing for predicting human behavior.

Fixed interval schedules. On a **fixed interval (FI) schedule**, reinforcement is available after a certain amount of time has passed since the last reinforcement. Thus, on an FI-2 schedule, reinforcement follows the first response an animal makes after 2 minutes have elapsed since the last reinforcement. Responses made during the 2-minute interval are "wasted;" that is, they elicit no reinforcement. After some experience with the schedule, the animal's pattern of responding includes a pause after each reinforcement and a gradual increase in its rate of responding as the interval ends. This pattern, called "scalloping," is evident in Figure 2.26.

The behavior generated by the FI schedule may be based in part on temporal discrimination. Animals tend to create an internal "clock" to monitor the interval between responses. A second influence on behavior is the distribution of reinforcement. On the FI schedule, responding that occurs early in the interval is not closely followed by reinforcement; thus the behavior is less likely to occur again. If the response occurs later in the interval, the closer temporal association with reinforcement increases the recurrence of the behavior. Thus, the

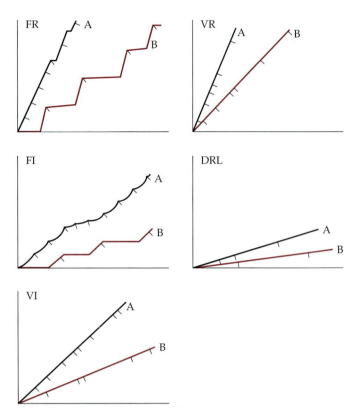

2.26 SAMPLE CUMULATIVE RECORDS OF RESPONDING maintained by different schedules of reinforcement. The abscissa represents the passage of time; the ordinate represents cumulative responding. Horizontal lines in the records indicate time when no responses occurred. Nonhorizontal portions (slopes) of the records demonstrate the rate of response; the steeper the slope, the greater the response rate. For each schedule, the ratios are smaller or the time intervals shorter for A responders than for B responders. Reinforcements are indicated by the short diagonal lines on the record. (After Carlton, 1983.)

responses of an experienced subject tend to be clustered at the end of the interval.

Differential reinforcement of low rates of responding. A modification of the FI schedule yields a schedule that produces **differential reinforcement of low rates of responding (DRL)**. In the DRL schedule, reinforcement is programmed to be available after a certain period of time has elapsed since the previous response. If a response occurs during this interval, however, not only is no reinforcement delivered, but the interval timer is reset and a new waiting period begins. If the animal's waiting time exceeds the specified period, a lever press produces reinforcement. Thus, the DRL schedule produces very low rates of responding. Animals need a large amount of training on this schedule before responding is stable.

Variable interval schedules. Another type of schedule is the **variable interval (VI) schedule**. Reinforcement following lever pressing under a VI schedule depends upon the time elapsed since the previous reinforcement. In contrast to the FI schedule, the interreinforcement intervals in the VI schedule vary around a mean value, which is used to describe the schedule. A VI-2 minute schedule, for example, has a mean interreinforcement time of 2 minutes. As you might suspect, the uncertainty of reinforcement inherent in this schedule produces a high and stable rate of responding. The VI schedule is frequently incorporated into multiple schedules (i.e., a combination of schedules that permits the study of several behaviors in the same animal) because drug-induced disruption of the stable response rate can be readily detected (see below). A second advantage is that the behavior is maintained over long periods of time with relatively few reinforcements, so motivation is not altered by delivery of many reinforcements in a short time.

Drug Effects and Baseline Response Rate

In Chapter 1 we emphasized the dose-dependent nature of drug effects as it relates to receptor occupancy. At this point it is important to extend our argument to include the idea that the characteristics of the behavior being measured can also interact with the dose of drug to determine drug effect. In particular, the rate of occurrence of the behavior is the dimension most often used when comparing drug effects on different behaviors. Any drug evaluation must consider both dose-dependent effects and rate-dependent effects.

One example of the interaction between dose and rate of behavior involves the CNS stimulant amphetamine. Dose-dependent effects have been well documented: increases in the rate of responding occur after low or moderate doses of amphetamine, but at higher doses, behavior tends to be depressed (Dews, 1958). In addition, the baseline rate of responding modifies the effects of amphetamine (Dews and Wenger, 1977). Clark and Steele (1966) showed that when the initial response rate is very low, amphetamine increases the rate of responding in a dose-dependent manner (Figure 2.27, curve A). When the initial response rate is moderate (as for an FI-4 minute schedule), low doses of amphetamine increase responding, and high doses decrease it (curve B). At doses of up to 1 mg/kg, the response rate increases, whereas from 1 to 4 mg/kg, a gradual decline in responding occurs. When the initial response rate is high (as for an FR-25 schedule), amphetamine tends to decrease the rate as a function of increasing dose (curve C). Thus, although amphetamine is ordinarily classified as a CNS stimulant, it is clear that its pharmacological effect is highly dependent on the rate of the behavior being observed.

Further examination of the interaction between the dose of amphetamine and the initial rate of behavior has led to the conclusion that rate dependency becomes increasingly significant as the dose is increased (Heffner,

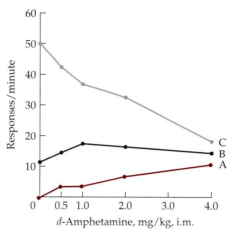

2.27 RESPONSE RATE–DRUG EFFECT INTERACTIONS. Mean rates of responding on three schedules of reinforcement are modified by the effects of *d*-amphetamine. Curve A illustrates the drug's effect on a low rate of responding with no reinforcement; curve B, responding at moderate rates under FI-4 minutes; curve C, responding at high rates under an FR-25 schedule. (After Clark and Steele, 1966.)

Drawbaugh, and Zigmond, 1974). In one series of experiments rats were trained on several different operant schedules to generate different baseline rates of responding before receiving different doses of amphetamine. Each point in Figure 2.28 represents the increase in responding over saline controls. The rate dependency is evident at all doses except 0.3 mg/kg; that is, the same dose of amphetamine had different effects on different baseline rates of behavior. Further, the interaction between dose and rate becomes more pronounced (as shown by the steeper slope and downward displacement) with higher doses. These results and many others clearly show that variables that modify behavior also contribute to drug effects, just as the type of drug and the dose of drug contribute to the overall effect. The importance of rate dependency is discussed in more depth by Carlton (1983) and others.

Many other CNS stimulants have been tested under the same conditions and the results compared with the effects of amphetamine. One striking finding is that nicotine has many of the same effects on schedule-controlled behavior as amphetamine, although it suppresses responding briefly after administration, unlike the latter drug. This similarity of action between the two drugs may have important implications about the biochemical and behavioral bases of abuse of this class of drugs.

Negative Reinforcement and Punishment

The simplest schedule of **negative reinforcement** involves the use of the lever press to terminate an aversive condition. Once again, an FR schedule can be used, so that after a given number of responses the negative reinforcer (usually electric shock) is terminated. An FI or VI

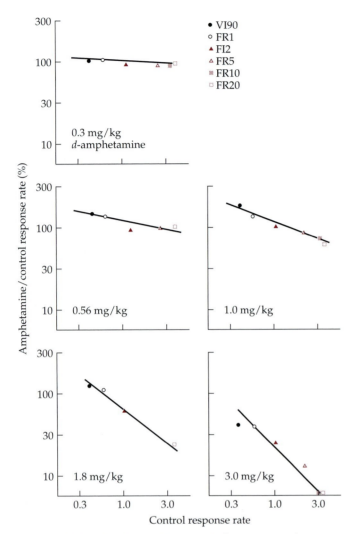

Legend:
- VI90
- FR1
- FI2
- FR5
- FR10
- FR20

0.3 mg/kg
d-amphetamine

0.56 mg/kg   1.0 mg/kg

1.8 mg/kg   3.0 mg/kg

Amphetamine/control response rate (%)

Control response rate

2.28 RATE DEPENDENCY FUNCTIONS demonstrating the interaction between dose of amphetamine and baseline rates of responding generated by several different schedules of reinforcement. Each data point represents the amphetamine-induced increase in responding over saline controls on a particular schedule of reinforcement. (After Heffner, Drawbaugh, and Zigmond, 1974.)

The intensity of the shock at this point indicates how much "pain" will be tolerated by the subject. The method is very sensitive even to mild analgesics such as aspirin. However, without an independent measure of behavioral depression, it is not clear whether a change in threshold is due to the test drug's analgesic effects or to general behavioral depression.

Multiple schedules.   **Multiple schedules** are created by combining two or more schedules in a regular pattern. The two schedules (e.g., FI and FR) are alternated during a test session, and each schedule is signaled by the appearance of a colored light or other cue. A typical multiple schedule might begin with a green light to signal an FI-2, which lasts for 20 minutes. At the end of that period, a red light signals the start of an FR-8, which lasts for 10 minutes. Several alternations between schedules may occur, and each time the animal adjusts its response rate to optimize reinforcement. The greatest advantage of a multiple schedule is that a drug effect can be tested on behaviors with different baseline rates. From our earlier discussion, it should be clear that ongoing behavior frequently modifies drug effects. One of the more popular multiple schedules is used in the Geller conflict procedure, described in Chapter 16.

Signaled avoidance–escape.   Another popular experimental design uses avoidance or postponement of noxious conditions rather than escape or termination. One of the best-known screening tests for psychotropic drugs is based on this type of behavior. In this test, called the **signaled avoidance–escape procedure**, a rat is placed in a box with a grid floor through which an electric shock can be delivered. A vertical climbing pole in the box provides a means of avoiding the shock. A trial consists of sounding a buzzer and subsequently delivering a foot shock. The rat can escape the shock by climbing the pole. After several pairings of buzzer and shock, the rat climbs the pole when the buzzer sounds. This response to the signal is referred to as the **conditioned avoidance response (CAR)**. If the rat fails to climb the pole when the buzzer sounds, it can climb the pole when the shock is delivered and thus escape.

When drug effects were tested using this design, it was found that drugs that act effectively in reducing symptoms of schizophrenia (such as the phenothiazines) blocked only the conditioned avoidance response. In contrast, other depressants of the CNS that are not effective against schizophrenia (such as the barbiturates) depressed the conditioned avoidance response but also depressed the escape response. Thus, the antischizophrenic drugs showed selective blocking action, whereas the others tested slowed all behavior.

Sidman avoidance procedure.   A variation on this method, the Sidman avoidance procedure or continuous avoidance procedure, uses no signal to mark the onset of

schedule can also be used, in which termination depends on a response occurring after an interval of time has elapsed.

Negative reinforcement techniques are a relatively new means of testing the analgesic properties of drugs. These methods may have an advantage over those previously described because they depend upon a learned response of the subject. The learned response may correlate better with the human response to pain, which certainly has a complex learned component based on previous experience. In an operant titration schedule test (Weiss and Laties, 1961), the animal is first trained to perform a particular operant response (most often a lever press) to eliminate a noxious stimulus such as foot shock. The experimenter then applies the nociceptive stimulus in increasing intensities up to the point at which the animal responds (the "aversive threshold").

shock (Sidman, 1953). Brief foot shocks are delivered to the animal at regularly spaced intervals. The delivery of shock can be delayed by a fixed time interval if the animal makes the appropriate response. For example, a shock can be presented every 5 seconds unless a lever press occurs. If the animal makes the response, no shock occurs again until 15 seconds after the response. By optimally spacing the lever pressing, an animal can avoid receiving any shocks. This behavioral test has not been used as frequently as the signaled avoidance test because training is significantly more difficult. The difficulty arises from the fact that when shock is applied, animals will frequently "freeze," behavior that is incompatible with lever pressing.

Conditioned emotional response. The "freezing" response itself has been used by other investigators as a behavioral measure of anxiety or fear. In these tests, an animal first develops regular responding based on an appropriate schedule. Once the trained behavior is stable, a signal is introduced and is followed by an electric shock that can neither be avoided nor escaped. The signal alone produces a suppression of the trained behavior after several pairings of signal and shock. This **conditioned emotional response (CER)** has been used to identify anxiety-reducing drugs because anxiolytics are highly effective in increasing behavior that is normally suppressed by punishment. Although this procedure is frequently used, several factors influence the degree of suppression of behavior and hence its usefulness as a screening device. These include the relative durations of the presence and absence of the preshock signal, the schedule of reinforcement used to maintain the behavior, and the previous experimental history of the subject (Kelleher and Morse, 1964).

Drugs Used as Discriminative Stimuli

A **discriminative stimulus** (usually designated S^D) is any stimulus that signals reinforcement for a subject performing an operant task. For example, in one experiment, a green light (the S^D) may signal that reinforcement is available following the appropriate response, and a red light may signal that reinforcement is unavailable regardless of the response made. The nonreinforcement condition (red light) is designated S^Δ. An animal that learns to press a lever in the presence of the green light but not the red light clearly can discriminate between the two lights, and its behavior is said to be "under stimulus control." The sensitivity of discrimination can be tested by presenting stimuli that vary in their similarity to the training S^D. As you would expect, the more similar a test stimulus is to the original training S^D, the greater the likelihood that the animal will respond. This phenomenon, called **stimulus generalization**, is shown graphically in Figure 2.29. In this experiment (Guttman and Kalish, 1956), pigeons were trained to peck at a translucent plastic disk of a particular spectral

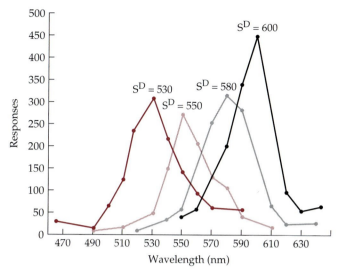

2.29 STIMULUS GENERALIZATION. Generalization curves for four groups of pigeons trained on a VI schedule to peck a particular wavelength (color) disk (S^D). The curve shows the mean number of responses made to the original training stimulus (S^D) and to each stimulus that varied from the original. (After Guttman and Kalish, 1956.)

wavelength (S^D). When they were tested with a range of colors varying 60 nm on either side of the S^D, the amount of pecking was related to the similarity of the test stimulus to the S^D. The more similar the wavelength (color), the greater the generalization to the S^D, and the more responses occurred.

Discrimination training allows the researcher to evaluate sensory processes in subjects that are unable to communicate verbally. Thus, color vision can be studied by training an animal to respond to one color and not to another. Furthermore, the effects of drugs on sensory perception can be tested with the same procedure.

Although discriminative stimuli are usually changes in the physical environment (e.g., lights, patterns, or tones), interoceptive stimuli have been found to be significant environmental cues as well. The ability of subjects to discriminate altered internal states has been utilized to study drug effects. In most such experiments, the subject is trained to emit one response (e.g., press the left lever of a pair) to obtain reinforcement in one drugged state and to make a different response (press the right lever) for reward in a nondrugged or different drugged state. The animal's response depends on its discriminating among internal cues produced by the drug. This procedure is referred to as **drug discrimination learning**.

Just as physical stimuli fall along a curve of stimulus generalization, so too do internal cues, including those associated with drug states. If an animal is trained to respond after 5 mg of morphine, maximum responding will occur at 5 mg, and the response rate will fall off in a predictable fashion as the dose deviates from 5 mg. The drug clearly provides some cue(s) that follows the laws of stimulus generalization. Following training with morphine as the cue(s), other drugs in the morphine class (the narcotics) can substitute for morphine as an S^D in the trained animals to a greater extent than nonnarcotic drugs that act on the CNS. For example, amphetamine or marijuana are both treated by the animals as S^Δ. The extent to which another drug can substitute for morphine as the S^D without loss of a sharp stimulus discrimination curve is an indication of how similar a state the new drug produces. In this way, novel drugs can be characterized by the extent of their generalization to the known drug.

The same operant technique can be used to identify the neurochemical basis for a given drug cue. Drugs that abolish or disrupt the cue can provide a hint about its mechanism. For instance, the drug cue can be challenged with increasing doses of a suspected antagonist until the cue has lost its effect. If the antagonist acts in a competitive manner with the drug cue, the dose–response curve will be parallel but shifted to the right. If the antagonist does not act specifically at the drug cue receptor site, then the dose–response shift will not be parallel. In the case of the morphine cue, a specific antagonist that is known to bind to the morphine receptor also disrupts the cue effects of morphine (Lal, Gianutsos, and Miksic, 1977).

These techniques can also be used to evaluate hypotheses regarding the mechanism of a drug's action. For example, the anxiolytic drug chlordiazepoxide (CDP; Librium) is believed to block the release of serotonin, a neurotransmitter, from axon terminals. If this is true, then serotonin agonists should diminish the responses to CDP. To test this hypothesis, one experiment used CDP as a discriminative stimulus in a two-lever Skinner box design. As the doses of the serotonin agonists rose, the rats pressed the CDP lever less and the saline lever more (Figure 2.30). Thus, these drugs, when administered with CDP, seem to diminish the cue value of the anxiolytic, suggesting that serotonin plays a role in the discriminative properties of CDP (McElroy and Feldman, unpublished).

To further evaluate the neurophysiological basis of a drug discrimination, the drug may be injected into discrete areas of the brain. Another approach to studying mechanisms of drug action is to mimic a drug cue by electrically stimulating a specific brain area. Alternatively, it should be possible to modify the cue by making specific brain lesions at the drug's site of action.

The use of drugs as discriminative stimuli provides a technique for identifying drug antagonists that can be used therapeutically. The discriminable stimulus properties of phencyclidine (PCP) have been studied in order to elucidate the biochemical basis of schizophrenia. PCP produces psychotic-like symptoms in some abusers and is readily trainable as a discriminative stimulus (Browne, 1982). Pharmacologically similar drugs, such as keta-

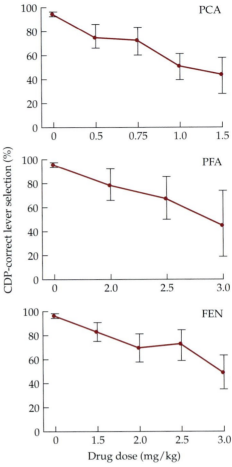

2.30 THE DISCRIMINATIVE PROPERTIES OF CDP (2.5 mg/kg) are blocked by drugs that enhance the release of serotonin from nerve terminals. As the dose of the drugs was increased, the animals responded less often to the CDP lever. CDP = chlordiazepoxide; PCA = *p*-chloroamphetamine; PFA = *p*-fluoroamphetamine; FEN = fenfluramine. Each bar represents the mean ± *SEM* for 10 rats.

mine, can mimic the PCP cue. However, a wide variety of agonists and antagonists of the principal CNS transmitters (e.g., norepinephrine, GABA, opiates, 5-HT, and others) failed to block or mimic the discriminative properties of PCP. Out of more than 40 drugs tested, only adenosine analogs antagonized the PCP cue. Although the mechanism of antagonism is unknown, the possibility of therapeutic effects of adenosine on long-term PCP-induced psychosis or schizophrenia must be investigated further.

The use of drug cue discrimination testing has increased over the last few years. It has been found useful in identifying new drugs that have therapeutic effects similar to those of known drugs and in examining the neurochemical basis of drug action. Goudie and Leathley (1993) provide an excellent description of basic methodology as well as an assessment of potential pitfalls.

Part II Summary

Behavioral pharmacology evaluates the effects of drugs on behavior. The testing is done in a controlled and systematic way to enhance the reliability and the validity of the results. The testing of drugs on animals under well-controlled conditions probably provides the most objective assessment of drug effects on behavior. Certainly, animal testing is not a perfect way to evaluate drugs designed to modify mood and thought processes in humans. Nevertheless, neurochemical and behavioral methods of determining drug action can provide significant information regarding the basis of effective drug therapy. Usually drugs are researched in humans after animal studies reveal no physiological or behavioral toxicity and establish an effective range of doses.

When studying the effects of drugs on animals, baseline behavior (behavior in the nondrugged state) is carefully assessed before behavior is examined in the drugged state in the same animals or in drugged animals that are carefully matched to the nondrugged controls. Primary evaluations are made using measures of possible drug-induced ataxia, tremors, general sedation, and so forth, as well as drug effects upon behaviors that require no training, such as locomotion, food and water ingestion, reactions to novel environments and noxious stimuli, and sleep. Secondary evaluations are made of the effects of drugs on more complex behaviors, for example, on anxiety and learning. Animals may also be trained in various ways to respond to food or liquid rewards, to sensory discrimination, or to pain avoidance using operant conditioning techniques. All of these techniques in behavioral pharmacology provide significant information on the interaction of drugs, brain chemistry, and behavior.

Chapter 3

Neurons and Glial Cells

To understand how drugs can affect behavior, we must know something about the chemistry of drug substances, how these chemical substances affect neural tissue, and how chemically induced neural changes lead to behavioral changes. Because nerve cells (**neurons**) are the point of contact for the molecules of psychotropic drugs, we present an overview in this chapter of the structure and function of these cells. Special emphasis has been placed on the genetically determined structure and function of neurons because drug molecules exert their effects on membrane and inner organelles that set in motion the series of events that ultimately lead to cellular changes and behavioral effects. In Chapter 5, the activity of neurons will be discussed in terms of their patterns of response among the structures of the nervous system whose functional anatomy is described in Chapter 4.

The nervous system has been systematically studied for centuries, but contemporary investigators, using techniques and instruments developed only recently, are providing us with prodigious amounts of new information about the functional significance of its parts in both healthy and dysfunctional states. The high resolution of the electron microscope permits the visualization of the outer and inner structures of neurons. Of special interest are neuronal membranes, which possess structures that mediate interactions among neurons. In most instances, the sites of drug action are the contact points on neurons, which are called **synapses** (Gr., "to touch together"). Some of the significant parts of synapses are proteins that can be chemically characterized, and the genes that program their synthesis have been determined in some cases.

Neuron Function

Neurons are the functional units of the CNS. These cells plus the **neuroglia**, which support neurons physiologically, make up the bulk of the brain and other parts of the CNS. Neuroglia will be described later, but first we will direct our attention to neurons. Neurons are distinctive in that their excitable membranes extend over the entire surface of the cell. Excitation of these membranes can be conveyed to adjacent cells, or it can be used to activate effector organs. Neurons usually communicate with each other by releasing chemical substances known as neurotransmitters. The cells of the endocrine glands also stimulate other cells by releasing chemical substances, called hormones, into the bloodstream, through which they are carried to receptor sites on target cells. Interneural communication, however, occurs more rapidly than hormonal communication, and it is more specific.

The key process of neural function is the way neurons influence one another through synaptic contacts. A neuron can be in contact with a few other neurons or with many thousands (divergence), or many different neurons can target a single cell to modulate the output of that cell (convergence). Neurons influence one another by the release of their various neurotransmitters—some that increase the output of the target cell and some that decrease it. A variety of nerve cells and neurotransmitters can be organized into specialized circuits because a given neurotransmitter will excite or inhibit some neurons, but not others.

Neural circuits may be as simple as a monosynaptic reflex loop that involves only one synapse between the sensory and the motor nerves (such as the circuit that causes extension of the lower leg in response to a slight knock below the knee), but it should be noted that the execution of the reflex response involves hundreds of sensory nerves, each of which synapses with one or more motor nerves. For more complicated activities there are polysynaptic circuits of unimaginable complexity involving sensorimotor and perceptual processes, memory, language, intellectual activities, and emotion. Try to imagine the neural response to the following stimulus: You won the lottery!

The effects of drugs on these circuits is our immediate concern in neuropsychopharmacology. For example,

consider some of the effects of amphetamine. This drug heightens arousal, reduces boredom, increases attention, and combats fatigue. Pharmacologically, amphetamine intensifies the action of two neurotransmitters, norepinephrine (NE) and dopamine (DA), in the nervous system. These neurotransmitters play a major role in the activity of the sympathetic nervous system as well as the CNS. Consequently, amphetamine elicits an alert, energetic, vigorous physiological state that sometimes allows behavior to exceed its normal capacity. The licit and illicit uses of amphetamine are discussed in Chapter 13.

Neuron Morphology

Neurons can be classified in several ways, but they are frequently classified according to the number of branches that extend from the cell body (Figure 3.1.) There are **unipolar**, **bipolar**, and **multipolar neurons**. Unipolar cells

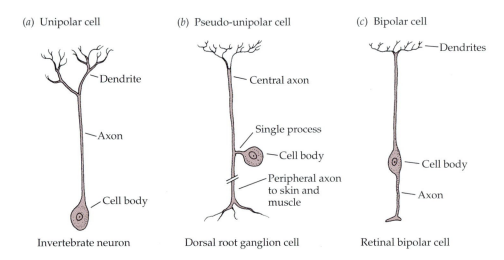

(a) Unipolar cell

Dendrite

Axon

Cell body

Invertebrate neuron

(b) Pseudo-unipolar cell

Central axon

Single process

Cell body

Peripheral axon to skin and muscle

Dorsal root ganglion cell

(c) Bipolar cell

Dendrites

Cell body

Axon

Retinal bipolar cell

(d) Three types of multipolar cells

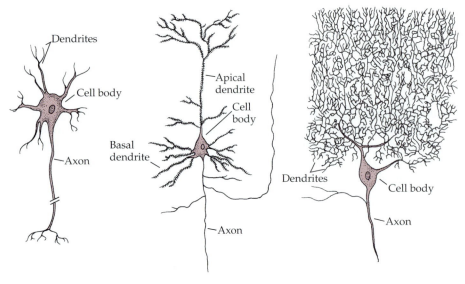

Dendrites

Cell body

Axon

Spinal motor neuron

Apical dendrite

Cell body

Basal dendrite

Axon

Hippocampal pyramidal cell

Dendrites

Cell body

Axon

Purkinje cell of cerebellum

3.1 NEURON CLASSIFICATION. (a) An invertebrate unipolar cell. (b) A pseudo-unipolar cell. (c) A retinal bipolar cell. (d, *left to right*) Three types of multipolar cells: a spinal motor neuron, a hippocampal pyramidal cell, and a Purkinje cell (shown in only one plane). (After Ramón y Cajal, 1933.)

(Figure 3.1*a*) are characteristic of invertebrate nervous systems, and though there are unipolar cells in some vertebrate ganglia, they need not concern us here.

Until recently, spinal sensory afferent neurons were also classed as unipolar cells because a single extension emerges from the cell body, as shown in Figure 3.1*b*. These neurons have a peripheral branch that conveys sensory information from the skin, muscles, and joints to the cell body and a central branch that conveys information from the cell body to the spinal cord. During fetal development these neurons develop as bipolar cells, but at a later stage the two branches fuse and emerge as a single process for a short distance from the cell body, then split into two processes, both of which function as axons: one goes to the periphery, and the other enters the spinal cord to communicate with other neurons involved with reflexes, sensory awareness, and motor control. These cells are now known as **pseudo-unipolar neurons**. Their clustered cell bodies form the **dorsal root ganglia** that lie adjacent to the spinal cord.

True bipolar neurons (Figure 3.1*c*) receive inputs from the sense organs of vision, hearing, and taste and from the vestibular apparatus. These neurons convey sensory information to the CNS, wherein the information is sent via multisynaptic routes to the various areas of the brain responsible for all of the manifestations of each of the sensory modalities. For example, sounds effect alertness and cause your head and body to turn toward the sound source. You may perceive the sounds as language or music that you recognize and sing along with, and you may recognize and respond to the sound of your name. Auditory stimuli originating in the cochlea are routed to a number of brain loci to produce all of these and other effects.

Multipolar neurons are the most common in the CNS. They have many short, branched dendrites, such as those of the spinal motor neurons that stimulate the muscles of the trunk, limbs, hands, and face (Figure 3.1*d*). Other neurons of this type are pyramidal cells, such as those found in the hippocampus or those in the motor cortex that mediate control of fine movements of the hand, and Purkinje cells from the cerebellum, which transmit the output from the cerebellum to the cerebellar deep nuclei for relay to the brain stem for muscle coordination. The elaborate branching of the dendritic tree of the Purkinje cell enormously increases its synaptic surface, making it possible for these cells to receive as many as 150,000 contacts from other cells. These cell types are described in more detail in later sections of this chapter.

Having classified neurons by their dendritic and axonal extensions, we have by no means eliminated other classifications using different criteria. Estimates of the number of different neuron types range from 1,000 to as high as 100,000. For example, neurons can be classified by the neurotransmitters and peptides they secrete, the types of receptors and ion channels they possess, their sensitivity to activating and inhibitory influences, and

the diameter of their axons and degree of myelination (discussed later in this chapter), which determines the speed of impulse conduction, or their susceptibility to genetically determined neural malfunctions. In succeeding chapters most of these factors will be encountered in explaining the effects of psychotropic drugs.

Microanatomy of Neurons

In this section we shall see that there is a wide variety of neuron specializations, but first we will describe the four major characteristic features of neurons, namely, the cell body, dendrites, axon, and presynaptic terminals. Because of the wide variety of neurons in the vertebrate nervous system, it is not possible to describe a single neuron that would include all the cytological features that exist. Therefore, we present a model neuron that possesses most of the characteristics typical of all neurons (Figure 3.2.) All of these characteristics will be described in detail in the following paragraphs.

The Cell Body

The metabolic center of a neuron is the cell body, frequently called the **soma**, which is enclosed by a plasma membrane that extends over the extensions of the soma that make up the dendrites, axon, and axon terminals. The interior of the soma, as in most eukaryotic cells, consists of cytoplasm, a gel within a microtrabecular lattice formed by the microtubules, filaments, and associated proteins that make up the cytoskeleton (Figure 3.3). These microstructures of the cytoplasm will be described in greater detail below.

The principal activities of the neuronal soma are energy-producing metabolism and the synthesis of most of the macromolecules used by the cell to maintain its structure and execute its particular functions. Thus, embedded within the neuronal cytoplasm are the organelles common to other cells, namely, the nucleus, nucleolus, endoplasmic reticulum, Golgi apparatus, mitochondria, and ribosomes. These cell inclusions, shown in Figure 3.4, participate in the expression of genetic information controlling the synthesis of cellular proteins and enzymes that are involved in energy production, growth, and the replacement of materials lost by injury or attrition. All in all, it is estimated that the genetic material in the nucleus of most cells in humans provides the blueprint for about 60,000 proteins that are needed to keep us alive and healthy. However, in most cells, including neurons, most of the genetic material is dormant, and only a small fraction is involved with the cells maintenance and function.

Here we may note that proteins may exist in many forms and perform many functions. For example, the protein hemoglobin has an oxygen transport function, insulin is a hormone that mediates sugar metabolism, snake venoms are toxins, α-keratin is the major component of hair and feathers, and choline acetyltransferase (ChAT) is an enzyme that catalyzes the formation of the

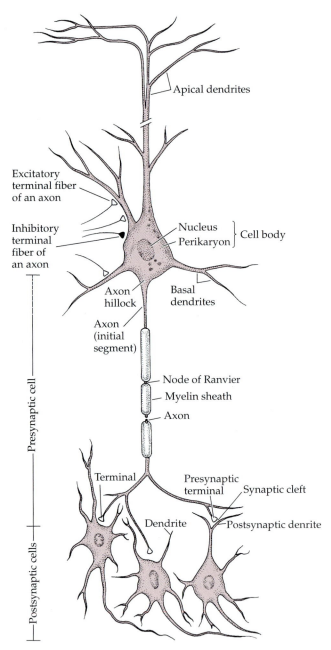

Apical dendrites

Excitatory
terminal fiber
of an axon

Inhibitory
terminal
fiber of
an axon

Nucleus
Perikaryon } Cell body

Axon
hillock

Basal
dendrites

Axon
(initial
segment)

Node of Ranvier

Myelin sheath

Axon

Presynaptic cell

Terminal

Presynaptic
terminal
Synaptic cleft

Dendrite

Postsynaptic denrite

Postsynaptic cells

3.2 A MULTIPOLAR VERTEBRATE NEURON. For illustrative purposes, the axon is shorter and thicker than that of an actual cell. Also, the internodal segments of the myelin sheath are shortened: normally they are 100 to 200 times longer than the axon diameter. (After Kandel, 1991.)

neurotransmitter acetylcholine from acetyl CoA and choline. Today more than 1,500 enzymes are known that catalyze thousands of chemical reactions in living tissue with high specificity and rapidity. The names of enzymes can often be recognized in print by the suffix *-ase* after the name of the substrate and the chemical process involved, as in *choline acetyltransferase*. But the names of many other enzymes, such as pepsin and trypsin, which catalyze the hydrolysis of proteins, are not informative as to the reaction catalyzed.

The Nucleus and Nucleolus

Depending upon the neuron type, the **nucleus** can be between 3 and 18 micrometers in diameter (micrometer, $\mu m = 10^{-6}$ m or 10^{-3} mm). It is centrally located and has a spherical shape. The principal component of the nucleus is deoxyribonucleic acid (DNA), the chemical substance of the chromosomes and genes. The genes are the source of the information that directs prenatal development and the postnatal management of all cell processes in the organism. Almost every cell in the body, with the exception of the gametes (sex cells) and nonnucleated cells such as blood platelets, has a full complement of genes. These genes direct the development of a new organism, but after the vertebrate offspring is physically free of its mother, only the parent cells (i.e., skin cells, liver cells, and muscle cells, but not neurons) replicate themselves during growth and the repair and renewal of tissues. Only a tiny fraction of the gene pool, however, controls postnatal cell multiplication and intracellular activities. There is further discussion of the mechanisms of genetic expression later in this chapter.

The **nucleolus** is found in the nuclei of all neurons, except some of the very smallest ones. It can be seen as a prominent, deeply stained spherical inclusion about one-third the size of the nucleus and does not have a limiting membrane. It is an assembly of duplicated genes constituted for the purpose of synthesizing ribosomal RNA (rRNA), which has a major role in protein synthesis that will be described below.

Although the information needed for the synthesis of protein macromolecules is encoded in the chromosomes within the cell's nucleus, the actual protein synthesis occurs in the cytoplasm. Therefore, the information in the chromosomes must be communicated to organelles in the cytoplasm. A number of different membranes associated with the nucleus play a role in protein production. From the inside out, the first membrane is the nuclear envelope, which surrounds the nucleus. The nuclear envelope is a double membrane that encloses an area known as the perinuclear cisterna. However, the layers of the envelope come together at intervals to form pores 65 nm in width, which allow the nucleoplasm to be in contact with the cytoplasm. Also, the outer layer of the nuclear envelope is contiguous with other types of membranes, those of the **endoplasmic reticulum (ER)**, **Golgi apparatus**, and **secretory granules**. Thus, the spaces within the nuclear envelope, the ER, and the Golgi apparatus are continuous and make up a system of sheets, sacs, and tubules where protein synthesis takes place. Still other membranes are those of the mitochondria and peroxisomes, which are discussed below. It should be noted that because the ER is extended in three dimensions, a thin slice of a cell cannot show that the parts of this organelle are all connected; in micrographs, pieces of the ER are visible, but appear as islands in the cytoplasm.

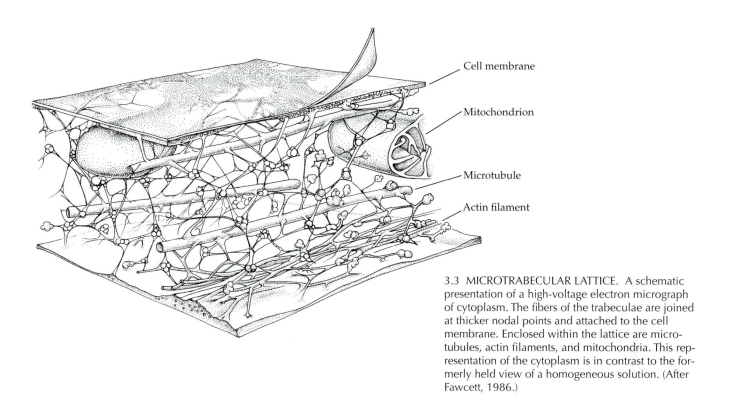

Cell membrane

Mitochondrion

Microtubule

Actin filament

3.3 MICROTRABECULAR LATTICE. A schematic presentation of a high-voltage electron micrograph of cytoplasm. The fibers of the trabeculae are joined at thicker nodal points and attached to the cell membrane. Enclosed within the lattice are microtubules, actin filaments, and mitochondria. This representation of the cytoplasm is in contrast to the formerly held view of a homogeneous solution. (After Fawcett, 1986.)

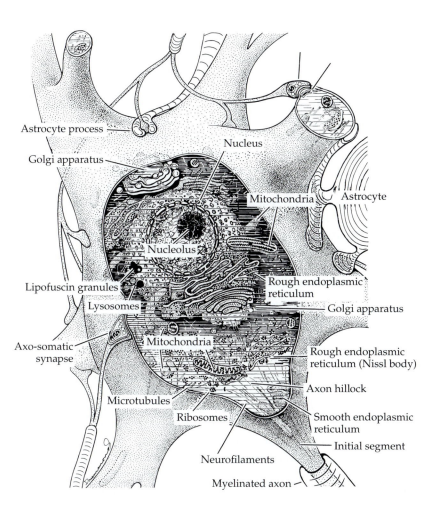

Astrocyte process

Golgi apparatus

Nucleus

Mitochondria

Astrocyte

Nucleolus

Lipofuscin granules

Lysosomes

Rough endoplasmic reticulum

Golgi apparatus

Axo-somatic synapse

Mitochondria

Rough endoplasmic reticulum (Nissl body)

Microtubules

Axon hillock

Ribosomes

Smooth endoplasmic reticulum

Initial segment

Neurofilaments

Myelinated axon

3.4 INTERNAL STRUCTURE OF A NEURONAL CELL BODY. This cutaway view reveals the cell inclusions, such as the nucleus and nucleolus, mitochondria, and the Golgi apparatus. Many axon terminals from other neurons form synapses upon the outer surface of the soma and upon the dendrites. In this illustration, their number is markedly reduced. Only one astrocyte process is shown; normally there might be hundreds. The initial segment of an axon is shown at the lower right, just above the first myelin segment. (From McGeer, Eccles, and McGeer, 1978, *Molecular Neurobiology of the Mammalian Brain*, © Plenum Press.)

Mitochondria

Mitochondria are synthesized in the cell soma by a self-duplicating fission resembling the reproductive style of bacteria. This is possible because mitochondria have their own special DNA, RNAs, and ribosomes that code for some of their properties and functions. This unique situation led to the proposal that mitochondria in the distant past had an independent existence like that of bacteria and were engulfed by eukaryotic cell membranes by the process of endocytosis. This notion is supported by the similarity of the structure and respiratory function of the inner mitochondrial membrane to that of the outer membrane of bacteria, and the good possibility that the outer mitochondrial membrane originated from the plasma membranes of early eukaryotes. In time, the mitochondria came to have a symbiotic relationship with eukaryotic cells, a relationship that came to be hereditary (see Wilson et al., 1973.) However, mitochondria are dependent upon nuclear DNA for coding some of their inner membrane proteins, such as those needed for replicating their own DNA and RNA. These proteins are synthesized by cytoplasmic ribosomes and transported into the mitochondria, as will be described below in more detail (Fawcett, 1986).

Each neuron contains several hundred mitochondria that are similar to those found in other organs. In neurons, they are elongated oval structures between 0.2 and 0.3 μm in diameter and 2 to 6 μm long. They are scattered throughout the somata, the axons, and even the narrowest branches of dendrites. They are most numerous in cell areas having high levels of energy consumption. In muscle cells, for example, mitochondria are clustered around the contractile elements. In neurons, they are numerous between the ER and the Golgi apparatus, and especially so in dendrites (see Figure 3.11) and axon terminals, where intense metabolic activity is associated with the synthesis, storage, release, and reuptake of neurotransmitters.

Glucose is the essential fuel for neurons, and it enters the soma after transport from the blood across the capillary endothelium. In the cytoplasm, a series of enzyme actions converts glucose to acetyl coenzyme A (acetyl CoA), which is then transported across the mitochondrial outer membrane to the inner membrane and the respiratory assemblies. There, acetyl CoA undergoes a series of transformations called the citric acid (or Krebs) cycle. Because it utilizes oxygen, this process is known as oxidative metabolism. Its end product is large amounts of **adenosine triphosphate (ATP)**, which contains high-energy phosphate bonds. For this reason, mitochondria are commonly known as the powerhouses of the cell.

ATP is transported from the mitochondria into the cytoplasm and diffuses throughout the cell, where it releases its stored energy for cellular functions. Energy consumption in the brain is higher per unit weight than in any other organ, and although the brain represents only about 2% of the total body weight, it accounts for 20% of the total body oxygen requirements. The metabolic rate varies among the different structures of the CNS, and is also dependent upon which areas are being stimulated. For example, olfactory stimulation in the rat elevates metabolism in the olfactory areas of the brain, and occluding the auditory canals with wax causes a 35% to 60% metabolic depression in the auditory areas of the brain (see Sokoloff, 1984.) Some toxic chemicals, such as 2,4-dinitrophenol (DNP), which is found in herbicides, disrupt oxidative metabolism and thus block ATP production in the mitochondria. This causes neuron function, as well as other cell functions, to fail. The virulent toxicity of cyanide is also due to its disruption of mitochondrial respiration (Klaassen, 1985).

ATP fuels three important cellular functions, namely, gene transcription and translation for the synthesis of chemical substances within the cell, transport across membranes, and mechanical work. Many cellular materials needed for the functions and maintenance of the cell are synthesized in the soma, and it takes mechanical work to transport these materials over comparatively long distances to where they are needed (Ochs, 1972; 1981). The excitability of neurons and the propagation of nerve impulses depends upon the active transport of ions across the plasma membrane. That is, ions from an area of low concentration must be carried across a membrane to an area of high concentration, another process that requires energy expenditure.

Beyond their classical role in the generation of ATP, many mitochondria in the brain and spinal cord also exhibit specialized functions related to neurotransmitter metabolism. Some of these mitochondria, which are concentrated in axon terminals, contain the enzyme monoamine oxidase (MAO) in their outer membrane. MAO plays an important role in the catabolism of monoamine transmitters such as dopamine, norepinephrine, and serotonin (see Chapters 8 and 9). MAO-bearing mitochondria are also found within glial cells and in some peripheral organs including the liver, kidneys, and intestines. Still other enzymes found in mitochondria participate in the metabolism of the amino acid transmitters glutamate and γ-aminobutyric acid (GABA) (see Chapter 10).

Peroxisomes

Another cellular inclusion in plant and animal cells, including neurons, are the **peroxisomes**, which are membrane-bounded vesicles related to mitochondria in that both utilize molecular oxygen. Whereas mitochondria are the major sites of oxygen consumption in the cell because they use it to oxidize glucose, peroxisomes contain enzymes that prevent the accumulation of the strong oxidizing agent hydrogen peroxide, H_2O_2, which is frequently generated by chemical reactions in cells. Half of the protein content of peroxisomes is the enzyme catalase, which degrades H_2O_2 to water and oxygen in order to prevent the injurious effects of high concentrations of H_2O_2 in plant and animal tissue.

Lysosomes and Endosomes

Two other kinds of cellular inclusions are found within the cytoplasm in a wide variety of animal cells. **Lyso-somes** are formed by budding off the Golgi apparatus in a variety of membrane-bound shapes and sizes, between 250 and 700 nm in diameter. They contain an aggregate of enzymes capable of digesting organic compounds that originate inside or outside the cell. For example, they are involved in converting proteins to amino acids and glycogen to glucose, the basic nutrient of neurons. They also serve as vesicles for reverse transport from axon terminals to the soma. Many lysosomes become degraded to lipofuscin granules, which accumulate as the organism ages and are regarded as neuronal refuse.

Endosomes are different from lysosomes. They originate by budding off the smooth ER, and their function is the delivery of vesicles that contain proteins and lipids for renewing the plasma membrane by bringing newly formed membranous constitutents to it and returning existing constituents back into the cell body to be recycled or removed (Schwartz, 1991b).

The Neuronal Cytoskeleton: Microtubules, Neurofilaments, and Actin Filaments

The cytoskeleton makes up about 20% of the protein content of a neuron by weight and plays significant roles in neuronal structure and function. It is made up of three components (Figure 3.5). **Microtubules (MTs)** are slender tubular structures (about 24 nm in diameter) of varying lengths made up of helical or spiral arrays of the neurotubule protein **tubulin**. MTs originate in the perikaryon adjacent to the nucleus and seem to resemble a long string of beads tightly wrapped around a cylinder. Some of the units seem to have a transitory existence, and some appear to be more stable. Microtubules are shown in Figure 3.5, at the shaded-color arrow.

Associated with MTs are at least ten different proteins called **microtubule-associated proteins (MAPs)** that are instrumental in MT growth and assembly, cross-linking of MTs together and with other filaments, and axonal transport. Some MAPs are found only in embryonic neurons during periods of rapid growth, and some are found only in the adult, which may account for their transient and stable forms. Further, MAPs having a comparatively large molecular weight and known as **MAP2** are found in the dendrites and cell bodies, whereas those of low molecular weight, known as **tau (τ)**, are confined to axons. In the cell body, the tubules tend to cross and interlace. In dendrites and axons they tend to run in parallel, cross-linked to each other and other filaments, but in dendrites they are more widely spaced. Also, the microtubules appear to have many projections or arms along their length, which play a role in cross-linkage and axonal transport.

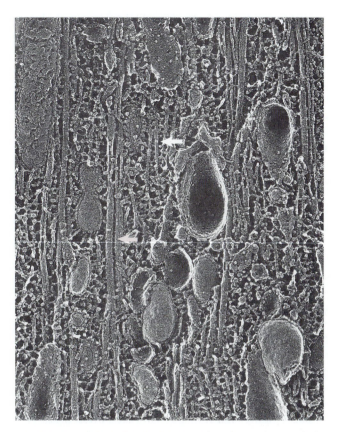

3.5 THE AXONAL CYTOSKELETON. This photomicrograph depicts a frog axon that was quickly frozen, fractured, etched, and then rotary shadowed and viewed in an electron microscope. A cross-linked network of microtubules (shaded color arrow) and neurofilaments (white arrow) fills the axon. Vesicles of various sizes and mitochondria are interspersed with the network. (From Hirokawa, 1982. Reproduced from *The Journal of Cell Biology*, 94:129–142, by copyright permission of The Rockefeller University Press.)

Neurofilaments are as long as, but only about a third of the diameter of, microtubules. They are made up of three different protein subunits, collectively termed the **neurofilament triplet proteins**. These proteins can serve as a marker specific for neurons because glial cell filaments contain different proteins. Also, in mammalian axons, neurofilaments are more abundant than microtubules, whereas the reverse is true in dendrites. Like the microtubules, the neurofilaments are oriented longitudinally, parallel to the axon's long axis.

Actin filaments are a type of microfilaments, and are so named because they contain a form of actin, one of the major contractile proteins of muscle. They are shorter than microtubules and neurofilaments and are not longitudinally aligned. Rather, they form a complex meshwork that resembles steel wool beneath the surface membrane. Here, the filaments are bundled together by actin-binding proteins that cross-link them to form a gel. Other proteins attach the filaments to the surface membrane or to other cytoskeletal proteins. The actin-binding proteins are regulated by a complex battery of proteins that presumably mediate changes in the cytoskeleton during cell movement.

The function of the microtubules, the neurofilaments, and the actin filaments has been the subject of many investigations, but questions still exist. They do not seem to be involved in the propagation of nerve impulses; that function is the property of the cell membrane. It does appear, however, that both microtubules and actin filaments play a significant role in maintaining the three-dimensional structure of neurons. This is borne out by the finding that the axoplasm of the squid giant axon retains its cylindrical shape even after being extruded from the plasma membrane (Vale, Banker, and Hall, 1992). Also, as we shall see in a later section, these structures have an important role in axonal transport.

Genetic Activity within Neurons

Cell division occurs constantly in most tissues to replace cells that have degenerated. It has been estimated that over seven years, the whole body, including all internal organs, is replaced. However, as mentioned earlier, cell replacement does not occur among mature neurons; consequently, the effects of injury or disease in neural tissue are more permanent than in other tissues. Nonetheless, there is evidence that transplants of fetal brain tissue can restore neurons lost to certain neuronal diseases (see Chapter 20).

Because of the absence of cell division, neuronal nuclear chromosomes are not arranged in compact units; rather, they exist in a relatively uncoiled state, giving the nucleus an amorphous appearance even at high levels of magnification with light microscopes. Surrounding the nucleus is the perikaryon (Gr., "around the nucleus"; see Figure 3.2), containing darkly staining Nissl granules, composed of ribosomes associated with the ER (see below).

Within the nucleus, strands of DNA make up the 23 pairs of chromosomes within which the genes of human cells are distributed. Each pair contains one chromosome contributed by the male parent and one contributed by the female parent. These genes, numbering over a million, make up the genomic code, which determines the development of the organism from a fertilized ovum to an independent member of the species. After the birth of the organism, some of the genes control the growth, differentiation, and maintenance of its cells.

Genes exist in many variations, known as **alleles**. For example, all humans have genes that determine that they will have hair on their heads. However, one parent may have fine, blond, curly hair and the other may have straight, brown, thick hair, each characteristic being determined by slightly different pairs of genes. During the formation of the gametes, ova and sperm, only half of each gene pair (one allele) will be included in each gamete, and which allele will be included in a given sperm cell or ovum is a matter of chance. The alleles received by each offspring will determine the color, shape, and texture of his or her hair.

Gene activation begins with the copying of certain genes that express a phenotype, such as a certain protein for membrane receptors or an enzyme to synthesize a secretory substance that is needed. Moreover, gene expression also regulates the amount of protein that is produced and the timing and the sequence of its appearance. Most important, however, is the general rule that proteins and enzymes are made only when they are needed. For example, the amino acid histidine is necessary for the viability of the bacterium *Escherichia coli*. When histidine is absent in the culture medium, all the required enzymes for making histidine from its precursors are synthesized by the cell. But when preformed histidine is added to the culture medium, the synthesis of the histidine-forming enzymes quickly stops.

DNA Structure

The details of DNA structure and function could easily fill a book the size of this one. Therefore, we can only present the barest outline of this subject within these pages.

A gene exerts its influence by using its part of a chromosome as a template to copy itself. The copy is then used to construct a phenotype, a chemical end product of gene expression such as an enzyme or structural protein. The copying process is known as **gene transcription**. Before describing the transcription process, we will briefly describe the chemical structure of DNA as it relates to genetic processes.

The information in chromosomes is coded in the form of combinations of four nucleotide bases. Two of the bases, cytosine and thymine, are pyrimidines; a third pyrimidine, uracil, substitutes for thymine during gene expression (see below). The two other bases, adenine and guanine, are purines. These five bases are known by their first letters: C, T, U, A, and G, respectively (Figure 3.6). Each of these bases is linked to a molecule of the sugar 2-deoxyribose, and the genetic code is written in combinations of these nucleotides arranged along the length of chromosomal DNA. Figure 3.7a shows how the bases are connected to the deoxyribose molecules and to each other along a DNA strand, which in a human may consist of 3 billion base pairs. The total length of all the DNA in a single human cell has been estimated to be 2 meters. Even the bacterium *E. coli*, which has only one chromosome, has 4.7 million base pairs that participate in expressing 3,000 different proteins.

As an example of the amount of information that can exist in a human chromosome made up of combinations of just four nucleotides, we can imagine that even if it had only the impossibly low number of one hundred bases, there would still be 4^{100} combinations of the four bases in that one chromosome. This arrangement makes it possible for hundreds of millions of genes to be made

Pyrimidine and the major pyrimidine bases.

Purine and the major purine bases.

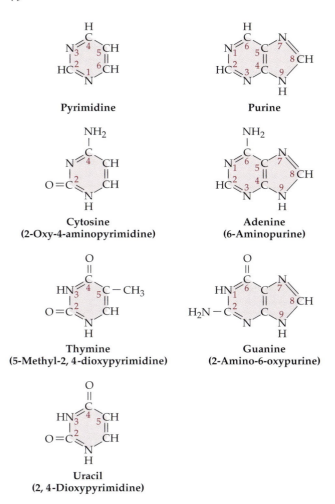

Pyrimidine

Cytosine
(2-Oxy-4-aminopyrimidine)

Thymine
(5-Methyl-2, 4-dioxypyrimidine)

Uracil
(2, 4-Dioxypyrimidine)

Purine

Adenine
(6-Aminopurine)

Guanine
(2-Amino-6-oxypurine)

3.6 THE NUCLEOTIDE BASES. These molecules attach to molecules of the sugar 2-deoxyribose to make up the chemical components of DNA and the genes. Careful scrutiny of these molecules reveals how chemically similar they are within a nucleotide class.

up of combinations of only four nucleotides. Nonetheless, 99.9% of all genes are the same in all humans (i.e., all humans have hearts, lungs, noses, body hair, and digestive systems with similar digestive enzymes). But because a single strand of DNA may have 100,000 genes, the number of combinations that can occur among the remaining 0.1% of genes that have multiple alleles is more than sufficient to account for the genetically determined differences among humans.

Each strand of DNA is paired with another strand, as shown in Figure 3.7*b*, and the bases of the two strands are paired in a complementary way throughout its length: adenine (A) is always paired with thymine (T), and guanine (G) is always paired with cytosine (C). The two strands are wrapped around each other in the form of a double-stranded helix, which resembles a spiral ladder with 2 million rungs. In the cell reproductive process

involving the copying of the whole chromosomes, the two strands are split apart and one is copied. It does not matter which strand is copied because each strand will always produce its complement from the free nucleotides in the nuclear sap to make up new double-stranded DNA molecules. If a cell such as a liver cell is to be replicated, its DNA is completely copied so that the daughter cells are all the same.

The Permanence of the Genetic Code

In practice, the arrangement of the bases is not a random process. The present form of DNA in a given species is the result of millions of years of evolution. In other words, if the phenotype expressed by the genes is able to survive in an environment that fosters the reproduction of the species, then that genotype will be conserved. Phenotypes that cannot survive become extinct along with their genes. Thus, the mere presence of a species in our time is testimony that its gene pool is favorable, and the surviving genotypes will be faithfully copied in future generations.

Mutations. Although permanence is a major attribute of genomes, changes in the genome (mutations) obviously had to occur to allow the development of new species. Stated another way, mutations are the raw material of evolution. It is presumed that mutations are most likely to occur as accidents during gene replication, but such accidents are relatively rare, occurring within an estimated range of less than once per 10,000 to once per 10 billion genes per DNA duplication, depending upon the organism and the particular genes. Even though humans have an estimated 10^{14} cells, with 4×10^9 base pairs per cell, which go through 10^{16} cell division cycles in a normal life span, the number of mutations is exceedingly small, largely because most cells have a DNA repair enzyme that corrects errors as they occur. Most mutations occur when one nucleotide substitutes for another, or when a nucleotide is added or deleted during the synthesis of a new DNA strand. It will be seen below how the addition or deletion of a single nucleotide among thousands in a gene can completely alter the genes expression.

Gene Transcription

For a cell to use its genetic plan for synthesizing needed proteins, the first step is the copying of the part of the chromosomal strand that serves as the genetic code for that protein. The copying process, known as **transcription**, starts with the action of an enzyme in the nucleus, **RNA polymerase**, which binds to a chromosome at a particular section known as the promoter. Proteins called transcription factors bind to nearby sites on the gene, thereby acting either to enhance or to suppress gene transcription. Several of these factors are discussed further in Chapter 6.

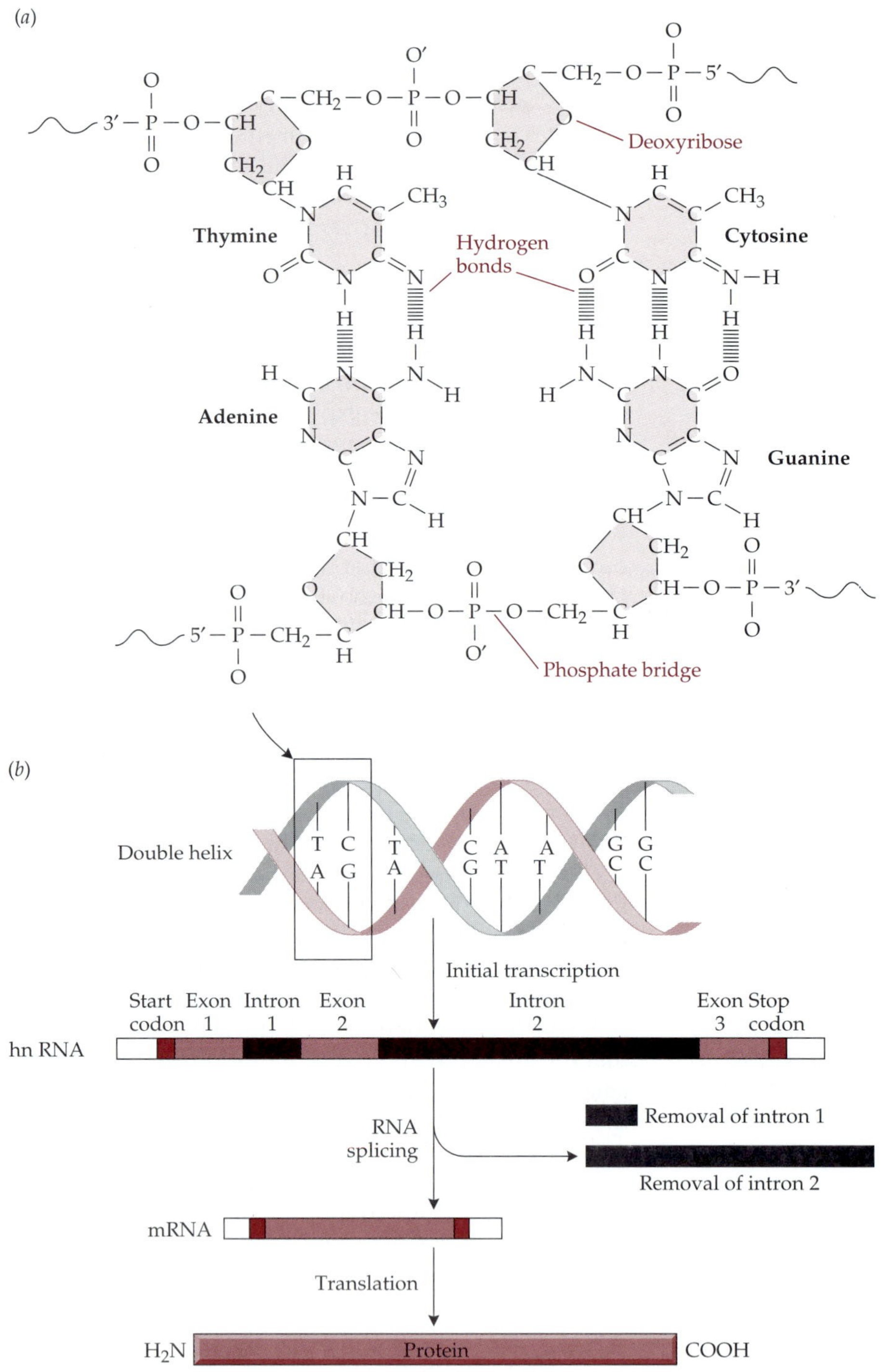

(a)

(b)

3.7 DNA: CHEMICAL STRUCTURE, TRANSCRIPTION, AND TRANSLATION. (a) Molecules of thymine and cytosine, each coupled to deoxyribose, are linked by a phosphate bridge. They are also linked by hydrogen bonds to similarly linked adenine and guanine, which are coupled to deoxyribose. (b) Initial transcription leads to heterogeneous nuclear RNA (hnRNA), which in this example contains two introns that are excised to form messenger RNA (mRNA).

If transcription begins, RNA polymerase briefly unwinds the DNA helix. One strand of the helix will serve as a template for synthesizing an RNA molecule complementary to that section of the chromosome. The new molecule is formed by the action of RNA polymerase, which moves along the DNA strand, matching a nucleotide to each particular base of the strand (e.g., matching G with the complementary base C, then moving along to T, which it will match with A, and so on), adding complementary bases one at a time until a terminator signal is reached. Thus, an exact copy of the *opposite* DNA strand is formed, except that the base thymine (T) is replaced by uracil (U), which fits better to the ribose that substitutes for 2-deoxyribose in RNA. At this point, the single-stranded complementary RNA chain is released; it is then known as a molecule of **heterogeneous nuclear RNA (hnRNA)**. Meanwhile, the double-stranded DNA is reconstituted by the action of the enzyme DNA polymerase.

At this stage, a given molecule of hnRNA in the nucleus may be 8,000 to 20,000 nucleotides long, whereas only 1,000 to 2,000 nucleotides may be sufficient for the synthesis of a particular protein. Thus, the hnRNA strand is cut and large interior sections, known as **introns,** are removed; the retained sections, known as **exons**, are then spliced back together to produce a mature messenger RNA. The mRNA is released into the cytoplasm, where it is suspended as long, straight strands. This process of cutting out introns contributes to the wide variability of mRNA because the size and location of introns can vary, as can the exons that are spliced together. Thus, a process of alternative mRNA splicing allows the same gene to code for two or more different (though related) proteins.

In the cytoplasm, the mRNA encounters ribosomes, which are macromolecular complexes of ribosomal RNA (rRNA) and proteins (Figure 3.8). As mentioned earlier, ribosomes are partly synthesized within the nucleolus from parts of DNA and proteins transferred from the cytosol. Their synthesis is catalyzed by RNA polymerase I. Situated around the nuclear membrane pores are specific receptors that bind to these cytosolic proteins and translocate them to the nucleus. Consequently there is two-way traffic in the pores of the nuclear envelope, with ribosomes coming out of the nucleus and cytosolic proteins going in. In the nucleolus, ribosomes are manufactured at different molecular weights depending on the amount of their associated proteins. They are produced in such prodigious amounts that rRNA is the most abundant RNA found in nerve cells, constituting 80–90% of the total RNA produced by the nucleus. Because such large amounts of rRNA are available to be acted upon by mRNA, a large multiplication of coded elements, which can contribute to a large increase in protein production, is possible. This is particularly true of secretory cells such as neurons.

Gene Translation

In the cytoplasm, ribosomes serve as workbenches for the assembly of proteins in the process known as translation. Proteins are made up of combinations of the 20 amino acids, which are synthesized and present in the cytoplasm (Table 3.1.) The mRNA code supplies the instructions for translation, and any ribosome can be used because the instructions are built into the structure of mRNA. Because mRNA is constructed of combinations of the nucleotide bases A, C, G, and U, the codes for the 20 amino acids must also consist of those bases. Also, because there are 20 amino acids and only four bases, combinations of bases must be used. If combinations of two bases were to be used, there could only be $4^2 = 16$ combinations. If three bases were to be used, there could be $4^3 = 64$ combinations, more than enough to identify 20 amino acids, and this most parsimonious system is the one that came into being. Thus, the codes that are used

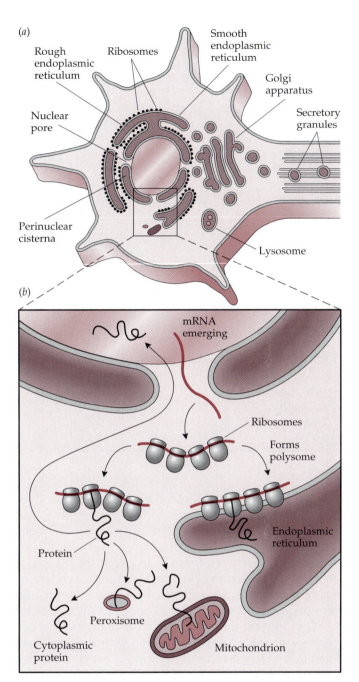

3.8 STRUCTURAL SITES FOR NEURONAL TRANSCRIPTION AND TRANSLATION. (*a*) The organelles responsible for the synthesis and processing of proteins. (*b*) Enlargement of (*a*) in the region of a nuclear pore. Messenger RNAs, transcribed from genomic DNA in the neuron nucleus, emerge from nuclear pores to form polysomes by attaching to ribosomes. (After Schwartz, 1991c.)

to specify amino acids for protein synthesis are triplet combinations of the bases, called codons, each of which translates into only one type of amino acid. For example, GCU is a code for alanine, GGU for glycine, and UAU for tyrosine (Table 3.2 contains the complete codon dictionary for all the amino acids).

Table 3.1   Amino Acid Symbols

Amino acid	One-letter symbol	Three-letter abbreviation
Alanine	A	Ala
Arginine	R	Arg
Asparagine	N	Asn
Aspartic acid	D	Asp
Asn + Asp	—	Asx
Cysteine	C	Cys
Glutamine	Q	Gln
Glutamic acid	E	Glu
Gln + Glu	—	Glx
Glycine	G	Gly
Histidine	H	His
Isoleucine	I	Ile
Leucine	L	Leu
Lysine	K	Lys
Methionine	M	Met
Phenylalanine	F	Phe
Proline	P	Pro
Serine	S	Ser
Threonine	T	Thr
Tryptophan	W	Trp
Tyrosine	Y	Tyr
Valine	V	Val

specific for both the amino acids and their corresponding tRNAs, one type for each of the 20 amino acids. One part of the tRNA molecule combines with the appropriate amino acid, and another part has a complementary triplet that combines with the mRNA codon for that amino acid.

As a ribosome moves along the mRNA template, it accepts the amino acid from the tRNA that binds to the codon and adds another link to the growing sequence of amino acids. The amino acids form peptide bonds with one another as they are added to the growing peptide chain. After the amino acid is added to the sequence, the tRNA is bumped off the end of the mRNA template as another tRNA appears to supply the next link for the peptide chain. The result of these activities is the formation of a particular polypeptide which, by a chemical self-initiated folding process, becomes a protein. In this manner the linear chains of bases in DNA are translated into three-dimensional proteins.

Here it should be noted that codons can be read accurately only if they are in the proper register because if one nucleotide is accidentally deleted or added, all the formulae for amino acids will be distorted. To provide an example, we will divide an mRNA message into triplets using commas, although there are no such divisions in reality. Thus, if the mRNA message is UCCCCAGC-CCAG . . . , the codon message would be UCC, CCA, GCC, CAG . . . . But if an extra G were added to the

Because there are potentially 64 codons and 20 amino acids, more than one and up to six codons can exist for one amino acid, and indeed they do. Only one codon, UGG, exists for tryptophan, and one, AUG, for methionine; however, there is no codon that specifies more than one amino acid. Furthermore, the codon for methionine, AUG, also signifies the operator site for augmenting transcription, and the codons UGA, UAA, and UAG signify the termination of a particular translation. In this way, mRNA translates its genetic information into protein structures, and every protein or enzyme requires a particular sequence of mRNA. The codons for amino acids are known to be identical in bacteria, humans, the tobacco plant, certain amphibians, and the guinea pig, and are probably universal for all species. This should not be too surprising because, as we noted above, there are many identical biological processes among virtually all living things.

The translation process begins when ribosomes bind to the mRNA strand and read the codons one at a time. However, protein synthesis also depends upon yet another form of RNA, known as **transfer RNA (tRNA)**, which is synthesized in the extranuclear region by RNA polymerase III. The action of tRNA follows the chemical activation of the amino acids by enzymes called aminoacyl-tRNA synthetases so that each amino acid will bond with its corresponding tRNA. These enzymes are highly

Table 3.2   The Codon Dictionary[a]

	U		C		A		G	
U	UUU	Phe	UCU	Ser	UAU	Tyr	UGU	Cys
	UUC	Phe	UCC	Ser	UAC	Tyr	UGC	Cys
	UUA	Leu	UCA	Ser	UAA	Ochre	UGA	
	UUG	Leu	UCG	Ser	UAG	Amber	UGC	Trp
C	CUU	Leu	CCU	Pro	CAU	His	CGU	Arg
	CUC	Leu	CCC	Pro	CAC	His	CGC	Arg
	CUA	Leu	CCA	Pro	CAA	Gln	CGA	Arg
	CUG	Leu	CCG	Pro	CAG	Gln	CGG	Arg
A	AUU	Ile	ACU	Thr	AAU	Asn	AGU	Ser
	AUC	Ile	ACC	Thr	AAC	Asn	AGC	Ser
	AUA	Ile	ACA	Thr	AAA	Lys	AGA	Arg
	AUG	Met	ACG	Thr	AAG	Lys	AGG	Arg
G	GUU	Val	GCU	Ala	GAU	Asp	GGU	Gly
	GUC	Val	GCC	Ala	GAC	Asp	GGC	Gly
	GUA	Val	GCA	Ala	GAA	Glu	GGA	Gly
	GUG	Val	GCG	Ala	GAG	Glu	GGG	Gly

[a]The third nucleotide of each codon is less specific than the first two. For example, CCU, CCC, CCA, and CCG all code for proline. But no codon designates more than one amino acid.

mRNA message in the seventh position (UCCCCA**G**GC-CCAG . . .), the codon message would then read UCC, CCA, **G**GC, CCA, G??, . . . , and this error would be perpetuated down the complete length of the mRNA strand, which may involve 2,000 nucleotide bases and over 600 codons. Thus, a protein would be made with a virtually random array of amino acids. If the needed protein was essential for survival, such an addition or loss of one nucleotide could be fatal for the organism. For example, if the protein were an enzyme needed to digest milk, a newborn infant in earlier times could have died of starvation or dehydration without any apparent reason.

Because most mRNA molecules are much longer than a ribosome, many ribosomes can read the codons of a single molecule of mRNA at the same time, one following another and forming an assemblage of a thread of mRNA studded with beadlike ribosomes trailing their growing polypeptide chains (see Figure 3.8*b*). These assemblages are known as **polyribosomes** or **polysomes** and are characteristic of cells that are actively synthesizing proteins.

Protein Destination

The class of protein formed by a polysome is determined by the information encoded in it by a particular mRNA. There are roughly three classes of proteins that are typically synthesized in neurons. Class 1, cytosolic proteins, are the most abundant proteins in the cell. They are formed in the cytosol and make up the cytoskeleton and the numerous enzymes that catalyze synthetic reactions in the cell. Class 2 proteins are also formed in the cytosol, but are later incorporated into the nucleus, mitochondria, and peroxisomes (see below). Other class 2 proteins located near the nuclear pores recognize, bind, and translocate some of these proteins from the cytoplasm into the cell nucleus. Proteins destined for the nucleus include enzymes such as RNA polymerase and various transcription factors that regulate gene expression. Class 3 proteins attach themselves to the membranes of the ER and the Golgi apparatus, where they undergo further processing to become secretory products and membrane constituents.

The Role of the Endoplasmic Reticulum

The ribosomes that bind to the ER do so as a result of the action of special proteins, interestingly known as **foldases** and **chaperonins**. These proteins cause a molecular conformation of the ribosomes that fosters binding to the ER. The ER is a continuation of the nuclear envelope that forms flattened sheets, which become studded with ribosomes. Because the ER is convoluted, in slices of a cell examined under the electron microscope, it appears as oval-shaped cisternae with rough surface membranes. Therefore, that part of the ER that binds ribosomes is known as the **rough endoplasmic reticulum** (**RER**). The bound ribosomes are easily identified when stained with basic histologic dyes and are known as Nissl granules after the histologist who first studied them in the 1890s. Nissl found that when protein synthesis occurs at high rates to restore protein loss due to attrition, disease, or injury, the granules appear to be finely divided and dispersed toward the cells membrane, a process known as chromatolysis. This phenomenon was used in some early efforts to locate the source of a neural tract in animals. In these experiments, the tract was severed, and after a time delay, serial sections of the suspected source of the tract were examined. Cells showing evidence of chromatolysis revealed the source of the severed tract.

The main part of the RER is found in the cell body of a neuron, and extensions are found in the dendrites and axon as well. Because parts of some neurons, such as axon terminals, can be very far from their cell bodies, the local presence of RER serves important functions in supplying these extended parts with enzymes, proteins for membrane repair, and secretory substances.

The structure and destination of the third class of proteins is determined by the treatment they undergo. For example, one function of the RER is the synthesis of secretory proteins, which comes about when nascent (newly formed) proteins are wholly translocated into the lumen of the RER. Within the lumen, the proteins undergo further processing, which may continue in the smooth ER (see below), the Golgi apparatus, and secretory granules before they become secretory proteins. In contrast, some proteins are only partly translocated into the lumen, while a part remains on the cytoplasmic side of the ER. This partial translocation results in an intrinsic protein. Such proteins, when translocated to plasma membranes, may become the receptors for neurotransmitters or form ion channels that mediate neuron functions (Schwartz, 1991c). The role of such proteins in the neurophysiological activity of neurons is discussed in Chapters 5 and 6.

The Smooth Endoplasmic Reticulum and the Golgi Apparatus

The part of the ER free of ribosomes is known as the **smooth endoplasmic reticulum** (**SER**). In neurons, it extends from the RER as a microtubular system that stretches from the soma into the axon and dendrites, and serves as a transport system for substances needed for the normal maintenance and function of these neuron extensions. The SER also serves as the site for the synthesis of lipids that are needed for the maintenance of cell membranes, endosomes, lysosomes, and the plasma membrane. New membrane and secretory proteins may begin synthesis in the RER and continue to the end of the SER, where pieces of the SER pinch off to form transport vesicles that shuttle with their contents to the Golgi apparatus.

The Golgi apparatus is a highly developed organelle found in the somata of virtually all neurons and secretory cells. Under the high-power magnification of the electron microscope, it appears to consist of a parallel array of about a half dozen flattened, interconnected membranous cisternae about 1 μm in diameter arranged in a stack. The stack has a *cis*, or convex, and a *trans*, or concave, surface, with the convex surface lying close to the RER. As shown in Figure 3.9, the lumens of the cisternae are narrower on the convex surface and become wider toward the concave surface, and the density of the internal contents also increases as the lumens grow wider. The contents of the cisternae are presumed to be proteins in different stages of processing, which would account for the differences found among the various layers in the chemical nature of the contents.

As mentioned earlier, the precursors of these proteins are formed in the RER and are carried toward the convex surface in small transport vesicles that seem to bud off from the SER and fuse together to form the outermost cisterna in the stack. Thus, as new cisternae are formed behind it, each cisterna progresses step by step toward the concave surface of the Golgi apparatus. During the course of migration through the stack, the proteins become more concentrated and undergo different biochemical modifications. These modifications include glycosylation (incorporation of sugar molecules), proteolysis (hydrolysis of proteins to simpler forms), sulfation (incorporation of or treatment by sulfate groups), phosphorylation (the addition of phosphate groups), and the addition of fatty acids. The enzymes that participate in these chemical transformations reside on the inner membranes of the cisternae, and the processes that occur depend upon the destination of the proteins.

Upon reaching the concave face of the Golgi apparatus, the cisternae round up into a number of small vacuoles containing the concentrated proteins. The vacuoles then coalesce to form a single large condensing vacuole, which, after more protein concentration, becomes a dense, spherical secretory granule. These granules are then transported to their destinations within the cell: the cell membrane, secretory vesicles, lysosomes, and so on (Fawcett, 1986; Rothman, 1981).

Dendrites

Dendrites, which were briefly described earlier, are the parts of the neuron that usually receive information from the axon terminals of other neurons. This is accomplished by an array of receptors on dendrite surfaces that react to transmitters released from the axon terminals of other neurons. Dendrites may consist of a single twiglike extension from the soma or a multibranched network capable of receiving inputs from literally thousands of other cells. For instance, an average spinal motor cell with a moderate-sized dendritic tree, both in the number of branches and their length, may receive about 10,000 contacts, 2,000 on the soma and 8,000 on

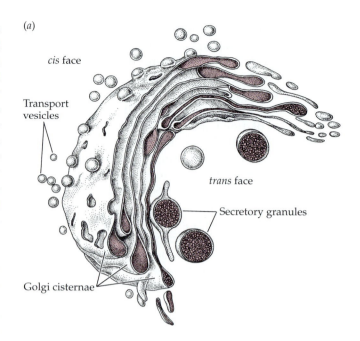

(*a*)

cis face

Transport vesicles

trans face

Secretory granules

Golgi cisternae

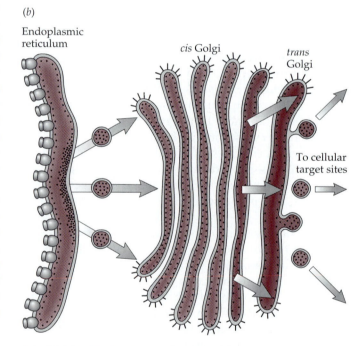

(*b*)

Endoplasmic reticulum

cis Golgi

trans Golgi

To cellular target sites

3.9 GOLGI APPARATUS. (*a*) This three-dimensional view shows transport vesicles from the smooth endoplasmic reticulum (SER) approaching and fusing with the convex or *cis* face, and secretory granules emanating from the concave or *trans* face. (*b*) The schematic representation illustrates the refining process of protein precursors from the SER. The increased density of the shading represents the progressive processing of the protein. The thick arrows represent the transport steps of the exported proteins through the Golgi compartments and then to appropriate target sites in the cell (thin arrows). The small black dots within the vesicles represent the ER proteins that are budded off and returned to the ER for recycling. (*a* after Fawcett, 1986; *b* after Rothman, 1981.)

the dendrites, whereas a Purkinje cell in the cerebellum may receive as many as 150,000 contacts. In the typical vertebrate neuron shown in Figure 3.2, the dendritic tree has a long, slender set of apical dendrites emerging from the soma apex, and several sets of stubbier basal dendrites emerging from the base of the cell.

In multibranched **dendritic trees**, the surfaces of the primary, secondary, and tertiary branches are mostly smooth, but they do have a few short projections about 1 to 2 μm in diameter, known as **spines**. In contrast, the more distal branches are covered with many of these spines, as shown in Figure 3.10. On pyramidal cells in the visual cortex of mice, the number of spines increases in an exponential fashion with distance from the cell body, and the spines account for 43% of the total soma–dendrite surface. The spines in the dendritic tree of a single Purkinje cell in the cerebellum of a cat, monkey, or human may number 100,000 or more and thus provide a combined synaptic surface of more than 400,000 μm².

The dendrites of various brain areas show considerable variation among their spines, from little more than an evagination from the dendrite to grapelike protrusions up to 5 μm long consisting of a short stem expanding into a terminal bulb. Also, spines may vary in size, shape, and style along the surface of a single dendrite. In some cases the shape and size of a spine may be specifically elaborated to match a particular kind of axon terminal (see Peters, Palay, and Webster, 1970.) Mitochondria are infrequently encountered within the spines, but they are very numerous in the growing tips of the dendrite (Figure 3.11). In some brain areas dendritic tips have been found that quickly enlarge and become filled with mitochondria and glycogen particles. The concentration of mitochondria may reach a level as high as 10

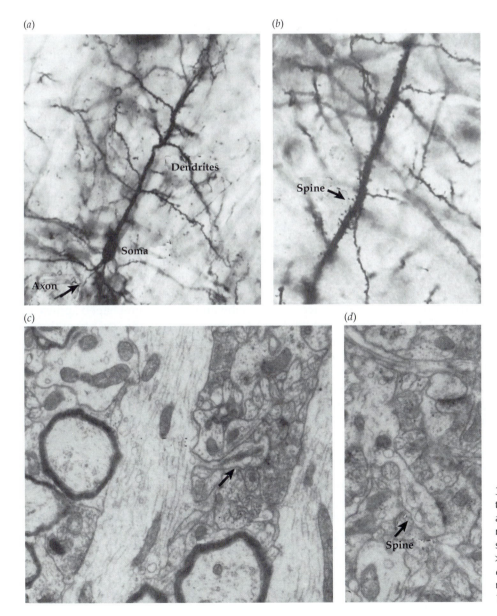

(a)

(b)

(c)

(d)

Dendrites

Spine

Soma

Axon

Spine

3.10 DENDRITIC TREES. The dendritic trees of neurons from the motor cortex of a rat are shown at different levels of magnification. (*a*) The entire cell with its soma, axon, and dendrites (Golgi stain ×100). (*b*) Dendritic spines (×250). (*c* and *d*) Dendritic spines as shown in electron micrographs (×30,000). (From Jacobson, 1972.)

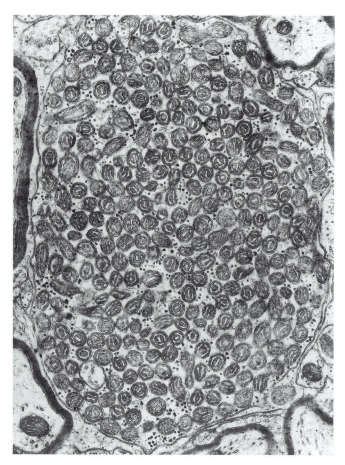

3.11 GROWING TIPS OF A DENDRITE. High concentrations of mitochondria are characteristic of areas with high levels of metabolism. (Magnification ×40,000.) (From Peters, Palay, and Webster, 1970.)

whereas the orientation is random in the dendrites. It will be seen later that this arrangement may be a determinant for the selective distribution of dendrite and axon protein materials. The neuron model shown in Figure 3.12 summarizes the distinguishing features of dendrites and axons.

Learning and Dendritic Changes

Environmental stimuli are believed to cause functional reorganization of neuronal networks in order to bring about behavioral adaptation (i.e., learning). A number of studies have suggested that stimulation-induced changes in dendrites and their spines may be significant factors in learning. For example, stimulation of a neural pathway in the hippocampus, the perforant pathway, resulted in the widening of dendritic spines in the neurons of the target area, and it was suggested that this morphological change was related to long-term increases in synaptic efficiency (Van Harreveld and Fifkova, 1975). Synaptic efficiency can be marked by lowered thresholds of activation, the release of increased amounts of neurotransmitters, or an increased density of axon terminals or dendrites. It has already been reported that there was more dendritic branching near the soma, and more spines on the pyramidal cells of the primary visual cortex, in rats that were exposed to a rich environment than in littermates that were exposed to an impoverished environment (Greenough, Juraska, and Volkmar, 1979; Rosenzweig, Bennett, and Diamond, 1972; Volkmar and Greenough, 1972).

Purpura (1974) found a correlation between the absence of normal dendritic spines and the presence of abnormal ones in the cortical neurons of some mentally retarded persons. Normal spines in general have a narrow neck and an ovoid bulb (see Figure 3.10d), and are divided into three types: thin, stubby, and mushroom-shaped. In mentally retarded persons, there is a marked absence of the stubby and mushroom-shaped spines, to an extent depending upon age and the severity of the retardation. Instead, there are many long, fine, and sometimes entangled spines with prominent terminal heads. It is possible that these abnormalities in the dendritic spines have profound effects on the ability of neurons to integrate their synaptic input. (See Svoboda, Tank, and Denk (1996) for recent research on dendritic spine function.)

Axons

Axons are the message-bearing parts of neurons that convey messages to the axon terminals. In some respects axons can be compared to telephone cables, but the analogy is limited because the signals transmitted via axons travel comparatively slowly (between 1 and 100 meters per second), whereas electrical signals in copper wires are conducted almost at the speed of light. Electrical conduction requires nothing more than two copper wires

units per μm^3. Axons and dendrites contain similar cytoskeletal elements: microtubules, neurofilaments, and actin filaments, but these elements do not enter the spines. The spines are filled with a fluffy material consisting of fine filaments.

Dendrites differ from axons in two other ways. We have already mentioned that MAPs of high molecular weight are found in dendrites, whereas those of low molecular weight are confined to axons. It is also known that ribosomes translating mRNA for the expression of the high molecular weight MAPs can be found in both the cell body and the dendrites, whereas mRNAs for the expression of tubulin for microtubules and the low molecular weight MAPs for the axons are confined to the cell body. Furthermore, microtubules are polarized, with plus (+) and minus (–) ends. Microtubules are polymers that grow by self-assembly, adding monomers at the (+) end and dropping monomers at the (–) end. In axons, the hydrolysis of ATP to ADP is required for the microtubules to polymerize at one end (+) and depolymerize at the other end (–). The (+) ends of the microtubules are mostly (about 90%) oriented toward the axon terminals,

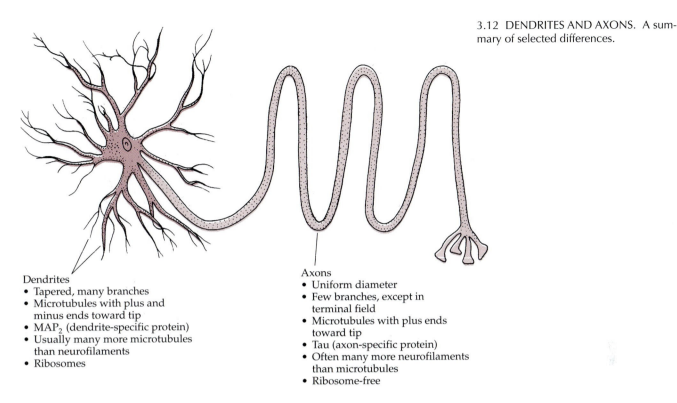

3.12 DENDRITES AND AXONS. A summary of selected differences.

Dendrites
- Tapered, many branches
- Microtubules with plus and minus ends toward tip
- MAP$_2$ (dendrite-specific protein)
- Usually many more microtubules than neurofilaments
- Ribosomes

Axons
- Uniform diameter
- Few branches, except in terminal field
- Microtubules with plus ends toward tip
- Tau (axon-specific protein)
- Often many more neurofilaments than microtubules
- Ribosome-free

and a power source such as a battery, and the cable is unaltered by the passage of the current bearing the message, except that the wire may become heated when large currents are introduced. In contrast, nerve impulse transmission by simple conduction, as occurs in wires, is severely limited because of the high resistance of nerve fibers and their leaky membranes. Rather, the message-bearing function of axons is due to built-in amplifying systems composed of special biological structures and chemical substances. The details of these systems are described in Chapter 5.

The axons of motor neurons, which emerge from cell bodies in the ventral horns of the spinal cord, are about 20 µm in diameter and arise from the **axon hillock** (see Figures 3.2 and 3.4). From this point, the axon is covered by a membrane known as the **axolemma** that is similar to the plasma membrane of the cell body. The axon hillock is free of ribosomes (Nissl granules) and other cellular inclusions, and the neurofilaments are clustered together in fascicles before proceeding along the axon proper. Motor neurons, which have relatively thick axons, have a specialized feature just beyond the axon hillock known as the **initial segment**, also shown in Figures 3.2 and 3.4. The diameter of this segment is reduced, and it too is free of ribosomes and other organelles. Functionally, the initial segment plays a significant role in the propagation of nerve signals. It is here that excitatory and inhibitory influences are summed, either to promote the onset of a nerve impulse or to impede it. Consequently, this part of the axon is sometimes known as the trigger zone.

Axon Dimensions

Axon lengths vary considerably. Some axons are quite short, extending only several cell body diameters, while others may extend several thousand cell body diameters. The phrenic nerve, which innervates the muscles of the respiratory diaphragm, originates from cell bodies in the brain stem near the base of the skull. In the giraffe, the axons of these cells terminate on the diaphragm, about 15 feet below the skull. In a 6-foot man, the axons that emerge from cell bodies in the lower spinal cord and extend to the muscle in the lower leg (the extensor hallucis longus) that extends the big toe may be 5,000 cell body diameters long. By comparison, if the cell body were as large as a football, the axon would extend the length of 15 football fields. Further, in some mature nerve cells, the volume of the axon may be hundreds or thousands of times that of the cell body. It is thus apparent that the transport of substances synthesized in the soma to distant parts of the neuron is a process of major physiological importance. Axonal transport is discussed in a later section.

The diameter of axons in the CNS is maintained throughout their length, but near the distal end the axons may divide into a few branches or into as many as a few thousand fine branches with terminal enlargements. These enlargements form synaptic connections to other neurons or effector organs. The axons of sympathetic or parasympathetic neurons have fine terminal branches with thousands of synaptic swellings (**synaptic varicosities**) along their length, many of which form junctions with effector cells.

Axon Collaterals

In some axons, branches known as axon collaterals originate from nodes of Ranvier (see below) and distribute nerve signals to alternative destinations. For example, branches may extend backward to influence the source of their own stimulation. These backward-running branches, known as **recurrent collaterals**, are diagrammed in Figure 3.13. Collaterals from motor neurons run backward to synapse on **Renshaw cells**, which in turn synapse back upon the same or other motor neurons. The Renshaw cells exert inhibitory effects upon the motor neurons, providing, in this case, negative feedback that prevents them from firing too often and thus distributing the workload more evenly within the neuron and muscle cell population.

Axonal Transport

An essential part of cell function is the transport of proteins, lipids, and vesicles to and from the plasma membrane and between the intracellular organelles such as the nucleus, the endoplasmic reticulum, the Golgi apparatus, and the small vesicles. The magnitude of this process is substantially increased in neurons because of the distances between the cell body and dendrites, and especially between the cell body and the axon terminals. Thus, the cell body has the prodigious task of manufacturing and delivering proteins and lipids to maintain dendrites and an axon that are 10,000 times greater in volume and 60,000 times greater in surface area than itself. The cell body continually makes these substances and delivers them to the dendrites and the farthest reaches of the axon via **anterograde** (forward) **axonal transport** (i.e., from the cell body to the axon terminals, or in the case of afferent somesthetic spinal neurons, from the cell body near the spinal cord to the sense organs in the skin.) The transported materials consist of cytoskeletal and soluble proteins, vesicles containing proteins for the growth and maintenance of the axolemma, mitochondria, and other proteins and enzymes needed for transmitter synthesis and secretion. Moreover, there is **retrograde axonal transport** of vesicle membrane material and excess or degenerated axon proteins from the axon terminals to the cell body via endosomes or other multivesicular bodies. Some vesicles at the axon terminals capture materials in the synaptic clefts and transport these substances to the cell body. Material returned to the cell body is either recycled or transferred to lysosomes for disposal.

The mechanical work of axonal transport utilizes the chemical energy of ATP generated within mitochondria, and there are putative targeting signals to direct the macromolecules to their appropriate destinations. For example, because axons and dendrites are different in structure and function, their protein requirements are also different. Consequently, sorting mechanisms are needed to separate the different vesicles and proteins that are bound for one domain or the other. This sorting process is described below.

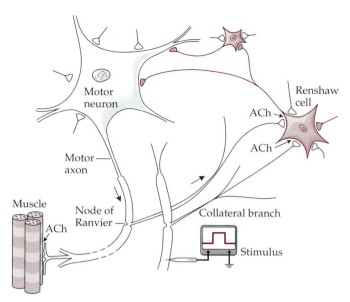

3.13 THE ROLE OF AXON COLLATERALS. Renshaw cells are found near motoneurons in the spinal cord. The motoneurons receive excitatory inputs from many sources (open axon terminals). Collateral fibers from the nodes of the motoneuron axons stimulate the Renshaw cells, the transmitter being acetylcholine (ACh). The Renshaw cell axons return to the motoneurons forming inhibitory synapses (solid terminals); the transmitter is glycine. (*Bottom*) a stimulus applied to the axon stimulates the Renshaw cell, which has a strong inhibitory action on motoneurons. Renshaw cells receive excitatory and inhibitory inputs from a number of sources. (After Eccles, 1967.)

Within axons, microtubules, in addition to serving a skeletal function, appear to provide one of the means of transport within the axon: that is, they appear to move through the cytoplasm in polymerized form toward the axon terminals (Ellisman, 1981; Thoenen and Kreutzberg, 1981). The means of this apparent movement is the addition of monomers of tubulin to the (+) end (facing the synaptic terminals), while monomers are dropped off at the (−) end (facing the cell body), a process known as treadmilling. This has not been proposed as the sole method of axonal transport, but the proposed transport role of the microtubules is buttressed by the finding that the alkaloids colchicine, found in the seeds of the autumn crocus, and vinblastine, obtained from periwinkle, bind and degrade tubulin and disrupt axonal transport.

The rate of axonal transport has been established in experiments in which axon materials were labeled and observed by electron microscopy at various stages of their passage along the axon. In an early experiment by Ochs (1972), the rate of axonal transport was measured by microinjecting radiolabeled amino acids into the fluid surrounding the dorsal root ganglia (DRG) in the lumbar region of the spinal cord of cats. (The DRG are made up of the cell bodies of sensory spinal nerves.) The amino acids were taken up by the cell bodies and incorporated into proteins, with different amino acids labeling different proteins. Then, after various time intervals, the distribution of radiolabeled proteins in successive segments cut from the peripheral end of sensory axons was measured. It was found that some of the proteins synthesized in the cell bodies moved along the axons at rates of 200–400 mm/day, termed **fast axonal anterograde transport**, whereas other materials were transported at much slower rates of 0.2 to 1 mm/day and 2 to 8 mm/day, termed **slow axonal transport**. At the highest rate of 400 mm/day, the materials would traverse an axon 35 mm long in about 2 hours, and at the slowest rate, it would take about half a year (Vale, Banker, and Hall, 1992). Other investigators identified four different rates depending upon the material being transported: for example, 0.21 mm/day for microtubules and neurofilaments; 28 mm/day for actin filaments, metabolic enzymes, and clathrin complex (see below); 50–100 mm/day for mitochondria; and 200–400 mm/day for small vesicles, neurotransmitters or their precursors, membrane proteins, and lipids (Lasek, 1980).

In another experiment, Grafstein and Forman (1980) injected radiolabeled amino acids into one eye of a goldfish, where the amino acids were taken up by the ganglion cells of the retina and incorporated into proteins of the optic nerves. These proteins were transported within the optic nerves to the tectum of the midbrain, which in fish is the terminal area of the optic nerves. After various time intervals, the fish were killed and the degree of radioactivity in the tectum was measured. The untreated eye served as a control; its branch of the optic nerve showed no labeled transport. The investigators estimated that the transport rate of labeled proteins was 10–50 mm/day when the fish were kept at room temperature. When the temperature was increased, the rate doubled or tripled with every increase of 10°C.

Once transport begins, it continues, at least for a time, even if the soma is severed from the axon. This finding indicates that transport is not dependent upon metabolism in the soma, which was once thought to provide a pressure front to push the axoplasm and its contents toward the axon terminals. Transport will occur even in an isolated segment of an axon, provided sufficient oxygen and calcium are available. An oxygen deficit, restricted to a small axon segment, will slow or completely block axonal transport through that segment, indicating that transport depends upon local oxidative metabolism. Calcium deficits, which interfere with the assembly of microtubules, reduce the amount of material that can be transported, but not the rate of transport. Calcium is also required in the soma for coupling the synthesized proteins to the transport mechanism (see Reinis and Goldman, 1982).

Fast axonal transport. Transport at the rate of 200–400 mm/day particularly requires energy supplied by ATP and oxygen. The materials that move at the fastest anterograde rate are mostly enzymes used in neurotransmitter synthesis and newly synthesized synaptic vesicles from the Golgi apparatus containing precursors of neurotransmitters . These vesicles are subject to anterograde transport only. At the axon terminals, the vesicles discharge their contents during synaptic activity and then are recycled; that is, they are refilled with transmitters over and over again within the terminal area. The vesicle membranes are maintained by the replacement of damaged or missing parts with new components arriving from the cell bodies. When they cannot be reused any longer, the vesicle remnants are returned to the cell bodies via retrograde transport in multivesicular bodies to be reduced to proteins or lipids for reuse, or to be disposed of by lysosomes. Also included in fast axonal transport are membrane proteins for the maintenance of the axolemma.

Vesicles moved by fast transport seem to move independently of the general flow, and if vesicles enter the axoplasm as a group, they become dispersed as they move along the axon. The vesicles also seem to move in jumps. Experiments using snail neurons show that the more crowded the vesicles are, the faster they move, and vice versa. This maintains a relatively constant rate of vesicle movement (Schwartz, 1980).

Mitochondria are transported in the anterograde direction at about 50–100 mm/day to wherever they are needed to provide the energy for nerve growth, impulse propagation, and synaptic activity. Degenerated mitochondria are subject to retrograde transport, either for recycling in the cell body or for elimination by the lysosomes.

Slow axonal transport. The bulk of the axoplasm moves by slow transport, at the rate of 1–10 mm/day, depending upon the axon length: the longer the axon, the faster the rate. As mentioned earlier, the axoplasm contains the fibrillar elements of the cytoskeleton, which include tubulin (the protein for microtubules), neurofilaments, and actin filaments, together with their associated proteins. These substances also mediate the movement of organelles from one region of the cell to another and anchor membrane constituents, such as receptors, at appropriate locations on the cells surface. Also, some proteins are needed to replace those that have been metabolized for energy production, to supply enzymes for mitochondrial activity, and to provide protein for nerve growth and general maintenance of nerve fibers. Also, some protein is released along with neurotransmitters, and this too must be replaced. Slow axonal transport accounts for 75% to 80% of the materials carried in the axon. The mechanism for slow transport is unknown, but it may depend on the movement of microtubules and other filaments by the treadmilling process (Schwartz, 1991c).

Retrograde axonal transport. Retrograde (reverse) axonal transport occurs at an average rate of about 24 mm/day. It is highly selective in what is transported, and moves far less material than is moved in the anterograde direction. Retrograde transport may convey subtances to the cell nucleus that regulate the synthesis and transport of proteins, lipids, and neurotransmitters toward the axon terminals (Ochs, 1975). It may also carry the signal for chromatolysis, the dispersion of Nissl granules that represents increased protein and lipid synthesis following axon injury.

Electron microscopic studies of ligated nerves have revealed that within hours, large numbers of vesicles and mitochondria accumulate on both sides of the ligation. This finding supports the notion that axonal organelles are being transported in both directions simultaneously. It also suggests that after prolonged synaptic activity at the axon terminals, synaptic vesicles ultimately need repair or replacement, so they are subject to retrograde transport to the cell body. Further, through the process of endocytosis, some proteins in the extracellular fluid are surrounded by the terminal membranes and drawn into the axoplasm for retrograde transport. Similarly, endosomes gather up excess membrane material for recycling or transfer to lysosomes for disposal. Thus, retrograde transport serves a scavenger function for axons.

Retrograde transport serves other functions as well. A peptide known as the **nerve growth factor** (**NGF**) is synthesized in the target cells of certain central and peripheral synapses, and can be taken up by the innervating axon terminals and carried back to the cell bodies, where it mediates neuron survival and growth. Thus, retrograde transport has a role in informing the cell body about events that occur at the distant terminals.

Retrograde transport can be utilized to determine the sources of axons that influence certain parts of the brain. The enzyme **horseradish peroxidase** (**HRP**) can be deposited in the target neural tissue, and if the cells are stimulated, HRP will be taken up by the terminal membranes and transported back to the cell bodies. Within a few days, this chemical treatment will yield a dark precipitate that can be visualized in the cell bodies of neurons whose terminals were exposed to the enzyme. For example, when HRP was deposited in the association cortex of a rhesus monkey, reaction products were observed in the nucleus of the basal forebrain two days later, thus affirming neural connections between these two areas. HRP and other substances are widely used for locating neuron sources because this method is faster and more accurate than the earlier method of sectioning axons and looking for Nissl chromatolysis in the cell bodies of the sectioned axons.

Retrograde transport may have negative consequences in that many neurotropic viruses and toxins gain access to the CNS in this manner. It has been found to be the means for the transport of viruses such as herpes simplex, rabies, and poliomyelitis, and for tetanus toxin. These substances are engulfed by terminal membranes, packaged in large vesicular organelles, and transported to the cell bodies, where the offending substances are released, usually resulting in cell death

(Schwartz, 1991c; see also Hammerschlag and Roberts, 1976; Schwartz, 1980; Schwartz, 1991c; Theodosis, 1979.)

Propelling mechanisms for fast axonal transport.   With the development of video microscopy, which enabled the detection of vesicles and individual microtubules, small organelles can be clearly seen moving bidirectionally at 1 to 5 µm/s in the squid giant axon, a rate consistent with fast axonal transport. Further, it was found that when the axoplasm was extruded from the axon onto a glass slide, organelle transport continued as long as ATP was supplied.

The force-generating mechanism for fast axonal transport was investigated by isolating the protein components of the axon and recombining them to reconstitute axonal transport in vitro. In this way, axoplasmic organelles isolated from squid axons were found to move along microtubules prepared from purified tubulin in the presence of ATP. Further, the motor for fast transport appeared to be attached to the organelles because the purified microtubules were devoid of their associated proteins. Moreover, it was found that factors in a soluble protein extract from the squid giant axon could bind to a glass slide, upon which microtubules could move along the glass surface. Latex microspheres (beads) could adsorb those protein factors and be transported along stationary microtubules, and after being injected into squid axons, the beads were transported along the axons. Because the transport of these beads and of organelles in vitro could be inhibited by the same pharmacological agents acting in vivo, it was proposed that the soluble protein motor that propelled the beads and organelles, and caused microtubules to move on glass, was the same in all instances.

These **motor** (force-generating) **proteins** were identified as **kinesin**, **dynein**, and **dynamin**. Kinesin and dynein are ATPases that are activated by binding to microtubules. Kinesin has a structure similar to that of myosin, a protein associated with muscle contraction, and cytoplasmic dynein is related to the motor proteins that power the movement of cilia (hairs) and flagella (tails), the motoric structures of one-celled organisms. Also, these two proteins occur widely in association with vesicles in eukaryotic cells, and mutants of the genes encoding these proteins led to deficient delivery of synaptic vesicles in axon terminals in *Drosophila*.

Dynamin differs from kinesin and dynein in that its energy source is guanosine triphosphate (GTP) rather than ATP and that in vitro, it forms cross-bridges between adjacent microtubules and induces sliding between them. Mutants of the gene that encodes dynamin prevent the formation of new synaptic vesicles, suggesting that dynamin has a role in vesicle recycling and other endocytotic activities.

About 20 years ago, electron microscopists observed cross-bridges between microtubules and vesicles that were thought to play a role in the movement of the vesicles. Kinesin has been suggested to form these cross-bridges, which have the appearance of little feet walking along the microtubules (Schwartz, 1991). Kinesin and dynein are currently thought to be unidirectional motors that move in opposite directions along microtubules—kinesin to the plus (+) end, and dynein to the minus (−) end. This hypothesis conveniently explains the bidirectional transport of vesicles within axons. Because 90% or more of the microtubules are oriented with their (+) ends toward the terminals, organelles bound with kinesin will be transported in an anterograde direction, and organelles destined for the cell body will be bound to the dynein motor.

For smooth operation, the proper motor must be attached to the proper organelles and activated. Latex spheres, which bind both kinesin and cytoplasmic dynein, frequently change the direction of their movement on microtubules. Thus, organelles, if they are to move in either direction, must incorporate both kinesin and dynein, as well as proteins that regulate motor attachment and activation (Figure 3.14). Axon organelles to be transported contain both motors, which are themselves transported and recycled. Kinesin must first be in position in or near the cell body, where it will bind to a vesicle and be activated for anterograde vesicle transport. The dynein protein is also bound to the vesicle, but presumably in an inactivated state. After the vesicle is carried to the axon terminal, the vesicle discharges its contents, kinesin becomes inactive, and dynein becomes active. The dyenin carries the empty vesicle and inactivated kinesin retrogradely to the cell body. When the vesicle reaches the cell body, dynein protein must again be inactivated so that it and the vesicle can be brought back to the terminal area. Thus, both types of motors are bound to vesicle membranes and undergo activation and inactivation, but the order is continually reversed so that only one motor is active at a time. Figure 3.14*a* is a schematic rendering of the processes involved in axonal transport.

Sorting and the destination of proteins. In the sections above describing axons and dendrites, a question was raised about the mechanism for the sorting and transport of proteins manufactured in the cell body that are specific for the dendrite/soma and axon domains. Dendrites are specialized for receiving signals that come from other cells; cell bodies manufacture the substances needed for cell maintenance and cell function; axons are specialized for the conduction of action potentials toward nerve terminals; and axon terminals are specialized for the synthesis and transport of proteins and enzymes and the release of neurotransmitters. How the various parts of the neuron are supplied with their respective needs may be explained as follows.

Both dendrites and axons have the same basic cytoskeletal components: microtubules, neurofilaments, and actin filaments. The structure and polarity of the microtubules supply the principal difference between axons

and dendrites that determines the destination of the substances needed by each part of the cell. It was mentioned earlier that 90% or more of the microtubules in axons are oriented with their plus (+) ends toward the axon terminals and their minus (−) ends toward the soma, and that in dendrites the orientation is random, either (+) or (−). It was also mentioned that mRNAs for heavy microtubule-associated proteins (MAP2) are found in the cell bodies and dendrites, and mRNAs for tubulin and lighter MAPs (tau) are confined to the cell bodies.

To explain the difference in the destinations of specific mRNAs for MAP2 and tau, it was proposed that the key again is the difference between the longitudinal orientation of microtubules in axons and dendrites. For example, any organelle in the cell body that is specified for transport toward the (−) ends of microtubules will be transported into dendrites, but not into axons. Thus, the microtubules and their intrinsic organization in axons and dendrites may determine the difference in the destinations of different neuronal proteins (see Vale, Banker, and Hall, 1992).

The Nerve Cell Membrane

As with all cells, a membrane covers the exterior surface of nerve cells, including the soma, the dendrites, and the axon. This membrane, about 8–10 nm thick, is called the **plasmalemma** to distinguish it from the membranes that surround the internal organelles of the cell. As mentioned earlier, the part of the membrane that covers the axon is known as the axolemma. In some axons, the axolemma is covered by a myelin sheath, but the membrane covering the dendrites and soma is not myelinated, nor are the nodes of Ranvier.

The plasmalemma serves as a sturdy envelope to keep needed substances in and unneeded substances out. It controls the passage of nutrients, as well as the amino acid precursors of neurotransmitters and proteins, into the cell. The membrane also permits the passage of waste products out of the cell and into the bloodstream, from which they are taken up by the kidneys or liver and excreted. Events within the cell, such as the production of proteins and lipids and their transport to where they are needed, all serve to maintain the normal structure and activity of the plasmalemma. The transmission of neuronal messages is determined by ion flow across the axolemma in axons, the details of which are discussed in Chapter 5.

Membrane Structure

Membranes are composed of two classes of molecules: lipids and proteins. Lipids (molecules that make up fats and waxes) provide the main structural characteristics of a membrane, and average about 40% of its dry weight. However, the ratio of lipid to protein in neuronal membranes varies according to the function of the membrane. For example, myelin sheaths have a very low protein

(a)

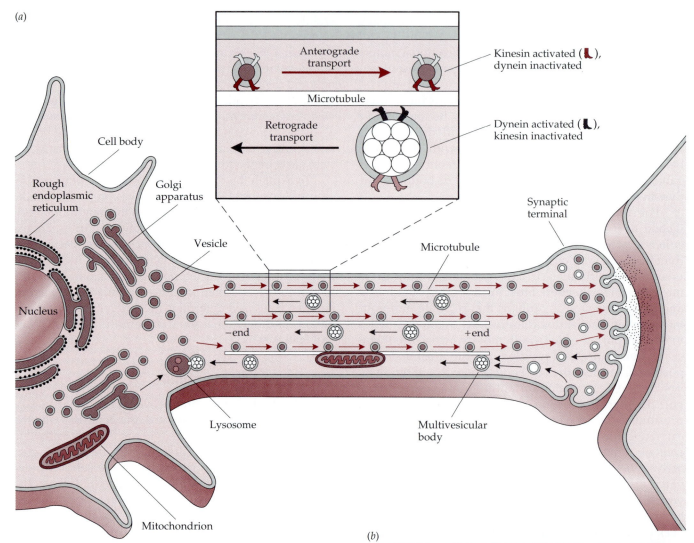

Anterograde
transport

Microtubule

Retrograde
transport

Kinesin activated (🔴),
dynein inactivated

Dynein activated (🔴),
kinesin inactivated

Cell body

Rough
endoplasmic
reticulum

Golgi
apparatus

Vesicle

Microtubule

Synaptic
terminal

Nucleus

−end

+end

Lysosome

Multivesicular
body

Mitochondrion

(b)

3.14 AXONAL TRANSPORT. (a) Anterograde transport supports
the transfer of substances synthesized by the ER and Golgi apparatus to distant parts of the axon membrane and to axon terminals.
Surplus membrane particles (proteins and lipids) at the synaptic
terminals are packaged into multivesicular bodies which return to
the cell body by retrograde transport for degradation by lysosomes. Mitochondria move in both directions to supply the energy demands of the cell wherever it is needed. Organelles bind
kinesin and dynein in the cell body, but dynein is inactive so kinesin mediates anterograde transport. At axon terminals, the
vesicular contents are released and kinesin presumably becomes
inactive. Dynein then becomes active and elicits retrograde transport (inset). After many cycles the organelles break down and are
disposed of by lysosomes; newly synthesized organelles take their
place. (b) A quick-freeze, deep-etched electron micrograph of a
nerve fiber in a rat spinal cord. Rod-shaped structures of kinesin
molecules bridge vesicular organelles and microtubules. There are
globular endings where the rods contact the microtubules (arrows). Bar = 100 nm. (a after Schwartz, 1980; Vale, Banker, and
Hall, 1992; b from Hirokawa et al., 1989, Cell, 56:867–878, ©
Cell Press.)

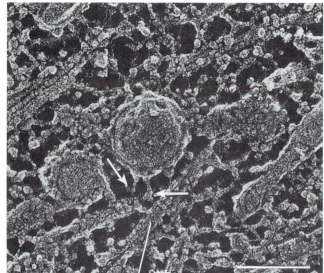

Microtubule

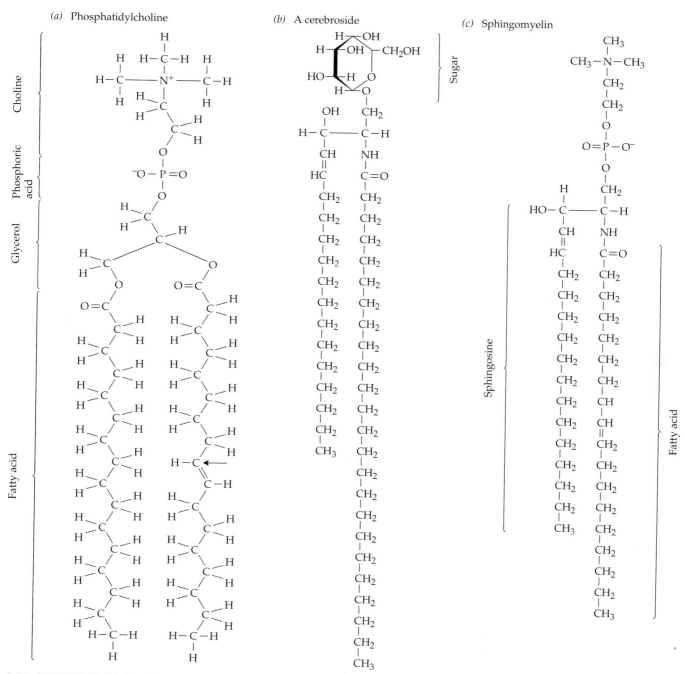

(a) Phosphatidylcholine   (b) A cerebroside   (c) Sphingomyelin

3.15 CONSTITUENTS OF LIPIDS. (*a*) A molecule of phosphatidylcholine. Note the negative charge on the phosphate group in the polar head. The fatty acid tail on the left is saturated, meaning that every carbon atom is linked to two or three hydrogen atoms. The tail on the right is unsaturated, with a double bond between carbon atoms at the point indicated by the arrow. (*b*) A cerebroside is a sphingolipid that contains a sugar molecule in addition to sphingosine and a fatty acid molecule. (*c*) Sphingomyelin is the most common and the simplest sphingolipid. It contains one molecule of the alcohol choline, a molecule of phosphoric acid, as well as sphingosine.

content, but their proteins are crucial for myelin formation, and myelin has a significant role in neuron functioning. In contrast, the plasmalemma itself has a high

protein content, which provides the machinery for nerve impulse transmission and transmembrane transport.

Membrane lipids. Membrane lipid molecules, with the exception of cholesterol, have three parts: a polar head (so designated because it carries a negative electric charge), a glycerol backbone, and two nonpolar fatty acid tails made up of long chain hydrocarbons similar to those in oil molecules. The polar head contains phosphates and other constituents; thus these lipids are called **phospholipids**. Figure 3.15*a* shows the molecular arrangement of the lipid molecule phosphatidylcholine, which is commonly found in neuronal membranes. Note the negative charge on the phosphate group (PO_4). Lipids known as **cerebrosides** (Figure 3.15*b*) are also found in the brain, and are most heavily concentrated in myelin sheaths. They contain both a sugar and an amino alcohol called **sphingosine**, and are classified both as **glycolipids** and as **sphingolipids**. **Sphingomyelin** is a lipid that is a constituent of myelin sheaths (Figure 3.15*c*). Other lipids known as **gangliosides** are found in the cytoplasmic membranes of nerve terminals. They have very large heads made up of complex sugars. They also have an affinity for calcium ions (Ca^{2+}), which play a significant role in membrane excitability at nerve terminals.

An important feature of lipids is the water solubility of the polar head, which is thus designated as **hydrophilic**. The fatty acid tails, on the other hand, are water insoluble and are designated as **hydrophobic**, a property that is exemplified by the insolubility of oils and waxes in water. Molecules with a hydrophilic and a hydrophobic end are called **amphipathic**; phospholipids and glycolipids are examples of amphipathic molecules. Because of the amphipathic nature of phospholipids, when they are placed in an aqueous medium, they spontaneously coalesce into an orderly bilayered alignment with the polar heads oriented toward the aqueous environment and the tails oriented toward each other, as shown in Figure 3.16. This arrangement forms the basic structure of biological membranes. In neuronal membranes, the lipid bilayer is about 4.5 nm thick and serves as the framework of the cell membrane as well as the anchoring structure for the proteins associated with the membrane.

Another important characteristic of membranes is their relative rigidity. A factor determining this rigidity is the extent of saturation of the fatty acid tails. *Saturation* in this context means the degree to which hydrogen atoms are linked to every carbon atom. An unsaturated condition exists when carbon atoms are linked by double bonds to other carbon atoms. The molecule of phosphatidylcholine shown in Figure 3.15*a* contains a saturated fatty acid tail on the left and an unsaturated tail on the right. When phospholipids are saturated, the fatty acid tails nest together and form a rigid structure. When double bonds are present, the resulting deformations interfere with orderly stacking, and the lipid layer is less rigid and more fluid (Figure 3.17). There is a relationship between the fluidity of the lipid layer and the rate of transfer of substances across the membrane. Experiments have shown that when the proportion of unsaturated fatty acids is high, transport across the membrane can be 20 times faster than when the proportion is low and the membrane is more rigid.

Lipid pathology.   A number of inherited neurological disorders are caused by pathologies of membrane lipids. The case of *shi/shi shivering* mice, described below, is an example of such a disease in animals. Examples of these disorders in humans are Gauchers, Niemann-Picks, and

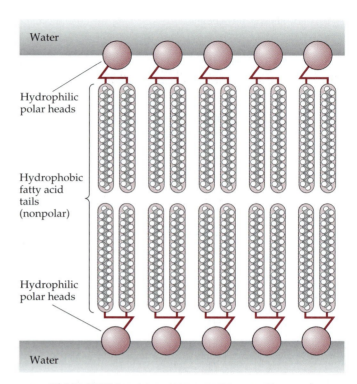

3.16 CROSS SECTION OF A LIPID MEMBRANE. The membrane is formed from two layers of amphipathic lipid molecules. The hydrophilic polar heads of the lipids face the aqueous solution on both sides of the membrane, whereas the hydrophobic nonpolar fatty acid tails face inward, toward each other.

Krabbes diseases, as well as Fabrys disease and Tay-Sachs disease. Known in humans as **lipidoses**, these pathologies are caused by the absence of genetically determined metabolizing enzymes, which allows a high accumulation of abnormal lipid metabolites that interferes with normal neural functions. In some cases, treatment is possible by supplying the missing enzyme. Usually the faulty gene is recessive, and if it is present in only one parent, none of their children will show any symptoms. But if each parent has one copy of the recessive gene, the chances are 1:4 that a child will have the disease. Detection of the faulty genes in the parents provides the basis of genetic counseling to minimize the passing on of the defects. The diseases can also be detected in utero, enabling the parents to consider terminating the pregnancy. Some of these diseases are largely confined to certain ethnic groups, or are sex-linked and occur primarily in males. Symptoms of some of them occur in infancy; in others, symptoms appear in the teen years. (See Brady, 1975 for an early review and more recent reviews on diagnosis and treatment by Beutler, 1993; and Hechtman and Kaplan, 1993.)

Membrane proteins.   Membrane proteins are of two types. **Extrinsic proteins** are located on either the inner or the outer membrane surface. **Intrinsic proteins** occupy positions either partially or completely within the lipid bilayer. An intrinsic protein may span the membrane

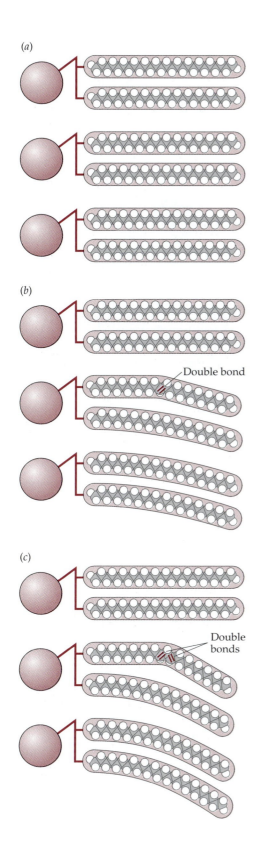

(a)

(b)

Double bond

(c)

Double bonds

3.17 EFFECTS OF VARIATION IN PHOSPHOLIPID FATTY ACID COMPOSITION. (a) If a lipid layer is composed entirely of saturated fatty acids, the fatty acid tails nest together to form rigid structures. (b) In unsaturated fatty acids, a double bond causes a deformation that interferes with the orderly stacking of the molecules and makes the fatty acid region more fluid. (c) When more double bonds are present, the deformations and resulting fluidity are greater still.

The stability of these molecules and their positions in the membrane depend upon their amphipathic character. The chains of amino acids that make up proteins are either hydrophilic or hydrophobic. Intrinsic proteins have a large proportion of hydrophobic amino acids, whereas extrinsic membrane proteins are mostly hydrophilic. Thus the lipid and the protein components of the membrane are attached to one another by both hydrophobic and hydrophilic interactions, which, along with other interactions, contribute to the stability of the membrane.

Extrinsic proteins may serve as enzymes, and on synaptic membranes, such enzymes break down some transmitter molecules, thus terminating their action. It has also been found that membrane lipids may activate or inactivate these enzymes. For example, the saturation of the fatty acids can alter the enzyme activity of adjacent proteins and thus alter synaptic events.

The intrinsic proteins that are embedded within the lipid matrix may form clusters or aggregates with similar or different proteins to form functional units. For example, some proteins on axon terminals take up neurotransmitters from synaptic clefts, thereby limiting their synaptic effects. Other protein carriers serve to transfer various water-soluble (polar) substances, such as sugars and amino acids, through the lipid bilayer into the nerve cell. This function is vital because these substances are excluded by the membrane, yet they are essential for cell viability and functioning.

Among the most important intrinsic membrane proteins in neurons are those involved in cell excitability and neural transmission. As we shall see in Chapter 5, many of these proteins are ion channels, controlled either by changes in the membrane voltage or by neurotransmitter binding. Other proteins function as pumps that move substances against concentration gradients or against an electric charge, as in the transport of a positively (+) charged ion into a similarly charged area. This process requires an energy source and is known as active transport (see below).

Transport across Membranes

The transport of substances across the plasma membranes of capillary endothelial cells within the brain is a vital process for supplying critical nutrients to brain cells as well as for removing metabolic waste products. As described in Chapter 1, the capillaries in organs other than the brain possess intercellular spaces and thinnings (fenestrations) that readily permit the diffusion of small

and protrude at both ends, as seen schematically in Figure 3.18. Such intrinsic proteins are amphipathic, as are the lipid molecules. Only part of the protein molecule is exposed to the aqueous environment within or outside of the cell; the rest is submerged in the oily medium formed by the fatty acid chains.

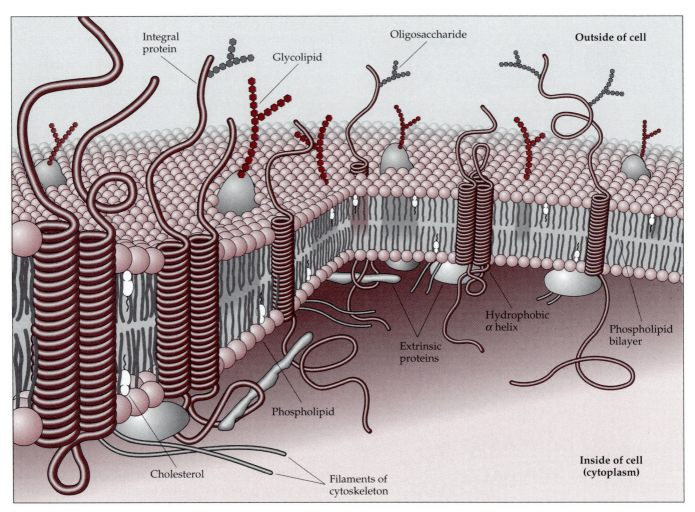

3.18 A BIOLOGICAL MEMBRANE. The membrane is formed by phospholipid molecules stacked side by side and tail to tail. Protein molecules are shown either penetrating into or through the lipid bilayer (intrinsic proteins), or attached to the bilayer without penetrating it (extrinsic proteins).

polar compounds and even macromolecules. In the brain, however, tight junctions between the endothelial cells (i.e., the blood–brain barrier) prohibit passage of these substances. Consequently, compounds must pass through the endothelial cell membrane either by passive diffusion (lipid-soluble compounds) or by some type of assisted transport mechanism (water-soluble compounds). Moreover, even after a substance has reached the intercellular fluid of the brain, it is faced with the problem of transport across neuronal and glial cell membranes. In this section, we will discuss some of the basic mechanisms involved in these transport functions.

Passive diffusion.   The process of passive diffusion was first discussed in Chapter 1, where we showed how the presence of a concentration gradient across a membrane causes a substance to move down that gradient until an equal concentration is established on both sides. This phe-

nomenon requires no energy to drive it, beyond whatever energy may have been expended to produce the original concentration gradient. On the other hand, the *rate* of transport, or the time to reach equilibrium, depends on a number of factors, including the molecular size and shape of the transported compound and its chemical properties and electric charge. Particularly important is the way these characteristics influence the compound's relative lipid versus water solubility. The high lipid content of membranes hampers the passive diffusion of water-soluble (i.e., polar) substances;* nevertheless, a number of these substances are observed to undergo high rates of transmembrane transport. This finding implies the existence of either membrane channels (pores) through which selected substances can pass, or other mechanisms that might rely on specific membrane proteins to facilitate the transport process. In the discussion below, we describe the basic types of transport proteins and their operation. The structure and functioning of membrane ion channels is taken up in detail in Chapter 5.

---

*It is noteworthy that water itself diffuses freely through membranes and thus is an exception to this general rule.

Membrane transport mediated by transporter proteins.
Intrinsic membrane proteins that are intimately involved in transport functions are usually termed **transporters**. These proteins possess a binding site for the transported substance. The substance being transported may be considered a substrate for the transport reaction in a manner analogous to the substrate of an enzymatic reaction.

Through a mechanism that is not yet fully understood, a substrate molecule binds to the transporter on the extracellular side of the membrane and then, following some kind of conformational change in the protein, the substrate is released into the cytoplasm of the cell. In the simplest case, which is termed **facilitated diffusion**, the transported compound moves down its concentration gradient, and binding of the substrate to the transporter protein is the only process needed to initiate the reaction. One important way of distinguishing between passive and facilitated diffusion depends on the fact that in the latter case, the density of the transporter protein in the membrane is a limiting factor with respect to the maximum rate of transport. With passive diffusion, one can raise the transport rate higher and higher by simply increasing the concentration of the substrate. With facilitated diffusion, however, increasing the concentration of the substrate eventually causes all of the transporter sites to be occupied, at which point the rate of transport reaches a maximum. This situation is very similar to the saturation of an enzyme by its substrate, and indeed, the relationship between substrate concentration and transport rate can be described by the same mathematical equation that characterizes the kinetics of enzyme catalysis (see below).

Carrier-mediated transport of one substance is often coupled to the transport of another (sometimes several) chemical species. In such cases, the cotransported molecule or ion is typically moving down a chemical and/or electrical gradient, which provides the energy necessary for transporting the substance of interest. When both substances are moving in the same direction across the membrane, the carrier is called a **symporter** (Figure 3.19). An **antiporter**, on the other hand, transports molecules or ions in opposite directions. In later chapters, we will see many examples of symporter and antiporter transport systems. For example, many transmitters are removed from the synaptic cleft by symporters that cotransport Na^+ ions. The presence of these ions is necessary for transport to occur, and the Na^+ electrochemical gradient across the membrane provides the necessary energy. In contrast, transmitters are generally accumulated by synaptic vesicles through a proton antiport system (i.e., H^+ ions, or protons, are concentrated within the vesicle interior, and transport of neurotransmitter molecules into the vesicle is coupled to outward transport of protons).

One final type of transport is termed **active transport**. In this case, transport of a substrate is directly linked with a chemical reaction that provides free energy to drive the process. As shown in Figure 3.19, ac-

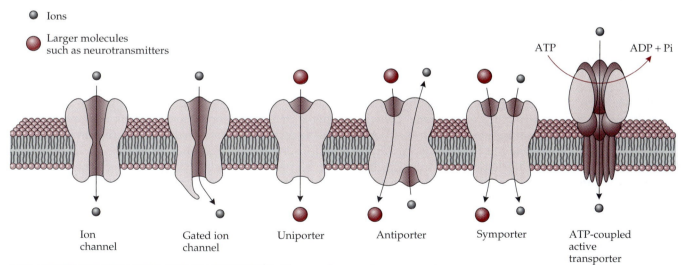

3.19 MEMBRANE CHANNELS AND TRANSPORTERS. The membranes of neurons and other cell types possess numerous proteins that participate in transport functions. Some of these are ion channels gated either by membrane voltage or by the binding of neurotransmitters or other ligands (see Chapter 5). Specific transporter proteins (uniporters) permit certain small hydrophilic molecules to move across the plasma membrane down a concentration gradient (facilitated diffusion). Transport may also be coupled to the movement of other substances (usually ions), either in the same direction across the membrane (symporters) or in the opposite direction (antiporters). Active transport is an energy-dependent process used to move ions or small molecules against a concentration gradient.

tive transport typically involves the hydrolysis of ATP, in which case the transport protein is called an ATPase. These enzymes are found in many kinds of cells, including neurons, and serve to stabilize ion concentrations both intracellularly and within the extracellular fluid (ECF). Perhaps the best-characterized active transport system in the brain is Na$^+$–K$^+$ATPase (also known as the Na$^+$–K$^+$ pump), which plays a vital role in the maintenance of the resting potential across the neuronal cell membrane (see Chapter 5). This enzyme also helps to regulate the composition of the brain ECF. For example, the concentration of K$^+$ ions in the ECF is maintained at a level about 40% lower than that in the blood plasma by an Na$^+$–K$^+$ATPase in the capillary endothelial cell membrane (i.e., K$^+$ is continuously pumped out of the ECF into the plasma). This process makes use of considerable amounts of ATP, supplied by the abundant mitochondria within the brain endothelial cells (Oldendorf, 1975).

Kinetics of transport.   The transport of a substance across a membrane is sometimes described as a high-affinity or low-affinity process. *Affinity* in this context refers to the interaction of a substrate with the carrier that transports it across the membrane. As mentioned above, the kinetics of membrane transport are analogous to those governing enzymatic reactions, and thus affinity in both cases can be expressed by the **Michaelis–Menten constant (K_m)**. In this instance, K_m is the extracellular concentration of a substrate that yields one-half of the **maximum velocity (V_{max})** of membrane transport of the substrate for a given amount of the transporter protein. It can be seen graphically in Figure 3.20 that as the substrate concentration increases, the transport velocity of the substrate also increases, but ultimately reaches a plateau. Once this plateau is reached, the rate of reaction cannot be increased by adding more substrate because the protein carrier is already saturated.

The shape of the curve in Figure 3.20 can be altered by decreasing the density of the transporter protein (lower V_{max}). Thus, comparing one substrate with another requires that the density of the protein carrier be kept constant. Likewise, differences in K_m are reflected in the slope of the curve (a lower K_m indicates greater affinity, which yields a steeper slope).

Some cells exhibit both high- and low-affinity transport of a given substrate. For example, the amino acids glycine and aspartic acid serve important physiological functions within most cells, but they both serve as neurotransmitters for some neurons as well. In these cells, two distinct transport affinities have been found. The high-affinity transport system associated with axon terminals takes up the amino acids that have been released as transmitters; the low-affinity system is usually associated with the uptake of amino acids for metabolic purposes (Snyder et al., 1973).

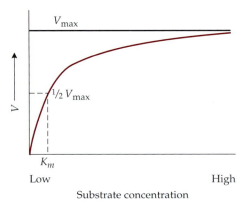

3.20. THE MICHAELIS–MENTEN CONSTANT (K_m). The curve shows how substrate concentration affects the reaction rate. K_m is the substrate concentration that yields one-half the maximum velocity (V_{max}) for the reaction being studied.

Exocytosis and endocytosis.   There are other mechanisms of active membrane transport. **Exocytosis** refers to the transfer of intracellular products such as neurotransmitters and peptides across the plasmalemma to the extracellular or synaptic space. When they are signaled to do so, the vesicles fuse to the terminal membranes and release their contents into the synaptic cleft (see Chapter 6). After exocytosis, most neurotransmitters are released from their postsynaptic receptors and are taken back into the axon terminals by high-affinity Na$^+$-dependent transporters that are specific for the neuron secreting that transmitter. In some instances transmitters are taken up by glia having similar high-affinity transporters. In both cases the transmitters are cotransported with Na$^+$, whose concentration gradient across the membrane provides the energy for uptake.

Endocytosis was mentioned earlier as a mechanism for transporting substances from the synaptic spaces back into the axon terminals for retrograde transport to the cell body. In one form of endocytosis, the vesicle membranes that adhered to the terminal membrane during exocytosis are retrieved from the terminal and used to form new vesicles. Some submicroscopic particles are enveloped by minute invaginations of the cell membrane, the edges of which fuse together. The resulting vesicles detach and move into the cytoplasm. Within the cytoplasm the vesicles lyse (dissolve), releasing their contents into the cytoplasm.

In a similar process, molecules attach to receptors that form pits, which later detach and form vesicles, the insides of which are lined with a carbohydrate-rich coat. This process is aided by a protein known as **clathrin**, which forms a latticelike cage or coat around the vesicle. Once these vesicles are internalized, the clathrin enclosures are shed, and the vesicles are transported to the cell body. There they may fuse with other vesicles to form endosomes and restore their particular contents, or they may fuse with lysosomes and undergo degradation. Some endosomes transport their protein contents to the cell membrane for membrane maintenance by the process of exocytosis described above, or transport proteins destined for secretion to the cell membrane, where they are released. Vesicles that become endosomes are also presumed to play a role in the selective uptake of nutritional or regulatory proteins (hormones) such as insulin. Now there is evidence suggesting that clathrin-coated vesicles are involved in the retrieval and recycling of the vesicle membranes that were added to the plasmalemma during exocytosis of transmitters (see Hall, 1992.)

Neuroglia

As we have shown, neurons are the functional units of the nervous system, but virtually all neurons are surrounded by functionally significant satellite cells called neuroglia, or simply glia. Glial cells fill in the spaces between nerve cells and outnumber nerve cells by at least 10:1, but being of smaller size, they make up only half of the brain volume. Glia were first described by Virchow (1860), who wrote that they make up a connective tissue that lies between neural elements and holds them together in a way different from other connective tissue. Virchow, therefore, named this tissue "neuro-glia" (nerve glue), a name that is somewhat appropriate because glia serve as supporting elements, providing firmness and structure to the brain. They also separate and occasionally insulate groups of neurons from one another. However, over the years, researchers have found that glia interact with neurons much more actively than originally thought. They take up many transmitters from the extracellular fluid, and they also possess receptors for a number of transmitters. There is also evidence that glia transfer nutrients and other materials between the neurons and the bloodstream (Lasek, Gainer, and Barker, 1977). Also, during development, certain classes of glial cells guide the migration of neurons and direct the outgrowth of axons (see Kandel, 1991e.) Glia are the source of a wide variety of tumors (gliomas) of the brain, the retina, and the spinal cord. This is probably due to the fact that glial cells undergo continuous mitotic division in the mature animal, which increases the chance of a gene mutation leading to uncontrolled glial growth, whereas neurons do not.

Based upon early studies of the unusually large glia in leech brains and later studies of amphibian and mammalian brains, the structural details of glia have been well established. Glia are metabolically active cells with the usual cell inclusions such as a nucleus, mitochondria, ER, ribosomes, and lysosomes. However, compared with neurons, the organelles in most glia are in scant supply. Glia resemble neurons in that they have numerous processes extending from the cell body, but they have nothing resembling axons. Glial cells may be coupled contiguously by low-resistance connections that allow direct passage of ions and small molecules between them. Neurons, however, are separated from glia by narrow fluid-filled intercellular spaces that prevent electrical currents generated by nerve impulses from affecting neighboring glia (see Figure 1.5; Nicholls, Martin, and Wallace, 1992).

There are two major types of glia in the CNS, **astrocytes** (Gr. *astron*, star; *kytos*, cell), and **oligodendrocytes** (Gr. *oligos*, few; *dendron*, tree; *kytos*, cell). The astrocytes are further subdivided into protoplasmic and fibrous astrocytes. The protoplasmic astrocytes have a relatively large nucleus, an abundant granular cytoplasm, and many thick processes that extend from the cell body (Figure 3.21a). The ends of these processes flatten out to form pedicles, or end-feet, that adhere to blood vessels and neurons, and on the CNS periphery, the pia mater, a thin membrane that invests the surface of the brain, brain stem, and spinal cord. These astrocytes are found within the gray matter of the nervous system, which consists largely of cell bodies, dendrites, and synapses.

The fibrous astrocytes are more prevalent among the bundles of myelinated nerve fibers that largely make up the white matter of the brain, and are distinguished by long, thin, smooth, infrequently branched extensions (Figure 3.21b). They, too, by way of pedicles, make contacts with capillaries and neurons, as shown in Figure 3.21e. In addition, the glial cytoplasm contains aggregations of densely packed slender protein filaments made up of **glial fibrillary acidic protein** (**GFAP**), a protein different from that of neurofilaments. In culture or tissue, antibodies to GFAP can be used to selectively stain and identify these cells.

Astrocytes, because of their high permeability, take up the excess K^+ that accumulates in the extracellular space during high rates of neuron activity. The astrocytes store the K^+, thereby protecting neurons from the depolarizing effects of high concentrations of these cations. The glia also take up an equal amount of Cl^- to maintain electrical neutrality. Astrocytes also join together to form sheets, or syncytia, that can take up excess K^+ at one site and deliver it to a distant site where K^+ concentration is low (Kandel, 1991e). An extended discussion of the role of potassium and sodium ions in nerve function appears in Chapter 5.

Oligodendrocytes resemble astrocytes in many respects, but they are smaller, they have smaller nuclei, and, as their name implies, they have few and slender branches (Figure 3.21c). On the other hand, compared with other glial types, the oligodendrocytes have a cytoplasm rich in ribosomes, a well-developed rough ER, a large Golgi apparatus, and numerous mitochondria. Microtubules are prominent in the oligodendrocyte soma and cell branches. These characteristics are in keeping with the myelin-synthesizing function of these cells, which will be described below.

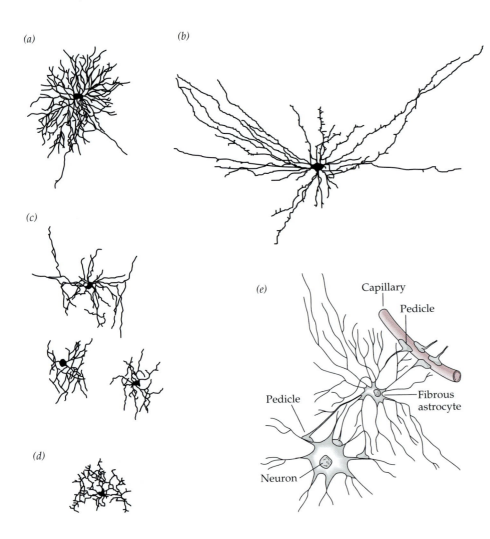

(a)

(b)

(c)

(d)

(e)

Capillary

Pedicle

Pedicle

Fibrous astrocyte

Neuron

3.21. NEUROGLIA. (*a–d*) Camera lucida drawings, all at the same magnification (×1,000). (*a*) A protoplasmic astrocyte. (*b*) A fibrous astrocyte. (*c*) Oligodendrocytes. (*d*) A microglial cell. (*e*) Fibrous astrocytes connect neurons to capillaries. (*a–d* after Jones and Cowan, 1983; *e* after Kandel, 1991e.)

The **microglia**, the smallest among the glia, have small, elongated nuclei surrounded by very little cytoplasmic fluid. They also have few branches that are short and twisted, and unlike the smooth branches of astrocytes, those of the microglia are covered with many tiny pointed spines (Figure 3.21*d*). These cells make up about 10% of all glia, and are scattered throughout the gray matter of the brain and spinal cord and to a lesser degree in the white matter. They proliferate rapidly near an inflammatory or degenerative lesion in the nervous system and migrate to the site of the injury, where they become phagocytes, or scavengers, that digest and remove the debris of dead or damaged cells. In experiments in which electrodes are implanted to record electrical activity in certain parts of the brains of living animals, it is necessary to examine the brain after the experiment to be certain that the electrode tip was in the designated place. Thus, the animal brains are treated with a substance that stains microglia black. When thin slices of the brain are examined and a thin line of black-stained microglia lining a gap in the tissue is found, it is a good indication that the gap was caused by the inserted electrode when the animal was alive. Glial cells likewise divide and occupy spaces vacated when neurons die during the natural process of aging. (For an extended discussion of neuroglia, see Kandel, 1991e; and Nicholls, Martin, and Wallace, 1992.)

Myelin and Myelination

Myelin is responsible for the white appearance of CNS tissue composed primarily of bundles of myelinated axon fibers (white matter). Myelin sheaths are found only in vertebrates, and only on some axons. Therefore, myelin is regarded as a relatively late development in the evolution of nervous systems. Myelin sheaths begin just beyond the initial segment and end at the terminals of the axon. A myelin sheath resembles an elongated tube that is segmented at regular intervals by unmyelinated sections known as the nodes of Ranvier (see Figure 3.2). It will be seen that the fatty structure and the segmented character of the myelin sheath serves to greatly increase the conduction velocity of nerve impulses.

Myelin is the product of two types of specialized glial cells known as **Schwann cells** in the peripheral nervous system (PNS) and **oligodendrocytes** in the CNS.

There are both myelinating and nonmyelinating Schwann cells, the latter type being found loosely wrapped around thin, nonmyelinated axon fibers such as those that make up the sympathetic trunk in the autonomic nervous system. Schwann cells have an additional function: If a peripheral nerve is severed, the distal end (the part between the cut and the periphery) degenerates, and the residues are consumed by phagocytes. However, the Schwann cells remain and form a cellular tube through which the regenerating axon will grow. Further, the interior of the tube provides a favorable surface for the adherence of the regenerating tip. In the CNS, severed or damaged axons do not regenerate, partly because oligodendrocytes do not support regrowth, and also because myelin in the CNS contains surface molecules that inhibit regrowth.

Because myelin is a product solely derived from the membranes of Schwann cells and oligodendrocytes, its chemistry is similar to that of the membranes of these cells. Myelin is made up of 70% lipid material (mainly cholesterol, phospholipids, and cerebrosides) and 30% protein, and therefore has a fatty consistency. These proportions vary to some degree depending upon the neuron type and the animal species. There are three types of myelin protein. **Protein zero (P_0)** is a major structural glycoprotein found only in myelin in the PNS. P_0 accounts for 50% of the protein in peripheral myelin sheaths, but it has not been detected within the CNS nor in the large number of Schwann cells that do not form myelin. Other functions of P_0 are described below. **Proteolipid protein (PLP)** is an integral membrane proteolipid in oligodendrocytes and myelin in the CNS. It accounts for about 50% of the myelin protein in the CNS, and small amounts, about 1%, in the PNS. It also plays a role in the myelinating process. **Myelin basic protein (MBP)** is actually a family of at least seven closely related proteins. They are not integral membrane proteins, and account for 30% of the myelin protein in the CNS and 5% to 15% of the myelin protein in the PNS. MBP proteins also have a role in myelin formation (see below.)

The high specificity of these proteins in the myelin formed by the two types of glial cells permits them to serve as markers for their myelin. This has been shown by Trapp and colleagues (1987) in their examination of the myelin of the trigeminal nerve of the rat. The motor branch of the trigeminal nerve originates from its nucleus of cell bodies in the pons and courses through white matter before emerging as a motor nerve for the muscles of the jaw. Thus, part of the nerve is within the CNS and part of the nerve is in the PNS. Using a radiolabeled DNA that detected the mRNAs for the three myelin proteins, it was found that before the CNS/PNS boundary in the CNS, the PLP gene was predominantly expressed. Beyond the boundary in the PNS, the gene for P_0 was exclusively expressed, and in both parts the MBP gene was expressed. This finding illustrates the strict dependency of myelin proteins on their respective glial cells.

It is also worth noting that MBP proteins are highly antigenic; that is, if they are injected into an animal, they produce a cellular autoimmune response characterized by a focal inflammation and demyelination in the CNS and the PNS. This response, referred to as **experimental autoimmune encephalomyelitis (EAE)**, was once considered a possible model for the study of multiple sclerosis (MS), a relatively common demyelinating disease in humans. MS manifests itself primarily as impaired sensory and motor performance due to the dysfunctional conduction of nerve impulses in demyelinated peripheral nerves and neural pathways in the CNS. However, MS clearly is a more heterogeneous and complex disease than EAE, and MBP autoreactivity is not thought to have a primary causative role in MS.

Myelin Formation

This subject has been intensely studied for over two decades and is extensively reviewed by Lemke (1992b). A first consideration is, What induces myelination? In peripheral sensory and motor neurons, there is a strong correlation between the axon circumference and myelination: small PNS axons (<1 µm in diameter) are rarely myelinated, whereas larger axons are always myelinated. The thickness of the myelin sheath is determined by the number of layers of Schwann cell membrane, and one lamella (layer) is added for every 0.2 µm increase in axon diameter. Moreover, experimental enlargement of axons can induce myelination in axons that are normally unmyelinated. These findings suggest that all axons possess a surface inducer whose concentration (per unit of membrane surface) is fixed, but that there is a threshold level of the inducer that triggers myelination by Schwann cells, and that the threshold level can be reached by enlarging the axon, which supplies more of the inducer.

Proliferation of Schwann cells is also driven by neurons. Schwann cells divide very slowly in certain cell cultures, but if Schwann cells are cocultured with sensory or sympathetic neurons, and there are cell–cell contacts, the Schwann cells undergo multiple rounds of cell division. Similarly, cell–cell contacts between axons and Schwann cells are necessary for the expression of certain proteins that participate in myelination.

When first formed, all nerve fibers are unmyelinated. In the human embryo, myelination begins at about the fourteenth week of intrauterine life and accelerates in the last trimester of pregnancy. In humans, myelination continues after birth; the myelination of the major descending neural pathways that mediate voluntary movements begins at birth and is usually completed 10 to 12 months postnatally, about the time when the infant starts to walk. Thereafter, as the brain and spinal cord grow by gene-governed processes, the myelin segments elongate along with the nerve fibers.

Along peripheral sensory or motor nerves, myelin is expressed by Schwann cells in the following way. In the first stage, axons stimulate Schwann cell proliferation, and the cells lie along the axons and form troughs by invagination. The presence of an axon causes the sides of a Schwann cell trough to wrap around the axon, and one edge of the flattened cell burrows under the opposite edge (Figure 3.22). The inside edge then expands and repeatedly curls around the axon, making layer after layer of myelin from the inside out. However, as this process proceeds, a slender extracellular space intervenes between the axolemma and the inner wrap of the myelin sheath (Bunge, Bunge, and Bates, 1989; Morell and Norton, 1980).

In the CNS, myelinization is much the same except that it is a product of oligodendrocytes rather than Schwann cells. However, there is a significant difference between these cells in that a single oligodendrocyte can send out as many as 50 strands and sheetlike extensions of its membrane to envelop nearby axons (Figure 3.23). Then, it is believed that the leading edges of all the membrane sheets continually curl around the axons, burrowing under the increasing layers of membrane (now myelin) so that the thickness of the myelin sheath grows from the inside out in a manner similar to that of the Schwann cells in the PNS.

Chemical Factors in Myelination

At the stage when one edge of the myelin-forming cell is burrowing under the edge on the opposite side, a strictly localized MBP membrane protein, **myelin-associated glycoprotein (MAG)**, is expressed at the juncture where the burrowing edge is encircling the axon, the area known as the **inner mesaxon**. MAG is a myelin-specific integral membrane protein expressed at low levels (about 1% of total protein) by both Schwann cells and oligodendrocytes. Despite the slender extracellular space that exists between the axolemma and the inner mesaxon, MAG molecules are said to promote an adhesion between the growing inner edge of the membrane and the axonal surface. (It has been proposed as an alternative explanation that the extracellular space may be a transient phenomenon.) Further, MAG expression can be detected in the earliest stages of peripheral myelination, before the appearance of any of the major myelin proteins. Thus, MAG appears to function as a mediator of the axon–glial adhesion events that precede myelination and to assist and direct the initial tucking under of the growing inner layer of myelin. Consistent with this notion, MAG can mediate an in vitro adhesion between cultured oligodendrocytes and neurons (see Lemke, 1992b.)

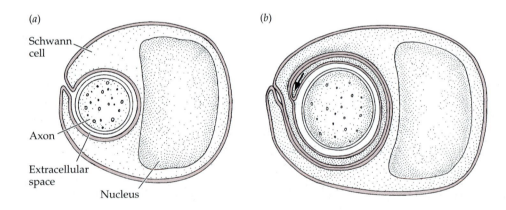

(a)

Schwann cell
Axon
Extracellular space
Nucleus

(b)

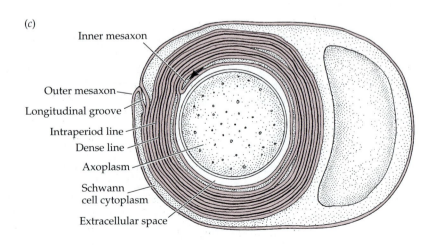

(c)

Inner mesaxon
Outer mesaxon
Longitudinal groove
Intraperiod line
Dense line
Axoplasm
Schwann cell cytoplasm
Extracellular space

3.22. MYELIN FORMATION ON PERIPHERAL AXONS. (*a*) The membrane of a Schwann cell encircles an axon. (*b*) The top part of the membrane burrows under the bottom part and completely encircles the axon. (*c*) The burrowing continues to encircle the axon and builds up many layers of myelin from the inside out (note the arrow in the leading edge). As the layers build up, the cytoplasm is squeezed out and the inner surfaces of membranes come together to form the dense line. When the outermost membrane surface of the newest ring and the next one come together, they form the intraperiod line. (After Morell and Norton, 1980.)

(a)

Node of
Ranvier

Nucleus

Oligodendrocyte

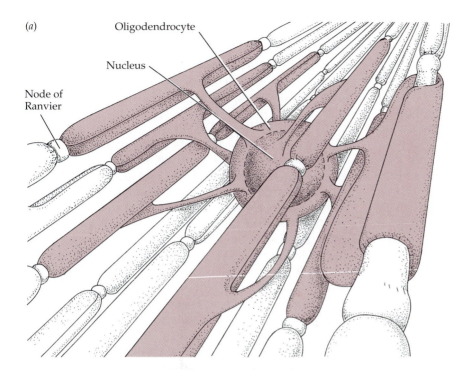

3.23. OLIGODENDROCYTES. (*a*) In the CNS, these glial cells send out kitelike sheets to envelop axons and form myelin sheaths in a manner similar to that of the Schwann cells. (*b*) An extraordinary view of oligodendrocytes beginning to myelinate axons in the corpus callosum of a 6-day-old rat. (*a* after Morell and Norton, 1980; scanning electron micrograph courtesy of Karen L. Valentino.)

(b)

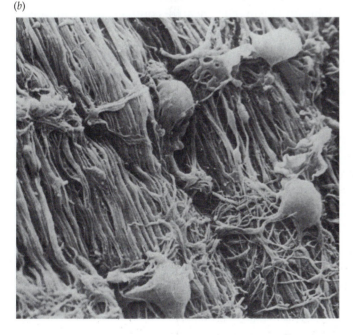

MAG is also of interest because of its chemical structure, which is closely related to that of a neural cell adhesion molecule known as N-CAM, a member of the neural cadherin family of cell surface proteins thought to be involved in cell–cell recognition. These molecules promote adhesion between cells when the same molecules appear on different cells that are close together, a process known as **homophilic interaction**. The early expression of MAG, its subcellular location, and its structural similarity to N-CAM suggest that MAG is an adhesion molecule important for the initiation and continuance of the myelinating process.

In peripheral nerve axons, the growth of the inner mesaxon is driven by rapid membrane biosynthesis as it continues to curl around the axon while continually insinuating itself under the growing layers of Schwann cell membrane (myelin). The layers of Schwann cell membrane become compacted, and the cytoplasm is squeezed toward the inner and outer mesaxons and the edges of the sheath. This compaction process is due, presumably, to the strong affinity of the P_0 membrane protein on the inside surface of the Schwann cell membrane for the same protein on the apposed inside membrane. To illustrate, if a part of the inside surface of a balloon had a strong affinity for the inside surface on the opposite side, the sides of the balloon would be drawn together, thereby squeezing the air to the edges of the balloon, which would become a two-layered rubber membrane with air-filled edges. In the same way, as the Schwann cell membrane curls around the axon, P_0 proteins pull the insides of the inner mesaxon membrane together, thereby squeezing the cytoplasm toward the inner and outer loops and the edges, leaving a double-layered membrane that appears in cross section as the **major dense lines**. Further, where the outer membrane surface of one myelin layer is fused with the outer surface of the next layer, an **intraperiod line** is formed, which under electron micrograph fixation conditions appears to be less tightly formed than the major dense lines (see Figure 3.22). Thus, the action of P_0 molecules is another case of homophilic interaction in which there is an adhesion between the same molecules in different areas within a cell, or different cells. Schwann cells grow and encircle adjacent axons, and under the effects of MAG and P_0 the growing edge is induced to burrow under the opposite edge, and forms from inside-out layers of lipid membrane (now called myelin). Oligodendrocytes function similarly in the CNS.

Nodes of Ranvier

As mentioned earlier, the myelin sheath along the axon is discontinuous; that is, it is made up of myelin segments. Each Schwann cell or oligodendrocyte extension forms a single sheath segment about 1 to 1.5 mm long. These segments are separated from one another by the **nodes of Ranvier**. In both the PNS and the CNS, the length of myelin segments is proportional to the thickness of the axon. On axons that range from 3 to 18 μm in diameter, the myelin segments range from 400 to 1,500 μm (0.4–1.5 mm) in length, with nodal intervals of about 4 μm of unmyelinated axolemma between segments.

The node results from the gradual thinning of the myelin sheets, and the rows of cytoplasmic swellings around the node make up the paranodal area. It is proposed that this appearance is the result of the following process: Assuming the buildup of myelin lamellae is from the inside out, it seems that the width of the inner mesaxon, attached to the axon, becomes more and more narrow with every wrap, so that the innermost lamella is the most narrow. By narrowing at the axon's surface, a space develops between neighboring segments (Figure 3.24). If this explanation is correct and if it were possible to unwrap a myelin segment in the PNS or CNS, the myelin segment would appear as an extended flattened sheet having a trapezoidal shape, with the outer and inner mesaxon parallel to each other and the sides converging toward each other from the outer to the inner mesaxon (Jones and Cowan, 1983).

The nodes are highly specialized areas of axons having high capacitance and low electrical resistance that contribute to the efficiency of transmitting action potentials from one end of an axon to the other (see Chapter 5). Also, within the axon at the nodes, a high concentration of mitochondria engages in high levels of metabolic activity to supply the energy needed for the propagation of nerve impulses, which are initiated and amplified at these points. Further, the axolemma at a node has a large concentration of sodium (Na^+) channels, which also have a role in the generation and propagation of nerve impulses. In addition, when myelinated axons branch, the branching occurs at a node.

Myelin Function

We have seen that each layer of myelin consists of double thicknesses of Schwann cell or oligodendrocyte membranes, each about 8.5 nm thick, forming a concentric insulating cover averaging about 4 μm thick. There may be only a few myelin layers or as many as 100, depending upon the thickness of the axon. Within certain limits, the thicker the myelin cover, the better it serves as an insulating material. As mentioned earlier, the presence of intersegmental nodes plays an important role in neuron function by greatly increasing the conduction velocity of nerve impulses, thereby more effectively serving the message-bearing function of the neuron. This subject is discussed in more detail in Chapter 5. The conduction speed of nerve impulses is proportional to axon diameter, but a myelinated axon of average radius (not including the myelin sheaths) conducts nerve impulses at a velocity approximately ten times that of an unmyelinated axon of the same diameter. Since the volume of an axon is directly related to the square of its radius, a myelinated axon occupies a volume 1/100th of that of an unmyelinated axon conducting impulses at a comparable speed. Invertebrates could evolve higher conduction rates by increasing their axonal radii, and in a small insect, two times practically nothing is still practically nothing, so an increase in axon size in these microscopic ranges would not be burdensome to the species. However, as vertebrates evolved with skulls that imposed limits on the housing of increasing numbers of rapidly conducting axons, available space for large axons would be seriously constrained. Thus, myelination of neuraxons is one of the highly significant advances in the evolution of vertebrates. (See Norton, 1976; Morell and Norton, 1980; Schwartz, 1980 and 1991a; Jones and Cowan, 1983; and Lemke, 1992b.)

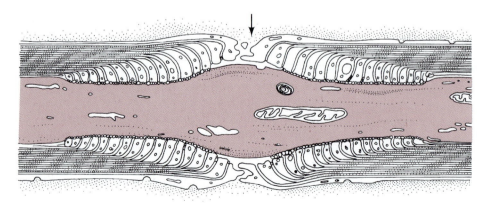

3.24 NODES OF RANVIER. A schematic drawing of a node of Ranvier in the PNS. At each myelin segment, the inner mesaxon narrows as it wraps around the axolemma which leads to the formation of bare axon between neighboring segments of myelin (arrow). The edges of the myelin lamellae (layers) become filled with cytoplasm as the top and bottom membranes are squeezed together. (After Jones and Cowan, 1983.)

Myelin Pathology

The critical role of myelin basic protein in myelin formation can be seen in mice that are homozygous for a mutant MBP gene called *shiverer (shi)* on chromosome 18. The mutation causes bodily shaking and intention tremors when the mouse instigates motor responses. These symptoms are traced to defective CNS myelinization, which also leads to increasingly frequent convulsions and premature death between 50 and 100 days postnatally. In these animals the myelin of peripheral axons appears to be normal, but CNS myelin is largely absent, and where it is present, it appears as abnormal whorls of membrane tightly compacted at the intraperiod line, but cytoplasm-rich and uncompacted at what would normally be the major dense line. Normally, MBP is exclusively located at the sites where it promotes adhesion between the sides of the oligodendrocyte membrane as it wraps around the axon, squeezing out the cytoplasm and forming the major dense line. But in *shi/shi* mice, the major dense line never forms. This is due to a specific 90% deficiency of MBP resulting from a large deletion of about 20,000 base pairs, which constitutes an 84% loss for the gene that expresses MBP protein. Furthermore, when the wild-type gene was injected into fertilized eggs of the *shiverer* mutant, the resultant transgenic mice expressed the wild-type gene at the right time, during the first month after birth, and produced about 20% of the normal amount of myelin basic protein. This resulted in enough of an improvement in the myelination of central neurons to prevent convulsions and give the mice a normal life span, even though they had occasional tremors. These results were definite proof that the mutant MBP gene *(shi)* was responsible for the shivering phenotype. This finding was the first transgenic replacement rescue of a mutant phenotype to be reported in vertebrates (Schwartz, 1991; for more details see Lemke, 1992.)

In conclusion, it can be asserted that myelin is an absolute requirement for the integrative functioning of higher nervous systems. The compelling evidence for this view is the omnipresence of myelin in its various forms in the nervous systems of vertebrates over millions of years, and the critically debilitating effects of inherited or acquired diseases in which the sheaths are imperfectly formed or disintegrate, as in multiple sclerosis.

Summary

The functional units of the nervous system are neurons. Neurons consist of three structural parts: the cell body, dendrites, and an axon. These structures are all covered by a membrane known as the plasmalemma, made up mostly of lipids along with a variety of membrane proteins. The plasmalemma prevents the intrusion into the cell of inappropriate or harmful substances. Oxygen and nutrients necessary for neuron maintenance and function pass through the membrane by a variety of transfer mechanisms, such as simple diffusion, facilitated diffusion, and active transport. Waste products are transported out of the cell in similar ways.

The cell body, with its nucleus of genetic material, directs the synthesis of proteins and lipids that interact with one another to maintain the structure and function of the neuron. Dendrites are the receiving ends of neurons that are stimulated by other neurons to initiate the formation of nerve impulses. Those impulses are transmitted by the axon to the axon terminals, where synaptic action conveys the neural message to postsynaptic neurons or to effector organs.

The internal organization of neurons consists of a protein-based cytoskeleton and organelles such as the endoplasmic reticulum, the Golgi apparatus, mitochondria, and a variety of vesicular bodies that are involved in the gene-controlled synthesis of proteins and lipids and their transport to the dendrites and axon for repair and growth. Neurons also synthesize their own specific neurotransmitters, which are bound within special vesicles that are transported to the axon terminals, where they release their contents when signaled to do so by nerve impulses.

Microtubules that are part of the cytoskeleton serve as tracks for anterograde transport of vesicles and other organelles toward the dendrites or axon terminals. Retrograde vesicle transport occurs simultaneously on the same or similar microtubules toward the cell body for vesicle repair and recycling or for transfer to lysosomes for digestion and disposal. These processes constitute mechanical work requiring energy, usually supplied by ATP generated within mitochondria.

Some groups of axons are covered with myelin sheaths, which significantly increase the velocity and efficiency of nerve impulse propagation while conserving space. The myelin sheaths are formed by glial cells: Schwann cells in the PNS and oligodendrocytes within the CNS. Other varieties of glial cells exist in close proximity to neurons and perform vital functions such as skeletal support, phagocytosis of injured and dead cells, and the uptake and supply of nutrients and some neurotransmitters.

Chapter 4

Functional Neuroanatomy

At the present time, a universally held tenet of neuroscience is that the various forms of brain function that lead to identifiable sensations, perceptions, visceral activities, overt behaviors, and cognitive functions are, to a significant degree, specifically localized anatomically in the nervous system. This was first appreciated toward the end of the nineteenth century when Fritsch and Hitzig in Germany startled the scientific community in 1870 by showing that they could produce characteristic leg movements in dogs by electrically stimulating certain regions of the brain. Also, there were reports that specific neural injuries due to accidents or disease caused specific psychological and behavioral deficits.

Pioneering research was being performed in the United States at about the same time by Herrick and Tite (1890) in which the motor cortex of animals was electrically stimulated to identify the areas that served various motor functions. (It is not known whether the Americans were familiar with the work of Fritsch and Hitzig.) After studies like these, it was proposed that it was now possible to specify which parts of the brain were responsible for the myriad of neurological symptoms observed in hospital patients, a proposal that caused a stir in the medical profession at the time (Herrick, 1893).

Beginning in the 1940s, some experiments with humans were performed during brain surgery to alleviate epilepsy. In the search for epileptic zones in the brain, different parts of the brain were electrically stimulated. Different areas were found to produce or inhibit muscular responses and speech, or the patients would describe specific feelings and thoughts during stimulation (Penfield and Rasmussen, 1950; Penfield and Roberts, 1959). However, results of animal experiments at that time by Lashley (1950) suggested that mental phenomena such as learning, thinking, and memory were dependent more on the amount of viable brain tissue than on any particular part of the brain.

For example, rats that had been blinded shortly after birth by enucleating their eyes were later trained to run in mazes of varying difficulty for food rewards. Such blinded rats learned the mazes almost as well as normal rats, indicating that visual cues were not important for the learning of this task. Other blinded rats had parts of the visual cortex removed in varying degrees before the learning trials, and some received similar lesions after the trials. The results showed that although vision was not critical, the lesions in the visual cortex prior to learning caused learning deficits, and lesions after learning caused deficits in remembering the mazes. Further, the magnitude of the deficits was correlated with lesion size rather than with lesion location, and was also positively correlated with maze difficulty. Based on these results, it was concluded that the visual cortex, aside from its role in vision, had a role in learning and memory, and that complex psychological phenomena are diffusely distributed in the brain. However, it was later argued that it is difficult to dissociate the effects of a lesion on memory or learning from its effects on other psychological processes such as perception, motivation, arousal, and lo-

111

comotor activity. Furthermore, lesion studies indicate only how behavior is altered by the lesion; they do not reveal the function of the damaged tissue (see Kupfermann, 1991d). Nonetheless, Lashley did discover that learning and memory processes are widely distributed in the brain despite the localization of some aspects of these processes.

Recent experiments have been more sophisticated in their means of ascertaining the neural locus for particular kinds of behavior. The song of male canaries, for example, is prominent in the spring, when a longer period of daylight leads to growth of the testes and secretion of the gonadal steroid testosterone, the male sex hormone that modulates sexual function. This hormone binds to and increases the size of the caudal nucleus of the ventral hyperstriatum (HVc) in the brain. This group of cells is an essential unit in a chain of nuclei that innervates the vocal organ, the syrinx, in the throat of birds (Arnold, 1985). Female canaries, which do not usually sing, have a similar HVc, albeit much smaller. In females, however, these brain cells permit the birds to identify the songs of male canaries and elicit courtship behavior indicating readiness to mate. This conclusion was made based on the finding that after damage to the HVc, female canaries still displayed courtship behavior with male canaries, but they also showed similar behavior with white-crowned sparrows, which have very different songs (Brenowitz, 1991; Nottebohm, 1979).

Recently, the functional specificity of some brain areas has been verified by positron emission tomography (PET) scanning. With this technique, one can observe changes in blood flow and metabolism in human brain areas associated with reading, speaking, and thinking. Further refinements in the technique have made it possible to distinguish among the effects in the visual cortex of the conditions of eyes closed, the presentation of a simple white light, a complex scene. PET scans showed a wider involvement of brain tissue as more information was being processed. Similarly, increasing involvement of brain tissue was seen in the auditory cortex when subjects heard nothing, when they listened to a story, or when they were told to remember certain phrases in the story. The last condition produced the widest area of increased metabolism in the auditory cortex as well as in the hippocampus, a part of the brain that is important for memory (Martin, Brust, and Hilal, 1991).

The nervous system can be thought of as an information input, processing, storage, retrieval, and output system. It deals with stimuli that arise from the internal environment of the body as well as stimuli from the external environment. These stimuli provide the information that is sent via the sensory nerves to the central nervous system (CNS), where it is routed to appropriate brain centers for processing into awareness of sensations and perceptions, for storage in memory, and for the elicitation of relevant motor responses.

Organization of the CNS

The CNS in vertebrate animals is made up of about 100 to 180 billion neurons, but it is not a homogeneous structure like the liver or the kidneys. Rather, there are about 10,000 different types of neurons, and clusters of similar neurons make up **nuclei**, which occupy specific areas in the CNS and have specific functions. These nuclei are functionally and anatomically distinct with respect to their inputs from hormones and from other nuclei, as well as outputs via their own axons to other neurons or to muscles and glands.

Some nuclei are related to sensory functions, such as the **dorsal column nuclei** (nucleus gracilis and cuneatus), which are located in the medulla (see below). These nuclei relay sensory information from ascending spinal tracts to higher centers such as the thalamus and cerebral cortex for conscious awareness and for storage as memory traces. Other nuclei mediate motor effects, such as the **oculomotor nuclei** in the midbrain, which control the muscles for eye movement. These nuclei are highly integrated with other nuclei, such as the **vestibular nuclei**, which contribute signals from the vestibular apparatus, near the inner ear. Thus, as we walk or run, our eye movements compensate for the up-and-down and side-to-side head movements so that we have a steady frontal view instead of a view that bounces left and right and up and down.

Furthermore, nuclei that are functionally related are juxtaposed to form subsystems that are integrated with other subsystems. For example, in humans, the thalamus, the cerebellum, and the basal ganglia are subsystems that interact to modulate motor activity, making movements accurate and coordinated. This integration allows us to walk, talk, and perform other skilled movements such as tying shoelaces or buttoning a shirt while being hardly aware of our actions. These simple acts would be very difficult if we had to think about each and every finger response to the touch signals that are involved, but because all of the delicate sequences are firmly bound in a kind of "motor memory," we can perform these functions even in the dark. Even though we know that the movements of an instrumental musician or an athlete must be coded in the nervous system, it is difficult to comprehend how the nerve impulse traffic can bring this about. On the other hand, almost all animal activity rests upon the same principles, and the activities of the virtuoso merely call our attention to those principles. Even understanding how an 18-month-old infant walks and runs tells us a great deal about the remarkable structure and efficiency of the nervous system.

A comprehensive description of the central nervous system and its functions would require many volumes, and our description is meant only to be relevant to the neuroanatomical structures we will mention frequently as they pertain to our foremost subject, psychopharmacology. With our descriptions, we have presented pictor-

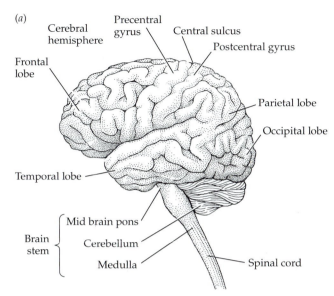

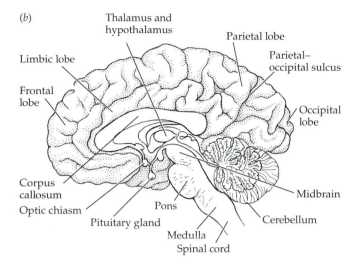

4.1 THE HUMAN CNS. (*a*) A lateral view. (*b*) A medial view.

ial illustrations of many neural structures and systems, but space limitations preclude the variety of views that are necessary for optimum visualization. These deficiencies can be overcome by referring to one of the many excellent atlases of neuroanatomy that are available.

Figure 4.1*a* is a lateral view of the human CNS; Figure 4.1*b* is a medial view showing internal brain structures that are hidden in the lateral view. These two figures should be carefully examined and referred to as we proceed with the topic of neuroanatomy. We will describe the function(s) of the various parts proceeding from the least complex structure, the spinal cord, to the more complex ones.

Part I
The Spinal Cord, Brain Stem, Diencephalon, Limbic System, and Basal Ganglia

The Spinal Cord

The spinal cord is a segmented column with 30 pairs of spinal nerves attached to it (one pair is shown in Figure 4.2*a*). Spinal nerves are made up of afferent and efferent neuraxons that form dorsal (sensory) and ventral (motor) roots. The dorsal roots originate from a cluster of cell bodies in the **dorsal root ganglion**. These nerves transmit somesthetic messages from the skin, muscles, tendons, and joints, and form synaptic connections with a variety of cells in the gray matter of the spinal cord (the H-shaped portion). The gray matter contains large numbers of glia and neuronal cell bodies, arranged in

functional nuclei (clusters) that extend longitudinally over many segments, forming cell columns.

Upon entering the spinal cord, the sensory nerves divide into three functional branches: one branch may ascend in the dorsal column to the brain stem (see Figure 4.2*b*[1]); other branches terminate locally in the spinal cord and form synapses in the gray matter (see Figure 4.2*b*[2 and 3]) either with spinal cells serving spinal reflexes or with cells that relay sensory signals in the white matter to upper levels of the cord for higher levels of coordination and conscious awareness of the sensory modalities. Other branches descend a few segments (see Figure 4.2*b*[4]) to coordinate upper and lower muscle systems.

The ascending and descending myelinated tracts in the white matter are named according to the direction that neural messages are transmitted within them—from one spinal cord level to another, or to upper relay points in the brain stem and the brain (see below). For example, sensory spinal nerves mediating touch and pain synapse with cells in the dorsal horn (see Figure 4.2*a*), whose axons cross to the opposite side and ascend as the anterior spinothalamic tract to the ventral posterolateral nucleus of the thalamus. In turn, the axons from the thalamus extend to their target area in the sensory areas of the brain (Figure 4.3).

In contrast, the sensory nerves mediating the sense of fine touch enter the spinal cord, and without synapse with other neurons, ascend as the fasciculus gracilis (from the lower trunk and limbs) and the fasciculus cuneatus (for the upper trunk and limbs), both of which make up the dorsal columns. In the brain stem, the fasciculus gracilis and the fasciculus cuneatus synapse with cells in the dorsal column nuclei (nuc. gracilis and cuneatus, respectively). The axons from these nuclei relay the sensory signals of fine touch across to the opposite side, where they join the fibers of the anterior spinothalamic tract to form the **medial lemniscus**, which projects to the thalamus and then to the sensory area of

(a)

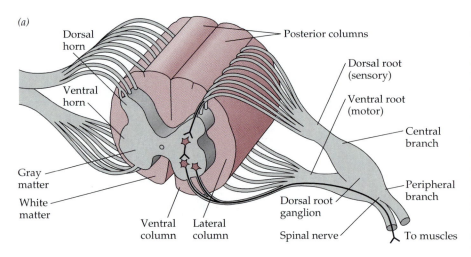

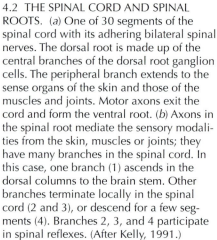

4.2 THE SPINAL CORD AND SPINAL ROOTS. (*a*) One of 30 segments of the spinal cord with its adhering bilateral spinal nerves. The dorsal root is made up of the central branches of the dorsal root ganglion cells. The peripheral branch extends to the sense organs of the skin and those of the muscles and joints. Motor axons exit the cord and form the ventral root. (*b*) Axons in the spinal root mediate the sensory modalities from the skin, muscles or joints; they have many branches in the spinal cord. In this case, one branch (1) ascends in the dorsal columns to the brain stem. Other branches terminate locally in the spinal cord (2 and 3), or descend for a few segments (4). Branches 2, 3, and 4 participate in spinal reflexes. (After Kelly, 1991.)

(b)

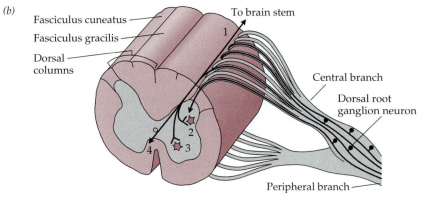

the brain. The direct route of this system partly explains the speed and the fine discrimination of this touch sense in contrast with the sense of pain or thermal sense, which are comparatively slow and diffuse because they synapse many times in their ascent to the brain. These pathways are examples of ascending tracts that form anatomically separate pathways for each of the different sensory modalities: light and fine touch, pressure, pain and thermal sense, and proprioception from muscles and tendons.

We have seen that almost all ascending sensory pathways, at one stage or another, cross to the white matter on the opposite side of the cord and ascend in that position to the brain. Similarly, movements of muscles on the right side of the body originate on the left side of the brain, since most descending pathways cross to the opposite side to effect motor responses. Consequently, there are a number of commissural fibers at most levels of the spinal cord, the brain stem, and the brain itself (note the internal arcuate fibers in Figure 4.3).

The descending tracts are named according to the origin and termination of their messages. For example, the corticospinal tract descends from the cerebral cortex to the spinal cord to stimulate the motor cells in the ventral horns of the spinal cord, whose axons transmit messages to the muscles of the trunk and extremities for the maintenance of posture, balance, and movement. In similar fashion the corticobulbar tract (the word *bulb* describes the medulla) descends from the cerebral cortex to terminate at various levels of the brain stem to stimulate motor nuclei of the cranial nerves. These nerves activate the voluntary muscles of the head, such as those that move the eyes and jaw, those involved in facial expression, and those used in the pharynx, larynx, and tongue for articulating speech. Other descending tracts, such as the cerebellospinal tract and the reticulospinal tract, branch off to the cranial motor nerves in their descent to the motor nerves of the spinal cord. Their function is the coordination of cranial and bodily musculature. The cranial and spinal motor nerves are the final common pathway to the skeletal muscles, and all the information about motor activity is transmitted via these nerves to the appropriate muscles. Thus, the overall function of the spinal cord is to receive coded information from the exteroceptors of the body via sensory nerves and process it in two ways. First, it integrates this information with motor nerves for spinal reflexes. If a barefoot person steps on a sharp stone with the left foot, sensory nerves are activated by nociceptors (pain sensors) on the foot and convey messages to the spinal cord to synapse with motor nerves that stimulate the ipsilateral (same side) flexor muscle, causing an immediate flexion of the left

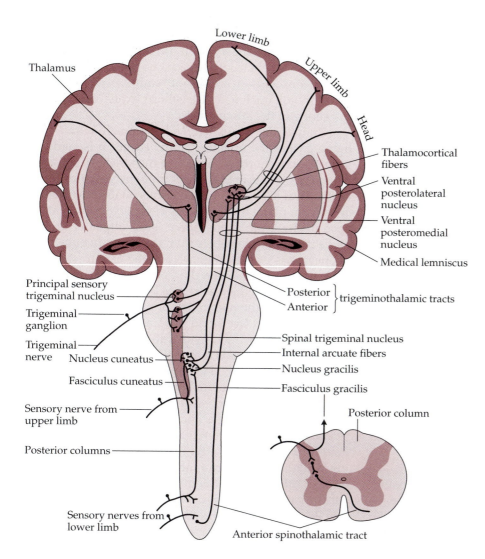

Thalamus

Lower limb

Upper limb

Head

Thalamocortical fibers

Ventral posterolateral nucleus

Ventral posteromedial nucleus

Medical lemniscus

Principal sensory trigeminal nucleus

Trigeminal ganglion

Trigeminal nerve

Nucleus cuneatus

Fasciculus cuneatus

Posterior
Anterior } trigeminothalamic tracts

Spinal trigeminal nucleus

Internal arcuate fibers

Nucleus gracilis

Fasciculus gracilis

Sensory nerve from upper limb

Posterior columns

Posterior column

Sensory nerves from lower limb

Anterior spinothalamic tract

4.3 THE DISCRIMINATIVE GENERAL SENSORY PATHWAYS: the anterior (ventral) spinothalamic tract, the posterior dorsal column–medial lemniscus pathway, and the trigeminothalamic pathway, which mediates touch sensibility for the head, face, and oral surfaces. Interneurons are omitted in some pathways. (After Noback and Demarest, 1977, *The Nervous System: Introduction and Review*, © Williams & Wilkins.)

leg to raise the foot from the stone. This action is called a flexion reflex.

But there is more to consider. With the flexing of the left leg, the contralateral (opposite side) extensor muscle reflexively contracts to extend and stiffen the right leg to support the body weight when the left leg is withdrawn from the ground. In addition, the lifting of the left leg with the flexor muscle cannot occur unless the opposing extensor muscle in the same leg is relaxed (inhibited). This occurs because the sensory message of pain is also carried to an interneuron that inhibits the left extensor muscle. The interneuron does that because its chemistry at the synapse is different from that of the excitatory synapse. Further, the extension of the right leg requires that the flexor muscle on the right leg be relaxed. These reflex reactions are known as **crossed extensor reflexes**.

The second function of the spinal cord is to relay information about the spinal activities (via ascending tracts) in the white matter to reach higher control centers such as the cerebellum and the brain, and to convey control signals (via descending tracts) back down the spinal cord to activate, for instance, the skeletal muscles of the trunk and forelimbs (arms) to coordinate arm and trunk movements to maintain balance. The ascending sensory tracts also activate higher centers such as the thalamus and cortex, necessary for the experience of pain and the emission of "ouch."

At this point, one might ask what determines which of the many reflex pathways is activated. The answer, of course, is that the nature of the stimulus determines the activated pathway—pain on the sole of the left foot elicits a left limb flexion and a right limb extension and stiffening. In contrast, slight pressure against the soles of the feet will elicit limb extension and stiffening. This is easily demonstrated with an infant about 6 months old. If you were to hold the infants' hands in your left hand, and with your right hand push gently against the soles of her feet while you lift her in the air, her legs will stiffen and she will assume a standing position.

Our description of spinal reflexes is markedly incomplete, because in reality hundreds of thousands of neurons would be involved in the described reflex, but it illustrates the fundamental nature of neural events. Behavior involves the stimulation of sense organs; the sense organs code a message that activates neurons; the neurons transmit the coded message to the spinal cord, where some motor neurons are activated and others are inhibited; the message is relayed to higher centers, resulting in finer control (that takes the immediate circumstances into account) and conscious awareness. In our example about the barefoot person above, the net result is this: the foot is removed from the offending stone without causing the person to topple over, the person perceives pain, and the details of the episode are remembered.

The Brain Stem

The brain stem can be subdivided, in ascending order, into the medulla, the pons and cerebellum, and the midbrain. As we discussed briefly above, in addition to the sensory and motor tracts in the brain stem, there are special sensory and motor nerves, known as **cranial nerves**, that mediate the special senses, such as vision, audition, taste, and smell (Figure 4.4). Some cranial nerves also mediate control of autonomic functions such as respiration, heart rate, and gastrointestinal (GI) functions. The functional anatomy of the autonomic nervous system will be described in more detail in a later section.

The Cranial Nerves

The cranial nerves provide the direct sensory inputs and efferent outputs of the brain stem. The afferent (sensory) cranial nerves mediate the special senses such as smell, vision, taste, hearing, and cutaneous senses from the head, face, and mouth, as well as inputs from internal organs of the chest and abdomen such as the heart, the respiratory organs, and the GI tract. The efferent (motor) cranial nerves exert control over the musculature of the head, such as the muscles of facial expression, the lower jaw and the tongue, and the larynx and pharynx (for speech), activate the salivary and lachrymal glands, and modulate the organs of the chest (heart and lungs) and abdomen (GI tract). (The pelvic organs—the bladder, colon, and reproductive organs—are controlled by pelvic nerves emanating from the lower levels of the spinal cord, which will be described in a later section.)

The basal view of the brain stem in Figure 4.4 shows the peripheral afferent and efferent branches of the cranial nerves. For convenience, the cranial nerves are identified by Roman numerals I through XII. The relative positions of the relay nuclei for the sensory cranial nerves are shown in black, while the cranial motor nuclei are shown in color. A summary of the functions of the cranial nerves is given in Table 4.1.

The axons from the cranial sensory relay nuclei project to the thalamus and brain for conscious sensations and to the cranial motor nuclei for reflexes. For example,

the sour taste of vinegar is mediated by the sensory branches of cranial nerves VII, IX, and X, which synapse in the solitary nucleus, whose axons project to the cortex for the conscious awareness of "sour," as well as to the facial motor nucleus (VII), whose axons mediate the puckering of the lips and face.

Cranial nerve I, which mediates smell, is shown as being part of the olfactory bulb because it is made up atypically of short projections of the olfactory sense organs. These short fibers project from the posterior recess of the nasal cavity through a porous bone structure (the cribriform plate) to synapse in the olfactory bulb at the base of the brain. Thus, there is no olfactory cranial nerve per se, and the fibers from the olfactory bulb to the deeper parts of the brain are defined as a tract, as are most fiber groups within the CNS, while fibers outside of the CNS are defined as nerves. Nonetheless, the olfactory tract from the bulb to the brain is often referred to as cranial nerve I (see Dodd and Castellucci, 1991).

The olfactory tract divides and forms synapses at a number of relay points that project to different terminations, indicating that olfactory information serves many functions, such as determining the acceptability of foods, territorial cues, cues for sexual expression, and identification of pack members and offspring. (Observe what your cat does when offered a novel morsel of food, and how your dog examines the territory during your morning walk.) It is the termination of the fibers in the orbitofrontal cortex that is involved with the conscious perception of smell. The orbitofrontal cortex is that part that lies over the eye sockets (orbits) in the skull; people with lesions in the orbitofrontal cortex are either anosmic or cannot discriminate between odors, nor can they identify objects by smell.

The optic nerve (N. II), which mediates vision, is also defined as a tract because the homologue of the sensory nerve is the microscopic layer of bipolar cells in the retina. The retinal rods and cones provide the input to the bipolar cells, which synapse with ganglion cells in the retina that give rise to the pathway to the brain. Thus, the pathway from the eye to the brain technically is also a tract. Further, after a short distance from the orbits, the nasal half of the visual fibers crosses to the opposite side in the so-called optic chiasm. This has led some anatomists to arbitrarily call the prechiasmatic fibers the optic nerve and the postchiasmatic fibers the optic tract. This arrangement also has no morphological basis.

The axons of the retinal ganglion cells enter the brain stem as the optic nerve (N. II) and synapse at their respective relay nuclei in the midbrain for reflexes (see below). Other optic fibers project to the lateral geniculate body of the thalamus and, via the optic radiations, to the occipital lobe for visual sensations and perceptions. Visual stimuli are projected from the retina to the Edinger–Westphal nucleus, whose axons make up a part of the oculomotor nucleus and cranial nerve III, for vi-

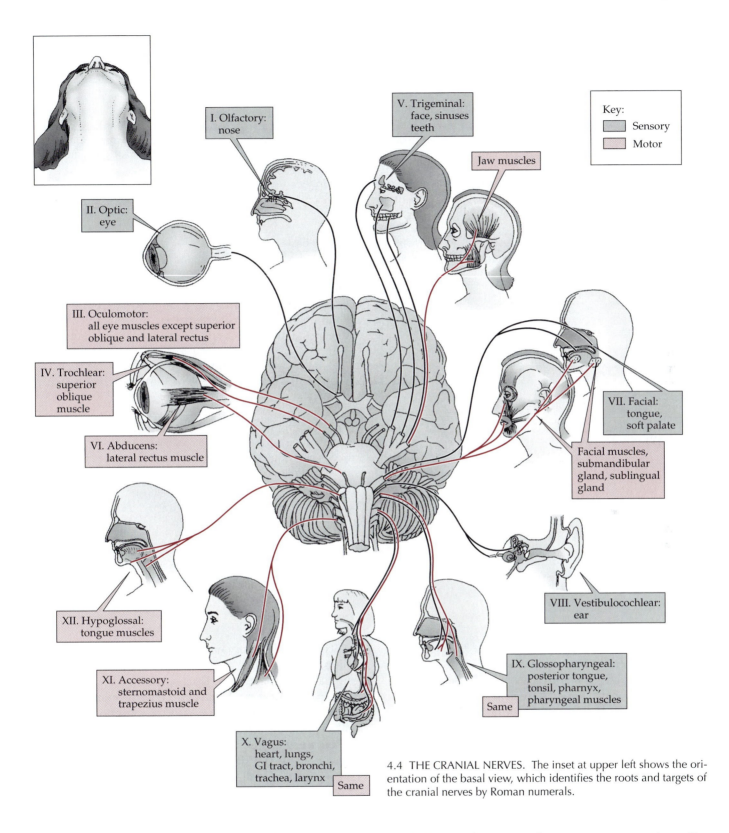

I. Olfactory: nose

II. Optic: eye

III. Oculomotor: all eye muscles except superior oblique and lateral rectus

IV. Trochlear: superior oblique muscle

VI. Abducens: lateral rectus muscle

XII. Hypoglossal: tongue muscles

XI. Accessory: sternomastoid and trapezius muscle

X. Vagus: heart, lungs, GI tract, bronchi, trachea, larynx

Same

V. Trigeminal: face, sinuses teeth

Jaw muscles

Key:

Sensory

Motor

VII. Facial: tongue, soft palate

Facial muscles, submandibular gland, sublingual gland

VIII. Vestibulocochlear: ear

IX. Glossopharyngeal: posterior tongue, tonsil, pharnyx, pharyngeal muscles

Same

4.4 THE CRANIAL NERVES. The inset at upper left shows the orientation of the basal view, which identifies the roots and targets of the cranial nerves by Roman numerals.

sual reflexes such as adjustments of pupil size, focus for near and far vision, and eye movement for tracking moving stimuli, reading, and maintaining a constant gaze when the head is moving.

From the occipital lobe, association fibers project to almost all other parts of the brain, adding visual input needed for reading, muscular movements, emotions, discrete recognition of objects, writing, and special forms of perception such as the recognition of faces. Also, auditory messages travel via N. VIII from the inner ear (the cochlea) to the cochlear nuclei for relay to reflex centers in the midbrain for startle reactions to sudden loud

Table 4.1 Functions of the Cranial Nerves

Cranial nerve	Type of nerve	Functions
Olfactory (I)	Sensory	Smell
Optic (II)	Sensory	Sight
Oculomotor (III)	Motor	Eye movements: innervates all extraocular muscles except the superior oblique and lateral rectus muscles (see N. IV and VI); innervates the striated muscle of the eyelid; mediates pupillary constriction and accommodation of the lens for near vision
Trochlear (IV)	Motor	Eye movements: innervates superior oblique muscle
Trigeminal (V)	Mixed	Sensory: mediates cutaneous and proprioceptive sensations from skin, muscles, and joints in the face and mouth, and sensory innervation of the teeth
		Motor: innervates muscles of mastication
Abducens (VI)	Motor	Eye movements: innervates lateral rectus muscle
Facial and intermediate (VII)	Mixed	Motor: innervates muscles of facial expression, lacrimal glands, salivary glands
		Sensory: mediates taste sensation from the anterior two-thirds of the tongue, and sensation from skin of external ear
Vestibulocochlear (VIII)	Sensory	Hearing, balance, postural reflexes, and orientation of the head in space
Glossopharyngeal (IX)	Mixed	Autonomic fibers innervate the parotid gland
		Swallowing: mediates visceral sensations from the palate and posterior one-third of the tongue
		Innervates the carotid body
		Innervates taste buds in posterior third of the tongue
Vagus (X)	Mixed	Autonomic fibers innervate smooth muscle in the heart, blood vessels, trachea, bronchi, esophagus, stomach, and intestine
		Innervates striated muscles in the larynx and pharynx and controls speech
		Mediates visceral sensation from the pharynx, larynx, thorax, and abdomen
		Innervates taste buds in the epiglottis
Spinal accessory (XI)	Motor	Motor innervation of the trapezius and sternocleidomastoid muscles
Hypoglossal (XII)	Motor	Motor innervation of the intrinsic muscles of the tongue

Source: After Role and Kelly, 1991.

sounds, or to the temporal lobes of the brain for conscious awareness and meaning of sounds in the environment and the perception of speech and music.

The other cranial nerves have features similar to those of spinal nerves; that is, the motor nerves emerge from motor nuclei in the brain stem (Figure 4.5). Also, some cranial nerves have sensory as well as motor functions (see Table 4.1). But some of the motor nerves are classed as special motor nerves because they mediate effects upon the heart and lungs and upon abdominal and other visceral organs (see below). It can be noted that the spinal accessory nerve (XI) is very similar anatomically and functionally to the spinal motor nerves, but because the motor outputs of this nerve are within the medulla, it is defined as a cranial motor nerve. This nerve controls the trapezius muscle, which raises the shoulder, and the sternocleidomastoid muscles, which are attached to the sternum of the chest and go around the head to the opposite mastoid processes behind the ears to turn the head horizontally.

The cranial sensory nerves, except those for smell and vision, have sensory ganglia similar to the dorsal root ganglia of the spinal cord. Thus, the cell bodies of the sensory division of nerve V make up the **trigeminal ganglion** (sometimes known as the Gasserian ganglion), and the cell bodies of the sensory branch of nerve VII make up the **geniculate ganglion**. For the auditory and vestibular branches of nerve VIII, the cell bodies are found in the **spiral ganglion** and **vestibular ganglion**, respectively.

Sensory data of touch, pain, heat, and cold from the head, face, and mouth are projected by the trigeminal nerve (V) to the trigeminal nucleus. They are then relayed to the facial motor nucleus (VII), for reflexes such as blinking in response to tactile stimulation of the cornea and facial responses to bad-tasting substances, as well as to the thalamus and brain for conscious sensations, as shown in Figure 4.3.

Taste messages from the tongue enter the brain stem via the sensory branches of nerves VII, IX, and X to

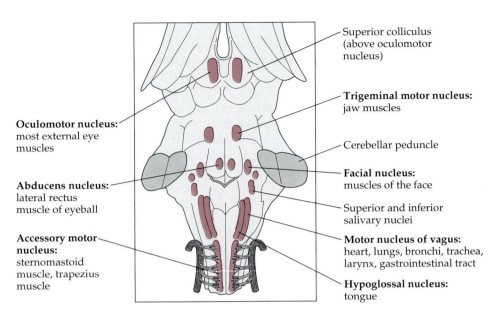

Oculomotor nucleus:
most external eye
muscles

Abducens nucleus:
lateral rectus
muscle of eyeball

Accessory motor
nucleus:
sternomastoid
muscle, trapezius
muscle

Superior colliculus
(above oculomotor
nucleus)

Trigeminal motor nucleus:
jaw muscles

Cerebellar peduncle

Facial nucleus:
muscles of the face

Superior and inferior
salivary nuclei

Motor nucleus of vagus:
heart, lungs, bronchi, trachea,
larynx, gastrointestinal tract

Hypoglossal nucleus:
tongue

4.5 MOTOR NUCLEI OF THE CRA-
NIAL MOTOR NERVES. With the cerebellum removed, the superior and inferior colliculi are seen on the dorsal
surface of the brain stem. The positions
of the motor nuclei of the cranial
nerves are also shown.

synapse at the solitary nucleus for relay to the salivary nuclei (VII and IX) for salivation, or to the thalamus and brain for conscious taste (see Table 4.1). Sensations from the GI tract, such as feelings of hunger or pain caused by abnormal distension or constriction of the intestines, are also projected to the solitary nucleus for relay to the brain. Thus, specific sensory information from the tactile or special senses is projected to sensory nuclei and relayed to specific motor nuclei for reflexes, or to the thalamus and brain for the conscious awareness of touch, pain and temperature, smell and taste, hearing, and vision.

The cranial nerves can also be classified as afferent or efferent, somatic or visceral, and special (for special senses) or general (for cutaneous senses). However, there is one class of motor fibers, **special visceral efferents**, that requires some explication. The special visceral motor fibers mediate the action of the facial muscles, the jaw, the neck, and the pharynx and larynx, all of which we perceive as being under voluntary control. But are they? A little introspection reveals that sometimes we cannot control our facial muscles when we experience a foul odor, hilarity, or grief or sadness, and the same is true of the larynx when we groan in pain, cry or shriek, or betray our emotions by the way we talk. Because these nerves and muscles evolved from the gill apparatus that provides for autonomic respiration in fishes, and are derived from our embryological gill arches (hence, *branchiomeric* "pertaining to the gills"), the nerves that mediate these responses are classed as special visceral efferents, suggesting that they are sometimes somatic and sometimes autonomic depending on their input (see Role and Kelly, 1991).

Thus, in the brain stem, there are sensorimotor reflexes mediated by the cranial nerves, there are outputs for "voluntary" or "visceral" control over some of the muscles of the head, and there are centers for the autonomic control of visceral activity such as salivation, respi-

ration, the heartbeat, and the activities of the GI tract. Most of these autonomic effects are mediated by the efferents of cranial nerve X, the **vagus nerve**. It will be seen below that this nerve makes up part of the cranial parasympathetic branch of the autonomic nervous system and is widely dispersed to the organs of the chest and abdominal cavity; hence its name, the vagus (wanderer).

An overall view of the function of the cranial nerves shows that they work in tandem in many intricate ways. The unifying structure for the interactions of the cranial nerves is the **medial longitudinal fasciculus** (MLF) (L. *fasciculus*, "small bundle"), a prominent nerve bundle in the brain stem that receives inputs from and provides outputs to virtually all cranial nerve sensory and motor nuclei, as well as those in the upper segments of the spinal cord for movement of the head and neck. Moreover, this system receives an input from the motor cortex via corticobulbar pathways for each of the cranial motor nerves for voluntary control during eating, facial expressions, and above all, speech. (*Bulb* is an archaic name for the brain stem.) Further, motor control of the bulbar motor nuclei is influenced by the cerebellum and basal ganglia, which modulate the control of voluntary motor effects. Thus, higher control centers and the MLF play a significant role in the reflex and voluntary interactions among the cranial nerves, such as taste–salivation reflexes, tongue–jaw–facial muscle interactions, pain–blinking–tears–facial–vocal responses, smell–facial expressions, smell–gastric (nausea) effects, vestibulooculomotor–head–trunk interactions, vestibulo–gastric sensations (nausea), auditory–oculomotor reactions (for sound localization), and many others.

The Cerebellum

The cerebellum constitutes about 10% of the total brain volume, yet it contains about half of all the neurons in the CNS. This structure is situated over the dorsal surface of the pons and is connected to the brain stem by three pairs of nerve bundles, the superior, middle, and inferior peduncles (peduncle, a stem or support) (Figure 4.6). It is highly organized into ten different lobules, each with an outer mantle (the cerebellar cortex), and each lobule mediates motor control over a different area of the body. In the cerebellar interior, there are four pairs of deep nuclei (the dentate, emboliform, globose, and fastigial), which receive the outflow from the cerebellum via the Purkinje cells of the cerebellar cortex and project it to various parts of the CNS.

There are three functional regions in the cerebellum: (1) the vestibulocerebellum, which is the oldest part of the cerebellum, (2) the spinocerebellum, and (3) the cerebrocerebellum, which is the most recent part. The **vestibulocerebellum** (the flocculonodular lobe) receives information from the semicircular canals and projects, along with the vestibular connection, to the vestibular nuclei. After the input from the cerebellum, the output of the vestibular nuclei is projected via the vestibulospinal tracts to the spinal cord to modulate postural reflexes. Further, the output from the vestibulocerebellum via the deep cerebellar nuclei (the dentate and fastigial

nuclei) is projected to the nuclei of the oculomotor nerves III, IV, and VI and to the MLF to modulate reflexive eye movements. Thus, this part of the cerebellum governs eye movement and body equilibrium during stance and gait. During any body movement, the vestibulocerebellum maintains a steady gaze and body equilibrium. Imagine a deer running through the woods to escape from a predator. It has to attend to its footing while dodging among the trees and boulders and making sharp turns to outrun its foe. This requires sharp visual constancy for the bounding animal, which must instantly decide where to put its feet down on its chosen path of escape.

The **spinocerebellum** is organized as a complete somatosensory map of the body and is located in the cerebellar vermis and the adjacent intermediate part of the cerebellar hemispheres. It receives its principal inputs from the muscles of the body by way of ascending spinocerebellar tracts, which originate from the nucleus dorsalis (Clarke's nucleus) in the spinal cord. It also receives information from the auditory, visual, and vestibular systems. The output of the spinocerebellum is localized in the deep cerebellar nuclei, from which some efferents

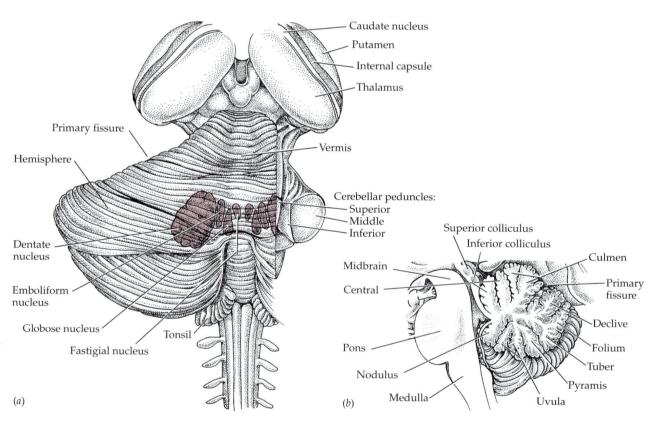

4.6 GROSS FEATURES OF THE CEREBELLUM. (*a*) A dorsal view, with the right hemisphere removed, showing the underlying cerebellar peduncles, which are made up of the input and output pathways of the cerebellum. The positions of the deep cerebellar nuclei are highlighted in color. (*b*) A midsagittal section showing the branching structure of the cerebellum and its relationship to the pons area of the brain stem.

emerge to ascend to the red nucleus (see below), from which the rubrospinal tract descends to the spinal cord to modulate voluntary movements. Its output also projects to the thalamus and motor cortex, which modulate the motor output via the corticospinal tracts.

The **cerebrocerebellum** (in the cerebellar hemispheres) receives its inputs from the sensory, motor, and parietal cortex by way of the relay nuclei in the pons. That is, these cortical areas give rise to corticopontine fibers that synapse in the pontine gray and are then projected laterally to the cerebellar hemispheres. From the cerebellar hemispheres, the output is projected to the cerebellar deep nuclei, then to the ventral lateral nucleus of the thalamus, and then as a feedback to the motor cortex. Functionally, this circuit forms a loop: cortex to pons to cerebellum to thalamus and back to cortex. This circuit, along with the cerebellorubral and rubrospinal system, plays a special role in planning and initiating movement.

Together, the inputs and the outputs of the subregions of the cerebellum indicate that it is able to compare internal feedback signals that reflect the *intended* movement with external feedback signals that reflect the *actual* movement. This control is thought to be dependent upon both information that the cerebellum receives from cortical motor areas about the intended motor command and feedback from the spinal cord and periphery, which provides details about the evolving movement. From the foregoing, it is possible to appreciate some of the important influences that bear upon the motor cells in the brain stem and spinal cord that mediate the great variety of muscular activity that is expressed as facial expression and speech, digital manipulation, arm and leg movements, and postural adjustments.

An overall view of the function of the cerebellum can be illustrated by a description of movement by a patient with a lesion in his right cerebellar hemisphere. He reported that the movements of his left arm were done subconsciously, but that he had to think out each movement of his right (affected) arm. Also, when he wanted to make a turn while walking, he had to come to a dead stop and think before he started to move again. Thus, it has been proposed that the "cerebellum spares us this mental task: A general movement command from the higher brain centers leaves the details of the execution of the movement to subcortical, notably cerebellar, control mechanisms." (For a review see Ghez, 1991.)

The Reticular Formation

The reticular formation might be called a brain stem accessory. It is an extension of the interneuronal networks of the spinal cord, but it is considerably more extensive. In the discussion of the spinal cord, it was noted that there are intricate arrangements of interneurons between the sensory inputs and the motor outputs of the spinal reflexes. These and other types of interneurons are said to be the building blocks of reflexes; that is, they are instrumental as to which sensory inputs are enhanced and which are suppressed, and which muscles contract or relax, in a wide variety of motor activities such as maintaining postures, rhythmic locomotor patterns in walking or running, and manipulative actions of the hands. Such intervention by interneurons is found almost everywhere in the CNS.

The reticular formation extends from the medulla to the red nucleus of the midbrain. It is made up of neurons organized in nuclear groups that distribute their axons widely in rostral and caudal directions, thereby forming widespread networks. Figure 4.7 represents a single neuron of the reticular formation of a 2-day-old rat. The relatively large cell bodies of these neurons lie in the gigantocellular nucleus of the pons, and the cell axon bifurcates into descending and ascending branches with many perpendicular collateral branches along its course. Thus, these neurons have multiple terminals permitting widespread interactions with other neurons. One estimate is that a single neuron in the reticular formation may have inputs from 4,000 other neurons (convergence), and may make contact with 25,000 other neurons (divergence).

Some of the inputs and outputs of the reticular formation are shown in Figure 4.8a and b, with the insets showing the origins and the positions of the ascending spinoreticular and the descending reticulospinal tracts. The inputs to these cells come from alternate ascending tracts in the spinal cord to make up a variety of spinoreticular pathways, including a large proportion of those that mediate pain. Other inputs that come from the nuclei of cranial nerves, especially the vestibular and cochlear nerves, mediate motor reflexes and an alerting function, respectively. The slightest rustle in the leaves will instantly alert an animal to the possible presence of a predator. There are also inputs from the cerebellum, the thalamus, and the frontal, motor, and sensory areas of cortex.

With respect to the outputs of the reticular formation, it is safe to say that reciprocal connections exist with virtually all of the input sources. Hence, branches of ascending sensory tracts terminate in the reticular formation, and descending axons from the reticular formation make up the reticulospinal tracts, which terminate on interneurons near the motor cells in the ventral horn of the spinal cord. Thus, reflex motor activities at the spinal level have a second order of modulation via the reticular formation and its descending tracts. This is illustrated by the finding that stimulating the pontine region of the reticular formation enhances extensor muscle tone, and that stimulating the reticular nuclei in the medulla exerts an inhibitory influence on extensor muscle tone.

The reticular formation has four major functions. First, the ascending connections to the thalamus and cor-

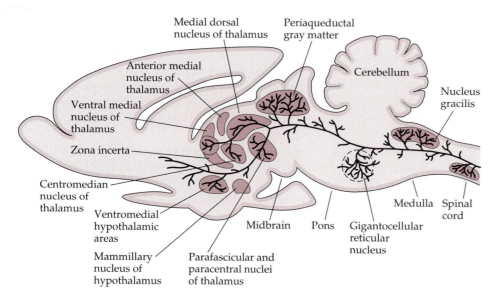

Medial dorsal
nucleus of thalamus

Periaqueductal
gray matter

Anterior medial
nucleus of
thalamus

Cerebellum

Nucleus
gracilis

Ventral medial
nucleus of
thalamus

Zona incerta

Centromedian
nucleus of
thalamus

Ventromedial
hypothalamic
areas

Midbrain   Pons

Medulla   Spinal
cord

Gigantocellular
reticular
nucleus

Mammillary
nucleus of
hypothalamus

Parafascicular and
paracentral nuclei
of thalamus

4.7 THE RETICULAR FORMATION. A neuron whose cell body lies in the nucleus giganto-cellularis of a 2-day-old rat illustrates the axonal divergence and widespread contact with other neurons that is characteristic of cells in the reticular formation.

tex serve as an activating system that regulates alertness. This conclusion is based on the finding that stimulating the reticular formation of a deeply anesthetized animal results in a change in the animal's electroencephalogram from a sleeping to a wakeful state. This activating and alerting function is particularly appropriate for the perception of pain because it signals something that requires immediate attention. It also contributes to the disagreeable nature of pain, since it cannot be easily ignored.

A second function of the reticular formation is the modulation of extensor muscle tone that was already mentioned. A third function is the modulation of heart rate and blood pressure. The carotid sinus is a receptor in the carotid artery that is sensitive to blood pressure changes. If the pressure increases, the receptor is activated and sends a neural message to a sensory nucleus in the brain stem (the solitary nucleus), which activates the vagus nerve, causing bradycardia (a slower heart rate), and inhibits certain sympathetic nerves that normally increase vascular tone. The fourth function is the attenuation of pain by a descending reticulospinal tract that terminates in the dorsal horn gray and diminishes the effects of pain-mediating sensory nerves of the spinal cord.

Thus, the reticular formation serves as a higher level of sensorimotor control that intervenes between the spinal cord and the brain. In addition, it channels sensory inputs to alert an organism and focus its attention according to its needs. It mediates cardiovascular effects and diminishes the perception of pain, which can lead to shock and paralysis instead of struggling if the pain is intense. All of these functions contribute to readiness and exertion to respond, which is especially valuable when responding to untoward events.

The Midbrain

At the midbrain, or mesencephalon, level of the brain stem, a horizontal section (Figure 4.9) shows a change in its overall shape because of the bundling of most of the descending tracts to form the cerebral peduncles (basis pedunculi or crus cerebri). Also found at this level of the brain stem are the already mentioned oculomotor nuclei (III) and the medial longitudinal fasciculus (MLF). An important level of motor control in the midbrain is the modulation of eye movements, which is centered in the superior colliculi (L. *colliculi*, "little hills") of the midbrain, which appear as swellings on the tectum (roof) (see Figure 4.9). There are several different types of eye movements, one of which holds images stable on the retina during brief head movements or sustained head rotation. Another, known as visual pursuit, holds the image of a moving target on the fovea. The third kind of movement occurs when scanning a view or reading. The perception is that the eyes move smoothly over the scene or along a line of print, but in reality, the eyes make little jerky movements with in-between pauses (saccades). Further, when looking to one side, one eye turns outward (pulled by the lateral rectus muscle) and the other eye turns inward (pulled by the medial rectus muscle) to a greater or lesser degree. In this case different muscles are coordinated for appropriate vergence.

The superior colliculi are made up of layers of cells that receive inputs from the retina, the visual cortex, the vestibular apparatus, the vestibulocerebellum of the cerebellum, the visual nucleus of the thalamus (the lateral

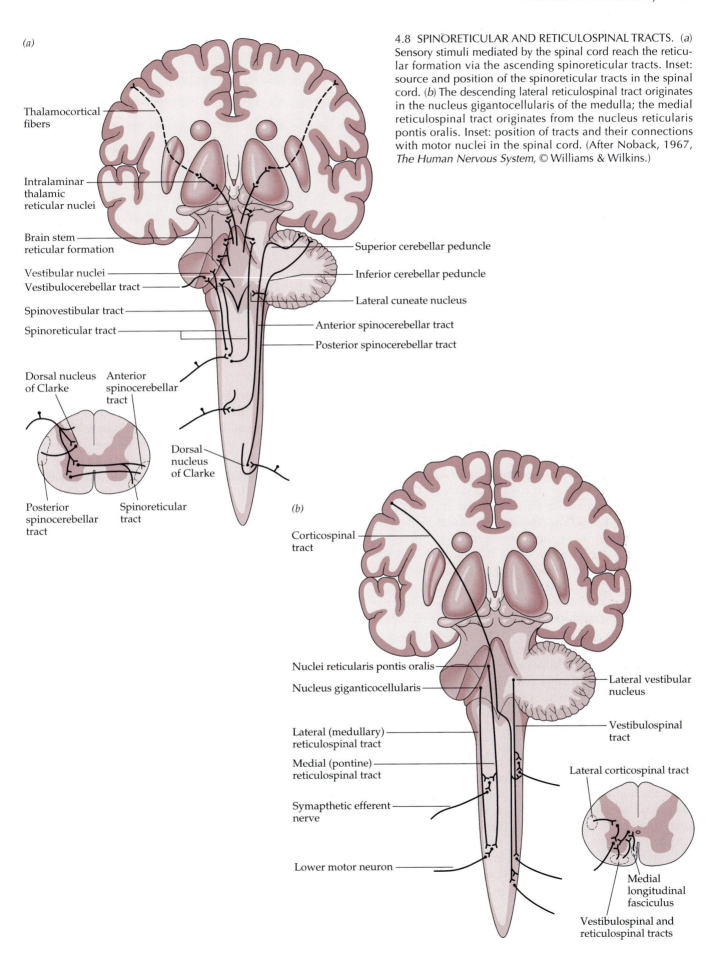

(a)

Thalamocortical fibers

Intralaminar thalamic reticular nuclei

Brain stem reticular formation

Vestibular nuclei

Vestibulocerebellar tract

Spinovestibular tract

Spinoreticular tract

Dorsal nucleus of Clarke

Anterior spinocerebellar tract

Posterior spinocerebellar tract

Spinoreticular tract

Superior cerebellar peduncle

Inferior cerebellar peduncle

Lateral cuneate nucleus

Anterior spinocerebellar tract

Posterior spinocerebellar tract

Dorsal nucleus of Clarke

4.8 SPINORETICULAR AND RETICULOSPINAL TRACTS. (a) Sensory stimuli mediated by the spinal cord reach the reticular formation via the ascending spinoreticular tracts. Inset: source and position of the spinoreticular tracts in the spinal cord. (b) The descending lateral reticulospinal tract originates in the nucleus gigantocellularis of the medulla; the medial reticulospinal tract originates from the nucleus reticularis pontis oralis. Inset: position of tracts and their connections with motor nuclei in the spinal cord. (After Noback, 1967, *The Human Nervous System*, © Williams & Wilkins.)

(b)

Corticospinal tract

Nuclei reticularis pontis oralis

Nucleus giganticocellularis

Lateral (medullary) reticulospinal tract

Medial (pontine) reticulospinal tract

Symapthetic efferent nerve

Lower motor neuron

Lateral vestibular nucleus

Vestibulospinal tract

Lateral corticospinal tract

Medial longitudinal fasciculus

Vestibulospinal and reticulospinal tracts

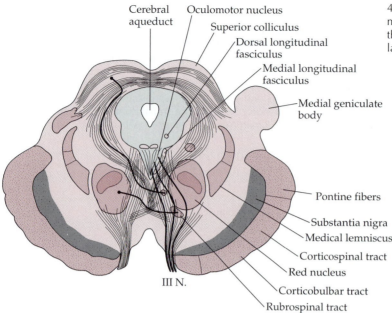

Cerebral aqueduct
Oculomotor nucleus
Superior colliculus
Dorsal longitudinal fasciculus
Medial longitudinal fasciculus
Medial geniculate body
Pontine fibers
Substantia nigra
Medical lemniscus
Corticospinal tract
Red nucleus
Corticobulbar tract
Rubrospinal tract
III N.

4.9 THE MIDBRAIN. A cross section through the human midbrain at the superior colliculus. The brachium (arm) of the inferior colliculus is its pathway to the medial geniculate body of the thalamus.

geniculate bodies), the reticular formation, and the basal ganglia. The outputs from these structures, of course, are channeled to the motor nuclei of cranial nerves III, IV, and VI, mediated by the integrating function of the MLF that was described earlier. The superior colliculi are also sensitive to auditory messages that signify sound locations. That is, the stimuli for a sound source on the right might be the difference in the time between the sound's stimulation of the far ear (the left) and the near ear (the right). In animals, these differences control the turning of the head and the positioning of the eyes toward the sound source. Recent evidence suggests that neurons in the superior colliculi send patterns of neural signals to a part of the auditory cortex that translates them into the position of the sound source (Middlebrooks et al., 1994). The control of eye movement, while very intricate, can be easily examined in detail by asking a person merely to look up, look down, look to the left, look to the right, and follow a moving finger. Many dysfunctions within the brain stem will be reflected by a lack of coordination of these eye movements. (For a detailed discussion of this subject, see Goldberg, Eggers, and Gowras, 1991.)

Slightly caudal to the superior colliculi are the inferior colliculi, which receive inputs from the ascending auditory fibers from the cochlear nuclei and relay the output to the auditory thalamus (the medial geniculate body or nucleus; see Figure 4.9) and then to the primary auditory cortex in the temporal lobe. There is also a feedback circuitry from the cortex back to the medial geniculate body, then to the inferior colliculi and from there back to the cochlea. These connections may be important for regulating attention to particular sounds by modulating the transduction mechanism in the inner ear (see J. P. Kelly, 1991a). An example of such regulation is sometimes

known as the "cocktail party effect;" that is, the ability, when in a crowd, to "tune out" all the loud conversation around yourself and to hear and process only the talk of the person with whom you are conversing. In most elderly persons, this effect is diminished, and the surrounding noise interferes with the desired conversation.

A prominent feature of the midbrain tegmentum is the **red nucleus**, which is regarded as part of the midbrain reticular formation, and is so named because of its rich vascularity. It is a prominent junction for tactile and proprioceptive inputs from the spinal cord, cerebellum, motor cortex, vestibular nuclei, superior colliculi, basal ganglia (see below), and the motor and parietal cortex. The output of the red nucleus is the rubrobulbar and rubrospinal tracts, which project mainly to the cranial motor nuclei and the motor nuclei of the spinal cord on a somatotopical basis; that is, the motor control of specific muscle groups is preserved from the motor cortex to the spinal levels. There are also some reciprocal fibers from the red nucleus back to the cerebellum and to the ventral lateral nucleus of the thalamus for relay to the motor cortex. Thus, the red nucleus is a prominent junction in a sensorimotor feedback loop originating in the spinal cord as the spinocerebellar tract, which projects proprioceptive information to the cerebellum, whose output projects to the red nucleus, which gives rise to the rubrospinal tract that modulates the spinal motor output to the somatic musculature.

Another feature of the midbrain is the substantia nigra (L., "black substance"), positioned in the dorsal area of the cerebral peduncles (see Figure 4.9). The darkly pigmented cells in this area have reciprocal inputs with the part of the basal ganglia known as the striatum via the nigrostriatal and the strionigral pathways. These pathways have significant effects upon motor systems, as we shall see below.

The Diencephalon

The diencephalon consists of the thalamus, epithalamus (which includes the habenula), subthalamic nucleus, and hypothalamus. It occupies a rostrolateral position at the top of the brain stem. Further, as shown in cross section in Figure 4.10, the diencephalon in mammals, and especially in humans, is covered and encircled by the cerebrum, which interacts with the thalamus to a high degree. The coronal section of a human brain through the diencephalon shows the position of the thalamus, which borders both sides of the third ventricle. Above the thalamus and adjoining the lateral ventricle is a part of the caudate nucleus, and lateral to the thalamus is the globus pallidus, both of which are parts of the basal ganglia and interact with the thalamus (see below).

Between the basal ganglia and the thalamus is the internal capsule, consisting of sensory fibers ascending from the thalamus to the sensory cortex and motor fibers descending from the motor cortex. Below the ventral border of the internal capsule and extending caudally into the cerebral peduncle of the midbrain is the subthalamic nucleus, which is an integral part of the basal ganglia (see below).

The Thalamus

Our discussion of the CNS up to this point has included many references to the thalamus as having nuclei that serve as synaptic relays of sensory and cerebellar information to the cerebral cortex. Figure 4.11 is a three-dimensional view of the thalamus on the left side of the brain, showing the approximate positions of the thalamic nuclei. (The medial thalamic nucleus, not shown, is joined to the medial nucleus on the opposite side by bridging fibers known as the massa intermedia.)

Relay nuclei. The thalamic nuclei are classified into two functional groups: relay nuclei and diffuse projection nuclei. The relay nuclei receive inputs of specific sensory modalities and project them to specific areas of the sensory cortex. For example, inputs of touch from the hand go via sensory spinal nerves to the spinal cord and ascend in the dorsal columns to the nuclei of the dorsal columns (e.g., nucleus gracilis and cuneatus) and from there to the thalamic ventral posterior lateral nucleus, from which the "touch" messages are relayed to the primary somatic sensory cortex in the postcentral gyrus (see Figure 4.3). Auditory inputs go to the medial geniculate body, and are relayed from there to the primary auditory cortex in the temporal lobe, whereas, as described above, visual inputs go to the lateral geniculate body and are relayed to the primary visual cortex in the occipital lobe. The thalamic medial dorsal nucleus is also a relay center. It is one of the structures that receives olfactory information from the olfactory tubercle, which in this case is relayed to the orbitofrontal cortex for conscious perception of smell. Thus, sensory functions to a great extent maintain their own identity and account for the specific sensory awareness of these stimuli; that is to say, there is no confusion between what is seen or heard and what is smelled.

However, sensory information is also channelled to other relay nuclei and brain areas for different effects.

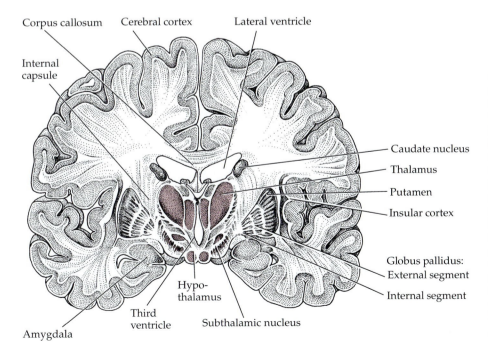

Corpus callosum   Cerebral cortex   Lateral ventricle

Internal capsule

Caudate nucleus

Thalamus

Putamen

Insular cortex

Globus pallidus:
External segment

Internal segment

Hypo-thalamus

Third ventricle   Subthalamic nucleus

Amygdala

4.10 THE DIENCEPHALON. A coronal section through the human diencephalon (*colored structures*) shows the highly developed cerebral hemispheres. The cortex (gray matter) follows the folded surface of the hemispheres. The thalamus forms the wall of the third ventricle and lies dorsal to the hypothalamus; the internal capsule separates the thalamus from the lenticular nucleus, which consists of the putamen and the globus pallidus and is part of the basal ganglia. Parts of the caudate and subthalamic nuclei are also shown. Beneath the cerebral cortex are the abundant bundles of ascending, descending, and commissural axons that interconnect all areas of the cortex, with the corpus callosum connecting the left and right hemispheres. (After Nieuwenhuys, Voogd, and van Huijzen, 1981.)

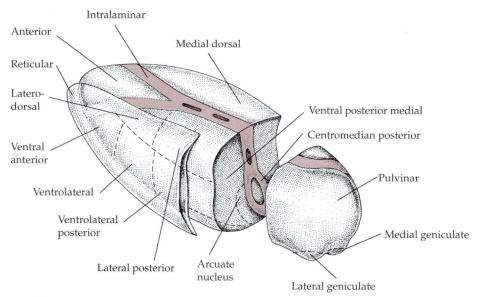

Anterior
Intralaminar
Medial dorsal
Reticular
Latero-dorsal
Ventral anterior
Ventrolateral
Ventrolateral posterior
Lateral posterior
Arcuate nucleus
Lateral geniculate
Ventral posterior medial
Centromedian posterior
Pulvinar
Medial geniculate

4.11 THE MAJOR NUCLEI OF THE THALAMUS.

For example, touch information is also projected from the thalamic lateral posterior nucleus to the **posterior parietal lobe**, which is an association area of the cortex. This makes it possible to put your hand in your pocket and recognize by touch that the size, mass, and shape of the object in your pocket is that of a dime, not a quarter, and is not enough for the parking meter. Also, visual data from the occipital lobe is projected to the pulvinar nucleus, which is the largest of the thalamic nuclei. This nucleus also receives visual data from the superior colliculi and has reciprocal connections to the temporal and parietal lobes. These connections give meaning to visual objects so that a key, a pencil, or a written telephone number are instantly recognized for what they are and what their functions are.

Diffuse projection nuclei. In contrast to the sensory relay nuclei, the diffuse projection nuclei (the midline, intralaminar, centromedian, and reticular nuclei) have more widespread connections and influence larger areas of the cerebral cortex, as well as the other nuclei of the thalamus itself. It will be seen that inputs from sensory, hypothalamic, and reticular systems to the diffuse projection system contribute to the integration and to the motivational aspects of the resulting behavior. The inputs to the diffuse projection nuclei are from branches of the spinothalamic tracts via the reticular formation, the hypothalamus, and the cerebral cortex via the basal ganglia; the outputs project back to the neural centers from which the inputs originated. Destruction of the intralaminar nuclei in animals results in temporary somnolence, lethargy, and minimal reactivity to noxious stimuli. Thus, the diffuse projection nuclei are presumed to regulate the overall level of excitability of different functional divisions of the cortex and the degree of arousal of the brain. The relationship between the thalamus and the basal ganglia will be described below.

The Hypothalamus and Limbic System

As shown in Figure 4.12*a*, the hypothalamus is an integral part of the diencephalon. It has connections with the thalamus as well as with the structures of the limbic system, of which it is also a part (see below). The function of the hypothalamus and the limbic system is to contribute to the constancy of the internal environment of the organism, a process known as homeostasis, and initiate behavior that contributes to the survival of the self and the species. Within the hypothalamus are a number of nuclei that respond to neural and hormonal signals related to heart rate, hunger, water balance, blood loss, body temperature, level of sex hormones in the blood, and needs associated with growth and procreation. These hypothalamic nuclei (Figure 4.12*b* and *c*) receive inputs from the primary olfactory cortex, the reticular formation, the hippocampus by way of the fornix and the mammillary bodies, the amygdala, the cingulate and parahippocampal gyri, and the neocortex. Most of the structures contributing inputs to the hypothalamus, with the exception of the neocortex, make up the limbic system.

In the limbic system, the amygdala has a prominent role. As shown in Figure 4.13*a*, it has two nuclear groups, the corticomedial and the basolateral nuclei. The corticomedial nucleus receives its major input from the olfactory bulbs via the lateral olfactory tract, and has interconnections with the contralateral amygdala and the ipsilateral basolateral group. Thus, the amygdala is intimately connected to the olfactory and limbic systems. These connections are particularly significant in animals

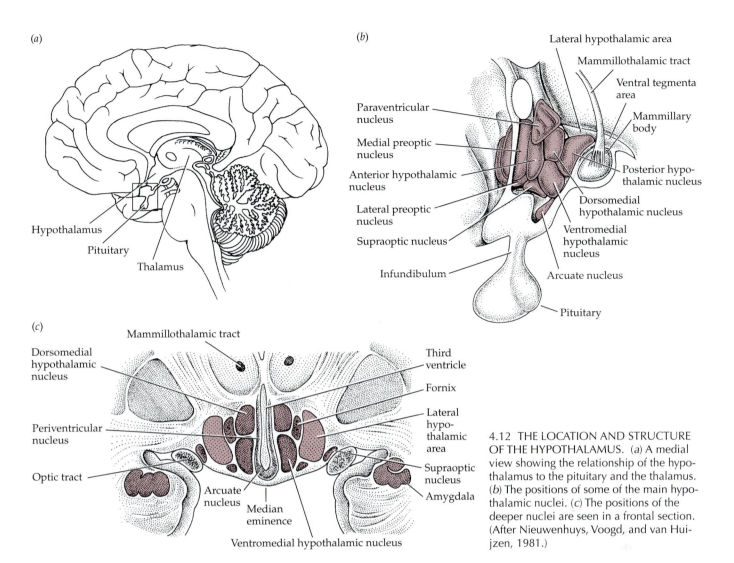

(a)

Hypothalamus
Pituitary
Thalamus

(b)

Lateral hypothalamic area
Mammillothalamic tract
Ventral tegmenta area
Mammillary body
Posterior hypo-thalamic nucleus
Dorsomedial hypothalamic nucleus
Ventromedial hypothalamic nucleus
Arcuate nucleus
Pituitary

Paraventricular nucleus
Medial preoptic nucleus
Anterior hypothalamic nucleus
Lateral preoptic nucleus
Supraoptic nucleus
Infundibulum

(c)

Mammillothalamic tract
Dorsomedial hypothalamic nucleus
Periventricular nucleus
Optic tract
Arcuate nucleus
Median eminence
Ventromedial hypothalamic nucleus
Third ventricle
Fornix
Lateral hypothalamic area
Supraoptic nucleus
Amygdala

4.12 THE LOCATION AND STRUCTURE OF THE HYPOTHALAMUS. (*a*) A medial view showing the relationship of the hypothalamus to the pituitary and the thalamus. (*b*) The positions of some of the main hypothalamic nuclei. (*c*) The positions of the deeper nuclei are seen in a frontal section. (After Nieuwenhuys, Voogd, and van Huijzen, 1981.)

that constantly monitor their environment for its olfactory content. The corticomedial cells project via the **stria terminalis** in a roundabout way to the septal region and the preoptic area of the hypothalamus on the same and opposite side (crossing over in the anterior commissure).

The basolateral group has many reciprocal interconnections with the cortex of the parahippocampal gyrus, which in turn has important connections with the neocortex of the temporal and the frontal lobe as well as the cingulate gyrus, as shown in Figure 4.13*b*. There are projections via the **ansa peduncularis** to the dorsomedial nucleus of the thalamus, which projects to association cortex; the ansa peduncularis projects as well to the hypothalamus and the septal region (see Figure 4.13*a*). The amygdala also receives inputs from other sensory sources, which are integrated and coordinated with autonomic and endocrine responses to provide the emotional tone to sensory inputs.

The outputs of the hypothalamus, as shown in Figure 4.13*c*, descend to the midbrain, pons, medulla, and spinal cord via the **medial forebrain bundle**, the **dorsal longitudinal fasciculus**, the **central tegmental tract**, and the **reticulospinal tract**, which activate the nuclei of the cranial efferent nerves such as V, VII, IX, and XII. These cranial nerves innervate the muscles of the face and head for eating, biting in defense, or killing prey, as well as emotional expression: whining for food or snarling, growling, and baring the teeth in defense of offspring or a food cache. Some of the branches of the vagus nerve (X) that energize the GI tract are also activated. Further, in the thoracic and lumbar segments of the spinal cord, cells in the lateral intermedial nucleus (nucleus intermediolateralis) are activated by the descending central tegmental tract. These cells energize the sympathetic nervous system, which mediates responses to fear or competition (higher blood pressure, faster heart and respiratory rate, perspiring, and release of epinephrine) that promote strength and stamina for fighting or flight (see the section on the autonomic nervous system below).

There are also hypothalamic outputs to the thalamus and the forebrain, and to the ventrally adjacent pituitary gland, whose hormones activate the gonads, the thyroid,

(a)

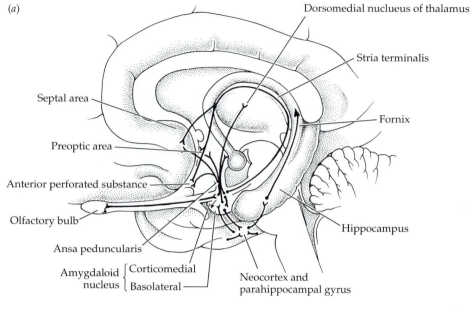

Dorsomedial nucleus of thalamus

Stria terminalis

Septal area

Fornix

Preoptic area

Anterior perforated substance

Olfactory bulb

Hippocampus

Ansa peduncularis

Amygdaloid { Corticomedial
nucleus { Basolateral

Neocortex and
parahippocampal gyrus

(b)

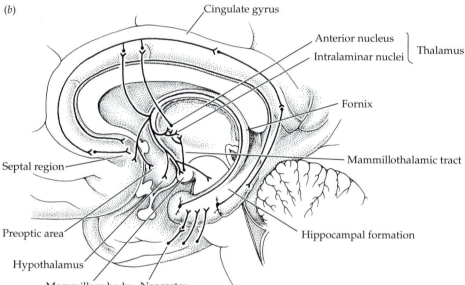

Cingulate gyrus

Anterior nucleus

Intralaminar nuclei } Thalamus

Fornix

Septal region

Mammillothalamic tract

Preoptic area

Hippocampal formation

Hypothalamus

Mammillary body   Neocortex

(c)

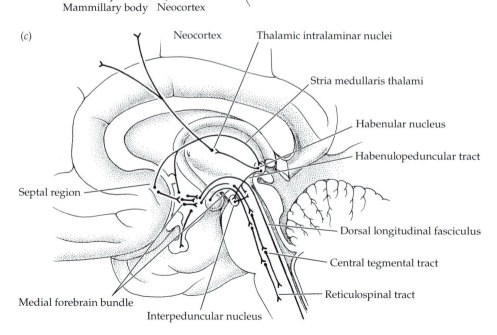

Neocortex   Thalamic intralaminar nuclei

Stria medullaris thalami

Habenular nucleus

Habenulopeduncular tract

Septal region

Dorsal longitudinal fasciculus

Central tegmental tract

Reticulospinal tract

Medial forebrain bundle

Interpeduncular nucleus

4.13 SCHEMA OF SOME CONNEC-
TIONS OF THE LIMBIC SYSTEM. (a)
The amygdaloid nucleus projects via
the stria terminalis and the ansa peduncularis to the septal area, the anterior
perforated substance, the hypothalamus, the contralateral amygdaloid nucleus, the dorsomedial nucleus of the
thalamus, and the cerebral cortex. (b)
There are also connections between the
hippocampus and the mammillary bodies via the fornix; from the mammillary
bodies to the anterior nucleus of the
thalamus via the mammillothalamic
tract; from the anterior nucleus to the
cingulate gyrus, and from the cingulate
gyrus back to the hippocampus. (c) The
outputs from the limbic system are projected from the septal region via the
stria medullaris thalami to the habenula
and then to the interpeduncular nucleus, or via the median forebrain bundle to the midbrain tegmentum. Both
systems contribute to the dorsal longitudinal fasciculus and the central tegmental tract, which project to the brain stem
and the spinal cord for the enactment
of motivated behavior. Major connections made by the descending tracts are
with the intermediolateral column in
the spinal cord. These connections
serve as the major inputs to the sympathetic nervous system. (After Noback,
1967, *The Human Nervous System,* ©
Williams & Wilkins.)

and the adrenal glands, which release hormones related to growth and metabolism. Thus, the hypothalamus is the key neuronal mechanism that acts directly upon the internal organs to maintain homeostasis by controlling the endocrine glands and the autonomic nervous system. Also, through its control and integration of emotions and motivated behavior, the hypothalamus acts indirectly to maintain homeostasis by providing motivating stimuli (such as hunger, thirst, or sexual arousal) so that animals (and humans) act on a challenging, changing, and oftentimes unpredictable environment. Such behavior that is immediately related to needs is regulated by what has come to be known as the **motivational system**, which in large part is synonymous with the limbic system (Kupfermann, 1991b,c).

Role in emotions.   As seen in Figure 4.13*b*, one of the structures of the limbic system is the cingulate gyrus. The cingulate gyrus covers the top of the brain stem and serves as a border between the brain stem and the cerebral hemispheres, and is part of the limbic lobe (L. *limbus*, "border"). The structures of the limbic lobe are the hippocampus, the mammillary bodies, the septal area, the habenula, the nucleus accumbens (a part of the striatum), the amygdala, which receives an important afferent input from the olfactory system, and the orbitofrontal cortex.

In 1937 James Papez proposed that the limbic lobe (i.e., the parahippocampal, the cingulate, and the subcallosal gyri) was part of a neural circuit that serves as the substrate for emotional expression, with the hypothalamus playing a significant role. He also proposed that because higher cognitive processes can affect emotions, the hypothalamus must have reciprocal communication with higher cortical centers. The so-called Papez circuit was elaborated from the findings of subsequent studies to bring other structures into the circuit, as shown in Figure 4.14.

Early experiments in the 1930s showed that by stimulating various areas of the hypothalamus in anesthetized animals via indwelling electrodes, it was possible to elicit autonomic responses such as alterations of heart rate, blood pressure, and gastrointestinal motility and bladder contractions. Hess (1954) improved the technique of hypothalamic stimulation by permanently fastening long, thin, flexible connecting cables to an animal's skull so that the stimulation effects could be observed in awake, freely mobile animals. He found that stimulation of certain parts of the hypothalamus produced characteristic constellations of responses making up organized forms of behavior. For example, stimulation of the lateral hypothalamus in cats elicited autonomic and somatic responses characteristic of anger: increased blood pressure, raised body hair, pupillary dilation, arched back, and raised tail.

Thus, it was proposed that the hypothalamus, in conjunction with limbic structures, integrates and coor-

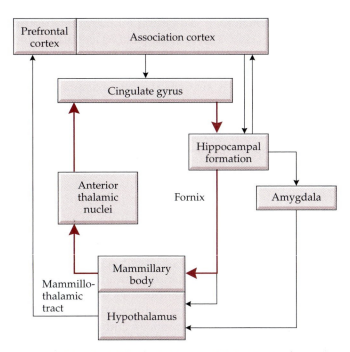

4.14 PROPOSED NEURAL CIRCUIT FOR EMOTION. The original Papez circuit is indicated by thick lines; more recent additions are in fine lines. The amygdala, along with the hypothalamus and the prefrontal cortex, are interconnected with limbic structures, and the reciprocal connections between the hippocampal formation and the association cortex are shown. (After Kupfermann, 1991).

dinates the behavioral expression of emotional states. This notion was supported by lesion and electrical stimulation studies that related various emotional states to different hypothalamic structures. For example, as mentioned above, electrical stimulation of the lateral hypothalamus elicited responses typical of anger, whereas lesions of the same area resulted in placidity. In contrast, animals having lesions in the medial hypothalamus became highly excitable and were easily triggered into aggressive responses. Further, Klüver and Bucy (1939) found that bilateral destruction of the temporal lobes, which include several limbic structures such as the hippocampus and the amygdala, produced dramatic changes in the emotional behavior of monkeys. Animals that were formerly quite wild became tame and showed remarkable oral tendencies in that they put all sorts of inappropriate objects in their mouths. They also showed inappropriate sexual tendencies, such as attempting to mate with a different species such as a chicken or with an inanimate object such as a teddy bear.

The connections between the limbic lobe, the hypothalamus, and other parts of the limbic system can be thought of as a "prewired," genetically determined system that manages internal processes as well as behaviors that promote the survival of the organism. This system is responsible for feelings of hunger and the behaviors that alleviate it, whether eating grass or meat, and the mechanisms by which food is digested for supplying useful energy. It is sensitive to an inadequate water balance and provides sensations of thirst that energize drinking behavior to restore the proper water balance in all tissues and body fluids. It also ensures the existence of the species by means of sex drives expressed toward conspecifics by courtship and reproductive behavior and parental behaviors such as nest building, brooding, feeding, nurturing (sometimes by both parents), and protecting the pups, cubs, chicks, or babies.

The Basal Ganglia

We have previously mentioned that the basal ganglia participate in the control of motor activity. Much of our knowledge of the motor functions of the basal ganglia first emerged from clinical observations that the motor dysfunctions of Parkinson's and Huntington's disease were related to postmortem findings of basal ganglia pathology. In contrast to dysfunction of the corticospinal systems, which results in spasticity and paralysis, basal ganglia dysfunction is characterized by tremor and involuntary movements, changes in posture and muscle tone, and poverty and slowness of movement without paralysis. Later, symptoms unrelated to movement, such as cognitive and affective disturbances, were found to be frequent accompaniments to the motor difficulties in Parkinson's disease, and in virtually all cases of Huntington's disease.

The four subcortical nuclei that make up the basal ganglia do not have direct input or output connections with the spinal cord. Rather, their primary input comes from the cerebral cortex, and their output is relayed through the thalamus and then back to the prefrontal, premotor, and motor cortices. The interconnected nuclei of the basal ganglia are shown in a three-dimensional view in Figure 4.15*a*. Figures 4.15*b* and *c* are schematic representations of coronal sections through the basal ganglia and the thalamus showing the major connections among the parts of these two systems. The lenticular (lens-shaped) nucleus is seen as consisting of the **putamen** and the **globus pallidus**, which is divided into external and internal segments (see Figure 4.15*c*). A section of the **caudate** (tail-like) **nucleus** and the subthalamic nucleus is also shown. Because the putamen and the globus pallidus are grouped together and referred to as the lenticular nucleus, the output pathways from these structures are conveniently known as lenticular fasciculi; and because the cells of the caudate nucleus and putamen are of the same type and the two nuclei are fused together anteriorly, they are known collectively as the **striatum** (i.e., striated), and their inputs and outputs are designated as **striatal** (e.g., "the corticostriate projection") (see below).

Figure 4.15*b* shows the major inputs to the striatum from the sensory and motor areas of the cerebral cortex, which make up the corticostriate projection, as well as the minor inputs from the diffuse projection centromedian nucleus of the thalamus. Figure 4.15*c* shows that there are reciprocal connections among the nuclei of the basal ganglia, and connections with the subthalamic nucleus and the substantia nigra. The major efferents from the basal ganglia, shown in Figure 4.15*c*, mainly arise from the globus pallidus, whose signals from the fibers ending in the external segment are relayed to the internal segment. The target area of the axons from the globus pallidus is the thalamus, especially the ventral lateral, the ventral anterior, and the centromedian nuclei, whose own outputs are projected back to the cortical areas that provided the inputs to the caudate in the first place.

These interconnections are summarized in Figure 4.16, which shows the source of the corticostriate projection as well as the reciprocal inputs between the putamen and the substantia nigra and between the centromedian nucleus and the putamen. In addition, there are reciprocal connections between the globus pallidus and the subthalamic nucleus (see below), and connections (not shown) from the globus pallidus to the medial dorsal thalamic nucleus, which projects to the amygdala, to other limbic structures, and to the frontal cortex.

The specificity of the motor, sensory, sensory association, and limbic cortex is maintained in the striatum, the globus pallidus, and the thalamus; hence the relay back to the cortex is to the specific sources in the cortex. By means of these connections, motor activity mediated by the corticobulbar and the corticospinal tracts is influenced by the loop from the cortex to the basal ganglia to the thalamus and back to the cortex.

Subthalamic and nigral effects.   The subthalamic nucleus, or subthalamus, is shown in Figure 4.16 as having reciprocal connections with the globus pallidus, but it also has an output to the ventral lateral and ventral anterior nuclei of the thalamus and thus to the premotor cortex, as well as to the red nucleus and the substantia nigra. Further, commissural connections are also made with the contralateral subthalamus, the globus pallidus, and the red nucleus.

The subthalamus thus serves as a relay in a circuit involving the basal ganglia that runs parallel to the corticospinal system, and is concerned with stabilizing cortically initiated motor responses. Interest in the subthalamus developed when it was found that it was involved in motor dysfunction. Lesions in the subthalamus or damage to its neural connection to the globus pallidus may be caused by stroke-induced blockage of its blood supply, or may occur in Huntington's disease when the activity of the subthalamus may be abnormally suppressed due to atrophy within the striatum (see below). Damage to the subthalamus itself leads to a form of hy-

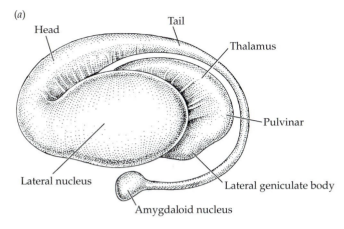

(a)

Head
Tail
Thalamus
Pulvinar
Lateral nucleus
Lateral geniculate body
Amygdaloid nucleus

4.15 GEOMETRY OF THE BASAL GANGLIA. (*a*) A lateral view of the lenticular and caudate nucleus and the thalamus within the left hemisphere of the human brain. (*b*) Some major connections among the basal ganglia, thalamus, and cerebral cortex. The cerebral cortex projects to the caudate and the putamen, which themselves are interconnected. The globus pallidus has reciprocal connections with the subthalamus, but the major output from the globus pallidus is to the ventral anterior nucleus which projects back to the cortex; a few pallidofugal fibers project to the ipsilateral and contralateral ventromedial nucleus of the hypothalamus. (*c*) Collaterals of the corticospinal and corticoreticular tracts project to the striatum (caudate and putamen), and to the red nucleus and substantia nigra, as does the output of the globus pallidus. The output from the red nucleus and the substantia nigra is projected to the centromedian and the ventral anterior nucleus of the thalamus, both of which project to the premotor cortex. (After Noback, 1967, *The Human Nervous System,* © Williams & Williams).

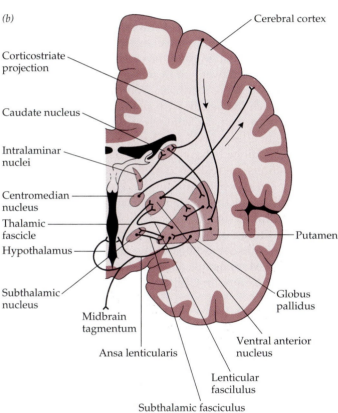

(b)

Cerebral cortex
Corticostriate projection
Caudate nucleus
Intralaminar nuclei
Centromedian nucleus
Thalamic fascicle
Hypothalamus
Subthalamic nucleus
Midbrain tagmentum
Ansa lenticularis
Lenticular fascilulus
Subthalamic fasciculus
Putamen
Globus pallidus
Ventral anterior nucleus

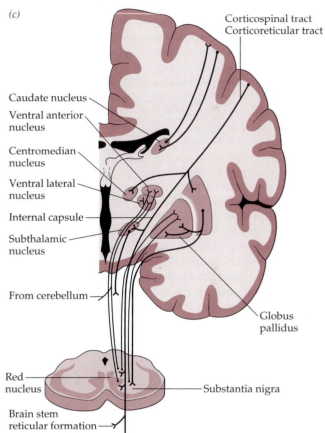

(c)

Corticospinal tract
Corticoreticular tract
Caudate nucleus
Ventral anterior nucleus
Centromedian nucleus
Ventral lateral nucleus
Internal capsule
Subthalamic nucleus
From cerebellum
Red nucleus
Brain stem reticular formation
Globus pallidus
Substantia nigra

perkinesia known as hemiballismus, which is characterized by sudden, involuntary, purposeless, violent, and forceful flinging movements, usually of the arm on the side opposite to the lesion. These movements persist during wakefulness, but disappear with sleep. These effects are presumed to be due to inadequate regulation and stabilization of the premotor cortical discharge.

With respect to the substantia nigra, as mentioned earlier, the cells in this area have reciprocal connections to the striatum, which have inhibitory effects on the motor activity of the trunk and extremities. In Parkin-

son's disease, dopamine-containing cells in the substantia nigra pars compacta atrophy, resulting in a loss of inhibition of the striatum and thereby increasing the striatal output to the thalamus. The consequence is tremor at rest (i.e., when no movement is involved), muscular rigidity, impaired postural reflexes (if standing patients close their eyes, they may fall down), and bradykinesia (abnormal slowness of movements). In Huntington's disease, cell loss (as much as 90%) occurs in the striatum, which leads to a suppression of the subthalamic nucleus and uncontrollable movement of the extremities, facial

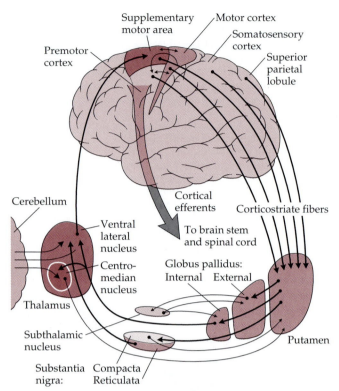

4.16 MAJOR CONNECTIONS BETWEEN THE CORTEX AND THE BASAL GANGLIA. The basal ganglia are part of a motor circuit that is a subcortical feedback loop from the motor and the somatosensory areas of the cortex to the thalamus and back to the cortex. Modulatory roles are played by the subthalamic nucleus and the substantia nigra. (After DeLong, 1974.)

contortions, and incomprehensible or absent speech. Further, in Huntington's disease, there is atrophy of the cells in the cortical areas that are modulated by the basal ganglia, resulting in the dementia that is characteristic of this disease.

Part I Summary

We may summarize this section by comparing the functions of the cerebellum with those of the basal ganglia. Both systems receive major projections from the sensory, motor, and prefrontal association areas of the cerebral cortex, and both project back to the cortex via the thalamus. However, there are differences, too: the cerebellum receives somatic sensory information directly from the spinal cord via spinocerebellar pathways, and it has many afferent and efferent connections with brain stem nuclei, such as the nuclei of the tegmentum and the reticular formation, the vestibular nuclei, and the red nucleus of the midbrain, which is the origin of the rubrospinal tract. Thus, the cerebellum has direct and indirect motor influences on mechanisms of the brain stem and spinal cord. In contrast, the basal ganglia have few direct connections with the brain stem and none at all with the spinal cord.

This difference suggests that the cerebellum can, in part, regulate the execution of movement in terms of the kinesthetic feedback from the skeletal musculature, whereas the basal ganglia are more involved with higher-order aspects of motor control, namely, the planning, timing, and execution of complex motor sequences that originate in the cortex. Such control might involve the timing of movement sequences during a 5-second gymnastic routine or the playing of a series of hundreds of musical notes within a few seconds. These sensorimotor feats would be impossible if it were necessary to pay attention to each and every movement or the playing of each and every note. Rather, a gymnastic routine or a musical presto resides in memory and is executed almost as a unit, much as one runs off a verbal response to "How are you?" with "I'm fine, thanks, and you?" In contrast, in performing novel or slower movement routines, the basal ganglia and the cerebellum may compare commands for movement from the premotor fields with the proprioceptive feedback from the evolving movement, which in speech, with practice, will be incorporated into a unit, as when learning the response to "Comment allez-vous?"

As mentioned above, the discovery that some motor dysfunctions are related to pathology of the basal ganglia has led to a better understanding of the functional mechanisms of this system, especially with regard to biochemical factors. In the case of Parkinson's disease, the symptoms appear to be related to the loss of dopaminergic cell bodies in the substantia nigra pars compacta. More details about this disease and its treatment can be found in Chapter 20.

Part II
The Cerebral Cortex

The Telencephalon

The telencephalon, also known as the cerebrum, consists of the cerebral hemispheres and the subcortical telencephalic nuclei of the hemispheres, namely, the basal ganglia, the hippocampus, and the amygdala (see Figures 4.1 and 4.2). The cerebrum is by far the largest part of the CNS in most mammals. In general, the evolution of brain size coincided with the evolution of cranium size, but ultimately cranium size was limited because the cranium must pass through the pelvic foramen during birth. Consequently, the brain evolved with gyri and sulci (convolutions and grooves), which allowed a greater surface area within the cranium than would be possible if the surface were smooth, just as a crumpled sheet of paper can be placed in a box smaller than one for a flat sheet. Moreover, there are many similarities in the patterns of grooves and convolutions among mammalian species that testify to the evolution of the verte-brate brain from its simplest to its most advanced form.

The Cerebral Cortex

The cerebral cortex is the source of the neural transac-tions that enhance memory, plasticity (i.e., learning new habits and discarding old ones), cognition, speech, and intellectual activity—attributes that are known as higher mental functions. The cortex covers the cerebral hemi-spheres as a dense layer consisting of a variety of neu-rons and glia. There are three phylogenetically old types of cortex: the archicortex, which makes up the hip-pocampus and the dentate gyrus; the paleocortex, com-prising the olfactory cortex, the piriform lobe, and parts of the parahippocampal gyrus; and the mesocortex, made up of other parts of the parahippocampal gyrus and the cingulate gyrus (see Figure 4.13*a* and *b*). It was seen in an earlier section that these older cortical areas are located deep in the mesial part of the temporal lobe, whereas the most phylogenetically recent cortex, the neocortex, covers the latest and largest parts of the cere-bral hemispheres; the neocortex constitutes 80–90% of the bulk of cortex in humans. It was also seen that the mesocortex (especially the cingulate gyrus) occupies an area between the neocortex and the archicortex and pale-ocortex.

In appearance, the neocortex is a gray mantle about 2–4 mm in thickness made up of about 10–15 billion neurons, which constitute about 40% of the brain by weight and about half of the neurons in the brain. It has been estimated that a piece of the cortex the size of a pinhead would contain 30,000 cells. In all, it is estimated that there are 100 billion neurons in the brain, each capa-ble of making 50,000 connections with other cells. A human fetus has an estimated 200 billion neurons, but half of them die off because either they fail to reach their appropriate target sites, or the neural inputs to the cells fail to materialize.

Neurons make connections most rapidly in younger brains, which is illustrated by the fact that children can rapidly acquire new languages, but after the age of about 16, an acquired new language will usually be spo-ken with a recognizable foreign accent. Further, in some circumstances, talented and highly motivated children can become prodigies in musical performance, mathe-matics, chess, and gymnastics to extraordinary degrees. Older brains maintain some flexibility during the whole life span, but the rapidity of establishing new neuronal interconnections and the ability to maintain them pro-gressively declines.

The cortex, if laid out flat, would have a surface area between 2,200 and 2,500 cm². Beneath the cortex, the un-derlying white matter consists of large bundles of axons, which are projections from the thalamus to the cortex and from the cortex, via the internal capsule, to the cere-bellum, the brain stem, and the spinal cord. Also, there are axon bundles that form interconnections among all areas of the cortex. Specifically, there are short association fibers connecting adjacent gyri and longer association bundles connecting distant cortical areas within the same hemisphere. There are also commissural or interhemi-spheric bundles connecting areas in one hemisphere with their counterparts in the opposite hemisphere. Many of these bundles are gathered together to form the corpus callosum and the anterior commissure; in the human brain, these principal interconnections between the hemi-spheres have about 300 million fibers (see Figure 4.10).

Function of the Corpus Callosum

For a long time, it seemed logical to assume that the cor-pus callosum served simply to unite the structures of both hemispheres. However, when the corpus callosum was completely sectioned in some patients to prevent the spread of epileptic loci from one hemisphere to the other, it came as a great surprise in early studies of these pa-tients that no functional alterations could be detected even after careful neurological and psychological exami-nations. Even complex activities such as piano and violin playing, typing, and writing could be performed with the same dexterity as prior to the sectioning of the cal-losal fibers.

Later studies with animals and humans utilized spe-cial techniques to provide a more accurate description of the functional role of this structure. In short, in patients with callosal sectioning, each hemisphere receives the same information about the world, which allows for in-tegrated function despite the absence of a direct inter-hemispheric communication. A deficit appears only when a function is virtually confined to one hemisphere, as is articulate speech, which is mediated by Broca's area, located only in the left hemisphere for right-handed individuals (see below).

Studies of epileptic patients that had undergone cal-losal sectioning showed that if a brief image of an object, such as a ball, was confined to the retina of both eyes so that it would be projected only to the *left* hemisphere, pa-tients reported that they had seen a ball. (To accomplish this, the patient looks straight ahead, and the image briefly appears on the right.) If the image was projected only to the *right* hemisphere, however, patients denied having seen anything, or guessed or confabulated. How-ever, if the patient could reach under a shelf to touch a number of objects, a ball could be selected to show what had been seen. Thus, the function of speech, which is confined to one hemisphere, was not accessible in the second case.

This finding illustrates that certain brain functions are not bilaterally distributed. This phenomenon also came to light in cases of stroke, in which speech was lost only if the left but not the right hemisphere was dam-aged. This is not to say that the right hemisphere is deficient, because for some functions, the right hemisphere is superior to the left, and normally, by way of the corpus callosum, the two sides work together, with the dominant side taking over for a particular function. This process works so well that it was discovered only recently that major differences in functions other than speech exist between the right and left hemispheres. (See Kupfermann, 1991d for further details and references.)

Cortical Cell Morphology

Though a primitive archicortex is found in the brains of reptiles, neocortex is an "organ" of mammals, and it has reached its peak development in primates, including humans. Nonetheless, parts of the mammalian cortex, including that of humans, consist of the phylogenetically older mesocortex that makes up the cingulate gyrus of the limbic lobe and accounts for about 10% of all cortex.

In most parts of the neocortex, its cytoarchitectural structure is characterized by a six-layered laminated pattern. However, there is considerable variation in the character of the cortical layers. That is, in the phylogenetically older brain areas, the cortex is thin, or has fewer than six layers (the limbic lobe has three layers), and in some areas there are no identifiable layers at all. Also, there is variation in the proportions of the kinds of cortical cells found in the various layers.

In the neocortex, layer 1 is made up mostly of glial cells, axons that run horizontally through the layer, and relatively few neurons, as shown in Figure 4.17. Layers 2–6 contain various proportions of two main classes of cells: pyramidal cells and several types of nonpyramidal

multipolar cells. The pyramidal cells, so named because of their shape, are the major output neurons of the cortex. Layer 2 contains small pyramidal cells, and layer 3 contains somewhat larger ones, which provide cortical outputs to other cortical regions. The largest pyramidal cells are found in layer 5 in the motor areas of the brain and are known as giant pyramidal or Betz cells (named after their discoverer). From the apex of the Betz cells, apical dendrites extend peripherally to layer 1 and intersect with the laterally running branches of axons in the upper layers. Among these branches reciprocal influences between these cells are expressed. Also, in layer 1, horizontal cells make connections between the tips of adjacent apical dendrites.

From the base of the pyramidal cell body, several basal dendrites spread laterally within the same layer and receive inputs from local granule and stellate cells, which serve as internuncial cells between the inputs—from other cortical areas and from the thalamus—and the pyramidal cells. The pyramidal cell axons exit from the base of the pyramidal cell bodies, but before leaving the gray matter, these axons give rise to an abundance of collaterals that extend back into the upper cortical layers (as recurrent collaterals) or horizontally (as intracortical association fibers) to synapse among adjacent stellate and Martinotti cells.

From the motor areas of the brain, the pyramidal cell axons pass through the gray matter via the **corona radiata** and the **internal capsule**, then through the cerebral peduncles of the midbrain to become the corticobulbar and corticospinal tracts (also known as the pyramidal

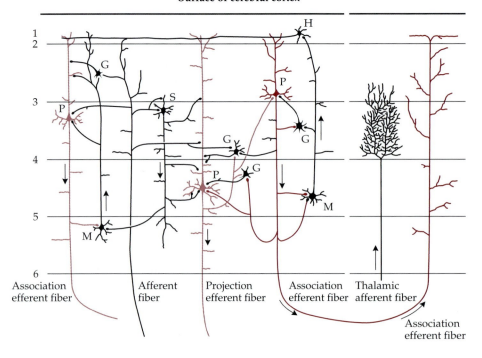

Surface of cerebral cortex

4.17 NEURONAL CONSTITUENTS OF THE NEOCORTEX. Afferent fibers to the cortex include thalamocortical fibers, commissural fibers, and association fibers. Stellate cells (S), Martinotti cells (M), and granule cells (G) are internuncial cells that connect with cells vertically or horizontally within the same layer or in different layers, as well as with other cells that are nearby or some distance away, even as far as the opposite hemisphere. Pyramidal cells (P) have long axons and mediate the outputs from the cortex to subcortical structures—the basal ganglia and the cerebellum—and the motor nuclei of the brain stem and spinal cord. (After Lorente de Nó, 1949.)

tracts). At various levels the axons leave the white matter and enter the gray matter to synapse within motor nuclei of the brain stem and spinal cord. Other parts of the corona radiata consist of fibers from other cortical areas that give rise to corticopontine fibers, which synapse in the pons with neurons of the pontocerebellar tracts, which are part of the feedback loops between the cortex and the cerebellum. Similarly, corticostriate fibers are part of the loop between the cortex and the basal ganglia. Further, as shown in Figure 4.17, pyramidal axons form association **efferent fibers** that enter the white matter and emerge elsewhere to become association **afferent fibers**, thereby establishing association loops with pyramidal cells elsewhere within the cortex.

Layer 4 is rich with stellate and granule cells, which receive the input to the cortex from thalamocortical fibers, association fibers, and commissural fibers. As shown in Figure 4.17, the terminals of the thalamic afferent fibers form a bushy cluster of highly subdivided dendrites, suggesting contacts with at least hundreds or thousands of stellate and granule cells. Some stellate and granule cells have axons that branch close to the cell body and rarely extend beyond layer 4, whereas other stellate cells have longer axons that extend to the deeper cortical layers. In layers 5 and 6, Martinotti cells, in contrast to pyramidal cells, have long axons that extend peripherally to synapse with neurons in the more superficial cortical layers 2 and 3; and in layer 6, pyramidal cells have axons that project back to the thalamus, thereby forming feedback loops between the cortex and thalamus.

Organization of the Cortex

Whereas the cortex is portrayed as being structurally organized in up to six horizontal layers parallel to the cortical surface, the functional units within the cortex are oriented vertically at right angles to the surface and extend from the surface of the brain down to the white matter. This columnar organization is present in virtually all sensory and motor areas of the cortex. Figure 4.18 represents a model of the columnar organization within the cortex and shows the typical arrangement of the pyramidal and the local internuncial cells (see Martin, 1991b).

The term "columnar organization" refers to the fact that cortical responses to sensory stimuli to the skin are recorded not by a lateral group of similar cells, but rather, among the cells within vertical columns. Furthermore, all neuron types within each column receive inputs from the same local area of skin. Thus, the neurons lying within the columns make up an elementary functional model of the cortex as a whole. A similar arrangement is found in the motor cortex as well as in all other sensory modalities.

Furthermore, columns in the somesthetic (primary sensory) areas of the brain have different columns for each submodality, such as touch, hair deflection on the hands, and steady pressure on the skin. However, the submodalities are combined and connected with other brain areas for the perception of objects. For example, when a familiar object is placed in the hand, it is instantly recognized without looking at it as a pen, a key,

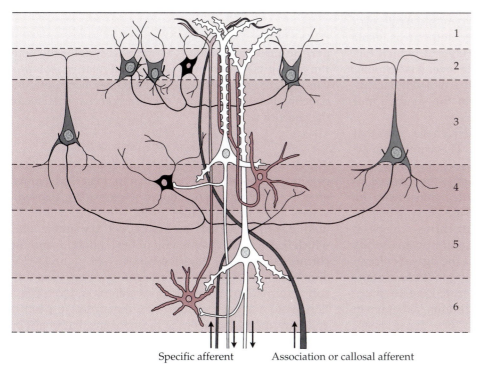

Specific afferent   Association or callosal afferent

4.18 A MODEL OF CORTICAL NEURONS ORGANIZED AS VERTICAL COLUMNS. In the sensory cortex, the stellate interneurons (colored) in layer 4 receive sensory inputs from the thalamus. The afferent associational and commissural (callosal) fibers from other cortical areas are directed to the more superficial layers 1 through 3. The pyramidal cells in layers 3 and 5 (white) receive multiple contacts from the cells in areas 1 through 4 and, as the output from the columns, have long axons that enter the white matter to send their influences to the motor cortex and related areas. In area 6, Martinotti cells (colored) receive inputs from the descending axons of the pyramidal cells and project in a reverse direction to the peripheral layers. Inhibitory basket stellate cells (black) also make connections with intracortical neurons (gray) in the more superficial layers. (After Szentágothai, 1969.)

or an apple, and one knows what it is used for. Similarly, all sensory systems engage the memory that gives meaning to what we see, hear, feel, taste, and smell. The processing of sensory information occurs in the upper cortical layers of nonpyramidal cells, whose output is projected via the pyramidal cells that make up the associational, commissural, and projection systems for the modulation and/or expression of sensorimotor activity and conscious awareness. (For a discussion of conscious awareness, see Kandel, 1991b.)

Cortical diversity. The thickness and the extent of the cortex is not the same for the various sensory and motor modalities, nor are the proportions of pyramidal and nonpyramidal cells the same in the various cortical layers. A number of investigators have labeled all areas of the cortex according to certain characteristics such as cell type, density, cell layering, input and output connections, and, most important, physiological function; as many as 200 identifiably distinct areas have been reported. However, the numbering system of Brodmann (1909), who described 52 areas, is still the most commonly used classification, even though later studies have led to subdivision of many of Brodmann's areas (Figure 4.19).

It was found that layer thickness varies with the functional nature of a given area. For instance, the thickness of layer 4 in a primary sensory area is expanded because there are abundant inputs from sensory relay nuclei of the thalamus, and this layer has a relatively high proportion of nonpyramidal cell bodies. The primary visual cortex in the occipital lobe, in particular, has a much expanded layer 4, which receives its inputs from the lateral geniculate body of the thalamus and is subdivided into four distinct sublayers; thus, the visual area is sometimes known as the striate cortex. Its pyramidal cells also project to many other brain areas. In motor areas, giant pyramidal cells are prominent in layer 5, which has many smaller pyramidal cells as well; layer 4 is virtually absent. In association cortex, the pattern of cellular layers is somewhere between those of the sensory and motor cortex.

The pyramidal cells in layers 3 and 5 have axons that are the outputs of the cortical areas. The axons emanating from layers 2 and 3 serve as association fibers between different cortical areas, or commissural fibers connecting to similar areas in the opposite hemisphere. The axons emanating from layers 5 and 6 are likely to be projection fibers either to subcortical structures—the basal ganglia or the ventral posterior lateral nucleus of the thalamus—or to the brain stem and the dorsal column nuclei to modulate the sensory input into those centers. Furthermore, basket cell axons connect to local internuncial neurons on the periphery of the column, as shown in Figure 4.18. The basket cell terminals form dense synaptic connections upon the internuncial somata and presumably exert an inhibitory effect on them to produce

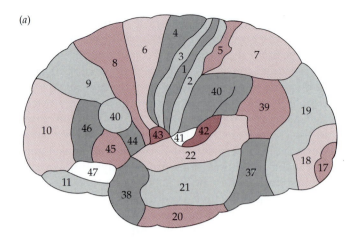

(a)

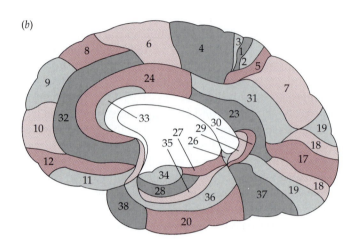

(b)

4.19 CYTOARCHITECTURAL MAPS OF THE HUMAN CEREBRAL CORTEX. (*a*) Lateral and (*b*) medial views of the human brain with numbers representing Brodmann's areas.

pericolumnar inhibition. This process enables the neurons in a given column to function in relative isolation from neighboring columns. Nonetheless, horizontal interaction between columns is a common characteristic of the neocortex.

Functional Localization in the Neocortex

The neocortex is divided into four lobes, the frontal, parietal, temporal, and occipital lobes, which are named after the overlying cranial bones (Figure 4.20). Two subsidiary lobes are the insular cortex, which lies within the medial wall of the sylvian fissure, and the limbic lobe, which lies over the rostral limit of the brain stem and the corpus callosum, as described above (see Figures 4.13*b* and 4.13*c*). All four lobes participate in integrating sensory information for conscious awareness and for projection to areas of cortical output for the control of posture and movement. Think of the mechanisms that might be active as a horse goes from a walk to a trot to a canter to a gallop, or as a child goes from a walk to a skip to a run.

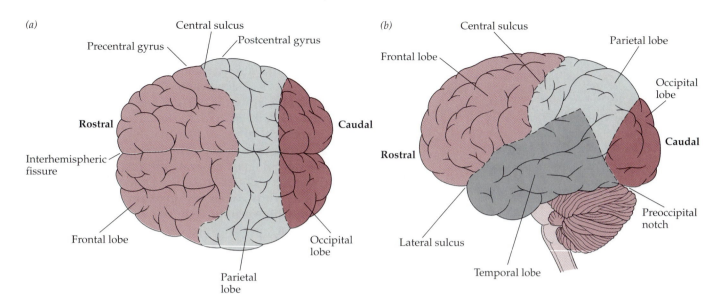

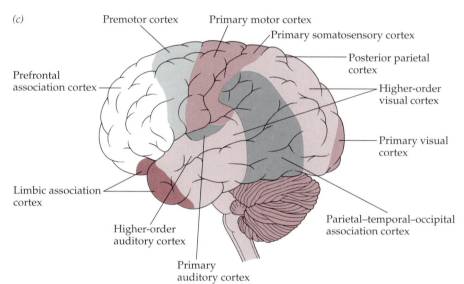

4.20 THE MAJOR DIVISIONS OF THE HUMAN CEREBRAL CORTEX. (*a*) As viewed from above, the left lobe (lower half) shows the major division of the lobes, and the right lobe (upper half) shows the boundaries of specific functional areas. (*b*) The lateral view also shows the division of the lobes and the specific functional areas. (*c*) A schematic drawing of the lateral surface of the human brain showing the juxtaposition of primary, higher-order, and association areas for vision, hearing, and motor activities.

Some parts of these lobes are more directly involved with either sensory information or motor output. The primary sensory areas respond to the sensory data relayed from the thalamus, and the primary motor areas are directly related to the motor neurons in the brain stem and spinal cord. As shown in Figure 4.20, the **primary somatic sensory cortex** lies in the postcentral gyrus, where it receives, with few interposed synapses, sensory information relayed from the thalamus for touch, kinesthesis, proprioception, pain, and temperature. (The anterior spinothalamic pathways for touch, pain, and thermal sense are shown in Figure 4.3.) The primary sensory area can be further subdivided quite specifically into portions that represent certain parts of the body. That is to say that when the face or a hand is touched, a certain area on the brain surface will be activated. Therefore, the body surface is represented by a somatotopic neural map in the somatosensory cortex. This representation does not have the

same proportions as the body. Rather, the size of a body area in the neural map is proportional to the density of the somatic sense organs and the cortical neurons that determine sensitivity at that position on the body. Therefore, as shown in Figure 4.21, the sensory homunculus, a graphic representation of the neural map in the primary sensory cortex, has a hand with an area that is about the same as that of the arm and trunk put together.

To explain these distortions, it has been found that the fingertips of humans have four types of sensory receptors that make up a total of about 2,500 receptors per square centimeter. These receptors are connected to 300 myelinated sensory axons per square centimeter. Also, each axon is activated by about 20 receptors, and each receptor connects to 2–5 axons. This overlapping arrangement promotes small, highly sensitive receptive fields of about 3–4 mm in diameter on the fingertips. On the trunk, the receptive fields are about 100 times larger

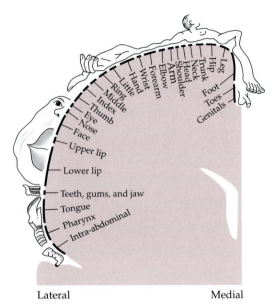

4.21 THE SENSORY HOMUNCULUS. The distribution of body parts in proportion to their representation in the primary somatosensory cortex (area 1) of the human. The exaggerated sizes of the foot, hand, face, lips, tongue, and pharynx reflect their more extensive sensory innervation. (After Penfield and Rasmussen, 1950.)

than on the fingertips, which means that about 100 times fewer sensory receptors and sensory axons go to the brain from a square centimeter of skin on the trunk. Consequently, large areas of skin on the trunk will be innervated by few cortical units and will take up little space on the cortex, whereas the cortical area for fingertips will be 100 times greater than that for the trunk. Thus, for the hand, the sensory representation can be so precise that a spot on the sensory cortex can be found that responds to the bending of a single hair on the back of the hand. The feel of a piece of silk is immediately detectible by the fingertips, but rubbing the silk on your back would tell you practically nothing. Reading braille is another example of the high degree of discrimination by touch that can be transmitted to the brain from the fingertips.

Moreover, there is evidence that suggests that there is an increased cortical representation of the index finger used by blind braille readers. This finding is among the evidence that has accumulated over the last few decades showing that special conditions can induce such plastic cortical reorganization, not only in primary somatic sensory cortex in the brains of braille readers, but also in other cortical areas in the mammalian central nervous system (Elbert et al., 1995).

In a recent study, magnetic resonance imaging (MRI) identified the representation of the fingers in the primary somatic sensory cortex when the fingertips of string players (violinists, cellists, and guitarists) were lightly stimulated. The primary somatic sensory cortex

representation for the thumb of the left hand and the digits of the right hand were similarly examined. The results showed that compared to the area for the right fingers, the right primary somatic sensory cortex area for the left fingers had significantly expanded by shifting toward the midsagittal plane, the region that represents the palm. Also, the shift for the left fifth digit (the pinkie) was somewhat greater than that for the left thumb, which corresponds to the diminished role of the thumb and the right fingers for string players. The strength of the response was also greater for the left than for the right digits. Thus, differences in expansion and strength of response between the right and left primary somatic sensory cortex in string players were marked in the absence of area shift for the fingers of nonstring-player controls. Further, the magnitude of change of the primary somatic sensory cortex for the left hand was correlated with the age at which the string players began the study of their instruments: the earlier they started, the greater the magnitude of expansion. These findings suggest that the representation of different parts of the body in the primary somatic sensory cortex of humans depends on use and changes to conform to the current needs and experiences of the individual (Elbert et al., 1995; Kandel and Jessell, 1991).

The output from the primary sensory cortex is mediated via pyramidal cell axons in layers 2, 3, and 5 that project via axon collaterals to adjacent nonpyramidal cells and other cortical areas in the same hemisphere (see below), and via interhemispheric fibers to the same areas in the opposite hemisphere. Also, some sensory outputs are projected back to the thalamus and the dorsal column nuclei in the brain stem to enhance the relay of some somesthetic information and to inhibit other information. The inhibitory feedback is especially useful for inhibiting responses from the weakly stimulated edges of strongly stimulated areas to increase the contrast between the two areas, which increases the perception of sharp contours and facilitates the perception of objects by touch.

Posteriorly adjacent to the primary sensory areas are the **secondary** and **tertiary sensory areas**. These higher-order areas, as well as the **posterior parietal association cortex**, receive inputs from the primary sensory areas, and are concerned with the more detailed analysis of sensation necessary for perception and the planning of movement. Whereas the primary sensory areas give rise to somatic sensations such as touch and proprioception, the secondary and tertiary areas are essential for the recognition and comprehension of weight, shape, texture, and form—and for the braille reader, language. Lesions in the posterior parietal cortex cause **astereognosis**, a loss of the ability to name an object held in the hand, even though there is no deficit in the somatosensory sensitivity of the hand. Also, these patients, with eyes closed, are unable to name the finger that has been touched by another person, though they can report that the touch was felt (Kandel and Jessell, 1991).

The **primary visual** (striate) **cortex** at the occipital pole is also surrounded by higher-order association cortex of the parietal and temporal lobes, which has connections with the prefrontal and frontal cortex. These association areas are concerned with optokinetic reflexes (turning the head toward a perceived movement in the periphery), integrating visual and auditory sensations, saccadic movements when reading or scanning a view, and smooth pursuit when eyes follow a moving object. The striate cortex (layer 6), the medial superior temporal areas, and the posterior parietal cortex mediate the smooth pursuit movements by projecting to the pons and cerebellum, which inform the system how fast the visual target is moving.

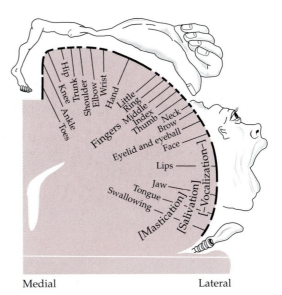

Medial   Lateral

4.22 THE MOTOR HOMUNCULUS. Motor projections from the brain to the body musculature are arranged in the cortex in somatotopic order. The comparative representation of body parts in the motor homunculus is similar to that of the sensory homunculus. (After Penfield and Rasmussen, 1950.)

Cortical Control of Movement

The motor homunculus shown in Figure 4.22 represents the proportional degree of control of the body parts exerted by the motor cortex. The amount of motor cortex the brain assigns to a body part is directly proportional to the relative variability and flexibility of movement of that body part, and the proportional distribution of the motor areas is, as expected, similar to that for the sensory cortex. Thus, in the motor cortex, relatively more space is devoted to hand and wrist movements than to those of the shoulder or elbow, and this translates to the high degree of fine motor control of the hand and digits (fingers). Also, this arrangement is the basis for the high degree of control of the muscles of facial expression and the oral musculature for language vocalization.

Postural control. Before or during a behavioral act, postural adjustments must take place. Posture refers to the orientation of the body in space before and during movements of any sort. Postural adjustments are essential because the slightest act may disturb the equilibrium of the body, resulting in a fall to the ground, especially in bipeds. For example, beginning to walk across the room requires that you lean forward and shift your weight toward the right as you raise your right foot for the first step, so that your weight is centered over the right foot as it hits the floor. If you did not shift your weight and tried to lift your left foot after placing your right foot, you could fall over backward. Thus, when walking, you are constantly shifting your weight from one foot to the other to maintain body equilibrium. (You will find that if you continually lean toward the right as you try to walk, your gait will be markedly disrupted and even painful after a few minutes.) Normally, this activity is automatic and requires no thought, although the shifting of weight is particularly noticeable when you are learning to skate or cross-country ski. A 1-year-old child obviously has automatic postural control by the time it can walk. One can readily observe the automatic nature of postural control by watching a toddler lean to the inside while running around a corner to offset the centrifugal force that would throw the body outward.

The postural adjustments necessary to support the body during movement utilize mechanisms quite different from those of voluntary movements, even though these processes are operative during voluntary body movements. Postural adjustment is largely controlled by local (i.e., spinal) reflexes and the so-called extrapyramidal systems mediated by the reticular formation, the basal ganglia, and the cerebellum. To illustrate, when standing in a moving bus and holding on to a support pole, one constantly makes postural adjustments as the bus starts, suddenly slows down, and goes around curves or corners. The cues that lead to the stabilizing of the body come from muscle **proprioceptors** that sense muscle stretch or tension, from **vestibular receptors** that sense sway through head motion, and from **visual inputs** that detect motion in the visual field. The muscle proprioceptors respond fastest, with a latency of about 70–100 ms; the others are slower by a factor of 2. These three mechanisms, which recruit the actions of the cerebellum and basal ganglia, induce the reflex responses that stabilize the body, and though there is some learning of how to stand in a moving bus, most of the responses are quite automatic. Nonetheless, special training is required for stabilizing the body for the execution of skilled movements or the use of the body in unusual ways, as in gymnastics and the extraordinary feats of some circus performers. Sometimes unusual postural adjustments are automatically made, such as the acquisition of "sea legs" when one must walk on a swaying

(a)

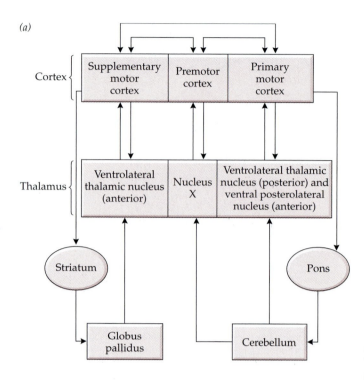

(b)

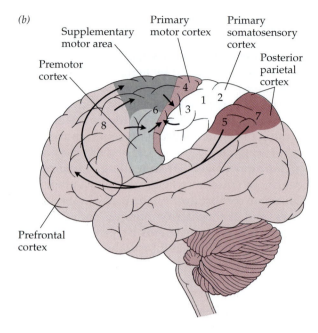

4.23 CORTICAL STRUCTURES AND INTERCONNECTIONS THAT MEDIATE VOLUNTARY MOVEMENTS. (*a*) A graphic representation of the interconnections among the cortical and subcortical structures, including the thalamus, striatum, globus pallidus, and the cerebellum. (*b*) The neuroanatomical areas and the major connection from the sensory association to the motor areas. The numbers indicate the Brodmann areas. (After Ghez, 1991.)

boat deck for an extended period. Within a few days the swaying is hardly noticeable, and for a day or two after leaving the ship, stationary sidewalks and floors occasionally feel as though they are moving like the boat deck.

Voluntary movement.   The major brain areas for the initiation and execution of voluntary behavior and their interconnections are illustrated in Figure 4.23. Figure 4.23*a* diagrams the relationships among the cortex and the subcortical structures, the thalamus, striatum, and globus pallidus, and the cerebellum. It is quite apparent that there are constant interactions that are responsible for the planning and the execution of voluntary movements and the constant monitoring of the movements as they progress. Figure 4.23*b* shows the positions of the primary motor cortex, the supplementary motor area, and the premotor cortex in the precentral gyrus of the left hemisphere of the human brain. Also shown are the inputs to the prefrontal cortex and the supplementary motor area from the posterior parietal cortex, which is a higher sensory association area that may initiate or monitor the effects of motor responses and modulate them for maximum effectiveness.

In the primary motor area (Brodmann's area 4), there are 30,000 prominent giant pyramidal cells as well as many more smaller pyramidal cells in cortical layer 5. The axons of these cells make up a portion of the million axons that emerge from area 4 and the supplementary motor area (area 6) to make up the corticobulbar and lateral corticospinal tracts (also known as the pyramidal tracts).

The supplementary motor cortex and the premotor cortex are instrumental in the initiation of movement, and the prefrontal association cortex functions as a planning center for a pattern of responses. As shown in Figure 4.23*b*, these areas receive inputs from the secondary and tertiary sensory areas, respectively (Brodmann areas 5 and 7), and project them to the primary motor area, area 4. These connections between the sensory cortex and the premotor and the prefrontal association cortex allow a more precise representation of sensory information to influence the execution of movement by the motor cortex. This can be demonstrated by the effects of electrical stimulation of the different motor areas. Stimulating a spot in the primary motor area results in discrete contralateral muscle contractions. In contrast, stimulation of the premotor area requires larger stimulus currents, which evoke coordinated contractions of muscles at more than one joint. Similar effects occur when stimulating the supplementary motor area, which evokes responses on both sides of the body as well. Thus, in executing a voluntary act, there is a constant interplay of sensory and motor influences. For example, if one enters a dark room and is searching for a wall switch to turn on the lights, what one touches and how the arm is extended will provide sensory data that will guide the arm and hand to the switch according to one's memories of it. On the first try, touching a picture frame will indicate that the hand is too high and too far, and further tries will occur until a protuberance on the wall is touched and is identified as the switch.

The concept of a cortical substrate for a planning or programming stage separate from the motor aspect of skilled movement is supported by many animal investigations. Whereas the comparative size of the primary motor cortex has remained relatively constant across primate evolution, the prefrontal and premotor areas increased about sixfold from the macaque monkey to humans. This increase is an indication of how much input of sensory perceptions and thought processes goes into the planning and execution of motor activity in humans. This is partly illustrated by the effects of lesions in any of the three cortical areas identified above. When monkeys received lesions in the primary motor cortex, the usual symptom was muscular weakness. Lesions in the premotor areas, however, impaired their ability to prepare an adequate strategy for movement. When monkeys with such lesions were presented with food behind a transparent screen, with openings at the sides of the screen, instead of reaching around the screen, they aimed straight at the food and bumped their hands into the screen over and over again. Furthermore, monkeys with lesions in the supplementary motor areas were unable to orient the hand and fingers appropriately to reach a peanut in a small well, nor could they use both hands effectively to obtain a morsel of food stuck in a hole in a thick piece of transparent plastic. Whereas a normal monkey would stick one finger into the hole and push, and with the other hand reach under the hole to catch the falling morsel, monkeys with a lesion in the supplementary premotor area pushed a finger into the hole from the top while pushing a finger of the other hand into the hole from the bottom (Brinkman, 1984).

The roles of these motor areas in humans were investigated in the following manner. While subjects performed simple motor tasks with one hand, their cerebral blood flow was monitored in the "hand" area on the opposite side of the brain. As the tasks increased in complexity, blood flow increased dramatically around the hand portions of both the primary motor and somatic sensory areas, but there was little spread to the lateral premotor areas. However, during complex movement sequences, such as trying to continuously touch the thumb with the fingers (index finger = 1, pinkie = 4) in the order 1–3–4–2 as fast as possible, increases in the subjects' blood flow were extended from the primary motor and somatic sensory areas to the supplementary motor area. And when the subjects were asked only to rehearse the sequence of finger movements mentally, blood flow increased only in the supplementary motor area (Roland et al., 1980).

Though the emphasis has been on human skills in the above discussion, other animals are not devoid of skilled movements. Watching a sparrow dart between tree branches and come to a dead stop on the perch of a bird feeder, or watching a spider building a web is enough to demonstrate that animals perform skilled motor activities. But highly skilled flying and web-building evolved over millions of years and are securely embedded in the genotype of the species. Skilled flying in birds is also a product of maturation and practice, but the rapidity of flight acquisition and the style of flight depends on a genetic substrate. In contrast, when motivated to do so, humans can, within a relatively short time, acquire skilled movements that demand the outer limits of neuromuscular capabilities. Animals can acquire and perform feats of considerable skill, but their execution of those skills is usually clumsy compared with their natural movements, and skills that involve high levels of digital dexterity and vocal language are virtually absent in nonhuman species. It is doubtful a chimpanzee could ever learn to button a shirt or tie a square knot. (See Ghez, 1991, for a review of voluntary movement.)

Voluntary acts involve the limbic lobe.   The limbic lobe also plays a role in voluntary acts. The limbic cortex includes the medial surface of the parietal lobe, the orbitofrontal cortex, the cingulate region, and the parahippocampal area (see Figure 4.13*b*). The limbic cortex receives sensory projections from the higher-order sensory cortices and adds memory, emotional, and motivational aspects to its projections to the prefrontal cortex for motor planning. Thus, for instance, a musician, an athlete, or a salesperson incorporates skill (motor and cognitive memories), zeal (motivation), and expressiveness (emotions) when playing an instrument, running a race, or presenting a product in a convincing way, all of which are accompanied by the autonomic counterparts of emotion: for example, the persuasive character of the salesperson's voice is enhanced by a higher pitch and loudness. Accordingly, we enjoy music played with passion, and we look for emotional themes in plays and films, because emotions are an intrinsic part of almost everything we do. However, in some cases, emotion must be controlled or suppressed according to propriety, style, or taste. In some cultures, things done passionately are appreciated most of the time; in other cultures, more control and a "low key" attitude is preferred. (See Ghez, 1991 for a review.)

Motivated behavior.   Functionally, the cerebral hemispheres carry out the highest level of sensorimotor coordination, and we have seen that an extensive area in the frontal lobe is given over to the planning and execution of fine motor skills. Such behavior is known as voluntary behavior. In contrast to reflexive behavior, voluntary behavior need not be preceded by external stimuli; rather, it feels as though thoughts may suffice to initiate behavior that emanates from the primary motor cortex.

First, it is important to understand what "voluntary" means in this context. It does not mean that there is a homunculus in the brain that tells the brain what to do. Nor does it mean that we initiate brain activity by an act of "will" independent of the brain. What "voluntary" does mean is that we are aware of what we are doing. We may or may not know, however, what stimuli initiated the behavior. For example, we may know why under certain circumstances we say, "Good morning," but we may not know why we eat some foods and reject others, or vigorously strive to win in competitive sports and games, often in the absence of tangible rewards. Consequently, it is becoming comfortable and convenient to describe voluntary behavior as "motivated" behavior and thereby avoid the former misconceptions or contrivances of "the inner voice" and "the will."

We know that food deprivation motivates hunting and eating, and that being too warm motivates moving into the shade. This view is compatible with the Skinnerian view that all "voluntary" behaviors are operants that were formed originally by trial and error, by imitation, or by instruction, and were followed by reinforcements such as food, the coolness of the shade, or merely achieving the intended effect or goal, such as the expected grade in an examination, learning to skillfully knit sweaters, or recognition and approval by others. More often than not, the reinforcement cannot be specifically identified. Thus, in contrast to reflexive behavior, motivated movement involves additional dimensions of neural control: awareness of goals and planning to achieve them. This may apply to the need for some drinking water and the effort to get it, or to the need for a house and the skills required at various stages to build it. Moreover, the effectiveness of voluntary movements improves with practice, which is the result of faster access to the choice of movements and a decrease in the time between successive muscle contractions. Observing the movements and skills of top athletes makes this abundantly clear. Their responses to a baseball, football, or tennis ball appear to be more like reflexes than voluntary acts that involve the identification and location of a target, a plan of action, and the execution of a series of movements of different muscles at different durations and forces.

Language Functions of the Cerebral Cortex

It is perhaps appropriate to cap our discussion of the CNS with the topic of speech and language. The critical mark of division between humans and animals is the human faculty of articulate speech and language. In animals, the absence of brain space for the acquisition of language and the paucity of vocal variations precludes anything resembling human language and speech. Moreover, human language is the crux of cognitive behavior. Words are the substance of thoughts, and thoughts, from the simplest through the most profound,

are the equivalent of talking to oneself. The origins and biomechanisms of speech and the structure and acquisition of language are subjects of huge proportions that cannot be presented here, but we can briefly describe the role of the cortex in this activity, and enthusiastically recommend the review of this subject by Mayeux and Kandel (1991).

Much of what is known about brain function has come from cases of brain insult caused by vascular damage, trauma, or tumor in specific regions of the brain, especially the cortex. This is particularly true of our understanding of language because there are no animal models of language, and experimental invasive investigations of human brains are impermissible. Nonetheless, there are cases in which abnormal brain tissue must be removed, and to spare cortical areas associated with speech, electrical probes are used to identify them. Also, noninvasive techniques such as PET scanning, which monitors blood flow in specific areas, are adding important data about the neural substrates of speech and language. Finally, there are 200,000 cases of aphasia (language deficiencies) resulting from head trauma and 100,000 cases due to stroke each year in the United States; such cases are a valuable source of data on the mechanisms of human language.

The earliest studies of aphasias discovered two brain areas in the frontal and temporal lobes that play crucial roles in language function, Broca's and Wernicke's areas (Figure 4.24). Paul Broca was a French neurologist who reported in 1861 that one of his patients understood language but could not speak in full sentences, had a vocabulary of not more than a few isolated words, and could not express his thoughts in writing. Postmortem examination of the patient's brain revealed a lesion in the posterior region of the frontal lobe of the left hemisphere; similar findings were reported in eight other aphasic patients. Thus, this brain area became known as Broca's area or convolution, and the symptoms are known as Broca's aphasia. Another symptom of Broca's aphasia is the absence of articles, adjectives, and adverbs. When asked to repeat "a large gray cat," a patient may only say "gray cat." Such patients have difficulty in reading aloud, and their writing is impaired, but they are aware of their difficulties.

In 1876, at the age of 26, Carl Wernicke reported the identification of a new type of aphasia characterized by impaired comprehension rather than impaired expression; that is, Wernicke's patients could speak but not understand. This dysfunction was traced to a lesion in the posterior part of the temporal lobe, now known as Wernicke's area, which is near the angular gyrus (the junction of the parietal and occipital lobes). In this and similar patients, speech was fluent and normal in rate, rhythm, and melody, but the comprehension of visual and auditory language was impaired by the use of wrong words or combinations of words. For example,

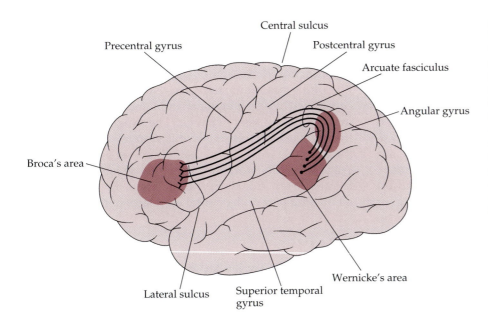

Precentral gyrus · Central sulcus · Postcentral gyrus · Arcuate fasciculus · Angular gyrus · Broca's area · Wernicke's area · Lateral sulcus · Superior temporal gyrus

4.24 SOME LANGUAGE CENTERS IN THE CEREBRAL CORTEX. The lateral view shows Wernicke's area, near the primary auditory cortex, which is important for understanding spoken language. It is also near the angular gyrus, which combines the auditory input with information from other senses. The arcuate fasciculus connects Wernicke's area with Broca's area, where grammatical speech is initiated, via the adjoining vocalization region of the motor area. Also, during the association tasks there is increased activity in the frontal lobe (area 47). (After Kandel, 1991a.)

when asked to describe a picture showing two boys stealing cookies behind a woman's back, a patient with Wernicke's aphasia replied, "Mother is away here working her work to get her better, but when she's looking the two boys looking in the other part. She's working another time." Or, when asked where he lived, another patient replied, "I came there before here and returned there."

Other patients added extra syllables and words to phrases, and some made up new words (neologisms). Such patients could not repeat words or phrases, and they had reading and writing disabilities. They were unaware of these deficits, probably because their inner language (thoughts) was similarly affected.

After further study, Wernicke (1908) proposed that Broca's area controls the motor program for coordinating mouth movements for speech, and, as shown in Figure 4.24, it is appropriately located immediately in front of the facial motor area that controls the mouth, tongue, palate, and vocal cords. In contrast, he attributed word perception, the sensory component of language, to the part of the temporal lobe that he had discovered. This area was also suitably juxtaposed with the higher-order auditory and visual cortices and the parietal–temporal–occipital association cortex, which integrates auditory, visual, and somatic sensation into complex perceptions. Thus, normally, the spoken word "tree" instantly conjures up the image of a tree and associations connected with "tree." However, visual information, such as written words, was later believed *not* to be conveyed to Wernicke's area and transformed into an auditory representation; rather, words that are read are separately processed by a modality-specific pathway to the anterior frontal cortex for word meaning, and by Broca's area for language expression by writing or reading aloud.

To reply to spoken language, the neural representation is relayed from Wernicke's to Broca's area via the arcuate fasciculus, where "the perception of language is translated into the grammatical structure of a phrase and where the memory of word articulation is stored. This information about the sound pattern of the phrase is then conveyed to the facial area of the motor cortex that controls articulation so that the word can be spoken" (Mayeux and Kandel, 1991). In the absence of Broca's area, this transformation cannot occur, and vocal speech is blocked. Further, if a lesion destroys part of the arcuate fasciculus, thus separating Wernicke's from Broca's area, a different aphasia syndrome appears. Known as **conduction aphasia**, it is due to loss of the connection between language comprehension and language expression, and is characterized by incorrect usage of words. Such patients can understand words that are heard and seen, but they cannot repeat simple phrases. They omit parts of words and substitute incorrect sounds in the words, and whereas they are painfully aware of their own errors, they are unable to correct them. Also, naming of objects is severely impaired, and reading aloud is abnormal, but patients can read silently with good comprehension. In these cases writing is also impaired; spelling is poor, with omissions, reversals, and substitutions of letters.

Here it should be noted that brain injuries leading to aphasia vary considerably among patients, and that the aphasias described above are illustrative of only a few typical types. There are many types of aphasia, and in most cases the brain damage is not clearly confined to Broca's or Wernicke's cortical convolutions, but rather, extends to lateral or deeper areas that involve other neurological functions. Moreover, aphasic patients, especially younger ones, frequently can recover a substantial degree of speech function, which suggests that the right side of the brain has the capacity to "take over" speech functions when the left hemisphere is disabled (Mayeux and Kandel, 1991).

Nonetheless, there is evidence for specific speech zones in the brain. Petersen and coworkers (1988), in PET scanning studies, examined changes in blood flow in various brain areas during language tasks. First, blood flow measurements were taken when subjects were passively presented with a word visually or auditorily and told to process the word but do nothing (sensory task). Second, subjects were told to repeat the word (output task), and third, they were asked to generate a use for the word (association task; e.g., to the word "cake," a response "eat" would be appropriate). The results of these tests supported the notion that there is modality-specific independence between the visual and auditory primary and secondary sensory areas, and specific sensory and motor areas, during the output task. Also, during the association task, there was an increased activation of the frontal lobe (area 47) and an unexplained bilateral activation in the anterior cingulate area of the limbic lobe.

Part II Summary

Electrical stimulation of the motor cortex showed that it is organized somatotopically, but it was later found that motor areas are not distribution centers for particular patterns of motor activity. Rather, the motor cortex has a modular organization, and in the primary motor areas, modules of columnar arrangements of neurons control the direction of particular limb movements. However, there are cortical neurons that control the most distal movements, those of the digits, by acting directly upon single muscles, whereas for the movement of the more proximal parts, the limbs, the directional signal is distributed through axon collaterals to many cortical neurons and spinal interneurons, producing facilitation and inhibition among the many synapses.

Further, the firing of individual cortical neurons encodes simple movement parameters such as the force or the change of force that is needed, and this process is continuously modulated by sensory feedback originating in the periphery and directed toward the many stages of reflexive control: the spinal cord, the reticular formation, the cerebellum, the thalamus, the basal ganglia, and the cortex itself. Thus, the sensory and motor processes are seen as being tightly interactive at all of these levels.

Also, it is evident that the interaction between the premotor and the parietal association areas is not totally dependent upon external stimulation; rather, it also reflects the subject's intentions, which stem from motivations. This aspect of movement is not concerned with the fine details of movement; here the concern is the more global aspects of motor tasks—the coordination of posture and the movements of different body parts that is a necessary antecedent for purposeful skillful movement. This sensorimotor plan seems to be universal among

vertebrates and rises to its zenith with the evolution of articulate speech in humans (see Ghez, 1991).

With the end of this brief section on the structure and function of the CNS, we turn now to an examination of the autonomic nervous system, which should be considered as a frequent instigator and modulator of somatically expressed behavior. The exogenous needs of the organism are sensed by this system, which controls the internal organs to maintain homeostasis. It also energizes the behaviors that satisfy those needs, and contributes to emotional expression. Thus, it will be seen as an integral part of the neural correlates of behavior.

Part III
The Autonomic Nervous System

The autonomic nervous system (ANS) consists of peripheral and central neuronal networks that modulate the functions of the internal (visceral) organs to achieve homeostasis. The ANS is essentially a nonvoluntary, self-regulating visceral sensorimotor system even though there is some degree of voluntary control.

Most visceral organs are under the control of both the parasympathetic and the sympathetic systems, as diagrammed in Figure 4.25. A major difference between the two systems, however, is the extent of their neuronal divergence. In the sympathetic system, the ratio of pre-

4.25 THE AUTONOMIC NERVOUS SYSTEM. *Parasympathetic system.* The parasympathetic nerves that innervate the autonomic organs and glands (thick black lines) emerge from parasympathetic cranial nuclei (III, VII, IX and X) and from sacral segments of the spinal cord. The preganglionic fibers of the cranial nerves synapse in peripheral ganglia near the innervated organs, and short postganglionic fibers (gray lines) extend to the autonomic effectors: intrinsic eye muscles; salivary and lachrymal glands; and the thoracic, abdominal, and pelvic organs. Pelvic nerves make up the sacral division of the parasympathetic nervous system and project to the colon, bladder, and sexual organs. *Sympathetic system.* Preganglionic sympathetic nerves (thin black lines emerging from the left and right of the spinal cord) arise from the intermediolateral nuclei of the thoraco-lumbar segments of the spinal cord (T1–L3) and synapse in the paravertebral chain ganglia. Some of the postganglionic fibers (black arrows on the left) join the spinal nerves and project to the microorgans of the skin: blood vessels, arrector pili muscles, and sweat glands. Ascending collateral axons in the sympathetic trunk synapse with sympathetic postganglionic axons that join cervical spinal nerves C1–C8 to innervate the microorgans of the head and neck. Similarly, descending collaterals in the trunk synapse with postganglionic connections that join spinal nerves L4–S5. Other sympathetic nerves pass through the paravertebral ganglia and synapse within the adrenal medulla or within the prevertebral ganglia giving rise to postganglionic fibers (colored lines) that project to the autonomic muscles and glands in the head, and to those in the thoracic, abdominal, and pelvic cavities. s.c.s.g. = superior cervical sympathetic ganglion; s.m.g. = superior mesenteric ganglion; i.m.g. = inferior mesenteric ganglion; m.c.g. = middle cervical ganglion; s.g. = stellate ganglion. (After Carlson, 1991.)

ganglionic to postganglionic fibers is 1:10, whereas in the parasympathetic system, the ratio is only 1:3. This difference accounts for the more diffuse and intense effects of the sympathetic system and the more specific and normalizing effects of the parasympathetic system. For example, the sympathetic system has a stronger and more widespread influence on autonomic activity during great effort, excitement, or stress by increasing respiration and heart rate, increasing the supply of blood glucose, increasing the release of adrenal hormones, and inhibiting gastrointestinal activity. In contrast, the parasympathetic system maintains more selective and moderate levels of autonomic activity with respect to the heart rate, blood pressure, and gastrointestinal activity.

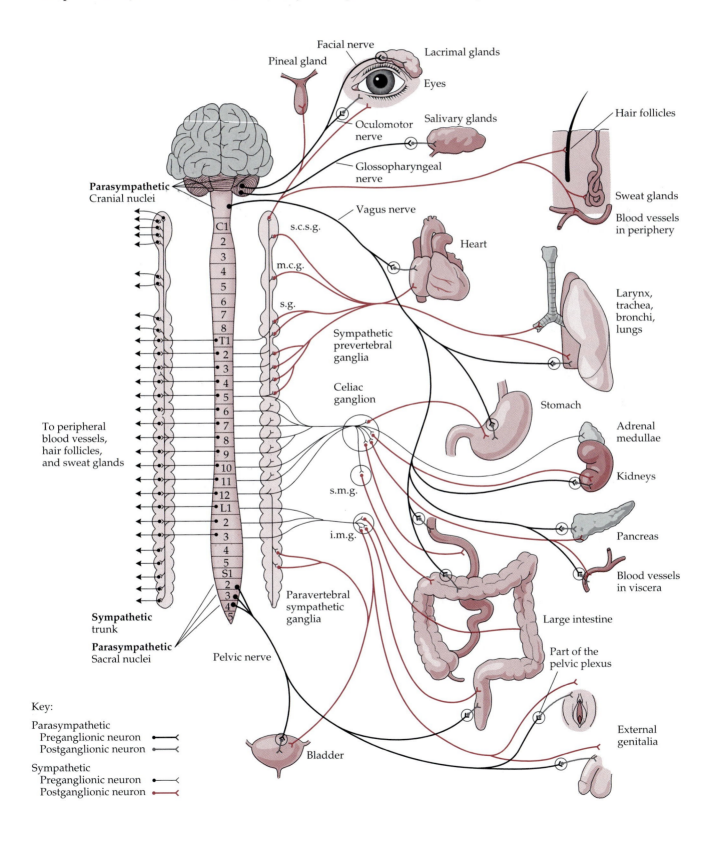

Thus, these two systems complement each other by means of an autonomous interplay that optimizes the functions of the organs of the thoracic and abdominal viscera according to the demands placed upon the organism (Dodd and Role, 1991).

The Enteric System

The enteric system is considered to be a part of the ANS, and though it is of minor interest here, it deserves brief mention. Sometimes known as the myenteric plexus, it exists throughout the length of the gastrointestinal (GI) tract from the esophagus to the anus. It is composed of an intertwining web of neurons located between the longitudinal and the circular muscle layers, which mediate peristalsis (gut motility). Its function is to provide "local" reflexes caused by stimuli arising from changes in the tension of the gut wall and in the chemical composition of the gut contents. The action of local areas of the plexus also influences GI blood vessel tone, gastric secretions, and fluid transport into the bloodstream.

The major role of the enteric system is characterized by the process of peristalsis. When food is thoroughly mixed with digestive juices in the stomach, a wave of stomach contractions propels the contents, known as chyme (a thick liquid mass of semidigested food), into the duodenum, the upper end of the small intestine. If the duodenum becomes filled to a certain extent, an enterogastric reflex is elicited that inhibits further peristaltic waves in the stomach and the flow of chyme into the duodenum. The stomach chyme is highly acidic, and it is normally neutralized by pancreatic juices in the duodenum. Acidic chyme is an irritant to the duodenum and elicits the enterogastric reflex in this way as well until the chyme acidity is neutralized. Also, when fats enter the small intestine, they stimulate the release of the hormone **cholecystokinin** from the duodenum. Cholecystokinin is absorbed into the bloodstream, and when carried to the stomach, it slows stomach peristalsis until the fats are thoroughly digested (see Chapter 11). This system is mostly self-regulated, but it does receive some excitatory input from the parasympathetic system and some inhibitory input from the sympathetic system.

The Parasympathetic System

The parasympathetic nervous system can be divided into cranial and sacral subdivisions. The generalized plan of parasympathetic innervation is illustrated in Figure 4.26: cells in the CNS give rise to axons that innervate parasympathetic ganglia and visceral organs. The cranial division is made up of cranial nerve axons that project to specific parasympathetic ganglia that lie close to the target organs. Postsynaptic cells in the ganglia project short postganglionic axons to the target glands and visceral organs. The particular cranial nerves and their specific ganglia are also shown in Figure 4.26. In the sacral division, axons making up splanchnic nerves emanate from the sacral spinal cord. The nuclei and ganglia of the parasympathetic nervous system and their target organs are listed in Table 4.2.

The cranial division.   The cranial division consists mainly of branches of four cranial efferent nerves whose nuclei are located in the brain stem (see the summary of the cranial nerves in Table 4.1). The Edinger–Westphal nucleus is the most rostral and is adjacent to the oculomotor nucleus (III) in the midbrain (see Figure 4.26). It contributes autonomic axons to the oculomotor nerve. These axons are known as preganglionic fibers because they terminate in the ciliary ganglion, which lies within the eye socket near the orbit (eyeball). From this ganglion, short postganglionic fibers project to the pupillary muscles that regulate the iris for pupil size according to light intensity, and to the ciliary muscles that alter the thickness of the lens to accommodate for near and far vision. This arrangement for the control of the autonomic activities associated with vision is similar to that for all other parasympathetic functions.

Other parasympathetic nerves are made up of the efferent branches of facial nerve VII emanating from the lacrimal nucleus and the superior salivary nucleus in the medulla to terminate in the **pterygopalatine** and **submandibular ganglia**. The postganglionic fibers control the lacrimal and mucous glands and the salivary glands, respectively. Similarly, parasympathetic efferent branches of the glossopharyngeal nerve (IX) emanate from the inferior salivary nucleus in the medulla to control, via the **otic ganglion**, other salivary and mucous glands in the oral cavity. The parasympathetic branches of these two nerves (VII and IX) also exert autonomic control of the lower two-thirds of the esophagus.

Parasympathetic branches of the vagus nerve (X) make up the fourth and most extensive group of parasympathetic efferents, which emerge from the **dorsal vagal nucleus** (also known as the dorsal efferent or motor nucleus) and **nucleus ambiguus** in the medulla. The emerging axons from these nuclei synapse with postganglionic cells in the **terminal ganglia** situated near or embedded within most organs of the viscera. The postganglionic cells in the terminal ganglia have short postganglionic fibers that innervate the organs of the thoracic and abdominal viscera (see Figure 4.26 for more details).

Stimulation of the nucleus ambiguus decreases the heart rate and cardiac contractility, resulting in a reduction of cardiac output. Activation of the dorsal vagal nucleus promotes the absorption of digested food by enhancing salivary, gastric, pancreatic, and intestinal secretions; it also increases peristalsis and promotes the relaxation of the pyloric sphincter that controls the passage of the stomach contents into the duodenum. Thus, we see that parasympathetic nerves may have either stimulating or inhibiting effects.

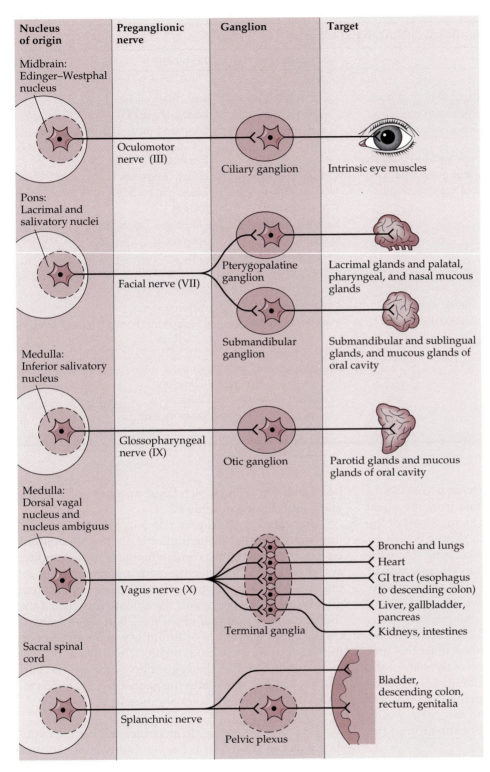

Nucleus of origin	Preganglionic nerve	Ganglion	Target
Midbrain: Edinger–Westphal nucleus	Oculomotor nerve (III)	Ciliary ganglion	Intrinsic eye muscles
Pons: Lacrimal and salivatory nuclei	Facial nerve (VII)	Pterygopalatine ganglion	Lacrimal glands and palatal, pharyngeal, and nasal mucous glands
		Submandibular ganglion	Submandibular and sublingual glands, and mucous glands of oral cavity
Medulla: Inferior salivatory nucleus	Glossopharyngeal nerve (IX)	Otic ganglion	Parotid glands and mucous glands of oral cavity
Medulla: Dorsal vagal nucleus and nucleus ambiguus	Vagus nerve (X)	Terminal ganglia	Bronchi and lungs / Heart / GI tract (esophagus to descending colon) / Liver, gallbladder, pancreas / Kidneys, intestines
Sacral spinal cord	Splanchnic nerve	Pelvic plexus	Bladder, descending colon, rectum, genitalia

4.26 THE PARASYMPATHETIC NERVOUS SYSTEM. Cranial nerves III, VII, IX, and X are preganglionic fibers to the terminal ganglia embedded within or lying near target organs. Short postganglionics nerves innervate the target sites. Sacral nerves project to the pelvic plexus or directly to pelvic organs.

Other fibers that are parts of cranial nerves VII, IX, and X emerge from the nucleus ambiguus, but most of these fibers, in contrast to those from the dorsal vagal nucleus, subserve voluntary activities such as the actions of the larynx and pharynx for speech, the intricate acts of swallowing, and the voluntary action of the upper third of the esophagus that accompanies swallowing. It should be further noted that some autonomic activities are partly under voluntary control, and that others can sometimes be conditioned. For example, we can voluntarily, within some limits, increase or decrease our respiratory rate and the volume of inspiration, and we can exert some control of the esophagus and the anal and bladder sphincters. But, for the most part, the ANS is self-regulated.

Table 4.2   The Autonomic Nervous System: Nuclei and Ganglia

Subsystem	Origin			Ganglion	Target site
Parasympathetic system					
Cranial division	N. III	Edinger–Westphal nucleus		Ciliary ganglion	Iris; ciliary muscles
	N. VII	Lacrimal nucleus		Pterygopalatine	Lacrimal gland
		Superior salivatory nucleus		Submandibular	Submandibular and sublingual glands
	N. IX	Inferior salivatory nucleus		Otic ganglion	Parotid salivary gland
	N. X	Nucleus ambiguus		Cardiac plexus	Heart, lungs, trachea
		Dorsal vagal nucleus		Hepatic plexus	Liver, gall bladder
				Renal plexus	Kidney
				Esophageal plexus	Esophagus, stomach
				Splenic plexus	Spleen
				Celiac plexus	Pancreas, intestine
Sacral division	Sacral spinal cord			Pelvic plexus	Bladder, descending colon, rectum, genital organs
Sympathetic system	Intermediolateral nucleus			Direct innervation	Adrenal gland
	Intermediolateral nucleus			Paravertebral ganglia	Cranial and thoracic organs, body wall
				Prevertebral ganglia	
				Celiac	Stomach, liver, pancreas, small intestine
				Aortico-renal	Kidney
				Superior mesenteric	Large intestine
				Inferior mesenteric	Large intestine, pelvic organs

The sacral division.   The sacral division consists of branches of the pelvic nerve emanating from the sacral parasympathetic nuclei in sacral segments S2–S4 of the spinal cord (see Figures 4.25 and 4.26.) These nerves innervate the smooth muscles of the descending colon, the rectum, the bladder, and the glands and vascular system of the male and female genitalia via the pelvic plexus nuclei lying near the respective pelvic organs. Visceral afferents from the bladder, rectum, and genital organs also project back to the spinal cord for autonomic reflexes, and for further projection to the thalamus and sensory cortex for conscious awareness of the state of the pelvic organs. For example, some of these sensory feedbacks provide sensations from the genital organs, and the sensations from the bladder and the colon which contribute to the voluntary control of function of the pelvic organs.

Parasympathetic postganglionic nuclei.   As described above, the efferent parasympathetic nerves of both divisions do not innervate the target areas directly. As can be seen in Figure 4.26, the autonomic efferent nerves synapse with aggregated neurons making up autonomic ganglia that lie near the target areas. Examples of these autonomic ganglia are the ciliary ganglion within the eye, the otic ganglion near the parotid salivary gland, and the ganglia of the coronary plexus that affect the

heart and lungs. Thus, each target area has its own ganglion, as indicated in Table 4.2.

The ganglion cells give rise to a network of short, fine, unmyelinated postganglionic fibers with **boutons en passant** (varicosities) containing the neurotransmitter **acetylcholine** (ACh), which spreads among receptors on the muscles of the iris, the cells of the salivary and tear glands, cardiac muscle, and the smooth muscles of the thoracic and abdominal viscera. ACh in these systems can be either excitatory or inhibitory depending upon the receptors on the various organs. Thus, it is somewhat inaccurate to say that the vagus nerve inhibits the heart when it actually stimulates the ganglion cells, which release ACh that inhibits coronary muscles.

Visceral afferent nerves.   In an earlier section, the hypothalamus was described as having a number of neuronal nuclei that respond to neural and hormonal signals related to the rate of the heartbeat, hunger, water balance, blood loss, body temperature, sex hormone concentrations, and needs associated with growth and procreation. Most of the inputs to these nuclei are hormonal or come from the limbic lobe and its ancillary neural structures; the major outputs are projected to the brain stem efferent nuclei, which give rise to the parasympathetic preganglionic fibers. In addition to this control system, there are a number of autonomic systems that are either self-modulating or able to elicit modulating influences from higher levels of the neuraxis. At the simplest level, the ANS is activated in obvious ways: bright light instigates pupil constriction, the smell and taste of food instigate salivary responses, corneal irritation or emotional expression elicits the release of tears, food in the stomach elicits the release of digestive enzymes and peristalsis, and high blood pressure elicits a decrease in the heart rate and the force of contraction.

These reactions are self-regulated partly by reflexive sensory feedback that is mediated by visceral afferent nerves. These nerves follow the same course in the body as the visceral efferent nerves, but the flow of information obviously is in the opposite direction. The cell bodies of these sensory nerves are in the nodose ganglion of the vagus nerve (X), and the sensory axons enter the brain stem as the solitary tract (fasciculus solitarius). This tract terminates in the **solitary nucleus** (also known as the parasolitary nucleus), which lies adjacent to the dorsal vagal nucleus and nucleus ambiguus (N.X; see Figure 4.5 and Table 4.2).

Along with the hypothalamus, the solitary nucleus is a major coordinating center for autonomic function. It consists of a long column of cells that receive visceral sensory information, including taste, and its output influences the adjacent dorsal vagal nucleus and nucleus ambiguus, which provide the principal autonomic outputs from the brain stem (Figure 4.27). Such autonomic reflex circuits are made up of sensory (visceral afferent) fibers from the heart, lungs, and the organs of the GI tract that project to cell groups within the solitary nucleus in a viscerotopic manner; that is, there are separate cell groups in the solitary nucleus for each organ. As mentioned above, the axons of these cell groups, in turn, project to and modulate those cell groups in the dorsal vagal nucleus that initiated the visceral activity in the first place.

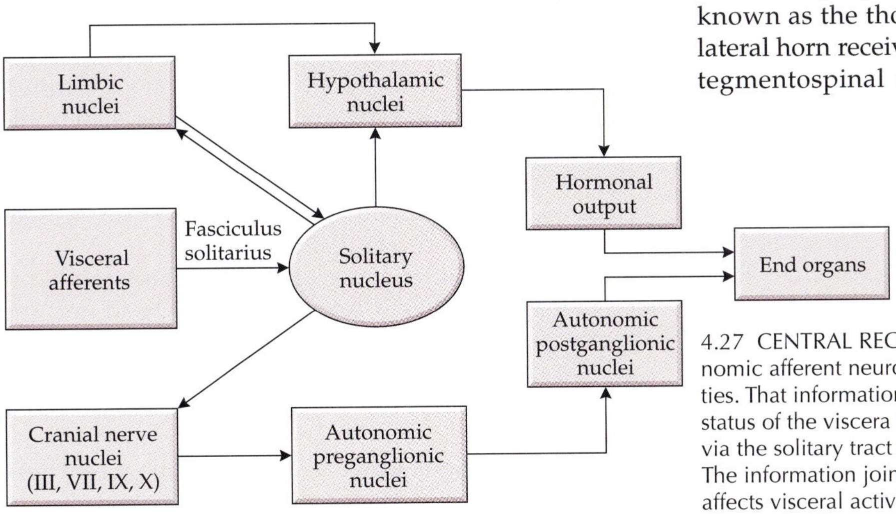

Further, the solitary nucleus coordinates elaborate homeostatic adjustments by transmitting visceral sensory information to the higher autonomic centers of the limbic system, such as the amygdala, the paraventricular nucleus of the hypothalamus, and the bed nucleus of the stria terminalis, which arises in the amygdala and projects to the hypothalamus and other brain stem and forebrain nuclei. These regions then relay the integrated information required for more complex autonomic control back to the solitary nucleus, the dorsal vagal nucleus, and other lower brain stem nuclei, as well as the spinal cord centers from which the sympathetic system originates. However, some of the solitary nuclear outputs inhibit the sympathetic centers to balance the execution of autonomic functions.

The solitary nucleus is also a major relay point for taste and sensory visceral stimuli, which are projected not only to the cranial nuclei for salivation, facial reflexes (puckering the mouth to sour tastes), and peristalsis, but also to the thalamus and sensory cortex for conscious sensations of taste and visceral sensations such as hunger, general malaise, indigestion, nausea, and pain from hyperacidity, or cramps from bowel distension. Nonetheless, for the most part, the GI tract functions without any conscious awareness; once food is swallowed, the GI tract executes the digestive process autonomously. The visceral afferents from the pelvic organs were described above in the section on the parasympathetic sacral division.

The Sympathetic System

The neurons making up the sympathetic division of the ANS are also shown in Figure 4.25. They consist, first, of preganglionic sympathetic nerves originating from cell bodies in the **intermediolateral nucleus** in the lateral horn of the spinal cord (Figure 4.28). The intermediolateral nucleus extends as a cell column from the first thoracic (T1) to the third lumbar (L3) segment of the spinal cord. Thus, the sympathetic division of the ANS is sometimes known as the thoracolumbar division. The cells of the lateral horn receive inputs from limbic structures via the tegmentospinal and reticulospinal tracts (see Figure

4.27 CENTRAL REGULATION OF AUTONOMIC OUTPUT. Autonomic afferent neurons supply information about visceral activities. That information is processed for reflexive responses, or the status of the viscera is monitored by the central autonomic circuits via the solitary tract (fasciculus solitarius) or the solitary nucleus. The information joins with the hypothalamic hormonal input that affects visceral activities in the end-organs in the thoracic, abdominal, and pelvic cavities. (After Loewy and Spyer, 1990.)

4.13). These inputs consist of information integrated by the hypothalamus and other limbic structures into a coherent pattern for autonomic responses.

The preganglionic sympathetic efferent axons that emerge from the lateral horn cells exit the spinal cord along with the ventral (motor) roots for a short distance before separating from them to enter the myelinated **white communicating rami** (communicating branches) that lead to the **sympathetic paravertebral ganglia** (also known as chain ganglia), which lie along both sides of the vertebral column (see Figure 4.25). Twenty-six pairs of these ganglia are arranged in a chainlike fashion and are interconnected by ascending presynaptic axon collaterals among the upper chain ganglia and by descending collaterals among the lower ones. The top ganglion in the chain is known as the superior cervical ganglion, the second is the middle cervical ganglion, and the third is the stellate ganglion.

Within the chain ganglia, some of the presynaptic neurons synapse with postganglionic neurons that recombine with the spinal nerves via the gray communicating rami (see Figure 4.28), and follow the spinal nerves to the body wall, where they energize peripheral autonomic effector microorgans such as hair follicles, sweat glands, and the smooth muscles of blood vessels in the skin. One instance of this system is illustrated in Figure 4.25. Preganglionic fibers enter the chain ganglia, where some fibers turn and ascend to the superior sympathetic ganglion. There, the fibers synapse with postganglionic cells whose axons project to the microorgans in the body wall. Even though there are only twenty-six chain ganglia and thirty pairs of spinal nerves, all spinal nerves contain sympathetic postganglionic components because the superior cervical ganglion supplies cervical spinal nerves C1 through C4, the middle cervical ganglion supplies nerves C5 and C6, and the stellate ganglion supplies nerves C7 and C8 (as shown in Figure 4.25). Thus, the peripheral vasculature, sweat glands, and hair follicles of the entire body wall are influenced by this system. The function of this part of the sympathetic system is to constrict peripheral blood vessels and fluff up body hair (fur and feathers in animals) when the body is cold, and to stimulate sweat glands (or panting) and dilate the blood vessels when the body is warm.

Another part of the sympathetic system is made up of postganglionic axons from the top three chain ganglia—the superior cervical, the middle cervical, and the stellate ganglion—and the first five thoracic chain ganglia. These axons project to intracranial blood vessels and to all organs and glands that are also innervated by the parasympathetic cranial nerves. One sympathetic pathway to the eye provides the stimulation of the pupillary muscles that causes pupil dilation during states of fear or emotion, whereas bright light stimulates the parasympathetic input to the pupillary muscles, causing pupil constriction. Other branches provide the

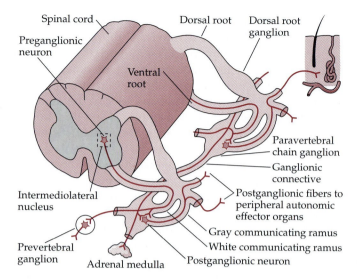

4.28 THE SYMPATHETIC NERVOUS SYSTEM. Preganglionic sympathetic nerves emerge from the intermediolateral nucleus of the spinal cord. The preganglionic nerves exit via the ventral root and the white rami to the chain ganglia. After synapse, some postganglionics reenter the spinal nerve via the gray rami and project with the spinal nerve to the body wall. Other preganglionics proceed from the chain ganglia without synapsing to the adrenal gland or to the prevertebral ganglia and effector organs. (After Loewy and Spyer, 1990.)

sympathetic input for the heart and lungs. For example, the sympathetic cardiac accelerator fibers that emanate from the top eight chain ganglia terminate upon specialized receptors on the heart wall that lie close to the pacemaker and modulate its inherent rhythm and thus the heart rate. Sympathetic postganglionics from the lower chain ganglia control the vasculature of the lower body and the organs in the pelvic viscera.

It should be evident that sympathetic system affects virtually all internal organs of the body, either by activating them or by inhibiting them. For example, whereas the parasympathetic system slows the heart and energizes the GI tract, the sympathetic system energizes the cardiovascular system and inhibits the GI tract. Furthermore, whereas the sympathetic system affects all of the internal organs at the same time in one way or the other, the parasympathetic system can act more selectively by promoting digestion without affecting the cardiovascular system or the salivary glands.

The sympathetic innervation of the abdominal organs differs somewhat from that of the head and the thoracic organs. The preganglionic axons for the abdominal organs emerge from the lateral horn and pass through the chain ganglia without synapse, then converge to form splanchnic nerves that terminate in the **prevertebral ganglia** (see Figure 4.25, Table 4.2). These ganglia are known as the celiac, the aorticorenal, the superior mesenteric, and the inferior mesenteric ganglia.

From these ganglia, long sympathetic postganglionics are projected to the organs of the abdominal viscera such as the stomach, kidneys, pancreas, gall bladder, liver, and intestines. They also supply sympathetic inputs to the pelvic organs: the descending colon, the urinary bladder, and the vasculature and smooth muscle of the internal and external genitalia. Thus, the sympathetic postganglionics are considerably longer than the postganglionic parasympathetic fibers, and travel in bundles from their respective prevertebral ganglia to their target sites.

An exception to the above arrangement is found in the paths of preganglionic fibers from the lower thoracic spinal nerves that pass through the chain ganglia and terminate directly upon the adrenal glands. When sympathetic preganglionic nerves stimulate the core of these glands, the adrenal medulla, they produce and release **epinephrine** and **norepinephrine** into the bloodstream. These compounds are neurotransmitters that are also produced in the CNS, and when they are released by the adrenal medulla, they supplement those substances of neural origin. They enhance sympathetic activity by directly activating a number of biological systems that are also under neuronal control, and though this hormonal control is slower, it is more sustained. A pedestrian crossing the street accelerates instantly when a car comes dangerously close, but the rapid heartbeat and respiration and trembling continue long after reaching the opposite side. Sympathetic responses to sustained threats include the acceleration of the heart and respiratory rates, diminished GI peristalsis, an increased release of glucose from the liver, an up to a 100% increase in basal metabolism, an increased release of epinephrine from the adrenal glands, and a shift in the blood circulation away from the abdominal viscera and toward the heart and somatic musculature. (Other neurotransmitters besides acetylcholine and norepinephrine also function within the autonomic nervous system. These include certain neuropeptides, which are discussed further in Chapter 11.)

Furthermore, because sympathetic effects tend to be diffuse and somewhat intense when the organism is exposed to stresses such as heat, cold, or predator threat, the limbic lobe activates the hypothalamus, which in turn activates the sympathetic system in its entirety, thereby dominating the autonomic system in using the body resources to withstand the threatening situation. This function is maximized by the high divergence of the sympathetic system, which was described at the beginning of this section.

The sympathetic sensory system. Finally, it is important to mention that all organs that are affected by sympathetic nerves also have sense organs that give rise to sympathetic afferent (sensory) nerves. These nerves project to the spinal cord where they synapse with visceral motor

nerves for visceral reflexes in ways similar to somatic spinal reflexes. A comparison between somatic and visceral reflexes is shown in Figure 4.29. The visceral sensory nerves follow the path of the sympathetic efferents in the opposite direction back to the white rami to enter the spinal sensory dorsal root ganglia. The axons of these cells synapse via short interneurons in the gray matter upon sympathetic preganglionic visceral neurons in the lateral horn, while some collateral fibers ascend to the thalamus and brain to provide some awareness of visceral function. The axons of the lateral horn cells emerge via the ventral roots and the white rami to synapse upon postganglionic cells in the chain ganglia or those in the prevertebral ganglia. The postganglionic fibers project to the visceral organs of origin, mostly the organs of the GI tract, while some project to the peripheral blood vessels and the microorgans of the skin. Also, collaterals of these nerves continue their course to the thalamus or nucleus solitarius and the limbic lobe for sensory awareness of visceral sensations such as hunger, feelings of malaise, discomfort, and pain. Further, as mentioned earlier, the cells in the intermediolateral gray in the lateral horn are under the influence of limbic structures so that emotional states can affect visceral organs.

In general, the relations between the sympathetic and parasympathetic systems can be summarized as follows:

1. Either system may be stimulatory or inhibitory on a particular organ.
2. When both systems act on an organ, their actions are usually opposed to one another.
3. Many of the visceral organs are predominantly controlled by one system or the other, and some organs are exclusively controlled by one system or the other.

Autonomic substrates for emotions. It should be noted that the solitary nucleus has reciprocal relationships with the limbic structures such as the hippocampus and the hypothalamus (see Figure 4.27). It is the head nucleus of the ANS and mediates many of the attributes of emotional behavior. Also, as mentioned earlier, there are inhibitory as well as excitatory effects on the sympathetic nervous system that are mediated via tegmental or reticular spinal tracts that project to the spinal origin of the sympathetic nervous system: the intermediolateral nucleus. The inhibitory effects may serve to balance the effects of the parasympathetic and sympathetic systems. On the other hand, the sympathetic nervous system plays a dominant role in emotional behavior that is mediated by connections between the solitary nucleus and the limbic lobe.

Figures 4.13c and 4.14 show some of the relationships between the limbic structures and their projections to the brain stem. What should be especially noted is the descending output from the hypothalamus to the brain

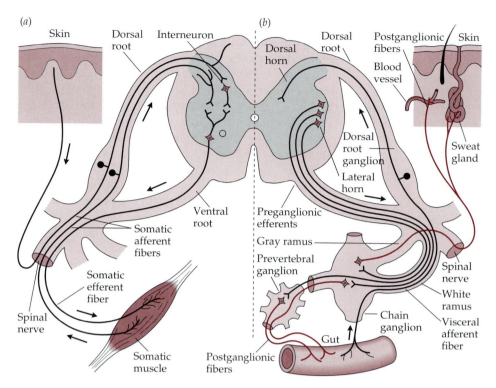

(a) Skin · Dorsal root · Interneuron · Dorsal horn · *(b)* Dorsal root · Postganglionic fibers · Skin · Blood vessel · Dorsal root ganglion · Lateral horn · Sweat gland · Ventral root · Preganglionic efferents · Gray ramus · Prevertebral ganglion · Somatic afferent fibers · Somatic efferent fiber · Spinal nerve · Spinal nerve · White ramus · Visceral afferent fiber · Chain ganglion · Gut · Somatic muscle · Postganglionic fibers · Somatic muscle

4.29 A COMPARISON BETWEEN SOMATIC AND VISCERAL SPINAL REFLEXES. (*a*) Somatic nerves. Somatic afferent fibers from sense organs in the skin or muscles enter the spinal cord via the dorsal roots and activate the efferent fibers (motor neurons) which exit via the ventral roots. (*b*) Visceral nerves. Sympathetic visceral afferents arise from sense organs of the viscera and enter the spinal cord via the white rami and dorsal roots, and the preganglionic sympathetic efferents exit via the ventral roots and white rami to project back to the paravertebral and prevertebral ganglia to synapse with postganglionics that project to the visceral organs of origin. Some postganglionics innervate the microorgans of the skin. The interneurons in the gray matter between the afferent and efferent neurons are not shown. (After Bloom and Fawcett, 1986.)

stem and spinal cord via the central tegmental tract (part of the reticular formation) and the dorsal longitudinal fasciculus (which originates in the limbic structures of the diencephalon). These descending tracts make synaptic contact with cranial nerve nuclei such as those of the facial nerve (VII), which mediate the facial expression of emotion with crying and tears, and the dorsal vagal nucleus and nucleus ambiguus (X), which modulate the heart rate and mediate the emotional responses of the thoracic and visceral organs. Thus, connections among the solitary nucleus, the cortex, and the limbic lobe allow the sight, smell, taste, or even the thought of food to lead to salivation; and scolding, conflict, shame, fear, or feelings of guilt can lead to tears, loss of appetite, indigestion, increased blood pressure and heart rate, and inhibition of the sacral parasympathetic control of sexual behavior.

Part III Summary

Parasympathetic activity is principally under the control of limbic structures of the diencephalon and the older parts of the cerebrum such as the limbic lobe and its accessory structures: the amygdala, the hippocampus, and the septal regions associated with olfactory stimuli. The output from these structures is projected via the medial forebrain bundle, the dorsal longitudinal fasciculus, and related pathways to the brain stem nuclei of cranial nerves III, VII, IX, and X, which supply parasympathetic innervation of the visceral organs.

Important elements of the ANS are the autonomic sympathetic and parasympathetic sensory afferent nerves. The sympathetic afferents modulate the sympathetic output, and the parasympathetic afferents supply information about the internal organs of the body to the solitary nucleus, which reflexly regulates the autonomic outflow from the parasympathetic brain stem nuclei. In addition, the solitary nucleus has reciprocal relations with the limbic lobe and the hypothalamus to form a central autonomic circuit that affects autonomic, hormonal, and behavioral activities. In this way, changes in the internal environment supply the instigating stimuli for motivated behavior and energize the efforts needed to restore homeostasis, with the highly divergent sympathetic system permitting the entire body to respond in energetic ways.

Sympathetic inputs to the visceral organs are energized in situations of stress as formulated by the limbic lobe and cerebral cortex, whose influence is promulgated via the hypothalamus and the tegmentospinal and reticulospinal tracts to the preganglionic sympathetic neurons in the lateral horn. These neurons activate postganglionic neurons that also make neuroeffector synapses on autonomic organs, but generally, the sympathetic autonomic responses are opposite to those elicited by the parasympathetic stimuli.

This arrangement is similar to that of the somatic motor system described earlier. That is, the spinal motor nerves activate the skeletal musculature to perform intricate motor skills, but the instructions for those skills have been formulated in great detail by the sensory and motor cortex and modulated by the cerebellum and the basal ganglia before being projected to the motor neurons of the spinal cord. Similarly, the limbic lobe signals sympathetic responses, which are projected via the tegmentospinal and reticulospinal tracts to the lateral horn of the spinal cord for the ultimate expression of the sympathetic response by the pre- and postganglionic sympathetic nerves. Further, parasympathetic and sympathetic local reflexes may "fine-tune" the autonomic responses just as somatic responses are fine-tuned by spinal reflexes.

To illustrate the function of the ANS in a simple case: A human newborn, only days old, wakes after a nap with cries and thrashing limbs. An offered nipple is readily drawn into the mouth and vigorously sucked. The infant has a "wired" program in the limbic lobe for an extremely intricate form of behavior initiated by "hunger" stimuli and mediated by somatic and visceral afferent and efferent cranial nerves. These nerves mediate a sense of hunger, vocalization, taste, and the tactile sensation of the nipple. This information is integrated and projected to the nerves mediating the oral musculature for sucking and swallowing until digestion and satiety signals terminate the behavior and restore sleep. Moreover, this behavior becomes more efficient after a few sessions, indicating maturation and learning.

Thus, we see that the autonomic and the somatic systems are continually interacting to convert the needs of the body (such as food and water) or of the species (sexual expression) into overt behaviors such as seeking or hunting for food or competing for sexual partners. Further, acts such as hunting or competing for partners, or defense against predators, are accompanied by high levels of sympathetic activity that increase the energy output and thus the probability of success. In humans, the awareness of these high levels of autonomic activity contributes in an important way to our feelings and emotions. Furthermore, in humans, these autonomic substrates may be aroused by symbolic stimuli that arise out of racial, ethnic, and political differences, frequently with catastrophic consequences.

This outline of the structure and function of the central and autonomic nervous system describes many structures that will be mentioned and discussed in future chapters. Understandably, our treatment of this subject is severely restricted by the amount of space available for this purpose. However, we have presented enough information so that the rationale, method, and consequences of chemical alterations of neural function will be more completely understood.

Chapter 5

Neurophysiological Mechanisms

Part I
Bioelectric Properties of Neurons

This chapter describes the electrochemical events that lead to the generation of nerve impulses, their propagation from one end of a neuron to the other, and the transfer of the impulse from one cell to another. A basic review of these processes will contribute to an understanding of drug actions on neural tissue.

Perhaps the very beginning of neurophysiology goes back to 1839 when Theodor Schwann extended the cell theory from plants to animals and discovered the peripheral glia that bear his name (see Chapter 3). Since then, Cajal, in 1887, mastered the Golgi stain to show the variation among neurons; Sherrington, in 1897, named the synapse; Bernstein, in 1902, proposed the membrane hypothesis; Adrian, in 1914, described the all-or-none principle in nerves; and Loewi and Dale, in 1921, in their Nobel Prize-winning work, demonstrated chemical neurotransmission at nerve–muscle synapses.

Jumping ahead to the mid-1930s, Dale and Feldberg demonstrated the release of acetylcholine in sympathetic ganglia, and teams of researchers set up laboratories in many countries to advance neuroscience. In Europe, this activity was interrupted by political extremism and World War II, but was resumed at an accelerated pace during the postwar years. In 1963, John C. Eccles, Alan L. Hodgkin, and Andrew F. Huxley were awarded the Nobel Prize in Physiology and Medicine for their contributions to the understanding of nerve function. In 1970, Julius Axelrod, Bernhard Katz, and Ulf von Euler were also awarded a Nobel Prize for their work in neurochemistry. Most recently, Bert Sakmann and Erwin Neher shared a 1991 Nobel Prize for their novel patch-clamp methods for investigating the molecular attributes of neuromuscular signal transmission. These researchers, as well as many others we did not name, made significant contributions to the foundations of contemporary neurophysiology.

In the present period of neuroscience, the mechanics of synaptic interaction and the analysis of neuronal connectivity are central to all theories of information processing by the nervous system. Further, we have entered a period of molecular neurobiology, which emphasizes the molecular basis of cellular and systemic function. This chapter presents a relatively brief overview of neural cell physiology, and many contemporary studies in molecular neurobiology are cited in this volume. (For an interesting historical review, see Horn, 1992.)

Neuron Excitability

In multicellular organisms, each cell population is dependent upon, and responds to the requirements of, other cell populations. Coordination is possible because chemical signals serve as messengers among the cell groups. Excitable cells respond to these chemical signals by way of molecular "antennae" (receptors) that are dispersed upon their surface membranes. For example, when stimulated, neurons generate and propagate nerve impulses, muscle cells contract, and glandular cells secrete. To illustrate, glucose, at high blood levels, stimulates receptors on the β-cells of the pancreas, causing a release of insulin, and this hormone in turn acts upon other cell membranes to initiate the transport of the glucose into the cells that need it. When the blood glucose level falls, the process is terminated.

The suckling reflex is an example of the coordination among neuronal and hormonal cell groups. When a mammalian offspring, such as a cub, pup, foal, calf, or infant stimulates tactile sense organs in the mother's nipple, the resulting nerve impulses are propagated to her brain, as shown in Figure 5.1. There, other nerve cells are stimulated, which send signals to neurosecretory cells in the hypothalamus. In turn, hypothalamic neurons release a hormone, oxytocin, which is transported via the cell axons to the posterior pituitary, where it is absorbed into a capillary system of the bloodstream and distributed throughout the body. In the mammary glands, oxytocin stimulates receptors on the myoepithelial cells that line the milk-collecting channels, causing them to contract and expel milk into the ducts leading to the nipple (see Chapter 11 for further details). In molecular terms, special receptors on the nipple, nerve cells, neurosecretory cells, and myoepithelial cells participate in a train of events that is started by suckling and ultimately ends with the satiety of the newborn.

Neurons, like many other plant and animal cells, have excitable cytoplasmic membranes. The membrane of a neuron covers the dendrites, cell bodies, and axons (the axolemma), and the stimulation of receptors on the neuronal surface can lead to nerve impulses that are propagated over the surface of the cell, including the entire length of the axolemma, whose surface may be 5,000 times greater than the surface of the cell soma. Stimulation of skeletal and cardiac muscle membranes also leads to excitation that spreads to adjacent areas, and similar events occur in the pituitary secretory cells and in the islet cells of the pancreas that secrete insulin. Indeed, the ability to generate and propagate impulses is a general characteristic of many different cells depending on their particular functions.

In the case of neurons, however, the propagation of nerve impulses to axon terminals, and the transfer of the signal to other neurons or effector organs, appears to be their sole function. Furthermore, sense organs on the skin, in muscle systems, and in the tissue of the special external sense organs are synaptically connected to sensory neurons. These neurons serve as transducers converting sensory stimuli into nerve impulses that lead to secretory activity and movement, conscious sensations, memory, and cognition. Whereas the conversion of nerve impulses into glandular secretion and muscle movement is generally well understood, the transduction of nerve

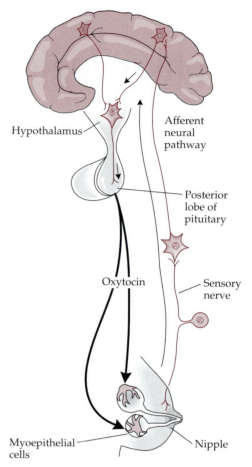

5.1 THE SUCKLING REFLEX. Stimulation of the nipples generates nerve impulses that pass to the central nervous system via sensory nerves. In the brain, these impulses are relayed to the hypothalamus, where they activate neurosecretory cells. When activated, these cells secrete oxytocin, which is conveyed via their axons to the posterior lobe of the pituitary. These axons terminate upon capillaries that absorb the oxytocin into the bloodstream. In the mammary glands, oxytocin causes the contraction of myoepithelial cells around the milk-collecting channels, expelling the milk. (After Fawcett, 1986.)

impulses into memory, sensory and perceptual awareness, and cognition is still a subject of intense speculation, even though the brain loci for these functions have been identified and much of the underlying molecular structure and physiology of the particular neurons have been determined.

The Membrane Resting Potential

The generation of a signal and its propagation from one part of a neuron to another depends upon a voltage difference between the outside and inside surfaces of the neuronal membrane. This voltage difference is known as the **resting potential**. The resting potential can be briefly modified by a variety of stimuli. When it is so modified, a signal, known as an **action potential**, is generated, which is propagated along the length of the axon to the axon terminals. This effect raises two questions: What is responsible for the resting potential, and how is the resting potential related to the generation of action potentials?

Early experiments in neurophysiology by John Z. Young in 1936, which led to an understanding of such phenomena as the resting potential, utilized the giant axon of squids and related species. In squids, this axon conducts nerve impulses to the jetlike apparatus that propels these creatures through the water. These axons, which were first thought to be veins, are between 0.5 and 1.0 mm in diameter, approximately 100 times thicker than the largest mammalian axons. They are large enough to allow the insertion of long electrodes, which can be used to measure the voltage difference between the inside and outside of an axon when it is at rest and when stimulated. Moreover, the absence of myelin on the axons of invertebrates further simplifies the interpretation of the recordings.

Later, in the 1950s, Alan Hodgkin and Andrew Huxley developed a method known as voltage clamping, which clearly identified the molecular events leading to resting and action potentials. (For an exposition of the voltage clamping technique, see Hall, 1992.) Microelectrode tips less than 0.5 μm in diameter, which can stimulate and measure voltage changes in axons only 10 μm in diameter, were subsequently developed. These microelectrode tips can be inserted through the axolemma, whose lipid layers naturally form a tight seal around it and allow the axon to function quite normally for several hours.

More recently, improved microelectrodes have been designed for use in new methods of recording electrical events in neurons, methods known as **patch clamping**. These methods allow measurements to be made from microscopic patches of neuronal surfaces instead of penetrating the axolemma with a pointed tip. A patch-clamp electrode consists of the fire-polished tip of a glass micropipette having a diameter of 1–5 μm. After the extracellular matrix, consisting of substances secreted by the cell, has been broken down and eliminated, the tip is brought into close contact with the cell surface. The contact between the tip of the pipette and the membrane surface can be secured by a gentle suction within the pipette, which induces an extremely strong and tight seal that has a gigaohm (10^{11} ohms) resistance between the pipette orifice and the lipid bilayer. This method causes less injury to the cell than penetration by a conventional microelectrode. Further, it can electrically isolate a small patch that may include only a single microscopic membrane channel so that measures of the small changes in resistance caused by the opening and closing of the single channel can be made (see Sakmann, 1992).

Figure 5.2*a* shows a patch-clamp pipette sealed against the membrane of a frog skeletal muscle fiber to isolate one acetylcholine (ACh) receptor. The pipette is filled with a physiological salt solution. A metal electrode connects the electrolyte to a special electric circuit that measures the current that flows through the membrane

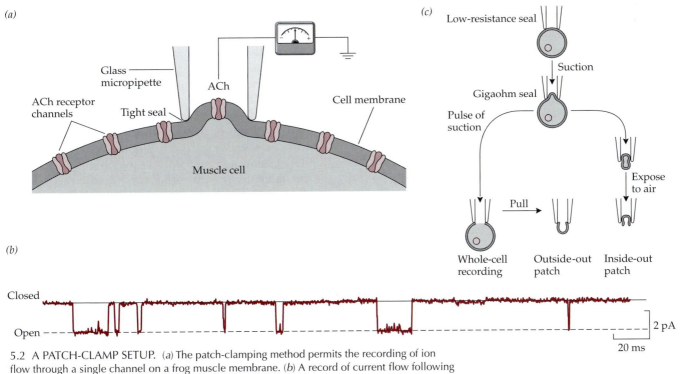

5.2 A PATCH-CLAMP SETUP. (*a*) The patch-clamping method permits the recording of ion flow through a single channel on a frog muscle membrane. (*b*) A record of current flow following channel opening and closing. The clarity of the on–off signal is a consequence of the isolation of the patch-clamped channel from other channels (*c*) Gigaohm seals permit four different methods of recording the electrical properties of membranes. (*b* after Sakmann, 1992; *c* after Hamill et al., 1981.)

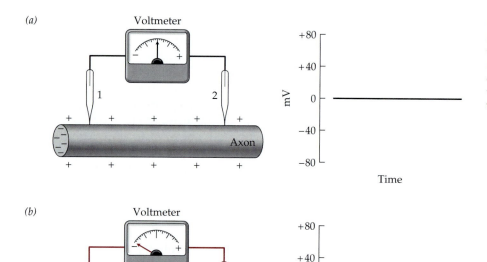

(a) Voltmeter

(b) Voltmeter

Axon

Electrode
inserted

Time

5.3 INTRACELLULAR RECORDING FROM A SQUID AXON. (a) Microelectrodes applied to the membrane surface record no voltage change. (b) When microelectrode 1 is inserted into the axoplasm, a voltage change is recorded. The graphs chart the voltage changes over time.

channels under the pipette tip (Figure 5.2b). This ion flow constitutes the electric current across the membrane.

The patch-clamp technique can also be used to pull a small piece of the membrane away from the cell by increasing the suction of the pipette (Figure 5.2c). This technique provides a low-resistance pathway into the cell interior. This preparation permits whole-cell recording when substances are diffused into the cell from an aqueous environment. In another procedure, a small patch of membrane can be removed from a cell. The membrane patch normally forms a closed vesicle after its detachment, but if it is exposed to air, the vesicle bursts, providing the pipette with an inside-out membrane patch that allows researchers to observe the effects of various electrical or chemical treatments on channels from the intracellular side. The results of such treatments are described in the following sections. (See Hamill, Marty, Neher, Sakmann, and Sigworth, 1981; and Sargent, 1992, for more details.)

Measurement of the Resting Potential

If two recording electrodes are separated and placed in contact with the outside surface of a squid axolemma in a seawater bath, no voltage is recorded (Figure 5.3a). However, if one of the electrodes is inserted into the axoplasm, a negative voltage difference of approximately 70 millivolts (−70 mV) between the interior and the exterior of the axolemma will be recorded (Figure 5.3b). This voltage across the membrane is the membrane resting potential, consisting of an excess of negatively charged

ions on the inner membrane surface and an excess of positive ions on the outer surface. The excesses of these ions represent a minuscule fraction of the total number of ions inside and outside the axolemma, and the voltage difference is almost insignificantly small. The membrane, however, is only about a millionth of a centimeter thick. Thus, the resting potential is equivalent to about 100,000 volts across a membranelike structure 1.0 cm thick. Further, it should be noted that −70 mV is only approximate; the resting potentials of most neurons range between −60 and −70 mV.

Figure 5.4 schematically shows the relative concentrations of different ions on either side of a squid axolemma in a seawater bath. Organic anions (A^-) are highly concentrated on the inner membrane surface but are virtually absent in the seawater because they are the product of the dissociation of cellular proteins along with aspartic, glutamic, and fumaric acids. In the natural state they are largely confined to the inner part of a cell because they are not able to pass through the axolemma to the outside due to their size and lipid insolubility. Potassium ion (K^+) concentration is 40 times greater inside the axon than outside, and the outside concentrations of sodium ions (Na^+) and chloride ions (Cl^-) are 9 and 13.5 times greater, respectively, than the inside concentrations.

Table 5.1 shows a comparison of experimentally determined ion concentrations in the cytosol and extracellular fluid of two large excitable cells from which measurements are relatively easy to obtain: a frog muscle

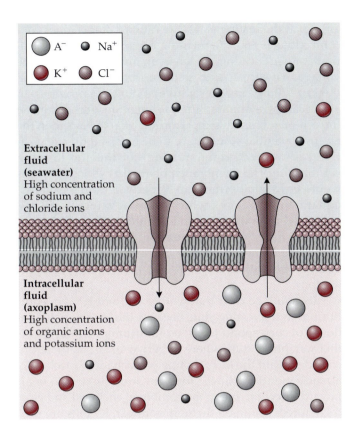

Extracellular
fluid
(seawater)
High concentration
of sodium and
chloride ions

Intracellular
fluid
(axoplasm)
High concentration
of organic anions
and potassium ions

5.4 ION DISTRIBUTIONS ACROSS A SQUID AXON. The shaded area represents a section of the membrane covering a squid axon that divides the intracellular from the extracellular fluid (seawater). In the fluid of the two compartments, various ion species are suspended. The greater intracellular concentration of K^+ induces it to flow out into the extracellular fluid, and the greater Na^+ concentration outside the cell induces it to flow inward. The membrane is impermeable to the organic anions (A^-), and the pores for Cl^- transport are not shown.

Establishment of the Resting Potential

We can now ask, how do these differential ion distributions and concentrations come to exist and create the resting potential? We can begin to answer this question by pointing out that ions diffuse freely in aqueous solutions. This is exemplified by the rapidity with which salt (NaCl) dissolves in water, forming ions of Na^+ and Cl^-. But ions rarely cross cell membranes because ions in solution are surrounded by adhering water molecules, which cannot penetrate the oily phospholipid bilayer that makes up the axolemma. (See Chapter 3 for a description of membrane constituents.) Considering this incompatibility alone, an ion is 10^{72} times more likely to be found in an aqueous solution than in a hydrocarbon environment. Thus, living cells, which depend upon the uptake and extrusion of a variety of ions and molecules, must have a means by which materials can pass in both directions through the confining cell membrane.

One mechanism for membrane transport is the presence of families of special channels in cell membranes. For ions such as K^+, Na^+, Cl^-, and some others that are characteristically present in the intracellular and extracellular compartments of nerve cells, transport through these channels is selective, allowing certain ions to pass into or out of the cell, but excluding others.

To explain the existence of neuronal membrane resting potentials, we will first mention a few facts about electricity in biological systems. In copper wires, electric currents are manifested by the movement of electrons

fiber and a squid giant axon in situ. The absolute values of these measurements were somewhat different from those obtained from squid axons in seawater, but the values for the axon of a squid, a marine animal, and muscle fibers from a frog, a freshwater species, were quite similar. As the table shows, for each ion, the ratios between inner and outer concentrations were about the same, and in the same direction. Also, it should be noted that the frog extracellular fluid contains organic anions, which have negligible effects on the resting potential, but whose negative charge within the axoplasm is a factor in determining the distribution of other ions to which the cell is permeable.

Table 5.1	Approximate Concentrations of the Major Ionic Constituents Inside and Outside Cells (mM)					
	Frog muscle fiber			Squid giant axon		
Ion	Intracellular	Extracellular	$E_{ion}{}^a$	Intracellular	Extracellular	$E_{ion}{}^a$
K^+	140	2.5	−102 mV	400	10	−93 mV
Na^+	10	120	+63 mV	50	460	+56 mV
Cl^-	1.5	77.5	−99 mV	100	540	−42 mV
Organic anions	86	40	—	360	—	—
Membrane potential (V_m)			−90 mV			−70 mV

$^a E_{ion}$ = equilibrium potential.
Sources: After Hodgkin, 1964; Katz, 1966.

that are part of the copper molecules, whereas in biological systems, electric currents are carried in ionic solutions by anions (–) and cations (+), with currents flowing (by convention) from + to –, or in the direction of cation movement. Thus, when cations flow into an axon, making the inside less negative (e.g., from –70 to –40 mV), we say that the membrane is **depolarized**,* and when cations flow out of an axon, making the interior more negative (e.g., from –70 to –90 mV), we say that the membrane is **hyperpolarized**.

It is also necessary to point out that two basic chemical conditions must be met for a resting potential to exist. First, both the intracellular and the extracellular environments have to be electrically neutral. That is, within both environments, every positive ion (e.g., K⁺ inside the cell) must be paired with a negative ion (e.g., organic anions and Cl⁻). Second, the cell has to be in osmotic balance with its environment. If the concentration of particles in solution is less within the cell than outside of the cell, water will leave the cell, causing the cell to shrink. If the particle concentration within the cell is greater than that outside the cell, water will enter the cell, causing the cell to swell until osmotic balance is achieved. It is sufficient to say here that the mechanisms underlying the establishment of the resting potential allow these chemical conditions to be satisfied.

As discussed earlier, in the resting state, the concentration of K⁺ is greater on the cytoplasmic side of the neuronal membrane than on the extracellular side, whereas the concentration of Na⁺ is greater outside than inside the membrane. These differences are due to the relative proportions of specific membrane channels through which these ions can pass, whether these channels are open or closed, and active pumping of ions across the membrane (see below). In the resting state, many K⁺ channels in neuronal membranes are always open, which allows K⁺ to move freely through them, whereas few of the limited Na⁺ channels are open, which limits Na⁺ passage into the cell. Indeed, the permeability of the membrane to the K⁺ ion is 100 times its permeability to the Na⁺ ion during the resting state. The cell membrane is also moderately permeable to Cl⁻ ions; however, there is no net Cl⁻ movement across the membrane because this ion is in equilibrium at the resting potential.

Two forces act upon each ion: a chemical force (the concentration gradient) and an electrical force corresponding to the voltage across the membrane (Figure 5.5). When these forces exactly counterbalance each other for a particular ion, there is no net movement of that ion across the membrane. In the case of Na⁺, for ex-

ample, in the resting state, the ratio of outer/inner concentrations is 460/50, forming a substantial concentration gradient driving the ion in an inward direction. The voltage that corresponds to the normal resting potential (–60 to –70 mV inside relative to outside) provides an electrical force oriented in the same direction. Hence, if the cell membrane were permeable *only* to Na⁺, then the electric potential would have to be reversed (inside positive with respect to the outside) for this ion to reach equilibrium. The membrane potential at which Na⁺ ions would be in equilibrium can be derived from the Nernst equation (see below), which yields a value of +56 mV measured from the inner to the outer surface. This voltage is termed the **equilibrium potential** for Na⁺ (E_{Na}). The same formulation can be used to show that the equilibrium potential for K⁺ (E_K) is –93 mV (see next section).

It should be clear that neither Na⁺ nor K⁺ is in equilibrium in the resting state because the resting potential does not correspond to the equilibrium potential for either ion, but is somewhere in between. Let us therefore consider again the forces acting on each ionic species. As already mentioned, Na⁺ ions are strongly driven in an inward direction due to the combined chemical and electrical forces acting on them. In contrast, K⁺ ions are propelled outward by their concentration gradient, but driven inward by the existing electrical gradient. The net effect is a small outward-directed force. As shown in Figure 5.5, the net flux for each ionic species is dependent on both the strength of the driving force and the relative permeability of the membrane to that species. Therefore, the low permeability to Na⁺ can be offset if the force tending to drive Na⁺ ions into the cell is sufficiently strong. The resting potential can thus be seen as the voltage at which the inward flux of Na⁺ equals the outward flux of K⁺ (i.e., equilibrium). Because permeability factors favor the influx of K⁺, the membrane voltage (V_R) at rest (–70 mV) is more like E_K (–93 mV) than E_{Na} (+56 mV). Thus, as a general rule, if the resting voltage (V_R) is determined by two or more species of ions, the influence of each species is determined both by its concentration inside and outside the cell and by the permeability of the membrane to that species.

Thus far, we have seen that permeability to Na⁺ is low despite the large chemical and electrical forces that could drive Na⁺ into the cell; and we have seen that permeability to K⁺ is high, but the driving force is low because the membrane potential (V_m) is very close to the equilibrium potential for K⁺ (E_K). Nonetheless, there is a steady flow of K⁺ out of the cell, and a steady flow of Na⁺ into the cell. Although the currents due to these steady ion leaks cancel each other out, over the long term, the inner concentration of potassium ($[K^+]_i$) could be depleted and inner sodium ($[Na^+]_i$) could increase, and this would cause the ion gradients to run down and

---

*It is conventional to say that the membrane is depolarized, but if this were literally true, there would be no membrane potential—the potential would be zero. Thus, "depolarized" only means less negative.

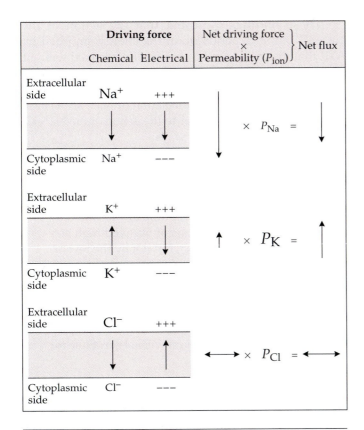

	Driving force		Net driving force × Permeability (P_{ion})	Net flux
	Chemical	Electrical		
Extracellular side	Na^+	+++		
Cytoplasmic side	Na^+	---	$\times\ P_{Na}\ =$	
Extracellular side	K^+	+++		
Cytoplasmic side	K^+	---	$\times\ P_K\ =$	
Extracellular side	Cl^-	+++		
Cytoplasmic side	Cl^-	---	$\times\ P_{Cl}\ =$	

Ion	Cytoplasm (mM)	Extracellular fluid (mM)	E_{ion} (mV)
K^+	400	20	–75
Na^+	50	440	+55
Cl^-	52	560	–60
A^-	385	—	—

5.5 DRIVING FORCE AND MEMBRANE PERMEABILITY DETERMINE ION FLUX. The movement of Na^+, K^+, and Cl^- ions across the neuronal membrane is determined jointly by the electrochemical forces acting on each ion and the permeability to that ion. The fluxes illustrated here pertain to a cell with a membrane potential of –60 mV under the ionic conditions shown in the table. The vertical arrows depict the strength of each force or ion flux, whereas the horizontal arrows indicate no net force or flux. (After Koester, 1991a.)

bring the membrane potential (V_m) close to zero. This dissipation of ionic gradients is prevented by the actions of the sodium–potassium pump, which extrudes Na^+ from the cell while taking in K^+ (see below).

The Nernst Equation

In 1888, the German physical chemist Walter Nernst established a mathematical description of the equilibrium potentials for the ions that contribute to the membrane resting potential. The Nernst equation for K^+ for the squid axon in seawater is as follows:

(5.1)
$$E_K = \frac{RT}{ZF} \ln \frac{[K^+]_o}{[K^+]_i}$$

where E_K = the equilibrium potential for K^+, R is the gas constant, T is the temperature in degrees Kelvin, Z is the valence of K^+, F is the Faraday constant of capacitance, and $[K^+]_o$ and $[K^+]_i$ are the outer and inner cellular concentrations of K^+.

For E_K, Z = +1, and at 25°C, RT/ZF = 26 mV. The constant for converting natural logarithms (ln) to base 10 logarithms is 2.3, and the outer/inner K^+ concentration, in mM, is 10/400. Thus,

(5.2)
$$E_K = 26\ mV \times 2.3 \log_{10} \frac{10}{400} = -93\ mV$$

The Nernst equation can be used to find the equilibrium potential of any ion present on both sides of a membrane that is permeable to that ion when the particular ion channel is open to allow maximum permeability of that ion. Thus, the Nernst equation for Na^+ is

(5.3)
$$E_{Na} = 26\ mV \times 2.3 \log_{10} \frac{440}{50} = +50\ mV$$

The Nernst equation can also be used for chloride ions, but membrane pores for Cl^- are always open, and the permeability to Cl^- is such that the inner and outer concentrations of Cl^- accommodate to the membrane resting potential by passive diffusion. That is, if the membrane potential is displaced (e.g., by an influx of Na^+) so that Cl^- is no longer in equilibrium, Cl^- will diffuse across the membrane until its concentration gradient matches the electrical gradient (resting potential) of the membrane. Thus, in this case, the membrane gradient determines the E_{Cl}, not the other way around. It should be noted, however, that in some instances, Cl^- is pumped out of or pumped into certain cells, and the reader will be informed when this condition exists.

Ion Involvement during Changes in Membrane Potentials

How many ions are involved during changes in membrane potentials? The greatest changes occur during the generation of action potentials, when the membrane potential may swing from –70 mV to as much as +50 mV. If relatively large numbers of ions were involved, their movement could have effects that would have to be evaluated. Calculations have shown, however, that if an axon 50 μm in diameter, having an internal KCl concentration of 100 mM, underwent an influx of Na^+ that changed the membrane potential by 100 mV, the total amount of K^+ within the cell would be 100,000 times greater than the efflux of K^+ needed to reverse the voltage change to –70 mV. Thus, in real cells, it is likely that electrical signals in the nervous system are effected by the movement of relatively few ions (see Hille 1992; Sargent, 1992).

The Sodium–Potassium Pump

As we have said, the membrane of a neuron, even at rest, is not static: K^+, Na^+, and Cl^- are constantly moving across the membrane. To maintain the appropriate inner and outer K^+ and Na^+ concentrations and preserve the resting potential, the **sodium–potassium pump** (also known simply as the Na^+–K^+ pump or the sodium pump) restores the concentration gradients by reversing the flow of potassium and sodium ions: it extrudes Na^+ from the cell while taking in K^+. Because the extruded Na^+ must flow against its high *extracellular* concentration, and K^+ must flow against its high *intracellular* concentration, the Na^+–K^+ pump requires energy to actively drive these fluxes.

Membrane pumps that transport substances against concentration gradients are intrinsic protein molecules that utilize energy supplied by adenosine triphosphate (ATP), the product of glucose metabolism in mitochondria (Figure 5.6). ATP is degraded by hydrolysis into adenosine diphosphate (ADP) and inorganic phosphate (P_i) by a number of ATP-degrading enzymes (ATPases). The enzyme in this case is activated by the presence of Na^+ and K^+. Further, although the Na^+–K^+ pump pumps Na^+ out of the cell and exchanges it for K^+ pumped into the cell, it is not a simple 1:1 exchange; rather, the ratio of Na^+ outflow to K^+ inflow is 3:2 (i.e., for every three Na^+ ions pumped out, two K^+ ions are pumped in). This exchange results in an outward current of one ionic charge per cycle and contributes about 7% to the internal negativity of the squid axon.

The action of the Na^+–K^+ pump was examined by injecting a radioactive isotope of sodium (^{24}Na) into a squid axon and then measuring the Na^+ efflux (see Nicholls, Martin, and Wallace, 1992). Under resting conditions there was continuous Na^+ movement out of the axon, and this Na^+ efflux could be modified in various ways.

1. Na^+ movement was blocked by poisons such as cyanide and dinitrophenol (DNP), which interfere with oxidative production of ATP.
2. Na^+ movement was also blocked by drugs such as ouabain (pronounced "wah′ bain"), which blocks the Na^+–K^+ pump without altering oxidative metabolism. Ouabain acts only if applied to the outside surface of the membrane, not the inside surface.
3. Na^+ movement is diminished by low external K^+, or blocked if K^+ is totally removed from the external bath fluid of the axon.
4. In addition to extruding Na^+, the axon also accumulates K^+, and this process is also blocked by cyanide and ouabain.
5. Lithium ions, which can substitute for Na^+ in producing action potentials, are not extruded from the cell by the Na^+–K^+ pump.

These findings indicated that the action of the Na^+–K^+ pump depends upon the energy supplied by ATP, that the pump can be specifically poisoned without altering the internal processes of the cell, and that K^+ and Na^+ themselves stimulate the pump in vital ways.

It was also found that the action of Na^+–K^+ ATPase in red blood cells was similar to the action of the Na^+–K^+ pump in neurons in several ways:

1. The optimal Na^+ and K^+ concentrations required for enzyme activity are the same as those for the Na^+–K^+ pump.
2. Both the ATPase and the pump are activated by high *inside* concentrations of Na^+ and high *outside* concentrations of K^+, but not by the reverse ratios.
3. In red blood cells, ouabain is also a highly specific blocker of ATPase.
4. The ionic specificity for the activation of ATPase is the same as for the activation of the pump in nerves. For instance, lithium will not substitute for sodium.

Highly purified Na^+–K^+-dependent ATPases have been isolated from a number of vertebrates and invertebrates, and they all bind three Na^+ and two K^+ ions for every molecule of ATP that is hydrolyzed. Further, as mentioned earlier, these enzymes are highly specific for Na^+—it is the only ion species that can be pumped out of the cell, and, among a number of substances that can be pumped into the cell, Na^+ is the only one that cannot. These and other findings also led to the conclusion that the actual pump is the Na^+–K^+-dependent ATPase itself.

The Na^+–K^+ pump is an integral membrane protein. It is a multimeric complex consisting of two different polypeptides: a transmembrane catalytic subunit (α) and a glycoprotein regulatory subunit (β). The structure of the holoenzyme is $\alpha_2\beta_2$, and it has a molecular weight of 270 kDa. The catalytic subunit has binding sites for Na^+ and ATP on its intracellular surface and sites for K^+ and ouabain on its extracellular surface. ATP transfers its terminal phosphate group to the catalytic subunit, forming a Na^+-dependent covalent intermediate, and protein phosphorylation changes the conformation of the complex, which leads to the removal of three Na^+ ions from the inside of the cell to the outside in exchange for two extracellular K^+ ions. The phosphorylated catalytic subunit is hydrolyzed in the presence of K^+ ions. Thus, the overall reaction results in the hydrolysis of ATP (see Koester, 1991a).

Na^+–K^+ pump density.   The density of pump sites in rabbit vagus nerves was ascertained by measuring the binding of radioactive ouabain that was just sufficient to block the pumps. Based on evidence that one molecule of ouabain will block one molecule of ATPase, it was de-

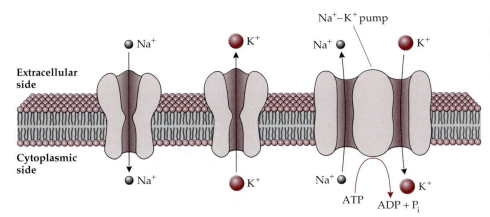

5.6 THE Na^+–K^+ PUMP. Passive Na^+ and K^+ fluxes into and out of a cell at rest are balanced by active transport in the opposite directions by the ATP-dependent Na^+–K^+ pump.

duced that there were 750 sites per square micrometer on the axon membrane (Nicholls, Martin, and Wallace, 1992).

Part I Summary

To briefly summarize, the resting potential of neuronal membranes is a product of membrane properties that account for differential permeability to and distribution of ion species and their electrostatic forces. Further, the distribution of ions and their concentrations activate an ATPase that serves as a pump that drives Na^+ and K^+ ions against their concentration gradients to maintain the appropriate membrane potential for the generation and propagation of action potentials.

Part II
Action Potentials: Development, Propagation, and Behavior

Determinants of Ion Permeability

Carrier Proteins

Having seen that differences in ion permeability have an effect upon the membrane potential, we now turn to the source of those differences. Disregarding the Na^+–K^+ pump for the moment, transport across membranes is accomplished in one of two ways. First, as described in Chapter 3, ions may simply diffuse along a concentration gradient through water-filled pores in neural membranes. Some ion channels are large integral membrane glycoproteins ranging in molecular weight from 25 kDa to 250 kDa and have a central aqueous pore that spans the entire thickness of the membrane. Second, ions can be transported across the membrane by carrier proteins, a process known as facilitated diffusion. In the latter case, an ion may bind to an intrinsic protein that is embedded in the membrane and has

polar (charged) binding sites, as well as nonpolar binding sites that are hydrophobic and therefore interactive with the lipid membrane. The protein subsequently translocates the ion binding site from the extracellular side of the membrane to the intracellular side, at which point the ion dissociates from the carrier. The maximum rate of carrier-mediated ion transfer, which is dependent upon the translocation rate of the carrier protein, is estimated to be about 10^5 ions per second. In another form of carrier-mediated transport, ions approach amphipathic membrane-spanning proteins, causing the protein to undergo a transformation that provides a pore for the ion.

Relatively simple molecules can serve as carriers to facilitate the movement of specific ions across membranes. For example, the antibiotic valinomycin can increase K^+ permeability when it is added to a membrane. Valinomycin forms a complex with K^+ at one surface, diffuses across the membrane, and releases the ion on the other side. With the rubidium ion (Rb^+), valinomycin will increase translocation by over 30,000 ions per second. Another antibiotic, gramicidin, forms a simple channel whose chemical and physical structures are known. Gramicidin is a polypeptide made up of fifteen hydrophobic amino acids with both NH_2 and COOH terminals blocked so that the molecule is uncharged and readily soluble in a phospholipid membrane. In a bilayer, the amino acids form an unusual helix around a stable aqueous pore through which small cations, but not anions, can pass. Hydrophobic amino acid residues are on the outside of the helix, and relatively polar residues line the pore. Two helices align head-to-head to form a dimer long enough (30 Å) to span the bilayer (Figure 5.7).

Some polypeptides in animal cells form transmembrane helices without a central pore, but several can associate to make a central pore. For example, a simple ion pore can be made by a 21-amino acid synthetic peptide consisting only of serine and leucine in the ratio 2:1. These amino acids can form a helix with the polar serine residues aligned along one side, and when presented to

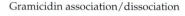

Gramicidin association/dissociation

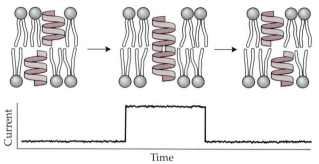

5.7 PROPOSED STRUCTURE OF A GRAMICIDIN CHANNEL. A functional channel is formed within a phospholipid membrane by end-to-end dimerization of two gramicidin peptides. (After Sawyer et al, 1989.)

a lipid bilayer membrane, six helices spontaneously assemble to form an aqueous pore lined by serine hydroxyl groups. The pore seems to have a diameter of 8 Å and is permeable to cations. This pore has an ion specificity and ion flow rate similar to that of an acetylcholine (ACh) receptor, suggesting that ion channels do not need to be complex molecules (Hall, 1992).

Thus, carrier molecules can have nonpolar, hydrophobic membrane-spanning regions that can interact with membrane lipids, as well as polar binding sites for attachment during transmembrane transport. Similarly, a membrane pore may be lined with nonpolar (hydrophobic) amino acids that interface with the lipid bilayer, and polar (hydrophilic) amino acids that face the central aqueous environment and form a channel favorable to charged ions. Whereas these two methods of ion transfer are different, the basic principle is the same: polar and nonpolar groups combine in a single molecule that adopts a configuration in a membrane that allows polar groups to interact with the ion while the nonpolar groups interact with the hydrophobic membrane interior.

Both mechanisms may be operative in establishing and maintaining membrane potentials, but the parameters of transmembrane ionic transport favor the pore principle for the following reasons. The main difference between carriers and pores is the velocity of ion flow. Carriers usually are complex molecules that are similar to enzymes with respect to the number of molecules they can process per active site per second. As mentioned above, when carrier-facilitated ion transport is dependent upon protein translocation, ion transport rates are limited to an estimated 10^5 ions per second, whereas transfer rates of 10^7 to 10^8 ions per second are commonplace and are attributed to ion transfer through channels. The diminished flow rate when carriers are involved is probably due to their relatively large size, which restricts their rate of conformational change. Just as, by analogy,

cars cross a river more rapidly by a tunnel than by a ferry, ions move more quickly through pores than by binding to carriers for ion transport (Hille, 1992).

Membrane Channels

Although membrane channels are not directly observable because of their submicroscopic size, much is known about them. We have already seen that membrane channels are more than passive holes in a membrane; rather, they are made up of polypeptides that are readily soluble in phospholipid membranes and come together to form integral proteins that traverse the cell membrane around an aqueous pore. These channels have three functions: they conduct ions; they recognize and select among specific ions; and they open and close in response to specific electrical, mechanical, or chemical signals. Further, there are many varieties of channels that function in different ways. Also, it is known that there is not just one type of K^+, Na^+, and Cl^- channel; rather, there are many subtypes of each, with K^+ channels being more diverse than the others. This variation suggests that signaling in the nervous system is quite varied and intricate.

The precise chemical and mechanical structures of some channels have been recently established to the point that it is now possible to extract them, purify and clone them, and insert them into lipid membranes, where they function normally (Catterall, 1988). Membrane channels from many species have been extensively studied, and their responses to electrical stimulation are virtually the same in mollusks (squid), annelids (marine worms), arthropods (lobster), and vertebrates (amphibians, birds, and mammals). Thus, it is supposed that channel design and function was already stabilized in the membranes of the common ancestor of these phyla 500 million years ago (Hille, 1992).

Figure 5.8 presents Hille's general model of a voltage-gated membrane channel as a transmembrane protein embedded in the lipid bilayer of a cell membrane. A water-filled pore runs through the center, and protein anchor attachments hold the channel in place by fastening to other membrane proteins or to the microtrabecular lattice, the skeletal structure inside the cell (see Chapter 3). The channel is a glycoprotein that has several thousand amino acids and hundreds of sugar molecules arranged on the outer surface. Hydrophilic amino acids line the inside of the pore, and hydrophobic ones form an interface with the lipid bilayer. The channel is somewhat wider than an ion except at one end, where a filter determines ion selectivity. The sensor and the gating mechanism are at the other end of the pore, and they serve to open and close the pore in response to signals from other cells (see below). Later in the chapter, we will discuss current information concerning the actual molecular structure of these channels.

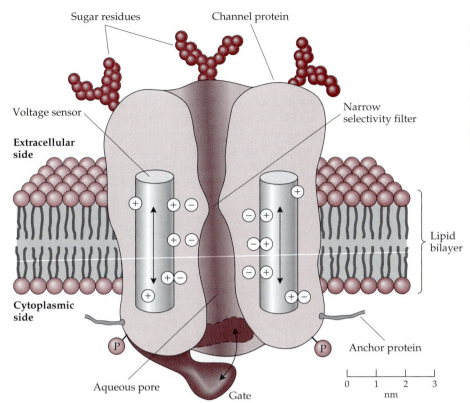

Sugar residues   Channel protein

Voltage sensor

Extracellular side

Narrow selectivity filter

Lipid bilayer

Cytoplasmic side

P   P   Anchor protein

Aqueous pore   Gate

0 1 2 3
nm

5.8 BASIC MODEL OF A VOLTAGE-GATED CHANNEL. The channel is characterized as a transmembrane macromolecule with a hole (pore) through its center. The external surface of the molecule is glycosylated. The functional regions—the selectivity filter, the gate, and the sensor—were initially deduced from the results of voltage-clamping experiments, but more recent studies have begun to elucidate their structural features. (After Hille, 1992.)

Channel Gating Mechanisms

Some channels are open all the time, but there are other channels that open or close as a function of electrical, mechanical, or chemical stimulation. This way of inducing channel transitions between open or closed states is known as **channel gating** and serves to control transmembrane movement of ions. In contrast, **passive diffusion** refers to ion movement through channels down concentration gradients or by electrostatic forces. During the signaling process in neurons, the gated channels have the determinant role, for they transiently alter channel availability for the flow of particular ions and thus briefly magnify changes in the membrane potential, which is the substrate for the initiation of action potentials.

Whereas relatively little is known about the actual gating mechanisms, it is safe to say that they involve conformational changes in channel structure. This notion is supported by high-resolution electron microscopy of gap junction types of ion channels (see below), which shows that the opening and closing of such channels involves a concerted twisting and tilting of six subunits that make up the channel.

Figure 5.9 is a schematic representation of four forms of channel gating (see Siegelbaum and Koester, 1991). As shown in Figure 5.9*a*, an extracellular molecule (called a ligand) can bind to a receptor molecule that constitutes all or part of the channel sensor. In such cases, binding of the ligand causes the channel to open.

The ligand may be a hormone, a drug, or a neurotransmitter released by another neuron. Many instances of ligand-gated channels will be presented in later chapters.

In certain other instances, intracellular molecules known as "second messengers" are activated by a drug or a neurotransmitter to start a cascade of chemical events, including, for example, an increase in calcium (Ca^{2+}) ions or the stimulation of cyclic adenosine monophosphate (cAMP) formation. In turn, these second messengers lead to the phosphorylation and dephosphorylation of some channel proteins and thus to the opening or closing of the channels (Figure 5.9*b*). Second messenger systems are discussed in detail in Chapter 6.

Voltage gating refers to the process whereby channel gates respond to voltage changes in the membranes to open and close pores to control ion flow. As shown in Figure 5.9*c*, a negatively charged cell interior will keep a channel closed, and a positively charged interior will open a channel; or, if the resting potential is reduced in magnitude (e.g., from −70 mV to −40 mV), sensors will respond by opening certain gates, whereas an increase in the membrane voltage (from −70 to −90 mV) will close them. In the case of voltage-gated Na^+ channels, pore opening and closing is due to changes in the membrane voltage that induce movements of a charged region of the channel back and forth through the electric field, which drives the channel through closed and open

(a)

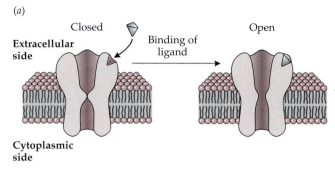

(b)

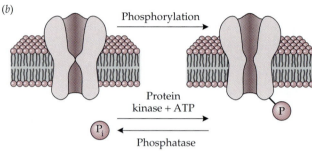

(c)

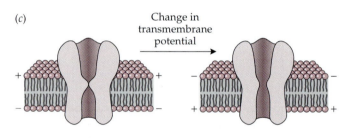

(d)

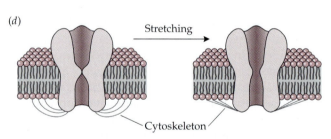

5.9 CHANNEL GATING IS CONTROLLED BY SEVERAL TYPES OF STIMULI. (*a*) A Ligand-gated channel opens in response to a ligand binding to its receptor. The energy from ligand binding drives channel gating toward an open state. (*b*) Protein phosphorylation and dephosphorylation regulates the opening and closing of some channels. The energy for channel opening comes from the transfer of the high-energy phosphate, P. (*c*) Changes in voltage can open and close some channels. The energy for channel gating comes from changes in the electric potential across the membrane. (*d*) Other channels are activated by stretch or pressure. The energy for gating may come from mechanical forces due to channel–cytoskeleton interactions. (After Siegelbaum and Koester, 1991.)

states. For mechanically activated channels (Figure 5.9*d*), the energy associated with membrane stretch is believed to be transferred to the channel through the cytoskeleton. (See Stevens, 1987; Siegelbaum and Koester, 1991).

The rate of transition from the closed to the open state depends upon the signals that gate the channel and can vary between a microsecond and a minute, but on average, a few milliseconds are required. Once a voltage-gated Na^+ channel is opened, it stays open for a few milliseconds, and after it closes, it stays closed for a few milliseconds. Ions pass through the channel in less than a microsecond in single file, at a rate as high as 100,000,000 per second. Further, under the influence of multiple regulators, ion channels can enter one of three possible states: closed and able to be activated (resting); open (active); and closed and not able to be activated (refractory). It will be seen that these different states play a role in the propagation of action potentials (see below).

Channel selectivity.   The voltage change necessary to open a gate may vary according to the sensitivity of the gate sensor, but ligand-gated channels are quite specific with respect to the ligands that they bind. For example, a channel sensor that binds and is activated by one neurotransmitter may be completely insensitive to another. This specificity is due to the chemistry of the receptor protein of the channel sensor. Moreover, once a gate is opened, either by a voltage change or by ligand binding, the channel itself exercises a degree of specificity as to which ion species can pass. For example, one type of open channel may allow free and rapid transit of sodium ions while severely restricting other ions; another may allow cations (+) to pass, but exclude anions (–). Also, when ion concentrations are high, there may be competition among and blockage by small ions. Further, selection for small ions can be made by certain channels that seem to narrow somewhere along their length to a diameter ranging between 3 and 7 Å, so that permeability to ions exceeding a certain size is cut off. To achieve selectivity between chemically similar ions whose radii may differ by only a few hundredths of a nanometer, such a passive sieving action would probably not be adequate, so other mechanisms come into play (see below).

On the other hand, the facts suggest that no channel is perfectly selective for a single ion. For example, several types of potassium channels pass at least four types of ions, and some sodium channels pass at least fourteen. Moreover, the calcium channels that play a significant role in synaptic transmission can pass at least eight. It is not likely that all ion types that pass through a single pore do so at the same rate, but the selectivity seems to be sufficient to provide the membrane with the appropriate electrical characteristics (Hille, 1992).

Channel identification.   Strong empirical support for different types of channels was found during investigations of the toxicity of certain substances. As Hille (1992) described, the toxic substances were "magic bullets" that contributed to our understanding of channel function. One such substance was tetrodotoxin (TTX), a paralytic poison found in the ovaries and liver of some puffer fish species of the order Tetraodontoformes. In Japanese cuisine, puffer fish is considered a delicacy, but if it is not prepared properly, eating it can be fatal. Studies had shown that TTX blocks impulse conduction in nerve and muscle cells, and in squid axons it was found to selectively block Na^+ channels without affecting K^+ channels (Narahashi, Moore, and Scott, 1964). The same effect was found in axons of other species.

At about the same time that TTX became known, another toxin with similar properties was discovered. Known as saxitoxin (STX), it is synthesized by microscopic marine organisms that multiply at an explosive rate under certain conditions and discolor the water with their reddish color, a phenomenon known as "red tide." The toxin accumulates in shellfish such as the clam *Saxidomus* (after which the toxin was named), and it is not destroyed by cooking the clams. Eating only one contaminated clam can be fatal. Thus, as toxins, TTX and STX are highly and equally potent, being fatally effective at nanomolar concentrations.

It is now established that TTX and STX act upon Na^+ channels on the extracellular side to prevent them from opening. Also, TTX and STX bind exclusively to the same receptor on the Na^+ channel, and to no other receptors, even at concentrations 10,000 times greater than the effective concentration for blocking Na^+ channels. The fact that the toxin is effective only on the outside of the cell suggests that its binding site is on the outer membrane surface, and that the pore need not be open for binding to occur. It is thus unlikely that the receptor is inside the pore. On the other hand, the stings of certain scorpions and sea anemones release neurotoxins that also affect Na^+ channels, but these toxins block receptors inside the pores, thus keeping the pores open and preventing the normal generation of action potentials. This causes pain, paralysis, and abnormal heart rhythms, and can lead to death by asphyxiation due to the blocking of the phrenic nerve, which activates the diaphragm (see Hille, 1992; Nicholls, Martin, and Wallace, 1992). Many more neurotoxins are now known that come from various plants and animals and have various effects upon neurons: inhibiting ion transport across membranes, blocking depolarization, or preventing repolarization, thereby either deactivating the axon or causing repetitive firing. Knowing the chemistry of these substances, where they bind on the channel proteins, and what effects they have tells us much about the nature of the channels (Catterall, 1988).

Potassium channels, too, can be specifically blocked by chemical substances. It has been known since the findings of Marshall (1913) and Burn and Dale (1915) that tetraethylammonium (TEA) blocks activity in the autonomic nervous system, but it was not known until the early 1970s that TEA selectively blocks K^+ channels, which have a significant role in autonomic systems (Hille, 1970; Armstrong and Hille, 1972). TEA is less potent than TTX and SXT, but it is effective in blocking K^+ channels in millimolar concentrations applied to the inner surface of the membrane. This was the expected finding because this channel and its gate control the outward flow (efflux) of K^+.

Several toxins have also been found that act on different kinds of K^+ channels. These include apamin, found in the venom of honeybees, noxioustoxin and charybdotoxin from scorpion venom, and dendrotoxin, which is found in the venom of the eastern green mamba snake (Castle, Haylett, and Jenkinson, 1989). Apamin selectively blocks an important class of Ca^{2+}-activated, voltage-independent K^+ channels. Such channels are involved in the hyperpolarizing afterpotential that typically follows an action potential (see below), as well as in neurotransmitter- and hormone-stimulated increases in K^+ permeability in many peripheral tissues. In contrast, noxioustoxin inhibits the voltage-dependent K^+ channel that underlies termination of the action potential (the so-called **delayed rectifier current**). The results of studies using channel-specific toxins have helped to confirm the hypothesis of specific openings in neural membranes with selective ionic permeability that contribute importantly to the signaling functions of such membranes.

Channel similarity and diversity. Experiments have shown that there is a remarkable similarity of function among different channels both within and between species. For example, when the activity of Na^+ channels was compared among frog muscle, frog nodes of Ranvier, crayfish axons, the human heart, and the squid axon, it was found that the time constants for activation (depolarization) and inactivation (repolarization) did not differ more than twofold. (The time constant is the time duration from the stimulus to two-thirds of the maximum depolarization or repolarization.)

Nevertheless, although the electrical properties of all Na^+ channels are very similar, pharmacological differences do exist. For example, vertebrate cardiac Na^+ channels are much less sensitive to the channel-blocker TTX than are vertebrate skeletal or nerve Na^+ channels. And, as expected, the Na^+ channels of puffer fish and other related forms are highly resistant to the toxin of their own making (Hille, 1992).

There is also considerable diversity among voltage-dependent K^+ channels. Some open after the membrane is depolarized, and some after hyperpolarization; some open rapidly, some slowly; and some are modulated by neurotransmitters or by "second messengers" (see Chapter 6). Also, some K^+ channels can be blocked by applying the chemical TEA (see above) to the inside of the membrane, and some by applying it to the outside, each with its own sensitivity. These electrical and pharmacological differences suggest that there may be several forms of K$^+$ channels in the same membrane with different functional roles (Hille, 1992).

Channel density.   Whereas channels play a vital role in membrane resting and action potentials, their concentration, compared with that of other membrane proteins, is rather small. The simplest way to count them is to label them with radioactive ligands and count the radioactive spots on photographic emulsion that has been in contact with the tissue sample. Another method is to compare the current flow through a single channel with the total current flow through a known area of membrane, usually 1 cm^2. Also, if the chemical composition of a channel is known, its physical size can be estimated. All of these methods must take a number of factors into account to arrive at probable estimates. (For details of the techniques, see Hille, 1992.) Using these methods, it was estimated that if channel molecules could be packed together side by side, their density would be about 52,000 per square micrometer. Measuring Na$^+$ channel density on unmyelinated axon membranes, however, revealed approximately 50–500 per square micrometer, and about 2,000 to as many as 12,000 per square micrometer were found at nodes of Ranvier, where action potentials are generated in myelinated axons (Ritchie and Rogart, 1977). With per channel flux rates being anywhere between 6 and 160 million ions per second, the question is not why there are so few, but rather, why there are so many (Hille, 1992).

Pore–ion dimensions and pore specificity.   First, we will assume that pore diameter and ion size can determine the ease with which ions can pass through pores. As described above, the organic anions (A$^-$) are excluded partly because of their size, and studies have shown that the monovalent ions Cs$^+$ and Rb$^+$ are also excluded from K$^+$ channels because of their size. There is a question, however, about why K$^+$ channels are so selective between K$^+$ and Na$^+$, preferring K$^+$ to Na$^+$ by ratios as high as 100:1, even though the two ions have the same shape and charge. Perhaps the explanation might be related to pore diameter and the relative sizes of K$^+$ and Na$^+$ ions.

It has been established that the diameter of the voltage-regulated K$^+$ channel is 3.3 Å. The diameter of K$^+$ ions is 2.66 Å, and that of Na$^+$ ions is 1.9 Å. Thus, even though K$^+$ ions are larger than Na$^+$ ions, the pore is, by far, more permeable to K$^+$. However, as mentioned earlier, water molecules, each of which have an overall size of 2.8 Å, bind to ions, and the adherence of these H$_2$O molecules changes the ion dimensions such that the diameters of the hydrated Na$^+$ and K$^+$ ions are 5.12 and 3.96 Å, respectively. Thus, hydrated Na$^+$ ions are larger than hydrated K$^+$ ions, and even larger than the K$^+$ pore diameter. Thus, at first glance, channel size would seem to be an important factor in determining selective per-

meability for K$^+$ among hydrated ions, and to explain the relative permeability to K$^+$, Na$^+$, and Cl$^-$, which is estimated to be 1.00:0.04:0.45.

However, before ions can enter a pore, they must get rid of their associated water molecules so that they can interact with the polar groups lining the pore, which determine which ion is to be transported and at what rate. Because large ions can shed their associated water molecules faster than small ions, the K$^+$ pore, which has *weak* polar sites, will prefer large ions to small ones. Thus, the speed of dehydration may be the selective factor for K$^+$ ions.

On the other hand, for Na$^+$ pores, which have a diameter of 4 Å and *strongly* charged polar sites, the interaction of dehydrated ions with the polar sites may be more important in determining the ion preference than the ease of dehydration. Consequently, it has been proposed that small ions have an advantage over large ones because they can get closer to the polar sites and interact with them more strongly. However, at the time of this writing, the structural details of Na$^+$ channels needed to evaluate this proposal are not known (see Hall, 1992).

Voltage-Gated Channels

Channel structure.   There are perhaps a dozen or more different types of channels in the membrane of a single neuron (Stevens, 1984; 1987). The structures of several types of ligand-gated channels that serve as neurotransmitter receptors are discussed in some of the chapters that follow. Here we will focus on the structures of the voltage-gated channels that are permeable to Na$^+$ and K$^+$. Current ideas about channel structure have been made possible by the cloning of channel protein genes, which was pioneered by the work of Numa and his colleagues on Na$^+$ channels (Noda, et al., 1983, Noda, Shimizu et al., 1986).

The properties of voltage-gated Na$^+$ channels were recently reviewed by Catterall (1993a,b). The overall structure of the voltage-gated Na$^+$ channel in the rat brain is illustrated in Figure 5.10. The channel consists of a large membrane-spanning α subunit (260 kDa molecular mass) as well as two smaller subunits designated β1 (36 kDa) and β2 (33 kDa). The α subunit contains an intrinsic pore and can form a functional ion channel when expressed alone in a cell (although certain channel properties are abnormal). This subunit also possesses binding sites for tetrodotoxin (TTX; see above) and α-scorpion toxins (ScTx). The β2 subunit is covalently linked to the α subunit by disulfide bonds (—S—S—), whereas the β1 subunit is associated noncovalently with the channel complex. The extracellular surface of each subunit possesses several sites for N-linked glycosylation (attachment of carbohydrate chains).

The amino acid sequences of Na$^+$ channel α subunits from two different sources, rat brain and the elec-

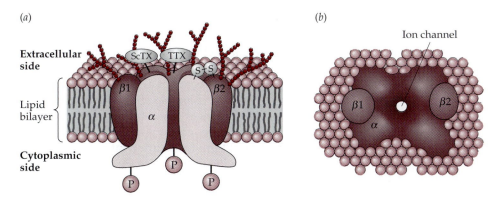

(a)

Extracellular side

Lipid bilayer

Cytoplasmic side

(b)

Ion channel

5.10 PROPOSED STRUCTURE OF THE VOLTAGE-DEPENDENT Na⁺ CHANNEL. (a) The channel is composed of three subunits, α, β1, and β2, with the α subunit forming the ion pore. TTX and ScTX indicate approximate binding sites for tetrodotoxin and certain scorpion toxins, respectively. Also shown is cyclic AMP–dependent phosphorylation of the α subunit (–P), a disulfide bond linking the α and the β2 subunits (—s—s—), and carbohydrate chains bound to the extracellular surface of each subunit. (b) A cross-sectional view of the channel through the α, β1, and β2 subunits (After Hille and Catterall, 1989).

troplax (electric organ) of the electric eel, have been deduced by cloning and sequencing a cDNA for each protein. cDNA (complementary DNA) can be synthesized from the messenger RNA coding for a given protein using molecular biological techniques. The general structure of the Na⁺ channel α subunit is shown in Figure 5.11. It can be seen that the protein contains four repeating domains (labeled I–IV), each of which is made up of six transmembrane (membrane-spanning) segments. These transmembrane segments exhibit considerable se-

quence homology—that is, similarity of amino acid composition and order.

Current structural models suggest that the four domains are arrayed together in the membrane such that certain of their transmembrane segments face inward to create the wall of the pore (thus, each domain provides a quarter of the wall; see Figure 5.10b). In considering which segments are involved, it is useful to view a closeup of one of the large domains (Figure 5.12). Experimental evidence indicates that transmembrane segments S5 and S6 are arrayed around the ion pore like the staves of a barrel (Catterall, 1993a,b). The short segments ss1 and ss2 are believed to form loops that enter the pore, where they help to determine the channel's ionic selectivity (see next section).

We can see from Figure 5.11 that the β1 subunit, which is not involved in the channel pore, possesses only a single transmembrane segment. Like the α subunit,

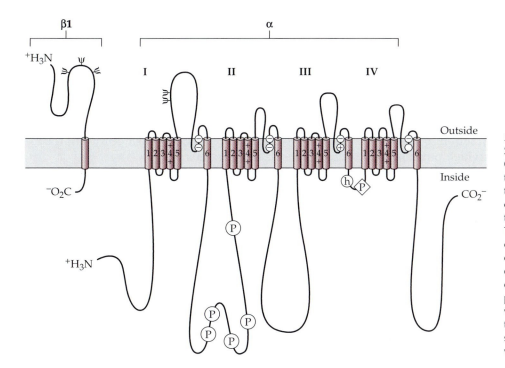

5.11 STRUCTURE OF THE α AND β1 SUBUNITS OF RAT BRAIN Na⁺ CHANNELS. The repeating domains of the α subunit are labeled I–IV. Putative transmembrane segments are depicted by cylinders. Small circles represent the positions of amino acid residues necessary for TTX binding (a "−" or "+" sign within the circle indicates that the amino acid is charged). Other features shown are sites of extracellular glycosylation (ψ), sites of cyclic AMP–dependent (P within a circle) phosphorylation and protein kinase C (P within a diamond) phosphorylation, and the locations of amino acid residues responsible for channel inactivation (h within a circle). (After Catterall, 1993a,b.)

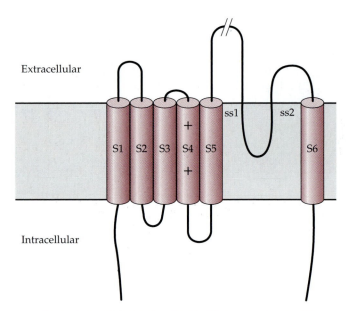

Extracellular

Intracellular

5.12 TRANSMEMBRANE SEGMENTS OF A VOLTAGE-GATED ION CHANNEL. Transmembrane segments S5 and S6 along with the short loop segments ss1 and ss2 are believed to make up the wall of the channel pore. Segment S4 contains a number of positively charged amino acid residues and is thought to serve as the channel's voltage sensor. (After Catterall, 1993b.)

however, it is heavily glycosylated. As of this writing, the primary structure of the β2 subunit is still unknown.

Information about the structure of voltage-gated K[+] channels first came from the molecular analysis of an interesting mutant form of the fruit fly, *Drosophila melanogaster*. A number of years ago, a mutation was discovered that causes flies to shake their legs vigorously when anesthetized (a behavior not seen in wild-type, i.e., normal, flies). Flies bearing this *Shaker* mutation also exhibit behavioral abnormalities when awake, such as antennal twitching, abdominal spasms, and scissoring of the wings. Studies in the laboratory of Jan and Jan (1994) resulted in the cloning of the *Shaker* gene, which was found to code for the α subunit of a major type of voltage-gated K[+] channel (Papazian et al., 1987). Because of the abnormal structure and function of these channels, *Shaker* flies show unusually long action potentials (Tanouye, Ferrus, and Fujita, 1981), which presumably are at least partly responsible for the aberrant behavioral characteristics described above.

The original *Shaker* experiments, along with many subsequent studies, have demonstrated that K[+] channel structure differs somewhat from that of voltage-gated Na[+] channels (reviewed by Catterall, 1993a; Jan and Jan, 1994). In K[+] channels, each α subunit consists of only a single domain containing the six transmembrane segments. Therefore, formation of the channel pore requires the participation of four α subunits rather than just one. Native (naturally occurring) channels also possess four β subunits (Jan and Jan, 1994).

Channel selectivity. Until fairly recently, there has been little direct information concerning which structural aspects of voltage-gated channels confer the ion selectivity discussed in earlier parts of this chapter. However, mutagenesis experiments directed at altering the amino acid composition of specific channel subunit regions indicate that the selectivity filters in many (perhaps all) channels are made up of structures called pore loops (reviewed by MacKinnon, 1995). Pore loops are relatively short segments of the channel subunit that extend into the pore, in this case, from the extracellular side of the membrane. In the case of voltage-gated Na[+] and K[+] channels, the pore loop corresponds to the short segments ss1 and ss2 depicted in Figure 5.12. Another view is presented in Figure 5.13. When, for example, the four α subunits that make up a K[+] channel combine within the membrane, the pore loops are arrayed as shown in Figure 5.13*b*. The exact manner in which these pore loops determine ion selectivity is not yet known; however, it seems likely that critical amino acids within the loop form specific binding sites for the ion(s) conducted by a given channel.

Channel activation and inactivation. As mentioned above, voltage-gated Na[+] and K[+] channels shift between three different states: resting (channel closed), activated (channel open), and inactivated (channel closed). As discussed later, transitions between these states are governed by the depolarization and repolarization of the cell membrane. With respect to channel activation, it is known that a protein capable of responding to alterations in membrane potential must contain amino acid residues inside the electric field (i.e., within the membrane) that are charged or at least possess a dipole (positive and negative ends). The region of the protein that includes these amino acids therefore constitutes the "voltage sensor" element of the channel. When the voltage across the membrane changes, as when an action potential sweeps down the axon, the altered electric field exerts a force on the voltage sensor to cause physical movement that in some way opens the pore. In the case of the Na[+] channel, early studies by Hodgkin and Huxley (1952) led to the hypothesis that channel activation requires movement of at least six positive charges from the cytoplasmic toward the extracellular side of the membrane.

Where is the putative voltage sensor located? It now seems likely that one critical region in both Na[+] and K[+] channels is the S4 transmembrane segment of the α subunit (Catterall, 1993a). This segment consists of a series of positively charged amino acid residues (mostly arginine) separated from each other by two hydrophobic residues. As with other membrane-spanning protein regions, S4 is presumed to assume a helical configuration within the lipid bilayer. Although several models have been proposed to account for depolarization-induced voltage sensor movement (e.g., the "sliding helix" or "helical screw" models), none has yet been confirmed experimentally.

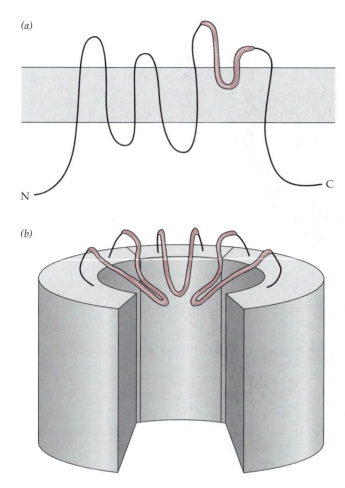

(a)

N   C

(b)

5.13 FORMATION OF ION CHANNEL SELECTIVITY FILTERS BY PORE LOOPS. (a) The region of a voltage-gated channel α subunit that constitutes the pore loop is shown by a colored segment (this region corresponds to intramembrane segments ss1 and ss2 of Figure 5.12.) (b) A voltage-gated K^+ channel is depicted with one of the four α subunits removed for visual clarity. The loops are shown arrayed around the ion pore and entering it from the extracellular side of the membrane. (After MacKinnon, 1995.)

Once a channel has been activated by the voltage sensor, the duration of channel opening is controlled by a separate mechanism called the "inactivation gate." The function of this gate is to bind to the cytoplasmic opening of the pore, thereby blocking ion flow. Inactivation is a rapid process, as shown by the fact that Na^+ channels remain open for only a few milliseconds following membrane depolarization. Although a gating mechanism is used to inactivate both Na^+ and K^+ channels, the structure of the gate differs in the two cases (Catterall, 1993a; Jan and Jan, 1994). For the Na^+ channel, the gate consists of a hinged-lid mechanism formed from the short cytoplasmic segment linking the α subunit domains III and IV (Figure 5.14a). In contrast, K^+ channels are believed to be inactivated by a ball-and-chain structure formed from the N-terminal region of the α subunit (Figure 5.14b). The "ball," which corresponds to approximately the first

20 amino acid residues of the protein, is tethered to the first transmembrane segment (S1) by a long "chain" of amino acids.

It is important to note that the processes of channel activation and inactivation interact with each other. Specifically, inactivation blocks activation by preventing the requisite charge movement within the protein. Furthermore, once channels have been inactivated following membrane depolarization and brief activation, the membrane must be repolarized to reverse the inactivation process and return the channels to their resting state.

The Generation and Propagation of Action Potentials

In the foregoing section, we drew attention to some of the electrical characteristics of neurons, especially those of neuronal membranes. We emphasized the importance of the distribution of different ion species on the outside and inside of the neuronal membrane that is the basis of the resting potential, and we mentioned that membrane resting potentials are the precursors of the generation of action potentials and their propagation to the axon terminals. However, before we describe the biomechanisms of action potentials, we shall describe some electrical phenomena related to neuron morphology that influence the probability of the occurrence of action potentials.

Passive Electrical Conduction by Neurons

Because membrane resting potentials, ion equilibrium potentials, and action potentials are expressed as electrical phenomena, there is a tendency to think of nerve impulses as being similar to electrical signals carried by telephone wires. Telephone messages are transduced to fluctuations in voltage, which are transmitted by metal wires passively in the sense that the wires do not supply the energy needed for the propagation of the signals. It is true that, as in wires, there is some passive conduction in nerves because their inner contents, the cytoplasm and axoplasm, are wet and contain salts in solution. However, Herman von Helmholtz, in 1850, measured the speed of nerve impulses in large nerves from a frog and found it to be about 40 m/s, nowhere near as fast as current traveling down a copper wire, which moves almost at the speed of light, about 300,000 km/s. This finding showed that neural messages, in the form of action potentials, could not be transmitted by nerves acting as passive conductors. In comparison with metal wires, nerves as conductors are 1 million to 100 million times slower and less efficient for the following reasons:

1. In a wire, the charges are carried by a large number of rapidly moving electrons, whereas in an axon, the charges are carried in the axoplasm by significantly fewer and slower-moving ions.

(a)

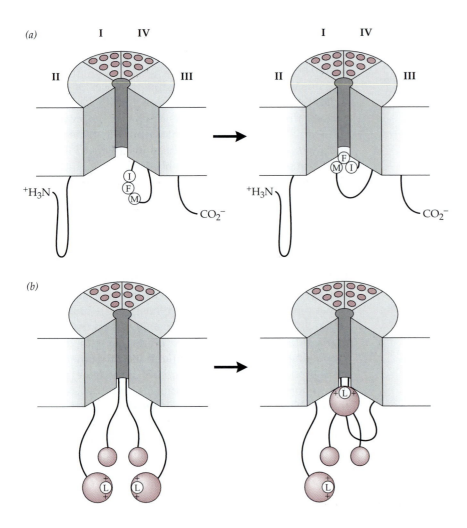

5.14 MECHANISMS OF Na⁺ AND K⁺ CHANNEL INACTIVATION. (a) A hinged-lid mechanism is thought to be responsible for fast Na⁺ channel inactivation. The hinge is made up of three amino acids, isoleucine (I), phenylalanine (F), and methionine (M). As shown, the hinge inactivates the channel by occluding the cytoplasmic opening of the pore. (b) K⁺ channels are thought to be inactivated by a ball-and-chain mechanism. Among the important amino acids constituting the ball are a leucine (L) at position 7 and several positively charged residues (+). (After Catterall, 1993a.)

2. Neuronal dendrites and some axons are exceedingly thin, ranging from 0.1 to 10 μm in diameter, which makes them highly resistive. The longer the dendrites, the more resistive they are because ions experience more collisions among themselves as they flow down the length of the dendrite. Thin wires are also resistive and will heat up and melt if high currents are applied to them.

3. The axolemma acts as a capacitor where the negative and positive charges are separated by the lipid bilayers and stored. Accordingly, before any current can flow along the axon interior, the capacitive elements have to be filled. This slows the generation and propagation of action potentials (see below).

4. The axolemma is only about 7.0 nm thick and is a poor insulator. Thus, there is considerable leakage of current, causing the amplitude of propagated voltage changes to rapidly dissipate with distance traveled along a dendrite or an axon. This is particularly true of unmyelinated axons.

Hodgkin (1964) compared electrical conduction in neurons with that in metal wires. He calculated that a nerve fiber with a diameter of 1.0 μm has an axial (longitudinal) resistance per unit length of 10 ohms/cm. Thus, an axon 1.0 meter in length would have the same resistivity as a 22-gauge copper wire 10^{10} miles in length—a distance roughly ten times that between the Earth and the planet Saturn.

These capacitive and resistive factors adversely affect the generation of neuronal potentials and the efficiency of signal propagation, but, on the other hand, they contribute to synaptic integration, the process by which a neuron sums all incoming signals—inhibitory as well as excitatory ones—that influence whether or not it will generate an action potential (see below). Accordingly, because neurons are poor passive conductors, their superb ability as signal carriers must depend upon other characteristics.

The Generation of Electrotonic Potentials

The generation and propagation of nerve signals in a squid giant axon serves as an excellent model because, as shown earlier, these neural phenomena are virtually the same in every known animal species. In the laboratory, a brief positive electrical stimulus applied to the axoplasm of a squid axon can evoke changes in the membrane potential that are identical to the changes that occur when appropriate ligands are bound to neuron receptors. This finding suggests that ligand binding and an electric pulse have the same ultimate effect on primary or postsynaptic neurons.

Figure 5.15*a* illustrates the method used in these experiments. Using microelectrodes, a short (1.0 ms) pulse of a weak positive (+) stimulus is applied to the cytoplasm of a squid axon. Adding a positive charge to the cytoplasm makes the axon interior less negative, changing it, for instance, from –70 to –60 mV. Further, the positive charge (carried by cations) passively spreads from the stimulus site to depolarize adjacent membrane sites in both directions from the injection site, while the stimulus site is restored to the membrane resting potential by the flow of negatively charged ions from adjacent areas to counteract the positive charge inserted into the axoplasm. These changes in the membrane potential are

recorded when the area of depolarization spreads past contact electrodes that are placed near the stimulating electrode and spaced a few centimeters apart. The contact electrodes are connected to two recording oscilloscopes (V_1 and V_2) serving as voltmeters. The voltage change induced in this manner is known as an **electrotonic potential** or **receptor potential**. The passive spread of the voltage change along the neuron is known as **electrotonic conduction**, and consists of the transmembrane passage of positive and negative ions during the depolarization and the repolarization that restores the resting potential.

If the electrodes are separated by 20 mm, and the axon is subjected to 1.0 ms positive stimuli of two different intensities (S_1 and S_2), the voltage recordings show depolarizations that are proportional to the stimulus intensity, and the deflections recorded at V_2 are smaller than those recorded at V_1 (Figure 5.15*b*). These findings illustrate the fact that although the membrane response passively spreads rapidly along the axon, the magnitude of the response is attenuated by distance. Figure 5.15*b* also shows that if the polarity of the stimulus pulse is reversed from positive to negative, the stimulus causes a hyperpolarization: that is, the stimulus increases the internal negativity of the axon from –70 to –80 mV at V_1, and from –70 to –75 mV at V_2. Further, the responses from V_2 are slightly delayed compared to those from V_1 because of the distance between R_1 and R_2.

Accordingly, because the amplitude of the membrane responses to depolarizing and hyperpolarizing stimuli is proportional to the stimulus intensity, these electrotonic potentials are characterized as **graded**, and because the amplitude of the elicited responses rapidly declines over distance, the responses are known as **decremental**. This latter phenomenon, as mentioned above, is attributed to the few charge carriers (ions) in the axoplasm, the longitudinal and membrane resistance of the neuron, and its leaky insulation.

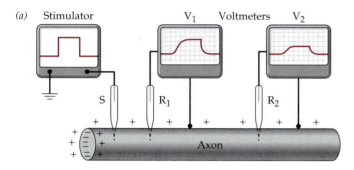

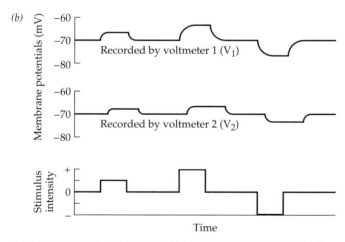

The length constant. Quantitatively, the factors that account for the voltage decrement determine the **length constant** of the nerve fiber, which is defined as the distance over which the stimulus-induced voltage change falls to $1/e$, or 37%, of its highest value at 0 distance (a 63% loss; Katz, 1966; $e = 2.72$ and is the base of the system of natural logarithms.) This effect can also be shown when a dendrite is stimulated for a few seconds to fill the capacitor so that the resistance is due to only the axial length of the dendrite. Figure 5.16*a* shows a current injected into the dendrite cytoplasm flowing out through membrane pores via several pathways along its length to a return electrode in the extracellular fluid. Also, it can be seen that more of the current flows across the membrane near the stimulus site than at more distant regions because the current follows the path of least resistance. The farther down the dendrite the voltage change (current) spreads, the more axial resistance it encounters,

5.15 ELECTRICAL STIMULATION AND RECORDING FROM A SQUID AXON. (*a*) The stimulators deliver a brief electric pulse via the stimulating electrode inserted into the axoplasm. Recording electrodes R_1 and R_2 detect voltage changes occurring across the axon membrane. The changes are displayed on the screens of oscilloscopes that serve as voltmeters (V_1 and V_2). (*b*) Effects of stimuli (*bottom trace*) applied to a squid axon: positive stimuli cause local potentials that are recorded as upward deflections by voltmeters V1 and V2 (*top traces*). The greater intensity of the second stimulus causes a greater local potential, but the potentials recorded by V2 are smaller than those recorded by V1, demonstrating that the evoked responses have diminished over distance. A negative stimulus is recorded as a downward deflection because it elicits a hyperpolarization of the membrane.

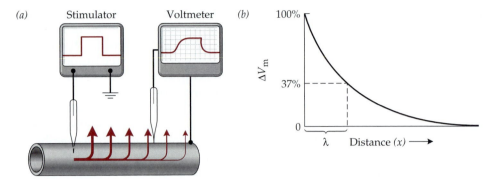

(a) Stimulator   Voltmeter   *(b)*

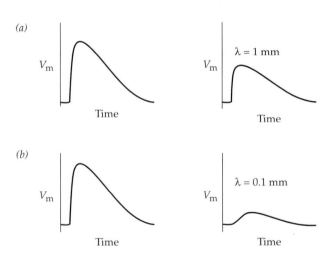

5.16 THE LENGTH CONSTANT OF LOCAL POTENTIALS. (*a*) When current is injected into a dendrite, ion flux across the membrane declines with increasing distance from the site of stimulation due to the resistive character of the nerve fiber. (*b*) This phenomenon causes the current-induced change in membrane potential (ΔV_m) to decay exponentially as a function of distance along the fiber. The rate of decay for a given fiber is expressed by the length constant (λ), which corresponds to the distance at which ΔV_m has reached a value of $1/e$ (37%) of its value at point 0 (the site of stimulation). (After Koester, 1991X.)

and the weaker is the current that exits to the return electrode. As seen in Figure 5.16*b*, the curve representing the relationship between current decay and distance along the dendrite has an exponential shape. The length constant, lambda, can be calculated as follows:

$$\lambda = \sqrt{r_m / r_a}$$

where λ = length constant, r_m = membrane resistance which is a constant, in ohms/cm, and r_a = the axial (longitudinal) resistance of the cytoplasmic core expressed in ohms/cm.

Here, the principal factor is the insulation of the membrane: the better the insulation (i.e., the higher r_m is), the lower the current leakage, and the better the conducting properties of the axial core (i.e., the lower r_a is), and the greater the length constant (λ) of the dendrite. In other words, with higher membrane insulation and lower electrical leakage, the current is able to spread farther along the inner conductive core before leakage becomes a significant factor. For dendrites and very thin axons, the length constant is short (about 0.2 mm); for the thickest axons, it may be as much as 10.0 mm. Thus, because response amplitude declines quite rapidly in thin, unmyelinated dendrites and axons, the membrane changes can only be detected close to the stimulus source. Therefore, graded potentials are sometimes designated **local potentials**. Also, because graded potentials are produced in dendrites as a consequence of synaptic action, they are also known as **synaptic potentials**.

Despite their wide variability, graded potentials play a significant role in determining the probability of signal-bearing action potentials. This role is illustrated in Figure 5.17, which shows the result of two neurons with different length constants receiving the same synaptic input. Cell *b* has thinner dendrites than cell *a*, resulting in a substantially shorter length constant. Consequently, the amplitude of the graded potential reach-

ing the trigger zone of cell *a* is much greater than the amplitude in cell *b*, and cell *a* is more likely to fire an action potential (see below).

The time constant.   Another significant parameter of electrotonic potentials is the membrane time constant, which is a function of the capacitance and the resistance of the cell membrane with respect to ion flow. Figure 5.18 shows the role of these circuit elements in current-induced changes in membrane potential. In this model, *C* represents the membrane capacitance, which is made up of the intracellular and extracellular surfaces of the membrane separated by the lipid bilayer. *R* is the sum of the pore

5.17 EFFECT OF THE LENGTH CONSTANT ON THE CONDUCTION OF SYNAPTIC POTENTIALS. (*a*) In a cell with a long length constant relative to the length of its dendrites, a synaptic potential generated in the dendrite (*left*) shows only a modest decay by the time it reaches the trigger zone of the cell's axon (*right*). (*b*) In contrast, a cell with the same dendritic length but with a short length constant (because the dendrites are thinner) exhibits much greater decay of synaptic potentials.

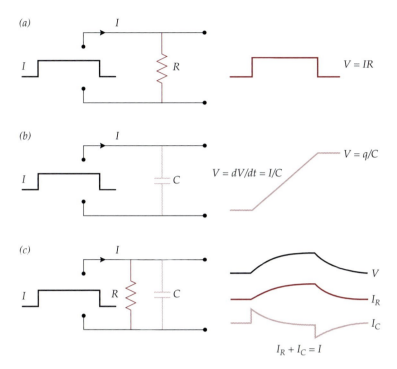

5.18 RESISTANCE AND CAPACITANCE DETERMINE CHANGES IN THE MEMBRANE POTENTIAL. (*a*) If a rectangular current pulse *I* is applied to a circuit with resistance (*R*) but no capacitance, the change in voltage (*V*) is proportional to the current and exhibits the same time course. (*b*) If the circuit instead possesses only a capacitive element (*C*), then the rate of change in the voltage (*dV/dt*) is proportional to the current. (*c*) Nerve fibers exhibit both resistance and capacitance. Consequently, an applied stimulus causes a rapid capacitative current (*IC*) followed by a slower resistive current (*IR*). At any point in time, the total membrane current (*Im*) = *IR* + *IC*. The membrane potential (*V*) shows an exponential rise characterized by a time constant (τ) = *RC* and a final value = *IR*. At the end of the current pulse, *V* declines exponentially as the membrane capicitance discharges through the resistance with an equal but opposite *IC* and *IR* and with the same time constant. (After Nicholls, Martin, and Wallace, 1992.)

resistances to nongated K^+, Na^+, and Cl^- ion fluxes. The membrane current (I_m) at any moment is the sum of the resistive current (I_R, which is carried by ions passing through the membrane channels) and the capacitive current (I_C); i.e., $I_m = I_R + I_C$. Moreover, from the laws of physics, the voltage across the two circuit elements R and C must be equal at all times.

When a rectangular current pulse (I) is injected into the cell, the change in membrane potential (V) lags behind the current pulse as shown in Figure 5.18c. This is because most of the initial current flows into the capacitative element of the membrane (note the almost instantaneous increase in I_C at the onset of the current pulse). As the pulse continues and the capacitor is charged, more and more of the current must flow through the membrane resistance to balance the voltage across the resistor with that of the capacitor (note the gradually increasing value of I_R). With more current flowing through the resistor, there is less current available for further charging the capacitor; thus the *rate of change* of V decreases over time. When V reaches its plateau value, all of the membrane current is flowing through the resistor. When the current is turned off at the end of the pulse, the capacitor discharges and drives the current back through the resistor to restore the resting potential as shown in Figure 5.18c.

The degree to which the change in membrane voltage lags behind the stimulus pulse is expressed as the membrane time constant, or tau (τ). Tau is equal to RC (the product of the resistance and capacitance of the membrane) and can be determined experimentally as the time required for the membrane potential to reach 63% of its final value. The time constants of different neurons typically range from 1 to 20 ms (see Koester, 1991).

The significance of the time constant can be seen in the process of **temporal integration**. Most synaptic potentials are caused by brief currents resulting from the opening of ligand-gated channels on postsynaptic dendrites. The time course of the event is a function of the membrane time constant. Individually, the postsynaptic excitatory potentials may be too small to trigger an action potential, but if the postsynaptic cell has a long membrane time constant, the synaptic potentials last long enough to overlap and add together, a process known as **temporal summation**. In this way, repeated weak stimuli can sum to reach the threshold for triggering an action potential (Figure 5.19).

The Mechanics of Action Potentials

Having discussed some of the factors that play a role in the generation of action potentials, we may now describe their immediate antecedents. A demonstration using the method illustrated in Figure 5.15a will show how action potentials are generated. An axon is first stimulated at a low voltage (S_1), followed 2 ms later by a second stimulus at a higher voltage (S_2). The membrane responses are recorded by two voltmeters, V_1 and V_2, spaced 20 mm apart (see Figure 5.15). The results of this procedure are shown in Figure 5.20. Here we see that the first stimulus (S_1) elicits a graded potential recorded by V_1, but not by V_2. The absence of a trace at V_2 is due to the length constant of the axon; that is, the response to the stimulus rapidly dissipates so that at V_2, 20 mm away from V_1, a response can no longer be generated.

The second stimulus (S_2) is stronger than S_1 and has a greater effect on the axon. First, at V_1, the membrane is depolarized to approximately –40 mV; then a sudden polarity reversal of the axon occurs as the voltage jumps from –40 to +45 mV. The polarity then reverses again and declines to a level slightly below that of the resting potential before returning to it. These voltage changes are the components of an action potential. The whole event occurs in approximately 1.0 ms in a squid axon and in half that time in mammalian neurons.

If the suprathreshold stimulus were significantly increased, the amplitude and duration of the action potential would be the same, except that the slope of the graded potential component would be steeper. Thus the action potential would occur sooner after the onset of the stimulus.

The voltmeter V_2 also records the action potential; and even though the local potential component is absent, the amplitude of the action potential is undiminished. Accordingly, action potentials are said to have an all-or-none quality—meaning that they appear with their full effect or not at all—and to be nondecremental.

Briefly, action potentials occur because ligand- or voltage-gated sodium channels open so that Na^+ flows down its concentration gradient through the membrane, reducing the internal negativity. This ion flow is equivalent to a flow of electricity through the membrane. If the effect were weak, it would be quickly counteracted by a K^+ efflux, which would return the resting potential to its original value (–70 mV). However, if the stimulus exceeds a threshold value at which there is more Na^+ influx than K^+ efflux, then more Na^+ channels open, increasing Na^+

influx and further decreasing internal negativity. Thus, a sufficiently large Na^+ influx, by itself, causes a voltage change in the membrane that serves as a stimulus for more channels to open. The net result is a regenerative influx of sodium, which means that the more Na^+ influx there is, the more Na^+ influx there will be.

At this juncture, some details of Na^+ and K^+ channel function should be reviewed. A comparison of voltage-gated Na^+ and K^+ channels reveals two similarities and two differences between them. They are similar in that both channel populations open in response to depolarizations of the membrane potential, and the greater the depolarization, the faster and the greater the extent (i.e., more channels) of the response. However, Na^+ channels open more rapidly than do K^+ channels, and they close more rapidly when the depolarizing pulse is brief. Also, even if the depolarization is maintained, the Na^+ channels begin to close or inactivate, thereby causing a decay of Na^+ influx. In contrast, K^+ channels remain open for as long as the depolarization persists.

Each Na^+ channel can exist in three different states that represent three different conformations of the Na^+ channel protein (see above): resting, activated, or inactivated. When the membrane is depolarized, the channel goes from the resting (closed) state to the activated (open) state. If the depolarization is brief, the channel goes directly back to the resting state, but if the depolarization is maintained, the channel goes to the inactivated (closed) state. Once this state is established, the channel cannot be activated (opened) by another depolarization. Only after repolarization can the inactivation be reversed and the channel revert to the resting state, in which it can again be activated by depolarization. These switches between states take time because channels leave the inactivated state slowly (Figure 5.21).

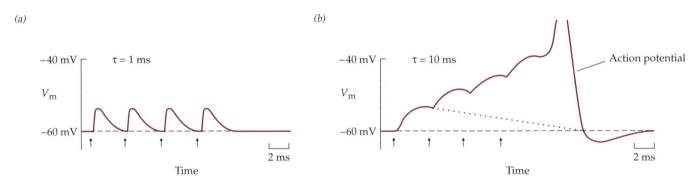

5.19 THE TIME CONSTANT AND TEMPORAL SUMMATION. Postsynaptic responses to repetitive synaptic stimulation are shown in two cells that differ in their membrane time constant (τ) (arrows indicate action potentials in the presynaptic cell). (a) In a cell with a small τ, even rapid synaptic stimulation (285 Hz, which corresponds to an interval of about 3.5 ms between action potentials) fails to generate a spike because each excitatory postsynaptic potential (EPSP) decays before the next one begins. (b) In a cell with a large τ, however, the EPSPs overlap sufficiently for the membrane threshold to be reached and a spike to be generated. The dotted line illustrates the slow rate of decay of a single EPSP in this cell.

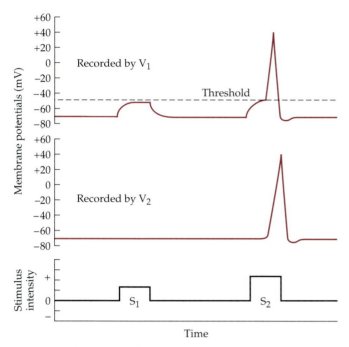

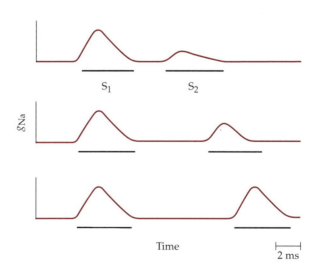

5.20 STIMULUS-EVOKED ACTION POTENTIALS. Using the procedure illustrated in Figure 5.15, recordings from V_1 show that stimulus S_1 elicits a local potential. The suprathreshold stimulus S_2 evokes an action potential. The recording from V_2 shows no response to S_1, indicating that the response decayed before it reached V_2, which is positioned 20 mm from V_1. However, the action potential is recorded by V_2 even though the local potential component was absent. Note the slight "undershoot" of the declining phase to –80 mV before returning to the resting potential.

These phenomena suggest that the Na$^+$ channel has two gates—an **activation gate** that is closed when the membrane is at its resting potential, and an **inactivation gate** that is open at the resting potential but closes slowly during depolarization—and that the channel conductance occurs only during the brief interval during depolarization when both gates are open. Repolarization reverses the two processes, and after the channel has returned to the resting state, it is again available for activation by depolarization (Koester, 1991).

Threshold mechanics. These observations indicate that if a depolarizing stimulus is strong enough, a threshold is crossed, bringing into play the series of events that produce the action potential. Experiments have shown that the increase in stimulus intensity needed to convert a graded potential to an action potential is only 1/5,000 over the subthreshold stimulus, and according to some calculations, the increase need only be 1×10^{-14} over the subthreshold stimulus (Brinley, 1974). In a recent review it was pointed out that the all-or-none phenomenon is universally applicable to all excitable cells despite the dozens of different voltage-gated ion channels that have been described. For virtually all nerve and muscle cells, a fraction of a millivolt may be the difference between a

subthreshold depolarizing stimulus and a stimulus that generates a full-scale action potential.

This phenomenon is perhaps all the more surprising because the Na$^+$ conductance is proportional to the number of Na$^+$ channels that are open, and increases in conductance occur in a strictly graded manner as depolarization increases. Specifically, with each increment of depolarization, the number of voltage-gated Na$^+$ channels that switch from the closed to the open state increases in a gradual fashion, thereby causing a gradual increase in Na$^+$ influx. Why, then, is there a threshold for action potential generation?

Close inspection shows that Na$^+$ conductance is not the sole element in this event. Whereas depolarization of the membrane does elicit inward flow of Na$^+$ (I_{Na}), it also increases two outward currents: that of K$^+$ (I_K) and that from normal leakage (I_l). As I_k and I_l increase with depolarization, they tend to resist the depolarizing action of Na$^+$ influx. However, the great driving force of the exterior Na$^+$ and the rapid kinetics of the Na$^+$ channel activation process ensure that the depolarization eventually will reach a point—the threshold—at which the increase in inward I_{Na} exceeds the increase in outward I_k and I_l and becomes regenerative. The threshold, $V\tau$, is therefore the specific value of V_m at which the net ionic current ($I_{Na} + I_k + I_l$) just changes from outward to inward, depositing positive charge on the inside of the membrane (Koester, 1991). Thus, it seems that the critical instant that corresponds to the crossing of the threshold is when enough Na$^+$ influx starts the regenerative process of recruiting more and more Na$^+$ channels be-

5.21 Na$^+$ CHANNEL ACTIVATION AND INACTIVATION. When the axonal membrane is depolarized (horizontal traces), Na$^+$ conductance (g_{Na}) rapidly increases but then declines due to rapid inactivation and closure of the Na$^+$ channels. The channels remain inactivated for a few milliseconds before changing to the resting state, from which they can be reactivated. Consequently, the fraction of channels activated by successive stimuli depends on the stimulus interval (compare second trace in each plot).

fore the start of K⁺ efflux and before the increase of normal current leakage.

During the development of the action potential, one might expect that the Na⁺ influx would continue until the internal voltage rises to a level at which further influx of Na⁺ is electrostatically repelled. For Na⁺, the necessary internal voltage would have to be about +50 mV, which is the equilibrium potential for Na⁺ (E_{Na}) (see above). However, before E_{Na} is reached, the slow-starting inactivation gates close the Na⁺ channels, thereby terminating Na⁺ influx. Also, soon after the start of Na⁺ influx, the gates of the K⁺ channels open and K⁺ efflux begins. This slows the rise of the membrane voltage and ultimately reverses the polarity toward the resting potential. At this point the membrane is impermeable to Na⁺ because the Na⁺ channels are in an inactivated (closed) state, but because K⁺ efflux lasts a little longer, there is a slight undershoot before the resting potential is restored. This short period of hyperpolarization is known as an **afterpotential**. All of these events take place within a few milliseconds.

Figure 5.22 shows the time course for the action potential and a comparison of the conductance of the Na⁺ and K⁺ ions. These curves, derived from the theory and experiments of A. L. Hodgkin and A. F. Huxley (1952), served as the cornerstone of subsequent neuroscience and won for them and J. C. Eccles (1964b) the Nobel Prize in 1963.

One consequence of action potentials is that for each response, there is a small gain of Na⁺ and a small loss of K⁺ from the axon. This is of little importance because, although the increase of Na⁺ influx is great, the duration of flow is short. Thus, a squid axon loses only about one-millionth of its K⁺ per nerve impulse, and this is quickly restored by the sodium–potassium pump. A very thin mammalian axon may lose as much as one-thousandth of its K⁺ content per impulse, but, as mentioned previously, the action of the sodium–potassium pump is accelerated by high internal concentrations of Na⁺ and high external concentrations of K⁺. So, even if thin axons fire hundreds of times per second over a sustained period, the internal concentrations of Na⁺ and K⁺ remain relatively constant.

To briefly summarize, action potentials occur when appropriate ligands bind to receptors on the soma or dendrites of a nerve cell and cause the opening of Na⁺ channels in the membrane, allowing an influx of Na⁺ ions that depolarizes the membrane. If the depolarization is of sufficient magnitude, voltage sensors open the gates of more Na⁺ channels in a regenerative way (i.e., as channels open, more adjacent channels will open) so that more Na⁺ flows down its concentration gradient into the cytoplasm. However, during the Na⁺ influx, the voltage change activates K⁺ channels and increases normal current leakage, resulting in the membrane's return to its resting potential.

Propagation of the Action Potential

Once an action potential has occurred, it is propagated without decrement to the axon terminals. This phenomenon can be explained by the fact that each action potential serves as the stimulus for an adjacent action potential; the energy for this occurrence arises from the axon and is not related to the original stimulus. A simple anal-

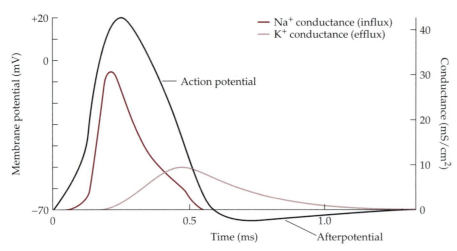

5.22 THE ACTION POTENTIAL IS A FUNCTION OF Na⁺ AND K⁺. The left ordinate is a scale of the membrane potential. The action potential begins at –70 mV and rises to about +20 mV due to the Na⁺ influx. The scale of conductance is indicated on the right ordinate. Just before Na⁺ conductance reaches its maximum, K⁺ efflux begins, arresting the rise of the action potential, and together with the fall in Na⁺ influx, brings the membrane voltage momentarily below –70 mV until K⁺ efflux ends. This increase in negative voltage is known as an afterpotential. (mS = milli-Siemens[unit of conductance].)

ogy illustrates this mechanism: One can ignite a fuse with a match. The burning fuse then ignites adjacent parts of the fuse if there is enough combustible material in the adjacent sections. The burning match does not now have anything to do with the propagation of the flame. The potential energy is in the fuse itself, and it will burn with equal intensity throughout its length. But one should not press this analogy too far: an action potential does not induce its own propagation by transferring heat to the adjacent sections. It does so by the spread of the depolarizing action of the sodium influx. It should be recalled that an action potential starts with a regenerative Na^+ influx, which makes the interior of the axon positive. The positive ions in the interior of the axon flow toward the negativity of the adjacent section and neutralize it, thus depolarizing the membrane at that site. There, the sodium channels open to start an action potential, which then depolarizes the next site, and so on to the axon terminal. In other words, the voltage change in the membrane caused by an action potential is sufficient to depolarize an adjacent site, initiating an action potential at that site, and this process continues throughout the length of the axon.

The known details of axon physiology are largely based upon studies of the axons from squid and other species, but the details are virtually the same for all species. However, it is likely that not all neural activity is dependent upon action potentials. In the brain, there are many areas where neurons are densely packed together, and communication between them is via extremely short extensions of their cell bodies. It is possible that passive spread of membrane depolarizations may be a sufficient mode of communication under these conditions (see Chapter 6).

Local anesthetics block impulse propagation. Local anesthetics such as procaine (Novocaine) and lidocaine (Xylocaine) exert their anesthetic effects by blocking Na^+ channels and thus the transmission of action potentials along axons. It is significant that fibers mediating pain impulses are blocked before fibers that mediate touch, kinesthetic, and motor impulses. This would suggest that these anesthetic drugs have a clinical specificity for "pain" fibers; however, these differential effects are actually due to the absence of myelinization on the very thinnest "pain" fibers, or the presence of many nodes of Ranvier in thinly myelinated fibers. Thus, the anesthetics gain greater access to the axolemmas of these fibers and exert the earliest and greatest effect on them. However, these drugs are highly lipid soluble, and, at sufficient doses, they will gain access to the larger myelinated sensory and motor nerves and will exert similar blocking effects. Indeed, anesthetics of this type are injected into the vertebral canal during spinal anesthesia at doses that block all sensory and motor function (Ritchie and Greene, 1985).

Propagation velocity. There is a wide range of propagation velocities for nerve impulses—from 1.0 to 100 m/s—all of which are considerably slower than the passive spread of graded membrane currents over very short distances. This relative slowness is explained by the time it takes to generate action potentials, and the wide range is due, in part, to the fact that propagation velocity in unmyelinated axons is proportional to the square root of the axon diameter. Thus, for example, increasing the diameter of an axon 16-fold would increase the velocity only 4-fold. However, axon diameter alone does not account for the variation in velocity; there are no axons in existence that could support the higher range of propagation velocity on the basis of axon diameter alone. A crab axon 30 μm in diameter, for example, conducts nerve impulses at 5 m/s. The axon would have to be 1.2 cm in diameter to conduct at 100 m/s if axon diameter were the only consideration.

The structure that accounts for the highest propagation velocities is the myelin sheath, which forms a segmented insulated cover around many axons (see Chapter 3). All fast-conducting axons are equipped with myelin. Myelin sheaths speed conduction in the following ways:

1. Myelin sheaths make the axon membrane less leaky, so that there is less decrement of passive currents over distance.
2. More important, the myelin sheath reduces the capacitive characteristics of the axolemma to less than 1% of the expected value, and this also prevents voltage loss over distance.
3. The sheath reduces the number of points where the axolemma is in contact with the extracellular fluid and where Na^+ influx occurs during action potentials. In myelinated fibers, contact occurs only at the intersegmental areas (the nodes of Ranvier). At the nodes, the total transmembrane resistance is low, the density of Na^+ channels is greatest (up to $12,000/\mu m^2$), and K^+ channels are almost completely absent. However, K^+ channels are well distributed in the internodal myelinated segments, where K^+ efflux occurs slowly, but at a rate sufficient to maintain the resting potential of the axons.

Accordingly, action potentials develop at the nodes and initiate the passive currents associated with the flow of Na^+ toward areas of negativity. In myelinated axons, this current flows quickly and efficiently (with little loss) to the next node, where depolarization of the axon membrane and a new action potential can occur. Because the nodes are relatively far apart (from 0.2 to 2 mm, which may be 100 times the axon diameter), the action potentials figuratively skip from node to node, a process called **saltatory conduction**. In contrast, action potentials in nonmyelinated axons are generated practically next to each other and proceed along the axon like a flame along a burning fuse (Figure 5.23). Thus, neural messages are transmitted much faster in myelinated axons because there are fewer points where action potentials are generated. An analogy would be to compare the speed of a local train stopping at every station with that of an express train stopping only at a few principal stations; the express reaches the end of the line much sooner.

An ancillary benefit of myelination is a reduction of the energy needed to get the message from one end of the axon to the other. With every action potential, energy is expended to restore the ions to their proper places and concentrations. Therefore, the fewer action potentials generated over the course of the axon, the less energy is expended. Consequently, myelinated neurons function more efficiently, even under conditions of great demand over a considerable period of time. In the human, myelination saves energy by a factor of about 5,000, and saves packing volume by a factor of 1,000 (Morell, 1978). This means that the human nervous system, in order to have the same capability without the benefit of myelin, would have to be 1,000 times larger.

Determinants and Effects of Nerve Impulse Frequency

For the most part, nervous systems are organized so that information is transmitted by a neural code that is expressed in terms of nerve impulse frequency. Throughout this section and the rest of this book, the reader should bear in mind that neural activity, like all other cell activities, is not an on–off phenomenon. Rather, neural activity is continuous and dynamic, and the

processes or substances that act on the system usually do so by increasing or decreasing nerve impulse frequency.

Nerve impulse frequency varies depending upon the duration and intensity of the stimulus and the neural system involved. It is a common observation that any stimulus, whether it be visual, auditory, olfactory, or pressure applied to the skin, can be perceived as having a finite duration and intensity (e.g., bright or dark, loud or soft, heavy or light). The effects of the stimulus are determined by (1) the duration of the stimulus, (2) the number of sense organs and neurons that are stimulated, and (3) the frequency of the nerve impulses that are generated. The effects of these factors are illustrated in Figure 5.24, which shows the patterns of action potentials generated by light stimuli focused on light-sensitive, densely pigmented organelles in the giant nerve cell bodies of *Aplysia* ganglia. The different effects are the function of different intensities and durations of the light stimuli.

Information Transmission

Action potentials, because they are propagated without decrement, are superbly suited for information transmission in the nervous system. However, because of their all-or-none nature, information about the intensity of a stimulus cannot be transmitted by an amplitude modulation (AM) of membrane potentials. Rather remarkably, information about the intensity of stimuli is transmitted by a frequency modulation (FM) of action potentials— the greater the stimulus intensity, or the more strongly a muscle acts or the more a gland secretes, the higher the sensory or the motor **nerve impulse frequency**.

The great advantage of this system is its high signal-to-noise ratio. The concept of the signal-to-noise ratio is best understood by comparing AM and FM radio trans-

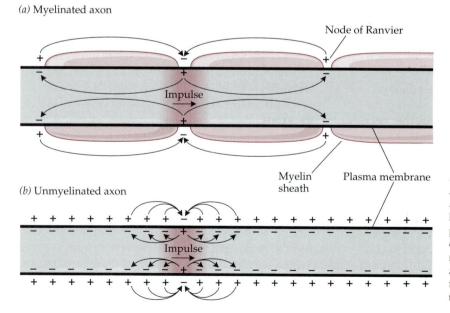

(a) Myelinated axon

Node of Ranvier

Impulse

Myelin sheath   Plasma membrane

(b) Unmyelinated axon

Impulse

5.23 ACTION POTENTIALS IN MYELINATED AND NONMYELINATED AXONS. In myelinated axons, Na$^+$ influx reverses the polarity of the membrane at a node of Ranvier. The positive ions move passively in the cytoplasm and extracellular fluid in either direction to the adjacent nodes, where the membrane becomes depolarized to initiate another action potential, and so on. In nonmyelinated fibers, the positive ions spread only a small distance away to depolarize the adjacent membrane.

mission during adverse conditions. AM radio stations transmit signals denoting speech or music by modulating the amplitude of a carrier wave of a given frequency to which the radio (receiver) is tuned. However, electrical storms and electronic devices near the receiver also radiate amplitude-modulated signals to which the receiver is sensitive, thereby creating static (noise). The signal, then, is distorted if the signal and the noise have the same intensity—a condition having a low signal-to-noise ratio, in this case 1:1. Turning up the volume does not improve matters because the noise as well as the signal becomes louder. In FM radio (and television), the signals are transmitted by varying the frequency of a carrier wave band, and FM receivers detect differences in the frequency, but not the amplitude, of the waves. Consequently, changes in the amplitude of the waves caused by electrical storms and electronic devices are undetected, so the speech, music, and television pictures being transmitted are minimally affected. In this case, the signal-to-noise ratio may be as high as 100:1.

In the nervous system, there are constant metabolic changes in neurons that cause slight changes in the resting potential. If the brain responded in some way to those changes, or if changes in intensity between slightly different stimuli also caused slight amplitude changes in axon potentials, neural messages would always be contaminated by physiological changes. However, because messages denoting changes in stimulus intensity are conveyed by changes in nerve impulse frequency, physiological membrane changes do not seriously affect them. In this case, the signal-to-noise ratio is very high, making it possible to detect stimulus differences that are exceedingly small. For example, a young person with healthy ears is able to detect the presence of a sound that causes a depression of the eardrum of less than the diameter of a hydrogen atom, and the tips of the hair cells in the cochlea need to move only 1–100 picometers (trillionths of a meter) to accomplish this.

Refractory Periods

Refractory periods are of two types, and both are important in the determination of impulse frequency. The **absolute refractory period** is the time interval during the course of an action potential when a second stimulus to the same cell receptor will not elicit another action potential. This time period coincides with the falling phase of the action potential caused by K^+ efflux. For example, if an adequate stimulus is applied to a motor neuron of a cat and a recording made of the axonic activity, the record will show that an action potential has occurred. However, if the stimulus is followed by a second stimulus (no matter how strong) within 0.7 ms of the first, there is no noticeable effect on the action potential, and no new response occurs. This "silent" period occurs because the Na^+ influx of the second stimulus is negated by the K^+ efflux following the first stimulus.

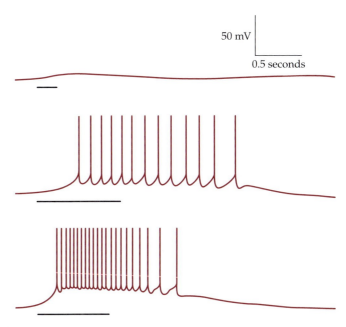

50 mV

0.5 seconds

5.24 PARAMETERS OF ACTION POTENTIAL FREQUENCY. The duration and intensity of stimuli affect the frequency of action potentials. The top trace shows the effect of a brief light stimulus of low intensity focused upon densely pigmented organelles in the giant nerve cells in *Aplysia* ganglia; only a local depolarization occurs. The middle trace shows the effect of a longer stimulus of greater intensity, which elicits a burst of action potentials. The bottom trace is the result of a stimulus of greater intensity but of shorter duration than the second; the frequency of action potentials is greater, but the burst duration is shorter. The ratio of the intensities of the stimuli (from top to bottom) is 0.05:0.2:2.0. (After Arvanitaki and Chalazonitis, 1961.)

If, on the other hand, the interval between the two stimuli is increased to 0.8 ms, a second action potential might immediately follow the first, but its amplitude might be slightly diminished. During this period, however, a normal action potential will occur if the stimulus is greater than normal. This period, known as the **relative refractory period**, or afterpotential, is a transient hyperpolarization or depolarization that may immediately follow an action potential. These refractory periods may appear in sequence, just one alone, or none at all, depending upon the animal and the type of neuron. An example is the undershoot (afterpotential) shown in Figure 5.22, during which the threshold is elevated because of an excess of K^+ efflux, which briefly hyperpolarizes the membrane. A stimulus arriving during that period would have to be stronger than normal to elicit another action potential on the axon. If the undershoot were followed by an elevation above the resting potential—an overshoot—the axon would then be in a supernormal state with a lower threshold. In this situation, a weaker than normal stimulus could excite the axon to fire an action potential. Normally, an interval of about 2–3 ms must elapse before a second action potential can be elicited after a preceding one.

Thus, after the onset of an action potential, there is a "silent" period during which the axon is unresponsive to stimuli, followed by a period during which the membrane is hyperpolarized and requires stronger than normal stimuli to generate action potentials, or is slightly depolarized and can generate action potentials after a weaker than normal stimulus. In these ways the relative refractory periods serve to modulate the thresholds for action potentials and thus decrease or increase the probability of the occurrence of successive action potentials.

The refractory periods also contribute to one-way impulse propagation by preventing action potentials from oscillating between adjacent points. As mentioned earlier, if an axon is stimulated near the middle of its length, the passive flow of Na^+ ions in the cytoplasm spreads and initiates action potentials in both directions from the stimulus point because axons are perfectly capable of propagating action potentials toward, as well as away from, the cell soma (see Figure 5.23). Accordingly, under normal conditions, after an action potential has been propagated from the cell body to the axon, another response at the previous site is not possible because it is in the absolute refractory phase and cannot be excited again so soon. Consequently, action potentials are propagated in one direction only.

Other factors may also influence the frequency of action potentials. For example, the design of a synaptic junction may influence the size of the membrane area that is exposed to a neurotransmitter, or inhibitory transmitters may be released from presynaptic axons. In general, the maximum rates for motor neurons are about 200–300 impulses/s, whereas rates as high as 1,600 impulses/s have been recorded from Renshaw cells, the interneurons found in the ventral horn of the spinal cord.

Impulse Transmission between Neurons

The earlier discussion of squid axon physiology might lead to the incorrect conclusion that if one axon terminal adequately stimulates another neuron, an action potential will be generated in the other neuron. It is very unlikely that action potentials are generated in this way because the effect occurring at any one terminal is too small. Microscopic examination shows that the dendrites and somata of neurons are covered by thousands of axon terminals from other neurons, and it is the interaction of the inputs from all of those terminals that determines whether or not action potentials will occur in the postsynaptic neuron.

Temporal and spatial summation.   As described above, Figure 5.19 illustrates how the time constant of a postsynaptic cell determines whether or not local depolarizations can sum to elicit an action potential in that cell (temporal summation). It has also been found that the magnitude of a depolarization at one synaptic junction is between 0.1 and 0.5 mV, whereas a depolarization of about 5.0 mV or more is necessary to trigger an action potential. In such a case, an adequate postsynaptic depolarization can be easily accomplished by the process of spatial summation. If a number of axon terminals clustered within a confined space on a postsynaptic neuron and all terminals are activated within a few milliseconds of one another, the stimulus effects will sum to form a suprathreshold stimulus adequate for generating an action potential in the recipient neuron. Thus, the spatial summation of nerve impulses is a significant factor in determining the adequacy of the signal for synaptic transmission.

Excitatory–inhibitory interactions.   Neurons do not only receive depolarizing or excitatory inputs, they also receive hyperpolarizing or inhibitory inputs. For example, as shown in Figure 5.25, the knee-jerk reflex involves both excitatory and inhibitory messages. A brisk tap on the patellar tendon will cause a free leg to extend because of the contraction of the extensor quadriceps muscle in the thigh. However, the leg will not move unless the flexor biceps femoralis muscle relaxes. Therefore, when an excitatory signal is sent to the quadriceps' motor neurons to contract the quadriceps, a concurrent hyperpolarizing inhibitory signal is sent to the biceps' motor neurons to relax the biceps. This type of inhibition occurs by way of interneurons similar to Renshaw cells.

Excitatory inputs cause a depolarization, or an **excitatory postsynaptic potential** (**EPSP**), on the membrane. This response is similar to the local potentials described earlier. In motor neurons, the amplitude of an EPSP is estimated to be about 0.1 mV. An inhibitory input causes a hyperpolarization, or an **inhibitory postsynaptic potential** (**IPSP**). The interaction between EPSPs and IPSPs determines whether or not action potentials are generated in the postsynaptic neuron, and if they are generated, how long they will continue.

The nature of the EPSP–IPSP interaction can be understood if we know how one nerve impulse at a synapse causes an EPSP and how another causes an IPSP. In general, the determinants are (1) the nature of the transmitter substance that is released from the axon terminals, and (2) the nature of the receptor sites on the postsynaptic membrane. We may simply mention that in the example cited above, the transmitter that transmits excitatory inputs to the quadriceps' motor neuron is glutamic acid, which opens Na^+ channels for depolarization, and the transmitter that transmits inhibitory inputs to the biceps' motor neuron is glycine, which opens Cl^- channels for an influx of chloride anions, which increase the intracellular negativity (hyperpolarization), making it more difficult for Na^+ to depolarize the membrane.

Figure 5.26 shows the effect of inhibitory neurons upon other neurons in the brain that spontaneously generate action potentials for extended periods, or when there is rapid alternation of finger movements during

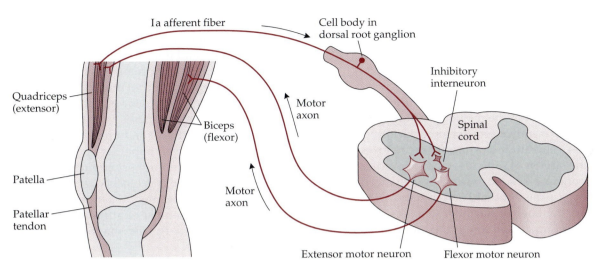

5.25 THE ROLE OF INHIBITORY NEURONS IN SPINAL REFLEXES. The afferent neuron from the stretch receptors of the quadriceps muscle (Ia afferent fiber) makes an excitatory connection with the motor neuron innervating the same muscle group. It also excites an inhibitory interneuron that, in turn, makes an inhibitory connection with the motor neuron innervating the antagonist muscle group, the biceps, whose relaxation permits the quadriceps muscle to extend the leg. (After Kandel and Schwartz, 1991.)

piano playing, or in the rapid back-and-forth movements of the elbow during tremolo violin bowing. The inhibitory neurons generate IPSPs that prevent the postsynaptic cell membranes from achieving threshold levels of depolarization (see Chapter 6 for more details). Thus, neurons have multiple receptor sites, each responding to different transmitters in different ways. Here it should be mentioned that a given neurotransmitter may not be solely excitatory or inhibitory; rather, in many instances, it can be excitatory or inhibitory depending upon the receptor upon which it acts. Neurotransmitters and their actions will be described in greater detail in Chapter 6, but here it must be emphasized that the type and number of axon terminals and receptor sites that are activated or inactivated determines the effect of a transmitter upon a neuron or an effector organ such as a muscle or a gland. If the excitatory influences dominate the inhibitory influences, it is likely that action potentials will occur, and effector organs will respond appropriately. If the inhibitory influences are dominant, the action potentials will be blocked, delayed, or reduced in frequency, and the effector organs will be less active.

Integration within a neuron.   Threshold differences for the generation of action potentials exist among motor neurons as well as among other neuron types. Eccles (1964b) recorded action potentials in motor neurons and found that the algebraic sum of EPSPs and IPSPs first influences the initial segment (IS) of the axon (see Figures 3.2 and 3.4). This area of the axon has a lower threshold than does the somatodendritic (SD) part of the cell, and serves as the trigger zone for action potentials. The

threshold at the IS ranges from 6 to 18 mV, whereas that at the SD ranges between 20 and 40 mV. In some motor neurons, the IS threshold may be half of the SD threshold, although in other neurons the difference is barely detectable. In most neurons, the initial segment is the site where the balance between excitation and inhibition is resolved. Functionally, at least in motor neurons that constitute the final neural pathway for action (behavior), this seems to be a more efficient system than one in

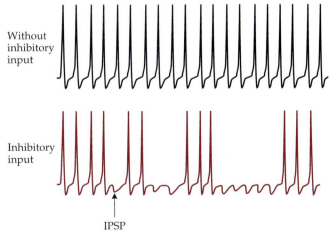

5.26. INHIBITION CAN SHAPE THE PATTERN OF ACTION POTENTIALS. The upper trace shows the repetitive firing pattern of a hypothetical neuron in the absence of inhibitory synaptic input. When inhibitory inputs are activated, however, the pattern of spiking is altered due to the generation of hyperpolarizing IPSPs. This process is sometimes called "sculpturing." (After Kandel and Schwartz, 1991.)

which determinations about action potentials occur simultaneously at different parts of the cell.

Part II Summary

We may summarize this section by describing the neuronal interactions involved in the relatively simple proprioceptive reflexes that utilize sensory proprioceptive and motor neurons to maintain posture. These reflexes are initiated by the stretch of muscles, whose spindles depolarize and generate graded responses, which, if strong enough, surpass the threshold and initiate action potentials at the trigger zone of sensory cell axons. The action potentials are propagated to the axon terminals, which synapse with motor neurons. If the graded EPSPs sum and overbalance IPSPs to surpass the threshold on the motor neurons, action potentials are generated and propagated in an all-or-none fashion to neuromuscular junctions. There, the motor nerve terminals release the neurotransmitter acetylcholine (ACh) in graded amounts that depend upon the rate of arrival of action potentials at the terminal. The ACh diffuses across the synaptic space, causing graded muscle contractions appropriate for the maintenance of body equilibrium.

Here we see the functional significance of local potentials that are initiated at the dendritic part of the sensory cell by the tens, hundreds, or even thousands of muscle spindles that impinge upon it. Starting at the dendritic site, the response of the sensory neuron is graded and integrative, and if it surpasses the membrane threshold, an all-or-none, nondecremental action potential is generated and propagated to the axon terminals. At the synapse with the motor neuron, the quantity of released transmitter is determined by the frequency of action potentials reaching the axon terminals; therefore, the effect upon the motor cell depends upon the algebraic sum of excitatory and inhibitory inputs to the cell. If the depolarization threshold is reached, action potentials are generated and propagated to a muscle that will contract, and the duration and strength of the response will again be determined by the magnitude of the graded transmitter release.

From the foregoing discussion, we have seen that frequency-modulated nerve impulses are the language of nerve function, and that neurotransmitters are the chemical links that activate neurosensory, neuroeffector, and neuro-neuronal connections. However, the determinants of the frequency-modulated message are graded sensory stimuli and graded synaptic voltages that are positive or negative, which in turn are guided by the length and time constants of neurons and the presence of afterpotentials. Further characteristics of neurotransmitters and their release, catabolism, and uptake will be discussed in the chapters that follow.

Chapter 6

Synaptic Structure and Function

In the preceding chapter our discussion centered around the initiation of nerve impulses (action potentials) and their propagation from one end of the nerve cell to the other. However, a behavioral response is the result of tens of thousands or millions of neurons interacting among themselves, resulting in the stimulation of effector organs such as muscles and glands. The process starts with interoceptive or exteroceptive stimuli acting on sense organs that activate sensory neurons. The frequency and duration of sense organ and sensory neuron responses are proportional to the intensity and persistence of the stimuli impinging upon the sense organs. The sensory neurons, via their axons, send messages to other neurons within the CNS that are parts of circuits of various types that may have enhancing, diminishing, prolonging, delaying, or timing effects. These circuits are combined into systems that produce sensory and perceptual effects, control reflexes, fixed action patterns, and learned responses. The sites on neurons whereby neurons stimulate one another are known as synapses, and it is at these loci that the specificity, plasticity, and variability of the nervous system is to be found.

Tanzi in 1893 was one of the earliest to propose that learning occurs as a result of modifications in the junctions between neurons (the term "synapse" appeared a few years later). This view, amply buttressed by decades of experiments and supporting data, is currently the most widely accepted hypothetical position on this subject. Briefly, this view holds that learning is the result of neural activity that alters the growth, number, structure, level of activity, and efficacy of synapses so that they act as switches either to facilitate or to inhibit the flow of nerve impulses from one area of the brain to another. For example, through innumerable co-occurrences of the sight or sound of cats and the word "cat," synapses are modified such that the mere sight of the word leads to action upon those synapses opening countless numbers of circuits that result in the reader's immediate subjective perception of the texture, scent, sounds, visual images, memory of events, and emotions associated with a particular animal.

Figure 6.1 illustrates the effect of experience on synaptic modification by comparing a synapse from the visual pathway of a normally reared dog with a synapse from a dog reared in darkness. The more elaborate surface of the synapse from the normal dog is better equipped to transmit messages than that from the visually deprived dog: there are more dendritic spines and contact areas, and more vesicles and mitochondria. The role of synapses in other types of behavior, particularly learning, will be discussed in more detail later in this chapter.

Psychotropic Drugs and Synapses

Drugs that affect mood and behavior have an affinity for receptors associated with neurons. These substances are known as **psychotropic drugs**, and synapses are the loci where most of the pharmacological responses occur

185

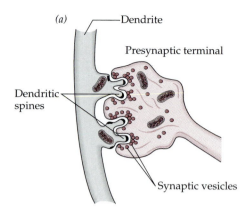

(*a*) — Dendrite

Presynaptic terminal

Dendritic spines

Synaptic vesicles

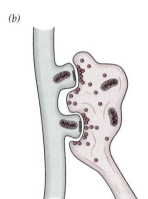

(*b*)

6.1 SYNAPTIC MODIFICATION due to light deprivation in the lateral geniculate nucleus of a dog. (*a*) A normal dog, and (*b*) a dog reared in darkness. The synapse from the normal dog is more elaborate than that of the dog reared in darkness. (After Shepherd, 1988.)

(Figure 6.2). At one time, psychotropic drugs were known as **sympathomimetics**, indicating that the drugs mimicked the action of the sympathetic nervous system, or **cholinomimetics**, indicating mimicry of the action of acetylcholine (ACh). Later, some drugs were classified as **analeptics**, meaning stimulants of the nervous system (e.g., caffeine and amphetamine), or as **neuroleptics**, meaning drugs that have overall beneficial effects upon the nervous systems of patients with mental disease. Later, as more precise anatomical and physiological information was obtained about the effects of drugs upon the nervous system, psychotropic drugs were described in terms of their affinity for synapses and the mechanism of action by which their effects upon these synapses occur. However, it should be mentioned that some psychotropic drugs do not act upon synapses. For example, as already mentioned, local anesthetics such as procaine and lidocaine block the conduction of action potentials, especially in the thinly or unmyelinated axons that characteristically mediate pain.

Yet, because most psychotropic drugs exert their effects on the degree or duration of synaptic activity, it is important that synaptic structure and function be clearly understood. Moreover, the fact that synapses are the sites of action of many drugs suggests that psychopathological states and some neurological diseases may be

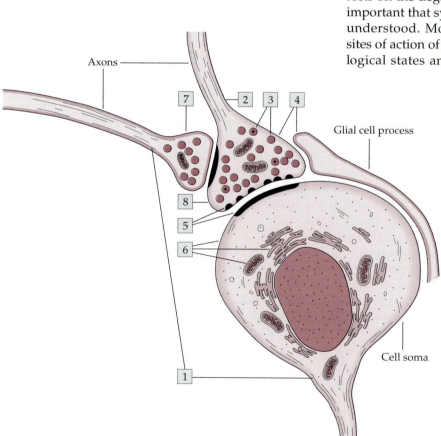

Axons

Glial cell process

Cell soma

6.2 DRUG-SENSITIVE SITES involved in synaptic transmission. A schematic view of some drug-sensitive sites in a variety of synapses. (All structures are greatly oversized.) In the center, a postsynaptic neuron receives upon its soma a presynaptic axon terminal. The presynaptic terminal is also in contact with an axoaxonic terminal (7). Drug-sensitive sites include: (1) microtubules responsible for anterograde and retrograde transport of macromolecules between the neuronal soma (cell body) and distal processes; (2) excitable membranes; (3) sites for the synthesis and storage of neurotransmitters; (4) sites for the active uptake of some transmitters into nerve terminals or glia; (5) sites for the release of transmitters and sites (receptors) that generate responses; (6) cytoplasmic organelles and postsynaptic membranes for maintenance of synaptic activity and for long-term mediation of altered physiological states; and (7) presynaptic receptors on adjacent presynaptic processes and (8) on nerve terminals (autoreceptors). (After Bloom, 1985a.)

traced to abnormal synaptic function. For example, the psychopathology of schizophrenia has been related to excessive activity of dopaminergic synapses in one part of the brain known as the nucleus accumbens. Whether this excessive activity is a primary or an ancillary cause of schizophrenia is not known, but it is significant that dopamine receptor blocking drugs relieve the symptoms of this disease (Snyder, Creese, and Burt, 1977; see Chapter 18). Also, the neurological symptoms of Parkinson's disease are related to deficits of dopamine synaptic activity in a different part of the brain known as the striatum, and drugs that increase dopaminergic activity in the striatum relieve these symptoms (see Chapter 20). Further, abnormal degeneration of neuromuscular junctions accounts for the extreme muscle weakness of a form of myasthenia gravis (Drachman, 1987), and certain drugs that potentiate the action of ACh, the neurotransmitter at these junctions, aid in the diagnosis and treatment of this illness. Thus, the development of synaptology has been beneficial in the treatment of some diseases that were formerly beyond any treatment. Further, the capacity for experimental control of neural function with psychotropic drugs has advanced our understanding of neural functions in highly significant ways.

Morphology of Synapses

The word "synapse" was coined in 1897 by Sir Charles Sherrington, a British neurophysiologist. He derived it from the Greek word *synapto*, which means "to clasp." Sherrington's research was limited by the relatively low resolution of the light microscope, but he was able to observe the bulbous expansions at the axon terminals that had been first described by Held in the same year. He later attributed the particular features of the reflex arc to the special structure of the opposing membranes of two neurons in close juxtaposition. There was a need to answer two questions: (1) why do nerve impulses pass in only one direction, from the sensory to the motor neurons, but not vice versa; and (2) why is there a 1–3 ms delay when a nerve impulse traverses a synapse—a distance of only about 20 nm, which would require only a tiny fraction of the delay if there were direct electrical coupling between the sensory and motor neurons? (Eccles, 1964b). An understanding of these phenomena developed slowly until the 1950s, when significant improvements in biotechnology allowed access to the molecular structure and function of the organelles in nerve cells and the recording of brain processes with noninvasive techniques.

Synaptic Ultrastructure

Most neuro-neuronal synaptic junctions in vertebrate brains consist of presynaptic elements known as **axon terminals** (bulbs, knobs, boutons) and postsynaptic receptor areas, which can be on the surfaces of dendritic spines, as shown in Figure 6.3, or on receptor sites on the somata of postsynaptic cells. An axon terminal can be as large as 5 μm, but most are between 1 and 2 μm in diameter and are surrounded by a thin membrane. A large number of mitochondria are usually seen within the cytoplasm, indicating a high level of metabolic activity.

Where the presynaptic and postsynaptic membranes come into apposition, there is a dark filamentous or granular material adhering to the presynaptic membrane and extending back into the adjacent cytoplasm, against which vesicles appear to congregate. Sometimes postsynaptic membranes also seem to be thickened with an electron-dense substance adhering to them (**postsynaptic density**). These dark materials may be limited to small areas with spaces in between, or may be continuous along the entire length of the junction.

Synaptic vesicles. The synaptic terminal contains large numbers of small, spherical saclike objects. These structures, which are called **synaptic vesicles**, are concentrated in the area where the presynaptic and postsynaptic membranes are separated only by the synaptic cleft. Descriptions of synaptic vesicles first appeared in the 1950s in the work of several laboratories (see below). In 1962, research by De Robertis and colleagues showed that the synaptosomal fraction of neural tissue containing the vesicles had the highest concentration of transmitter substance—in their case, ACh. Because vesicles are fre-

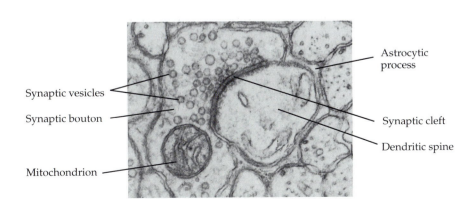

Synaptic vesicles

Synaptic bouton

Mitochondrion

Astrocytic process

Synaptic cleft

Dendritic spine

6.3 AN AXODENDRITIC SYNAPSE. A dendritic spine from a Purkinje cell in the rhesus monkey cerebellum is capped by an axon terminal showing typical features: numerous vesicles and a mitochondrion. Note the postsynaptic density underlying the postsynaptic membrane. (From Peters, Palay, and Webster, 1991.)

(a)   Spherical agranular vesicles   Spherical granular vesicles

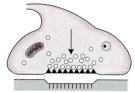 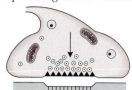

Flattened vesicles

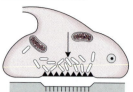

6.4 VESICLE VARIETIES. *(a)* A schematic representation of three main types of synaptic vesicles. *(b)* A reciprocal junction, with vesicles present on both sides of the synaptic cleft. (After Bodian, 1962.)

(b)   Reciprocal junction

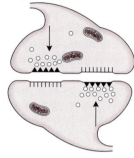

quently found in secretory cells, this finding ultimately led to the conclusion that all transmitters might be sequestered within vesicles.

Evidence suggests that vesicles, at least in part, are formed in the perikaryon by the Golgi apparatus and rapidly transported (200–400 mm/day) along microtubules to the axon terminals (see Chapter 3). There is also evidence that new vesicles are formed by a process of endocytosis, whereby pieces of vesicular membranes that are attached to the presynaptic membrane are detached and recycled into newly filled vesicles—all of this taking place within the cytoplasm of the axon terminal (see below).

Vesicles exist in a variety of appearances and sizes. Most common are small vesicles (40–60 nm in diameter) that are clear, or agranular, under the electron microscope (Figure 6.4*a*). In some cells (e.g., ganglionic neurons of the parasympathetic nervous system), these vesicles contain ACh. Clear vesicles of this size in other neurons may contain amino acids that also serve as neurotransmitters (e.g., glutamate or γ-aminobutyric acid, GABA). A second type of vesicle of small to medium size (80–100 nm) is referred to as granular because of an electron-dense core that is seen under the electron microscope. These granular vesicles are associated with catecholamines and serotonin, which are neurotransmitters known as biogenic amines. Large granular vesicles (100–160 nm) contain peptides, a more recently identified class of neurotransmitters. Because granular and agranular vesicles sometimes appear in the same axon terminal, there may be more than one transmitter in a terminal (one so-called "classical" neurotransmitter and one or more neuroactive peptides), or the different vesicle types may represent stages in neurotransmitter synthesis (Marshall, 1974; also see Chapter 11).

Vesicles are enclosed by a thin (8 nm) membrane that differs in its protein and lipid constituents from the plasma membrane. Calcium (Ca^{2+}) ions are necessary for the release of neurotransmitters from vesicles, as evidenced by the finding of Ca^{2+} binding sites on vesicle membranes and by many physiological experiments that have shown that synaptic transmission cannot occur in the absence of Ca^{2+} (see below).

The presence of synaptic vesicles on only one side of the synaptic cleft has become for all practical purposes an identifying marker for presynaptic elements. However, **reciprocal junctions** have been described in which vesicles are found on both sides of the synaptic cleft, clustered at one edge of the synapse on one side of the cleft and at the other edge on the other side (Figure 6.4*b*). In this arrangement, synaptic action could go in either direction; in some instances, the action may be excitatory in one direction and inhibitory in the opposite direction (Mountcastle and Baldessarini, 1974).

Synaptic release sites.   With the aid of a method called the freeze-fracture technique, which we will describe later on, Akert, Peper, and Sandri (1975) observed some ultrastructural features that they incorporated into a model of the neuro-neuronal synapse (Figure 6.5). The axon terminal has a presynaptic membrane with dense structures reaching into the cytoplasm, a feature of synaptic membranes that was described earlier. These areas of the terminal, which contain the sites of vesicle attachment and transmitter release, are known as **active zones**. Synaptic vesicles form a hexagonal array around the dense projections. The dense structures seem to have pits (**synaptopores**, more recently called **fusion pores**) through which the vesicles may discharge their contents into the synaptic cleft. The postsynaptic membrane beneath the synaptic knob appears to be encrusted with fine particles, which may be the postsynaptic receptor sites or other membrane proteins. Also shown is the subsynaptic web that De Robertis (1967) described. However, it is not seen in some preparations and may be an artifact of the drying process for electron micrography.

The synaptic cleft.   The synaptic cleft lies between the presynaptic axon terminal and the postsynaptic membrane and has a width ranging from 10 to 50 nm depending upon the material studied. The width of the cleft for mammalian motor neurons in the spinal cord

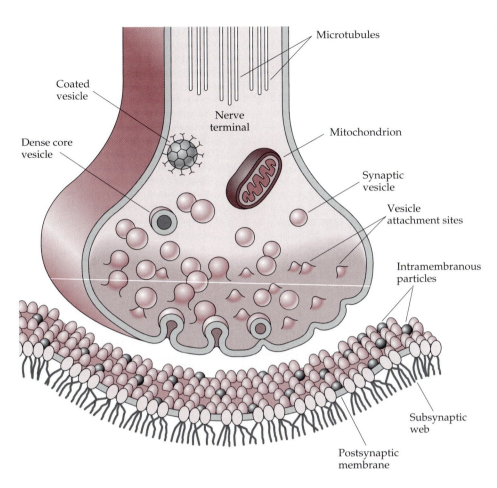

Coated vesicle

Microtubules

Nerve terminal

Dense core vesicle

Mitochondrion

Synaptic vesicle

Vesicle attachment sites

Intramembranous particles

Subsynaptic web

Postsynaptic membrane

6.5 A NEURO-NEURONAL SYNAPSE. This model was constructed after an examination of the internal and the external aspects of a synapse in the CNS. Vesicles surround dense structures (not shown), and discharge their contents through the pits of the vesicle attachment sites. The particle aggregation on the postsynaptic membrane may be postsynaptic receptor sites. The connection between the subsynaptic web and the particles is hypothetical. (After Akert, Peper, and Sandri, 1975.)

ranges from 20 to 30 nm. The cleft is continuous with the extracellular fluid, which serves as a low-resistance conduit for shunting stray ionic currents away from the postsynaptic surface. The cleft has sometimes been characterized as having intersynaptic filaments that serve to attach the pre- and postsynaptic membranes and perhaps to guide transmitter molecules to their receptor sites (De Robertis, 1967). Using immunocytochemical techniques, many workers have observed that the synaptic cleft contains a material of intermediate density sometimes referred to as **synaptic gap substance** (Pappas, 1975). This material is made up of many different proteins and sugars in the form of mucopolysaccharides and glycoproteins. It has been suggested that this material may bind the membranes together and impede the diffusion of transmitter molecules away from the synaptic cleft. This suggestion seems reasonable because mucopolysaccharides are known to form chemical bonds with water to produce mucilaginous and lubricating fluids such as those found in mucous secretions and in intercellular spaces.

A number of different glycoproteins (proteins with carbohydrate attachments) are also found on synaptic membranes. Associated with these proteins are enzymes such as glycosyl transferases, which can rapidly modify the structure of these proteins, and exoglycosidases,

which can degrade them. Furthermore, glycoproteins on membranes are known to be **autoimmunologically active**, meaning that they can cause antibody production. The glycoproteins serve as an antigen and trigger antibody production in other cells. These autoantibodies interact with the antigen to form autoimmune complexes that result in adhesions between cells. Therefore, within the CNS, glycoproteins may play a role in intercellular recognition during synaptogenesis—that is, when the developing CNS is forming genetically determined synaptic connections (Roseman, 1974; Quarles, 1975). The role of glycoproteins in synaptic function is the object of continuing studies (see Jessell, 1991).

Synaptosomes. Synapses can also be studied biochemically by means of isolated pinched-off nerve endings called **synaptosomes**. These structures can be prepared by a process of subcellular fractionation. The simplest type of subcellular fractionation involves suspending a small amount of ground-up neural tissue in a liquid medium in a small test tube. The homogenate is then centrifuged (spun around) at increasing speeds to create strong centrifugal forces on the contents of the tube. At lower speeds, only the heaviest particles are forced to the bottom of the tube, where they form a pellet consisting of membrane fragments and cell nuclei. The liquid above

Rat cerebral cortex homogenized and centrifuged

Sucrose gradient

Low-density sediment

Intermediate-density sediment

High-density sediment

Myelin sheath fragments

Synaptosomes

Mitochondria

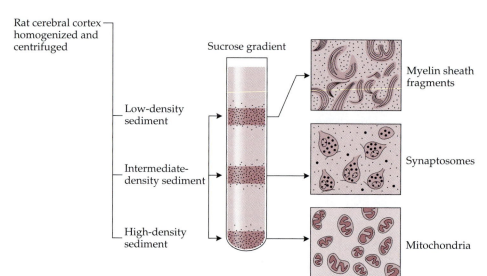

6.6 SUBCELLULAR FRACTIONATION OF BRAIN TISSUE USING SUCROSE GRADIENTS. After the tissue is homogenized, it is centrifuged at an intermediate speed. The sediment separated from the cytoplasm is then placed in a tube containing layered sucrose solutions of increasing density (density increases from the top to the bottom of the tube). After high-speed centrifugation, the lightest subfraction, containing myelin sheath fragments, remains near the top, a heavier subfraction containing synaptosomes and vesicles is found near the middle, and the heaviest particles (the mitochondria) are found at the bottom.

the pellet (called the supernatant) is then drawn off, placed in another tube, and spun at a higher speed. This sediments some of the lighter elements into a pellet containing mitochondria, synaptosomes, and pieces of the endoplasmic reticulum. Again, the fluid above the pellet is drawn off and spun at even higher speeds, and so on, step by step, until the fluid is completely cleared of any cell fragments and organelles. At this point, the supernatant contains small molecules and soluble proteins from the tissue and is called **cytosol**. This process of subcellular fractionation thus separates and partially purifies all the cell parts.

One disadvantage of the above procedure is that the synaptosomes obtained are contaminated with mitochondria and other subcellular elements. To obtain a higher-purity synaptosomal fraction, one can use a variation of the fractionation technique involving sucrose gradients. Basically, a tube is filled with layers of sucrose solutions of varying concentration and density, with the densest layer on the bottom and the least dense on the top. Even when spun at high speeds, the separation of the sucrose layers remains largely intact. When the pellet from a preliminary, intermediate-speed spin is placed on the top layer and centrifuged for 20 minutes at increasing speeds to create centrifugal forces up to $100,000 \times g$,* the cell particles are forced down through the sucrose levels until the density of the particle matches that of the sucrose solution (Figure 6.6). Among the tissue fragments found in sucrose layers of intermediate density are the synaptosomes. When these particles are examined under the electron microscope, they are found to consist of torn-off axon terminals that are often attached to portions of the postsynaptic membrane (i.e., to parts of the dendritic spines). When the axonal stumps of the synaptosomes are separated from the axons, they are sealed off by the natural adhesive action of the lipid bilayers, thereby keeping the synaptosomal contents intact. The synaptosomes may be drawn off and lysed (broken up) so that their contents can be examined. Lysis is usually carried out by osmotic shock, after which the lysed material is suspended and centrifuged again to separate the synaptosomal contents (e.g., the vesicles, synaptic membranes, and unspecified microsomes). The constituents of synaptosomes are verified by electron microscopy and by the use of various biochemical analytic techniques. Alternatively, the synaptosomes may be used in their intact state to study processes such as neurotransmitter synthesis, release, and reuptake.

Quantitative Considerations

Synaptic junctions usually occur on the dendrites and somata of neurons. However, somata and glial cell bodies make up only about 5% of the gray matter of the CNS; the rest consists of neuronal axons, dendrites, and associated blood capillaries. Consequently, effective neural control of the organism is managed at synapses that constitute a small proportion of the bulk of the CNS.

The number of synaptic terminals terminating on a single receptive cell varies enormously, depending upon cellular features such as size, extent of the dendritic tree, and function. In the case of sensory bipolar neurons (such as those in the retina), a single axon of a bipolar cell may provide the only input to the next cell (the ganglion cell). On the other hand, a single motor neuron in the spinal cord may receive as many as 16,000 synaptic terminals (boutons). Figure 6.7 is a drawing made from a series of micrographs of a motor neuron showing the soma completely covered by axon terminals from a variety of sources. Judging by size alone, there seem to be at

---

*In this context, "g" refers to an acceleration equivalent to that produced by the Earth's gravitational force.

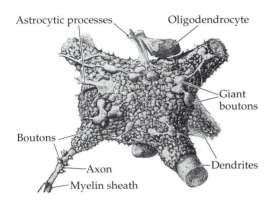

Astrocytic processes   Oligodendrocyte

Giant boutons

Boutons

Axon

Myelin sheath

Dendrites

6.7 SYNAPSES ON THE SURFACE OF A MOTOR NEURON. This figure is a reconstruction based upon serial sections seen in electron micrographs. Note that the surface of the cell and dendrites are completely covered with synaptic boutons of different sizes. (From Poritsky, 1969.)

least five distinct types of terminals, possibly representing terminals that are excitatory or inhibitory, terminals from recurrent collaterals, terminals having one type of transmitter or another, and so on. Presumably, each type comes from a different system having a specific function, such as maintaining muscle tone, exerting postural control, enabling reflexes in response to pain, facilitating excitatory and inhibitory influences upon intersegmental, crossed, and reciprocal reflexes for locomotion, modulations by the cerebellum and the corpus striatum, and cortical influence for fine skilled movements. It has been estimated that 20,000 terminals can influence a single pyramidal cell. Pyramidal cells provide the major output from the cerebral cortex and influence fine motor activity during skilled movements. There are also an estimated 200,000 synapses on the dendritic tree of each Purkinje cell of the human cerebellar cortex; these cells modulate muscle tone and coordinate the somatic musculature. Thus, there is extreme variety and complexity in the input and output to these systems and the interactions within them.

Qualitative Considerations

Electron microscopic studies of synaptic junctions have revealed a wide variety of forms. An extensive description of even a small number of these would be beyond the scope of this book. A few examples of types of synapses are presented here to illustrate their variety and to demonstrate the possible structural and functional relationships. Within the CNS there are generally three types of synaptic linkages: axon terminals that join dendritic trunks or spines (**axodendritic**), those that join the cytoplasmic membranes of cell bodies (**axosomatic**), and those that join other axon terminals (**axoaxonic**) (Figure 6.8). More recently, synapses have been found between adjacent dendrites, obviously referred to as **dendrodendritic**, and rare forms such as **somatosomatic**,

somatodendritic, **dendrosomatic**, and **dendroaxonic** have been found in vertebrate brains.

In addition to these organizational features of synapses, other details have been described. Early studies by Gray (1959) showed synapses that differed in the widths and lengths of their synaptic clefts, as well as in membrane thickenings (whether they were uniform or broken up, or whether the thickenings were on the pre- or postsynaptic membrane or both; and, if the thickenings were on both sides, whether they were the same or different). Also, there seemed to be differences in synaptic vesicles—there were spherical, flat, and elliptical ones, but the shapes seemed to depend upon the substances used to prepare them for microscopic viewing. Nevertheless, attempts were made to ascribe functional differences related to vesicle shape; for example, it was proposed that spherical vesicles were excitatory whereas flattened one were inhibitory (McGeer, Hattori, and McGeer, 1975). However, spherical and flattened vesicles have been found together in the same terminal, and synaptic excitability probably has less to do with vesicle shape than with the nature of the transmitter and the postsynaptic receptors.

One thing is certain, however: It is probably rare that a single synapse operates in isolation in the brain. Rather, one synapse usually operates within a large pattern of interconnecting synapses. This is graphically illustrated in Figure 6.9, a reconstruction of an electron microscopic view of synapses around a dendrite in the pulvinar of a monkey. The pulvinar is a nucleus in the posterior thalamus that receives auditory, visual, and somesthetic inputs from other parts of the thalamus. The pulvinar projects its axons to the posterior parietal and temporal lobes of the brain and to **extrastriate cortex** (areas surrounding the striate or optic cortex). Thus, this structure seems to integrate auditory, visual, and somesthetic impulses for projection to the association areas of the brain, where meaningfulness of stimuli is perceived. A person with a lesion in the extrastriate cortex that disconnects the visual cortex from the association areas of the brain may be shown a key and, though he sees it, cannot name it or say what it is used for. He may ask if it is a toy, something to eat, or something to wear, and he may be surprised to be told that it is used to open a door. However, if it is placed in his hand, he may readily identify it. Thus, in this case, the visual concept of the object was poorly associated with its use, but the tactile associations were intact. It is also interesting to note that *d*-lysergic acid diethylamide (LSD-25) binds to receptors mediating visual impulses in the thalamus, which may have a bearing on the bizarre visual perceptions that follow ingestion of this substance. These examples illustrate the morphological complexity that underlies behavior. This morphological complexity is probably the rule rather than the exception in vertebrate brains, and it points to the enormous task of describing the neural

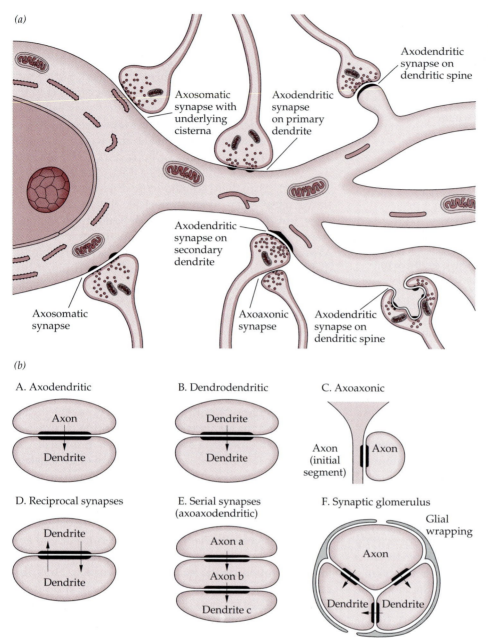

(a)

Axosomatic synapse with underlying cisterna

Axodendritic synapse on primary dendrite

Axodendritic synapse on dendritic spine

Axodendritic synapse on secondary dendrite

Axosomatic synapse

Axoaxonic synapse

Axodendritic synapse on dendritic spine

(b)

A. Axodendritic

Axon

Dendrite

B. Dendrodendritic

Dendrite

Dendrite

C. Axoaxonic

Axon (initial segment)

Axon

D. Reciprocal synapses

Dendrite

Dendrite

E. Serial synapses (axoaxodendritic)

Axon a

Axon b

Dendrite c

F. Synaptic glomerulus

Glial wrapping

Axon

Dendrite   Dendrite

6.8 VARIETIES OF SYNAPSES made by axon terminals on the various parts of neurons. (*b*) A schematic rendering of synapse varieties, including some not shown in *a*. (*a* after Fawcett, 1986; *b* after Shepherd, 1988.)

substrates of even the simplest of behavioral events. Yet it is still possible, as we shall see, to find or make chemical entities (drugs) that are reasonably specific in their behavioral effects.

Axoaxonic Synapses and Presynaptic Inhibition

One type of axoaxonic synaptic junction deserves special mention. As illustrated in Figure 6.10, an inhibitory axon terminal (I) forms a synaptic junction upon an excitatory axon terminal (E). The E-terminal is from a primary sensory neuron, and it normally produces EPSPs on the postsynaptic membrane of a secondary neuron in the spinal cord. Secondary neurons send their messages to motor neurons of the spinal cord for reflex responses, or to higher centers in the brain stem or forebrain for sen-

sory awareness and for fine motor control. From these higher centers, modulating neurons send axons down to the spinal cord, where they form axoaxonic synapses with E-terminals as shown. The effect of transmission at these synapses is to inhibit transmitter release from the E-terminals. This phenomenon is called **presynaptic inhibition** because the modulating effect is exerted upon the presynaptic rather than the postsynaptic membrane.

Presynaptic inhibition can occur through at least two different mechanisms. One well-known mechanism involves the release of GABA from the I-terminal onto the E-terminal, which produces increased activity of chloride (Cl^-) channels in the E-terminal. Increased Cl^- conductance in this particular system slightly depolarizes the membrane by about 10 mV (from a resting potential of −

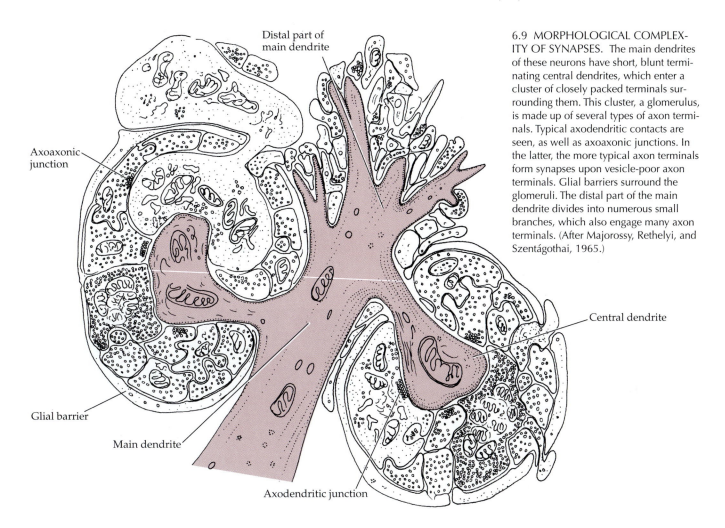

Distal part of
main dendrite

Axoaxonic
junction

Glial barrier

Main dendrite

Axodendritic junction

Central dendrite

6.9 MORPHOLOGICAL COMPLEX-
ITY OF SYNAPSES. The main dendrites
of these neurons have short, blunt terminating central dendrites, which enter a
cluster of closely packed terminals surrounding them. This cluster, a glomerulus,
is made up of several types of axon terminals. Typical axodendritic contacts are
seen, as well as axoaxonic junctions. In
the latter, the more typical axon terminals
form synapses upon vesicle-poor axon
terminals. Glial barriers surround the
glomeruli. The distal part of the main
dendrite divides into numerous small
branches, which also engage many axon
terminals. (After Majorossy, Rethelyi, and
Szentágothai, 1965.)

70 mV to a new potential of –60 mV). This depolarization is called a **conditioning stimulus**. If an action potential arrives at the E-terminal shortly after the conditioning stimulus, the magnitude of the action potential is diminished because it starts from a lower resting potential; therefore the amplitude range of the action potential is from –60 to +45 mV rather than from –70 to +45 mV. This causes a smaller output of neurotransmitter from the E-terminal and a smaller effect (i.e., a smaller EPSP) on the postsynaptic neuron. An alternative mechanism involves a GABA-mediated enhancement of the potassium (K$^+$) channels that terminate the action potential. Decreased

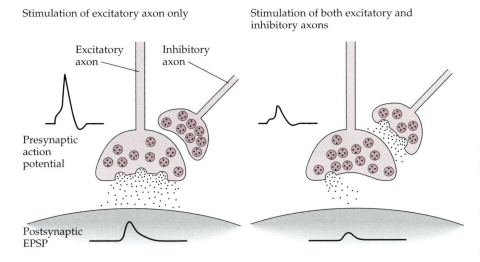

Stimulation of excitatory axon only

Stimulation of both excitatory and
inhibitory axons

Excitatory
axon

Inhibitory
axon

Presynaptic
action
potential

Postsynaptic
EPSP

6.10 PRESYNAPTIC INHIBITION. The
presynaptic terminal of the excitatory axon is
from a spinal sensory neuron. The descending
inhibitory axon originates in higher centers:
the brain stem or the cerebrum. The inhibitory
terminal modulates the presynaptic output of
the excitatory terminal by slightly depolarizing
it. This process is thus known as presynaptic
inhibition. (After Hall, 1992.)

action potential duration decreases transmitter release by reducing the influx of Ca^{2+} into the terminal.

Should a number of axoaxonic endings be activated on primary sensory terminals, there can be a significant decrease in the number of action potentials generated by secondary neurons, thereby reducing the effect of sensory stimuli on the nervous system. Muscle relaxant drugs such as diazepam (Valium) provide relief from muscle spasms by enhancing this mechanism. At higher doses, however, diazepam may also cause incoordination.

Neuroeffector Junctions

Neuroeffector junctions are somewhat different from synapses because here neurons have direct effects upon muscles and glands, with behavior as the end result. Before the neural message is sent to a neuroeffector junction, the force of the response has been predetermined by the activity of the circuits and systems at "higher" levels, and it is expressed in terms of the frequency of nerve impulses directed at appropriate effectors. Within the body this determines the force and frequency of the heartbeat or the release of epinephrine (adrenaline) from the adrenal gland, or in the case of the peripheral effectors, the speed of locomotion or the degree of perspiring. Once the neural message is delivered, the only modification that can occur depends on the state of the effector organ—whether or not the muscle is fatigued or the glandular products are depleted. (It should be mentioned, however, that there are such things as local reflexes that probably occur without the intervention of the CNS. For example, applying heat or an irritant to the skin leads to dilatation of blood vessels and a reddening of the skin, and stretching of the intestine can cause a local reflex contraction of the intestinal muscles (i.e., cramps.)

Autonomic neuroeffectors.

Autonomic neuroeffectors.   As previously discussed in Chapter 4, one type of neuroeffector junction is found at the terminals of the autonomic nerves, which activate smooth muscles and glands such as the muscles of the gastrointestinal tract, the smooth muscles of the iris for pupil dilation and constriction, and salivary and tear glands. The axons of these nerves divide into as many as a few thousand fine branches along which numerous swellings, or varicosities, are serially arranged and separated by short lengths (2–3 μm) of the axon. The varicosities contain neurotransmitters—usually acetylcholine (ACh) in parasympathetic fibers and norepinephrine (NE) in sympathetic fibers.

Fluorescent micrographs of the sympathetic innervation of mesenteric veins from the intestines of a sheep show typical smooth muscle innervation (Figure 6.11). The finely branched axons lie along the smooth muscle membrane, sometimes within depressions or furrows on the surface of the muscle cell. The varicosities form synapses *en passage* at many points along the axon, releas-

ing their neurotransmitter to initiate widespread control of the blood circulation in the intestines (Marshall, 1974). This type of synaptic arrangement is also found in the CNS. It has been estimated that one cell body may give rise to 500,000 terminals of this type, thereby influencing activity in widespread areas of the brain.

Neuromuscular junctions.   Different features can be noted at neuromuscular junctions (i.e., the connections between axon terminals and striated muscle fibers). Figure 6.12 is a three-dimensional drawing of a motor neuron axon terminal, known as a motor end plate, lying next to the muscle membrane within an invagination known as the **synaptic trough**. The floor of the trough is further invaginated by a series of **subneural clefts** or

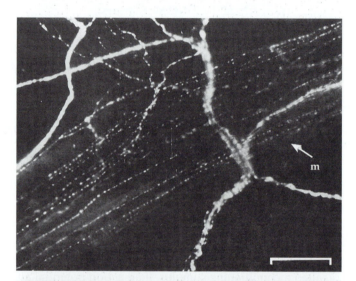

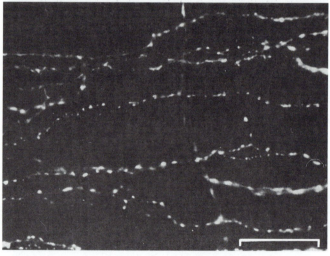

6.11 SYNAPSES "EN PASSAGE." Norepinephrine-containing nerve fibers visualized by formaldehyde-induced histofluorescence are shown innervating smooth muscle (m) in the lung of a lizard (*top*) and in the sheep mesenteric vein (*bottom*). The fibers contain beadlike swellings or varicosities that form synaptic junctions with thousands of smooth muscle cells. Bars = 100 μm (*top*) and 50 μm (*bottom*). (From Burnstock, 1970.)

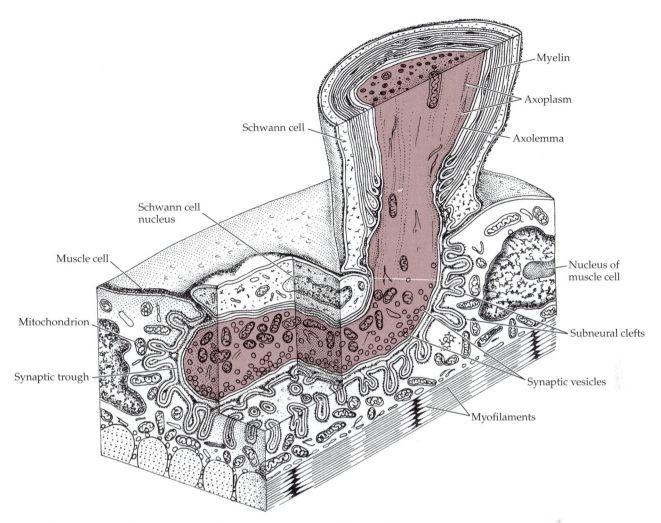

Myelin

Axoplasm

Axolemma

Schwann cell

Schwann cell nucleus

Muscle cell

Mitochondrion

Synaptic trough

Nucleus of muscle cell

Subneural clefts

Synaptic vesicles

Myofilaments

6.12 A NEUROMUSCULAR JUNCTION. Neuro-neuronal synapses have much in common with neuromuscular junctions, but neuronal postsynaptic membranes have no basal lamina or subneural clefts. (After Fawcett, 1986.)

junctional folds, which substantially increase the synaptic surface and widen its exposure to the transmitter, thereby increasing the efficiency of the transmission process. It is estimated that each presynaptic vesicle contains up to 10,000 ACh molecules, and that within one neuromuscular junction in the human deltoid muscle there are 2.1×10^7 synaptic sites (Drachman, 1987).

Figure 6.13 shows a three-dimensional model of a highly magnified neuromuscular junction of a frog. The model was constructed after analysis of electron micrographs of material prepared by the **freeze-fracture technique**. In this method tissue is rapidly frozen in liquid nitrogen and cracked in a vacuum using a blade cooled to −196°C. The fractures frequently follow a path of least resistance, which in membranes is between the two hydrophobic regions of the lipid bilayer (Akert et al., 1969). Thus, the fractures occur within the bilayers of the membranes themselves rather than between the pre- and postsynaptic membranes. The tissue is then prepared for examination with an electron microscope. This method gives a view into the interior of a membrane and reveals many synaptic features (Nicholls, Martin, and Wallace, 1992). On the cytoplasmic side of the presynaptic membrane, the vesicles are lined up along both sides of transverse bars of electron-dense material. This material may serve as recognition sites for vesicle binding (Heuser and Reese, 1977) and makes up the active zones where neurotransmitters are released. There are about 50 closely apposed vesicles per terminal bar and about 500 such bars in each neuromuscular junction (Heuser, 1976). The vesicles are fused to the presynaptic membrane over synaptopores, through which the neurotransmitter may be released into the synaptic cleft. The inner leaflet of the presynaptic membrane contains particles that protrude into pits in the outer leaflet of the membrane that faces the synaptic cleft. These pits may be Ca^{2+} channels (Heuser, 1976).

The postsynaptic membrane includes junctional folds that are opposite the active zones of the presynaptic membrane. The neurotransmitter molecules diffuse

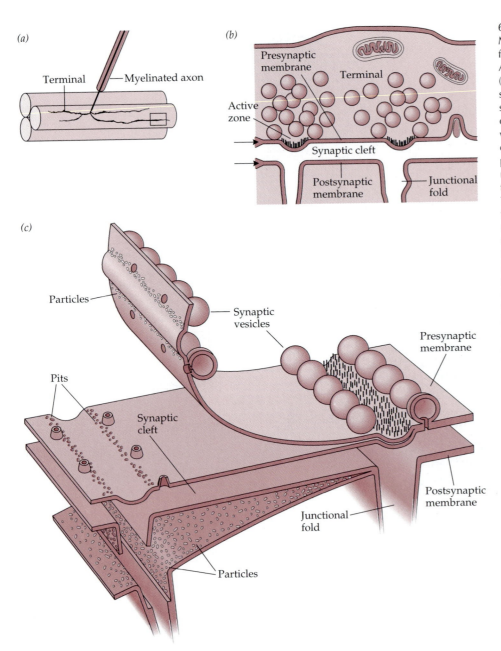

6.13 FEATURES OF THE NEURO-MUSCULAR JUNCTION revealed by freeze-fracture electron microscopy. (a) An entire frog neuromuscular junction. (b) A longitudinal section through the shaded portion of the nerve terminal shown in a. (c) Three-dimensional view of pre- and postsynaptic membranes with active zones and immediately adjacent rows of synaptic vesicles. The plasma membranes are split at the arrows shown in b to illustrate structures that can be seen after freeze-fracture. The cytoplasmic leaflet of the presynaptic membrane at the active zone shows on its fracture face protruding particles whose counterparts are seen as pits on the fracture face of the outer membrane leaflet. Vesicles that fuse with the presynaptic membrane give rise to characteristic protrusions and pores in the fracture faces. The fractured postsynaptic membrane in the region of the subneural clefts shows a high concentration of particles on the cytoplasmic leaflet. The particles are probably ACh receptors. (After Nicholls, Martin, and Wallace, 1992.)

into these invaginations, which enlarge the area of neurotransmitter contact. The particles seen between the layers of the postsynaptic membrane are thought to be related to membrane proteins, but their exact identity has not been determined (Robertson, 1975).

There are many drugs that can alter the activity of neuroeffector junctions, and their effects can be psychologically important. For example, epinephrine is sometimes injected to block the symptoms of an acute allergic reaction, but the patient may experience an increase in blood pressure and tachycardia (increased heart rate), a condition that could be extremely frightening to anyone treated with this drug. In this case, the fear is a secondary effect of the drug because epinephrine does not pass the blood–brain barrier. From a psychopharmacological view, neuroeffector drugs are important because some of these drugs also affect neurons in the CNS, and their mechanisms of action are the same in the CNS.

Gap Junctions

Gap junctions differ from regular synaptic junctions by the close apposition of their pre- and postsynaptic membranes: 2 nm, compared with 20 nm in regular synapses (Nicholls, Martin, and Wallace, 1992). More importantly, local potentials are conducted across these junctions without the benefit of chemical transmitters and with no appreciable synaptic delay. This is possible because the electrical resistance between the closely apposed membranes is significantly less than that between the membranes of an ordinary synapse, and there is virtually no loss of current into the extracellular space. Furshpan and Potter (1959) described the activity of electrical synapses

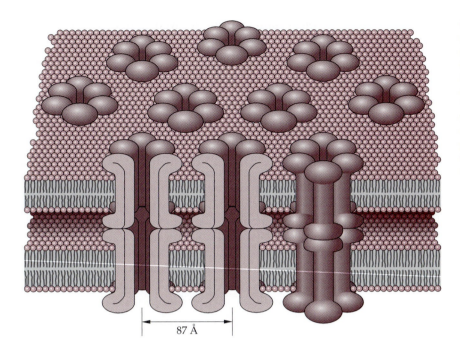

6.14 GAP JUNCTION CHANNELS. The channels shown here connect the lipid bilayers of two cells. The channel in each cell consists of six subunits of a protein called connexin that together form a connexon, which joins a similar unit of another cell, forming an aqueous pore connecting their cytoplasmic compartments. Presumably the pore may close by a twisting of one connexon that causes the six subunits to pinch together. This drawing was reconstructed from electron microscope and X-ray diffraction images. (After Hille, 1992.)

after studying those that mediate the rapid tail-flip movement that is a defensive swimming reflex in crayfish. The threshold for passage of local potentials across gap junctions is in the submillivolt range, as compared with a range of 20–100 mV in chemically mediated synapses.

Some gap junctions are polarized, thereby rectifying synaptic currents that then flow in one direction, whereas other junctions are not polarized, allowing current to flow in either direction. Gap junctions also exist between neurons and glia, with the latter serving as a buffer to take up neurotransmitters or their metabolites as well as surplus Na^+, K^+, or Ca^{2+} ions. This finding supports the idea that some gap junctions are characterized by connecting channels through which small molecules can pass (Figure 6.14). Further support comes from the finding that a fluorescent dye injected into one cell can spread to many other cells. This suggests that the free flow of some cytoplasmic molecules among a large assembly of cells may bring them all under similar influences (Loewenstein, 1981). Such channels are not always open. The flow through them may be dependent upon membrane potential differences, and they may close in response to other chemical factors. Also, gap junctions between dendrites permit a rapid transfer of excitation through a group of neurons, permitting them to respond in unison. Motor neurons controlling fine movements in some fishes are coupled electrically, as are the electric organs of *Torpedo californica*, an electric ray that stuns prey or intruders with electric shocks. Gap junctions are a common form of interneuronal connection in invertebrates and lower vertebrates, and they have been found at many sites in mammalian brains (see Kandel, Siegelbaum, and Schwartz, 1991). Electrical transmission over

gap junctions is not modified by drugs such as curare (a drug that blocks neuromuscular junctions) or neostigmine (a drug that intensifies the action of ACh). In some synapses, part of the interface between the pre- and postsynaptic membrane is made up of a chemical synapse, and another part has a gap junction. These synapses are known as **mixed junctions**. Gap junctions unquestionably play important roles in neural activity; however, their direct relevance to neuropharmacological effects is unknown.

Neurochemistry of Synaptic Transmission

In 1877, Du Bois-Reymond reported that transmission from one neuron to another could occur either chemically or electrically, and it is true that both mechanisms occur in nervous systems. However, much evidence clearly shows that the preponderance of synaptic action in warm-blooded animals is chemically mediated. The accumulation of this evidence was, perhaps first of all, dependent upon refinements in the design and construction of microelectrodes, electrical stimulators, amplifiers, and recording equipment such as the cathode ray oscilloscope (Minz, 1955).

When experimenters tried to determine whether synaptic stimulation was electrical or chemical, the following facts emerged.

1. After a presynaptic element was stimulated, there was a short delay (about 0.3 ms) before the postsynaptic element showed a response. This delay was too long to support the hypothesis that an electric pulse passed directly from one cell to the next.

2. When a postsynaptic element was stimulated, a response was not recorded in the presynaptic element. This finding indicated that the synapses were polarized; that is, that the signal passed only from the presynaptic to the postsynaptic membrane. It also suggested that some intervening mechanism existed between the cells that transmitted the pulse from one cell to the other.

3. Stimulation of the presynaptic element could result in an inhibitory influence on the postsynaptic element rather than an excitatory one. This would be difficult to explain in terms of a direct passage of the electrical event since nerve impulses are of only one kind and would not be likely to excite some neurons and inhibit others.

4. There was no relationship between the magnitude of the presynaptic electrical event and the postsynaptic one. That is, the presynaptic event might be either smaller or larger than the postsynaptic event. From an electrical standpoint, it would be easy to explain a slight decrement, but more difficult to explain an increment, in the absence of some intervening process.

All of the facts listed above are in complete harmony with the chemical hypothesis of synaptic transmission:

1. The synaptic delay of 0.3 ms has been calculated to be an appropriate length of time for the release and transport of a transmitter substance across a gap of 20 nm, the width of the synaptic space.

2. The fact that stimulation of the postsynaptic element does not produce a response in the presynaptic element is compatible with transmitter release occurring only at axon terminals.

3. Excitation and inhibition caused by identical nerve impulses are compatible with the idea that nerve impulses occurring in one axon terminal might cause a release of an inhibitory transmitter, whereas in a different terminal there might be a release of an excitatory transmitter. It is also true that the same transmitter may be excitatory on some cells and inhibitory on others due to differences in the receptors of the affected cells.

4. Finally, the fact that there is no correlation between the magnitude of the presynaptic and the postsynaptic electrical discharge speaks strongly for an intervening process whereby a small electrical signal may cause the release of enough chemical transmitter to produce a much larger electrical response in the postsynaptic cell. Also, a strong presynaptic response might result in a weak postsynaptic response if the release of the presynaptic transmitter were inhibited in some way, such as by presynaptic inhibition, or if the transmitter were somewhat depleted.

The Identification of Neurotransmitters

During the time when synaptic action was becoming better understood, attempts were also being made to identify the chemical substances that might be the transmitters. Early in the twentieth century, Elliott (1904, 1905) suggested that nerves of the sympathetic nervous system stimulate the heart and constrict blood vessels by liberating epinephrine on the effector organs. This conclusion was based on his own and earlier observations by Langley in 1901 that direct application of the hormone from the adrenal gland (epinephrine) to cardiovascular muscles had the same effect as direct stimulation of the nerves to those muscles (Langley, 1921).

In 1906, Dixon proposed that parasympathetic nerves released a substance that was equivalent to muscarine, a substance obtained from the mushroom *Amanita muscaria*, because muscarine caused the same effect as that obtained by stimulating parasympathetic nerves. For example, stimulating the vagus nerve led to stimulation of the gastrointestinal tract in the same way that muscarine does. In 1921 Otto Loewi performed a simple but effective experiment that demonstrated that a neurotransmitter is released from the vagus nerve when it is stimulated, and thus proved that Dixon was correct. There are a number of versions of how Loewi came to do his famous experiment, and one of them includes the following account. Loewi wanted to find out whether synapses were chemical or electrical. One night he had a dream of how to do an experiment, whereupon he got up and made some notes about it. However, in the morning, he could not decipher what he had written. The next night he had the dream again, and this time he took no chances—he got out of bed at 3:00 A.M. and hurried to the laboratory (Cotman and McGaugh, 1980; McLennan, 1970).

Loewi was aware that stimulation of the cardiac nerve (a branch of the vagus) arrested heart contractions and that these effects persisted for a short time after the electrical stimulation ceased. Loewi suspected that the explanation for this effect was that stimulating the nerve caused the release of some substance that continued to inhibit the force of the heartbeat. He now thought that if he electrically stimulated the cardiac nerve of a frog to arrest its heartbeat and at the same time dripped some Ringer's solution over the heart and collected it, he might be able to collect something that was released from the nerve endings. If he then dripped the collected solution over a second heart, it should respond in the same way as the first (Figure 6.15). It should be mentioned that a heart taken from a frog will continue to beat for a long time, at least long enough for an experiment like this to be done.

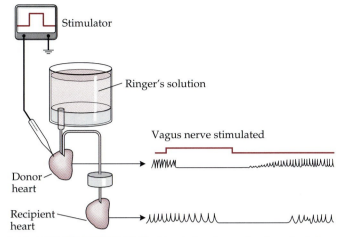

6.15 LOEWI'S EXPERIMENT. Stimulating the cardiac branch of the vagus nerve of a donor frog heart arrested the heartbeat. Ringer's solution perfusing the donor heart was transferred to the recipient heart. After 15 seconds, the beat in the second heart was also arrested.

As the figure shows, stimulating the vagus nerve innervating the first heart caused an arrest of the heartbeat in the first heart. When the Ringer's solution flowed from the first to the second heart, after a brief delay, the beat in the second heart was arrested. Thus, something in the perfusate caused the reaction in the second heart. In a way, Loewi was fortunate because it was unlikely that enough vagus secretion would have been released and captured to affect the second heart (Cotman and McGaugh, 1980). Later, in a similar experiment, the sympathetic accelerator nerve of the first heart was stimulated, producing a tachycardia (increased heart rate). During the heart perfusions, the second heart also showed a tachycardia. Thus, there was little doubt that stimulation of the nerves of the heart caused the release of an inhibitory or excitatory substance that could mimic the action of the nerves.

Loewi called the inhibitor material *"Vagusstoff,"* meaning substance or material from the vagus. He did not realize that this substance was actually ACh, even though this transmitter was first synthesized in 1867 and its biological action was known as far back as 1906. In 1914, Dale noted that applying ACh to the nerves mimicked the effects of stimulating the parasympathetic fibers. Many subsequent experiments revealed similarities between ACh and Vagusstoff, yet there was a reluctance to accept them as identical because it had not been shown that ACh was a constituent of the body. Finally, in 1929, ACh was isolated from spleen extracts, and the parallel action of both substances removed all doubt that Vagusstoff was ACh (see McLennan, 1970). Later it was established that ACh was also the transmitter substance that acted on glands and on smooth and striated muscles (Dale, Feldberg, and Vogt, 1936).

In the case of the excitatory transmitter, Loewi first referred to it as *"Acceleranzstoff,"* but later correctly identified the substance as epinephrine. It was not known until 25 years later that the epinephrine transmitter in a frog heart is unusual, NE being the transmitter in most other species (von Euler, 1971).

Neurotransmitters within the CNS. From the foregoing, we have seen that early knowledge of neurotransmitters came from experiments on synapses in the peripheral nervous system. Neurotransmitters were first identified at neuromuscular junctions such as those on the smooth muscles of the viscera, the cardiac muscles, and the striated skeletal muscles, and at synapses in the para- and prevertebral ganglia. Analysis at these structures was relatively easy because of their accessibility, and the transmitter was almost always ACh, although it was found many years later that neuroactive peptides were also present in these terminals (see Chapter 11). It is also quite clear that the transmitter at the terminals of sympathetic nerves is in almost all instances NE (see Chapter 8).

Within the CNS, however, a given cell may be acted upon by a wide variety of terminals having different transmitters. Electron micrographs show that a single motor neuron in a cat may have as many as 16,000 synaptic contacts. This makes identification of a particular transmitter acting on that cell rather difficult. Also, whereas samples of transmitter metabolites that can help to identify the transmitter can be easily collected in peripheral synapses, this becomes more difficult in the CNS. Furthermore, if the effectiveness of a suspected transmitter were tested by applying it directly to a brain site, the transmitter might have an indirect effect on the brain site by causing local vasoconstriction and ischemia (limited blood supply) and thereby altering the function at that site. In this case, one could be misled into thinking that the suspected transmitter influenced behavior by directly modifying brain function.

Criteria for neurotransmitters. For the above reasons, a set of criteria that must be met before a substance can be designated as a neurotransmitter has been proposed (Werman, 1966). However, in many instances, even if all the criteria cannot be met, there is enough evidence to support a transmitter role for a given substance. The proposed criteria are:

1. The presynaptic terminal should contain a store of the suspected transmitter substance, preferably in a bound or sequestered form. However, quantification of the store during a period of low impulse traffic should show an abundance of the substance, whereas during high impulse traffic there might be a severe depletion of the store.
2. The effects of application of a suspected transmitter substance to a synapse should mimic the effects caused by stimulation of the presynaptic terminal at that synapse. That is, a recording of the effects of iontophoretic applications of a suspected transmitter should compare favor-

ably with the effects obtained by electrically stimulating the presynaptic elements if the applied substance and the natural transmitter are the same.

3. Conversely, if a drug is known to block the action of a transmitter, it should have the same effect on the same transmitter from an exogenous source.

4. A mechanism must exist for the synthesis of the transmitter. Therefore, the precursors and the appropriate enzymes should be present in the presynaptic terminal.

5. A mechanism must exist for inactivating the transmitter, such as a catabolic enzyme to degrade the transmitter, or an active reuptake system in the presynaptic terminal or in adjacent glial elements.

With these criteria in mind, many transmitters have been identified with a fair degree of certainty. First, it should be noted that transmitters cannot always be classified as excitatory or inhibitory because the receptor often determines what the response will be, and whether it will be fast or slow, or of short or long duration. In addition, other compounds have been found that seem to influence synaptic events in perhaps less direct ways. These substances, called **neuromodulators**, may act in a hormonelike manner. They are not responsible for the direct transfer of nerve impulses from one neuron to another; rather, their release from neurons, glia, or other secretory cells may alter the action of neurotransmitters by enhancing, reducing, or prolonging their effectiveness. They may do this by influencing neurotransmitter synthesis, release, receptor interactions, reuptake, and metabolism (Zigmond, 1985). For example, glucocorticoids, which are secreted by the adrenal gland, and neuropeptides, which are released by neuroendocrine cells, influence the rate of synthesis of NE by controlling the activity of its synthesizing enzyme, tyrosine hydroxylase (see Chapter 8). Thus it can be seen how stress, leading to adrenal activity and thus to steroid and neuropeptide release, can increase the availability of NE, which is a crucial transmitter for sympathetic activity associated with emergency reactions.

Furthermore, the specificity of release of neurotransmitters is not as strict as was once thought. There is evidence that more than one transmitter and a large variety of peptides are not only released by the same axon terminal, but can even occupy the same vesicles (see Chapter 11). Table 6.1 lists the "classical" neurotransmitters, a number of important neuropeptides, and a variety of other neurotransmitter or neuromodulatory substances. Of these, subsequent chapters will focus mainly on ACh, NE, dopamine (DA), epinephrine, serotonin (5-HT), histamine, glutamate, aspartate, GABA, glycine, and a few of the neuropeptides.

What is perhaps most remarkable is that as varied as vertebrates and invertebrates are, virtually all of them share the same neurotransmitters in their nervous systems (Shepherd, 1988). The remarkable conservation of this chemical code for synaptic transmission, as well as the chemical code for genetic transmission, over millions of years of organic evolution illustrates the vigor of these codes and their effectiveness for the adaptation of most living species to their environment.

The Chemical Structure of Neurotransmitters

The chemical structure of all known and suspected neurotransmitters is well established. Except for the neuropeptides, most of them are small, water-soluble molecules containing amine and (in the case of amino acid transmitters) carboxyl groups. These chemical groups cause the transmitters to be ionized at physiological pH, which reduces their tendency to diffuse through the membranes that are responsible for the blood–brain barrier (see Chapter 1). Thus, central (within the CNS) and peripheral transmitter pools are generally independent of each other (see Scheller and Hall, 1992).

A considerable amount of research has been devoted to studying the origins and synthesis of synaptic transmitters. The importance of these findings is reflected in the fact that a number of the principal scientists involved became Nobel laureates in medicine. The significance of their work lay in their descriptions of the chemistry of brain function, which opened the possibility that brain function could be altered by pharmacological agents. Drugs then became tools for brain research. These new tools had the advantage of exerting mostly reversible effects in freely moving animals. In some cases, drug research complemented other forms of brain research, such as electrical stimulation of the brain via implanted electrodes, with effects from one method increasing the understanding of effects from the other. The consequence of this research was an ability to understand the mechanisms of action of newly discovered psychotropic agents and to design better ones for clinical chemopsychotherapy. These subjects will be elaborated upon in succeeding chapters.

The nonpeptide neurotransmitters are synthesized largely from dietary precursors such as choline, certain amino acids, glucose, and fatty acids. Most of these substances are able to enter the brain from the circulatory system by passing the blood–brain barrier. After these substances diffuse into neurons, some transmitter synthesis occurs in the perikarya, after which the transmitters are enclosed in vesicles for transport to the axon terminals. In this form the transmitters are shielded from metabolizing enzymes. Transmitter-synthesizing enzymes are actually concentrated most heavily in the nerve terminals. The highest rate of synthesis thus occurs within the terminals, accompanied by vesicle recycling and refilling. Some neurotransmitters require a number of synthesizing enzymes, whereas others, such

Table 6.1 Substances Found to Have Neurotransmitter or Neuromodulatory Properties

Phenethylamines and derivatives	**Neuropeptides**
Dopamine (DA)	Enkephalins
Norepinephrine (NE)	β-Endorphin
Epinephrine (EPI)	Dynorphin
Tyramine	Vasopressin
Octopamine	Oxytocin
Phenethylamine	Substance P
Phenylethanolamine	Cholecystokinin (CCK)
Dimethoxyphenylethylamine (DMPEA)	Neurotensin
	Vasoactive intestinal peptide (VIP)
Tetrahydroisoquinolines	Somatostatin
Indoleamines	Neuropeptide Y (NPY)
Serotonin (5-HT)	Galanin
Tryptamine	Angiotensin
Melatonin	Atrial natriuretic factor
Dimethyltryptamine (DMT)	Delta sleep factor
5-Methoxytryptamine	Thyrotropin-releasing hormone (TRH)
5-Methoxydimethyltryptamine (bufotenine)	Corticotropin-releasing factor (CRF)
	Gonadotropin-releasing hormone (GnRH)
Tryptolines	Adrenocorticotropic hormone (ACTH)
Cholinergics	Melanocyte-stimulating hormone (MSH)
Acetylcholine (ACh)	**Nonpeptide Hormones**
Choline	Estrogens
Amino acids, analogs, and nucleosides/nucleotides	Androgens
	Progestins
Glutamate	Corticosteroids
Aspartate	Thyroid hormones
Glycine	
γ-Aminobutyric acid (GABA)	
γ-Hydroxybutyrate (GHB)	
Histamine	
Taurine	
Adenosine	
Adenosine triphosphate (ATP)	

as some of the amino acid transmitters, are regular cellular constituents and require no further treatment. In contrast, neuropeptides are synthesized in the cell body as large protein precursors, after which the active peptide is liberated from its precursor. The details of synthesis for most of the better-known transmitters and peptides are discussed in succeeding chapters.

Neurotransmitter Release

The source of released neurotransmitter. Neurotransmitter molecules are released from nerve endings at a low level spontaneously (i.e., in the absence of neuronal activity) and at higher levels upon stimulation. Spontaneous release takes place continuously and emanates at least in part from the cytoplasmic compartment of the cell. Cytoplasmic release may occur as a result of trans-

mitter leakage across the cell membrane or, in some cases, as a function of reverse transport by membrane carrier proteins (Levi and Raiteri, 1993). Examples of carrier-mediated release are presented for catecholamines and 5-HT in Chapters 8 and 9.

Neural signaling generally does not make use of the continuous transmitter leakage described above, but rather, involves a process known as **quantal release**. This phenomenon was first demonstrated in the classic experiments by Fatt and Katz (1952) that demonstrated the existence of spontaneous synaptic events (i.e., miniature end-plate potentials) at the frog neuromuscular junction. The amplitude distribution of these potentials suggested that they corresponded to the release of preformed packets of neurotransmitter—in this case, ACh. Each packet of transmitter molecules came to be called a **quantum** (see Chapter 7 for more details). Moreover, stimulation

(a)   *(b)*

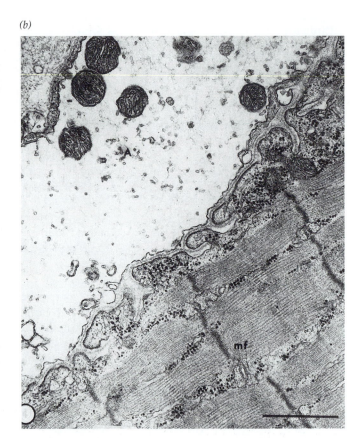

6.16 VESICLE DEPLETION from a frog neuromuscular junction. (*a*) Electron micrograph of a control preparation in Ringer's solution containing curare (30 µg/ml) to block muscle contraction. The motor nerve terminal contains many synaptic vesicles and mitochondria. Active zones (arrows) are seen as the electron-dense areas on the presynaptic membranes opposite the openings of the junctional folds. Glial cell processes are interposed between the terminal and the end-plate membrane (×34,000). (*b*) Electron micrograph of a preparation stimulated for 8 hours. Note that the axon ending appears swollen, and few vesicles are visible (×30,000). (From Ceccarelli, Hurlbut, and Mauro, 1972. Reproduced from *The Journal of Cell Biology*, 54:30–38, by copyright permission of The Rockefeller University Press.)

of the motor nerve caused a much greater release of neurotransmitter quanta than occurred spontaneously.

Just a few years after these observations, several research groups reported the first observations of neural tissue at the electron microscopic level. When nerve endings were visualized, they were found to contain large numbers of saclike objects that came to be called synaptic vesicles (De Robertis and Bennett, 1955; Palade, 1954; Palay, 1956). As the vesicles were large enough to hold the estimated number of transmitter molecules in a quantum (on the order of 1,000 to 10,000) and were obviously well positioned for transmitter storage and release, it was tempting to speculate that they were indeed the source of stimulus-induced quantal release.

The neuromuscular junction continued to be a favorite preparation for studying transmitter release, and a variety of biochemical experiments seemed to support the vesicular hypothesis. For example, when neuromuscular junctions were treated with the ACh-releasing toxin black widow spider venom (BWSV), the muscle initially responded violently to the venom, as it was suddenly ex-

posed to a tremendous amount of neurotransmitter. Within 10 to 15 minutes, however, the muscle became quiescent, presumably due to ACh depletion. Electron microscopic examination of the neuromuscular junctions at this time showed a corresponding depletion of vesicles, suggesting that release had occurred from the vesicular compartment (Clark, Hurlbut, and Mauro, 1972). Other preparations given intense, long-lasting electrical stimulation similarly exhibited a marked reduction in release along with a severe loss of synaptic vesicles (Figure 6.16; Ceccarelli, Hurlbut, and Mauro, 1972).

Although the above results were intriguing, they were obtained under nonphysiological conditions and were therefore subject to criticism. Furthermore, no one had yet achieved an actual visualization of vesicular release. This goal was accomplished just a few years later by Heuser and coworkers, again using the frog neuromuscular junction (Heuser, 1977). The investigators stimulated junctions in the presence of 4-aminopyridine, a drug that blocks K^+ channels, thus prolonging action potential duration and increasing transmitter release by almost a hundredfold. Following a single electrical stimulus, the tissue was slammed onto a copper block cooled to a temperature of 4°K (4 degrees above absolute zero!) by liquid helium. This procedure was shown to freeze the superficial (topmost) 15 μm of muscle within no more than 0.3 milliseconds. When preparations treated in this manner were sectioned for electron microscopic examination, they revealed striking images of vesicles that appeared to be caught in the act of fusing with the nerve terminal membrane and releasing their transmitter contents into the synaptic cleft (Figure 6.17). This process of fusion and release is called **exocytosis**.

Despite the attractiveness of the vesicular hypothesis, certain phenomena remain to be fully explained by this theory. These include fluctuations in quantal size, the mechanism of vesicle fusion, the fate of the vesicle membrane following release, and the rapidity of the release process (Oorschott and Jones, 1987; Vautrin, 1994). Some of these issues are discussed further below. It should be noted that alternatives to the vesicular hypothesis have been proposed and are still put forward by a few investigators. In particular, Dunant, Israël, and their collaborators have published a number of studies dealing with ACh release from the nerves innervating the electric organ of the electric fish *Torpedo* (reviewed by Dunant, 1986). Their experiments consistently found that stimulation of these nerve fibers led to a reduction in the ACh content of the cytoplasmic compartment (measured following subcellular fractionation of the tissue), whereas vesicular ACh generally remained stable. These results were interpreted to mean that stimulated or quantal release emanates from the nerve terminal cytoplasm rather than from the vesicles. A membrane protein named "mediatophore" was later isolated and proposed as the mediator of the cytoplasmic releasing mechanism (Dunant and Israël, 1993). As for the purpose of the synaptic vesicles, these researchers suggested that vesicular ACh serves as a reserve pool for replenishing the releasable cytoplasmic pool under conditions of prolonged activity. The vesicles were also hypothesized to take up Ca^{2+} from the nerve terminal cytoplasm following transmitter release (see below for a discussion of the role of Ca^{2+} in the release process) and secrete it from the nerve terminal by exocytosis (thus, the exocytotic profiles captured by Heuser and Reese were suggested to reflect Ca^{2+} rather than transmitter release).

Despite the questions raised above and the apparent contrary evidence obtained in some studies of *Torpedo*, few investigators seriously doubt the vesicular hypothesis of transmitter release. This is partly due to strong support gathered from two model systems not yet mentioned: the hypothalamic magnocellular neurosecretory system and the adrenal medullary chromaffin cells. The magnocellular system, which will be described in more detail in Chapter 11, comprises two clusters of neurons in the hypothalamus that send their axons to the posterior lobe of the pituitary gland. The cells synthesize two

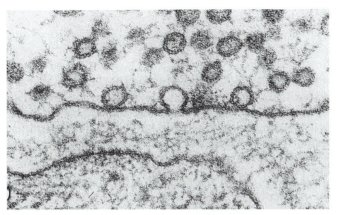

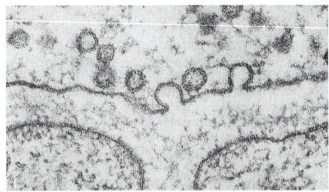

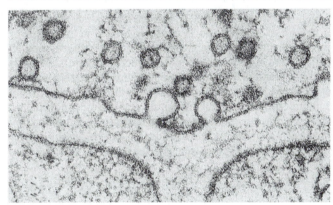

6.17 EXOCYTOSIS at the frog neuromuscular junction. Three electron micrographs of frog neuromuscular junctions are shown at high magnification (×145,000). A single electrical stimulus was applied to the motor nerve, after which the tissue was frozen extremely rapidly. The drug 4-aminopyridine was used to prolong action potential duration, thereby greatly increasing transmitter release from the terminals. In each micrograph, several vesicles are seen fused with the presynaptic membrane, presumably in the act of exocytosis. Such fusion events occurred only at the active zones opposite the junctional folds of the motor end plate. (From Heuser, 1977.)

peptide hormones, vasopressin (also known as antidiuretic hormone) and oxytocin, which are released into the circulation in response to appropriate physiological stimulation. These peptides, along with associated proteins called neurophysins, are found in storage granules (similar to vesicles but larger) in the axon terminals. When the vasopressin or oxytocin nerve cells are stimulated, peptide and neurophysin molecules are released from the nerve endings in the same proportion in which they are found in the storage granules (White et al., 1985). This fact, along with the fact that little, if any, peptide or neurophysin is even present outside of the granules, provides powerful evidence that release must be occurring from the vesicular compartment.

Adrenal medullary chromaffin cells are derived embryologically from neural tissue and possess many of the biochemical properties of catecholamine neurons. These cells synthesize epinephrine and NE, which are again stored inside large secretory granules. There are a number of other substances inside these granules, including the NE-synthesizing enzyme dopamine β-hydroxylase (DBH). Some of this DBH is free within the granule, while the remainder of the enzyme is bound to the inside of the granule membrane. When chromaffin cells are stimulated, the release of catecholamines is accompanied by a co-release of the unbound DBH within the granules. Furthermore, the DBH formerly bound to the inside of the granule membrane can then be seen on the outer surface of the chromaffin cells using immunohistochemical staining procedures (Dowd et al., 1983; Winkler, Sietzen, and Schober, 1987). These observations strongly suggest that the chromaffin granules must fuse with the cell membrane (i.e., undergo exocytosis) in order for catecholamine release to occur.

Because electron micrographs of synaptic junctions typically show large numbers of vesicles near active zones (which represent release sites), it is often assumed that each action potential causes the exocytosis of many vesicles. However, in at least some well-studied systems, a nerve impulse seems to stimulate release from no more than one vesicle in a given active zone (Korn et al., 1994). Furthermore, even this seemingly meager result is not invariable; that is, there is a significant possibility that *not even one* vesicle at the active zone will fuse with the membrane in response to any given stimulus. In circuits that exhibit this property, a possible mechanism of synapse strengthening is an increase in the probability of transmitter release when action potentials invade the presynaptic terminals (for further discussion, see the section on long-term potentiation in Chapter 10).

Synaptic vesicle recycling.   A large body of evidence indicates that synaptic vesicle membranes are retrieved and recycled in the normal process of neurotransmission. One interesting system demonstrating the importance of vesicle recycling is the temperature-sensitive *shibire* (*shi*) mutation of the fruit fly *Drosophila melanogaster*. The *shi* gene codes for the protein dynamin, which was mentioned in Chapter 3 as an important factor in the recycling process. When *shi* flies are exposed to a temperature of 29°C, vesicle recycling appears to be completely blocked. Within 10 minutes at that temperature, synaptic vesicles are almost entirely missing from motor nerve endings, and the amplitude of postsynaptic

muscle potentials is similarly reduced by over 90% (Koenig, Kosaka, and Ikeda, 1989). Besides supplying material for vesicle resynthesis, recycling prevents the continuous growth of the nerve terminal membrane. For example, Maddrell and Nordmann (1979) estimated that if the fused vesicles from the neurosecretory nerve endings in the posterior pituitary gland were not removed from the terminal membrane, the membrane area would increase by 16% in 1 day under basal (unstimulated) conditions and by as much as 100% in 1 hour under conditions of maximal stimulation.

In a number of vesicle recycling studies, the enzyme horseradish peroxidase (HRP) has been used as a tracer substance due to its ready detectability with a simple staining technique. When neuromuscular junction preparations were caused to undergo high rates of quantal release for prolonged periods of time with HRP present in the extracellular medium, many synaptic vesicles were later found to be loaded with the enzyme (reviewed by Valtorta et al., 1990). This finding has been construed to indicate the occurrence of endocytosis, a process involving invagination and pinching off of the cell membrane that captures some of the extracellular fluid. Endocytosis and vesicle recycling appear to occur relatively rapidly. Recent studies using advanced optical techniques suggest that a complete round of transmitter release, recycling of the vesicle, and repriming (preparation for a second release event) takes place within approximately 1 minute (Betz and Bewick, 1992; Ryan et al., 1993).

In the early studies of Heuser's group (Heuser and Reese, 1973; Heuser, 1977), prolonged motor neuron stimulation led not only to a depletion of the normal synaptic vesicles, but also to an increase in so-called **coated vesicles**. The "coating" that gave rise to this name is an electron-dense material on the outside of the vesicle membrane that is composed mainly of a protein called clathrin. A clathrin coating was also sometimes observed on membranous profiles of endoplasmic reticulum (ER) in the nerve terminal (called cisternae). After a certain amount of time had elapsed, the coated vesicles were reduced in number, while the normal vesicular complement was regained. These observations led to the widely accepted model of vesicle recycling shown in Figure 6.18. According to this hypothesis, clathrin plays an important role in the endocytotic retrieval of vesicle membrane components from the nerve terminal plasma membrane. The resulting coated vesicles are transported to the cisternae, where they fuse with the ER membrane. Finally, new vesicles are formed by budding off from the cisternae, after which they are loaded with neurotransmitter molecules.

The model just presented assumes that following exocytosis, the vesicle membrane flattens into the plane of the nerve terminal membrane. This would seemingly allow for mixing of the constituents of the two mem-

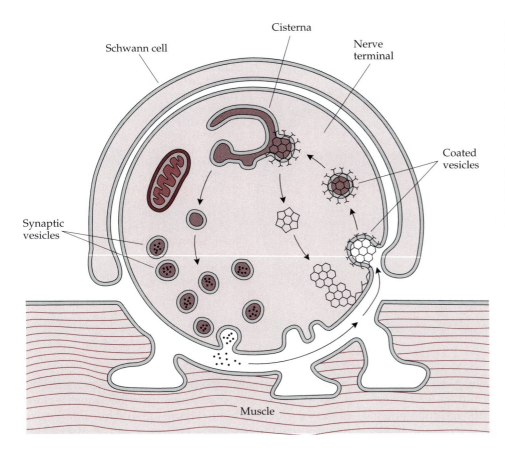

Cisterna

Schwann cell

Nerve terminal

Coated vesicles

Synaptic vesicles

Muscle

6.18 SYNAPTIC VESICLE RECYCLING. In Heuser and Reese's model of synaptic vesicle recycling (based on their studies of the frog neuromuscular junction), following exocytosis, the vesicle membrane flattens into the plane of the nerve terminal membrane. At sites distant from the active zones, retrieval of vesicle membrane components occurs by a process of endocytosis and formation of clathrin-coated vesicles. The coated vesicles subsequently fuse with cisternae of the endoplasmic reticulum. Finally, new vesicles bud off the cisternae and become available for transmitter refilling and release. (After Heuser and Reese, 1973.)

branes, yet vesicles and nerve terminal membranes retain a different composition of both proteins and lipids. Consequently, some investigators have suggested that vesicles do *not* always undergo collapse following membrane fusion and the opening of a fusion pore (see below). Rather, the pore might close and the vesicle detach from its release site without flattening (Nordmann and Artault, 1992; see also Valtorta et al., 1990). Such a process would still allow extracellular HRP to enter the vesicle interior, and it would have the advantage of not requiring a specialized mechanism for selectively retrieving vesicle proteins or lipids after possible mixing with the nerve terminal membrane. Perhaps both recycling mechanisms occur, with various factors such as cell type and firing rate determining which mechanism predominates.

Mechanisms of exocytosis. The ability of action potentials to trigger neurotransmitter release from nerve terminals is called **excitation–secretion coupling**. The immediate stimulus for vesicle fusion and exocytosis is the opening of voltage-gated Ca^{2+} channels in the terminal membrane (reviewed by Smith and Augustine, 1988). These channels are present at particularly high densities near active zones, thereby giving rise to large and rapid increases in local Ca^{2+} concentration (Llinás, Sugimori, and Silver, 1992). Several structurally and pharmacologically distinct Ca^{2+} channels are expressed in the nervous system; however, the most recent information indicates

that only N-type and P-type channels participate in the stimulation of transmitter release (Dunlap, Luebke, and Turner, 1995).

Whereas the Ca^{2+} requirement for transmitter release has been known for many years, the molecular targets of Ca^{2+} action have been more difficult to elucidate. Over the past several years, however, enough progress has been made in this area that a tentative (though still incomplete) scheme can now be offered. First, it is currently believed that a protein called **synapsin I** helps to regulate the availability of synaptic vesicles for exocytosis (Greengard et al., 1993). Biochemical studies on several synaptic systems suggest that only a small fraction of vesicles (called the readily releasable pool) is capable of participating in the release process at any time. The remaining vesicles constitute the reserve pool, from which vesicles can be mobilized for release (see the discussion of ACh release in Chapter 7). Under resting conditions, most vesicles appear to be linked to actin filaments of the nerve terminal cytoskeleton (Figure 6.19). This association is thought to be one of the characteristics of the reserve pool, as actin-linked vesicles presumably cannot undergo exocytosis. The linkage between vesicles and actin is mediated by synapsin I, a protein that is bound to the outside of the vesicle membrane. In the presence of Ca^{2+}, however, synapsin I can be phosphorylated by the enzyme Ca^{2+}/calmodulin-dependent protein kinase II (CaM-K II; for further details, see the section below on second messenger

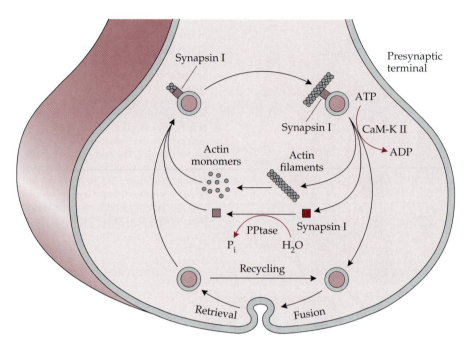

6.19 MODEL OF SYNAPSIN I ACTION IN REGULATING SYNAPTIC VESICLE AVAILABILITY FOR EXOCYTOSIS. When the neuron is inactive, synaptic vesicles are thought to be cross-linked to cytoskeletal actin filaments by synapsin I. Under this condition, the vesicles are unavailable for transmitter release (reserve pool). Ca^{2+} activation of CaM-K II causes phosphorylation of synapsin I, thereby dissociating the vesicles from the filamentous network. The vesicles are now capable of participating in exocytosis (releasable pool). Following membrane fusion and retrieval, some vesicles may be recycled within the releasable pool. Alternatively, dephosphorylation of synapsin I by phosphoprotein phosphatase (PPtase) permits vesicles to return to their actin cross-linked state and reenter the reserve pool. P_i = inorganic phosphate. (After Greengard et al., 1993.)

systems). In its phosphorylated state, synapsin I exhibits a reduced affinity for actin, thereby permitting the release of vesicles from the cytoskeletal matrix and their entry into the readily releasable pool. Subsequent dephosphorylation of synapsin I causes a reassociation of vesicles with actin filaments (Greengard et al., 1993).

It is still not entirely clear how vesicles undergo membrane fusion and release once they are liberated from the cytoskeleton. We know that the process is extremely rapid, taking only 0.1–1.0 ms following Ca^{2+} influx (Smith and Augustine, 1988). This finding strongly suggests that the machinery for exocytosis is preassembled at the release site, awaiting the necessary ionic signal. Once such an assembly is in place, the major task is to bring the vesicle and nerve terminal membranes into extremely close proximity. If the membranes are under curvature or high tension at that point, they will apparently fuse spontaneously due to hydrophobic interactions between the lipid bilayers (Helm and Israelachvili, 1993). This same tension then leads to the creation of a fusion pore, a small opening in the fused membranes through which the vesicle contents begin to emerge. Studies of several model systems point to the formation of such a pore as a critical step in the secretory process (reviewed by Monck and Fernandez, 1994). Fusion pores often flicker open and closed several times before expanding irreversibly to release the entire vesicle contents (reminiscent of the flickering of voltage-gated channels). On other occasions, the pore may open and then either close immediately so that no release occurs, or close after a brief period, during which partial release occurs.

A recently presented model for membrane fusion and pore formation is shown in Figure 6.20. Electron microscopic examination of secretory cells (including neurons) indicates that fusion pore formation is preceded by a "dimpling" of the plasma membrane that brings it close to the vesicle membrane (Figure 6.20a). This dimpling is hypothesized to be directed by a scaffold of specialized proteins that pulls the plasma membrane inward and brings it into the necessary proximity with the vesicle membrane. When the two membranes are separated by less than 2 nm, the lipid bilayers fuse due to the action of the hydrophobic force mentioned above. Alternatively, it is possible that one or more "fusion proteins" are necessary to mediate the interaction between the membranes. In either case, the fusion pore then begins to form, exposing the vesicle interior to the extracellular fluid and permitting the initiation of release (Figure 6.20b). However, neurotransmitter molecules are not free to simply diffuse through the newly opened pore because the transmitter is packaged in a condensed gel matrix composed mainly of proteoglycans. (Proteoglycans are large molecules, each of which consists of a protein core to which many complex carbohydrate chains are linked.) Consequently, this matrix must decondense before the transmitter can be liberated from within the vesicle.

The major remaining step is to identify and characterize the proteins required for exocytosis. According to the model just presented, some of these proteins would be structural components of the scaffold, others would mediate the interactions of the scaffold with the vesicle and plasma membranes, and still others might be needed for scaffold activation (i.e., to initiate dimple formation and subsequent membrane fusion). Many proteins are found in nerve endings, some of which are specific either to the synaptic vesicle membrane or to the plasma membrane of the terminal. Of particular interest are proteins that bind either Ca^{2+} or guanine nucleotides such as guanosine triphosphate (GTP), as

(a)

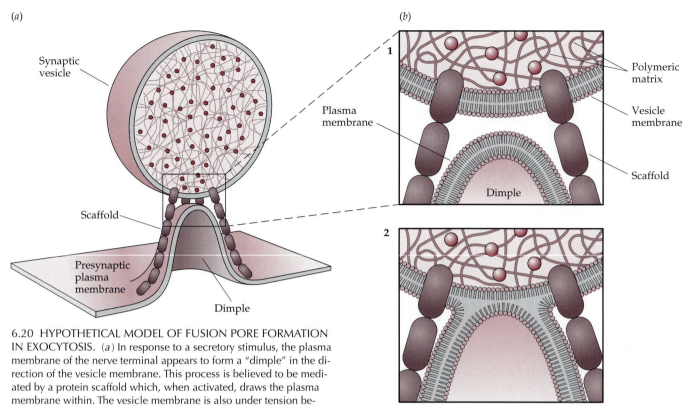

Synaptic vesicle

Scaffold

Presynaptic plasma membrane

Dimple

(b)

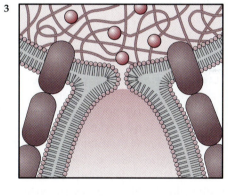

Plasma membrane

Polymeric matrix

Vesicle membrane

Scaffold

Dimple

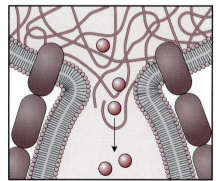

6.20 HYPOTHETICAL MODEL OF FUSION PORE FORMATION IN EXOCYTOSIS. (*a*) In response to a secretory stimulus, the plasma membrane of the nerve terminal appears to form a "dimple" in the direction of the vesicle membrane. This process is believed to be mediated by a protein scaffold which, when activated, draws the plasma membrane within. The vesicle membrane is also under tension because of its interactions with a polymeric matrix of proteoglycans and other substances within the vesicle interior. (*b*) When the plasma membrane and vesicular membranes are sufficiently close to each other (1), fusion of the lipid bilayers takes place (2). Continuing stresses on the membrane lead to the formation of a small fusion pore (3), which is followed by pore expansion and release of neurotransmitter from the vesicle matrix (4). (After Monck and Fernandez, 1994.)

these substances function together to regulate exocytotic activity.

Figure 6.21 depicts some of the proteins that are currently candidates for participation in the exocytotic mechanism (Thiel, 1995). Synaptobrevin, a vesicle membrane protein, forms complexes with the terminal membrane proteins syntaxin and SNAP-25 (synaptosomal-associated protein of 25-kDa molecular weight). Together, these proteins may be involved in vesicle docking and/or fusion. Another important participant in this process is a second complex composed of NSF (*N*-ethylmaleimide-sensitive fusion protein) and the NSF-attachment proteins α/β- and γ-SNAP. This group of soluble proteins is believed to interact in some way with the synaptobrevin/syntaxin/SNAP-25 complex to trigger exocytosis. Synaptotagmin is another vesicle membrane protein that can interact with synaptobrevin/syntaxin/SNAP-25 and also with nerve terminal Ca^{2+} channels and membrane proteins called neurexins. Synaptotagmin is believed to be an important Ca^{2+} sensor in the exocytotic machinery. It appears to inhibit spontaneous fusion under resting conditions (low Ca^{2+} levels) and may also help to instigate fusion in the presence of a Ca^{2+} signal (Littleton and Bellen, 1995).

Munc-18 is another candidate protein, although less is known about its role. Finally, it is appropriate to mention rab3, a GTP-binding protein that is potentially involved in the exocytotic protein scaffold (see Figure 7.4; Monck and Fernandez, 1994).

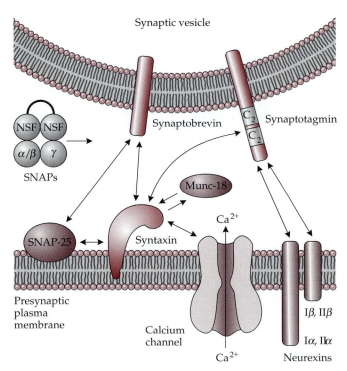

6.21 NERVE TERMINAL PROTEINS THAT MAY BE INVOLVED IN THE EXOCYTOTIC MECHANISM include vesicle membrane proteins such as synaptobrevin and synaptotagmin, the plasma membrane proteins syntaxin and SNAP-25, and the soluble proteins NSF and α/β- and γ-SNAP. (After Thiel, 1995.)

In summary, neurotransmitters are stored in synaptic vesicles and released via a Ca^{2+}-dependent exocytotic process. Following release, vesicles are rapidly recycled and returned to the releasable pool. A phosphoprotein called synapsin I that is bound to the outside of the vesicle membrane appears to play an important role in regulating vesicle availability for release. The process of exocytosis is still not fully understood; however, it is thought to involve the rapid fusion of the vesicle and nerve terminal membranes, followed by the development of a fusion pore and the release of neurotransmitter. A protein scaffold is probably required to bring the two membranes into close proximity so that fusion can take place. A number of proteins in the nerve terminal have recently been identified as likely candidates for participation in scaffold formation and as mediators of vesicle docking and fusion.

Neurotransmitter Receptors and Signal Transduction Mechanisms

The Concept of Receptor Subtypes

All transmitter systems that have been extensively studied to date have been found to possess more than one type of receptor. Often there are multiple levels of recep-

tor diversity. For example, cholinergic receptors are broadly categorized as either nicotinic or muscarinic; however, there are further subtypes within each of these general classes. In the case of closely related receptor subtypes that are coded by distinct genes, it is highly likely that the subtypes evolved from a common ancestral form through a process of gene duplication followed by mutation and recombination. Additionally, multiple receptor subtypes can be created from a single gene product by a process called alternative mRNA splicing, which was discussed in Chapter 3. For many years, knowledge of receptor diversity was based entirely on pharmacological analysis—that is, the ability of certain drugs to selectively activate or inhibit some, but not all, of the actions of a neurotransmitter. In recent years, however, gene cloning studies have verified the existence of many proposed receptor subtypes and have even demonstrated the presence of subtypes not previously detected by pharmacological investigation. We can only speculate as to the selection pressures underlying the evolution of receptor diversity; however, Schofield, Shivers, and Seeburg (1990) have proposed that one important advantage of such diversity is the increased information handling capacity (i.e., plasticity) it confers upon the nervous system.

The existence of multiple receptor subtypes for a given transmitter has as least two important implications. First, as we shall see, a variety of signal transduction mechanisms are available by which receptors can influence postsynaptic activity. If some of the receptors for a transmitter use distinct transduction mechanisms, then that transmitter can evoke a variety of excitatory or inhibitory responses in its postsynaptic targets, depending on which receptor subtype is present on each target cell. Second, although a neurotransmitter obviously recognizes and activates all of its receptor subtypes, the unique structure of each subtype allows for the development of synthetic compounds that exhibit selectivity for one (or some) subtype(s) versus others. Selective agonists and antagonists are useful not only for identifying and characterizing different receptor subtypes, but also for determining their involvement in behavioral and physiological functions.

Receptor Superfamilies

Neurotransmitter receptors fall into two distinct superfamilies of membrane proteins: **ligand-gated channels (LGCs)** and **G protein–coupled receptors (GPCRs)**. These will be described separately because each superfamily has a distinct type of structure and mechanism of action.

Ligand-gated channels. LGCs are large proteins thought to be composed of five subunits that assemble in the membrane. The prototype of this group is the nicotinic cholinergic receptor, which is discussed in detail in Chapter 7. LGCs tend to exhibit considerable heterogeneity in their subunit composition, thereby leading to variation in function. One receptor subtype for the inhibitory amino acid transmitter GABA, for example, is called $GABA_A$. Although all $GABA_A$ receptors are members of the LGC superfamily and function in the same general manner, ethanol (ethyl alcohol) enhances the action of some $GABA_A$ receptors that possess a particular type of subunit, whereas other $GABA_A$ receptors lacking that subunit are insensitive to ethanol (see Chapter 10).

As suggested by their name, LGCs contain a neurotransmitter binding site and an intrinsic ion channel that is gated by the transmitter. This type of mechanism is therefore sometimes called **ionotropic transmission**. Whether receptor activation depolarizes or hyperpolarizes the postsynaptic membrane depends on the ionic permeability of the channel. Some LGCs, such as nicotinic receptors, certain receptors for the amino acid transmitter glutamate, and an LGC for 5-HT called the $5\text{-}HT_3$ receptor, possess nonspecific univalent cation channels that cause depolarization due to Na^+ influx across the membrane. Another type of glutamate receptor called the NMDA receptor is additionally permeable to Ca^{2+}, which can serve as a second messenger (see below). In contrast, the channels associated with $GABA_A$ receptors, as well as with those for another inhibitory amino acid transmitter called glycine, are permeable to Cl^- ions. Passage of these ions across the membrane usually leads to hyperpolarization and thus an inhibition of cell firing.

Besides the recognition site for the neurotransmitter, some LGCs are known to possess additional binding sites capable of modulating receptor function. For example, in later chapters we shall see that $GABA_A$ receptor functioning is enhanced by benzodiazepine and barbiturate drugs acting at allosteric binding sites on the receptor complex. NMDA receptors, on the other hand, are inhibited by phencyclidine (PCP) and related drugs. These compounds are believed to bind to a site within the channel, effectively blocking ion flow across the membrane.

Because of the close linkage between receptor activation and ion channel opening, LGCs operate with a very short latency (i.e., a few milliseconds). Dissociation of the transmitter from the receptor likewise causes rapid channel closing. Consequently, such receptors are well suited for fast signaling within the nervous system. One other noteworthy feature of many LGCs is their rapid desensitization (loss of activity) when continuously exposed to the transmitter or an agonist drug (see Ochoa, Chattopadhyay, and McNamee, 1989). This process may limit the extent of postsynaptic responding under conditions in which presynaptic elements are highly active for a period of time.

G protein–coupled receptors. GPCRs differ from LGCs both structurally and functionally. These receptors consist of a single subunit that, in all known cases, is predicted to contain seven membrane-spanning (i.e., transmembrane) regions. GPCRs include the muscarinic ACh receptors, all known DA receptors, all known adrenergic receptors, all 5-HT receptors except for $5\text{-}HT_3$, the so-called metabotropic receptors for glutamate, $GABA_B$ receptors, histamine receptors, cannabinoid receptors, and all known receptors for neuropeptides.

As implied by their name, GPCRs operate by coupling to members of a family of membrane proteins called **G proteins**. G proteins are so named because their functioning is regulated in part by the binding of guanyl nucleotides such as GTP and guanosine diphosphate (GDP). It is important to note that these G proteins differ from the presynaptic GTP-binding proteins implicated in exocytosis (see next section for more information). Each type of GPCR selectively interacts with some G proteins but not others, which partly accounts for the specificity of cellular actions produced by different members of this receptor superfamily.

Once a G protein molecule has been activated by coupling to an agonist-stimulated receptor, the G protein stimulates one or more types of membrane **effectors** that mediate the cellular response. In most cases, these effectors are enzymes that participate in second messenger synthesis or degradation (see below). The second messengers can then influence a variety of cell processes, including transmembrane ion conductances by various voltage-gated channels. However, we shall see that in some cases the effectors may be the ion channels themselves. This dual mechanism of G protein–coupled signal transduction is diagrammed in Figure 6.22.

Cellular effects mediated by second messengers have latencies measured in hundreds of milliseconds, and these effects may outlast the initiating synaptic event by seconds or even minutes. Second messenger systems are thus best suited for slow but sustained signaling or for modulating the influence of fast neurotransmitters. In contrast, direct modulation of ion channels by G proteins occurs with a somewhat shorter latency, although signaling by this mechanism is still much slower than that mediated by LGCs.

Structure and Mechanism of G Proteins

As noted above, G proteins mediate the interaction between GPCRs and various membrane effectors. In sensory receptor cells, they play a similar role in the transduction of visual, olfactory, and gustatory stimuli. Since the late 1970s, a great deal has been learned about the structure and mechanism of action of G proteins. All G proteins have a common structure containing three subunits termed α, β, and γ. The α subunit contains the guanyl nucleotide binding site and plays the major role in G protein specificity. To date, researchers have found 20 distinct α subunits and have organized them into four subfamilies based on sequence homology (i.e., sim-

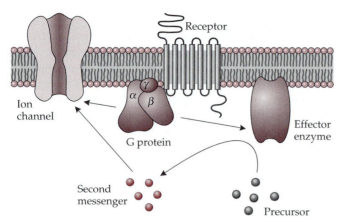

6.22 DUAL MECHANISM OF G PROTEIN–COUPLED SIGNAL TRANSDUCTION. Receptor-activated G proteins may stimulate effector enzymes to alter levels of second messengers that regulate ion channels, or alternatively, the G protein may influence ion channel function via direct interaction with the channel. (After Sternweis and Pang, 1990.)

ilarity of amino acid sequence): α_s, $\alpha_{i/o}$, α_q, and α_{12}. Five different β subunits and eight γ subunits have also been identified (Offermanns and Schultz, 1994). G proteins are named on the basis of their α subunits; hence, G_s is the generic name for any G protein containing an α_s subunit.

The mechanism of G protein action is shown in Figure 6.23. When the G protein is inactive, all of the subunits are bound together as a heterotrimer, and the guanyl nucleotide binding site is occupied by GDP. Activation of the G protein is triggered by the binding of an agonist (A) to the receptor (R). This results in an interaction between the agonist–receptor complex and the G

protein, which in turn promotes a magnesium (Mg^{2+})-dependent exchange of GTP for GDP on the α subunit. The α subunit then dissociates from the β and γ subunits, which remain together as a dimer. Early studies seemed to indicate that only the α subunit was responsible for effector (E) activation; however, more recent research has provided a number of examples of activation by βγ dimers (Clapham and Neer, 1993). The functional activity of the G protein is terminated by the hydrolysis of GTP to GDP by the α subunit, which serves as its own GTPase. The α subunit, with GDP once again present in the guanyl nucleotide binding site, then reassociates with the βγ dimer, and the cycle begins anew.

Table 6.2 provides a listing of some of the best-characterized G proteins. The first G proteins to be identified, G_s and G_i, were named on the basis of their effects on adenylyl cyclase, the enzyme that catalyzes synthesis of the second messenger cyclic AMP (cAMP): adenylyl cyclase is stimulated by G_s, but inhibited by G_i. Another G protein that stimulates adenylyl cyclase is G_{olf}, a member of the G_s subfamily specific to olfactory sensory neurons that transduces odorant information in those cells (Jones and Reed, 1989). Still other G proteins, such as G_q, G_t, and G_o, have little effect on adenylyl cyclase one way or the other. G_q stimulates the enzyme phospholipase C, thereby triggering the phosphoinositide second messenger system, as described later. G_t, which is sometimes called transducin, is found in retinal rod and cone cells, where it participates in the transduction of light input into membrane electrophysiological changes. Finally, G_o, which is one of the most widespread G proteins in the brain, appears to function by directly opening or closing various ion channels (see below) (Birnbaumer, Abramowitz, and Brown, 1990).

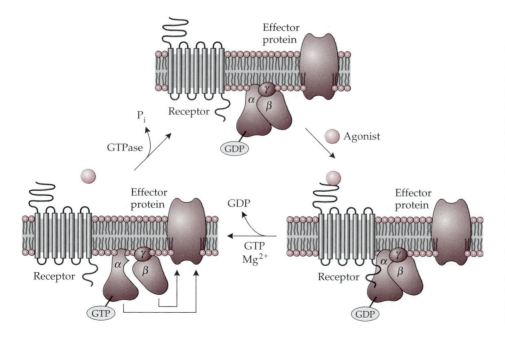

6.23 MECHANISM OF G PROTEIN ACTION. G proteins are heterotrimers (i.e., composed of three different components) of α, β, and γ subunits. The α subunit possesses a binding site for guanyl nucleotides. In the inactive state (top), all three subunits are present, and the guanyl binding site is occupied by GDP. Interaction of the G protein with an agonist-stimulated receptor (bottom right) leads to the replacement of GDP with GTP and dissociation of the α subunit from the remaining βγ dimer (bottom left). The α subunit, and in some cases the βγ subunits, stimulate various effector proteins in the cell membrane. The system returns to the resting state by α subunit–mediated hydrolysis of GTP to GDP, followed by a reassociation of all three subunits. (After Clapham and Neer, 1993.)

Table 6.2	G Proteins Involved in Neurotransmission	
G protein	Second messenger action	Toxin sensitivity
G_s	↑Adenylyl cyclase	Cholera
G_i	↓Adenylyl cyclase	Pertussis
G_q	↑Phospholipase C	—
G_{olf}	↑Adenylyl cyclase (olfactory)	Cholera
G_t	↑cGMP phosphodiesterase (retina)	Cholera, pertussis
G_o	None	Pertussis

The identification and study of G proteins has been greatly facilitated by the use of two toxins that selectively ADP-ribosylate various α subunits. ADP-ribosylation refers to the covalent transfer of an ADP-ribose unit from nicotinamide adenine dinucleotide (NAD^+) to the G protein. One of the toxins with this capability is cholera toxin, which is produced by the bacterium *Vibrio cholerae*. As shown in Table 6.2, cholera toxin ADP-ribosylates G_s, G_t, and G_{olf}. The effect in each case is to block the GTPase activity of the α subunit and hence to persistently activate it. In cells of the intestinal mucosa, this results in an abnormally high concentration of cAMP (due to continuous stimulation of adenylyl cyclase by G_s), which causes increased Na^+ and water transport into the gut, thereby leading to the massive diarrhea that is characteristic of cholera.

The other toxin used to study G proteins is pertussis toxin, which is made by the bacterium responsible for whooping cough, *Bordetella pertussis*. Pertussis toxin ADP-ribosylates G_i, G_o, and G_t (note that G_t is a substrate for both cholera and pertussis toxins), whereas G_q is insensitive to both toxins. Pertussis toxin produces a different effect than cholera toxin because the ADP-ribose group is attached to a different site on the α subunit. More specifically, in this case the G protein is inactivated because its ability to interact with receptors is blocked. How this effect is related to the symptoms of whooping cough has not yet been determined. The important point for researchers is that when a new G protein is discovered, its relationship to previously identified family members can be ascertained in part by its susceptibility to either cholera or pertussis toxin.

Continuous exposure of cells to a receptor agonist is well known to cause a down-regulation of GPCR function. As discussed in Chapter 8 for the β-adrenergic receptor, this process is generally thought to involve the uncoupling of receptors from G proteins and possibly also receptor degradation or at least removal from the membrane. Recent studies have indicated that agonist treatment can also lead to down-regulation of G proteins (Milligan, 1993). This new level of analysis has just

begun to be explored by researchers interested in drug effects on neuronal signaling and the pathological processes underlying various psychiatric and neurological diseases (Manji, 1992).

Direct Interactions of G Proteins with Ion Channels

G proteins were first discovered in relation to their involvement in second messenger functions. However, experimental findings suggest that in some cases, G proteins may directly influence ion channels without the need for an intervening second messenger (in such cases, the channel itself is the effector, rather than an enzyme). Let us consider one type of experiment that has provided support for this mode of G protein action. Assume that in normal whole-cell preparations a particular transmitter or agonist drug either enhances or inhibits the action of some ion channel. To test for the possible involvement of a second messenger in this effect, researchers may investigate the action of the transmitter or drug on cells in a liquid-filled bath (Figure 6.24). In this case, each cell to be studied is impaled with a patch micropipette, which isolates one or a few channels from the rest of the membrane and enables researchers to measure the ionic currents carried by the isolated channel(s) (see Chapter 5). An agonist applied to the bath stimulates receptors located outside of the pipette, but not those present within the small patch of membrane containing the channels being analyzed. If the agonist still influences channel functioning in the patch, then we infer that a second messenger diffusing through the cytoplasm of the cell mediates the interaction between the receptors and the channels. If, on the other hand, the agonist has no effect on channel activity, then a diffusible second messenger is presumably not involved in the process. This second type of modulation, which requires interaction of the channels with an activating or inhibiting factor within the membrane, is sometimes termed **membrane-delimited**.

Of course, the point of this discussion is the hypothesis that activated G protein subunits serve as the mediating factors in membrane-delimited channel modulation. Before this hypothesis can be considered fully validated, it is necessary to rigorously exclude the possible involvement of lipid-soluble second messengers (e.g., arachidonic acid and some of its metabolites; see below) that remain within the membrane instead of diffusing through the cytoplasm. Nevertheless, the notion of direct G protein–ion channel interactions has become fairly well accepted in a few well-studied systems (reviewed by Clapham, 1994; Hille, 1994). One example is the inward-rectifying K^+ channel found in cardiac atrial cells and in many types of neurons. Whereas most voltage-gated ion channels are closed at the resting potential and tend to open when the membrane depolarizes, the conductance of inward-rectifying channels increases with hyperpolarization and decreases with depolariza-

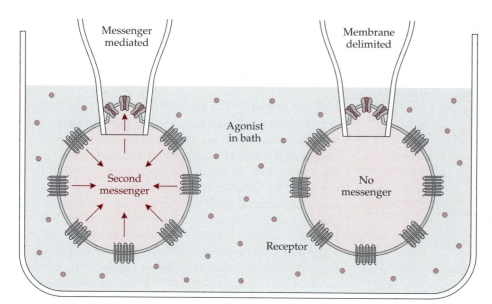

6.24 DETERMINING G PROTEIN IN-FLUENCE ON ION CHANNELS. Cells in a liquid-filled bath are impaled with a patch micropipette in order to isolate individual channels in the cell membrane. Membrane receptors known to modulate those channels are stimulated by the application of an agonist drug to the bath. If a diffusible second messenger mediates this effect, the channels within the confines of the pipette will be influenced as usual (*left*). If no diffusible messenger is involved (the effect is membrane delimited), channel functioning will not be altered by the application of agonist to the bath (*right*). (After Hille, 1994.)

tion (Hille, 1992). Inward-rectifying K$^+$ channels are activated by a pertussis toxin-sensitive G protein (possibly G$_o$) that can be coupled (depending on the cell type) to cholinergic muscarinic M$_2$, adrenergic α_2, dopaminergic D$_2$, serotonergic 5-HT$_1$, GABA$_B$, opioid μ and δ, histamine, and somatostatin (a neuropeptide) receptors (North, 1989; North et al., 1987). This mechanism mediates the ability of ACh, released from parasympathetic (vagal) nerve endings, to cause a slowing of the heart rate by hyperpolarizing pacemaker cells of the sino- and atrioventricular nodes and the atria. Inhibitory postsynaptic potentials are likewise produced in neurons by activation of inward-rectifying K$^+$ channels. Another likely instance of direct G protein modulation is that of N-type Ca^{2+} channels. These channels are involved in spike-frequency adaptation (afterhyperpolarization) and in transmitter release at nerve terminals. A pertussis toxin–sensitive G protein (again probably G$_o$) inhibits N-type Ca^{2+} channel conductance in sympathetic neurons as well as in cells of the dorsal root ganglia (Hille, 1994).

It should also be noted that G protein coupling and second messenger systems may sometimes act synergistically to regulate channel activity. For example, there is evidence that G$_s$ may stimulate the opening of L-type Ca^{2+} channels via both second messenger–mediated phosphorylation (see below) and direct interaction of G protein subunits with the channel (Clapham, 1994).

Receptor Tyrosine Kinases

Receptor tyrosine kinases represent a third receptor superfamily that is not involved in neurotransmission, but is important in the functioning of various growth factors and neurotrophins. The neurotrophins, which include nerve growth factor (NGF), brain-derived neurotropic factor (BDNF), neurotrophin-3 (NT-3), and NT-4/5, are thought to play important roles in neural development as well as in the functioning of the adult nervous system. Receptor tyrosine kinases possess a single transmembrane domain, an extracellular domain that contains the neurotrophin binding site, and a cytoplasmic domain. When activated, the cytoplasmic domain phosphorylates various substrate proteins (including the receptor itself) on specific tyrosine residues. For more information on the mechanism of action of neurotrophins and receptor tyrosine kinases, the reader is referred to reviews by Eide, Lowenstein, and Reichardt (1993), and Schlessinger and Ullrich (1992).

Second Messenger Systems

Chemical substances that transmit information between cells (i.e., neurotransmitters and hormones) often exert their effects by altering the concentration of some physiologically active compound within the receiving cell. This process is sometimes referred to as **metabotropic transmission** (because it involves more elaborate metabolic processes than the simpler ionotropic transmission), and the mediating substances are called **second messengers**. According to the terminology that has developed, the original signaling agent traveling from one cell to the other is termed the first messenger, while the intracellular compound that mediates the effect of the first messenger is considered the second messenger.

Second messengers typically function by activating enzymes known as **protein kinases** that catalyze the phosphorylation of various substrate proteins (Figure 6.25). These reactions consist of the transfer of phosphate (PO$_4$$^{2-}$) groups from ATP to one or more hydroxyl (OH) groups of serine, threonine, or tyrosine residues in the amino acid chain of the protein (note, however, that the phosphorylation reactions associated with second mes-

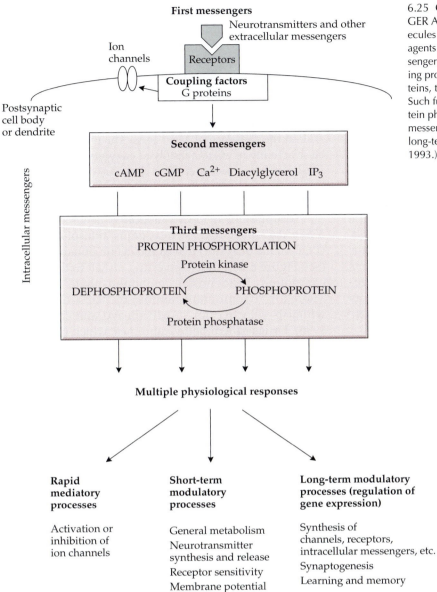

First messengers

Neurotransmitters and other extracellular messengers

Ion channels

Receptors

Coupling factors
G proteins

Postsynaptic cell body or dendrite

Intracellular messengers

Second messengers

cAMP   cGMP   Ca²⁺   Diacylglycerol   IP₃

Third messengers
PROTEIN PHOSPHORYLATION

Protein kinase

DEPHOSPHOPROTEIN   PHOSPHOPROTEIN

Protein phosphatase

Multiple physiological responses

Rapid mediatory processes

Activation or inhibition of ion channels

Short-term modulatory processes

General metabolism
Neurotransmitter synthesis and release
Receptor sensitivity
Membrane potential
Short-term memory

Long-term modulatory processes (regulation of gene expression)

Synthesis of channels, receptors, intracellular messengers, etc.
Synaptogenesis
Learning and memory

6.25 GENERAL MECHANISM OF SECOND MESSENGER ACTION. Second messengers are intracellular molecules or ions that are regulated by extracellular signaling agents such as neurotransmitters and hormones (first messengers). Second messengers typically operate by activating protein kinases that phosphorylate various target proteins, thereby altering the functioning of these proteins. Such functional effects are subsequently reversed by protein phosphatase–mediated dephosphorylation. Second messengers modulate a wide range of both rapid and long-term neuronal processes. (After Hyman and Nestler, 1993.)

senger signaling occur only on serine or threonine residues). The importance of this process stems from the fact that addition of the electrically charged phosphate groups alters the conformation (three-dimensional structure) of the affected protein, with an associated change in its biological activity. If the protein is an enzyme, for example, then its catalytic activity might be either increased or reduced in the phosphorylated state.

It is also necessary to return phosphorylated proteins to their unphosphorylated state. This process, called dephosphorylation, is accomplished by a class of enzymes known as **phosphoprotein phosphatases**. Dephosphorylation terminates the cellular effects of second messengers by reversing the phosphorylation-induced changes in protein function. Calcineurin is an example of

a phosphoprotein phosphatase which, in this case, is activated by Ca²⁺ ions.

As shown in Figure 6.25, second messenger signaling can produce varying effects ranging from rapid changes in ion channel activity to long-term neuronal modulation involving altered gene expression. In the sections below, we shall discuss the major second messenger systems in the nervous system and the mechanisms by which they influence brain function.

Cyclic AMP

The first substance to be called a second messenger was discovered by the late E. W. Sutherland, for which he received a Nobel Prize in 1971. Sutherland was interested in how, in times of stress, epinephrine stimulates glycogenolysis, the conversion of glycogen to glucose in liver and muscle cells. In these cells, glycogen is the storage form of carbohydrates, and the conversion reaction is crucial for providing glucose as a source of energy when it is needed. It had previously been established that glycogen breakdown is catalyzed by the enzyme phosphorylase. Sutherland and his colleagues determined that epinephrine stimulates the conversion of the relatively inactive form of this enzyme, phosphorylase b, to the more active form, phosphorylase a. More importantly, they found that this effect required the synthesis of a small, heat-stable molecule within the cell that they subsequently determined to be the nucleotide cyclic adenosine 3',5'-monophosphate (cyclic AMP, or **cAMP**) (see Robison, Butcher, and Sutherland, 1971). Researchers soon found this substance in virtually all animal species, including unicellular organisms and bacteria. Its role is modulation of the many homeostatic processes governed by the endocrine system as well as the responses to many transmitters in the nervous system.

Synthesis and degradation.   Cyclic AMP and the related compound cyclic guanosine 3',5'-monophosphate (**cGMP**) are synthesized from the nucleotides adenosine triphos-

phate (ATP) and guanosine triphosphate (GTP), respectively (Figure 6.26). In the case of cAMP, the reaction is catalyzed by the enzyme adenylyl cyclase. The brain is an unusually rich source of this enzyme, exhibiting higher activity than any other organ. When a neurotransmitter molecule or other agonist binds to an adenylyl cyclase–coupled receptor, the agonist–receptor complex activates G_s, which then stimulates the enzyme to form cAMP from ATP in the presence of Mg^{2+} ions. The term adenylyl cyclase actually refers to a family of enzymes, of which eight members have been identified thus far (designated types 1–8) (Iyengar, 1993). All are membrane glycoproteins, and all have been found in the brain.

Termination of cAMP action is accomplished by 3',5'-cAMP phosphodiesterase, or just phosphodiesterase (PDE). This enzyme cleaves the cyclic phosphate bond (see Figure 6.26), thus converting cAMP to the inactive compound 5'-adenosine monophosphate (5'-AMP). There are five different families of PDEs, only one of which is selective for cAMP (Beavo and Reifsnyder, 1990). Drugs called methylxanthines, which include caffeine and theophylline, inhibit cAMP hydrolysis by PDE. An early theory of caffeine action postulated that its behavior-stimulating effects are mediated by inhibition of PDE, with a resultant increase in cellular cAMP levels.

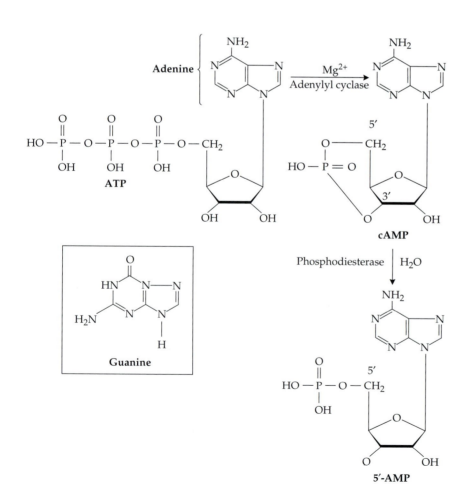

6.26 SYNTHESIS OF CYCLIC AMP. Adenylyl cyclase converts adenosine triphosphate (ATP) into cyclic AMP. Phosphodiesterase converts cAMP into the inert compound 5'-AMP. Cyclic GMP undergoes similar reactions, but guanine is substituted for the adenine moiety.

However, subsequent research has supported an alternative mode of action that is discussed in Chapter 14.

Mechanism of action.   Sutherland's pioneering studies on the regulation of glycogenolysis showed that the cAMP-mediated stimulation of glycogen phosphorylase occurred as a result of phosphorylation of the enzyme. The particular protein kinase responsible for this effect came to be known as the cAMP-dependent protein kinase (also known as protein kinase A or PKA). When epinephrine stimulates adenylyl cyclase in a liver cell, therefore, the resulting increase in cAMP concentration stimulates PKA, which ultimately results in the phosphorylation and activation of the glycogen-degrading enzyme.

PKA is found primarily in the cytoplasmic compartment. The mechanism of PKA activation is illustrated in Figure 6.27. As shown, the enzyme contains two catalytic subunits, each of which is linked noncovalently to a regulatory subunit. Each regulatory subunit contains two high-affinity binding sites for cAMP. When all four sites are occupied, the catalytic subunits are activated by dissociating from the regulatory subunits. The enzyme returns to the inactive state by dissociation of cAMP from the regulatory subunits and their reassociation with the catalytic subunits (Scott, 1991).

An impressive array of different proteins are phosphorylated by PKA, including many voltage-gated channels (e.g., Na^+ channels, Ca^{2+}-dependent K^+ channels, and L-type Ca^{2+} channels), LGC receptors (such as nicotinic, $GABA_A$, and non-NMDA glutamate receptors), Na^+–K^+ ATPase, synapsins I and II, β-adrenergic receptors, and the catecholamine-synthesizing enzyme tyrosine hydroxylase (see Levitan, 1994, for a review of channel phosphorylation). In this way, cAMP is intimately involved in the control of ion fluxes across the membrane, neurotransmitter release processes, and the functioning of catecholamine systems. This second messenger also plays an important role in the mechanisms by which neurotransmitters alter neuronal gene regulation, a topic that is discussed in a later section.

Cyclic GMP

The other important cyclic nucleotide second messenger is cyclic GMP (**cGMP**). This compound was discovered in 1963 by Ashman and colleagues, but for many years it took a back seat to cAMP in terms of interest and recognition. However, the recent discoveries discussed below have finally brought cGMP into the forefront of neuropharmacological research.

Synthesis and degradation.   Cyclic GMP is synthesized from guanosine triphosphate (GTP) by guanylyl cyclase. Two general forms of this enzyme have been found, a membrane-bound form and a soluble (cytoplasmic) form. Membrane-bound guanylyl cyclases serve as re-

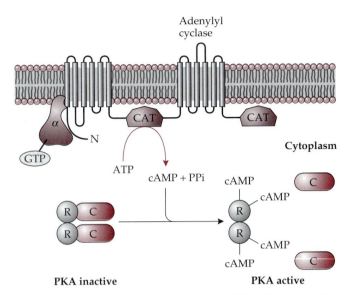

6.27 STRUCTURE AND MECHANISM OF ADENYLYL CYCLASE AND cAMP-DEPENDENT PROTEIN KINASE A (PKA). Adenylyl cyclase is a membrane glycoprotein possessing a total of 12 transmembrane domains (depicted as lines passing through the membrane) and two catalytic domains (CAT) within the cytoplasm. This enzyme converts ATP to cAMP upon stimulation by the α subunit of G_S. In the inactive state, PKA is a complex of two catalytic subunits (C) bound to two regulatory subunits (R) that inhibit catalytic activity. When two molecules of cAMP bind to each of the regulatory subunits, the catalytic subunits dissociate from the complex and are free to phosphorylate various target proteins. (After Nicholls, 1994.)

ceptors for certain peptides such that the extracellular domain of the receptor possesses the peptide binding site, whereas a part of the cytoplasmic domain contains the catalytic region responsible for synthesizing cGMP (Schulz, Yuen, and Garbers, 1991; Yuen and Garbers, 1992). Among the most interesting compounds that function via this mechanism are the natriuretic peptides. The first-discovered member of this family was atrial natriuretic peptide (ANP), a hormone produced by cells of the atrium in response to elevated blood pressure. Following its release into the bloodstream, ANP travels to the kidneys, where it stimulates water loss (diuresis) and Na^+ excretion (natriuresis). Two related peptides, brain natriuretic peptide (BNP) and C-type natriuretic peptide (CNP), were subsequently identified. Although ANP and BNP are present mainly in the heart, CNP is highly localized to the nervous system, where it presumably serves a signaling function.

The soluble form of guanylyl cyclase operates in a completely different manner. The functioning of this enzyme was first elucidated in smooth muscle cells that regulate arterial blood flow. ACh and a variety of other substances had long been known to produce vascular smooth muscle relaxation and consequently vasodilation; however, the mechanism by which this occurred was unclear. Then Furchgott and Zawadzki (1980) published a classic paper demonstrating that the presence of endothelial cells (cells that form blood vessel walls) was necessary for the relaxant effect of ACh. Subsequent studies showed that a highly labile (i.e., short-lived) chemical factor mediated the interaction between the endothelia and the smooth muscle cells (Furchgott, 1984). As its chemical identity was not yet known, this compound was initially called endothelium-derived relaxing factor (EDRF). The next important step was the discovery that EDRF acted by stimulating the soluble form of guanylyl cyclase (Rapoport and Murad, 1983); however, this still left the nature of EDRF itself undisclosed. The final key to the puzzle came from the work of several laboratories demonstrating that EDRF was a gaseous substance, nitric oxide (NO) (reviewed by Moncada et al., 1991). The relationship between cGMP and NO is discussed in the next section.

Like cAMP, cGMP is degraded by PDE, in this case, to 5'-guanosine monophosphate (5'-GMP). One family of cGMP-specific PDEs has been studied most intensively in the retina due to its role in sensory mechanisms (Beavo and Reifsnyder, 1990; see below).

cGMP and nitric oxide. The chemistry of NO must be discussed before we can consider its relationship with cGMP. NO is synthesized according to the reaction shown in Figure 6.28. The enzyme nitric oxide synthase (NOS) reacts with the amino acid arginine to yield citrulline and NO. This enzyme is activated by Ca^{2+} and the Ca^{2+}-binding protein calmodulin (see below). Within a few seconds or less, NO is eliminated by reaction with O_2 to yield NO_2 and NO_3.

Although NOS was first studied in endothelial cells, it has since been found in many brain regions. In some of these areas, NOS is found in various interneurons, but not in long axon projection pathways. Such a pattern has been observed in (1) the cerebellar cortex, in which the basket and granule cells, but not the Purkinje cells, are NOS-positive; (2) the cerebral cortex and hippocampus, in which NOS is absent from pyramidal cells but is present in scattered interneurons in various layers; and (3) the striatum, in which the medium spiny projection neurons lack NOS, but the enzyme is found in a population of aspiny interneurons (Vincent and Hope, 1992). In the cerebellum and hippocampus, Garthwaite (1991) demonstrated that Ca^{2+} activation of NOS is probably mediated by excitatory amino acid stimulation of NMDA receptors.

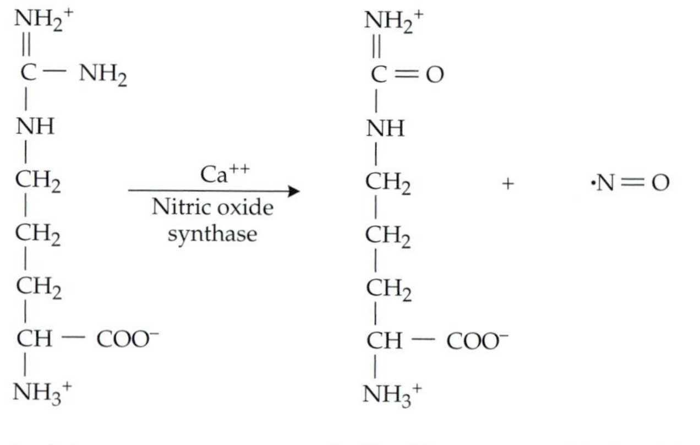

As mentioned earlier, NO operates by increasing intracellular cGMP levels through activation of the soluble form of guanylyl cyclase. This enzyme has a heme (iron-binding) moiety in its core, and the activational effect occurs through binding of NO to the heme–iron complex. A close relationship between NO and soluble guanylyl cyclase in the brain is supported by the similar regional distribution of NOS staining and staining for cGMP following stimulation of NO synthesis (Southam and Garthwaite, 1993). On the other hand, staining is not usually found in the same cells within a given area. In most cases, either NOS is found in postsynaptic cells and cGMP in presynaptic elements, or the reverse. These and other findings strongly suggest that NO diffuses from its site of origin to target cells, where it activates guanylyl cyclase (Figure 6.29).

Several features of transmission by NO are unique as compared with other intercellular messengers. First, due to its high membrane permeability, NO cannot be packaged or stored in any vesicular (or other) structure. It must instead be made and released upon demand. Second, rapid diffusion of NO, along with the lack of any known uptake mechanism, may permit the gas to diffuse for relatively (on a cellular scale) long distances and consequently to act on distant targets (Wood and Garthwaite, 1994). Finally, as already mentioned, NO is able to directly stimulate second messenger synthesis without the intervention of a membrane receptor.

Mechanisms of action. Cyclic GMP modulates cellular functioning through at least three distinct mechanisms (Lincoln and Cornwell, 1993). First, there are two types of cGMP-dependent protein kinase (protein kinase G, or PKG). Type I is a soluble form of the enzyme, whereas type II is membrane-bound (Francis and Corbin, 1994). Type I, which is the more widespread form, has been detected in the brain (mainly the cerebellum), lung, smooth muscle, and platelets. Second, ion channels in retinal photoreceptor cells (i.e., rods and cones) are directly gated by cGMP without an intervening phosphorylation step. This mechanism is discussed in the next section. Finally, certain types of PDE are either activated or inhibited by cGMP (Beavo and Reifsnyder, 1990). This permits an interaction between the cAMP and cGMP signal transduction systems. For example, in some types of cells, cGMP reduces the effects of cAMP by stimulating PDE-mediated cAMP breakdown (Lincoln and Cornwell, 1993).

6.28 SYNTHESIS OF NITRIC OXIDE.

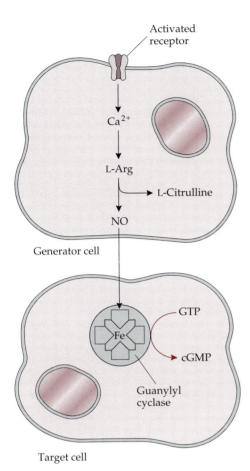

6.29 INTERCELLULAR SIGNALING BY NITRIC OXIDE. The first step in NO signaling is an elevation of cytoplasmic Ca^{2+} levels by the opening of ligand- or voltage-gated Ca^{2+} channels. This causes the generation of NO from the amino acid L-arginine (L-Arg) by the Ca^{2+}-activated enzyme nitric oxide synthase. NO then diffuses out of the generator cell to target cells, where it stimulates cGMP synthesis by soluble guanylyl cyclase. (After Kennedy, 1992.)

Role of cGMP in photoreceptor signal transduction. On a molecular level, the cellular effects of cGMP are perhaps best understood in the retinal photoreceptor cells called rods (similar processes also occur in the cones). Rods are extremely sensitive to light (they can be excited by a single photon), and a great deal of research has been performed in order to understand the mechanism by which light stimulation is transduced into a change in the electrical activity of the cell (reviewed by McNaughton, 1990). Studies indicate that in a dark-adapted rod, the outer segment (where signal transduction occurs) contains unusually high concentrations of cGMP because PDE activity is suppressed by the binding of inhibitory subunits. Moreover, the plasma membrane contains an unusual type of cation channel, permeable mainly to Na^+ and Ca^{2+} ions, that is gated directly by cGMP without the intervening step of kinase-mediated phosphorylation. That is, the channel is opened by binding with cGMP itself (Lincoln and Cornwell, 1993). (Another example of a cyclic nucleotide-gated ion channel has been

found in olfactory receptors, where cAMP rather than cGMP stimulates the opening of a membrane cation channel (Ronnett and Snyder, 1992).)

Because of the influence of cGMP, the cation channels are maintained in an open state in the absence of light. The resulting inward Na^+ current (sometimes called the "dark current") leads to a partial depolarization of the rod membrane to approximately −40 mV (the membrane potential would otherwise be at about −80 mV due to the efflux of K^+ through K^+ channels in the inner segment of the cell). This modest activation is sufficient to cause continuous transmitter (in this case, glutamate) release from the secretory terminals of the rods while they are in darkness (Figure 6.30*a*).

The first step in the phototransduction process involves a pigment protein known as rhodopsin that is present in the outer segment. Rhodopsin has the same general structural features as neurotransmitter GPCRs, that is, a single subunit with seven putative transmembrane domains. When light strikes a rod, rhodopsin molecules absorb the photons and, as a result, alter their three-dimensional conformation to an activated state. The activated rhodopsin in turn activates the retina-specific G protein G_t (also called transducin). Transducin then removes the inhibitory influence on PDE, resulting in a rapid decrease in cGMP levels (Figure 6.30*b*). This leads to a closure of the Na^+ channels, decreased Na^+ current across the cell membrane, and a hyperpolarization of the cell (McNaughton, 1990).

The photoreceptor system provides a good illustration of the tremendous signal amplification that can occur in G protein–coupled systems. This amplification is a multistage process because a single receptor can activate many G protein molecules, which can, in turn, stimulate many effector enzyme molecules in the membrane before they become inactivated. Each effector enzyme molecule then catalyzes the synthesis or degradation of many second messenger molecules before its action is terminated. In the specific case of photoreception in rod cells, a single photon striking a rhodopsin molecule has been estimated to activate several hundred transducin molecules, resulting eventually in the PDE-catalyzed breakdown of as many as 1 million cGMP molecules (Kühn and Wilden, 1987).

Calcium and Calmodulin

The concentration of free cytoplasmic Ca^{2+} in most neurons is estimated to be approximately 100 nM. Under resting conditions, this concentration is maintained by Ca^{2+}–Mg^{2+} ATPases (i.e., Ca^{2+} pumps) that transport the ion either out of the cell through the plasma membrane or into intracellular storage compartments (mainly the ER). However, cytoplasmic Ca^{2+} levels can be rapidly elevated by several mechanisms, notably influx through voltage-gated Ca^{2+} channels, influx through NMDA channels, and/or release from the ER. In such cases,

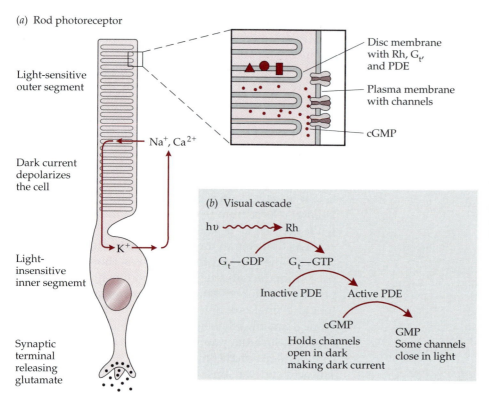

(a) Rod photoreceptor

Light-sensitive outer segment

Dark current depolarizes the cell

Light-insensitive inner segmemt

Synaptic terminal releasing glutamate

Na⁺, Ca²⁺

K⁺

Disc membrane with Rh, G$_t$, and PDE

Plasma membrane with channels

cGMP

(b) Visual cascade

$h\upsilon$ ⟿ Rh

G$_t$—GDP   G$_t$—GTP

Inactive PDE   Active PDE

cGMP   GMP

Holds channels open in dark making dark current

Some channels close in light

6.30 PHOTOTRANSDUCTION IN RETINAL RODS. (a) The anatomy of a vertebrate rod. In the absence of light, the rod membrane is partially depolarized due to an open cation channel. The disc membrane (shown magnified at the upper right) contains high concentrations of the rod photopigment rhodopsin (Rh), the G protein transducin (G$_t$), and a cGMP phosphodiesterase (PDE). (b) Absorption of light ($h\upsilon$) by Rh initiates a cascade involving activation of G$_t$, stimulation of PDE, and cation channel closing due to the rapid reduction in cGMP levels. These events cause membrane hyperpolarization and a reduction in transmitter (glutamate) release by the rod. (After Hille, 1992.)

Ca^{2+} can act as a second messenger to alter a variety of intracellular functions (Ghosh and Greenberg, 1995).

Most second messenger functions of Ca^{2+} require its interaction with an intracellular Ca^{2+}-binding protein known as **calmodulin** (Gnegy, 1993). (Various neurons have also been found to possess other Ca^{2+}-binding proteins, including parvalbumin, calbindin, or calretinin (Baimbridge et al., 1992). However, unlike calmodulin, the function of these proteins is still unknown.) Calmodulin has been found in virtually all nucleated cells—from one-celled organisms and plant cells to human brain cells. The protein has a molecular weight of approximately 17 kDa and comprises a single polypeptide chain. Structurally, calmodulin is dumbbell-shaped, with globular regions at each end that are joined by a long α–helical domain (Babu et al., 1985). Each globular region contains two binding sites for Ca^{2+} ions, and the protein is activated when all four sites are occupied.

Some of the proteins regulated by the Ca^{2+}/calmodulin complex (CaM) are listed in Table 6.3. Thus, a rise in intracellular Ca^{2+} concentration can activate enzymes that are involved in cAMP synthesis and degradation, NO synthesis, and protein dephosphorylation. CaM also triggers a negative feedback system that tends to reduce Ca^{2+} levels by activating membrane Ca^{2+}–Mg^{2+} ATPase. Binding of CaM to various cytoskeletal proteins seems to

Table 6.3 Some Ca²⁺/Calmodulin (CaM)-Regulated Proteins	
Protein category	**Protein**
Enzymes	CaM-dependent kinases
	Adenylyl cyclase (types 1 and 3)
	Cyclic nucleotide phosphodiesterase (specific CaM-dependent forms)
	Nitric oxide synthase
	Calcineurin (CaM-dependent phosphoprotein phosphatase)
	Ca²⁺–Mg²⁺ ATPase
Cytoskeletal proteins	Tubulin
	Microtubule-associated protein-2 (MAP-2)
	Tau
	Fodrin

alter cytoskeletal structure, which may then affect cell shape, motility, secretion, or transport (Gnegy, 1993).

Among the enzymes stimulated by CaM are five different protein kinases, the most important of which is Ca^{2+}/calmodulin-dependent protein kinase II (**CaM-K II**); sometimes also called the multifunctional CaM kinase because of its widespread effects. CaM-K II is highly enriched in the brain, where it is present throughout neurons, but particularly in postsynaptic densities. Proteins phosphorylated by CaM-K II include tyrosine hydroxylase, tryptophan hydroxylase, $GABA_A$ receptors, synapsin I, PDE, calcineurin, phospholipase A_2, MAP-2, and neurofilament proteins (Schulman and Hanson, 1993). Therefore, like cAMP, CaM participates in many features of synaptic transmission, both pre- and postsynaptically.

An interesting feature of CaM-K II enables it to act as a kind of "molecular switch." When activated, the enzyme can engage in autophosphorylation (i.e., phosphorylation of itself) (Figure 6.31; Schulman and Hanson, 1993). This "turns on the switch" by causing the kinase to become temporarily independent of Ca^{2+}. Eventually, the switch is turned off when the kinase becomes dephosphorylated. Some investigators have hypothesized that conversion of CaM-K II, and possibly other kinases, to a stimulation-independent state may play a role in long-term potentiation or other forms of neuronal plasticity (see Chapter 10).

Phosphoinositide-Derived Second Messengers

Phosphoinositides are a class of phospholipids that includes the monophosphorylated compound phosphatidylinositol (**PI**), as well as the polyphosphoinositides phosphatidylinositol 4-monophosphate (**PIP**) and phosphatidylinositol 4,5-bisphosphate (**PIP$_2$**). Phosphatidylinositol 4,5-bisphosphate is formed by the se-

Phosphatidylinositol (PI)

Phosphatidylinositol 4,5-bisphosphate (PIP$_2$)

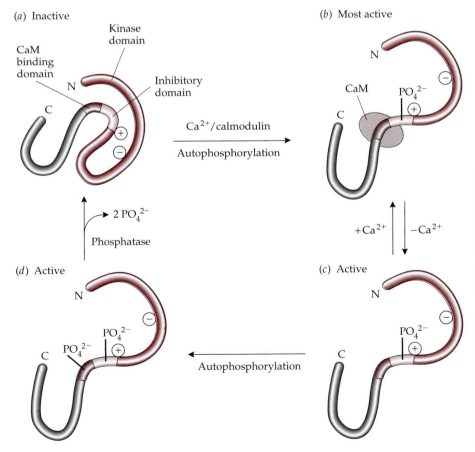

(a) Inactive

(b) Most active

Ca^{2+}/calmodulin

Autophosphorylation

(d) Active

(c) Active

Autophosphorylation

Phosphatase

$+Ca^{2+}$ $-Ca^{2+}$

6.31 CaM-K II AS A MOLECULAR SWITCH. (*a*) In the absence of Ca^{2+}/calmodulin (CaM), the active site of CaM-K II (kinase domain) is inhibited by binding of the inhibitory domain. (*b*) Binding of CaM to its recognition site alters the enzyme's conformation, leading to phosphorylation of substrate proteins, including CaM-K II itself (this occurs at a threonine residue at position 286). (*c*) When the intracellular Ca^{2+} level falls, CaM dissociates from the enzyme; however, the phosphorylated threonine prevents reassociation of the inhibitory domain with the active site. Kinase activity is now partially independent of Ca^{2+} (the "switch" is on). (*d*) Autophosphorylation may now occur at a site within the CaM binding domain, which causes the enzyme to be completely insensitive to CaM. Finally, CaM-K II is dephosphorylated by phosphatases, returning it to its inactive state. (From Kennedy, 1992.)

quential phosphorylation of PI and PIP, with ATP as usual providing the phosphate groups (see Fisher, Heacock, and Agranoff, 1992, for a detailed discussion of phosphoinositide biochemistry). Although these lipids are found in the membranes of many if not all, cells, the first indication that they might play a role in signal transmission came from the work of Hokin and Hokin (1953), who demonstrated that ACh stimulated the incorporation of radiolabeled phosphate into phospholipids in pancreatic cells. A great deal of subsequent research has demonstrated that two breakdown products of PIP_2, namely, diacylglycerol (**DAG**) and inositol 1,4,5-trisphosphate (**IP_3**), serve as second messengers in many neuronal and nonneuronal cells (Berridge, 1993; Furuichi and Mikoshiba, 1995).

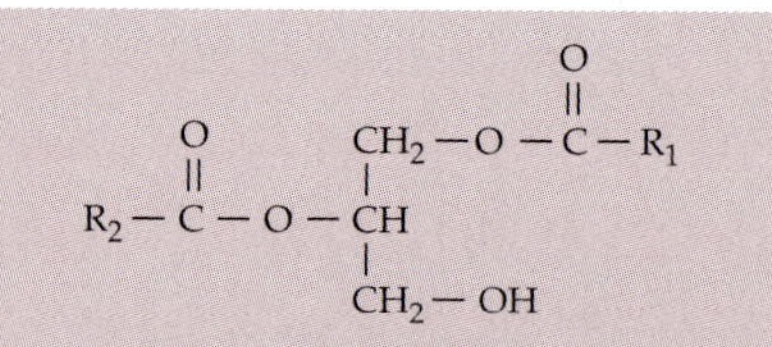

Diacylglycerol (DAG)

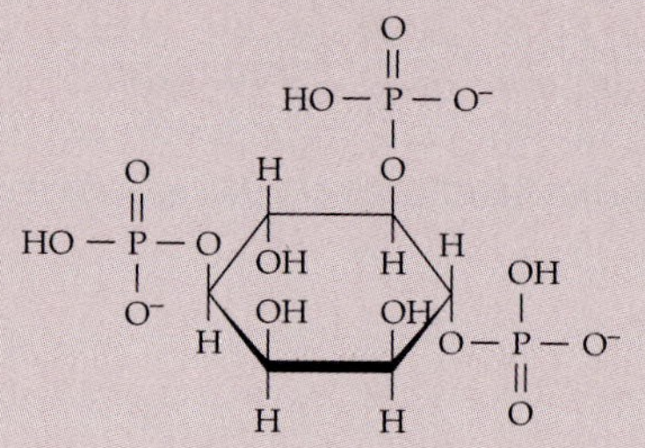

Inositol 1,4,5-trisphosphate (IP_3)

The production and mechanisms of action of these second messengers are illustrated in Figure 6.32. A number of different neurotransmitter receptors (including cholinergic muscarinic, α-adrenergic, 5-HT_2 serotonergic, and metabotropic glutamate receptors) and neuropeptide receptors (including vasopressin, substance P, and cholecystokinin receptors), as well as photic stimuli in photoreceptors and odorant stimuli in olfactory receptors, are coupled to G proteins that stimulate the $\beta 1$ isozyme of phospholipase C (PLC). (Isozymes are distinct molecular forms of an enzyme that may vary in substrate specificity, regulatory mechanisms, and other important properties.) As shown in the figure, a second PLC isozyme (PLC-$\gamma 1$) can be activated by receptor tyrosine kinases (see above). PLC is a general type of membrane enzyme that hydrolyzes the phosphate ester bond of phospholipids. Because the $\beta 1$ and $\gamma 1$ isozymes are relatively selective for polyphosphoinositides, they are sometimes called phosphoinositidases. When these enzymes act on PIP_2 in the cell membrane, they cleave the phospholipid into IP_3 and DAG, each of which has a distinct second messenger function.

Due to its strong electrical charge and its resulting poor lipid solubility, IP_3 leaves the plasma membrane and enters the cytoplasm of the cell, where it binds to a specific receptor on the membrane of the ER and stimulates the release of Ca^{2+} ions from the ER storage compartment. The increased levels of Ca^{2+} (which might be considered a third messenger in this context!) may then activate a number of Ca^{2+}-dependent functions in the cell, including those involving the participation of calmodulin.

The other second messenger, DAG, remains in the membrane, where it plays an important role in stimulating the activity of protein kinase C (PKC). PKC represents a family of enzymes activated by certain membrane lipids. Some PKC isozymes (α, β, and γ) are also Ca^{2+}-dependent, and these will be the focus of the remaining discussion. Prior to cell stimulation, PKC is found in an inactive state in the cytoplasm. When the intracellular Ca^{2+} concentration is raised by the mobilizing effects of IP_3 and/or by the opening of membrane Ca^{2+} channels, the kinase translocates to the cell membrane. There it is activated by binding to phospholipids (preferentially phosphatidylserine) in a Ca^{2+}-dependent manner. Furthermore, such binding is strongly stimulated by DAG, which is therefore necessary for full activation of the enzyme (Huang and Huang, 1993; Tanaka and Nishizuka, 1994). The synergistic action of IP_3/Ca^{2+} and DAG in stimulating PKC activity is certainly one of the interesting features of this second messenger system. DAG stimulation of PKC is terminated by metabolism of the compound and eventual resynthesis of PIP_2. However, PKC can be persistently activated by a group of compounds called phorbol esters, which mimic the effects of DAG but with a greater potency and slower rate of metabolism. Phorbol 12-myristate 13-acetate (PMA) is one example of a phorbol ester. These compounds have been extremely useful in studying the relationship between polyphosphoinositides and PKC regulation.

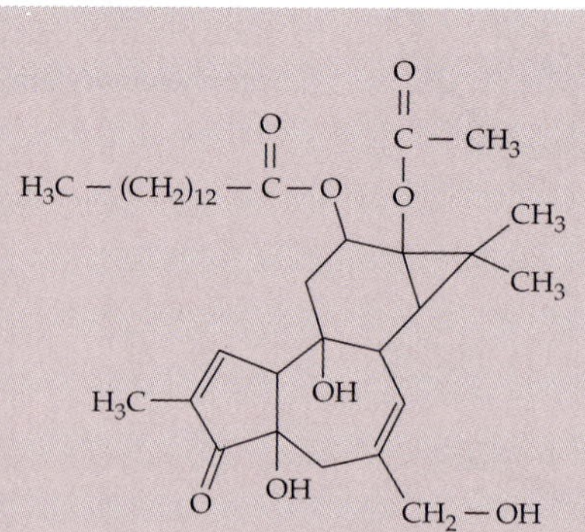

PMA

Many important neural proteins are substrates for PKC. Ion channels subject to PKC phosphorylation include voltage-gated Na^+ channels, Ca^{2+}-dependent K^+ channels, nicotinic receptors, $GABA_A$ receptors, and

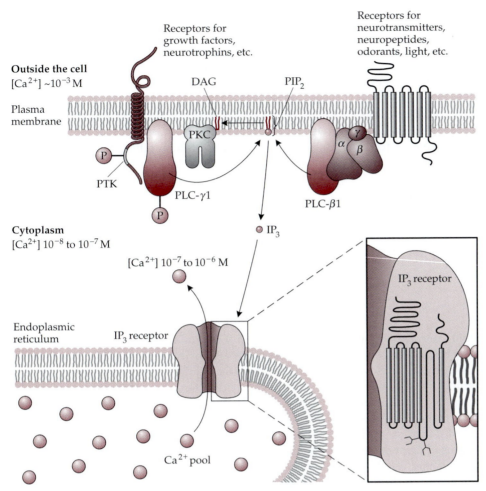

6.32 FORMATION AND ACTION OF SECOND MESSENGERS DERIVED FROM PIP_2. PIP_2 is a membrane phospholipid that can be hydrolyzed by two different forms of phospholipase C (PLC), one coupled to certain G proteins and the other activated by neurotrophin-stimulated protein tyrosine kinase (PTK) receptors. PIP_2 hydrolysis liberates two second messengers, diacylglycerol (DAG) and inositol trisphosphate (IP_3). DAG remains in the membrane, where it stimulates protein kinase C (PKC). IP_3 diffuses into the cytoplasm, where it releases Ca^{2+} from the endoplasmic reticulum by binding to a specific receptor on the ER membrane. The Ca^{2+} concentration is typically in the millimolar range (10^{-3} M) outside of the plasma membrane, but much lower (10^{-8}–10^{-7} M) in the cytoplasm. Release of Ca^{2+} from the ER can elevate intracellular concentration to a range (10^{-7}–10^{-6} M) that activates Ca^{2+}-dependent processes. (From Furuichi and Mikoshiba, 1995.)

NMDA receptors. Another interesting substrate is growth-associated protein 43 (GAP-43; also called protein B-50 or neuromodulin by some investigators). This protein is highly concentrated in growth cones in the developing nervous system and in nerve terminals in adult animals. Although the exact function of GAP-43 is still not known, it is thought to play multiple roles in neuronal development, plasticity, and possibly also transmitter release (Benfenati and Valtorta, 1993; Coggins and Zwiers, 1991). Indeed, several studies found enhanced phosphorylation of GAP-43 under conditions of heightened release.

It was noted earlier that CaM-K II can become stimulus-independent through a process of autophosphory-lation. To some extent, an analogous mechanism may occur with PKC. Prolonged stimulation of PKC appears to cause a temporary insertion of the enzyme into the plasma membrane that reduces its dependence on DAG and Ca^{2+} for activation (Huang and Huang, 1993).

Messenger Substances Related to Arachidonic Acid

Arachidonic acid (AA) is an unsaturated fatty acid commonly found in the 2-position of membrane phospholipids. It is readily liberated from these lipids by the action of phospholipase A_2, although it can also be generated through other mechanisms. Once released, AA can undergo an extremely complex series of metabolic reactions that result in the formation of many biologically active compounds. Figure 6.33 lists the major families of these AA derivatives, which collectively are referred to as **eicosanoids**. Eicosanoids can act as second messengers by influencing the cell in which they are formed, or they can subserve a first messenger function by diffusing to neighboring cells as NO does. Evidence has been accumulating suggesting that various eicosanoids may participate in both transmitter release and signal transduction mechanisms in some neuronal systems (reviewed by Shimizu and Wolfe, 1990).

$$H_2C \begin{cases} CH = CH - CH_2 - CH = CH - (CH_2)_3 - \overset{\displaystyle O}{\overset{\|}{C}} - OH \\ CH = CH - CH_2 - CH = CH - (CH_2)_3 - CH_3 \end{cases}$$

Arachidonic acid

Divergence and Convergence of Transmitter Action

Why do some cells exhibit a particular response to a given neurotransmitter or hormone, while other cells show a different response or none at all? In other cases, how do different transmitters stimulate the same response in a target cell? These phenomena are sometimes termed **divergence** and **convergence** of transmitter action, respectively (for example, see McCormick and Williamson, 1989). To account for instances of divergence or convergence, we must consider the mechanisms that underlie cellular responses to signaling agents. It should be clear from the information presented above that the response properties of a given cell depend upon its complement of receptors, G proteins, and effectors. To take an example of divergent responses, both liver cells and adipocytes (fat cells) possess β-adrenergic receptors coupled to G_s and to adenylyl cyclase. However, because the effector systems in these cells differ, the liver cells respond to epinephrine with a glycogenolytic response, whereas the adipocytes react by increasing their lipolytic (fat breakdown) activity. An example of response convergence is found in hippocampal pyramidal neurons,

which exhibit a K^+-mediated hyperpolarization following the application of either 5-HT or GABA. Evidence suggests that 5-HT_{1A} and $GABA_B$ receptors in the membranes of these cells are both coupled to the same pertussis toxin–sensitive G protein, which then activates an inward-rectifying K^+ channel in the membrane (Nicoll, 1988). In this case, therefore, response characteristics are determined by the possession of multiple receptor types coupled to the same G protein/effector mechanism.

Neurotransmitters and Gene Regulation in the Nervous System

The final topic to be covered in our discussion of neurotransmitter mechanisms is the regulation of gene activity. Endocrinologists have known for many years that certain hormones, such as gonadal and adrenal steroids, affect their target cells primarily by altering the transcription of various genes in those cells. Changes in gene transcription lead to alterations in the rates of synthesis or (less frequently) degradation of various cellular proteins. There is now growing evidence that neurotransmitters can similarly regulate gene expression, a process that may well be important in learning and memory as well as in long-lasting adaptive responses to drugs and other external agents.

Two phases of gene activation are triggered by synaptic input, as described by Armstrong and Montminy (1993). The initial phase is characterized by induction of **immediate–early genes** (**IEGs**; they are sometimes also called "early-response genes"). IEGs are usually expressed only at low levels in the absence of cellular excitation. When synaptic inputs are active, however, they are rapidly, though transiently, induced (e.g., mRNA levels may be significantly increased within 15 minutes, but remain elevated for only 30–60 minutes). Most IEGs code for nuclear proteins, several of which are discussed below.

The second phase of synaptic gene activation is the induction of "late-onset genes." As we shall see, these genes are slower to respond to stimulation because their

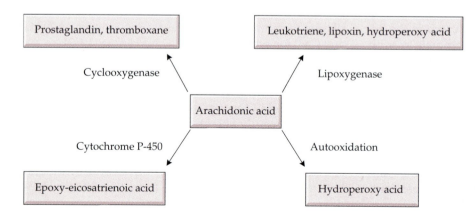

6.33 EICOSANOIDS THAT PARTICIPATE IN ARACHIDONIC ACID-MEDIATED SIGNALING. Following its release from membrane phospholipids, arachidonic acid (AA) is converted to a number of biologically active compounds by the enzymes cyclooxygenase, cytochrome P-450, and lipoxygenase. It can also be converted to hydroperoxy acid by nonenzymatic autooxidation. These compounds, which are collectively called eicosanoids, function as second or third messengers in AA signaling systems. (After Shimizu and Wolfe, 1990.)

induction is dependent on the action of IEG proteins. Although many important neuronal genes are undoubtedly subject to late-onset synaptic regulation, only a few examples have been well characterized. Among these are the genes for tyrosine hydroxylase and for several neuropeptides such as substance P (Armstrong and Montminy, 1993; also see Chapter 8 for further discussion).

Transcription factors and gene regulation. Neurotransmitters alter gene expression by means of a complex mechanism involving second messengers and a family of proteins known as **transcription factors**. Molecular biologists have known for some time that most genes contain several distinct regions with differing functions. One of these, obviously, is the coding region specifying the nucleotide sequence of the RNA transcribed from that gene. However, "upstream"* from the coding region is the so-called promoter region, within which are DNA sequences that serve as binding sites for transcription factors. Several broad families of transcription factors have been identified, with exotic names such as leucine-zipper, zinc-finger, and helix-loop-helix proteins, all of which refer to structural features that help mediate the interaction of the transcription factor with its DNA binding site (for more information, readers are advised to consult a contemporary biochemistry or molecular biology text such as Watson et al., 1992). The important point here is that binding of a transcription factor to a gene regulatory site either enhances or suppresses transcription of that gene.

As mentioned above, second messengers are linked with transcription factors in the neurotransmitter control of gene expression. For example, transcriptional activation by cAMP is mediated by a regulatory site in the promoter region called the cAMP response element (CRE), a short sequence of DNA containing only eight nucleotides (5'-TGACGTCA-3'). The first step, as illustrated in Figure 6.34, is cAMP formation and activation of PKA, as described earlier. In this case, however, some of the activated catalytic subunits of PKA enter the cell nucleus, where they phosphorylate a nuclear protein called cAMP response element binding protein (CREB) (Vallejo, 1994). CREB is a transcription factor that binds to the CRE, thereby enhancing transcription of the downstream gene. Interestingly, CREB can be phosphorylated by other kinases besides PKA, which allows multiple extracellular signaling pathways to converge on the same target gene(s) in a given cell (Figure 6.35).

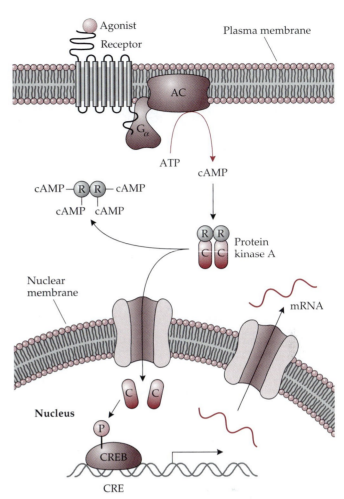

6.34 REGULATION OF GENE TRANSCRIPTION BY cAMP. Protein kinase A is activated as described in 6.28. After dissociating from the regulatory domains (R) of the enzyme, the catalytic subunits (C) are translocated into the cell nucleus, where they phosphorylate a transcription factor called cAMP response element binding protein (CREB). CREB stimulates transcription of target genes by binding to cAMP response elements (CREs) in the promoter regions of those genes. (After Vallejo, 1994.)

Role of c-fos *and other IEGs.* Transcription factors often function in a cascade. Thus, CREB and various other transcription factors induce a group of IEGs that includes *c-fos, fos B, c-jun, jun B, zif-268,* and others (Morgan and Curran, 1989a; Sagar and Sharp, 1993). The products of these IEGs are themselves transcription factors that play important roles in neuronal gene regulation. We will focus on the Fos and Jun families, which are among the best characterized IEGs.

The IEG *c-fos* is a **proto-oncogene**, which means that it is the normal cellular counterpart of a related gene that is present in certain cancer-causing viruses. The transcription factor encoded by the *c-fos* gene is called Fos. Its location and regulation in the brain have been studied using a variety of techniques, including immunohistochemistry for Fos protein and either Northern blotting or

---

*The linear sequence of a DNA strand is conventionally depicted with the 5'-end to the left and the 3'-end to the right. RNA transcription correspondingly proceeds in the 5'- to 3'- direction. If one region of DNA is located closer than another to the 5'-end of the strand, it is termed "upstream" from the second region. Conversely, a region located closer to the 3'-end is termed "downstream."

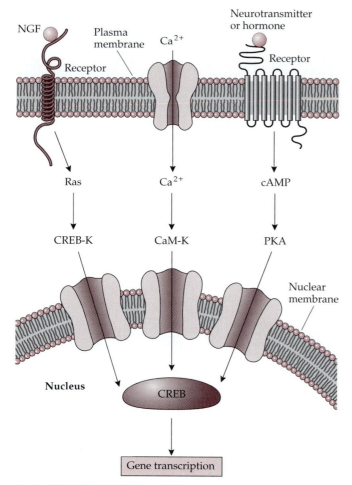

6.35 CONVERGENCE OF MULTIPLE SIGNALING PATHWAYS ON CREB. CREB is phosphorylated not only by cAMP-dependent protein kinase (PKA), but also by CaM kinases (CaM-K) and by a specific CREB kinase (CREB-K). CREB-K is activated by the action of certain growth factors, such as nerve growth factor (NGF), on their membrane receptors. The growth factor pathway is dependent on an intermediary guanyl nucleotide–binding protein known as Ras. (After Vallejo, 1994.)

in situ hybridization histochemistry for *c-fos* mRNA. As is the case for IEGs generally, levels of Fos protein and *c-fos* mRNA in most neurons are low in the absence of stimulation. However, stimuli that increase the appropriate second messengers (e.g., cAMP or Ca^{2+}) can rapidly induce Fos expression through the action of CREB and several other transcription factors known to participate in *c-fos* gene regulation. Depending on the neuronal population under investigation, such stimuli may be environmental or pharmacological. In this way, *c-fos* and other IEGs can serve as markers of neuronal activation (Morgan and Curran, 1989; Sagar and Sharp, 1993). Other research suggests that IEGs may play an important role in mechanisms of neural plasticity and learning (Abraham, Dragunow, and Tate, 1991).

The mechanism of action of Fos is shown in Figure 6.36. Fos, Jun (which is the product of another proto-

oncogene called *c-jun*), and related proteins belong to the leucine-zipper family of transcription factors. The leucine-zipper structure allows Fos and Jun to bind together to form a heterodimer (a unit made up of two different proteins) that binds to a DNA regulatory sequence known as AP-1. Dimers can also be formed by several related proteins within the Fos and Jun families such as Jun-B and Fra-1 (Fos-related antigen-1). Like CRE, the activated AP-1 site then stimulates transcription of the downstream gene. Figure 6.37 presents a simplified summary of the overall sequence of events, beginning with receptor activation and culminating in the modulation of target genes in the cell. As shown in the figure, as many as four different levels of messengers may participate in this process.

Fos expression has been of particular interest to neuropharmacologists because of its sensitivity to many different drugs. Fos induction in particular brain regions has been reported in response to amphetamine and cocaine (Graybiel, Moratalla, and Robertson, 1990), neuroleptic drugs such as haloperidol (Dragunow et al., 1990), morphine (Liu, Nickolenko, and Sharp, 1994), caffeine (Nakajima et al., 1989), nicotine (Kiba and Jayaraman, 1994), and tetrahydrocannabinol (THC), the active ingredient of marijuana (Mailleux et al., 1994). In the striatum, dopamine D_1 receptor-mediated CREB phosphorylation seems to play an important role in the Fos response to amphetamine (Konradi et al., 1994). Fos and other IEG proteins are therefore useful tools in helping us to understand the mechanisms of drug and neurotransmitter regulation of gene expression in the nervous system.

Termination of Transmitter Action

Each action potential is a discrete event having the capability of provoking transmitter release from nerve endings. If the process of synaptic transmission is to follow, there must be some mechanism for terminating the postsynaptic signal generated by the previous release event. To some extent, transmitter molecules can simply diffuse away from their receptor sites in the synaptic cleft. However, it is unlikely that such a passive process could serve as the sole mechanism of signal termination. Instead, there are two basic types of active processes that affect the availability of transmitter molecules to receptors, thereby regulating the time course of synaptic activity. One of these mechanisms is enzymatic degradation of the transmitter. Although catabolic processes occur for all neurotransmitters, such processes are most important for actual signal termination in the cases of ACh (particularly well studied at the neuromuscular junction) and the neuropeptide transmitters (see Chapters 7 and 11).

The other important mechanism is clearance from the extracellular space by active uptake processes. Cellular uptake of neurotransmitters is mediated by plasma

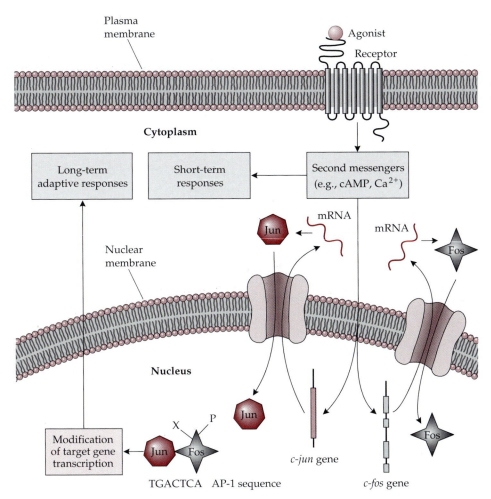

6.36 REGULATION OF GENE TRAN-SCRIPTION BY IMMEDIATE–EARLY GENES. Second messengers such as cAMP and Ca^{2+} stimulate IEGs such as *c-fos* and *c-jun*. The corresponding proteins, Fos and Jun, are synthesized in the cell cytoplasm and then translocated to the nucleus. Fos, Jun, and several related proteins form dimers that bind to the AP-1 sequence of target genes, thus altering the transcriptional activity of those genes. (After Morgan and Curran, 1989a.)

membrane proteins known as transporters (see Chapter 3). The neurotransmitter may be taken up into the cell that originally released it (often called "reuptake"), into other nerve cells, or sometimes into nearby glial cells (specifically astrocytes). Evidence for a neuronal uptake mechanism was found during the pioneering work of Axelrod and his colleages on the transmitter characteristics of NE (Axelrod, 1971). They discovered that intravenous injection of radioactive (tritiated) norepinephrine ([^{3}H]NE) into cats was followed by a rapid but unequal distribution of this substance in the tissues. Relatively little was found in brain tissue, suggesting that the blood–brain barrier prevented the transfer of NE from the bloodstream to brain tissue. On the other hand, [^{3}H]NE was selectively taken up by sympathetic nerve endings on cardiac muscle, the spleen, and other organs that receive a heavy sympathetic innervation. Also, when the tissues were examined 2 hours after the injection of [^{3}H]NE, they had almost the same level of NE as that found in subjects that had been sacrificed only 2 minutes after the injection. This finding showed that NE was rapidly taken up by sympathetic nerve terminals and then sequestered in some way to prevent its metab-

olism (presumably repackaged into synaptic vesicles). The uptake mechanism was found to be an active Na^+- and K^+-dependent transport system that can take up NE against concentration gradients as high as 10,000:1.

Much subsequent research has shown that uptake plays an important role in transmitter inactivation, not only for NE but also for DA, 5-HT, and amino acid transmitters such as glutamate, GABA, and glycine. As we shall see in subsequent chapters, different transporters have evolved for each of these neurotransmitters. However, most of them function by means of the same type of mechanism first discovered for the NE transporter by Axelrod's group.

Autoreceptors and Heteroreceptors

In our descriptions of synapses, we have usually indicated that neurotransmitters exert their chemical effects on receptors situated on the postsynaptic membranes of adjacent neurons or cells of glands and muscles. However, it is now well known that receptors on the cell's own axon terminals are responsive to the cell's own transmitter; these kinds of receptors also exist on the

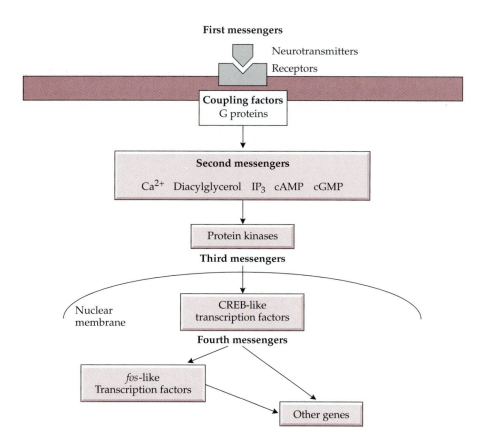

First messengers

Neurotransmitters

Receptors

Coupling factors
G proteins

Second messengers

Ca²⁺   Diacylglycerol   IP₃   cAMP   cGMP

Protein kinases

Third messengers

Nuclear
membrane

CREB-like
transcription factors

Fourth messengers

fos-like
Transcription factors

Other genes

6.37 SUMMARY OF TRANSCRIPTIONAL REGULATION BY NEUROTRANSMITTERS. This diagram summarizes the overall biochemical cascade by which neurotransmitters and other first messenger substances alter gene transcription in the nervous system. (After Hyman and Nestler, 1993.)

membrane of the soma and its dendrites. The term **autoreceptors** was coined by Carlsson (1975a) to define receptors that respond to the neuron's own neurotransmitter, regardless of their location at a given synapse. The first autoreceptor discovered was the α₂-adrenoceptor, which was found to inhibit NE release from sympathetic nerve endings. Many subsequent studies have shown that autoreceptors for various transmitters are widely distributed in both CNS and peripheral nerve tissues (for review, see Starke, Göthert, and Kilbinger, 1989).

The term "presynaptic autoreceptor" signifies a receptor on an axon terminal through which the neuron's own transmitter can influence terminal function. Presynaptic autoreceptors are usually characterized as exerting an inhibitory effect on transmitter release, although they may also suppress local transmitter synthesis. Release inhibition has been linked with inhibition of action potential-evoked Ca²⁺ influx into the nerve terminals (e.g., Mulder et al., 1984) and with enhanced K⁺ efflux from the terminals (Billingsley, Galloway, and Roth, 1984). Autoreceptors on the cell body and/or dendrites are termed "somadendritic," or "somatodendritic," autoreceptors. Somatodendritic autoreceptors can be activated by transmitter released either from recurrent axon collaterals or from the soma and dendrites themselves. These autoreceptors function differently from presynaptic autoreceptors in that they inhibit the rate of cell firing. Of course, a secondary consequence of a lower firing rate

is reduced transmitter release at the terminals, so overall neurotransmission is diminished in both cases.

Autoreceptors can be thought of as serving a negative feedback function in neuronal regulation. That is, when there is a high concentration of a neurotransmitter in the synaptic cleft, autoreceptor activation may lead to down-regulation of release and/or synthesis so that postsynaptic receptor sites are not overstimulated. Alternatively, autoreceptor activation is minimal when cells are quiescent, thereby allowing release to occur when the cells subsequently receive excitatory afferent input.

Although we usually think of agonist or antagonist drugs as affecting postsynaptic receptors, autoreceptors are also important targets of drug action. For example, very low doses of clonidine exert a sedative effect in rodents that may be due to stimulation of α₂-adrenoceptors on noradrenergic neurons of the locus coeruleus. Another example comes from the DA system, in which certain compounds (e.g., apomorphine) seem to have a higher affinity for presynaptic autoreceptors than for the postsynaptic DA receptors. Consequently, very low doses of such compounds diminish dopaminergic neurotransmission by selectively activating autoreceptors, whereas somewhat higher doses stimulate dopaminergic functions by acting directly on the postsynaptic receptors (for further discussion, see Chapter 8). Finally, it should be mentioned that, like postsynaptic receptors, autoreceptors can exhibit sensitization or desensitization in response to persistent antagonist or agonist stimulation. Indeed, the delayed therapeutic response to 5-HT-selective antidepressants such as fluoxetine (Prozac) may be related to the time needed for 5-HT autoreceptors to desensitize in response to drug treatment (Blier and de Montigny, 1994).

Whereas autoreceptors on a nerve terminal are receptors for the neurotransmitter released by that cell, one may also find presynaptic receptors for other transmitters. Such receptors are called **heteroreceptors** to distinguish them from autoreceptors. Unlike autoreceptors, which are usually inhibitory, heteroreceptors may either inhibit or stimulate transmitter release. Many examples of heteroreceptors have now been identified (see Kalsner and Westfall, 1990), suggesting that local modulation of transmitter release (i.e., at the synapse) may, in some cases, be as important as modulation via traditional axodendritic and axosomatic synaptic connections.

Synaptic Plasticity

Reflexive and Instinctive Behaviors

The nervous system is designed to mediate the adaptation of organisms to environmental changes as well as to changes within the organism. Many responses are carried out reflexively via genetically determined "prewired" circuits; examples include the knee-jerk, eyeblink, and startle reflexes, patterns of emotional expression, salivation to the smell of food, and the various forms of locomotion. Other responses, such as sexual activity, migration, and hibernation, are also "prewired" but are activated periodically. For example, during hormone-induced estrus, a female rat will display lordosis, the copulatory stance of arching her back and moving her tail to one side, when a male rat mounts her and grasps her flanks. During anestrus, the female will generally fight off a mounting male. It has been proposed that most, if not all, of these behaviors occur because of changes in the neural circuitry brought on by the periodic release of hormones. This proposal is supported by the finding that estrogens, gonadal hormones that elicit

lordosis in female rats, are taken up by cells in the brain that directly control this behavior. Evidence that the sexual response is governed by those cells was supplied by the rapid occurrence of lordosis when small amounts of estrogens were injected directly into a cluster of those cells in ovariectomized rats (McEwen et al., 1979; McEwen, 1980).

Many recent studies have supplied more direct evidence that hormones exert their effects by directly modifying synaptic morphology. For example, there are clusters of motor neuron cell bodies in the spinal cord of the male rat that take up androgens (e.g., testosterone) and whose axons innervate the left and right bulbocavernosus muscles, which are exclusively attached to the penis and control it during copulation. These cell bodies are designated the spinal nucleus of the bulbocavernosus (SNB). The SNB was identified by injecting HRP directly into the bulbocavernosus muscle, where it was taken up by the nerve terminals and transported by retrograde axoplasmic flow to the SNB in the spinal cord, where it could be revealed by special staining for HRP.

The lengths and distributions of the dendritic trees from HRP-containing SNB cells were compared among normal rats, rats that were castrated 6 weeks before HRP injection, and castrated rats that had received testosterone during the 6-week waiting period. The study also included control groups that were sham-operated and received placebos instead of testosterone. As shown in Figure 6.38, it was found that the SNB dendritic tree from a rat 6 weeks after castration was reduced by 56% compared with that from a normal rat, and that this effect was completely reversed if a castrated rat was given 4 weeks of testosterone treatment (Kurz, Sengelaub, and Arnold, 1986). These findings illustrate the effect of testosterone on the plasticity of neurons intimately related to sexual activity.

Other studies investigated the effect of sex hormones on cell groupings in the brain associated with bird song (Arnold, 1985; Arnold et al., 1987). These studies for the most part were done with male birds because in most species only males sing; in those species in which females

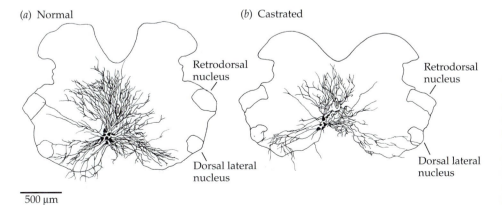

(a) Normal   (b) Castrated

Retrodorsal nucleus

Dorsal lateral nucleus

500 μm

6.38 ANDROGEN-INDUCED SYNAPTIC MODIFICATION. Camera lucida composites of HRP-labeled dendritic trees and left spinal nuclei of the bulbocavernosus (SNB) of a normal male rat (a) and a castrated male (b). Motoneuronal somata (dark bodies) are shown to indicate the location of the SNB. Scale bar = 500 μm. (After Kurz, Sengelaub, and Arnold, 1986.)

sing, most of them sing less than males and have less complicated songs. Learning plays a role in singing, as evidenced by the absence of singing in birds that were deafened before they began to sing. Among songbird species, the neuron clusters in the song systems in the brain are larger in male birds than in females, and the difference is inversely proportional to the singing behavior of the female; that is, the male–female difference is large in species in which the female sings little or not at all, and small in species in which the female sings almost as much as the male. The volume of the cell groups is determined by the size and number of the cells and their axons and the size of the dendritic trees.

That hormone-induced synaptic plasticity is a significant determinant of bird song is borne out by the following evidence:

1. The neurons that constitute much of the song system take up and bind androgens (testosterone).
2. Castrated male birds stop singing, and singing resumes after treatment with androgens. Treating female birds with androgens causes some of them to sing, but the songs differ from those of males and are much simpler. However, androgen treatment of females from some species causes significant increases in their song systems, and the birds sing well-developed songs.
3. In the spring, when androgen levels are high, the volume of male song systems increases by as much as 77% to 99%, singing increases, and more syllables are added to the song. In fall and winter, when androgen levels are low, the song systems decline in size due to dendritic shortening and loss of synapses. These changes result in diminished vocal motor coordination, very little singing, and the dropping of syllables from the song.

This evidence indicates that the uptake of androgens stimulates dendritic growth, which promotes singing and facilitates the acquisition of new motor patterns and new auditory–motor integrations that are needed for the learning and elaboration of songs. Thus, four variables covary with the seasons: androgen levels, size of brain centers and their synapses associated with bird song, amount of singing, and the complexity of the song that is sung. The periodicity of singing by songbirds is an expression of behavior determined by seasonal changes; for example, more daylight causes increased hormone synthesis and release, and thus synaptic modifications in the brain. (See Cotman, 1985, for a review.)

Learning

Yet another category of behavior consists of conditioned responses to environmental stimuli encountered during the experiences of the organism, which, of course, is learning. It is to be emphasized that learning basically is a genetically determined mechanism whereby a response that has a favorable outcome is likely to be repeated, and this mechanism is just as surely traceable to neurochemical events as any other behavioral mechanism (Skinner, 1966, 1981; Thompson, 1986; Black et al., 1987).

Most responses that occur do not fall easily into one of the three somewhat arbitrarily defined categories of reflexes, instinctual responses, and learned behaviors. Rather, responses that seem to fit best in one category are most often influenced by mechanisms in each of the other categories, so it is almost impossible to say for a given response what determinants are foremost. For example, crying may be a response to the word "No" from the mother rather than to physical discomfort, salivation may occur at the thought of a favorite restaurant, and running can be made more efficient by training and practice. Thus, neurally mediated adaptation to the environment occurs via "prewired" circuits, circuits periodically activated by hormonal influences, and learning, which is the establishment of new circuits or the modification of old ones. All of these factors interact with one another to a lesser or greater extent depending upon the phyletic level of the organism.

The most extraordinary feat of all surely is human articulate speech. It embodies intricate circuits that manipulate the vocal apparatus, a short-term memory that stores what was just said or heard, and a long-term memory of virtually limitless capacity for words, written or spoken, with all their synonyms, antonyms, homonyms, homophones (to, two, and too), rules for plurals, metaphors, idioms, slang, spelling, pronunciation, and so on. Considered as an information processing system, language for the communicator involves the taking of a complex web of ideas, feelings, and associations and reducing it to a string of words, which are articulated in a linear fashion to a listener, who recognizes individual words, classifies them as parts of speech ("can" as a noun or verb), determines the grammatical role each word is playing (subject or object, verb or adjective), links the words into phrases, clauses, and sentences, keeps track of pronouns and what they refer to, and follows chains of inference—all simultaneously (see Waldrop, 1987). This process, characteristic of all humans, is the capstone of reflex, prewired circuitry, and an ever-expanding learned memory, all of which seems to be possible because of the stability and the plasticity of synapses.

Mechanisms of Synaptic Plasticity

Synaptic plasticity and learning.   Over the lifetimes of higher forms, such as mammals and especially humans, reflexes and instincts are continually overlaid by learning, indicating that the nervous systems of these animals have an enormous capacity for continued modification. The current view is that these changes are the result of

(a)

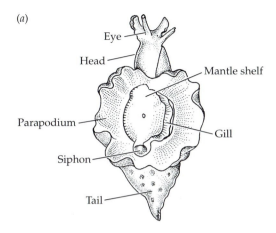

(b)

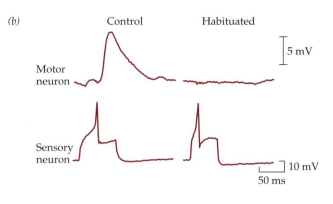

(c)

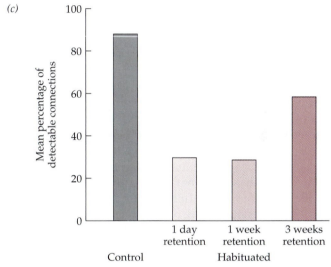

6.39 LONG-TERM HABITUATION. (*a*) A dorsal view of *Aplysia*. The parapodia have been peeled back to partially expose the mantle, gill, and siphon. (*b*) A comparison of synaptic potentials in a siphon sensory neuron and a gill motor neuron in a control (untrained) animal and in an animal subjected to long-term habituation, recorded 1 week after training. The synaptic potential in the motor neuron is still undetectable in the habituated animal. (*c*) The mean percentages of detectable connections in habituated animals at several time intervals after long-term habituation training. (After Kandel, 1991b.)

synaptic plasticity, as already mentioned above. This view has been buttressed by a wealth of findings obtained in studies of the CNS in very simple invertebrate organisms, whose limited behavioral repertoire can be linked to specific neural systems.

One of the most valuable models for studying synaptic mechanisms of learning is the sea slug *Aplysia*. Early studies by Bailey and Chen (1983) demonstrated that novel but innocuous tactile stimuli applied to the tail or siphon of *Aplysia* instantly led to gill withdrawal, but that after repeated trials, the behavioral effect disappeared. This decrease in behavioral response, which is called **habituation**, was still present to some degree 3 weeks later (Figure 6.39). This finding suggested that the synaptic connections between the sensory and motor nerves had lost their efficacy. In other tests, tactile stimuli applied to the siphon were preceded by a brief shock to the tail. Thereafter, the tactile stimuli by themselves elicited strong withdrawal effects of significantly longer duration, an effect known as **sensitization** (Figure 6.40). This finding suggested that the sensory–motor synapses had been strengthened. Staining the neurons involved in these phenomena with HRP and examining the synaptic terminals with an electron microscope revealed that the cells of habituated animals had fewer, and that those of sensitized animals had more, presynaptic terminals than those of control animals (Figure 6.41). Thus, whereas cell growth is characteristic of increased synaptic sensitivity, the opposite is true of long-term habituation, in which there is neuronal regression and pruning of as many as a third of the synaptic terminals per neuron.

Because *Aplysia* has such a primitive nervous system, the individual neurons involved in sensitization have been identified and studied. Kandel and coworkers (Kandel, 1976; 1979; Kandel and Schwartz, 1982; Kandel et al., 1987) found that noxious stimulation of the tail causes specific interneurons to release 5-HT from axoaxonic synapses on the presynaptic endings of sensory neurons. The transmitter activates a cascade of adenylyl cyclase and cAMP-dependent protein kinase. The resulting phosphorylation of K^+ channels in the terminals inhibits channel opening, thereby slowing repolarization of the membrane after action potentials have occurred. This reduced rate of repolarization allows more Ca^{2+} to enter the terminals, thereby increasing transmitter release from the sensory neurons and increasing the sensitivity of the reflexive circuit. Also, cAMP has another effect: it activates a protein kinase that mobilizes more of the transmitter, thus maintaining the increased level of transmitter release. These findings were further supported in a study demonstrating enhanced transmitter release from individual sensory neurons following sensitization training (Dale, Schacher, and Kandel, 1988). Thus, learning and memory are now, to some extent, understood as an increase in synaptic efficiency, a concept that squares with other examples of neural plasticity.

6.40 LONG-TERM SENSITIZATION. (*a*) Synaptic potentials in an *Aplysia* siphon sensory neuron and a gill motor neuron in a control animal and in an an animal that received long-term sensitization training, recorded 1 day after the end of training. (*b*) Group data for animals receiving long-term sensitization training, illustrating median time to siphon withdrawal for the control and experimental groups. (Pre = score before training; Post = score after training.) The experimental group was tested 1 day after the end of training. (*c*) Median values of the synaptic potential from siphon sensory neuron to gill motor neuron for the control group and for sensitized animals 1 day after the end of training. (After Kandel, 1991b.)

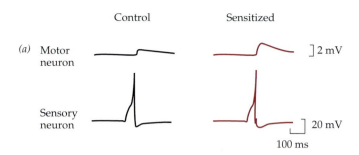

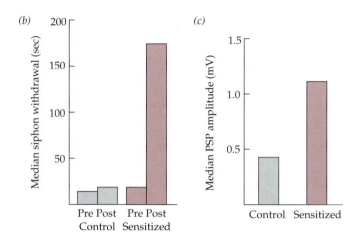

The potential role of synaptic plasticity in behavioral flexibility is best exemplified in the human nervous system, which contains an estimated 10^{11} neurons, each possessing approximately 10^4 interconnections. While many of the connections (synapses) are probably immutable, only a small fraction would need to be temporarily or permanently modifiable to ensure that expansion of the behavioral repertoire by learning could never outgrow the system's capacity for information storage.

Synaptic loss and remodeling. For many years the accepted view has been that there is no neuronal division in the CNS, and thus, after an injury, disease, or normal attrition, lost neurons are not replaced, although glia do reproduce. It is also true that nerve tracts in the CNS that are severed or severely injured do not repair themselves, although this does occur in peripheral nerves if the severed ends can be brought together. Now, however, there is a growing body of evidence that the loss of function following substantial neuron loss or denervation can be at least partially reversed through synaptic changes that occur naturally, or that can be induced either by chemical means or by transplantation of neural tissue.

Research over a number of years has demonstrated that cell loss from lesions or disease can be compensated by transplanting fetal tissue close to the receptors that would normally be innervated by the lost cells. The transplanted cells may either form synapses with the target cells or help to restore function by releasing neurotransmitters or trophic factors that diffuse to their sites of action (see Cotman and Nieto-Sampedro, 1984; and Cotman, 1985 for reviews). Survival of a transplant depends on the characteristics of the transplanted tissue as

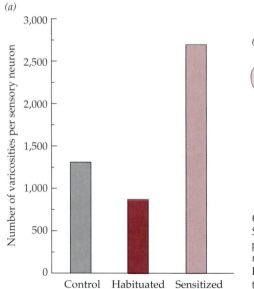

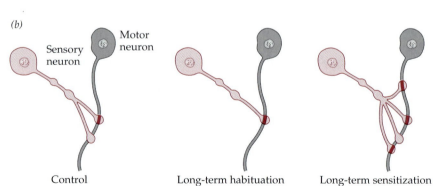

6.41 LONG-TERM HABITUATION AND SENSITIZATION ARE ACCOMPANIED BY STRUCTURAL CHANGES in the presynaptic terminals of sensory neurons. (*a*) Comparisons of structural features among control, habituated, and sensitized *Aplysia*. The number of presynaptic terminal varicosities is highest among sensitized animals. (*b*) Long-term habituation leads to a loss of synapses, and long-term sensitization leads to their increase. (After Kandel, 1991b.)

well as on the area of the brain in which it is placed (Bohn, 1987). Specific instances of this therapeutic approach will be described in the discussion of Parkinson's and Alzheimer's diseases in Chapter 20.

Perhaps equally dramatic is the finding that synaptic remodeling is a naturally occurring phenomenon in the mature nervous system. As the nervous system is constantly engaged in information processing, synaptic turnover is probably an ongoing process, even in the absence of injury or experimental intervention (Wolff et al., 1995). Even peripheral neurons that are not usually considered to be involved in learning mechanisms may undergo synaptic remodeling over time. This has been shown in an elegant series of studies by Purves and his colleagues, who directly imaged changes in the synaptic connectivity of individual autonomic ganglion cells in adult mice (Purves, Voyvodic, and Yawo, 1987). Specifically, the investigators studied the parasympathetic ganglia lying on the salivary glands, which are easily accessible for visual examination. The ganglion cells receive innervation from cranial parasympathetic nerves (VII and IX) and, via very short axons, activate the gland cells to secrete saliva. Under anesthesia, the glands were exposed, and the presynaptic terminals on the ganglionic neurons were stained and photographed. After intervals of 1 hour, 1 week, and 3 weeks, the glands were reexposed, and the terminals of the same cells were again stained and photographed. Comparisons between the original distribution of the terminals and the distribution after 1 hour showed little change; however, there were marked deviations after intervals of 1 and 3 weeks. This finding indicated that even in adult animals there is an ongoing rearrangement of interneuronal synapses in the nervous system (Purves, Voyvodic, and Yawo, 1987).

We have now seen examples of both structural and functional alterations in synaptic connectivity. Some of these changes may be induced by experience (i.e., learning), others by hormonal mechanisms, and still others cannot be traced to any specific stimulus. Such continuous synaptic remodeling may be critical in permitting expansion of the behavioral repertoire. Finally, synaptic reorganization is also an important adaptive response to injury or disease, although it is rarely able to fully compensate for the insult. However, the possibility that synaptic loss can be repaired by therapeutically inducing new synaptic connectivity has produced new hope for individuals suffering neurological damage.

Summary

Synaptic action is an intricate cascade of chemical events whereby sense organs, neurons, and effector organs communicate with one another. The language for most of these interactions is the frequency-modulated action potentials that are generated by the responses of sense organs, and then transferred from neuron to neuron or from neuron to effector organ at synaptic junctions. A stimulus–response event may involve only one synaptic step interposed between the sensory and the motor neurons, as in the case of a stretch reflex. More complicated reflexes, such as a cough or a sneeze, involve a bewildering array of tens of thousands or more synaptic connections that make an appropriate response possible.

In vertebrate nervous systems, synaptic transmission is largely a chemical process involving substances called neurotransmitters. A variety of transmitters have been characterized, ranging from small molecules such as amines and amino acids to moderately sized peptides. Neurotransmitter molecules are packaged into several different types of storage vesicles or granules, and are released into the synaptic cleft by a Ca^{2+}-dependent process of exocytosis. Because of the rapidity of this process, investigators now believe that transmitter release can occur only by means of a preformed releasing mechanism acting on vesicles that are already docked at release sites in the nerve terminal. Several vesicle and nerve terminal membrane proteins have recently been identified that may participate in various aspects of vesicle docking, membrane fusion, and the opening of a fusion pore to permit transmitter release. Evidence suggests that following exocytosis, vesicles are fairly rapidly recycled and become available for refilling with the neurotransmitter.

Despite the diversity of transmitter structure, all neurotransmitters function to influence the excitability of target cells (either postsynaptic neurons or effector organs) by somehow modulating the activity of ion channels and pumps in the cell membrane. The mechanisms underlying such modulation are related to the structural and functional features of the two neurotransmitter receptor superfamilies. Ligand-gated channel receptors contain an intrinsic channel that is rapidly opened in response to transmitter binding, whereas G protein–coupled receptors (GPCRs) activate G proteins in the membrane, which then stimulate various membrane effector proteins.

GPCRs sometimes directly influence channel gating without the intervention of any diffusible second messenger. Often, however, the membrane effectors are enzymes involved in second messenger synthesis or degradation. The major second messengers in the nervous system are cAMP, cGMP, Ca^{2+}, IP_3, and DAG (derived from the PI system), and possibly some of the metabolites of AA. Many actions of Ca^{2+} require the participation of calmodulin, an intracellular Ca^{2+}-binding protein. Also of interest is the gaseous messenger NO, which has been closely linked to cGMP in some systems due to its activating effect on the soluble form of guanylyl cyclase.

Most of the effects of second messenger substances occur through the activation of several protein kinases, notably PKA, PKG, CaM-K II, and PKC. Phosphorylation by these kinases alters the functioning of many different target proteins, including a number of voltage-gated channels, LGCs and GPCRs, ion pumps, enzymes, cytoskeletal proteins, and certain nuclear proteins, including transcription factors. Phosphatases are responsible for reversing these effects by causing protein dephosphorylation.

As we have seen, neurotransmitters do not merely cause rapid, short-term changes in postsynaptic activity. By means of second messengers and various transcription factors, they also give rise to longer-term changes in nerve cells by altering gene expression. Immediate-early genes like *c-fos* are of particular interest because they can serve as useful markers of neuronal activation, and also because their protein products (e.g., Fos protein) are themselves transcription factors that stimulate the expression of other genes involved in cellular functioning.

Following transmitter release, the signal is terminated either by enzymatic degradation of the transmitter (ACh and peptides) or by cellular uptake. Uptake can occur against a steep concentration gradient and is mediated by specific Na^+-dependent transporter proteins in the plasma membrane of neurons and sometimes also glial cells. When transmitter reuptake into the nerve terminal occurs, some of the transmitter reenters vesicles and is reutilized. Ultimately, transmitter molecules are catabolized by intracellular enzymes, after which the metabolic products enter the bloodstream to be cleared by the kidneys.

In addition to the usual postsynaptic receptor sites, many neurons possess autoreceptors on their somata, dendrites, and terminal membranes that respond to the cell's own transmitter. Some of these receptors initiate inhibitory feedback by reducing transmitter synthesis and release; others are activated by axon collaterals that regulate firing rates in the parent cell or in adjacent ones. Some autoreceptors seem to be pharmacologically distinguishable from postsynaptic receptors for that transmitter, thus allowing for the development of selective pharmacological agonists or antagonists. Also present are heteroreceptors, which are presynaptic release-modulating receptors that recognize a transmitter different from the one produced by that cell. Both autoreceptors and heteroreceptors are important regulators of synaptic activity.

Synaptic plasticity is a persistent ongoing characteristic of neurons that has a central role in behavioral modification. For example, hormones lead to the expansion of dendritic trees and form new synapses in special neuronal centers as illustrated by changes in bird behavior during springtime. The extra daylight increases sex hormone synthesis, which causes dendritic expansion in a certain brain center that is responsible for the onset and continuous expression of bird song. These changes are completely reversible when the hormonal influence abates. Learning can be defined as the result of experiences that overlay reflexes and instinctual behavior, and this, too, is traceable to the addition of new synaptic components to genetically determined ("prewired") circuits.

In higher vertebrates, new neurons do not replace neurons lost by attrition, accidents, or disease. However, many functions are maintained at least to some degree by the formation of new synaptic connections among surviving cells. Synaptogenesis can in some cases be instigated by chemical means, and grafting of embryonic tissue into some diseased areas will stimulate appropriate synapse formation and restore function. Advances in these techniques may prove to have important clinical significance.

Neurotransmitter Systems

Chapter 7

Acetylcholine

Although acetylcholine (ACh) was first synthesized in 1867, its biological importance was not known for many years thereafter. Nevertheless, as discussed in the previous chapter, ACh holds a central place in neuropharmacology because it was the first neurotransmitter to be identified. Dale (1914) noted that the effects of applying ACh mimicked the effects of stimulating parasympathetic nerves. This observation was followed by Loewi's (1921) famous studies demonstrating vagal release of a chemical substance that slowed the heart rate (though Loewi did not initially know that the substance involved was ACh). Finally, Dale and colleagues (1936) chemically identified ACh as the neurotransmitter at the skeletal neuromuscular junction. Despite these early discoveries, ACh proved to be a difficult compound to study, which resulted in comparatively slow progress for many years (Minz, 1955).*

In this chapter, we shall present a broad overview of **cholinergic** (the word "cholinergic" is the adjectival form of the term "acetylcholine") neurochemistry, pharmacology, anatomy, and function. In Part I, we shall introduce the chemistry of ACh synthesis and its control, followed by a consideration of ACh release, ACh catabolism, and the effects of drugs that alter these processes. In Part II, we shall discuss the anatomy and physiology of cholinergic systems, beginning with the distribution of central and peripheral (outside the CNS) pathways utilizing ACh as a transmitter. Knowing the anatomy of cholinergic neural systems provides important clues and insights into the neurochemical antecedents of the behavior that is controlled by these systems. Next, we shall describe the varieties of cholinergic receptors, their mechanisms of action within synapses and neuroeffector junctions, and the pharmacology of cholinergic receptor agonists and antagonists. Finally, in Part III, we shall discuss the role of ACh in several important behaviors.

Part I
Acetylcholine Neurochemistry: Synthesis, Storage, Release, and Inactivation

Acetylcholine is a small molecule with a relatively simple chemical structure. One of its noteworthy features is the positively charged nitrogen atom with four attached methyl groups. This nitrogen is termed a quaternary nitrogen, and ACh is thus classified as a **quaternary amine**. Many other neurotransmitters are also amines, although not usually of this type.

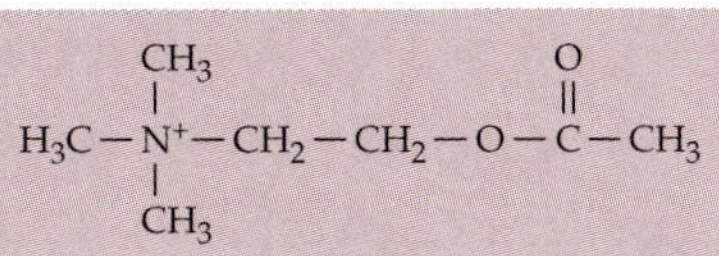

$$H_3C-\overset{\overset{\displaystyle CH_3}{|}}{\underset{\underset{\displaystyle CH_3}{|}}{N^+}}-CH_2-CH_2-O-\overset{\overset{\displaystyle O}{||}}{C}-CH_3$$

Acetylcholine

---

*Readers interested in learning more about the history of research on ACh are referred to the recent review by Karczmar (1993).

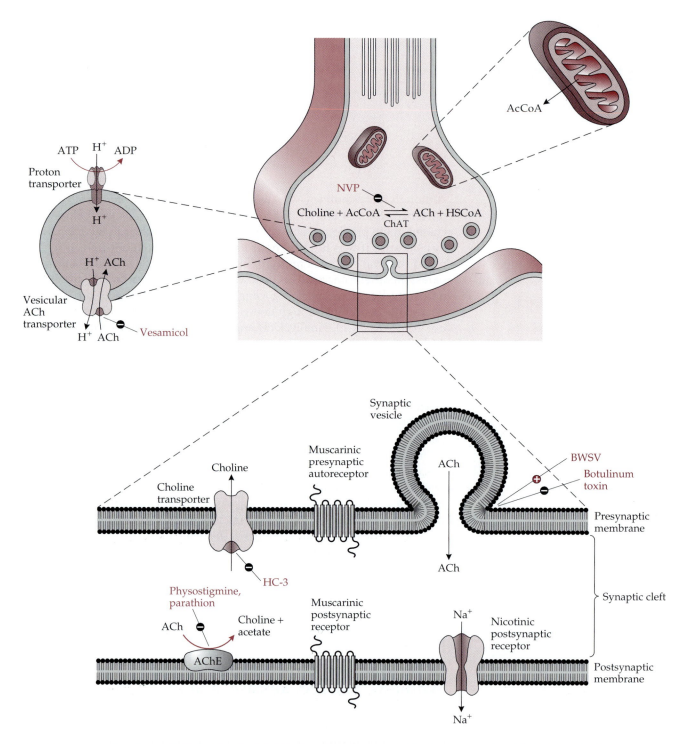

Receptor subtype	Agonists	Antagonists
Nicotinic	Nicotine, methylcarbachol, DMPP	D-Tubocurarine, gallamine, mecamylamine, hexamethonium
Muscarinic	Muscarine, pilocarpine, oxotremorine	Atropine, scopolamine, pirenzepine (M1-selective), AF-DX 116 (M2-selective)

7.1 THE CHOLINERGIC SYNAPSE illustrating the processes of acetylcholine (ACh) synthesis and metabolism, presynaptic choline uptake, and vesicular ACh uptake and release. Pre- and postsynaptic ACh receptors and sites of action of some cholinergic drugs are also shown. The table lists important cholinergic receptor agonists and antagonists. See the text for details and explanations of the abbreviations.

Figure 7.1 is a schematic diagram of a cholinergic neuron and synapse. It depicts the chemical processes of ACh synthesis, release, recapture, and metabolism, as well as the sites of action of some cholinergic drugs. Reference to this figure while reading the succeeding sections will facilitate understanding of the material.

Acetylcholine Synthesis

Choline Acetyltransferase

Acetylcholine is synthesized in a single reaction from the precursors **acetyl coenzyme A (acetyl CoA)** and **choline** (Figure 7.2). The reaction is reversible, although the equilibrium is strongly shifted to the right in favor of ACh formation. Acetylcholine synthesis is catalyzed by the enzyme **choline acetyltransferase (ChAT)**, which in the older literature was sometimes referred to as choline acetylase. Free coenzyme A (HS-CoA) is generated as a by-product of the reaction.

A number of nonneuronal sources of ChAT have been reported, including bacteria, certain plants, sperm cells, and placenta (for a review, see Salvaterra and Vaughn, 1989). However, within the nervous system, ChAT is considered to be a selective marker for cholinergic neurons. ChAT has proved to be a difficult enzyme to characterize, in part because of its low abundance. Most of the biochemical studies have suggested that ChAT is a globular protein with a single subunit and a molecular weight ranging from 67–75 kDa depending on the species (Salvaterra and Vaughn, 1989). The recent cloning of the rat ChAT gene (Hahn et al., 1992) should provide significant help in the further characterization of this enzyme. There is also evidence that ChAT can be phosphorylated, although researchers are just beginning to determine what role this process may play in the normal regulation of ACh synthesis (Rylett and Schmidt, 1993).

ChAT is synthesized in the rough endoplasmic reticulum of the perikaryon and transported via axoplasmic transport to the axon terminals. Following homogenization and differential centrifugation of cholinergic tissue, ChAT is found primarily in synaptosomes (pinched-off nerve endings; see Chapter 6). Most ChAT is thought to exist freely in the nerve terminal cytoplasm, although there is evidence for a small amount of membrane-bound enzyme that may or may not be physiologically important (reviewed by Wu and Hersh, 1994). The tissue concentration of ChAT in any particular region of the nervous system roughly parallels the density of ACh terminals in that region. Thus, there is a large concentration of the enzyme in the caudate nucleus and very little in the cerebellum (see Part II for the anatomy of central cholinergic systems). Also, the enzyme is abundant in ventral spinal roots, which contain the axons of cholinergic motor neurons, but there is very little in the dorsal sensory roots, which contain noncholinergic sensory axons. Consequently, one study showed a 450-fold difference in the ACh synthesis rate between the ventral and dorsal spinal roots: 10.8 versus 0.025 mg ACh formed per gram of tissue per hour (Marchbanks, 1975).

The Sources of Acetylcholine Precursors

Coenzyme A. Coenzyme A is found within mitochondria and contains the purine nucleotide base adenine, the vitamin pantothenic acid, and other chemical groups. The sulfhydryl group at the bottom of the hydrocarbon chain is the site of attachment of the acetyl group to form acetyl CoA.

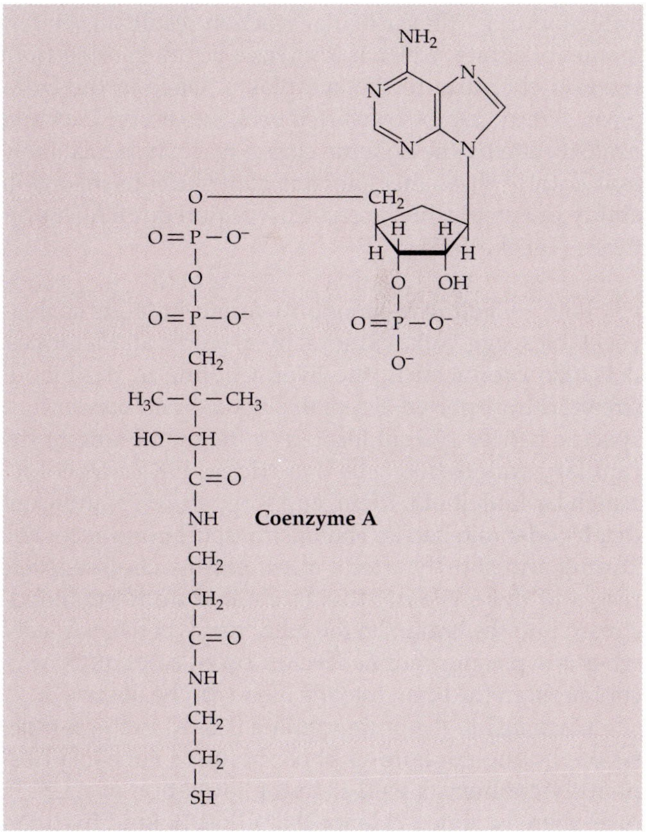

Coenzyme A

7.2 SYNTHESIS OF ACETYLCHOLINE.

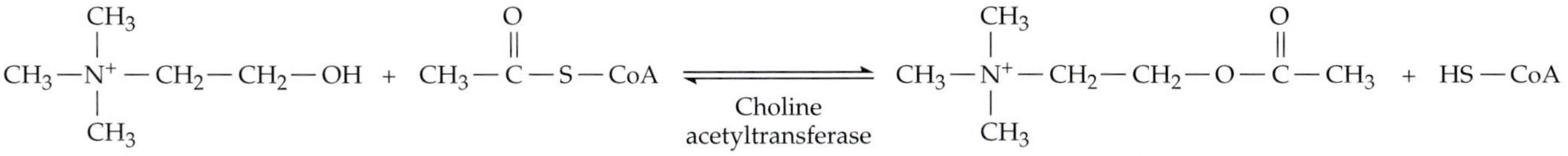

Acetyl CoA.   Acetyl CoA is synthesized mainly by the pyruvate dehydrogenase complex, which is located in the mitochondrial matrix of virtually all cells. Pyruvate, of course, is derived from the early stages of glucose catabolism, a process known as glycolysis. Most of the acetyl CoA generated from pyruvate feeds into the mitochondrial citric acid cycle (also called the tricarboxylic acid or Krebs cycle), which is the principal pathway by which energy (ATP) is generated aerobically from the metabolism of carbohydrates. In cholinergic neurons, some of the acetyl CoA must be transported across the mitochondrial membranes in order to participate in the formation of ACh; however, the mechanism of transport is still not well defined. One possibility is direct transmembrane passage of acetyl CoA to the cytoplasm. Although the inner mitochondrial membrane is generally considered to be impermeable to charged species as large as acetyl CoA, evidence exists for a Ca^{2+}-dependent mechanism that can stimulate the efflux of acetyl CoA from mitochondria (Benjamin and Quastel, 1981). Alternatively, acetyl groups can be transferred from acetyl CoA to acceptors such as oxaloacetate inside the mitochondria. This particular reaction results in the formation of citrate, which is known to be transported from the mitochondria to the cytoplasm. Once in the cytoplasm, citrate can be converted back into acetyl CoA and oxaloacetate by the enzyme citrate lyase. It seems likely that both of these mechanisms contribute to the availability of cytoplasmic acetyl CoA required for ACh synthesis (Tuček, 1985).

Choline.   Choline is commonly found in foods such as vegetables, egg yolk, kidneys, liver, seeds, and legumes. It is also produced in the liver. Choline in the bloodstream is transported across the blood–brain barrier by a specific carrier system located in the membrane of the capillary endothelial cells (Pardridge, 1984). Recent research by Löffelholz, Klein, and Köppen (1993) indicates that blood–brain barrier choline transport is bidirectional. During and shortly after a meal, plasma choline levels rise, and there is a net flux of choline from the bloodstream into the brain. On the other hand, between meals, when the plasma choline level is lower, a net outflow of choline from the brain into the blood can be observed.

Once inside the brain, choline is used in the synthesis of choline-containing phospholipids such as phosphatidylcholine, as well as in the formation of ACh. In turn, there is some evidence that phospholipid hydrolysis may contribute to the pool of choline used for ACh synthesis in cholinergic neurons (Blusztajn et al., 1987). Finally, a major source of choline for the synthesis of ACh comes from previously released ACh that has been degraded in the synaptic cleft by the enzyme acetylcholinesterase (see below). Cholinergic neurons possess a carrier-mediated, Na^+-dependent, high-affinity uptake mechanism for recapturing choline from the extracellular fluid (Yamamura and Snyder, 1973). This mechanism is estimated to recycle 35% to 50% of the liberated choline back into ACh synthesis. Some investigators have proposed that the high-affinity choline uptake process may be directly coupled to ACh synthesis; however, Tuček (1985) has argued against this hypothesis. Choline uptake also occurs via a low-affinity uptake mechanism. This system is present in all cells, including cholinergic neurons, and is presumed to supply choline for the synthesis of phospholipids.

Regulation of Acetylcholine Synthesis

Multiple factors are thought to be involved in the regulation of ACh synthesis, including (1) product inhibition, (2) mass action, (3) acetyl CoA and choline availability, and (4) neuronal activity (see Tuček, 1985; Salvaterra and Vaughn, 1989). These factors interact in complex ways, as we shall see in the following discussion.

First, several studies in the 1970s indicated that ChAT is subject to feedback or product inhibition (Salvaterra and Vaughn, 1989). That is, increasing concentrations of the reaction product, ACh, lead to a progressive inhibition of enzyme activity. This occurs by the following mechanism: Acetylcholine synthesis is activated by the binding of the substrates (acetyl CoA and choline) to the ChAT molecule. The product, ACh, also binds to ChAT, but at a different site from the substrates. Acetylcholine interaction with ChAT is thought to alter the three-dimensional conformation of the enzyme, thereby reducing its catalytic activity. The ACh binding site on the ChAT molecule is known as an **allosteric** site (Gr., "other space or site"). Allosteric mechanisms have likewise been found to operate with many other enzymes, including some other neurotransmitter-synthesizing enzymes.

Principles of mass action also pertain to the regulation of ACh synthesis. If we assume that the reaction catalyzed by ChAT is maintained close to its equilibrium position in cholinergic nerve terminals, then the law of mass action predicts that the concentration of ACh will depend on the amounts of the other reactants (i.e., choline, acetyl CoA, and coenzyme A) present in the nerve terminal. Consequently, the rate of ACh formation is sensitive to the concentrations of the precursors, such as choline. It is clear that high-affinity choline uptake is crucial for ACh synthesis, as drugs such as hemicholinium-3 that block this transport system strongly inhibit ACh formation (see below). Somewhat more controversial are studies attempting to enhance choline availability by administering exogenous choline either via injection or as dietary supplements. Although some studies have reported that acute treatment with choline elevates brain ACh, these findings have generally been obtained in animals previously subjected either to overall food restriction or to selective choline deprivation (Wecker, 1990). Nondeprived animals given supplemental choline generally do not show elevated brain ACh under "resting" conditions. However, choline administration has proved successful in preventing ACh depletion under various conditions of heightened ACh release. These observations have led to a model in which the level of ACh is normally maintained by a balance between ACh synthesis and ACh release (Wecker, 1990). When ACh release is stimulated, for example, by increased neuronal activity, synthesis may temporarily lag behind release, thus causing a depletion of ACh in the nerve terminal. Under these conditions, choline administration seems capable of enhancing ACh synthesis and reinstating normal concentrations of the neurotransmitter.

As just mentioned, stimulation of cholinergic cells may produce a temporary reduction in ACh levels. Yet even without choline supplementation, such activation stimulates ACh synthesis in an attempt to maintain adequate stores of the neurotransmitter. There are a number of possible mechanisms that might contribute to this response (Tuček, 1985). First, it is reasonable to assume that when synaptic release is accelerated, ACh will be transferred at an increasing rate from the cytoplasm (where it is synthesized by ChAT) to the vesicles. Given the reversibility of the synthetic reaction, the law of mass action dictates that a decrease in the concentration of ACh accessible to ChAT will drive the reaction to the right, that is, in the direction of enhanced ACh formation. Second, the maximum velocity (V_{max}) of the high-affinity choline uptake system is increased by neuronal activity (Rylett and Schmidt, 1993). Several different mechanisms have been hypothesized to account for this phenomenon, including stimulation of carrier efficiency, an increase in the density or turnover of functional transporters, or an increase in transporter availability. With respect to the last possibility, there is some evidence that ACh in the nerve terminal cytoplasm can bind to the choline transporter and briefly immobilize it in an inward-facing direction. If so, then activity-dependent reductions in cytoplasmic ACh would remove this inhibition, thereby enhancing the rate of choline uptake. Third, released ACh is rapidly broken down in the synaptic cleft (or neuromuscular junction) by the enzyme acetylcholinesterase (see below) to produce free choline and acetate. This increases the extracellular concentration of choline, thus contributing further to choline transport into the nerve terminal. Finally, neurotransmitter release is triggered by a large influx of Ca^{2+} ions into the terminal. If, as mentioned earlier, the direct transport of acetyl CoA from mitochondria to the cytoplasm is Ca^{2+}-dependent, then this process might be accelerated under conditions of neural activity.

Throughout this section, we have seen that the formation of ACh is thought to be controlled largely by changes in the concentrations of its precursors, choline and acetyl CoA. This raises the question of whether ChAT is saturated with these compounds, either under resting conditions or under conditions of heightened activity. The term *saturation* was previously introduced in Chapter 2 to refer to the progressive occupation of a receptor site as the concentration of the ligand (e.g., a neurotransmitter or drug) binding to that receptor was gradually increased. In an analogous way, the binding of a substrate to an enzyme displays saturation kinetics. Consequently, when the point of saturation is reached, further increases in the concentration of that substrate produce no additional change in the rate of the enzymatic reaction.

According to results summarized by Tuček (1985), brain ChAT has been reported to have a K_m (the substrate concentration yielding half-maximal reaction velocity) for choline ranging from 0.4–1.0 mM, and a K_m for acetyl CoA of 7–46 µM. On the other hand, the cytoplasmic concentrations of choline and acetyl CoA in a cholinergic nerve terminal are estimated to be approximately 0.05 mM and 5 µM, respectively. This indicates that ChAT is probably not nearly saturated by either choline or acetyl CoA in vivo, which is consistent with the notion that ACh synthesis is regulated by the availability of these precursors.

Acetylcholine Storage and Release

Miniature End-Plate Potentials

While studying the electrical characteristics of frog muscle fiber end plates, Fatt and Katz (1952) found that microelectrodes inserted near the end plates enabled them to record small, random, and apparently spontaneous depolarizations of the muscle cell membrane having an amplitude between 0.5 and 1.0 mV (Figure 7.3). Because these spontaneous membrane responses were smaller than synaptically induced end-plate potentials (EPPs), they were named **miniature end-plate potentials (MEPPs)**. Additional studies showed that the MEPP rate was increased by depolarizing the presynaptic membrane, decreased by hyperpolarizing it, and abolished by botulinum toxin, a drug that blocks ACh release.

These and other observations led to the conclusion that each MEPP represented the spontaneous release of an individual packet (termed a "quantum") of ACh from the nerve terminal. Even though MEPPs varied somewhat in amplitude, it was assumed that the quanta were of equal size and that such amplitude differences were the result of variable micropipette placement in relation to the region of maximum ACh receptor density. (In vertebrate subsynaptic membranes, the receptor density is $10,000/\mu m^2$, whereas in the extrasynaptic region it is only $5/\mu m^2$; see Fertuck and Salpeter, 1974). By determining how many iontophoretically applied ACh molecules were necessary to evoke a MEPP-sized response, it was estimated that each quantum corresponded to between 1,000 and 10,000 molecules of ACh. Finally, ACh quanta were presumed to be the building blocks of the EPPs evoked by synaptic stimulation.

(a)

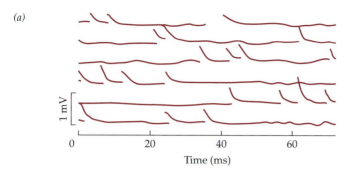

(b)

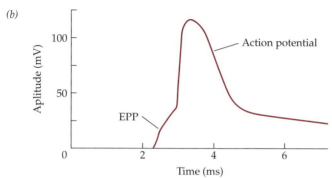

7.3 MINIATURE END-PLATE POTENTIALS (MEPPs) at a frog neuromuscular junction (a; the tracings are all part of a single continuous record from one preparation). These responses are due to the spontaneous release of single packets (quanta) of ACh from the motor nerve terminal. The small amplitude of each MEPP (less than 1 mV) contrasts with the much larger, stimulus-evoked endplate potentials (EPPs) that can elicit a muscle action potential (b; note the differences in voltage and time scales). (After Nicholls, Martin, and Wallace, 1992.)

It should be noted that the phenomenon of quantal release is not unique to the cholinergic system. Rather, this process appears to occur at diverse types of synapses and is probably characteristic of all chemically mediated neurotransmission (Nicholls, Martin, and Wallace, 1992).

Nonquantal acetylcholine release.   Not all ACh release occurs in a quantal manner. Acetylcholine is steadily released from the cytoplasm of nerve terminals at neuromuscular junctions as well as in the brain. This process, which is not dependent on calcium, was first thought to represent passive diffusion of ACh across the axonal membrane. More recent findings, however, suggest that nonquantal ACh release may be carrier-mediated (e.g., see Ivy and Carroll, 1988). The amount of ACh released in this manner has only a small effect on the postsynaptic membrane potential; however, it could influence other processes within the target muscle or nerve cell (Thesleff, 1986).

The Source of Quantally Released Acetylcholine

Spontaneous and stimulus-evoked quantal release of ACh raise a number of interesting and important questions. The most controversial of these concerns the source of the quantally released transmitter. Through early studies using the electron microscope, synaptic vesicles were discovered at about the same time as quantal ACh release. Under these conditions, it was quite natural to associate the two phenomena with each other; that is, to hypothesize that ACh is stored in synaptic vesicles and that the quantal unit represents

the amount of transmitter released from a single vesicle. Thus was born the **vesicle hypothesis** of neurotransmitter release. Much evidence favors this view, with respect to both ACh and other transmitters (Oorschot and Jones, 1987; Rash, Walrond, and Morita, 1988). However, over the years, some research groups have presented findings that argue for the cytoplasmic rather than the vesicular compartment as the source of released ACh (reviewed by Dunant and Israël, 1993). Several of these arguments are discussed in Chapter 6, and hence we will not repeat them here. Suffice it to say, however, that the great majority of neuropharmacologists adhere to the vesicle hypothesis based on the weight of the available evidence.

Cholinergic Vesicles and Biochemical Pools of Acetylcholine

The electric organs of electric fishes and rays are derivatives of muscle tissue and receive a massive cholinergic innervation. Hence, ACh-containing vesicles can be obtained in large numbers from these organs. Rays of the genus *Torpedo* have been particular favorites in the study of cholinergic vesicles. The vesicles obtained from the *Torpedo* electric organ are large: 90 nm in diameter as compared with 50 nm for typical mammalian cholinergic vesicles. Figure 7.4 presents a schematic diagram of some of the major vesicle constituents. Within the vesicles, ACh is present at a very high concentration, estimated at almost 1 M (Whittaker, 1987). It is important to recognize, however, that a number of other constituents are also present and are released into the extracellular fluid upon vesicle exocytosis. These include various nucleotides such as ATP, ADP, and GTP, as well as Ca^{2+} ions. The vesicle membrane also contains a large number of proteins, several of which serve important transport functions. Other vesicle membrane proteins such as synapsin I, synaptophysin, synaptobrevin (VAMP), and synaptotagmin are believed to play important roles in various aspects of the exocytotic process (e.g., vesicle docking or fusion; see Chapter 6 for more details).

A specific **vesicular ACh transporter (VAChT)** is responsible for carrying ACh from the cytoplasm into the vesicle (reviewed by Usdin et al., 1995; also see Figure 7.4). VAChT is an antiporter (see Chapter 3) that couples ACh entry into the vesicle with proton (H^+) efflux. This

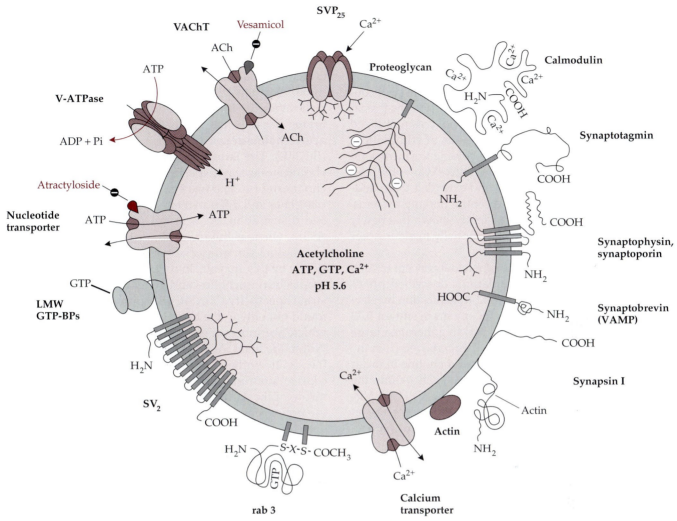

7.4 MAJOR CONSTITUENTS OF CHOLINERGIC VESICLES. The interior of cholinergic vesicles contains ACh, nucleotides such as ATP and GTP, and Ca²⁺ ions, and is maintained at an acidic pH. A number of proteins have been found in the vesicle membrane, including transporters of ACh, nucleotides, various ions, and also several proteins thought to play important roles in the process of exocytosis. (After Zimmermann et al., 1993.)

type of mechanism is used for other transmitters as well, and is discussed in greater detail in Chapter 8. A novel and unexpected feature of VAChT is that its gene is contained within the first intron of the ChAT gene (Usdin et al., 1995). Consequently, cholinergic neurons probably synthesize ChAT and VAChT in a coordinated manner in response to various demands. Vesicular ACh transport is potently inhibited by the drug vesamicol, which has played an important role in studying the mechanism of uptake.

The general view among neurochemists is that cholinergic vesicles originate in the cell body and are then transported to the nerve terminals. After releasing their contents, the vesicles are recycled, probably by an endocytotic process, and then refilled with transmitter.

Extensive studies by Whittaker, Zimmermann, and their colleagues have demonstrated the presence of two

populations of cholinergic vesicles having distinct physical properties (Whittaker, 1987; Zimmermann et al., 1993). The vesicles in one population (designated VP₁) are larger and less dense than those in the other (designated VP₂). Based on a number of findings, these investigators have proposed that VP₁ represents reserve or resting vesicles, whereas VP₂ comprises a population of recycling vesicles. It is possible that the smaller size of the VP₂ vesicles is due to incomplete refilling with ACh, whereas their increased density may be related to osmotic dehydration.

The concept of physically distinct populations of cholinergic vesicles is based on physical separation techniques such as density gradient centrifugation. However, biochemical and pharmacological studies have likewise given rise to the notion of *functional* pools of ACh. This approach can be traced back to the now classic studies of Birks and MacIntosh (1961), who examined the dynamics of ACh synthesis and release in the isolated and perfused superior cervical ganglion of cats. They interpreted the results in terms of a readily releasable pool of ACh and a larger component that they called the reserve pool. The readily releasable pool contained the ACh that was first liberated when the preparation was stimulated. The reserve pool was mobilized and released following longer periods of stimulation. Using more modern techniques involving the incorporation of radiolabeled precursors into ACh, other researchers have since confirmed and extended these findings in both the peripheral and central nervous systems. In particular, studies have consistently shown that newly synthesized ACh is released preferentially to older stores of the transmitter.

It is tempting to relate the functional concept of ACh pools to the two vesicle populations described previously. Whittaker (1987) addressed this question by electrically stimulating *Torpedo* electric organs in situ for 3.33 hours at a low frequency (0.15 Hz) to generate a large VP_2 population. The organs were then removed from the subjects and perfused with deuterated choline in order to label the pool of newly synthesized ACh. Within the first few hours after perfusion, both the VP_1 and VP_2 vesicular populations could be isolated; however, the labeled ACh was found almost exclusively in the presumptively recycling VP_2 vesicles. After a 16-hour rest period, however, the VP_2 population had disappeared, and the labeled ACh was now present in VP_1.

These findings and others by Zimmermann et al. (1993) support the idea that newly synthesized ACh, which preferentially enters the readily releasable pool, is associated primarily with the recycling vesicle population under conditions of prolonged nerve stimulation. Upon recovery, these vesicles reenter the reserve population, thus accounting for the later presence of labeled ACh in VP_1. Whether this model applies equally well to shorter periods of neural activity remains to be determined.

Acetylcholine Inactivation

Cholinesterases

There is meager evidence of uptake of ACh into any part of nerve cells. Thus, ACh degradation and diffusion out of the synaptic cleft are the principal mechanisms for ter-

minating its synaptic action. Figure 7.5 presents the biochemical reaction involving the hydrolytic breakdown of ACh. Enzymes responsible for catalyzing this reaction are generically known as cholinesterases because they cleave the ester linkage between the choline and acetate moieties of the ACh molecule. As summarized in a recent review by Massoulié and coworkers (1993), vertebrates possess two distinct types of cholinesterases: **acetylcholinesterase** (**AChE**) and butyrylcholinesterase (BuChE). The latter is sometimes also called pseudocholinesterase, nonspecific cholinesterase, or simply cholinesterase. The two enzymes are encoded by separate genes and differ in their substrate specificity and tissue distribution. ACh is the preferred substrate for AChE, whereas butyrylcholine and other choline- and noncholine-containing esters are hydrolyzed more slowly by this enzyme. In contrast, BuChE effectively degrades butyrylcholine and generally exhibits less substrate specificity than AChE. High levels of AChE are found not only in the brain but also in striated muscles, which are innervated by cholinergic motor neurons. Within the brain, AChE is generally found in cholinergic (i.e., ACh-synthesizing) or cholinoceptive (i.e., ACh-receptive) neurons, although some exceptions exist (see below). Like AChE, BuChE is present in muscle and in the brain (mainly in glial cells); however, it can also be detected in the liver, placenta, and blood plasma. All evidence points to AChE as the key enzyme for inactivating ACh at synapses and neuromotor junctions; hence the remainder of the discussion will focus on this enzyme.

Properties of Acetylcholinesterase

AChE is a glycoprotein (a sugar-containing protein) made up of one or more subunits, each with a molecular weight of 70–80 kDa, depending on the species. As illustrated in Figure 7.6, the various forms of AChE can be subdivided into heteromeric and homomeric families. This diversity is produced by alternative mRNA splicing of a single gene product (see Chapters 3 and 11 for a description of this process; the figure notes which exons are involved in this process). An additional nomenclature system distinguishes between globular (G) and asymmetric (A) forms of the enzyme, and also utilizes a number following the letter to denote the number of subunits present in each form.

The asymmetric form of AChE is so named because it possesses a tail made up of three collagen filaments

7.5 HYDROLYSIS OF ACETYLCHOLINE BY CHOLINESTERASE.

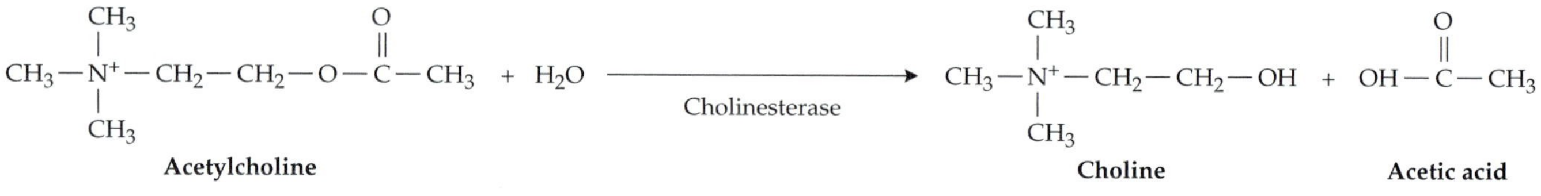

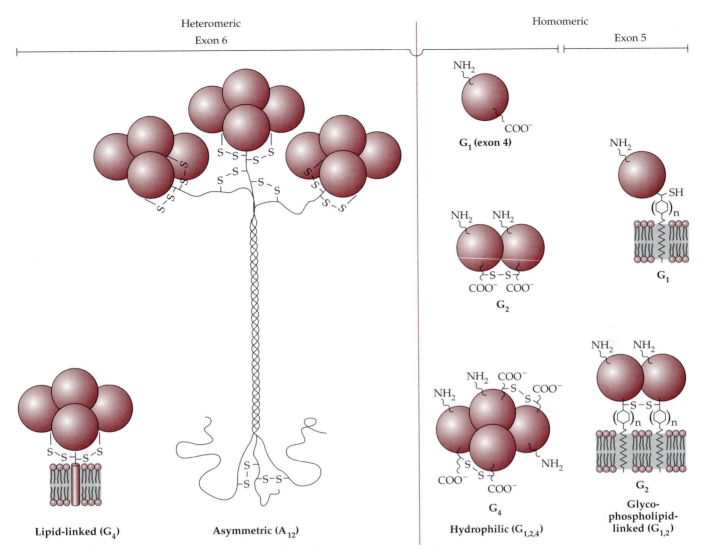

7.6 STRUCTURES OF THE VARIOUS MOLECULAR SPECIES OF ACETYLCHOLINESTERASE.
AChE can be divided into heteromeric and homomeric families, as well as into globular (G) and asymmetric (A) forms that vary in their subcellular localization. The number following the letter denotes the number of subunits contained in that form. The hydrophilic G forms are present in the cytoplasm, the lipid-linked G forms are anchored to the plasma membrane, and A_{12} is attached to the extracellular matrix by a helical collagen-containing tail. (After Taylor and Radić, 1994.)

wound in a helical arrangement. As shown in the figure, disulfide bonds (—S—S—) play a role in linking the subunits to each other and also to the tail. This form of AChE is found mainly at the neuromuscular junction, where it is secreted by muscle and nerve cells. The enzyme molecules then become tethered to the extracellular matrix by means of their collagenous tails (Massoulié et al., 1993).

The globular forms are even more complex due to their heterogeneity. For example, G_1 and G_2 each have two variants, a hydrophilic form found in the cytoplasm and a glycophospholipid-linked form that is anchored to the cell membrane. G_4 also exists in two forms, a homomeric hydrophilic form and a heteromeric form with a

lipid membrane anchor (Taylor and Radić, 1994). It is likely that in the brain, ACh released into the synaptic cleft is degraded mainly by the membrane-bound forms of G_1, G_2, and G_4. A_{12} is presumably a major participant in ACh breakdown at the neuromuscular junction. Finally, the soluble globular forms of the enzyme are well positioned to degrade excess intracellular ACh.

AChE is one of only a few enzymes that have attained near catalytic perfection; that is, ACh molecules are hydrolyzed almost as rapidly as they can diffuse to the active site of the enzyme. In quantitative terms, AChE has a turnover number of 14,000 (Voet and Voet, 1990), which means that 14,000 molecules of ACh are hydrolyzed per second by each enzyme molecule under conditions of full saturation. This corresponds to a turnover time per substrate molecule of approximately 70 μsec. On the other hand, in vitro studies have shown that extremely high ACh concentrations actually reduce the rate of enzymatic activity. Whether this phenomenon, which is termed excess substrate inhibition, also occurs in vivo is not entirely clear. However, it conceivably could serve as a mechanism to retard the speed of ACh inactivation in cases in which prolonged stimulation of the postsynaptic cell is necessary.

AChE is one of the most extensively studied enzymes with respect to its mechanism of action.* The active site of AChE comprises two subsites critical for its functioning. One of these has traditionally been termed the anionic subsite because it was hypothesized to consist of one or more negatively charged groups that electrostatically interacted with the positively charged quaternary nitrogen of the substrate. However, recent studies indicate that hydrophobic interactions may play an equally, if not more, important role in binding this part of the substrate to the enzyme molecule. The other region of the active site is the so-called esteratic subsite, which possesses a serine residue that is responsible for driving the hydrolytic reaction. Following binding of ACh to the active site of AChE, this reaction occurs in two steps as follows. In the first step, the ester bond of the ACh molecule is broken, and choline is released into the surrounding medium, where it can be taken up by the presynaptic nerve terminal. The acetate group becomes covalently bound to the above-mentioned serine, resulting in an acetylated enzyme as a transient intermediate in the reaction. In the second step, a molecule of water rapidly reacts with this unstable intermediate to liberate the acetate group and regenerate the active enzyme.

$$E^*ACh \rightarrow E^*A + choline$$

$$E^*A + H_2O \rightarrow E + acetate$$

where E^*A = acetylated enzyme.

Noncholinergic Functions of Acetylcholinesterase

Although we usually think of AChE only in the context of cholinergic neurotransmission, there is considerable evidence that this protein may also serve other functions. First, substantial AChE activity is found in the various major classes of blood cells, including erythrocytes (red cells), lymphocytes (white cells), and platelets. It is unlikely that the purpose of AChE in these cells is to break down ACh. Second, during development, AChE (but not ChAT) is transiently expressed at high levels in

thalamocortical projection neurons and in their termination areas of the sensory cortex (Robertson and Yu, 1993). These observations suggest a possible developmental role for AChE apart from its well-known function in terminating ACh action. Third, even in the adult brain, AChE in certain areas displays properties that are inconsistent with its usual role. This has been shown most clearly in the substantia nigra, where substantial amounts of soluble AChE appear to be released from the somata and dendrites of the nigrostriatal dopamine cells (Appleyard, 1992; Greenfield, 1991). These cells also exhibit somatodendritic dopamine release, and it is possible that the two substances are co-released from the same subcellular compartment (possibly the smooth endoplasmic reticulum). Although the nigra does receive a cholinergic input, the pathway is sparse and therefore would not require the high levels of AChE shown to be present.

To elucidate the possible function of AChE in the substantia nigra, Greenfield and her coworkers infused various cholinesterase preparations into this area in guinea pigs (see Greenfield, 1991). Infusion of purified AChE from electric eel caused a hyperpolarization of the nigrostriatal cells, which was due to an opening of membrane K^+ channels. Prior inactivation of AChE by the irreversible inhibitor Soman failed to block this effect, whereas infusion of BuChE rather than AChE produced no change in cellular membrane potential. Other studies using freely moving animals (guinea pigs and rats) demonstrated a certain correlation between behavioral activity and nigral AChE release. Finally, nigral infusions of AChE, but not BuChE, evoked behavioral responses often associated with striatal activation, such as locomotion, stereotyped behaviors, chewing movements, and contralateral circling (i.e., circling away from the treated side of the brain). Taken together, these results indicate that AChE can exert novel electrophysiological and behavioral effects that are independent of its enzymatic properties. It has been hypothesized that such effects reflect an enhancement of the sensitivity of nigrostriatal dopamine neurons to afferent stimulation (Appleyard, 1992; Greenfield, 1991).

Drugs That Affect Acetylcholine Synthesis, Storage, Release, and Inactivation

Drugs That Block Acetylcholine Synthesis

The synthesizing enzyme ChAT would seem to be an obvious site at which to interfere with ACh formation. However, only a few ChAT inhibitors have been found, and even those are not very selective in their action. Two ChAT inhibitors are the styrylpyridine derivative 4(1-naphthylvinyl)pyridine (NVP) and a compound called juglone (5-hydroxy-1,4-napthoquinone) that is found in

---

*We will comment only briefly on this topic, although interested readers are referred to Massoulié et al. (1993) and Taylor and Radić (1994) for further information.

walnut hulls (Goldberg, Satama, and Blum, 1971; Haubrich and Wang, 1976).

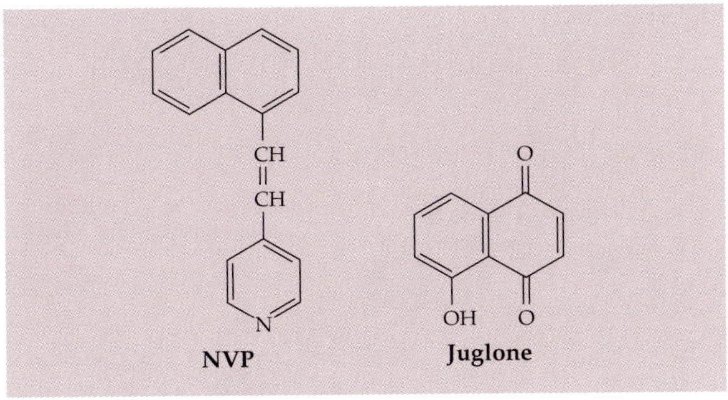

NVP Juglone

An alternative method of blocking ACh synthesis is to inhibit high-affinity choline uptake by the cholinergic nerve terminals. Two drugs that work this way are hemicholinium-3 (HC-3) and triethylcholine (TEC). It is inter-

Hemicholinium-3 (HC-3)

Triethylcholine (TEC)

esting to note that synaptic vesicles can still be observed in the nerve terminals of HC-3-treated motor neurons, although the vesicles have been depleted of their ACh content (Ceccarelli and Hurlbut, 1975). In vivo, HC-3 seems to block ACh synthesis more effectively than ChAT inhibitors, which is consistent with the notion that the rate of ACh formation generally depends more on the velocity of choline uptake than on ChAT availability. To affect central cholinergic functioning, however, HC-3 must be injected directly into the brain because its two charged quaternary nitrogen groups restrict its ability to cross the blood–brain barrier.

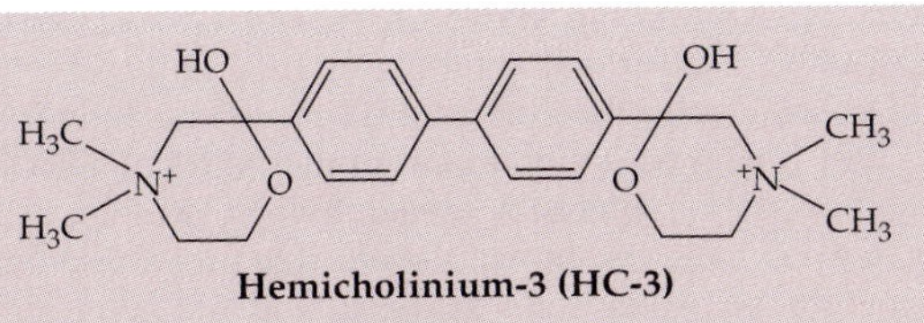

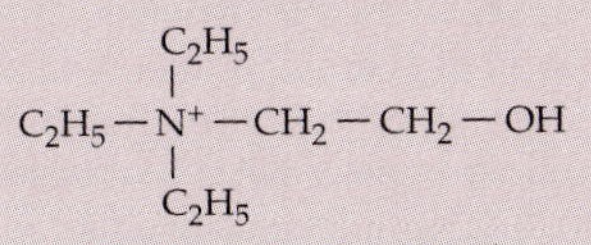

Drugs That Affect Acetylcholine Storage and Release

A major advance in ACh pharmacology was made several years ago when Parsons and his colleagues discovered a compound called AH5183 or vesamicol (2-(4-phenylpiperidino) cyclohexanol), which selectively inhibits the vesicular ACh transporter. The ability of this drug to block ACh storage can be seen at the neuromuscular junction using a model system such as the mouse phrenic nerve–hemidiaphragm preparation. Rapid stimulation of the tissue had no effect on subsequent MEPP amplitude under normal conditions. However, when vesamicol was present during the period of stimulation,

subsequent MEPP amplitude was reduced due to the inhibition of vesicle refilling and consequent decrease in quantal size (Marshall and Parsons, 1987).

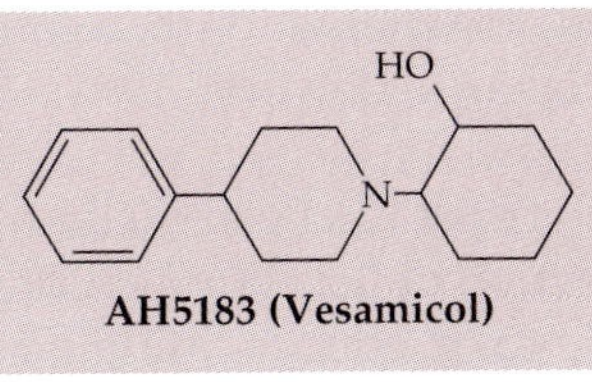

AH5183 (Vesamicol)

A number of animal and bacterial toxins have dramatic effects on ACh release. One of these is α-latrotoxin, a 130-kDa protein present in the venom of the black widow spider, *Latrodectus mactans*. The toxin is not specific to cholinergic neurons, but rather induces neurotransmitter release from most, if not all, peripheral nerve cells. α-Latrotoxin accomplishes this effect by binding to terminal membranes, where it acts as a potent ionophore for divalent cations. Consequently, large amounts of Ca^{2+} enter the terminal, causing massive exocytosis followed by vesicle depletion and blockade of neurotransmission (Chiappinelli, 1989). At the frog neuromuscular junction, black widow spider venom causes a marked rise and then a fall in MEPP frequency (Nastuk, 1974). The rise in MEPP frequency reflects the initial stimulating (i.e., ACh-releasing) effect of the latrotoxin, and the fall in frequency is due to the subsequent depletion of synaptic vesicles.

Also of great interest are the toxins produced by the clostridial bacteria *Clostridium botulinum* and *Clostridium tetani*. *Clostridium botulinum* produces a family of seven toxins termed botulinum toxins A–G. Each is synthesized as a single large protein, which is then cleaved to yield a heavy chain (100 kDa) and a light chain (50 kDa) that are joined by a disulfide bond. Botulinum toxin powerfully inhibits the release of ACh, and as a consequence it is extraordinarily toxic. The estimated lethal dose in humans is 0.3 µg; in other words, 1 gram (equivalent to the weight of three aspirin tablets) is enough to kill about 350,000 individuals.

Botulinum toxins A, B, and E are most frequently implicated in botulism poisoning. The primary symptom of this disorder is muscular paralysis, which results in death by asphyxiation. The clostridial bacteria do not grow in the presence of oxygen; however, they can thrive in an anaerobic environment such as a sealed food can. Fortunately, the bacteria are inactivated by heating, and thus botulism poisoning is rare.

Tetanus toxin, which is produced by *Clostridium tetani*, is chemically similar to botulinum toxin. This substance is responsible for tetanus poisoning, which is estimated to kill over a million people per year worldwide (Bagetta, Nisticò, and Bowery, 1991). The symptoms of tetanus were first described by Hippocrates over 2,000 years ago, and consist of spastic paralysis, severe convulsions, and other EEG abnormalities. Whereas botulinum toxin is most potent at blocking release from cholinergic nerve terminals, tetanus toxin is relatively nonselective. In fact, blockade of GABA and glycine release at spinal inhibitory synapses is thought to be responsible for the spastic paralysis associated with tetanus poisoning (Bagetta, Nisticò, and Bowery, 1991; Mellanby and Green, 1981).

Considerable effort has been made to delineate the mechanisms of action of botulinum and tetanus toxins. In both cases, the toxic effect is initiated by a two-step process involving binding to the nerve cell membrane followed by internalization of the toxin molecule. Once inside the nerve terminal, the toxins not only act locally to block transmitter release, but can also be transported back to the cell body by the axonal retrograde transport system (Bagetta, Nisticò, and Bowery, 1991).

The mechanism underlying release inhibition is just beginning to be understood. An early report by Kao, Drachman, and Price (1976) indicated that botulinum toxin did not work by blocking Ca^{2+} entry into the nerve terminal, nor did it interfere with vesicular storage of ACh. Based on an observed clumping of synaptic vesicles, these investigators instead suggested that the toxin interferes in some fashion with a membrane component of vesicle release. Recent research has shown this to be a remarkable insight. The first breakthrough in delineating the mechanism of action of clostridial toxins came from Montecucco and colleagues (Schiavo et al., 1992), who showed that botulinum toxin B and tetanus toxin both exhibit specific proteolytic (protein-degrading) activity toward the synaptic vesicle membrane protein synaptobrevin-2. This protein, also known as VAMP-2, is believed to play a critical role in exocytosis, possibly by helping to mediate the initial step of vesicle docking with the nerve terminal membrane (Barinaga, 1993; Südhof and Jahn, 1991). Toxin-induced inhibition of ACh release from identified cholinergic neurons of the sea slug *Aplysia californica* was markedly delayed by the addition of peptides that block the toxins' proteolytic activity. This finding supports the hypothesis that botulinum toxin B and tetanus toxin prevent transmitter release by inactivating synaptobrevin-2. On the other hand, separate experiments with botulinum toxins A and E found no effect on synaptobrevin-2, suggesting that these substances might influence a different component of the releasing mechanism. Indeed, subsequent studies have indicated that at least three different proteins thought to be involved in vesicle exocytosis are targets for various clostridial neurotoxins (Blasi et al., 1993; Huttner, 1993; Wonnacott and Dajas, 1994; Figure 7.7).

Drugs That Affect Acetylcholine Inactivation

Anticholinesterase (anti-AChE) agents increase the duration of action of endogenous ACh at cholinergic receptor sites by blocking ACh hydrolysis by AChE. In most cases, this is accomplished by competing with ACh for

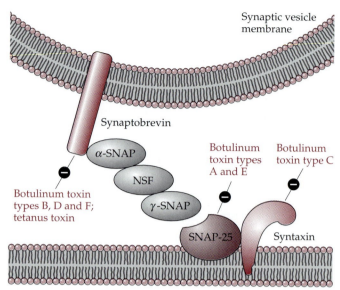

7.7 MOLECULAR MECHANISMS OF ACTION OF CLOSTRIDIAL NEUROTOXINS. Clostridial neurotoxins are a group of related bacterial toxins responsible for botulism poisoning and for tetanus. They are all potent neurotransmitter release-inhibiting agents that exert their effects by breaking down proteins required for vesicle exocytosis. As shown, the affected proteins include the vesicle membrane protein synaptobrevin and two nerve terminal membrane proteins, SNAP-25 and syntaxin. These three proteins are shown in a hypothetical arrangement with several soluble proteins (α-SNAP, γ-SNAP, and NSF) also thought to play necessary roles in the exocytotic process. SNAP = synaptosomal-associated protein; NSF, N-ethylmaleimide-sensitive factor. (After Wonnacott and Dajas, 1994.)

access to the active site on the AChE molecule. The actions of a particular anti-AChE compound depend on a variety of factors, including whether the drug crosses the blood–brain barrier, whether its effects are reversible or irreversible, and the rate of clearance of the drug.

Reversible acetylcholinesterase inhibitors. Some anti-AChE drugs are considered reversible inhibitors because they bind to the enzyme for a limited period of time. We will discuss only a few such drugs, although interested readers are referred to Taylor (1985b) for a more comprehensive listing. One well-known reversible anti-AChE compound is edrophonium (Tensilon), which is particularly short-acting because of its rapid elimination by the kidneys. Edrophonium is sometimes used in the diagno-

Edrophonium

sis of **myasthenia gravis**, a crippling autoimmune disorder characterized by muscular weakness due to a progressive loss of ACh receptor sites on the muscle membrane (Drachman, 1987). Blockade of ACh hydrolysis by edrophonium causes a sudden increase in muscle action potentials and muscle strength upon exertion.

One of the earliest reversible anti-AChE agents was found in the Calabar bean, the seed of a climbing woody plant named *Physostigma venenosum* Balfour that grows in the Calabar region of Nigeria. The beans were used for many years by the local peoples as an ordeal poison

Physostigmine

in trials for witchcraft. The active ingredient was extracted in 1864 and given the name physostigmine. Physostigmine (Eserine) crosses the blood–brain barrier and thus exerts central effects. Accidental poisoning produces slurred speech and confusion, loss of reflexes and convulsions, coma, and death. These effects can be countered with high doses of atropine, a drug that blocks muscarinic ACh receptors (see below for a discussion of cholinergic receptor subtypes). In 1877, physostigmine was first used therapeutically in the treatment of glaucoma by direct application to the eye, and it is still used for this purpose today.

Neostigmine (Prostigmin) is a synthetic analog of physostigmine that was introduced in 1931. In contrast to physostigmine, neostigmine does not pass the blood–brain barrier because of its charged quaternary nitrogen group. On the other hand, this structure confers upon

Neostigmine

the molecule a weak agonist action at some cholinergic receptors. Neostigmine is useful for stimulating the organs of the gastrointestinal tract when there is a loss of tone due to disease, injury, or surgery. It is also effective in treating myasthenia gravis because it potentiates the action of ACh on the few receptors that are left. Finally, it can serve as an antidote for curare poisoning by providing more ACh to compete with the curare molecules (as described below, curare is a nicotinic cholinergic receptor blocker). Because neostigmine does not pass the blood–

brain barrier, these beneficial effects occur without psychotropic side effects.

Both physostigmine and neostigmine are alternative AChE substrates that form a carbamylated enzyme complex with the serine residue at the active site. (Carbamylation is the formation of a compound with a carbamate ester group [NH_2—CO–].) Whereas the acetylated enzyme formed by the interaction of ACh with AChE is rapidly hydrolyzed, carbamylated enzyme complexes are broken down a million times more slowly because of their greater stability. Carbamylating inhibitors such as physostigmine and neostigmine thus show a prolonged duration of action compared with edrophonium.

Irreversible acetylcholinesterase inhibitors. A number of synthetic organophosphorus compounds can be considered irreversible acetylcholinesterase inhibitors. Such compounds form highly stable phosphorylated complexes with AChE that resist hydrolytic cleavage for many hours or even longer. The longest-lasting of these agents are thus essentially irreversible, which means that AChE activity reappears only gradually over a period of days or weeks as new enzyme molecules are synthesized (Koelle, 1975a; Marx, 1980).

One of the earliest organophosphorus compounds was synthesized in 1854, 10 years before the isolation of physostigmine. The commercial potential of these agents, however, dates from a 1932 German publication by Lange and Krueger describing persistent blurred vision and choking sensations following inhalation of one of these compounds (cited in Koelle, 1975a). Because of the role of ACh in insect neurotransmission, other German investigators then began looking into these compounds as possible insecticides. This led to the development of parathion (Taylor, 1985b), which soon became the most widely used product of this class. However,

Parathion

parathion proved to be very toxic to animals and humans, and was responsible for more lethal poisonings than any other compound in use at that time. It therefore gave way to malathion, which had good insecticidal properties yet was rapidly broken down to inactive metabolites in mammals and birds.

Prior to and during World War II, several anti-AChE agents were secretly produced by Schrader's group in Germany as chemical warfare agents. These compounds, which were called Sarin, Soman, and Tabun, had even greater toxicity than parathion. Over 10,000 tons of Tabun was manufactured by Germany, although it was fortunately never used. The Allied countries also

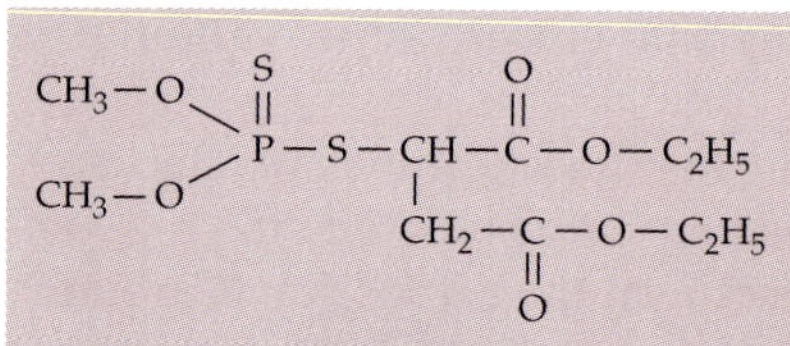

Malathion

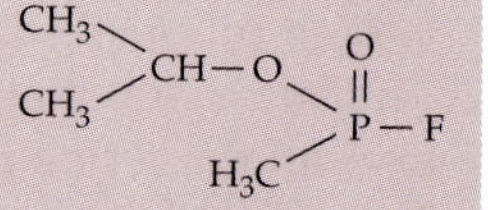

Sarin

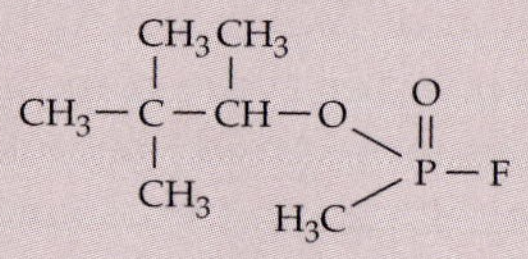

Soman

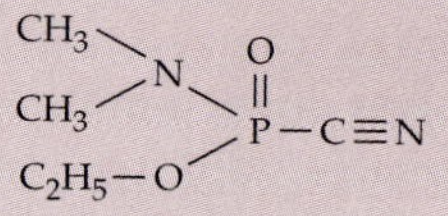

Tabun

searched for chemical warfare agents, leading to the development of diisopropylfluorophosphate (DFP) for deployment if chemical warfare had ensued.

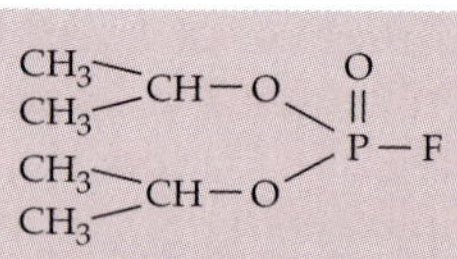

Diisopropyl fluorophosphate (DFP)

These organophosphorus "nerve gases" can be stored as liquids and released as a vapor cloud or spray. After contacting the skin or being inhaled into the pulmonary alveoli, they rapidly penetrate into the bloodstream due to their high lipid solubility. For the same reason, passage across the blood–brain barrier occurs readily. Inactivation of both peripheral and central AChE leads to a rapid accumulation of ACh in the autonomic nervous system, at neuromuscular junctions, and at cholinergic synapses in the CNS. This accumulation causes a wide variety of symptoms such as intense sweating, filling of bronchial passages with mucus, bronchial constriction, dimmed vision, uncontrollable vomiting and defecation, convulsions, and ultimately paralysis and asphyxiation from respiratory failure. As little as 1 mg or less of Sarin or Soman are thought to be lethal (Meselson and Robinson, 1980). Fortunately, substances such as pralidoxime (pyridine-2-aldoxime methiodide) and trimedoxime have been developed that can serve as effective antidotes by breaking the phosphate–enzyme bond, thus regenerating the active enzyme.

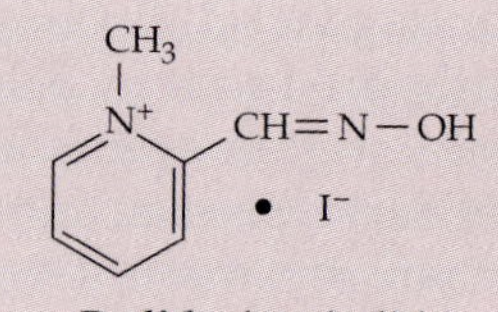

Pralidoxime iodide

Part I Summary

Acetylcholine is formed in a single, reversible reaction involving the condensation of choline and acetyl CoA. The reaction is catalyzed by the enzyme ChAT, which is concentrated in the cytoplasm of cholinergic nerve terminals. Acetyl CoA is formed in mitochondria as a byproduct of glycolysis. Choline is obtained from the ingestion of dietary lipids and can also be made by the liver. All cells possess a low-affinity choline uptake system used in the synthesis of choline-containing phospholipids. Cholinergic neurons, however, also exhibit a Na^+-dependent, high-affinity uptake mechanism that provides choline for ACh formation. The rate of ACh formation is governed by several factors, including product inhibition of ChAT, mass action, availability of the choline and acetyl CoA precursors, and neuronal activity. When ACh release is stimulated by increased neuronal activity, synthesis may temporarily lag behind release, thus causing a depletion of ACh in the nerve terminal. Under these conditions, choline administration can enhance ACh synthesis and reinstate normal concentrations of the neurotransmitter.

Early electrophysiological studies of the neuromuscular junction demonstrated the existence of small, spontaneous depolarizations of the muscle cell membrane. These so-called MEPPs were shown to result from the release of single packets (quanta) of ACh from the presynaptic nerve terminal. Most investigators believe that such quantal release of ACh is mediated by exocytosis of ACh-containing vesicles found within the terminals. In addition, a steady nonquantal release of ACh occurs from the cytoplasmic compartment. Cholinergic vesicles contain a number of other substances, including various nucleotides as well as Ca^{2+} ions, that are released exocytotically along with ACh. The vesicles appear to exist in two physically distinct populations, recycling and resting (or reserve). These populations may be related to the two functional pools of ACh that have been described, namely, the readily releasable pool versus the storage or reserve pool. Newly synthesized ACh preferentially enters the readily releasable pool.

Acetylcholine inactivation is mediated by rapid hydrolysis by the enzymes AChE and, to a lesser extent, BuChE. AChE molecules are composed of one or more globular subunits that can exist in numerous forms. Some of these forms are soluble, others are bound to cell membranes, and one possesses a collagenous tail that binds to the extracellular matrix. AChE is one of the fastest enzymes known, thus leading to extremely rapid termination of ACh action. The reaction works by a two-step mechanism involving the formation of an acetylated enzyme as a transient intermediate, followed by addition of water to regenerate the active enzyme molecule. Various studies have indicated that AChE may also serve functions unrelated to the inactivation of ACh, including the modulation of dopaminergic cell excitability in the substantia nigra.

A variety of drugs interfere with ACh synthesis, storage, release, or inactivation. ACh synthesis can be inhibited by blocking ChAT with NVP or juglone, or by preventing high-affinity choline uptake with HC-3. Vesamicol is a novel drug that selectively inhibits ACh transport into synaptic vesicles. Acetylcholine release is affected by several naturally occurring toxins, such as α-latrotoxin (one of the active ingredients of black widow spider venom), which stimulates vesicle exocytosis, and botulinum and tetanus toxins, which inhibit ACh release. Finally, cholinergic activity can be enhanced by various AChE inhibitors. These include the reversible inhibitors edrophonium, physostigmine, and neostigmine, as well as the highly toxic irreversible organophosphorus compounds Sarin, Soman, Tabun, and DFP.

Part II
Anatomy and Physiology of Cholinergic Systems

Distribution of Cholinergic Neurons and Their Connections

Cholinergic neurons are found in numerous locations throughout the PNS and CNS. We will begin this section with a description of centrally located cholinergic neurons and their connections, followed by a brief summary of peripheral cholinergic systems.

Cholinergic Systems within the CNS

ACh as a central neurotransmitter. Although ACh was one of the first neurotransmitters identified in peripheral nerves, its presence in the CNS was not verified until somewhat later. In 1936, Quastel's group demonstrated the synthesis of ACh in brain slices. This was followed by studies by MacIntosh and his colleagues showing that ACh was distributed heterogeneously in the brain and that the substance could be released from the cerebral cortex in vivo (MacIntosh, 1941; MacIntosh and Oborin, 1953). The first convincing evidence for a neurotransmitter action of ACh in the CNS was provided by Curtis and Eccles in 1958. These investigators showed that stimulating the axons of spinal motor neurons caused retrograde action potentials to be sent back to the motor neurons and, via axon collaterals, activation of local interneurons known as Renshaw cells (see Figure 3.13). Because the neurotransmitter released by these motor neurons at the neuromuscular junction is ACh, the transmitter released upon the Renshaw cells was

also assumed to be ACh. This hypothesis was subsequently confirmed by various pharmacological studies on the motor neuron–Renshaw cell synapses.

Identifying cholinergic circuits in the CNS. Major progress in identifying cholinergic pathways within the CNS was not made until the locations of the ACh-containing cell bodies and their projections could be visualized. Initial attempts to stain for ACh itself proved disappointing, so researchers turned to other markers associated with cholinergic neurons. This led to the development and widespread use of histochemical techniques for staining AChE. By examining patterns of AChE staining in normal animals versus animals given lesions in specific brain areas, Lewis and Shute (1978) were particularly successful in mapping putative cholinergic pathways. However, there are several major problems with the use of AChE as a marker for ACh. First, not all ACh-synthesizing cells have been shown to possess AChE. Second, as we saw earlier, AChE is usually present postsynaptically at cholinergic junctions. Finally, as we also saw earlier, AChE may serve certain cellular functions not associated with ACh at all.

The most important advance in ACh localization occurred with the development of staining procedures for ChAT. As the ACh-synthesizing enzyme, ChAT is a more logical choice than AChE as a selective marker for cholinergic neurons in the brain. Choline acetyltransferase staining is accomplished by the technique of immunohistochemistry, which involves the use of specific antibodies to the substance being visualized (see Chapter 2). Whereas the first anti-ChAT antibodies suffered from a lack of requisite specificity, these problems were later overcome, and the procedure is now performed routinely.*

Location of Cholinergic Cell Groups and Pathways in the Brain

Woolf (1991) recently reviewed the available information on central cholinergic pathways based on ChAT immunohistochemistry. Figure 7.8 illustrates the distribution of ChAT-immunoreactive neurons and their projections in the rat brain. As emphasized by Woolf and others, the cholinergic cell bodies form a continuum that reaches from the caudate–putamen in the telencephalon to motor neurons in the spinal cord. Nevertheless, it is possible to delineate clusters of these cell groups and their corresponding axonal projections.

Interneurons of the striatal complex. Numerous large, aspiny (i.e., lacking dendritic spines) cholinergic neurons are found in all parts of the striatal complex, including the caudate–putamen, nucleus accumbens, olfactory tu-

---

*The interested reader is referred to Wainer et al., 1984, for more information on this topic.

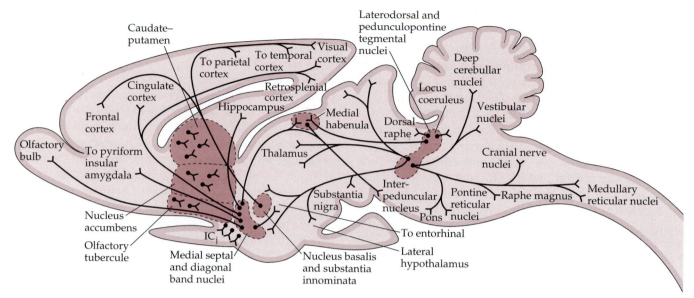

7.8 DISTRIBUTION OF CHOLINERGIC CELL GROUPS AND PROJECTIONS IN THE RAT BRAIN. Locations of choline acetyltransferase-containing cell bodies and dendrites in a parasagittal section through the rat brain (shaded areas) and major projections of the cholinergic cell groups. Note that the basal forebrain cholinergic cell groups project to the neocortex and to functionally interrelated limbic structures such as the hippocampus, whereas most subcortical areas are innervated by cholinergic neurons of the pontomesencephalic system. (After Woolf, 1991.)

bercle, and the islands of Calleja. These cells serve as interneurons: short-axoned cells that participate in local circuits. The cholinergic neurons of the caudate–putamen synapse on the medium-sized spiny output neurons of the striatum, and they receive glutamatergic afferents from the neocortex and a dopaminergic input from the substantia nigra. These cholinergic cells play an important role in the functioning of the extrapyramidal motor system.

Projection neurons of the basal forebrain.   The basal forebrain of mammals contains a major cholinergic projection system with cell groups located in a number of areas. As an alternative to traditional anatomical terminology, Mesulam and his colleagues have proposed a system in which groups of cholinergic projection neurons are named by the designation "Ch" followed by a number (see Wainer et al., 1984). We will therefore identify cell groups using both types of nomenclature where appropriate.

The most rostral cholinergic cell groups of the basal forebrain are located in the medial septal nucleus (Ch1) and the vertical limb nucleus of the diagonal band of Broca (Ch2). These cells send major projections to the hippocampus and to the limbic cortex. An intermediate group of cholinergic neurons is found in the horizontal limb nucleus of the diagonal band (Ch3) and the magnocellular preoptic area. Axons of these cells terminate in

the olfactory bulbs, amygdala, and limbic cortex. The most caudal portion of this system is represented by cells in the nucleus basalis, the substantia innominata, and the nucleus ansa reticularis (Ch4). These neurons innervate all parts of the neocortex, synapsing preferentially on pyramidal cells of cortical layer 5. As discussed below, the basal forebrain cholinergic neurons appear to play an important role in memory and other cognitive functions.

Neurons of the diencephalon.   Within the diencephalon, cholinergic neurons have been observed in several hypothalamic nuclei as well as in the medial habenula. Axons of cells in the medial habenula enter the fasciculus retroflexus and terminate in the interpeduncular nucleus. Projections of the hypothalamic cholinergic neurons are less well known. Some fibers are presumed to act locally in the regulation of neuroendocrine function, whereas others may contribute to the neocortical cholinergic innervation.

Pontomesencephalic cell groups.   Within the caudal mesencephalic and rostral pontine tegmentum, cholinergic neurons are found in the pedunculopontine tegmental nucleus (Ch5), the dorsolateral tegmental nucleus (Ch6), and the parabigeminal nucleus. From the pedunculopontine tegmental nucleus, there are widespread projections to the tectum (especially to the superior colliculus), thalamus (especially to the posterior and the mediodorsal nuclei), globus pallidus, interpeduncular nucleus, substantia nigra, locus coeruleus, raphe nuclei, deep cerebellar nuclei, reticular formation, and the motor nuclei of cranial nerves III–VII and IX–XII. Cholinergic neurons of the dorsolateral tegmental nucleus tend to send their fibers to the same regions as the cells of the pedunculopontine tegmental nucleus, although the detailed distribution of fibers from the two cell groups varies considerably. Finally, the parabigeminal cell cluster projects mainly to the superior colliculus and the dorsal lateral geniculate nucleus of the thalamus.

Neurons of the medulla.   Scattered cholinergic neurons have been found in the prepositus hypoglossal nucleus and nearby areas of the medullary tegmentum. These cells are thought to innervate the cerebellar cortex and the nucleus of cranial nerve VII.

Peripheral Cholinergic Systems

Spinal and cranial motor neurons.   Acetylcholine is synthesized in spinal and cranial motor neurons whose somata are located in the spinal cord and brain stem respectively, and whose axons transport the transmitter to neuromuscular junctions affecting the skeletal musculature of the body and head. For example, motor neurons of the spinal cord are responsible for the movement of the limbs and the trunk, whereas cranial motor neurons control eye movements (oculomotor [III], trochlear [IV], and abducens [VI] nerves), movements of the jaw (trigeminal [V] nerve), facial muscles (facial [VII] nerve), and the tongue (hypoglossal [XII] nerve). All of these motor neurons secrete ACh at their axon terminals. The motor neuron cell bodies are located in the ventral horns of the spinal gray matter, and are stimulated or inhibited by a variety of reflex inputs as well as by signals from higher centers such as the cerebral cortex, cerebellum, and hypothalamus.

The parasympathetic system.   Acetylcholine plays a prominent role as a neurotransmitter in both the parasympathetic and sympathetic branches of the autonomic nervous system. The reader will recall from Chapter 4 that axons within the autonomic nervous system are characterized by their relationship to the autonomic ganglia. In the parasympathetic system, for example, axons emanating from the brain (i.e., the cranial nerves) and from parasympathetic nuclei in the sacral region of the spinal cord are considered preganglionic fibers. In contrast, the short axons traveling from the parasympathetic ganglion cells to the gland or smooth muscle cells are the postganglionic fibers (see Figure 4.25). Both types of fibers release ACh at their terminals. Thus, the preganglionic fibers make cholinergic synapses with the ganglionic neurons, which in turn release ACh at their endings.

The sympathetic system.   Like those of the parasympathetic system, the preganglionic sympathetic fibers are cholinergic. The postganglionic sympathetic fibers, however, are all noradrenergic (they release norepinephrine; see Chapter 8) except for those fibers that activate the sweat glands, which are cholinergic.

Acetylcholine Receptors

Acetylcholine Receptor Subtypes

For each of the many neurotransmitters that have been identified, there typically seem to be several chemically distinct membrane receptors, which are known as **receptor subtypes**. Further complicating the picture is the fact that many receptors are coupled to multiple signal transduction mechanisms in the same or in different cells. This diversity of signaling processes allows the same neurotransmitter to cause membrane depolarization in one target cell but hyperpolarization in another. Likewise, the membrane response to a transmitter may develop and decay in a few milliseconds, or it may appear only after hundreds of milliseconds and persist for minutes. The existence of receptor subtypes allows for the discovery or creation of drug agonists or antagonists that selectively mimic or block a specific subset of responses to a given transmitter. Receptor subtype–selective agonists and antagonists can be of tremendous value, both clinically and in the experimental analysis of drug action. For many years, pharmacologists had to infer the existence of receptor subtypes based solely on drug selectivity in binding experiments or various functional assays. However, the application of modern biochemical and molecular biological techniques has, in many cases, allowed for the direct demonstration of the genes and corresponding proteins that give rise to a family of receptor subtypes.

Early studies by Langley (1906), Dale (1914), and others showed that some effects of peripherally administered ACh were mimicked by muscarine, an alkaloid found in the fly agaric mushroom (*Amanita muscaria*), whereas other effects were mimicked by nicotine, an alkaloid from the tobacco plant *Nicotiana tabacum*. (Alkaloids are nitrogen-containing compounds, usually bitter-tasting, that are typically of plant origin.) These findings led to the concept of two subtypes of cholinergic receptors, termed **muscarinic** and **nicotinic receptors**. These two receptor subtypes could be further differentiated in terms of their electrophysiological effects as well as the ability of certain drugs to act as selective antagonists. Nicotinic responses are always excitatory, occur very rapidly (within a few milliseconds), and can be blocked by *d*-tubocurarine, the active ingredient in the poison curare. In contrast, muscarinic responses can be either excitatory or inhibitory, have a longer latency of onset (usually at least 100 ms), and can be blocked by atropine or scopolamine. More recent research has shown that nicotinic receptors belong to the superfamily of ligand-gated channels, whereas muscarinic receptors belong to the superfamily of G protein–coupled receptors (see Chapter 6 for an introduction to these two receptor superfamilies). Furthermore, it is quite clear that multiple subtypes exist for both nicotinic and muscarinic receptors. Thus, there are two whole families of cholinergic receptors, the members of which differ from one another in their chemical structure as well as in their mechanism of action and localization in the nervous system. These topics will be taken up in greater detail in the sections that follow.

Nicotinic Receptors

Structure and function.   After many years of intense investigation, the cholinergic nicotinic receptor is probably the most thoroughly characterized neurotransmitter receptor. The first step in this process was isolation and purification of the receptor. The electric organs of the electric ray *Torpedo* and the Amazonian eel *Electrophorus* were an ideal source of tissue for this purpose because of their massive cholinergic innervation and dense concentration of nicotinic receptors. *Torpedo* electroplaques (the cells of the electric organ) are extremely large cells (dimensions: 5 mm × 5 mm × 0.02 mm), and one face of each electroplaque receives synaptic contacts over as much as 50% of its surface area (Cohen and Changeux, 1975). Another critical tool proved to be the venom of the banded krait (*Bungarus multicinctus*), a snake found in Taiwan. Lee (1972) had discovered that the toxicity of the venom was due mainly to the presence of a small polypeptide, which became known as α-bungarotoxin, that binds selectively and virtually irreversibly to nicotinic receptors. Consequently, cholinergic transmission is blocked at neuromuscular junctions, leading to death by paralysis and asphyxiation. Investigators used α-bungarotoxin as a tag for the nicotinic receptor, which made it possible to identify, extract, and purify the receptor protein from electric organs (see reviews by Changeux, Devillers-Thiéry, and Chemouilli, 1984; Changeux, 1993).

The electric organ nicotinic receptor is made up of four glycoprotein subunits designated α, β, γ, and δ. Two α subunits and one each of the others are clustered together in the membrane to form a pentameric (five-membered) structure with a total molecular mass of 280–290 kDa (Figure 7.9a, inset). The subunits surround a central pore 0.65 nm in diameter that serves as a channel for small cations. Consequently, the opening of the channel by ACh permits the passage of K^+ and especially Na^+ ions because of the strong Na^+ electrochemical gradient across the membrane. The resulting inward current depolarizes the membrane and results in a fast excitatory postsynaptic or end-plate potential. Binding sites for both ACh and α-bungarotoxin have been localized mainly to the two α subunits. Both sites must be occupied by ACh for the ion channel to open; however, fulfillment of this requirement is helped by the fact that the two sites show **positive cooperativity**. Cooperativity is a phenomenon whereby the binding of a neurotransmitter or drug to one receptive site influences the affinity of that substance for another site on the same receptor com-

plex. Cooperativity can be either positive, as in the present example, or negative, in which case ligand binding to the first site diminishes, rather than enhances, binding of another ligand molecule to the second site.

Recent studies have made remarkable progress in elucidating the organization and function of the nicotinic receptor at the molecular level (Changeux, 1990, 1993). As illustrated in Figure 7.9a, each of the receptor subunits contains a large hydrophilic domain at the amino (NH_2) terminal end of the protein. This region of the molecule is located on the extracellular side of the membrane, and recent studies strongly suggest that the ACh binding site is formed by several loops of the α subunit hydrophilic domain (Figure 7.9a and b); there may also be a contribution of negatively charged amino acids from the γ and δ subunits (Czajkowski, Kaufmann, and Karlin, 1993). These negative charges would form electrostatic interactions with the positively charged quaternary nitrogen group of ACh.

In addition to the hydrophilic domain, each subunit also contains four domains (designated M1–M4) consisting largely of hydrophobic amino acids. These domains are thought to be transmembrane (membrane-spanning) domains of the receptor, as shown in Figure 7.9a. Of particular interest are the M2 segments contributed by each subunit because these five domains constitute the ion channel of the receptor (Figure 7.9c). Certain amino acids of the M2 domain form negatively charged rings that presumably attract cations into the channel. Leucine residues (labeled L in the figure) form an additional uncharged ring at the center of the channel that is involved in closing the channel when the receptor is desensitized (see below).

Muscle and neuronal nicotinic receptors.   Further complexity is added to the structure of nicotinic receptors when we consider vertebrate muscle and nerve cells. Studies performed in the mid-1980s demonstrated the existence of a novel nicotinic receptor subunit that was

7.9 STRUCTURE OF THE ELECTRIC ORGAN NICOTINIC RECEPTOR. (a) The nicotinic receptor is made up of four glycoprotein subunits designated α, β, γ, and δ. Two α subunits and one each of the others are clustered together in the membrane to form a pentameric structure (inset). Each subunit possesses an extracellular hydrophilic domain as well as four hydrophobic domains (M1–M4) that presumably form helical membrane-spanning coils. (b) The ACh binding site is believed to consist primarily of amino acids in the α subunit hydrophilic domain. (c) Evidence indicates that the receptor-associated ion channel is formed by the M2 segments from each subunit (inset). The M2 segments contribute several rings of negatively charged amino acids as well as a ring of leucine (L) residues thought to be involved in receptor desensitization (note that only two M2 segments are shown here for the sake of clarity). The letters in b and c correspond to the standard amino acid abbreviations that may be found in Table 3.1. (After Changeux, 1993.)

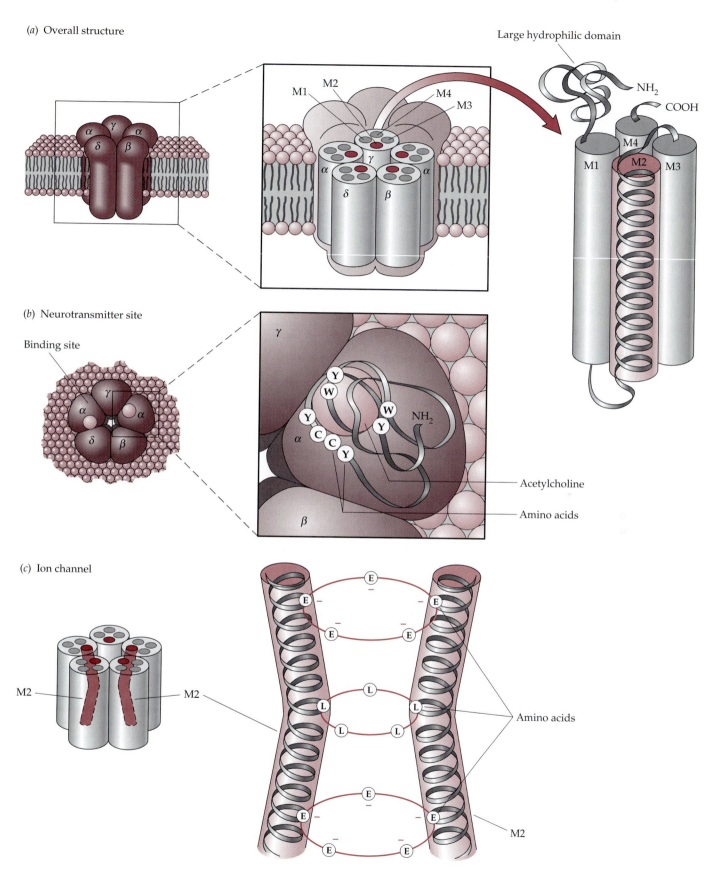

(a) Overall structure

Large hydrophilic domain

NH₂

COOH

M1 M2 M3 M4

(b) Neurotransmitter site

Binding site

Acetylcholine

Amino acids

(c) Ion channel

M2

M2

Amino acids

M2

designated ε (Schuetze, 1986). The ε subunit is homologous to the γ subunit and was found to substitute for it in the skeletal muscles of adult rats and cows. Interestingly, these species express the γ subunit during fetal development, but later switch to the ε subunit to yield an $\alpha_2\beta\epsilon\delta$ subunit composition (Brenner, 1991; Schuetze, 1986). Whether this is a universal developmental pattern in vertebrates remains to be determined. It should be noted that even the α, β, γ, and δ subunits of vertebrate muscle are not identical to the corresponding subunits found in the *Torpedo* electric organ. Nevertheless, there is substantial homology of the amino acid sequences across these tissues, indicating that the proteins are members of the same family and function in an analogous manner (Changeux, Devillers-Thiéry, and Chemouilli, 1984; Conti-Tronconi et al., 1982).

Neuronal nicotinic receptors exhibit both similarities to and differences from the receptors found in striated muscle. For example, neuronal receptors probably have the same basic type of pentameric structure; however, their subunit composition differs from that of muscle nicotinic receptors. Specifically, neuronal nicotinic receptors appear to consist of two families of subunits: α subunits, of which there are at least eight different isoforms present in rat brain (α2–α9; muscle α is considered α1), and β subunits, of which three different isoforms have been detected thus far (β2–β4; muscle β is β1) (Clarke, 1993; Decker et al., 1995; Patrick et al., 1993). The neuronal α subunits possess the ACh binding site and are homologous to muscle α subunits, whereas the neuronal β subunits share structural and functional properties with muscle β subunits. The most likely stoichiometry of neuronal nicotinic receptors is two α subunits plus three β subunits (Sargent, 1993). No homologues to the muscle γ, δ, or ε subunits have been found in neurons.

There is clear evidence for multiple subtypes of neuronal nicotinic receptors. One obvious way to distinguish between these subtypes is on the basis of their subunit composition (i.e., which α and β isoforms are present in the receptor complex). Eight different subunit combinations have been detected thus far, although more will almost certainly be found in the future. The known subtypes differ from one another in their sensitivity to various nicotinic agonists and antagonists, indicating that subunit composition has functional consequences for receptor action (Patrick et al., 1993; Sargent, 1993). An alternative approach to studying nicotinic receptor diversity is through the use of ligand binding techniques. Binding studies with brain tissue have identified two pharmacologically distinguishable classes of nicotinic receptors. One class binds labeled agonists (e.g., [³H]nicotine and [³H]ACh) with high affinity but does not bind α-bungarotoxin, whereas the other has a high affinity for α-bungarotoxin but a low affinity for agonists. Molecular biological studies have indicated that the agonist-preferring receptors possess the α4 subunit (usually in conjunc-

tion with β2), whereas α-bungarotoxin binding is conferred by the α7 subunit (Clarke, 1993). Continuing work at the molecular level will be needed to determine how many different receptor subtypes (in terms of subunit composition) are actually expressed in nervous tissue (see Vernallis, Conroy, and Berg, 1993).

Nicotinic receptor regulation. Expression and functioning of the nicotinic receptor is regulated by a number of important mechanisms. In this section we will focus on two such mechanisms: receptor desensitization, and receptor changes in response to tissue innervation and denervation.

Desensitization refers to a process by which repeated or prolonged exposure of a receptor to agonist stimulation causes the receptor to become temporarily refractory to further activation. In the case of the nicotinic receptor, continuous application of ACh or another agonist for a short period of time leads to a reduction in subsequent receptor-mediated channel opening. This phenomenon was first demonstrated for the neuromuscular junction by Katz and Thesleff (1957); however, it also occurs in electric organs and neurons.

Current ideas concerning the mechanisms of nicotinic receptor desensitization are reviewed by Léna and Changeux (1993) and Ochoa, Chattopadhyay, and McNamee (1989). The basis for desensitization is the concept of the receptor as an allosteric protein that can assume multiple conformational states with differing properties. Figure 7.10 presents the most popular model of the receptor, which proposes at least four such interconvertible states: a resting state (R) in which no agonist is present and the channel is closed; an agonist-induced active state (A) in which channel opening occurs; a rapidly formed (less than 1 second) intermediate state of desensitization (I); and a more slowly formed (seconds to minutes) and completely desensitized state (D). A few features of this model should be noted. First, in the rapidly desensitized state (I), transmembrane ion flux is reduced by 250-fold compared with the active state, whereas channel opening is virtually abolished in the slowly desensitized state (D). Second, even in the absence of an agonist, the receptor is hypothesized to be in equilibrium between the resting and desensitized states. This hypothesis has been confirmed in the case of *Torpedo*, in which 20% of the receptors were found to be in the D conformation with no agonist present. Third, the affinity of the receptor for agonists varies depending on its state. In particular, the two desensitized states exhibit a much higher affinity for ACh than do A or R.

Desensitization is an intrinsic property of the nicotinic receptor protein, which means that it requires no external mechanism. Nevertheless, a number of factors modulate the rates at which desensitization and resensitization occur. For example, desensitization is promoted by receptor phosphorylation via cAMP-dependent pro-

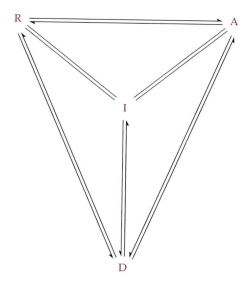

7.10 MODEL OF NICOTINIC RECEPTOR DESENSITIZATION. Nicotinic receptors exist in at least four interconvertible states: resting (R), active (A), rapidly desensitized or intermediate (I), and slowly desensitized (D). These states are in equilibrium in the membrane even in the absence of an agonist. (After Ochoa, Chattopadhyay, and McNamee, 1989.)

tein kinase, protein kinase C, a tyrosine kinase, and possibly also a Ca^{2+}-calmodulin-dependent kinase. Moreover, there exist various noncompetitive nicotinic antagonists (see below) that, in addition to inhibiting receptor functioning, also stabilize the desensitized (D) state of the receptor (Léna and Changeux, 1993; Ochoa, Chattopadhyay, and McNamee, 1989).

Studies performed on muscle nicotinic receptors have demonstrated another type of regulation that is me-

diated by the motor nerves (Brenner, 1991). As mentioned earlier, receptors found in fetal muscle cells prior to neural innervation have a $\alpha_2\beta\gamma\delta$ subunit composition. These receptors are spread over the entire length of the developing muscle fibers (myotubes) and exhibit a rapid turnover ($t_{\frac{1}{2}} \approx 1$ day). Furthermore, the channels formed by these receptors show relatively long opening times but a somewhat low current amplitude. When a motor nerve innervates a myotube, however, a number of striking changes take place. The cell membrane beneath the nerve terminal, which will become the end-plate region, begins to undergo multiple infoldings. Expression of the γ receptor subunit is suppressed, whereas ε subunit expression is induced. This leads to the formation of adult-type nicotinic receptors that exhibit briefer channel opening and a higher-amplitude current flow. The biological half-life of the receptors is increased ($t_{\frac{1}{2}} \approx 10$ days), and the receptors become concentrated almost exclusively in the end-plate region. These responses to innervation are illustrated schematically in Figure 7.11. A protein called agrin that is synthesized and released from the motor neuron appears to be responsible for the clustering of the cholinergic receptors at the neuromuscular junction. For further information, readers are referred to recent reviews by Nastuk and Fallon (1993) and Patthy and Nikolics (1993).

One reason for discussing the development of the muscle nicotinic receptor is its relevance for understanding the events that occur when an adult muscle is denervated. Surgically cutting the incoming motor nerve fibers results in a degeneration of the nerve terminals and a loss of release of ACh and other factors (e.g., agrin) present in the terminals. This leads to a reappearance of

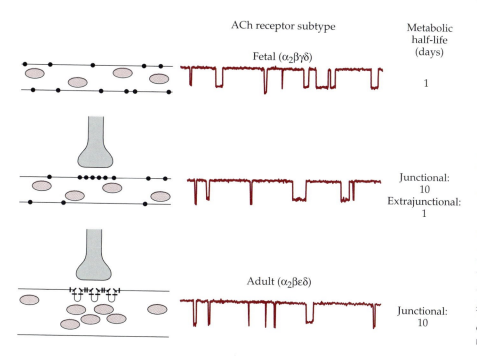

7.11 CHANGES IN THE LOCALIZATION AND PROPERTIES OF MUSCLE NICOTINIC RECEPTORS DURING DEVELOPMENT. Prior to innervation by motor nerve terminals, receptors are distributed along the entire surface of the muscle cells (*top panel*). These receptors possess the fetal subunit composition and mediate responses with relatively low amplitudes and long channel opening times. Innervation causes a switch to a pattern in which adult-type receptors (different subunit composition and channel properties) are clustered almost exclusively under neuromuscular junctions (*middle and bottom panels*). These events are accompanied by an increase in receptor half-life from approximately 1 to 10 days. (After Brenner, 1991.)

fetal-type nicotinic receptors which, as before, are distributed over the entire surface of the muscle cell membrane. Functionally, these events cause the muscle to become **supersensitive** to applied ACh or other agonists (Thesleff and Sellin, 1980). Another factor contributing to denervation supersensitivity is the lack of AChE activity in the extrajunctional region of the membrane. As might be expected, when the muscle is eventually reinnervated by a new nerve fiber, all of the above-mentioned events are reversed, and the muscle again becomes sensitive to ACh only in the end-plate region.

It should be mentioned here that receptor supersensitivity is not restricted to muscle cells, nor is it unique to the cholinergic system. Central neural pathways for many transmitters display this phenomenon when access of the transmitter to the receptors has been prevented. Furthermore, lesioning of the presynaptic neurons or transection of their fibers are not the only ways to produce supersensitivity in the postsynaptic target cells. "Pharmacological denervation" by means of receptor blockers or drugs that inhibit transmitter synthesis can also produce receptor changes that result in supersensitivity.

Muscarinic Receptors

General features. Despite the fact that they both evolved to mediate cholinergic transmission, muscarinic and nicotinic receptors differ tremendously in their structural and functional characteristics. Unlike nicotinic receptors, muscarinic receptors all belong to the G protein–coupled receptor superfamily. Thus, all muscarinic receptors share the general structural features of this superfamily, namely, a single amino acid chain with seven putative transmembrane domains. Furthermore, all synaptic responses mediated by muscarinic receptors are carried out through the activation of specific G proteins in the cell membrane. Finally, muscarinic responses show both a slower onset and a slower offset than nicotinic responses because of the actions of the G proteins and, in some cases, various second messenger systems. These and other aspects of muscarinic receptor functioning are explored further in the next several sections.

Subtypes. The notion of multiple muscarinic receptor subtypes was proposed a number of years ago (for review, see Hulme, Birdsall, and Buckley, 1990). This idea was based on the discovery of compounds that antagonized certain muscarinic responses more potently than others. Of particular importance was a cholinergic antagonist called pirenzepine that selectively blocked a population of neuronal muscarinic receptors while exhibiting a much lower affinity for muscarinic receptors found in heart and smooth muscle. The pirenzepine-sensitive receptors were named the M1 subtype (Hammer et al., 1980) (not to be confused with the M1 transmembrane

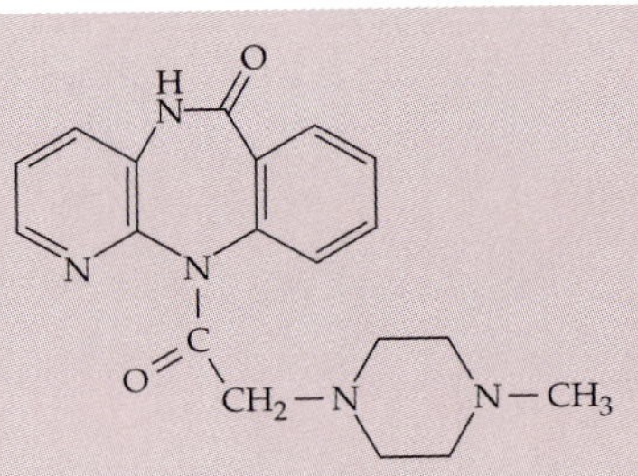

Pirenzepine

domains of nicotinic receptor subunits). Subsequent studies showed that the non-M1 receptors could be subdivided into two groups. Receptors found in the heart (M2) had a relatively high affinity for the pirenzepine analog 11-[[2-[(diethylamino)methyl]-1-piperidinyl]-acetyl]-5,11-dihydro-6H-pyrido[2,3-*b*][1,4]benzodiazepin-6-one (AF-DX 116), but relatively low affinities for the antagonists hexahydrosiladifenidol (HHSiD) and 4-diphenylacetoxy-N-methylpiperidine methiodide (4-DAMP). In contrast, M3 receptors present in ileum

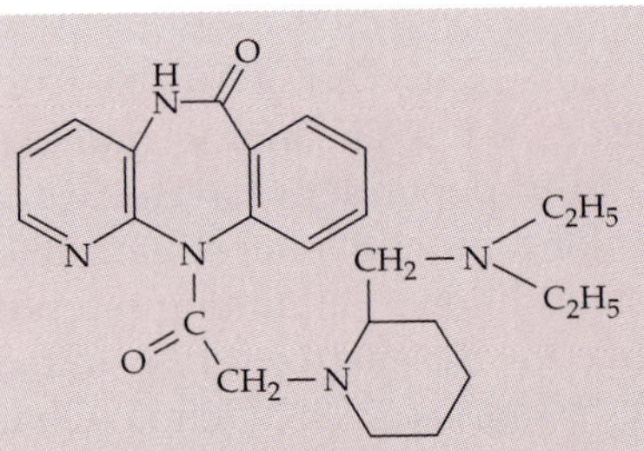

AF-DX 116

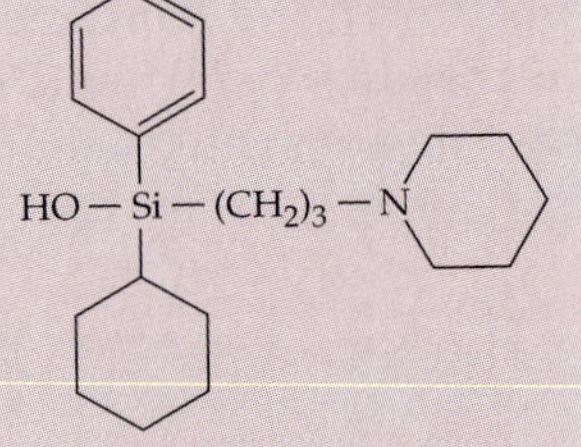

HHSiD

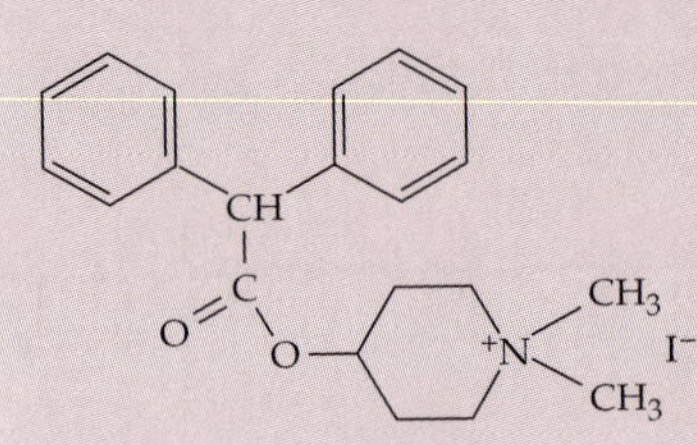

4-DAMP

and secretory glands (e.g., pancreas) exhibited a lower affinity for AF-DX 116, but higher affinities for HHSiD and 4-DAMP, compared to the M2 receptors (Hulme, Birdsall, and Buckley, 1990; Waelbroeck et al., 1990). Further studies then provided evidence for a fourth subtype, M4, located in both neuronal and nonneuronal cells (Lazareno, Buckley, and Roberts, 1990; Waelbroeck et al., 1990). Putative M4 receptors in rat striatum have binding properties that are similar to those of peripheral M3 receptors with respect to pirenzepine, AF-DX 116, HHSiD, and 4-DAMP. However, the M4 sites exhibit significantly higher affinities for two other muscarinic antagonists, himbacine and methoctramine (Waelbroeck et al., 1990).

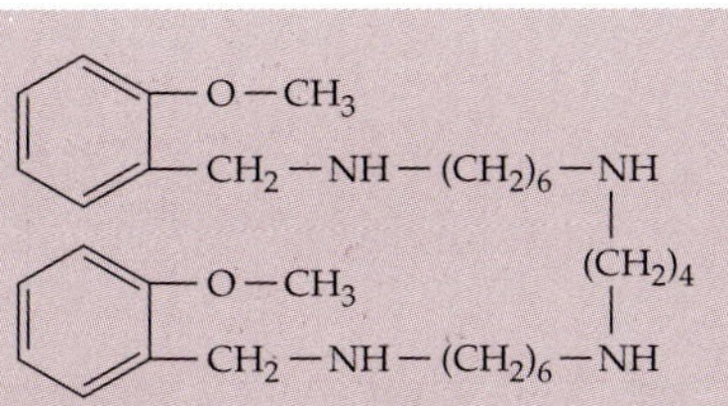

Methoctramine

Elucidation of the molecular biology of muscarinic receptors began in 1986 when Numa and coworkers reported cloning the first two genes for these receptors (Kubo, Fukuda et al., 1986; Kubo, Maeda et al., 1986). It is now clear that there are at least five different muscarinic receptor genes, conventionally denoted *m1–m5* (Bonner, 1989; Buckley, 1990; Richards, 1991). The proteins encoded by genes *m1*, *m2*, and *m3* appear to correspond to the M1, M2, and M3 receptors, respectively, determined through traditional pharmacological approaches.* The *m4* gene likewise probably codes for the M4 receptor (Lazareno, Buckley, and Roberts, 1990; Waelbroeck et al., 1990); however, at the time of this writing, the putative M5 receptor had not yet been pharmacologically identified in tissue binding studies.

To provide some understanding of the general structure of muscarinic receptors, the amino acid sequence and predicted structure of the rat m3 receptor are shown in Figure 7.12. Note the above-mentioned seven transmembrane domains, sites for N-glycosylation at the N-terminus, and the large third cytoplasmic loop (i3), which is characteristic of all muscarinic receptors and which appears to play an important role in receptor interactions with G proteins. Not shown are the potential phosphorylation sites in the cytoplasmic domains, particularly i3. Muscarinic receptor phosphorylation is stimulated by agonist exposure and may play an important role in receptor desensitization (Hosey, 1992; Wess, 1993a).

The transmembrane segments, which exhibit considerable sequence homology across the different muscarinic subtypes, are thought to be tightly packed together in the membrane, where they form a pocket for ACh binding. Amino acids predicted to interact directly with the neurotransmitter are shown in color. Of particular importance is the aspartate residue in transmembrane domain III (D147), which is conserved not only across all muscarinic receptors but also across the various G protein–coupled receptors for dopamine, norepinephrine, and serotonin. This negatively charged amino acid is critical for interacting with the positively charged nitrogen found in ACh as well as in the other transmitters mentioned (Wess, 1993a,b).

Mechanisms. The discussion of synaptic signaling in Chapter 6 pointed out that receptor-activated G proteins can either interact directly with ion channels or alter the cellular concentrations of second messengers such as cAMP, cGMP, Ca^{2+}, or inositol trisphosphate (IP_3) and diacylglycerol (DAG), the two products of phosphoinositide (PI) hydrolysis. To determine which of these mechanisms are used by different muscarinic receptor subtypes, numerous studies have been performed using not only "native" receptors (i.e., the receptors normally found in various neuronal and nonneuronal cell populations) but also individual genetically identified receptor subtypes introduced into cells that normally do not express those particular proteins.[†]

Table 7.1 is a summary of the effector mechanisms described thus far for the five cloned muscarinic receptor subtypes (for review, see Hulme, Birdsall, and Buckley, 1990; Jones, 1993). We can see that the five subtypes can be broken down into two separate families, one represented by the odd-numbered receptors m1, m3, and m5, and the other consisting of the even-numbered receptors m2 and m4. One of the most important effects of m1 family activation is PI hydrolysis, which occurs through activation of a specific phospholipase C by one or more pertussis toxin–insensitive G proteins. The two second messengers generated from PI, namely IP_3 and DAG, stimulate protein kinase C and elevate intracellular Ca^{2+} levels. Increased Ca^{2+} concentrations can in turn activate Ca^{2+}-dependent K^+ and Cl^- channels. An unexpected finding was that the odd-numbered muscarinic receptors can increase cAMP levels in several different cell types. Baumgold (1992) has hypothesized that this may be due to a novel mechanism involving stimulation of adenylyl cyclase by the $\beta\gamma$ subunits of G_q, the same G protein responsible for muscarinic receptor–mediated PI hydrolysis (see Chapter 6 for a more detailed discussion of G proteins and second messenger systems).

The m2 and m4 receptor subtypes are best known for their ability to inhibit adenylyl cyclase activity via the G

---

*Throughout this discussion lowercase letters will refer to both muscarinic receptor genes (e.g., m1) and the proteins encoded by these genes (e.g., m1); uppercase letters, for example, M1, will refer to receptors distinguished by pharmacological means. This distinction is only for methodological clarity and does not imply a difference between the two categories of receptors.

[†]The two principal methods for accomplishing the expression of a foreign protein are (1) transfection of cultured cells with the cloned gene for the protein, and (2) injection of frog oocytes (eggs) with the mRNA for the protein. In both cases, successful introduction of the genetic material leads to cellular synthesis of the specified protein, which can then be tested for its functional properties. For further information on these techniques, see Milner and Sutcliffe (1988) or Watson et al. (1992).

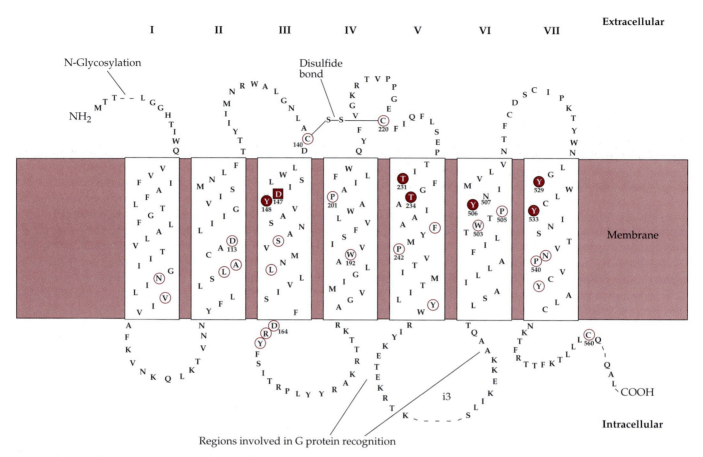

7.12 STRUCTURE OF THE RAT M3 MUSCARINIC RECEPTOR.
Like other G protein–coupled receptors, the m3 receptor consists of an extracellular amino terminus, seven putative transmembrane domains (I–VII), and an intracellular carboxy terminus. The amino acid residues shown in color are thought to participate in ACh binding. Other notable features of the receptor are sites for N-glycosylation on the amino terminal domain, regions of the third intracellular loop (i3) involved in G protein interaction, and a disulfide bond linking the second and third extracellular loops. Note that the dashed lines denote long segments of amino acids that are not shown. (After Wess, 1993b.)

protein G_i or in some cases possibly G_o. The resulting reduction in cAMP levels has been linked to inhibition of Ca^{2+} currents in cardiac muscle by muscarinic receptors.

Potassium channels are important targets of muscarinic receptor action. For example, receptors of the m1 family have been shown to inhibit a voltage-sensitive K^+ current known as the M-current ("M" for muscarinic). Although some M-channels are open at the normal resting potential, others begin to open as the membrane becomes depolarized due to excitatory synaptic input. The increased K^+ efflux through the M-channels tends to counteract the change in membrane potential. However, when the M-channels are inactivated by cholinergic stimulation, the result is a slow depolarization of the cell and a facilitation of synaptically induced repetitive firing. In contrast, m2 and m4 cause a rapid inhibitory

postsynaptic potential (IPSP) by triggering an inward-rectifying K^+ current.* This effect appears to be mediated by direct interaction of a receptor-coupled G protein with the ion channel (Hille, 1992).

One possible type of muscarinic mechanism not shown in the table involves cyclic guanosine monophosphate (cGMP). Although there is a long history of work implicating cGMP in muscarinic receptor action (see McKinney and Richelson, 1989), the manner in which ACh stimulates the formation of this second messenger is not well understood. Recent advances in cGMP research, however, have begun to shed light on this problem. Specifically, it appears that ACh-mediated increases in intracellular Ca^{2+} can trigger the synthesis of the novel gaseous messenger nitric oxide (NO), which in turn stimulates guanylyl cyclase activity and cGMP formation (see Chapter 6). One place in which this mechanism may operate is the striatum, where the NO-synthesizing enzyme nitric oxidase synthase (NOS) is present in a population of interneurons and where ACh and muscarinic agonists produce a Ca^{2+}-dependent stimula-

---

*Inward-rectifying K^+ channels are defined by their unusual voltage dependency: When the cell membrane is hyperpolarized, they open to allow an inward flow of K^+ ions, but when the membrane is depolarized, the channels close (see Hille, 1992).

Table 7.1 Effector Mechanisms Associated with Specific Muscarinic Receptor Subtypes[a]

Subtype	Mechanism
m1, m3, m5	Stimulate PI hydrolysis
	Increase intracellular Ca^{2+}
	Increase cAMP levels
	Release arachidonic acid
	Inhibit M-current (K^+)
	Activate Ca^{2+}-dependent K^+ and Cl^- currents
m2, m4	Inhibit adenylyl cyclase
	Stimulate inward-rectified K^+ current
	Inhibit Ca^{2+} currents

[a]Not all reported effects of muscarinic receptor activation are shown here (see text).
Source: After Richards, 1991; Hulme, Birdsall, and Buckley, 1990.

tion of cGMP formation (Vincent and Hope, 1992). The receptor subtype(s) mediating this effect remains to be determined; however, members of the m1 family are reasonable candidates due to their ability to activate PI hydrolysis and mobilize intracellular Ca^{2+}.

In closing, some of the major features of muscarinic receptor signaling mechanisms may be summarized as follows. First, a given receptor subtype can couple to multiple G proteins and influence multiple effector mechanisms. Second, muscarinic receptor-dependent processes in different cell populations depend not only on which subtypes are present, but also on the G proteins and effector systems expressed in each case. Third, although it was not emphasized earlier, it is important to recognize that the separation of subtypes into odd- and even-numbered is not complete. For example, a weak stimulation of PI hydrolysis has been reported for m2 and m4 under certain conditions. Nevertheless, the notion of two subtype families remains a useful way of categorizing most of the effects of these receptors.

Localization and Physiological Effects of Nicotinic and Muscarinic Receptors

Peripheral effects. Table 7.2 lists the distribution of nicotinic and muscarinic receptors in various peripheral neurons and effector organs. As already described, nicotinic receptors on striated muscles mediate the contractile effects of ACh on this tissue. Nicotinic receptors on postganglionic autonomic neurons and the catecholamine-secreting cells of the adrenal medulla are responsible for fast excitatory responses to the cholinergic inputs to these cells.

The muscarinic receptor responses of the heart, other parasympathetically innervated organs, and postganglionic neurons are more complex because of the above-mentioned presence of multiple receptor subtypes and signal transduction mechanisms. Inhibitory muscarinic responses are found in the heart, whereas the effects on most smooth muscles are excitatory. Cardiac muscle expresses predominantly (perhaps exclusively) the m2 muscarinic receptor subtype. Stimulation of these receptors by vagally released ACh has a dual effect: (1) inhibition of adenylyl cyclase, which decreases a voltage-gated Ca^{2+} current due to reduced phosphorylation of the Ca^{2+} channel, and (2) stimulation of an inward-rectifying K^+ current, which is mediated by direct action of a receptor-coupled G protein (i.e., no second messenger is involved) (Goyal, 1989). Together, these effects lead to a slowing of heart rate and a decrease in the strength of contraction.

Smooth muscles express members of both muscarinic receptor families, particularly m2 and m3 (Goyal, 1989). Thus, the previously mentioned excitatory effects of ACh on smooth muscle are mediated by a diverse set of mechanisms. These include (1) activation of a nonselective cation current, (2) activation of Cl^- currents, (3) inhibition of the M-current and other K^+ currents, and (4) mobilization of intracellular Ca^{2+} (Sims and Janssen, 1993). Moreover, the depolarization resulting from any of these processes may also open voltage-

Table 7.2 Distribution of Nicotinic and Muscarinic Receptors in Peripheral Neurons and Effector Organs

Receptor type	Distribution
Nicotinic	All striated muscles
	Postganglionic sympathetic and parasympathetic neurons[a]
	Adrenomedullary chromaffin cells[a]
Muscarinic	Parasympathetically innervated cardiac and smooth muscles (heart, iris, stomach, bronchioles, intestines, bladder, urogenital organs, etc.)
	Salivary, tear, and sweat glands

[a]These cells also possess muscarinic receptors.

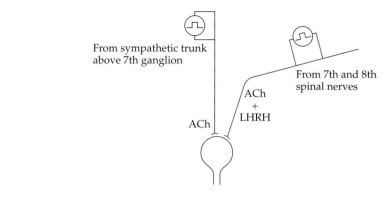

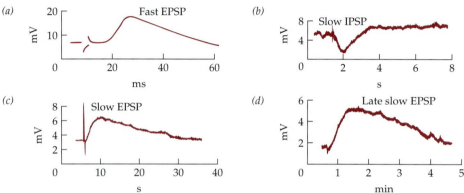

(a) Fast EPSP

(b) Slow IPSP

(c) Slow EPSP

(d) Late slow EPSP

7.13 SYNAPTIC RESPONSES ELICITED IN BULLFROG SYMPATHETIC GANGLIA. (*a*) Stimulating the preganglionic fiber once elicits a fast EPSP due to nicotinic receptor activation. Repetitive stimulation gives rise to a variety of additional responses including (*b*) a slow IPSP mediated by muscarinic receptors (to obtain this record, the fast EPSP was blocked with a nicotinic antagonist), (*c*) a muscarinic receptor-dependent slow EPSP that follows the first two responses and lasts for approximately 30 seconds, and (*d*) a late slow EPSP attributable to the release of a neuropeptide analogous to the mammalian hormone LHRH. (After Nicholls, Martin, and Wallace, 1992.)

sensitive Ca^{2+} channels, resulting in an increased contractile response.

In addition to possessing nicotinic receptors, neurons of autonomic ganglia have been reported to express mRNAs for muscarinic receptors m1, m2, m3, and m4 (Buckley, 1990). These cells provide a good example of the various synaptic responses that can be elicited by different cholinergic receptor subtypes. As shown in Figure 7.13, stimulation of the preganglionic cholinergic fibers innervating the bullfrog sympathetic ganglion can give rise to three different cellular responses: a fast EPSP, a slow IPSP, and a slow EPSP (Nicholls, Martin, and Wallace, 1992). (The late slow EPSP shown in *d* is due to an LHRH-like neuropeptide and is discussed further in Chapter 11.) Pharmacological investigations have shown that the fast EPSP is mediated by nicotinic receptors on the ganglionic neurons. The slow IPSP is due to an increase in K^+ efflux and is probably mediated by muscarinic m2 receptors. Finally, the slow EPSP is caused by an inactivation of M-channels, probably through the action of m1 or m3 receptors (Goyal, 1989). The muscarinic responses occur only with repetitive stimulation of the preganglionic fibers. This finding might indicate that the muscarinic system in these neurons is less sensitive than the nicotinic system. Alternatively, the muscarinic receptors on the cell membrane might be farther removed from the sites of ACh release, allowing for more AChE-catalyzed breakdown of the transmitter before it can reach the receptor-rich areas.

Central effects. In this section, we will focus initially on muscarinic receptors, as most of the known cellular effects of ACh in the CNS have been ascribed to muscarinic receptor activation. Autoradiographic studies have been used to determine the central distribution of M1 and M2 receptor subtypes (reviewed by Quirion et al., 1993) and more recently the M3 muscarinic receptor (Zubieta and Frey, 1993). However, the selectivity of the drugs available for this purpose is not sufficient to permit complete confidence in this approach. Hence, several laboratories have undertaken the development of subtype-specific muscarinic receptor antibodies raised against recombinant receptor proteins (this was possible, of course, because of the prior cloning of the *m1–m5* genes). Use of the resulting antibodies in immunohistochemical and immunoprecipitation studies has enabled researchers to determine the relative density of each receptor subtype in various brain regions.

Based on immunoprecipitation studies, Wolfe and coworkers observed the following regional distribution of muscarinic receptor subtypes in the rat brain. High levels of m1 receptors were found in the neocortex, hippocampus, striatum, and olfactory tubercles, but low levels were found in the diencephalon, the pons and medulla, and the cerebellum (Wall, Yasuda, Hory et al., 1991). A different pattern was obtained for the m2 receptor. Compared with m1, this subtype showed higher levels in the pons and medulla and in the cerebellum, but lower levels in all forebrain areas (Li et al., 1991).

Amounts of m3 muscarinic receptors were lower than either m1 or m2 in all brain areas except for the cerebellum (Wall, Yasuda, Li et al., 1991). Distribution of m4 was similar to that of m1, except that the striatum showed particularly high levels of this subtype (Yasuda et al., 1993). Finally, the level of m5 receptors was low in all brain areas examined (Yasuda et al., 1993).

Levey and coworkers (Hersch et al., 1994; Levey et al., 1991) used subtype-specific antibodies to examine the localization of muscarinic receptors by immunohistochemistry. In addition, a number of studies have been published concerning the distribution of muscarinic mRNAs in various brain areas (e.g., Brann, Buckley, and Bonner, 1988; Buckley, Bonner, and Brann, 1988; Vilaro et al., 1991; Weiner, Levey, and Brann, 1990). Table 7.3 provides a comparison of the regional variation in receptor subtypes found using immunochemical approaches (immunoprecipitation and immunohistochemistry), in situ hybridization for receptor mRNAs, and receptor binding studies. In general, the patterns of relative density match up rather well, although some differences in the distribution of receptor proteins and of mRNAs can be expected due to the fact that mRNA is located in or near the cell body, whereas many receptors are found on distal dendrites or on nerve terminals. Several other summary conclusions may also be drawn from this comparison. First, for reasons yet to be determined, it appears that the level of m3 receptor protein does not match the expression of the *m3* gene in some brain areas. Second, in forebrain cholinergic projection areas such as the neocortex and hippocampus, muscarinic receptors are largely of the m1, m2, and m4 subtypes. Finally, areas containing dense concentrations of cholinergic cell bodies, such as the basal forebrain and motor neuron groups, almost exclusively exhibit m2 receptors. This is consistent with the notion that some m2 receptors act as release-modulating autoreceptors (see below).

As summarized in recent reviews by Krnjević (1993) and McKinney (1993), the central electrophysiological effects of muscarinic receptor activation are largely excitatory and are typically related to a reduction in K^+ currents. Studies in the cerebral cortex have shown this effect to be mediated by a receptor with a high affinity for pirenzepine, presumably M1 (Hulme, Birdsall, and Buckley, 1990). Early research reported that only 20–30% of cortical neurons were responsive to applied ACh; however, these experiments looked only at changes in spontaneous firing rate. Later work demonstrated that in many more cases, ACh was able to enhance responsiveness to other excitatory inputs active at the same time (Rasmusson, 1993). This phenomenon, which is known as **heterosynaptic facilitation**, enables the ascending cholinergic projections to the cortex to amplify the effects of sensory input in various cortical areas. As discussed below, heterosynaptic facilitation may play an important role in the cognitive effects of ACh and cholinergic drugs.

In the hippocampus, ACh facilitates excitatory responses produced by activation of the NMDA-type glutamate receptor (see Chapter 10). In this case, the effect is dependent on M1-stimulated PI hydrolysis. Two examples of central inhibitory muscarinic effects are (1) an increase in K^+ currents in some brain stem areas, and (2) a decrease in Ca^{2+} currents in the hippocampus (Krnjević, 1993). These responses are most likely mediated by M2 or possibly M4 receptors.

The distribution of central nicotinic receptors has been mapped autoradiographically using labeled agonists and antagonists. High-affinity agonist binding sites are found in the neocortex (particularly layers 3 and 4), the molecular layer of the hippocampal dentate gyrus, various motor and sensory nuclei of the thalamus, the medial habenula, the interpeduncular nucleus, the outermost layers of the superior colliculus, the substantia nigra pars compacta, and the ventral tegmental area

Table 7.3 Distribution of Muscarinic Receptor Subtypes in Rat Brain: Comparative Receptor Protein Immunoreactivity, mRNA Levels, and Pharmacological Binding Sites[a]

Brain region	Receptor protein (immunohistochemistry)[b]				Receptor mRNA levels (in situ hybridization)[b]				Receptor binding (autoradiography)[c]	
	m1	m2	m3	m4	m1	m2	m3	m4	M1	M2
Neocortex	+++	++	+	++	+++	++	++	+	+++	++
Hippocampus	+++	++	+	++	+++	+	++	++	+++	++
Striatum	+++	++	+	+++	+++	++	−	+++	+++	+
Basal forebrain	−	+++	ND	−	−	+++	+	+	−	+++
Thalamus	+	+++	+	+	+	+++	++	+	+	++
Motor neurons	−	+++	ND	−	−	+++	−	−	−	+++

[a]Indices of relative density: −, extremely low or undetectable; +, low; ++, moderate; +++, high; ND, not determined.
[b]m5 immunoreactively and mRNA are undetectable or low in all of the listed areas.
[c]Neither M3 nor M4 receptor binding are shown because of uncertainties in the distribution of these pharmacologically defined subtypes.
Source: After Levey et al., 1991, based on data from the references cited in the text.

(Luetje, Patrick, and Séguéla, 1990). Although most of these receptors are probably postsynaptic, some appear to be located on nerve terminals, where they may regulate the release of ACh (autoreceptors) or possibly other neurotransmitters (heteroreceptors) (Sargent, 1993; see next section).

α-Bungarotoxin-labeled binding sites have a somewhat different distribution than those labeled with agonists. These sites are concentrated in neocortical layers 1 and 6, the hippocampus, the hypothalamus, the interpeduncular nucleus, and the superior and inferior colliculi (Clarke, 1993; Luetje, Patrick, and Séguéla, 1990). Although it is beyond the scope of this book, information on receptor subunit expression in these different regions can be obtained from the cited references.

As mentioned earlier, most of the electrophysiological responses to ACh by central neurons have been ascribed to actions on muscarinic receptors. Nevertheless, nicotinic receptors have been implicated in a few instances. The earliest report of a central nicotinic-type action came from the classic work of Eccles, Fatt, and Koketsu (1954) on the Renshaw cells of the spinal cord. Since that time, excitatory cholinergic responses with a nicotinic pharmacology have been demonstrated in virtually all brain areas that possess nicotinic receptor binding sites (Clarke, 1993; Luetje, Patrick, and Séguéla, 1990). Although the role of these receptors in normal cholinergic physiology is not yet fully understood, behavioral effects of central nicotinic receptor stimulation have now been described (see Decker et al., 1995).

Regulation of Neurotransmitter Release by Cholinergic Autoreceptors and Heteroreceptors

The cholinergic system provides important examples of the pharmacological concepts of autoreceptors and heteroreceptors. The definitions and historical background of these concepts can be found in Kalsner (1990), Koelle (1990), and Starke, Göthert, and Kilbinger (1989) (see also Chapter 6). Autoreceptors are presynaptic receptors through which cells may regulate their own electrophysiological activity, neurotransmitter synthesis, and transmitter release. Autoreceptors capable of influencing cell firing (generally in an inhibitory way) are located on the soma or dendrites of the cell. In contrast, synthesis- and release-modulating autoreceptors are appropriately located on the nerve terminals. Heteroreceptors are receptors located on nerve terminals that enable one transmitter to alter the release of another. In principle, this may occur either by means of axoaxonic synapses or through the action of transmitter molecules that have reached the nerve terminal via nonclassical mechanisms (e.g., release from nearby dendrites, or release at a distant site followed by diffusion through the extracellular space).

The presence of cholinergic autoreceptors in the brain and PNS has been demonstrated many times using various tissue preparations such as tissue slices and synaptosomes. In a typical experiment, the tissue is preincubated with a radiolabeled ACh precursor (for example, [^{3}H]choline), and then depolarization-induced release of labeled ACh is measured. The existence of an autoreceptor can be inferred if (1) the addition of exogenous unlabeled ACh or an ACh agonist inhibits (or stimulates) release of the labeled transmitter in a dose-dependent manner, and (2) the modulatory effect can be reversed by treatment with an ACh antagonist. Evidence for release-inhibiting autoreceptors has been found for cholinergic neurons projecting to the cortex, hippocampus, and other brain areas, for postganglionic cholinergic neurons innervating various peripheral organs, and for motor neurons innervating striated muscles and fish electric organs (reviewed by Grimm et al., 1994; Starke, Göthert, and Kilbinger, 1989). As shown in Figure 7.14, ACh autoreceptors generally exhibit a muscarinic pharmacology, although the subtype(s) involved has not been clearly delineated. Muscarinic autoreceptors have usually been considered to be of the M2 subtype because of their insensitivity to the M1-selective antagonist pirenzepine. Furthermore, as mentioned above, m2 receptors and mRNA are present at high levels in cholinergic neurons, where they are well situated to serve an autoreceptor role. However, recent pharmacological studies have not all been consistent with this view. For example, experiments on the hippocampal autoreceptor suggest an M4 pharmacology (McKinney, Miller, and Aagaard, 1993). Moreover, autoreceptors mediating inhibition of ACh release at the circular muscle of the guinea pig ileum may be of the M1 subtype (Kilbinger, Dietrich, and von Bardeleben, 1992). Thus, the identity of muscarinic autoreceptors must be determined for each system under investigation.

Muscarinic heteroreceptors are also found in the brain and periphery (Grimm et al., 1994). For example, some of the M1 receptors in the striatum appear to be located on the terminals of the dopaminergic nigrostriatal pathway. Stimulation of these receptors by ACh increases dopamine release from the terminals. Another example relates to the important cholinergic pathway from the septum to the hippocampus. Release of the excitatory amino acids glutamate and aspartate (see Chapter 10) from hippocampal nerve endings is inhibited by ACh. This effect is antagonized by AF-DX 116, but not by pirenzepine, which indicates a non-M1 pharmacology (Raiteri, Marchi, and Paudice, 1990).

Finally, it should be noted that various studies have presented evidence for nicotinic autoreceptors and heteroreceptors (Clarke, 1993; Starke, Göthert, and Kilbinger, 1989). In contrast to the muscarinic type, nicotinic autoreceptors usually enhance, rather than inhibit, ACh release. Wessler (1989) has shown that nicotinic autoreceptors at the neuromuscular junction are activated only upon repetitive stimulation, thereby serving to enhance ACh availability at times of vigorous muscular activity

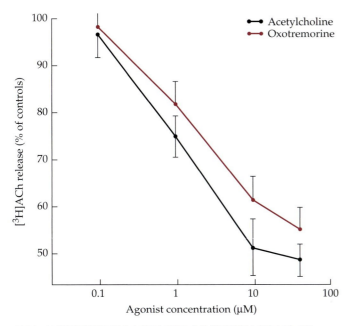

7.14 AUTORECEPTOR-MEDIATED INHIBITION OF ACh RE-
LEASE FROM RAT HIPPOCAMPAL SYNAPTOSOMES. Synaptosomes were preincubated with [^{3}H]choline to label internal ACh
stores. Release of [^{3}H]ACh was evoked by exposure to elevated
levels of K^+, which depolarizes the synaptosomal membranes.
Such release was inhibited in a dose-dependent manner by the
presence of unlabeled ACh or the muscarinic agonist oxotremorine. (After Raiteri, Marchi, and Paudice, 1990.)

when the motor neurons would be continuously active.
On the other hand, there is a safety valve built into this
positive feedback system because the receptors desensitize when exposed to ACh for several minutes.

Drugs That Affect Cholinergic Receptors

A summary of some important cholinergic receptor agonists and antagonists is given in Table 7.4. These and
other drugs are discussed in detail in the next few sections.

General Cholinergic Agonists

The synthetic ACh analogs carbachol (carbamyl choline)
and methacholine (Provocholine) are general cholinomimetic (ACh-mimicking) agents, although they have
been used primarily for their muscarinic receptor-related

functions. Both compounds are resistant to hydrolysis by
cholinesterases, which enhances their biological potency.
Furthermore, they show little penetration of the
blood–brain barrier and therefore exert no central effects
unless applied directly to the CNS. Methacholine has potent bronchoconstrictor properties and thus is sometimes
administered in inhalant form to test for bronchial hyperreactivity.

Nicotinic Agonists and Antagonists

Nicotine, of course, is the classic nicotinic agonist. We
will not discuss the pharmacology of nicotine here, since
this substance will be taken up in detail in Chapter 14.
However, other cholinergic agonists with nicotinic receptor selectivity have been identified. One such agent,
methylcarbachol, has been useful as a ligand in nicotinic
receptor binding studies (Boksa and Quirion, 1987). The
compound dimethylphenylpiperazinium (DMPP) is an
agonist with some selectivity for neuronal nicotinic receptors. Another group of compounds, including succinylcholine, decamethonium, and a substance called

anatoxin-a, exerts potent depolarizing effects on striated
muscles. Initial muscular contraction is followed rapidly
by a depolarization block of the cells that renders them
unresponsive to ACh. Because of this property, succinylcholine has proved useful as a muscle relaxant in certain

Table 7.4   Some Important Cholinergic Receptor Agonists and Antagonists

Drug	Action
Carbachol	General cholinergic agonist
Methacholine	General cholinergic agonist
Nicotine	Nicotinic agonist
DMPP	Neuronal nicotinic receptor agonist
Succinylcholine	Muscle nicotinic agonist (depolarization block)
Decamethonium	Muscle nicotinic agonist (depolarization block)
D-Tubocurarine	Nicotinic antagonist (preference for muscle)
Gallamine	Nicotinic antagonist (preference for muscle)
Hexamethonium	Nicotinic antagonist (preference for ganglia)
Mecamylamine	Nicotinic antagonist (preference for ganglia)
Muscarine	Muscarinic agonist
Pilocarpine	Muscarinic agonist
Oxotremorine	Muscarinic agonist
McN-A-343	M1 muscarinic agonist
Atropine	Muscarinic antagonist
Scopolamine	Muscarinic antagonist
QNB	Muscarinic antagonist (receptor binding studies)
Pirenzepine	M1 muscarinic antagonist
AF-DX 116	M2 muscarinic antagonist

surgical procedures. Anatoxin-a is a novel poison produced by the blue-green alga *Anabaena flos-aquae*. It is a potent agonist at both neuronal and muscle nicotinic receptors, and is responsible for occasional deaths of livestock and waterfowl in various parts of the world (Carmichael, Biggs, and Gorham, 1975; Chiang, Butler, and Brown, 1991; Wonnacott et al., 1991).

Nicotinic antagonists can be loosely divided into two groups: neuromuscular blocking agents and ganglionic blockers (Taylor 1985c,d). One of the most extensively studied antagonists at neuromuscular nicotinic receptors

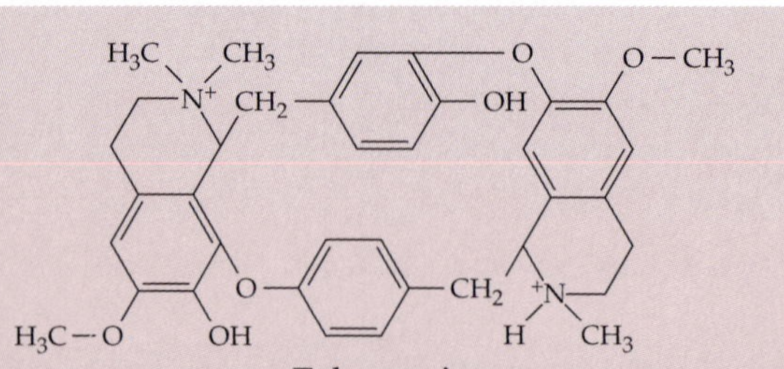

D-Tubocurarine

is *d*-tubocurarine (Chiappinelli, 1989). This substance also blocks ganglionic nicotinic receptors, but with less potency than at neuromuscular junctions. It apparently does not cross the blood–brain barrier and thus exerts no effects on central nicotinic receptors. D-Tubocurarine is the principal active ingredient of curare, a poison obtained from the tropical plant *Chondrodendron tomentosum*. Long before its discovery by pharmacologists, curare was being

used by South American Indians as an arrow poison for hunting. D-Tubocurarine acts by competitively binding to and blocking the nicotinic neuromuscular receptor sites. Because the binding is not irreversible, curare poisoning can be treated with an anti-AChE drug such as neostigmine, which overcomes the competitive inhibition by increasing junctional ACh concentrations.

A number of synthetic curare-type drugs, such as gallamine (Flaxedil), pancuronium (Pavulon), and dihydro-β-erythroidine, have been developed. Like D-tubocurarine, these compounds are competitive antagonists at muscle nicotinic receptors; however, they vary in their potency, duration of action, and side effects. Clinically,

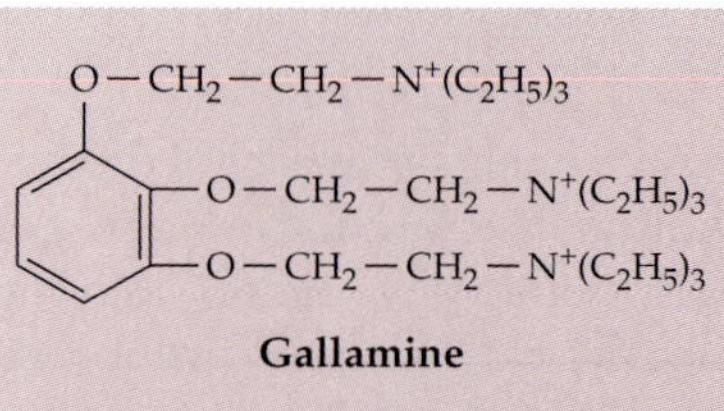

Gallamine

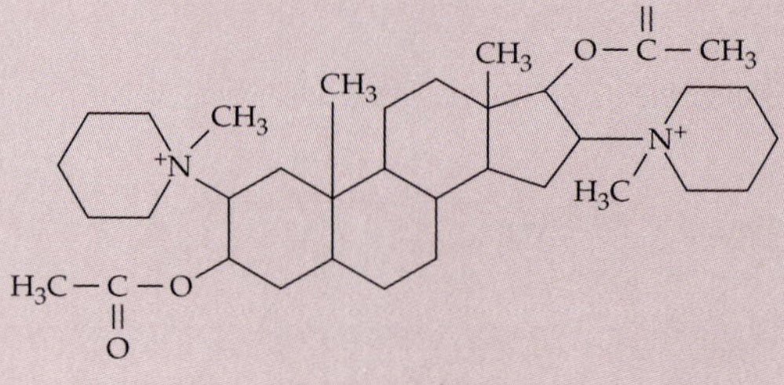

Pancuronium

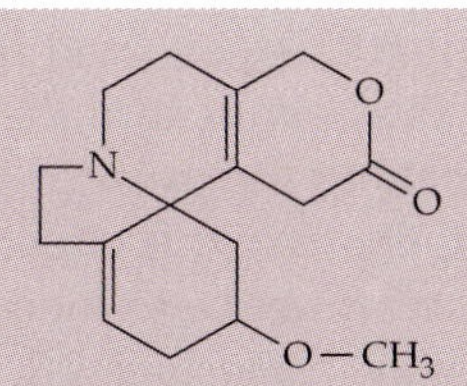

Dihydro-β-erythroidine

Muscarine

they are given intravenously to obtain muscular relaxation during surgery (especially during abdominal surgery) as well as during resetting of dislocated joints and aligning of broken bones. They have also been used as premedications to prevent the dislocations and bone fractures that can occur in patients undergoing electroconvulsive shock therapy for depression. In the case of gallamine, it should be noted that this compound exhibits muscarinic M2 antagonism in addition to its neuromuscular blocking effects.

Hexamethonium and mecamylamine (Inversine) are two well-known drugs that preferentially block nicotinic receptors at autonomic ganglia as compared with neuromuscular junction receptors. Because these substances can pass the blood–brain barrier, their affinity for neu-

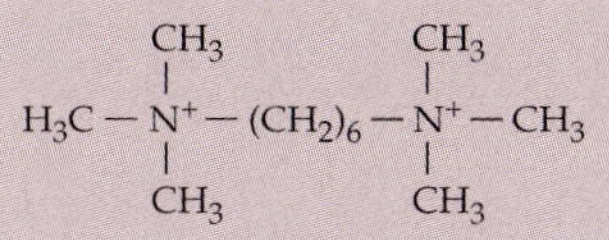

Hexamethonium **Mecamylamine**

ronal nicotinic receptors means that they also antagonize the actions of centrally acting nicotinic drugs. Ganglionic blocking agents were designed for controlling autonomic dysfunctions such as gastrointestinal hypermotility or cardiovascular hypertension. Unfortunately, the side effects of these drugs were quite pronounced. Therefore, although mecamylamine is still sometimes prescribed for severe cases of essential hypertension, the ganglionic blockers have generally been superseded by newer, more selective agents (see Taylor, 1985c).

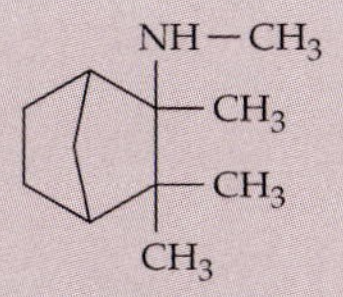

Muscarinic Agonists and Antagonists

Muscarine, pilocarpine, arecoline, and oxotremorine represent muscarinic agonists with varying degrees of selectivity (Taylor, 1985b). Because these substances have strong effects on structures innervated by postganglionic parasympathetic neurons, they are sometimes called **parasympathomimetic agents**. Some muscarinic agonists have clinical value, whereas others are mainly used experimentally.

Muscarine is a toxic alkaloid that was first extracted from the mushroom *Amanita muscaria* in 1869. Other mushrooms of the genera *Clitocybe* and *Inocybe* have even greater concentrations of this toxin. Muscarine has no therapeutic application, although it has had some use

as a pharmacological tool. In cases of accidental ingestion of muscarine-bearing mushrooms, the victim exhibits exaggerated autonomic responses such as marked lacrimation (tearing), salivation, sweating, pinpoint pupils, severe abdominal pain due to strong contractions of the smooth muscles of the viscera, painful diarrhea, cardiovascular collapse, coma, convulsions, and eventually death. Fortunately, these effects can be reversed by the muscarinic antagonist atropine, which displaces muscarine from its receptor sites and can reverse its effects even in severe cases of intoxication.*

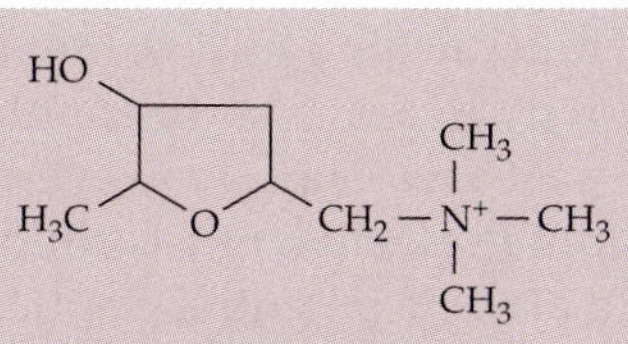

Other muscarinic agonists include the synthetic drugs oxotremorine and *cis*-dioxolane, as well as two naturally occurring compounds: pilocarpine, from the leaves of the South American shrub *Pilocarpus jaborandi*, and arecoline, found in the seeds of the betel nut palm *Areca catechu*. These substances exert many of the same parasympathomimetic effects as muscarine, particularly with respect to stimulating the secretion of sweat and saliva.

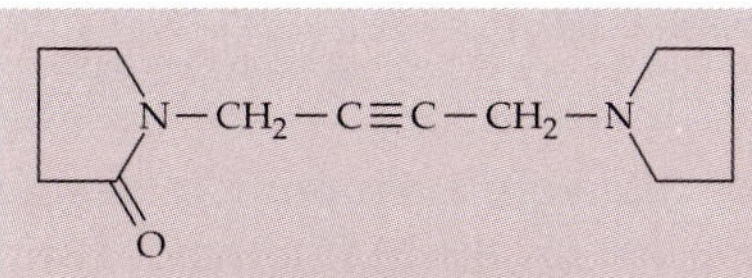

Oxotremorine

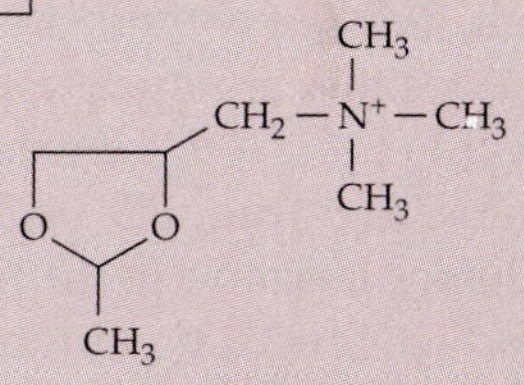

cis-**Dioxolane**

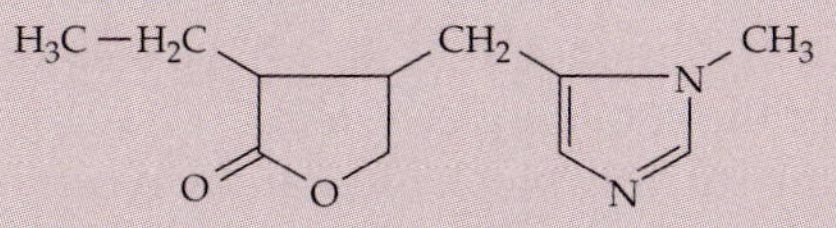

Pilocarpine

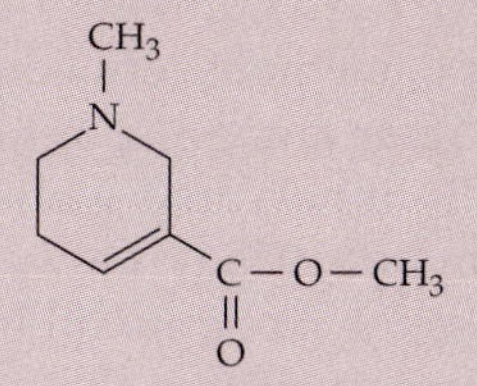

Arecoline

---

*Consumption of *Amanita muscaria* also leads to hallucinations and other effects due to the presence of the GABA agonist muscimol as well as ibotenic acid (which is metabolized to muscimol in the body). This mushroom reputedly got its colloquial name "fly agaric" because it has an intoxicating, even lethal, effect on flies that are attracted to and ingest its contents (Siegel, 1989).

None of the muscarinic agonists mentioned above show great selectivity in terms of different receptor subtypes. Over the past few years, however, interest has grown in developing selective muscarinic agonists for clinical use. One area of potential application is Alzheimer's disease (Davis et al., 1993; Palacios, Boddeke, and Pombo-Villar, 1991), in which the progressive decline in cognitive functioning (i.e., dementia) has been attributed at least partly to damage to the cholinergic innervation of the cerebral cortex and hippocampus (see below and Chapter 20). Selective M1 agonists might be particularly helpful in this situation, because this receptor subtype is much more prevalent in the CNS (including the cortex and hippocampus; see Table 7.3) than in peripheral organs. Beneficial behavioral effects might thus be achieved without the autonomic side effects that usually hinder the use of muscarinic agents. One extensively characterized M1 muscarinic agonist is 4-(3-chlorophenylcarbamoyl-oxy)2-butynyltrimethylammonium chloride, which was originally synthesized by the McNeil pharmaceutical company and designated McN-A-343. However, the selectivity of this compound is not

McN-A-343

high, and researchers are therefore attempting to design analogs that are more specific for the M1 subtype (Lambrecht et al., 1993). Parke-Davis has also developed an interesting drug, PD 142505, which has been reported to enhance learning performance in mice at low doses that produce few or no autonomic cholinergic effects (Davis et al., 1993). It remains to be determined whether selective M1 agonists will prove beneficial in Alzheimer's disease or other types of dementia that may have a significant involvement of the cholinergic system.

Drugs that competitively block muscarinic receptors have been known for many years. Muscarinic blockers are sometimes termed **parasympatholytic agents** because of their antagonism to ACh action at parasympathetically innervated glands and visceral smooth muscles (Taylor, 1985a). However, many of these drugs easily pass the blood–brain barrier and thus affect cholinergic synapses within the CNS. Two important naturally occurring muscarinic antagonists are atropine (hyoscamine) and the closely related scopolamine (hyoscine). These substances are alkaloids found in a group of plants that includes the deadly nightshade (*Atropa belladonna*), henbane (*Hyoscyamus niger*), and members of the genus *Datura*. Because of the systemic toxicity of muscarinic antagonists, extracts of the deadly nightshade were used during the Middle Ages as a poison to settle matters in many political and family intrigues. A

cosmetic use of the plant also evolved in which women instilled the juice of the berries into their eyes to cause pupil dilation (by blocking the muscarinic effects on the constrictor muscles of the iris); this effect was considered to make the user more attractive to men. Thus, the taxonomic designation *Atropa belladonna* reflects both the poisonous character of the plant and its use in beautification: *bella donna* means "beautiful woman" in Latin, whereas Atropos was the eldest of the Three Fates in Greek mythology, whose duty it was to cut the thread of life at the appropriate time.

Atropine

Scopolamine

Atropine passes the blood–brain barrier and, at low doses, mildly stimulates the brain stem and higher cerebral centers. Its effect on the vagus nerve causes a slight transitory increase in heart and respiration rate. At toxic doses, the CNS effects include restlessness, irritability, disorientation, hallucinations, or delirium. With still higher doses, stimulation gives way to depression, coma, and eventually death by respiratory paralysis. Compared with atropine, scopolamine has a shorter duration of action and is more potent in producing CNS depression. Scopolamine in therapeutic doses produces drowsiness, euphoria, amnesia, fatigue, and dreamless sleep. It has sometimes been used along with narcotics as a pre-anesthetic medication prior to surgery or alone prior to childbirth to produce "twilight sleep," a condition characterized by drowsiness and amnesia for events occurring during the duration of the drug action (Weiner, 1985a; see the discussion of ACh and memory below).

Antimuscarinic drugs have been used for a century or more to control dysfunctions of parasympathetically innervated organs. The desire to improve specificity of action at selected sites has led to the development of synthetic compounds such as dicyclomine (Bentyl), a GI tract antispasmodic agent useful in the treatment of irritable bowel syndrome, as well as isopropamide (Darbid), glycopyrrolate (Robinul), and clidinium bromide (Quarzan), all of which are prescribed as adjunctive agents in the treatment of peptic ulcers. Two useful atropine and scopolamine congeners are the *N*-methylated derivatives atropine methylnitrate and methscopolamine bromide. These drugs exert peripheral effects similar to those of their parent compounds, but show few central effects due to lack of penetration across the blood–brain barrier. In addition to their therapeutic applications in anesthesia and as decongestants, the methylated compounds have frequently been used experimentally to determine whether the behavioral effects of atropine or scopolamine in animals can be attributed to the peripheral autonomic effects of these drugs.

Labeling of muscarinic receptors for purposes of membrane binding or autoradiographic analysis has typically been accomplished using either [³H]methscopolamine or another nonspecific muscarinic antagonist, [³H]quinuclidinyl benzilate (QNB). Either ligand can be

QNB

used alone to label all pharmacologically known muscarinic receptors, or some degree of subtype selectivity can be obtained by blocking the binding to one or more subtypes through the addition of an appropriate nonradioactive antagonist such as pirenzepine (see Cortés et al., 1986, and Mash and Potter, 1986, for two examples of this approach).

In concluding this section, it is important to mention the issue of subtype-selective muscarinic antagonists. Because of the general lack of agonists that discriminate between various muscarinic receptor subtypes, the major advances that have been made in muscarinic receptor pharmacology have involved the development of antagonists with varying degrees of specificity. The M1 antagonist pirenzepine and its congener telenzepine remain among the most selective compounds available to pharmacologists. As discussed earlier, some other partially

Telenzepine

selective muscarinic antagonists are AF-DX 116, HHSiD, 4-DAMP, himbacine, and methoctramine (see Hulme, Birdsall, and Buckley, 1990, for subtype specificity profiles). Efforts are particularly being made to develop more specific M2 antagonists for the treatment of Alzheimer's disease (Doods et al., 1993), with the premise that blockade of central M2 autoreceptors might increase ACh release and thus improve cognitive functioning.

Part II Summary

Acetylcholine is widely distributed in the peripheral and central nervous systems. It is used as a transmitter by motor neurons found in the ventral horn of the spinal cord and in cranial nerves III, IV, V, VI, VII, and XII. Consequently, ACh is released at neuromuscular junctions, where it acts to stimulate muscular contraction. Acetylcholine also plays a prominent role in the autonomic nervous system as the principal transmitter released by the parasympathetic and sympathetic preganglionic fibers, as well as by most of the parasympathetic postganglionic fibers. Parasympathetically innervated glands and smooth muscles may be either stimulated or inhibited by ACh, depending on the actions of the cholinergic receptors present in each tissue.

Cholinergic neurons in the brain can be divided into several groups. Within the striatal complex (caudate–putamen, nucleus accumbens, and olfactory tubercle) are large numbers of cholinergic interneurons that play an important role in the functioning of the extrapyramidal motor system. A widely studied group of ACh-containing projection neurons is present in the basal forebrain, particularly in the nucleus basalis, medial septal nucleus, vertical and horizontal limb nuclei of the diagonal band, and the substantia innominata. These cells innervate the cerebral cortex and the hippocampus, and they are thought to be involved in various aspects of learning, memory, and attentional processes. The other two major cholinergic cell groups are found in the diencephalon (medial habenula and several hypothalamic nuclei) and in the pontomesencephalon (pedunculopontine and dorsolateral tegmental nuclei). The medial habenula projects to the interpeduncular nucleus, whereas the pontomesencephalic cholinergic neurons exhibit widespread projections to many subcortical structures.

As is the case for most (if not all) neurotransmitters, multiple subtypes of ACh receptors have been identified. The most basic division is into nicotinic and muscarinic receptors, which were so named because of their differential sensitivity to the plant alkaloids nicotine and muscarine. These subtypes can be further discriminated in several other ways: nicotinic responses are very rapid, always excitatory, and are blocked by D-tubocurarine, whereas muscarinic responses are somewhat slower, may be either excitatory or inhibitory, and are antagonized by atropine and scopolamine. Moreover, nicotinic receptors belong to the superfamily of ligand-gated channels, but muscarinic receptors are coupled to G proteins, which accounts for their diversity of effects and longer latency of action.

A wide variety of drugs act as agonists or antagonists at ACh receptors. Two general cholinergic agonists are carbachol and methacholine. Nicotine, of course, is the classic nicotinic agonist. Several other nicotinic agonists, namely succinylcholine, decamethonium, and the algal toxin anatoxin-a paradoxically lead to muscle relaxation because they produce such a prolonged excitation of the muscle cells that the cells undergo a so-called depolarization block until the drug is cleared. Nicotinic antagonists can be subdivided into compounds that preferentially block neuromuscular transmission and compounds that preferentially block ganglionic nicotinic receptors. Among the former are the naturally occurring poison D-tubocurarine as well as the synthetic agents gallamine, pancuronium, and dihydro-β-erythroidine. Hexamethonium and mecamylamine represent two well-known ganglionic blockers, although these compounds differ in that mecamylamine, but not hexamethonium, crosses the blood–brain barrier to antagonize central nicotinic receptors.

With regard to muscarinic receptors, important agonists (besides muscarine itself) are pilocarpine, arecoline, oxotremorine, and cis-dioxolane. Unfortunately, few agonists with high subtype selectivity are currently available for either research or clinical use. Somewhat more progress has been made in the case of muscarinic antagonists. Nonspecific muscarinic antagonists include atropine and scopolamine, two closely related plant alkaloids, and the synthetic compound QNB, which has been used in radiolabeled form to identify muscarinic receptors in membrane binding and autoradiographic studies. Several antagonist drugs have been developed that show varying degrees of selectivity for specific muscarinic receptor subtypes. Two M1-selective antagonists, pirenzepine and telenzepine, have been particularly valuable in studies of muscarinic receptor pharmacology. Other drugs such as AF-DX 116, HHSiD, 4-DAMP, and methoctramine have been used to discriminate between the various non-M1 subtypes. Current research is aimed at finding subtype-selective muscarinic agonists and antagonists that will specifically enhance central cholinergic activity with a minimum of peripheral side effects. It is hoped that such drugs may be useful in the treatment of Alzheimer's disease and other forms of dementia that may involve deficits in ACh functioning.

Part III
Behavioral Functions of Acetylcholine

Acetylcholine has been implicated in virtually every imaginable aspect of behavioral and physiological regulation, including aggressive behavior, sensory processing, biorhythms, ingestive behavior, learning and memory, thermoregulation, sleep and arousal, and sexual behavior. Due to space limitations, we will discuss only a few of these topics. In any case, it is important to emphasize that no transmitter system operates in isolation; rather, there are physiological interactions among all neurochemically specified systems. Thus, ACh is not the only, nor perhaps even the principal, neurotransmitter that is involved in these behavioral phenomena; all have multiple neurochemical determinants.

The Role of Acetylcholine in Sleep and Arousal

Acetylcholine and Ascending Arousal Systems

Electrophysiological studies carried out in the 1940s and 1950s led to the concept of an ascending reticular activating system (ARAS) that plays a critical role in the maintenance of cortical arousal and behavioral waking (Jasper et al., 1958). This system consists of a diffuse collection of neurons in the core of the brain stem, ranging from the medulla up through the pons and midbrain. Functionally, the ARAS serves to gate sensory inputs, to modulate neural transmission to caudal centers involved in the control of spinal effector mechanisms and visceral functions, and to modulate neural transmission in the ascending tracts that influence "a spectrum of states of consciousness from deep coma through a series of sleeping states to maximal vigilance" (Scheibel and Scheibel, 1967). Reticular activation produces a low-voltage, desynchronized cortical EEG, which is the same pattern observed during normal behavioral arousal (see the next section).

Numerous studies have shown that cholinergic agonists and antagonists increase and decrease cortical arousal, respectively (Vanderwolf, 1992). Furthermore, the transition from sleep to waking is associated with heightened activity in both brain stem and basal forebrain cholinergic neurons. What role do these cells play in the regulation of cortical activation and behavioral arousal? First, we must consider the anatomy of the reticular activating system. The fibers comprising the ARAS ascend via two pathways: a dorsal pathway that synapses in the thalamus, and a ventral pathway that passes through the subthalamus and hypothalamus to terminate in the nucleus basalis, substantia innominata, septum, and the nuclei of the diagonal band. The astute reader will recognize the latter group of structures as containing large numbers of cholinergic neurons that project massively to the cerebral cortex and hippocampus. Thus, the cholinergic cell groups of the basal forebrain participate in a multisynaptic pathway by which the ventrally coursing reticular fibers help to modulate cortical excitability (Jones, 1990).

Acetylcholine is likewise involved in the dorsal part of the ARAS. Brain stem cholinergic cells in the pedunculopontine and laterodorsal tegmental nuclei (PPT and LDT) are critical contributors to the reticular innervation of the thalamus. Part of this innervation is distributed to nuclei of the nonspecific thalamocortical system, which stimulates arousal via widespread projections to the cortex. Other cholinergic fibers synapse in thalamic relay nuclei such as the dorsal lateral geniculate nucleus (LGNd), the thalamic way station for visual input. McCormick (1992) recently reviewed studies showing that application of ACh to neurons of the cat LGNd shifted the cells from a rhythmic burst firing pattern to a pattern of tonic, single-spike firing (Figure 7.15). The significance of this change is that the cells are more responsive to afferent (sensory) input when in the tonic firing mode.

To summarize, cholinergic neurons of the pontomesencephalon and basal forebrain play a central role in the functioning of the ARAS and in the modulation of cortical excitability and sensory processing. These effects are accomplished partly by means of direct cortical projections, and partly through synaptic connections with various nuclei of the thalamus.

Acetylcholine and Sleep

Sleep is defined not only by a behavioral state of somnolence, but also by the presence of characteristic electrophysiological signs in the cortex and other brain areas. Thus, although sleep is definitely present throughout the mammalian order, it is not clear whether the states of torpor shown by many lower orders should be considered true sleep. The development of the electroencephalograph (EEG) in the 1920s and 1930s—generally credited to Hans Berger (Brazier, 1961)—enabled the establishment of EEG correlates for waking and sleep states. Recordings from the parietal or occipital lobes of a person at rest with eyes closed show a rather rhythmic fluctuation of 8–12 Hz at a moderate amplitude, 20–30 µV. This wave pattern is called the alpha rhythm (Figure 7.16). If the person is attentive to the features of the environment or tries to solve mental problems in arithmetic, the recording changes to a desynchronized pattern with lower amplitudes, 5–10 µV, and higher frequencies between 13 and 30 Hz. This pattern is known as the beta rhythm. As an individual relaxes and falls asleep, the recording pattern progresses through four stages of increased synchrony and amplitude from 1–4 Hz at 30–150 µV, collectively called the delta rhythms.

The delta rhythms occur during a sleep state known as slow-wave sleep (SWS), which is a rather profound, but dreamless, sleep. Typically after about 90 minutes of SWS, there is an abrupt change in the EEG record of the sleeping person: the EEG becomes desynchronized, with lower amplitudes resembling the EEG of an alert and active state. However, this state, which is called rapid eye movement (REM) or paradoxical sleep, is actually a deeper sleep state than SWS in terms of the individual's arousability. In addition to the low-voltage cortical EEG pattern, REM sleep is characterized by the occurrence of phasic eye movements (from which the name REM sleep is derived), continuous bursts of high-voltage electrical activity in the pontine reticular formation, lateral geniculate body, and occipital cortex (hence these bursts are called ponto-geniculo-occipital, or PGO, waves), and a tonic suppression of muscle tone. In humans, most dreaming occurs during REM sleep. During a typical night, there are four or five REM sleep epochs that alter-

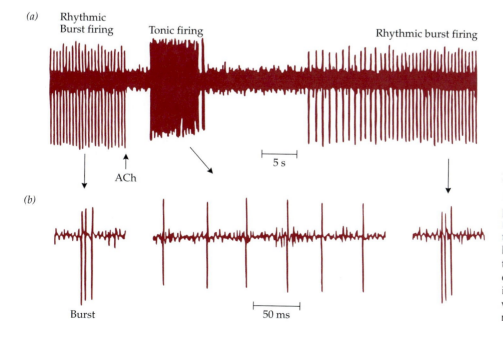

7.15 EFFECTS OF ACETYLCHOLINE APPLICATION ON CELL FIRING IN THE CAT DORSAL LATERAL GENICULATE NUCLEUS. (*a*) ACh was applied in vitro to a presumptive sensory relay neuron in the cat LGNd. The pattern of rhythmic bursting was inhibited by ACh, after which the cell entered a tonic (single-spike) firing mode. As this effect dissipated, the cell returned to its former state. (*b*) Some of the individual action potentials are shown in more detail. (After McCormick, 1992.)

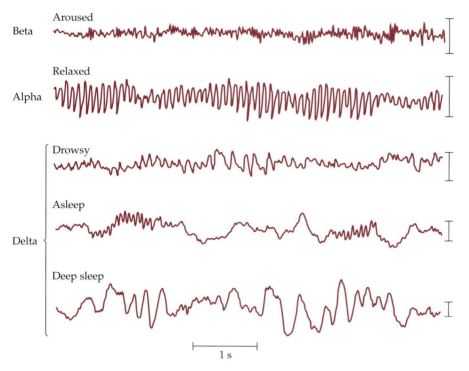

Beta — Aroused

Alpha — Relaxed

Delta {
Drowsy

Asleep

Deep sleep
}

1 s

7.16 EEG RECORDS DURING AROUSAL AND SLEEP. Typical EEG records from normal humans during arousal (beta waves), quiet relaxation (alpha waves), and stages of sleep (delta waves). Delta waves are often classed into four levels rather than the three shown here. The vertical lines at the end of the tracings indicate a calibration of 50 µV. (After Penfield and Jasper, 1954.)

nate with periods of SWS. The total amount of sleep time spent in REM sleep is approximately 20%.

Early theories posited that the brain is largely quiescent during sleep, and that sleep is caused simply by a diminution of activity in the neural systems responsible for maintaining an aroused, wakeful state. However, the presence of PGO waves and an active, desynchronized cortical EEG during REM sleep are inconsistent with this hypothesis. Furthermore, researchers began to discover mechanisms that directly regulate the different stages of sleep.

A major advance in our understanding of sleep mechanisms occurred in the 1960s, when the French physiologist Michel Jouvet and others found that lesions placed in the dorsolateral pons selectively suppressed REM sleep in cats (Jouvet, 1969). Because the lesions impinged on the locus coeruleus, a pontine structure densely packed with norepinephrine-containing cells (see Chapter 8), Jouvet originally hypothesized that these noradrenergic cells were critically involved in triggering the onset of REM sleep. However, the locus coeruleus is very small, and Jouvet's lesions inevitably damaged other cell groups as well as nerve fibers passing through the region.

Subsequent studies therefore began to implicate other transmitters, particularly ACh. A number of experiments showed that either full-blown REM sleep or specific REM sleep components could be elicited by microinjection of carbachol, more selective muscarinic agonists such as oxotremorine, or the AChE inhibitor neostigmine directly into the medial pontine reticular formation (reviewed by Hobson, Lydic, and Baghdoyan,

1986; Velazquez-Moctezuma, Shiromani, and Gillin, 1990). The effect of these cholinomimetic agents could be blocked by local administration of atropine or scopolamine. In humans, intravenous administration of arecoline or physostigmine during SWS was reported to cause the onset of REM sleep. The REM-inducing effect of arecoline could be blocked by pretreatment with scopolamine, but not with methscopolamine, which does not cross the blood–brain barrier (Gillin et al., 1993).

The above studies suggest an important role for muscarinic receptors in mediating the cholinergic regulation of REM sleep, although the identity of the relevant subtype(s) is still under investigation. Imeri and colleagues (1994) reported that direct application into the pontine reticular nucleus of an M2 antagonist (methoctramine), but not an M1 or an M3 antagonist, antagonized the REM sleep-inducing effect of carbachol. On the other hand, some other findings have implicated M1 receptors in the response to carbachol (see Gillin et al., 1993). Even nicotinic receptors may be involved, although further studies are needed to confirm this idea.

What anatomical circuitry underlies the action of ACh in REM sleep? The available evidence points to the pontine cell groups PPT and LDT as the location of the cholinergic cells involved in the circuit. Thus, Steriade and his coworkers found increased rates of cell firing in these areas both before and during REM sleep (Steriade and McCarley, 1990). In addition, lesioning of these cell groups caused a significant reduction in the occurrence of REM sleep in cats (Webster and Jones, 1988). Cholinergic fibers from PPT and LDT probably project to several different sites to mediate the various features of

REM sleep. One projection is presumably to the medial pontine reticular formation, the location at which cholinergic agonists have been found to induce REM sleep. The function of the cholinoceptive cells in the medial pons has not yet been determined. As discussed previously, other fibers from PPT and LDT ascend to the thalamus to innervate various thalamic nuclei, including the lateral geniculate. These projections are likely to be important in the generation of the low-voltage, fast cortical activity (see previous section) and the PGO waves that occur during REM sleep. Yet another pathway to the tectum (colliculi) may be responsible for producing the characteristic rapid eye movements for which this sleep stage is named (Webster and Jones, 1988).

In concluding this section, it is important to note that ACh is, of course, not the only neurotransmitter involved in REM sleep regulation. Indeed, Hobson, Lydic, and Baghdoyan (1986) have put forth an interesting theory that the onset and offset of REM sleep are governed by reciprocal interactions between a REM-on system, which includes the cholinergic components described above, and a REM-off system that includes noradrenergic and serotonergic cell groups in the brain stem. Whether or not this theory is confirmed, the stages of sleep are undoubtedly controlled by a complex circuit involving many neurotransmitters.

Cognitive Functions of Acetylcholine

Of the various functions that have been hypothesized for ACh, one of the most interesting and at times controversial is its proposed role in learning, memory, and other cognitive processes. In presenting this research, we will begin with a review of the effects of cholinergic drugs on learning and memory in animal studies as well as in humans. The following section will focus on the nucleus basalis, a cholinergic cell group that has been implicated in the cognitive deficits observed in Alzheimer's disease.

Effects of Cholinergic Drugs on Learning, Memory, and Attention

Animal studies.   Blockade of muscarinic receptors by atropine or scopolamine has been shown to interfere with the acquisition and maintenance of many different kinds of learning tasks (see reviews by Hagan and Morris, 1987; Spencer and Lal, 1983). Many of the early studies used traditional paradigms such as classical conditioning, discrimination learning, and passive and active avoidance learning. For example, experiments on classical conditioning of the rabbit nictitating membrane found that muscarinic antagonists impaired both acquisition and expression of the conditioned response while having little or no effect on the unconditioned responses. In addition, visual and auditory discrimination studies

were done in which rats were trained to perform a response (e.g., a lever press) in the presence of one stimulus, and either to perform a different response to a second stimulus (go/go discrimination) or to withhold the response when the second stimulus was presented (go/no go discrimination). Scopolamine was generally found to decrease the rate of correct responding, which is indicative of reduced stimulus control over the behavior (Spencer and Lal, 1983).

Another popular test procedure is the passive avoidance paradigm. Here, foot shock is used to train animals to withhold a prepotent response such as stepping off a platform or moving from a brightly lit to a dark compartment. One training trial is generally sufficient to produce considerable avoidance when the animal is tested at a later time (usually after 24 hours). Administration of scopolamine before the initial training trial led to decreased response latencies (i.e., poorer performance) on the subsequent test trial. However, treatment with the anti-AChE drug physostigmine unexpectedly had a similar effect, which may indicate that any disruption of normal cholinergic functioning impairs performance on this task.

Based on their review of the early literature, Spencer and Lal (1983) hypothesized that antimuscarinic agents primarily interfere with input (encoding) and output (retrieval) mechanisms involved in memory storage. However, some of the behavioral paradigms used to study the role of ACh present interpretative problems. For example, deficient performance on avoidance tasks may be due to altered activity levels rather than disruption of cognitive mechanisms. Therefore, investigators have developed more sophisticated tasks to assess drug effects on learning and memory processes.

One such task is the Morris water maze, which consists of a large circular pool filled with water that has been made opaque with milk powder (Morris, 1984; see Chapter 2). At the beginning of each trial, the subject is placed in the pool at one of several starting locations, usually arranged around the edge of the tank. Just below the surface is a small platform upon which the subject can stand in order to stop swimming and escape from the water. The platform is neither visible, nor does it emit any other cues discernible from a distance. Yet after a number of training trials, subjects can reliably swim in a fairly direct path to the platform from any of the starting locations. How is this accomplished? The apparatus is maintained in a room containing various large, stationary objects that can be seen by the subjects in the pool. These objects serve as visual cues that enable the subjects to determine their position relative to the submerged platform by a process that has been termed "place" or "spatial navigational" learning. Various procedures are available to determine whether the subjects are actually using this type of strategy in order to locate the position of the platform (Morris, 1984).

Blockade of muscarinic receptors by atropine or scopolamine or of neuronal nicotinic receptors by mecamylamine has been shown to impair rat place learning in the water maze (McNamara and Skelton, 1993). Detailed information is not yet available concerning the location and identity of the cholinergic receptors involved in place learning. However, because the peripherally acting drugs atropine methylnitrate and hexamethonium had no effect on learning (McNamara and Skelton, 1993), it is clear that the critical receptors are located within the CNS. With regard to muscarinic receptor subtypes, one study implicated M1 receptors by showing deficits following intracerebroventricular administration of a low dose of pirenzepine (Hagan and Morris, 1987).

Cholinergic interference with place learning is not necessarily at the level of learning or memory mechanisms per se. One alternative interpretation is suggested by a study done by Whishaw and Tomie (1987). In this experiment, rats were trained on two different tasks: a standard single-platform task in which the platform was submerged under the surface of the water, and a two-platform task in which both platforms were above the surface (and hence visible), but only one platform was correct because the other sank when the rat attempted to mount it. During the acquisition phase, the animals were given pretraining injections of either atropine or saline. Atropine-treated rats exhibited poorer acquisition of both tasks compared with control subjects (Figure 7.17). However, the controls, but not the treated animals, showed greater ease in performing the two-platform task than the single-platform task, indicating that the drug produced relatively more impairment in the former situation. In the two-platform task, distal room cues are necessary to distinguish which goal is correct. The authors hypothesize that cholinergic blockade disrupts a sensorimotor subsystem necessary for normal place navigation using distal cues. If the atropine-treated subjects were thus forced to rely more on proximate cues (the sight of the two platforms), they might be expected to initially approach the correct and incorrect platforms with roughly equal frequency. This would result in a partial reinforcement schedule that would retard the rate at which a new, distal cue–based, strategy would be implemented.

Another novel task is the delayed matching-to-position (DMTP) test (Dunnett, 1985). On each trial of this task, a rat in a Skinner box is first presented with one of two retractable levers. The rat presses the lever, after which it is retracted. In the second part of the trial, a delay is introduced by requiring the rat to poke its nose against a flap on a food tray for a variable period of time. Finally, both levers are reintroduced, and the rat must press the same lever that was presented before in order to receive reinforcement. This task was designed to assess "working memory," which refers to the encoding of task-specific information over short periods of time (e.g., within a single trial or test session). It is particularly useful in differentiating between memory-specific effects of a treatment and sensory or motor effects. An impairment in memory (as opposed to sensorimotor functioning) is implied if a given treatment causes response errors at long, but not short, time delays. In the present instance, systemic administration of scopolamine to animals learning the DMTP task led to significant performance deficits (Dawson, Heyes, and Iversen, 1992). However, the impairment was equivalent after short and long delays, thus failing to meet the criterion of a delay-dependent effect. This finding raises the possibility that muscarinic receptor blockade may disrupt some aspect of sensory processing or attention rather than working memory.

Human studies.   Earlier in the chapter, we mentioned that when scopolamine was given to surgical patients as a preanesthetic medication, the patients frequently had no recollection of subsequent events (e.g., transfer to the operating room, being prepared for the surgery, and so forth). Because other medications are often also administered in this situation, it is difficult to isolate the possible role of ACh in this type of amnesia. However, a number of controlled studies have been performed involving treatment of normal subjects with somewhat lower doses of scopolamine. As reviewed by Polster (1993) and by Rusted and Warburton (1989), this research has consistently shown that muscarinic receptor antagonism causes deficits in certain types of memory. One way to analyze memory processes is to distinguish between short-term and long-term memory. Most studies have suggested that scopolamine interferes with the transfer of information from short-term stores to long-term memory, although short-term memory itself may be impaired under conditions of heavy processing demands (Rusted and Warburton, 1989). In recent years, various theoretical models have divided long-term memory into several component processes (Tulving, 1987). One such scheme differentiates between declarative memory, which refers to memory of facts and events, and procedural memory, which refers to complex learned stimulus–response associations and motor skills (Squire, 1986). Whereas declarative memory is explicit (i.e., accessible to one's awareness) and can readily be verbalized, procedural memory is implicit and is expressed only in task performance. Nissen, Knopman, and Schachter (1987) reported findings consistent with the hypothesis that scopolamine primarily affects declarative and not procedural memory (also see Polster, 1993).

Does ACh play any role in attentional processes? Studies addressing this question indeed found that scopolamine impaired performance on several types of attentional tasks, including tests of sustained attention as well as perceptual intrusion paradigms (e.g., the Stroop test) (Rusted and Warburton, 1989). Thus, ACh

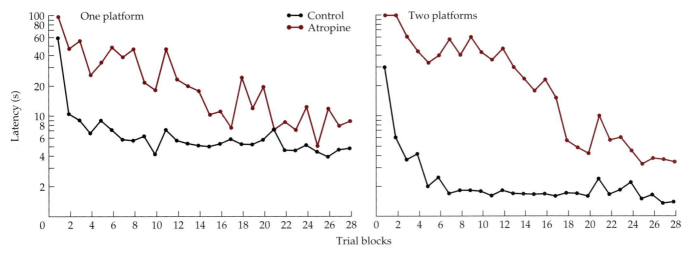

7.17 INFLUENCE OF ATROPINE ON TWO SPATIAL LEARNING TASKS in the water maze. Rats were trained on either a single-platform task in which the platform was submerged under the surface of the water, or a two-platform task in which both platforms were above the surface, but only one was correct because the other sank when mounted. Subjects were trained using two four-trial blocks per day for 14 days. Before each session, the animals were injected with either atropine sulfate (50 mg/kg) or saline. Compared with controls, atropine-treated rats exhibited significantly poorer acquisition of both tasks. (After Whishaw and Tomie, 1987.)

acting through muscarinic receptors has consistently been shown to help mediate several important cognitive processes, including attention and long-term (mainly declarative) memory.

Acetylcholine, Aging, and Memory

Aging in both humans and animals is often accompanied by declines in memory and other cognitive functions (although there are important individual differences in this regard; see Rapp and Amaral, 1992). Since this was long considered a "normal" and inevitable part of growing old, it was given little attention by neuroscientists until the 1970s, when several laboratories first reported that patients suffering from Alzheimer's disease exhibit large deficits in cortical, hippocampal, and striatal ACh levels and ChAT activity (Bartus et al., 1982, 1985). Detailed coverage of Alzheimer's disease can be found in Chapter 20. It is sufficient to mention here that this dreadful disorder is characterized by profound dementia, meaning a loss of memory, language, and other cognitive abilities. At the same time that Alzheimer's patients were being investigated, some (though not all) studies reported decreases in forebrain ChAT activity and muscarinic receptor binding in aged but healthy humans and laboratory animals (Bartus et al., 1982; Morgan and May, 1990). Considering these findings along with the pharmacological evidence described above, Bartus and others hypothesized a central role for ACh in aging-related memory deficits (Bartus et al., 1982).

On its face, the cholinergic hypothesis of memory dysfunction seems quite attractive, and it continues to spur considerable clinical as well as preclinical research. However, a number of criticisms have recently been raised against this theory. For example, Fibiger (1991) points out that the effects of scopolamine treatment on normal subjects may not mimic the characteristics of Alzheimer's disease as well as previously thought. Other experiments failed to find a correlation between the degree of memory impairment and the loss of septal ChAT-positive neurons in aged rhesus monkeys (Rapp and Amaral, 1992). Finally, Sarter (1991) notes that a large array of cholinomimetic agents have been examined for potential cognition-enhancing effects in animal models and, in some case, human clinical trials. The types of drugs tested include ACh precursors, muscarinic and nicotinic agonists, AChE inhibitors, and various putative ACh-releasing compounds. Although most of these drugs yielded positive results in animal testing, clinical trials have been largely disappointing (see Chapter 20). Such findings raise questions both about the cholinergic hypothesis and about the validity of the preclinical procedures used to screen these agents. Nevertheless, as our understanding of ACh receptor subtypes progresses and as more selective agonists and antagonists are developed, it may yet prove possible to improve cognitive performance in elderly (perhaps even demented) individuals through drugs that act on the cholinergic system.

Role of the Basal Forebrain Cholinergic System

What cell groups and pathways might be involved in the effects of cholinergic drugs on learning and memory, and in the hypothesized role of ACh in age-related cognitive deficits? Logically, the most likely candidate is the basal forebrain cholinergic system because it provides the main ACh innervation of the neocortex and limbic system. Furthermore, in Alzheimer's patients, the cortical ChAT deficit mentioned above is caused by a severe reduction in the number of basal forebrain cholinergic neurons. Investigators have particularly focused on the nucleus basalis of Meynert (NBM), which contains about 400,000 to 500,000 large ChAT-positive cells. These cells send widespread projections to the frontal, temporal, and parietal lobes, thus supplying about 70% to 80% of the entire cortical cholinergic innervation.

Because of the putative relationship between the loss of NBM cells and Alzheimer's-associated cognitive deficits, researchers suggested that lesioning this structure in primates or its rodent analog (the nucleus basalis magnocellularis) might provide an animal model of Alzheimer's dementia. Such lesions are typically produced by locally infusing an excitotoxic amino acid such as ibotenic acid. As described in Chapter 10, this treatment specifically destroys cells while sparing fibers passing through the area. Dozens of studies have been performed comparing lesioned to control subjects on a variety of learning paradigms, including discrimination tasks, passive and active avoidance tasks, delayed matching-to-sample tasks, and spatial tasks such as the radial arm maze and the Morris water maze. The results have overwhelmingly demonstrated lesion-induced deficits in task acquisition (learning) and retention (memory) (Dekker, Connor, and Thal, 1991). Damage to the nucleus basalis was shown to impair both types of memory typically studied in animal experiments: working memory, which was mentioned previously, and reference memory, which involves general task information that does not change between trials.

In a number of cases, stimulating cholinergic activity by means of the AChE inhibitor physostigmine improved performance in subjects with nucleus basalis lesions (Dekker, Connor, and Thal, 1991). This seemed to confirm the view that the lesion-induced deficits were due to the loss of cholinergic neurons. Several years ago, however, Dunnett and his colleagues made a striking observation. Like other research groups, they found that ibotenic acid lesions of the nucleus basalis led to impaired performance on a number of learning tasks. However, when they instead produced the lesions with another excitotoxin called quisqualic acid, in almost all cases few or no deficits were observed, despite the fact that ChAT was depleted to a greater extent than with ibotenic acid administration (Dunnett et al., 1987). Since that time, additional studies by Dunnett's group as well as by other investigators have confirmed that quisqualic acid lesions yield more damage to the cholinergic system (as assessed by ChAT measurements) but fewer behav-

ioral deficits than lesions made by ibotenic acid (Dunnett, Everitt, and Robbins, 1991).

To understand how ibotenic and quisqualic acids could produce differing behavioral effects, we must consider the anatomy of the nucleus basalis and the nature of excitotoxins. The cholinergic cells of the nucleus basalis are found in close proximity to the globus pallidus (Richardson and DeLong, 1988). This proximity is important because substances like ibotenic and quisqualic acid are relatively nonselective cellular toxins; that is, they are not specific to cholinergic neurons. Hence, noncholinergic cells in the globus pallidus and neighboring areas are also subject to destruction by excitotoxic lesions. For reasons that are not yet fully clear, ibotenic acid seems to damage certain noncholinergic cells that are spared by quisqualic acid. Although different hypotheses have been put forward as to the identity of those cells (Dunnett, Everitt, and Robbins, 1991; Wenk, 1993), growing evidence indicates that their loss (rather than the loss of nucleus basalis cholinergic neurons) is responsible for many of the effects of ibotenic acid–induced basal forebrain lesions. Such findings raise doubts concerning the putative role of the nucleus basalis in learning and memory.

In contrast, ibotenic and quisqualic acid lesions were approximately equivalent in disrupting performance on a five-choice serial reaction time task (Robbins, Everitt et al., 1989). This task requires rats to discriminate the spatial positions of brief visual events and is thought to assess attentional processes. Recent experiments investigating whether ACh is involved in these lesion-induced deficits showed that (1) the effects of quisqualic acid lesions could be ameliorated by grafts of ACh-rich fetal brain tissue, (2) deficits produced by lesioning with another excitotoxin, AMPA, were reversed by physostigmine treatment, and (3) similar physostigmine-reversible impairment was produced by the choline uptake inhibitor hemicholinium-3 (Muir et al., 1993; Figure 7.18). In accordance with findings presented earlier, these results are consistent with a possible role of the nucleus basalis cholinergic cells in attentional processes and arousal (Richardson and DeLong, 1988). Several investigators have similarly concluded that basal forebrain lesions in monkeys mimic the attentional rather than the memory losses observed in Alzheimer's patients (Voytko et al., 1994; Wenk, 1993).

Although the behavioral role of the nucleus basalis cholinergic neurons has been studied largely by means of the excitotoxic lesion methods described above, a novel lesioning approach has been developed that is more selective for these cells. Basal forebrain cholinergic neurons express a low-affinity receptor for nerve growth factor (NGF), a well-known neurotrophic factor (Yan and Johnson, 1989). Wiley, Oeltmann, and Lappi (1991) produced a monoclonal antibody (designated 192 IgG) to

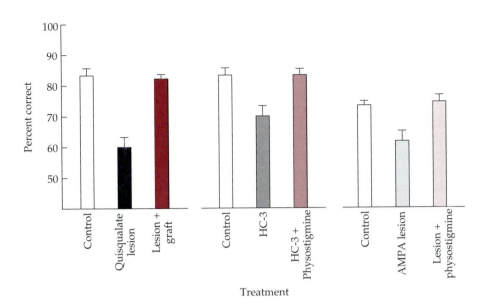

7.18 EFFECTS OF CHOLINERGIC MANIPULATIONS ON THE PERFORMANCE OF RATS IN A VISUAL ATTENTION TASK. (*a*) Quisqualic acid lesions of the nucleus basalis produced performance deficits that were reduced by grafting ACh-rich fetal brain tissue into the fronto-parietal cortex. (*b*) The effects of nucleus basalis lesions were mimicked by treatment with the choline uptake inhibitor hemicholinium-3 (HC-3) and alleviated by coadministration of the AChE inhibitor physostigmine. (*c*) Similar results were produced by lesioning with another excitotoxin, AMPA. (After Muir et al., 1993.)

the rat low-affinity NGF receptor and conjugated it to the ribosome-inactivating cytotoxin saporin. When the antibody–toxin conjugate is administered either intracerebroventricularly or directly into the basal forebrain, it undergoes binding to cholinergic nerve terminals, internalization, and retrograde transport to the cholinergic cell bodies where it causes cell death (Book, Wiley, and Schweitzer, 1992; Thomas, Book, and Schweitzer, 1991).

Several studies have investigated Morris water maze learning in rats with 192 IgG–saporin lesions of the basal forebrain cholinergic system. When rats were given intracerebroventricular injections of the immunotoxin, they subsequently showed deficits in water maze learning (Leanza et al., 1995; Nilsson et al., 1992). When the toxin was infused directly into the nucleus basalis, however, some investigators found an impairment on this task (Berger-Sweeney et al., 1994), whereas others did not (Baxter, Bucci et al., 1995). The reason for these discrepant results is not clear, although one factor may be differences in the extent of toxin-induced damage either to the forebrain cholinergic neurons or to other brain areas (see discussion in Baxter, Bucci et al., 1995). Thus, issues of lesion specificity must be dealt with in order for the 192 IgG–saporin immunotoxin approach to provide useful information about the role of ACh in learning and memory.

If Alzheimer's disease is ever to be treated effectively, we must understand the source of the profound cognitive deficits associated with this disorder. In the last several sections of this chapter, we have seen that simplistic hypotheses concerning the cognitive functions of ACh have recently come into question. Cholinergic systems undoubtedly participate somehow in the processes of attention, learning, and memory. Nevertheless, it must be kept in mind that ACh does not influence these processes in isolation, but rather, interacts with a number of other important transmitters such as norepinephrine, dopamine, serotonin, GABA, and various neuropeptides (Decker and McGaugh, 1991).

Part III Summary

One important behavioral role proposed for ACh is that of regulating states of arousal and sleep. Several lines of evidence suggest that ACh may play a central role in the ascending reticular activating system, a complex brain stem circuit involved in stimulating cortical arousal (EEG desynchronization) and behavioral states of waking and attention. The normal transition from sleep to waking is associated with increased firing of both brain stem and basal forebrain cholinergic neurons. Furthermore, pharmacological stimulation of cholinergic activity leads to increased cortical arousal. These effects are mediated by both the basal forebrain cell group and the cholinergic neurons of the pontomesencephalon. Indeed, one of the specific functions of the latter system is to enhance sensory input by heightening the responsivity of thalamic relay neurons.

Acetylcholine has additionally been implicated in triggering the state of sleep called REM sleep. REM sleep is characterized by a fast, low-voltage cortical EEG pattern, phasic eye movements, PGO waves, a tonic suppression of muscle tone, and the occurrence of dreaming in humans. In cats (the preferred animal subject for sleep research), REM sleep, or at least some of its components, can be elicited by administering a muscarinic agonist or an AChE inhibitor directly into the medial pontine reticular formation. Human studies have reported reduced latencies to enter REM sleep following intravenous injection of arecoline or physostigmine. Treatment with muscarinic antagonists prevented the REM sleep effect in both feline and human experiments. The pontomesencephalic cholinergic cell groups PPT and LDT again are likely to be the source of the cholinergic regulation of REM sleep, particularly with respect to generating cortical EEG desynchronization, rapid eye movements, and PGO waves.

A second important function of ACh concerns cognitive processes such as learning, memory, and attention. Animal studies have consistently shown that muscarinic receptor blockade can impair both the acquisition and the retention of various learned tasks. Scopolamine administration to humans similarly has been reported to impair long-term memory, particularly declarative memory.

Patients with Alzheimer's disease suffer from dementia, which refers to profound deficits in cognitive functioning, including memory. Examination of Alzheimer's patients' brains revealed a severe loss of cholinergic neurons in the nucleus basalis and a concomitant depletion of forebrain ACh. Similiar, but less severe effects have sometimes been found in aged, non-Alzheimer's brains. Moreover, animal studies showed that excitotoxic lesions of the nucleus basalis led to deficits in learning and memory. Together, these findings led to the cholinergic hypothesis of memory impairment in aging (and particularly in Alzheimer's disease). Subsequent studies, however, have cast some doubt on this simple hypothesis, both with respect to the presumptive role of the nucleus basalis and with respect to the effects produced by cholinergic blockade or damage. One alternative possibility supported by both animal and human experiments is that the major effect of the forebrain cholinergic projection is to stimulate attentional processes rather than to facilitate learning or memory per se.

Continuing research should help to sort out the exact nature of the cognitive functions influenced by ACh. The attentional hypothesis is intriguing because it seems to integrate the roles of this neurotransmitter in sensory processing and in learning and memory. On the other hand, it would be premature to conclude that ACh plays no role in the associative aspects of learning or in information storage. As this work progresses, we hope that appropriate cholinergic agents will be found that can reverse, at least to some extent, the devastating loss of cognitive abilities seen in Alzheimer's patients.

Chapter 8

Catecholamines

The catecholamines belong to the wider group of neurotransmitters called **monoamines**, that is, compounds possessing a single amine ($-NH_2$) group. More specifically, catecholamines contain a nucleus of catechol (a benzene ring possessing two adjacent hydroxyl groups) and a side chain of ethylamine or one of its derivatives. By far the most important catecholamines are **dopamine (DA)**, **norepinephrine (NE)**, and **epinephrine (EPI)**. EPI and NE are

Catechol nucleus

Dopamine
(3,4-Dihydroxyphenylethylamine)

Norepinephrine
(Noradrenaline)

Epinephrine
(Adrenaline)

sometimes called adrenaline and noradrenaline, respectively. "Adrenaline" is derived from the Latin *ad ren,* which means "near the kidney," whereas "epinephrine" comes from the Greek *epi nephros,* meaning "upon the kidney." These names refer to the fact that EPI and NE were first discovered in the adrenal glands, which are indeed situated just above the kidneys. The adjective forms for these substances are **adrenergic** and **noradrenergic**, although the term "adrenergic" is sometimes used broadly to refer to NE- as well as EPI-related features. The adjective form for DA is **dopaminergic**.

Catecholamine neurotransmitters were first found in the autonomic nervous system. Classic experiments by Walter Cannon and his associates had shown that a substance that they called "sympathin" was released upon stimulation of sympathetic nerves (Cannon and Uridil, 1921). Twenty-five years later, this substance was identified as NE by von Euler (1946b). Soon thereafter, NE was also found in the brain (Holtz, 1950), although its presence there was initially thought to be associated strictly with the autonomic fibers innervating the smooth muscles of the cerebral blood vessels. Marthe Vogt, however, made the important discovery that the distribution of NE in the brain was not correlated with the distribution of blood vessels, suggesting that NE might be a transmitter within central neurons (Vogt, 1954).

Part I
Catecholamine Neurochemistry: Synthesis, Storage, Release, and Inactivation

The synthetic pathway for catecholamines was first predicted by Blaschko (1939), who correctly proposed that DA was a precursor for NE and EPI. No independent role for DA was considered until Carlsson and his coworkers found large amounts of this substance in the basal ganglia and implicated it in the parkinsonian-like symptoms produced by reserpine (a catecholamine-depleting drug) (Carlsson, 1959; also see review by Carlsson, 1987b). By the 1960s, a group of Swedish investigators had developed histofluorescence staining techniques that allowed the visualization of catecholamine-containing cell bodies and fibers throughout the brain (reviewed by Carlsson, 1987b; also see Part II of this chapter). This development led to an explosion of research on the localization of catecholamine systems and paved the way for other experiments demonstrating the synthesis, uptake and storage, release, degradation, and functional effects of these neurotransmitters. Although EPI serves as a neurotransmitter for a small number of neurons, it is best known as a hormone secreted by the adrenal medulla. Therefore, the main emphasis in this chapter will be on DA and NE.

Figures 8.1 and 8.2 illustrate a dopaminergic synapse and a noradrenergic synapse respectively. Some of the processes illustrated in these figures, such as neurotransmitter synthesis, release, reuptake, and catabolism, are discussed in the current part of the chapter. Receptor mechanisms, on the other hand, are discussed in later parts that focus specifically on the dopaminergic and noradrenergic systems.

Basic Aspects of Catecholamine Synthesis

As shown in Figure 8.3, the synthesis of catecholamine neurotransmitters occurs in several steps. The precursor for all of the catecholamines is tyrosine, an aromatic amino acid (i.e., one whose side chain contains a benzene ring) derived from dietary protein. Tyrosine is also synthesized in the liver by the enzyme phenylalanine hydroxylase; however, this pathway normally serves as the first step in the degradation and elimination of excess phenylalanine. Individuals born with a genetic deficiency of phenylalanine hydroxylase suffer from a disorder called phenylketonuria (PKU).* Such individuals

exhibit a large buildup of phenylalanine which, if left untreated, causes mental retardation and other deleterious effects.

In the following sections, we will describe each step in the synthetic pathway, summarize the basic properties of all the enzymes involved, and indicate which drugs affect these enzymes. The discussion will then conclude with a consideration of the regulatory mechanisms believed to govern rates of catecholamine synthesis.

Tyrosine Hydroxylase

The first step in catecholamine synthesis is the hydroxylation of L-tyrosine to L-3,4-dihydroxyphenylalanine (L-DOPA).[2] This reaction is catalyzed by the enzyme tyrosine 3-monooxygenase, which is usually called tyrosine hydroxylase (TH). Tyrosine hydroxylase was first characterized in the adrenal medulla by Nagatsu, Levitt, and Udenfriend (1964). The complete reaction is illustrated in Figure 8.4. The oxygen and hydrogen atoms constituting the new hydroxyl group are donated by molecular oxygen (O_2) and by a reduced pteridine cofactor (tetrahydrobiopterin; BH_4), respectively. Besides DOPA,[†] the other reaction products are H_2O and the oxidized pteridine quinonoid dihydrobiopterin (DH_2). Tetrahydrobiopterin is subsequently regenerated from DH_2, NADH, and H^+ by the enzyme dihydropteridine reductase (DPR) (Kaufman, 1977).

The characteristics of TH are summarized in reviews by Kuhn and Lovenberg (1983), Nagatsu (1991), and Zigmond, Schwarzschild, and Rittenhouse (1989). The enzyme appears to exist in both soluble (cytoplasmic) and particulate (membrane-bound) forms, although research has focused primarily on soluble TH. Most studies indicate that native TH is made up of four identical subunits, each with a molecular weight of approximately 60 kDa. The enzyme contains Fe^{2+} ions, which are required for its activity. Tyrosine hydroxylase is encoded by a single gene, although Nagatsu's group has shown that in humans, the primary transcript of the gene yields four distinct mRNAs due to alternative mRNA splicing (Nagatsu, 1991). Thus, tyrosine hydroxylation is actually catalyzed by four isoforms of TH that differ from one another in terms of their kinetic properties.

Tyrosine hydroxylase is the rate-limiting enzyme in catecholamine synthesis, presumably because its maximum velocity is slower than that of any of the other enzymes in the synthetic pathway. Consequently, the activity of TH governs the overall rate of formation of all of the catecholamines. One consequence of this fact is that the most effective method for inhibiting catecholamine synthesis is to block TH. Pharmacological inhibitors of

---

*Phenylketonuria is so-named because the accumulated *phenyl*alanine is eventually metabolized to the *ketone*-containing compound phenylpyruvic acid, which is then excreted in the *urine*. The disorder can be managed by permanently reducing phenylalanine consumption.

[†]When we use the term "DOPA," it should be considered to mean L-DOPA, which is the biologically active isomer.

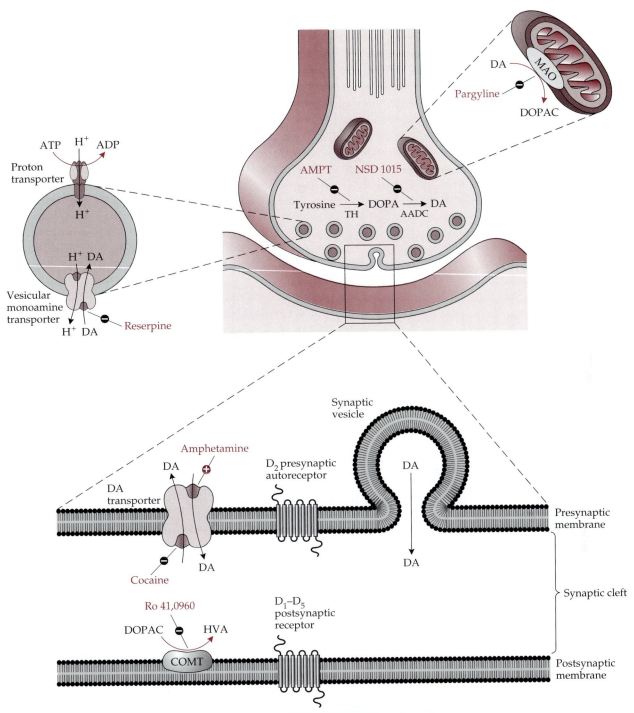

8.1 THE DOPAMINERGIC SYNAPSE illustrating the processes of dopamine (DA) synthesis and metabolism, presynaptic and vesicular DA uptake, and vesicular DA release. Pre- and postsynaptic DA receptors and sites of action of some dopaminergic drugs are also shown. The table lists important dopaminergic agonists and antagonists. See the text for details and explanations of the abbreviations.

Receptor subtype	Agonists	Antagonists
D_1	SKF 38393, SKF 82526 (fenol-dopam), dihydrexidine	SCH 23390, NNC-112, SCH 39166
D_2	Apomorphine, bromocriptine, quinpirole, pergolide	Haloperidol, sulpiride, spiperone, YM-09151-2
D_3	Quinpirole, pergolide	S 14297
D_4		Clozapine

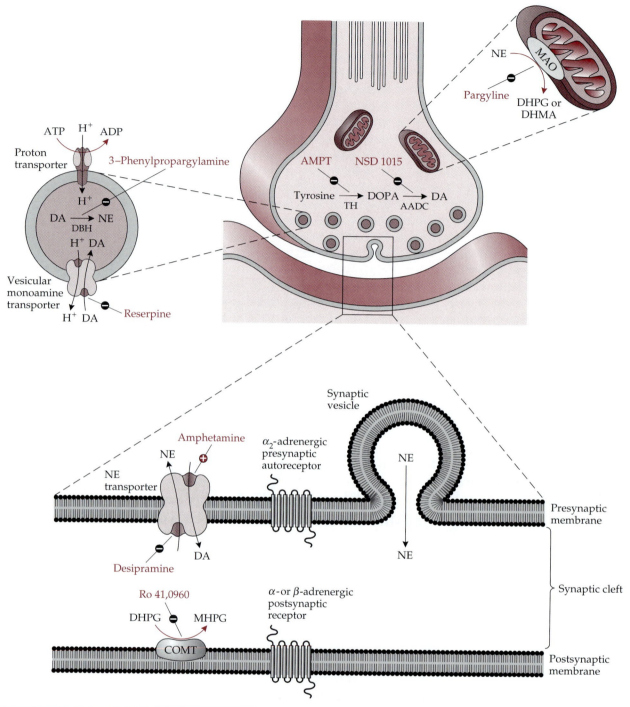

Receptor subtype	Agonists	Antagonists
α_1	Phenylephrine, methoxamine	Prazosin, WB-4101, phenoxybenzamine
α_2	Clonidine, B-HT 920	Yohimbine, rauwolscine, idazoxan
General β	Isoproterenol, albuterol	Propranolol, alprenolol, pindolol
β_1	Denopamine, xamoterol	Atenolol, bisopropolol
β_2	Procaterol	ICI-118,551
β_3	BRL 37344, CL 316,243	

8.2 THE NORADRENERGIC SYNAPSE illustrating the processes of norepinephrine (NE) synthesis and metabolism, presynaptic and vesicular NE uptake, and vesicular NE release. Pre- and postsynaptic adrenergic receptors and sites of some noradrenergic drugs are also shown. The table lists important noradrenergic receptor agonists and antagonists. See the text for details and explanations of abbreviations.

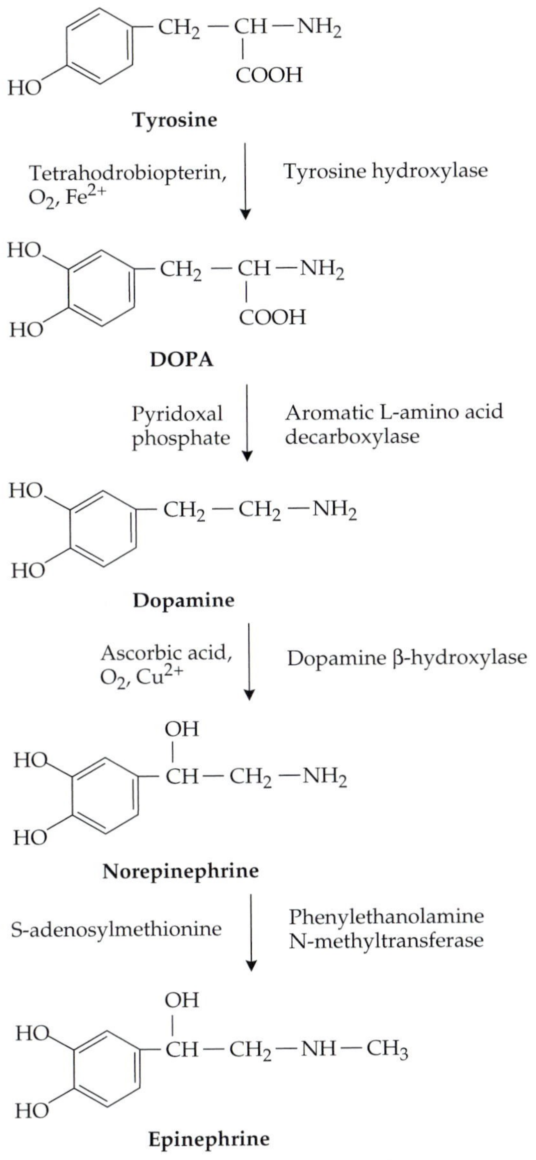

Tyrosine

Tetrahodrobiopterin, O_2, Fe^{2+} | Tyrosine hydroxylase

DOPA

Pyridoxal phosphate | Aromatic L-amino acid decarboxylase

Dopamine

Ascorbic acid, O_2, Cu^{2+} | Dopamine β-hydroxylase

Norepinephrine

S-adenosylmethionine | Phenylethanolamine N-methyltransferase

Epinephrine

8.3 SYNTHESIS OF THE CATECHOLAMINE TRANSMITTERS. The synthesizing enzymes are shown to the right of each arrow; enzyme cofactors are shown to the left.

TH generally act by one of three mechanisms: (1) chelation of Fe^{2+} ions, (2) competition at the pteridine cofactor binding site, or (3) competition at the tyrosine binding site (Moore and Dominic, 1971). The most popular TH inhibitor is a drug called α-methyl-*p*-tyrosine (AMPT), which falls into the third category. Over the years, AMPT has proved useful in the experimental depletion of DA and NE in neuropharmacological studies. Nevertheless, it does have at least two important drawbacks: it depletes both central and peripheral catecholamines when given systemically, and, because it blocks TH, it is not selective in terms of which catecholamines it affects. In humans, AMPT (trade name Demser) is sometimes used therapeutically in the treatment of pheochromocytomas, catecholamine-secreting tumors of the adrenal

glands. Unfortunately, the drug produces unwanted sedative effects in most patients because of its central catecholamine-depleting action.

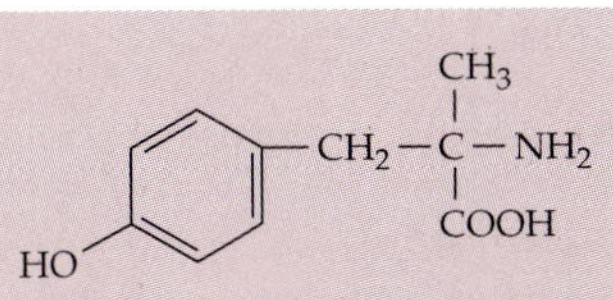

α-Methyl-*p*-Tyrosine (AMPT)

Aromatic Amino Acid Decarboxylase

The second step in catecholamine synthesis involves the formation of DA from DOPA (see Figure 8.3). This occurs via removal of the carboxyl group from the α-carbon on the side chain, with the consequent liberation of free carbon dioxide (CO_2). DOPA decarboxylation is catalyzed by the enzyme aromatic L-amino acid decarboxylase (AADC), a soluble protein that requires pyridoxal 5′-phosphate (derived from pyridoxine, which is vitamin B_6) as a cofactor. In DA neurons, this is the final step in the biosynthetic pathway.

As implied by its name, AADC acts on a variety of aromatic amino acids besides DOPA. For example, tyrosine can be decarboxylated to form tyramine (Figure 8.5), which in turn can be taken up by catecholaminergic nerve terminals and released as a so-called "false transmitter" (particularly in individuals being treated with a monoamine oxidase inhibitor). It should also be noted that AADC is found in many tissues besides the brain, including the liver, stomach, and kidneys. The presence of the enzyme outside of the nervous system suggests additional, as yet unknown, functions not related to catecholamine synthesis. Aromatic amino acid decarboxylase can be inhibited by several drugs, most notably α-methyl-dopa-hydrazine (carbidopa) and 3-hydroxybenzyl-hydrazine (NSD 1015). Enzyme inhibition by either of these

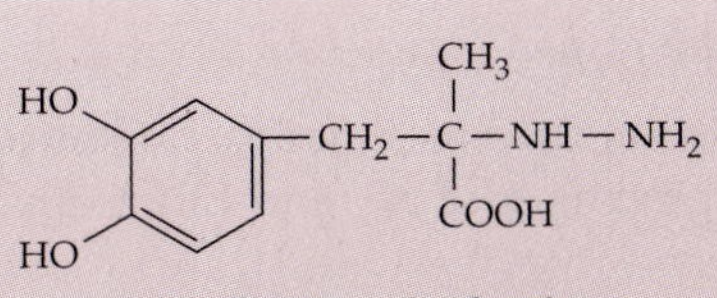

α-Methyldopa-hydrazine

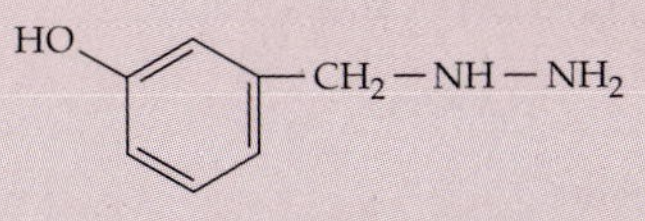

3-Hydroxybenzyl-hydrazine

compounds causes an accumulation of DOPA in the brain, which forms the basis of a valuable method for estimating the rate of TH activity in vivo (see below).

Because brain concentrations of DOPA are quite low in the absence of an AADC inhibitor, DOPA has traditionally been considered an inactive intermediate that is

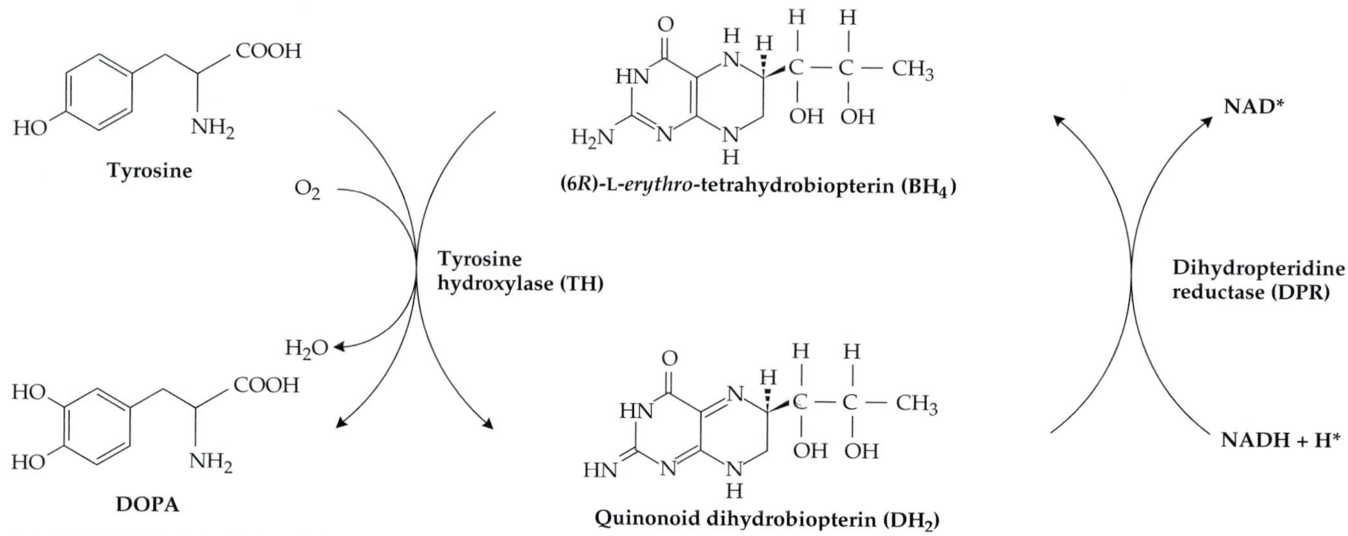

8.4 MECHANISM OF TYROSINE HYDROXYLATION. Tyrosine hydroxylation to DOPA is catalyzed by the enzyme tyrosine hydroxylase using molecular oxygen and tetrahydrobiopterin (BH_4) as cofactors. Because BH_4 is converted to quinonoid dihydrobiopterin in the course of the reaction, it must subsequently be regenerated by the action of dihydropteridine reductase. (After Nagatsu and Ichinose, 1991.)

present only briefly in the course of catecholamine synthesis. However, Goshima, Kubo, and Misu (1988) found that depolarization of superfused rat striatal slices caused a Ca^{2+}-dependent release of DOPA in addition to DA. The function of this released DOPA is not yet clear, although there is some evidence that it can modulate the release of DA (Misu and Goshima, 1993). Finally, several studies have reported the presence in brain of "L-DOPA neurons," meaning neurons that stain for DOPA but not DA, or that stain for TH but not AADC or the NE-synthesizing enzyme dopamine β-hydroxylase (Kitahama et al., 1990; Komori, Fujii, and Nagatsu, 1991; Meister et al., 1988). These results raise the intriguing possibility that DOPA may act as a neurotransmitter or neuromodulator under some circumstances.

Dopamine β-Hydroxylase

In addition to its role as a neurotransmitter, DA also serves as the precursor of NE and EPI. Cells that synthe-

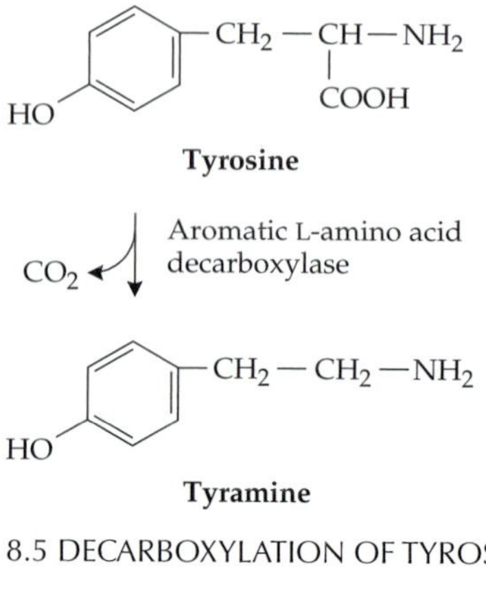

8.5 DECARBOXYLATION OF TYROSINE TO FORM TYRAMINE.

size either of these catecholamines thus possess an enzyme, dopamine β-hydroxylase (DBH), that converts DA to NE. Dopamine β-hydroxylase is a 290 kDa glycoprotein made up of four subunits, each with a molecular weight of 70–75 kDA (Stewart and Klinman, 1988). The enzyme contains Cu^{2+} ions (probably two per subunit), which are necessary for its activity. Ascorbic acid (vitamin C), which serves as an electron donor, is also required, as is molecular oxygen (see Figure 8.3). In the course of the reaction, ascorbate is oxidized to semihydroascorbate, which is subsequently reduced back to ascorbate by the action of cytochrome b-561 (Diliberto, Daniels, and Viveros, 1991).

The most detailed analyses of DBH have been carried out using adrenal chromaffin cells. These cells, which are found in the adrenal medulla (the interior part of the adrenal gland), have the same embryological origin as the sympathetic ganglionic neurons. Like sympathetic neurons, they synthesize and secrete catecholamines. Unlike neurons, however, chromaffin cells do not have any axons or dendrites, but instead secrete either NE or EPI into the general circulation as hormones. Cell fractionation studies have shown that DBH is located within the chromaffin granules, large secretory granules analogous to the synaptic vesicles of noradrenergic neurons (Winkler, Apps, and Fischer-Colbrie, 1986). Hence, DA must be transported from the cytoplasm of the cell into the granules in order to be converted to NE (this transport process will be taken up in more detail later). An interesting feature of DBH localization is that roughly half of the enzyme is soluble within the interior of the granule, whereas the remaining half is bound to the inward-facing side of the granule membrane (Winkler, Apps, and Fischer-Colbrie, 1986). The mechanism by which these two forms of DBH are generated has not yet been determined, although recent evidence suggests that both are encoded by the same mRNA (Lewis and Asnani, 1992). Unbound DBH is secreted along with NE or EPI and other soluble constituents when the chromaffin cell granule or noradrenergic vesicle is stimulated to release its contents. Indeed, some of the DBH released from the adrenal glands or from sympathetic neurons finds its way to the bloodstream, where it can be detected by various techniques (Goldstein et al., 1974; Lovenberg et al., 1974).

Because DBH is a Cu^{2+}-containing enzyme, it can be inhibited by drugs that act as Cu^{2+} chelating agents. (**Chelating agents** are compounds that bind metal ions, thereby rendering them incapable of participating in biological reactions.) Among the compounds within this category are diethyldithiocarbamate (DDC), disulfiram (tetraethylthiuram disulfide), and FLA 63 (bis-1-methyl-4-homopiperazinylthiocarbonyl disulfide). These drugs

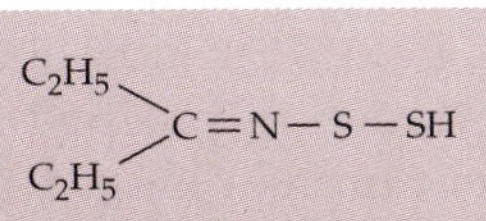

Diethyldithiocarbamate

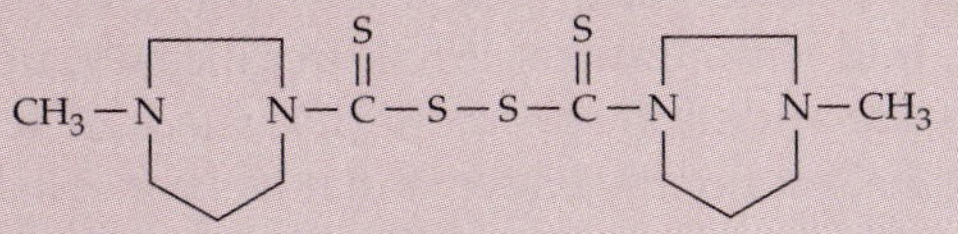

FLA 63

are not selective for DBH, however, because they also inhibit other Cu^{2+}-containing enzymes. Therefore, DBH inhibitors that work by other mechanisms are more valuable for both experimental and clinical purposes. One such agent is fusaric acid, an antibiotic produced by the fungus *Fusarium heterosporium*. Injection of this com-

Fusaric acid

pound into rabbits produced a marked inhibition of DBH activity, as well as reductions in both central and peripheral NE and EPI concentrations (Nagatsu et al., 1970). Finally, 3-phenylpropargylamine and 2-(2-thienyl)-allylamine represent prototypical members of a family of time-dependent, mechanism-based DBH inhibitors (Bargar et al., 1986). These compounds serve as DBH sub-

3-Phenylpropargylamine

strates, but in the process they are converted to inhibitors of the enzyme. Thus, drug administration is followed by a delayed but steadily growing reduction in DBH activity. Such time-dependent DBH inhibitors are capable of reducing blood pressure in a strain of genetically hypertensive rats and thus may eventually prove to have some clinical usefulness in treating hypertension in humans.

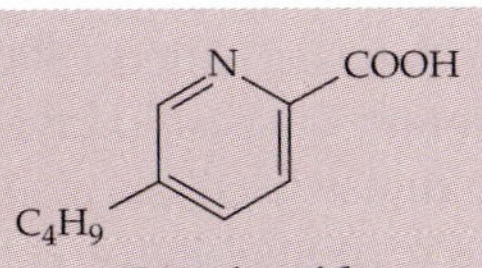

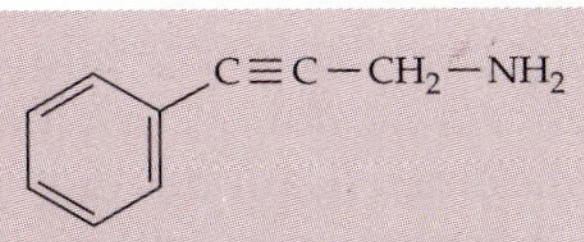

Phenylethanolamine N-Methyltransferase
Although all chromaffin cells synthesize NE, only a modest percentage of them release it as their secretory product. Most chromaffin cells, as well as a small number of neurons in the hindbrain, synthesize EPI from NE by a process of *N*-methylation (see Figure 8.3). Formation of EPI is catalyzed by an enzyme that reacts broadly with a range of phenylethanolamine derivatives and hence is called phenylethanolamine N-methyltransferase (PNMT). The methyl group for the reaction is provided by S-adenosylmethionine (SAM), which is the standard donor for most methylation reactions. Phenylethanolamine *N*-methyltransferase is a soluble, 30 kDa enzyme comprising a single subunit (Nagatsu, 1991).

Regulation of Catecholamine Synthesis
Catecholamine synthesis is regulated by a bewildering variety of processes, many of which operate via the rate-limiting enzyme TH. Thus, much of the discussion that follows will focus on alterations in TH activity. Some of the factors that regulate catecholamine synthesis operate very rapidly (within seconds or less), thereby allowing cells to respond to short-term needs. Other factors mediate alterations in catecholamine synthetic capacity over longer intervals (i.e., hours to days). Because different mechanisms are involved in acute and in long-term regulation, we will take these up in separate sections. It should also be noted that studies on the control of catecholamine synthesis have used a number of different model systems, including adrenal medullary chromaffin cells, pheochromocytoma cells, sympathetic noradrenergic neurons, noradrenergic neurons of the locus coeruleus, and nigrostriatal dopaminergic neurons. Consequently, we will generally identify the system used for any specific study cited; however, we will also combine the results freely, as similar regulatory mechanisms have been observed in most of these systems.

Acute Regulation of Tyrosine Hydroxylase
End-product inhibition. Early studies on the properties of TH found that enzyme activity could be inhibited in vitro by the addition of catecholamines, the "end products" of the synthetic pathway. This phenomenon thus came to be known as **end-product inhibition**, and was postulated to be an important mechanism in the regulation of catecholamine synthesis (see review by Masser-

ano et al., 1989). End-product inhibition is presumably mediated by the pool of catecholamines that is readily accessible to TH. According to the most commonly discussed scenario, end-product inhibition is maximal when neuronal activity and transmitter release are low, thereby leading to a high catecholamine concentration in the TH-accessible pool. In contrast, stimulation of transmitter release necessitates vesicle refilling, thus depleting the TH-accessible pool, reducing end-product inhibition, and enhancing TH activity (Masserano et al., 1989).

Initial experiments on the possible mechanisms of end-product inhibition showed that the effect of catecholamines could be reduced by increasing the concentration of the enzyme's pteridine cofactor. However, investigators have disagreed as to whether the catecholamine–pteridine interaction is competitive (Udenfriend, Zaltzman-Nirenberg, and Nagatsu, 1965), which would suggest that both bind to the same site on the enzyme molecule, or noncompetitive (Kaufman, 1973), which would indicate binding to different sites on the enzyme.

Despite this point of contention, recent studies have helped to clarify how end-product inhibition operates. Andersson and coworkers (1988) found that highly purified TH from bovine adrenal glands contained NE and EPI bound to the iron held within the enzyme. Moreover, the presence of catecholamines rendered the enzyme relatively inactive at physiological pH. Dopamine was likewise shown to bind to rat striatal TH (Okuno and Fujisawa, 1985) and to recombinant TH derived from rat PC12 pheochromocytoma cells (Ribeiro et al., 1992). These findings support the classic idea that under normal conditions, some proportion of the TH present in neurons and chromaffin cells is inactive due to the inhibitory effect of bound catecholamines. However, a new twist to the story is that this inactive TH is not activated by the simple release-dependent depletion of catecholamines, as suggested earlier. Rather, phosphorylation of TH by cyclic AMP (cAMP)-dependent protein kinase causes a liberation of the bound catecholamine and consequently an increase in enzyme activity at physiological pH (Haavik, Martinez, and Flatmark, 1990; Okuno and Fujisawa, 1985; Ribeiro et al., 1992). Tyrosine hydroxylase regulation by phosphorylation will be discussed in greater detail below.

Stimulation-induced activation.

A series of experiments by Roth and his colleagues in the early 1970s demonstrated that TH activity was enhanced following electrical stimulation of sympathetic nerve fibers, central noradrenergic neurons, and central dopaminergic neurons. Investigation of the kinetic properties of TH from stimulated preparations revealed a lower K_m (i.e., a higher affinity) for both tyrosine and the pteridine cofactor and a higher K_i (i.e., a reduced inhibitory potency) for catecholamines as compared with TH from unstimulated preparations (Morgenroth, Boadle-Biber, and Roth, 1974;

Murrin, Morgenroth, and Roth, 1976; Roth, Morgenroth, and Salzman, 1975). Studies by other investigators have generally replicated the changes in cofactor K_m and catecholamine K_i, but not the altered affinity for tyrosine (reviewed by Zigmond, Schwarzschild, and Rittenhouse, 1989). Furthermore, in many of these later studies, the V_{max} of the reaction was found to be increased by stimulation. Thus, neural activity increases the rate of tyrosine hydroxylation by reducing the influence of end-product inhibition and probably also by increasing the maximum velocity of the reaction. Mechanisms that may underlie these effects are considered in the following section.

Activation by phosphorylation.

Another important factor in the acute regulation of TH is phosphorylation by various protein kinases. Initial studies showed that TH could be phosphorylated by cAMP-dependent protein kinase (protein kinase A, or PKA), and that such phosphorylation led to a rapid activation of the enzyme (Edelman et al., 1978; Joh, Park, and Reis, 1978; Yamauchi and Fujisawa, 1979). Subsequent work demonstrated phosphorylation of purified TH by Ca^{2+}/calmodulin-dependent protein kinase, protein kinase C, and cyclic GMP (cGMP)-dependent protein kinase (reviewed by Masserano et al., 1989; Zigmond, Schwarzschild, and Rittenhouse, 1989). In all cases, phosphate groups are added to specific serine residues within the N-terminal part of the enzyme that has come to be called the "regulatory domain" of TH. The C-terminal part of the enzyme is responsible for its catalytic activity and hence is called the "catalytic domain."

Experiments using intact bovine adrenomedullary cells and rat PC12 cells have shown a more restrictive pattern of TH phosphorylation than observed with purified enzyme under cell-free conditions. Specifically, TH within intact cells is phosphorylated at serine 40 by PKA, at serine 19 by Ca^{2+}/calmodulin-dependent protein kinase II (CaM-K II), and at serine 31 by a novel family of protein kinases called ERKs (extracellular signal-regulated protein kinases) (Haycock, 1990, 1993; Figure 8.6). Protein kinase C (PKC) also plays an important role because it is responsible for activating ERKs in response to neurotransmitter or hormonal stimulation.

Phosphorylation at serine 31 has thus far been found to produce only a small change in TH activity (Haycock et al., 1992); however, phosphorylation at serines 19 and 40 both yield a clear activation of the enzyme (Masserano et al., 1989). Interestingly, the nature of the effect and the underlying mechanism is different in each case. Cyclic AMP-mediated phosphorylation increases the affinity of TH for its pteridine cofactor, and in some experiments has also been found to increase the V_{max} of the reaction (Zigmond, Schwarzschild, and Rittenhouse, 1989). These effects do not occur when the enzyme is free of catecholamines (Daubner et al., 1992; Ribeiro et al., 1992), which is consistent with the previously men-

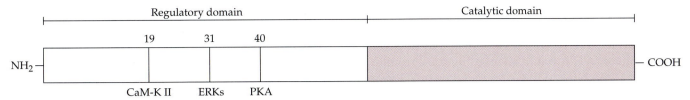

8.6 SITES OF TYROSINE HYDROXYLASE PHOSPHORYLATION. Tyrosine hydroxylase (TH) possesses two distinct domains: a catalytic domain that carries out the enzyme's catalytic function, and a regulatory domain, which contains several serine residues that are subject to phosphorylation. Within intact cells, TH phosphorylation occurs principally at serines 19, 31, and 40 via the actions of Ca^{2+}/calmodulin-dependent protein kinase II (CaM-K II), extracellular signal-regulated protein kinases (ERKs), and cAMP-dependent protein kinase (protein kinase A; PKA), respectively.

tioned notion that cAMP activates TH by causing a dissociation of iron-bound catecholamines. In contrast, phosphorylation of TH by CaM-K II has no effect by itself on enzyme function. Rather, activation of the phosphorylated enzyme requires the additional presence of a 70 kDa activator protein (Atkinson et al., 1987; Ichimura et al., 1987). In the presence of this protein, the V_{max} of the reaction is significantly increased, but there is no change in enzyme affinity for the cofactor.

Which of the receptors found on adrenal chromaffin and PC12 cells participate in the process of TH phosphorylation? Figure 8.7 illustrates one possible scheme that is consistent with the currently available evidence. The adrenal medulla is innervated by the splanchnic nerves,

preganglionic fibers of the sympathetic nervous system. Activity in these fibers causes a release of acetylcholine (ACh) and vasoactive intestinal peptide (VIP), a neuropeptide present in the nerve endings along with ACh (Hökfelt et al., 1980). The resulting stimulation of nicotinic cholinergic receptors depolarizes the cells, leading to an opening of voltage-dependent Ca^{2+} channels, activation of CaM-K II, and phosphorylation of TH at serine 19. As described in the previous chapter, muscarinic receptor stimulation causes phosphoinositide breakdown, thereby liberating the second messengers inositol trisphosphate (IP_3) and diacylglycerol (DAG) and activating PKC. According to recent work, PKC in this situation triggers a biochemical cascade that leads to the acti-

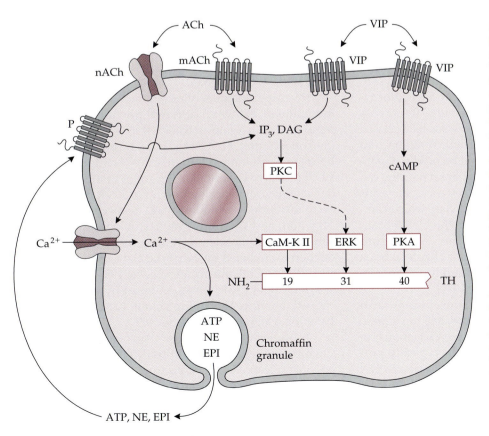

8.7 REGULATION OF TYROSINE HYDROXYLASE PHOSPHORYLATION IN ADRENAL CHROMAFFIN CELLS. When stimulated, axon terminals from the splanchnic nerves release acetylcholine (ACh) and vasoactive intestinal peptide (VIP [*top*]). Cholinergic activation of nicotinic receptors (nACh) depolarizes the chromaffin cells, thereby opening voltage-gated Ca^{2+} channels, activating CaM-K II and phosphorylating TH at serine 19. Simultaneous stimulation of muscarinic cholinergic receptors (mACh) activates the phosphosinositide second messenger system, leading to phosphorylation at serine 31 via the action of protein kinase C (PKC), which triggers a biochemical cascade (*dashed line*) that leads to the activation of ERK. VIP also appears to stimulate two different types of receptors, one of which acts through the phosphoinositide system while the other enhances TH phosphorylation at serine 40 by elevating cAMP and activating PKA. Finally, ATP co-released with the catecholamines may also be involved due to its stimulation of P2 purinergic receptors (P) in the cell membrane. (After Haycock, 1993.)

vation of ERK and TH phosphorylation at serine 31. One type of VIP receptor operates by the same pathway, as do P2 purinergic receptors (P) stimulated by adenosine triphosphate (ATP) that is released by the chromaffin cells along with NE and EPI. A second type of VIP receptor activates TH by stimulating the formation of cAMP, which in turn activates PKA and causes phosphorylation of the enzyme at serine 40 (Tischler et al., 1985).

It would be useful to be able to apply these findings to central noradrenergic and dopaminergic neurons in terms of whether TH in these cells is phosphorylated at the same serine residues by means of the same second messenger systems. Haycock and Haycock (1991) addressed this question by electrically stimulating the rat nigrostriatal tract, a massive dopaminergic pathway projecting to the corpus striatum (see Part II). Such treatment indeed caused the phosphorylation of striatal TH at the identical positions reported in the studies on adrenal chromaffin cells. Additional in vitro experiments using synaptosomes prepared from striatum suggested that phosphorylation is carried out by the same group of protein kinases mentioned above. Thus, it appears that similar mechanisms of TH phosphorylation occur in adrenal cells and in central catecholaminergic neurons. Furthermore, phosphorylation by several second messenger systems acting together appears to be sufficient to reproduce the activating effects of electrical stimulation on TH.

Regulation by changes in substrate availability. As in the case of choline acetyltransferase and ACh synthesis discussed in Chapter 7, we may address the issue of substrate regulation of catecholamine synthesis by first considering whether the local concentration of tyrosine is high enough to saturate TH. According to in vivo estimates of tyrosine concentrations as well as the K_m for tyrosine, it appears that TH is approximately 70% to 80% saturated under resting conditions (see Sved, 1983). Based on these findings, the rate of tyrosine hydroxylation, and hence catecholamine synthesis, should be mildly dependent on changes in tyrosine availability. Brain tyrosine can be decreased by treating animals with certain amino acids such as phenylalanine, valine, or tryptophan, which compete with tyrosine for transport across the blood–brain barrier (the role of this large neutral amino acid carrier system is discussed further in the next chapter). Such treatment has indeed been shown to retard the rate of catecholamine synthesis (Wurtman et al., 1974).

The apparent lack of TH saturation in vivo also means that it should theoretically be possible to increase catecholamine synthesis by administering exogenous tyrosine. In practice, tyrosine treatment has typically produced either no change or at most a 15% increase in DA synthesis or turnover (measured in whole brain or corpus striatum) when no attempt was made to accelerate the firing rate of the cells (Sved, 1983). In contrast, there is general agreement that when the firing rate is high, tyrosine supplementation leads to more substantial increases in DA synthesis and turnover. For the nigrostriatal system, this principle has been demonstrated using pharmacological techniques to enhance neuronal firing (Milner and Wurtman, 1986; Sved, 1983). There are also at least two different dopaminergic cell populations that are normally sensitive to tyrosine availability. One population consists of midbrain DA neurons that project to the prefrontal cortex and that exhibit higher rates of spontaneous activity than the nigrostriatal cells (Tam, Nobufumi, and Roth, 1987). Another consists of retinal DA-containing neurons, which fire more rapidly when stimulated by light (i.e., during the daytime) than in the dark. During the light period only, these cells respond to changes in tyrosine levels by altering their rate of DA synthesis (Fernstrom and Fernstrom, 1994).

Long-Term Regulation of Tyrosine Hydroxylase: Trans-Synaptic Induction

In the late 1960s and early 1970s, several laboratories reported that various stressors, including cold exposure, insulin-induced hypoglycemia, immobilization, and treatment with the amine-depleting drug reserpine (which stimulates sympathetic outflow by reducing blood pressure), all increased TH activity in the adrenal medulla and in the superior cervical ganglion, a commonly studied sympathetic ganglion (Kvetňanský, Weise, and Kopin, 1970; Thoenen, 1970; Thoenen, Mueller, and Axelrod, 1969). This effect could be blocked by prior denervation of the adrenal glands or the superior cervical ganglion (above references), indicating that the stress-related change in TH is mediated trans-synaptically (i.e., by neural activity in the fibers innervating these tissues) (Figure 8.8).

Investigators quickly recognized that **trans-synaptic induction** of TH was a different phenomenon than the rapid type of enzyme activation that is dependent on TH phosphorylation. First, trans-synaptic induction required hours to occur, rather than minutes (Guidotti and Costa, 1977; Fluharty et al., 1983). Second, TH induction could be prevented by blocking protein or RNA synthesis with cycloheximide or actinomycin D, respectively, (Mueller, Thoenen, and Axelrod, 1969). This observation led to subsequent studies demonstrating that trans-synaptic induction is mediated by enhanced transcription of the TH gene (Black, Chikaraishi, and Lewis, 1985; Stachowiak et al., 1985; Tank et al., 1985), followed by synthesis of increased amounts of enzyme protein (Chuang and Costa, 1974; Joh, Geghman, and Reis, 1973).

To determine the mechanisms involved in trans-synaptic induction of TH, initial studies focused on the possible role of ACh released from preganglionic cholinergic fibers. Indeed, trans-synaptic induction in the adrenal gland was found to be significantly attenuated, although not totally abolished, by pretreating subjects

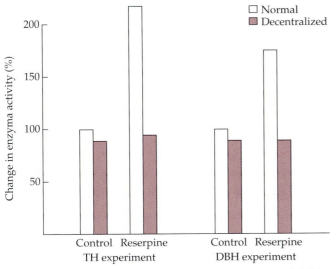

8.8 TRANS-SYNAPTIC INDUCTION OF TYROSINE HYDROXY-LASE AND DOPAMINE β-HYDROXYLASE IN THE SUPERIOR CERVICAL GANGLION. Reserpine was administered to rats either as a single 5 mg/kg dose (TH experiment) or as three doses of 2.5 mg/kg given on alternate days (DBH experiment). In the normal superior cervical ganglion, activities of both enzymes were elevated 24 hours after the last injection. This effect was completely blocked by prior denervation (decentralization) of the ganglion. (After Axelrod, 1971.)

with the ganglionic nicotinic receptor antagonists hexamethonium, mecamylamine, or chlorisondamine (Guidotti and Costa, 1974; Stachowiak, Stricker et al., 1988). Other experiments demonstrated induction of adrenal TH following the injection of nicotine (Slotkin and Seidler, 1975). This effect was completely blocked by nicotinic antagonists if the glands had previously been denervated, but only a partial inhibition occurred if the nerve supply was intact (Fossom, Carlson, and Tank, 1991; Fossom, Sterling, and Tank, 1991). These results indicate that systemically administered nicotine acts at two sites to cause TH induction: (1) directly on adrenal chromaffin cell nicotinic receptors (the only site of action in the denervated preparation), and (2) at higher levels of the nervous system to trigger activity in the splanchnic nerve (which is an additional site of action in the intact preparation). Moreover, because nicotinic antagonists failed to completely block TH induction when the splanchnic nerve was undamaged, the nerve must release one or more substances besides ACh that participate in the induction process. One candidate substance is VIP, which was mentioned earlier as a neuropeptide present with ACh in preganglionic fibers. Recent research indicates that VIP can increase TH mRNA levels either alone or in conjunction with ACh, thus implicating this peptide in the process of trans-synaptic induction (Olasmaa et al., 1991; Wessels-Reiker et al., 1991).

Cyclic AMP is one of the second messengers that have been implicated in stimulating TH gene transcrip-

tion. Early experiments by Guidotti and Costa (1973, 1974) showed that reserpine, cold exposure, and the cholinergic agonist carbachol all caused a transient rise in cAMP levels in adrenal chromaffin cells. This increase in cAMP was followed by a biochemical cascade consisting of (1) an increased concentration of catalytic subunits of protein kinase A (PKA) in the cytosol, (2) a shift of PKA catalytic activity from the cytosol to the nuclear fraction, indicating translocation of catalytic subunits to the nucleus, (3) increased synthesis of polyadenylated RNA,* and (4) increased TH synthesis and enzymatic activity (Guidotti and Costa, 1977; Figure 8.9). These correlational findings were consistent with the hypothesis that activation of the cAMP second messenger system plays an important role in trans-synaptic TH induction. Later research supported this notion by showing that treatment of pheochromocytoma cells with forskolin, a drug that stimulates adenylyl cyclase, or with the cAMP analogs 8-bromo cAMP or dibutyryl cAMP enhanced TH gene transcription (Lewis et al., 1983; Tank, Curella, and Ham, 1986). Recent evidence unexpectedly indicates that cAMP and PKA may even participate in the basal (i.e., noninduced) rate of TH gene transcription (Kim, Lee et al., 1993; Kim, Park et al. 1993).

Other second messenger systems to consider with regard to trans-synaptic TH induction are the phosphoinositide/protein kinase C (PKC) system as well as Ca^{2+} and CaM-K II. Protein kinase C can be activated by a family of compounds known as phorbol esters (see Chapter 6). When PC12 cells were treated with the phorbol ester tetradecanoyl-12,13-phorbol acetate (TPA), TH gene transcription was stimulated (Vyas, Biguet, and Mallet, 1990). Preliminary findings are consistent with the possibility that PKC may participate in the process of trans-synaptic induction (Icard-Liepkalns et al., 1992). As presented earlier in Figure 8.7, researchers have identified several signaling pathways by which PKA and PKC can be activated in chromaffin cells. It is possible that trans-synaptic induction involves both of these kinases and their associated second messenger systems. On the other hand, there is currently little or no evidence favoring a role for CaM-K II.

Studies aimed at determining whether reserpine-mediated TH induction occurs in the CNS surprisingly showed striking differences between different cell groups. Thus, a single high dose of reserpine produced marked and long-lasting increases in TH mRNA levels and enzyme activity in the noradrenergic cells of the locus coeruleus, a modest increase in TH mRNA in the dopaminergic cells of the ventral tegmental area, but no

*In the process of gene transcription, newly formed RNA molecules are usually modified by the addition of a long tail made up of adenylate residues (hence the term polyadenylate or, more usually, poly-A RNA). Mature mRNA molecules still contain this tail, which serves to increase their stability.

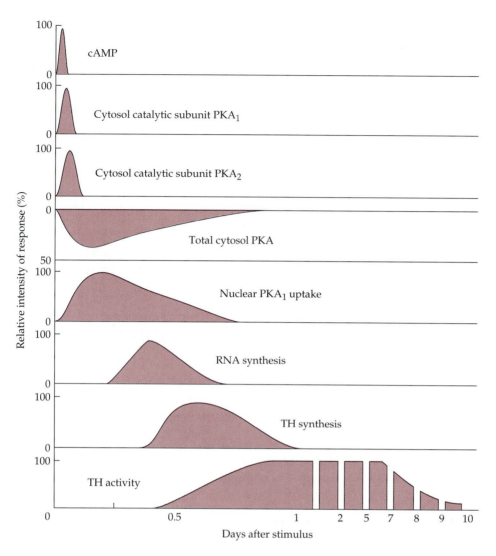

8.9 BIOCHEMICAL CASCADE IN-VOLVED IN TRANS-SYNAPTIC IN-DUCTION OF TYROSINE HYDROXY-LASE IN ADRENAL CHROMAFFIN CELLS. Application of an appropriate stimulus such as reserpine injection, cold exposure, or treatment with the cholinergic agonist carbachol leads to a rapid but transient (about 90 min) elevation in chromaffin cell cAMP levels. This is followed sequentially by increases in the catalytic subunits of PKA types 1 and 2, nuclear PKA$_1$ uptake, synthesis of polyadenylated RNA, and enhanced synthesis of TH. TH enzymatic activity remains elevated for approximately 1 week. (After Guidotti and Costa, 1977.)

change at all in the dopaminergic cells of the substantia nigra (Biguet et al., 1986; Pasinetti et al., 1990; Reis, Joh, and Ross, 1975; Zigmond, Schon, and Iversen, 1974). Figure 8.10 illustrates the comparative effects of reserpine treatment on the locus coeruleus, substantia nigra, and adrenal glands. The reasons for the differential responses of the above-mentioned cell populations have not yet been determined.

Regulation of Dopamine β-Hydroxylase and Phenylethanolamine N-Methyltransferase

Trans-synaptic induction by reserpine is not restricted to TH, but also occurs for DBH and PNMT (Axelrod, 1971; Reis, Joh, and Ross, 1975; Wessel and Joh, 1992). As shown in Figure 8.8, the elevation in DBH activity is dependent on an intact innervation, just as in the case of TH. Moreover, some of the same mechanisms may be involved in the induction process, as cAMP has been found to increase DBH mRNA levels in pheochromocytoma cells (McMahon and Sabban, 1992). With respect to PNMT induction in chromaffin cells, the stimulatory effect of

acetylcholine interestingly seems to be mediated by both nicotinic and muscarinic receptors acting through different signal transduction mechanisms (Evinger et al., 1994).

Another type of regulation is exerted by glucocorticoids, hormones made by the cortex (outer part) of the adrenal glands. Secretion of these hormones is enhanced by physical and psychological stressors, and they play a complex role in the adaptive physiological responses to stressful stimulation (Munck, Guyre, and Holbrook, 1984). Glucocorticoids have been shown to induce TH, DBH, and PNMT in chromaffin and pheochromocytoma cells (Ciaranello, Wooten, and Axelrod, 1975; Kim, Park, and Joh, 1993; Stachowiak, Rigual et al., 1988). Indeed, chromaffin cells are normally exposed to very high levels of glucocorticoids because the glucocorticoid-synthesizing tissue of the adrenal glands (adrenal cortex) encases the chromaffin tissue (adrenal medulla), and the adrenomedullary blood supply is derived largely from the adrenocortical venous effluent. The influence of glucocorticoids on PNMT is mediated by two different mechanisms: (1) increased transcription of the PNMT

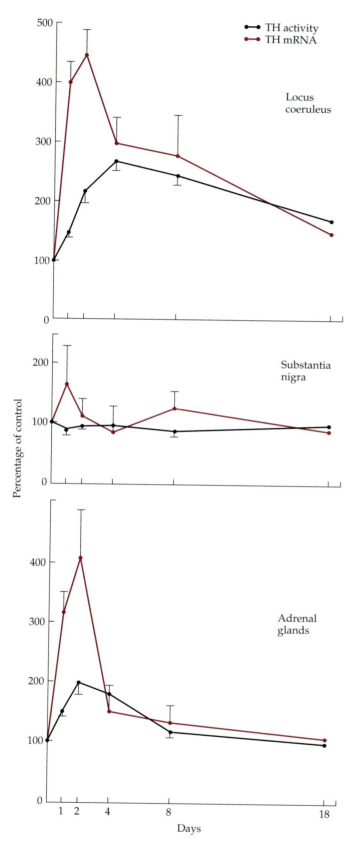

8.10 RESERPINE-INDUCED TRANS-SYNAPTIC INDUCTION OF TYROSINE HYDROXYLASE IN THE LOCUS COERULEUS, SUBSTANTIA NIGRA, AND ADRENAL GLANDS. Changes in TH enzymatic activity and TH mRNA levels were examined in rats following a single dose of reserpine (10 mg/kg). The results show the presence of trans-synaptic induction in the locus coeruleus and adrenal glands, but no significant effect in the substantia nigra. (After Biguet et al., 1986.)

gene (Evinger et al., 1992), and (2) a reduced rate of PNMT degradation due to enhanced levels of the cofactor *S*-adenosylmethionine (Ciaranello, 1978; Wong, Zager, and Ciaranello, 1982).

Summary of Catecholamine Synthesis Regulation

Tyrosine hydroxylase activity is acutely regulated by several processes acting together to coordinate the rate of catecholamine synthesis with ongoing neural and secretory activity. Early studies of TH regulation focused on the ability of catecholamines to inhibit enzyme activity (end-product inhibition) and of electrical stimulation to activate the enzyme. Kinetic studies showed that stimulation-induced activation is associated with a decreased K_m for the pteridine cofactor, an increased K_i for enzyme inhibition by catecholamines, and an increased V_{max} for the reaction. These phenomena can be explained in part by the ability of TH to adopt two distinct states: a relatively inactive state caused by the binding of catecholamines to iron within the enzyme, and a catalytically active state in which catecholamine is not present. Conversion of TH from the inactive to the active state is greatly accelerated by cAMP/protein kinase A–mediated phosphorylation of the enzyme at the serine 40 residue. Tyrosine hydroxylase can also be phosphorylated at serine 19 by CaM-K II, and at serine 31 by extracellular signal-regulated protein kinases, which in turn are activated by protein kinase C. All three reactions are enhanced by stimulation, although current evidence suggests that PKA- and CaM-K II–mediated phosphorylation are most important for activating TH under these conditions. Tyrosine hydroxylase activity is also subject to some degree of modulation by changes in tyrosine availability; however, because the enzyme is thought to be approximately 70% to 80% saturated with substrate under resting conditions, tyrosine is usually not rate-limiting unless the cells are firing at a high rate.

Long-term regulation of TH occurs via trans-synaptic induction, a process shown to occur in the adrenal medulla, sympathetic ganglia, and the noradrenergic neurons of the locus coeruleus. Trans-synaptic induction refers to increased TH gene transcription and synthesis of enzyme molecules following stressful stimuli such as reserpine administration, cold exposure, or physical immobilization. Elimination of synaptic input or blockade of the appropriate neurotransmitter receptors prevents TH induction, thus demonstrating the trans-synaptic nature of the phenomenon. In the adrenal medulla, ACh and the colocalized neuropeptide VIP are two likely mediators of trans-synaptic induction. The intracellular mechanisms underlying this process are not yet understood; however, some evidence suggests the possible involvement of PKA, PKC, and perhaps even glucocorticoid hormones.

DBH and PNMT are subject to trans-synaptic induction similar to that of TH. In addition, levels of these enzymes are increased by glucocorticoid hormones. In particular, the synthesis of EPI by adrenomedullary chromaffin cells is dependent on stimulation of PNMT gene transcription and stabilization of the enzyme by glucocorticoids from the cortical part of the adrenal gland. Thus, although TH is still considered the focal point of catecholamine synthesis regulation, particularly within central catecholaminergic neurons, we should not ignore potentially important changes in the other synthetic enzymes.

Catecholamine Storage and Release

Catecholamine Storage Mechanisms

Once catecholamines have been synthesized, they are packaged in granules or vesicles for subsequent release. Catecholamine storage mechanisms have been studied most extensively in adrenal chromaffin cells and in sympathetic neurons; hence these model systems will be emphasized in the present discussion. As mentioned earlier, chromaffin cells possess large numbers of storage granules about 300 nm in diameter that are called chromaffin granules (reviewed by Winkler, Apps, and Fischer-Colbrie, 1986; Winkler, Sietzen, and Schober, 1987). The major soluble constituents of these granules and an estimate of each one's relative abundance are shown in Table 8.1. In addition to the obvious presence of catecholamines, chromaffin granules also contain nucleotides (mainly ATP), ascorbic acid, Ca^{2+} ions, a family of glycoproteins called chromogranins, a small number of DBH molecules, enkephalin peptides (see Chapter 12), and another peptide called neuropeptide Y. The chromogranins probably contribute significantly to the electron-dense (i.e., darkly staining) core of the granules as seen in electron micrographs (Winkler, Apps, and Fischer-Colbrie, 1986). The roles of DBH and ascorbic acid in NE synthesis were discussed earlier; however, the physiological roles of the remaining granule constituents are still being investigated.

The life cycle of chromaffin granules is diagrammed in Figure 8.11. The protein precursors of the chromogranins, enkephalins, and also neuropeptide Y (which is not shown in the figure) are synthesized in the smooth endoplasmic reticulum (see Chapter 11 for a more detailed discussion of protein and peptide synthesis). These substances are packaged into vesicle-like struc-

Table 8.1	Relative Quantities of Secretory Constituents of a Single Bovine Chromaffin Granule
Constituent	**Number of molecules**
Catecholamines	3×10^6
Nucleotides	930,000
Ascorbic acid	120,000
Calcium	90,000
Chromogranin A	5,000
Chromogranin B	80
Chromogranin C	?
Dopamine β-hydroxylase	140
Total enkephalin equivalents	4,000
Neuropeptide Y	428

Source: After Winkler, Sietzen, and Schober, 1987.

tures and transported to the Golgi apparatus for post-translational modification by the addition of phosphate (PO_4), sulfate (SO_4), and carbohydrate groups. As in the case of other secretory granules, chromaffin granules then form by budding off from the Golgi apparatus. ATP synthesized in mitochondria is transported into the granules, along with DA synthesized in the cytoplasm of the cell. As described earlier, DA is converted into NE within the chromaffin granules. In EPI-secreting chromaffin cells, NE must return to the cytoplasm in order to be *N*-methylated by PNMT (Corcoran, Wilson, and Kirshner, 1984). The resulting EPI is then taken back up into the granule by the same mechanism that transports DA. After exocytosis, it is believed that the granule membrane constituents are retrieved from the chromaffin cell membrane and possibly recycled for use in the formation of new granules.

Sympathetic neurons possess two types of dense-core vesicles, large and small. The large vesicles seem to contain most, if not all, of the same substances present within chromaffin granules (Winkler, Sietzen, and Schober, 1987). The small vesicles can take up catecholamines and can synthesize NE; however, they contain no chromogranins or peptides. One interesting, though as yet unsubstantiated, hypothesis is that the small dense-core vesicles of sympathetic nerve terminals arise locally from the recycling of large vesicles following exocytosis (Smith, 1978).

Among the processes mentioned above, the transport of catecholamines into the secretory granules is of obvious importance. The mechanism underlying this process is illustrated schematically in Figure 8.12. The granule membrane possesses an ATPase that translocates protons (H^+ ions) from the cytoplasm of the cell into the interior of the granule (Johnson, 1987). This process causes the formation of a pH gradient across the granule membrane (an inside pH of about 5.5 compared with a cytoplasmic pH of

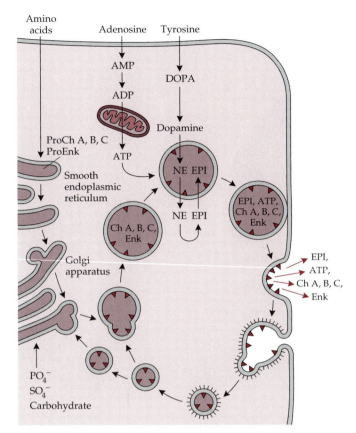

8.11 LIFE CYCLE OF CHROMAFFIN GRANULES. Precursor proteins for the chromogranins (ProCh) and enkephalins (ProEnk) are synthesized from amino acids and then enter the smooth endoplasmic reticulum. They are subsequently transported to the Golgi apparatus, the site of posttranslational modifications such as addition of phosphate, sulfate, and carbohydrate groups. New chromaffin granules containing these proteins and peptides bud off from the Golgi apparatus and then are filled with EPI, NE, and ATP. Following release by exocytosis, the granule cell membrane is retrieved and recycled. Membrane-bound DBH molecules are shown as small triangles. (After Winkler, Sietzen, and Schober, 1987.)

in noradrenergic, dopaminergic, and serotonergic cell groups in the brain, indicating that this one protein is probably responsible for accumulating all three amines in synaptic vesicles (Erickson, Eiden, and Hoffman, 1992). Adrenal chromaffin cells, however, expressed a different, though closely related, transporter protein (Liu et al., 1992). Thus, at least two monoamine vesicular transporters exist, one that is specific for neurons and another that is present in chromaffin cells.

Both the neuronal vesicle and chromaffin granule catecholamine transporters can be inhibited by several important drugs. The best known of these are tetrabenazine (Nitoman), a synthetic compound, and reserpine (Serpasil), an alkaloid derived from the roots of *Rauwolfia serpentina* (snake root). In India and other parts

Tetrabenazine

Reserpine

of Asia, *Rauwolfia* has been known for centuries for its medicinal properties. By the 1940s, Indian physicians had recognized two distinctive properties of *Rauwolfia*, a hypotensive (blood pressure–lowering) effect and a sedating effect, and had begun using the substance in clinical practice. In 1953, treatment of Indian psychiatric patients with *Rauwolfia* came to the attention of the American psychiatrist Nathan Kline by way of an article in the *New York Times* (see Caldwell, 1970). Kline was initially quite interested, since chlorpromazine had just been introduced and psychiatrists were excited about the prospect of finding other new agents for treating psychotic patients. But the hypotensive action of reserpine proved to be a troublesome side effect, and furthermore, the drug was soon recognized to be a less effective antipsychotic agent than chlorpromazine and other phenothiazines (see Chapter 18). Reserpine was therefore relegated to the prescription list of antihypertensive agents, although even here it has been largely supplanted by new agents.

approximately 7) as well as a transmembrane electric potential (the inside is electropositive compared with the cytoplasm). This combined electrochemical gradient is used by a membrane transport protein to take up catecholamines from the cytoplasm into the granules. Like the acetylcholine transport protein found in the membrane of cholinergic vesicles, the catecholamine vesicular transporter functions as a proton antiporter (Figure 8.12). This mechanism is so efficient that it is estimated to be capable of producing a 135,000:1 gradient of catecholamines across the chromaffin cell membrane (i.e., a granule concentration 135,000 times higher than the concentration in the cell cytoplasm) (Johnson, 1987).

Cloning studies have recently identified the rat (Erickson, Eiden, and Hoffman, 1992; Liu et al., 1992) and human (Erickson and Eiden, 1993; Surratt et al., 1993) vesicular transporters. The same transporter was found

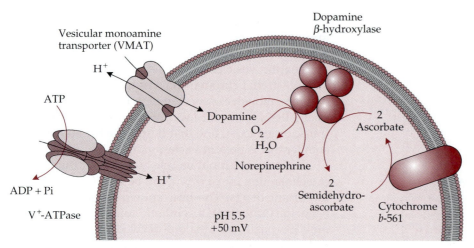

8.12 UPTAKE AND HYDROXYLATION OF CATECHOLAMINES BY CHROMAFFIN GRAN-ULES. Chromaffin granule membranes possess an ATPase that translocates protons (H^+ ions) into the interior of the granule. This process acidifies the granule (pH of approximately 5.5) and also creates a transmembrane electrical potential of about 50 mV. The cate-cholamine transporter uses the resulting electrochemical gradient across the membrane to concentrate catecholamines within the granule. The transporter functions as a proton an-tiporter, meaning that a proton is carried out of the granule for each molecule of cate-cholamine that is carried inside. Inside the granule, DA is hydroxylated to NE by a mecha-nism described earlier in the text. (After Winkler, Apps, and Fischer-Colbrie, 1986.)

Reserpine and tetrabenazine both bind to sites on the vesicle and chromaffin granule transporters. These compounds (when radioactively labeled) can therefore be used as probes for visualizing the location of monoamine storage vesicles (Henry and Scherman, 1989; Kilbourn et al., 1993). As a consequence of their binding to the transporters, catecholamine and 5-HT accumulation are blocked. By preventing the storage of newly formed transmitter molecules, vesicular uptake inhibitors initially stimulate catecholamine and 5-HT release. This is soon followed by a profound transmitter depletion, which, in the case of reserpine, lasts for several days. A classic study by Carlsson, Lindqvist, and Magnusson (1957) showed that DOPA antagonized reserpine-induced behavioral depression, whereas 5-hydroxytryptophan (the precursor of 5-HT) did not. This effect of DOPA is probably attributable to DA synthesis from DOPA as NE synthesis is inhibited due to lack of access of DA to intravesicular DBH.

Questions concerning the dynamics of catecholamine storage in CNS neurons have been difficult to address. For example, how rapidly do vesicles fill with transmitter? How much transmitter turnover occurs in vesicles due to normal leakage and refilling? A recent study by Floor and colleagues (1995) has begun to approach these issues by examining radiolabeled DA uptake and efflux from a brain synaptic vesicle preparation in vitro. Considerable exchange occurred between vesicular and extravesicular DA, with a turnover half-time of minutes under the conditions of the experiment. If these results are representative of the situation in vivo, then the vesicular pool of DA (see below) may be quite labile.

Catecholamine Release

Stimulus-evoked release of catecholamines has been shown to occur through the mechanism of vesicular exocytosis. The classic work leading to this conclusion was performed using adrenal chromaffin cells and sympathetic noradrenergic neurons (reviewed by Trifaró, Vitale, and Del Castillo, 1992). One of the fundamental pieces of evidence obtained from chromaffin cells was that cell stimulation caused the release not only of catecholamines but also of other granular constituents such as chromogranins, nucleotides, and DBH. In contrast to chromogranins and DBH, no lactate dehydrogenase (a cytoplasmic enzyme) was detected outside the stimulated chromaffin cells, suggesting an absence of release from the cytoplasmic compartment. More recently, sophisticated optical techniques have enabled investigators to directly visualize the exocytosis of individual chromaffin granules in living chromaffin cells (Terakawa et al., 1991). Stimulation of sympathetic neurons likewise causes vesicle exocytosis, as indicated by the release of chromogranins and DBH (Trifaró, Vitale, and Del Castillo, 1992) as well as by electron microscopic evidence for fusion of vesicles with the nerve terminal membrane (Thureson-Klein, 1983). In other experiments, animals were given reserpine along with a monoamine oxidase inhibitor to deplete vesicular NE while allowing it to accumulate in the nerve terminal cytoplasm. Under these conditions, little or no NE release occurred when the sympathetic fibers were subsequently stimulated (Trifaró, Vitale, and Del Castillo, 1992).

Dopamine release has been studied mainly in the CNS using tissue slices or synaptosomes, and more recently by means of in vivo techniques such as microdialysis and voltammetry (see Chapter 2). As discussed in Chapter 6, exocytosis is known to be triggered by a large influx of Ca²⁺ into the nerve terminal or cell. Hence, pharmacological studies using any of the above preparations generally infer the presence of an exocytotic process if release is Ca²⁺-dependent and is sensitive to blockade of Na⁺ channels by tetrodotoxin (TTX) (opening of the Ca²⁺ channels requires membrane depolarization mediated by voltage-gated Na⁺ channels). Both in vivo and in vitro, depolarizing stimuli indeed cause a release of DA that possesses the above characteristics (Arbuthnott, Fairbrother, and Butcher, 1990; Raiteri et al., 1979). However, a second type of DA release has been identified that is Ca²⁺-independent but can be inhibited by drugs that block the DA transporter protein that is present in the cell membrane (Raiteri et al., 1979). As described in a later section, the normal function of cell membrane transporters (which should not be confused with the vesicular transporters discussed earlier) is to take up catecholamines from the synaptic cleft following release. Under certain conditions, however, both the DA and NE transporters can operate in a reverse direction, thus releasing these neurotransmitters from the nerve terminal cytoplasm (Arbuthnott, Fairbrother, and Butcher, 1990; Raiteri et al., 1979; Trendelenburg, 1991). Indeed, drugs that release catecholamines typically operate through reversal of the membrane carrier.

Numerous studies have suggested that DA exists in several distinct compartments or pools within the nerve terminal (Ewing, Bigelow, and Wightman, 1983; Justice, Nicolaysen, and Michael, 1988; McMillen, German, and Shore, 1980). In general, these experiments indicate that newly synthesized DA is preferentially released, and that this readily releasable pool can be replenished by a pool of previously stored transmitter. These two pools are usually assumed to be vesicular in origin. There must also be a cytoplasmic pool of DA that is presumably replenished by DA uptake and that is the source of DA release via reverse transport. Various models have been developed to account for these findings, one of which is shown in Figure 8.13. Among the important features of this particular model are the idea that DA synthesis feeds directly into the readily releasable vesicular pool, and that each pool is in equilibrium with the others. It should be noted that alternative models have been proposed, including one in which newly synthesized DA initially enters a primary cytoplasmic pool (Leviel, Gobert, and Guibert, 1989). Thus, some of the details of neurotransmitter disposition in catecholaminergic nerve terminals remain uncertain at this time.

Catecholamine release is potently stimulated by the behaviorally arousing drugs amphetamine and methylphenidate. To some extent, these compounds may release catecholamines from different intracellular compartments because reserpine blocks methylphenidate-induced, but not amphetamine-induced, DA release (see McMillen, German, and Shore, 1980). The biochemical

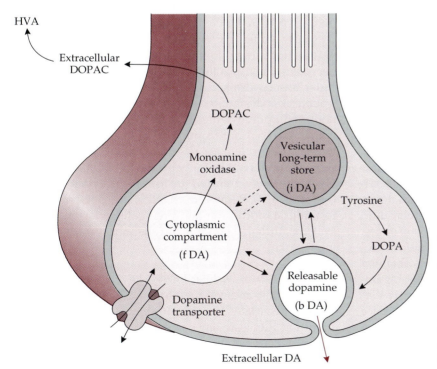

8.13 HYPOTHETICAL MODEL OF DOPAMINE POOLS WITHIN A DOPAMINERGIC NERVE TERMINAL. According to the model illustrated, DA synthesis feeds directly into a releasable bound (vesicular) pool (bDA), which is in equilibrium with a pool of free (cytoplasmic) DA (fDA) and an inactive bound pool (iDA). An alternative model involves the entry of newly synthesized DA into the cytoplasmic pool before it is taken up into vesicles. (After Arbuthnott, Fairbrother, and Butcher, 1990.)

mechanisms of action of these drugs are discussed further in Chapter 13.

Catecholamine Inactivation

Unlike ACh, which is rapidly degraded by a simple enzymatic process, catecholamines are subject to multiple routes of inactivation. Following release, both DA and NE are taken back up into the nerve terminal by means of the cell membrane transporters mentioned just above (see cover illustration). In addition, several important enzymes participate in catecholamine breakdown, both within and outside nerve cells. These processes are discussed in the next several sections.

Catecholamine Uptake

The general features of biogenic amine (i.e., catecholamines and 5-HT) uptake are reviewed by Graham and Langer (1992) (also see Horn, 1990, for a more specific review of DA uptake). Biogenic amine uptake is Na^+- and Cl^--dependent, and in fact these ions are believed to be cotransported across the membrane along with DA or NE (Krueger, 1990; Sammet and Graefe, 1979). Because the transport mechanism must take up catecholamines against a concentration gradient, it requires a source of metabolic energy. This energy is provided by the transmembrane Na^+ electrochemical gradient, which contrasts with the use of a proton gradient to accumulate catecholamines within vesicles and chromaffin granules. The formation and maintenance of the Na^+ gradient is accomplished by membrane Na^+–K^+ ATPase (the sodium–potassium pump). Hence, inhibition of this enzyme by ouabain potently inhibits catecholamine uptake. Researchers have generally assumed that at least part of the recaptured catecholamine is repackaged into vesicles for later release, but the proportion of transmitter subject to such recycling is difficult to determine.

Recent exciting work by the research group of Caron and colleagues has shown that the plasma membrane DA transporter plays a critical role in modulating synaptic DA concentrations (Giros et al., 1996). The investigators created a mutant strain of mice lacking a functional gene for the DA transporter (i.e., a "gene knockout") and compared this strain with normal control mice with respect to their neurochemical and behavioral characteristics. One experiment used cyclic voltammetry to determine the rate of DA removal from the extracellular fluid following stimulus-evoked DA release in tissue slices. DA clearance was complete within 1 s in the control slices, whereas clearance took 100 s in the slices obtained from the DA transporter knockout mice. This finding implies that extracellular DA levels are persistently elevated in the absence of active uptake. The knockout mice also showed substantial reductions in DA synthesis and in D_1 and D_2 receptor gene expression, which are thought to be adaptive responses aimed at reducing

dopaminergic activity. Yet despite these attempts to compensate for the lack of the transporter by down-regulating other parts of the dopaminergic system, the knockout mice still showed a behavioral syndrome of hyperlocomotion. Synaptic uptake, therefore, serves a vital function in regulating DA neurotransmission.

Although the basic features of catecholamine uptake have been known for many years, the structures of the transporters themselves have been determined only within the past few years through molecular biological techniques. The DA and NE transporters were found to be members of a novel family of membrane proteins that also includes the transporters for 5-HT, glutamate, and γ-aminobutyric acid (GABA) (reviewed by Amara and Kuhar, 1993; Uhl, 1992). These neurotransmitter transporters are all glycoproteins with molecular weights ranging from about 60–85 kDa, and they are all thought to possess 12 transmembrane domains, as shown in Figure 8.14 for the DA transporter. As we shall see in the next section, one reason for the current excitement about catecholamine transporter structure and function is that these proteins mediate the actions of many important psychoactive drugs.

A certain degree of uptake specificity is conferred upon dopaminergic and noradrenergic neurons by the fact that each cell type seems to express only the gene for its own transporter (Amara and Kuhar, 1993). However, the transporters themselves do not exhibit a high degree of specificity for their respective transmitters. Such lack of specificity accounts for the finding of Di Chiara and colleagues (1992) that significant DA uptake into noradrenergic nerve terminals may occur in the rat prefrontal cortex, an area where NE levels and the density of noradrenergic innervation are much higher than those of DA (Slopsema, Van der Gugten, and De Bruin, 1982).

Early studies performed on sympathetic noradrenergic junctions found that in addition to NE uptake by the nerve terminals, postjunctional smooth muscle and glandular tissues also accumulated NE. This extraneuronal uptake was designated $Uptake_2$ to differentiate it from neuronal uptake (which was termed $Uptake_1$). $Uptake_2$ was found to differ from $Uptake_1$ in several respects: it was less dependent on Na^+, had a lower affinity for NE, showed no stereoselectivity for the (−) and (+) isomers of NE, and was inhibited by different types of drugs (Iversen, 1974). Because most attention has been directed to understanding the neuronal catecholamine uptake systems, little is known about the mechanism underlying $Uptake_2$.

Catecholamine Uptake Inhibitors

The vesicular and cell membrane catecholamine transporters possess different pharmacological properties such that the vesicular uptake inhibitor tetrabenazine does not block synaptic catecholamine reuptake (Rostène et al., 1992). On the other hand, synaptic catecholamine

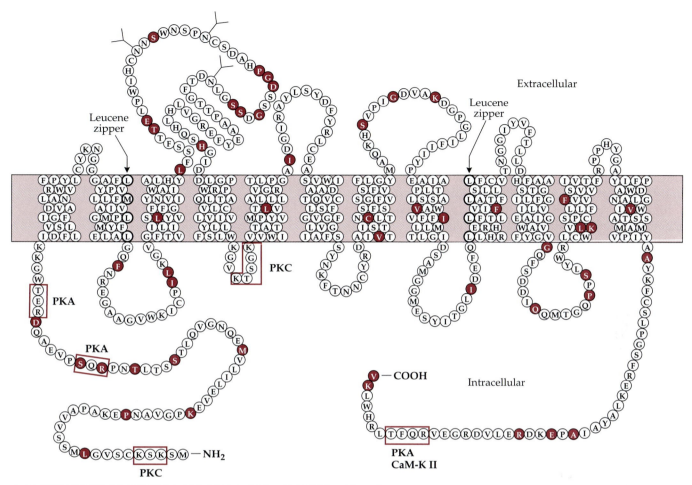

8.14 STRUCTURE OF THE HUMAN DOPAMINE TRANSPORTER. Like other transporters for amine neurotransmitters, the DA transporter possesses 12 putative transmembrane domains. Other features shown include three potential glycosylation sites on the second extracellular loop (Y-shaped symbols), as well as sites for phosphorylation by protein kinase A (PKA), protein kinase C (PKC), and Ca^{2+}-calmodulin-dependent protein kinase II (CaM-K II). The amino acid residues shown in black are those that differ in the rat DA transporter. These represent only 8% of the total amino acids, indicating a high degree of sequence homology between the human and rat proteins. (After Giros and Caron, 1993.)

reuptake can be inhibited by a wide variety of other drugs, such as cocaine, amphetamine, methylphenidate, mazindol, and nomifensine. Cocaine and amphetamine are roughly equipotent as NE and DA uptake blockers; however, the other compounds mentioned exhibit (to varying degrees) greater potency at the NE than at the

Cocaine

Amphetamine

Methylphenidate

Mazindol

Nomifensine

DA transporter (Richelson and Pfenning, 1984). Furthermore, cocaine and mazindol show the least selectivity within this group because both drugs are also effective 5-HT uptake inhibitors (Heikkila, Cabbat, and Mytilineou, 1977; Richelson and Pfenning, 1984).

As a group, the tricyclic antidepressant drugs inhibit NE, but not DA, uptake (see Chapter 19). Among the tricyclics, imipramine and amitriptyline inhibit 5-HT as well as NE uptake, whereas desipramine, protriptyline, and nortriptyline show relatively good selectivity for NE (Richelson and Pfenning, 1984). The novel nontricyclic antidepressant nisoxetine is also a selective NE uptake inhibitor. Indeed, [^{3}H]nisoxetine is a good ligand for membrane binding and autoradiographic studies of the NE transporter (Tejani-Butt, 1992).

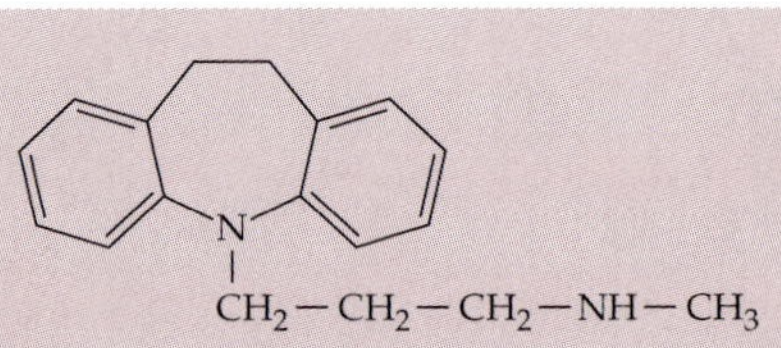

Desipramine

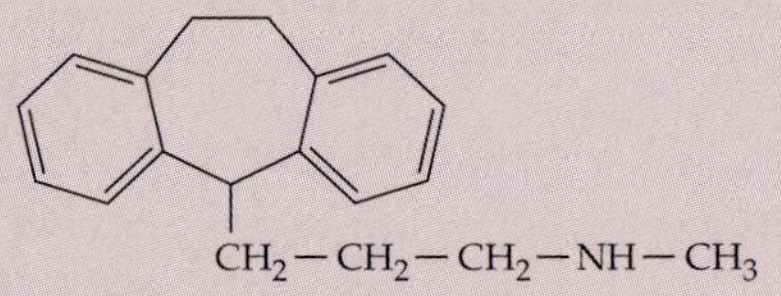

Protriptyline

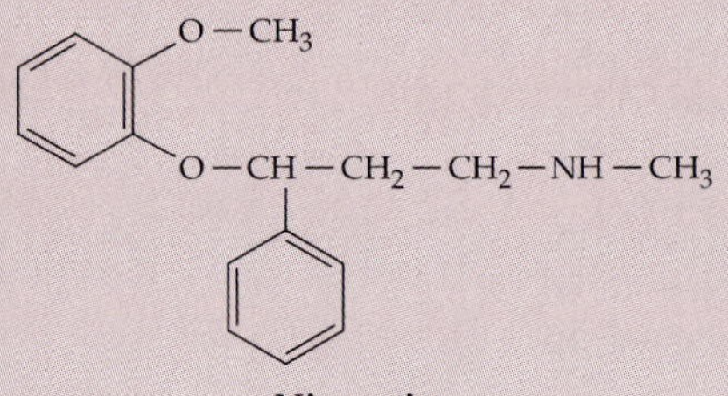

Nisoxetine

Some relatively selective DA uptake inhibitors are benztropine and a family of piperazine compounds that includes GBR 12909, GBR 12935, and GBR 12783 (Andersen, 1989; Van der Zee et al., 1980). [^{3}H]GBR 12935 has proved useful in studying the binding characteristics and localization of the DA transporter (Richfield, 1991).

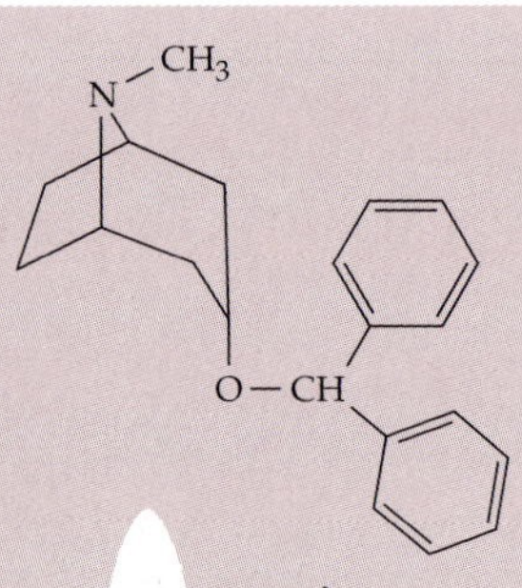

Benztropine

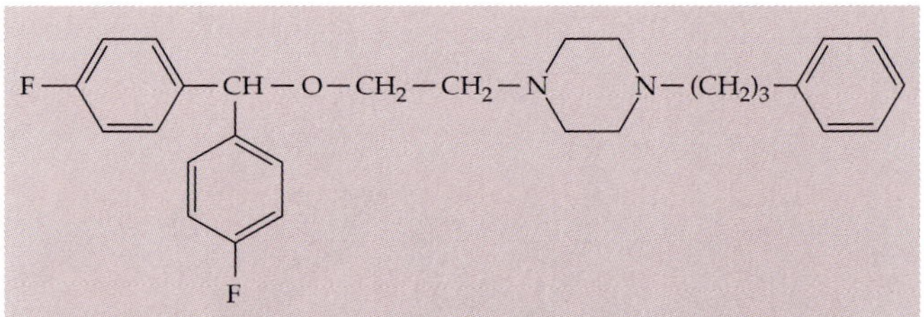

GBR 12909

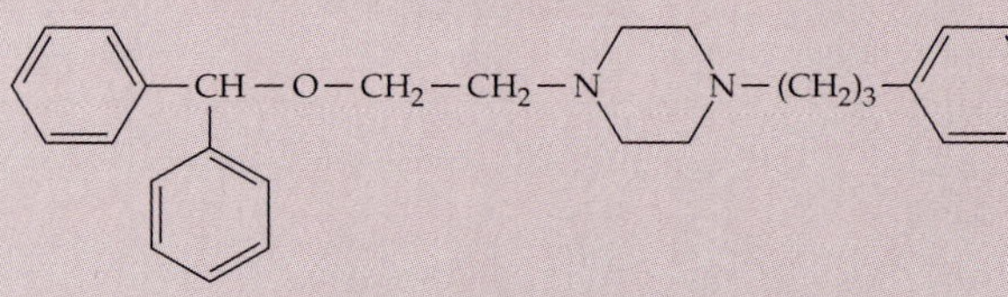

GBR 12935

Because reuptake plays an important role in clearing catecholamines from the extracellular fluid, drugs that inhibit reuptake cause increased extracellular catecholamine levels and enhance the various functions mediated by these transmitters. Dopamine and NE uptake inhibitors thus have powerful psychological and physiological effects, some of which are covered in later chapters that discuss the actions of cocaine (Chapter 13) and antidepressant drugs (Chapter 19).

Catabolism of Catecholamines

Although uptake is an effective method of terminating the synaptic actions of catecholamines, degradative processes must also exist to prevent excessive catecholamine accumulation. The catabolism of catecholamines primarily involves two enzymes, catechol-*O*-methyltransferase (COMT) and monoamine oxidase (MAO). We will describe the characteristics of these enzymes and then summarize the overall pathways of DA and NE breakdown. Finally, we will consider the significance of metabolite measurements for assessing the activity of dopaminergic and noradrenergic systems.

COMT.   COMT is a Mg^{2+}-dependent enzyme that catalyzes the transfer of a methyl group from *S*-adenosylmethionine (SAM) to the 3-position hydroxyl group of many catecholic compounds (Figure 8.15; see Kopin, 1985, for review). COMT is found not only in the brain but also in a variety of other tissues including liver, kidney, and heart. The enzyme exists in both a soluble and a membrane-bound form. The soluble form of COMT predominates in the brain and in virtually all other organs, although the membrane-bound form has a much higher affinity for catecholamines and hence would be active at considerably lower transmitter concentrations (Rivett, Francis, and Roth, 1983b). Immunohistochemical studies have found brain COMT only in nonneuronal cells such as glia, the ependymal cells forming the walls of the cerebral ventricles, and the cerebrospinal fluid–secreting cells of the choroid plexus (Kaplan, Hartman, and Crev-

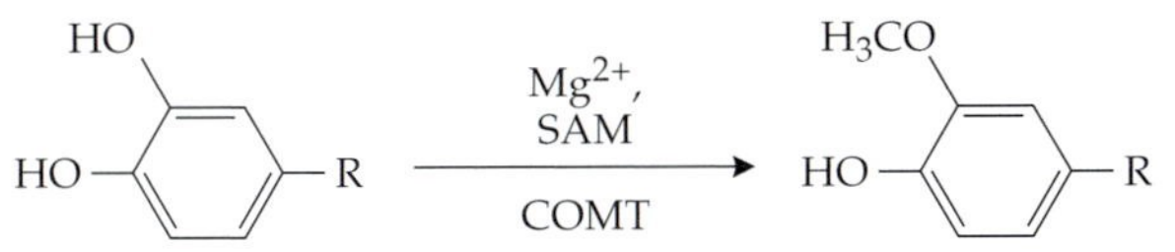

8.15 THE BIOCHEMICAL REACTION CATALYZED BY COMT.

Entacapone

eling, 1979). On the other hand, Rivett, Francis, and Roth (1983a) observed that destruction of rat striatal neurons by local injection of the neurotoxin kainic acid caused a large increase in the activity of soluble COMT (presumably due to lesion-induced gliosis), but a *decrease* in the activity of membrane-bound COMT. Hence, it is possible that the immunohistochemical approach detected only the glial-associated soluble form of the enzyme and not the sparser membrane-bound enzyme, which might be at least partially associated with neurons.

Certain catechol compounds inhibit COMT activity, but these drugs have not found widespread use either experimentally or therapeutically because *O*-methylation is a relatively minor factor in catecholamine dynamics. Tropolone and pyrogallol are considered the classic COMT inhibitors. These drugs, however, have

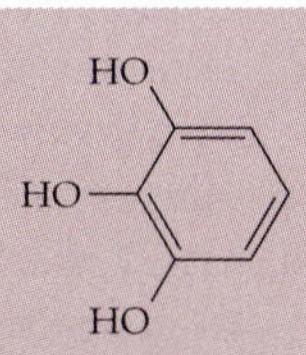

Pyrogallol

largely been supplanted by newer nitrocatechol derivatives such as Ro 41,0960 (2'-fluoro-3,4-dihydroxy-5-nitrobenzophenone), OR-462 (3-(3,4-dihydroxy-5-benzylidine)-2,4-pentanedione), and entacapone. OR-462 and entacapone have been characterized as peripherally acting COMT inhibitors (Nissinen et al., 1988; Törnwall et al., 1994), whereas Ro 41,0960 is also effective in blocking brain COMT (Männistö et al., 1988). In rats, these compounds increased the bioavailability and behavioral

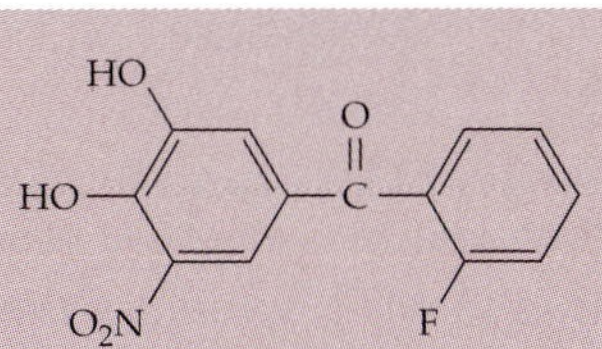

Ro 41,0960

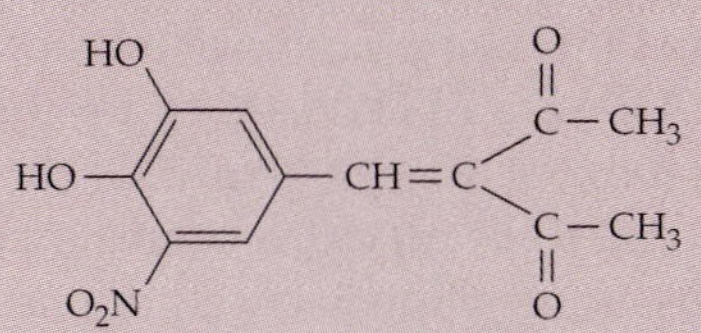

OR-462

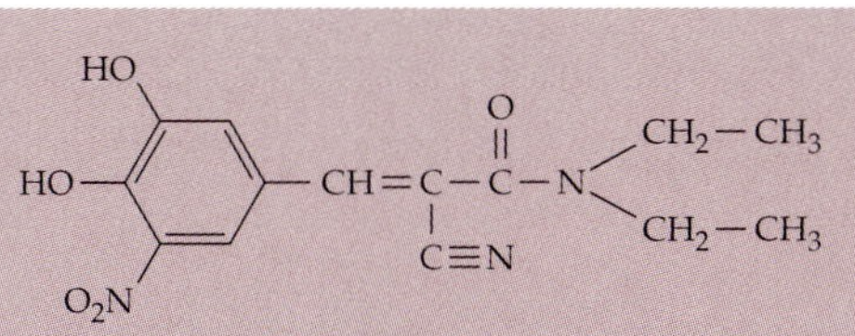

effects of systemically administered L-DOPA by blocking its metabolism to 3-*O*-methyl DOPA. Such results suggest that treatment with a COMT inhibitor might potentiate the therapeutic efficacy of L-DOPA in Parkinson's disease, an idea that has been supported in preliminary clinical trials with entacapone and another nitrocatechol compound called tolcapone (Männistö, 1994; see Chapter 20).

MAO. MAO catalyzes the oxidative deamination of a variety of monoamines using flavin adenine dinucleotide (FAD) as a cofactor (Kopin, 1985). The overall reaction, which is shown in Figure 8.16, additionally requires water and molecular oxygen. The reaction products include an aldehyde formed from the original primary amine as well as ammonia and hydrogen peroxide.

MAO is found throughout the body, with the highest levels in the liver and kidney. In the brain, MAO activity is present in both neurons and glial cells. The enzyme is located on the outer membranes of mitochondria, which (given the large numbers of mitochondria usually present in nerve endings) makes it well situated to catabolize catecholamine molecules in the nerve terminal cytoplasm.

Two forms of MAO have been identified, MAO-A and MAO-B (reviewed by Berry, Juorio, and Paterson, 1994a). The distinction between these forms was originally based on differences in inhibitor sensitivity and in substrate specificity. The compounds clorgyline and deprenyl are selective inhibitors of MAO-A and MAO-B, respectively. With respect to substrate specificity, 5-HT, NE, and EPI are preferentially deaminated by MAO-A in vitro, β-phenylethylamine and benzylamine are preferred substrates for MAO-B, and DA does not distinguish much between the two forms. Later work confirmed that MAO-A activity and MAO-B activity are due to two separate enzymes, each encoded by its own gene (Bach et al., 1988).

Histochemical studies have indicated that MAO-A is the predominant form of the enzyme in the noradrenergic neurons of the locus coeruleus (Berry, Juorio, and Paterson, 1994a). Other experiments using selective inhibitors of MAO-A or MAO-B have demonstrated that deamination of DA and NE in rats is carried out primarily by MAO-A (Butcher et al., 1990; Fagervall and Ross, 1986). On the other hand, the relative importance of these two isozymes in human catecholamine metabolism has not been clarified.

$$R-CH_2-NH_2 + O_2 + H_2O \xrightarrow[\text{MAO}]{\text{FAD}} R-CH=O + NH_3 + H_2O_2$$

8.16 THE BIOCHEMICAL REACTION CATALYZED BY MAO.

MAO inhibitors.   The discovery of the MAO inhibitors (MAOIs) is described in Chapter 19, although we will discuss some of their properties here. The early MAOIs included iproniazid (Marsilid), isocarboxazid (Marplan), phenelzine (Nardil), tranylcypromine (Parnate), and pargyline. With the exception of pargyline (which has some selectivity for MAO-B at low doses), these compounds are all nonselective with respect to MAO isoforms. Moreover, they are all "suicide substrates" of MAO,

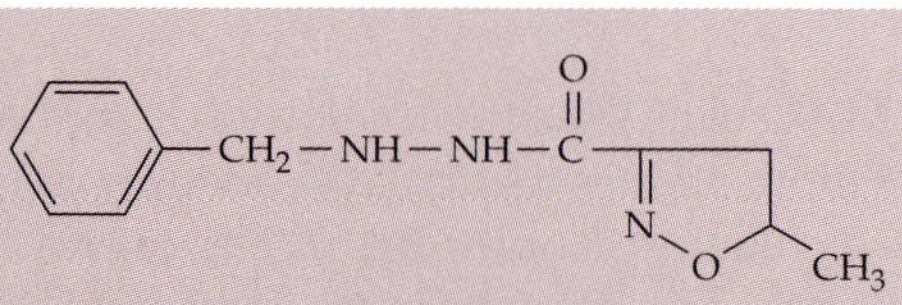

Isocarboxazid

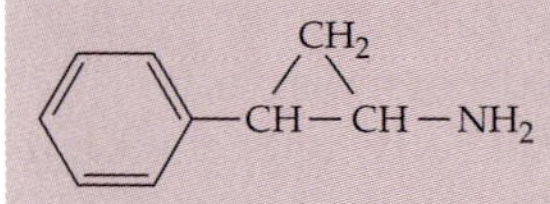

Tranylcypromine

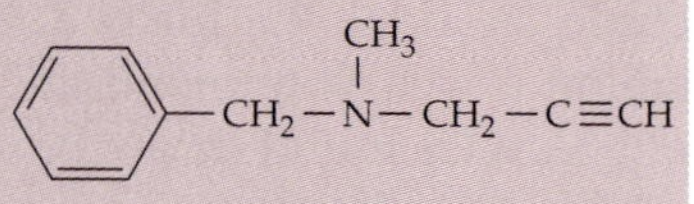

Pargyline

being converted to products that bind irreversibly to the enzyme. Hence, the inhibitory effect of a single dose is long-lasting, and the restoration of enzyme activity depends upon synthesis of new MAO molecules. In animal studies, MAOIs have been found to increase brain levels of biogenic amines, decrease brain and urine levels of deaminated metabolites, and increase brain and urine levels of O-methylated metabolites (see below). These drugs also cause behavioral excitement when given in conjunction with a monoamine precursor (e.g., L-DOPA) or with reserpine.

Later developments in MAO pharmacology have included the discovery of the selective, but still irreversible, inhibitors mentioned above, clorgyline and deprenyl. Even more important for antidepressant use has been the development of reversible MAO-A–selective inhibitors

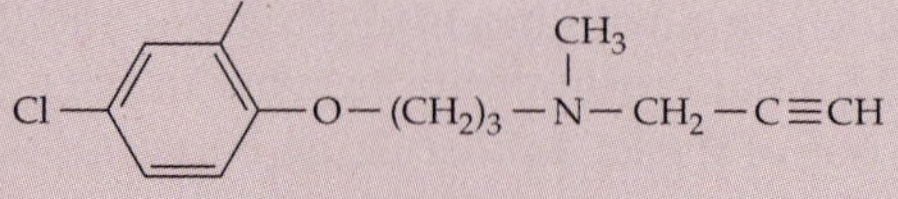

Clorgyline

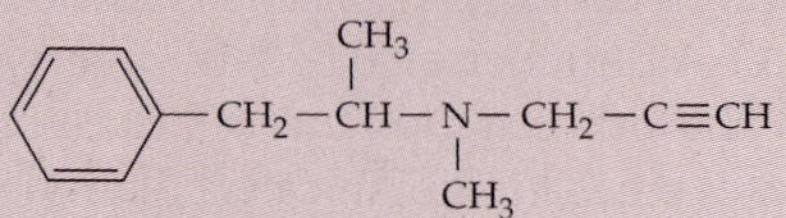

Deprenyl

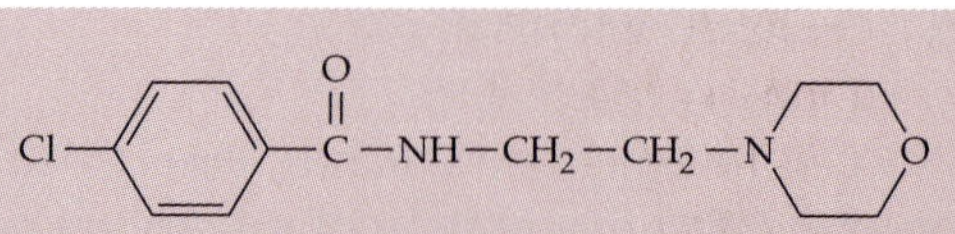

Moclobemide

such as moclobemide (Aurorix) (Pinder and Wieringa, 1993). Compared with the older irreversible MAO inhibitors, these compounds are significantly less likely to produce the diet-related hypertensive crisis known as the "tyramine–cheese reaction" (see Chapter 19).

Pathways of dopamine catabolism.   The major pathways of DA catabolism are shown in Figure 8.17. It can be seen that two alternative pathways are available, depending on whether the first step is catalyzed by MAO or COMT. Westerink (1985) has estimated that in the rat corpus striatum, about 90% of DA catabolism begins with oxidative deamination by MAO. The immediate product of this reaction, 3,4-dihydroxyphenylacetaldehyde (DHPA), is rapidly oxidized to 3,4-dihydroxyphenylacetic acid (DOPAC) by the nonspecific enzyme aldehyde dehydrogenase. About 40% of this DOPAC is eventually eliminated from the brain without being further metabolized by COMT. However, the other 60% is O-methylated to yield homovanillic acid (HVA). Both DOPAC and HVA enter the cerebrospinal fluid (CSF), from which they are actively transported out of the brain into the bloodstream for eventual excretion. This transport system, which operates on a variety of organic acids, can be blocked by the drug probenecid. The alternative path-

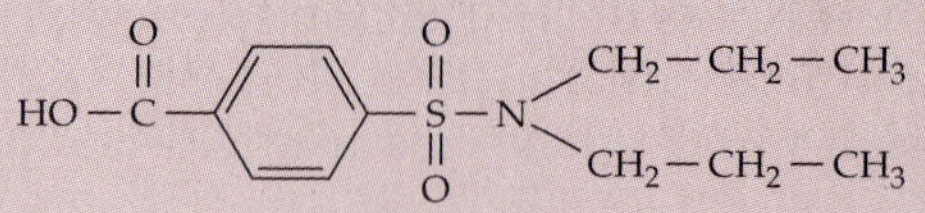

Probenecid

way that begins with COMT (and that constitutes about 10% of total DA catabolism) gives rise initially to 3-methoxytyramine (3-MT), which is then converted to HVA by MAO and aldehyde dehydrogenase. Tissue levels of 3-MT are normally quite low, suggesting that deamination of this compound occurs rapidly.

In rats, DOPAC and HVA are by far the most significant DA metabolites quantitatively. Of these, DOPAC is often considered to be an index of intraneuronal DA catabolism. This assumption is based in part on the observation that reserpine, which presumably stimulates intraneuronal catecholamine breakdown due to its blockade of vesicular storage, causes an initial surge in

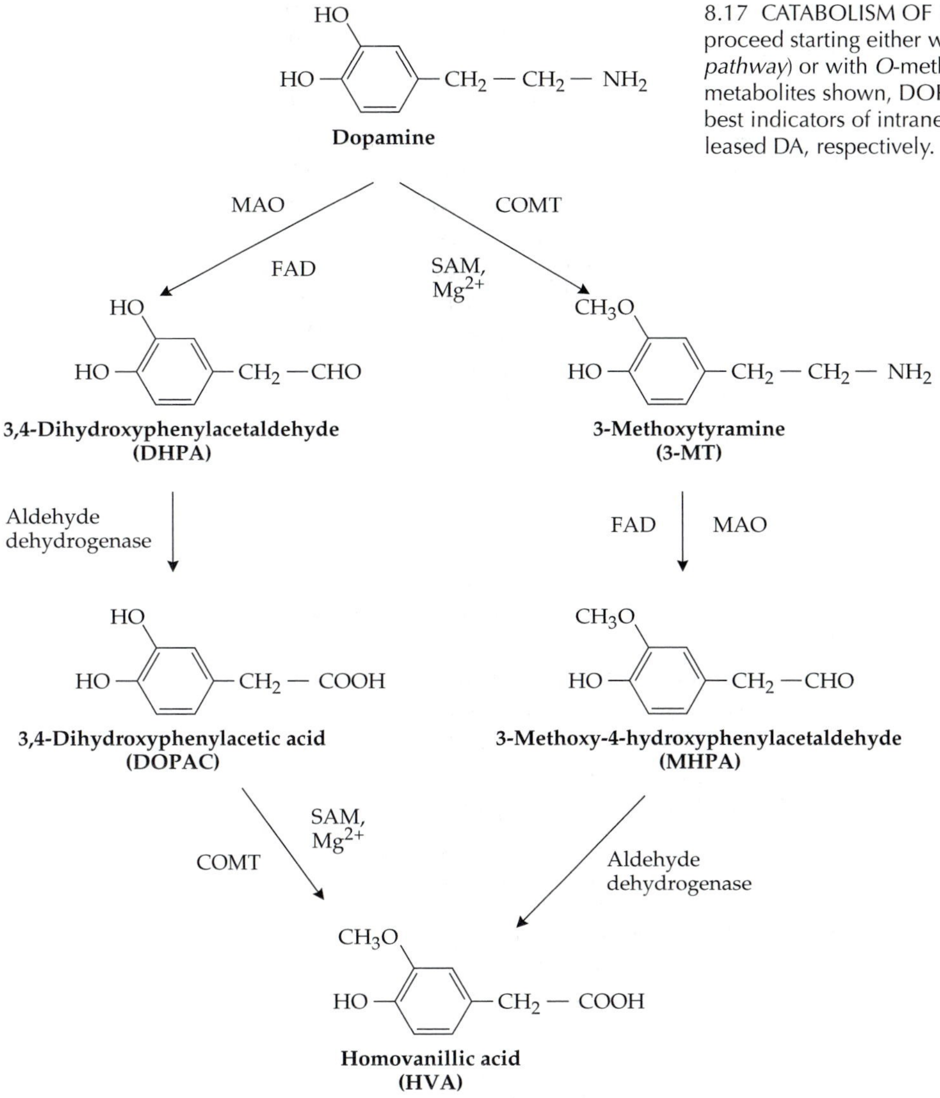

8.17 CATABOLISM OF DOPAMINE. Dopamine catabolism can proceed starting either with oxidative deamination by MAO (*left pathway*) or with *O*-methylation by COMT (*right pathway*). Of the metabolites shown, DOPAC and 3-MT are often considered the best indicators of intraneuronal catabolism and catabolism of released DA, respectively.

striatal DOPAC levels (Westerink, 1985). HVA is also transiently elevated by reserpine, which is not surprising in view of the fact that most HVA is generated from DOPAC. In contrast to these results, reserpine produces a striking *decrease* in striatal 3-MT, which is consistent with the idea that COMT (and hence 3-MT formation) is mainly located extraneuronally. Of course, DA must first be released from the nerve terminals in order to gain access to these extraneuronal sites. Consequently, several investigators have suggested that of the metabolites mentioned above, 3-MT is the best indicator of DA release despite its low steady-state concentration compared with DOPAC or HVA (Brown et al., 1991; Wood and Altar, 1988).

It should also be noted that in rats, a large proportion of DOPAC and HVA is conjugated with sulfate by the enzyme phenolsulfotransferase (Kopin, 1985). DOPAC sulfate and HVA sulfate are found in substantial concentrations in the brain, CSF, and urine, and they must be accounted for if one wishes to measure total

DOPAC and HVA production. On the other hand, sulfation of DOPAC and HVA represents only a minor metabolic pathway in dogs and primates (including humans).

Pathways of norepinephrine catabolism. The principal pathways of NE catabolism are shown in Figure 8.18. Its similarity to DA breakdown is apparent in that degradation may begin either with deamination or *O*-methylation. One important difference between NE and DA catabolism, however, is that in the case of NE, the aldehyde intermediates that are produced by MAO (3,4-dihydroxyphenylglycoaldehyde and 3-methoxy-4-hydroxyphenylglycoaldehyde, abbreviated DHPGA and MHPGA, respectively) can either be oxidized to acids (which parallels the situation for DA) or reduced to glycols. Aldehyde reduction is catalyzed by the enzyme aldehyde reductase.

Patterns of NE metabolites differ among animal species as well as with the tissue or fluid compartment being examined. Conjugated DHPG and MHPG are both

8.18 CATABOLISM OF NOREPINEPHRINE. Like DA, NE catabolism follows multiple pathways depending on whether the process begins with deamination (*left pathway*), or *O*-methylation (*right pathway*). In addition, however, the aldehyde products of MAO (DHPGA and MHPGA) may either be reduced to DHPG and MHPG or oxidized to DHMA and VMA.

found in various areas of the rat brain (Elsworth, Roth, and Redmond, 1983). Following probenecid administration to block efflux of these compounds from the brain, conjugated DHPG accumulated at a faster rate than conjugated MHPG, suggesting that DHPG levels may provide the best measure of central NE metabolism in rats (Li, Warsh, and Godse, 1983). On the other hand, much of the DHPG must later be *O*-methylated, because conjugated MHPG is the main urinary NE metabolite found in this species (Kopin, 1985). The pattern of NE metabolites found in humans likewise differs among CSF, plasma, and urine. In CSF, one finds a high concentration of MHPG (most of which is unconjugated), modest amounts of DHPG and 3,4-dihydroxymandelic acid (DHMA), and a low level of vanillylmandelic acid (VMA) (Elsworth, Roth, and Redmond, 1983; Kopin, 1985). The

major urinary NE metabolite, however, is VMA. Also present in urine are significant levels of conjugated MHPG, and lesser amounts of normetanephrine (NMN), DHPG, and DHMA. Finally, plasma shows a pattern of metabolites intermediate between that of CSF and that of the urine.

Because MHPG is the principal NE metabolite found in human CSF, whereas large amounts of VMA are found in the urine, it was formerly thought that the levels of these two compounds provided good estimates of brain and peripheral NE metabolism, respectively (see Demet and Halaris, 1979). However, considerable quantities of MHPG are generated in the peripheral nervous system (Izzo, Horwitz, and Keiser, 1979), and there is also evidence for significant conversion of plasma MHPG to VMA prior to excretion (Blombery et al., 1980;

Mårdh, Sjöquist, and Änggård, 1981). Hence, it is an oversimplification to associate plasma or urinary MHPG with brain NE metabolism and VMA with peripheral degradation.

Measurement of Catecholamine Turnover

Even though stimulation of a neuronal pathway can increase the neurotransmitter synthesis rate within that pathway, tissue concentrations of the neurotransmitter may show little change if the rate of transmitter catabolism increases to a similar degree. Hence, measures of neurotransmitter concentration are often of little utility in determining whether a particular pharmacological or environmental manipulation has influenced the activity of that transmitter system. A better approach is to obtain some index of the rate of usage of the neurotransmitter, which is usually called **turnover**. Depending on what is being measured, "turnover" may refer to the rate of transmitter synthesis, catabolism, or sometimes release. In the remainder of this section, we will summarize some of the major approaches developed to study turnover in catecholamine systems.

Turnover studies in experimental animals such as rats typically involve direct brain measurements of one or more variables (for review, see Sharman, 1981). One of the simplest approaches is to determine the whole-brain or (preferably) regional concentration of HVA or DOPAC in the case of DA, or DHPG or MHPG in the case of NE. If transmitter concentrations are also measured, it is possible to calculate metabolite/transmitter ratios such as HVA/DA or DHPG/NE. Changes in metabolite concentrations or, in the second case, metabolite/transmitter ratios are thought to reflect altered turnover. Alternatively, appropriate drugs may be used to isolate a particular step in the catecholamine biosynthetic or degradative pathway, thus providing an estimate of the rate of flux through that step. Examples of this general approach include (1) inhibiting TH with AMPT and then determining the rate of DA or NE degradation by examining the subsequent decline in transmitter concentration over time (Javoy and Glowinski, 1971; Widerlöv and Lewander, 1978), (2) inhibiting AADC with NSD 1015 or another suitable compound and then determining the rate of tyrosine hydroxylation by measuring DOPA accumulation (Broadhurst and Briley, 1988; Carlsson et al., 1972), and (3) blocking efflux of the sulfate conjugates of DOPAC, HVA, DHPG, and MHPG with probenecid and measuring their accumulation within the brain (Elchisak, Maas, and Roth, 1977; Meek and Neff, 1973). Finally, isotopic methods can be used in which [³H]tyrosine is administered and the rate of formation of [³H]DA or [³H]NE is determined (Costa, Groppetti, and Naimzada, 1972).

Although each of these approaches has advantages and disadvantages, most investigators currently use either assessment of metabolite levels or ratios, catecholamine disappearance rate following TH inhibition,

or DOPA accumulation rate following AADC inhibition. Measurement of catecholamine metabolites is easily accomplished and does not involve any interference with the system dynamics. On the other hand, metabolite concentration data must be interpreted cautiously because the presence of intraneuronal catabolism (mainly by MAO) raises questions about the relationship between metabolite formation and catecholamine release or utilization (Commissiong, 1985). The two remaining approaches can be criticized because their validity rests in part on the assumption that catecholamine degradation or synthesis will not be affected by disruption of the normal biochemical pathways. Nevertheless, the DOPA accumulation method has become particularly attractive because it can be combined with microdialysis to assess in vivo rates of tyrosine hydroxylation in freely moving subjects (Westerink and De Vries, 1991).

In humans, studies of catecholamine turnover have relied mainly on the measurement of metabolite concentrations in plasma, urine, or in some cases CSF (e.g., within psychiatric populations). Plasma and urinary metabolite levels, particularly those of NE, are difficult to interpret with respect to the relative contributions of central versus peripheral metabolism. This may not always be a serious problem in that animal studies have found evidence for parallel activation of central and peripheral noradrenergic neurons under at least some conditions (Elam et al., 1984). CSF measurements have generally been considered more straightforward, under the assumption that CSF catecholamine metabolites are derived entirely from the brain and therefore accurately reflect central catecholamine turnover. However, this assumption may not be completely true for MHPG due to exchange between the CSF and plasma compartments (Kopin, 1985). Readers interested in obtaining a current perspective on the usefulness of CSF monoamine metabolite concentrations are referred to an excellent commentary by Potter and Manji (1993).

Catecholamine Neurotoxins

Neuropsychopharmacology, like other branches of neuroscience research, depends heavily on information gleaned from lesion studies. Early researchers had to rely entirely on physical lesioning techniques involving the application of electric current, heat, cold, suction, or knife cuts to specific parts of the brain. These relatively crude techniques destroy all cells alike regardless of their basic phenotype (neurons vs. glia) or, in the case of neurons, neurotransmitter expression. Imagine, then, the value of obtaining a chemical toxin that selectively damages neurons expressing a particular neurotransmitter or family of transmitters. Such was the case when Thoenen and Tranzer (1968) and Ungerstedt (1968) first reported the toxic effects of 6-hydroxydopamine (6-OHDA) on sympathetic neurons and central catecholaminergic neurons respectively. 6-Hydroxydopamine is a DA analog that is taken up by DA and NE neurons via the plasma membrane transporters. When high doses are given systemically to adult animals, the terminals, but not the cell bod-

6-Hydroxydopamine (6-OHDA)

ies, of the noradrenergic sympathetic neurons rapidly degenerate (Thoenen and Tranzer, 1968). The damage is not permanent, however, and the terminals eventually regenerate. In contrast, 6-OHDA administration to neonates causes a long-lasting and virtually complete loss of sympathetic cell bodies as well as fibers (Angeletti, 1971). Thus, 6-OHDA can be used to produce either a temporary or a permanent "chemical sympathectomy," depending on when the drug is administered.

6-Hydroxydopamine does not readily cross the blood–brain barrier; hence central catecholamine systems are largely spared by peripheral injections of the neurotoxin. Intracerebroventricular or intracisternal 6-OHDA administration, however, leads to nerve terminal degeneration and profound neurotransmitter depletion in areas innervated by dopaminergic and noradrenergic fibers (Bloom et al., 1969; Ungerstedt, 1968). Unlike the periphery, these areas show little regeneration of the lost nerve endings. When 6-OHDA is administered intracerebroventricularly or intracisternally, relative selectivity for the DA system can be conferred by pretreating subjects with the NE uptake blocker desipramine. However, even greater selectivity and effectiveness are obtained when the neurotoxin is delivered directly into a targeted area. It is even possible to lesion catecholaminergic cell bodies (e.g., the dopaminergic neurons of the substantia nigra) by local injection of 6-OHDA in their vicinity. Regional administration is also preferable because 6-OHDA can produce some damage to serotonergic nerve terminals.

Animals with bilateral 6-OHDA lesions of the nigrostriatal system display a characteristic behavioral syndrome involving adipsia (lack of drinking), aphagia (lack of eating), hypokinesia (reduced movement), decreased exploratory behavior, and a general inability to initiate activity (Ungerstedt, 1971a). The motor deficits closely resemble some of the symptoms observed in Parkinsons's disease, which is not surprising because the nigrostriatal pathway is the primary site of damage in this disorder (see Chapter 20). On the other hand, the motivational changes are reminiscent of those found with lateral hypothalamic lesions. Indeed, typical lateral hypothalamic lesions produce significant damage to the nigrostriatal system, which accounts for the similarity between the two syndromes (Marshall, Richardson, and Teitelbaum, 1974).

The relative specificity of 6-OHDA for catecholaminergic neurons is almost certainly related to its interaction with the DA and NE transporters. However, the mechanism underlying its toxicity is still unresolved despite many years of study. 6-OHDA can undergo auto-oxidation and cyclization to form 5,6-dihydroxyindole, which may mediate the destructive effects of the parent compound. Alternatively, hydrogen peroxide or

5,6-Hydroxyindole

free radicals formed in the auto-oxidation process could play a critical role in 6-OHDA toxicity (reviewed by Kopin, 1987).

A more specific toxin for noradrenergic neurons is the compound N-(2-chloroethyl-)N-ethyl-2-bromobenzylamine (DSP-4) (Jonsson et al., 1981; Ross, 1976). The exact mechanism of DSP-4 action remains unknown; however, it is thought to interact initially with NE uptake sites on the nerve terminals (Dudley, Howard, and Cho, 1990). When administered systemically to rats,

DSP-4

DSP-4 damages both central and peripheral noradrenergic nerve endings, although the peripheral systems recover more quickly and completely (Hallman, Sundström, and Jonsson, 1984; Jaim-Etcheverry and Zieher, 1980). Within the brain, areas innervated by the locus coeruleus (see Part II) show the greatest NE depletion (Jonsson et al., 1981). The neurotransmitter selectivity of DSP-4 is relatively good, although the drug has been reported to produce some minor changes in DA and 5-HT (Hallman, Sundström, and Jonsson, 1984).

Finally, we should mention the most recently discovered catecholamine (particularly DA) neurotoxin, 1-methyl-4-phenyl-1,2,3,6-tetrahydropyridine (MPTP). Because this compound has played an important role in the development of new theories concerning the etiology of Parkinson's disease, it will be covered in detail in Chapter 20.

Part I Summary

The catecholamines are a group of important neurotransmitters and hormones consisting of NE, EPI, and DA. These substances are synthesized in a multistep pathway beginning with the enzyme tyrosine hydroxylase (TH). Other enzymes involved in catecholamine biosynthesis are aromatic L-amino acid decarboxylase (AADC), dopamine β-hydroxylase (DBH), and phenylethanolamine N-methyltransferase (PNMT).

The rate of catecholamine synthesis is regulated by altering the activity of TH, which is the rate-limiting enzyme in the pathway. Tyrosine hydroxylase is subject to end-product inhibition, a process in which catecholamines bind tightly to the enzyme and block the action of the pteridine cofactor. On the other hand, activity in catecholaminergic cells reduces end-product inhibition and also appears to increase the V_{max} of the reaction. These effects may be mediated through TH phosphorylation by several different protein kinases: cAMP-dependent protein kinase A (PKA), Cam-K II, and extracellular signal-regulated protein kinases (ERKs). Furthermore, when catecholaminergic neurons are firing at a high rate, precursor availability may become a rate-limiting factor, and hence transmitter synthesis can be enhanced by providing exogenous tyrosine to the cells.

In addition to the rapid regulatory mechanisms mentioned above, catecholamine synthetic enzymes (particularly TH) also exhibit a longer-term enhancement in response to stressors such as cold exposure, hypoglycemia, and reserpine treatment. This phenomenon, which is called trans-synaptic induction, has been demonstrated in the adrenal medulla, in sympathetic ganglia, and in some catecholaminergic cell groups within the brain. Trans-synaptic induction causes an increase in TH enzyme activity due to increased gene transcription and synthesis of new enzyme protein.

Catecholamines are stored in dense-core vesicles within catecholaminergic neurons and in larger chromaffin granules within the adrenomedullary chromaffin cells. Chromaffin granules also contain many other constituents, including ATP, ascorbic acid, Ca^{2+}, several neuropeptides, DBH, and other proteins called chromogranins. The presence of DBH means that NE synthesis occurs within the interior of the granules. Catecholamines are carried across the chromaffin granule membrane by a specific transporter protein that functions as a proton antiport system. The transporter can be inhibited by reserpine, which causes a rapid depletion of catecholamines by preventing their sequestration from intracellular metabolizing enzymes such as monoamine oxidase.

Catecholamine release occurs through a Ca^{2+}-dependent, exocytotic mechanism. The principal evidence for this comes from studies on chromaffin cells and sympathetic ganglia. Within dopaminergic nerve terminals, the transmitter is thought to exist within several distinct compartments or pools. Dopamine is preferentially released from the newly synthesized pool, which is then replenished from a pool of previously stored transmitter. Certain psychostimulants such as amphetamine and methylphenidate are potent catecholamine releasers.

After catecholamines have been released synaptically, transmitter action is terminated by efflux from the synaptic cleft and by reuptake into the presynaptic nerve terminal. The reuptake process is mediated by specific Na^+-dependent membrane transporters for DA and for NE/EPI. Cocaine, amphetamine, and methylphenidate are among the drugs that inhibit both DA and NE reuptake. Tricyclic antidepressants block the NE, but not the DA, transporter, whereas other compounds have been developed with the opposite selectivity.

Catecholamines are also inactivated metabolically by the actions of MAO and COMT. Two isoforms of MAO (MAO-A and MAO-B) have been identified that differ in their substrate specificity and sensitivity to the inhibitors clorgyline (MAO-A) and deprenyl (MAO-B). However, MAO-A appears to be the most important for catecholamine metabolism in vivo. The major DA metabolites are DOPAC and HVA, although a third compound, 3-MT, may be a better indicator of the amount of DA released. Patterns of NE metabolism are more complicated, as they vary considerably among animal species and with the tissue or fluid compartment being studied. In humans, for example, MHPG is the principal metabolite in CSF, whereas VMA is the major compound found in urine.

Levels of catecholamine metabolites or metabolite/ transmitter ratios are frequently used as indices of catecholamine turnover. However, a number of other methods are available that isolate a particular step in the catecholamine biosynthetic or degradative pathway. One recent approach that has gained some popularity is the use of microdialysis to measure in vivo rates of DOPA accumulation following administration of an AADC inhibitor.

Also useful to neuropharmacologists are toxins that selectively lesion catecholaminergic nerve terminals or cell bodies. The classic general catecholaminergic neurotoxin is 6-OHDA, which can be given systemically to destroy sympathetic nerve endings or introduced directly into the brain to lesion specific terminal areas or cell groups. A different compound, DSP-4, has been found to act as a selective neurotoxin for noradrenergic nerve terminals in the brain. A third, recently discovered neurotoxin, called MPTP, has proved important in the study of Parkinson's disease, and therefore will be discussed in Chapter 20.

Part II
Dopamine Systems: Anatomy, Physiology, and Behavior

Distribution of Dopamine Neurons in the Nervous System

Methods Used to Map Dopaminergic Pathways

By the late 1950s and early 1960s, NE and EPI were well established as humoral agents in the adrenal medulla and sympathetic nervous system, yet their status as central transmitters (as well as that of DA) was just beginning to be acknowledged. This situation changed dramatically with the discovery of a fluorescence histochemical method that enabled researchers to visualize the locations of catecholaminergic (and also serotonergic) cell bodies and fibers throughout the brain. Although the process underlying this method was discovered by Eränkö in 1955, the method was subsequently perfected by Falck, Hillarp, and their collaborators (Falck et al., 1962) and thus came to be known as the Falck-Hillarp fluorescence technique. The technique consisted of treating tissues with formaldehyde vapor to produce catecholamine condensation products called isoquinolines (see Chapter 2 for more information). The specific compound formed from dopamine and formaldehyde vapor condensation is called 3,4-dihydroisoquinoline. When illuminated by ultraviolet light, this

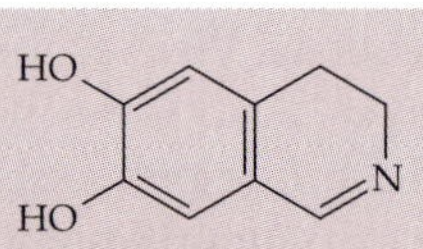

3,4-Dihydroisoquinoline

product emits a bright green fluorescent glow. It is possible under the appropriate conditions to discriminate between the presence of NE, EPI, and DA (Eränkö, 1976). A later refinement of the technique involved treatment of the tissue with glyoxylic acid rather than formaldehyde, which provided a more intense fluorophore and thus increased sensitivity (Lindvall and Björklund, 1974b). The histochemical fluorescence method provided basic information on the localization of catecholamine cell bodies and nerve terminals in the brain (Dahlström and Fuxe, 1964; Fuxe, 1965), and this approach was subsequently combined with other techniques to permit the first mapping of DA and NE pathways (Ungerstedt, 1971c). The procedures involved in applying the formaldehyde and glyoxylic acid methods are reviewed in Fuxe and Jonsson (1973) and Lindvall and Björklund (1974a) respectively.

Although histochemical fluorescence is still occasionally used in catecholamine localization studies, it has been largely supplanted by immunohistochemical staining for catecholamine-synthesizing enzymes and, more recently, the transmitters themselves. Thus, dopaminergic cell bodies and pathways have been mapped using antibodies against TH (even though the enzyme is present in all catecholaminergic cells) (Hökfelt, Johansson, and Goldstein, 1984a) or against DA (Decavel et al., 1987; Geffard et al., 1984). Other localization methods that deserve mention include light or electron microscopic autoradiography following exposure of tissues to [³H]DA (Descarries et al., 1980), and electron microscopic visualization of 5-hydroxydopamine, a false transmitter taken up by DA nerve endings (Arluison, Agid, and Javoy, 1978).

Anatomy of Central Dopaminergic Systems

In their classic mapping studies of central monoaminergic cell groups, Dahlström and Fuxe (1964) designated the various dopaminergic and noradrenergic cell groups with the letter A, the serotonergic cell groups with the letter B (see Chapter 9), and the adrenergic cell groups with the letter C. According to current nomenclature, groups A1–A7 are noradrenergic, A8–A15 are dopaminergic, and C1–C3 are adrenergic.

Dopamine is estimated to constitute as much as 80% of the total brain catecholamine content. However, the total number of DA cells is rather small: no more than a million cells in the entire human brain, as compared with 10 billion cells in the cortex alone. Dopamine-containing nerve cells are found in relatively rostral parts of the brain (i.e., the midbrain, hypothalamus, and olfactory bulbs) compared with adrenergic and noradrenergic cells. The locations of these cells and their ascending and descending projections are presented in Figure 8.19 and summarized in Table 8.2. In the figure and in the discussion that follows, we will distinguish between several different forebrain projections from the mesencephalic (midbrain) DA cell groups. However, it should be noted that some investigators have argued in favor of a collective mesotelencephalic DA system based on the substantial degree of overlap observed among the mesencephalic cell groups as well as their projection fields (Roth, Wolf, and Deutch, 1987).

The mesostriatal system. The mesostriatal system originates from cells in the substantia nigra (SN), particularly the pars compacta of the SN (A9), the ventral tegmental area (VTA; A10), and the A8 group located caudal to A9 and partly in the retrorubral nucleus. The dorsal component of this system, which is sometimes called the nigrostriatal pathway, ascends via the medial forebrain bundle and then the internal capsule to innervate the caudate nucleus, the putamen (the caudate and putamen are fused in rodents, but not in primates), and the globus pallidus* (Figure 8.19a) (Fuxe et al., 1985). In rats, there are an estimated 10,000 DA cell bodies in the A9 cell group on one side of the brain (German and Manaye, 1993); however, a single axon from one of these cells may branch so many times that it ultimately gives rise to thousands of synaptic boutons in the striatum (Andén et al., 1966). Many of these synaptic connections are made with the medium-sized, spiny (i.e., possessing dendritic spines) neurons that give rise to the output pathways of the striatum (Freund, Powell, and Smith, 1984). Researchers have also known for many years that DA in-

---

*The caudate and putamen together comprise the neostriatum, which is often shortened simply to "striatum." The neostriatum plus the globus pallidus make up the corpus striatum (striated body). The striated appearance of this structure is due to the presence of ascending and descending fibers of the internal capsule.

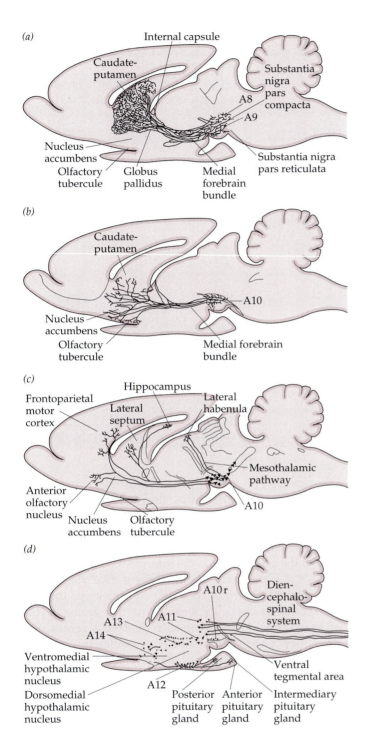

(a)

Internal capsule

Caudate-putamen

Substantia nigra pars compacta

A8

A9

Nucleus accumbens

Olfactory tubercule

Globus pallidus

Medial forebrain bundle

Substantia nigra pars reticulata

(b)

Caudate-putamen

A10

Nucleus accumbens

Olfactory tubercule

Medial forebrain bundle

(c)

Hippocampus

Frontoparietal motor cortex

Lateral septum

Lateral habenula

Mesothalamic pathway

A10

Anterior olfactory nucleus

Nucleus accumbens

Olfactory tubercule

(d)

A10r

Dien-cephalo-spinal system

A13

A11

A14

Ventromedial hypothalamic nucleus

A12

Ventral tegmental area

Dorsomedial hypothalamic nucleus

Posterior pituitary gland

Anterior pituitary gland

Intermediary pituitary gland

8.19 DOPAMINERGIC PATHWAYS IN THE RAT BRAIN. Dopaminergic cell bodies are represented by triangles and axonal fibers by solid lines. (*a*) Dorsal mesostriatal (nigrostriatal) system. (*b*) Ventral mesostriatal (mesolimbic) system. (*c*) Mesolimbocortical and mesodiencephalic (mesothalamic) systems. (*d*) Periventricular, diencephalospinal, incertohypothalamic, and tuberohypophyseal systems. Groups A8–A15 represent dopaminergic cell groups. (After Fuxe et al., 1985.)

An interesting feature of the nigrostriatal system is its relationship to the striatal "patch" and "matrix" compartments. These terms refer to a neurochemical differentiation of the striatum in which there are patches containing a high density of µ-opiate receptors (see Chapter 12) but low levels of acetylcholinesterase, embedded in a matrix characterized by low µ-receptor binding, higher amounts of acetylcholinesterase, and the presence of neurons containing a 28-kDa Ca^{2+}-binding protein called calbindin (reviewed by Gerfen, 1992). The patch and matrix compartments have somewhat different afferent and efferent connections. Thus, DA neurons projecting to the patch compartment are located in the ventral part of the SN pars compacta and the SN pars reticulata, whereas the dopaminergic innervation of the matrix arises mainly from the dorsal SN pars compacta, the VTA, and the A8 cell group.

The mesostriatal system also possesses a ventral component that innervates the nucleus accumbens, olfactory tubercles, and medial caudate–putamen (Figure 8.19*b*; Fuxe et al., 1985). Some authors include this pathway as part of the mesolimbic DA system, which is discussed in the next section. Dopamine projections to the nucleus accumbens are thought to play a critical role in the reinforcing properties of psychostimulants and possibly other drugs of abuse as well (Chapter 13).

The mesolimbocortical system. A second major dopaminergic system, termed the mesolimbocortical system, originates primarily in A10, with smaller contributions from A9 and A8. This system projects to the septum, amygdala, hippocampus, nucleus of the diagonal band, anterior olfactory nucleus, and limbic cortical areas (Figure 8.19*c*; Fuxe et al., 1985). As mentioned above, the nucleus accumbens and olfactory tubercles are sometimes placed within this grouping. Details of the cortical DA projections in rats and primates are summarized in Berger, Gaspar, and Verney (1991). As discussed in Chapter 18, the mesolimbocortical DA system is the system hypothesized to be hyperactive in the classic DA theory of schizophrenia.

The mesodiencephalic and mesopontine systems. Two other DA systems also originate in the midbrain. One is the mesodiencephalic (sometimes also called the mesothalamic) system, which projects to the subthalamic nu-

hibits large, aspiny cholinergic interneurons in the striatum; however, it is still not clear whether this inhibition is mediated by standard axodendritic or axosomatic synapses or by axoaxonic contacts (Stoof et al., 1992). The nigrostriatal pathway is vitally important in motor control, and degeneration of this system is the key feature of Parkinson's disease. The motor functions of the nigrostriatal pathway and its relationship to Parkinson's's disease are discussed in Chapter 20.

Table 8.2   Central Dopamine-Containing Neuronal Systems

System	Cells of Origin	Projections
Mesostriatal system	Substantia nigra (A9), ventral tegmental area (A10), retrorubral nucleus (A8)	Nucleus caudatus–putamen, globus pallidus, nucleus accumbens
Mesolimbocortical system (mesocortical system)	Ventral tegmental area, substantia nigra, retrorubral nucleus	Forebrain limbic and cortical areas as indicated in Table 8.3
Mesodiencephalic system	Substantia nigra, ventral tegmental area	Subthalamic nucleus, lateral habenula
Mesopontine system	Substantia nigra, ventral tegmental area	Locus coeruleus
Diencephalospinal system	Dorsal and posterior hypothalamus, zona incerta, caudal thalamus (A11)	Spinal cord
Periventricular system	Mesencephalic periaqueductal gray, periventricular gray of caudal thalamus (A11)	Periaqueductal gray, medial thalamus and hypothalamus
Incertohypothalamic system	Zona incerta, periventricular hypo-thalamus (A11, A13, A14) septum	Zona incerta, anterior, medial preoptic and periventricular hypothalamus,
Tuberohypophyseal system	Arcuate and periventricular hypo-thalamic nuclei (A12, A14)	Median eminence, intermediate and posterior lobes of the pituitary
Periglomerular dopamine neurons	Olfactory bulb (A15)	Dendritic processes into olfactory glomeruli
Retinal dopamine system	Mainly in the inner nuclear layer of the retina	Local dendritic projections

Source: After Lindvall and Björklund, 1983.

cleus and the habenula (Figure 8.19c). The second is the mesopontine system, which connects the A9 and A10 cell groups to the locus coeruleus, a major noradrenergic structure in the pons (not shown in the figure). Table 8.3 summarizes the origins and terminal areas of all of the mesencephalic DA systems.

The periventricular and diencephalospinal systems. Additional DA pathways emanate from A11, which is a cell group rostral to A10 that is located in the periventricular gray of the posterior and dorsal hypothalamus and the caudal thalamus (Figure 8.19d). Local projections of A11 to medial thalamic and hypothalamic nuclei constitute the periventricular DA system. Collateral branches of some of these fibers form the diencephalospinal DA system, which descends via the dorsal longitudinal fasciculus and terminates in the spinal dorsal gray (laminae I–IV) and the intermediolateral cell columns (the location of sympathetic preganglionic neurons). Dual innervation of hypothalamic and sympathetic preganglionic cell groups by A11 dopaminergic neurons may permit integrated control of the central and autonomic components of complex motivated behaviors such as food consumption or sexual behavior.

The incertohypothalamic and tuberohypophyseal systems. The incertohypothalamic system arises mainly in the A13 cell group found in the zona incerta (Figure 8.19d). Fibers

of this system project locally as well as to the anterior and periventricular hypothalamus, the medial preoptic area, and the septum. The tuberohypophyseal system emanates from the A12 group located in the periventricular and arcuate nuclei of the hypothalamus (Figure 8.19d). Some of the cells project to the intermediate and posterior lobes of the pituitary gland. Others give rise to the tuberoinfundibular DA tract, which projects to the median eminence of the hypothalamus. The axons of this pathway do not form synapses in the median eminence; rather, they release DA into the perivascular spaces of the capillary plexus of the hypothalamic–hypophyseal portal system (see Chapter 11). Dopamine taken up by these capillaries is transported to the anterior pituitary gland, where it acts on cells called lactotrophs to inhibit the release of prolactin, a hormone that stimulates milk production in lactating mammals. The tuberoinfundibular neurons help to regulate this process by releasing more DA when serum prolactin levels are high and less DA when the levels are low (Moore and Demarest, 1984).

Olfactory and retinal dopamine neurons. Of the DA cell groups originally identified by Dahlström and Fuxe, the most rostral is the A15 group, located in the olfactory bulbs. This group consists of periglomerular cells that regulate the olfactory glomeruli by means of dendritic interactions (Shepard and Greer, 1990). In various species, DA is also present in retinal amacrine or interplexiform cells, where it exerts numerous effects on retinal functioning (Djamgoz and Wagner, 1992).

Peripheral Dopaminergic Systems

Although NE has long been known as an important transmitter in the peripheral nervous system (see below), the presence of peripheral dopaminergic neurons has been less widely appreciated. Considering various organ systems, the best evidence for a DA innervation comes from the kidney, where the function of DA is to stimulate renal vasodilation and inhibit Na^+ and water reabsorption (Bell, 1989). Dopamine is also synthesized by a population of small, intensely fluorescent (SIF) cells in sympathetic ganglia (Elfvin, Lindh, and Hökfelt, 1993). SIF cells generally serve either as interneurons within the ganglia or as endocrine-like cells. Dopamine released from SIF cells appears to act as a modulator to produce a long-lasting enhancement of the muscarinic slow EPSPs and IPSPs that were described in Chapter 7 (Grace and Bunney, 1985; Libet, 1992).

Fine Structure of Dopamine Synapses: Implications for Dopaminergic Neurotransmission

Dopaminergic (and also noradrenergic) fibers display a characteristic varicose appearance in their terminal arborization (Maley et al., 1990). The varicosities (intermittent swellings along the fiber, much like beads on a string) contain a high density of synaptic vesicles and are believed to be the major sites of transmitter synthesis and release. It is important to consider whether or not DA varicosities show the membrane specializations usually indicative of synaptic contacts. Agnati, Fuxe, and their colleagues (1990) have proposed the existence of two distinct types of chemical communication in the CNS: wiring transmission (WT) and volume transmission (VT). According to this model, WT is a fast, point-to-point transmission of information mediated by traditional synaptic contacts. As we shall see in Chapter 10, the amino acid transmitters glutamic acid and GABA are the workhorses for WT in vertebrate brains. In contrast, VT is a slower, more diffuse mechanism of signaling that operates at a distance from the site of release and hence does not require the presence of classic synaptic specializations.

With respect to DA, the majority of DA-immunoreactive nerve terminals in both cortical and subcortical areas show synaptic specializations (Maley et al., 1990; Parnavelas and Papadopoulos, 1989). Although this finding is consistent with the notion that DA operates via WT, recent evidence suggests that significant efflux may occur from the synaptic cleft following DA release (Garris et al., 1994). This efflux could permit transmitter effects in areas distinct from the sites of release. Such a possibility is supported by the recent findings of Smiley and colleagues (1994), who used antibodies to the DA D_1 receptor along with electron microscopy to determine the ultrastructural localization of this receptor in monkey cerebral cortex.

Table 8.3 Origins of Different Projections from the Mesencephalic Dopamine Neuron Systems

Terminal area	Origin[a]
Globus pallidus	A9
Nucleus accumbens	A10, medial A9, (A8)
Nucleus caudatus–putamen	A9
Ventral part	A8
Anteromedial part	A10 [lateral part]
Olfactory bulb	A10, medial A9
Anterior olfactory nuclei	A10, medial A9
Olfactory tubercle	A10 [lateral part]
Islands of Calleja	A9, (A10)
Lateral septal nucleus	A10 [medial part]
Interstitial nucleus of the stria terminalis	A10
Pyriform cortex	A10, medial A9
Amygdala	A10, medial A9
Ventral entorhinal cortex	A10 [lateral part], (A8)
Hippocampus	A10, A9
Suprarhinal cortex	Dorsolateral A10
Pregenual anteromedial cortex	A10 [medial part]
Supragenual anteromedial cortex	A9
Perirhinal cortex	Lateral A10, A9
Lateral habenular nucleus	Medial A10
Subthalamic nucleus	A9
Locus coeruleus	A10, A9

[a]Brackets denote the predominant location of cells of origin within a nucleus; parentheses denote minor projection.
Source: After Lindvall and Björklund, 1983.

Immunoreactivity was typically observed in dendritic spines receiving asymmetric synapses (asymmetric synapses are those that display a pronounced postsynaptic density); however, the staining was generally *not* in the immediate vicinity of presumptive transmitter release sites. Thus, even when DA is released at a classic synaptic structure, some diffusion may occur before the transmitter reaches its site of action.

Coexistence of Dopamine with Other Transmitters

In rats, many of the mesencephalic DA neurons also contain one or both of the neuropeptides cholecystokinin (CCK) and neurotensin (NT) (Hökfelt et al., 1987). It is likely that these peptides are stored in the large dense-core vesicles, but not the smaller vesicles found in DA nerve terminals. Such differential storage is consistent with the finding that stimulation of the mesocortical pathway at a low frequency selectively released DA, but not NT, in the rat prefrontal cortex (Bean and Roth, 1991). Higher frequencies, on the other hand, did result in significant peptide release. When co-released with DA, CCK and NT have been found to exert complex actions both postsynaptically (Deutch and Zahm, 1992) and presynaptically in terms of reciprocal modulation of the release process (e.g., Bean, During, and Roth, 1990; Marshall et al., 1991). The general features of neuropeptide colocalization with classical transmitters are discussed further in Chapter 11.

Electrophysiology of Dopaminergic Neurons

The electrophysiological properties of midbrain DA neurons have been extensively studied (see Chiodo, 1988). These cells alternate between a state of spontaneous activity and a silent state that is due to temporary hyperpolarization. Moreover, when the cells are active, they may be in either a single-spike or a bursting mode. The single-spike mode consists of a relatively regular firing pattern with an average frequency of 4–6 Hz, whereas the bursting mode consists of clusters of 3 to 10 action potentials each, with a decrease in spike amplitude and an increase in interspike intervals as the burst progresses. These characteristics are illustrated in Figure 8.20. During spontaneous activity in one cell, neighboring cells sometimes fire in synchrony with the driving neuron. This is indicative of electrical coupling between the cells, which is mediated by the existence of intercellular gap junctions. Burst firing may play an important role in DA-mediated synaptic transmission, at least for the midbrain dopaminergic systems. This conclusion stems from evidence that the amount of DA released per spike is much greater for bursts than for single action potentials (Gonon et al., 1991).

Dopamine cell firing can be influenced by several different factors. For example, the compound γ-butyrolactone (GBL) is widely used experimentally to inhibit impulse flow in DA neurons. Dopamine receptor agonists and indirect agonists such as amphetamine also suppress the activity of these cells, whereas firing rate is enhanced by DA antagonists (Chiodo, 1988). The effects

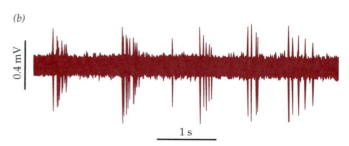

γ-**Butyrolactone**

of dopaminergic drugs are mediated in part by somatodendritic autoreceptors (see below) as well as by the action of a long-loop negative feedback pathway from the striatum to the substantia nigra (SN) (Bunney and Aghajanian, 1978a). A variety of sensory stimuli also inhibit the spontaneous activity of midbrain DA neurons (Chiodo, 1988).

Dopamine Receptors

Modern DA receptor research began in the early 1970s with the discovery of DA-stimulated adenylyl cyclase activity (Kebabian, Petzold, and Greengard, 1972) and

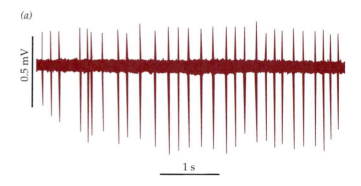

(a)

0.5 mV

1 s

(b)

0.4 mV

1 s

8.20 FIRING PATTERNS OF DOPAMINERGIC NEURONS IN THE RAT SUBSTANTIA NIGRA. Electrophysiological recordings were made from putative dopaminergic cells in the substantia nigra of freely moving rats. (*a*) Single-spike pattern of activity (overall firing rate = 5.6 spikes/s). (*b*) Burst pattern of activity with decreasing spike amplitude within each burst (overall firing rate = 5.8 spikes/s). Not shown are other cells that oscillate between single-spiking and burst firing. (After Freeman, Meltzer, and Bunney, 1985.)

the advent of binding studies using radiolabeled DA or DA antagonists (reviewed by Seeman and Grigoriadis, 1987). Biochemical evidence for two distinct DA receptors was first provided by Garau and coworkers (1978) and Titeler and coworkers (1978), and was followed shortly thereafter by the designation of these subtypes as D_1 and D_2 (Kebabian and Calne, 1979).

Although the DA receptor story underwent some turmoil during the 1980s, D_1 and D_2 continued to be recognized as authentic subtypes. Gradually, however, pharmacological evidence began accumulating that further receptor subtypes probably existed (see Andersen et al., 1990). A major breakthrough occurred with the cloning and characterization of a novel DA receptor that was designated D_3 (Sokoloff et al., 1990). Since then, molecular biology has continued to hold center stage as the DA receptor family has grown to at least six members.

The pharmacology and molecular biology of DA receptors is summarized in a number of recent reviews (Civelli, Bunzow, and Grandy, 1993; De Keyser, 1993; Jackson and Westlind-Danielsson, 1994; O'Dowd, 1993; Seeman and Van Tol, 1994). All of the known DA receptors belong to the G protein–coupled receptor superfamily. Five basic subtypes have been well characterized, designated D_1 through D_5. The sixth member of the family arises from the fact that the D_2 receptor exists in two isoforms (see below). There are important similarities between the D_1 and D_5 subtypes and between the D_2, D_3, and D_4 subtypes; hence the discussion below is organized on the basis of D_1-like and D_2-like receptor subfamilies.

The D_1-Like Receptor Subfamily

D_1 receptors. The D_1 receptor was first distinguished by virtue of its ability to stimulate adenylyl cyclase activity and then later by means of binding studies differentiating it from the D_2 subtype. The gene for the D_1 receptor was cloned independently by three different laboratory groups and was found to encode a protein of 446 amino acids (Dearry et al., 1990; Sunahara et al., 1990; Zhou et al., 1990). As in the case of other G protein–coupled receptors, the structure of the D_1 receptor suggests the presence of seven membrane-spanning domains.

A number of DA agonists have been developed that discriminate between D_1 receptors and members of the D_2 subfamily. Among the most widely used D_1-selective agonists are members of a family of 1-phenyl-tetrahydrobenzazepines, including the prototypical compound SKF 38393 (1-phenyl-2,3,4,5-tetrahydro-7,8-dihydroxy-(1H)-3-benzazepine) along with a variety of congeners such as SKF 81297, SKF 82958, and SKF 82526 (fenoldopam) (Andersen and Jansen, 1990). Dihydrexidine is a recently introduced nonbenzazepine DA agonist that exhibits moderate selectivity between D_1 and D_2 receptors (Brewster et al., 1990). Some of the benzazepine compounds, such as SKF 38393 and SKF 82526, are only partial D_1 agonists, as assessed by the stimulation of D_1-

sensitive adenylyl cyclase (Andersen and Jansen, 1990). This means that the maximal effectiveness of these drugs is less than that of DA itself.

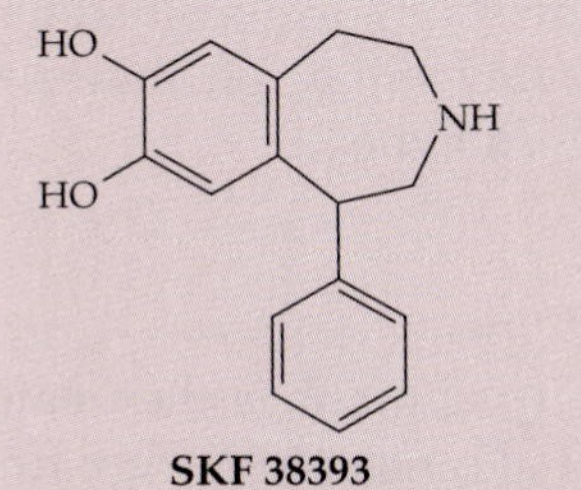

Several substituted benzazepines act as D_1 receptor antagonists rather than agonists. The best-known of these compounds are SCH 23390 (3-methyl-1-phenyl-2,3,4,5-tetrahydro-7-chloro-8-hydroxy-(1H)-3-benzazepine) and its brominated analog SKF 83566 (Hyttel, 1983). More recently introduced D_1 antagonists include the benzazepine derivatives NNC-112 (previously called NO-112) (3-methyl-1-(7-benzofuranyl)-2,3,4,5-tetrahydro-8-chloro-7-hydroxy-(1H)-3-benzazepine) and NNC-756 (NO-756) (Andersen et al., 1992), and the benzonaphthazepine SCH 39166 (Chipkin et al., 1988). The benzazepine-derived D_1 antagonists such as SCH 23390 also have a measurable affinity for 5-HT$_2$ receptors, which should particularly be taken into account in the performance of receptor binding assays (Bischoff et al., 1986).

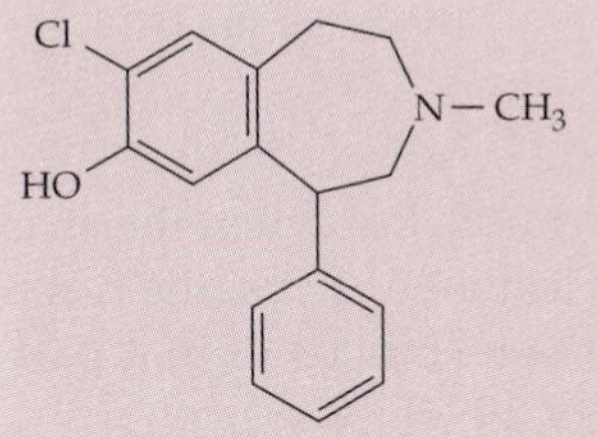

SCH 23390 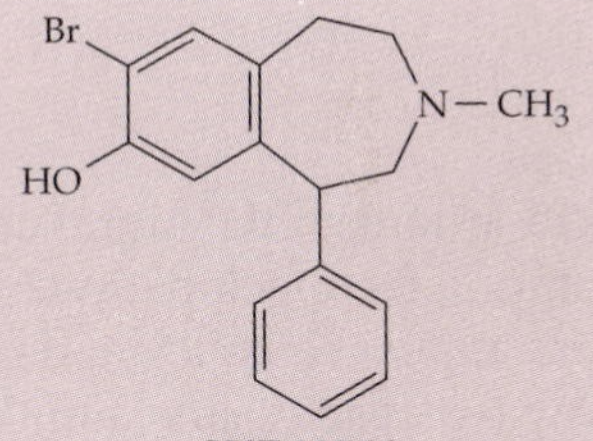   **SKF 83566**

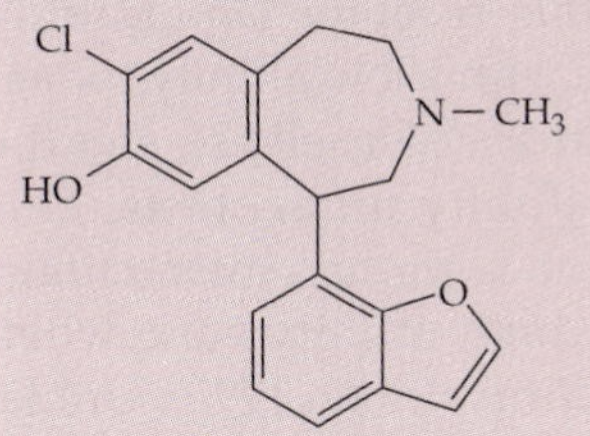

NNC-112 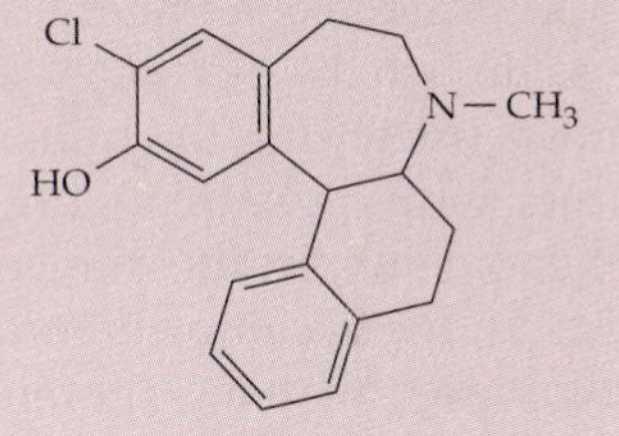   **SCH 39166**

The distribution of D_1 receptors in the rat brain has been mapped by means of in vitro autoradiography using several different agonists and antagonists (Boyson, McGonigle, and Molinoff, 1986; Dawson et al., 1986; Wamsley, Alburges, McQuade et al., 1992). The highest receptor densities were found in the termination areas of the mesostriatal system—namely, the caudate–putamen, nucleus accumbens, and olfactory tubercle—and in the substantia nigra. Intermediate levels of receptor binding occurred in the ventral pallidum, entopeduncular nucleus, and some of the nuclei of the amygdala. Low D_1 receptor levels were found in the neocortex, thalamus, cerebellum, hippocampus, septum, and most areas of the hypothalamus. Comparative studies on several different species, including humans, showed a high concentration of D_1 receptors within the mesostriatal systems of all the species, but some differences in other brain areas (Camps, Kelly, and Palacios, 1990). In rats, D_1 receptor binding in the substantia nigra is not affected by kainic

SKF 38393   **SKF 81297**

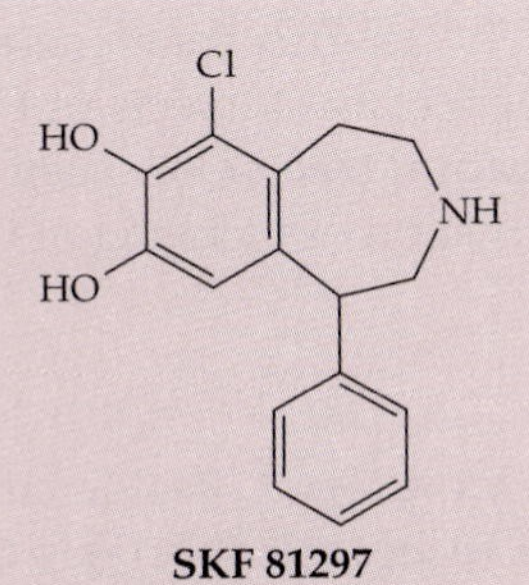

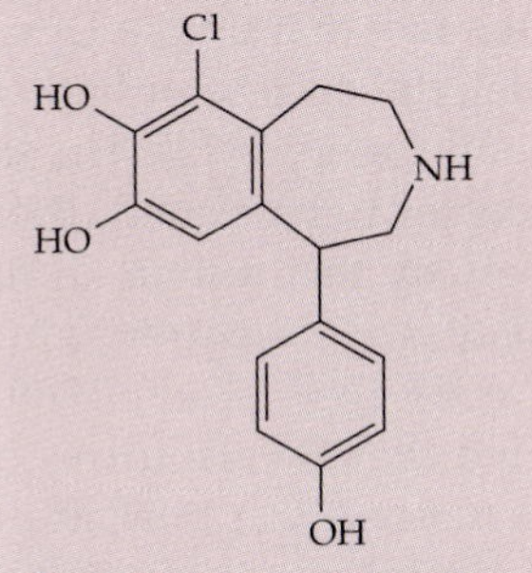

SKF 82526 (Fenoldopam)   **Dihydrexidine**

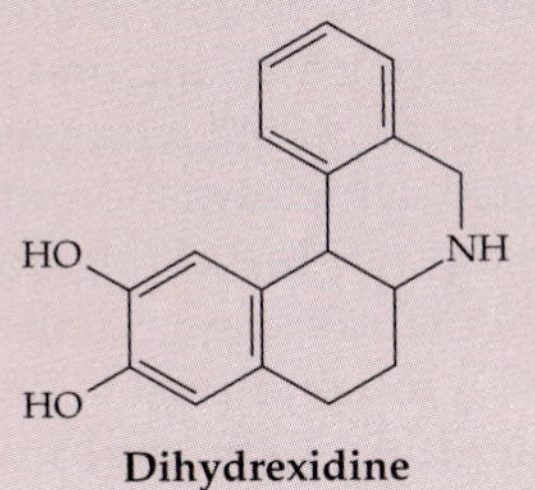

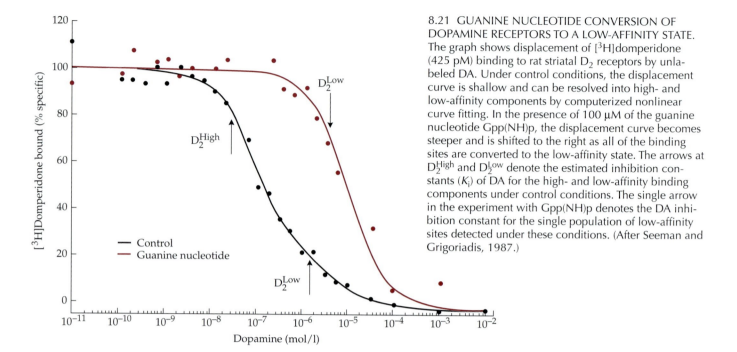

8.21 GUANINE NUCLEOTIDE CONVERSION OF DOPAMINE RECEPTORS TO A LOW-AFFINITY STATE. The graph shows displacement of [^{3}H]domperidone (425 pM) binding to rat striatal D_2 receptors by unlabeled DA. Under control conditions, the displacement curve is shallow and can be resolved into high- and low-affinity components by computerized nonlinear curve fitting. In the presence of 100 μM of the guanine nucleotide Gpp(NH)p, the displacement curve becomes steeper and is shifted to the right as all of the binding sites are converted to the low-affinity state. The arrows at D_2^{High} and D_2^{Low} denote the estimated inhibition constants (K_i) of DA for the high- and low-affinity binding components under control conditions. The single arrow in the experiment with Gpp(NH)p denotes the DA inhibition constant for the single population of low-affinity sites detected under these conditions. (After Seeman and Grigoriadis, 1987.)

acid lesions of the nigral cells, but is lost when the striatonigral feedback pathway is lesioned. Thus, the receptors appear to be located on the terminals of that pathway (see also Ariano and Sibley, 1994).

We mentioned above that DA receptors are coupled to G proteins. Members of this receptor superfamily exist in two distinct states: one with a low affinity for agonists (including the transmitters themselves), and the other with a relatively high affinity for agonists. This phenomenon is due to receptor–G protein interactions; that is, the receptor is in the high-affinity state when complexed with a G protein (Birnbaumer, 1990). Unlike agonists, antagonist drugs do not differentiate between the two states of the receptor. In binding studies, the addition of a nonhydrolyzable GTP analog such as 5′-guanylylimidodiphosphate (Gpp(NH)p) promotes conversion of the high-affinity to the low-affinity state by increasing the rate of dissociation of the receptor–G protein complex (Figure 8.21).* This technique therefore can be used to obtain evidence that a particular receptor is coupled to G proteins.

D_5 receptors.   Currently the only other known member of the D_1 receptor subfamily is the D_5 receptor (Sunahara et al., 1991; Weinshank et al., 1991). Some investigators have used the terminology D_{1A} and D_{1B} to refer to the D_1 and D_5 receptors, respectively. The D_5 receptor is grouped with D_1 because the two receptors have significant amino acid sequence homology, have very similar pharmacological profiles, and both stimulate the forma-

tion of cAMP. It is interesting to note that in the case of humans, but not rats, the D_5 receptor exhibits a tenfold higher affinity for DA than the D_1 receptor (Sunahara et al., 1991; Weinshank et al., 1991).

Because of the pharmacological similarity of the D_1 and D_5 receptors, the so-called D_1-selective agonists and antagonists available at this time also affect D_5 receptors. On the other hand, D_5 receptors appear to be present at very low levels in the brain. In situ hybridization studies have generally found D_5 mRNA only in the hippocampus, the hypothalamus, and the parafascicular nucleus of the thalamus (Meador-Woodruff et al., 1992; Tiberi et al., 1991). This sparseness of D_5 receptors means that in practice, most effects of D_1 agonist or antagonist administration (see below) can probably still be attributed to activation or blocking of the D_1 subtype.

The D_2-Like Receptor Subfamily

D_2 receptors.   Besides the D_1 receptor, the other major DA receptor subtype is the D_2. D_2 receptors were first identified on the basis of their high affinity for antipsychotic (neuroleptic) drugs and the fact that unlike D_1 receptors, they either inhibited adenylyl cyclase or had no effect on its activity (Kebabian and Calne, 1979). The rat D_2 receptor was the first DA receptor to be cloned (Bunzow et al., 1988), followed closely by the human D_2 receptor, which was found to possess 96% sequence homology with the rat receptor (Dal Toso et al., 1989). Other studies soon demonstrated that two isoforms of the D_2 receptor exist in both rats (Giros et al., 1989; Monsma et al., 1989) and humans (Dal Toso et al., 1989). These isoforms, which are produced from the same gene by alternative mRNA splicing, differ with respect to the

---

*Although this figure is based on studies of the D_2 receptor (see below), the technique can be applied to the D_1-like family as well.

presence or absence of a stretch of 29 amino acids located in the third cytoplasmic loop of the receptor (Figure 8.22). The longer and shorter forms are designated D_{2L} and D_{2S} respectively. Although there is currently no evidence for any important pharmacological or functional differences between D_{2L} and D_{2S}, the third cytoplasmic loop is involved in receptor–G protein interactions and could therefore behave differently in the two receptor isoforms.

A variety of D_2 agonists and antagonists have been developed for experimental and clinical use. Bromocriptine (which is an ergot derivative), LY-171555 (also called quinpirole), and apomorphine are some well-known D_2 receptor agonists. Apomorphine is a morphine analog and, like morphine, it can cause nausea and emesis (vomiting). Thus, apomorphine has long been used as an emetic after oral ingestion of certain poisons or drug overdosage. Its mode of action is to stimulate D_2 recep-

tors in the chemical trigger zone of the medulla. Fortunately for animal researchers, rats are incapable of vomiting and hence are good subjects for the use of apomorphine in neuropharmacological studies. Although apomorphine's behavioral effects seem to reflect primarily D_2 receptor activation (see below), the drug is actually not as selective for D_2 over D_1 receptors as some of its analogs, such as 10,11-dihydroxy-*N*-propyl-noraporphine or 2,10,11-trihydroxy-*N*-propyl-noraporphine (Andersen and Jansen, 1990; Gao et al., 1990). Finally, pergolide is another D_2 agonist that possesses some D_1 activity as well (Fuller and Clemens, 1991).

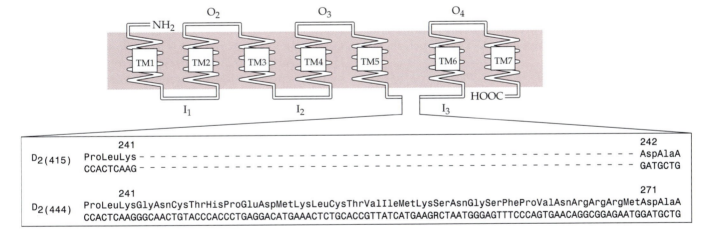

8.22 STRUCTURAL DIFFERENCE BETWEEN THE SHORT AND LONG FORMS OF THE DOPAMINE D_2 RECEPTOR. The rat D_2 receptor exists in two isoforms, a short form consisting of 415 amino acids (termed D_{2S} or $D_{2(415)}$) and a long form consisting of 444 amino acids (termed D_{2L} or $D_{2(444)}$). These isoforms are produced from the same gene by alternative mRNA splicing and differ only with respect to the presence or absence of a 29-amino acid sequence located in the third cytoplasmic (intracellular) loop of the receptor. The extra sequence is depicted in terms of nucleotides from the receptor cDNA and the predicted amino acid sequence. I and O denote the intracellular and extracellular loops, respectively; putative transmembrane domains are denoted by Mb. (After Giros et al., 1989.)

The classic antipsychotic drugs are DA receptor antagonists that possess varying degrees of selectivity for D_2 as compared with D_1 receptors. Members of this group with a high degree of selectivity include haloperidol, pimozide, raclopride, and sulpiride (Meltzer, Matsubara, and Lee, 1989; Schwartz, Giros et al., 1993). The

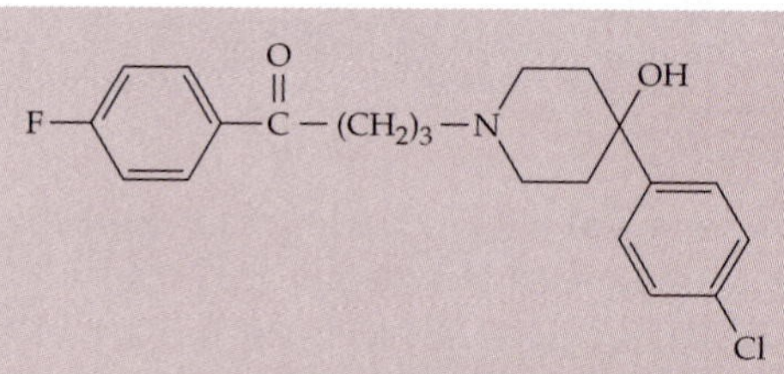

Haloperidol

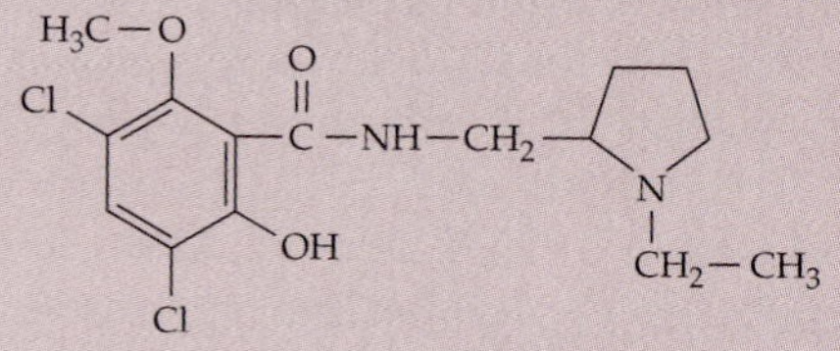

Raclopride

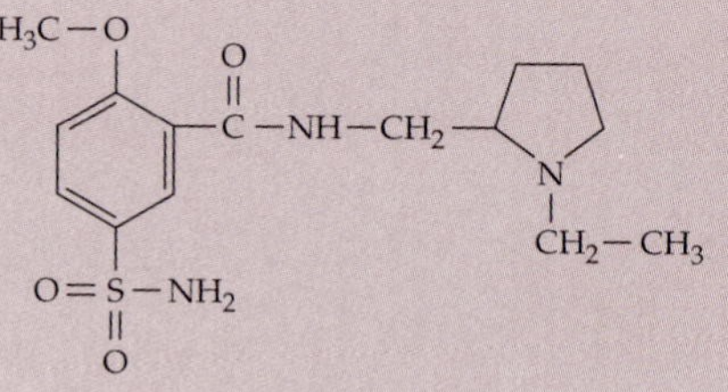

Sulpiride

use of these drugs in the treatment of schizophrenia is discussed in Chapter 18. Some other important D_2 antagonists are spiperone (which is also called spiroperidol), YM-09151-2 (cis-*N*-(1-benzyl-2-methyl-pyrrolidin-3-yl)-5-chloro-2-methoxy-4-methylaminobenzamide), and domperidone. The last compound blocks only peripheral

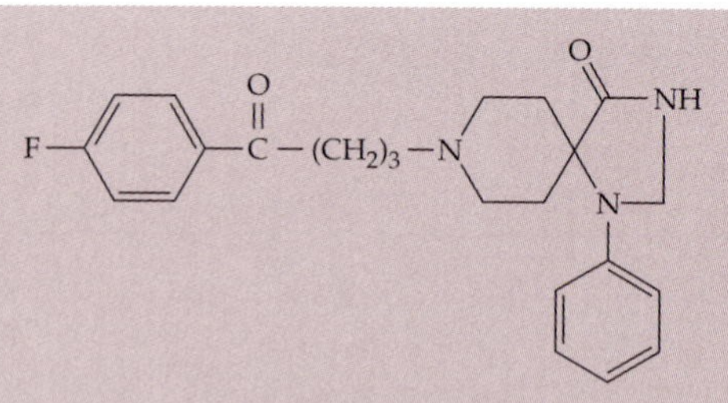

Spiperone

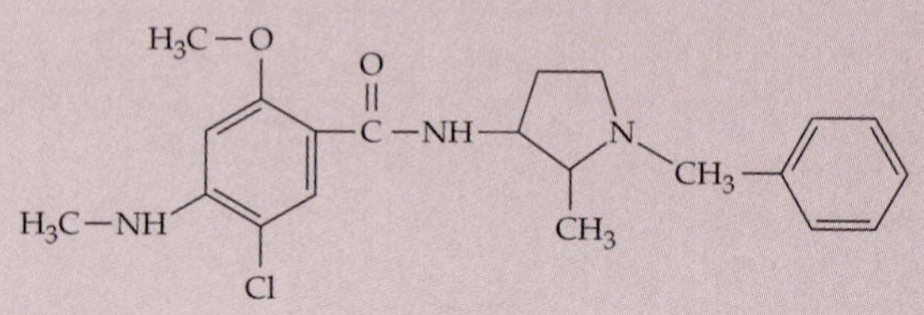

YM-09151-2

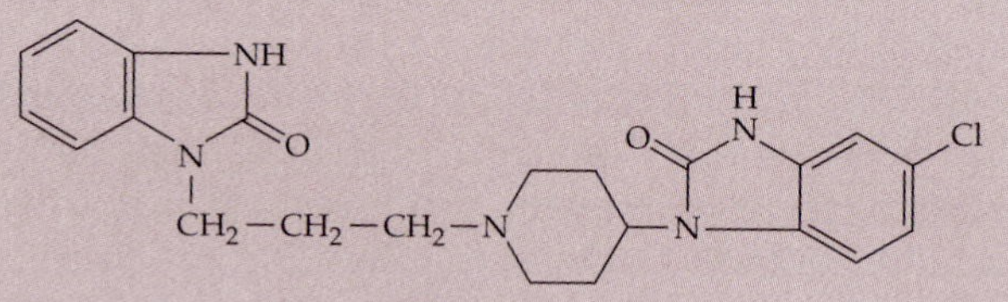

Domperidone

D_2 receptors because of its lack of penetrance across the blood–brain barrier (Laduron and Leysen, 1979).

Like the D_1 subtype, D_2 receptors display a widespread but heterogeneous distribution in the brain. In rats, the highest levels of D_2 receptor binding have been detected in the caudate–putamen, nucleus accumbens, olfactory tubercle, substantia nigra pars compacta, and the glomerular layer of the olfactory bulbs (Boyson, McGonigle, and Molinoff, 1986; Charuchinda et al., 1987; Gehlert and Wamsley, 1985). Intermediate receptor levels were found in the central nucleus of the amygdala, lateral septum, superior colliculus, molecular layer of the hippocampus, and the entorhinal cortex. It is interesting to note that in virtually all areas in which D_1 and D_2 receptor densities were directly compared, levels of D_1 receptors were distinctly greater (Boyson, McGonigle, and Molinoff, 1986).

The localization of DA receptors on striatal output neurons has recently been a matter of some contention. These cells fall into two broad classes that differ in their projections and neuropeptide content (although both classes contain GABA as their classical transmitter). Striatonigral cells send their axons to the substantia nigra and typically contain the peptides substance P and dynorphin, whereas striatopallidal cells project to the globus pallidus and entopeduncular nucleus and usually contain enkephalin (Gerfen, 1992). In situ hybridization studies by Gerfen and his colleagues have suggested that DA receptor gene expression is likewise segregated, with D_1 mRNA being found almost exclusively in substance P neurons and D_2 mRNA present in enkephalin neurons (Gerfen et al., 1990). This interesting hypothesis has potentially important implications for understanding the effect of DA on striatal functioning. However, electrophysiological and single-cell mRNA amplification experiments by Surmeier and colleagues (1993) indicate colocalization of D_1 and D_2 receptors in a substantial majority of striatal output neurons. This issue therefore requires further investigation.

Within the pituitary gland, D_2 receptors are located on the membranes of the lactotrophs, where they mediate the inhibitory effect of DA on prolactin secretion. In vivo D_2 receptor blockade produced by antagonist treatment of laboratory animals can therefore be assessed by measuring the subsequent rise in circulating prolactin levels. Furthermore, the D_2 agonist bromocriptine (Parlodel) has been used clinically in the treatment of hyperprolactinemia (excessive blood prolactin levels) (Kebabian and Calne, 1979). This problem not only arises in some types of pathologies, but can also be induced by long-term treatment with neuroleptic drugs. Disinhibition of prolactin release in female patients being treated with phenothiazines (one of the major categories of neuroleptics) causes a substantial incidence of galactorrhea, a distressing seepage of breast milk (Bianchine, 1985; Rubin, 1987). This effect has even been reported in 10% of male patients receiving this treatment. Although treatment with bromocriptine does not completely eliminate galactorrhea in all cases, the severity of the disorder can be diminished.

D₃ and D₄ receptors. The second member of the D_2 receptor subfamily to be discovered was the D_3 receptor (Sokoloff et al., 1990). D_3 receptor pharmacology is not unlike that of D_2 receptors; however, some important distinctions should be noted. A few of the previously mentioned D_2 agonists, particularly quinpirole and pergolide, actually have a higher potency at the D_3 subtype. The compound 7-OH-DPAT (7-hydroxy-N-N-di-n-propyl-2-aminotetralin) is even more D_3-selective in receptor binding studies (Lévesque et al., 1992), and this drug has been used to investigate the possible behavioral and physiological effects of D_3 receptor activation (see below).

7-OH-DPAT

Among DA receptor antagonists, haloperidol, spiperone, and domperidone all exhibit a modest 10- to 20-fold selectivity for D_2 over D_3 receptors, whereas many other antagonists are even less selective (Sokoloff et al., 1990). A novel naphthofurane compound, (+)-S 14297 ((+)-[7-(N,N-dipropylamino)-5,6,7,8-tetrahydronaphtho(2,3b)dihydro,2,3-furane]), is the first reported selective D_3 antagonist, with a 200-fold greater affinity for cloned human D_3 than for D_2 receptors (Millan et al., 1994).

The highest density of D_3 receptor binding and mRNA is found in the islands of Calleja, dense clusters of small granular neurons located mainly within the olfactory tubercles (Lévesque et al., 1992; Mengod et al., 1992; Sokoloff et al., 1990). Other areas of D_3 receptor concentration include the anterior nucleus accumbens, the olfactory tubercles (outside of the islands), the bed nucleus of the stria terminalis, and the molecular layer of lobules 9 and 10 of the cerebellum. Although the striatum has generally been reported to exhibit minimal levels of D_3 receptor gene expression, immunohistochemical experiments using antibodies directed against this receptor showed staining of many medium-sized striatal neurons (Ariano and Sibley, 1994).

Yet another D_2-like receptor has been cloned from human and rat tissues and named the D_4 receptor (K. L. O'Malley et al., 1992; Van Tol et al., 1991). There appear to be multiple genetic variants of this receptor in the human population, although the functional significance of such variation remains to be established (Van Tol et al., 1992). In monkeys, rats, and/or mice, D_4 receptor mRNA has been identified in the frontal cortex, hypothalamus, thalamus, midbrain, medulla, amygdala, olfactory bulbs, and retina (Cohen et al., 1992; K. L. O'Malley et al., 1992; Van Tol et al., 1991). Only low levels were found in the striatum. However, the rat heart was shown to possess much larger amounts of D_4 receptor mRNA than the nervous system, suggesting that this receptor subtype may at least partially mediate the positive inotropic effect (increased strength of contraction) of D_2-like agonists on heart muscle (Zhao, Fennell, and Abel, 1990).

One of the most interesting features of the D_3 and D_4 receptor subtypes is their potential role in the etiology of schizophrenia and the action of antipsychotic drugs. In the case of the D_3 receptor, this notion is based on the high affinity of classic neuroleptic drugs for this receptor, as well as its presence in the "limbic" part of the striatal complex (i.e., nucleus accumbens and olfactory tubercles) (Schwartz et al., 1993). In contrast, the D_4 receptor is important because it is a potential site of action of clozapine, an atypical antipsychotic drug that is clinically effective in some patients who are not responsive to classic neuroleptic drugs (Seeman, 1992; Van Tol et al., 1991; see also Chapter 18). These are certainly intriguing ideas; however, they will remain largely speculative until more supporting evidence has been provided.

Dopamine Receptor Mechanisms

Electrophysiological effects. The effects of DA itself and of selective agonists and antagonists on the electrophysiological activity of striatal neurons have been extensively studied. The results have been quite complicated and somewhat inconsistent; nevertheless, we will present the findings from a few representative experiments. In iontophoretic studies, very low ejection currents of DA or the selective D_1 agonist SKF 38393 had no effect on the spontaneous activity of striatal neurons, but potentiated the increase in firing produced by the excitatory amino acid glutamate (Chiodo and Berger, 1986; Hu and Wang, 1988). This type of neuromodulatory action may be a mechanism whereby DA from the nigrostriatal pathway can enhance the excitatory glutamatergic input from the neocortex to the striatum (the corticostriatal pathway). At high ejection currents, both DA and selective D_1 or D_2 agonists mainly exert an inhibitory effect on spontaneous and glutamate-evoked nerve cell firing

(Hu and Wang, 1988; Shen, Asdourian, and Chiodo, 1992). However, there is also evidence that more moderate stimulation of D_2 receptors can elicit an excitatory rather than an inhibitory response (Akaike et al., 1987; Shen, Asdourian, and Chiodo, 1992). Further studies are necessary to determine how these different electrophysiological effects relate to the behavioral correlates of DA as discussed in later sections.

Signal transduction mechanisms. As mentioned earlier, a characteristic feature of the D_1 receptor subtype is its ability to increase adenylyl cyclase activity and hence cAMP formation by coupling to the stimulatory G protein G_s (Stoof and Kebabian, 1981; Zhou et al., 1990). There is also evidence that a D_1-like receptor can activate the phosphoinositide second messenger system (Mahan et al., 1990; Undie and Friedman, 1990). However, this receptor does not appear to be either the D_1 or the D_5 subtype (U. B. Pedersen et al., 1994), and thus may be a family member whose gene has not yet been identified.

The functional significance of these second messenger effects remains to be determined. For example, in comparisons between various partial and full D_1 agonists, efficacy in activating adenylyl cyclase was not clearly related to either inhibition of firing of nucleus accumbens neurons (Johansen, Hu, and White, 1991) or stimulation of several D_1-mediated behaviors (Arnt, Hyttel, and Sánchez, 1992; see section on receptor–behavior relationships below). On the other hand, at least one function has been demonstrated at the biochemical level: in neurons containing D_1 receptors, activation of cAMP-dependent protein kinase (PKA) by DA stimulates phosphorylation of a protein called DARPP-32 (*d*opamine and cAMP-regulated *p*hospho*p*rotein, 32-kDa

molecular weight) (reviewed by Hemmings et al., 1987). DARPP-32 is a potent inhibitor of protein phosphatase-1, one of a family of enzymes that dephosphorylates proteins that have been phosphorylated by protein kinases (including PKA). Hence, as shown in Figure 8.23, D_1 receptor–mediated phosphorylation of DARPP-32 may act as a kind of positive feedback mechanism by delaying the inactivation (i.e., dephosphorylation) of other cellular proteins (designated by "X" in the figure) that have been phosphorylated in response to DA.

Several different second messenger systems seem to participate in D_2 receptor signal transduction. The classic mechanism in both neurons and pituitary lactotrophs, of course, is that of inhibiting cAMP formation (Stoof and Kebabian, 1981; Vallar and Meldolesi, 1989). This effect is most easily demonstrated when adenylyl cyclase has been previously stimulated by another receptor system or by treatment with forskolin, a compound that directly activates the enzyme. D_2 receptors also influence the release of arachidonic acid (AA) from phospholipids. AA is an unsaturated fatty acid present in many phospholipids that, once liberated by the activation of phospholipase A_2, can serve many cellular functions (see Chapter 6). D_2 agonists have been reported to potentiate Ca^{2+}-evoked AA release in cultured striatal neurons (Schinelli, Paolillo, and Corona, 1994) and in Chinese hamster ovary (CHO) cells transfected with the D_2 receptor gene (Piomelli et al., 1991). In the striatal cell model, D_1 receptor stimulation reduced AA release, acting in an opposite manner to the D_2 receptor. However, in CHO cells coexpressing both D_1 and D_2 receptors, D_1 agonist treatment had no effect by itself, but produced a synergistic enhancement of AA release when given along with a D_2 agonist. The reason for this discrepancy in the effects of D_1 receptors on AA release is not yet known. Finally, some investigators have reported that striatal D_2 receptors inhibit phosphoinositide hydrolysis (Pizzi et al., 1988); however, this finding has been challenged by other researchers (Rubinstein and Hitzemann, 1990).

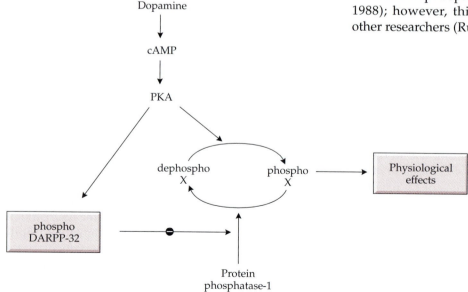

8.23 POTENTIATION OF CELLULAR DOPAMINERGIC EFFECTS BY DARPP-32. DARPP-32 is a protein found in cells containing D_1 receptors. When phosphorylated by cAMP-dependent protein kinase (PKA), DARPP-32 can inhibit the action of protein phosphatase-1, an enzyme that dephosphorylates some proteins (X) that have also been phosphorylated by PKA. In this way, DARPP-32 may facilitate various effects of DA that are mediated by D_1 receptors and the activation of PKA. (After Hemmings et al., 1987.)

The effects of D_2 receptors on ion channels should also be mentioned. These receptors have been found to activate K^+ channels in lactotrophs (Vallar and Meldolesi, 1989), DA neurons in the substantia nigra (Lacey, Mercuri, and North, 1987), and striatal neurons (Freedman and Weight, 1988). Increased opening of K^+ channels leads to membrane hyperpolarization and a consequent decrease in cell excitability. In lactotrophs, D_2 receptors additionally reduce intracellular Ca^{2+} concentrations, which could be secondary to the hyperpolarizing effect and/or could involve a direct action on Ca^{2+} channels (Vallar and Meldolesi, 1989).

Signal transduction mechanisms associated with the D_3, D_4, and D_5 receptors have only begun to be studied. When investigators first cloned the D_3 receptor, they failed to observe any guanine nucleotide–induced shift in agonist binding affinity (Sokoloff et al., 1990). This finding was interpreted to mean that unlike other DA receptors, the D_3 subtype might not be G protein–coupled. Nevertheless, recent studies have demonstrated that D_3 receptors can couple to G proteins, exhibit high-affinity and low-affinity agonist binding states, and inhibit adenylyl cyclase activity (Chio, Lajiness, and Huff, 1994). D_4 receptors also inhibit adenylyl cyclase (Cohen et al., 1992), whereas D_5 receptors stimulate cAMP formation (Sunahara et al., 1991). Table 8.4 summarizes the signal transduction mechanisms and other features of each DA receptor subtype.

Dopamine Autoreceptors

The previous sections have been concerned mainly with DA receptors located postsynaptically. DA autoreceptors are also found on the terminals, cell bodies, and dendrites of dopaminergic neurons (for review, see Mercuri, Calabresi, and Bernardi, 1992; Starke, Göthert, and Kilbinger, 1989). Activation of presynaptic (terminal) DA autoreceptors inhibits both DA synthesis and release. On the other hand, somatodendritic DA autoreceptors cause a reduction in cell firing, which secondarily reduces transmitter release in terminal areas (Santiago and Westerink, 1991). One might wonder how autoreceptors located in the soma or dendritic area of the cell have access to DA under normal circumstances. There is strong evidence, however, that dendrites of dopaminergic cells in the substantia nigra release DA (Cheramy, Leviel, and Glowinski, 1981), and that such release is similar in some ways to striatal release in that it can be stimulated by membrane depolarization or amphetamine administration, and inhibited by tetrodotoxin-induced blockade of Na^+ channels (Robertson, Damsma, and Fibiger, 1991; Santiago and Westerink, 1992). Dendritic DA release can thus be presumed to provide a source of stimulation of somatodendritic autoreceptors, thereby modulating neuronal impulse flow and terminal DA release (Santiago and Westerink, 1991).

Most early studies suggested that DA autoreceptor effects are mediated by receptors with a D_2-like rather than a D_1-like pharmacology (Morelli, Mennini, and Di Chiara, 1988; Starke, Göthert, and Kilbinger, 1989). Although the identity of these autoreceptors is still under investigation, there is considerable evidence that their pharmacology is distinct from that of classic postsynaptic D_2 receptors. For example, low doses of apomorphine preferentially stimulate autoreceptors, and other (more

Table 8.4 Properties of Dopamine Receptor Subtypes

	Amino acids		Signal transduction mechanisms	Regional enrichment
	Human	Rat		
D_1-like family				
D_1	446	446	↑cAMP	Caudate–putamen, nucleus accumbens, olfactory tubercles
D_5	477	475	↑cAMP	Hippocampus, hypothalamus
D_2-like family				
D_{2S}/D_{2L}	414/443	415/444	↓cAMP, ↑AA, ↑K^+, ↓Ca^{2+}	Caudate–putamen, nucleus accumbens, olfactory tubercles
D_3	400	446	↓cAMP	Islands of Calleja, olfactory tubercles, nucleus accumbens
D_4	387	368	↓cAMP	Frontal cortex, diencephalon, brain stem

selective) D_2 agonists similarly appear to be more potent at autoreceptors than at postsynaptic receptor sites (see Drukarch and Stoof, 1990). A novel benzamide compound, CGP 2545A (*N*-(diethylamino-ethyl)-4-chloro-5-cyano-2-methoxy-benzamide HCl), was recently introduced as a D_2-like antagonist that preferentially blocks DA autoreceptors as compared with postsynaptic receptor sites (Bischoff et al., 1994).

CGP 25454A

In light of the recent discovery of new subtypes within the D_2 family, it has become necessary for researchers to reexamine the question of DA autoreceptor identity. Indeed, recent results suggest that D_3 receptors might function as both release- and synthesis-inhibiting autoreceptors in some systems (Meller et al., 1993; Tang, Todd, and O'Malley, 1994). The exact subtype identity of DA autoreceptors (D_2 vs. D_3) is thus unclear at present.

Current findings indicate that the action of both somatodendritic autoreceptors and presynaptic release-inhibiting autoreceptors is mediated by increased opening of K^+ channels (Chiodo, 1992; Zahniser, Cass, and Fitzpatrick, 1992), which hyperpolarizes the cell membrane, thereby decreasing cell firing (somatodendritic autoreceptors) and DA release (presynaptic autoreceptors). In contrast, autoreceptor-mediated inhibition of DA synthesis seems to occur via a reduction in cAMP-dependent activation of TH in the nerve terminals (Onali, Mosca, and Olianas, 1992; Strait and Kuczenski, 1986).

It is important to note that autoreceptors are not found in all DA systems. In rats, for example, autoreceptors appear to be present on most ascending dopaminergic projections except for those terminating in the prefrontal and cingulate cortices (Figure 8.24; Roth, 1984). This difference may contribute to the higher firing rates of mesoprefrontal and mesocingulate fibers as compared with those of the mesostriatal system. Meador-Woodruff, Damask, and Watson (1994) also reported that, unlike rats, monkeys and humans showed no detectable expression of either D_2 or D_3 receptor mRNA in neurons of the ventral tegmental area (A10). The possibility thus exists that in primates, all of the pathways arising from this dopaminergic cell group have little or no autoreceptor activity.

The D_2 Receptor and Dopaminergic Behavioral Supersensitivity

Denervation of the mesostriatal system has been known for many years to produce behavioral supersensitivity to DA receptor stimulation. One approach to studying supersensitivity involves using the DA agonist apomorphine, which, when given to intact rats at a dose of 1–10 mg/kg, produces a syndrome of **stereotyped behavior** consisting of continuous sniffing, snout contact with the ground, forward movement, circling/pivoting, and (depending on dose and other factors) biting, licking, and gnawing (Mason, 1984; Szechtman et al., 1985). These stereotypies are intensified in rats with bilateral 6-OHDA lesions in various parts of the mesostriatal system, indicating that the DA receptors have become more sensitive to apomorphine stimulation (Fink and Smith, 1980; Kelly, Seviour, and Iversen, 1975).

A different approach was used by Ungerstedt (1971b), who created *unilateral* lesions of the nigrostriatal pathway by infusing 6-OHDA directly into the substan-

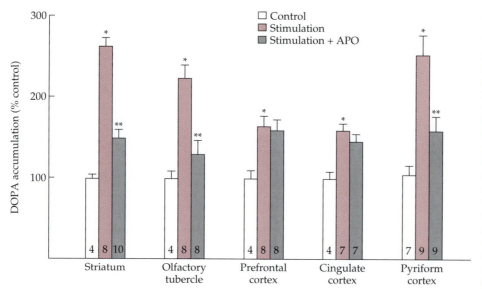

8.24 REGIONAL DISTRIBUTION OF DOPAMINE TERMINAL AUTORECEPTORS. Rats were administered the aromatic L-amino acid decarboxylase inhibitor Ro 4-4602 and then subjected to stimulation of midbrain DA neurons for 20 minutes at 15 Hz. DOPA accumulation (an index of TH activity) was enhanced by electrical stimulation in all brain regions. Apomorphine (APO) (100 µg/kg i.v.) suppressed this enhancement in most cases, but not in the prefrontal and cingulate cortices, indicating a lack of terminal synthesis-inhibiting autoreceptors in those areas. The number within each bar denotes the number of animals in that condition. (*, significantly different from sham control [$p < .01$]; **, significantly different from stimulation alone [$p < .01$]). (From Roth, 1984.)

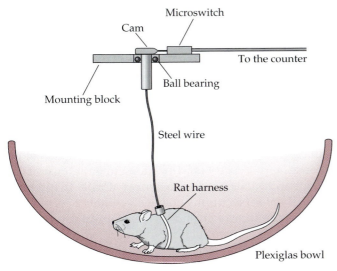

8.25 THE ROTOMETER. A wire connected to a harness fitted to the rat's chest extends to a swivel switch and a counter that records circling behavior. The hemisphere-shaped bowl encourages circling behavior in animals with unilateral striatal lesions. (After Ungerstedt, 1971b.)

tia nigra on only one side of the brain. The effect of such a lesion was a postural asymmetry in which the rat leaned and moved toward the lesioned side due to the dominance of the untreated side. Rotational behavior was quantified by a novel apparatus called a rotometer (Figure 8.25). The importance of DA in this phenomenon was demonstrated by the finding that administration of the DA-releasing drug amphetamine greatly increased ipsilateral rotation (i.e., toward the lesioned side; Figure

8.26). However, subsequent treatment of the animals with apomorphine or with L-DOPA evoked a strong rotational response in the *contralateral* direction. This finding indicated that the denervated side was more sensitive to direct stimulation than the undamaged side, again presumably because of the loss of DA input.

Apomorphine-induced rotation in lesioned animals could be almost completely blocked by haloperidol, suggesting that the behavior is dependent on D_2 receptor activation (Ungerstedt, 1971). Subsequent studies by Creese, Burt, and Snyder (1977) showed that unilateral nigrostriatal tract lesions led to an increased density ("up-regulation") of D_2 receptor binding sites in the denervated striatum. Likewise, chronic treatment with neuroleptic drugs (which block D_2 receptors) was found to produce heightened behavioral sensitivity to dopaminergic agonists as well as increased striatal D_2 receptor density (Burt, Creese, and Snyder, 1977). Together, these findings seemed to provide strong evidence that D_2 receptor up-regulation could account for the behavioral supersensitivity associated with striatal denervation or chronic receptor blockade.

More recent research has further examined the biochemical and functional aspects of this up-regulation phenomenon. For example, several experiments have found that levels of D_2 mRNA in the striatum are elevated following chronic neuroleptic administration, indicating a role for increased transcription of the receptor gene (Martres et al., 1992; Rogue et al., 1991). In addition, LaHoste and Marshall (1989) have provided evidence that the effects of a 6-OHDA lesion and D_2 antagonist treatment on striatal D_2 receptor density are nonadditive. This finding suggests that a common mech-

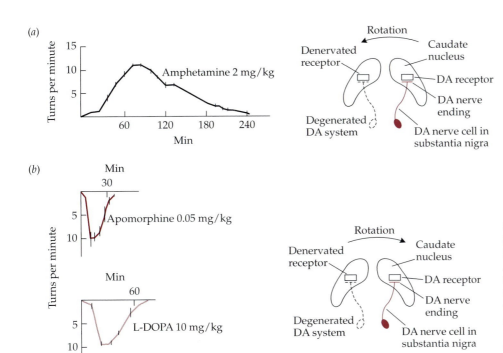

8.26 DRUG-INDUCED ROTATIONAL BEHAVIOR IN RATS WITH UNILATERAL NIGROSTRIATAL LESIONS. (*a*) Amphetamine (which releases DA from the undamaged nigrostriatal nerve terminals) causes the animal to rotate toward the side with the lesion. (*b*) Apomorphine and L-DOPA both cause rotation away from the lesioned side by stimulating supersensitive DA receptors on that side. (After Ungerstedt, 1974b.)

anism underlies receptor up-regulation in response to both manipulations. On the other hand, studies of the 6-OHDA lesion model have found that such up-regulation is quantitatively insufficient to account for the accompanying behavioral supersensitivity (Mandel et al., 1993) and have shown other types of dissociations between receptor density and behavior (LaHoste and Marshall, 1992; Mileson, Lewis, and Mailman, 1991). We must therefore conclude that supersensitivity following nigrostriatal lesions involves not only an increase in the number of D_2 receptors but also changes in other cellular properties, probably involving postreceptor signal transduction mechanisms.

Behavioral Effects of Selective Dopamine Receptor Agonists and Antagonists

The studies described in the previous section began to demonstrate some of the effects of DA receptor activation on motoric behaviors. However, as mentioned before, apomorphine is a relatively nonselective agonist and therefore is not suitable for determining the behavioral roles of specific DA receptor subtypes. If we look back to the early 1980s when the simple D_1/D_2 classification still dominated DA receptor theorizing, it is interesting to note that virtually all behavioral functions of DA were ascribed to D_2 receptors only (Seeman, 1980). This was due primarily to the fact that the behavioral potency of most DA agonists and antagonists known at that time correlated much more strongly with their affinities for D_2 than for D_1 receptors. Later studies, however, clearly demonstrated that appropriate systemic doses of the D_1 agonist SKF 38393 caused a robust stimulation of grooming behavior in rats (Molloy and Waddington, 1984; Wachtel, Brooderson, and White, 1992). SKF 38393-induced grooming in mice was inhibited by the intracerebroventricular injection of antisense oligodeoxynucleotides* to D_1 receptor mRNA (Figure 8.27; Zhang, Zhou, and Weiss, 1994). Furthermore, direct infusion of D_1 agonists into the striatum or nucleus accumbens could also elicit various patterns of hyperactivity and stereotyped behavior (Bordi and Meller, 1989; Meyer, Van Hartesveldt, and Potter, 1993). These results, as well as those of other studies, have convincingly demonstrated the functional relevance of central D_1 receptors.

Moderate to high doses of D_2-like agonists such as quinpirole or RU 24213 have been reported to produce increased locomotion, sniffing, and snout contact (Eilam

---

*An antisense oligonucleotide is a short nucleotide sequence synthesized to be complementary to a portion of a particular mRNA. When the oligonucleotide is taken up by a cell, it hybridizes with that mRNA, thus blocking translation of the mRNA to protein (called "translational arrest") and also enhancing its breakdown by RNase H. This technique is well suited to investigating the consequences of reversibly (since the oligonucleotide molecules are degraded soon after administration) inhibiting the synthesis of a specific gene product. For more information, see Pilowsky, Suzuki, and Minson (1994).

et al., 1992; Molloy et al., 1986; Walters et al., 1987). These behaviors are reminiscent of those observed following apomorphine administration, although the effects seem to be less robust. An important and unexpected finding concerning D_2 agonist effects is that they can be blocked not only by administration of a D_2 antagonist, but also by a D_1 antagonist or by depletion of endogenous DA (Waddington, 1986; Walters et al., 1987). Moreover, combined administration of D_1 and D_2 agonists, either systemically or directly into the striatum, causes much more intense stereotyped behavior than either agonist alone (Bordi and Meller, 1989; Walters et al., 1987). Interestingly, there is electrophysiological evidence for similar synergistic effects of D_1 and D_2 receptors on neuronal firing in the basal ganglia (Carlson, Bergstrom, and Walters, 1987; Wachtel et al., 1989). Such results have given rise to the hypothesis of D_1/D_2 synergism, which states that D_1 receptor occupancy is necessary for the full expression of D_2 receptor–mediated effects (for review, see Clark and White, 1987; Waddington and Daly, 1993). Although many findings support this hypothesis, it is important to note that for some behaviors, D_1 and D_2 receptors appear to function in an oppositional rather than a synergistic manner (Daly and Waddington, 1992; Eilam et al., 1992).

The typical effect of administering a DA receptor antagonist is a suppression of spontaneous exploratory and locomotor behavior and the elicitation of a state known as **catalepsy** (Mason, 1984). Catalepsy refers to a marked difficulty in initiating voluntary motor activity, usually demonstrated experimentally by showing that the subject does not change position when placed in an awkward, presumably uncomfortable posture. Nevertheless, the subject is not asleep, and in fact can be aroused to move by an appropriate stimulus. For example, an early experiment by Feldman and Lewis (1962) studied the cataleptic effect on rats of 5 mg/kg of the neuroleptic drug chlorpromazine. When placed on a small grid, the animals sprawled in a lifeless manner and were described as "skins filled with sand." But when a mild gridshock was applied, they stood up, faced a pair of windows, and jumped over an 8-inch space toward the appropriate window, which they pushed open to reach a platform and a food reward.

Catalepsy can be elicited by selective antagonists of both D_1 and D_2 receptors (Wanibuchi and Usuda, 1990). Moreover, receptors in the striatum appear to play an important role in both cases (Fletcher and Starr, 1988; Sanberg, 1980). These results are reasonably consistent with the prevailing hypothesis of D_1/D_2 receptor synergism and indicate that normal motor functioning requires continued activity at both subtypes in the striatum.

The potential behavioral and physiological effects of D_3 receptor activation have mainly been examined using the partially selective agonist 7-OH-DPAT. This compound has generally been found to produce dose-depen-

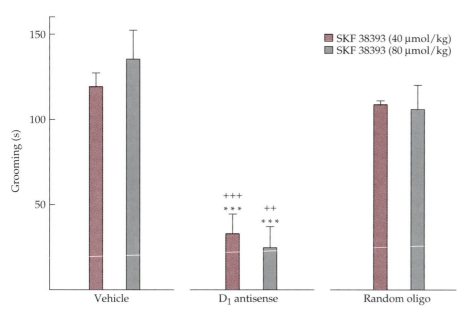

8.27 INHIBITION OF DRUG-INDUCED GROOMING BEHAVIOR BY D₁ RECEPTOR ANTISENSE OLIGONUCLEOTIDES. Mice were injected i.c.v. with the injection vehicle (artificial CSF) alone, D_1 antisense oligonucleotides, or a random oligonucleotide twice daily for 7 days. Subjects were then challenged with a single injection of the D_1 agonist SKF 38393 (40 or 80 μmol/kg s.c.) and behaviorally scored for a total of 5 minutes (300 seconds) spread over a 60-minute test period. Drug-induced grooming behavior was significantly inhibited by the D_1 antisense, but not by the random oligonucleotide. (***$p < .001$ versus vehicle group; ++$p < .01$ and +++$p < .001$ versus the random oligonucleotide-treated group.) (After Zhang, Zhou, and Weiss, 1994.)

dent, biphasic effects on spontaneous sniffing and locomotor activity in rats: behaviors were inhibited at low doses, but stimulated at higher doses (Daly and Waddington, 1993; McElroy et al., 1993). Like apomorphine, 7-OH-DPAT at high doses promoted contralateral rotational behavior in animals with unilateral nigrostriatial 6-OHDA lesions. These findings suggest that D_3 receptors were selectively stimulated at low doses, and that higher doses led to additional stimulation of D_2 receptors. If so, then the D_3 subtype might be inhibitory with respect to locomotor activity (also see Waters et al., 1994). It is possible that D_3 receptor activation reduces activity due to an autoreceptor function; however, various findings argue against this hypothesis (Svensson et al., 1994). Finally, Millan and coworkers (1994) recently reported that 7-OH-DPAT induced hypothermia that could be completely blocked by the D_3 antagonist S 14297. Therefore, current evidence indicates that postsynaptic D_3 receptors are involved in at least the regulation of locomotor behavior and body temperature.

The Role of Dopamine in Motivational Processes

There is a tremendously rich literature concerning the role of DA in many different behavioral processes. Attempting to review this entire body of information is obviously beyond the scope of this volume. We have already devoted some attention to the involvement of DA in motoric functioning, and this topic is taken up further in the discussion of Parkinson's disease in Chapter 20. Moreover, Chapters 13 and 18 provide extensive coverage of DA in relation to psychomotor stimulant action and the etiology of schizophrenia. In the final part of this section, we consider some general aspects of how DA may be involved in mechanisms of motivation, particularly with respect to the neural mechanisms underlying reward and reinforcement.

Basic Concepts of Motivation: Reward and Reinforcement

Physiological psychologists and psychopharmacologists often use the terms "reward" and "reinforcement" interchangeably. However, as White (1989) has pointed out, these terms have different historical origins and somewhat different meanings. When properly used, *reward* refers to the notion of pleasure (as discussed in hedonic theories of psychology and philosophy) and is operationally defined by approach behavior. That is, rewarding stimuli are those that are actively sought out and contacted by humans and animals. The principle of "reinforcement" originates in Thorndike's law of effect and the later work of B. F. Skinner. In these theories, "reinforcement" refers to the ability of certain events to strengthen preceding stimulus–response (or, in some cases, stimulus–stimulus) associations. Reinforcing events *may* also be rewarding, but there is no necessary connection between the two concepts.

In 1954, Olds and Milner published a classic paper describing a phenomenon whereby direct electrical stimulation of the septal area and several other brain areas evoked both a rewarding effect (animals would approach a part of their environment in order to receive such stimulation) and a reinforcing effect (brain stimulation supported the learning of an instrumental task such as lever pressing) in the subjects. Many investigators have postulated that the neural circuitry involved in intracranial self-stimulation (ICSS) may also underlie natural biological rewards such as food, water, and sex (e.g., see Stellar and Stellar, 1985). There has also been a concerted effort to determine what regions elicit ICSS and which transmitters might participate in this phenomenon. As we shall see in the next section, DA has been a featured player in studies of ICSS pharmacology.

Dopamine and Brain Self-Stimulation

Although a surprisingly large number of brain areas elicit ICSS (Wise and Rompre, 1989), the "hottest" area is generally considered to be the medial forebrain bundle (MFB). The MFB is a large collection of ascending and descending pathways that passes through the lateral region of the hypothalamus. To ascertain which areas of the brain are activated when rats self-stimulate via electrodes in the MFB, Gallistel and coworkers (Gallistel, 1983; Yadin, Guarini, and Gallistel, 1983) used the technique of 2-deoxyglucose (2-DG) autoradiography. As described in Chapter 2, this procedure enables researchers to map brain regions that are metabolically activated by specific pharmacological, physiological, or behavioral stimuli. The autoradiographic results indicated that the ventral tegmental area (VTA) was one of the major regions activated during self-stimulation of either the anterior or posterior MFB. As we learned earlier, the VTA is the source of ascending dopaminergic fibers that terminate in the nucleus accumbens and other limbic and cortical areas (mesolimbocortical system). Other investigators have shown that ICSS can be elicited by electrodes implanted directly in or near the VTA (Wise and Rompre, 1989). Moreover, stimulation of rewarding sites in the VTA has recently been demonstrated to cause enhanced DA release in the nucleus accumbens (Figure 8.28; Fiorino et al., 1993). Together, these results support the notion that at least one pathway for ICSS involves the mesolimbic DA system from the VTA to the nucleus accumbens.

Pharmacological studies have provided further evidence that DA is important in MFB self-stimulation. However, experiments that simply look at the influence of drugs on self-stimulation rates must be interpreted with caution because many compounds exert motoric effects that might strongly influence an animal's bar-pressing ability. Consequently, researchers have devised several methods to study the influence of drugs on ICSS reward while controlling for such possible side effects. One such approach is the autotitration, or set–reset, technique developed a number of years ago by Stein and Ray (1959). In this procedure, either the intensity or the frequency of the stimulating current is reduced by a predetermined amount after a given number of lever presses (e.g., five). At any time, the subject may leave the stimulation lever temporarily and move to another lever in a different part of the cage that *resets* the current to its original parameters. The current intensity or frequency at which resetting occurs thus provides an index of the reward threshold for that subject under the existing experimental conditions. As summarized in Stellar and Stellar (1985), the DA-releasing drug amphetamine has

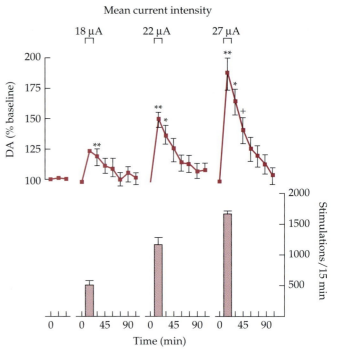

8.28 EFFECTS OF ELECTRICAL SELF-STIMULATION OF THE VENTRAL TEGMENTAL AREA ON EXTRACELLULAR DOPAMINE IN THE NUCLEUS ACCUMBENS. In vivo microdialysis was used to assess extracellular DA levels in the nucleus accumbens of rats during intracranial self-stimulation of the ventral tegmental area. Dopamine levels were monitored before, during, and after 15-minute bouts of stimulation at three different current intensities (18–27 µA). Increasing current intensity led to enhanced rates of self-stimulation (right ordinate) and elevated DA concentrations in the nucleus accumbens. (After Fiorino et al., 1993.)

been found to decrease the reset threshold, indicating an increase in the rewarding value of the stimulation. In contrast, DA receptor antagonists elevated this threshold, suggesting a reduction in stimulus reward.

Another widely used paradigm is the curve-shift procedure. This technique relies on the observation that if one holds either current intensity or frequency constant, increasing the value of the other parameter leads to an increased response rate up to some maximum that varies partly as a function of brain area. Curve-shifting refers to treatment-induced changes in this relationship between the frequency (or intensity) of electrical stimulation and the animal's rate of responding. Drugs that enhance the rewarding effect of the stimulation shift the curve to the left (i.e., subjects press the lever more vigorously at a given frequency), whereas drugs that reduce reward efficacy cause a rightward shift in the curve. The results have been similar to those of the autotitration procedure: amphetamine has been shown to cause a curve shift to the left, whereas DA receptor antagonists have the opposite effect (Wise and Rompre, 1989).

Together, the above findings strongly implicate DA in the rewarding effects of ICSS in the MFB. The mesolimbic dopaminergic pathway originating in the VTA may play a particularly important role in this process. The specific receptor(s) involved in DA-mediated reward is still unclear, especially in light of the various subtypes now known to exist and the relative lack of selective agonists and antagonists discriminating between them. Nevertheless, research to date suggests that both D_1- and D_2-like receptors may participate in the rewarding properties of self-stimulation (Nakajima, 1989; Nakajima, Liu, and Lau, 1993). Finally, it is important to keep in mind the cautionary comments of Wise and Rompre (1989), who point out that DA is not the only transmitter involved in ICSS, and that the midbrain DA neurons do not represent a final common pathway for either brain stimulation or other types of rewards.

Self-Administration of and Place Conditioning with Dopaminergic Drugs

One of the most powerful tools for ascertaining the reinforcing (and perhaps also rewarding) properties of drugs is the technique of drug self-administration by animal subjects. If an animal will learn to press a lever or perform some other operant response in order to receive an injection of a particular substance, then that substance is by definition reinforcing to the subject. Moreover, if the subject consumes the drug to the point of intoxication, endures aversive stimuli in order to obtain the drug, or forgoes standard biological rewards such as food and water in favor of continued drug self-administration, we may well surmise that the drug has significant rewarding properties.

Various types of dopaminergic agonists are self-administered by rats and monkeys, leading to the conclusion that these agents are reinforcing and possibly also rewarding. The most robust self-administration is found with the DA-releasing and reuptake-inhibiting drug amphetamine and the DA reuptake inhibitor cocaine. These compounds are discussed in detail in Chapter 13. Self-administration has also been reported for the DA reuptake inhibitors GBR 12909, nomifensine, and mazindol (Bergman et al., 1989; Howell and Byrd, 1991; Roberts, 1993) and for the D_2 receptor–preferring agonists apomorphine and bromocriptine (Woolverton, Goldberg, and Ginos, 1984). On the other hand, the D_1-selective agonist SKF 38393 did not support self-administration when tested in rhesus monkeys previously trained to self-administer either amphetamine or cocaine (Woolverton, Goldberg, and Ginos, 1984).

Place conditioning is another method of studying the rewarding or aversive effects of drugs (Van der Kooy, 1987). In this technique, animals are given several conditioning trials (one per day) in which either a drug or the injection vehicle is administered. Following the injection, the subject is confined for some period of time (e.g., 30 min) to one of the compartments of a two-compartment apparatus. The two compartments are constructed with distinctly different sensory characteristics, such as light versus dark walls or smooth floor versus rough floor. Drug and vehicle injections are always paired with different compartments so that the animal has an opportunity to associate drug-induced changes in internal state with the sensory cues provided by the apparatus. Finally, a test session is performed in which the animal is given free access to both compartments and the time spent in each one is measured. A rewarding drug such as morphine increases the amount of time spent in the compartment with which it was paired (**conditioned place preference**), whereas aversive drugs such as lithium chloride decrease the time spent in the compartment paired with them (**conditioned place avoidance**).

White, Packard, and Hiroi (1991) used this procedure to examine the effects of the D_1 agonist SKF 38393 and the D_2 agonist quinpirole injected either intraperitoneally or directly into the nucleus accumbens. When administered systemically, SKF 38393 elicited a conditioned place avoidance, and quinpirole produced only a weak conditioned place preference. On the other hand, infusion of either drug into the nucleus accumbens led to strong place preferences (Figure 8.29). Based on these interesting results, the authors proposed that both D_1 and D_2 receptor activation in the nucleus accumbens are rewarding, whereas activation of D_1 and possibly also D_2 receptors at one or more locations outside of this area (central or peripheral) produces aversive effects in the animal.

We have seen that, like ICSS, self-administration and place conditioning studies support a role for DA in reinforcement and reward. In addition, the nucleus accumbens continues to be a prominent area in terms of mediating these effects. In the final part of this section, we will briefly consider some of the theoretical positions that have been advanced to explain the involvement of DA in learning and motivation.

Dopamine in Learning and Motivation: Theoretical Formulations

Much of the current thinking about DA's role in learning and motivation has been influenced by a seminal paper published by Mogenson, Jones, and Yim in 1980. These authors proposed that the nucleus accumbens serves as a critical interface between the limbic and motor systems, thus linking motivation with action. In this model, the VTA–accumbens dopaminergic pathway is seen as part of a gating mechanism that governs the translation of motive states into overt motor responses.

Robbins, Cador, and colleagues (1989) seem to agree at least partially with the formulation of Mogenson, Jones, and Yim (1980), although they place particular emphasis on limbic–ventral striatal interactions in the process of conditioned reinforcement. Moreover, Robbins, Cador, and colleagues also bring into play the appetitive and consummatory aspects of motivation. A typical motivational sequence directed toward some goal

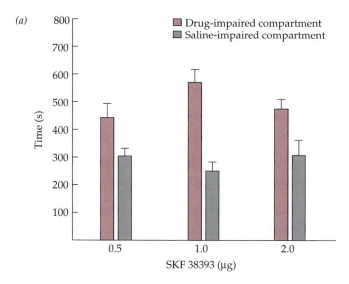

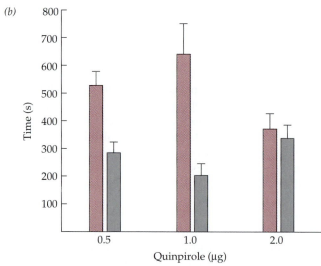

8.29 PLACE CONDITIONING WITH DOPAMINE AGONISTS INFUSED INTO THE NUCLEUS ACCUMBENS. Rats were given twelve daily place conditioning sessions in an apparatus with two compartments that differed in their sensory properties. On 6 alternating days, each animal was given an intra-accumbens infusion of a DA agonist (the D_1 receptor agonist SKF 38393 or the D_2 agonist quinpirole) and then sequestered for 30 minutes in one of the compartments. On the other 6 days, a saline control infusion was administered and the animal was sequestered in the other compartment. On the test day, the animal was given free access to both compartments, and the time spent in each was measured during a 20-minute test session. The drug-paired side was significantly preferred for all doses of SKF 38393 and for all but the highest dose of quinpirole. (After White, Packard, and Hiroi, 1991.)

object (e.g., food) begins with an appetitive phase, which consists of a potentially variable behavior pattern that enables the organism to approach and contact the goal. The appetitive phase is generally characterized by behavioral excitation, sometimes in the form of heightened locomotor activity. Interaction of the subject with the goal object is "consummated" during the subsequent consummatory phase, which tends to be more stereotyped in nature. Dopamine in the ventral striatum (particularly the nucleus accumbens) seems to be important in the appetitive aspects of motivation. For example, food-deprived rats with 6-OHDA lesions in the nucleus accumbens fail to show the normal increase in locomotor activity when presented with food. Female subjects with similar lesions show a selective loss of so-called proceptive behaviors (hopping, darting, and ear-wiggling) that represent appetitive sexual responses, whereas their consummatory response (lordosis) is unimpaired. In contrast, the dorsal striatum (caudate–putamen) seems to be more involved in the consummatory phase of motivated behavioral sequences (Robbins et al., 1989).

Blackburn, Pfaus, and Phillips (1992) have reviewed studies of dopaminergic functioning in feeding, male sexual behavior, and defensive behavior. These authors concur with Robbins et al. that DA is more important for appetitive than for consummatory behaviors. However, the major point of their article is their two-pronged theory of DA action: (1) motivationally relevant stimuli elicit heightened forebrain dopaminergic activity, and (2) the effect of this increased DA release is to prepare the organism to respond behaviorally to significant environmental stimuli that may be forthcoming.

Salamone (1992) has argued that DA in the striatum and nucleus accumbens modulates the effectiveness of certain sensory, associative, and affective processes to alter complex motor functions. In Salamone's terms, lesioning or otherwise interfering with the ascending dopaminergic pathways leads to a "subcortical apraxia" characterized by a dissociation of complex stimulus and motor processes. *Apraxia* is a neurological term for the inability to carry out purposeful action even though sensory and motor functions are still present, and indeed, basic sensory and motor capabilities remain relatively unaffected following damage to the DA system. Finally, Miller, Wickens, and Beninger (1990) propose that DA has two broad types of behavioral actions: (1) a performance activating effect, and (2) an ability to serve as an internal reward signal. Furthermore, they argue that the performance-related actions of DA are mediated primarily by D_2 receptors, whereas the reward properties occur mainly via the D_1 subtype with some modulation by D_2.

This brief survey has shown that forebrain DA is generally considered to subserve broad functions related to motivation and learning. Some investigators have emphasized traditional views of separate motoric (striatally mediated) and reward (accumbens-mediated) functions of DA. However, there seems to be a recent trend toward recognizing that DA may be most important in the integration of sensory, motivational, and motor functions. Further research should permit an even greater refinement of our ideas about the behavioral aspects of this important transmitter.

Part II Summary

Dopamine pathways were originally mapped using the Falck-Hillarp fluorescence technique; however, this technique has been largely supplanted by immunohistochemical staining for TH or for DA itself. Dopamine-containing cell groups in the brain were designated A8–A15 in classic histofluorescence mapping studies. The largest ascending pathway is the mesostriatal system, which originates in the pars compacta of the substantia nigra (A9), the ventral tegmental area (A10), and the A8 group. The dorsal (nigrostriatal) component of this system send fibers to the corpus striatum, while a ventral component terminates in the nucleus accumbens and olfactory tubercles. The mesolimbocortical system, which is derived mainly from A10, projects to the septum, amygdala, hippocampus, nucleus of the diagonal band, and limbic cortical areas. Other well-characterized dopaminergic pathways include the mesodiencephalic, mesopontine, diencephalospinal, periventricular, incertohypothalamic, and tuberohypophyseal systems. Together, these pathways innervate the subthalamic nucleus, habenula, locus coeruleus, various medial thalamic and hypothalamic nuclei, the medial preoptic area, median eminence of the hypothalamus, spinal dorsal gray and intermediolateral cell columns, and the intermediate and posterior lobes of the pituitary gland. Locally projecting dopaminergic neurons are also located in the olfactory bulbs and retina. The mesencephalic DA cells are well known to contain the colocalized neuropeptides CCK and NT. These peptides act reciprocally with DA to regulate release at the nerve endings.

Mesencephalic dopaminergic neurons alternate between a state of spontaneous activity and a silent state that is due to temporary hyperpolarization. When active, the cells may be in either single-spike or bursting mode. Dopamine is released from varicosities along the nerve fibers, most of which appear to form specialized synaptic contacts with their target cells. The rate of cell firing and the amount of DA released can be inhibited by the drug GBL as well as by various DA agonists. The effects of dopaminergic drugs on nigral cell firing are mediated by somatodendritic autoreceptors and by the activation of a long-loop negative feedback pathway from the striatum.

Dopamine receptors all belong the G protein–coupled receptor superfamily. There are five basic subtypes of DA receptors that have been designated D_1 through D_5. Based on their structure, pharmacology, and signal transduction mechanisms, the various subtypes can be grouped into a subfamily of D_1-like receptors (D_1 and D_5) and a subfamily of D_2-like receptors (D_2, D_3, and D_4). Agonists for the D_1 subfamily include SKF 38393, SKF 81297, fenoldopam, and dihydrexidine. D_1-like antagonists include SCH 23390, SKF 83566, NNC-112, and SCH 39166. Bromocriptine, quinpirole, and apomorphine are some important D_2-like agonists, whereas antagonists at this subtype include the antipsychotic drugs haloperidol, raclopride, and sulpiride, as well as spiperone, YM-09151-2, and domperidone. Very high densities of both D_1 and D_2 receptors are found in the substantia nigra and in the termination areas of the mesostriatal system, namely, the caudate–putamen, nucleus accumbens, and olfactory tubercles. Most other brain regions exhibit intermediate or low DA receptor levels. D_3 receptors are found mainly in the nucleus accumbens, olfactory tubercles (particularly in the islands of Calleja), and the bed nucleus of the stria terminalis. The striatum shows only a low level of D_3 receptor gene expression, although striatal receptors have been observed using immunohistochemistry. D_4 receptors exhibit a fairly broad distribution in the brain (although striatal levels are again low); however, D_5 receptors are present only sparsely. The atypical antipsychotic drug clozapine has an especially high affinity for D_4 receptors, although it remains to be determined whether this subtype actually represents the therapeutic site of action of clozapine or any other antipsychotic agent.

D_1 and D_5 receptors stimulate adenylyl cyclase activity and cAMP formation, whereas all members of the D_2 subfamily inhibit adenylyl cyclase. D_2 receptors also potentiate Ca^{2+}-evoked release of arachidonic acid, increase K^+ channel opening, and (in some cells) decrease intracellular Ca^{2+} concentrations. In electrophysiological studies, low levels of DA or the selective D_1 agonist SKF 38393 have been reported to potentiate the stimulatory effect of glutamate on striatal neurons. In contrast, higher levels of DA or D_1 agonists typically inhibit spontaneous or evoked striatal cell firing.

Dopamine synthesis and release are regulated by inhibitory autoreceptors located on the terminals of most dopaminergic neurons. There are also somatodendritic DA autoreceptors that reduce the rate of cell firing. Both types of autoreceptors exhibit a D_2-like pharmacology, and both act by opening K^+ channels and thus hyperpolarizing the cell membrane.

When rats are given 6-OHDA lesions of the mesostriatal system, they show a behavioral supersensitivity to DA receptor stimulation. With bilateral lesions, for example, subjects show intensified stereotyped behaviors in response to apomorphine administration. When lesions are performed unilaterally, on the other hand, supersensitivity can be demonstrated in terms of contralateral rotational behavior following apomorphine administration. These effects are mediated partially, though not entirely, by an up-regulation of striatal D_2 receptors.

Subtype-selective DA receptor agonists and antagonists have been used to elucidate some of the behavioral functions subserved by D_1, D_2, and D_3 receptors. The most pronounced effect of D_1 agonists in rats is to stimulate grooming behavior. In contrast, D_2 receptor activation has been reported to produce hyperlocomotion, sniffing, and snout contact with the ground. Evidence from several sources suggests that the full expression of D_2-mediated effects requires concurrent occupancy of D_1 receptors (D_1/D_2 synergism). Both D_1 and D_2 antagonists produce a state of catalepsy, which appears to be due to blockade of DA receptors in the striatum. D_3 receptor activation has been associated with reduced locomotor activity and hypothermia.

Beyond its obvious effects on motoric function, DA has also been implicated in motivational processes such as reward and reinforcement. Dopaminergic pathways, particularly the ascending projections of the ventral tegmental area to the nucleus accumbens, are important in the mechanism of brain self-stimulation. The reinforcing and rewarding effects of general DA agonists as well as D_2-selective drugs have also been demonstrated using the techniques of drug self-administration and place conditioning. Based on these and other findings, various researchers have theorized that DA may play a central role in the integration of sensory, motivational, and motor functions. Future studies should permit a further elucidation of the behavioral functions of this neurotransmitter.

Part III
Norepinephrine and Epinephrine Systems: Anatomy, Physiology, and Behavior

Distribution of Noradrenergic and Adrenergic Neurons in the Nervous System

Methods Used to Map
Noradrenergic and Adrenergic Pathways

As in the case of DA, neuronal cell groups and fibers containing NE and EPI were first visualized by means of fluorescence histochemistry and are now usually studied immunohistochemically. Cells that are immunoreactive for the NE-synthesizing enzyme dopamine β-hydroxylase (DBH) but negative for the EPI-synthesizing enzyme phenylethanolamine N-methyltransferase (PNMT) can generally be considered noradrenergic, whereas cells containing PNMT (and presumably also TH and DBH) are assumed to use EPI as their transmitter (Hökfelt, Johansson, and Goldstein, 1984a).

Anatomy of Central Noradrenergic Systems

Figure 8.30 depicts a sagittal view of the noradrenergic system of the rat brain. The cell body aggregations are numbered according to the schema of Dahlström and Fuxe (1964) mentioned earlier. Their original nomenclature has undergone some modification because, for example, the populations of some cell clusters were later deemed too small for them to be designated specific nuclear groups (e.g., A3 is now considered to be part of A1). As shown, the nuclei of origin for the NE system are in the pons and medulla. According to Lindvall and Björklund (1983), the nuclei consist of three main groupings: (1) the locus coeruleus complex (A6) and its caudal extension (the A4 group of Dahlström and Fuxe); (2) the lateral tegmental cell system, which is divided into a pontine group (A5 and A7, which together are sometimes called the subcoeruleus group) and a medullary group (A1); and (3) a dorsal medullary group (A2). The projections of these cell groups are summarized in Tables 8.5 and 8.6, and are further described in the sections below.

The locus coeruleus complex.
The locus coeruleus (LC) is the most important noradrenergic nucleus even though it comprises only about 1,600 cells on each side in the rat brain (Rogawski, 1985). Its axons project rostrally as the dorsal noradrenergic bundle (Figure 8.30), dorsally into the cerebellum, and caudally into the spinal cord. Some of these axons bifurcate near the cell body

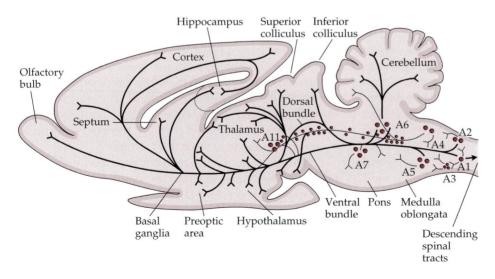

8.30 THE NORADRENERGIC SYSTEM IN THE RAT BRAIN. The projections of noradrenergic neurons are shown in a sagittal view. Clusters of cell bodies are shown as dots and are differentiated by numbers prefixed by the letter A, according to the schema of Dahlström and Fuxe. (After Cotman and McGaugh, 1980.)

Table 8.5 Origins of Projections from Noradrenergic Neurons in the Principal Locus Coeruleus

Terminal area	Origin within the nucleus[a]
Hippocampus	Intermediate-dorsal
Septum	Dorsal
Cerebellum	All regions
Hypothalamus	Anterior–(posterior)–intermediate–dorsal
Thalamus	(Anterior)–posterior–intermediate–dorsal
Neocortex	Intermediate–dorsal
Amygdala/pyriform cortex	Intermediate–dorsal
Spinal cord	Ventral

[a]Parentheses denote minor projection. Anterior part comprises one intermediate and one dorsal portion. Posterior part consists of ventral, intermediate, and dorsal portions.
Source: After Lindvall and Björklund, 1983.

and project both rostrally and caudally. The LC innervates virtually all parts of the telencephalon and diencephalon, including the neocortex, hippocampus, amygdala, septum, thalamus, and hypothalamus. The nerve fibers become so highly ramified in their terminal areas that each axon may branch as many as 100,000 times, creating a terminal plexus having an estimated total length of about 30 cm (Moore and Bloom, 1979). Although investigators once thought that each LC neuron innervated multiple brain areas, subsequent retrograde tracing methods have shown that at least some cells project almost exclusively to specific structures, such as the septum, hypothalamus, or spinal cord.

Noradrenergic fibers from the LC are found in all layers of the neocortex, although the relative density of these fibers differs in each layer, depending on the cortical region and the species. Squirrel monkey visual cortex, for example, exhibits the greatest fiber densities in layers 3, 5, and 6 (Morrison et al., 1982), whereas the noradrenergic innervation of rat cortex is most prominent in layers 1, 4, 5, and 6 (Morrison et al., 1978). Of particular interest is the presence in the rat brain of long, tangentially oriented fibers in layers 1 and 6. This pattern of innervation potentially enables the LC to synchronously modulate cellular activity across wide expanses of cortical tissue.

Table 8.6 Origins of Projections from the Noradrenergic Lateral Tegmental and Dorsal Medullary Neurons

Terminal area	Origin
Spinal cord	A5, A7
Nucleus tractus solitarius and dorsal vagal complex	A1, A2
Spinal sensory trigeminal nucleus	A1, A5
Locus coeruleus	A1, A2, A7
Parabrachial nucleus	A1
Dorsal raphe nucleus	A1
Medial preoptic area	A1, A2
Paraventricular hypothalamic nucleus	A1, A2
Supraoptic nucleus	A1, A2
Dorsomedial hypothalamic nucleus	A1, A2
Ventromedial hypothalamic nucleus	A1, A2
Anterior, lateral, and posterior hypothalamic areas	A1, A2
Median eminence	A1, A2
Arcuate nucleus	A1, A2
Septum	A1, A2
Amygdala	A1, A2

Source: After Lindvall and Björklund, 1983.

The lateral tegmental system.   Axons of the lateral tegmental cell system (particularly from A5 and A7) course caudally to the spinal cord. These fibers terminate in the intermediolateral cell columns of the thoracic and upper lumbar cord, which are the locations of the cell bodies of most of the sympathetic preganglionic neurons (recall that the sympathetic branch is sometimes termed the thoracolumbar system). The axons form inhibitory synaptic connections with these cells, thereby providing a mechanism by which the central noradrenergic system regulates cardiovascular and visceral function (Guyenet and Cabot, 1981; also see later section on the therapeutic use of adrenergic drugs). The rostral projections of A5, A7, and A1 together make up the ventral noradrenergic bundle (see Figure 8.30), which terminates in the hypothalamus and other diencephalic structures. The connections between the diencephalon (especially the hypothalamus) and the peripheral sympathetic system mediated via these noradrenergic cell groups are the basis for integration of the central and peripheral NE systems.

The dorsal medullary group.   From A2, fibers project to the nearby nucleus of tractus solitarius in the medulla. Cells of this nucleus receive gustatory and visceral sensory inputs and relay this information to the thalamus for sensory awareness as well as to the cranial nerve nuclei of the glossopharyngeal (IX), facial (VII), and trigeminal (V) nerves, which are involved in salivation, mastication, and swallowing. A2 fibers also project to the dorsal vagal complex (the principal source of cranial parasympathetic projections to the visceral organs) and, along with axons from A5, A7, and A1, innervate other primary motor and visceral nuclei of the cranial nerves (Lindvall and Björklund, 1983). Thus the A2 group serves as an adjunct to the descending branches of the lateral tegmental cell system by providing inputs to the cranial parasympathetic system.

Fine structure of noradrenergic synapses.   The terminals of LC fibers are extremely fine and give rise to intensely fluorescent varicosities about 1 μm in diameter. The varicosities contain a large number of small synaptic vesicles and a smaller number of large, electron-dense granules (Maley et al., 1990). The characteristics of cortical noradrenergic transmission are still under investigation. Descarries, Séguéla, and Watkins (1991) have suggested that noradrenergic terminals in the rat neocortex form a considerably smaller proportion of synaptic contacts than do dopaminergic fibers. This difference might be associated with a more spatially diffuse action of NE following its release (i.e., "volume transmission," as discussed above in Part II). However, the view that cortical NE terminals are mainly nonjunctional and that the transmitter is released in a nonsynaptic manner has been challenged by other investigators (e.g., Parnavelas and Papadopoulos, 1989). On the other hand, recent results indicate that in the upper layers of the cingulate and sensory cortex, NE uptake is minimal and transmitter molecules may diffuse for relatively long distances (up to 100 μm) following release (Mitchell, Oke, and Adams, 1994).

Anatomy of Central Adrenergic Systems

As mentioned earlier, the localization of EPI-containing cells and pathways in the nervous system was made possible by the development of immunohistochemical techniques for labeling PNMT. In the rat, cells containing the highest PNMT activity are localized in two clusters within the medullary reticular formation, designated C1 and C2 (Hökfelt, Johansson, and Goldstein, 1984a). The C1 cell group is found in the ventrolateral medulla and appears as a rostral extension of the A1 noradrenergic group. Axons from this group project as ascending and descending bundles. The ascending fibers join the medial forebrain bundle (which also contains the dorsal and ventral noradrenergic bundles) to innervate the periaqueductal central gray, various hypothalamic nuclei, and olfactory centers. Most of the descending fibers terminate in the lateral sympathetic horn at the thoracic and lumbar levels of the spinal cord. The C2 group lies dorsomedially under the floor of the fourth ventricle. Terminals from these cells have been found in the dorsal motor nucleus of the vagus nerve and in the nucleus of tractus solitarius, a pattern that is similar to the projections of the A2 dorsal medullary noradrenergic cell group. Thus, the adrenergic system may participate in the coordination of eating and visceral activities. In particular, there is substantial evidence of a role for central EPI in blood pressure regulation (Hökfelt, Johansson, and Goldstein, 1984a).

Norepinephrine and Epinephrine in the Peripheral Nervous System

Most of the primary neurons of the sympathetic ganglia are noradrenergic and are responsible for the autonomic actions of NE discussed later. A small percentage of these cells, however (located mainly in the paravertebral ganglia), appear to be cholinergic instead (Elfvin, Lindh, and Hökfelt, 1993). The sweat glands in particular are innervated by cholinergic sympathetic fibers, a condition conferred upon the ganglionic neurons by the glands themselves (Landis, 1990).

As we have discussed earlier, the chromaffin cells of the adrenal medulla represent another population of peripheral NE- and EPI-containing cells. The adrenal medulla is essentially a specialized sympathetic ganglion, as the cells exhibit an adrenergic or noradrenergic phenotype and are innervated by preganglionic sympathetic fibers from the splanchnic nerve. Finally, some of the SIF cells in sympathetic ganglia may use EPI rather than DA as their neurotransmitter (Elfvin, Lindh, and Hökfelt, 1993).

Coexistence of Norepinephrine with Other Transmitters

Like DA, NE has been found to coexist with various other neurotransmitters and modulators, depending in part on the species. Noradrenergic neurons in the LC have been reported to show immunoreactive staining for enkephalin (cats), vasopressin (rats), and especially a peptide called neuropeptide Y (NPY) (rats and humans) (reviewed by Hökfelt et al., 1987). NPY is likewise found in primary sympathetic neurons, and studies by Bartfai and colleagues (1988) have shown that NE and NPY inhibit each other's release at sympathetic nerve endings (Figure 8.31). Finally, we noted previously in this chapter that catecholaminergic vesicles contain ATP along with their other constituents. It is interesting to note that this substance seems to act as yet another cotransmitter when released with NE by sympathetic neurons (Burnstock, 1990a; von Kügelgen and Starke, 1991).

Electrophysiology of Noradrenergic Neurons

In rats, the firing rate of LC neurons (all of which are noradrenergic in this species) varies in a consistent way as a function of the sleep–waking cycle. During active waking, the cells discharge at a rate of approximately 2 Hz (Aston-Jones and Bloom, 1981a). Firing decreases to an average rate of less than 1 Hz during slow-wave sleep (SWS), whereas the cells are almost completely silent during rapid eye movement (REM) sleep. Changes in cell firing actually precede alterations in sleep–waking state, suggesting their involvement in the mechanisms controlling these states. In addition to the variation related to the sleep–waking cycle, the firing rate of LC cells changes as a function of behavioral activity and sensory input. For example, neuronal discharge was found to be reduced during certain specific behaviors, such as grooming or consumption of a sweetened water solution (Aston-Jones and Bloom, 1981a). In contrast, auditory, visual, or somatosensory stimuli all elicited biphasic responses consisting of a brief burst of firing followed by a more prolonged interval of decreased activity (Aston-Jones and Bloom, 1981b). In a subsequent section, we will consider the implications of these findings for the behavioral functions of NE and the LC.

Adrenergic Receptors

The receptors for NE and EPI are called adrenergic receptors (an alternative term is "adrenoceptors"). Like DA receptors, the adrenergic receptors all belong to the G protein–coupled receptor superfamily. However, they serve a broader role by mediating both the neurotransmitter (mainly NE) and hormonal (mainly EPI) actions of the catecholamines.

Early studies of sympathetically innervated peripheral organs suggested the existence of two major types of adrenergic receptors differentiated on the basis of their responses to sympathomimetic drugs such as isoproterenol (ISO) as well as to adrenergic antagonists such as phentolamine and propranolol. Ahlquist (1948, 1979) designated these receptor subtypes as alpha (α) and beta (β). In terms of agonist potencies, α-receptors showed a rank ordering of NE $\approx$ EPI > ISO, whereas β-receptors displayed the opposite ranking, namely, ISO > EPI $\approx$ NE. Moreover, α-receptors were found to be blocked by phentolamine, whereas β-receptors were blocked by propranolol.

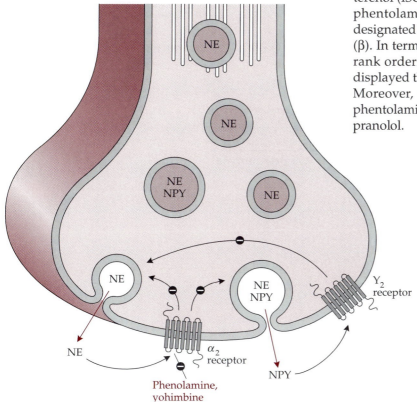

8.31 RECIPROCAL REGULATION OF NEUROTRANSMITTER RELEASE BY NOREPINEPHRINE AND NEUROPEPTIDE Y. NE and NPY are colocalized in sympathetic nerve terminals from rat and mouse vas deferens and pig splenic nerve. Noradrenergic stimulation of terminal α_2-receptors inhibits release of both NE and NPY (this effect is blocked by the α_2-antagonists phentolamine and yohimbine). NPY reciprocally inhibits NE release, probably via action on Y_2 receptors. Note that different populations of vesicles exist in these terminals, some containing both transmitters and some containing only one or the other (see Chapter 11 for further discussion of transmitter–peptide colocalization). (After Bartfai et al., 1988.)

The major peripheral actions of adrenergic receptors are shown in Table 8.7. In terms of their effects on smooth muscle, α-receptors are typically excitatory and β-receptors inhibitory. For example, EPI and other general adrenergic agonists (e.g., ephedrine) that activate both α- and β-receptors are sometimes used in the treatment of bronchial asthma. Stimulation of the α-receptors causes contraction of vascular smooth muscle in the bronchial lining, thus reducing congestion and edema (tissue swelling) by restricting blood flow to the tissue. On the other hand, β-receptor stimulation leads to relaxation of the bronchial muscles, providing a wider airway (see below for a more detailed discussion of the therapeutic uses of adrenergic drugs).

Receptor binding and, more recently, molecular biological approaches have clearly shown that the simple designation of adrenoreceptors as α or β is inadequate. Rather, there are multiple subtypes within each general family that differ in their amino acid sequences, localization in brain and peripheral organs, and functional effects (see Bylund et al., 1994). These various subtypes are discussed in the sections that follow.

α-Adrenergic Receptors

The characteristics of the α-receptor family have been described in several reviews (Bylund et al., 1994; Minneman and Esbenshade, 1994; Ruffolo, Stadel, and Hieble, 1994). The subclassification of α-receptors was begun many years ago when investigators discovered that α-receptor antagonists enhanced the stimulation-induced overflow of NE at sympathetic junctions. This effect was suspected to be due to the blockade of presynaptic autoreceptors that normally exerted an inhibitory effect on NE release (see the section on autoreceptors below). Subsequent studies indicated that postsynaptic and presynaptic α-re-

ceptors had distinctive pharmacological characteristics, leading to Langer's (1974) proposal that the postsynaptic receptor be designated α₁ and the presynaptic autoreceptor be designated α₂. Later α-receptor subtypes came to be defined pharmacologically when some α₂-receptors were found to be located postsynaptically rather than presynaptically. According to current criteria, α₁-receptors are characterized by a high sensitivity to the agonists phenylephrine, methoxamine, and cirazoline, and to the antagonists WB-4101, prazosin, phenoxybenzamine, and corynanthine (Ruffolo et al., 1991). The α₂-receptors are activated by α-methyl-norepinephrine, clonidine, B-HT

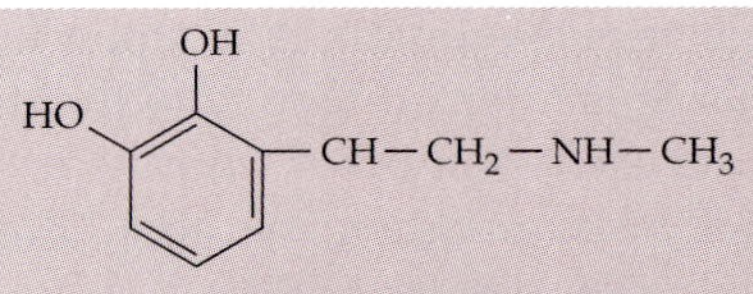

Phenylephrine

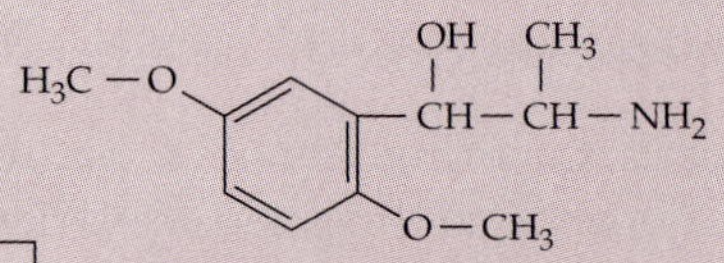

Methoxamine

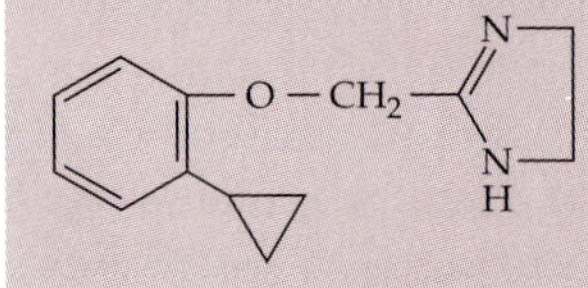

Cirazoline

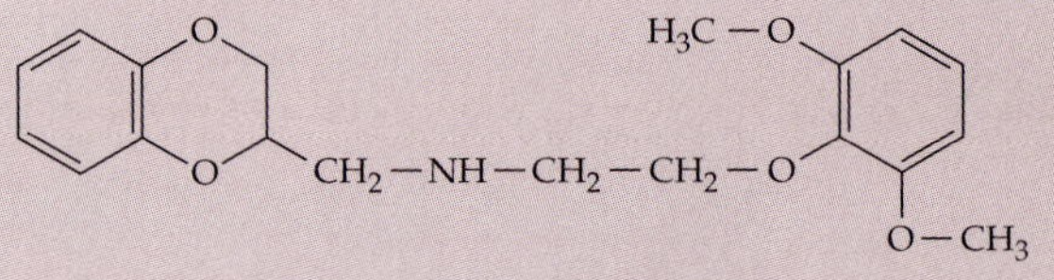

WB-4101

Table 8.7   Location and Physiological Actions of α and β Adrenergic Receptors

Location	Action	Receptor subtype
Heart	Increased rate and force of contraction	β
Blood vessels	Constriction	α
	Dilation	β
Tracheal and bronchial smooth muscle	Relaxation	β
Uterine smooth muscle	Contraction	α
Bladder	Contraction	α
	Relaxation	β
Spleen	Contraction	α
	Relaxation	β
Iris	Pupil dilation	α
Adipose tissue	Increased lipolysis	β

Source: After Bradford, 1986.

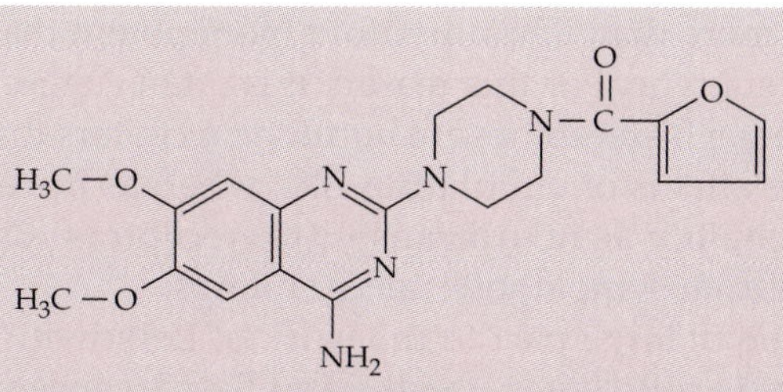

Prazosin

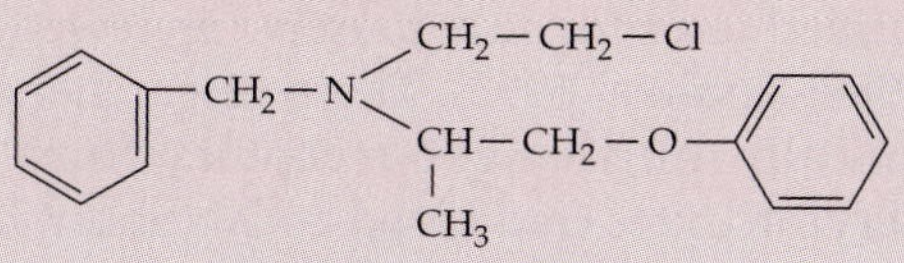

Phenoxybenzamine

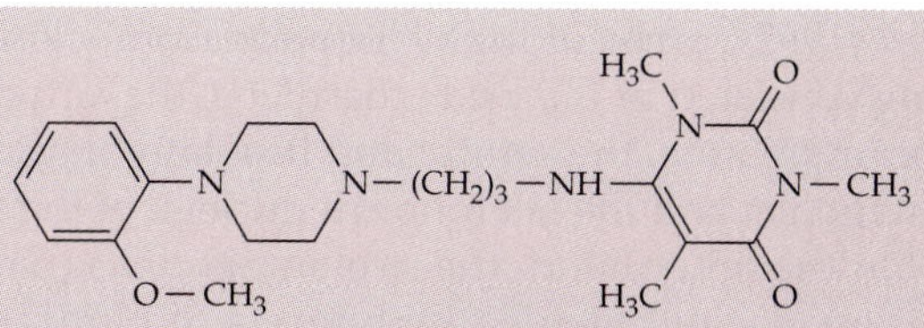

5-Methylurapidil

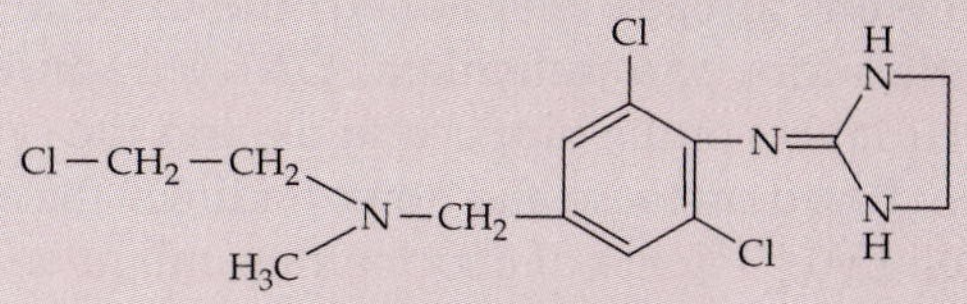

Chloroethylclonidine

920, and UK-14,304, and are blocked by yohimbine, rauwolscine, and idazoxan.

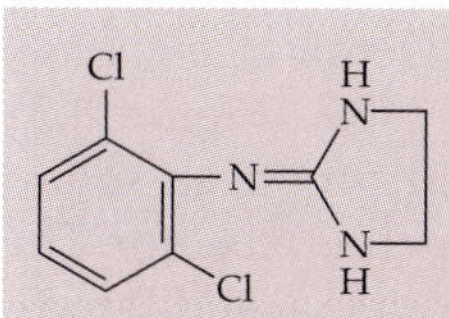

Clonidine

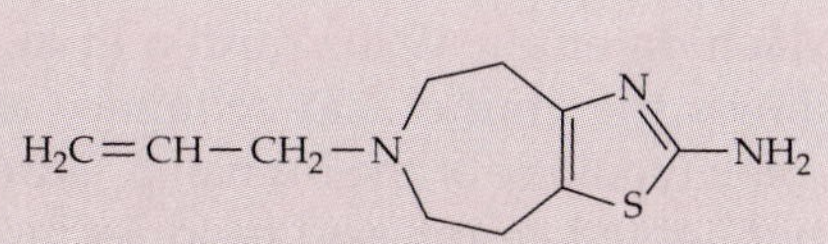

B-HT 920

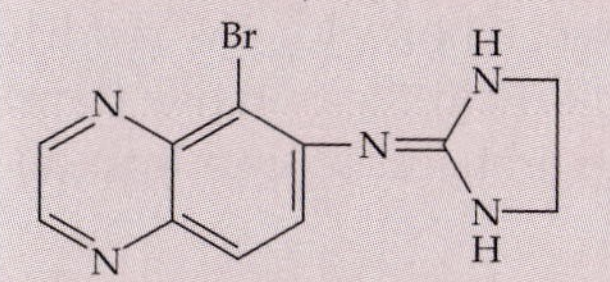

UK-14, 304

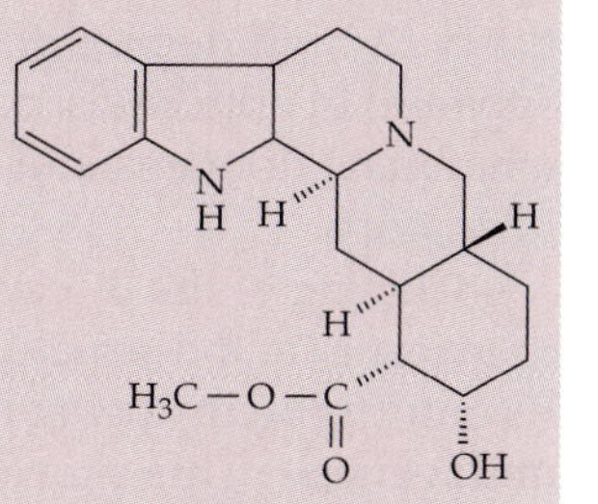

Yohimbine

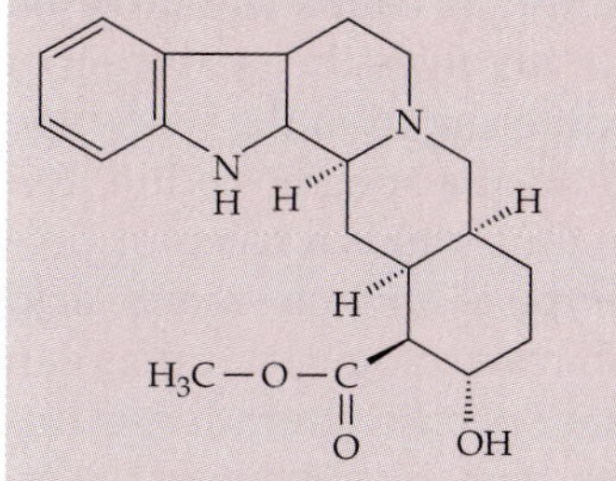

Rauwolscine

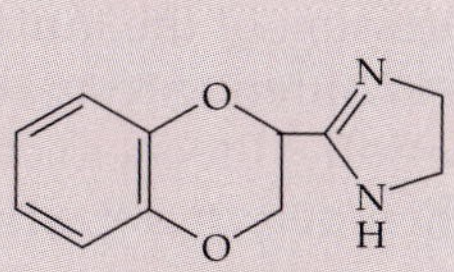

Idazoxan

α₁-Receptors. Pharmacological studies carried out in the early 1980s showed that the α_1-antagonists WB-4101 and phentolamine bound with differing affinities to two distinguishable sites in the rat brain (Battaglia et al., 1983; Morrow and Creese, 1986). The higher-affinity site was called α_{1A}, while the lower-affinity site was called α_{1B}. Currently, the best pharmacological criteria for defining α_{1A}-receptors are a high affinity for another antagonist, 5-methylurapidil, along with resistance to inactivation by the irreversible alklylating agent chloroethylclonidine (CEC) (Ruffolo, Stadel, and Hieble, 1994). In contrast, α_{1B}-receptors have a low affinity for 5-methylurapidil but high sensitivity to CEC. Both subtypes are present throughout the rat CNS; however, α_{1A}-receptors (defined

by high affinity for WB-4101 and resistance to CEC inactivation) were found to predominate in the hippocampus, pons–medulla, and spinal cord, whereas the α_{1B} subtype (lower affinity for WB-4104 and sensitivity to CEC) was the major form detected in the cerebral cortex, thalamus, hypothalamus, and cerebellum (Wilson and Minneman, 1989). Approximately equal levels of α_{1A}- and α_{1B}-receptors were found in the caudate–putamen.

Receptor cloning studies have thus far identified three α_1-receptor subtypes. A nomenclature committee of the International Union of Pharmacology (IUPHAR) recently recommended that these recombinant receptors be designated α_{1a}, α_{1b}, and α_{1d} (the α_{1c} designation has been eliminated due to an unfortunate confusion in the literature; Hiebel et al., 1995). The α_{1a}- and α_{1b}-receptors are thought to correspond to the pharmacologically defined α_{1A}- and α_{1B}-receptors respectively, whereas α_{1d} corresponds to a novel α_{1D}-receptor found in the rat aorta (Saussy et al., 1994).

α₂-Receptors. As in the case of α_1-receptors, α_2-receptor heterogeneity was originally described in terms of two subtypes (reviewed by Bylund et al., 1994). This initial classification was based on the observation that α_2-receptors in human blood platelets had a low affinity for prazosin (which was not unexpected, given that prazosin is generally considered an α_1-antagonist), whereas the α_2-receptors in neonatal rat lung had a considerably higher affinity for prazosin. The platelet and lung receptors were called α_{2A} and α_{2B} respectively, and both subtypes were detected in brain tissues. Subsequent pharmacological research demonstrated the presence of additional subtypes termed α_{2C} and α_{2D} (Bylund et al., 1994; Ruffolo, Stadel, and Hieble, 1994). Furthermore, cloned receptors corresponding to the pharmacologically defined α_2 subtypes have been isolated in several species.

Autoradiographic localization of α_2-receptors in the brain has been accomplished using the agonist [³H]para-aminoclonidine as well as several different antagonists such as [³H]idazoxan and [³H]rauwolscine. In experiments reported by Wamsley, Alburges, Hunt, and

Bylund (1992), areas of high [³H]para-aminoclonidine binding consisted of the locus coeruleus, the amygdalo-hippocampal area, the central and basolateral nuclei of the amygdala, and the laterodorsal nucleus of the thalamus. On the other hand, the two antagonists (particularly rauwolscine) yielded high levels of binding in a wider range of brain areas. These included (in addition to the regions already mentioned) the dentate gyrus, substantia nigra pars reticulata, CA1 pyramidal and molecular layers of the hippocampus, and the caudate–putamen. Based on these and other findings, the authors suggested that [³H]para-aminoclonidine might be preferentially labeling the α_{2A}-receptor subtype, whereas [³H]rauwolscine appeared to label one or more subtypes besides α_{2A}.

Recent in situ hybridization studies examined the distribution of mRNAs for the rat α_{2A}-, α_{2B}-, and α_{2C}-receptor genes (Nicholas, Pieribone, and Hökfelt, 1993a; Scheinin et al., 1994). Although we will not present detailed results here, it is worth noting that α_{2A}- and α_{2C}-receptor mRNAs were widely but disparately distributed in the brain. In contrast, α_{2B}-receptor mRNA was detected only in the thalamus, although it was also found outside of the brain in the kidney. The LC contained mainly α_{2A} mRNA, suggesting that this subtype may serve as the autoreceptor in noradrenergic neurons.

β-Adrenergic Receptors

The family of β-adrenergic receptors is currently divided into three subtypes designated β_1, β_2, and β_3 (Bylund et al., 1994; Hieble and Ruffolo, 1991b). The β_1 and β_2 subtypes are the best understood, and we will discuss these first.

β_1- and β_2-receptors.

The initial proposal of a distinction between β_1- and β_2-receptors was made by Lands and coworkers (1967). These investigators studied the potencies of a series of sympathomimetic phenylethylamine compounds to elicit β-adrenoceptor-mediated responses in four different peripheral tissues, each in a different species. The responses studied were (1) lipolysis (fat breakdown) in rat adipose tissue, (2) heart rate stimulation in rabbits, (3) bronchodilation (widening of the airways) in guinea pigs, and (4) vasodepression (reduced blood pressure) in dogs. The results clearly showed that the relative drug potencies were organized into two clusters based on the response being measured. That is, relative potencies to elicit responses 1 and 2 were well correlated, as were potencies to elicit responses 3 and 4 (both $r \geq 0.95$). Potencies across these two groups, however (e.g., between 1 and 3 or 1 and 4), were poorly correlated (all $r < 0.35$). These findings suggested that responses 3 and 4 were mediated by a different receptor subtype (β_2) than responses 1 and 2 (β_1). Of particular importance was the finding that NE and EPI have approximately equal potency at β_1-adrenoceptors, whereas

EPI is more than a hundredfold more potent than NE at the β_2 subtype. For this reason, it is often suggested that peripheral β_2-receptors are hormone receptors that mediate the effects of circulating EPI, whereas β_1-receptors serve mainly as neurotransmitter receptors for NE released from sympathetic nerve endings.

Due in large part to the work of Lefkowitz, Caron, and their colleagues, the β_1- and β_2-adrenoceptors are probably the best-characterized members of the G protein–coupled receptor superfamily (reviewed by Frielle et al., 1988; Kobilka, 1992). These researchers began by biochemically purifying β-receptors from frog and turkey erythrocytes (red blood cells) (Shorr, Lefkowitz, and Caron 1981; Shorr et al., 1982) and subsequently from hamster, guinea pig, and rat lungs (Benovic et al., 1984). By 1990, various laboratories had cloned the genes for the human β_1- and β_2-receptors (Frielle et al., 1987; Kobilka et al., 1987) and for the corresponding receptors of several nonhuman species (e.g., Dixon et al., 1986; Machida et al., 1990; Yarden et al., 1986). Figure 8.32 shows the amino acid sequence and proposed membrane typology of the human β_1-adrenergic receptor. The highlighted amino acid residues in panels A and B indicate points of homology with the avian (turkey erythrocyte) β-receptor and with the human β_2-receptor, respectively. A high degree of sequence homology is readily apparent in both cases, particularly in the putative transmembrane domains and in the first and second intracellular loops.

Cloning of the β-receptor genes has made it possible to investigate the structure–function relationships of the receptor proteins using a technique called **site-directed mutagenesis**. This procedure involves the synthesis of various mutant genes, each differing from the wild-type (i.e., normally occurring) gene at a specific codon. Expression of the mutant gene thus yields a receptor protein differing from the wild-type at only one amino acid residue. Biochemical and pharmacological studies can then determine whether that specific alteration influences agonist or antagonist binding, interaction of the receptor with G proteins, and so forth. This procedure has been exploited particularly in the case of the β_2-receptor (reviewed by Ostrowski et al., 1992). Site-directed mutagenesis studies have shown that an aspartic acid residue at position 113 in transmembrane domain III plays an important role in the binding of both agonists and antagonists. Because the side chain of aspartic acid is negatively charged, it is presumed to interact electrostatically with the positively charged amine group of the catecholamines.* This notion is supported by the fact that an acidic amino acid is present at the equivalent position of

---

*Based on measured pK_a values of 8.59 and 8.53 for EPI and NE respectively (Mack and Bönisch, 1979), it can be calculated that about 93% to 94% of both catecholamines will be protonated (i. e., have an H^+ ion bound to the amine group) at physiological pH of 7.4.

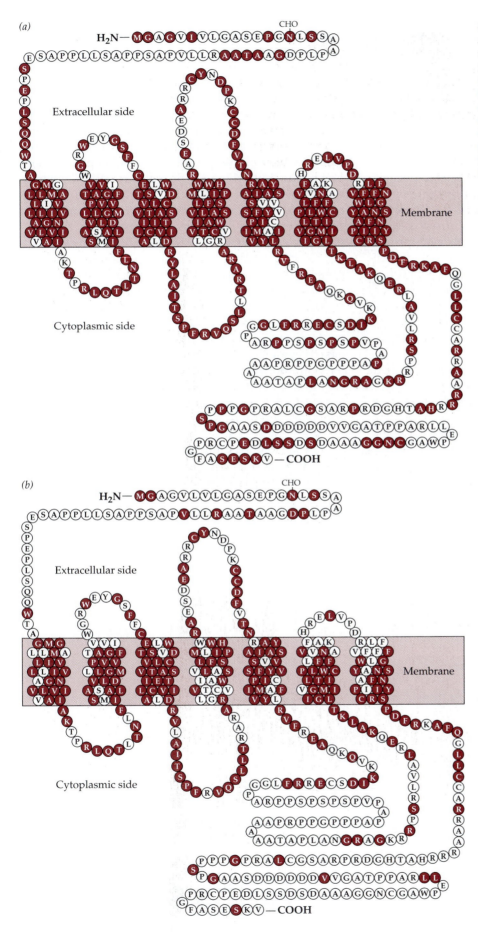

(a)

(b)

8.32 STRUCTURE OF THE HUMAN β₁-ADRENERGIC RECEPTOR. The amino acid sequence and hypothesized membrane organization of the human β₁-receptor are shown in both panels. (a) Amino acid residues identical to those of the avian β-receptor are highlighted. (b) Residues identical to those of the human β₂-receptor are highlighted. In both cases, note the high degree of sequence homology, particularly in the putative transmembrane domains. (After Frielle et al., 1988.)

all G protein–coupled receptors for biogenic amines. Also important for agonist binding are two serine residues at positions 204 and 207 of transmembrane domain V. These residues are believed to form hydrogen bonds with the two hydroxyl groups of the catechol ring of EPI, NE, and other agonist compounds. Taken together, these findings suggest a receptor model in which the agonist binding site is located within the core of the receptor, as shown in Figure 8.33.

Early studies by Palacios and Kuhar (1980, 1983) examined the distribution of β-adrenergic receptors in rat brain by means of in vitro autoradiography with [³H]dihydroalprenolol. β-receptor binding showed a widespread distribution, with particularly high levels present in the nucleus accumbens, caudate–putamen, globus pallidus, olfactory tubercles, layers 1–3 of the cerebral cortex, the molecular and Purkinje cell layers of the cerebellum, the dentate gyrus and CA1 pyramidal cell fields of the hippocampal formation, certain thalamic nuclei, the substantia nigra, and the locus coeruleus. Rainbow, Parsons, and Wolfe (1984) subsequently mapped the location of β₁- and β₂-receptor subtypes by labeling brain sections with the nonselective compound [¹²⁵I]pindolol while blocking either β₁ binding with the selective antagonist ICI-89,406 or β₂ binding with the complementary drug ICI-118,551. The results showed that β₁-receptors predominated (≥ 65% of total β-receptor binding) in most layers of the cerebral cortex, the lateral dorsal and medial dorsal nuclei of the thalamus, the dentate gyrus and CA1 cell field, the caudate–putamen, and the globus pallidus. The β₂ subtype was enriched in the cerebellum (> 90% of the total) and in the central, paraventricular, and reticular nuclei of the thalamus. Other areas examined showed a fairly even distribution of β₁- versus β₂-receptors.

As in the case of α-adrenergic receptors, researchers have recently begun to determine the distribution of mRNAs for β₁- and β₂-receptors using in situ hybridization (Nicholas, Pieribone, and Hökfelt, 1993b). Some similarities were found between the locations of receptor mRNAs and the pattern of labeling previously reported using receptor binding methods. For example, the cerebral cortex showed mainly β₁-receptor mRNA, whereas the cerebellum displayed mRNA exclusively for the β₂-receptor. On the other hand, the relative absence of mRNA for either β-receptor subtype in the caudate–putamen contrasts with previous evidence for substantial receptor labeling (particularly β₁) in this area. It is possible that most striatal β-receptors reside on the terminals of pathways whose cell bodies lie outside of the striatum (e.g., corticostriatal or thalamostriatal pathways). Alternatively, results from the binding studies might represent an interaction of the ligands with some non-receptor site present in this area. The latter possibility is in line with the fact that the striatum has only a very sparse noradrenergic innervation and hence would not normally be expected to possess substantial levels of adrenergic receptors.

With respect to β-receptor pharmacology, isoproterenol and albuterol (also called salbutamol) are general agonist drugs, while propranolol, alprenolol, and pindolol are examples of nonselective β-antagonists. β₁-selective agonists include denopamine, xamoterol, and Ro-363, whereas procaterol (OPC-2009) and sulfonterol are two β₂-agonists. Selective antagonists at the β₁ subtype are atenolol, bisoprolol, and CGP-20712A; the major β₂-selective antagonist is ICI-118,551 (Hieble and Ruffolo, 1991b).

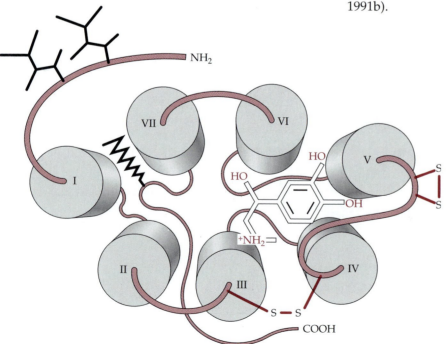

8.33 PROPOSED BINDING SITE FOR EPINEPHRINE IN THE β₂-ADRENERGIC RECEPTOR. The binding site for EPI (and presumably also NE) in the β₂-receptor is thought to reside within the membrane, in a cleft formed by transmembrane (TM) domains III, IV, V, and VI. Site-directed mutagenesis experiments have implicated an aspartic acid residue in TM III in binding the positively charged amine group of the transmitter, while serine residues in TM V are believed to form hydrogen bonds with the hydroxyl groups on the phenyl ring. (After Ostrowski et al., 1992.)

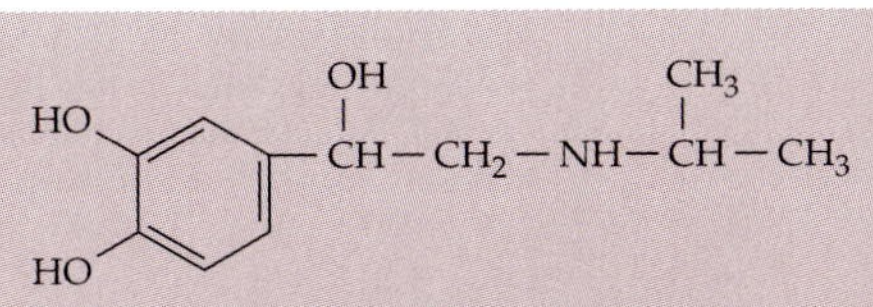

Isoproterenol

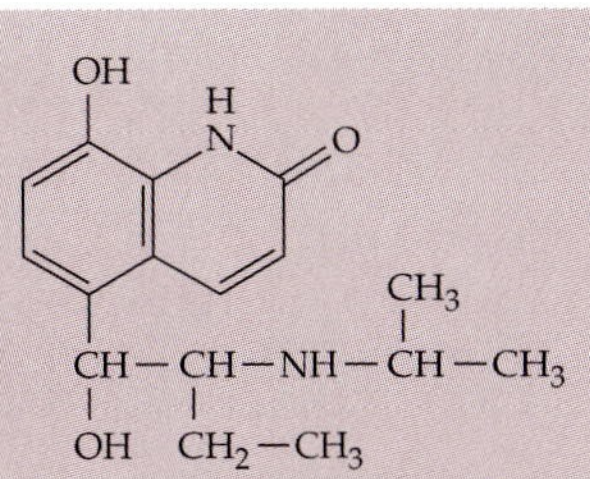

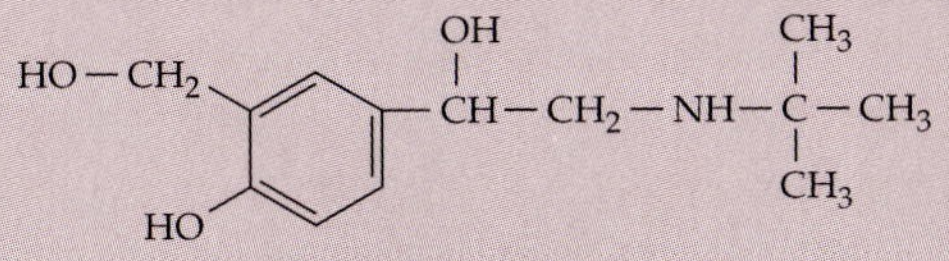

Albuterol (Salbutamol)

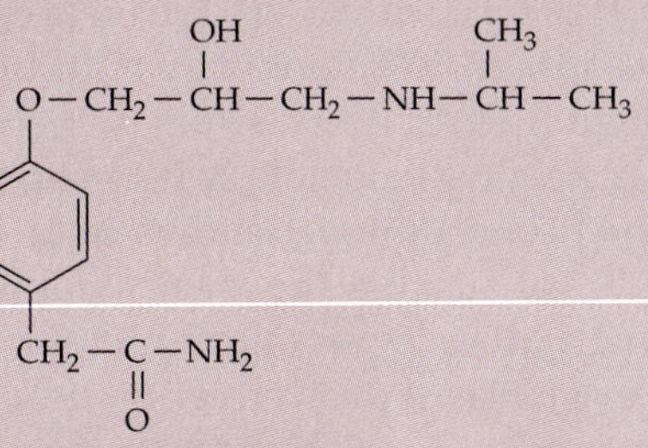

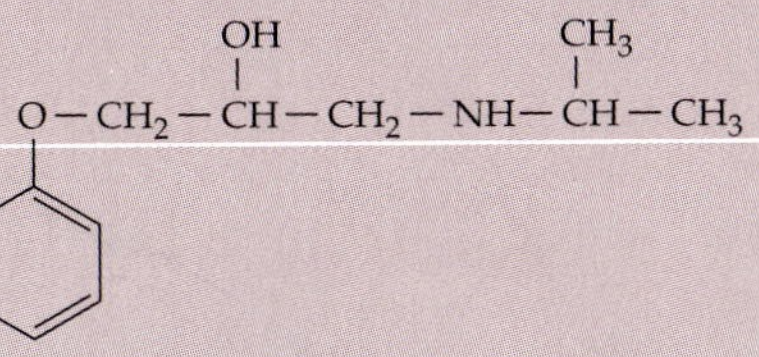

Propranolol

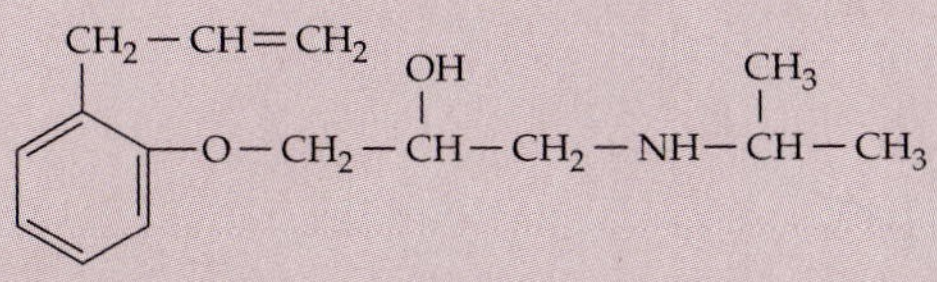

Alprenolol

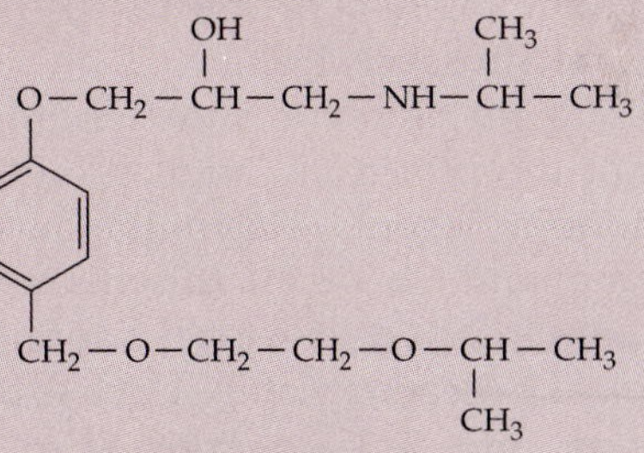

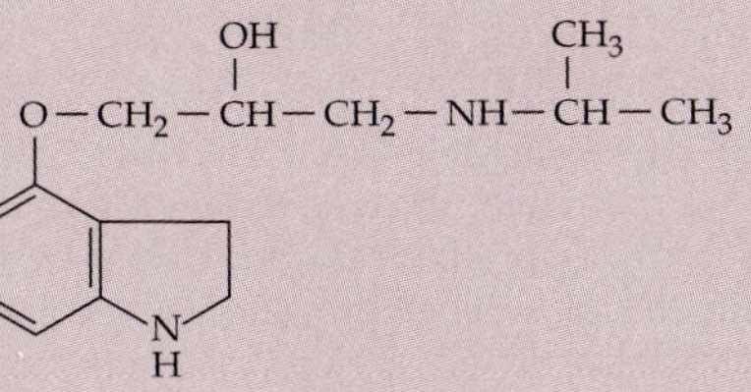

Pindolol

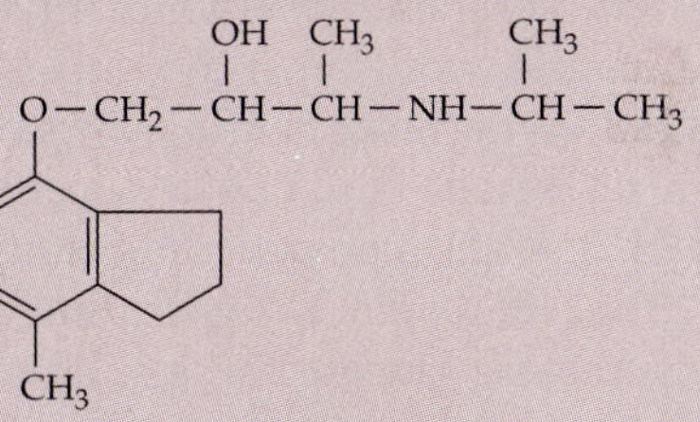

Denopamine

Xamoterol

Procaterol

Atenolol

Bisopropolol

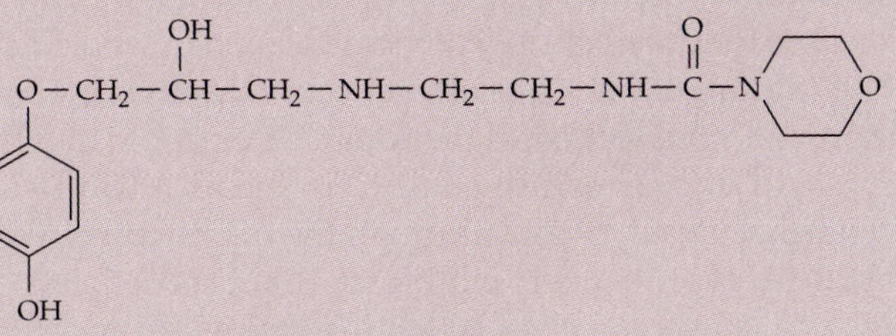

ICI-118, 551

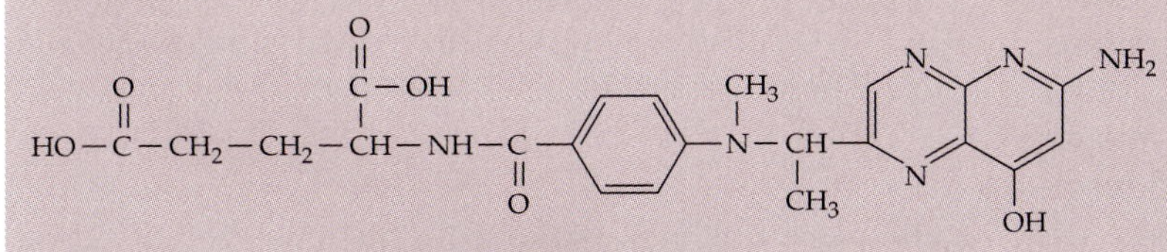

β₃-Receptors. Norepinephrine release from sympathetic nerve endings stimulates lipolysis and thermogenesis (heat production) in brown adipose tissue (a specialized tissue that differs from the typical white adipose tissue). This effect is mediated by β-receptors in the adipocytes. However, studies by Arch and coworkers (1984) at Beecham Pharmaceuticals in England found that the standard β-adrenoceptor agonists isoprenaline, salbutamol, and fenoterol were all relatively weak in terms of their lipolytic activity compared with their potency in stimulating heart rate (β₁) or bronchodilation (β₂) in rats. Even more important, a series of novel compounds synthesized at Beecham (e.g., BRL 37344) exhibited the opposite profile: strong lipolytic activity but weak effects in the standard tests of β₁- and β₂-receptor activity. These findings suggested the existence of an atypical β-adrenoceptor with pharmacological properties distinct from those of the classic β₁- and β₂-receptors.

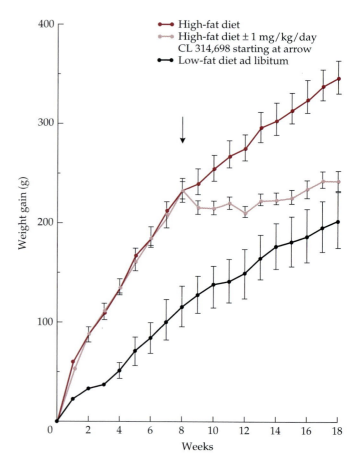

BRL 37344

Five years later, a group in France cloned the gene for a novel human β-receptor that they designated β₃ (Emorine et al., 1989). The amino acid sequence of this receptor displays 45% to 50% homology with the previously cloned human β₁- and β₂-receptors (which is similar to the degree of sequence homology between β₁ and β₂). In addition, the β₃-receptor was shown to be highly sensitive to BRL 37344, just like the atypical rat receptor studied previously. More recent studies have generally confirmed the existence of the β₃-receptor in several human tissues (adipose tissue, gall bladder, and colon), and have additionally shown that the atypical β-receptor of rats is the species homologue of the human β₃-receptor (Emorine, Blin, and Strosberg, 1994).

Because of the lipolytic and thermogenic consequences of β₃-receptor stimulation, β₃-agonists are potential antiobesity agents. This notion has been tested with the compound CL 316,243 (disodium (R,R)-5-[2[[2-(3-chlorophenyl)-2-hydroxyethyl]-amino]propyl]-1,3-benzodioxole-2,2-dicarboxylate), which is even more β₃-selective than BRL 37344 (Largis et al., 1994). The physiological effects of CL 316,243 were examined in the obese *(ob/ob)* and diabetic *(db/db)* mutant mouse strains, both of which suffer from hyperglycemia (elevated blood glucose levels), hyperinsulinemia (elevated insulin levels), insulin resistance, and obesity. Animals were administered CL 314,698, a prodrug that is rapidly metabolized to CL 316,243 in vivo. Drug treatment significantly decreased circulating glucose and insulin concentrations, and also reduced body weight gain (Largis et al., 1994). Moreover, the drug also inhibited weight gain in a rat model of dietary obesity (Figure 8.34). CL 316,243 represents a new generation of potential antiobesity agents that work on peripheral metabolic processes rather than on the central mechanisms of hunger and satiety. The compound is currently in phase II clinical trials.

CL 316, 243

8.34 INHIBITION OF WEIGHT GAIN BY A β₃-ADRENORECEPTOR AGONIST IN A RAT MODEL OF DIETARY OBESITY. Rats were fed either a normal lab chow diet (low fat) or a high-fat diet (33% calories from fat) for 18 weeks (the data shown represent the results from the 25% of subjects that showed the greatest weight gain in response to the dietary manipulation). Beginning at 8 weeks, the high-fat group was restricted to 25 grams of food per day, and half of the subjects were given daily doses in the food of 1 mg/kg CL 314,698, a prodrug of the β₃-receptor agonist CL 316,243. Drug treatment significantly blocked further weight gain in the high-fat diet animals. (After Largis et al., 1994.)

Adrenergic Receptor Mechanisms

Electrophysiological effects.   Activation of α₁-receptors in a variety of brain regions (e.g., cerebral cortex, lateral geniculate nucleus, supraoptic nucleus, dorsal raphe, and dorsal motor nucleus of the vagus) causes a slow depolarization, thereby increasing cell excitability (for review, see McCormick, 1991; Nicoll, Malenka, and Kauer, 1990) (Figure 8.35*a*). This effect occurs through the inhibition of a non-voltage-dependent K⁺ current (I_{KL}) that is present under resting conditions and contributes to the normal "leak" of ions through the membrane. In contrast, α₂-receptors exert inhibitory (hyperpolarizing) effects as a consequence of activating an inward-rectifying K⁺ current (I_{KG}). This is the same ionic response that is associated with D₂ receptors (see above) and certain muscarinic receptors (Chapter 7) as well as with 5-HT₁ₐ, GABAᵦ, and several other neurotransmitter receptors (McCormick, 1991). α₂-Receptors also block Ca²⁺ currents in some cells, although the mechanism underlying this action is still uncertain.

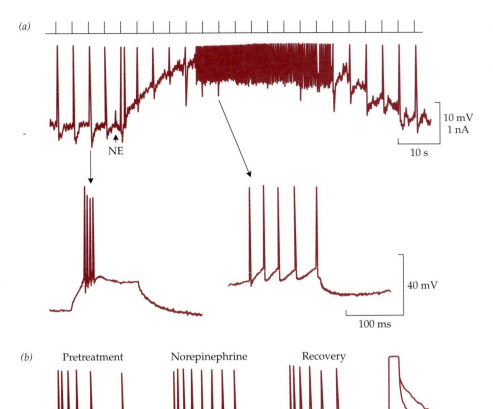

(a)

NE

10 mV
1 nA

10 s

40 mV

100 ms

(b) Pretreatment   Norepinephrine   Recovery

NE

8.35 ELECTROPHYSIOLOGICAL ACTIONS OF α- AND β-ADRENORECEPTORS. (*a*) Activation of α_1-receptors on a cat thalamic relay neuron by local application of NE (upper trace) leads to a slow membrane depolarization that causes the cell to shift from a burst firing to a single-spike firing mode (lower traces). (*b*) Application of NE to a human neocortical neuron decreases the slow afterhyperpolarization current (I_{AHP}), thereby reducing spike-frequency adaptation (first panel, pretreatment recording; second panel, NE treatment; third panel, recovery period; fourth panel, plot of NE-induced reduction in I_{AHP}). (*a* after McCormick and Prince, 1988; *b* after McCormick and Williamson, 1989.)

Effects of β_1- and β_2-receptor activation have not been differentiated and hence will be discussed together. In cells of the cerebral cortex and hippocampus, β-receptor activation leads to the suppression of the slow afterhyperpolarization current (I_{AHP}) (McCormick, 1991; Nicoll, Malenka, and Kauer, 1990). The I_{AHP} is a Ca^{2+}-activated K^+ current that reduces the rate of action potential generation during constant depolarization (this process is also known as spike frequency adaptation). Consequently, the effect of inhibiting I_{AHP} is to increase the rate of cell firing under conditions of high excitation (Figure 8.35*b*). Two other responses produced by β-receptors are a stimulation of Ca^{2+} currents in dentate granule cells and the enhancement of a hyperpolarization-activated cation current (I_h) in the thalamus. The latter effect occurs in conjunction with the previously mentioned excitatory effect of α_1 activation, and would be expected to further enhance cell excitability by decreasing the ability of inhibitory inputs to hyperpolarize the cells.

Second messenger systems. Second messenger systems involved in α-receptor responses have been reviewed by Exton (1985) and more recently by Ruffolo, Stadel, and Hieble (1994). There is a general consensus that almost all effects of α_1-receptor activation result from increased cytoplasmic Ca^{2+} levels. This increase is accomplished through G protein–mediated stimulation of phospholipase C activity, which leads to production of the second messengers inositol trisphosphate (IP_3) and diacylglycerol (DAG) via the phosphoinositide second messenger system. As described earlier in Chapter 6, IP_3 stimulates Ca^{2+} release from storage in the smooth endoplasmic reticulum. Diacylglycerol, which remains in the cell membrane, enhances the activity of protein kinase C. It can also become phosphorylated to phosphatidic acid (PA), which acts as a Ca^{2+} ionophore and thus permits the entry of extracellular Ca^{2+} into the cell. Once inside the cell, Ca^{2+} ions interact with calmodulin and other Ca^{2+}-binding proteins to elicit various biochemical responses. According to experiments summarized by Ruffolo, Stadel, and Hieble (1994), contractions of smooth muscle produced by α_1-receptor activation can be accounted for by a combination of IP_3- and DAG/PA-mediated increases in cytoplasmic Ca^{2+} concentrations. However, the relationship between Ca^{2+} and/or protein kinase C stimulation and the electrophysiological effects of α_1-receptors on neurons remains to be clarified.

The α_2- and β-receptors are differentially coupled to adenylyl cyclase and the formation of cAMP. All β-receptors (including β_3) are positively coupled to adenylyl cyclase via G_s, whereas α_2-receptors inhibit the enzyme through the action of G_i. It is worth noting that the β-adrenoceptor/adenylyl cyclase system was the first transmembrane signaling mechanism to be fully identified in terms of its components and to be reconstituted in vitro (see Levitzki, 1988). Indeed, this system continues

Table 8.8	Mechanisms Associated with Adrenergic Receptor Subtypes		
	Mechanism		
Receptor subtype	Second messenger(s)	Ionic responses	Major neuronal effects
α_1	↑ PI system; ↑Ca^{2+}	↓I_{KL}; ↓I_A	Slow depolarization
α_2	↓ cAMP	↑I_{KG}; ↓Ca^{2+}	Slow hyperpolarizaton
β (β_1 and β_2)	↑ cAMP	↓I_{AHP}; ↑I_h; ↑I_{Ca2+}	↓ Spike frequency adaptation

to represent a most valuable paradigm for the ongoing investigation of the G protein–coupled receptor superfamily (Kobilka, 1992).

There is some evidence for a relationship between cAMP and the electrophysiological actions ascribed to β-receptor stimulation. More specifically, all three of the β-receptor responses described in the previous section can be mimicked by application of 8-bromo-cAMP or the adenylyl cyclase-stimulating drug forskolin (McCormick, 1991). Unfortunately, it is not as clear whether reduction in cAMP levels can account for the effects of α_2-receptor occupancy. Of course, in the case of both α-receptor subtypes, some responses may well be mediated by direct coupling of receptor-activated G proteins with ion channels without the intervention of any second messenger. A summary of adrenergic receptor mechanisms is presented in Table 8.8.

Adrenergic Autoreceptors

The action of release-inhibiting autoreceptors on the terminals of noradrenergic neurons has been demonstrated in many sympathetically innervated organs as well as in various brain regions receiving noradrenergic input (Langer and Arbilla, 1990; Starke, Göthert, and Kilbinger, 1989). In the early 1970s, several research groups independently showed that α-receptor agonists reduced stimulation-induced NE overflow from isolated perfused tissues, whereas α-receptor antagonists tended to increase NE overflow following nerve stimulation (Farnebo and Hamberger, 1971; Langer et al., 1971; Starke, 1971). Subsequent work has shown that the autoreceptor mediating this effect is almost always of the α_2 subtype. Autoreceptors in the brain and most peripheral tissues have thus far been found to exhibit an α_{2A} pharmacology, although the receptors present in rat atria appear to be α_{2B} (Alberts, 1993). The mechanism underlying autoreceptor-mediated release inhibition has not yet been resolved. One possibility is a reduction in depolarization-evoked Ca^{2+} entry into the nerve terminal, although an alternative hypothesis is terminal hyperpolarization via increased K^+ conductance (Starke, Göthert, and Kilbinger, 1989).

At least some sympathetic nerve endings also seem to possess β_2-receptors that stimulate rather than inhibit NE release. Given the particular sensitivity of the β_2 subtype to EPI as compared with NE, these stimulatory autoreceptors may serve as a mechanism by which in-creased adrenal EPI secretion (triggered, for example, by stress) enhances sympathetic noradrenergic activity.

It is easy to make the uncritical assumption that if presynaptic autoreceptors are present, they must exert a tonic brake on NE release. However, it might be the case that "autoinhibition" of release (i.e., previously released NE suppressing subsequent release from the same terminal) comes into play only under certain circumstances. Angus, Dyke, and Korner (1990) tested this notion by looking for evidence of such autoinhibition in several different tissues (for example, rat and guinea pig right atria and rat mesenteric arteries) under various stimulation conditions. These researchers found that in the atrium, reuptake seemed to limit the availability of NE for stimulating the α_2-autoreceptors unless the nerves were strongly stimulated to evoke a near-maximal cardiac response. In mesenteric arteries, however, autoinhibition of NE release was more prominent, and reuptake appeared to play a much smaller role. It is quite possible, therefore, that the importance of autoreceptors for regulating NE release varies as a function of the density of the receptors and/or their proximity to release sites, the activity of local reuptake systems, and, of course, the rate of firing of the presynaptic fibers (Angus, Dyke, and Korner, 1990).

In concluding this section, two other autoreceptor functions should be noted. First, somatodendritic α_2-autoreceptors have been found in cells of the locus coeruleus (Cederbaum and Aghajanian, 1977). Like the somatodendritic DA autoreceptors, these autoreceptors inhibit firing by increasing K^+ conductance, thus hyperpolarizing the cell (Aghajanian and van der Maelen, 1982). Somatodendritic autoreceptors in the locus coeruleus may be activated by NE released from axon collaterals within this area (Aghajanian, Cederbaum, and Wang, 1977). Second, in contrast to DA, relatively little attention has been paid to the possibility that presynaptic adrenergic autoreceptors might inhibit NE synthesis as well as release. Nevertheless, one study has found evidence for α_2-autoreceptor inhibition of tyrosine hydroxylase activity in vivo in hypothalamus and cerebral cortex, but not in corpus striatum (Pi and García-Sevilla, 1992).

Adrenergic Receptors in Nonneuronal Cells

Adrenergic receptors are obviously present in the organs and tissues that receive a sympathetic innervation. However, these receptors have also been discovered in several cell types where their occurrence is less predictable. First, a considerable literature has developed demonstrating the presence of adrenergic receptors on glial cells, specifically astrocytes (reviewed by Salm and McCarthy, 1992; Stone and Ariano, 1989). Receptor binding and other pharmacological studies performed on cultured astroglia have shown that these cells possess α_1-, α_2-, β_1-, and perhaps also β_2-receptors. The receptors respond to NE and other adrenergic agonists, and they are coupled to the same second messenger systems described earlier. A study of rat brain β-receptor immunostaining at the electron microscopic level supported the in vitro studies by finding immunoreactivity in glial cell processes in addition to neuronal fibers and postsynaptic densities (Aoki, Joh, and Pickel, 1987). Furthermore, at least one function of astroglial β-receptors appears to be the stimulation of glycogenolysis to increase glucose availability (for the astrocytes themselves and/or for neighboring neurons) when needed (Salm and McCarthy, 1992; Stone and Ariano, 1989). Thus, the presence of adrenergic receptors in neuroglia seems well established by most criteria. More controversial, however, is the hypothesis advanced by some investigators that glial β-receptors predominate over neuronal receptors, at least in some brain areas. Stone and coworkers (1992), for example, have presented intriguing evidence that β-receptor-mediated cAMP formation in rat forebrain may occur primarily in glial cells. As astrocytes can apparently release cAMP following β-receptor activation (Rosenberg and Dichter, 1989; Stone and John, 1991), perhaps these cells are responsible for the cAMP-dependent β-receptor effects on neuronal excitability described above. This is a highly speculative idea, but one that merits further study.

Also of interest to neuropharmacologists is the presence of adrenergic receptors in blood cells. Blood platelets possess functional α_2-receptors (Hourani and Cusack, 1991), whereas β_2-receptors have been found in mononuclear leukocytes (white blood cells), mainly lymphocytes (Landmann, 1992). Because these cells can be obtained in relatively large quantities by the simple procedure of blood drawing, they represent the most readily available source of human adrenergic receptors for study. One use of blood cell adrenergic receptors has been in psychiatry, in which investigators have attempted to determine whether adrenergic receptor function is altered in patients suffering from affective disorders or schizophrenia, and whether treatment with psychiatric medications produces changes in these receptors. Psychophysiological researchers have also been interested in the effects of various stressors on blood cell receptors as models of adrenergic function.*

---

*Although space considerations do not permit a detailed discussion of this work, interested readers are referred to recent reviews by Hudson and colleagues (1993), Potter and Manji (1994a), and Mills and Dimsdale (1993).

β-Receptor Regulation

Receptor desensitization. The β-receptors, particularly β_2, have been extensively studied as a model of receptor regulation. Numerous studies have shown that exposure of cells to an appropriate agonist causes a rapid (seconds to minutes) reduction in β-receptor responsivity. This desensitization is related to the uncoupling of the receptor from G_s and adenylyl cyclase (for review, see Hausdorff, Caron, and Lefkowitz, 1990; Kobilka, 1992). The principal mechanism underlying β-receptor desensitization is phosphorylation of the receptor, as illustrated in Figure 8.36. Regions of the third intracellular loop and the proximal region of the intracellular carboxy (C) terminal tail are known to be important for interaction of the receptor with G_s. Each of these regions possesses a site that can be phosphorylated by cAMP-dependent protein kinase (protein kinase A; PKA). Hence, when β-receptors are exposed to low concentrations (nanomolar range) of agonist, the resulting PKA activation by cAMP leads to phosphorylation of one or both of these sites. This causes a significant, though incomplete, disruption of the interaction between the receptor and the α_s subunit of G_s. Such "partial desensitization" is manifested as a decrease in the potency of agonists to stimulate adenylyl cyclase (a rightward shift in the dose–response curve). At higher agonist doses (micromolar range), a second protein kinase is also activated that is more specific for the β-receptor. This enzyme, which is called β-adrenergic receptor kinase (βARK), phosphorylates several sites on the distal portion of the receptor's C-terminal. In conjunction with an additional 48-kDa protein called β-arrestin, this process results in complete uncoupling and desensitization of the receptor. Nevertheless, uncoupling is not an irreversible process; removal of the agonist results in rapid dephosphorylation of the receptor and a return of normal sensitivity (resensitization).

At the same time that receptor phosphorylation is occurring, continuous agonist exposure also causes a sequestration of receptor molecules in a compartment less accessible to hydrophilic (but not hydrophobic) ligands. Lefkowitz and his colleagues have theorized that receptors are removed from the membrane and internalized in some intracellular compartment (Sibley, Nambi, and Lefkowitz, 1985), although other interpretations are also possible. Recent experiments by the Lefkowitz group found that blocking receptor sequestration had little effect on receptor desensitization, but completely blocked normal resensitization (Yu, Lefkowitz, and Hausdorff, 1993). Hence, sequestration may be important in the processes of receptor dephosphorylation and restoration of normal function (Figure 8.37).

Receptor down-regulation and up-regulation. When β-receptors are exposed to agonists for a longer period of time (>1–2 hours), a second type of reduced sensitivity occurs that is called down-regulation. Down-regulation

8.36 MECHANISM OF AGONIST-INDUCED β-RECEPTOR DESEN-
SITIZATION. Activation of G_s following agonist binding stimulates
cAMP synthesis by adenylyl cyclase. This activates protein kinase
A, which phosphorylates one or both of two sites on the β-receptor
that are implicated in receptor coupling to α_s (the α subunit of G_s).
At high (micromolar) agonist concentrations, β-adrenoceptor kinase
(βARK) is also activated, which results in phosphorylation of sites in
the distal region of the C-terminus of the receptor. Uncoupling of
the receptor from α_s, and hence desensitization, is produced by
both kinases, although the action of βARK is thought to involve an
additional contribution from a 48-kDa arrestin-like protein. (After
Lefkowitz, Hausdorff, and Caron, 1990.)

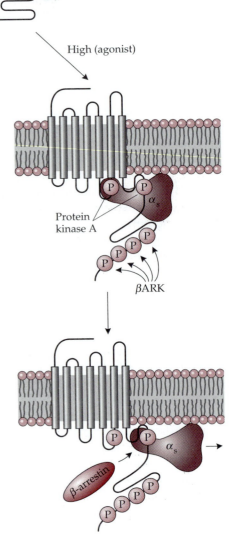

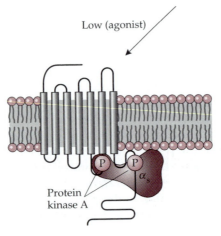

is characterized by a loss of receptor binding sites, not
merely an uncoupling of the receptors from adenylyl cyclase. Down-regulation of β-receptors is accomplished
through several processes, including increased degradation of the receptor protein and decreased levels of receptor mRNA (Collins, 1993; Collins, Caron, and
Lefkowitz, 1991). Interestingly, short-term activation of
β-receptors actually increases rather than decreases transcription of the β-receptor gene by means of a cAMP-dependent mechanism (Collins et al., 1990). Such a positive
feedback system may be important in providing a balance against the desensitizing effect of agonist-induced
receptor uncoupling.

In addition to the above-mentioned mechanisms of
β-receptor desensitization and down-regulation, these receptors can also be up-regulated under certain conditions. For example, destruction of catecholaminergic
nerve terminals by intracerebroventricular administration
of 6-OHDA led to increased β-receptor binding, although
the effect was not uniform across brain areas or receptor
subtypes (Johnson, Wolfe, and Molinoff, 1989). Some regions showed significant increases in both β_1- and β_2-re-
ceptors (e.g., the cingulate and motor cortex, the CA1 and
CA3 regions of the hippocampus, the medial central and
lateral central nuclei of the thalamus, and the granule cell
and molecular layers of the cerebellum). In other brain
areas, there was an increase in either β_1- or β_2-receptor
densities, but not both. Like many other receptors, therefore, β-receptors respond to denervation by up-regulation. The reason for the regional and subtype specificity
of this response, however, is still not understood.

Therapeutic Use of Adrenergic Drugs

The functional consequences of adrenergic receptor activity have led to the widespread clinical use of various
adrenoceptor agonists and antagonists. While some of
these applications are related to activation or blockade of
central receptor populations, many others are based on
peripheral adrenoceptor physiology (see Table 8.7). As
described below, the catecholamines themselves have
long been used in medical practice; however, many important clinical advances have been predicated on the
development of receptor subtype-selective drugs.

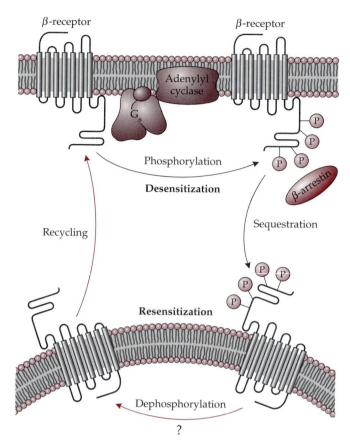

8.37 HYPOTHESIZED ROLE OF SEQUESTRATION IN β-RECEPTOR DESENSITIZATION AND RESENSITIZATION. β-Receptors that have been uncoupled from G_s (desensitized) by phosphorylation are believed to be sequestered away from the plasma membrane in a vesicle-like compartment. The receptors may be resensitized by dephosphorylation, after which they could presumably be recycled back to the cell membrane for further participation in cell signaling. (After Yu, Lefkowitz, and Hausdorff, 1993.)

Use of Catecholamines as Drugs

Epinephrine and NE have some therapeutic utility, although their usefulness is limited in part by their rapid degradation by liver MAO and COMT. Neither drug is efficacious when taken orally (due to both gastrointestinal and hepatic metabolism); however, both can be given intramuscularly or intravenously if highly diluted (1:1,000 or 1:10,000) and slowly administered. The therapeutic usefulness of EPI comes into play when an immediate and strong sympathomimetic effect is needed. Examples of such uses include intravenous injection to counteract shock-induced hypotension or to provide rapid relief from strong allergic reactions, intracardial administration to aid in cardiac resuscitation, inhalation from a nebulizer to relax bronchial smooth muscle and widen the airways during respiratory distress caused by an acute asthma attack, and application to the eyes to reduce intraocular pressure in cases of glaucoma (Weiner, 1985c). Because of its potent vasoconstrictive properties, EPI is also commonly coadministered with local anesthetics to prolong their action by delaying their absorp-

tion into the bloodstream. Thus, EPI is used to enhance peripheral sympathetic activity for short durations in acute situations. None of these treatment modes have CNS effects because EPI does not pass the blood–brain barrier. Nevertheless, an emergency dose of EPI can produce restlessness, apprehension, tremor, and headache that are secondary to the profound cardiorespiratory and other peripheral effects of the compound.

Norepinephrine (Levophed) differs from EPI in its potency for stimulating α- and β_2-receptors. Epinephrine and NE are approximately equipotent at β_1 cardiac receptors, but NE has little effect on β_2-receptors and is somewhat less potent than EPI on α-receptors in most organs. Clinically, NE is currently used mainly for the control of blood pressure in certain hypotensive conditions.

Adrenergic Agonists

Selective stimulation of α_1-receptors is of value in several clinical situations. For example, the α_1-agonist methoxamine (Vasoxyl) is used for the maintenance of adequate blood pressure during anesthesia. Another α_1-agonist, phenylephrine, is the active ingredient in the well-known cold medication Neosynephrine. This drug is used as a nasal spray to constrict the blood vessels and reduce inflamed and swollen nasal membranes resulting from colds and allergies. In the form of eye drops, it is also used to stimulate α-receptors of the iris to dilate the pupil during ophthalmoscopic examinations or before intraocular surgery.

Several clinical applications have been found for α-receptor agonists, most notably in the treatment of hypertension. One drug used in this way is α-methyl-DOPA (Aldomet). Besides acting as an inhibitor of aromatic L-amino acid decarboxylase, this compound is converted in the brain to α-methyl-NE, which is a relatively selective α_2-agonist. Another widely used antihypertensive agent is the classic α_2-receptor agonist clonidine (Catapres). Evidence indicates that the therapeutic effect of clonidine (and presumably that of α-methyl-DOPA) is mediated by central α_2-receptors situated in the caudal brain stem (reviewed by Ruffolo et al., 1993). Activation of these receptors, which may be postsynaptic, inhibits sympathetic outflow and stimulates parasympathetic outflow, thereby causing reductions in blood pressure and heart rate.

α-Methyl-DOPA

Other clinical uses of clonidine are in the management of drug (particularly opiate) withdrawal symptoms, to reduce intraocular pressure in glaucoma, and as an analgesic agent (Buccafusco, 1992; Ruffolo et al., 1993). One of the commonly reported side effects of clonidine is sedation, which may be related to activation of α_2-autoreceptors and a consequent inhibition of locus coeruleus cell firing and NE release (see below for a discussion of the role of the locus coeruleus in arousal). Although sleepiness may be an annoying side effect in patients taking clonidine for hypertension, it has led to the development of this drug as an adjunct to general anesthesia.

Numerous effects on sympathetic end-organs have been associated with β-receptors (see Table 8.7). These effects include increased rate (positive chronotropic effect) and force (positive inotropic effect) of heart contraction, general vasodilation, and relaxation of smooth muscle in the respiratory, gastrointestinal, and urogenital systems (Hieble and Ruffolo, 1991a). One of the important clinical applications of these effects is in the relief of bronchospasm related to asthma or other conditions. Although the classic nonselective β-receptor agonist isoproterenol (Isuprel) is still sometimes used in this context, it has been largely supplanted by other compounds such as albuterol (Ventolin) and metaproterenol (Metaprel). These drugs are partially β_2-selective, and as a result, they are somewhat more effective in relaxing tracheal and bronchial smooth muscle (β_2 more important than β_1) but exert less of an effect on the heart (mainly β_1).

Adrenergic Antagonists

Adrenergic antagonists have also proved useful in certain therapeutic settings. For example, the atypical antidepressant mianserin has α_2-antagonist properties, although it also exerts other neurochemical effects that may well contribute to its therapeutic efficacy. Nevertheless, pharmaceutical companies are developing and testing more selective α_2-blockers for possible use as antidepressants (Pinder and Wieringa, 1993). Interestingly, the α_2-antagonist yohimbine (Yohimex) appears to aid in the treatment of certain types of male sexual impotence. This compound increases parasympathetic and decreases sympathetic activity, which is thought to stimulate penile blood inflow and/or inhibit blood outflow (Ruffolo et al., 1993).

Propranolol (Inderal) and other nonselective β-receptor antagonists such as pindolol (Visken) and timolol (Blocadren) are used medicinally for a variety of cardiac conditions such as hypertension, angina pectoris (severe heart pain), and cardiac arrhythmias. In addition, β-blockers have been found to reduce heart attack recurrence in patients surviving an initial myocardial infarction (occlusion of the coronary arteries) (Kolata, 1981b). It is worth noting that greater cardioselectivity (and hence fewer side effects) can be achieved by blocking only β_1-receptors, which has led to the clinical introduction of β_1-antagonists such as atenolol (Tenormin), betaxolol (Kerlone), bisoprolol (Zebeta), and metoprolol (Lopressor). Finally, propranolol and other β-blockers have also found use in the treatment of generalized anxiety disorder, perhaps because of their ability to inhibit some of the autonomic symptoms of strong anxiety such as palpitations, flushing, and tachycardia (Tyrer, 1992).

Behavioral Functions of Norepinephrine

Like DA, NE is involved in more areas of behavioral regulation than can conveniently be discussed here. Therefore, in this concluding section, we shall consider the functional role of NE in two behavioral processes that have been extensively studied: (1) attention and arousal and (2) feeding behavior.

The Role of Norepinephrine in Attention, Arousal, and Vigilance

As described in a previous section, the small complement of neurons in the locus coeruleus (LC) provides virtually the entire noradrenergic innervation of the telencephalon. To quote Berridge, Arnsten, and Foote (1993), "The LC constitutes a system in which alterations in activity of a very small number of neurons can be broadcast to vast brain regions and neuronal populations of immense number" (p. 558). What purpose might such a system serve? Recall that the activity of LC neurons varies with the sleep–waking cycle, with the cells becoming virtually silent during REM sleep (Aston-Jones and Bloom, 1981a). Because various sensory stimuli were found to trigger bursts of LC cell firing (Aston-Jones and Bloom, 1981b), one might conclude that the function of the telencephalic noradrenergic system is to increase the overall level of arousal. In apparent support of this hypothesis, pharmacological activation of the LC was reported to elicit forebrain EEG activation in anesthetized rats (Berridge and Foote, 1991). However, at least one major problem with such a theory is that LC neurons are inhibited not only during REM sleep, but also during maintenance behaviors such as grooming and ingestive behavior (Aston-Jones and Bloom, 1981a). It is difficult to argue that animals are not aroused during the performance of such behaviors.

An alternative hypothesis proposed by Aston-Jones (1985) suggests that the LC does not regulate arousal, but rather the related phenomenon of **vigilance**. Vigilance is defined as a high level of attentiveness and behavioral responsivity to environmental stimuli. According to this notion, then, LC activity is inhibited during low-vigilance states such as sleep or maintenance (vegetative) behaviors. This inhibition allows the neural programs associated with such states to be carried out uninterrupted. However, when the organism is exposed to a strong stimulus that elicits an alerting response, LC neurons are strongly (albeit briefly) activated, thus preparing various brain areas for the necessary sensory processing and initiation of adaptive behavioral responses (Figure 8.38).

Substantial evidence has accumulated in support of this hypothesis of LC function. First, application of NE to cortical and hippocampal neurons often reduces neuronal responsiveness to weak synaptic inputs while maintaining or even enhancing responses to strong inputs (Aston-Jones, 1985). In this manner, noradrenergic system activity enhances the "signal-to-noise" ratio of target cells in the telencephalon, priming them to react to the most potent stimuli currently impinging on the organism. Second, in cynomolgus monkeys performing a vigilance task, LC neurons were selectively activated by presentation of the target stimulus (Aston-Jones et al., 1994). Third, the LC appears to play an important role in generating the P300 component of event-related potentials (ERPs) in squirrel monkeys (see Berridge, Arnsten, and Foote, 1993). Event-related potentials are signal components extracted from EEG recordings that are time-locked with respect to sensory, motor, or cognitive events (hence P300 means a positive-going waveform occurring approximately 300 ms after the triggering event). Because the P300 component in both humans and nonhuman primates has been associated with attentional mechanisms, involvement of the LC in its production fits well with the vigilance hypothesis. Finally, a number of behavioral studies have demonstrated that LC lesions or forebrain NE depletion produce performance deficits on learning tasks in which the animal must make a difficult sensory discrimination or when irrelevant (distracting) stimuli are presented during learning (Aston-Jones, 1985; Berridge, Arnsten, and Foote, 1993). Pharmacological studies suggest that α_2-receptors may be important in at least some of the cognitive/attentional functions of NE (Coull, 1994).

As a final point, it is interesting to note that retrograde tracing as well as electrophysiological experiments by Aston-Jones and coworkers (1986) found only two structures in the entire brain that provided major excitatory synaptic inputs to the LC: the nucleus paragigantocellularis (PGi) and the nucleus prepositus hypoglossi (PrH), both of which are located in the rostral medulla. The PGi was found to be particularly important in mediating the excitatory effects of various polymodal and noxious environmental stimuli on LC activity. Furthermore, additional connections from the PGi to the intermediolateral cell columns indicate that this nucleus may coregulate the LC and the sympathetic preganglionic neurons. These findings suggest that although the LC is influenced by diverse sensory and behavioral events, information about such events is preprocessed and is relayed to the noradrenergic system via a common pathway. Moreover, even though the LC affects widespread areas of the forebrain, there is no evidence of a reciprocal forebrain control mechanism.

Regulation of Hunger and Feeding Behavior

Feeding behavior is under complex neuroanatomical and neurochemical control. This should come as no surprise, considering that the system underlying this behavior must carefully integrate a variety of internal (i.e., metabolic) and external stimuli, and must further provide appropriate signals for both short-term and long-term regulation of ingestion. Although a number of different neurotransmitters and neuropeptides participate in the control of feeding and body weight regulation (Leibowitz, 1986, 1992), NE seems to play a pivotal role in this process. In order to fully understand the research on NE and feeding, it is first necessary to be aware of some of the relevant lesion studies that have attempted to delineate the neural (particularly hypothalamic) substrates underlying this behavior.

Classic experiments in the early 1940s showed that bilateral damage to the ventromedial area of the rat hypothalamus (VMH) caused a large increase in food intake (hyperphagia) and body weight gain (Brobeck, Tep-

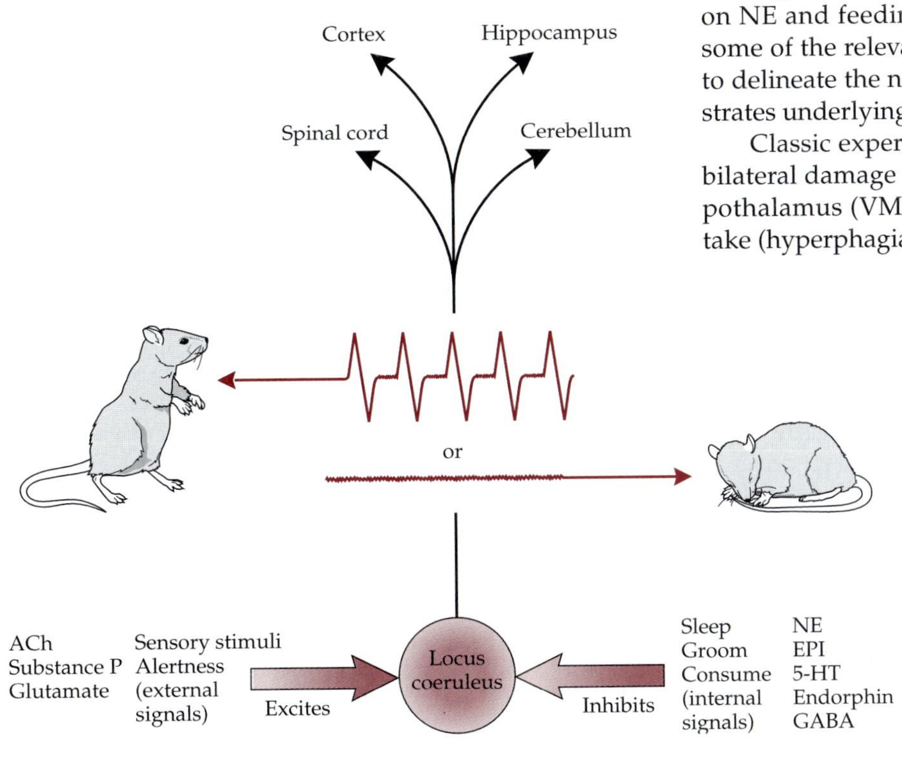

8.38 PROPOSED VIGILANCE FUNCTION OF THE LOCUS COERULEUS. The firing of LC neurons is activated by arousing sensory stimuli and inhibited during the performance of maintenance functions such as sleeping, grooming, and ingestive behaviors. From these and other findings, Aston-Jones has hypothesized that NE plays an important role in vigilance; that is, attentiveness to salient and relevant external stimuli. The structures shown at the top of the figure represent some of the projection areas of LC neurons (After Aston-Jones, 1985.)

perman, and Long, 1943; Hetherington and Ranson, 1940). These findings were initially interpreted to mean that the VMH is a "satiety center," the loss of which causes unabated hunger and hence overeating (Stellar, 1954). This view has been criticized on a number of grounds (see, for example, Powley, 1977); however, the important point here is that the work of Gold and colleagues (Gold, 1973; Gold et al., 1977) demonstrated that the hyperphagic and obesity-producing effects of typical, large VMH lesions are at least partly dependent on the destruction of a fiber pathway passing through that area. Moreover, this pathway was shown to originate in a nearby part of the hypothalamus, namely, the paraventricular nucleus (PVN). Studies conducted prior to that time had already shown that NE and other noradrenergic agonists injected directly into the hypothalamus of rats could elicit a robust eating response, even in previously satiated animals (Leibowitz, 1974a). Using a microinjection technique, Leibowitz (1978) then found that the PVN was the most sensitive site for noradrenergic stimulation of eating. These results fit well with the findings of Gold et al. and helped to establish NE and the PVN as important factors in the control of food intake.

The stimulatory effect of PVN NE on feeding is mediated by α_2-receptors, because it can be mimicked by the α_2-agonist clonidine and blocked by the administration of α_2-antagonists (reviewed by Wellman et al., 1993). The α_2-receptors appear to be postsynaptic and to mediate an inhibitory effect of NE on cells in the PVN (see the section above on the electrophysiological actions of adrenergic receptors). Studies by Leibowitz's group (Leibowitz, 1986, 1992) have identified a number of other important characteristics of this noradrenergic feeding system. First, if animals are allowed to select among pure macronutrient sources, activation of PVN α_2-receptors causes a rather specific enhancement of carbohydrate ingestion with little or no change in protein or fat consumption. Second, meal size and duration (rather than number of meals) are enhanced, which may indicate that the normal satiating effect of carbohydrates has been reduced. Third, NE concentration and α_2-receptor density in the PVN exhibit a circadian rhythm, with the highest levels occurring at the beginning of the dark period of the day–night cycle. In nocturnal species such as rats, this peak corresponds to a time of low energy stores and the onset of the primary period of food intake. Fourth, the influence of NE is potentiated by the neuropeptide NPY and also by corticosterone, an adrenal steroid hormone. The reader will recall that NPY is colocalized with NE in many noradrenergic fibers from the LC and is co-released from these fibers during periods of high activity. Corticosteroids have long been known to play an important physiological role in regulating carbohydrate metabolism. Finally, like NE, NPY and corticosterone exhibit circadian rhythms in phase with the onset of eating behavior. The relationships between these variables are illustrated in Figure 8.39. Such findings suggest that in rats, NE and NPY in the PVN may contribute importantly to the marked increase in carbohydrate consumption displayed at the onset of the dark phase of the light–dark cycle.

Although researchers have most extensively studied the role of hypothalamic α_2-receptors in eating behavior,

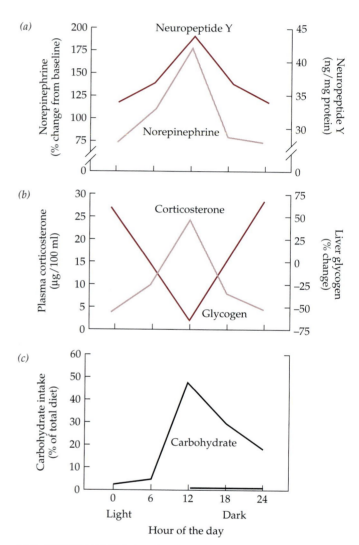

8.39 CIRCADIAN RHYTHMS OF NEUROTRANSMITTERS AND HORMONES IN RELATIONSHIP TO CARBOHYDRATE INTAKE. Application of NE to the paraventricular nucleus (PVN) of the hypothalamus stimulates eating behavior in rats. This effect is potentiated by neuropeptide Y (NPY) and the adrenal hormone corticosterone. (a) In normal untreated subjects, NE and NPY levels in the PVN exhibit a circadian rhythm with a peak at the beginning of the dark phase of the light–dark cycle (during which most food intake occurs). (b) At the same time, plasma corticosterone is also peaking, but liver glycogen stores are low. (c) Carbohydrate intake, which will replenish liver glycogen, is maximal at the beginning of the dark period. Although correlational, these results are consistent with the possibility that NE, NPY, and corticosterone are normally involved in stimulating food (particularly carbohydrate) ingestion at the onset of darkness in rats. (After Liebowitz, 1992.)

Wellman and colleagues (1993) have reviewed evidence for α_1-receptors in the PVN that suppress, rather than stimulate, food intake. Based on the overall α-receptor findings, Wellman and colleagues propose that a subset of PVN neurons gives rise to a descending inhibitory pathway that suppresses brain stem feeding centers. Excitatory α_1-receptors stimulate these neurons, thereby reducing subsequent food intake. However, the activation of inhibitory α_2-receptors on the cell membrane releases the brain stem feeding mechanism from the tonic braking effect of the PVN, thus allowing food intake to occur. The circadian rhythm in PVN α_2-receptors might help to explain how the balance between α_2-mediated eating and α_1-mediated intake suppression can vary across the sleep–waking cycle. However, the model still fails to account for the apparent macronutrient (i.e., carbohydrate) selectivity of the α_2-receptor system.

Part III Summary

Noradrenergic neurons are located in the pons and medulla and can be organized into three main clusters: the locus coeruleus complex (cell groups A6 and A4), the lateral tegmental system (groups A5, A7, and A1), and a dorsal medullary group (A2). The LC, which is the most prominent noradrenergic nucleus, projects rostrally to virtually all regions of the telencephalon and diencephalon, dorsally to the cerebellum, and caudally to the spinal cord. This broad innervation indicates that the LC is well situated to modulate a variety of important behavioral and physiological processes. One of the functions of the lateral tegmental system and dorsal medullary group is to provide noradrenergic input to the brain stem and spinal nuclei that control autonomic function. Noradrenergic neurons give rise to fine varicose fibers in their terminal areas. The existence of synaptic contacts associated with NE-containing varicosities has been a matter of some controversy.

In addition to the above-mentioned systems in the CNS, there also exist peripheral noradrenergic cells as well as central and peripheral cells that synthesize and release EPI. In the periphery, catecholaminergic cells are found in sympathetic ganglia (noradrenergic principal ganglion cells and adrenergic SIF cells) and in the adrenal medulla. The coexistence of NE and EPI with various neuropeptides such as enkephalin and NPY has been demonstrated in all of these cell types.

Adrenoceptors are divided into two broad families: α-receptors, which are relatively insensitive to the classic adrenergic agonist isoproterenol, and β-receptors, which are potently stimulated by that compound. Pharmacological and receptor cloning studies have given rise to further subdivision of these main groupings into α_1 (divided yet again into α_{1A}, α_{1B}, and α_{1D}), α_2 (α_{2A}, α_{2B}, etc.), and β_1, β_2, and β_3 subtypes (the last of which seems to be found only in certain peripheral organs). EPI has a much greater affinity than NE for β_2-receptors, which has suggested to some investigators that at least in peripheral tissues, this subtype may function mainly as a receptor for circulating EPI released from the adrenal gland. Some α_2-receptors are found on the terminals of central and peripheral noradrenergic fibers, where they serve as release-inhibiting autoreceptors. Somatodendritic α_2-autoreceptors inhibit the firing of LC neurons much like the D_2-autoreceptors found in the substantia nigra.

The α_1-receptors exert an excitatory postsynaptic effect by inhibiting a non-voltage-dependent K^+ current and thus eliciting a slow membrane depolarization. In contrast, α_2-receptors hyperpolarize the cell membrane by activating an inward-rectifying K^+ current. With respect to second messenger systems, α_1-receptors stimulate the phosphoinositide second messenger system and increase intracellular Ca^{2+} concentrations, whereas α_2-receptors inhibit cAMP formation. Activation of either β_1- or β_2-receptors increases cell excitability by inhibiting the slow afterhyperpolarization current. This effect seems to be related to activation of adenylyl cyclase and enhancement of cAMP synthesis.

It is worth noting that astrocytes possess both α- and β-receptors. Furthermore, astrocytic β-receptors are positively coupled to adenylyl cyclase and appear to stimulate glycogenolysis when activated. Neuropharmacologists are also interested in α_2-receptors on blood platelets and β_2-receptors on lymphocytes because these cells represent a readily available source of human adrenergic receptors for study and may reflect the status of central receptor populations.

When β-receptors are continuously exposed to an agonist, they rapidly desensitize due to an uncoupling of the receptor from G_s and adenylyl cyclase. This phenomenon is caused by phosphorylation of the receptor by two protein kinases, protein kinase A (PKA) and a separate β-adrenergic receptor kinase (βARK). Longer periods of agonist exposure (>1–2 hours) lead to down-regulation in which receptor binding sites are lost. Several processes contribute to β-receptor down-regulation, including decreased levels of receptor mRNA and increased receptor degradation. Along with the phenomena of desensitization and down-regulation, β-receptors also exhibit up-regulation in response to 6-OHDA-induced denervation.

Receptor subtype-selective adrenergic drugs have found widespread clinical usage. For example, because of their vasoconstrictive effects, α_1-agonists may be used for the maintenance of adequate blood pressure during anesthesia and for the relief of nasal congestion. In contrast, α_2-agonists are administered in the treatment of hypertension. The α_2-agonist clonidine is also used in the management of drug withdrawal symptoms, for the treatment of glaucoma, and even as an analgesic agent. β_2-agonists have proved particularly valuable in producing bronchial relaxation in people suffering from asthma or certain other respiratory disorders. Finally, β-receptor blockers are used clinically in the treatment of various cardiac conditions and also to reduce some of the somatic symptoms associated with strong anxiety.

Electrophysiological and behavioral studies of the LC suggest that this noradrenergic cell group plays an important role in processes of attention, arousal, and vigilance. First, recording of LC neurons in unrestrained rats has shown that the cells fire at a slower rate during SWS than during waking and become almost completely silent during REM sleep. Moreover, cell firing is also inhibited during the performance of maintenance behaviors such as grooming, but it is robustly stimulated by sensory stimuli of almost every modality. Other experiments have found that (1) application of NE to cortical and hippocampal neurons enhanced the overall "signal-to-noise" ratio of cellular responsivity, (2) the LC is involved in generation of the P300 component of event-related potentials, and (3) LC lesions or forebrain NE depletion produce learning deficits in tasks requiring a high level of attention. Based on these findings, Aston-Jones has proposed that the LC noradrenergic system regulates an organism's level of vigilance; that is, attention and behavioral reactivity to salient external stimuli.

Norepinephrine also seems to be critically involved in processes of hunger and satiety. Studies by Leibowitz and others have found that NE in the paraventricular nucleus (PVN) of the hypothalamus acts on α_2-receptors to stimulate eating behavior even in previously satiated animals. This effect is manifested by increases in meal size and duration, and is directed primarily to carbohydrate consumption rather than protein or fat. Neuropeptide Y (NPY), a peptide colocalized with NE in many noradrenergic fibers, potentiates the influence of NE on feeding. Furthermore, NE and NPY concentrations, as well as the density of α_2-receptors in the PVN, exhibit a circadian rhythm in which the peak coincides with the beginning of the dark period, when rats normally begin their main period of daily food consumption. Finally, there is some evidence that activation of PVN α_1-receptors suppresses rather than enhances eating behavior. Thus, NE in the PVN appears to exert complex effects on food intake that vary depending on the receptor subtype involved.

Chapter 9

Serotonin

The discovery of serotonin can be traced to its presence in the blood and in the gastrointestinal tract. As far back as 1868, investigators knew that the serum of clotted blood contained a factor capable of producing vasoconstriction. The identity of this factor, however, remained unknown for many years. Beginning in the 1930s, Page and his colleagues began to look for vasoconstrictive, blood-borne substances that might be responsible for cardiovascular hypertension. Turning their attention to the still-unidentified serum factor, they eventually isolated it and named it *serotonin* to indicate its origin from blood *serum* and its effect on vascular muscle *tone* (Rapport, Green, and Page, 1948). Meanwhile, Erspamer had independently discovered a substance in gastric mucosa that likewise exerted a contractile effect on vascular and other smooth muscles (Erspamer, 1940). This substance was initially called "enteramine" because it was secreted by enterochromaffin cells of the gastrointestinal tract. Later, enteramine and serotonin were found to be identical (Erspamer and Asero, 1952), and this compound is now referred to exclusively as serotonin.

Further investigation demonstrated the presence of this substance in the blood and intestinal tract of virtually every vertebrate species, as well as in the tissues of numerous invertebrates such as sea anemones, planarians, leeches, lobsters, crabs, octopuses, squids, wasps, and scorpions (Essman, 1978). It is also found in many plants and fruits, particularly pineapples and bananas.

Studies with humans, dogs, and rats showed that serotonin is widely distributed in different organ systems (Twarog and Page, 1953). It is found not only in blood serum and in the digestive tract, but also in the spleen, liver, lungs, and skin. Most important to neuropharmacologists, it is also present in the nervous system. Ninety percent of the serotonin in the human body is believed to exist in the mucous membranes of the gastrointestinal system, 8% to 10% in the blood platelets (which release their serotonin during the clotting process), and 1% to 2% in the central nervous system. Another notable location of high serotonin concentrations is the pineal gland, where the compound serves as a precursor for the pineal hormone melatonin.

The discovery of serotonin in the nervous system naturally raised the possibility that the compound might serve as a neurotransmitter. Welsh found several molluscan preparations, such as the *Venus mercenaria* clam heart, to be exquisitely sensitive to serotonin, and he subsequently proposed a neurohumoral role for this substance in invertebrates (Welsh, 1957). Meanwhile, other investigators reported that the potent hallucinogenic drug lysergic acid diethylamide (LSD) antagonized the contractile effect of serotonin on smooth muscle (Gaddum, 1953), that the early antipsychotic drug reserpine significantly reduced brain serotonin content (Pletscher, Shore, and Brodie, 1955), and that platelet serotonin levels were altered by the antidepressants imipramine and iproniazid (Marshall et al., 1960).

These findings sparked tremendous interest in the possible involvement of serotonin in abnormal behavioral functioning and in the actions of psychotropic drugs that either induce or ameliorate such abnormalities. Nevertheless, the acceptance of serotonin as a bona fide transmitter did not come until (1) the substance was shown to be unevenly distributed in the brain and then later visualized within specific populations of nerve cells and their projections; (2) metabolic pathways for its synthesis and inactivation were demonstrated in the brain; (3) it was shown to be released under physiological conditions; and (4) it was found to mimic the action of the endogenous transmitter at identified synapses. As we shall see, a prodigious amount of research carried out over the past 30 years has clearly established serotonin as a major neurotransmitter subserving a number of important physiological and psychological functions. Readers interested in a broad survey of the serotonergic system are referred to the recent review by Jacobs and Azmitia (1992).

Part I
Serotonin Neurochemistry: Synthesis, Storage, Release, and Inactivation

Shortly after the discovery of serotonin, its chemical identity was elucidated and the compound was synthesized. Serotonin is an indolealkylamine that is chemically designated 3-(2-aminoethyl)indol-5-ol, but ordinarily goes by the name **5-hydroxytryptamine (5-HT)**. The chemical structure of 5-HT reveals its close relationship to the amino acid tryptophan, which serves as the dietary precursor of the neurotransmitter.

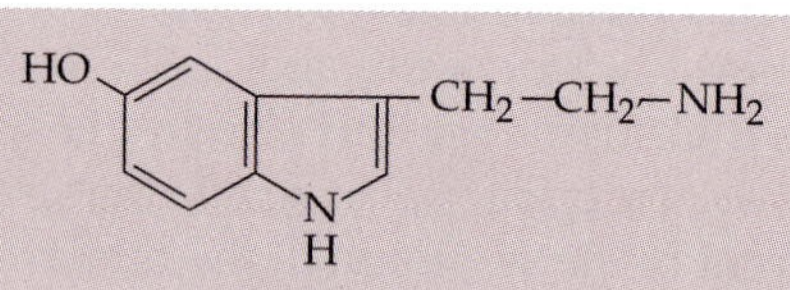

Serotonin

Figure 9.1 diagrams an idealized serotonergic nerve terminal and synapse. Included in the diagram are some of the important processes that occur at these terminals, including synthesis of 5-HT, transport of 5-HT into synaptic vesicles, release of 5-HT, interaction of 5-HT with postsynaptic receptors, and 5-HT reuptake and metabolism. Also shown are a few of the drugs that can interact with these processes. In general, substances that stimulate release, block reuptake, or inhibit metabolism of 5-HT act acutely as serotonergic agonists, whereas compounds that block 5-HT synthesis or disrupt its storage function as serotonergic antagonists. Of course, serotonergic functioning can also be influenced by drugs that act directly on the postsynaptic receptors.

Serotonin Synthesis

Tryptophan Hydroxylase

The pathway for 5-HT synthesis and degradation is shown in Figure 9.2. The first, and rate-limiting, step in the pathway involves hydroxylation of L-tryptophan in the 5-position to form 5-hydroxytryptophan (5-HTP). This reaction is catalyzed by the enzyme tryptophan-5'-monooxygenase, commonly known as tryptophan hydroxylase. In the nervous system, this enzyme is specifically localized in serotonergic neurons and serves as a marker for such cells. The reaction catalyzed by tryptophan hydroxylase requires a reduced pterin cofactor and molecular oxygen. The cofactor in vivo is tetrahydrobiopterin (BH_4), although the synthetic cofactors 6-methyl-tetrahydropterin ($6-MPH_4$) and 6,7-dimethyl-tetrahydropterin ($DMPH_4$) are sometimes used to assay enzyme activity experimentally.

The mRNAs coding for tryptophan hydroxylase in the rat brain and pineal gland have been characterized (Darmon et al., 1988; Kim et al., 1991). Messenger RNAs from the two tissues encode an identical protein with a molecular weight of approximately 51 kDa. This protein probably represents the basic subunit of the enzyme, since previous biochemical studies suggest that native tryptophan hydroxylase consists of four subunits with a full molecular weight of over 200 kDa (Kuhn and Lovenberg, 1983). The presence of the same tryptophan hydroxylase mRNA in both the brain and the pineal gland is somewhat surprising, considering that many differences in its enzymatic properties have been found in the two tissues. This finding raises the possibility of differential posttranslational modification of the enzyme in different cell types.

Tryptophan hydroxylase is synthesized in serotonergic nerve cell bodies and undergoes axonal transport to the nerve terminals, where most of the 5-HT synthesis occurs (Meek and Neff, 1972). Following subcellular fractionation of pig brain stem, about 65% of the enzyme activity was found in the particulate fraction and 25% in the soluble fraction (Moussa, Youdim, and Bourgoin, 1974). Given the presence of synaptosomes in the particulate fraction, this distribution is consistent with a high concentration of tryptophan hydroxylase in serotonergic nerve endings.

Tryptophan Hydroxylase Inhibitors

Several drugs have been discovered that inhibit tryptophan hydroxylase and consequently lead to a depletion of 5-HT. These drugs include 6-fluorotryptophan, α-*n*-propyldopacetamide (H22/54), and *p*-chloroamphetamine (PCA), which is better known as a 5-HT releasing agent (see below). The classic tryptophan hydroxylase inhibitor, however, is *p*-chlorophenylalanine (PCPA), a drug that has been used in numerous studies elucidating

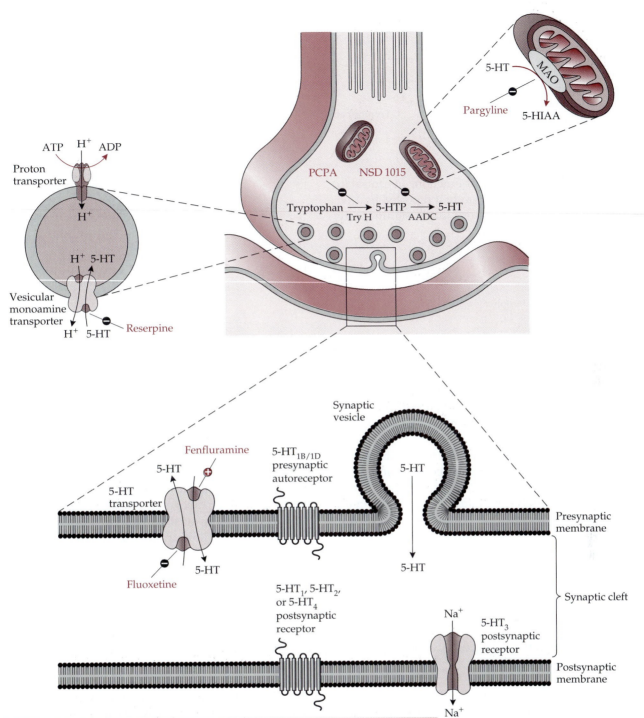

Receptor subtype	Agonists	Antagonists
5-HT$_{1A}$	8-OH-DPAT, buspirone, ipsapirone	SDZ 216-525, WAY-100135
5-HT$_{1B}$	CP-93,129, RU 24969, m-CPP	5-(Nonyloxy)tryptamine, sumatriptan
5-HT$_2$	DOM, MK212 (partially 5-HT$_{2B}$-selective), *m*-CPP (partially 5-HT$_{2C}$-selective)	Ketanserin, ritanserin, mesulergine (partially 5-HT$_{2C}$-selective)
5-HT$_3$	*m*-Chlorophenylbiguanide	Ondansetron
5-HT$_4$	n-Butyl renzapride	GR113808

9.1 THE SEROTONERGIC SYNAPSE, illustrating the processes of serotonin (5-HT) synthesis and metabolism, presynaptic and vesicular 5-HT uptake, and vesicular 5-HT release. Pre- and postsynaptic 5-HT receptors and sites of action of some serotonergic drugs are also shown. The table lists some important serotonergic agonists and antagonists. See the text for details and explanations of the abbreviations.

9.2 SYNTHESIS OF SEROTONIN.
Serotonin (5-HT) is synthesized from the amino acid tryptophan in two steps catalyzed by the enzymes tryptophan hydroxylase and aromatic L-amino acid decarboxylase. The cofactor for each reaction is also shown.

the behavioral and physiological functions of central 5-HT. The properties of PCPA were first reported by Koe and Weissman (1966), who found that it significantly

depleted stores of 5-HT and its metabolite 5-HIAA in the brain, peripheral tissues, and blood. They also reported that PCPA blocked the increase in brain 5-HT induced by pargyline (a monoamine oxidase inhibitor) and by tryptophan loading. Tryptophan uptake was not prevented, however, suggesting that PCPA acts on the hydroxylating enzyme itself.

PCPA acts in two stages. The first stage of inhibition occurs rapidly and may result from competition of the drug with tryptophan for the substrate binding site. However, this competitive inhibition declines over a period of hours as brain levels of PCPA fall. The second, longer-lasting stage of tryptophan hydroxylase inhibition comes into play within 1 day following PCPA treatment. This irreversible inhibition prevents replenishment of 5-HT until sufficient amounts of new enzyme have been synthesized by the serotonergic neurons (Sanders-Bush, Gallagher, and Sulser, 1974). Indeed, brain 5-HT levels in rats may be depressed by 80% to 90% and may not return to normal for as long as 2 weeks following a single 300 mg/kg dose of PCPA.

5-Hydroxytryptophan Decarboxylation

The product of tryptophan hydroxylation—namely, 5-HTP—undergoes rapid decarboxylation to form 5-HT. This step is analogous to the decarboxylation of DOPA to form dopamine. Some early studies (for example, Sims and Bloom, 1973) suggested the existence of a specific 5-HTP decarboxylase, distinct from the decarboxylating enzyme present in catecholaminergic cells. The current view, however, is that aromatic L-amino acid decarboxylase (AADC) catalyzes both reactions. There may be isoforms of AADC that differ in their activity toward 5-HTP and DOPA (Boadle-Biber, 1993), thus accounting for the earlier controversy. As mentioned in the previous chapter, AADC is a soluble protein that requires pyridoxal 5′-phosphate as a cofactor. The rapid rate of 5-HTP

decarboxylation means that only low concentrations of this intermediate are present in the brain under normal circumstances. Like DOPA, however, 5-HTP accumulates following injection of the AADC inhibitor NSD 1015, which can be useful in assessing tryptophan hydroxylation rates in vivo (see below).

In the brain, one would expect to find AADC activity in serotonin- and catecholamine-containing neurons because of its obligatory role in the synthesis of these neurotransmitters. Jaeger and her colleagues confirmed this prediction for most monoaminergic cell groups by means of AADC immunohistochemistry (Jaeger, Ruggiero, Albert, Park, et al. 1984). However, these investigators also found evidence for AADC-immunoreactive neurons that were negative for both tyrosine hydroxylase and 5-HT. It is tempting to speculate that such cells may directly decarboxylate certain amino acids without prior hydroxylation. For example, the decarboxylation of tryptophan, tyrosine, and phenylalanine leads to the formation of tryptamine, p-tyramine, and β-phenylethylamine, respectively. These so-called "trace amines" are all found in the brain and have been postulated, in certain instances, to serve as either neurotransmitters or neuromodulators (Dabadie, Mons, and Geffard, 1990; Dyck, 1989; Paterson, Juorio, and Boulton, 1990).

Regulation of Serotonin Synthesis

Tryptophan hydroxylase activation.   As in the case of the catecholamine transmitters (see Chapter 8), a number of control mechanisms operate to regulate 5-HT synthesis (Boadle-Biber, 1993). Some of these involve alterations in the activation state of tryptophan hydroxylase, which is not surprising given that this enzyme is the rate-limiting step in the biosynthetic pathway. To begin, there is considerable evidence that tryptophan hydroxylase activity and the rate of 5-HT formation are governed by the level of firing in serotonergic neurons. Electrical stimulation increases both tryptophan hydroxylase activity (Boadle-Biber et al., 1986; Figure 9.3) and in vivo conversion of tryptophan to 5-HTP (Duda and Moore, 1985). Depolarization-induced activation of tryptophan hydroxylase appears to be calcium-dependent and to involve phosphorylation of the enzyme by Ca^{2+}/calmodulin-dependent protein kinase II (CaM-K II) (Boadle-Biber and Phan, 1987; Kuhn and Lovenberg, 1982). The kinetic effects of depolarization or direct enzyme phosphorylation have been a matter of contention. Various investigators have reported increases in the maximum velocity of the reaction (V_{max}), decreases in the Michaelis constant (K_m) (and hence increases in the affinity) for the substrate and/or pterin cofactor, or combinations of both V_{max} and K_m changes (Boadle-Biber et al., 1986; Kuhn and Lovenberg, 1982, 1983).

A role for cyclic AMP (cAMP) in tryptophan hydroxylase activation has not been definitely established at this time. However, studies by Fujisawa and colleagues suggest that phosphorylation of the enzyme by cAMP-dependent protein kinase produces a significant stimulatory effect (Makita, Okuno, and Fujisawa, 1990). This research group has also shown that both Ca^{2+}/calmodulin-mediated and cAMP-mediated stimulation of tryptophan hydroxylase require a so-called "activator protein," which was characterized several years ago (Ichimura et al., 1987; Makita, Okuno, and Fujisawa, 1990).

Regulation of serotonin synthesis by firing rate also operates in the opposite direction—namely, during reductions in neuronal activity. Research in this area has recently been facilitated by the use of the drug 8-hydroxy-2-(di-*n*-propylamino)-tetralin (8-OH-DPAT), a potent agonist at 5-HT$_{1A}$ receptors. Somatodendritic 5-HT autoreceptors appear to be of the 5-HT$_{1A}$ subtype (see below), and stimulation of these receptors consequently suppresses the firing of serotonergic neurons. Several studies have demonstrated that 8-OH-DPAT administration inhibits 5-HT synthesis, presumably due to the drug's influence on cellular activity (Fernstrom, Massoudi, and Fernstrom, 1990; Invernizzi et al., 1991). Although the mechanism underlying this effect has not yet been determined, the results are consistent with a reduction in the V_{max} of tryptophan hydroxylase (Fernstrom, Massoudi, and Fernstrom, 1990). Perhaps the phosphorylation state of the enzyme is reduced when neuronal firing diminishes, thus accounting for the kinetic change hypothesized by these investigators.

Chapter 8 discussed the importance of end-product inhibition of tyrosine hydroxylase by catecholamines such as norepinephrine (NE) and dopamine (DA). However, there is no convincing evidence that a similar process normally occurs with 5-HT and tryptophan hydroxylase.

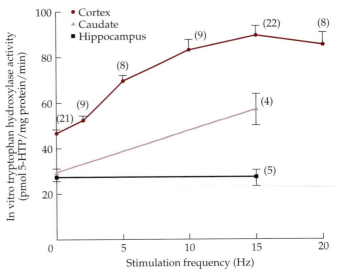

9.3 EFFECT OF ELECTRICAL STIMULATION ON TRYPTOPHAN HYDROXYLASE ACTIVITY. The serotonergic neuron-containing dorsal raphe nucleus was stimulated in anesthetized rats at the frequencies shown. Brain tissues were removed and assayed for tryptophan hydroxylase activity in both stimulated animals and sham-stimulated controls (0 Hz). Neuronal activation resulted in a significant increase in enzyme activity in the cerebral cortex and caudate nucleus, both of which receive projections from the dorsal raphe. The hippocampus, which is innervated by a different serotonergic cell group, was unaffected by the treatment. The values in parentheses represent the numbers of animals tested in each condition. (After Boadle-Biber et al., 1986.)

Tryptophan availability. The issue of enzyme saturation and its relationship to neurotransmitter synthesis was first considered with respect to acetylcholine formation (see Chapter 7), and then further developed in the case of tyrosine hydroxylase and catecholamine synthesis (Chapter 8). The analogous question for 5-HT is whether tryptophan hydroxylase is saturated with its substrates (tryptophan and oxygen) and cofactor (BH$_4$), and consequently, whether changes in the levels of these compounds in vivo alter the rate of 5-HT synthesis. Here we will discuss tryptophan only, although BH$_4$ and oxygen availability may also influence tryptophan hydroxylation (Boadle-Biber, 1993).

Using the natural cofactor of tryptophan hydroxylase (i.e., BH$_4$), investigators have reported K_m values as low as 14 µM for tryptophan (reviewed by Kuhn, Wolf, and Youdim, 1986). Furthermore, by pharmacologically manipulating brain tryptophan concentrations and measuring the corresponding changes in rates of tryptophan hydroxylation, Carlsson and Lindqvist (1978) determined an in vivo K_m of approximately 25 µM. If tryptophan hydroxylase in serotonergic nerve terminals is normally exposed to tryptophan concentrations that are below, or do not greatly exceed, the estimated K_m value, then changes in tryptophan availability should lead to significant alterations in 5-HT synthesis. The concentration of tryptophan in rat brain ranges from 10 to 30 μM, depending on the area (Leathwood, 1987). Given that these values are close to the apparent K_m, it would appear that tryptophan hydroxylase is not saturated with tryptophan.

Before this assumption is accepted uncritically, however, it is important to note that *tissue* measurements generally involve a mixture of both serotonergic and nonserotonergic cells. Do such measurements accurately reflect the concentration of tryptophan within serotonergic neurons? All cells in the brain must take up tryptophan for incorporation into cellular proteins. It is not entirely clear, however, whether the same tryptophan uptake process is used for protein synthesis and for 5-HT formation. Two distinct transport systems for tryptophan have been described in brain slices and synaptosomes. One is a high-affinity, low-capacity system, whereas the other has low affinity and high capacity. The low-affinity mechanism may simply represent passive diffusion of tryptophan across the cell membrane (Denizeau and Sourkes, 1977). Moreover, Mandell and Knapp (1977) found that the high-affinity system had greater selectivity for tryptophan and appeared to be closely linked to the process of tryptophan hydroxylation. If this high-affinity system were unique to serotonergic neurons, then these cells might be able to achieve higher intracellular concentrations of tryptophan than other brain cells. However, the regional distribution of high-affinity tryptophan uptake did not closely parallel other markers of serotonergic function (Mandell and Knapp, 1977), and lesion studies attempting to link the high-affinity uptake system with serotonergic pathways yielded conflicting results (Denizeau and Sourkes, 1978; Kuhar, Roth, and Aghajanian, 1972). Current evidence, therefore, does not support the existence of a specialized tryptophan uptake system in serotonergic nerve terminals.

Given the above considerations, it is reasonable to conclude that tryptophan hydroxylase is not saturated in vivo and that 5-HT synthesis is regulated partially by the level of brain tryptophan. This was confirmed over 20 years ago by Fernstrom and Wurtman (1971), who demonstrated that a single intraperitoneal injection of tryptophan at a dose of 12.5 mg/kg or higher elevated not only plasma and brain tryptophan concentrations, but also brain 5-HT levels in rats. There is now ample evidence from several different species, including humans, that increasing the availability of tryptophan increases the rate of 5-HT formation (Diksic et al., 1991; Gillman et al., 1981; Lookingland et al., 1986; Westerink and De Vries, 1991). It is possible that the extra 5-HT synthesized following tryptophan loading is simply metabolized intraneuronally, and some investigators have indeed argued that tryptophan administration does not lead to increased 5-HT release (see Kuhn, Wolf, and Youdim, 1986). However, recent work suggests that tryptophan-

induced enhancement of 5-HT synthesis is accompanied by a Ca^{2+}-dependent, tetrodotoxin-sensitive stimulation of 5-HT release, and therefore is functionally relevant for the organism (Carboni et al., 1989; Schaechter and Wurtman, 1989; Westerink and De Vries, 1991). Figure 9.4 presents results from cerebral microdialysis showing a stimulation of both synthesis and release of 5-HT following systemic tryptophan injection.

Dietary manipulations.   Tryptophan is an essential amino acid, which means that it cannot be synthesized by humans and therefore must be supplied in the diet. Given the fact that tryptophan administration can stimulate 5-HT synthesis and release, is it possible that brain 5-HT metabolism might be affected by what we eat? Animal and plant proteins provide the major source of tryptophan in our diet. One might expect, therefore, that brain 5-HT would be elevated following ingestion of a high-protein meal. However, when previously fasted rats were fed a meal containing significant amounts of

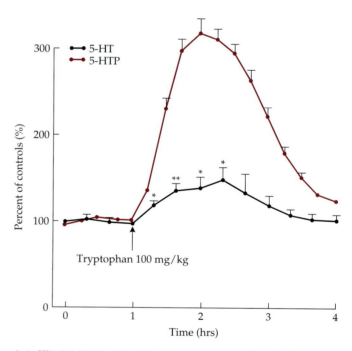

9.4 STIMULATION OF SEROTONIN SYNTHESIS AND RELEASE BY TRYPTOPHAN ADMINISTRATION. Rats were implanted with microdialysis probes in the caudate nucleus (striatum). For the synthesis experiments, the aromatic amino acid decarboxylase inhibitor NSD 1015 (10 μM) was infused through the probe to permit accumulation and efflux of 5-HTP as a measure of in vivo tryptophan hydroxylation rate. To examine 5-HT release, NSD 1015 was omitted. However, in this case, the perfusate contained the 5-HT uptake inhibitor imipramine (30 μM) to increase the basal concentration of extracellular 5-HT to a detectable level. When subjects were injected intraperitoneally with tryptophan (arrow), there was a significant augmentation of tryptophan hydroxylation and 5-HT release lasting over 1 hour (*$p < .05$, **$p < .01$ compared with basal values of 5-HT). (After Westerink and De Vries, 1991.)

the protein casein, brain tryptophan and 5-HT concentrations did not rise, even though the level of tryptophan in the plasma was elevated following the meal (Fernstrom and Wurtman, 1972a).

To find out why protein ingestion failed to increase brain 5-HT synthesis, Fernstrom and Wurtman fed some animals mixtures of tryptophan and other pure amino acids. Under these conditions, the tryptophan-induced rise in brain tryptophan and 5-HT was blocked by inclusion of the amino acids leucine, isoleucine, valine, phenylalanine, and tyrosine. These so-called large neutral amino acids (LNAA) share a common blood–brain barrier transport system with tryptophan (Pardridge, 1984). Consequently, the investigators proposed that when circulating tryptophan levels are increased along with levels of other amino acids (as following a protein-containing meal), competition for the LNAA transport system prevents the extra tryptophan from entering the brain and stimulating 5-HT formation. According to this view, it is the *ratio* between tryptophan and the sum of the competing amino acids, not tryptophan concentration alone, that is important in determining the rate of 5-HT synthesis (Figure 9.5).

Fernstrom and Wurtman (1972a) did not merely show that brain 5-HT concentrations are not elevated by protein ingestion. They also made the intriguing observation that 5-HT can be increased by a high-carbohydrate, low-protein meal! This phenomenon can be explained by the joint influence of two factors: the effect of carbohydrates on insulin secretion, and tryptophan binding to blood albumin. In a fasted animal or human, intake of carbohydrates (sugar or starches) provokes a surge of insulin secretion. The insulin, in turn, stimulates transport of sugar, free fatty acids, and amino acids from the plasma into various tissues such as skeletal muscle. Plasma concentrations of leucine, isoleucine, valine, phenylalanine, and tyrosine therefore decline under these conditions. In contrast, the plasma tryptophan concentration following insulin administration either does not change (Daniel et al., 1981) or actually increases (Fernstrom and Wurtman, 1972b). This probably occurs because 80% to 90% of circulating tryptophan is bound (noncovalently) to blood albumin, and this protein-bound fraction is not readily transported into peripheral tissues. Other amino acids do not share this property, and therefore can be influenced by changes in insulin levels. It can readily be seen that by stimulating insulin release, a high-carbohydrate meal will increase the value of the critical fraction—plasma tryptophan concentration divided by the sum of the concentrations of the competing amino acids—thereby facilitating tryptophan entry into the brain and increasing brain 5-HT synthesis (see Figure 9.5).

Most studies on the relationship between diet and 5-HT have examined the effect of varying only a single meal. However, Fernstrom and Fernstrom (1995) recently investigated the influence of sequential meals on

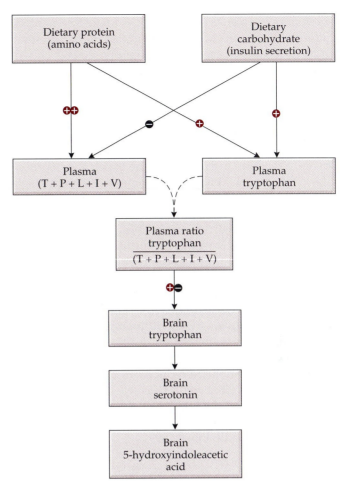

9.5 PROPOSED MODEL OF DIET-INDUCED CHANGES IN BRAIN SEROTONIN SYNTHESIS. According to this model, diet-induced alterations in the ratio of the plasma tryptophan concentration to the sum of the concentrations of tyrosine (T), phenylalanine (P), leucine (L), isoleucine (I), and valine (V) lead to increased or decreased brain tryptophan and 5-HT levels. (After Fernstrom and Wurtman, 1972a.)

brain tryptophan concentration and 5-HT synthesis in previously fasted rats. The results showed that if a protein-containing meal was followed by a carbohydrate-only meal, the second meal could stimulate brain 5-HT synthesis as long as a sufficient interval (in this case, 3 hours) was allowed to elapse between feedings. On the other hand, when a carbohydrate-only meal was followed by a protein-containing meal 2 hours later, the carbohydrate-induced stimulation of 5-HT synthesis was reversed by the second meal. These results are important in showing that the effects of diet extend beyond a single feeding period.

The discovery that meal composition can significantly influence neurotransmitter synthesis was a startling revelation. Researchers had previously assumed that signaling mechanisms in the brain would be relatively impervious to the vagaries of one's diet (Fernstrom and Wurtman, 1974). Indeed, the purpose of the serotonergic system's responsiveness to dietary manipulations still remains to be demonstrated, although some provocative hypotheses have been proposed (which will be discussed later in the chapter). Nevertheless, the excitement surrounding this link between 5-HT and food intake must be tempered by several considerations. Most of the results cited above were obtained from previously fasted rats fed a single meal high in carbohydrates but low in protein. If the rats are not fasted ahead of time to lower circulating insulin levels, the experiments probably will not work as indicated (some investigators have even found that tryptophan loading is not very effective in stimulating 5-HT release unless subjects are previously food-deprived: Schwartz, Hernandez, and Hoebel, 1990b). The same is true if the animals are fed a more balanced meal containing both carbohydrate and protein, because the added competing amino acids from the dietary protein will negate the effect of the meal-induced insulin surge. Finally, studies have shown that brain 5-HT is unrelated to long-term differences in dietary protein content unless the protein level is extremely low. Under such a situation of protein malnourishment, brain 5-HT concentrations are reduced rather than elevated (see Fernstrom, 1988a, 1990). Thus, we must be very cautious not to extend the relationship between meal composition and 5-HT synthesis beyond a very restricted set of conditions (Boadle-Biber, 1993).

Serotonin Storage and Release

Mechanisms of Storage and Release

Although some 5-HT is present in the cytoplasm of serotonergic cell bodies and nerve terminals, most of the neurotransmitter is stored in vesicles. Identified serotonergic nerve terminals have generally been found to contain many large dense-core vesicles 70–120 nm in diameter, as well as some 40–60 nm electron-lucent (clear) vesicles (Maley et al., 1990). The transmitter is believed to be stored in the large dense-core granules, which leaves the function of the smaller, clear vesicles in question. As mentioned in the previous chapter, 5-HT is accumulated in storage vesicles via a membrane transporter that appears to be identical to that found in catecholaminergic neurons. Consequently, reserpine and tetrabenazine block 5-HT vesicular uptake and deplete brain 5-HT as well as DA and NE.

Brain serotonergic neurons, as well as peripheral 5-HT-concentrating cells that originate embryologically from the neural crest, contain a protein that binds 5-HT with high affinity (Tamir and Gershon, 1990). This serotonin-binding protein (SBP) exists in three forms, with apparent molecular weights of 45, 56, and 68 kDa. Recent findings suggest that the 45-kDa SBP is selectively packaged in secretory vesicles and is released with 5-HT in the process of exocytosis (Tamir et al., 1994).

Metabolic studies suggest that two different pools of 5-HT are present in the serotonergic neurons (Morot-Gaudry, Bourgoin, and Hamon, 1981; Tracqui et al., 1983). A small pool comprising 10% to 25% of brain 5-HT, which is considered to be the functional pool, contains the newly synthesized and preferentially released transmitter. In contrast, a large pool containing 75% to 90% of the total neuronal 5-HT content is thought of as a storage or reserve pool. The problem with this view, however, is that no one has yet successfully linked these biochemically defined compartments with actual physical sites of 5-HT occupancy such as the cytoplasm or vesicles.

The mechanism of 5-HT release is usually assumed to be exocytosis (for review, see Sanders-Bush and Martin, 1982), although the evidence for this hypothesis is not as complete as for the model systems discussed in Chapter 6. Evoked 5-HT release, measured either in vitro from brain slices or in vivo by means of cerebral microdialysis, is sensitive to the sodium (Na^+) channel blocker tetrodotoxin and to the presence of Ca^{2+} ions (Auerbach, Minzenberg, and Wilkinson, 1989; Carboni et al., 1989; Schaechter and Wurtman, 1989; Sharp, Bramwell, Clark, et al., 1989). These properties are consistent with, but do not prove, an exocytotic mechanism. One of the most convincing means of demonstrating such a mechanism is to show the co-release of one or more substances present with the transmitter inside the storage vesicles. For example, co-release of 5-HT and SBP has been demonstrated in several types of 5-HT-containing cells (Jonakait et al., 1979; Tamir et al., 1994). Co-release of 5-HT with other vesicular components has also been studied in blood platelets, which are discussed in a later section, and parafollicular cells of the thyroid gland. These cells, which are neural crest–derived and which express many of the characteristics of serotonergic neurons, possess secretory granules that contain 5-HT and SBP along with the peptide hormone calcitonin (Barasch et al., 1987). Given that exocytosis is the accepted mechanism for peptide secretion (see Chapter 11), we may surmise that 5-HT is likewise released exocytotically from the parafollicular cells. These model systems thus provide some indication that 5-HT is not only stored in vesicles, but is also physiologically released from the vesicular pool by a process of exocytosis.

Serotonin-Releasing Drugs

A number of drugs have been found that stimulate 5-HT release. Reserpine and tetrabenazine possess this action, although the effect is secondary to their disruption of vesicular storage. More important both experimentally and clinically are the substituted amphetamines. D-amphetamine and methamphetamine were described in Chapter 8 as classic catecholamine-releasing agents. Various substituents on the phenyl ring give rise to drugs with potent 5-HT-releasing properties, such as *p*-chloroamphetamine (PCA), *p*-fluoroamphetamine, *p*-chloromethamphetamine, *p*-methoxyamphetamine, and fenfluramine. These agents act as serotonergic agonists, although their effects are blocked by pretreatment with the tryptophan hydroxylase inhibitor PCPA and are thus dependent on endogenous 5-HT.

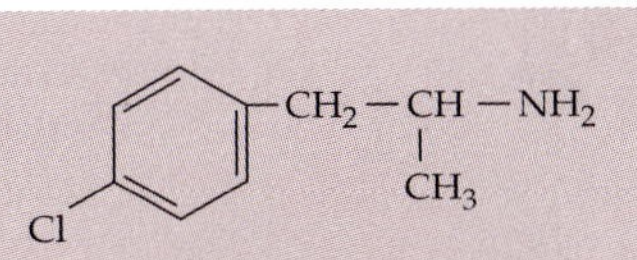

p-Chloroamphetamine

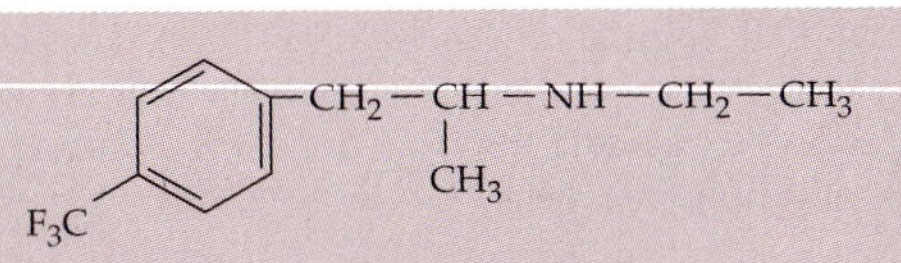

though their effects are blocked by pretreatment with the tryptophan hydroxylase inhibitor PCPA and are thus dependent on endogenous 5-HT.

Fenfluramine

The best-characterized and most widely used 5-HT-releasing drugs are PCA and fenfluramine. Both compounds stimulate a variety of serotonergic behavioral and physiological functions, and both have been used extensively in animal studies (Fuller, 1992). Fenfluramine is also used clinically as an appetite suppressant because of the influence of 5-HT on food intake (see below). This is despite the fact that in certain animal models, PCA and fenfluramine exert toxic effects on certain serotonergic neurons, thus leading to long-lasting reductions in brain 5-HT levels. The neurotoxicity of these drugs is discussed in more detail in a later section.

Current evidence indicates that substituted amphetamines induce 5-HT release mainly by a nonexocytotic mechanism (Carboni and Di Chiara, 1989). Consistent with this view, vesicular disruption by reserpine failed to prevent behavioral activation following systemic PCA treatment, despite 90% to 95% reductions in 5-HT concentrations in serotonergic projection areas (Kuhn, Wolf, and Youdim, 1985). The parent compound of PCA, amphetamine, has similarly been shown to release DA from a reserpine-resistant pool (Langer and Arbilla, 1984). Based on these results, it is likely that fenfluramine, PCA, and related compounds release 5-HT from the cytoplasmic compartment. The mechanism of release may be transporter-mediated exchange, in which the membrane 5-HT uptake system (see below) transports the drug into the nerve cell and carries 5-HT from the inside to the outside (Gu and Azmitia, 1993; Rudnick and Wall, 1992). This hypothesis is consistent with earlier observations that the action of 5-HT releasers can be prevented by pretreatment with drugs that inhibit synaptic 5-HT reuptake (Sanders-Bush and Martin, 1982). Such reverse transport of a neurotransmitter has been strongly implicated in the catecholamine-releasing effects of amphetamine (see discussion in Chapter 13).

Regulation of Serotonin Release by Autoreceptors

As in the case of many other transmitters, 5-HT release is regulated by the action of inhibitory autoreceptors (see reviews by Göthert, 1990; Sharp and Hjorth, 1990; Starke, Göthert, and Kilbinger, 1989). The idea that autoreceptors might exist on serotonergic neurons began with studies in the 1960s and 1970s showing that lysergic acid diethylamide (LSD), an agonist at certain 5-HT receptor subtypes, has a direct and potent inhibitory effect on the firing of these cells (Aghajanian, 1981). This suppression of serotonergic activity also causes a reduction in 5-HT release from terminal areas (Göthert, 1990). Further experiments established that other serotonergic agonists, including 5-HT itself, similarly inhibit 5-HT release. Release inhibition by 5-HT agonists was shown to be receptor-mediated because it could be blocked by the 5-HT receptor antagonist metitepine (also called methiothepin) (Starke, Göthert, and Kilbinger, 1989).

Like the DA cells of the substantia nigra, serotonergic neurons possess both somatodendritic and presynaptic autoreceptors. The somatodendritic autoreceptors suppress cell firing and are thought to play a role in collateral inhibition among serotonergic neurons (Aghajanian, 1981). By inhibiting neuronal activity, somatodendritic autoreceptors also lead to reductions in 5-HT synthesis and release in the areas to which the cells project. Presynaptic autoreceptors can inhibit 5-HT release and possibly also synthesis in the nerve terminals (Sawada and Nagatsu, 1986); however, they are not believed to influence cell firing. Interestingly, these two types of autoreceptors differ not only in their location and action, but also in their pharmacological characteristics. For example, the 5-HT$_{1A}$ agonist 8-OH-DPAT, which was discussed earlier in terms of its inhibitory effect on 5-HT synthesis, also inhibits 5-HT release. This compound is effective when administered systemically or infused into serotonergic cell body areas such as the dorsal raphe nucleus, but not when infused into a projection area such as the hippocampus. In contrast, the 5-HT$_{1B}$ agonists 5-methoxy-3(1,2,3,6-tetrahydropyridin-4-yl)-1H-indole (RU 24969) and 3-(1,2,5,6-tetrahydropyrid-4-yl)pyrrolo-[3,2-b]pyrid-5-one (CP-93,129) potently inhibit 5-HT release when infused into the rat hippocampus (Hjorth and Tao, 1991; Sharp and Hjorth, 1990). These and other studies strongly suggest that somatodendritic autoreceptors are of the 5-HT$_{1A}$ subtype, whereas presynaptic autoreceptors are of either the 5-HT$_{1B}$ subtype (rat and mouse brain) or the 5-HT$_{1D}$ subtype (pig, guinea pig, and probably human brain) (Göthert, 1990; Sharp and Hjorth, 1990; Figure 9.6).

Several drugs seem to be effective as autoreceptor antagonists. The classic blocking agent at terminal autoreceptors is metitepine (Starke, Göthert, and Kilbinger, 1989), although this compound is a nonselective 5-HT$_1$ antagonist and thus may also affect somatodendritic autoreceptors in some cases (Becquet, Faudon, and Hery,

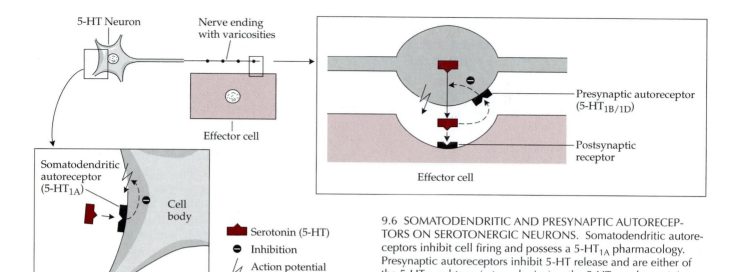

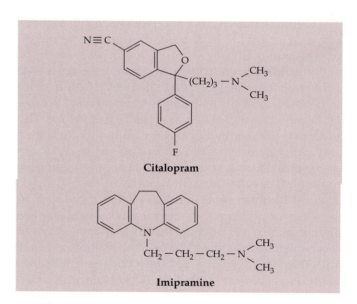

9.6 SOMATODENDRITIC AND PRESYNAPTIC AUTORECEPTORS ON SEROTONERGIC NEURONS. Somatodendritic autoreceptors inhibit cell firing and possess a 5-HT$_{1A}$ pharmacology. Presynaptic autoreceptors inhibit 5-HT release and are either of the 5-HT$_{1B}$ subtype (rats and mice) or the 5-HT$_{1D}$ subtype (pigs, guinea pigs, and humans). (After Göthert, 1990.)

1990). Certain β-adrenergic blockers such as pindolol, cyanopindolol, and propranolol can also be used as serotonergic autoreceptor antagonists because of their 5-HT$_1$ receptor-blocking properties. However, these drugs lack selectivity toward different 5-HT$_1$ receptors and thus block both somatodendritic (Sharp and Hjorth, 1990) and presynaptic (Schlicker, Göthert, and Hillenbrand, 1985) autoreceptors.

Some information is available concerning the mechanism of action of 5-HT autoreceptors. Stimulation of somatodendritic autoreceptors has been reported to inhibit firing by hyperpolarizing the cell, probably through an increase in membrane potassium (K$^+$) conductance (Aghajanian and Lakoski, 1984). In contrast, presynaptic autoreceptors do not alter impulse transmission, but rather inhibit some aspect of stimulus–secretion coupling of transmitter release. Göthert (1980) hypothesized that presynaptic 5-HT autoreceptors operate by modifying the influx of Ca^{2+} through voltage-dependent Ca^{2+} channels. Cyclic AMP may also play a role in this process, as both 5-HT$_{1B}$ and 5-HT$_{1D}$ receptors have been reported to inhibit the activity of adenylyl cyclase. Differences in the mechanisms needed to modulate impulse flow and transmitter release may help to explain why distinct 5-HT receptor subtypes are required for these purposes.

Serotonergic autoreceptors appear to respond to chronic changes in extracellular 5-HT concentrations. Repeated administration of the 5-HT uptake inhibitors citalopram and imipramine caused a functional desensitization of both presynaptic and somatodendritic autoreceptors (Chaput, de Montigny, and Blier, 1986; Moret and Briley, 1990), as well as a decreased density of 5-HT$_{1B}$ receptors (Johanning, Plenge, and Mellerup, 1992). As imipramine and citalopram are known for their efficacy as antidepressants, these results raise interesting questions concerning the possible role of autoreceptor changes in antidepressant action.

The final point to be touched on here concerns the physiological importance of autoreceptor function. Together, the somatodendritic and presynaptic autoreceptors are positioned to provide an exquisite negative feedback system modulating several key processes in cellular serotonergic activity. To what extent does such modulation occur in vivo under physiological conditions? There is no doubt that autoreceptor agonists such as 8-OH-DPAT and RU 24969 can inhibit 5-HT release, but the effects of exogenous drugs do not tell us how much of a signal is normally generated by endogenous 5-HT acting on the same receptors. This difference can be seen in the results of Sharp, Bramwell, Clark and coworkers (1989), who found that pindolol did not influence basal 5-HT release in the rat hippocampus, but attenuated the release-inhibiting effect of 8-OH-DPAT. Becquet, Faudon, and Hery (1990) have suggested that somatodendritic autoreceptors in the cat dorsal raphe nucleus are not tonically activated. Likewise, there might be little stimulation of presynaptic autoreceptors under resting conditions due to rapid removal of 5-HT by the synaptic reuptake system (see the next section) (Wolf and Kuhn, 1990). On the other hand, perhaps behavioral or physiological challenges that stimulate 5-HT release bring the autoreceptor system into play. To resolve these questions, further studies using microdialysis are needed to determine whether locally applied autoreceptor blockers cause an increased release of 5-HT in either untreated or appropriately challenged animals.

Serotonin Inactivation

Serotonin Uptake

Termination of the effects of synaptically released 5-HT occurs largely by means of a reuptake process that presumably allows at least some of the transmitter to be recycled for further use. Uptake is mediated by a transporter protein found in the plasma membrane of serotonergic neurons. The uptake process displays saturability, a high affinity for 5-HT, Na^+ dependence, and a requirement for metabolic energy (Graham and Langer, 1992). As would be expected for a carrier-mediated mechanism (as opposed to simple diffusion), 5-HT uptake also shows structural specificity and can be selectively inhibited by a number of different drugs (see next section).

Serotonin uptake in the brain has been studied largely in vitro, using brain slice and synaptosomal preparations. As summarized in Ross (1982), the K_m value for 5-HT is typically about 0.05–0.1 µM for synaptosomes, compared with 0.1–0.5 µM for slices. The potencies of uptake inhibitors are also found to be higher in studies using synaptosomes. The reason for these differences is not yet known, but could be related to diffusional barriers in the slice preparation or to accumulation of the transmitter in nonserotonergic compartments in the tissue.

The 5-HT uptake system operates by the same type of mechanism used to transport catecholamines, choline, and amino acid neurotransmitters across the plasma membrane. The driving force for transport is the Na^+ electrochemical gradient across the membrane. Thus, 5-HT uptake can be inhibited by ouabain, a drug that blocks the membrane Na^+–K^+ ATPase (sodium–potassium pump) responsible for maintaining this gradient. The current functional model of the transport process, which is summarized in Marcusson and Ross (1990), is presented in Figure 9.7. According to this model, Na^+ binds to the carrier protein, followed by 5-HT in its protonated form. Although chloride (Cl^-) ions are not required for 5-HT binding, they are necessary for net transport to occur. After translocation of the carrier in the cell membrane, 5-HT and the cotransported ions dissociate from their respective binding sites. Potassium then binds to the carrier, leading to translocation of the binding complex back to the exterior of the membrane, where the cycle can repeat. Most researchers currently believe that uptake-inhibiting drugs bind to the same site on the transport complex as 5-HT itself (Graham et al., 1989; Marcusson and Ross, 1990).

Until just a few years ago, little was known about the structural characteristics of the transporter protein itself. However, the transporter gene has now been cloned from rat brain (Blakely et al., 1991), rat basophilic leukemia cells (Hoffman, Mezey, and Brownstein, 1991), human brain (Lesch, Wolozin, Estler et al., 1993), and human placenta (Ramamoorthy et al., 1993). In most cases, identity as a bona fide 5-HT transporter was confirmed by demonstrating that 5-HT uptake with the appropriate biochemical and pharmacological properties could be conferred upon nonserotonergic cells by transfecting the cells with the gene in question. Examination of the predicted amino acid sequences of these transporters showed that the rat and human proteins are quite similar in their sequences, and also that the 5-HT transporter exhibits significant amino acid homology with other re-

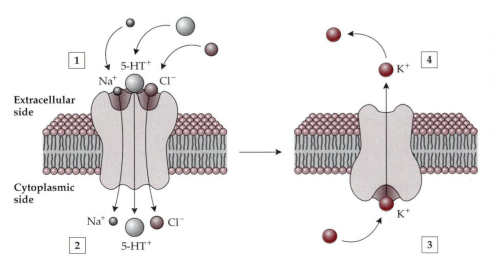

9.7 HYPOTHESIZED MECHANISM OF SEROTONIN TRANSPORT ACROSS THE PLASMA MEMBRANE. Serotonin uptake is a carrier-mediated process requiring the presence of Na^+ and Cl^- ions. Sodium binds first to the carrier, followed by 5-HT (1). Chloride is needed for transport but not for transmitter binding. The carrier is translocated in the membrane by an unknown mechanism, after which 5-HT and the ions dissociate from their binding sites (2). Potassium then binds to the carrier (3), is translocated to the outside of the membrane (4), and dissociates from the carrier to complete the cycle. (After Marcusson and Ross, 1990.)

cently identified transporters for NE, DA, and γ-aminobutyric acid (GABA). The 5-HT transporter further possesses 12 putative transmembrane domains and is considered to belong to the transporter protein superfamily described in Chapter 8 (Amara and Kuhar, 1993).

Although high-affinity 5-HT uptake is often thought of as specific to serotonergic neurons, the 5-HT transporter is also found in placenta, lung, and blood platelets (see below; Ramamoorthy et al., 1993). Even within the brain, this property may not be unique to serotonergic neurons, as astrocytes have been shown to accumulate [^{3}H]5-HT both in tissue culture and in vivo (Anderson, McFarland, and Kimelberg, 1992; Kimelberg, 1986). Astrocytic processes lie in close proximity to nerve terminals, which may allow for astrocytic uptake of 5-HT that escapes the neuronal reuptake process. Furthermore, the presence of monoamine oxidase in astrocytes (see the section on 5-HT metabolism below) means that 5-HT taken up by these cells can be inactivated and subsequently cleared from the brain.

Serotonin Uptake Inhibitors

During the 1960s, researchers discovered that the tricyclic antidepressant imipramine blocks 5-HT as well as NE uptake. Since that time, there has been a great deal of interest in the possible role of 5-HT in clinical depression, and much effort has been expended to develop drugs that are **selective 5-HT uptake inhibitors** (Lemberger, Fuller, and Zerbe, 1985).

Among the 5-HT uptake inhibitors, fluoxetine provides a particularly interesting case study. This compound, which was developed in the 1970s by Fuller, Wong, and their colleagues at the Lilly pharmaceutical company, belongs to a group of phenoxyphenylpropanamines that also includes the NE uptake blocker nisoxetine (see Fuller, Wong, and Robertson, 1991). The

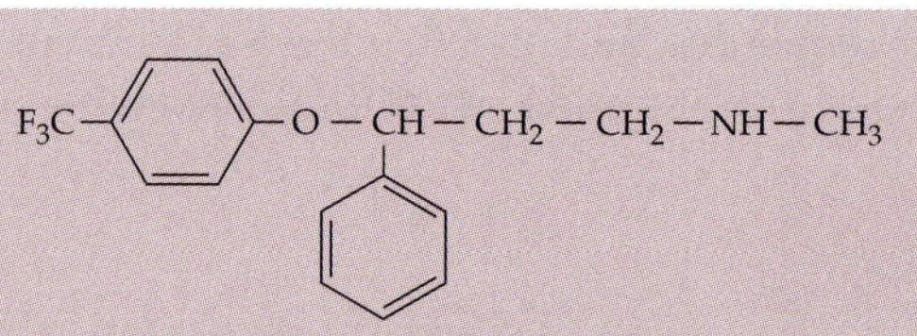

Fluoxetine

selectivity of fluoxetine in blocking 5-HT versus NE uptake is quite good, with IC_{50} values (the concentration required to inhibit 50% of the specific uptake) of 70 and 10,000 nM, respectively. Structure–activity studies have shown that the trifluoromethyl group is one of the features of the molecule that is important for its potency and selectivity. Fluoxetine displays only a weak affinity for most 5-HT receptor subtypes, thereby supporting its specificity for reuptake inhibition (Wong, Threlkeld, and Robertson, 1991). In recent years, fluoxetine was introduced into clinical practice on the basis of extensive animal experimentation and clinical trials establishing its

efficacy in the treatment of depression (Fuller, Wong, and Robertson, 1991; Hall, 1988). The drug is now a very widely used antidepressant under the trade name Prozac (see Chapter 19 for a further discussion of the 5-HT hypothesis of depression).

Blockade of synaptic reuptake increases extracellular concentrations of 5-HT, thereby stimulating many behavioral and physiological functions mediated by this transmitter (Fuller and Wong, 1990; Fuller, 1994). A few of these functions are described in Part III of this chapter. Another effect of uptake inhibition is the exertion of negative feedback on the serotonergic neurons, presumably via activation of the autoreceptors discussed earlier. Consequently, uptake inhibitors such as fluoxetine and citalopram suppress serotonergic neuronal firing (Chaput, Blier, and de Montigny, 1986; Rigdon and Wang, 1991) and decrease 5-HT synthesis and turnover (Fuller and Wong, 1990). These effects are thought to be mediated by 5-HT autoreceptors because autoreceptor blockade was found to potentiate citalopram-induced increases in extracellular 5-HT levels (Hjorth, 1993).

The 5-HT transporter protein has sufficient affinity for uptake inhibitors to enable binding studies to be performed. Such studies were first carried out with [^{3}H]-imipramine and have since been extended to more potent and selective compounds such as [^{3}H]paroxetine and [^{3}H]citalopram (Hrdina, 1986; Marcusson and Ross, 1990). Studies using these compounds have been useful

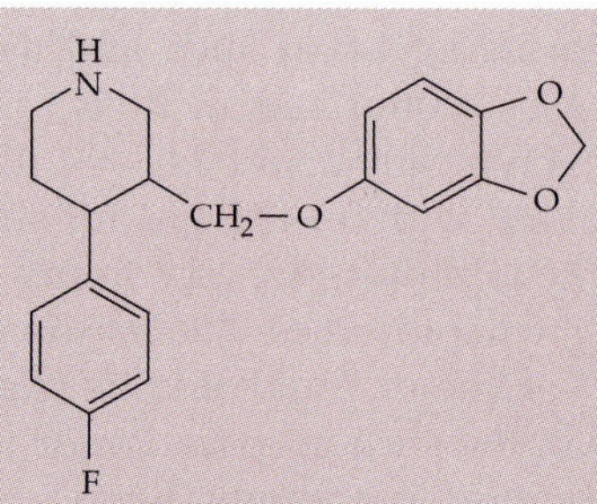

Paroxetine

in characterizing the 5-HT transporter and also in mapping its distribution in the brain by means of in vitro autoradiography (see Color Plate 1).

Metabolism of Serotonin

In nervous tissues, 5-HT is metabolized by oxidative deamination. The reaction is catalyzed by monoamine oxidase (MAO), the same mitochondrial enzyme that is instrumental in catecholamine degradation. As shown in Figure 9.8, the product of MAO action on 5-HT is 5-hydroxyindoleacetaldehyde. This compound is rapidly oxidized by aldehyde dehydrogenase to 5-hydroxyindoleacetic acid (5-HIAA), which is considered the primary metabolite of 5-HT. 5-HIAA diffuses out of the nerve cell and soon enters the cerebrospinal fluid (CSF). Humans show considerable interindividual variability in CSF 5-HIAA concentrations, and the level seen in a

HO — [indole ring] — CH$_2$—CH$_2$—NH$_2$ + O$_2$ + H$_2$O

5-Hydroxytryptamine

| Monoamine oxidase (MAO) | Flavin adenine dinucleotide (FAD) |

HO — [indole ring] — $CH_2-\overset{O}{\overset{\|}{C}}-H$ + NH$_3$ + H$_2$O$_2$

5-Hydroxyindoleacetaldehyde

| H$_2$O, NAD$^+$ | Aldehyde dehydrogenase |

HO — [indole ring] — $CH_2-\overset{O}{\overset{\|}{C}}-OH$

**5-Hydroxyindoleacetic acid
(5-HIAA)**

9.8 CATABOLISM OF SEROTONIN. Serotonin is initially catabolized by the mitochondrial enzyme monoamine oxidase (MAO) to yield the intermediate 5-hydroxyindoleacetaldehyde. This compound is then rapidly converted to 5-hydroxyindoleacetic acid (5-HIAA) by the enzyme aldehyde dehydrogenase.

given subject can change significantly over a period of days (Hildebrand et al., 1990). 5-HIAA is eventually eliminated from the brain by a probenecid-sensitive acid transport mechanism in the choroid plexus (see Chapter 8). Probenecid-induced accumulation of 5-HIAA in the brain is the basis of an early method of estimating 5-HT turnover (Curzon, 1981); however, the method has certain weaknesses and is therefore little used at the present time.

As mentioned in Chapter 8, two different MAO isozymes have been identified, MAO-A and MAO-B (Bach et al., 1988). In vitro studies indicated that the K_m of rat brain MAO-A for 5-HT was approximately tenfold lower than that of MAO-B (Fowler and Ross, 1984). With 5-HT as the substrate, the V_{max} of MAO-A was likewise found to be much higher than the V_{max} of MAO-B. Thus arose the idea that 5-HT is preferentially metabolized by MAO-A compared with MAO-B. This hypothesis was tested by examining changes in extracellular 5-HIAA in the rat striatum following treatment with the selective MAO inhibitors clorgyline (MAO-A) or deprenyl (MAO-B) (Kato et al., 1986). Extracellular 5-HIAA concentrations declined only after clorgyline treatment, which supports the notion that MAO-A is the physiologically relevant MAO isozyme in 5-HT metabolism. Similar conclusions were drawn from experiments on rat hypothalamus and spinal cord (Azzaro et al., 1988; Fagervall and Ross, 1986). The problem with this view is that immunocytochemical and histochemical localization studies have identified MAO-B, but not MAO-A, in serotonergic neurons of the rat (Levitt, Pintar, and Breakefield, 1982; Willoughby, Glover, and Sandler, 1988), cat (Kitahama et al., 1986), monkey (Westlund et al., 1985), and human (Konradi et al., 1988; Westlund et al., 1988) brain. If the in vitro affinity of MAO-B for 5-HT is reflective of its in vivo affinity, then the cytoplasmic concentration of 5-HT must presumably rise to a high level before significant deamination takes place within serotonergic cells. Perhaps such a situation is necessary to promote vesicular uptake and storage over immediate degradation and elimination. Until these issues are resolved, the relative importance of MAO-A and MAO-B for 5-HT catabolism in vivo will remain uncertain.

Measurement of Serotonin Turnover

As in the case of the catecholamines, a number of methods have been developed to estimate regional rates of 5-HT turnover. One of the earliest methods was to inject subjects with radiolabeled tryptophan and then measure the rate of formation of labeled 5-HT (Curzon, 1981). Diksic and colleagues recently introduced a novel variation on this theme that involves administering labeled α-methyltryptophan, a tryptophan analog that acts as a substrate for tryptophan hydroxylase (Diksic et al., 1990; Nagahiro et al., 1990). Accumulation of the product, α-methylserotonin, can be measured either in dissected brain tissues or by autoradiography, which provides excellent anatomic resolution. Moreover, the use of a positron-emitting isotope such as ^{11}C allows this method to be used for in vivo imaging of 5-HT synthesis by means of positron emission tomography (PET) (Diksic, 1992; Diksic et al., 1991).

Besides the probenecid method mentioned in the previous section, various other nonisotopic methods have been used to estimate 5-HT turnover. These methods include (1) measuring the ratio of 5-HIAA to 5-HT, (2) measuring the rate of accumulation of 5-HTP following injection of an AADC inhibitor such as NSD 1015, and (3) measuring the rate of 5-HT accumulation or the rate of 5-HIAA decline following MAO inhibition by pargyline (Curzon, 1981). Although the first approach has been popular because of its simplicity and because it involves no pharmacological manipulation of the system, one should remember that turnover studies are usually aimed at providing a biochemical index of synaptic activity. As a consequence of the intracellular location of MAO, significant amounts of 5-HIAA are generated from 5-HT that was never released. This lack of coupling between 5-HT release and metabolism means that changes in 5-HIAA production do not necessarily reflect synaptic activity in the serotonergic system (Auerbach,

Minzenberg, and Wilkinson, 1989; Commissiong, 1985; Kuhn, Wolf, and Youdim, 1986).

With regard to the second and third approaches mentioned above, experiments by Shannon, Gunnet, and Moore (1986) supported the NSD 1015 method over the pargyline method by showing that only the former was sensitive to changes in serotonergic cell activity. Use of an AADC inhibitor is particularly attractive to researchers specifically interested in assessing the rate of tryptophan hydroxylation in vivo. This approach initially involved measuring 5-HTP levels in dissected brain areas (Duda and Moore, 1985); however, investigators more recently have administered NSD 1015 directly into the brain using in vivo microdialysis and then measured 5-HTP in the dialysate fractions (Westerink and De Vries, 1991). In this way, one can determine changes in tryptophan hydroxylation rates in freely moving animals not subjected to AADC inhibition throughout the brain and the rest of the body.

Serotonin Neurotoxins

Much of our knowledge of the anatomy, physiology, and behavioral role of serotonergic systems comes from the use of toxic agents that damage or destroy serotonergic neurons (Baumgarten et al., 1982). The first 5-HT-selective neurotoxins to be discovered were the 5-HT analogs 5,6-dihydroxytryptamine (5,6-DHT) and 5,7-dihydroxytryptamine (5,7-DHT). These compounds, which were

5,6-Dihydroxytryptamine

5,7-Dihydroxytryptamine

first introduced and studied by Baumgarten, Björklund, and their colleagues, caused reductions in brain 5-HT concentration, tryptophan hydroxylase activity, and 5-HT uptake when administered intracerebroventricularly (Baumgarten et al., 1978). Histological studies revealed terminal degeneration in 5-HT projection areas, although the serotonergic cell bodies appeared to be largely spared by these neurotoxins.

A number of characteristics of 5,6-DHT- or 5,7-DHT-induced lesions have been established. First, early experiments showed extensive regrowth of fibers (sprouting) after 5,6-DHT administration, but a less pronounced response following 5,7-DHT administration (Baumgarten

et al., 1974). Partly for this reason, and also because 5,6-DHT is less specific in its cytotoxic action, 5,7-DHT quickly became the favored 5-HT neurotoxin. Second, even 5,7-DHT is not totally selective for serotonergic neurons because it also damages noradrenergic systems to some extent. Fortunately, this problem can be overcome by pretreating animals with the NE uptake inhibitor desipramine (Björklund, Baumgarten, and Rensch, 1975). Third, as mentioned earlier, 5,7-DHT primarily damages the serotonergic nerve terminals when given to adult subjects. Neurotoxin treatment accordingly leads to a much greater depletion of 5-HT in forebrain projection areas than in the midbrain and hindbrain regions where the serotonergic cell bodies reside. However, Towle and colleagues (1984) reported an extensive, long-lasting destruction of serotonergic neurons when 5,7-DHT was given neonatally (day 3 postnatal) rather than in adulthood. This approach can be useful to investigators who wish to study the behavioral or physiological characteristics of animals that are almost completely devoid of central serotonergic activity. Fourth, the behavioral effects of 5,7-DHT vary as a function of time after administration (Gately, Segal, and Geyer, 1986), presumably due to a combination of sprouting-related reinnervation and compensatory mechanisms triggered by the loss of serotonergic inputs. One such compensatory mechanism appears to be the development of supersensitivity to 5-HT agonists (Trulson, Eubanks, and Jacobs, 1976). Finally, although the mechanism of 5,7-DHT action is not completely understood, recent experiments suggest that the compound may be oxidized intracellularly to several by-products, which then proceed to damage the neuron by a complex series of biochemical reactions (Tabatabaie et al., 1993).

Various amphetamine derivatives constitute an entirely different group of 5-HT neurotoxins. These substances include the halogenated compounds PCA and fenfluramine, as well as the drugs methamphetamine, 3,4-methylenedioxyamphetamine (MDA), and 3,4-methylenedioxymethamphetamine (MDMA). All of these drugs have at least some degree of 5-HT releasing activity, as we have previously seen for PCA and fenfluramine. MDA and MDMA exert a complex spectrum of behavioral actions. They are hallucinogenic at high doses; however, at lower doses, they have been reported to induce a subjective state of well-being, a sense of closeness to other individuals, and feelings of enhanced insight (Liester et al., 1992). Such properties have led some clinicians to propose the use of these drugs as pharmacological adjuncts in psychotherapy (Eisner, 1989; Grob et al., 1992). However, the therapeutic use of MDA and MDMA has been discouraged not only because of their potential neurotoxicity, but also because they have a high abuse potential. MDMA, for example, is self-administered by animals (Lamb and Griffiths, 1987) and is heavily abused in some circles under the street names "ecstasy" or "Adam" (see Chapter 17 for a further discussion of MDA, MDMA, and related hallucinogens). Moreover, recent case studies have reported instances of MDMA-precipitated panic disorder in recreational users (Pallanti and Mazzi, 1992).

The serotonergic neurotoxicity of MDA, MDMA, and PCA has been demonstrated using both biochemical (De Souza, Battaglia, and Insel, 1990; Gibb et al., 1990; Insel et al., 1989) and histological (Molliver et al., 1990) methods. The histological studies have indicated that these compounds are more selective in their toxic action than 5,7-DHT. Specifically, they seem to spare ascending serotonergic projections from the median raphe nucleus while causing a loss of fine axon endings that arise from the dorsal raphe nucleus and terminate in the neocortex and other forebrain areas. Figure 9.9 illustrates the loss of 5-HT-immunoreactive fibers in the rat parietal cortex following multiple doses of either PCA or MDA.

Evidence for fenfluramine neurotoxicity has been more controversial. Early reports by Harvey and coworkers (Harvey, 1978) indicated that fenfluramine and PCA damaged cells in the B9 cell group (see Part II on the anatomy of the serotonergic system); however, their findings were not replicated by other laboratories. Nevertheless, more recent studies have found evidence for reduced forebrain 5-HT concentrations, uptake sites, and immunoreactive fibers in several animal species following chronic fenfluramine treatment (McCann, Hatzidimitriou, et al., 1994; Ricaurte et al., 1991; Rowland et al.,

1993; Zaczek et al., 1990). Whether these findings denote actual damage to serotonergic neurons or a long-lasting depletion of 5-HT without structural damage remains to be clarified.

It is important to know under what conditions, if any, the substituted amphetamines may be neurotoxic in humans as well as in the nonhuman species that have been tested thus far. This is particularly true for fenfluramine, which has seen widespread clinical use as an appetite suppressant. Despite the above-mentioned studies in laboratory animals, a number of arguments have been raised against the notion that fenfluramine poses a hazard to human users, and many issues remain to be resolved (see Kalia, 1991, and also letters to the editor in the February 8, 1992 issue of *The Lancet*, vol. 339, pp. 359–361). With respect to MDA and MDMA, the possibility of human neurotoxicity should be investigated to determine whether chronic abusers are at risk for brain damage, particularly as nonhuman primates seem to be even more vulnerable to these compounds than rats (Ricaurte et al., 1988, 1992; Scanzello et al., 1993). Although histological examination of the brains of chronic MDMA abusers has not yet been carried out, initial biochemical studies have revealed lower CSF 5-HIAA levels in such individuals than in control subjects (McCann, Ridenour, et al., 1994; Ricaurte et al., 1990). These results suggest a reduction in serotonergic activity following long-term MDMA exposure; however, more research is clearly needed before firm conclusions can be drawn.

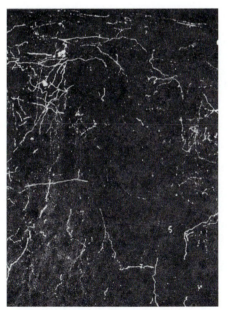
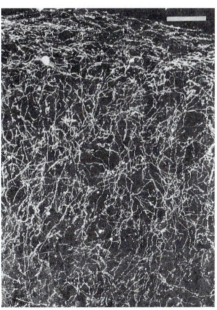
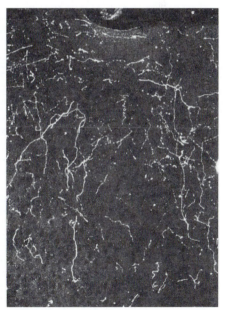

PCA   Control   MDA

9.9 PCA- AND MDA-INDUCED DEGENERATION OF SEROTONERGIC FIBERS IN THE RAT PARIETAL CORTEX. Dark-field photomicrographs show 5-HT immunoreactive nerve fibers in control animals and in animals treated 2 weeks earlier with PCA (2 × 10 mg/kg) or MDA (2 × 20 mg/kg/day for 4 days). Scale bar = 100 μm. (From Molliver et al., 1990, *Ann. N.Y. Acad. Sci.*)

Blood Platelets as a Model for Serotonergic Neurons

The ultimate aim of neuropharmacology is to understand drug action in the human nervous system; however, human studies in this area face a variety of practical and ethical problems. First, there are few opportunities to obtain brain tissue for direct measurements of neurochemical variables. Even when postmortem samples are available, this approach has a number of obvious limitations. Second, although we have seen that CSF samples are sometimes collected for measurement of 5-HIAA and other transmitter metabolites, metabolite levels do not always yield an accurate picture of transmitter turnover. Furthermore, CSF measurements cannot provide information concerning neurotransmitter receptors or uptake processes. Finally, because of its invasiveness and the slight possibility of spinal damage, collection of CSF is often difficult to justify unless the subject already needs a spinal tap for medical reasons.

These problems point out the need for more accessible model systems with which to study human neuropharmacology. For the serotonergic system, an interesting and widely used model turns out to be the blood platelet (Da Prada et al., 1988; Stahl, 1985). Platelets do not possess tryptophan hydroxylase, hence they cannot synthesize 5-HT. However, they express a number of other 5-HT-related characteristics, including 5-HT uptake, 5-HT$_{2A}$ receptors on their surface, and the presence of MAO-B. By means of their uptake system, platelets avidly accumulate 5-HT that has been secreted into the bloodstream by the enterochromaffin cells of the gut. The platelet 5-HT transporter appears to be the same as the neuronal transporter (Lesch, Wolozin, Murphy et al., 1993), and in fact has provided much of our current information concerning the mechanism of transport (Marcusson and Ross, 1990). Platelet 5-HT$_{2A}$ receptors are likewise identical to the receptors found in the frontal cortex (Cook et al., 1994). Following uptake, 5-HT is stored in dense-core granules until its release when the platelet is activated. Serotonin is one of a number of mediators that work synergistically to trigger the processes of platelet secretion, aggregation, and ultimately clot formation (De Clerck and De Chaffoy de Courcells, 1990; Holmsen, 1985). The effect of 5-HT on these processes is mediated by the above-mentioned 5-HT$_{2A}$ receptors. A summary of the serotonergic mechanisms found in platelets is given in Figure 9.10.

The use of platelets in neuropharmacology dates back to the 1950s, when reserpine was found to cause a depletion of platelet 5-HT content (see Pletscher, 1988, for review). Since that time, the platelet model has provided a veritable bonanza for biological psychiatrists and for neuropharmacologists interested in monitoring

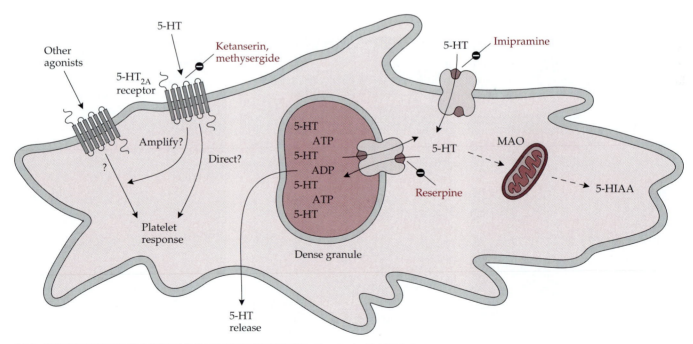

9.10 SEROTONERGIC FUNCTIONS IN BLOOD PLATELETS. Serotonin (5-HT) is transported into platelets by a membrane transporter that is sensitive to imipramine. Inside the platelet, the transmitter is taken up into dense-core granules, where it is stored with ATP, ADP, and divalent metal cations such as Ca^{2+} or Mg^{2+}. Following exocytotic release, 5-HT acts on 5-HT$_{2A}$ receptors to enhance platelet aggregation. 5-HT is also degraded intracellularly by monoamine oxidase (MAO). (After Holmsen, 1985.)

the cellular effects of clinical agents, particularly antidepressants (Lingjærde, 1990). Platelet MAO activity has also been studied extensively as a possible trait marker for various psychopathological states. Because platelet MAO and brain MAO-B are encoded by the same gene and appear to be identical proteins (Chen, Wu, and Shih, 1993), researchers have assumed that platelet MAO differences between psychologically normal and abnormal individuals might reflect differences in the brain enzyme. Murphy and Wyatt (1972) first reported that MAO activity was abnormally low in platelets obtained from chronic schizophrenics. Although this finding has been replicated in many (though not all) subsequent studies, it is not specific to schizophrenia. Low MAO has also been associated with bipolar affective disorder, suicidality, and alcoholism (Belmaker, 1984; Wirz-Justice, 1988; Youdim, 1988). This lack of specificity, as well as the possibility of environmentally induced changes in enzyme activity, raises important questions concerning the meaning of platelet MAO differences. Thus, platelet measurements are useful for certain purposes; however, the limitations associated with studying a peripheral, nonnucleated, and, of course, nonneuronal cell type must always be kept in mind.

Part I Summary

Serotonin is an indolealkylamine that is found not only in the nervous system but also in many other tissues, such as blood platelets. Serotonin is synthesized from the amino acid tryptophan in a two-step process catalyzed by the enzymes tryptophan hydroxylase and AADC. These enzymes can be inhibited by the drugs PCPA and NSD 1015, respectively. Tryptophan hydroxylation, which is the rate-limiting step in the synthetic pathway, is regulated by a number of factors, including neuronal firing rate and substrate availability. Dietary studies have shown that brain tryptophan and 5-HT concentrations in previously fasted subjects can be elevated by ingestion of a high-carbohydrate, low-protein meal.

Serotonin is stored in vesicles that accumulate in the varicosities of serotonergic nerve fibers. Normal stimulus-evoked release probably occurs through a vesicular exocytotic mechanism, although drugs like PCA and fenfluramine may release 5-HT from a cytoplasmic compartment. Transmitter release can be inhibited by 5-HT_{1A} somatodendritic autoreceptors that suppress serotonergic cell firing, and also by 5-HT_{1B} or 5-HT_{1D} presynaptic autoreceptors that act locally on the releasing mechanism. Serotonin in the synaptic cleft is transported back into the nerve terminal by a reuptake mechanism that is inhibited by fluoxetine and some tricyclic antidepressants. Intracellular degradation occurs through the action of MAO. Serotonin turnover can be estimated by several techniques, including measurement of the rate of

accumulation of the intermediate 5-HTP following inhibition of AADC by NSD 1015.

A number of compounds have been found that exert toxic effects on serotonergic neurons. Of these, 5,7-DHT has proved particularly useful in experimental work. The substituted amphetamines such as PCA, MDMA, and possibly also fenfluramine likewise exhibit significant 5-HT neurotoxicity.

Part II
Anatomy and Physiology of Serotonergic Systems

Distribution of Serotonin Neurons in the Nervous System

The earliest maps of serotonergic neurons and fibers in the brain were produced by applying the formaldehyde-induced fluorescence method to 5-HT (Dahlström and Fuxe, 1964; Dahlström and Fuxe, 1965; Fuxe, 1965). This technique involves an interaction of 5-HT with formaldehyde to yield a fluorescent condensation product that has been identified as 6-hydroxy-3,4-dihydro-β-carboline (also called 5-hydroxytryptoline). In contrast to the blue-green formaldehyde-induced fluorescence of catecho-

6-Hydroxy-3,4-dihydro-β-carboline

lamines, this compound appears yellow under UV light, thus allowing for a differentiation between serotonergic and catecholaminergic pathways. Unfortunately, the 5-HT fluorophore has a lower intensity of emission than the catecholamine fluorophore, and it also decomposes rapidly when activated. For these reasons, investigators have sometimes increased the yield of 5-HT by various pharmacological means (for example, administering an MAO inhibitor) or eliminated interfering catecholamines by pretreatment with 6-hydroxydopamine. In addition, suspected serotonergic terminals can be verified by determining whether they disappear following administration of 5,7-DHT.

Although the histochemical fluorescence method was extremely important in establishing the principal serotonergic cell groups and their projection areas, this approach continued to suffer from problems of sensitivity and specificity. A more detailed mapping of the serotonergic system has therefore relied on the implementation of new procedures, including autoradiography following in vivo or in vitro application of [³H]5-HT, immunohistochemistry for tryptophan hydroxylase, and finally, immunohistochemistry for 5-HT itself. Although each technique has certain advantages and disadvantages (see Consolazione and Cuello, 1982), they have all contributed to the mapping of the serotonergic system and in most instances have led to similar conclusions regarding the location of 5-HT-containing cell bodies and fibers.

Serotonergic Pathways in the Brain

In their pioneering studies, Dahlström and Fuxe (1964) described nine 5-HT-containing cell groups, which they designated Bl–B9 (Figure 9.11). As indicated in Table 9.1, most of these groups are associated with the raphe nuclei and the reticular region of the lower brain stem. The largest cluster of serotonergic neurons is found in the dorsal raphe nucleus; this cluster has been estimated to contain approximately 24,000 cells in cats and about 165,000 cells in humans (Törk, 1990). Nevertheless, all of the serotonergic neurons combined make up only a minuscule fraction of the full complement of nerve cells in the brain.

It is important to be aware of the distinctions between the raphe nuclei, which are defined according to classic neuroanatomical criteria, and the cell clusters that are identified histochemically as serotonergic. First, in many cases the serotonergic neurons extend beyond the boundaries of the corresponding raphe nucleus, particularly in the lateral dimension. Second, not all of the neurons in the raphe system contain 5-HT. In most of the

raphe nuclei, the majority of the cells are nonserotonergic (Nieuwenhuys, 1985).

The serotonergic neurons of the brain stem are conveniently divided into a caudal system and a rostral system, as described by Törk (1990). The caudal system consists of the B1–B4 cell groups, which are located in the median and paramedian regions of the medulla and caudal pons. The axons of these cells descend to the spinal cord along several pathways (Figure 9.12). Some serotonergic fibers (mainly from the nucleus raphe magnus, B3) travel in the dorsolateral fasciculus and terminate in the dorsal horn gray matter, particularly in laminae I and II. A second descending projection from the nucleus raphe pallidus (B1) and the nucleus raphe obscurus (B2 and B4) terminates on the motor neurons of the ventral horn. Finally, serotonergic neurons of the rostral ventrolateral medulla (part of B3) innervate preganglionic sympathetic cells in the intermediolateral columns of the thoracic spinal cord (Törk, 1990). These pathways largely mediate the varied roles of 5-HT in sensory, motor, and autonomic functioning.

The rostral 5-HT system comprises the B5–B9 cell groups, which are associated with raphe nuclei of the rostral pons and mesencephalon as well as with the caudal linear nucleus, the nucleus pontis oralis, and the supralemniscal region (see Table 9.1). Early studies showed that the dorsal and median raphe nuclei together account for about 80% of the forebrain serotonergic terminals, and therefore can be considered the major source of

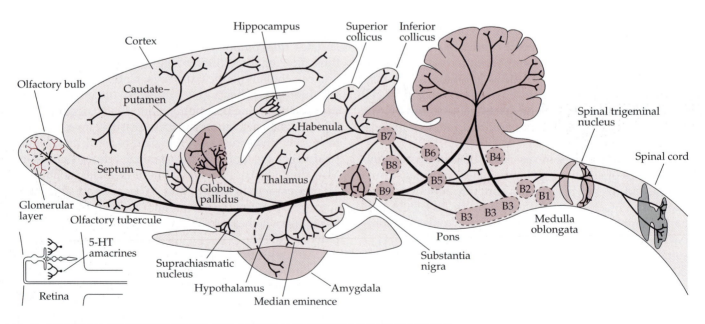

9.11 LOCATION OF SEROTONERGIC CELL BODIES AND PATHWAYS IN THE RAT CNS. Serotonergic cell bodies are located within the B cell groups of Dahlström and Fuxe (1964), from which they project caudally to the spinal cord and rostrally to many forebrain structures. 5-HT-immunoreactive amacrine cells have also been found in the retina. (After Consolazione and Cuello, 1982.)

Table 9.1 Relationship between Anatomical Structures and Dahlström and Fuxe's System for Designating Serotonergic Cell Groups[a]

5-HT cell group	Anatomical structure(s)
B1	Raphe pallidus nucleus
	Caudal ventrolateral medulla
B2	Raphe obscurus nucleus
B3	Raphe magnus nucleus
	Rostral ventrolateral medulla
	Lateral paragigantocellular reticular nucleus
B4	Raphe obscurus nucleus, dorsolateral part
B5	Median raphe nucleus, caudal part
B6	Dorsal raphe nucleus, caudal part
B7	Dorsal raphe nucleus principal, rostral part
B8	Median raphe nucleus, rostral main part
	Caudal linear nucleus
	Nucleus pontis oralis
B9	Nucleus pontis oralis
	Supralemniscal region

[a]These designations are based on Törk (1990). Other sources may define serotonergic cell groups somewhat differently; for example, the term nucleus raphe pontis has often been used to designate the anatomical structure associated with the B4 or B5 cell group.

tex. The cortical serotonergic projections display a nonuniform laminar distribution and in some cases seem to be complementary to the noradrenergic system. This is particularly evident in the primate visual cortex, where layer 4 displays a very high density of serotonergic terminals but receives only a sparse noradrenergic input (Morrison et al., 1982).

The dorsal ascending pathway emanates mainly from B7 and B8. It sends fibers to the mesencephalic gray as well as to the inferior and superior colliculi. Most of the axons of the dorsal pathway ultimately enter the medial forebrain bundle, where they join the ventral pathway to form a combined ascending system.

Two other serotonergic projection systems have been identified in the brain (Nieuwenhuys, 1985). The first is

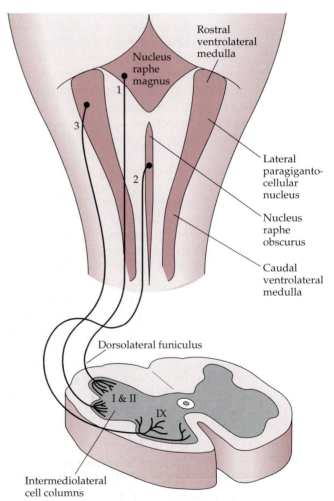

9.12 SEROTONERGIC PROJECTIONS TO THE SPINAL CORD. Three major descending pathways are illustrated: (1) from the nucleus raphe magnus via the dorsolateral funiculus to laminae I and II of the dorsal horn, (2) from the nucleus raphe obscurus to lamina IX of the ventral horn, and (3) from the rostral ventrolateral medulla and the lateral paragigantocellular reticular nucleus to the intermediolateral cell columns of the spinal cord. Projections from the caudal ventrolateral medulla are not known at present. (After Törk, 1990.)

the forebrain innervation (Azmitia, 1978). More detailed analyses have found that the rostral 5-HT system gives rise to two distinct ascending projections, termed the ventral and dorsal pathways (Nieuwenhuys, 1985).

The ventral ascending pathway originates primarily from the B6–B8 cell groups and supplies projections to numerous parts of the diencephalon, basal ganglia, limbic system, and cortex. Serotonergic fibers pass through the midbrain, where they innervate the substantia nigra, ventral tegmental area, and interpeduncular nucleus. A major part of the ventral pathway enters the medial forebrain bundle, from which fibers branch off in several directions. Diencephalic projections terminate in the medial habenula, various thalamic nuclei, the mammillary body, many hypothalamic areas (particularly the posterior hypothalamus and the ventromedial and suprachiasmatic nuclei), and the medial and lateral preoptic areas. Other fibers innervate the dorsal and ventral striatum (caudate–putamen and nucleus accumbens), limbic structures such as the amygdaloid complex, hippocampal formation, and septal nuclei (both medial and lateral), parts of the olfactory system including the anterior olfactory nucleus, olfactory tubercle, and the glomerular layer of the olfactory bulb, and all regions of the neocor-

a major pathway to the cerebellum that terminates in both the cerebellar cortex and the deep cerebellar nuclei. This projection has contributions from a number of serotonergic cell groups, most notably B2, B3, and B5. The second is a widespread system that innervates a number of structures in the pons and medulla. These structures include the locus coeruleus, dorsal tegmental nucleus, inferior olivary nucleus, nucleus solitarius, the rhombencephalic reticular formation, and several cranial nerve nuclei including the nucleus of the trigeminal nerve. It should be noted that connections between some of the raphe nuclei have also been demonstrated.

Fine structure of serotonergic fibers.   The sites of 5-HT release are varicosities (swellings) that occur in large numbers along the length of serotonergic fibers in terminal areas. These varicosities contain the vesicles responsible for 5-HT storage and release (see the earlier section on storage and release mechanisms). Anatomic studies have established the existence of two types of serotonergic axons in the forebrain. The most numerous are thin, extensively branched fibers with small fusiform (spindle-shaped) varicosities. The second type of serotonergic fiber starts out as a thick, nonvaricose axon. In the terminal areas, these axons branch out to form thinner fibers possessing larger, spherical or oval varicosities that give the fiber a beaded appearance (Figure 9.13).

The two types of 5-HT-containing axons appear to emanate from different cell groups, thereby forming the basis of two distinct projection systems (Kosofsky and Molliver, 1987; Mulligan and Törk, 1988). As shown in Figure 9.14, the so-called "**D system**" originates in the dorsal raphe nucleus and consists of fine fibers with fusiform varicosities. The "**M system**," which consists of the second type of serotonergic axon, has its origin in the median raphe nucleus. Both systems are extensively represented in most areas of the neocortex. However, some of the other brain regions studied thus far have shown a predominance of one system or the other. For example, the striatum and frontal cortex are innervated primarily by D fibers, whereas the hippocampal formation and septum receive input mainly through the M system (see Figure 9.14; Molliver, 1987; Törk, 1990). Another important point to mention is that the D system is more vulnerable than the M system to the neurotoxic actions of substituted amphetamines such as PCA and MDMA. This difference is manifested in the selective toxicity mentioned in the previous discussion of these compounds.

Although it is widely accepted that 5-HT release occurs from the varicosities found in both fiber systems, the extent to which these varicosities form conventional synaptic connections with target dendrites and/or somata is not as clear. Early studies were carried out by administering radiolabeled 5-HT and then performing autoradiography at the electron microscopic level to

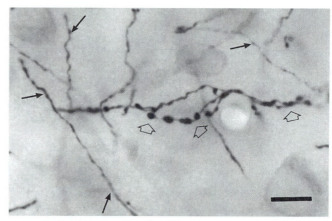

9.13 TWO SEROTONERGIC FIBER TYPES DEMONSTRATED IMMUNOCYTOCHEMICALLY. Light microscopic examination of 5-HT-immunoreactive fibers in the forebrain reveals the existence of two fiber types. Some fibers bear small fusiform varicosities (narrow, solid arrows), whereas other fibers display much larger varicosities, which give them a beaded appearance (wide, open arrows). Scale bar = 10 μm. (From Törk, 1990, *Ann. N.Y. Acad. Sci.*)

identify serotonergic terminals. When individual varicosities labeled in this manner were followed through their entire extent in serial sections, most investigators found that conventional synaptic arrangements (that is, with visible postsynaptic densities or other types of membrane specialization) were observed only infrequently (reviewed by Descarries, Séguéla, and Watkins, 1991; Maley et al., 1990). These findings led to the idea that 5-HT might typically operate at a distance from its sites of release, possibly serving as a neuromodulator to regulate the actions of more conventional transmitters (see Chapter 11 for a more extensive discussion of neuromodulation). On the other hand, two later studies using 5-HT immunocytochemistry have found a much higher incidence of conventional synaptic junctions by serotonergic terminals (Maley et al., 1990; Parnavelas and Papadopoulos, 1989). A resolution to this problem may be forthcoming from the D and M systems just described. Preliminary evidence suggests that M fibers make a much higher percentage of conventional synaptic contacts than do fibers of the D system, which could explain the observation of both junctional and nonjunctional arrangements in dually innervated areas like the neocortex (see Figure 9.14; Törk, 1990). If these findings are confirmed, and if it is also established that 5-HT released from terminals originating in the dorsal raphe nucleus exerts "action at a distance," then the distinction between the D and M systems should take on great significance for understanding the functional mechanisms of serotonergic transmission.

Coexistence of serotonin with other transmitters.   Several instances have been found in which 5-HT coexists with other transmitters in the same cells. For example,

9.14 DUAL SEROTONERGIC FIBER SYSTEM PROJECTING TO THE FORE-BRAIN. The two types of fibers illustrated in 9.13 arise from distinct cell groups in the brain stem. The thin, varicose fiber system (D system) arises from the dorsal raphe nucleus, whereas the beaded fibers (M system) originate in the median raphe nucleus. The D system branches diffusely in its target areas and appears to make few classical synaptic contacts. In contrast, the M system forms extensive pericellular arrays ("baskets") with typical morphological synaptic contacts. As indicated, some brain regions (e.g., cerebral cortex) are innervated by both systems, whereas others receive input primarily from either the D system (striatum) or the M system (dentate gyrus). (After Törk, 1990.)

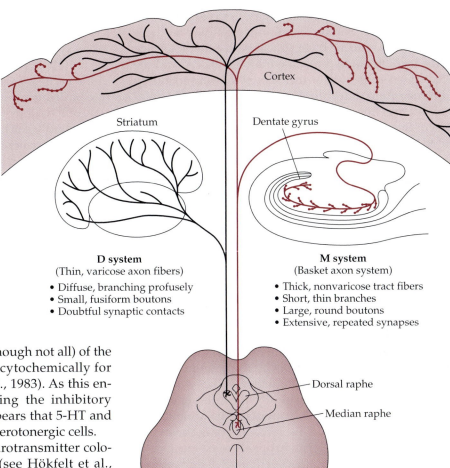

throughout the raphe nuclei, some (though not all) of the serotonergic neurons stain immunocytochemically for glutamate decarboxylase (Belin et al., 1983). As this enzyme is responsible for synthesizing the inhibitory amino acid transmitter GABA, it appears that 5-HT and GABA are colocalized in a subset of serotonergic cells.

As discussed in Chapter 11, neurotransmitter colocalization often involves peptides (see Hökfelt et al., 1987, for review), and this is true for 5-HT. The most extensively studied case of 5-HT–peptide coexistence involves the descending serotonergic pathway that terminates in the ventral horn of the spinal cord. At least some of these fibers and the cells from which they arise contain the peptides substance P (SP) and thyrotropin-releasing hormone (TRH) in addition to 5-HT (Johansson et al., 1981). Immunocytochemical studies have indicated that 5-HT and SP are stored together in large dense-core vesicles (Pelletier, Steinbusch, and Verhofstad, 1981), and are therefore presumably co-released upon nerve stimulation. On the other hand, Bartfai and colleagues reported that a low dose of PCA caused a depletion of 5-HT, but not SP, in the spinal cord, which suggested to them that these two substances are present in separate vesicular populations (Bartfai et al., 1986, 1988). However, because PCA does not release 5-HT by an exocytotic mechanism, it is likely that these results reflect selective displacement of 5-HT from the vesicles and subsequent release from the cytoplasmic compartment. Nevertheless, we cannot rule out the possibility that some vesicles contain 5-HT but no coexisting peptides.

Regardless of the intracellular relationship between 5-HT and SP, these transmitters seem to be involved in substantial cross-regulation of release (see Bartfai et al., 1988). In slices of rat spinal cord, 5-HT enhanced the evoked release of SP through a receptor with 5-HT$_2$

pharmacology. SP correspondingly promoted 5-HT release, and also antagonized the release-inhibiting effects of presynaptic serotonergic autoreceptors. Such positive feedback loops may play an important role in augmenting neurotransmitter action under conditions of relatively low neuronal activity.

Location of Other Serotonergic Cells

Serotonergic neurons or neuron-related cells are found in several locations other than the brain. As noted above in Figure 9.11, some of the amacrine cells of the retina may use 5-HT as a transmitter. Serotonin is prominent in the frog retina, but less so in some of the other species that have been examined (Osborne, 1982). Serotonergic neurons have also been found in the enteric nervous system, which is a part of the autonomic system that serves the gastrointestinal tract (for review, see Gershon, 1982). Finally, Holzwarth and Brownfield (1985) found biochemical and immunohistochemical evidence for the presence of 5-HT in rat adrenomedullary chromaffin cells, which are normally thought of for their synthesis and secretion of the catecholamines epinephrine and norepinephrine. Serotonin immunoreactivity in these cells could be reduced by treatment with either reserpine or the tryptophan hydroxylase inhibitor PCPA, and the effect of reserpine was further shown to be reversible by administration of tryptophan along with the MAO inhibitor pargyline. Staining was found in approximately 75% of the chromaffin cells, which interestingly turned out to be the same subset of cells that were immunopositive for the epinephrine-synthesizing enzyme PNMT. Although it is possible that 5-HT is taken up by chromaffin cells from the circulation (Kent and Coupland, 1984), Delarue et al. (1992) recently reported evidence for de novo 5-HT synthesis by frog interrenal tissue (the amphibian homologue of the mammalian adrenal gland). Regardless of its origin, 5-HT in the adrenal glands appears to function as a regulator of corticosteroid hormone secretion (Delarue et al., 1988).

Electrophysiology of Serotonergic Neurons

The serotonergic neurons of the rat brain raphe nuclei give rise to fine (0.15–1.5 µm in diameter), unmyelinated axons that exhibit a slow conduction velocity of about 0.5–1.5 m/s. Electrophysiologically, the cells are characterized by a regular and slow spontaneous firing rate of about 0.5–2.5 spikes/s. This autoactivity is consistent among the various nuclei and appears to be intrinsic to the cells. It has been found as early as 3–4 days before birth and can even be observed in serotonergic tissue in vitro (Jacobs, Wilkinson, and Fornal, 1990).

Knowledge concerning the electrophysiological properties of serotonergic neurons has proved useful in unraveling the role of these cells in various behavioral functions. In order to correlate behavioral changes with alterations in firing rate, it is necessary to record from awake, behaving animals. For the serotonergic system, much of the research of this kind has been performed by Jacobs and his coworkers. These investigators have primarily studied the activity of single units in the dorsal

raphe nucleus of freely moving cats. Although nonserotonergic as well as serotonergic cells are found in the raphe system, various lines of evidence indicated that the units being examined were indeed serotonergic. One of the earliest conclusions from this work was that the rate of firing varies systematically with the behavioral state of the subject. As shown in Figure 9.15, the cells fire most rapidly during active waking (waking with gross body movements), a bit more slowly during quiet waking, much more slowly during slow-wave sleep, and virtually not at all during REM sleep (Jacobs and Fornal, 1993). These findings suggest a possible relationship between motor activity and the rate of dorsal raphe cell firing, particularly since REM sleep is characterized by atonia of the major skeletal muscle groups (see Chapter 7). Such a relationship is further supported by studies on cats with bilateral lesions of the pontine tegmentum. Such lesions block the atonia normally associated with REM sleep, causing the animals to display overt behavior during REM epochs. Although dorsal raphe units in these subjects still showed an overall decrease in activity during REM sleep, the cells exhibited bursts of firing correlated with gross body movements.

Various studies have demonstrated further complexity in the behavioral functions of serotonergic neurons. Specifically, some dorsal raphe neurons are activated by repetitive movements such as treadmill walking, chewing, or grooming with the tongue. Conversely, cell firing seems to be suppressed when the animal orients to a strong sensory stimulus (Jacobs and Fornal, 1993; Figure 9.16). Still other experiments subjected cats to a variety of perturbing stimuli including (1) noise stress for 15 minutes, (2) restraint stress for 15 minutes, (3) exposure to a dog for 5 minutes, (4) several types of painful stimuli, (5) increases in body temperature, (6) hypo- or hypertension produced by appropriate drug treatments, and (7) hypo- or hyperglycemia consequent to insulin or glucose administration. Amazingly, none of the above manipulations produced significant alterations in the firing of serotonergic neurons (Jacobs, Wilkinson, and Fornal, 1990).

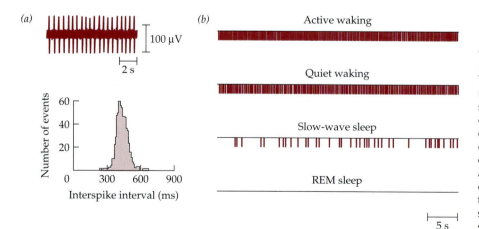

9.15 SINGLE-UNIT ACTIVITY IN THE CAT DORSAL RAPHE NUCLEUS AS A FUNCTION OF BEHAVIORAL STATE. Single-unit activity was recorded in dorsal raphe serotonergic neurons of freely moving cats. (a) During waking, the cells fire at an extremely regular rate, as shown by the oscilloscope tracing (top) and the histogram of interspike intervals (bottom). (b) Unit activity varies across the sleep–waking cycle. The cells fire most rapidly during active waking but are almost completely silent during rapid eye movement (REM) sleep. (After Jacobs and Fornal, 1993.)

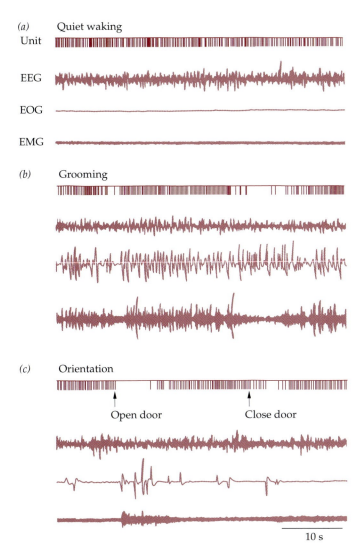

(a) Quiet waking
Unit

EEG

EOG

EMG

(b) Grooming

(c) Orientation

Open door   Close door

10 s

9.16 DORSAL RAPHE UNIT ACTIVITY IN RELATION TO MOTOR AND SENSORY ACTIVATION. In comparison with quiet waking (*a*), firing of dorsal raphe neurons is stimulated when a cat engages in self-grooming (*b*), but is suppressed during sensory orientation (*c*). The tracings below the unit recordings show cortical EEG, eye movements (EOG: electro-oculogram), and muscle activity (EMG: electromyogram). (After Jacobs and Fornal, 1993.)

Based on these and other findings, Jacobs and Fornal (1993) recently hypothesized that the principal function of brain 5-HT is to facilitate motor output while suppressing the ongoing processing of sensory input. This would explain why the raphe cells fire vigorously during states of behavioral activation but are inhibited either when the motor system is quiescent (e.g., during REM sleep) or when sensory processing takes precedence (e.g., during an orienting response). The results described above further suggest that some cells may be linked to the activity of so-called "central pattern generators," circuits that produce rhythmic behaviors such as chewing and walking. Indeed, 5-HT has been shown to initiate or modulate rhythmic motor programs not only

in cats but also in tadpoles, lampreys, neonatal rats, and rabbits (see Wallis, 1994).

Although this hypothesis accounts for many of Jacobs's findings, it seemingly fails to explain many neurochemical and pharmacological studies implicating 5-HT in nociception (perception of painful stimuli), thermoregulation, cardiovascular function, ingestive behaviors, reproduction, aggression, and stress (a few of these topics are taken up in Part III of this chapter). It is possible that these pharmacological studies are artifactual and that 5-HT plays a more limited, perhaps permissive, role in behavioral regulation than previously believed. A second possibility is that serotonergic control is exerted to a large extent by presynaptic modulation of 5-HT release, thus bypassing the need for changes in cell firing. However, Jacobs, Wilkinson, and Fornal (1990) present some limited evidence against this notion. A third possibility relates to the D and M systems described above. By choosing to study the dorsal raphe nucleus, from which the D system originates, Jacobs and colleagues have focused on one part of the serotonergic system that may act broadly to modulate basic motor and sensory processes. This still leaves open the possibility that serotonergic projections from the median raphe nucleus (M system) might serve other behavioral and physiological functions not addressed in Jacobs and Fornal's hypothesis.

Serotonin Receptors

Serotonin Receptor Subtypes

Any attempt to provide a comprehensive account of 5-HT receptors at this time must be made with caution. In recent years, serotonergic receptor subtypes have proliferated more rapidly than the proverbial rabbit, and it is likely that further subtypes await discovery by enterprising pharmacologists and molecular biologists. Nevertheless, some important organizing principles have been discovered. First, almost all of the known 5-HT receptor subtypes belong to the G protein–coupled superfamily. As we have seen in previous chapters, this knowledge provides us with important information concerning the general structure and operation of these receptors. Second, as would be expected, the 5-HT receptors are linked to multiple signal transduction mechanisms. As we shall see, the transduction mechanisms used by particular subtypes have been helpful in differentiating several related families of 5-HT receptors. Third, it is important to note that the $5-HT_3$ receptor does not fit into this general category, but rather is a ligand-gated channel. Finally, although we will be discussing each 5-HT receptor subtype individually, there is considerable evidence that different subtypes may interact with one another in mediating the various behavioral effects of 5-HT (Glennon, Darmani, and Martin, 1991).

We shall begin our discussion of 5-HT receptors by presenting a brief history of the early research in this area. This will be followed by more detailed information concerning the structural, pharmacological, and functional characteristics of the various serotonergic receptor subtypes.

Early studies. The first suggestion of multiple subtypes of serotonergic receptors came from the work of Gaddum and Picarelli (1957), who were studying the contractile effect of 5-HT on the isolated guinea pig ileum. They observed that this response was partially antagonized by either morphine or Dibenzyline (phenoxybenzamine) given alone. However, the effect of 5-HT could be completely blocked by combining appropriate doses of the two drugs. Gaddum and Picarelli proposed that their results were due to the existence of two different serotonergic receptors, which they named the M (morphine) and D (Dibenzyline) receptors. The M receptor was also sensitive to atropine and cocaine, whereas the D receptor could be blocked by LSD. It was hypothesized that the M receptors were located on the neurons innervating the ileum, whereas the D receptors were present on the ileal smooth muscle itself.

Although problems soon arose in applying this classification system to serotonergic receptors in the brain, no alternative was available until 1979, when Peroutka and Snyder published a landmark paper suggesting the existence of two receptor subtypes in brain tissue based on radioligand binding studies. When 5-HT receptors in rat frontal cortex were labeled with either tritiated serotonin, LSD, or spiperone, displacement of the binding by varying concentrations of unlabeled drugs depended on which ligand was used (Figure 9.17). Based on the relative potency of each unlabeled competitor and the shapes of the displacement curves, Peroutka and Snyder concluded that [³H]5-HT and [³H]spiperone label distinct populations of serotonergic receptors in the frontal cortex. These were designated 5-HT$_1$ and 5-HT$_2$ receptors, respectively. It was proposed that LSD has a similar affinity for each receptor subtype and thus labels both. This hypothesis was further supported by saturation analyses yielding B_{max} values of about 10 pmol/g tissue for [³H]5-HT or [³H]spiperone, but a B_{max} of approximately 20 pmol/g tissue for [³H]LSD (Peroutka and Snyder, 1979).

The current classification system. Further advances in 5-HT pharmacology led to the subsequent adoption of a nomenclature system involving three major classes of 5-HT receptors: 5-HT$_1$ (with multiple subtypes within this category), 5-HT$_2$, and 5-HT$_3$ (Bradley et al., 1986; Zifa and Fillion, 1992). However, even this more elaborate system proved insufficient, particularly as molecular biologists have cloned a number of novel 5-HT receptor subtypes in just the past few years. Consequently, the current

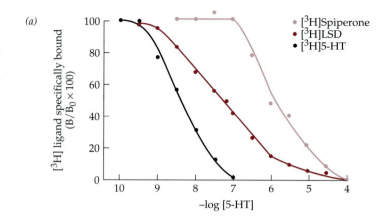

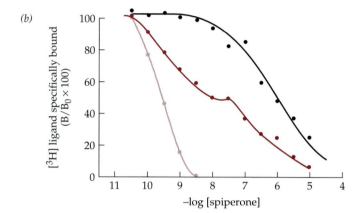

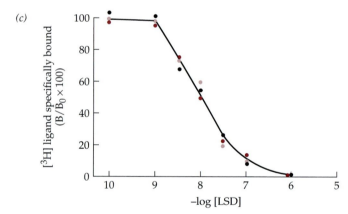

9.17 INHIBITION OF BINDING TO RAT FRONTAL CORTEX SEROTONERGIC RECEPTORS LABELED WITH [³H]5-HT, [³H]SPIPERONE, AND [³H]LSD. The potency of unlabeled 5-HT, spiperone, and LSD in displacing binding to serotonergic receptors varied depending on which ligand was used to label the receptors. These results led to the hypothesis of two receptor subtypes, 5-HT$_1$ (5-HT-preferring) and 5-HT$_2$ (spiperone-preferring). (After Peroutka and Snyder, 1979, 1982.)

classification system recognized by the International Union of Pharmacology (IUPHAR) includes a family of 5-HT$_1$ receptors, a family of 5-HT$_2$ receptors, and separate 5-HT$_3$, 5-HT$_4$, 5-HT$_5$, 5-HT$_6$, and 5-HT$_7$ subtypes (reviewed by Hoyer et al., 1994). There are also several "orphan" 5-HT receptors not yet characterized well enough to be included in the formal nomenclature. Counting all members of the 5-HT$_1$ and 5-HT$_2$ receptor families along with the other characterized and "orphan" receptors, there are already at least 18 known or proposed 5-HT receptor subtypes! In the present chapter, we will focus on the 5-HT$_1$ through 5-HT$_4$ subtypes, as the newer receptors have not yet been studied as thoroughly.

5-HT$_1$ Receptors

In the original binding study of Peroutka and Snyder (1979), 5-HT$_1$ sites were identified by a high affinity for radiolabeled 5-HT. This has remained one of the defining characteristics of the 5-HT$_1$ receptor subtype. However, pharmacological and molecular cloning studies have demonstrated a need for further subdivisions of this category. As shown in Table 9.2, there are currently five known 5-HT$_1$ receptor subtypes, designated 1A, 1B, 1D, 1E, and 1F. Until recently, there was also a 5-HT$_{1C}$ subtype; however, by most criteria, this receptor belongs to the 5-HT$_2$ family and thus has been renamed 5-HT$_{2C}$ (see below). It can be seen from the table that selective agonists and particularly antagonists are available for only a few of the 5-HT$_1$ subtypes. However, several additional drugs are available that can at least differentiate between the 5-HT$_1$ family and other serotonergic receptors. These drugs include the general 5-HT$_1$ agonist 5-carboxamidotryptamine (5-CT) and the general antagonist metitepin.

5-HT$_{1A}$ receptors.

The structure of the rat 5-HT$_{1A}$ receptor is shown in Figure 9.18. The receptor protein is predicted to have the usual seven transmembrane domains of a G protein–coupled receptor. In fact, the similarity within this superfamily is shown by the large number of amino acid residues this protein shares with the hamster β$_2$-adrenergic receptor (shown in color). The figure also illustrates some other notable features of the 5-HT$_{1A}$ receptor, including sites for N-linked glycosylation (i.e., asparagine [N] residues where sugars can be attached) at the C-terminal end, putative phosphoryla-

tion sites on serine (S) and threonine (T) residues in the second and third intracellular loops, and a cysteine (C) residue at the N-terminal end that represents a putative attachment site for a molecule of the fatty acid palmitate.

Pharmacologically, the 5-HT$_{1A}$ receptor is the best-characterized member of the 5-HT$_1$ family because of the availability of several selective agonists. These drugs include the tetralin compound 8-OH-DPAT and the azapirone derivatives ipsapirone, buspirone, and gepirone. Autoradiography using these drugs has revealed high densities of 5-HT$_{1A}$ binding in the hippocampus (particularly CA1 and the dentate gyrus), lateral septum, central amygdala, and frontal and entorhinal cortices. The

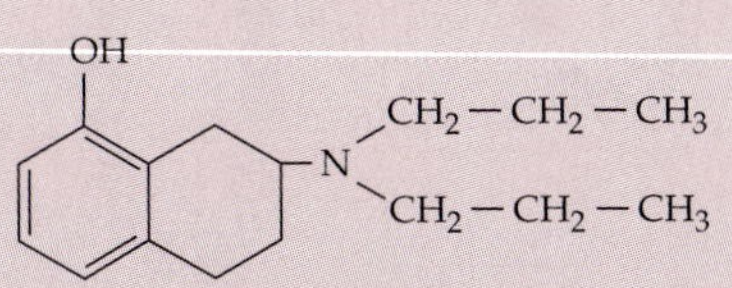

8-OH-DPAT

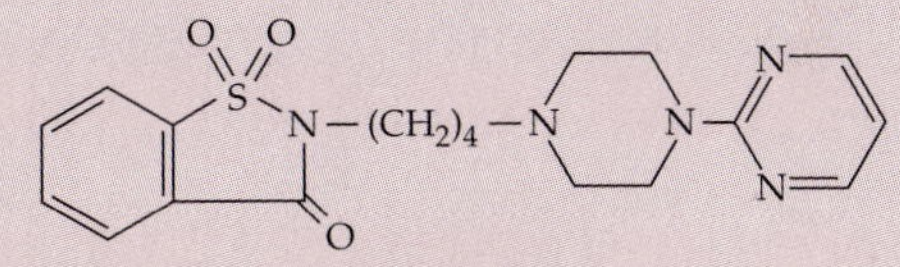

Ipsapirone

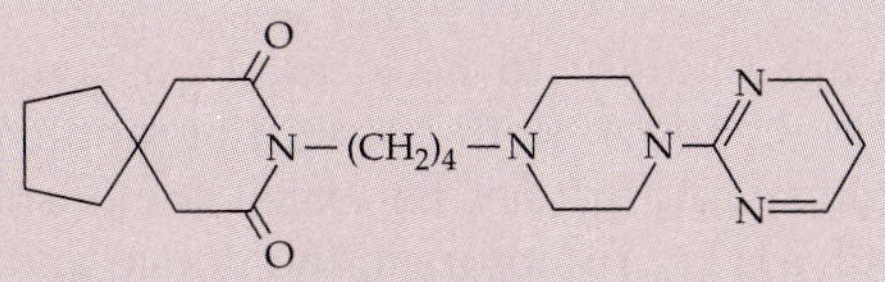

Buspirone

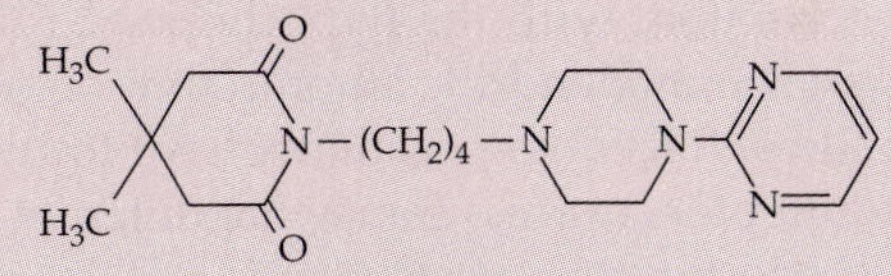

Gepirone

Table 9.2 Pharmacology of 5-HT$_1$ Receptors

Receptor subtype	Pharmacological properties			
	Agonists	Antagonists	Radioligands	Effector pathways
5-HT$_{1A}$	8-OH-DPAT, ipsapirone	SDZ 216-525, WAY-100135	[^{3}H]8-OH-DPAT	↓ cAMP, ↑ K$^+$ channel
5-HT$_{1B}$	CP-93,129		[^{125}I]GTI, [^{3}H]CP-96,501	↓ cAMP
5-HT$_{1D}$	Sumatriptan, 5-(Nonyloxy)tryptamine		[^{125}I]GTI	↓ cAMP
5-HT$_{1E}$				↓ cAMP
5-HT$_{1F}$				↓ cAMP

Source: After Humphrey, Hartig, and Hoyer, 1993.

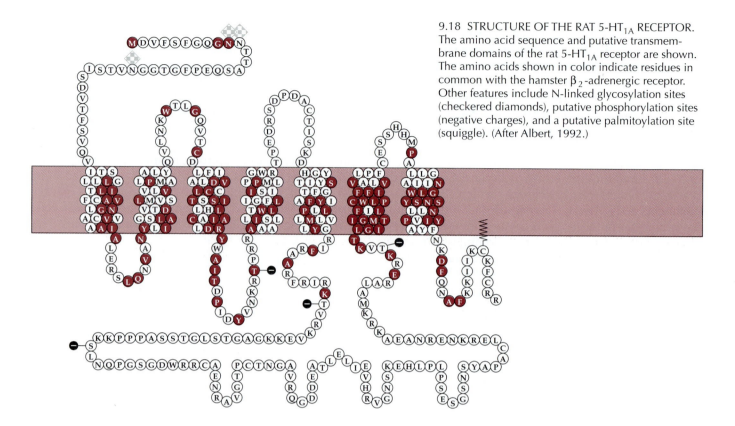

9.18 STRUCTURE OF THE RAT 5-HT$_{1A}$ RECEPTOR. The amino acid sequence and putative transmembrane domains of the rat 5-HT$_{1A}$ receptor are shown. The amino acids shown in color indicate residues in common with the hamster β$_2$-adrenergic receptor. Other features include N-linked glycosylation sites (checkered diamonds), putative phosphorylation sites (negative charges), and a putative palmitoylation site (squiggle). (After Albert, 1992.)

receptors are thought to be located postsynaptically (Hamon et al., 1990). Both autoradiographic and immunohistochemical studies have also demonstrated the presence of 5-HT$_{1A}$ receptors in the dorsal and median raphe nuclei (Hamon et al., 1990; Sotelo et al., 1990), which is consistent with the hypothesized role of this subtype as a somatodendritic autoreceptor on serotonergic cell bodies. Recent experiments have found that 5-HT$_{1A}$ autoreceptors express somewhat different pharmacological properties than postsynaptic 5-HT$_{1A}$ receptors, and may therefore represent a distinctive subtype (de Montigny and Blier, 1992).

The behavioral functions of 5-HT$_{1A}$ receptors have been studied by examining the effects of 8-OH-DPAT and the 5-HT$_{1A}$-specific azapirones. Systemic administration of these compounds to laboratory animals leads to hyperphagia, hypothermia, and various behavioral effects predictive of an anxiolytic (antianxiety) action in humans (Barrett and Vanover, 1993; Glennon, 1990b; Lucki, 1992). In fact, buspirone (trade name Buspar) is already in clinical use as an anxiolytic (see Chapter 16), while other 5-HT$_{1A}$ drugs are currently under development for this purpose. Buspirone and the other azapirones produce less sedation and have less abuse potential than the benzodiazepines, although their therapeutic action takes longer to develop (Barrett and Vanover, 1993; Lader, 1991). Interestingly, these compounds also appear to have antidepressant efficacy and may eventually prove useful in that role as well.

Another consequence of 5-HT$_{1A}$ agonist administration is the so-called "5-HT syndrome." Studies in the 1960s and 1970s found that a specific constellation of behavioral effects was produced in rats given a 5-HT precursor such as L-tryptophan (with an MAO inhibitor) or 5-hydroxytryptophan (with or without an MAO inhibitor), a 5-HT releasing drug such as fenfluramine or PCA, or the direct 5-HT receptor agonist 5-methoxy-N,N-dimethyltryptamine. This syndrome typically consisted of (1) resting tremor, (2) muscular hypertonicity or rigidity, (3) reciprocal treading of the forepaws, (4) hindlimb abduction (forceful splaying out of the hindlimbs), (5) lateral head weaving, (6) Straub (rigidly arched) tail, and other components such as low body posture, head shaking, hyperactivity, hyperreactivity, and salivation (Jacobs, 1976). Although the 5-HT syndrome has been studied mainly in animals, there is evidence that a human analogue with symptoms such as myoclonus (repetitive muscle spasms), tremor, ataxia, akathisia (extreme restlessness), hyperreflexia, diaphoresis (sweating), and delirium may occur following ingestion of an overdose of a 5-HT uptake inhibitor or various combinations of L-tryptophan, a 5-HT uptake inhibitor, and/or an MAO inhibitor (reviewed by Lejoyeux, Adès, and Rouillon, 1994). In extreme cases, the syndrome can be fatal. Pharmacological studies have suggested that activation of postsynaptic 5-HT$_{1A}$ receptors, perhaps in the lower brain stem or spinal cord, is responsible for producing the behavioral effects associated with the 5-HT syndrome (Lucki, 1992). It is important to note, however, that while 8-OH-DPAT elicits the full 5-HT syndrome, buspirone and other azapirones given alone elicit only a few components of the syndrome, notably low body posture and hindlimb abduction. On the other hand, pretreatment with any of these compounds blocks the ability of 8-OH-DPAT to produce the full syndrome. These findings indicate that, at least for this behavioral paradigm, 8-OH-DPAT acts as a full agonist, whereas the azapirones act as partial agonists at the 5-HT$_{1A}$ receptor. As we can see from this example, **full agonists** elicit the maximum effect in a given functional assay with no antagonist action, whereas **partial agonists** elicit weaker or incomplete effects (regardless of dose), and also show some degree of antagonist activity by their ability to block the effects of full agonists.

Before leaving the topic of 5-HT$_{1A}$ receptors, we should mention that two selective antagonists, methyl 4-{4-[4-(1,1,3-trioxo-2H-1,2-benzoisothiazol-2-yl)butyl]-1-piperazinyl}1H-indole-2-carboxylate (SDZ 216-525) and (S)-N-tert-butyl-3-(4-(2-methoxyphenyl)piperazin-1-yl)-2-phenylpropanamide (WAY-100135) have recently been introduced (Cliffe et al., 1993; Schoeffter et al., 1993).

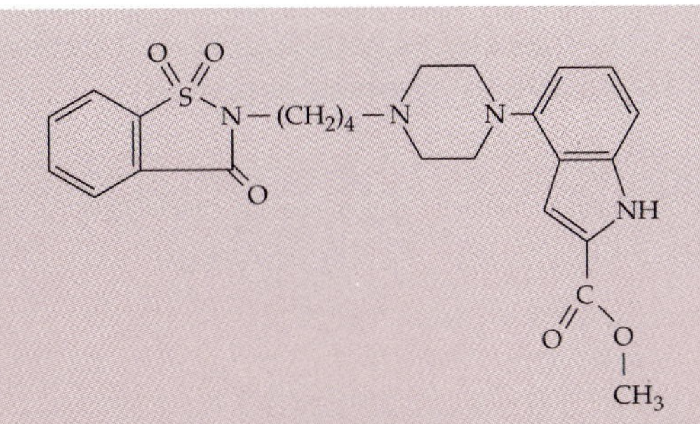

SDZ 216-525

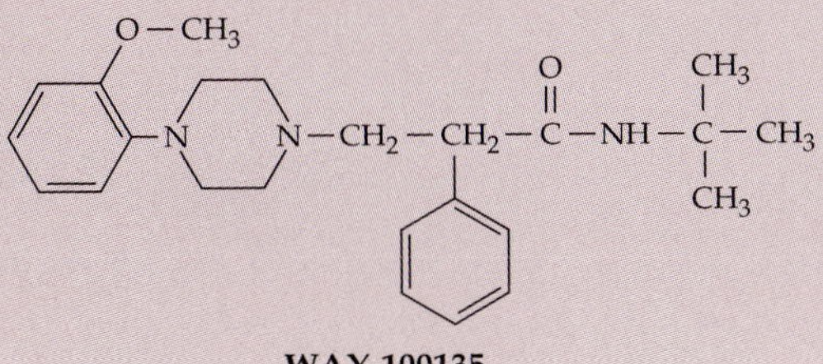

WAY-100135

Along with the agonists just discussed, these compounds should prove valuable in the continuing efforts to characterize the behavioral and physiological functions of the 5-HT$_{1A}$ receptor subtype.

5-HT$_{1B}$ and 5-HT$_{1D}$ receptors. The 5-HT$_{1B}$ and 5-HT$_{1D}$ receptors together constitute a small family of related subtypes that vary with the species (Hartig, Branchek, and Weinshank, 1992). For example, rats express both subtypes (Hamblin et al., 1992), whereas humans do not express 5-HT$_{1B}$ receptors, but rather, show two variants of the 5-HT$_{1D}$ subtype termed 5-HT$_{1D\alpha}$ and 5-HT$_{1D\beta}$ (Weinshank et al., 1992). The structural and pharmaco-

logical relationships within this family have proved quite interesting. The human 5-HT$_{1D\alpha}$ and 5-HT$_{1D\beta}$ receptors are virtually identical with respect to their pharmacological properties, yet not nearly as similar in their amino acid sequences. In contrast, the rat 5-HT$_{1B}$ and human 5-HT$_{1D\beta}$ receptors are very similar structurally (>90% amino acid homology); however, they exhibit quite distinctive pharmacological characteristics.* Recent studies have in fact shown that a change in only one amino acid in the seventh transmembrane domain is sufficient to account for the pharmacological differences between the rat and human receptors (Oksenberg et al., 1992; Parker et al., 1993). This finding provides a powerful example of the fact that substantial regions of a receptor protein may not be critical to its functional properties (e.g., human 5-HT$_{1D\alpha}$ vs. 5-HT$_{1D\beta}$), yet a small alteration in another region of the receptor can lead to significant pharmacological changes (human 5-HT$_{1D\beta}$ vs. rat 5-HT$_{1B}$).

Investigators at the Pfizer pharmaceutical company have developed a group of specific 5-HT$_{1B}$ agonists consisting of 3-(1,2,5,6-tetrahydropyrid-4-yl)pyrrolo[3,2-b]pyrid-5-one (CP-93,129), 3-(1,2,5,6-tetrahydropyrid-4-yl)-5-propoxypyrrolo[3,2-b]pyridine (CP-94,253), and 3-(1,2,5,6-tetrahydropyrid-4-yl)-5-propoxyindole (CP-96,501) (Koe et al., 1992; Macor et al., 1990). Other, less selective agonists include RU 24969, 1-[3-(trifluoromethyl)phenyl]piperazine (TFMPP), and 1-(3-chlorophenyl)piperazine (*m*-CPP), which is a metabolite of the antidepressant trazodone (Middlemiss and Tricklebank, 1992). At the present time, no selective 5-HT$_{1B}$ antagonists have yet been developed.

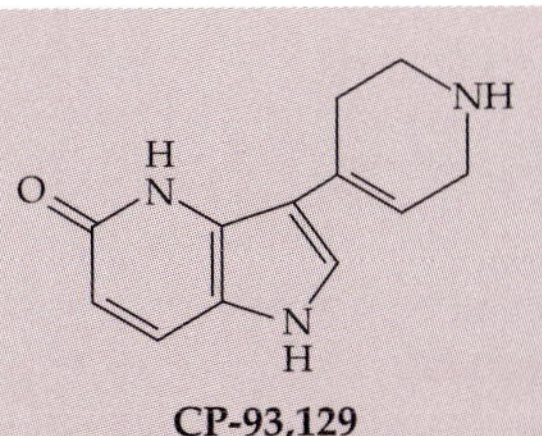

CP-93,129

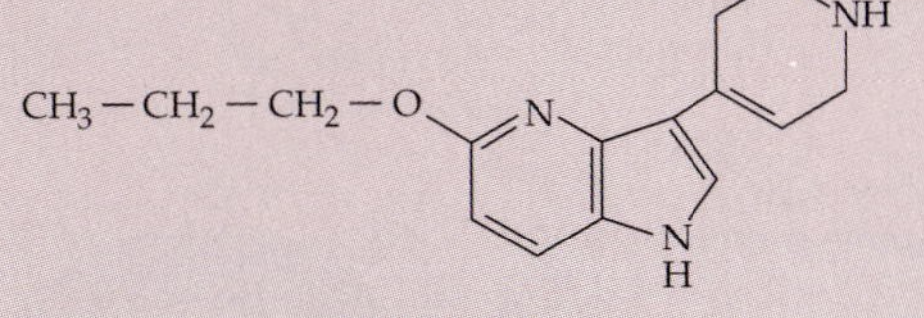

CP-94,253

*The close structural similarity between the human 5-HT$_{1D\beta}$ and the rat 5-HT$_{1B}$ receptor has led some investigators to likewise designate the human receptor as a 5-HT$_{1B}$ subtype. This designation, however, is inconsistent with the pharmacology of this receptor, which is clearly 5-HT$_{1D}$-like. As the 5-HT receptor subtypes have traditionally been distinguished by their *pharmacological* properties, we have chosen to adopt the 5-HT$_{1D\alpha}$/5-HT$_{1D\beta}$ convention (see Humphrey, Hartig, and Hoyer, 1993).

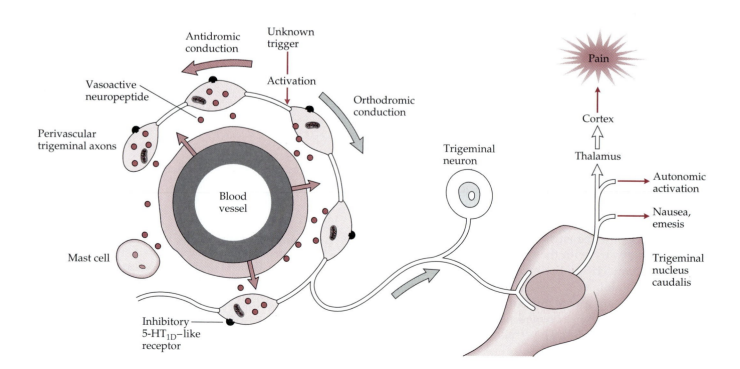

CP-96,501

RU 24969

TFMPP

m-CPP

densities were found in the substantia nigra, dorsal subiculum, globus pallidus, superficial layer of the superior colliculus, caudate–putamen, and central gray. 5-HT_{1B} receptors may be important in the enhanced locomotor activity, hypophagia (reduced food intake), and hypothermia observed following RU 24969 or CP-94,253 administration (reviewed by Chopin, Moret, and Briley, 1994).

Although 5-HT_{1D} receptors are present at low levels in the rat brain (Bruinvels, Palacios, and Hoyer, 1993), they are quantitatively much more important in other species (e.g., humans) that do not express the 5-HT_{1B} subtype. Autoradiography with [^{125}I]GTI, which labels 5-HT_{1D} as well as 5-HT_{1B} receptor sites, has revealed high densities in the substantia nigra, globus pallidus, caudate, putamen, and nucleus accumbens of the human brain (Palacios et al., 1992).

5-HT_{1D} receptor pharmacology is not yet well developed, although Glennon and coworkers (1994) recently published a preliminary evaluation of 5-(nonyloxy)tryptamine, a putative high-affinity 5-$HT_{1D\beta}$ receptor agonist. A better-known, though less selective, 5-HT_{1D} agonist is sumatriptan (Imitrex). This compound is currently in clinical use as an antimigraine medication (The Sumatriptan Auto-Injector Study Group, 1991). Migraine headaches are known to involve distension of large cranial

Autoradiographic localization of 5-HT_{1B} receptors in the rat brain has been accomplished using [^{3}H]CP-96,501 (Lebel and Koe, 1992) and also with the compound 5-O-carboxamidomethylglycyl[^{125}I]tyrosinamide-tryptamine ([^{125}I]GTI; Boulenguez et al., 1992). The highest receptor

[^{125}I]GTI

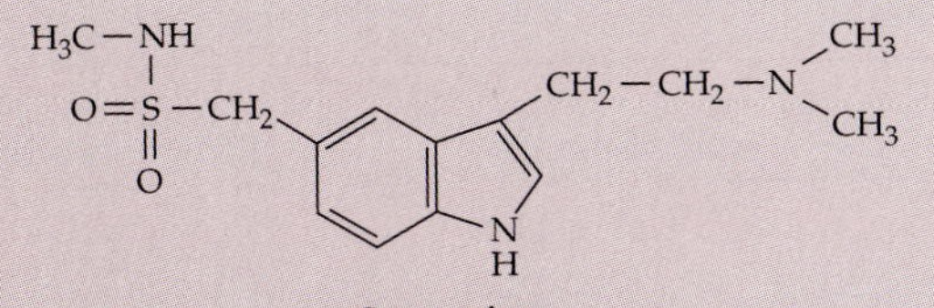

Sumatriptan

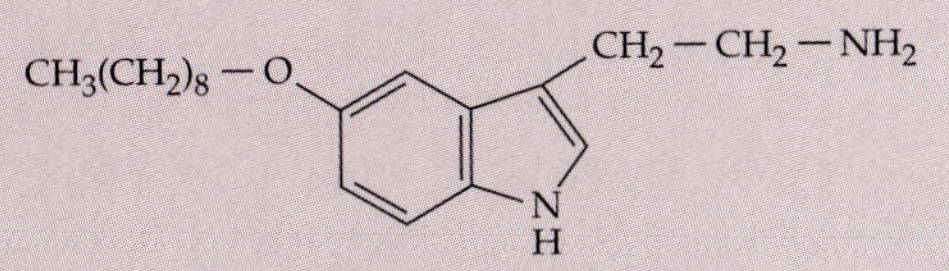

5-(Nonyloxy)tryptamine

blood vessels, and one hypothesized mechanism of sumatriptan's effects is constriction of those vessels by acting directly on vascular 5-HT_{1D} receptors (Humphrey and Feniuk, 1991). An alternative hypothesis is based on data suggesting that migraine headaches are initiated when some as yet unknown mechanism stimulates perivascular trigeminal nerve axons in the meninges to release vasoactive neuropeptides such as substance P and calcitonin gene-related peptide (CGRP) from their terminals. These peptides cause vasodilation, plasma extravasation (leakage of plasma into the tissue), and release of inflammatory mediators from nearby mast cells (Moskowitz, 1992; Figure 9.19). The inflammatory response is spread along the nerve fibers, resulting in the transmission of pain messages to the thalamus and cortex. According to this model, sumatriptan alleviates headache symptoms by blocking peptide release via presynaptic 5-HT_{1D}-like heteroreceptors located on the trigeminal nerve terminals.

5-HT_{1E} and 5-HT_{1F} receptors. Additional 5-HT receptors have been cloned that possess the basic 5-HT_1 pharmacology, yet are distinct from the previously described subtypes (Adham et al., 1993; Lovenberg et al., 1993); hence, these receptors have been designated 5-HT_{1E} and 5-HT_{1F}. The 5-HT_{1F} subtype appears to be particularly concentrated in the hippocampus, cortex, and dorsal raphe nucleus. Little is currently known about the function of these receptors, and no selective agonists or antagonists have yet been developed.

◄ 9.19 HYPOTHETICAL MECHANISM OF MIGRAINE HEADACHE INDUCTION AND SITE OF SUMATRIPTAN ACTION. Recent studies suggest that the primary cause of migraine headache is neurogenic inflammation triggered by unknown causes. According to this hypothesis, perivascular trigeminal nerve axons within the meninges are stimulated to release neuropeptides, which cause vasodilation, plasma extravasation, and secretion of inflammatory mediators by mast cells. The inflammatory response is spread along the nerve fibers by ortho- and antidromic conduction, ultimately resulting in the transmission of pain impulses to higher brain centers. Sumatriptan is believed to inhibit neuropeptide release from the nerve terminals by acting on 5-HT_{1D} heteroreceptors. (After Moskowitz, 1992.)

5-HT_2 Receptors

The 5-HT_2 subtype constitutes another 5-HT receptor family. Its pharmacological features are presented in Table 9.3 (for review, see Baxter, Kennett et al., 1995; Hoyer et al., 1994). Within this family, the 5-HT_{2A} subtype represents the "classic" 5-HT_2 receptor and additionally corresponds to the peripheral D receptor of Gaddum and Picarelli (see above). As mentioned earlier, the 5-HT_{2C} receptor was originally designated 5-HT_{1C}; however, we anticipate that the new and more appropriate nomenclature will soon become commonplace. The most recent addition to the 5-HT_2 receptor family is 5-HT_{2B}.

No agonists have yet been developed that are highly selective for individual members of the 5-HT_2 family, although MK212 (6-chloro-2-(1-piperazinyl)pyrazine) and *m*-CPP exhibit some selectivity for 5-HT_{2B} and 5-HT_{2C} receptors as compared with 5-HT_{2A} (note, however, that *m*-CPP is a partial rather than a full agonist). General agonists for the 5-HT_2 receptor family include the 5-HT analog α-methyl-5-HT and the phenylalkylamines DOM, DOI, and DOB (1-(2,5-dimethoxy-4-methylphenyl)-2-aminopropane and its iodinated and brominated analogs). LSD also exerts 5-HT_2 agonist effects in

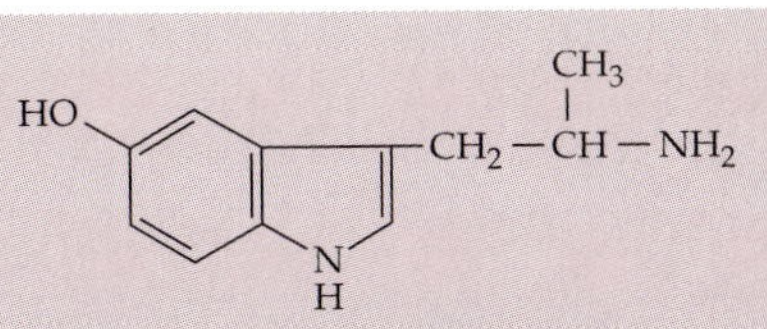

α-Methyl-5-HT

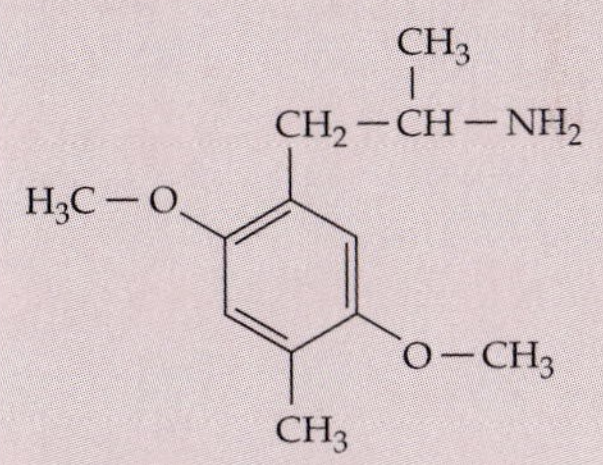

DOM

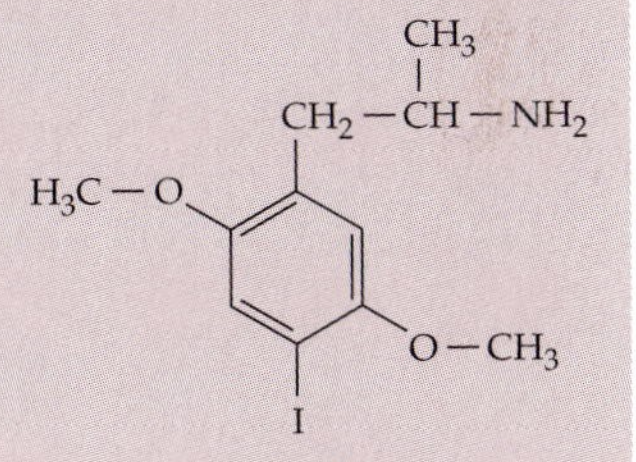

DOI

some model systems, although the pharmacology of this compound is quite complicated. DOM, DOB, DOI, and of course LSD all exert hallucinogenic effects, which has led to a 5-HT_2 receptor theory of hallucinogenic action (Glennon, 1990a; see also Chapter 17).

A number of potent 5-HT_2 antagonists have been developed, including ketanserin, ritanserin, mesulergine, 4-isopropyl-7-methyl-9-(2-hydroxy-1-methylpropoxycarbonyl-4,6,6A,7,8,9,10A-octahydroinodolo(4,3FG) quinolone (LY-53857), pirenperone, and pipamperone (Leysen, 1990; Middlemiss and Tricklebank, 1992). These compounds exhibit varying affinities for the various 5-HT_2 subtypes, with ritanserin showing modest selectivity for 5-HT_{2A} and mesulergine slight selectivity for 5-HT_{2C}. Although ketanserin was one of the first 5-HT_2 antagonists to be developed, its selectivity is compromised somewhat because it also has moderate affinity

Table 9.3 Pharmacology of 5-HT$_2$, 5-HT$_3$, and 5-HT$_4$ Receptors

Receptor subtype	Agonists	Antagonists	Radioligands	Effector pathways
5-HT$_{2A}$	α-Methyl-5-HT,	Ketanserin, ritanserin, LY-53857	[^{3}H]Ketanserin	↑ IP$_3$/DAG
5-HT$_{2B}$	α-Methyl-5-HT, m-CPP,[a] MK212	SB 200646A, LY-53857		↑ IP$_3$/DAG
5-HT$_{2C}$	α-Methyl-5-HT m-CPP,[a] MK212	SB 200646A, mesulergine, LY-53857	[^{3}H]Mesulergine	↑ IP$_3$/DAG
5-HT$_3$	2-Methyl-5-HT, m-chlorophenyl-biguanide	Tropisetron, ondansetron, granisetron	[^{3}H]GR65630, [^{3}H]zacopride	Cation channel
5-HT$_4$	5-Methoxytryptamine, SB 205149, BIMU8	GR113808, RS 23597-190	[^{3}H]GR113808	↑ cAMP

[a]m-CPP is a partial agonist at 5-HT$_{2B}$ and 5-HT$_{2C}$ receptors.

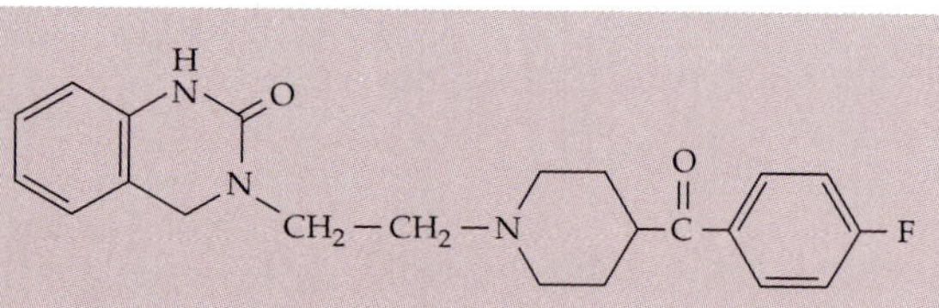

Ketanserin

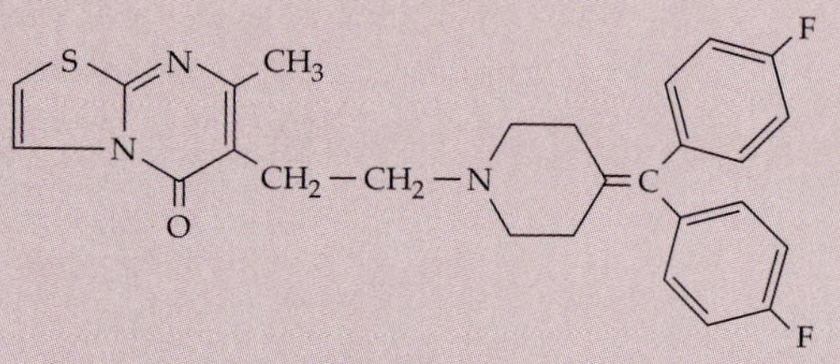

Ritanserin

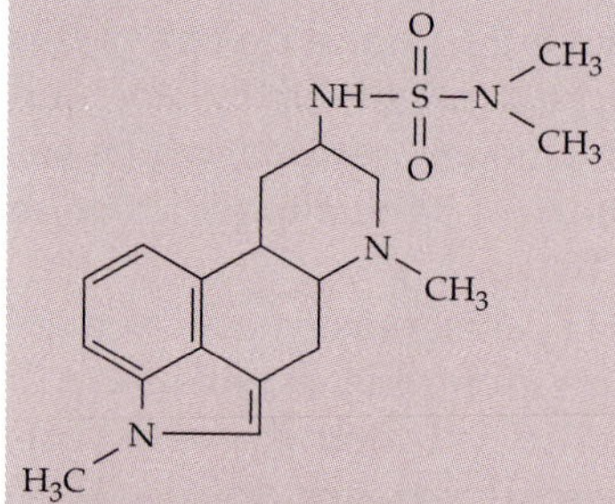

Mesulergine

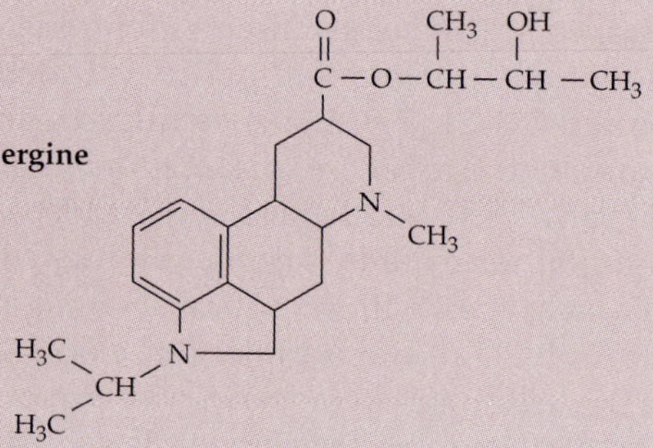

LY-53857

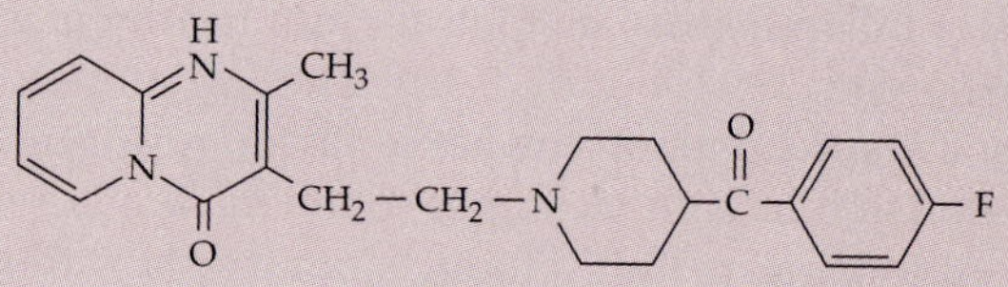

Pirenperone

for α$_1$-adrenergic and H$_1$-histaminergic receptors. More recently, researchers have developed a novel 5-HT$_{2B/2C}$ antagonist, N-(1-methyl-5-indolyl)-N'-(3-pyridyl)urea (SB 200646A) (Forbes et al., 1993), which is proving useful in determining whether particular 5-HT$_2$ effects are mediated by the 5-HT$_{2A}$ subtype or by either 5-HT$_{2B}$ or 5-HT$_{2C}$ receptors.

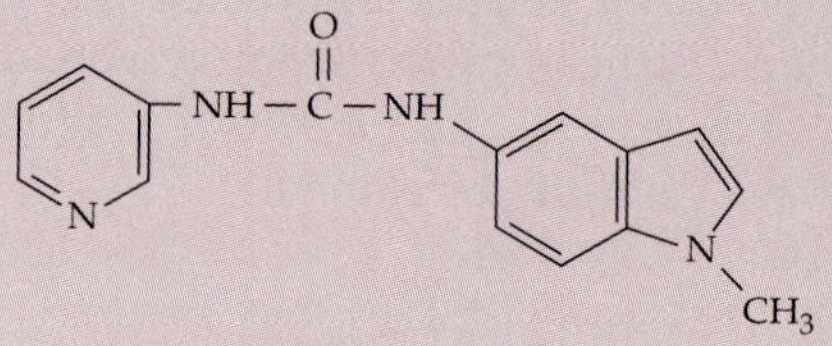

SB 200646A

Autoradiographic mapping of 5-HT$_2$ binding sites in the rat brain has demonstrated particularly high receptor densities in the claustrum, nucleus accumbens, olfactory tubercle, piriform cortex, and layers 1 and 4 of the neocortex (Malgouris, Flamand, and Doble, 1993; Pazos, Cortés, and Palacios, 1985). 5-HT$_2$ ligands tagged with positron-emitting isotopes have also been used for positron emission tomographic (PET) scanning of 5-HT$_2$ receptors in vivo (Hartig and Lever, 1990). 5-HT$_{2C}$ receptors can be labeled relatively selectively with [³H]mesulergine, although care must be taken to minimize binding to other 5-HT$_2$ subtypes.

The functional properties of the 5-HT$_2$ receptor family have been studied by observing which effects of nonspecific serotonergic agonists could be blocked by general 5-HT$_2$ receptor antagonists. Thus, compounds such as ketanserin, ritanserin, and pirenperone were found to antagonize tryptamine-induced tremors and clonic seizures, 5-HTP-induced head twitches and "wet-dog" shakes, behavioral effects of LSD and the hallucinogenic phenylalkylamines, serotonergic stimulation of blood platelet aggregation, and constriction of vascular and bronchial smooth muscle produced by 5-HT administration (Awouters, 1985; Glennon, 1990). However, delineating which 5-HT$_2$ receptor subtypes are involved in these responses (particularly the behavioral effects) has been difficult due to the lack of subtype-selective antagonists. Head twitches and "wet-dog" shakes are among the motor responses generally considered to involve the "classic" 5-HT$_2$ (i.e., 5-HT$_{2A}$) receptor (Koek, Jackson, and Colpaert, 1992; Zifa and Fillion, 1992). For the 5-HT$_{2C}$ and 5-HT$_{2B}$ receptor subtypes, information has been obtained from the behavioral effects of certain agonist drugs, particularly TFMPP (mentioned earlier as a putative 5-HT$_{1B}$ agonist) and *m*-CPP (a mixed 5-HT$_{1B/2B,2C}$ agonist). When administered to rats, these compounds cause reduced locomotor activity, hypophagia, penile erections, and anxiogenic-like behavioral responses (Berendsen, Jenck, and Broekkamp, 1990; Curzon and Kennett, 1990; Koek, Jackson, and Colpaert, 1992). Such effects are blocked by the relatively selective 5-HT$_{2B,2C}$ antagonist SB 2006465A, suggesting an involvement of either or both of these receptor subtypes (Baxter, Kennett et al., 1995).

In certain cases, the physiological action of a particular 5-HT$_2$ receptor subtype can be readily defined because of its selective localization in a specific tissue. For example, 5-HT$_{2C}$ receptors were first discovered in the choroid plexus, where they are expressed at high levels by the choroidal epithelial cells and may be involved in the inhibition of CSF production by CSF-borne 5-HT (Hartig et al., 1990). 5-HT$_{2B}$ receptors are present in a number of peripheral organs, and they are known to mediate the contractile effect of 5-HT on the rat fundus (part of the stomach) (Hoyer et al., 1994). Messenger RNA for the 5-HT$_{2B}$ receptor has been found in the human brain (Kursar et al., 1994), but may be present only at low levels in the rat brain (see Hoyer et al., 1994). These findings have obvious implications for whether any behavioral effects of serotonergic agonists can be attributed to 5-HT$_{2B}$ receptor activation, although it is still premature to dismiss a possible contribution of this subtype.

It is interesting to note that 5-HT$_2$ receptor blockade in animals and humans *not* treated previously with a serotonergic agonist was found to have few effects other than increasing the ratio of slow-wave to rapid-eye-movement sleep and (in rats) reducing fear responses to aversive stimuli (Leysen, 1990). Based on these observations, Leysen (1990) hypothesized that 5-HT$_2$-mediated effects come into play only during brief periods of the normal sleep–waking cycle or during certain physiological challenges, as seen in the serotonergic enhancement of blood clotting following injury-induced release of platelet 5-HT.

5-HT$_2$ receptors exhibit unusual regulatory responses to changes in 5-HT availability. As we have seen in previous chapters, neurotransmitter receptors are often up-regulated following denervation, transmitter synthesis inhibition, or chronic pharmacological blockade. Conversely, down-regulation is a frequent occurrence in response to chronic agonist administration. In the case of 5-HT$_2$ receptors, rapid down-regulation has usually been observed in response to 5-HT agonist treatment. However, neither lesions of serotonergic neurons nor 5-HT synthesis inhibition seem to alter 5-HT$_2$ receptor density (Leysen, 1990; Sanders-Bush, 1990). Leysen (1990) has hypothesized that 5-HT$_2$ receptors normally receive little synaptic stimulation and thus might normally be in a state of supersensitivity. If so, this would account for the lack of further increases in receptor density as a consequence of denervation. Leysen's theory also explains why so few effects are observed following acute 5-HT$_2$ receptor blockade.

5-HT$_2$ receptors also show an anomalous response to antagonist treatment. A number of studies have demonstrated that repeated administration of 5-HT$_2$ antagonists produces a *down-regulation* of both receptor binding and gene expression, rather than the expected up-regulation (Pranzatelli, Murthy, and Tailor, 1993; Sanders-Bush, 1990; Toth and Shenk, 1994). Although the mechanism underlying this response is still not known, a possible explanation comes from recent findings of Barker et al. (1994). Over the past few years, instances have been found in which G protein–coupled receptors exhibited constitutive activity—that is, stimulation of second messenger systems in the absence of an applied agonist, which is apparently due to a low level of G protein activation produced by unbound receptor. The results of Barker et al. demonstrated the presence of such constitutive activity in cells transfected with the 5-HT$_{2C}$ receptor (in this case, the receptor is positively coupled to the phosphoinositide second messenger, and therefore phosphoinositide turnover was measured as an index of receptor activity). A true neutral antagonist should have no effect on constitutive receptor activity, since this activity occurs independently of agonist treatment. However, the researchers found that a number of drugs traditionally considered to be 5-HT$_2$ antagonists (e.g., ketanserin, mianserin, and mesulergine) unexpectedly *reduced* phosphoinositide turnover even without agonist treatment. A drug acting in this manner is classified as an **inverse agonist** rather than an antagonist because it does show intrinsic efficacy at the receptor, although the direction of the drug effect is opposite to that shown by normal agonists (see Chapter 10 for a discussion of inverse agonists for a ligand-gated channel, the GABA$_A$ receptor). Of particular interest here is that all inverse agonists tested by Barker et al. also caused a down-regulation of the 5-HT$_{2C}$ receptor. In contrast, the LSD analog 2-bromolysergic acid diethylamide (BOL), which acted as a pure antagonist because it had no effect on constitutive receptor activity but blocked agonist-induced phosphoinositide turnover, failed to alter 5-HT$_{2C}$ receptor binding. These results suggest that down-regulation of 5-HT$_2$ receptors by so-called antagonists may be related to the activity of these drugs as inverse agonists rather than as classic neutral antagonists.

5-HT$_3$ Receptors

The 5-HT$_3$ receptor is unique among the currently known subtypes. Specifically, 5-HT$_3$ receptors are *not* coupled to G proteins or second messenger systems, but instead belong to the ligand-gated channel superfamily. These receptors exhibit many structural and functional similarities to the nicotinic cholinergic receptor, and they mediate the same type of rapid, excitatory electrophysiological response (Peters, Malone, and Lambert, 1992). Interestingly, the 5-HT$_3$ subtype was actually one of the first 5-HT receptors identified, since it corresponds to Gaddum and Picarelli's morphine-sensitive M receptor.

Despite its early discovery, little research was performed on the 5-HT$_3$ receptor for over 20 years due to a lack of specific agonists or antagonists. Since the early to middle 1980s, however, the introduction of a number of selective agonists and antagonists has led to a growing understanding of the functions of this receptor subtype (Kilpatrick, Bunce, and Tyers, 1990; Middlemiss and Tricklebank, 1992). Potent 5-HT$_3$ agonists include 2-methyl-5-HT, phenylbiguanide, and *m*-chlorophenylbiguanide, the last of which is thought to possess the greatest combination of potency and selectivity. Some of the more important 5-HT$_3$ antagonists are ondansetron, granisetron, tropisetron, ICS 205-930, and MDL 72222, which was developed from cocaine (a weak, nonspecific 5-HT$_3$ antagonist).

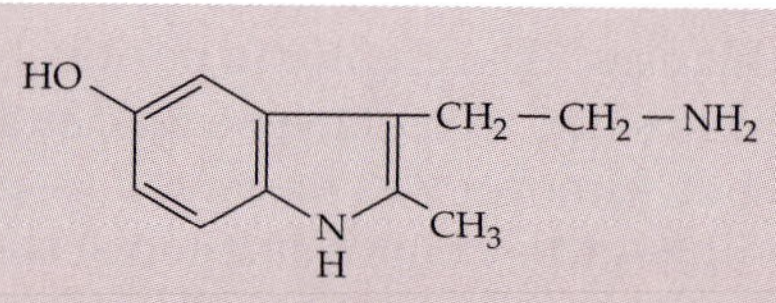

Ondansetron

Granisetron

MDL 72222

2-Methyl-5-HT

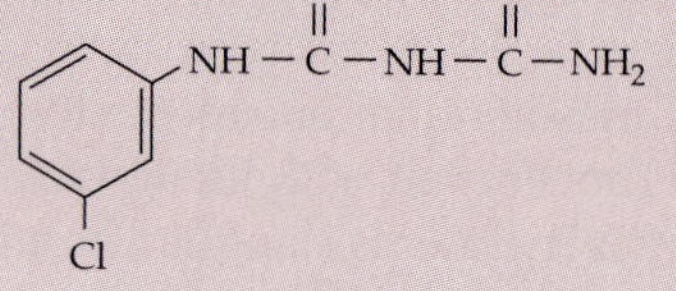

***m*-Chlorophenylbiguanide**

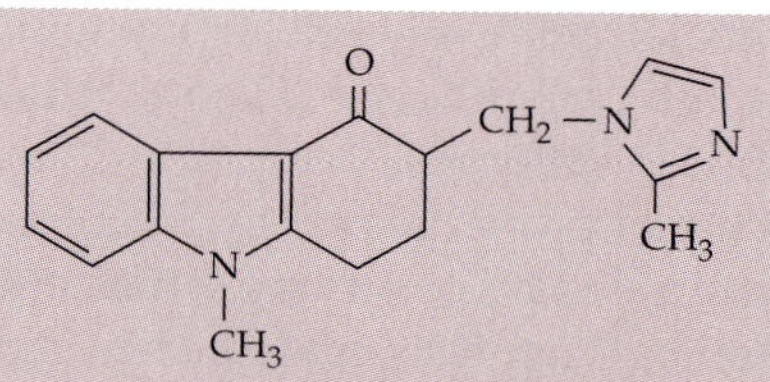

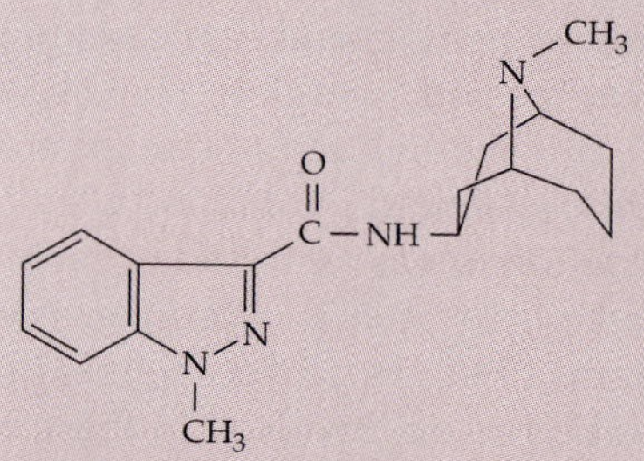

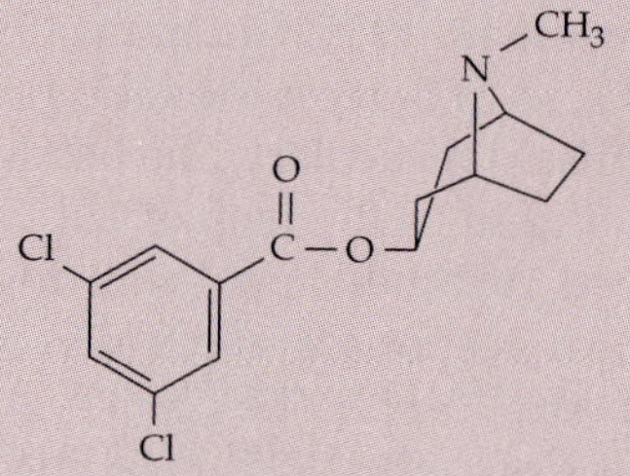

Physiological studies indicate a widespread distribution of 5-HT$_3$ receptors in the peripheral nervous system (Kilpatrick, Bunce, and Tyers, 1990). Serotonergic effects thought to be mediated by this receptor subtype have been found in the sensory system, the sympathetic and parasympathetic branches of the autonomic nervous system, and the enteric nervous system (which is not surprising in view of the original discovery of M receptors in the guinea pig intestine). 5-HT$_3$ receptors have likewise been detected in the brain, with the highest densities found in the area postrema, the entorhinal cortex, the amygdala, and certain brain stem nuclei, including the nucleus of the solitary tract and the vagal and the trigeminal nerve nuclei (Kilpatrick, Bunce, and Tyers, 1990; Hoyer, 1990). Particularly low levels of binding were reported in the cerebellum, striatum, hypothalamus, and thalamus.

Recent studies of 5-HT$_3$ receptor function have revealed significant activity in a remarkable variety of test systems, including hyperlocomotion triggered by DA agonists in the nucleus accumbens, various models of anxiety, tests of pain sensitivity, measures of food intake, drug withdrawal syndromes, and nausea and emesis (vomiting), which is induced by drug or radiation treatment (Barnes, Barnes, and Cooper, 1992; Costall, 1993; Greenshaw, 1993). Here we will briefly discuss the role of 5-HT$_3$ receptors in the control of treatment-induced emesis, as some of the other behaviors mentioned are covered below in Part III.

The possibility that 5-HT$_3$-acting compounds might influence emetic responses was suggested by the recognition that metoclopramide, an agent that had been used to control drug- and radiation-induced emesis for a number of years, had significant 5-HT$_3$ antagonist potency in addition to its well-known DA D$_2$ receptor blocking action. When more selective 5-HT$_3$ antagonists were developed and tested in various animal models, they were found to possess potent antiemetic properties (Kilpatrick, Bunce, and Tyers, 1990). Human clinical trials subsequently confirmed the usefulness of 5-HT$_3$ antagonists such as ondansetron (Zofran) and granisetron in preventing postoperative nausea and emesis (Russell and Kenny, 1992; Scuderi et al., 1993) as well as emetic responses to chemotherapy and radiation treatment (Falkson and van Zyl, 1989; Hunter et al., 1991). As these drugs exhibit few adverse side effects compared with metoclopramide and other formerly used agents, their introduction into the clinical realm represents a significant advance in medical care.

Figure 9.20 illustrates the probable mechanism of action of 5-HT$_3$ receptor antagonists in preventing nausea and vomiting due to chemotherapy or radiation (Tyers and Freeman, 1992). Sensory fibers of the vagus nerve project from the gastrointestinal mucosa to the brain stem vomiting system, which consists of the dorsovagal nucleus, the nucleus of the solitary tract, and the area postrema. Cytotoxic anticancer drugs or radiation treatments are thought to provoke gastrointestinal enterochromaffin cells to release 5-HT, which then stimulates 5-HT$_3$ receptors on the nearby vagal afferents. The resulting vagal activation triggers an emetic response from the vomiting system. According to the model shown in the figure, 5-HT$_3$ antagonists not only block the effect of 5-HT in the GI tract, but may also act on presynaptic 5-HT$_3$ receptors to inhibit neurotransmitter release by the vagus nerve.

5-HT$_4$ Receptors

Several years ago, Dumuis and colleagues (1988) reported on a novel 5-HT receptor in mouse collicular neurons that stimulated the formation of cAMP and that exhibited a pharmacology unlike that of the known 5-HT$_1$, 5-HT$_2$, or 5-HT$_3$ receptors. On the basis of these findings, the receptor was considered to represent a new 5-HT receptor subtype and was designated 5-HT$_4$ (Bockaert et al., 1992). Since then, several laboratories have cloned other 5-HT receptors positively coupled to adenylyl cyclase (Bard et al., 1993; Ruat et al., 1993; Shen et al., 1993); however, it remains to be seen whether these receptors, together with 5-HT$_4$, can be considered a new family of 5-HT receptors.

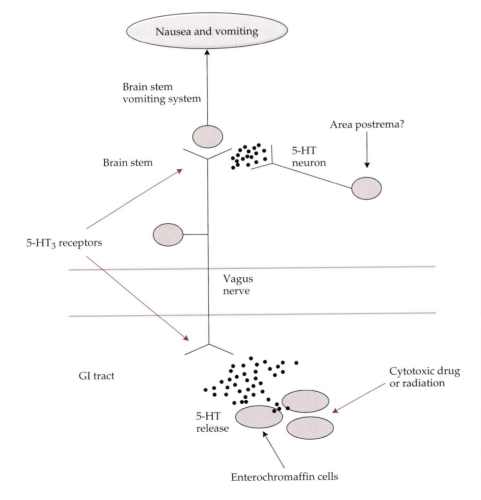

9.20 MECHANISMS UNDERLYING THE ANTIEMETIC ACTION OF 5-HT$_3$ RECEPTOR ANTAGONISTS. Cytotoxic drug or radiation treatments are believed to cause the release of 5-HT from enterochromaffin cells in the GI tract. Activation of 5-HT$_3$ receptors on vagal afferents stimulates these fibers to trigger an emetic response by the brain stem vomiting system. 5-HT$_3$ antagonists could act to block the initial activation of the vagus nerve and/or to inhibit neurotransmitter release via presynaptic 5-HT$_3$ receptors located on the vagal nerve fibers. (After Tyers and Freeman, 1992.)

It has proved difficult to find drugs that are selective for the 5-HT$_4$ receptor; however, the situation has been improving. The best agonist developed to date is n-butyl renzapride (SB 205149; Baxter et al., 1993), followed by members of the benzimidazolone family such as (endo-N-8-methyl-8-azabicyclo[3.2.1]oct-3-yl)-2,3-dihydro-3-isopropyl-2-oxo-1H-benzimadazol-1-carboxamide (BIMU8). Useful antagonists include [1-[2-[(methylsulfonyl)amino]ethyl]-4-piperidinyl]methyl-1-methyl-1H-indole-3-carboxylate (GR113808), 3-(piperidin-1-yl)propyl-4-amino-5-chloro-2-methoxybenzoate (RS 23597-190), and 2-methoxy-4-amino-5-chloro-benzoic acid 2-(diethylamino) ethyl ester (SDZ20557).

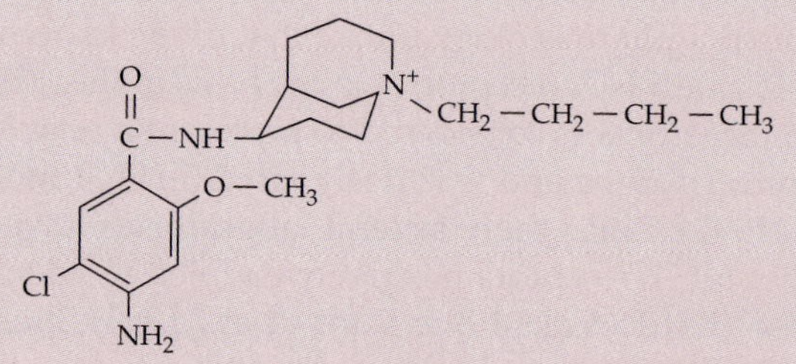

n-Butyl Renzapride

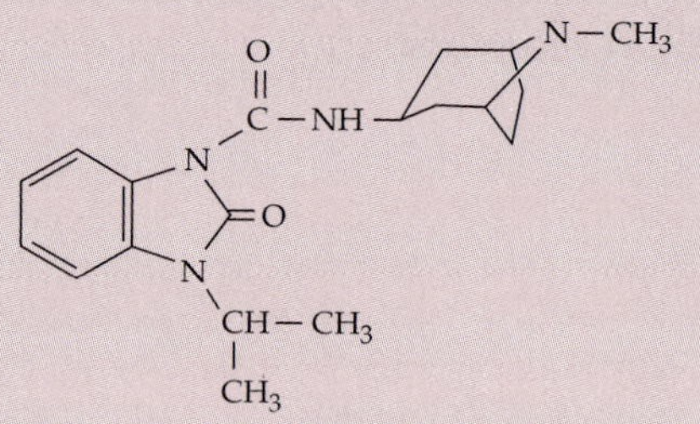

BIMU8

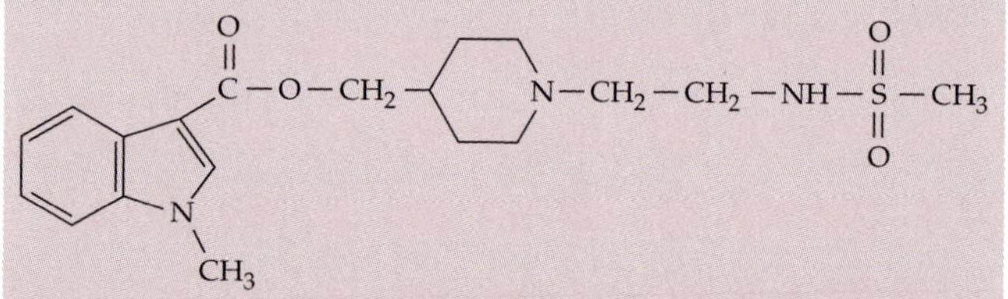

GR113808

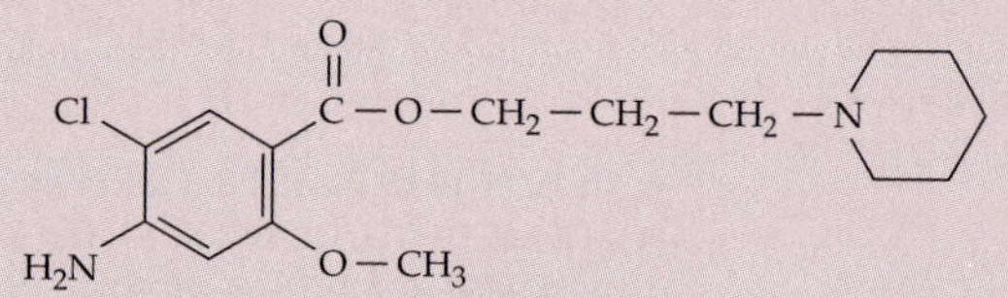

RS 23597-190

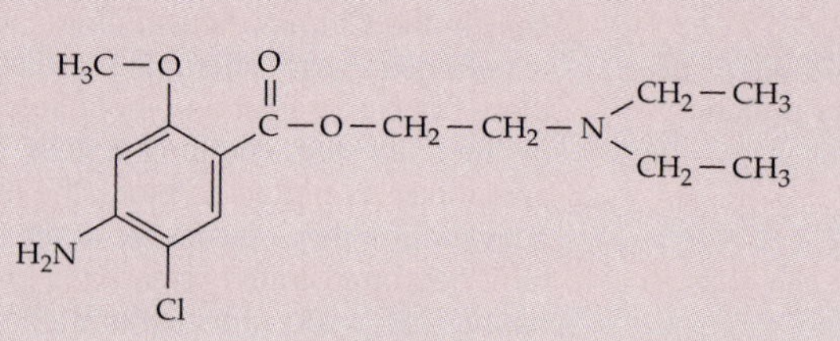

SDZ205557

Peripherally, 5-HT$_4$ receptors have been identified in guinea pig ileum, pig and human heart, and rat esophagus, where they mediate a variety of excitatory and inhibitory responses (Bockaert et al., 1992; Ford and Clarke, 1993). Mapping studies in rat, guinea pig, and human brain have reported the highest receptor densities in the globus pallidus, olfactory tubercles, substantia nigra, and caudate nucleus. Intermediate levels were found in the hippocampus, and low levels were found in the neocortex (Grossman, Kilpatrick, and Bunce, 1993; Waeber et al., 1993). At the present time, we know little about the participation of 5-HT$_4$ receptors in behavioral regulation. However, Costall and Naylor (1993) recently presented evidence that the 5-HT$_4$ subtype, in addition to 5-HT$_{1A}$ and 5-HT$_3$ receptors, may play a role in mediating the effects of 5-HT on anxiety.

Serotonin Receptor Mechanisms

The effector mechanisms used by various 5-HT receptor subtypes have been reviewed by Andrade and Chaput (1991), Bobker and Williams (1990), Cornfield and Nelson (1991), and Hoyer and Schoeffter (1991). Here we will focus on the 5-HT$_1$, 5-HT$_2$, and 5-HT$_4$ subtypes, since the mechanism of action of 5-HT$_3$ receptors was discussed earlier.

As shown in Table 9.2, 5-HT$_1$ receptors are all negatively coupled to adenylyl cyclase and cAMP formation. The functional consequences of this effect have not yet been determined. However, the 5-HT$_{1A}$ receptor subtype has also been shown to produce a membrane hyperpolarization and an inhibition of cell firing in the rat hippocampus and cortex (Andrade, 1992; Andrade and Chaput, 1991). This effect is independent of cAMP, and is caused instead by activation of a pertussis toxin–sensitive G protein directly coupled to the opening of a K$^+$ channel. In hippocampal pyramidal neurons, this K$^+$ channel may be the same one regulated by the GABA$_B$ receptor (Figure 9.21; see also Chapter 10).

As mentioned earlier, some 5-HT$_{1B}$ and 5-HT$_{1D}$ receptors are thought to act as presynaptic autoreceptors on serotonergic nerve terminals. There is evidence that 5-HT can also inhibit the release of other neurotransmitters via 5-HT$_{1B}$ and 5-HT$_{1D}$ receptors located on nonserotonergic endings (Bobker and Williams, 1990; Hen, 1992). The mechanism underlying these effects is still unknown.

5-HT$_2$ receptors have no effect on the cAMP system, but instead activate the phosphoinositide (PI) second messenger system (see Table 9.3). As discussed in previous chapters, the products of PI hydrolysis, namely, inositol trisphosphate (IP$_3$) and diacylglycerol (DAG), elevate intracellular Ca^{2+} levels and stimulate protein kinase C. Electrophysiologically, 5-HT$_2$ receptors increase cell excitability and firing rate by decreasing resting K$^+$ conductance and hence depolarizing the cell membrane (Andrade and Chaput, 1991; Panicker, Parker,

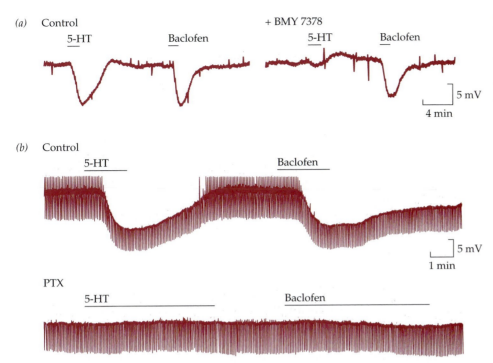

(a) Control   + BMY 7378

5-HT   Baclofen   5-HT   Baclofen

5 mV

4 min

(b) Control

5-HT   Baclofen

5 mV

1 min

PTX

5-HT   Baclofen

9.21 HYPERPOLARIZATION OF HIP-POCAMPAL CA1 PYRAMIDAL CELLS BY 5-HT$_{1A}$ RECEPTOR ACTIVATION. (*a*) The pyramidal cell membrane is hyperpolarized by administration of either 5-HT (30 µM) or the GABA$_B$ receptor agonist baclofen (30 µM). The response to 5-HT is selectively blocked by the 5-HT$_{1A}$ antagonist BMY 7378. (*b*) Effects of both 5-HT and baclofen are completely inhibited by pertussis toxin (PTX), indicating mediation of both responses by a PTX-sensitive G protein. (After Andrade and Chaput, 1991.)

and Miledi, 1991). One functional role of these receptors may be to mediate cortical desynchronization produced by application of a noxious sensory stimulus (Neuman and Zebrowska, 1992). It is also interesting to note that rat cortical neurons coexpress 5-HT$_{1A}$ and 5-HT$_2$ receptors. Due to the complex relationship between the electrophysiological effects of these receptor subtypes, the net effect of 5-HT is to reduce the effectiveness of weak excitatory inputs to the cells but to greatly enhance the effectiveness of strong inputs (Andrade, 1992).

The 5-HT$_4$ receptor was the first subtype found to be positively coupled to adenylyl cyclase. The resulting increase in cAMP and activation of cAMP-dependent protein kinase (protein kinase A) inhibits certain K$^+$ channels, thereby causing a slow depolarization of the cell (Bockaert et al., 1992). In some systems, this depolarization has been observed to open voltage-sensitive Ca^{2+} channels and to stimulate neurotransmitter release.

Part II Summary

Serotonin-containing neurons are found primarily in the raphe nuclei of the brain stem. These cells give rise to ascending and descending pathways that innervate large areas of the brain and spinal cord. Recent anatomical studies suggest that the dorsal and median raphe nuclei give rise to distinctive forebrain terminal systems designated D and M, although the functional significance of these systems is not yet known.

Electrophysiological work by Jacobs and colleagues has shown that dorsal raphe neurons in cats typically fire at a very regular rate. Firing rate is highest when the animals are awake, lower during slow-wave sleep, and almost completely abolished during REM sleep. These cells also tend to be activated during repetitive movements and inhibited by strong sensory stimuli. Based on these findings, Jacobs has hypothesized that the serotonergic system facilitates motor output while suppressing ongoing sensory processing.

The well-characterized 5-HT receptor subtypes consist of a family of 5-HT$_1$ receptors (5-HT$_{1A}$, 5-HT$_{1B}$, 5-HT$_{1D}$, 5-HT$_{1E}$, and 5-HT$_{1F}$), a family of 5-HT$_2$ receptors (5-HT$_{2A-C}$), 5-HT$_3$ receptors, and 5-HT$_4$ receptors. Selective agonists have been identified for some 5-HT receptor subtypes, such as 8-OH-DPAT and ipsapirone for 5-HT$_{1A}$, CP-93,129 for 5-HT$_{1B}$, sumatriptan for 5-HT$_{1D}$, α-methyl-5-HT for 5-HT$_2$, *m*-chlorophenyl-biguanide for 5-HT$_3$, and SB 205149 and BIMU8 for 5-HT$_4$ receptors. Relatively selective antagonists include SDZ 216-525 and WAY-100135 for 5-HT$_{1A}$, ketanserin and ritanserin for 5-HT$_{2A}$, mesulergine for 5-HT$_{2C}$, ondansetron and granisetron for 5-HT$_3$, and GR113808 for 5-HT$_4$ receptors. Sumatriptan has been introduced clinically for the treatment of migraine headaches, whereas ondansetron is effective in counteracting nausea and vomiting associated with chemotherapy, radiation therapy, and general surgery.

5-HT$_1$, 5-HT$_2$, and 5-HT$_4$ receptors all belong to the G protein-coupled superfamily and mediate either excitatory or inhibitory electrophysiological effects. In contrast, 5-HT$_3$ receptors directly gate a membrane cation channel, thus leading only to fast excitatory responses. 5-HT$_1$ receptors inhibit the formation of cAMP, whereas 5-HT$_4$ receptors stimulate cAMP synthesis. Members of the 5-HT$_2$ family all stimulate the PI second messenger system.

Part III
Behavioral Functions of Serotonin

Since its discovery in the nervous system in the early 1950s, 5-HT has been implicated in the regulation of virtually every kind of behavior. This is not surprising for a transmitter with such a widespread distribution in the brain, spinal cord, and peripheral nervous system. The sheer amount of reported research on serotonergic functions precludes exhaustive coverage in this section. We have therefore chosen to analyze in detail the possible involvement of 5-HT in three areas: hunger and body weight regulation, aggression and suicidality, and obsessive–compulsive disorder. The roles of 5-HT in alcohol abuse, anxiety, and affective disorders are taken up in Chapters 15, 16, and 19, respectively.

Feeding Behavior and Body Weight Regulation

Serotonin undeniably influences various aspects of food intake. The more difficult question to answer concerns the nature of its effect(s). Changes in serotonergic activity might conceivably alter the physiological substrates of meal initiation ("hunger" signals), the physiological substrates of meal termination ("satiety" signals), the mechanisms that regulate macronutrient choice, the sensory perception of food, the motor components of food ingestion, and so on. We can see, therefore, that the question before us is much more complicated than "Does 5-HT cause organisms to increase or decrease their food intake?" although this is obviously one question among many that might be raised. Our analysis of 5-HT and feeding behavior will accordingly be divided into three parts. The first section will consider changes in brain serotonergic activity associated with food intake. Next, the effects of serotonergic drugs on various aspects of feeding behavior will be discussed. The final section will deal with the possible relationship between 5-HT and overeating and obesity.

Changes in Serotonergic Activity Associated with Feeding

The pharmacological studies to be discussed in the following section provide powerful evidence that *perturbing* normal serotonergic functioning can alter feeding behavior. It is at least equally important to determine whether changes in the *spontaneous* activity of serotonergic neurons can be observed during the presentation of food stimuli, during the occurrence of ingestive behavior, or as a consequence of postingestive events.

Only recently have researchers begun to investigate whether the firing of serotonergic neurons is related to feeding behavior. One approach has been to study the influence of serotonergic afferents on the activity of rat lateral hypothalamic neurons that are sensitive to the presence of glucose. Experiments by Kai, Oomura, and

Shimizu (1988) indicated that approximately 75% of such cells receive a 5-HT$_1$ receptor-mediated inhibitory input from the dorsal raphe, suggesting that 5-HT may modulate the hypothalamic system involved in glucose detection and the initiation and termination of eating. Equally important are in vivo microdialysis studies demonstrating increased 5-HT release in both the medial and lateral hypothalamus during exposure to food stimuli and during the subsequent period of food intake, but not after termination of eating (Schwartz, Hernandez, and Hoebel, 1990a). Although the functional role of 5-HT in feeding cannot be ascertained from these findings alone, they do suggest that serotonergic projections to the hypothalamus are activated during the preingestive and ingestive phases of a meal.

Studies concerning postingestive effects on the serotonergic system have focused on the "carbohydrate connection" discussed above in Part I. Ingestion by rats of a high-carbohydrate, low-protein meal can elevate brain tryptophan concentrations and stimulate 5-HT synthesis and release. Because this effect requires fairly strict experimental conditions, including prior fasting by the subjects, its relevance for understanding patterns of human food intake is questionable. Nevertheless, we shall consider the hypothesis of a feedback loop between 5-HT and carbohydrate craving.

Effects of Serotonergic Drugs on Food Intake

Pharmacological manipulations of the serotonergic system in both laboratory animals (usually rats) and humans have been remarkably consistent in showing that increasing serotonergic activity (e.g., by administering 5-HT precursors, releasing or reuptake inhibiting agents, or direct receptor agonists) generally leads to a suppression of food intake and, if drugs are administered chronically, weight loss (see reviews by Blundell, 1991; Nathan and Rolland, 1987). 5-HT$_{1B}$ and 5-HT$_2$ receptors may be involved in these effects, as feeding is inhibited by both RU 24969 (5-HT$_{1B}$ agonist) and DOI (5-HT$_2$ agonist) (Bovetto and Richard, 1995). Furthermore, the 5-HT$_{1B}$ receptors are thought to be postsynaptic (rather than autoreceptors) because the anorectic effect of RU 24969 is not abolished by depleting brain 5-HT with PCPA (Kennett, Dourish, and Curzon, 1987). On the other hand, treatment with the 5-HT$_{1A}$ agonists 8-OH-DPAT, ipsapirone, or buspirone causes increased food intake (hyperphagia) in freely fed rats (Dourish et al., 1986; Lucki, 1992). This effect appears to be due to stimulation of 5-HT$_{1A}$ somatodendritic autoreceptors, with a consequent inhibition of raphe unit firing and a decreased release of 5-HT in critical forebrain target areas. The ability of autoreceptor activation to enhance food intake has important theoretical implications because it suggests that under normal conditions, 5-HT may exert a tonic inhibitory influence on some aspect of food motivation.

The site of action of 5-HT in regulating feeding behavior has not yet been determined, although, not surprisingly, the hypothalamus has received much attention in this regard. Several studies indicated that microinjection of 5-HT itself or of various direct or indirect 5-HT agonists into the medial hypothalamus caused reductions in food intake (Hutson, Donohoe, and Curzon, 1988; Leibowitz, Weiss, and Suh, 1990; Weiss et al., 1986). The paraventricular nucleus (PVN) seemed to be the critical site of action of these centrally administered drugs. On the other hand, later work from Coscina's laboratory found little change in eating behavior following medial hypothalamic injections of the 5-HT$_1$ agonists RU 24969 or TFMPP, nor were the behavioral effects of peripherally administered serotonergic drugs abolished by PVN lesions (Fletcher et al., 1992, 1993). Hence, questions still remain concerning the possible role of the PVN or other medial hypothalamic sites in the serotonergic control of eating behavior.

Anorectic effects of fenfluramine.   Although many serotonergic agonists have anorectic (appetite suppressant) effects, the most widely studied of these agents has been fenfluramine. As described earlier, this compound is a halogenated amphetamine derivative with potent 5-HT-releasing and uptake-inhibiting properties. Acute fenfluramine administration reduces subsequent food intake in a number of animal species (Rowland and Carlton, 1986). Although the most common test situation has involved measuring consumption after a period of deprivation, fenfluramine is also effective in other paradigms, such as tail pinch–induced eating and consumption in a "dessert test." The latter is an interesting model in which nondeprived rats develop a tendency to ingest large amounts of a highly palatable food (for example, sweetened milk) when given brief access to this "dessert" on a daily basis.

Fenfluramine, and more recently the uptake inhibitor fluoxetine, have proved useful as weight control treatments in humans (Blundell and Hill, 1991; Fuller and Wong, 1989). In studies reviewed by Blundell and Hill (1991), fenfluramine significantly inhibited food intake in both lean and obese subjects over periods ranging from 1 day to 6 months. The degree of intake suppression typically ranged from 11% to about 25%, depending on the test situation. D,L-fenfluramine, the racemic mixture of the steroisomers, has been available clinically for a number of years under the trade name Pondimin. The Food and Drug Administration has recently approved use of the pure D-isomer, dexfenfluramine, which will be marketed as Redux.

Because many subjects regain much, if not all, of their lost weight following cessation of fenfluramine treatment, Weintraub and his colleagues carried out an important study examining the efficacy and safety (in terms of bothersome side effects) of long-term fenflur-amine treatment. The initial subject population consisted of 121 obese individuals ranging in age from 18–60 years old. During the course of the 3-year study, all subjects were given regular sessions of behavior modification, received dietary counseling to assist in restricting their caloric intake, and were maintained on an exercise regimen. During various phases of the investigation, individuals received either placebo or a combination of 60 mg D,L-fenfluramine hydrochloride (in an extended release formula) and 15 mg phentermine resin (Ionamin). Phentermine is also an anorectic agent, although it is thought to act through catecholamine systems rather than through 5-HT. The drugs were administered together in this trial for two reasons. First, it was hoped that greater appetite suppression would be achieved with the combination than with either compound alone because the two drugs act through different neurochemical mechanisms and may also affect different subjective aspects of hunger and satiety. Second, one of the troublesome side effects of fenfluramine is drowsiness; however, phentermine is a behavioral stimulant and was therefore expected to counteract this effect when given concurrently.

The results of the study were published in a series of nine consecutive articles in *Clinical Pharmacology and Therapeutics* (see Weintraub, 1992a,b, and succeeding papers). The first phase of the study was conducted over 34 weeks, and consisted of a double-blind comparison of fenfluramine/phentermine versus placebo. As shown in Figure 9.22, drug treatment along with behavior modification, dietary counseling, and exercise was substantially more effective in inducing weight loss than the behavioral methods alone (Weintraub et al., 1992). However, as other investigators had previously reported, a plateau effect occurred in which the subjects' weight stabilized (albeit at a lower level than before) despite continuing treatment. This effect has typically been considered evidence of tolerance to the anorectic effect of fenfluramine; however, Weintraub points out that true tolerance should result in weight regain, rather than stabilization. This distinction is supported by the observation that at various points during the study when individuals were taken off the drugs, they usually showed substantial weight increases that at least sometimes could be reversed by reinstatement of drug treatment.

Weintraub (1992b) concludes that the combination of fenfluramine and phentermine can be helpful in long-term weight control when combined with a regimen of behavioral modification, dietary counseling, and exercise. Adverse side effects were tolerable for most individuals, and were somewhat reduced in magnitude over time. It is important to note, however, that some individuals were not helped by this treatment program. Moreover, anorectic drugs such as fenfluramine and phentermine do not *cure* obesity in the sense that antibiotics cure an infection. Thus, like antihypertensive medications or

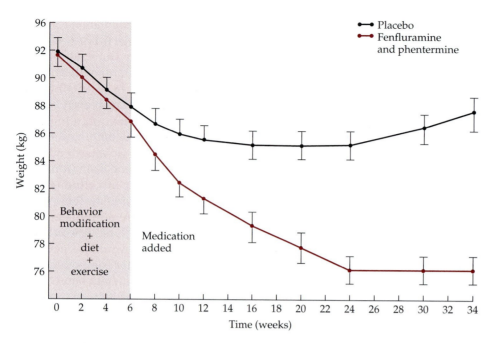

9.22 EFFECTS OF FENFLURAMINE AND PHENTERMINE ON BODY WEIGHT OF OBESE HUMAN SUBJECTS. Obese men and women were entered into a program of behavior modification, dietary counseling, and exercise. After 6 weeks, some subjects (n = 58) were started on daily treatment with 60 mg fenfluramine and 15 mg phentermine. The remaining subjects (n = 54) were given placebo in a double-blind procedure. Significantly greater weight loss occurred with drug treatment than with placebo. (After Weintraub et al., 1992.)

drugs used to lower blood cholesterol, these compounds might have to be taken indefinitely by the patient in order to maintain therapeutic efficacy.

What is the mechanism of fenfluramine action? From a psychological standpoint, drug-treated individuals typically report lower subjective hunger ratings and higher ratings of "fullness" than people given placebo (Figure 9.23). This effect is translated behaviorally into decreased meal size and an inhibition of eating between meals (i.e, snacking) (Blundell and Hill, 1991; Rowland and Carlton, 1986). Blundell and his colleagues have interpreted these findings to mean that fenfluramine somehow enhances the satiating effects of food. Release of brain 5-HT certainly plays some role in this process, as Leibowitz and Shor-Posner (1986) showed that direct administration of fenfluramine into the medial hypothalamus reduced food intake in rats. On the other hand, there is evidence that the drug can also act peripherally to slow the rate of gastric emptying (Davies et al., 1983), which in turn might intensify and prolong satiety signals arising from the stomach (Deutsch, 1983b). Finally, fenfluramine potently stimulates thermogenesis (heat production) in rats (Rothwell and Le Feuvre, 1992), and may exert a similar, though weaker, effect in humans (Schutz et al., 1992).

Thus, central and peripheral mechanisms probably interact to mediate the anorectic effect of fenfluramine. Appetite suppression is clearly the most important factor in the drug's ability to promote weight loss in humans, although increased metabolic activity might also contribute to a small extent.

Serotonin and Obesity

Beyond its apparent role in regulating normal food intake, 5-HT has been linked to obesity in a particular sub-

set of overweight individuals who specifically crave carbohydrates (Wurtman and Wurtman, 1988; Wurtman, 1990). Such individuals reportedly exhibit relatively normal mealtime food intake, but overeat in the form of large snacks typically consisting of low-protein but high-carbohydrate or high-carbohydrate/high-fat items. Research on obese "carbohydrate cravers" revealed that fenfluramine selectively inhibited the intake of carbohydrate-rich snacks as well as carbohydrate intake during meals (Wurtman et al., 1981, 1993). As we saw in Part I of this chapter, ingestion by fasted rats of a high-carbohydrate, low-protein meal elevates brain tryptophan and stimulates brain 5-HT synthesis and release. Combining these findings with the notion that 5-HT selectively modulates carbohydrate consumption led to the theory that a feedback loop exists between serotonergic activity and carbohydrate ingestion. This theory posits that a high level of carbohydrate ingestion enhances 5-HT release, which consequently diminishes the desire for carbohydrates in the following meal (see Fernstrom, 1988a). Abnormal craving for carbohydrates (with a consequent tendency toward obesity) is presumably caused by a chronic deficiency in central serotonergic activity.

This theory is an attractive one because it seems to describe how normal carbohydrate consumption might be regulated by a neurochemical sensing mechanism, and how a derangement of this mechanism could result in a certain type of obesity. However, there are several theoretical and empirical problems with the theory. First, the discussion of dietary carbohydrates and brain 5-HT in Part I pointed out the difficulties involved in extrapolating from the results of single high-carbohydrate/low-protein meals given to previously fasted subjects. This problem raises doubts about the extent to which brain 5-

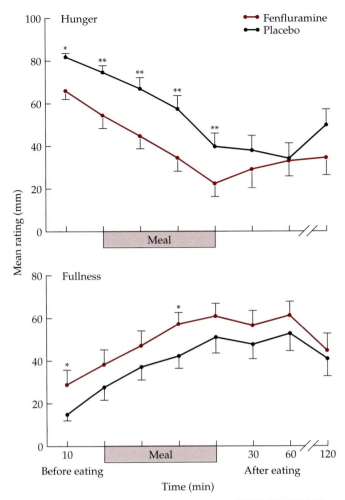

9.23 EFFECTS OF FENFLURAMINE ON SUBJECTIVE RATINGS OF HUNGER AND FULLNESS. Normal-weight women were given 30 mg of dexfenfluramine or placebo orally, 3 hours before a meal. Hunger and fullness ratings were made using a visual analog scale. Before and during the meal, drug-treated subjects showed significantly lower hunger ratings and higher fullness ratings compared with subjects given placebo (*$p < .05$; **$p < .01$). (After Blundell and Hill, 1991.)

HT in humans is regulated by carbohydrate consumption under real-life situations. Second, it is important to consider whether fenfluramine (and hence 5-HT) really exerts a selective effect on carbohydrate consumption. In rat studies, fenfluramine suppressed carbohydrate intake while sparing protein intake under some conditions, but not others (Blundell and Hill, 1989; Lawton and Blundell, 1992; Luo and Li, 1992), suggesting that any macronutrient-selective effect of 5-HT on eating behavior is probably subtle. Finally, in a critique of the 5-HT–carbohydrate feedback loop theory, Fernstrom (1988b) points out that human studies on snacking behavior have failed to control for the sensory and hedonic (pleasurable) qualities of the available food items. For this reason, questions persist about whether the existence of true carbohydrate cravers has yet been proved.

Serotonin and Aggression

Aggression is another important behavior influenced by 5-HT. The relationship between 5-HT and aggression has been investigated in both animals and humans, although the forms of aggressive behavior studied in each case are typically different. Consequently, the animal and human literature will be presented separately, followed by an attempt to identify possible unifying principles and avenues for future research.

The Role of Serotonin in Animal Aggression

Types and models of aggression.   One of the problems associated with identifying the neurobiological substrates of aggression is defining the behavior itself. Because of the diversity of the behavior patterns normally labeled aggressive, it is useful (if not absolutely necessary) to distinguish between different types of aggressive interactions. One of the earliest and most influential typologies of aggression was proposed by Moyer (1968), who argued the importance of defining various types of aggression operationally and of relating each type to its underlying physiological mechanisms. Moyer's typology consisted of predatory, intermale, fear-induced, irritable, territorial, maternal, and instrumental aggression. Although this system had great heuristic value, it also suffered from various problems. Consequently, alternative typologies have been proposed, such as Brain's (1981) classification scheme of predatory attack, self-defensive behaviors, parental defensive behaviors, and social conflict. Furthermore, because threatening and/or violent encounters between individuals involve not only attacks but also defensive maneuvers and withdrawal or fleeing, it is often valuable to use the term "agonistic behavior," which subsumes the latter categories in a clearer way than does the term "aggression."

Historically, quite a wide range of animal models have been used to study the pharmacology of aggression. Some of these, like muricide (mouse-killing) by rats or shock-elicited fighting, have virtually disappeared because they fail to meet current ethical standards of animal research. In rodents, the most widely used test situations still in use include the following: (1) isolation-induced aggression (housing a male rat or mouse in isolation for several weeks and then testing its response to an intruder), (2) resident–intruder aggression (similar to the above except that the male is housed socially with one or more females), (3) maternal aggression (defense of the young by a lactating female), and (4) brain stimulation-induced aggression (aggressive behavior elicited by direct electrical stimulation of appropriate brain areas, usually in the hypothalamus) (Koolhaas and Bohus, 1991; Olivier and Mos, 1992). Aggression in primate species is usually evaluated by examining agonistic interactions and dominance-related behaviors within a

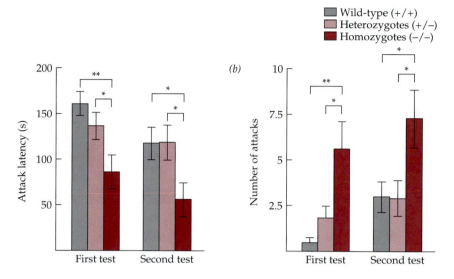

9.24 ISOLATION-INDUCED AGGRESSION IN MUTANT MICE LACKING THE 5-HT$_{1B}$ RECEPTOR. Male mice were isolated for 4 weeks and then tested at 12–14 weeks of age for their aggressive responses to an intruder male. Three strains of animals were tested: wild-type mice, mutant mice homozygous for deletion of the 5-HT$_{1B}$ receptor gene, and heterozygous mice expressing one copy of the gene. In two tests conducted 1 week apart, the homozygous males exhibited (a) a decreased latency to attack the intruder and (b) an increased number of attacks (*p < .05; **p < .01). (After Saudou et al., 1994.)

social group. When evaluating results obtained in a particular test situation, it is important to note that various forms of aggression may differ in their underlying neural and endocrine mechanisms and may thus be differentially affected by a given experimental manipulation. In pharmacological studies, one must also consider that drugs can act both centrally and peripherally to influence aggressive responding, and that the environmental and social consequences of altered agonistic behavior can feed back on the CNS to change subsequent drug sensitivity (Miczek, DeBold, and Thompson, 1984). Finally, determining whether a drug specifically affects aggressive interactions may require that investigators monitor other behaviors occurring concurrently in the test situation. The study of the effects of drugs on a broad range of species-typical behaviors is sometimes termed "ethopharmacology."

Pharmacological studies in rodents. Many studies in rodents indicate that pharmacological enhancement of serotonergic activity tends to suppress aggressive behavior (Miczek, Mos, and Olivier, 1989; Olivier and Mos, 1992). In the case of isolation-induced aggression, this phenomenon was first demonstrated over 30 years ago by Yen, Stranger, and Millman (1959). More recent experiments have examined the effects of various receptor agonists in the same paradigm. Thus, inhibition of isolation-induced aggression can be produced by 5-HT$_{1A}$ agonists such as 8-OH-DPAT and by mixed 5-HT$_{1B/2C}$ agonists such as RU 24969, TFMPP, and *m*-CPP (Bell and Hobson, 1994; Sánchez et al., 1993; White, Kucharik, and Moyer, 1991). It is not clear whether the effects of 5-HT$_{1A}$-active agents are mediated by postsynaptic receptors or by somatodendritic autoreceptors.

Other aggression paradigms have yielded somewhat different results. Mos, Olivier, and Tulp (1992) examined the influence of serotonergic agonists on resident–intruder and maternal aggression in rats. In their studies, 5-HT$_{1A}$ agonists suppressed aggression primarily at relatively high doses that also produced signs of inactivity or sedation. In contrast, TFMPP, RU 24969, and another mixed agonist, eltoprazine, showed a more selective behavioral profile with marked decreases in the incidence of aggressive interactions, increases in exploration, and little or no change in the amount of time spent inactive. Kruk (1991) likewise reported that TFMPP, but not 8-OH-DPAT, inhibited aggression produced by hypothalamic stimulation. Thus, it appears that in rodent studies, mixed 5-HT$_{1B/2C}$ agonists show the most consistent anti-aggression properties.

Recent research specifically supports a role for 5-HT$_{1B}$ receptors in suppressing isolation-induced aggression. In this work, a mutant mouse strain lacking the 5-HT$_{1B}$ receptor gene was developed (Saudou et al., 1994). When adult males of this strain were isolated and then tested for their aggressive responses to an intruder male, they showed a marked decrease in attack latency and a substantial increase in number of attacks (Figure 9.24).

Pharmacological studies in nonhuman primates. The ability of several types of serotonergic agonists to inhibit aggression in rodents suggests that serotonergic activity in vivo should be negatively correlated with aggression or related behaviors. Such a relationship has been demonstrated in studies of male rhesus monkeys by Linnoila and colleagues (Higley et al., 1992; Mehlman et al., 1994). These researchers have been investigating a large group of free-ranging monkeys living on Morgan Island, a 475-acre sea island located off the coast of South Carolina. Juvenile and adolescent males from this population were observed behaviorally and were also subjected to CSF sampling for the purpose of measuring 5-HIAA concentrations as an index of central 5-HT turnover. Level of aggressivity was significantly negatively correlated with

CSF 5-HIAA, but not with the NE metabolite 3-methoxy-4-hydroxyphenylglycol (MHPG) or the DA metabolite homovanillic acid (HVA). Low 5-HIAA also predicted a high level of risk-taking behavior. Consequently, the authors argued that low 5-HT turnover is more closely related to a lack of impulse control (manifested in part by inappropriately high levels of aggression) than to aggressivity per se (see also the discussion of human behavior below).

Another line of research has been conducted on male vervet monkeys by Raleigh and coworkers. These animals were maintained in groups containing multiple adult males and females along with their offspring. Within each group, one male is normally dominant over the other males, as assessed by the outcome of agonistic encounters. The attainment of a dominant rank by a particular male appears to depend on several factors, including affiliative interactions with females in the group. Consequently, social status is not positively correlated with level of aggressiveness in this case.

The investigators first showed that whole-blood 5-HT levels in dominant male vervets were almost twice as high as those of lower-ranking males in the same groups (Raleigh et al., 1984). Spontaneous changes in the dominance hierarchy were accompanied by parallel alterations in whole-blood 5-HT; that is, newly dominant males showed elevations in 5-HT, whereas reduced 5-HT concentrations were observed in newly subordinate subjects. Most strikingly, when changes in group hierarchy were induced experimentally by removal and subsequent replacement of the dominant male, blood 5-HT levels again shifted in accordance with social status.

Subsequent experiments investigated the behavioral effects of various drugs that act on the serotonergic system (Raleigh et al., 1991). Initial dominance rankings were obtained in 12 groups of monkeys, after which the dominant male in each group was temporarily removed and one of the two remaining subordinate males was randomly chosen for drug treatment. Treated males received tryptophan, fluoxetine, fenfluramine, or cyproheptadine for a period of 4 weeks, followed by 4 weeks of injection vehicle alone. Tryptophan and fluoxetine were both considered serotonergic agonists due to their ability to increase synaptic 5-HT concentrations (although by different mechanisms). Cyproheptadine and fenfluramine were both considered 5-HT antagonists, cyproheptadine because it is a 5-HT receptor blocker and fenfluramine because it depletes 5-HT when given chronically. The other subordinate male in each group (the referent male) was given vehicle injections only. During the drug treatment phase, the subjects were observed for changes in their social behavior, and determinations were made as to whether one of the males attained dominant status over the other. The originally dominant male was then returned to the group and allowed to regain his initial rank. Next, a second removal

and treatment period was instituted using a crossover procedure in which the original agonist-treated (tryptophan or fluoxetine) subjects now received an antagonist (cyproheptadine or fenfluramine), and vice versa.

The results of treating male vervet monkeys with these serotonergic drugs were quite striking. In every instance, subjects given an agonist drug became dominant over the referent males they were paired with, whereas subjects given serotonergic antagonists became subordinate to the referent males. Because a crossover design was used, this means that the *same subjects* attained the opposite status in treatment phases 1 and 2, depending on which type of drug they received in each phase. The effects of these drugs on aggressive behavior were equally noteworthy. The serotonergic agonists significantly decreased the rate of initiation of aggressive events, whereas the antagonist drugs increased the incidence of aggressiveness (Figure 9.25). These results are consistent with the rodent studies discussed earlier, and also demonstrate the above-mentioned distinction between overt aggressiveness and the attainment of a dominant rank in male vervet monkeys.

The finding that treatment with serotonergic agonists promotes the attainment of a high social rank when the group hierarchy has been disrupted nicely parallels the earlier observation of high 5-HT concentrations in the dominant males. However, legitimate concerns might be raised concerning the use of whole-blood 5-HT levels, which primarily represent 5-HT synthesized in the gut and then taken up by platelets. Therefore, an additional experiment was performed, which showed that

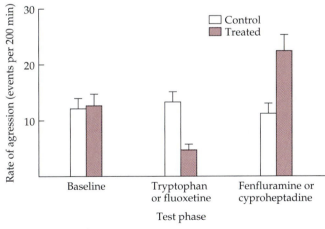

9.25 EFFECTS OF SEROTONERGIC AGONIST OR ANTAGONIST TREATMENT ON AGGRESSIVE BEHAVIOR IN MALE VERVET MONKEYS. Subjects were given either serotonergic agonists (tryptophan or fluoxetine) or serotonergic antagonists (cyproheptadine or fenfluramine). Drug-treated subjects displayed altered levels of aggressiveness compared with baseline conditions, whereas no changes were noted in vehicle-treated referent males. Data were combined for the two agonists and antagonists for presentation purposes and are expressed as the mean ± *SEM* number of aggressive events per 200 minutes. (After Raleigh et al., 1991.)

chronic fenfluramine treatment reduced 5-HT concentrations in both brain and blood and also lowered the levels of 5-HIAA in brain and cerebrospinal fluid (CSF) (Brammer et al., 1991). Based on these findings, the authors concluded that changes in whole-blood 5-HT do reflect changes in brain 5-HT, and that the behavioral effects of fenfluramine on aggression and social rank are mediated by central serotonergic systems.

Serotonin and Human Aggression

For more than 20 years, biological psychiatrists have been exploring the possible relationship between 5-HT and human aggressiveness (see reviews by Åsberg et al., 1987; Brown and Linnoila, 1990; Coccaro, 1992). This line of inquiry began with an early paper by Shaw, Camps, and Eccleston (1967), which was followed by additional studies reporting reduced concentrations of 5-HT and/or 5-HIAA in postmortem brain tissues of suicide victims. Åsberg and her colleagues in Sweden further noted particularly low CSF 5-HIAA concentrations in clinically depressed patients who had a history of suicide attempts (Åsberg, Träskman, and Thorén, 1976). This finding has since been replicated several times, although conflicting results have been reported by some investigators. Additional studies from several laboratories demonstrated reduced binding of [3H]imipramine, a tricyclic antidepressant that labels the 5-HT transporter on serotonergic nerve terminals, in the brains of suicide victims (see Åsberg et al., 1987; Nordström and Åsberg, 1992).

Low levels of brain 5-HT, CSF 5-HIAA, and imipramine binding sites are all consistent with a deficiency on the presynaptic side of serotonergic synapses. However, there have also been several reports of elevated 5-HT$_2$ receptor binding in the frontal cortex of suicide victims (Nordström and Åsberg, 1992). Increased 5-HT$_2$ receptor density could be a secondary consequence of decreased 5-HT availability, although it should be recalled that many studies have failed to observe the expected up-regulation of 5-HT$_2$ receptors in animals subjected to serotonergic denervation or synthesis inhibition (see Part II). Thus far, the alteration in serotonergic receptors appears to be specific to the 5-HT$_2$ subtype, as a recent study found no overall changes in frontal cortical 5-HT$_{1A}$ binding sites in suicide victims as compared with controls (Matsubara, Arora, and Meltzer, 1991).

Why should abnormalities in the serotonergic system of suicidal individuals shed light on the relationship between this neurotransmitter and aggressiveness? One possible answer lies in the long-standing view among many psychiatrists that suicide and violence toward others represent different manifestations of the same underlying aggressive tendency. One need not subscribe to this theory, however, to link 5-HT with human aggressiveness and violence. For example, Åsberg's group found that among suicide victims and attempters, low CSF 5-HIAA occurred mainly among individuals who

attempted to take or actually took their own lives by violent means such as firearms or jumping from heights rather than by ingesting poison or taking a drug overdose (Åsberg et al., 1987). Furthermore, in a study in which a group of psychiatric patients was tested on one psychological scale designed to measure suicide risk and another scale measuring the risk of violent behavior, scores on the two scales were found to be positively correlated (Plutchik and van Praag, 1989).

Considering aggression rather than suicidality, an impressive number of studies have found an inverse relationship between CSF 5-HIAA concentrations and various measures of aggressive behavior or mood. In one study of normal adults (both males and females), 5-HIAA values were negatively correlated with scores on the "urge to act out hostility" subscale of the Hostility and Direction of Hostility Questionnaire (Roy, Adinoff, and Linnoila, 1988). Within populations of psychiatric patients, most studies have reported a relationship between low CSF 5-HIAA levels and either high aggression ratings on psychological scales or a prior history of aggressive behavior (Brown et al., 1981; Brown et al., 1982; Kruesi, 1989; Lidberg et al., 1985). Levels of other CSF monoamine metabolites generally were found either not to correlate with aggression indices or (in a few cases regarding MHPG) to display a positive rather than a negative correlation. In many instances, low 5-HIAA seems to be linked particularly to impulsive, antisocial aggressiveness (reviewed by Linnoila et al., 1993). This association may actually begin in childhood, as relatively low CSF 5-HIAA levels have been reported in children and adolescents (age 6.3 to 17.4 years) with disruptive behavior disorder (Kruesi et al., 1990).

One useful alternative to studying CSF monoamine metabolites is to examine the effects of selective drugs on circulating hormone concentrations. The results are then used as an index of the status of the neurotransmitter system(s) acted on by a given agent. In the case of 5-HT and aggression, this approach is exemplified by the work of Coccaro and colleagues (1989), who investigated the prolactin response to a challenge dose of fenfluramine in male patients with affective or personality disorders and in normal male controls. Overall, the patient group displayed an attenuated prolactin response to fenfluramine, a 5-HT-releasing/reuptake-inhibiting drug. Most importantly, however, the subgroup with personality disorders exhibited a significant negative correlation between the change in prolactin concentration and measures of irritable, impulsive aggression (Figure 9.26). By implying an inverse relationship between serotonergic activity and impulsive aggression, these findings further support the results of the CSF 5-HIAA studies described above.

The most interesting recent development in the study of 5-HT and aggression comes from the Netherlands, where a kindred that carries a mutation in the gene for MAO-A has been discovered (Brunner, Nelen,

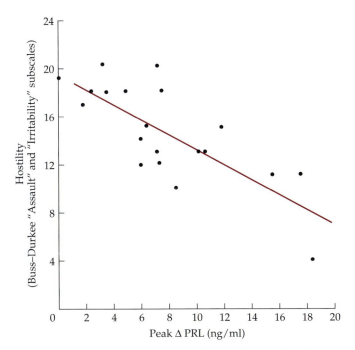

9.26 NEGATIVE CORRELATION BETWEEN PROLACTIN RE-
SPONSES TO FENFLURAMINE TREATMENT AND IRRITABLE AG-
GRESSION IN MALE PATIENTS WITH PERSONALITY DISOR-
DERS. Male patients with diagnoses of DSM-III personality
disorders were given a single challenge dose of fenfluramine (60
mg), after which hourly blood samples were collected and prolactin (PRL) levels measured for the next 5 hours. Peak Δ PRL values (maximum plasma PRL concentration minus the average baseline value) were negatively correlated with the patients' summed
scores on the Assault and Irritability subscales of the Buss–Durkee
Hostility Inventory ($n = 20$, $r = .77$, $p = .0002$). (After Coccaro,
1989; original data from Coccaro et al., 1989.)

van Zandvoort et al., 1993). Because the gene is located
on the X chromosome and the mutation is recessive, only
males that possess the mutant gene show phenotypic
changes. Biochemically, affected individuals displayed a
virtual absence of MAO-A activity, along with large reductions in the urinary excretion of 5-HIAA as well as
the catecholamine metabolites HVA, MHPG, and vanillylmandelic acid (VMA) (Brunner, Nelen, van Zandvoort
et al., 1993; Brunner, Nelen, Breakefield et al., 1993). Behaviorally, these same individuals showed borderline
mental retardation and a high incidence of impulsive
and aggressive acts, including violent assault, arson, and
sexual abuse and rape (Brunner, Nelen, Breakefield et al.,
1993). This appears to be the first documented instance
of a single-gene mutation in humans that links neurotransmitter functioning with social behavior. Of additional interest is the recent report of a transgenic mouse
strain created to mimic this congenital absence of MAO-
A (Cases et al., 1995). These mutant mice exhibited a
number of behavioral abnormalities, one of which was
enhanced male aggressiveness in the standard isolation
test situation. Although these results are quite fascinat-

ing, they are somewhat difficult to interpret because the
subjects showed 5-HT immunoreactivity in anomalous
cellular locations and also suffered from abnormal cortical development.

A number of issues remain to be resolved in the
study of 5-HT and aggression in humans. It is fair to
state, based on the research findings discussed above,
that aggressiveness per se is not the critical feature associated with low CSF 5-HIAA levels. It seems more likely
that serotonergic dysfunction leads to a psychopathological syndrome manifested variously as hyperirritability,
impulsivity, exaggerated stimulus reactivity, depressed
mood, and/or heightened anxiety (Apter et al., 1990;
Coccaro, 1992; Spoont, 1992). Such underlying psychopathology might then manifest itself in aggressive impulses directed either toward the self (suicidality) or toward others. Despite its attractiveness, however, this
hypothesis is far from substantiated at the present time.
Furthermore, new questions have been raised by the recent discovery of a genetic mutation associated with loss
of MAO-A activity, reduced 5-HIAA formation, and
heightened impulsivity and aggressiveness. Researchers
had previously assumed that low CSF 5-HIAA concentrations indicated a reduced rate of 5-HT turnover (i.e.,
serotonergic hypoactivity). However, we must now consider the possibility that decreases in 5-HIAA levels are
due to deficient MAO activity (though not necessarily
from a mutation per se), which could mean that 5-HT
levels are actually *elevated* in these individuals. These
questions can presumably be resolved by assessing multiple measures of serotonergic functioning, not just 5-
HIAA, in future studies.

Is There a Link between Animal and Human Research?

The majority of both animal and human studies has
shown that increased serotonergic functioning is associated with decreased aggressiveness, whereas heightened
aggressive behavior is found under conditions of reduced serotonergic activity. These analogous findings,
unfortunately, are not by themselves sufficient to ensure
that animal research will ultimately enhance our understanding of human aggressiveness. For example, some
animal models of aggression, such as muricide in rats
and other examples of predatory aggression, do not have
obvious parallels in human behavior. Such models are
therefore questionable, at least on the basis of face validity (although if there were a common underlying neurochemistry for all types of aggression, such lack of face
validity would prove unimportant). On the other hand,
isolation-induced aggression in animals may share some
similarities with irritable or impulsive aggression in humans, thus serving as a better model for neurochemical
research. Finally, as we saw at the conclusion of the previous section, abnormal serotonergic activity in humans
may be more predictive of impulsive personality distur-

bances, anxiety, and/or depression than of aggression dysfunction. Can this idea be related to the findings from animal studies of 5-HT and behavior? Soubrié (1986) has attempted to forge such a link by hypothesizing a critical role for 5-HT in fundamental processes of behavioral (impulse) control in both humans and animals. Whether or not Soubrié's hypothesis proves to be correct, it serves as a valuable paradigm for anyone attempting to integrate the broad literature on 5-HT and aggression.

Serotonin and Obsessive–Compulsive Disorder

Many drugs used in the treatment of psychiatric patients have potent effects on the serotonergic system. Accordingly, in later chapters, we shall consider the role of 5-HT in affective disorders and in the genesis of anxiety. Recent research suggests the possible involvement of this neurotransmitter in yet another type of disorder, namely, **obsessive–compulsive disorder (OCD)**. According to the *Diagnostic and Statistical Manual of Mental Disorders, Fourth Edition* (DSM-IV) (American Psychiatric Association, 1994), OCD is characterized by the presence of recurrent obsessions and/or compulsions that are severe enough to interfere with the individual's daily functioning or to cause significant psychological distress. Obsessions are defined as incessant, intrusive thoughts or impulses, usually of some senseless or even repugnant act (e.g., killing a loved one). The individual experiences extreme guilt or shame over the obsessive ideation and attempts to ignore or suppress it. In practice, however, this proves impossible. Compulsions are repetitive acts, often performed in a ritualized or stereotypic manner, generally thought to occur in response to an obsession (e.g., compulsive hand washing due to fear of germs). Attempts to resist the compulsion lead to heightened anxiety, even dread. Thus, a person with OCD must continue to perform these behavioral rituals, despite knowing that they are groundless and feeling great embarrassment and humiliation.

OCD has traditionally been considered an anxiety disorder, and it is categorized as such in the DSM-IV. However, some investigators have begun to question this view. At a behavioral level, ethological analyses have attempted to relate OCD either to displacement or stereotypic activities in animals (Insel, 1988) or to self-protective, species-typical behaviors that have been released from normal control mechanisms by some pathological process (Rapoport, 1991). With respect to therapeutic interventions, OCD typically resists treatment with either benzodiazepines, which are used in generalized anxiety disorder, or standard tricyclic antidepressants such as imipramine, which have some efficacy in the treatment of panic disorder (Murphy, Pigott, and Insel, 1990). Finally, neurological and brain imaging studies point to a

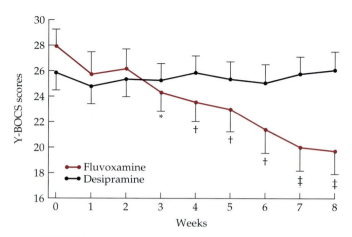

9.27 EFFECTIVENESS OF FLUVOXAMINE VERSUS DESIPRAMINE IN REDUCING OBSESSIVE–COMPULSIVE SYMPTOMATOLOGY. Male and female patients diagnosed with OCD were treated for 8 weeks either with the 5-HT uptake inhibitor fluvoxamine ($n = 21$) or the NE uptake inhibitor desipramine ($n = 19$). Doses began at 50 mg daily and were gradually increased to a maximum of 300 mg. Severity of OCD symptoms was measured by the Yale–Brown Obsessive Compulsive Scale (Y-BOCS; $*p < .02$, $†p < .10$; $‡p < .001$ compared with baseline (week 0) rating. (After Goodman et al., 1990.)

possible involvement of the basal ganglia, the thalamus, and the orbital and prefrontal cortices (Azari et al., 1993; Insel, 1992a). Although this work is still in its infancy, it suggests that a unique biological substrate for OCD may be identified as further research is performed.

Evidence for serotonergic involvement in OCD stems largely from the therapeutic effectiveness of selective 5-HT uptake inhibitors in this disorder. The relatively 5-HT-selective tricyclic antidepressant clomipramine (also known as chlorimipramine; trade name, Anafranil) and the nontricyclic 5-HT uptake inhibitors fluoxetine (Prozac), sertraline (Zoloft), and fluvoxamine (Luvox) all display substantial clinical efficacy in OCD (Fineberg et al., 1992; Wood, Tollefson, and Birkett, 1993). Moreover, the NE-selective tricyclic antidepressant desipramine does not alleviate OCD symptoms (Figure 9.27).

The fact that 5-HT uptake inhibitors can alleviate some of the symptoms of OCD does not prove that this disorder stems from an abnormality in serotonergic functioning. Recent work has therefore attempted to assess the responsivity of the serotonergic system in OCD patients by means of pharmacological challenges. Several behavioral studies found a transient exacerbation of obsessive–compulsive symptomatology in at least some currently unmedicated OCD patients given the 5-HT agonist *m*-CPP (Hollander et al., 1992; Murphy et al., 1989). In some cases, OCD patients also exhibited a blunted prolactin response to either *m*-CPP or fenfluramine administration as compared with controls (Hewlett et al., 1992; Hollander et al., 1992). Although not all studies have reported these effects (e.g., McBride et al., 1992), the results nonetheless provide some of the first direct evidence for 5-HT dysfunction in OCD. Further research is obviously needed to pinpoint the nature of this abnormality.

Despite the usefulness of 5-HT uptake inhibitors in treating OCD, these drugs by no means eliminate all symptomatology. Therefore, other transmitters, such as DA, could also be involved in this disorder (Goodman et al., 1990). Moreover, a lag of several weeks usually occurs between the beginning of drug treatment and the onset of significant clinical improvement. This delay is reminiscent of the therapeutic lag associated with antidepressant action, and it suggests that secondary drug effects on neurotransmitter receptors and second messenger systems (e.g., development of subsensitivity?) may be more important than the primary uptake blocking effects for therapeutic efficacy.

Part III Summary

Despite its presence in only a tiny fraction of all the neurons in the brain, 5-HT is clearly involved in some of the most basic elements of behavioral and physiological control. It has an inhibitory effect on food intake, possibly by enhancing mechanisms of satiety. For this reason, serotonergic agonists such as fenfluramine are used as anorectic agents in the treatment of obesity. In addition, 5-HT may regulate impulsivity or some related psychological trait, such that abnormally low serotonergic activity results in suicidality or pathological aggression. A kindred was recently discovered in the Netherlands in which some of the men are characterized by borderline mental retardation, irritability, and impulsive aggressiveness. The affected individuals were found to suffer from a rare mutation that completely eliminated their MAO-A activity, thus leading to low 5-HIAA excretion. Finally, 5-HT has been implicated in the etiology of obsessive–compulsive disorder because selective 5-HT, but not NE, uptake inhibitors show therapeutic efficacy in this disorder. The role of 5-HT in other psychopathological disorders is discussed in later chapters.

Chapter 10

The Amino Acid Neurotransmitters and Histamine

Part I
Excitatory Amino Acids: Glutamate and Aspartate

Although the classical neurotransmitters discussed in previous chapters, such as acetylcholine, serotonin, and the catecholamines, are extremely important in behavioral regulation and in the actions of psychotropic drugs, they are nevertheless used by only a small proportion of the neurons in the brain. What substances, then, serve as neurotransmitters for the remaining populations of nerve cells? Since the 1950s, evidence has been accumulating indicating that the most widely used neurotransmitters belong to a class of compounds known as **amino acids**. We previously encountered several amino acids that served important roles as precursors for catecholamine and serotonin synthesis. This chapter will explore a number of other amino acids that act directly as neurotransmitters themselves.

Amino Acids

Amino acids are small molecules that possess the general structure shown in Figure 10.1a. At physiological pH, amino acids exist primarily in the ionized form. Molecules such as these that carry both a positive and a negative charge are termed **zwitterions**. The —R group is called the **side chain**, and differs for each type of amino acid. The smallest side chain is simply a hydrogen atom (—H), which yields the amino acid glycine. If the side chain contains a carboxyl group (—COOH), then the resulting amino acid is acidic because the carboxyl hydrogen will tend to dissociate at physiological pH (Figure 10.1b). As we shall see, the acidic amino acids glutamic acid and aspartic acid are important excitatory neurotransmitters. Conversely, if the side chain contains an amine group (—NH$_2$), the amino acid is basic because the amine group will tend to pick up a proton (hydrogen atom) at physiological pH. Another property of amino acids derives from the fact that the so-called α carbon atom (the carbon atom to which the side chain is bonded) is asymmetric. This means that the four chemical groups arrayed around that atom can exist in two different configurations, called **isomers**, that are mirror images of each other. Conventional biochemical nomenclature refers to these isomeric forms as L- and D-amino acids. The L-form predominates in vivo and typically has maximum biological activity (for example, only L-amino acids are incorporated into proteins).

All cells in the body contain high concentrations of various amino acids because of the crucial role these compounds play in protein synthesis and in certain aspects of intermediary metabolism. We may ask, therefore, why some amino acids are also used in neurotransmitter-related functions. There is no clear answer to this question, except to ascribe such multiplicity of function to the biochemical economy of the body. Examples of a similar economy will be found in Chapter 11, in which it will be seen that a number of small peptides serve both as hormones and as neurotransmitters or neuromodulators.

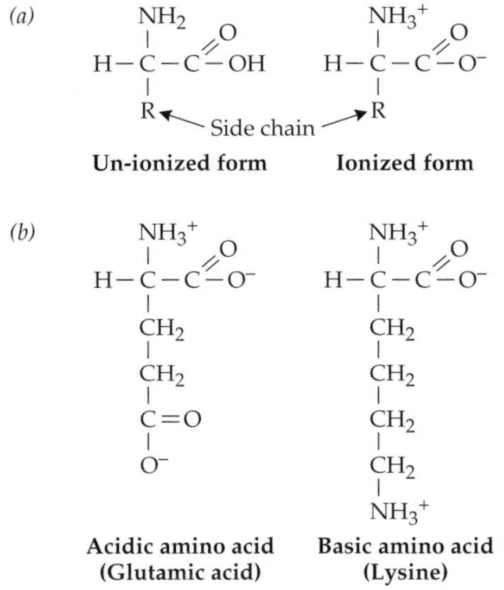

(a)

Un-ionized form   Ionized form

(b)

Acidic amino acid   Basic amino acid
(Glutamic acid)   (Lysine)

10.1 STRUCTURE OF AMINO ACIDS. (a) The general structure of amino acids in their un-ionized and ionized forms. (b) Examples of an acidic and a basic amino acid.

Glutamate and Aspartate as Neurotransmitters

Glutamate and **aspartate** (throughout the remainder of the chapter, glutamic acid and aspartic acid will be referred to by the terms for their ionized forms, namely, glutamate and aspartate) are nonessential amino acids, which means that they can be readily synthesized by the body and therefore are not required in the diet. They are the most abundant free amino acids in the mammalian brain. In the cat brain, for example, glutamate and aspartate are found at concentrations of 186 and 114 mg/100 g tissue, respectively, compared with only 24 mg/100 g tissue for glycine (Tallan, Moore, and Stein, 1954). One of the earliest reports of glutamate action in the nervous system concerned its possible use as a transmitter at the crayfish neuromuscular junction (Van Harreveld, 1959), and indeed, this role for glutamate is now well established in many crustaceans and insects. Although the excitatory properties of glutamate in vertebrates were first described by Hayashi (1954), these studies were carried out by grossly applying the substance to the exposed cerebral cortex. More detailed analyses of glutamate and aspartate actions in the vertebrate nervous system began in the late 1950s and early 1960s when David Curtis and his colleagues devised iontophoretic techniques to deliver minute amounts of glutamate, aspartate, and various glutamate or aspartate analogs directly to the outer surfaces of nerve cells and to record the electrophysiological responses to these compounds. Curtis's group and several other laboratories soon reported that nerve cells in the spinal cord, as well as in virtually every region of the brain, could be strongly depolarized (hence, excited) by the iontophoretic application of glutamate,

aspartate, or a number of amino acid analogs (see Orrego and Villanueva, 1993). Ironically, these early results were in a sense "too good" for investigators to accept the amino acids as neurotransmitters because the compounds seemed to lack the regional specificity expected of a chemical signaling agent. Furthermore, in some experiments, D-glutamate was unexpectedly found to be nearly as potent as the L-isomer in causing neuronal depolarization. This finding implied a lack of **stereoselectivity**, a concept that was first discussed in Chapter 2 in relation to drug–receptor interactions. Given these and other considerations, it is perhaps not surprising that Curtis and Koizumi (1961) concluded that "the excitation produced by this [glutamate] and other closely related dicarboxylic amino acids is unrelated to synaptic excitatory mechanisms." Nevertheless, it is now widely acknowledged that glutamate is a bona fide transmitter in the vertebrate nervous system, and in fact is considered to be *the* principal transmitter for fast excitatory signaling (Orrego and Villanueva, 1993). Hence, we shall focus primarily on glutamate here, although we shall review some evidence that aspartate may also serve a neurotransmitter function.

Figure 10.2 illustrates the primary features of a glutamatergic synapse. In contrast to the neurotransmitter systems presented in previous chapters, glutamate neurons seem to operate in close cooperation with neighboring astrocytes, which accumulate extracellular glutamate, store it as glutamine, and then release it for conversion back to glutamate by the nerve cells. Details of these processes are discussed in the sections that follow.

Synthesis and Metabolism of Glutamate and Aspartate

Synthesis

Glutamate can be synthesized via a number of different biochemical reactions; however, biochemical studies indicate that the carbon skeleton of most glutamate molecules is derived from the normal oxidative metabolism of glucose (glycolysis) (Peng et al., 1993). This process involves the breakdown of glucose to pyruvate, the conversion of pyruvate to acetyl coenzyme A (acetyl CoA), and the subsequent entry of acetyl CoA into the citric acid cycle. One of the key constituents of the citric acid cycle, α-ketoglutarate (α-KG; also called 2-oxoglutarate), can then be converted to glutamate by means of a reaction called **transamination**. A number of enzymes, collectively called aminotransferases, can transfer an amino group from a donor amino acid to one of several acceptor molecules. When the acceptor is α-KG, as is most commonly the case, a molecule of glutamate is formed (Figure 10.3a). The enzymes catalyzing these reactions use pyridoxal phosphate (a form of vitamin B_6) as a cofactor and are named according to the identity of the

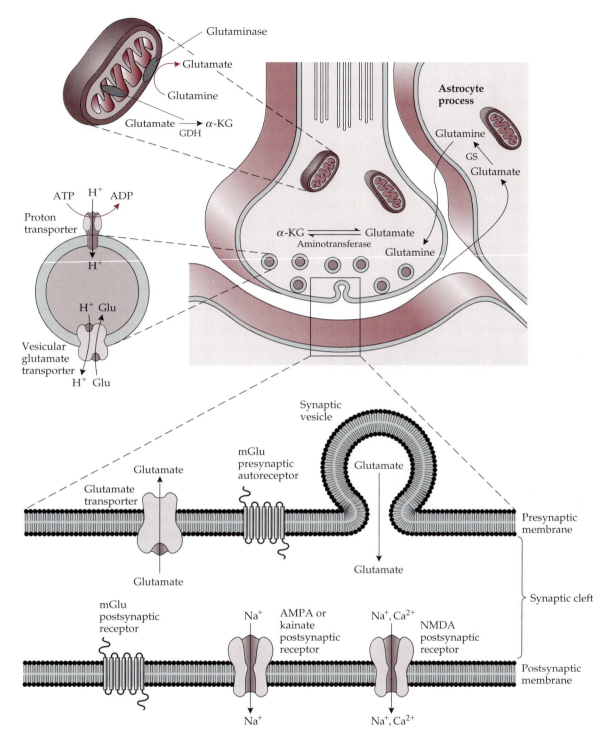

Receptor	Agonists	Antagonists
AMPA/Kainate	AMPA, kainic acid, quisqualic acid, domoic acid	CNQX, NBQX
NMDA	NMDA	CPP, D-AP5 (D-APV), D-AP7
Metabotropic	Quisqualic acid, *trans*-ACPD, L-AP4	α-Methyl-4-carboxyphenyl glycine

10.2. THE GLUTAMATERGIC SYNAPSE, illustrating the processes of glutamate synthesis and metabolism, neuronal and glial glutamate uptake, and vesicular glutamate uptake and release. Pre- and postsynaptic excitatory amino acid receptors are also shown. The table lists important glutamatergic receptor agonists and antagonists. See the text for details and explanations of the abbreviations.

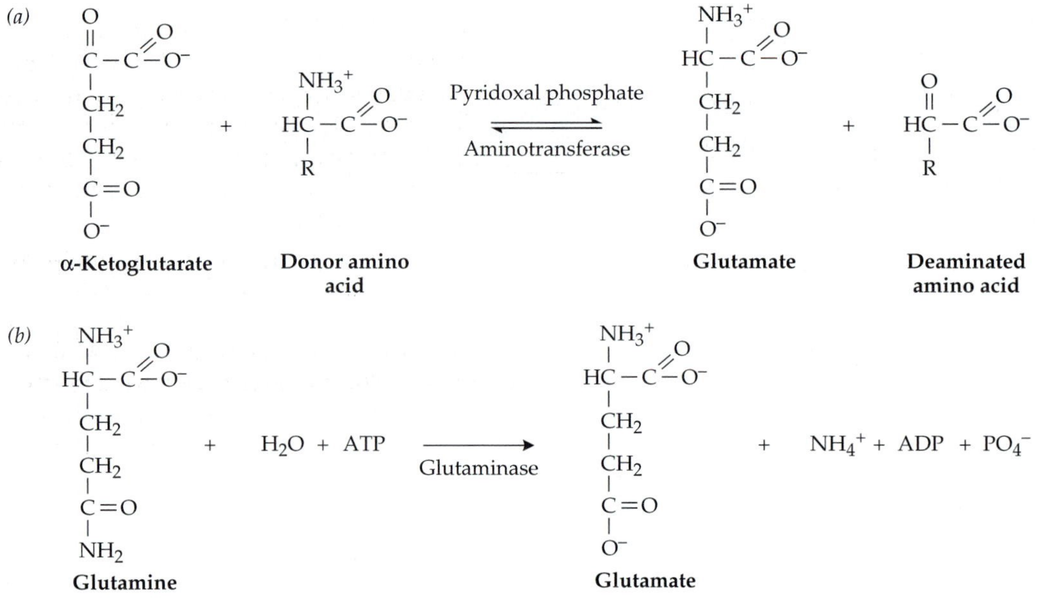

(a)

α-Ketoglutarate   +   Donor amino acid $\xrightleftharpoons[\text{Aminotransferase}]{\text{Pyridoxal phosphate}}$ Glutamate   +   Deaminated amino acid

(b)

Glutamine   + H_2O + ATP $\xrightarrow{\text{Glutaminase}}$ Glutamate   + NH_4^+ + ADP + PO_4^-

10.3 PATHWAYS OF GLUTAMATE SYNTHESIS. Glutamate is synthesized in neural tissues by two major pathways: (a) from α-ketoglutarate and donor amino acids by means of transamination, and (b) from glutamine by the action of the enzyme glutaminase.

donor amino acid in each instance. In the brain, it appears that alanine aminotransferase (which uses alanine as the amino group donor) is the most important enzyme participating in glutamate formation via transamination (Peng et al., 1993).

Another important pathway of glutamate synthesis involves its formation from glutamine via phosphate-activated glutaminase, a mitochondrial enzyme that requires ATP for its activity (Figure 10.3b). Indeed, Hamberger and his colleagues (1979) showed a number of years ago that glutamate molecules destined for release are preferentially formed from glutamine. Glutamate formation by glutaminase appears to be regulated by product inhibition of the enzyme. Both of the products of the reaction, glutamate and, to a lesser extent, ammonia, exert an inhibitory effect on glutaminase activity. This product inhibition may be a mechanism for retarding glutamate formation when intraterminal concentrations are sufficient for current synaptic activity.

The glutamine cycle. It is important to realize that unlike the glucose-to-glutamate pathway described above, the formation of glutamate from glutamine does not represent any *net* synthesis of additional glutamate molecules. This is because the glutamine itself must first be synthesized from glutamate by means of another enzyme called glutamine synthetase. What, then, is the purpose of these metabolic interconversions (i.e., glutamate → glutamine → glutamate)? First, glutamine is a synaptically inactive compound and is therefore thought to serve as a convenient storage reservoir for glutamate. Second, immunohistochemical studies have demonstrated staining for glutamine synthetase in astrocytes (and, in some cases, oligodendrocytes), but not in neurons (Norenberg, 1979; Tansey, Farooq, and Cammer,

1991). Of particular interest is the presence of glutamine synthetase immunoreactivity within fine astrocytic processes that lie in close proximity to synaptic endings (Derouiche and Frotscher, 1991). Because astrocytes possess a membrane transport mechanism for glutamate (see below for more details), these cells are well positioned to take up synaptically released glutamate and convert it to glutamine. On the other hand, several studies indicate that glutaminase is enriched in nerve endings (e.g., Ward and Bradford, 1979), although it is also found in astroglia. The differential localization of these enzymes has led to the concept of a "glutamine cycle" (Nicklas, Zeevalk, and Hyndman, 1987) in which some of the glutamate released from glutamatergic (glutamate-using) neurons is taken up by neighboring astrocytes, converted into glutamine for temporary storage, and then later transported out of the glial cells by diffusion and taken up by the nerve endings for conversion back to glutamate. Peng and colleagues (1993) have summarized recent information indicating that α-KG and alanine may also be supplied to neurons by astrocytes for conversion to glutamate (Figure 10.4). Unlike neurons, astrocytes possess the enzyme pyruvate carboxylase, which enables them to use the citric acid cycle for extra α-KG production by means of CO_2 condensation with pyruvate.

Glutamate compartments. As mentioned earlier, high concentrations of glutamate are found in all cells. It is logical to assume that glutamatergic neurons, which possess a specialized ability to store and release glutamate as a neurotransmitter (see below), must also possess a mechanism for separating (i.e., compartmentalizing) their neurotransmitter-designated glutamate from the more general pool of glutamate used for other metabolic

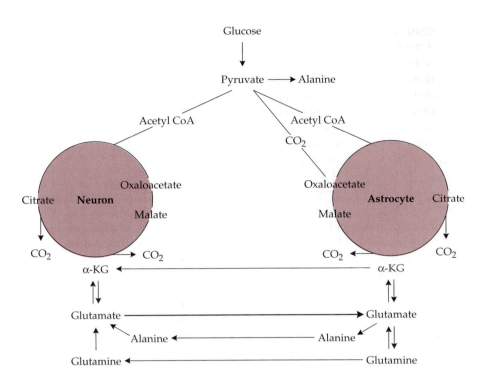

10.4 BIOCHEMICAL PATHWAYS OF GLUTAMATE SYNTHESIS AND STORAGE IN NEURONS AND ASTROCYTES. In both neurons and astrocytes, glucose is converted to pyruvate by the process of glycolysis. Pyruvate is then transaminated to alanine or, more typically, enters the citric acid cycle either following conversion to acetyl CoA or by condensation with CO_2 to generate oxaloacetate. The latter reaction is catalyzed by the enzyme pyruvate carboxylase, which is present in astrocytes but not in neurons. Glutamate is formed in part from α-ketoglutarate (α-KG) by transamination. Following synaptic release, some neuronal glutamate is accumulated by astrocytes (heavy arrow), where it can be converted to glutamine for storage. Glutamine and possibly alanine are released by astrocytes and taken up by neurons for glutamate synthesis. (After Peng et al., 1993.)

functions. The concept of multiple glutamate "pools" in the brain has indeed been proposed, based in part on the rates of conversion of various radiolabeled precursors to radioactive glutamate (Fonnum, 1984). To summarize a complex literature, there appear to be at least two such metabolic compartments for glutamate, which have been designated the large and small compartments based on the proportion of the total glutamate pool that is ascribed to each compartment. The glutamine synthesis rate is high in the small compartment but low in the large. Therefore, the small compartment is thought to correspond to glutamate metabolism taking place in astrocytes. The large compartment is rapidly replenished by glucose breakdown (probably mainly through transamination) and may correspond to metabolic activity occurring in nerve cells. Further compartmentation within glutamatergic neurons remains to be established.

Catabolism

The pathways for glutamate catabolism are closely related to those involved in its synthesis. For example, one obvious means of inactivating glutamate is through conversion to glutamine in astrocytes as part of the glutamine cycle discussed above. Second, it should be apparent that when any transamination reaction occurs from right to left, a molecule of glutamate will be converted to α-KG (see Figure 10.3). Interestingly, this direction of transamination provides a major pathway for aspartate synthesis, which may be important in neurons using aspartate as a transmitter. Finally, glutamate can be converted to α-KG through a different reaction that uses the enzyme glutamate dehydrogenase (GDH) (Figure 10.5). This reaction requires either a cofactor of nicotinamide adenine dinucleotide (NAD^+) or its phosphorylated form ($NADP^+$).

10.5 GLUTAMATE CATABOLISM. One route of glutamate catabolism is oxidative deamination by the enzyme glutamate dehydrogenase (GDH).

Storage, Release, and Uptake of Glutamate and Aspartate

Vesicular Storage and Release

Many studies have demonstrated Ca^{2+}-dependent release of glutamate and of aspartate in vivo as well as in vitro from brain slices and synaptosomes (see Nicholls, 1989, for a review of the synaptosomal work). However, the intracellular source of these released amino acids has been somewhat controversial. Early studies measuring the amino acid content of synaptic vesicles prepared from brain tissue failed to find clear evidence for vesicular storage of glutamate or aspartate. However, more recent research has demonstrated the existence of such storage, at least for glutamate (Storm-Mathisen and Ottersen, 1990). As summarized in several reviews (Maycox, Hell, and Jahn, 1990; Nicholls and Attwell, 1990), vesicle loading is accomplished by means of an energy-dependent transport system that is distinct from the axon terminal uptake system (see below). The vesicular transporter has a high specificity for L-glutamate and, like the vesicular transporters described in earlier chapters, functions as a proton antiport system. The ability of vesicles to take up and store glutamate supports the likelihood of its release by an exocytotic mechanism, but additional evidence is still needed to confirm this hypothesis.

Synaptic Uptake

As in the case of the monoamine transmitters, rapid inactivation of released amino acids is accomplished through an uptake mechanism (see Figure 10.2). The synaptic uptake system for excitatory amino acids is characterized by a high affinity (K_m approximately 10–40 μM) (Erecińska, 1987) compared with that of the vesicular glutamate transporter ($K_m \approx$ 1–2 mM; Naito and Ueda, 1985). On the other hand, the uptake system has very low specificity and readily transports L-glutamate, L- and D-aspartate, cysteate, and several other acidic amino acids. D-glutamate, the aspartate analog N-methyl-D-aspartate, and the excitotoxic glutamate analog kainic acid (see below) are not, however, transported by this system (Erecińska, 1987). A number of studies have demonstrated reductions in glutamate uptake following lesions of presumed glutamatergic pathways, suggesting that such uptake is closely associated with glutamatergic nerve terminals (Fonnum, 1984).

The synaptic glutamate uptake system must be able to maintain an estimated 1,000–10,000-fold concentration difference between the cytoplasm of the glutamatergic neuron and the extracellular space. It has been known for some time that this is accomplished by linking uptake to the Na^+ electrochemical gradient across the neuronal membrane. This electrochemical gradient represents the joint contributions of the Na^+ concentration gradient and the electrical potential across the mem-brane. There is substantial evidence that Na^+ ions are co-transported with glutamate with a stoichiometry of two or three Na^+ per molecule of glutamate (Erecińska, 1987; Nicholls and Attwell, 1990). As with other Na^+-dependent transport processes, therefore, amino acid uptake into nerve endings does not directly require ATP. However, energy is indirectly used because the membrane Na^+–K^+ ATPase is required to maintain the transmembrane Na^+ concentration gradient.

In 1992, three different laboratories reported the cloning of a high-affinity glutamate transporter (for review, see Kanai, Smith, and Hediger, 1993). Each transport protein proved to have a distinct structure and localization. One glutamate transporter is present in many neurons (as well as in cells of various peripheral tissues), the second is found mainly in Bergmann glia of the cerebellar cortex, and the third is localized specifically in astrocytes throughout the brain (Kanai, Smith, and Hediger, 1993; Rothstein et al., 1994). Immunohistochemical studies at the electron microscopic level found particularly dense glutamate transporter staining in fine astrocytic processes (Danbolt, Storm-Mathisen, and Kanner, 1992). This finding is reminiscent of the localization of glutamine synthetase, and thus further supports the notion that astrocytes accumulate synaptically released glutamate and convert it to glutamine for storage.

Localization of Glutamatergic and Aspartatergic Pathways

The localization of neuronal pathways using excitatory amino acids as their transmitter has proceeded more slowly than for many other transmitters. This slow rate of progress is directly attributable to technical difficulties. For a number of years, there were no histochemical or immunohistochemical methods for the visualization of glutamatergic or aspartatergic pathways. Researchers therefore had to depend on such indirect approaches as lesioning a proposed source of glutamate-containing fibers and then looking for reductions in glutamate uptake or Ca^{2+}-dependent release in the hypothesized terminal areas. Because glutamate and aspartate are found everywhere in the brain due to their roles in intermediary metabolism and protein synthesis, it might be expected that immunohistochemical staining for these amino acids would label all cells and hence would be useless for pathway mapping purposes. However, anti-glutamate and anti-aspartate antibodies have been raised that do selectively stain certain neuronal populations such as pyramidal cells in the neocortex. It has been argued, therefore, that immunohistochemistry can be successfully used to localize glutamatergic and aspartatergic cell bodies and nerve terminals in the CNS (Conti et al., 1987; Dori, Petrou, and Parnavelas, 1989).

Using the various procedures described above, many pathways have been tentatively identified as using acidic amino acids (in most cases glutamate) as their neurotransmitter. In the brain, glutamate is very likely used by a number of descending pathways originating from neocortical pyramidal cells (including the corticostriate pathway as well as projections to a variety of limbic, diencephalic, and brain stem structures), by several intrahippocampal and hippocampal projection pathways, by the parallel fibers of the cerebellar cortex that convey information from the granule to the Purkinje cells, and by other pathways (Figure 10.6) (Fonnum, 1984; Nieuwenhuys, 1985). In the spinal cord, there is considerable evidence that glutamate is the transmitter used by excitatory interneurons as well as by many (if not all) terminals of primary afferent neurons (Broman, Anderson, and Ottersen, 1993; Watkins, 1984).

Although aspartate, like glutamate, has potent excitatory effects on many neurons, the case for aspartate as a neurotransmitter in specific pathways has been less

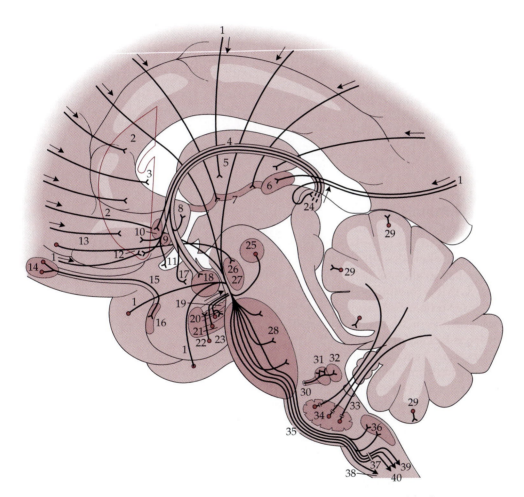

10.6 PROPOSED PATHWAYS USING ACIDIC AMINO ACID TRANSMITTERS. Either glutamate or aspartate is thought to serve as the neurotransmitter for the indicated pathways. Key: 1 = fibers from the neocortex; 2 = caudate nucleus; 3 = putamen; 4 = fornix; 5 = thalamus; 6 = lateral geniculate body; 7 = reticular thalamic nucleus; 8 = bed nucleus of the stria terminalis; 9 = anterior commissure; 10 = lateral septum; 11 = diagonal band; 12 = nucleus accumbens; 13 = fibers from the rostral and medial prefrontal cortex; 14 = olfactory bulb; 15 = lateral olfactory tract; 16 = prepyriform cortex; 17 = mediobasal hypothalamus; 18 = mammillary bodies; 19 = dentate gyrus; 20 = Ammon's horn of the hippocampal formation; 21 = subiculum; 22 = perforant path; 23 = parahippocampal gyrus; 24 = superior colliculus; 25 = red nucleus; 26 = substantia nigra; 27 = cerebral peduncles; 28 = pons; 29 = granule cells, giving rise to the parallel fibers; 30 = cochlear nerve (cranial nerve VIII); 31 = ventral cochlear nucleus; 32 = dorsal cochlear nucleus; 33 = olivocerebellar tract; 34 = inferior olive; 35 = pyramids; 36 = medial cuneate nucleus (and nucleus gracilis); 37 = decussation of the pyramidal tract; 38 = anterior pyramidal tract; 39 = lateral pyramidal tract; 40 = spinal cord. (After Nieuwenhuys, 1985.)

clear. Nevertheless, various findings indicate that aspartate may be present as a neurotransmitter in certain cortical and hippocampal pathways (Dori et al., 1992; Fleck et al., 1993), in the climbing fibers that originate in the inferior olive of the medulla and synapse on the cerebellar Purkinje cells (Wiklund, Toggenburger, and Cuénod, 1982), and in some primary afferent neurons (Tracey et al., 1991).

Excitatory Amino Acid Receptors

In most cases, the neural receptors stimulated by glutamate or aspartate evoke excitatory postsynaptic potentials (EPSPs) when stimulated. At one time it was thought that a single receptor type was sufficient to account for this effect. However, a large number of pharmacological studies using various agonists, antagonists, and in some cases modulatory substances subsequently led to the current view that there are at least four different subtypes of excitatory amino acid receptors (Table 10.1; reviewed by Gasic and Hollmann, 1992; Sommer and Seeburg, 1992).

Ionotropic Receptors

The first three excitatory amino acid receptor subtypes to be characterized are termed the **AMPA**, **kainate**, and **NMDA receptors**. These subtypes are all ionotropic receptors, which means that they belong to the ligand-gated channel receptor superfamily. Furthermore, they are all named after pharmacological agonists to which they respond relatively selectively. AMPA (α-amino-3-hydroxy-5-methyl-4-isoxazole proprionic acid) and NMDA (N-methyl-D-aspartic acid) are synthetic amino acid analogs, whereas kainic acid was isolated from the seaweed *Digenea simplex*. Other important agonists for these receptors include quisqualic acid (from the plant genus *Quisqualis*), which preferentially activates non-NMDA (particularly AMPA) receptors; domoic acid, a potent kainate receptor agonist responsible for a rare neurotoxicity caused by eating contaminated mussels (Perl et al., 1990; Stewart et al., 1990); and ibotenic acid, which is relatively selective for the NMDA receptor. It is generally presumed that glutamate (or aspartate) is the

normal endogenous ligand for all of these receptors. In some cases, however, alternatives have been proposed, such as cysteic and homocysteic acid, both of which are sulfur-containing amino acids with neuroexcitatory properties.

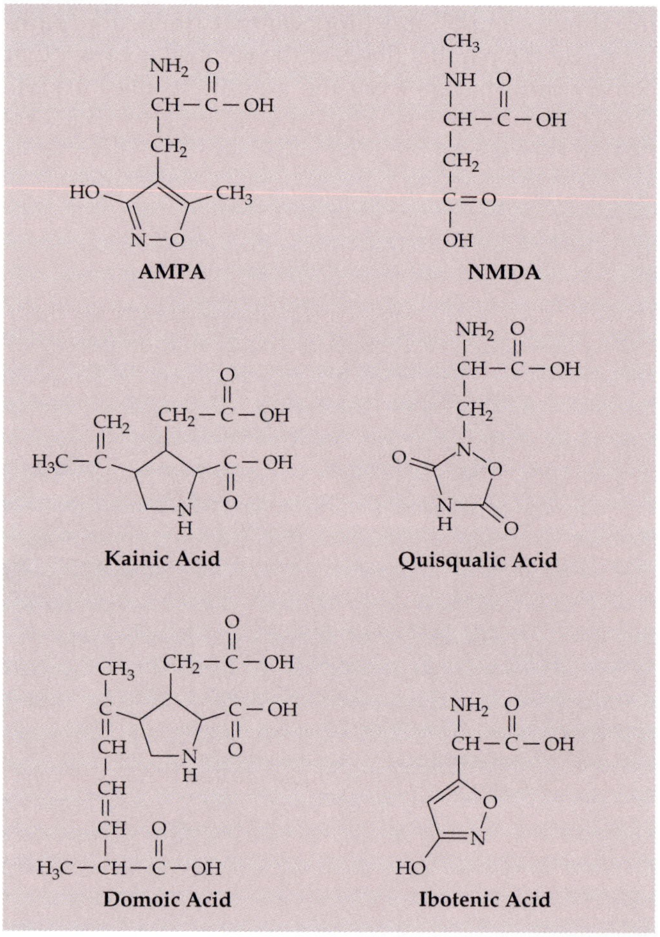

AMPA

NMDA

Kainic Acid

Quisqualic Acid

Domoic Acid

Ibotenic Acid

The discovery of selective antagonists has also been instrumental in elucidating the various classes of excitatory amino acid receptors. Competitive antagonists for the NMDA receptor including 3-(($\pm$,-2-carboxypiperazin-4-yl)propyl-1-phosphonic acid (CPP), 2-amino-5-phosphonovaleric acid (D-AP5; sometimes also called APV), and 2-amino-7-phosphonoheptanoic acid (D-AP7). It has

Table 10.1   Structural and Functional Properties of Excitatory Amino Acid Receptors

Receptor subtype	Properties				
	Superfamily	Genes		Cation selectivity	Second messengers
AMPA	Ligand-gated channel	*GluR1–GluR4*		Na$^+$, K$^+$	
Kainate	Ligand-gated channel	*GluR5–GluR7, KA1, KA2*		Na$^+$, K$^+$	
NMDA	Ligand-gated channel	*NR1, NR2A–NR2D*		Na$^+$, K$^+$, Ca^{2+}	
Metabotropic	G protein-coupled receptor	*mGluR1–mGluR7*			IP$_3$, DAG, cAMP

proved more difficult to find equally selective blockers for AMPA and kainate receptors. Based on receptor binding as well as electrophysiological studies, 6-cyano-7-nitroquinoxaline-2,3-dione (CNQX), 6,7-dinitroquinoxaline-2,3-dione (DNQX), and 6-nitro-sulfamoyl-benzo(f)-quinoxaline-2,3-dione (NBQX) are considered general, competitive non-NMDA antagonists with some selectivity for AMPA over kainate receptors (Cunningham, Ferkany, and Enna, 1993; Johnson and Koerner, 1988). Greater AMPA receptor selectivity has been proposed for two recently developed compounds, YM900 and LY215490 (Ornstein et al., 1993). One additional drug of interest is GYKI52466, which is a novel 2,3-benzodiazepine that acts as a noncompetitive AMPA/kainate antagonist (Rogawski, 1993). This compound differs structurally and functionally from the better-known 1,4-benzodiazepines discussed in Chapter 16.

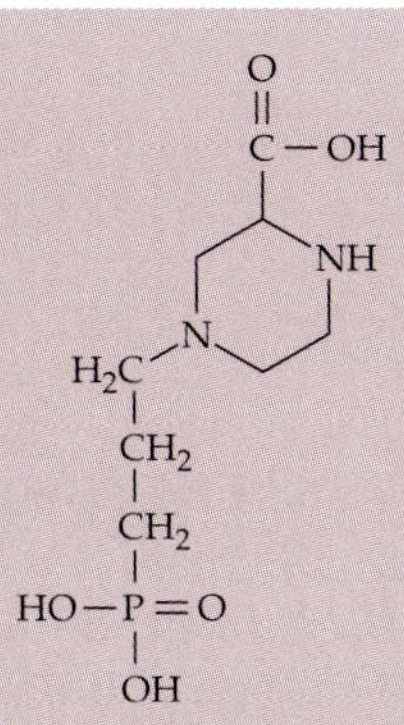

CPP

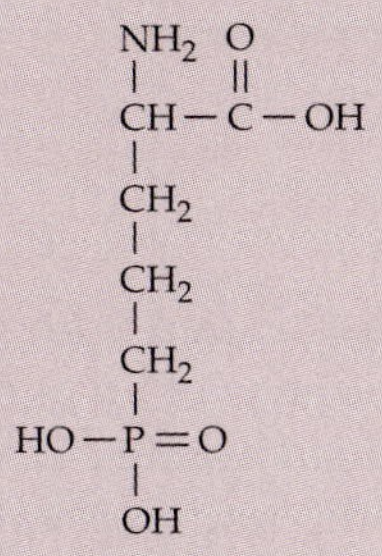

D-AP5

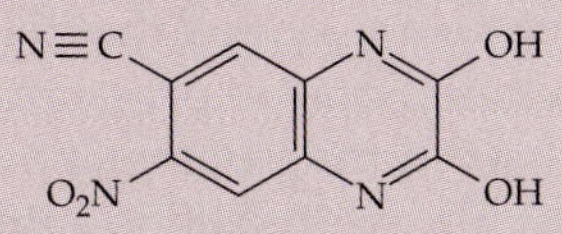

CNQX

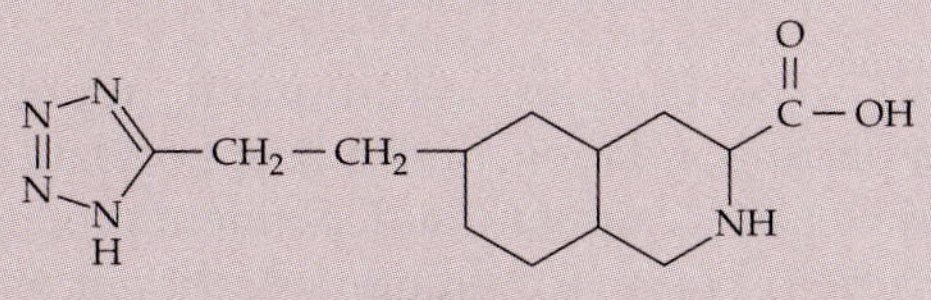

LY215490

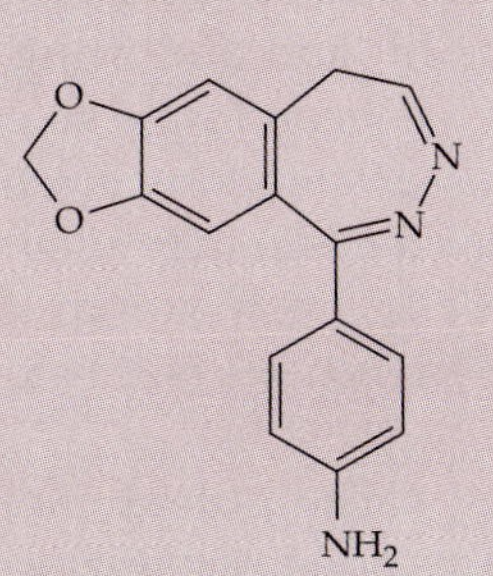

GYKI52466

AMPA receptor structure and function. AMPA receptors are associated with a cation channel that is nonselective with respect to Na^+ and K^+ ions, but in most cases is im-

permeable to Ca^{2+}. AMPA receptor-mediated currents exhibit very fast kinetics, meaning that they show a rapid onset, offset, and desensitization. Furthermore, AMPA-mediated responses are widely distributed in the brain, and this receptor subtype is considered to be the workhorse for fast excitatory signaling in the CNS (Seeburg, 1993).

Over the past few years, the cloning of a number of glutamate receptor genes has led to rapid progress in characterizing these receptors. At the time of this writing, 16 different subunits for ionotropic glutamate receptors have been cloned (reviewed by Hollmann and Heinemann, 1994; Schoepfer et al., 1994). Four of these subunits, termed GluR1–GluR4 (or GluRA–GluRD by some investigators), are involved in the AMPA subtype (Bettler and Mulle, 1995). These subunits are similar to one another in structure, and each codes for a protein containing approximately 900 amino acids. It is not yet clear whether naturally occurring receptor complexes are homomeric (combinations of the same subunit), heteromeric (combinations of two or more different subunits), or both. Although cells can make homomeric AMPA-type receptor channels when provided with only one type of subunit (Boulter et al., 1990; Keinänen et al., 1990), the classes of neurons examined to date all express at least two different subunits (Seeburg, 1993). This finding suggests that native receptors are typically heteromeric.

Another important finding is that the typical lack of Ca^{2+} permeability of AMPA receptors depends on the presence of a GluR2 subunit that has undergone post-transcriptional RNA editing. There is a CAG (cytosine–adenine–guanine) codon in GluR1, GluR2, GluR3, and GluR4 transcripts that codes for a glutamine residue (designated Q in the single-letter abbreviation system) located in a region between the putative second and third transmembrane domains of each subunit (see below). Channels assembled from subunits containing this glutamine residue exhibit a high permeability to Ca^{2+}. In adult animals, however, the CAG codon of the GluR2 transcript is virtually always edited to CGG, which codes for arginine (R) (Bettler and Mulle, 1995). This simple substitution of arginine for glutamine at one position of the GluR2 subunit greatly reduces Ca^{2+} permeability of channels containing this subunit (Hume, Dingledine, and Heinemann, 1991; Verdoorn et al., 1991). Q/R editing of GluR1, GluR3, or GluR4 transcripts has not been found. Consequently, the low Ca^{2+} permeability of most native AMPA receptor channels implies that GluR2 is a typical constituent of these receptors. A few cell populations, however, possess atypical AMPA receptors that lack the GluR2 subunit and that display a high permeability to Ca^{2+} (Bochet et al., 1994; Hollman, Hartley, and Heinemann, 1991).

The subunits of other ionotropic receptors (most notably the nicotinic cholinergic receptor) possess a struc-

(a)   (b)

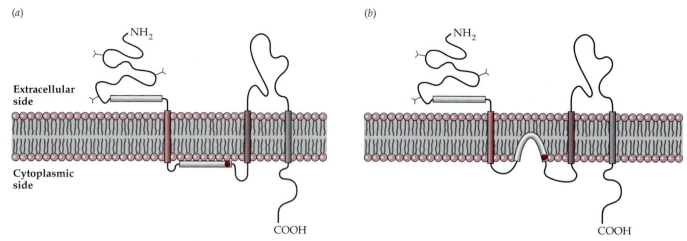

10.7 HYPOTHETICAL TOPOLOGY OF GLUTAMATE RECEPTOR SUBUNIT 1 (GluR1).
GluR1 possesses five hydrophobic regions, as shown by the various cylindrical structures.
Previous models of GluR1 topology proposed that four of these regions were membrane-
spanning domains, consistent with the structure of nicotinic cholinergic receptor subunits.
New findings, however, suggest that GluR1 has only three transmembrane domains (TMDs).
The region formerly believed to constitute TMDII is now thought either to be positioned
near the intracellular face of the membrane (a) or to loop into and out of the membrane
without fully traversing it (b). The large dot shown within this region identifies the Q/R editing site described earlier. (After Hollmann, Maron, and Heinemann, 1994.)

ture that is consistent with the existence of four membrane-spanning regions (transmembrane domains).
When researchers first examined the amino acid sequences of the AMPA receptor subunits, they concluded
that these subunits assumed a similar conformation.
However, subsequent findings began to raise questions
about this model. Recently, a group of researchers led by
Stephen Heinemann has provided strong evidence that
GluR1 (and, by inference, the other three subunits) possesses only three transmembrane domains (Hollmann,
Maron, and Heinemann, 1994). The region of the protein
formerly thought to be the second transmembrane domain (out of a putative four) is now hypothesized either
to be entirely outside of the membrane or to loop into
and out of the membrane instead of traversing it (Figure
10.7). If verified, this new model will have important
consequences not only for the understanding of glutamate receptor functioning, but also because it signifies a
new family of receptor proteins with a novel structure.

AMPA receptor regulation.   AMPA receptor structure
and function are regulated by several different processes.
First, it should be noted that each of the AMPA-related
subunits (GluR1–GluR4) occurs in two forms, called
"flip" and "flop," that arise from alternative mRNA
splicing (Sommer et al., 1990). Flip and flop subunits
vary only with respect to a sequence of 38 amino acid
residues near the last transmembrane domain of the protein. This difference, however, causes a significant
change in receptor properties. Ion currents associated
with flip subunits show slower desensitization than

those associated with flop subunits, and in the continuous presence of an agonist, flip subunits display a low-
level steady-state current (Figure 10.8). In the adult rat
brain, flip and flop vary somewhat in their cellular expression, particularly in the hippocampus, cerebral cortex, and cerebellum (Seeburg, 1993; Sommer et al., 1990).
Other studies have demonstrated that the two forms differ in their developmental expression. Flip subunits
begin to be expressed during prenatal development and
persist throughout life, whereas flop subunits do not appear until after birth (Monyer, Seeburg, and Wisden,
1991).

AMPA receptors are additionally regulated by
means of phosphorylation. Such phosphorylation can be
catalyzed by Ca^{2+}/calmodulin-dependent protein kinase
and by protein kinase C, but apparently not by cAMP-
dependent protein kinase (McGlade-McCulloh et al.,
1993; Tan, Wenthold, and Soderling, 1994). Moreover,
phosphorylation has been found to enhance the amplitude of receptor-associated ion currents, suggesting that
this regulatory mechanism may play a role in processes
of synaptic plasticity, such as long-term potentiation,
that involve AMPA receptors (see below).

Kainate receptors.   The potent excitatory compound
kainic acid produces nondesensitizing currents when applied to AMPA receptors. There are other receptors in the
brain, however, that bind kainic acid and that rapidly desensitize when exposed to this agonist (Figure 10.8).
Such receptors constitute the kainate subtype of excitatory amino acid receptor.

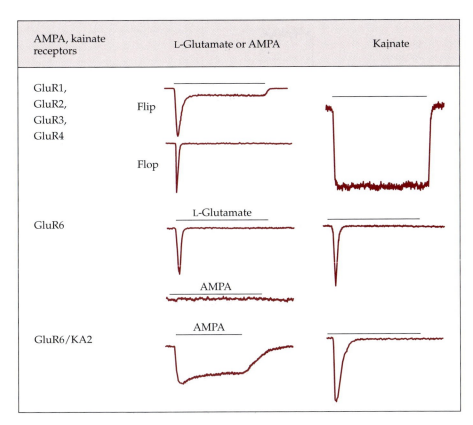

10.8 MEMBRANE CURRENTS EVOKED BY THE APPLICATION OF GLUTAMATE RECEPTOR AGONISTS TO SPECIFIC RECEPTOR SUBUNITS. Subunits of non-NMDA glutamate receptors were expressed in human embryonic kidney cells, and the cells were then exposed to glutamate, AMPA, or kainate. AMPA-type receptor channels were formed in cells expressing GluR1, GluR2, GluR3, or GluR4. Such channels mediate rapidly desensitizing currents in response to glutamate or AMPA application, but nondesensitizing responses to kainate. In contrast, GluR6, expressed alone or in combination with KA2 subunits, formed kainate-type receptor channels that desensitized in response to kainate application but showed either no response (GluR6) or a nondesensitizing response (GluR6/KA2) to AMPA. Horizontal bars denote the period of agonist application (2 s for kainate on AMPA receptors, 300 ms in all other cases). (After Seeburg, 1993.)

Kainate receptors can be formed from five different subunits designated GluR5, GluR6, GluR7, KA1, and KA2 (Bettler and Mulle, 1995; Seeburg, 1993). Various types of neurons in the hippocampus and cerebellar cortex seem to express differing combinations of these subunits, although the precise composition of native kainate receptors remains to be determined. Like AMPA receptors, kainate receptors appear to be regulated by phosphorylation (Henley, 1994).

NMDA receptor structure and function. Several authors have recently reviewed the properties of the NMDA receptor subtype (McBain and Mayer, 1994; Scatton, 1993). Compared with AMPA and kainate receptors, NMDA receptor channels exhibit slower kinetics, and they also show significant permeability to Ca^{2+} ions as well as to Na^+ and K^+. Consequently, NMDA receptor stimulation can activate Ca^{2+}-mediated functions that are unaffected by the action of AMPA or kainate receptors. Early studies of the NMDA receptor revealed another critical property; namely, that the receptor is subject to a voltage-dependent blockade by relatively low concentrations of Mg^{2+}. More specifically, when the cell membrane is at the resting potential, NMDA receptors are only weakly affected by agonists (e.g., glutamate or NMDA) when Mg^{2+} is also present at submillimolar concentrations. When the membrane has been depolarized, however, the Mg^{2+} block is removed. Figure 10.9 presents patch-clamp recordings showing current flow through a single

NMDA receptor channel under varying conditions of Mg^{2+} concentration and membrane potential. When the membrane was at its resting potential, increasing the Mg^{2+} concentration to 10 µM or higher produced a flickering effect in which current flow repeatedly started and stopped (Ascher and Nowak, 1988). This effect is thought to be due to rapid binding and dissociation of Mg^{2+} ions at a site deep within the channel itself. However, when the cell was depolarized to +40 mV, even 100 µM Mg^{2+} had no inhibitory effect on current flow, apparently because the affinity of the binding site for Mg^{2+} progressively decreases as depolarization is increased (Mayer, Vyklicky, and Sernagor, 1989). Because this Mg^{2+} block occurs at concentrations at or below those normally found in the brain, it is clear that NMDA receptors can be only minimally activated by agonists unless the cell has previously been stimulated so that it is already in a depolarized state.

The NMDA receptor exhibits another important property: the simple amino acid glycine binds to a separate recognition site on the receptor complex and in effect acts as an obligatory co-agonist (Johnson and Ascher, 1987). That is, both the glutamate and glycine sites must be occupied for activation of the receptor. Local changes in extracellular glycine levels could therefore serve as a modulatory influence on NMDA receptor function (Kemp and Leeson, 1993). It should be noted that the glycine binding site on the NMDA receptor complex is distinct from the classic strychnine-sensitive receptor that

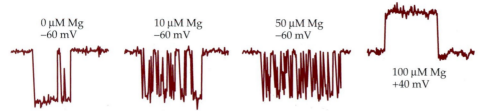

0 µM Mg
−60 mV

10 µM Mg
−60 mV

50 µM Mg
−60 mV

100 µM Mg
+40 mV

10.9 EFFECT OF MAGNESIUM ON NMDA-MEDIATED IONIC CURRENTS. Cultured mouse neurons were exposed to 10 µM NMDA, and single-channel currents were measured by patch clamping. The three recordings on the left show the results obtained at various concentrations of Mg^{2+} (0–50 µM) when the membrane potential was at −60 mV (near the resting potential). Current flow through the NMDA receptor channel is indicated by a downward deflection in the trace. Note that as the Mg^{2+} concentration is increased, a flickering phenomenon is observed that represents rapid onset and offset of current flow through the channel. The recording on the right was obtained in the presence of 100 µM Mg^{2+} when the membrane potential was held at +40 mV. Under these depolarizing conditions, no flickering was observed even though the Mg^{2+} concentration was high. (After Ascher and Nowak, 1988.)

mediates glycine's actions as an inhibitory transmitter (see Part III of this chapter). Indeed, the NMDA receptor–associated glycine site exhibits a unique pharmacology, with the compounds hydroxyethylvinyl glycine and 1-amino-1-carboxycyclopropane acting as agonists at this site, and various kynurenic acid derivatives such as 7-chloro-5-iodokynurenic acid acting as antagonists (Kemp and Leeson, 1993). An unusual naturally occurring ago-

1-Amino-1-Carboxycyclopropane

7-Chloro-5-iodokynurenic acid

nist at the NMDA receptor-associated glycine site is D-serine. D-serine, but not L-serine, binds to this site with an affinity equal to that of glycine itself (see Wood, 1995). Moreover, most regions of the rat brain possess sufficient concentrations of D-serine for this compound to be considered along with glycine as a potential co-agonist with glutamate at the NMDA receptor.

Because the concentration of glycine in the cerebrospinal fluid is much greater than its apparent dissociation constant (K_d) for the glycine/D-serine site on the NMDA receptor, many investigators have assumed that this site must be saturated under normal conditions. Some electrophysiological studies have provided support for this hypothesis (Kemp and Leeson, 1993). But

experiments on NMDA receptor–stimulated cGMP formation in the cerebellum and hippocampus found that cGMP synthesis can be augmented by local administration of either glycine or D-serine (Wood, 1995). These findings suggest that the glycine/D-serine site on the NMDA receptor may not be saturated, at least in the two brain areas studied. Changes in glycine or D-serine availability could therefore interact with glutamate in regulating NMDA receptor activity. Because of the important role of NMDA receptors in various physiological and pathological functions (see below), the glycine site is likely to be an important target for future therapeutic drug development.

Yet another regulatory site on the NMDA receptor is recognized by the dissociative anesthetics phencyclidine (PCP) and ketamine. In the early 1980s, Lodge and his coworkers discovered that these compounds selectively antagonize excitatory responses to NMDA, but not to quisqualate (which stimulates AMPA receptors) or kainate (Anis et al., 1983; Lodge and Anis, 1982). Such inhibition is noncompetitive, indicating that it is mediated by a site distinct from the agonist (i.e., glutamate) binding site on the receptor. Subsequent research demonstrated the existence of a unique recognition site for PCP, ketamine, and several other noncompetitive antagonists such as the drug MK-801 (also known as dizocilpine), and further showed that drug binding to this site was enhanced by NMDA agonists and by glycine (Wood et al., 1990). Some of the properties of NMDA receptor inhibition by dissociative anesthetics resemble those of inhibition by Mg^{2+}. For example, in both cases the effect is voltage dependent. In addition, although the PCP binding site on the receptor is distinct from the Mg^{2+} site, it also appears to be located on the inside of the cation channel. Support for such localization comes from studies demonstrating that both the blocking action of PCP and ketamine and subsequent recovery from blockade are "use dependent" (Mayer, Vyklicky, and Sernagor, 1989; Wood et al., 1990). That is, the receptor must be stimulated by an NMDA agonist in order for an initial PCP effect to occur, and once the receptor is blocked, alleviation of this effect again requires exposure of the receptor to agonist stimulation. From these observations, we can envision a scenario in which PCP molecules must enter an open NMDA receptor ion channel in order to interact with their binding site on the receptor, and if the channel then closes, the drug remains trapped within the interior of the channel. Modulation of NMDA receptor function probably accounts for many of the psychological and behavioral properties of dissociative anesthetics. The pharmacology of PCP and related drugs is discussed in greater detail in Chapter 17.

Finally, there are two other modulatory sites associated with the NMDA receptor complex. One site binds zinc (Zn^{2+}) ions, thereby producing a voltage-independent block of NMDA responses (Mayer, Vyklicky, and Sernagor, 1989). Zinc may play a particularly important role in regulating NMDA receptor activity in pathways containing high levels of this ion (e.g., the hippocampal mossy fibers). The other site is a polyamine site at which spermine and spermidine (compounds that are normally considered to be important for tissue growth and development) act to facilitate NMDA receptor-mediated transmission. This facilitation is accomplished, at least in part, by increasing the affinity of the receptor for glycine (Ransom and Deschenes, 1990). Thus, the NMDA receptor is a complex molecular structure with modulatory binding sites for a number of different compounds and ions. A schematic illustration of this structure is shown in Figure 10.10.

The genetics of the NMDA receptor has proved to be as complicated as its pharmacology (reviewed by McBain and Mayer, 1994; Seeburg, 1993). The first NMDA receptor subunit to be cloned was designated NMDAR1 (now usually shortened to NR1). Subsequent studies showed that at least nine different isoforms of this protein are created by alternative mRNA splicing. Furthermore, there exists a family of four additional subunits (named NR2A–NR2D) that are structurally similar to one another but exhibit relatively little sequence homology to NR1. Homomeric NMDA receptors can be formed from NR1 subunits alone, although this is not the case for members of the NR2 family. Even so, the assembly and functioning of such homomers seems to be inefficient, and it therefore seems likely that native NMDA receptors are usually (if not always) some type of heteromeric combination of NR1 and NR2 subunits. Indeed, NMDA receptor pharmacology and channel properties both vary depending on which NR2 isoform (A–D) is present, suggesting that NMDA receptor function in different cell populations is probably regulated by expression of this subunit (Buller et al., 1994; McBain and Mayer, 1994).

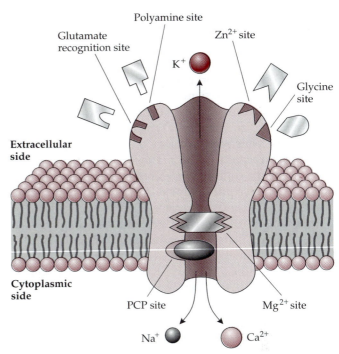

10.10 SCHEMATIC REPRESENTATION OF THE NMDA RECEPTOR COMPLEX. The NMDA receptor complex possesses a glutamate recognition site to which receptor agonists and competitive antagonists bind, as well as other binding sites for glycine, polyamines such as spermine and spermidine, phencyclidine (PCP) and related drugs, Mg^{2+}, and Zn^{2+}. Channel opening permits an influx of Na^+ and Ca^{2+} ions, and an efflux of K^+ ions. (After Scatton, 1993.)

Ca^{2+}-dependent processes activated by NMDA receptors. A critical difference between the NMDA receptor and the AMPA and kainate receptors is that the Ca^{2+} influx caused by NMDA receptor activation triggers a number of Ca^{2+}-dependent processes. Among the most prominent of these are stimulation of Ca^{2+}/calmodulin-dependent protein kinase II, stimulation of the phosphoinositol second messenger system and protein kinase C, liberation of arachidonic acid due to the action of phospholipase A_2, and increased activity of the polyamine synthesizing enzyme ornithine decarboxylase. As we shall see below, some of these effects are critically involved in the roles of NMDA receptors in various physiological and pathological processes. Furthermore, activation of protein kinase C, activation of ornithine decarboxylase, and arachidonic acid synthesis all seem to function in a positive feedback loop to enhance NMDA receptor functioning (Scatton, 1993).

Yet another important consequence of NMDA receptor–mediated Ca^{2+} influx is stimulation of nitric oxide (NO) formation by nitric oxide synthase. As discussed in Chapter 6, NO is a novel gaseous messenger that can rapidly diffuse across cell membranes to increase cGMP synthesis in nearby target cells. This process is responsible for the well-known ability of NMDA receptor activation to cause elevated cGMP levels in the cerebellar cortex (Garthwaite, 1991).

Metabotropic Receptors

In 1985, Sladeczek and coworkers reported that a novel glutamate receptor stimulated phospholipase C and phosphoinositide turnover in cultured striatal neurons. Although this receptor was sensitive to quisqualate, in other respects its pharmacology differed from that of the ionotropic receptor family. These and other findings gave rise to the concept of metabotropic glutamate receptors, that is, receptors coupled to G proteins and operating through second messenger systems (see Table 10.1). The discovery of the rigid glutamate analog *trans*-1-aminocyclopentane-1,3-dicarboxylic acid (*trans*-ACPD) as a selective metabotropic receptor agonist (Palmer, Monaghan, and Cotman, 1989) was particularly helpful in identifying these receptors. Recent work has demonstrated that certain phenylglycine derivatives such as α-methyl-4-carboxyphenylglycine are selective metabotropic receptor antagonists (Watkins and Collingridge, 1994).

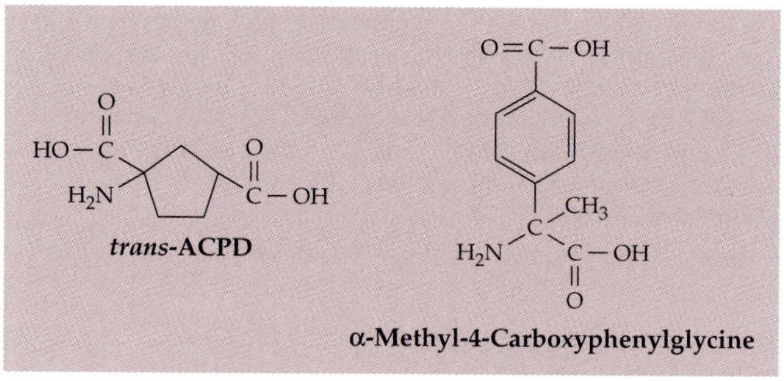

trans-ACPD

α-Methyl-4-Carboxyphenylglycine

Genetic studies indicate the existence of seven different metabotropic receptors designated mGluR1 through mGluR7 (reviewed by Bockaert, Pin, and Fagni, 1993; Schoepp, 1994; Schoepp and Conn, 1993). Alternative mRNA splicing further gives rise to three isoforms of mGluR1 (α, β, and c) and two isoforms of mGluR5 (a and b). All metabotropic glutamate receptors are thought to conform to the standard seven-transmembrane-domain topology of the G protein–coupled receptor superfamily; however, they are structurally distinct in several ways from other known members of this superfamily. One of their interesting properties is an extremely large N-terminal region that may contain the agonist binding site. This contrasts with the monoamine receptors, in which the agonist site is believed to exist in a cleft within the transmembrane region.

The metabotropic receptors can conveniently be divided into three groups based on similarity of amino acid sequence, pharmacology, and second messenger coupling (Schoepp, 1994). The first group, which consists of mGluR1 and mGluR5, is sensitive to *trans*-ACPD and quisqualate and is positively coupled to the phosphoinositide second messenger system. The second group,

which consists of mGluR2 and mGluR3, is sensitive to *trans*-ACPD, but not quisqualate. These receptors inhibit cAMP formation when activated. The third group consists of mGluR4, mGluR6, and mGluR7. Although these receptors likewise are negatively coupled to adenylyl cyclase, they exhibit a unique pharmacology in that they do not respond to *trans*-ACPD or quisqualate, but rather are sensitive to the phosphorylated amino acids L-2-amino-4-phosphonobutyrate (L-AP4) and L-serine-*O*-phosphate (L-SOP). When investigators first discovered

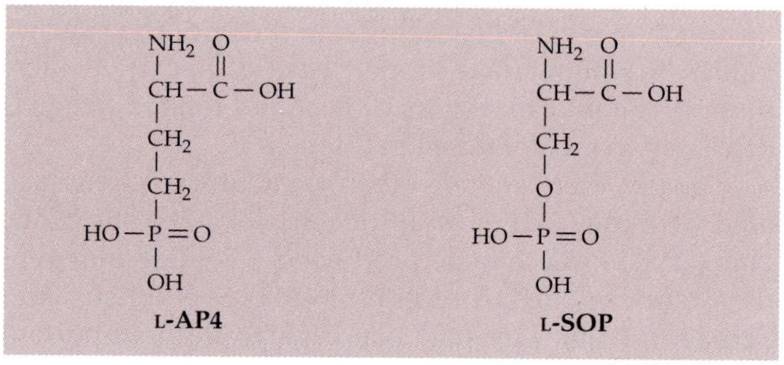

L-AP4

L-SOP

this glutamate receptor subtype based on its unusual pharmacological properties, its relationship to the other metabotropic receptors was not realized, and it was termed the L-AP4 receptor (Johnson and Koerner, 1988). It is now known that some L-AP4-sensitive metabotropic receptors act as presynaptic autoreceptors that suppress glutamatergic activity by inhibiting glutamate release (Schoepp, 1994).

Distribution of Excitatory Amino Acid Receptors

The distribution of excitatory amino acid receptors has been studied using in vitro autoradiographic binding studies and, more recently, immunohistochemistry for specific subunits and in situ hybridization for subunit mRNAs. AMPA and kainate binding sites can be visualized directly using [^{3}H]AMPA and [^{3}H]kainate, respectively, whereas NMDA sites can be labeled with the antagonists [^{3}H]CPP or [^{3}H]MK-801, or with [^{3}H]glutamate in the presence of unlabeled quisqualate and kainate (to occlude binding of the ligand to other receptive sites). Mapping studies applied to the rat brain have revealed a widespread distribution of NMDA receptors, with a particularly high density in the cortex (especially layers 1 through 3), hippocampal formation, basal ganglia, and lateral septum (Figure 10.11). AMPA receptors tend to be found in many of the same regions as the NMDA receptors. On the other hand, kainate receptors have a distinctly different distribution. There are a number of areas, such as the mammillary bodies and deep cortical layers, that are rich in kainate receptors but have a low density of NMDA sites. Furthermore, in the hippocampus, which contains large numbers of both NMDA and kainate binding sites, the laminar distribution of the two receptor types is complementary rather than overlapping (Monaghan, Bridges, and Cotman,

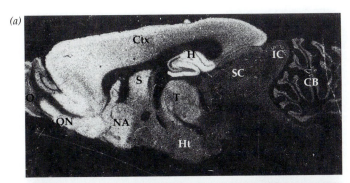

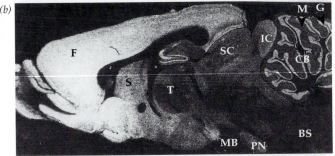

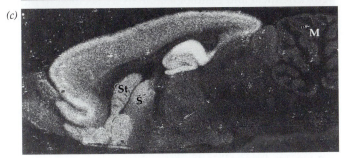

10.11 DISTRIBUTION OF EXCITATORY AMINO ACID RECEPTORS IN THE RAT BRAIN. Localization of different receptor subtypes is demonstrated by autoradiograms of (a) NMDA-sensitive [³H]glutamate, (b) [³H]kainate, and (c) [³H]AMPA binding sites. Light areas show higher levels of binding. BS = brain stem; CB = cerebellum; Ctx = cerebral cortex; F = frontal cortex; G = granule cell layer; H = hippocampus; Ht = hypothalamus; IC = inferior colliculus; M = molecular layer; MB = mammillary bodies; NA = nucleus accumbens; O = olfactory bulb; ON = anterior olfactory nuclei; S = septum; SC = superior colliculus; St = striatum; T = thalamus. (From Monaghan, Bridges, and Cotman, 1989; courtesy of Dan Monaghan.)

1989). Information concerning the immunohistochemical staining patterns for specific AMPA, kainate, and NMDA receptor subunits may be found in several papers by Petralia and his colleagues (Petralia and Wenthold, 1992; Petralia, Wang, and Wenthold, 1994a,b; Petralia, Yokotani, and Wenthold, 1994).

The phosphoinositide-coupled metabotropic receptor mGluR1α has also been localized using immunohistochemistry. Although immunoreactivity for this receptor was observed in many brain areas, staining was particularly intense in the olfactory bulbs, parts of the hippocampal formation, globus pallidus, thalamus, substantia nigra, superior colliculus, and cerebellum (Martin

et al., 1992). The distribution of the receptor can provide some clues to its potential function. Thus, mutant mice lacking mGluR1 expression (i.e., mGluR1 "knockout mice") were recently reported to exhibit significant deficits in motor coordination (probably based at least partly on cerebellar dysfunction) and in spatial learning (possibly hippocampus-related) (Conquet et al., 1994).

Many neurons are likely to possess both ionotropic and metabotropic receptors. One cell type in which this occurs is the Purkinje cells of the cerebellar cortex, which receive multiple glutamatergic inputs from the climbing and parallel fibers. Interestingly, electron microscopic studies indicated that AMPA receptors at these synapses are present in the main body of the synapse, near the transmitter release sites, whereas mGluR1α staining was found only at the edge of the synapse (Nusser et al., 1994). This finding raises the intriguing possibility that the ionotropic receptors at these synapses can respond to low levels of glutamate release, whereas the metabotropic receptors (because of their peripheral location) may respond only when the amount of transmitter released is high.

We noted earlier that glutamate appears to be an important transmitter for primary sensory neurons. Various studies have suggested that several glutamate receptor subtypes are also present in other parts of the peripheral nervous system, including both sympathetic and parasympathetic ganglia (Erdö, 1991). Further research is needed to clarify the possible role of excitatory amino acids in peripheral neurotransmission.

The Role of Excitatory Amino Acids in Neural and Behavioral Functions

Excitatory amino acids have been implicated in numerous physiological and behavioral processes. Due to space limitations, we have chosen to focus here on two of these processes that have received particular attention in recent years. The first is the ability of glutamate and related compounds to cause neuronal damage or death, and the possible role of this phenomenon in various types of neuropathology. The second is the role of excitatory amino acids in the cellular mechanisms thought to underlie learning and memory.

Amino Acid Excitotoxicity

The discovery of excitotoxicity. In 1957, Lucas and Newhouse reported the discovery that the sodium salt of glutamic acid, monosodium glutamate (MSG), could cause retinal damage in mice following subcutaneous administration. The effect occurred rapidly, beginning within 30 minutes of treatment, and could also be produced in an attenuated form by injection of sodium aspartate. Moreover, infant mice appeared to be more vulnerable than adults to this toxic action of MSG.

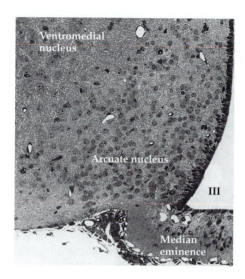
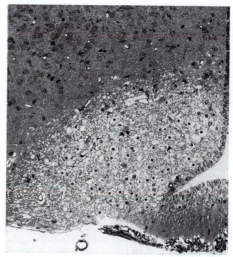

10.12 ARCUATE NUCLEUS DAMAGE FOLLOWING SUBCUTANEOUS IN-JECTION OF MONOSODIUM GLUTA-MATE (*Left*) The arcuate nucleus of the hypothalamus of an untreated 10-day-old mouse. This nucleus forms an arch-like structure situated on either side of the third ventricle, dorsal to the median eminence. (*Right*) Damage to the arcu-ate nucleus is revealed by the loss of cell staining in a littermate subject in-jected 6 hours earlier with MSG. Note the lack of apparent injury in areas out-side of the arcuate nucleus. (From Ol-ney, Ho, and Rhee, 1976. Courtesy of John Olney; reproduced with premis-sion from the *Journal of Neuropathol-ogy and Experimental Neurology*.)

Twelve years later, Olney (1969) presented the first evidence that MSG also produces brain damage in neonatal mice. The effect was confined to a few specific subcortical areas, and was particularly marked in the ar-cuate nucleus of the hypothalamus, which appeared to be completely destroyed (Figure 10.12). These hypothal-amic lesions were further found to produce severe en-docrine dysfunction in adulthood, as indicated by stunted skeletal growth, extreme obesity, and (particu-larly in females) reproductive abnormalities.

The areas damaged by systemic MSG either lack a blood–brain barrier or are near the ventricular system. This pattern suggested that access of the amino acid to the tissue, rather than a selective vulnerability of certain cell populations, was the major determinant of regional toxicity. Later studies showed a close relationship be-tween the excitant properties of various amino acids and their neurotoxicity in the MSG model, and also demon-strated ultrastructurally that postsynaptic (i.e., dendritic and somatic), but not presynaptic, sites exhibited patho-logical changes following amino acid treatment (Olney, Ho, and Rhee, 1971). Thus arose the **excitotoxicity hy-pothesis**, which proposed that the effects produced by glutamate and related excitatory amino acids are caused by a prolonged depolarization of receptive neurons that in some way leads to their eventual damage or death. Current theories on how this may happen are presented later in this section.

Amino acid neurotoxins as pharmacological tools.   A few years after the advent of the excitotoxicity hypothe-sis, the powerful depolarizing agent kainate was tested and was also found to possess potent neurotoxic proper-ties (Olney, Rhee, and Ho, 1974). A series of subsequent studies performed by Schwarcz, Coyle, and their col-leagues (see Coyle, 1983, for review) demonstrated simi-larities between the neuropathology observed in Hunt-ington's disease (see below) and the effects of kainate produced by infusion directly into the corpus striatum (rather than subcutaneous injection) in adult rats. Both neurochemical and histological analyses seemed to indi-cate that kainate administered in this manner lesioned only cells intrinsic to the striatum, sparing incoming axons and nerve terminals. A separate report by Simson and colleagues (1977) presented evidence that MSG in-fused into the hypothalamus likewise destroyed cell bodies, but not axons of passage.

These findings ushered in an important new tech-nology in the fields of neuropharmacology and physio-logical psychology. The electrolytic and thermal tech-niques traditionally used to destroy neurons in a specific brain structure have always suffered from inter-pretive problems because the behavioral or physiologi-cal effects of the lesion might actually result from dam-age to axon fibers passing through that structure. Chemical neurotoxic lesions, on the other hand, are thought to provide unambiguous evidence of local cel-lular contributions to a given neural function. As sum-marized by Contestabile and colleagues (1984), this as-sumption may be overly simplistic in some cases. Kainate, for example, has sometimes been found to pro-duce damage in areas distant from the site of infusion. Such remote lesions have been observed mainly in the hippocampus and amygdala, and appear to be due to seizure activity induced by the treatment. Nevertheless, chemical lesioning with excitatory amino acids has been widely adopted as an alternative to physical lesioning techniques. The amino acid of choice for this purpose is generally considered to be ibotenate. This compound is considerably more toxic than glutamate, and while it is less potent than kainate, it does not share the latter's undesirable side effects.

Mechanisms of excitotoxicity.   Using the immature retina as a model system, early studies of the mecha-nisms underlying excitotoxic cell damage showed that one of the earliest observable responses is massive swelling of neuronal dendrites and cell bodies (reviewed by Rothman and Olney, 1987). Actual cell lysis (bursting) can occur when the excitatory amino acid exposure is prolonged. These observations indicated that large amounts of water were being pulled osmotically into affected cells, presumably due to ion fluxes occurring during the extended period of depolarization. It should be recalled that one effect of opening the channels linked to AMPA and kainate receptors is an influx of cations (mostly Na^+) into the cell. In addition, it is likely that a prolonged depolarization also drives chloride (Cl^-) ions into the cell by altering the Cl^- electrochemical gradient across the membrane. Eventually, the growing accumulation of ions in the interior of the cell draws water across the membrane to restore osmotic equilibrium.

Although osmotic swelling may contribute to some of the neuronal loss associated with excitatory amino acid administration, it is not the most important factor. Studies carried out over the past 10 years by Choi and his colleagues have demonstrated the presence of a *delayed* neurotoxic effect of excitatory amino acids applied to cultured neocortical neurons (see Choi, 1992; Coyle et al., 1991). This effect can be produced by exposing the cells to 10 mM glutamate for as little as 5 minutes. Over the next 24 hours, the cells exhibit morphological and biochemical signs of disintegration. Pharmacological experiments demonstrated that the delayed neurotoxic effect of glutamate could be elicited by selective NMDA receptor activation and was dependent on the presence of Ca^{2+} in the culture medium. Brief glutamate treatment in the absence of extracellular Ca^{2+} caused a temporary swelling, but the cells subsequently recovered.

According to current theorizing, therefore, intense glutamate exposure leads to Na^+ influx due to the activation of both NMDA and non-NMDA receptors, thereby producing the early osmotic phase of cell damage. The NMDA receptor-mediated increase in intracellular Ca^{2+} is largely responsible for triggering the delayed pathological reaction. Schoepp and Conn (1993) have theorized that metabotropic receptors could also contribute to neurotoxicity by their ability to enhance NMDA receptor function through phosphorylation of the receptor. On the other hand, intracellular Ca^{2+} levels can be elevated through processes in addition to NMDA receptor activation, such as opening of voltage-gated Ca^{2+} channels, passive leakage of Ca^{2+} across the cell membrane due to osmotic distension and instability, and mobilization of Ca^{2+} from intracellular stores (Choi, 1992; Mody and MacDonald, 1995). Possible mechanisms underlying Ca^{2+}-mediated neuropathology are discussed in the next section. Finally, it should be noted that kainate-induced neuronal damage may be subserved by a different mechanism, at least in some cases, since kainate neurotoxicity in cultured cerebellar neurons is dependent on Cl^- ions, but not on Na^+ or Ca^{2+} (Coyle et al., 1991).

Excitotoxicity and human neurological disorders. When the excitotoxicity hypothesis was first proposed by Olney, Ho, and Rhee (1971), they speculated that endogenous amino acids might play a role in the genesis of certain human neurological or psychological disorders. Recent work has gone a long way toward confirming this idea, at least with respect to the cell loss observed in several different types of brain trauma and disease. Our discussion here will focus on the possible involvement of excitatory amino acids in cell death that occurs due to **cerebral ischemia** (disruption of blood flow to all or a part of the brain), **hypoxia** (reduction in oxygen availability), and **epilepsy** (a neurological disorder characterized by recurrent neuronal hyperactivity and seizures). We shall also briefly discuss Huntington's disease and amyotrophic lateral sclerosis, two important degenerative disorders.

Cerebral ischemia can result from several different events. Any prolonged stoppage of the heart, whether due to a heart attack or any other reason, will obviously halt blood flow to the entire brain. This condition is termed global ischemia. Focal ischemia, on the other hand, refers to a regionally specific loss of blood flow because of a stroke—that is, the occlusion (blockage) or hemorrhaging of a blood vessel supplying that region. Ischemia is obviously accompanied by hypoxia, because oxygen is carried to all tissues by way of the bloodstream. However, there are additional causes of hypoxia, such as asphyxia and carbon monoxide poisoning. In cases of global ischemia or hypoxia, irreversible brain damage is generally thought to occur within 5–8 minutes. Yet even after this long a period of oxygen deprivation, many neurons and other brain cells appear histologically normal until many hours later. This finding suggests that much of the brain damage following a severe stroke or heart attack occurs after the actual ischemic episode. Similar observations have been made with respect to focal ischemic events. Such events give rise to several zones of damage, including a central zone of maximum insult, in which the neurons may not be salvageable, and a bordering "penumbra," where some minimal blood flow remains and where irreversible damage probably has not yet occurred.

For many years, medical personnel felt relatively little urgency in treating ischemia/hypoxia-related brain damage because little could be done to slow or prevent the continuing course of cell loss. However, studies concerning the involvement of excitatory amino acids in ischemic injury raise hopes that appropriate therapeutic interventions can be found. Several minutes into an ischemic episode, there is an abrupt rise in extracellular K^+ concentration and a concomitant fall in extracellular Na^+ (Szatkowski and Attwell, 1994). The increase in extracellular K^+ results in a rapid cellular depolarization termed "anoxic depolarization." These changes in ionic and voltage gradients across the nerve cell membrane

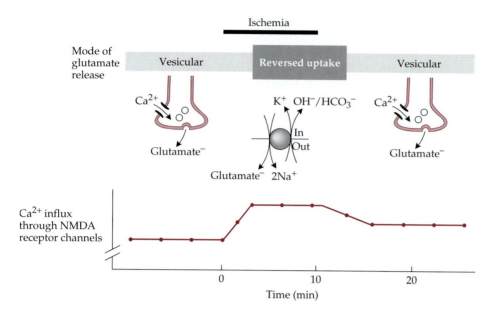

10.13 POSTULATED CHANGES IN GLUTAMATE RELEASE AND NMDA CHANNEL ACTIVATION DURING BRAIN ISCHEMIA. Some evidence suggests that glutamate release during an ischemic episode is Ca^{2+}-independent and nonexocytotic. According to this hypothesis, anoxic depolarization leads to a reversed action of the plasma membrane glutamate transporter. Exposure to glutamate during membrane depolarization causes an opening of NMDA receptor channels and an influx of Ca^{2+} into the cell. Ca^{2+} entry persists even when oxygenation is restored due to an apparent potentiation of NMDA channel activity. (After Szatkowski and Attwell, 1994.)

are thought to cause a reversal of the glutamate transporter, which leads to a massive Ca^{2+}-independent release of glutamate. Following the reestablishment of blood flow, ionic gradients are restored, extracellular glutamate levels decline, and glutamate release presumably returns to its normal Ca^{2+}-dependent, exocytotic mode. Yet a number of studies have demonstrated that NMDA receptor antagonists can attenuate neuronal damage when given during this postischemic period (e.g., Steinberg, Saleh, and Kunis, 1988).

How can we explain this puzzling finding? As summarized by Szatkowski and Attwell (1994), NMDA receptor currents appear to be enhanced following ischemic insult, perhaps through a mechanism like that responsible for the phenomenon of long-term potentiation (see below). Szatkowski and Attwell propose that such enhancement leads to a prolonged period of increased Ca^{2+} influx (Figure 10.13), thereby triggering delayed neuronal death as described earlier. Because of this focus on the possible role of NMDA receptors in ischemic/hypoxic brain damage, various types of NMDA receptor antagonists are presently either in clinical trials or being considered for clinical testing. These compounds include CGS19755 (a competitive NMDA receptor antagonist), felbamate (an antagonist at the glycine site on the NMDA receptor), ifenprodil and eliprodil (polyamine site antagonists), and dextrorphan, dextromethorphan, memantine, remacemide, and CNS 1102 (open-channel NMDA receptor blockers) (Lipton and Rosenberg, 1994; Scatton, 1994).

How does intracellular Ca^{2+} precipitate neuronal damage and death in cases of ischemia or other excitotoxicity? Some of the processes currently thought to be involved in this phenomenon are summarized in Figure 10.14. One possibility is that accumulation of excess Ca^{2+} by mitochondria injures these critical energy-producing organelles. Another important route of damage appears to be the stimulation of various Ca^{2+}-activated catabolic enzymes, including certain proteolytic (i.e., protein-degrading) enzymes, phospholipases, and endonucleases that can break down cellular DNA (Choi, 1992; Lipton and Rosenberg, 1994). Activation of phospholipase A_2, for example, stimulates the release of arachidonic acid, which in turn can lead to the formation of free radicals (highly reactive chemical species containing an unpaired electron) and oxidative cell damage. Nitric oxide, which as we saw earlier is sometimes synthesized as a consequence of NMDA receptor activity, can also participate in the generation of harmful free radicals (Coyle and Puttfarcken, 1993). Despite the large amount of evidence implicating Ca^{2+} in glutamate neurotoxicity, it should be noted that producing an equivalent elevation of intracellular Ca^{2+} by other methods causes less damage than is caused by glutamate stimulation (Lipton and Rosenberg, 1994). It is possible that the intracellular location of Ca^{2+} influx is important, or that other factors participate along with Ca^{2+} to produce delayed neurotoxicity.

Epilepsy is another disorder in which brain damage may sometimes occur through an excitotoxic mechanism. In 1880, W. Sommer discovered an area of the hippocampus that is vulnerable to injury in patients suffering from recurrent and/or prolonged seizures (status epilepticus). This region, which is called "Sommer's sector," consists of the pyramidal cell fields in the subiculum and in the CA1 region of Ammon's horn (Figure 10.15; more detail on hippocampal anatomy and circuitry will be presented in the section below on excitatory amino acids and learning). The CA1 pyramidal neurons are also among the brain cells most vulnerable to ischemic insult. Autoradiographic studies have shown that Sommer's sector in the human hippocampus contains a very high density of NMDA receptors (Geddes et al., 1986). In the rat, in which measurements have been made in a greater number of areas, the hippocampal CA1 region possesses the

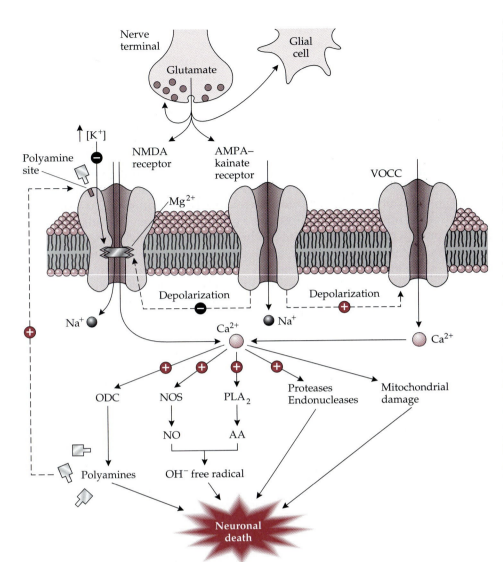

10.14 BIOCHEMICAL PROCESSES HYPOTHESIZED TO UNDERLIE IS-CHEMIC NEURONAL INJURY AND DEATH. Reduced cellular energy metabolism during ischemia causes increased release and decreased reuptake of glutamate, as well as increased extracellular K^+ concentrations due to inhibition of the Na^+–K^+ ATPase. Neurons are strongly depolarized by glutamate stimulation of AMPA and kainate receptors and by exposure to the elevated extracellular K^+ levels. Persistent glutamate activation of NMDA receptors with simultaneous membrane depolarization leads to a prolonged opening of NMDA receptor channels, permitting massive Ca^{2+} influx across the membrane. Depolarization is also thought to cause additional Ca^{2+} entry into the cell through voltage-operated Ca^{2+} channels (VOCC). Elevated intracellular Ca^{2+} levels activate a variety of Ca^{2+}-dependent processes, including specific proteases and endonucleases; phospholipase A_2 (PLA_2), which liberates arachidonic acid (AA) from membrane lipids; nitric oxide synthase (NOS), which catalyzes the formation of nitric oxide (NO); and ornithine decarboxylase (ODC), which mediates polyamine biosynthesis. Ca^{2+} accumulation in mitochondria can also lead to severe damage to these organelles. (After Scatton, 1994.)

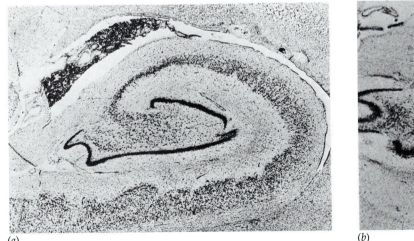

(a)

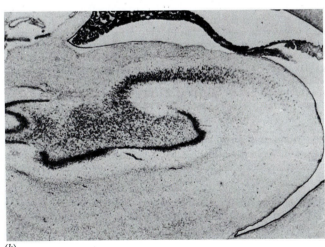

(b)

10.15 LOSS OF NEURONS IN THE SOMMER SECTOR OF THE HIPPOCAMPUS PRODUCED BY EPILEPSY. Pyramidal neurons in the Sommer sector of the hippocampal formation (CA1 and the subiculum) are vulnerable to loss as a result of epilepsy. Compare the absence of cell staining toward the right-hand side and the bottom of the photomicrograph in an epileptic with the appearance of the hippocampus in a normal brain (b). (From Corsellis and Bruton, 1983, *Advances in Neurology*, © Raven Press.)

highest density of NMDA receptors in the entire brain (Monaghan and Cotman, 1985). Excitotoxicity involving both NMDA and non-NMDA receptors may thus play an important role in both seizure-induced and ischemic brain damage (Meldrum, 1991).

We will conclude this section with a brief discussion of possible excitotoxic mechanisms in Huntington's disease and in amyotrophic lateral sclerosis (ALS). Huntington's disease is an inherited neurodegenerative disorder characterized by massive neuronal loss in the corpus striatum. In the early stages of the disease, typically beginning during middle age, the patient begins to exhibit involuntary and irregular limb movements. (The other name for this disorder is Huntington's chorea, which comes from the Greek word for "dance.") As time goes on, the movement disorder worsens, the patient becomes cognitively impaired, and death finally ensues. The striatum receives a massive glutamate projection from the neocortex and possesses a high overall density of excitatory amino acid receptor sites (both NMDA and non-NMDA). Many of these receptors are present on the medium spiny striatal output neurons, which are among the first cells to be destroyed as the disease progresses. The first evidence for an involvement of excitatory amino acids in Huntington's disease was provided by Coyle and Schwarcz (1976), who reported that excitotoxic lesions of the striatum (performed initially with kainate) could mimic many of the neurochemical and histopathological features of the disorder. Some investigators have suggested that quinolinic acid, an excitatory amino acid formed endogenously from tryptophan, produces an even better model of Huntington's disease when given intrastriatally to animals (see DiFiglia, 1990; Olney, 1989). It is still unclear whether excitotoxic pro-

Quinolinic acid

cesses are even responsible for the cell death in Huntington's disease, much less whether quinolinic acid might behave as an endogenous excitotoxin. However, investigators are continuing to explore this possibility.

ALS ("Lou Gehrig's disease") is a progressive degenerative disorder characterized by the loss of motor neurons in the spinal cord and brain stem. The disease begins with symptoms of mild weakness, followed later by paralysis, muscle wasting, respiratory depression, and eventually death (usually within 2 to 5 years following diagnosis). The mechanism underlying the motor neuron destruction has remained obscure until recently. One important factor in ALS pathogenesis is now known to be a deficit in superoxide dismutase, which is one of several enzymes involved in the elimination of free radicals (see Chapter 20 for a further discussion of free-radical generation and removal). Recent findings suggest that glutamate toxicity may also participate in motor neuron loss. For example, studies by Rothstein and co-workers suggest that ALS patients suffer from a defect in glutamate reuptake. Compared with control subjects, these patients show increased CSF glutamate concentrations and decreased high-affinity glutamate uptake in the spinal cord and the motor and somatosensory cortices (Rothstein et al., 1990; Rothstein, Martin, and Kuncl, 1992). One possible problem in linking ALS with excitotoxic mechanisms is that such mechanisms have generally been considered to act relatively quickly, which does not fit the slower degenerative pattern of ALS. However, Rothstein's group recently reported that chronic blockade of glutamate transport by the selective uptake inhibitor threohydroxyaspartate caused a gradual loss of motor neurons from neonatal rat spinal cord cultures (Rothstein et al., 1993). Together, these results suggest that therapeutic interventions targeted at the glutamate system might have some efficacy in retarding the progress of ALS. One such drug currently being tested is riluzole (2-amino-6-(trifluoromethoxy)benzothiazole), a putative inhibitor of glutamate release. Recent

Riluzole

studies by European investigators found that riluzole treatment generally slowed down the loss of muscular function in ALS patients and also produced a modest increase in life span (Bensimon et al., 1994; Lacomblez et al., 1996). These results demonstrate the feasibility of pharmacotherapy for ALS, although we must continue to search for more effective drugs.

Excitatory Amino Acids, Synaptic Plasticity, and Learning

One of the great challenges facing neuroscientists is to understand how nervous systems process, store, and retrieve the information necessary for an organism's well-being and survival. Here, of course, we are referring to the mechanisms underlying learning and memory. Biochemical and pharmacological approaches to this problem have concentrated on determining what transmitters and receptor types might be used by neurons participating in a "learning circuit," as well as on identifying the second messenger systems or other mediating mechanisms that might be involved at the molecular level. Because of the vast complexity and enormous number of neurons present in an entire vertebrate nervous system, this type of research is conducted most profitably with simpler models involving either invertebrate systems or isolated parts of a vertebrate brain. An important example of the latter type of model is the hippocampal slice preparation, in which investigators have demonstrated an important form of neural plasticity that appears to be learning-related. We will first introduce this phenomenon, which is called **long-term potentiation (LTP)**, and then discuss evidence that glutamate and several of its receptor subtypes are intimately involved in LTP induction.

Long-term potentiation. Long-term potentiation refers to a persistent (at least 1 hour) increase in EPSP amplitude at a synapse that is typically induced by brief, high-frequency afferent stimulation. Prolonged low-frequency stimulation can produce a related phenomenon termed **long-term depression (LTD)**, which involves a reduction in synaptic efficacy. Space considerations preclude further discussion of LTD, but several recent reviews are available to interested readers (Artola and Singer, 1993; Christie, Kerr, and Abraham, 1994; Linden, 1994; Malenka, 1995).

Long-term potentiation has been found in a number of different brain areas (e.g., see Tsumoto, 1992), although the phenomenon is most easily demonstrated in the hippocampus, in which it was first discovered by Bliss and Lomo (1973). Hippocampal LTP can be induced in vivo, in which case the effect lasts for days or weeks. However, the biochemical and physiological mechanisms underlying LTP have primarily been studied in vitro using the hippocampal slice preparation. Hippocampal slice studies are performed by making transverse sections (typically around 200 μm in thickness) through a freshly removed hippocampus and maintaining the slices for the next several hours in a physiological medium while various experimental manipulations are carried out. The internal circuitry of the hippocampus, which is illustrated in Figure 10.16, is preserved in such slices. Long-term potentiation can be induced at all of the principal excitatory hippocampal pathways, including (1) the perforant path from the entorhinal cortex to the granule neurons of the dentate gyrus, (2) the mossy fibers connecting the dentate granule cells to the CA3 pyramidal neurons of Ammon's horn, (3) the Schaffer collaterals from area CA3 to CA1, and (4) the commissural projection to CA1 from the contralateral hippocampus. Postsynaptic responses may be recorded either intracellularly as individual excitatory postsynaptic potentials (EPSPs) or extracellularly as population EPSPs. In a typical experiment involving LTP induction in the Schaffer collateral/commissural pathways, a stimulating electrode is placed in the vicinity of the afferent fibers, and a recording electrode is placed either inside a CA1 pyramidal cell for intracellular EPSP measurements or in one of the dendritic field regions to obtain extracellular EPSPs. As can be seen in Figure 10.16, extracellular potentials are available from either

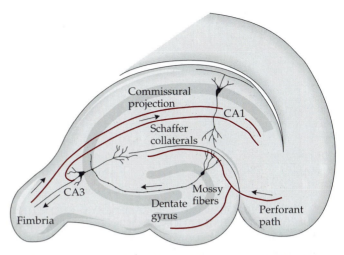

10.16 EXCITATORY PATHWAYS USED TO STUDY LONG-TERM POTENTIATION IN HIPPOCAMPAL SLICES. Input from the entorhinal cortex via the perforant path eventually reaches the hippocampal CA1 pyramidal neurons through a multisynaptic pathway. Long-term potentiation (LTP) can be demonstrated at these synapses, all of which are believed to use an excitatory amino acid (probably glutamate) as their transmitter. (After Collingridge and Bliss, 1987.)

the basal dendrites in the stratum oriens (upward-facing in this diagram) or the apical dendrites in the stratum radiatum (the downward-facing dendritic tree).

Long-term potentiation is most commonly induced by means of a single brief train of electrical pulses of 100–400 Hz (stimuli/s). This type of stimulus is termed "tetanic" because similar high-frequency activation of muscle fibers produces a sustained maximum contraction of the muscle called a tetanus. Tetanic stimuli applied, for example, to the Schaffer collateral/commissural pathway can give rise to several different types of response facilitation (Figure 10.17). One type of facilitation, called **post-tetanic potentiation** (PTP), is extremely transitory and reflects an increase in neurotransmitter release with no change in postsynaptic sensitivity. This phenomenon can be demonstrated experimentally with very brief tetanic stimuli applied in the presence of an NMDA receptor blocker (NMDA receptors are not required for PTP but do play an essential role in other forms of response facilitation). If NMDA receptor activation is permitted, tetanic stimuli can elicit a somewhat longer-lasting synaptic enhancement, called **short-term potentiation (STP)**, or a full-fledged LTP, which may remain stable for several hours in vitro. The intensity and pattern of the stimulation determine whether STP or LTP is induced, with STP generally being associated with weaker stimuli that presumably activate fewer afferent fibers. Mechanistically, however, the relationship between these two phenomena remains unresolved. For example, it is possible that (1) STP is mechanistically distinct from LTP; (2) STP is a necessary, but not sufficient, condition for the manifestation of LTP (i.e., LTP might

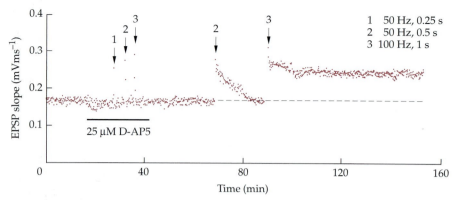

10.17 DIFFERENT FORMS OF HIPPOCAMPAL SYNAPTIC POTENTIATION EVOKED BY HIGH-FREQUENCY STIMULATION. A rat hippocampal slice preparation was subjected to three different tetanic stimuli (1–3) with the indicated frequency and duration parameters. In the presence of the NMDA receptor antagonist D-AP5, all stimuli produced only a short-lived (30–40 s) increase in synaptic strength (measured as the initial slope of the field EPSP in CA1), known as a post-tetanic potentiation (PTP). Following D-AP5 washout, a second application of stimulus 2 produced short-term potentiation (STP), whereas stimulus 3 was sufficient to produce a longer-lasting synaptic enhancement (long-term potentiation; LTP). (After Malenka and Nicoll, 1993; Malenka, 1991.)

require some additional intracellular event not present following STP production); or (3) STP and LTP are triggered by essentially the same mechanisms, but STP is shorter-lived because stabilization of synaptic enhancement requires threshold activation of one or more biochemical processes that occur only with stronger afferent stimulation (Hanse and Gustafsson, 1994; Malenka and Nicoll, 1993).

Mechanisms underlying long-term potentiation. The characteristics of hippocampal LTP and theories about its underlying mechanisms have been discussed in recent reviews (Bliss and Collingridge, 1993; Malenka, 1995). In considering the mechanisms of LTP, it is useful to distinguish between an "induction" phase, involving the initial processes required to trigger LTP, and a subsequent "maintenance" or "expression" phase, during which synaptic facilitation is sustained. As mentioned above, LTP induction requires a stimulus burst of a certain minimum intensity and duration. The reason for this can be understood by comparing the consequences of applying a single electrical stimulus versus a typical tetanic stimulus train. Activation of the Schaffer collateral/commissural pathway by a single electrical stimulus releases glutamate from that pathway's excitatory nerve terminals, but it simultaneously provokes activity in GABAergic interneurons (local inhibitory neurons that use γ-aminobutyric acid [GABA] as their transmitter). Glutamate stimulation of postsynaptic AMPA receptors causes a rapid EPSP, but this is quickly followed by an inhibitory postsynaptic potential (IPSP) produced by GABA's actions on the same cells. NMDA receptors respond more slowly than AMPA receptors, in part because they must overcome the voltage-dependent channel blockade by Mg^{2+} ions described earlier. Moreover, when the channels do begin to open due to the combination of glutamate stimulation and AMPA receptor-mediated membrane depolarization, they are thought to quickly reclose due to GABAergic hyperpolarization of the cell membrane and reinstatement of the Mg^{2+} blockade. Overall current flow through these channels is therefore limited following single stimuli or weak stimulus trains.

A somewhat different scenario occurs, however, following the application of strong, high-frequency stimulation. In this case, repeated excitation of the afferent fibers causes a greater and more sustained release of glutamate, which activates both the AMPA and NMDA receptors. There is also evidence for a depression of GABAergic activity that is thought to be mediated by $GABA_B$ autoreceptors (see Part II of this chapter for a discussion of GABA and its receptor subtypes). Consequently, the postsynaptic elements respond with a prolonged depolarization, which permits the opening of NMDA-gated channels and an influx of Ca^{2+} ions (Bliss and Collingridge, 1993).

Numerous pharmacological blocking experiments have demonstrated that NMDA receptor activity is an absolute requirement for LTP induction (Bliss and Collingridge, 1993; Malenka, 1995). The role of AMPA receptors during the induction phase is principally that of mediating the membrane depolarization needed to permit NMDA channel opening. Several recent studies, however, indicate an important role for metabotropic glutamate receptors as well (Ben-Ari and Ariksztejn, 1995). For example, the metabotropic receptor agonist *trans*-ACPD was found to induce LTP under certain conditions, and the selective antagonist α-methyl-4-carboxyphenylglycine was able to inhibit both tetanus-induced and *trans*-ACPD-induced LTP in the hippocampus (Watkins and Collingridge, 1994).

The high Ca^{2+} permeability of NMDA receptor channels compared with that of most AMPA receptors strongly suggests that an elevation of intracellular Ca^{2+} is a critical aspect of LTP induction. Indeed, this hypothesis has been supported by studies involving the imaging of Ca^{2+} concentration changes within dendritic processes and spines (Bliss and Collingridge, 1993). It now appears that the rise in Ca^{2+} mediated by NMDA receptor activation is augmented by Ca^{2+} mobilization from intracellular stores. This mobilization is probably mediated, at least in part, by metabotropic glutamate receptors coupled to the phosphoinositide second messenger system.

The expression phase of LTP has been a source of major controversy over the past few years. In particular, different research groups have found conflicting evidence regarding whether the locus of LTP expression is mainly presynaptic, mainly postsynaptic, or both pre- and postsynaptic (reviewed by Bliss and Collingridge, 1993; Malinow, 1994). In the hippocampal pathways usually studied in LTP research, synaptic transmission is erratic in that presynaptic action potentials often fail to elicit a detectable postsynaptic response. This has usually been interpreted as a failure of transmitter release from the nerve terminal. The proposed presynaptic change in LTP can be described in terms of increased probability of transmitter release at an individual synapse, or alternatively, increased quantal content (i.e., the average number of neurotransmitter quanta released per stimulus) across many synapses (Bekkers and

Stevens, 1990; Liao, Jones, and Malinow, 1992; Stevens and Wang, 1994). On the postsynaptic side, several groups have found evidence for increased quantal size (i.e., the amplitude of the response to a single quantum) instead of (Foster and McNaughton, 1991; Manabe and Nicoll, 1994; Manabe, Renner, and Nicoll, 1992) or in addition to (Liao, Jones, and Malinow, 1992) a change in quantal content. Enhanced postsynaptic sensitivity could be related to phosphorylation-mediated stimulation of AMPA receptor function (McGlade-McCulloh et al., 1993; Tan, Wenthold, and Soderling, 1994) and/or an increase in receptor density (Maren et al., 1993). Liao, Hessler, and Malinow (1995) recently presented evidence that prior to LTP induction, a substantial proportion of the glutamatergic synapses in the hippocampal CA1 region possess functional NMDA receptors but lack functional AMPA receptors. This circumstance provides an alternative *postsynaptic* explanation for the previously mentioned transmission failure at some hippocampal synapses, because single stimulus pulses should produce little or no postsynaptic response in the absence of AMPA receptor–mediated membrane depolarization. Following LTP induction, however, Liao and colleagues observed AMPA receptor–mediated responses at previously silent synapses. Enhanced postsynaptic responses were also found at some synapses that appeared to possess functional AMPA receptors before LTP. The investigators hypothesize that Ca^{2+} influx caused by tetanus-induced NMDA receptor stimulation somehow causes the addition of functional AMPA receptors, either through activation of previously nonfunctional receptors or through insertion of sequestered receptors into the postsynaptic membrane (Figure 10.18). According to this

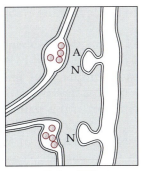
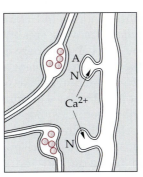
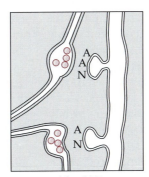
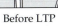

| Before LTP | LTP induction | After LTP |

10.18 PROPOSED POSTSYNAPTIC MECHANISM OF HIPPOCAMPAL LTP. Recent evidence suggests that many glutamatergic synapses in the hippocampal CA1 region possess functional NMDA receptors (N) but no functional AMPA receptors (A) (*left panel, bottom*). Stimulation conditions that trigger Ca^{2+} entry into the postsynaptic cell and that consequently induce LTP (*middle panel*) cause the appearance of AMPA-mediated responses at these previously silent synapses (*right panel, bottom*) and also enhance such responses at synapses that previously showed AMPA-mediated transmission (*right panel, top*). These results could be explained by activation of previously nonfunctional AMPA receptors or by insertion of sequestered AMPA receptors into the postsynaptic membrane. (After Liao, Hessler, and Malinow, 1995.)

view, there is no need to invoke increased neurotransmitter release to explain the basic phenomena of LTP. Nevertheless, because the question of pre- versus postsynaptic changes in LTP has not yet been resolved, in the following discussion of biochemical mechanisms we will assume that both types of changes occur.

LTP-associated changes in synaptic function are believed to stem from a Ca^{2+}-dependent biochemical cascade precipitated by NMDA receptor channel activation and augmented, as discussed above, by mobilization of intracellular Ca^{2+} stores. Although the details of this cascade are still being investigated, much attention has been paid to the possible roles of protein kinase C (PKC) and Ca^{2+}/calmodulin-dependent protein kinase II (CaM-K II). Both kinases are activated by tetanic stimulation (Fukunaga et al., 1993; Klann, Chen, and Sweatt, 1993), and inhibitors of either kinase can block LTP (Malenka et al., 1989; Malinow, Schulman, and Tsien, 1989). Additional support for the involvement of CaM-K II in LTP has come from studies using gene "knockout" techniques. Silva, Stevens, and coworkers (1992) created mutant mice deficient in one of the major isoforms of CaM-K II and then tested whether hippocampal neurons in these subjects showed normal LTP. Most neurons tested did not exhibit LTP, and furthermore, behavioral testing showed that the mice were impaired in their spatial learning capabilities (Silva, Paylor et al., 1992; see below for a discussion of the relationship between LTP and learning). The evidence presented above certainly points to a significant role for CaM-K II and PKC in LTP, but the exact nature of this role is still unclear. One interesting hypothesis is that the long duration of LTP is due to the transformation of both kinases to a state of persistent activation. For example, CaM-K II can phosphorylate itself ("autophosphorylation"), thereby becoming temporarily independent of calmodulin (see Chapter 6). Some results are consistent with the hypothesis of persistent kinase activation, but the evidence is not yet conclusive (see Malenka, 1995). Figure 10.19 illustrates how glutamate receptor activation of various protein kinases might trigger postsynaptic mechanisms involved in LTP.

Finally, it is important to return our attention briefly to the presynaptic side of the process. As mentioned above, LTP has been associated not only with an increase in postsynaptic sensitivity, but also with enhanced glutamate release from the presynaptic terminals. Moreover, the presynaptic effect is dependent on the activation of postsynaptic NMDA receptors, which strongly suggests that some type of retrograde messenger (generated as a consequence of this NMDA receptor activity) is sent from the postsynaptic elements back to the nerve terminals (Figure 10.19). One of the first retrograde messengers to be proposed was arachidonic acid, although more recently nitric oxide (NO) has become the favored candidate messenger substance. NO is formed by the Ca^{2+}/calmodulin-dependent enzyme NO synthase (NOS) and is released by cells in response to NMDA receptor activation (see Chapter 6). In some experiments, LTP induction has been blocked by inhibiting NOS or by scavenging NO after its release (Bliss and Collingridge, 1993; Malenka, 1995). The results, however, are not completely consistent with NO being a necessary factor in the LTP process. Furthermore, several other compounds, including carbon monoxide and a lipid called platelet-activating factor, also possess some of the characteristics of an LTP retrograde messenger. Hence, further research is required to resolve the important question of whether a retrograde messenger participates in LTP, and if so, the identity of this messenger.

NMDA receptors, LTP, and learning. We have seen that LTP is a neurophysiological, rather than a behavioral, process. What relevance, if any, does this process have for learning and memory? Many types of learning are associative in nature, meaning that the organism learns to associate stimuli with one another and with specific responses and reinforcers. Over 40 years ago, the psychologist Donald Hebb proposed that the neural mechanism underlying learning might be an increased transmission efficiency at certain synapses induced by repetitive, synchronous activation of the pre- and postsynaptic cells (Hebb, 1949). This hypothesis implies an associative mechanism because neurons are rarely driven by a single input. Thus, synchronous activation on both sides of a synapse would typically require that the presynaptic cell in question be repeatedly excited at the same time that other inputs to the postsynaptic cell are also firing. Researchers have long searched for such "Hebbian" synapses in view of their potential involvement in learning or memory processes. As reviewed by Maren and Baudry (1995), the discovery of NMDA receptors and their apparent role in LTP now suggests that the Hebbian synapse may be a reality.

The critical link between LTP and the Hebbian synapse is the existence of an associative form of LTP. Tetanic stimulation of "weak" synaptic inputs may fail to elicit LTP. Identical stimulation of those inputs, however, may produce synaptic potentiation if it is paired temporally with the activation of a "strong" input to the same postsynaptic cells (Figure 10.20) (Malenka, 1995). It should not be difficult to imagine the probable role of NMDA receptors in associative LTP. Stimulating a weak input alone is unlikely to cause sufficient NMDA receptor activation to trigger LTP induction. Simultaneous excitation of the postsynaptic cell by another afferent source, however, would cause sufficient depolarization to unblock the NMDA receptors and allow LTP to occur.

A direct relationship between LTP (and Hebbian synapses) and learning has yet to be firmly established. However, Morris and his coworkers reported that chronic intracerebroventricular infusion of the NMDA

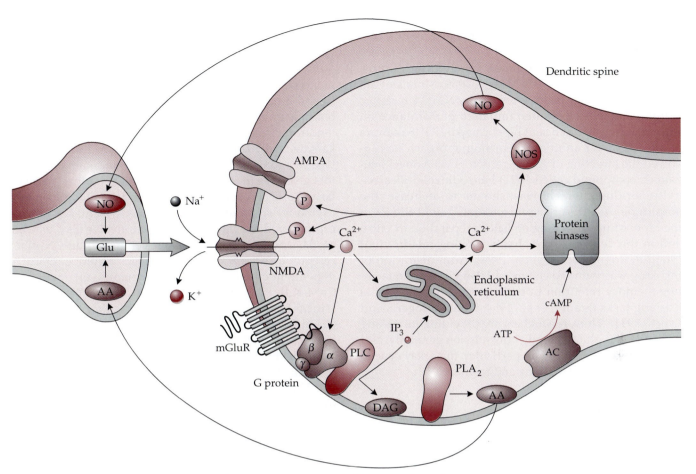

10.19 POSSIBLE MECHANISMS UNDERLYING LTP INDUCTION AND MAINTENANCE BY GLUTAMATE RECEPTOR ACTIVATION. LTP induction requires glutamate-stimulated Ca^{2+} influx through NMDA receptor channels. This process may be augmented by metabotropic glutamate receptor (mGluR) activation of phospholipase C (PLC), leading to inositol trisphosphate (IP_3) liberation and Ca^{2+} release from intracellular stores. LTP maintenance may involve the activation of protein kinases stimulated by Ca^{2+} and possibly other second messengers, including arachidonic acid (AA; liberated by phospholipase A_2 [PLA_2]) and cyclic AMP (cAMP; produced by adenylyl cyclase [AC]). These kinases phosphorylate several target proteins, probably including AMPA and NMDA receptors. There is some evidence that the biochemical cascade occurring postsynaptically also leads to the formation of one or more retrograde messengers, which may include nitric oxide (synthesized by nitric oxide synthase [NOS]) or arachidonic acid. (After Bliss and Collingridge, 1993.)

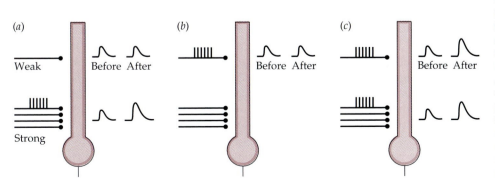

10.20 ASSOCIATIVE LTP. The three panels illustrate the consequences of applying a tetanic stimulus to synaptic inputs differing in strength. A tetanus elicits LTP when applied to a strong input alone (*a*), but not when applied to a weak input alone (*b*) (note the amplitude of the excitatory postsynaptic potentials elicited by test stimuli). However, when a tetanic stimulus is applied to both inputs simultaneously (*c*), it gives rise to LTP in both. This phenomenon, which is called associative LTP, supports the contention that LTP represents a neural mechanism underlying learning. (After Malenka, 1995; Nicoll, Kauer, and Malenka, 1988.)

receptor antagonist D-AP5 (which blocks LTP in vitro and in vivo) selectively disrupted the acquisition of a spatial navigation task, a type of learning that is dependent on normal hippocampal functioning (Davis, Butcher, and Morris, 1992; Morris, 1989; Morris et al., 1986). Mutant mice lacking one of the NMDA receptor subunits likewise exhibited impaired performance on this task as well as deficient hippocampal LTP (Sakimura et al., 1995). Yet another interesting approach has involved the targeting of AMPA receptors via a novel benzamide compound called 1-(1,3-benzodioxol-5-ylcarbonyl)piperidine, which was shown to increase the amplitude of AMPA receptor-mediated field EPSPs in the hippocampal CA1 region (slice preparation in vitro) and in the dentate gyrus (freely moving rats in vivo) (Stäubli, Rogers, and Lynch, 1994). Administration of this drug was found to enhance LTP in vivo and to facilitate memory retention in both spatial and nonspatial learning tasks (Stäubli et al., 1994; Stäubli, Rogers, and Lynch, 1994). Thus, researchers are providing increasing evidence that glutamatergic transmission generally, and glutamate-mediated LTP in particular, may play crucial roles in processes of learning and memory.

Part I Summary

Starting from a humble beginning, the excitatory amino acids glutamate and (to a lesser extent) aspartate have come to be seen as major players in the neurochemistry and pharmacology of behavior. The carbon skeleton of glutamate comes primarily from the oxidative metabolism of glucose (glycolysis) and the subsequent transamination of α-ketoglutarate. Following its release, some glutamate is taken up by astroglial cells and converted to the inactive compound glutamine by the enzyme glutamine synthetase. Glial cells apparently store glutamine and release it for reutilization by neurons following reconversion to glutamate by phosphate-activated glutaminase.

Glutamate synthesized in nerve terminals is stored in vesicles and is thought to be released by exocytosis. Following release, glutamate is taken up from the synaptic cleft by a Na^+-dependent process. Three different glutamate transporters have been cloned, one that is present in many neurons (as well as in various peripheral nonneuronal cells), a second that is found mainly in Bergmann glia of the cerebellar cortex, and a third that is localized specifically in astrocytes.

Although several putative aspartatergic pathways have been identified, there is generally stronger evidence for the use of glutamate as an excitatory transmitter in the brain and spinal cord. Identified glutamatergic pathways in the brain include various projections of neocortical pyramidal cells, several intrahippocampal and hippocampal projection pathways, and the parallel fibers of the cerebellar cortex. In the spinal cord, gluta-

mate is believed to serve as a transmitter used by excitatory interneurons as well as by many primary afferent neurons.

Excitatory amino acid receptors are divided into two major classes: ionotropic receptors, which belong to the ligand-gated channel receptor superfamily, and metabotropic receptors, which are coupled to G proteins. The ionotropic receptors are further subdivided into AMPA, kainate, and NMDA receptors, each named for its prototypical agonist. Activation of AMPA and kainate receptors gives rise to fast EPSPs, and these receptors (particularly the AMPA subtype) play a fundamental role in fast excitatory signaling in the nervous system. NMDA receptors mediate slower EPSPs that involve Ca^{2+} as well as Na^+ and K^+ fluxes across the cell membrane. NMDA receptor activation thereby stimulates a number of Ca^{2+}-dependent enyzmes in the postsynaptic cell, including CaM-K II, PKC, phospholipase A_2, and NOS. Another critical feature of NMDA receptors is that the receptor channel is subject to a voltage-dependent block by Mg^{2+} ions. Thus, the cell membrane must be depolarized (for example, by AMPA receptor activation) before NMDA receptor channel opening can occur.

Thus far, seven different metabotropic receptors (mGluR1–mGluR7) have been cloned. They fall into three different groups based on second messenger system coupling (i.e., stimulation of the phosphoinositide system vs. inhibition of cAMP synthesis) and pharmacology. Certain metabotropic receptors that are stimulated by the drug L-AP4 appear to function as release-inhibiting autoreceptors.

Continuous exposure of neurons to high levels of glutamate or other excitatory amino acids for several minutes can produce delayed toxic effects and even cell death. This phenomenon of excitotoxicity has been exploited as a research tool to selectively destroy neurons in a brain area while sparing glial cells and fibers of passage. There has also been considerable clinical interest in the possibility that excitotoxic mechanisms, particularly involving NMDA receptors and Ca^{2+} ions, may underlie the cell loss observed in cerebral ischemia, severe epilepsy, Huntington's disease, and amyotrophic lateral sclerosis. Various glutamate antagonists are currently being tested for their clinical efficacy in treating some of these disorders.

Finally, several types of glutamate receptors, including NMDA, AMPA, and metabotropic receptors, play critical roles in a form of synaptic enhancement called long-term potentiation (LTP). LTP, which has been studied most extensively in the hippocampus, is produced by a brief burst of high-frequency stimulation and is manifested by a persistent enhancement of the synaptic response. Most evidence indicates that LTP involves both an increase in presynaptic glutamate release and an increased sensitivity of the postsynaptic cells. These effects are dependent on activation of postsynaptic CaM-K II and PKC, and probably also require the action of one or more retrograde messengers such as NO or arachidonic acid. Although LTP is typically studied in vitro, it also occurs in vivo, where it may underlie certain forms of learning.

Part II
Inhibitory Amino Acids: GABA

In Part I of this chapter, we saw that certain amino acids, such as glutamate and aspartate, play a dominant role in fast excitatory transmission in the central nervous system. Inhibitory transmission is equally important in behavioral control mechanisms. The significance of neural inhibition is evident from the fact that blocking the action of either of the two major inhibitory amino acid transmitters leads to convulsions and even death. These two substances are γ-aminobutyric acid (**GABA**), the subject of Part II, and glycine, which is discussed in Part III.

The Discovery of GABA and Its Identification as a Neurotransmitter

The discovery of GABA in brain tissue was made independently by Eugene Roberts and by Jorge Awapara, along with their respective colleagues (Awapara et al., 1950; Roberts and Frankel, 1950). In addition to publishing their findings, both Roberts and Awapara attended the 1950 meeting of the Federation of American Societies for Experimental Biology to report on their work. As described by McGeer, Eccles, and McGeer (1978), the two investigators happened to share a room at the meeting, thereby becoming aware of their joint discovery. It was decided at that time that Roberts would continue to pursue research on GABA while Awapara would work on taurine, another amino acid that had been found in high quantities in brain tissue.

Interest in GABA as a possible neurotransmitter grew tremendously in the 1950s and 1960s. Results from a number of laboratories suggested that this substance might play an important role in inhibitory transmission in both vertebrates and invertebrates. Working with lobsters, Kravitz and coworkers showed that inhibitory fibers contained significant amounts of GABA, whereas the GABA content of motor (excitatory) fibers was extremely low or even undetectable (Kravitz, Kuffler, and Potter, 1963). These investigators subsequently demonstrated a Ca^{2+}-dependent release of GABA upon stimulation of inhibitory axons innervating the opener muscles of the claws (Otsuka et al., 1966). In the mammalian nervous system, much attention was focused on the Purkinje cells of the cerebellum, which send an inhibitory projection to the giant Deiter's cells of the lateral vestibular nucleus. Studies by Obata and others (Obata and Takeda, 1969; Obata et al., 1967) showed that increased GABA levels were found in the fourth ventricle when the cerebellar cortex (where the Purkinje cells are located) was stimulated, and that iontophoretic application of GABA to the Deiter's neurons mimicked the inhibitory effect of Purkinje cell activity. The use of GABA by Purkinje cells was finally confirmed by the demonstration of the presence of the GABA-synthesizing enzyme glutamate decarboxylase (see below) in their axon terminals (McLaughlin et al., 1974; Saito et al., 1974). At the present time, GABA is well established as a transmitter in the nervous systems of both nonhuman animals and humans (e.g., McCormick, 1989).

Synthesis and Metabolism of GABA

GABA is synthesized in a single step catalyzed by the enzyme glutamate decarboxylase (GAD). This enzyme converts L-glutamate to GABA and CO_2, using pyridoxal phosphate as a cofactor (Figure 10.21). Thus, the pathways for glutamate synthesis that were discussed

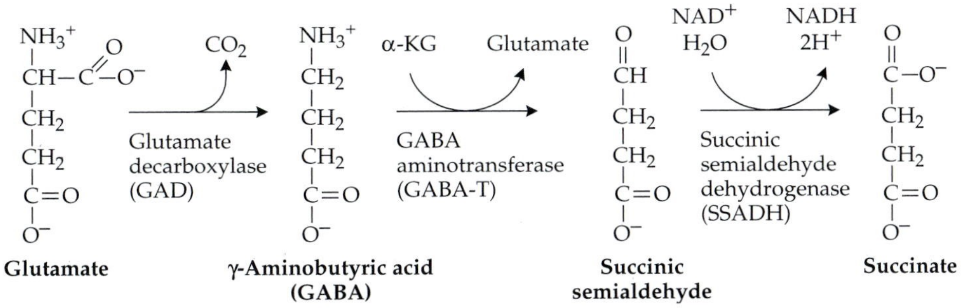

10.21 GABA SYNTHESIS AND METABOLISM. GABA is synthesized from glutamate by the enzyme glutamate decarboxylase (GAD). The breakdown of GABA is catalyzed by GABA aminotransferase (GABA-T), which forms succinic semialdehyde and regenerates the precursor glutamate from α-ketoglutarate (α-KG). Most of the succinic semialdehyde is converted to succinate, a citric acid cycle intermediate. This pathway is therefore often called the GABA shunt because it provides an alternate route (other than the citric acid cycle) by which succinate can be formed from α-KG.

earlier are also important in GABAergic neurons, particularly the conversion of glutamine to glutamate (Peng et al., 1993). Subcellular fractionation studies have shown that GAD is highly enriched in synaptosomes, where it is found in the cytoplasm. The synaptosomal localization of this enzyme indicates that GABA synthesis occurs primarily in axon terminals rather than in other parts of the cell.

The structural and functional characteristics of GAD have been summarized in several reviews (Erlander and Tobin, 1991; Martin and Rimvall, 1993). In rats and humans, two different forms of GAD are found, one with a molecular weight of 65 kDa (GAD_{65}) and another with a molecular weight of 67 kDa (GAD_{67}). These isoenzymes are encoded by different genes and exhibit over 90% amino acid sequence homology across the two species (Bu et al., 1992; Erlander et al., 1991). Although both GAD_{65} and GAD_{67} are found in nerve endings, the former is particularly enriched in terminals and thus may be somewhat more important for GABAergic transmission.

The catabolism of GABA is initiated by the enzyme GABA aminotransferase (previously called GABA transaminase, hence the abbreviation GABA-T). This enzyme operates like other aminotransferases discussed above, transferring the amino group from GABA to α-KG. The products of the reaction are succinic semialdehyde and glutamate (see Figure 10.21). Thus, the breakdown of GABA leads directly to the regeneration of its precursor, which also occurs in the case of choline liberation due to acetylcholine hydrolysis. GABA-T is a mitochondrial enzyme with a molecular weight of 109 kDa. Like GAD, it requires pyridoxal phosphate as a cofactor. GABA-T has been detected in GABAergic neurons as well as in glial cells (astrocytes). The enzyme is thus found in locations where it can inactivate synaptically released GABA and metabolize excess transmitter that is present outside of synaptic vesicles.

The succinic semialdehyde formed by GABA-T is quickly oxidized to succinate by the mitochondrial enzyme succinic semialdehyde dehydrogenase (SSADH). Hence, the net effect of synthesizing and metabolizing a molecule of GABA is to convert a molecule of α-KG to succinate (since the glutamate used in the initial step is subsequently regenerated). However, succinate is also made from α-KG in the normal course of the citric acid cycle, although the pathway involved is obviously different. This means that GABA synthesis and catabolism results in the "shunting" of α-KG → succinate conversion from the citric acid cycle to this alternate pathway. For this reason, the reaction sequence shown in Figure 10.21 is often called the GABA shunt. Turnover studies suggest that approximately 8% to 10% of overall brain glucose metabolism is funneled through the GABA shunt (Balazs et al., 1970; Baxter, 1976).

The overall cellular scheme for GABA metabolism is summarized in Figure 10.22. The full GABA shunt is operative in GABAergic neurons by virtue of their possession of GAD, GABA-T, and SSADH. However, astrocytes have also been found to contain GABA-T and SSADH. Thus, the GABA shunt also takes place in glial cells, although here the shunt is dependent on the uptake of extracellular GABA (see below) and recycling of the glutamate back to neurons via glutamine.

Regulation of GABA Synthesis

Although the control of GABA synthesis rate is not yet fully understood, the estimated rate in vivo is very low compared with the maximum possible rate determined by measuring total GAD activity (reviewed by Martin and Rimvall, 1993). Therefore, it appears that excess synthetic capacity is present that could provide for increased GABA formation when needed. As in the case of glutamate, overall GABA synthesis can be separated into two functional compartments: a "transmitter" compartment thought to represent GABA formation in GABAergic nerve terminals, and a "metabolic" compartment associated with perikarya and dendrites that may represent the utilization of GABA as an intermediate in energy metabolism (Martin and Rimvall, 1993). Approximately 50% of total GABA synthesis has been attributed to each compartment.

Changes in glutamate concentration in GABAergic nerve terminals could alter GABA synthesis if GAD is not normally saturated with this substrate. The overall rat brain tissue level of glutamate is almost 10 mM, which is much higher than the estimated K_m of GAD for glutamate (on the order of 0.2 to 1.2 mM) (Martin and Rimvall, 1993). If GAD in nerve cells were actually exposed to 10 mM glutamate, the enzyme would be totally saturated with substrate, and small to moderate changes in glutamate availability would have no effect on the rate of GABA formation. Various lines of evidence, however, suggest that the glutamate concentration in GABAergic neurons is much lower than in many other cell types. Nevertheless, researchers are still uncertain as to whether GAD is typically saturated with glutamate in vivo, and there is currently no indication that glutamate levels regulate GABA synthesis under physiological conditions.

Although precursor availability may not play an important role in GABA formation, this process may be regulated in a complex manner by other factors acting on GAD. In order for GAD to catalyze the decarboxylation of glutamate to GABA, it must first bind the cofactor pyridoxal phosphate. The complex formed by enzyme and cofactor is called a **holoenzyme**, whereas the term **apoenzyme** is used to denote the inactive form of the enzyme that lacks bound cofactor. Martin and his colleagues have demonstrated the existence of a regulatory cycle in which GAD is converted back and forth be-

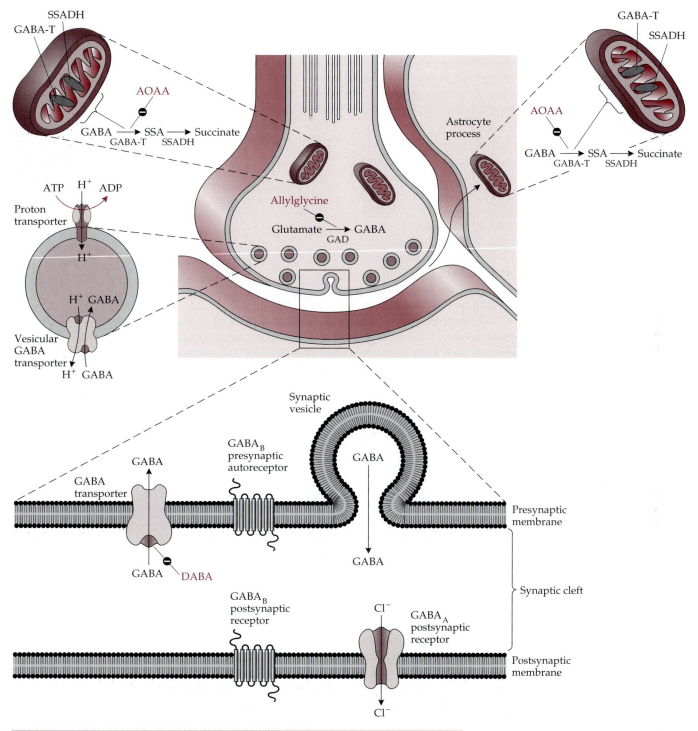

10.22. THE GABAERGIC SYNAPSE, illustrating the processes of γ-aminobutyric acid (GABA) synthesis and metabolism, neuronal and glial GABA uptake, and vesicular GABA uptake and release. Pre- and postsynaptic GABA receptors and sites of action of some GABAergic drugs are also shown. The table lists important GABAergic receptor agonists and antagonists. See the text for details and explanations of the abbreviations.

Receptor subtype	Agonists	Antagonists
GABA$_A$	Muscimol, THIP, isoguvacine	Bicuculline, pentylene-tetrazol, picrotoxin
GABA$_B$	Baclofen, saclofen	Phaclofen, 2-Hydroxysaclofen

tween the apoenzyme and holoenzyme forms (Martin, 1987; Martin and Rimvall, 1993). Of total tissue GAD, at least 50% exists as apoenzyme, thus representing a reserve pool of GABA synthetic capacity. Furthermore, the majority of this apoenzyme consists of GAD_{65}, which is the nerve terminal-enriched isoenzyme. Altering the dynamics of the apoenzyme–holoenzyme cycle is an obvious means of regulating GABA formation, and various studies have indicated that adenosine triphosphate (ATP) stimulates the conversion of holo-GAD to apo-GAD. Pyridoxal phosphate could also play a role in this process; however, intracellular levels of this compound may not vary much unless the individual is suffering from a vitamin B_6 deficiency (as mentioned in Part I, pyridoxal phosphate is a form of vitamin B_6). Finally, the concentration of cytoplasmic GABA might be important because GABA promotes the conversion of holo-GAD to apo-GAD. In a separate mechanism, GABA also acts as a competitive inhibitor at the glutamate binding site on the enzyme. Both of these processes represent ways in which GABA could exert negative feedback on its own synthesis, although the existence of such inhibition remains to be shown in vivo (Martin and Rimvall, 1993).

Drugs That Affect GABA Synthesis and Metabolism

As we have seen in previous chapters, the synthesis of certain neurotransmitters can be increased by administering their biochemical precursors. This strategy, however, has yielded negative results when applied to GABA (Manyam, 1987). Neither glutamate nor glutamine treatment reliably alters brain GABA concentrations. The ineffectiveness of glutamate could theoretically be explained by its poor penetration across the blood–brain barrier. Glutamine, however, is more lipophilic and does enter the brain from the circulation. An alternative explanation is that GAD is, in fact, normally saturated with its substrate, thus rendering changes in glutamate availability inconsequential.

Reductions in brain GABA can be produced by blocking GAD, although the drugs available for this purpose are not entirely specific. In general, drugs that inhibit GAD do so by interfering with the cofactor pyridoxal phosphate. Because many enzymes utilize this cofactor, such drugs may affect a number of neurochemical reactions. Nevertheless, the compounds allylglycine, L-glutamate-γ-hydrazide, and 3-mercaptoproprionic acid are considered somewhat selective for GAD inhibition. Other anti-pyridoxal phosphate compounds that block GABA synthesis include thiosemicarbazide and isoniazide. Drugs such as these that reduce GABA availability invariably cause convulsions when given at sufficient doses. This effect indicates that inhibitory GABAergic synapses must play a critical role in modulating overall brain excitability, a concept that we will return to in the discussion of epilepsy below.

Although GABA levels are not readily affected by precursor administration, they can be elevated by drugs that block GABA-T. Aminooxyacetic acid (AOAA), γ-acetylenic GABA, γ-vinyl GABA (vigabatrin), ethanolamine-O-sulfate (EOS), and 5-amino-1,3-cyclohexadienecarboxylic acid (gabaculine) are all well-known GABA-T inhibitors. Gottesfeld, Kelly, and Renaud (1972) provided direct evidence that AOAA enhances the inhibitory action of GABA by demonstrating that within 1 hour of injecting the drug intraperitoneally in cats, cortical neurons were significantly more sensitive to iontophoretically applied GABA, and the duration of inhibition due to synaptically released GABA was prolonged. As would be expected, GABA-T blockers exhibit sedative and anticonvulsant properties. In fact, vigabatrin has recently been introduced clinically for the treatment of epilepsy (see the section below on GABA and epilepsy).

Storage, Release, and Uptake of GABA

Vesicular Storage and Release

As in the case of glutamate and aspartate, early reports questioned whether GABA was present in sufficiently high concentrations in purified synaptic vesicles to support the hypothesis of vesicular storage and release of this transmitter. More recent studies have demonstrated that GABA can be transported into vesicles by a process that is pharmacologically distinct from the synaptic membrane uptake system (Burger et al., 1991; Maycox, Hell, and Jahn, 1990). GABA can also be released from synaptosomes in a Ca^{2+}-dependent manner (Nicholls, 1989). These observations are fully consistent with the view that GABA (and, by analogy, other amino acid neurotransmitters) is released from synaptic vesicles by an exocytotic process. However, without the type of supportive evidence that is available for the model systems discussed in Chapter 6, we cannot rule out the possibility that vesicles serve merely as a storage depot and that the release compartment is actually the nerve terminal cytoplasm. The widespread utilization of exocytosis for secretion both in the nervous system and in other secretory tissues argues that this mechanism is probably used here as well. Nevertheless, in the following section on synaptic uptake, we shall see that a small amount of GABA may also be released nonexocytotically when the nerve terminal is depolarized.

In vitro experiments with brain slices and synaptosomal preparations have indicated the existence of release-inhibiting GABA autoreceptors (Waldmeier and Baumann, 1990). The pharmacology of these autoreceptors indicates that they are of the $GABA_B$ receptor subtype (see below). However, experiments performed in vivo have yet to confirm the functioning of GABA autoreceptors under normal physiological conditions.

Release of both GABA and glycine is blocked by tetanus toxin, which causes acute convulsions followed by a spastic paralysis. The mechanism of action of this toxin was discussed previously in Chapter 7.

Synaptic Uptake

The removal of GABA from the synaptic cleft involves uptake of the transmitter into both neurons and astrocytes. Kinetic measurements of GABA uptake indicate the existence of separate high- and low-affinity components. Most laboratories have reported K_m values in the range of 5–40 μM for high-affinity transport, and considerably higher values for low-affinity transport (Erecińska, 1987; Seiler and Lajtha, 1987). The high-affinity uptake system clearly must be involved in the removal of synaptically released GABA, given its ability to function at relatively low concentrations of the neurotransmitter. In contrast, the involvement of the low-affinity system is difficult to ascertain without knowing the range of extracellular GABA concentrations reached under physiological conditions.

High-affinity GABA uptake is Na^+-dependent, like that of glutamate and other transmitters. The driving force behind the transport process is the Na^+ electrochemical gradient across the cell membrane. It is interesting to note that when a nerve terminal is depolarized by an action potential, the electrochemical gradient driving GABA transport is briefly reversed, so that GABA *efflux*, rather than influx, is favored. As the transport system can apparently carry GABA in both directions, it is distinctly possible that neural activity may release some GABA by a transporter-mediated, nonexocytotic mechanism (Nicholls, 1989). Once the nerve terminal is repolarized, GABA uptake would be expected to resume.

Several studies have found that chloride (Cl^-) ions also stimulate GABA uptake. Kanner and colleagues purified a high-affinity GABA transporter and found it to be a glycoprotein with an apparent molecular weight of approximately 80,000 (Radian, Bendahan, and Kanner, 1986). A reconstituted system with the purified transporter showed an absolute dependence on both Na^+ and Cl^- ions, which supports the contention that these species are cotransported with GABA. The stoichiometry of transport is most likely 2 Na^+:1 Cl^-:1 GABA (Kanner, 1983).

Within the past few years, researchers have cloned the genes for two different GABA transporters, GAT-A (also called GAT-1; Guastella et al., 1990) and GAT-B (Clark et al., 1992). There are significant regional differences in the expression of these transporters, with high mRNA levels of GAT-A, but not GAT-B, observed in the neocortex, hippocampus, striatum, and cerebellar cortex. At the cellular level, in situ hybridization studies found predominant expression of GAT-B in neurons (Clark et al., 1992), whereas immunohistochemical staining indicated the presence of GAT-A in both GABAergic nerve terminal membranes and glial cell processes (Radian et al., 1990). However, it is difficult at present to rule out the possibility of a glial-specific GABA transporter, distinct from GAT-A but similar enough antigenically to have been recognized by the anti-GAT-A antibody.

GABA uptake can be blocked by a number of drugs, such as 2,4-diaminobutyric acid (DABA), 2-hydroxy-GABA (2-OH-GABA), *cis*-3-aminocyclohexane-carboxylic acid (ACHC), nipecotic acid, and β-alanine. Many of

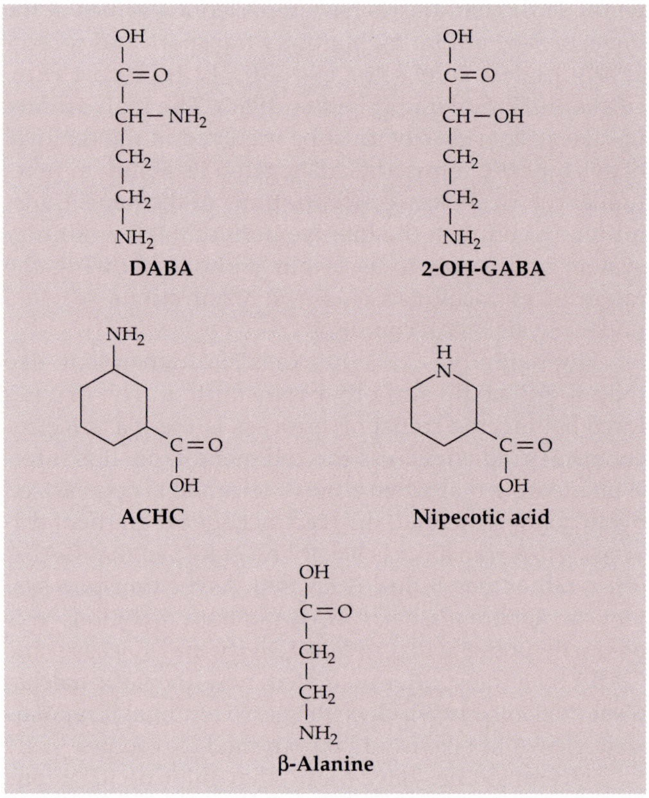

OH
|
C=O
|
CH—NH₂
|
CH₂
|
CH₂
|
NH₂

DABA

OH
|
C=O
|
CH—OH
|
CH₂
|
CH₂
|
NH₂

2-OH-GABA

NH₂

C=O
|
OH

ACHC

H
N

C=O
|
OH

Nipecotic acid

OH
|
C=O
|
CH₂
|
CH₂
|
NH₂

β-Alanine

these compounds differentially inhibit GAT-A versus GAT-B. For example, ACHC inhibits GAT-A much more potently than GAT-B, whereas the opposite selectivity is exhibited by β-alanine (Clark et al., 1992). The ability of β-alanine to block a neuronal GABA transporter was unexpected, given that this compound has usually been considered an inhibitor of glial uptake. Thus, additional research is needed to confirm the identity of the glial GABA transporter(s) and to identify new drugs that differentiate between neuronal and glial transporters.

GABA Distribution

To the neuropharmacologist or neurochemist, the widespread distribution of GABA across living organisms may be surprising. According to Davidson (1976), GAD activity is found in almost every class of organism, including green plants. In fact, glutamate decarboxylation was apparently first reported in squash in a 1937 Japanese botanical journal. One notable location of GABA outside of the brain is the insulin-secreting β-cells of the endocrine pancreas. These cells possess GAD activity, synthesize GABA, and store it in small vesicles (similar if not identical to synaptic vesicles) distinct from the larger insulin-containing secretory granules (Reetz et al., 1991). The function of GABA in this system is to inhibit secretion of the hormone glucagon (which generally functions in an opposite manner to insulin) by the neighboring pancreatic α-cells (Rorsman et al., 1989). Further-

more, pancreatic GAD may play an important role in the development of type 1 (insulin-dependent) diabetes mellitus. This form of diabetes is an autoimmune disorder characterized by an immune system attack (for unknown reasons) on the pancreatic β-cells. Recent findings indicate that the earliest detectable autoantibodies in type 1 diabetes are directed against GAD, suggesting that this protein is somehow involved in initiating the autoimmune reaction (Kaufman and Tobin, 1993). This work opens the way for possible novel immunotherapies to block the progression of the disease.

Anatomy of GABA Pathways

CNS pathways. The investigation of GABA pathways has been greatly facilitated by the finding that, at least in the CNS, GAD is a specific marker for GABAergic neurons. Thus, antibodies raised against GAD can be used in immunohistochemical procedures to map the distribution of GABA-containing cell bodies and nerve terminals. This approach was first adopted by Roberts's group to study GABAergic systems in the cerebellum (McLaughlin et al., 1974; Saito et al., 1974). Readers interested in detailed information concerning the distribution of GAD in the rat brain and spinal cord are referred to the excellent atlas of GAD immunohistochemistry prepared by Mugnaini and Oertel (1985).

The anatomy of GABAergic pathways in the CNS has been elucidated not only by immunostaining for GAD, but also by GABA immunohistochemistry and by histochemical staining for GABA-T. Figure 10.23 presents a comparison of all three methods. Although GABA-T is present in astrocytes as well as in neurons, Nagai and coworkers (1984) developed a method of preferentially staining the nerve cells. Using this procedure, these investigators found that all cell groups in the rat brain known to exhibit GAD immunoreactivity also stained positively for GABA-T. On the other hand, certain cell populations not previously identified as GABAergic also displayed GABA-T histochemical activity. Given that any staining technique has a finite sensitivity, it is possible that neurons positive for GABA-T but not for GAD might still possess the latter enzyme, but at a level below the limit of the immunohistochemical procedure used. Results with GAD, however, should generally be given priority over other approaches, considering that cells expressing this enzyme presumably synthesize GABA and therefore can be considered GABAergic (as long as other criteria, such as physiological release, are ultimately satisfied). In contrast, it is possible that some neurons expressing GABA-T do not use GABA as their transmitter, just as acetylcholinesterase activity can be found in some cells that are not cholinergic.

Using the above-described histochemical procedures as well as GABA uptake and release experiments, inves-

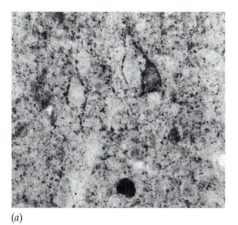
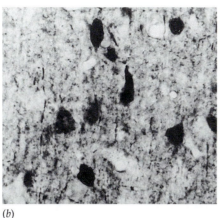
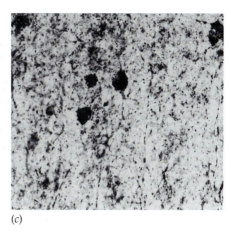

(a)　　　　　　　　　　　　(b)　　　　　　　　　　　　(c)

10.23 HISTOCHEMICAL LOCALIZATION OF GABAERGIC STRUCTURES. The localization of GABAergic cells, fibers, and terminals in the rat cerebral cortex demonstrated by three different methods: (a) GAD immunohistochemistry, (b) GABA immunohistochemistry, and (c) GABA-T histochemistry. Cell body and fiber staining appear to be most intense in *b* and *c*, whereas GABAergic nerve terminals are best stained in *a*. (Photomicrographs by H. Tago and H. Kimura; courtesy of P. L. McGeer.)

tigators have identified many cell groups and pathways in the brain as being GABAergic (Figure 10.24). In fact, it has been estimated that as many as 10% to 40% of the nerve terminals in the cerebral cortex, hippocampus, and substantia nigra may use GABA as their transmitter (Fonnum, 1987). Other brain areas known to be rich in GABA are the cerebellum, striatum, globus pallidus, and olfactory bulbs. The importance of GABA-mediated inhibitory neurotransmission in the cerebellar cortex has been particularly well established. GABA is the transmitter used by the locally projecting Golgi, stellate, and basket cells, as well as by the Purkinje cells that give rise to the output pathways from the cerebellar cortex to the deep cerebellar nuclei and the lateral vestibular nucleus in the brain stem.

GABA also plays a vital role in the spinal cord. GABAergic cells have been found throughout the spinal gray matter except for motor neuron regions (Nieuwenhuys, 1985). Functionally, there is evidence for involvement of this transmitter in both pre- and postsynaptic inhibition, as well as in a phenomenon known as presynaptic facilitation. Some of these effects of GABA in the spinal cord are discussed in greater detail below.

PNS pathways. GABA is found in the PNS as well as in the CNS. There is convincing evidence for the presence of GABAergic neurons in the myenteric plexus of the gut (see Chapter 4), and this transmitter may also be involved in the functional regulation of the heart, reproductive system, gallbladder, and the urinary bladder (Tanaka, 1985). The presence of GABAergic cells and/or terminals associated with these organs is probably responsible for the various peripheral effects produced by systemic administration of GABA-modulating drugs.

GABA$_A$ Receptors

At the majority of vertebrate GABAergic synapses, the effect of the transmitter is to increase Cl$^-$ conductance across the membrane (Harris and Allan, 1985). This leads to a rapid hyperpolarization of the postsynaptic cell, which accounts for GABA's inhibitory action. The Cl$^-$-dependent effects of GABA are generally mediated by a receptor complex called the GABA$_A$ receptor. GABA$_A$ receptors contain a Cl$^-$ channel that is an integral part of the complex, in a manner analogous to the nicotinic cholinergic receptor, the ionotropic glutamate receptors discussed in Part I of this chapter, and the glycine receptor (see Part III below). There is a significant amount of amino acid sequence homology among the receptors in this group, which led to the concept of the ligand-gated channel superfamily (Schofield et al., 1987).

The ionic specificity of the GABA$_A$ receptor-associated channel has been determined by means of permeability experiments. Although the channel effectively excludes cations, it is permeable to a number of anions besides Cl$^-$, including polyatomic species such as formate, bicarbonate, and acetate (reviewed by Kaila, 1994). Nevertheless, Cl$^-$ is the principal anion conducted by this channel under normal conditions. The permeability sequence found for the GABA$_A$ receptor channel is consistent with an effective pore diameter of approximately 0.5 nm (5 Å).

Pharmacology of the GABA$_A$ Receptor Complex

The GABA$_A$ receptor is similar to the glutamate NMDA receptor in its complexity. Besides the obvious binding site for GABA, the receptor complex possesses a number of other sites, as shown schematically in Figure 10.25

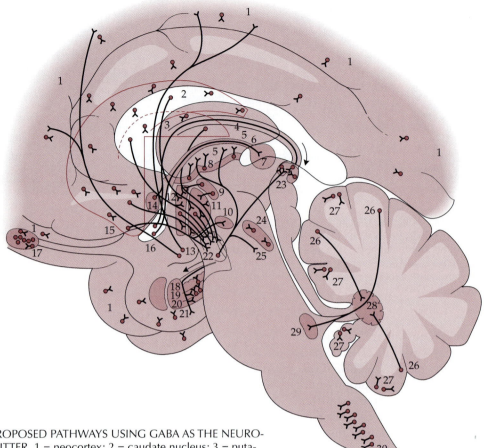

10.24 PROPOSED PATHWAYS USING GABA AS THE NEURO-TRANSMITTER. 1 = neocortex; 2 = caudate nucleus; 3 = putamen; 4 = fornix; 5 = thalamus; 6 = stria medullaris; 7 = medial habenular nucleus; 8 = reticular thalamic nucleus; 9 = subthalamic nucleus; 10 = ventral tegmental area; 11 = medial globus pallidus; 12 = lateral globus pallidus; 13 = GABA-containing cell groups in the caudal hypothalamus; 14 = medial septal nucleus; 15 = nucleus accumbens; 16 = nucleus of the diagonal band; 17 = olfactory bulb; 18 = dentate gyrus; 19 = Ammon's horn of the hippocampal formation; 20 = subiculum; 21 = entorhinal cortex; 22 = substantia nigra; 23 = superior colliculus; 24 = dorsal raphe nucleus; 25 = midbrain tegmentum; 26 = Purkinje cells; 27 = Golgi, stellate, and basket cells; 28 = central cerebellar nucleus; 29 = lateral vestibular nucleus; 30 = spinal cord. (After Nieuwenhuys, 1985.)

(see review by Sieghart, 1995). Several drugs function as agonists or antagonists at the GABA binding site. The classic GABA$_A$ agonist is a drug called muscimol, which in tritiated form can also be used to label the receptor for biochemical or autoradiographic study. Muscimol is a

degradation product of ibotenic acid from the mushroom *Amanita muscaria*. These substances attract flies and make them stuporous; hence the name of the mushroom, "fly" *(muscaria) Amanita*. When given to humans at relatively high doses, muscimol causes an intoxication characterized by hyperthermia (elevated body temperature), pupil dilatation, elevation of mood, difficulties in concentration, panilopia (endless repetitions of visions seen minutes before), anorexia (loss of appetite), ataxia, catalepsy, and hallucinations. These effects, which are similar to those experienced after ingestion of psychedelic drugs such as LSD, may be due to a GABA$_A$ receptor-mediated inhibition of serotonin release. Other agonists at the GABA binding site include the muscimol analog 4,5,6,7-tetrahydroisoxazolo[5,4-c]pyridin-3-ol (THIP) and isoguvacine.

Muscimol

THIP

Isoguvacine

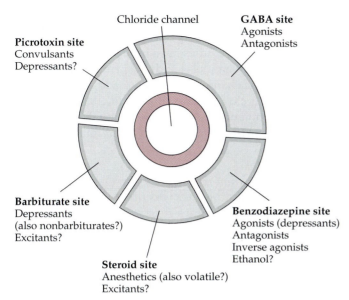

GABA site
Agonists
Antagonists

Picrotoxin site
Convulsants
Depressants?

Chloride channel

Barbiturate site
Depressants
(also nonbarbiturates?)
Excitants?

Steroid site
Anesthetics (also volatile?)
Excitants?

Benzodiazepine site
Agonists (depressants)
Antagonists
Inverse agonists
Ethanol?

10.25 SCHEMATIC MODEL OF THE GABA$_A$ RECEPTOR COMPLEX. As shown in this model, the GABA$_A$ receptor complex exhibits a GABA binding site that mediates the effects of agonists and competitive antagonists, a Cl$^-$ channel, and modulatory binding sites for benzodiazepines, barbiturates, picrotoxin, and anesthetic steroids. (The model is not meant to reflect the subunit structure of the receptor.) (After Olsen et al., 1991.)

The best-known competitive antagonist for the GABA$_A$ receptor is bicuculline. This substance is an alkaloid derived from *Dicentra cucullaria* and related plants. It blocks GABA-induced inhibition of Deiter's cells as well as of many cortical neurons, and has a potent convulsant effect when given systemically. These observations attest to the importance of GABA$_A$ receptors in mediating synaptic inhibition throughout the brain.

Bicuculline

It has been appreciated for a number of years that some GABA antagonists do not interact with the GABA binding site itself, but rather with separate sites on or near the Cl$^-$ channel. Such noncompetitive antagonists block GABA-mediated Cl$^-$ flux, and therefore act as potent convulsants just as the competitive blocker bicuculline does. One well-known drug of this type is the synthetic CNS stimulant pentylenetetrazol (Metrazol). For a time, pentylenetetrazol was widely used in convulsant therapy for psychiatric depression; however, it was

Pentylenetetrazol

eventually supplanted by antidepressant drug treatment (or occasionally electroshock therapy). Nevertheless, pentylenetetrazol is still sometimes used experimentally to induce seizures in animal subjects. A naturally occurring noncompetitive GABA antagonist is picrotoxin (picrotoxin actually contains two compounds, picrotin and the active ingredient picrotoxinin) which is found in the seeds of the East Indian shrub *Animirta cocculus*. The site

Picrotoxinin

on the GABA$_A$ receptor complex that is recognized by pentylenetetrazol, picrotoxin, and related drugs can be specifically labeled either with [^{3}H]α-dihydropicrotoxinin or with the more recently developed compound [^{35}S]-t-butylbicyclophosphorothionate (TBPS). TBPS is one of a group of drugs known as cage convulsants due to their unique molecular structure.

TBPS

Benzodiazepines and the GABA$_A$ Receptor

Sedative–hypnotic (relaxing and sleep-inducing) and anxiolytic (antianxiety) drugs are of great importance to psychopharmacologists both theoretically and clinically. Two classes of these agents, benzodiazepines (BDZs) and barbiturates, will be introduced in this chapter because their primary mechanism of action involves allosteric modulation of the GABA$_A$ receptor complex (Macdonald and Olsen, 1994). Readers are referred to Chapter 16 for a more detailed discussion of sedative–hypnotic and anxiolytic drugs, along with the chemical structures of many of the specific compounds mentioned below.

The BDZs include some of the best-known and most widely prescribed psychotropic drugs, such as diazepam (Valium), chlordiazepoxide (Librium), and flurazepam

(Dalmane). In addition to their sedative, hypnotic, and anxiolytic effects, these compounds also exhibit muscle relaxant and anticonvulsant properties. Some of the first evidence supporting an important role for GABA in the effects of the BDZs was reported over 20 years ago by research groups headed by Costa (Costa, Guidotti, and Mao, 1975) and by Haefely (Haefely et al., 1975). The idea of a BDZ–GABA interaction was subsequently strengthened by experiments using cultured neurons from embryonic chick (Choi, Farb, and Fischbach, 1977) and fetal mouse spinal cords (Macdonald and Barker, 1978a). In both systems, chlordiazepoxide was found to potentiate postsynaptic responses to GABA, but not to glycine. This observation was important because, as we shall discuss below, glycine is an important inhibitory transmitter in the spinal cord and had been thought by some investigators to mediate BDZ actions. Chlordiazepoxide exerted little, if any, effect of its own when applied in the absence of GABA. Moreover, although BDZ administration enhanced the size of the postsynaptic potential at submaximum doses of GABA, the peak response to the transmitter was unaffected. In general, the potentiating effects of BDZs on GABA-mediated functions are apparent only when GABAergic transmission is not maximally activated. As shown in Figure 10.26, this pattern can be represented by a shift of the agonist dose–response curve to the left without a change in the maximum response.

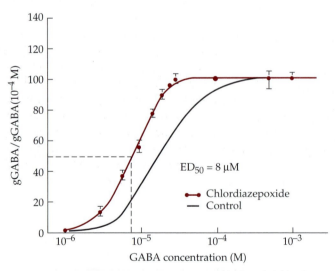

10.26 BENZODIAZEPINE-INDUCED SHIFT IN THE GABA DOSE–RESPONSE CURVE. GABA-stimulated Cl⁻ conductance was measured in cultured chick spinal cord neurons in the presence or absence of the BDZ chlordiazepoxide. Because the data were obtained in separate studies, the control dose–response curve was normalized to the same maximum as the curve obtained in the presence of chlordiazepoxide for comparative purposes. Under these conditions, it can be seen that BDZs shift the GABA dose–response curve to the left, but do not affect the maximum responsiveness. Bars represent *SEM*. (After Farrant, Gibbs, and Farb, 1990.)

The effects of BDZs are mediated by increased GABA-stimulated current flow across the cell membrane. Patch-clamp studies have indicated that activated GABA$_A$ receptor channels conduct current in a bursting pattern, with the channel cycling back and forth between an open and a closed state (Bormann, 1988; Mathers, 1987). The action of BDZs on these channels is complex, but may primarily involve an increased rate of channel opening.

The BDZ binding site on the GABA$_A$ receptor.   The discovery of BDZ binding sites was first reported independently by Squires and Braestrup (Braestrup and Squires, 1977; Squires and Braestrup, 1977) and by Möhler and Okada (1977a). Using rat brain membranes, these researchers found high-affinity binding sites for [³H]diazepam that were saturable, stereospecific, and unevenly distributed across different brain regions. The highest levels of binding were found in the cerebral cortex and hypothalamus, slightly lower levels in the cerebellum, midbrain, and hippocampus, and the lowest levels in the striatum and pons–medulla. Subcellular fractionation showed that the greatest density of binding sites was in the synaptosomal fraction, which would be expected of a neurotransmitter-related receptor. Most importantly in terms of establishing these binding sites as bona fide receptors, there was a very high positive correlation (approximately .9) between the ability of different BDZs to displace [³H]diazepam and their pharmacological potency in the cat muscle relaxant test (a test predictive of anxiolytic and anticonvulsant activity) (Figure 10.27). Such a relationship between binding affinity and behavioral or physiological activity is critical for verifying that the binding site under investigation is actually responsible for mediating the relevant drug actions. Other studies have demonstrated a high density of BDZ receptors (sometimes abbreviated BZ or ω receptors)* in human cortical tissue, as well as a significant positive correlation between BDZ binding affinities and clinical potency as indicated by recommended daily dosages (Braestrup, Albrechtsen, and Squires, 1977). These findings further establish the involvement of BZ receptors in the clinical effects of these drugs.

A number of binding studies have shown that the presence of a GABA$_A$ agonist in the incubation medium increases the apparent affinity of the BZ receptor for ligands such as [³H]diazepam (Karobath and Sperk, 1979; Tallman, Thomas, and Gallagher, 1978). This effect can be produced by GABA itself as well as by the more selective drug muscimol, and is blocked by the competitive GABA$_A$ antagonist bicuculline. The modulation of BZ receptors by GABA suggested that there might be some type of coupling between their respective binding sites

---

*Although "benzodiazepine" is usually abbreviated "BDZ," "BZ" is often used in reference to receptors, and we use it here in that regard.

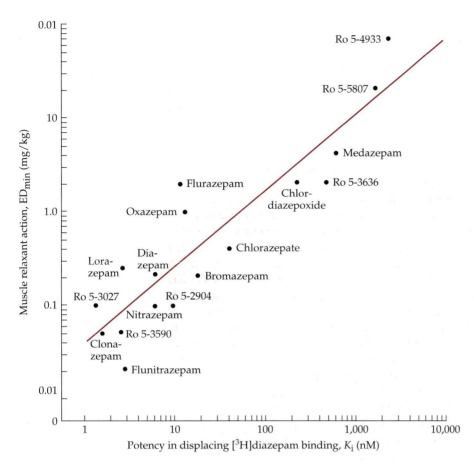

10.27 CORRELATION BETWEEN RECEPTOR AFFINITY AND BEHAVIORAL POTENCY AMONG VARIOUS BENZODIAZEPINES. Benzodiazepines were tested for their potency (K_i) in displacing [^{3}H]diazepam from specific BDZ binding sites on rat cerebral cortical membranes. The resulting values were highly correlated (r = .905, p < .0001) with the behavioral potency of the same drugs (ED$_{min}$) in the cat muscle relaxant test. (After Möhler and Okada, 1977a.)

in the membrane. This notion was further supported by localization studies showing that the distribution of BZ receptors, determined either immunohistochemically or autoradiographically, corresponds closely to the distribution of GABA$_A$ receptors as determined by [^{3}H]muscimol autoradiography (Schoch et al., 1985) (Figure 10.28). The structural relationship between BDZ and GABA binding sites in the GABA$_A$ receptor complex is still under investigation, as we shall see below.

Pharmacology of benzodiazepine receptors. Students of pharmacology are routinely introduced to the concepts of receptor agonists and antagonists. As discussed previously in this book, agonists stimulate the "normal" function of the receptor when they bind (such compounds are said to exhibit "positive efficacy" at that receptor). Antagonists, on the other hand, are compounds that may inhibit the influence of agonists by competing for the agonist binding site, but have no effect in the absence of an agonist (this is termed "zero efficacy"). A third important type of receptor–ligand interaction has also been discovered, namely, inverse agonism. As mentioned in Chapter 9, an inverse agonist is a compound that interacts with the receptor to produce functional effects opposite to those produced by traditional agonists (using the previous terminology, this is called "negative efficacy").

The first instance of inverse agonism to be discovered for a ligand-gated channel involved the BZ receptor on the GABA$_A$ receptor complex (since that time, the same concept has also been applied to G protein–coupled receptors; see Milligan, Bond, and Lee, 1995 and also Chapter 9). The classic BDZs diazepam and chlordiazepoxide represent typical drugs with positive efficacy, displaying an anxiolytic, sedative–hypnotic, muscle relaxant, and anticonvulsant profile. Antagonists have likewise been found that are able to block these effects, but have little efficacy of their own. One such drug is the imidazodiazepine Ro 15-1788 (flumazenil), a compound that has been used clinically to reverse the effects of BDZ overdose and to hasten recovery from anesthetic treatments involving the use of BDZs (Haefely, 1989). The first inverse agonists to be discovered were methyl-β-carboline-3-carboxylate (β-CCM) and methyl-6,7-dimethoxy-4-ethyl-β-carboline-3-carboxylate (DMCM), which produced convulsant and anxiogenic (anxiety-promoting) effects when given alone (Braestrup et al., 1984; Haefely, 1989). The behavioral properties of β-CCM and DMCM are blocked by Ro 15-1788, indicating that these compounds indeed interact with BZ receptors. Researchers believe that normal and inverse BDZ agonists are able to induce their disparate effects by allosterically modulating the GABA$_A$ receptor complex in

10.28 COLOCALIZATION OF BENZODIAZEPINE AND GABA$_A$ RECEPTORS IN RAT AND HUMAN BRAIN. Benzodiazepine receptor localization was determined by means of immunohistochemistry with the monoclonal antibody (mAb) bd-17 (*a* and *d*) or autoradiography with [^{3}H]Ro 15-1788 (*b* and *e*). The distribution of BDZ receptors closely parallels that of GABA$_A$ receptors mapped by [^{3}H]muscimol autoradiography (panels *c* and *f*). *a–c* show parasagittal sections through the rat brain; *d–f* show coronal sections through the human hippocampus. Scale bar = 2 mm. (After Schoch et al., 1985; courtesy of Grayson Richards.)

the opposite manner. According to this scheme, normal agonists positively modulate the GABA$_A$ receptor complex and thus potentiate GABA action, whereas inverse agonists negatively modulate the receptor and therefore lead to heightened anxiety and brain excitability (much like competitive GABA antagonists).

Although the results of early studies on the binding of radioactively labeled BDZs ([^{3}H]diazepam or [^{3}H]flunitrazepam) to brain cell membranes were consistent with a homogenous population of receptors, subsequent research with a group of drugs known as triazolopyridazines (especially the prototypical compound CL 218,872) suggested the existence of at least two BZ receptor subtypes (BZ$_1$ and BZ$_2$: Lippa, Meyerson, and Beer, 1982). According to the proposed model, BZ$_1$ receptors had a high affinity for both BDZs and triazolopyri-

dazines, and were thought to be most important in the anxiolytic effects of BDZs. BZ$_2$ receptors had a high affinity for BDZs, but not for triazolopyridazines, and were believed to be more involved in the sedative–hypnotic effects of BDZs. Although it had much heuristic value, this hypothesis unfortunately has not held up in the light of subsequent research. Moreover, it is now clear that the BZ$_2$ receptor subtype is pharmacologically heterogeneous and is associated structurally with several different isoforms of one of the GABA$_A$ receptor subunits (see below; Doble and Martin, 1992; Sanger et al., 1994).

There is an additional type of BDZ binding site, the so-called "peripheral-type" BZ receptor. This binding site was so named because it was initially discovered in the kidney and was later found to be present in several other peripheral tissues such as the adrenal glands and testes (Anholt, 1986). Peripheral-type BZ receptors have also been identified in the brain, where they are found particularly in glial cells. These sites have a structure different from that of BZ_1 and BZ_2 receptors, and they are not associated with the $GABA_A$ receptor complex (Parola, Yamamura, and Laird, 1993). Furthermore, although BDZs bind to peripheral-type BZ receptors with varying affinities, the pharmacological profile of these receptors differs from that of the central receptors. On the other hand, several nonBDZ compounds, such as the isoquinoline PK 11195, selectively bind to peripheral-type BZ receptors.

PK 11195

Peripheral-type BZ receptors are located subcellularly on the outer membranes of mitochondria, rather than on the cell membrane as in the case of BZ_1 and BZ_2 receptors. While their function is not known for all cell types, there is strong evidence that in steroid hormone-producing organs such as the ovaries, testes, and adrenal cortex, mitochondrial BZ receptors are involved in the transport of cholesterol (the precursor for steroid biosynthesis) from the outer to the inner mitochondrial membrane (Papadopoulos, 1993). This role is an important one because cholesterol transport is the rate-limiting step in steroid formation. Mitochondrial BZ receptors in the brain may be involved in the synthesis of "neurosteroids" (see below) and may further participate in various behavioral and physiological processes (Gavish et al., 1992; Papadopoulos, 1993).

In concluding this discussion, it is important to mention the question of the endogenous ligand(s) for both the GABA receptor–coupled and mitochondrial BZ receptors. In contrast to the GABA recognition site on the $GABA_A$ receptor complex (for which the endogenous ligand is obviously GABA), the nature of the endogenous ligand has not been resolved for either type of BZ receptor. This question is taken up later in Chapter 16.

Barbiturates and the $GABA_A$ Receptor

Like BDZs, barbiturate drugs such as phenobarbital and pentobarbital exert sedative–hypnotic, anxiolytic, and anticonvulsant actions in animals and humans (see Chapter 16). Electrophysiologically, the effects of these anesthetic barbiturates may be related to a depression of excitatory synaptic transmission at various sites in the

CNS (Willow and Johnston, 1983). At the molecular level, given the similarity in pharmacological profile between the barbiturates and the BDZs, it is not surprising that the barbiturates also powerfully potentiate GABAergic transmission via $GABA_A$ receptors. At low to moderate doses, barbiturates enhance postsynaptic responses to GABA, mainly by increasing the mean open time of $GABA_A$ receptor-coupled Cl^- channels (Macdonald et al., 1988). At high doses, barbiturates can act as GABA mimetics and directly open those channels.

It is clear from a number of studies that barbiturates influence $GABA_A$ receptor function by interacting with a distinct site on the receptor complex (Macdonald and Olsen, 1994). Occupation of this site by barbiturates and certain other CNS depressants allosterically enhances ligand binding to the GABA and BDZ recognition sites, and inhibits binding at the picrotoxin site. When the ability of different barbiturates to enhance [^{3}H]diazepam binding was related to their anesthetic potency, a correlation coefficient of over 0.95 was obtained (Leeb-Lundberg, Snowman, and Olsen, 1980). This finding lends important support to the notion that the barbiturate-related site on the $GABA_A$ receptor complex is a valid barbiturate receptor, and underscores the relevance of GABAergic regulation for the physiological and behavioral effects of these drugs. On the other hand, little attention has yet been directed to the normal role of this site (in the absence of drug treatment) and what its endogenous ligand(s) might be.

Steroid Hormones and the $GABA_A$ Receptor

Steroids are lipophilic hormones that are synthesized from cholesterol in the gonads and the adrenal cortex. The classic receptors for these compounds are located intracellularly, in the nuclear or cytoplasmic compartment. Cells containing such receptors are found in many organs, including the brain, where steroid-sensitive neurons are heavily concentrated in discrete regions such as the hypothalamus/preoptic area (receptors for estrogens and androgens) and the hippocampus (receptors for adrenocortical steroids) (Warembourg, 1985). Steroid hormones are best known for their ability to regulate the transcription of specific genes in target cell populations. These transcriptional effects are mediated by the above-mentioned intracellular receptors and occur over periods of minutes to hours.

The view that the neural action of steroids is limited to a slow transcriptional mechanism has been repeatedly challenged by electrophysiological studies showing that many of these compounds rapidly alter neuronal firing when applied to cells iontophoretically. Such electrophysiological effects seem to be more compatible with a membrane site of action than with an intracellular effect involving delayed changes in gene expression. Furthermore, certain steroids and steroid metabolites have been shown to act as sedative–hypnotic and anesthetic agents when administered systemically. Since the early 1980s, several research groups have accumulated evidence that these compounds exert modulatory effects on the GABA$_A$ receptor complex (reviewed by Lambert et al., 1995; Paul and Purdy, 1992). Of particular interest are the reduced progesterone metabolite 3α-hydroxy-5α-pregnan-20-one (3α-hydroxy-dihydroprogesterone, or 3α-OH-DHP) and the reduced deoxycorticosterone metabolite 3α,21-dihydroxy-5α-pregnan-20-one (allo-tetrahydrodeoxycorticosterone, or THDOC). Both com-

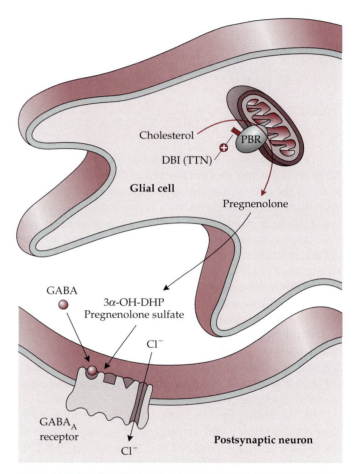

pounds enhanced the binding of [^{3}H]BDZs to the BZ site on the receptor, but inhibited binding of [^{35}S]TBPS to the convulsant site. They also potentiated GABA synaptic action on hippocampal and spinal cord neurons, and they stimulated Cl$^-$ uptake into synaptosomes and into cells transfected with GABA$_A$ receptor subunits. This pattern of effects is remarkably similar to the pharmacological profile of barbiturates. Other steroids, such as the sulfate esters of pregnenolone and dehydroepiandrosterone, inhibit rather than facilitate GABA$_A$ receptor function, thereby exerting excitatory (proconvulsant) rather than sedative effects in animals (Paul and Purdy, 1992). Together, these results indicate that certain steroids and steroid metabolites may be endogenous modulators of the GABA$_A$ receptor complex.

Swim stress in rats was reported to increase brain concentrations of 3α-OH-DHP and THDOC to the range of 10–30 nM, which is sufficient to enhance GABA$_A$ receptor–mediated functioning (Purdy et al., 1991). Surgical removal of steroid-synthesizing endocrine glands diminished, but did not eliminate, the presence of 3α-OH-DHP in the brain, whereas THDOC could no longer be detected. This finding is consistent with biochemical evidence that glial cells can synthesize 3α-OH-DHP de novo from cholesterol, whereas brain THDOC comes either directly from the plasma or is synthesized via reduction of blood-borne deoxycorticosterone (Paul and Purdy, 1992; Robel and Baulieu, 1994).

The term "neurosteroids" has been used to denote neuroactive steroidal substances formed in the brain (Baulieu, 1981). The current model for the role of glial-derived neurosteroids in modulating neuronal GABA$_A$

receptors is shown in Figure 10.29. The mitochondrial BZ receptors described above are well positioned to stimulate neurosteroid synthesis by glial cells. Possible endogenous ligands for those receptors are a family of peptides that includes diazepam binding inhibitor (DBI) and a smaller fragment of DBI (DBI$_{17-50}$) called triakontatetraneuropeptide (TTN) (see Chapter 16).

Ethanol and the GABA$_A$ Receptor

Although ethanol is covered extensively in Chapter 15, it will be discussed briefly here in terms of its effects on amino acid neurotransmitter receptors. Early theorizing on the mechanism of ethanol's sedative–hypnotic effects focused on the ability of this compound to diffuse non-

10.29 HYPOTHESIZED ROLE OF PERIPHERAL-TYPE BENZODI-AZEPINE RECEPTORS AND NEUROSTEROIDS IN MODULATING THE GABA$_A$ RECEPTOR. Peripheral-type BDZ receptors (PBR) located in the mitochondria of glial cells are thought to be activated by one or more endogenous ligands, which may include diazepam binding inhibitor (DBI) or a smaller fragment of DBI known as triakontatetraneuropeptide (TTN). Activation of PBR enhances the conversion of cholesterol to pregnenolone, which then serves as a precursor for the synthesis of neurosteroids such as 3α-hydroxy-dihydroprogesterone (3α-OH-DHP) and pregnenolone sulfate. When released from the glial cells, neurosteroids can positively or negatively modulate the activity of GABA$_A$ receptor–coupled Cl$^-$ channels. (After Papadopoulos, 1993.)

specifically into nerve cell membranes, thereby disordering the lipid bilayer and increasing membrane fluidity. However, there is now considerable evidence that ethanol exerts rather selective effects on a variety of ligand-gated channels, including the GABA$_A$, NMDA, glycine, nicotinic, and 5-HT$_3$ receptors (see Criswell et al., 1993).

In the case of the GABA$_A$ receptor, ethanol has been reported to enhance receptor-activated Cl$^-$ currents and thus synaptic inhibition (Mehta and Ticku, 1988; Palmer and Hoffer, 1990). Interestingly, there are important regional differences in the mechanisms of ethanol potentiation of GABA$_A$ receptor–mediated responses, as well as the sensitivity to such potentiation. For example, ethanol was found to enhance cellular responses to GABA application in the neocortex, medial septum, inferior colliculus, substantia nigra pars reticulata, ventral pallidum, diagonal band of Broca, cerebellum, and spinal cord, but not in the hippocampus or ventral tegmental area (Criswell et al., 1993; Palmer and Hoffer, 1990; Soldo, Proctor, and Dunwiddie, 1994). Such regional differences in ethanol responsivity have been attributed to structural variations in the GABA$_A$ receptor complex that appear to influence sensitivity to the drug (see next section).

The functional importance of ethanol's action on GABAergic transmission was tested in a novel way by the use of genetically unique strains of mice. Long-sleep (LS) and short-sleep (SS) mice differ markedly in their susceptibility to the sedative–hypnotic effects of ethanol, and this disparity is thought to be related to strain differences in the GABA$_A$ receptor complex. Wafford et al. (1990) extracted mRNA from the brains of LS and SS mice and expressed the mRNA in *Xenopus* oocytes. When the influence of ethanol on GABA$_A$ receptor responses was then tested in this system, ethanol potentiated the effect of GABA application on LS mRNA-injected oocytes; however, ethanol actually antagonized GABA responses in oocytes expressing receptors from SS mice. In contrast, ethanol inhibition of NMDA-mediated excitatory responses was comparable in the two groups. Thus, differences in GABA$_A$ receptor sensitivity to ethanol may play an important role in the behavioral differences between LS and SS mice.

Structure of the GABA$_A$ Receptor Complex

In recent years, the application of sophisticated biochemical and molecular biological techniques has led to rapid progress in the structural analysis of the GABA$_A$ receptor complex (reviewed by Lüddens, Korpi, and Seeburg, 1995; Macdonald and Olsen, 1994). Four different families of receptor subunits have been identified, most with more than one isoform. These subunits are designated α (6 isoforms), β (4 isoforms), γ (3 isoforms), and δ (1 isoform). Several subunits, including the γ2 subunit also exhibit alternative mRNA splicing. In the latter case, there are two splice variants that differ with respect to the presence (γ2L) or absence (γ2S) of 24 nucleotides coding

for eight amino acids located in the intracellular loop between the third and fourth transmembrane domains (Whiting, McKernan, and Iversen, 1990).

Purified GABA$_A$ receptors exhibit a five-fold symmetry, suggesting a pentameric structure analogous to that of the nicotinic cholinergic receptor (Nayeem et al., 1994). The receptor complex formed from the five subunits gives rise to the receptor-associated Cl$^-$ channel, and also possesses the various modulatory binding sites described above. The receptor protein is glycosylated and has an apparent molecular weight of about 275 kDa. Figure 10.30 depicts a hypothetical model of the receptor in which the second membrane-spanning domains of each subunit form the channel wall (as in the nicotinic receptor). GABA$_A$ receptors exhibit substantial heterogeneity in terms of ion channel properties and modulation by drugs. For example, some receptors do not possess the BZ binding site and thus are not responsive to BDZs (Gallager and Tallman, 1990), whereas others lack sensitivity to ethanol (Criswell et al., 1993). As described below, these variations in the effectiveness of modulatory compounds are thought to be related to differences in the subunit composition of the receptor.

Early studies found that GABA-sensitive ion channels could be formed in cells expressing only one type of receptor subunit (α, β, or γ), and that the responses of such homomeric receptors were blocked by bicuculline or picrotoxin and were potentiated by barbiturates (Blair et al., 1988; Pritchett et al., 1988; Shivers et al., 1989). Nevertheless, subsequent research has indicated that most (if not all) native receptors are heteromeric complexes. Based on current evidence, the most likely stoichiometry is 2 α subunits, 1 β subunit, and 2 γ subunits, although some receptors seem to contain 1 or 2 δ subunits in place of either or both of the γ subunits (Barnard, 1995). There is considerable regional heterogeneity in subunit expression (Persohn, Malherbe, and Richards, 1992; Wisden et al., 1992), suggesting variation in receptor subunit composition among different cell types.

Barnard (1995) has shown that approximately 850 subunit combinations are possible in theory (given the multiple isoforms), but the number of different GABA$_A$ receptors constructed naturally is probably more limited. One limiting factor in receptor heterogeneity may be the preferential assembly of particular subunit combinations. For example, Angelotti and Macdonald (1993) transfected mouse L929 fibroblast cells with cDNAs for either the α1 and β1 subunits together or γ2S along with α1 and β1. Although functional α1β1-containing GABA$_A$ receptors could be formed in the absence of γ2S, assembly of α1β1γ2S receptors was strongly preferred when all three subunits were coexpressed.

There is no definitive information yet available on the subunit composition of native GABA$_A$ receptors. Subunit colocalization studies, however, have provided data regarding the relative abundance of different sub-

(a)

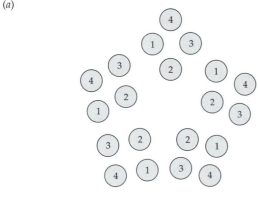

(b)

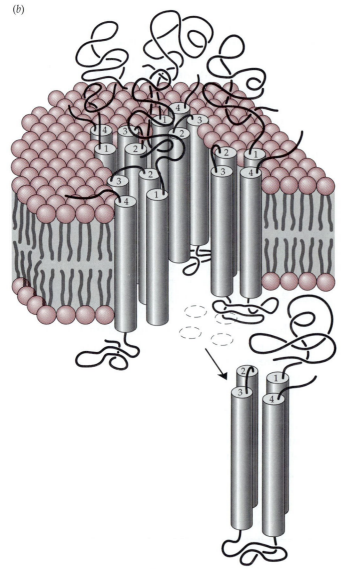

10.30 THE GABA_A RECEPTOR COMPLEX is believed to be composed of five subunits, each with four putative transmembrane domains (cylinders numbered 1–4). (a) A plan view from above, which shows that the second membrane-spanning regions of each subunit are thought to form the wall of the Cl⁻ channel (in a pattern analogous to the structure of the nicotinic cholinergic receptor). (b) The positions of the five subunits in the membrane, with one subunit displaced for greater clarity. (After Macdonald and Olsen, 1994.)

unit combinations as well as their regional and (in some cases) cellular distribution (McKernan and Whiting, 1996; Table 10.2). The most common subunit combination in the rat brain is α1β2γ2. If the stoichiometry proposed earlier is correct, then the receptors formed from these subunits consist of α1 (2), β2 (1), and γ2 (2). Other combinations are less abundant and more restricted in their distribution. It should be noted that the γ1 subunit is present in only a small minority of the native GABA_A receptors. Another important point concerns the localization of the α6 subunit, which has been found only in cerebellar granule cells (Lüddens et al., 1990).

The sensitivity of GABA_A receptors to BDZs and related compounds has been linked to particular subunits. High-affinity BDZ binding and functional sensitivity to BDZs requires the presence of a γ subunit (particularly γ2) along with α and β subunits (Pritchett et al., 1989). Moreover, Figure 10.31 shows that BZ receptor pharmacology depends mainly on the combination of α and γ subunits expressed in the cell. Coexpression of α4 or α6 subunits with the γ2 subunit in certain thalamic neurons (α4) or cerebellar granule cells (α6) leads to the formation of novel BZ receptors that exhibit a high affinity for the partial inverse agonist Ro 15-4513, but a relatively low affinity for diazepam and other typical BZ agonists (Barnard, 1995; Lüddens, Korpi, and Seeburg, 1995). Standard diazepam-sensitive BZ receptors, which contain α1, α2, α3, or α5 subunits can be subdivided based on their sensitivity to the sedative–hypnotic imidazopyridine zolpidem (Ambien) and their affinity for CL 218,872. Most of these receptors are zolpidem-sensitive (see Figure 10.31) and correspond to the pharmacologically defined BZ_1 and BZ_2 subtypes. The remaining subtypes exhibit atypical pharmacological characteristics and a limited distribution in the brain.

The localization of ethanol-sensitive GABA_A receptors has been reported to correlate closely with brain regions showing high zolpidem binding (Criswell et al., 1993). Those areas of the brain (see the section on ethanol above) were further found to preferentially express α1, β2, and γ2 subunits, suggesting that receptor complexes formed from this combination exhibit both BZ_1 binding sites and ethanol sensitivity. Additional information has been presented by Wafford et al. (1991), who found that ethanol enhancement of GABA_A receptor function occurred in the presence of the γ2L, but not the γ2S, splice variant.

Smith and Olsen (1995) recently reviewed the results of site-directed mutagenesis and affinity labeling studies that have begun to indicate which regions of the GABA_A receptor complex normally form the GABA and BDZ binding sites. In heteromeric receptors expressing α1, β2, and γ2 subunits, it appears that amino acid residues from the β2 and α1 subunits are necessary for normal GABA activation of the receptor (Figure 10.32). In contrast, BDZ modulation of the receptor seems to involve

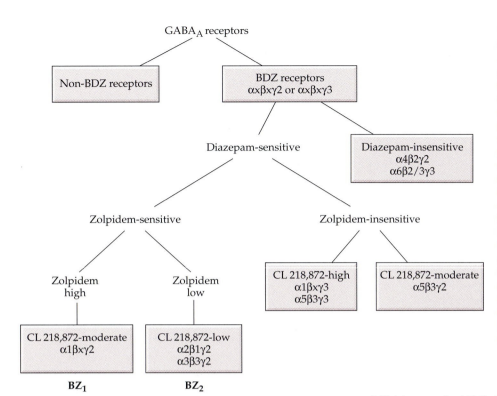

10.31 PROPOSED SUBUNIT COM-POSITION OF GABA$_A$–BENZODI-AZEPINE RECEPTOR SUBTYPES. Ben-zodiazepine recognition sites are only found in GABA$_A$ receptor complexes containing γ2 or γ3 subunits along with α and β. A few classes of neurons ex-press novel diazepam-insensitive BDZ receptors that are associated with the presence of α4 or α6 subunits. Other α subunits give rise to the more typical diazepam-sensitive BDZ receptors, al-though these can be subdivided based on their sensitivity to the nonBDZ seda-tive–hypnotic compound zolpidem. Pharmacologically defined BZ$_1$ recep-tors, which exhibit a high sensitivity to zolpidem and moderate affinity for the triazolopyridazine CL 218,872, contain a combination of α1, β, and γ2 sub-units. BZ$_2$ receptors contain an α2 or α3 subunit and are characterized by a lower sensitivity to zolpidem and a low affinity for CL 218,872. (After Lüddens, Korpi, and Seeburg, 1995).

regions of the γ2 and α1 subunits, which is consistent with the findings mentioned above.

Regulation of GABA$_A$ Receptors

The β subunit of the GABA$_A$ receptor possesses sites for phosphorylation by cAMP-dependent protein kinase and by protein kinase C (PKC) (Browning et al., 1993). The γ2L subunit also has a phosphorylation site for PKC

(Whiting et al., 1990). In all cases, subunit phosphoryla-tion is associated with a reduction in the amplitude of receptor-activated currents (Krishek et al., 1994; Moss et al., 1992). Second messenger–mediated phosphorylation may therefore play an important role in regulating GABA$_A$ receptor functioning in vivo. Moreover, Wafford and coworkers (1991) have hypothesized that the pres-ence of the PKC phosphorylation site in the γ2L, but not the γ2S, splice variant may somehow be related to the ethanol sensitivity of receptors containing γ2L.

Table 10.2	Colocalization of GABA$_A$ Receptor Subunits in the Rat Brain	
Subunit combination	Relative abundance (%)	Location[a]
α1β2γ2	43	Present in most brain areas; specific cell types include hippocampal and cortical interneu-rons, and cerebellar Purkinje cells
α2β2/3γ2	18	Hippocampal pyramidal cells and spinal cord motor neurons
α3βxγ2/γ3	17	Cholinergic and monoaminergic neurons
α2βxγ1	8	Limbic system structures and Bergmann glia of the cerebellum
α5β3γ2/γ3	4	Mainly found in hippocampal pyramidal cells
α6βγ2	2	Cerebellar granule cells
α6βδ	2	Cerebellar granule cells
α4βδ	3	Thalamus and hippocampal dentate gyrus
Other minor subtypes	3	Varied distribution

[a]Subunit location reflects current data and should not be considered comprehensive. Other minor subtypes include α1α6βγ2, α1α3βγ2, α2α3βγ2, and α5βγ2δ.
Source: After McKernan and Whiting, 1996.

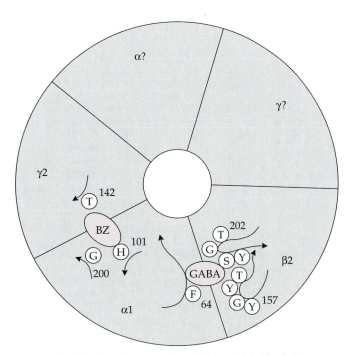

10.32 AMINO ACID RESIDUES IMPLICATED IN GABA AND BENZODIAZEPINE BINDING TO THE GABA_A RECEPTOR. The amino acid residues shown are believed to participate in GABA and BDZ binding based on site-directed mutagenesis and affinity labeling experiments. Amino acids are numbered according to their sequence position, and the arrows indicate the direction of each part of the polypeptide chain of a given subunit. (See Table 3.1 for a key to the one-letter amino acid abbreviations.) This information was obtained from studies on cells coexpressing α1, β2, and γ2 subunits; other subunits may not yield identical results. The additional α and γ subunits (with question marks) are shown for illustrative purposes only, as the stoichiometry of native GABA_A receptors is still under investigation. (After Smith and Olsen, 1995.)

GABA_B Receptors

Until the early 1980s, it was generally believed that all GABA responses in the nervous system were mediated by a single type of receptor. However, Bowery and colleagues discovered that GABA can presynaptically inhibit the release of other neurotransmitters in a manner that is not blocked by bicuculline (see Bowery, 1989, for review). Furthermore, this effect is mimicked by the drug (–)β-p-chlorophenyl GABA (baclofen), which has little potency at "classic" GABA receptor sites. Upon demonstrating the presence of bicuculline-insensitive binding sites for labeled baclofen in brain tissue, Hill and Bowery (1981) called these sites GABA_B receptors, in contrast to the previously identified bicuculline-sensitive sites that were termed GABA_A receptors. Autoradiographic mapping has revealed a different distribution of the two receptor types in the brain, with the heaviest concentrations of GABA_B receptors in the molecular layer of the cerebellum, layers 1–3 of the cerebral cortex, the superior colliculus, and the interpeduncular nucleus (Chu et al., 1990; Gehlert, Yamamura, and Wamsley, 1985). At the cellular level, GABA_B receptors have been found both pre- and postsynaptically.

Pharmacology of GABA_B Receptors

A number of drugs have been identified that are selective agonists of the GABA_B receptor. These drugs include the previously mentioned baclofen, saclofen, and 3-aminopropyl phosphinic acid (3-APPA). Under the trade name Lioresal, baclofen has been used for a number of years as a muscle relaxant and antispastic agent (see Wojcik and Holopainen, 1992). The first reported

Baclofen   **Saclofen**

3-APPA

GABA_B antagonists were phaclofen and 2-hydroxysaclofen; however, these compounds exhibited few central effects in vivo because of poor penetration across the blood–brain barrier. Olpe and colleagues (1990) subsequently introduced CGP 35348, a 3-aminopropyl-phosphinic acid derivative that antagonized electrophysiological responses to iontophoretically applied baclofen when given systemically. This prototype compound has now given rise to an entire family of centrally active GABA_B receptor blockers (see Bittiger et al., 1993).

Phaclofen   **2-Hydroxysaclofen**

CGP 35348

GABA_B Receptor Mechanisms

As of this writing, the GABA_B receptor has not yet been cloned. However, all available evidence indicates that the receptor functions through the activation of one or more G proteins, and therefore belongs to the G protein–coupled receptor superfamily. Additional pharmacological studies suggest the existence of multiple receptor subtypes. Although all GABA_B receptors respond to 3-APPA, some have been found to be relatively insensitive to baclofen (Bonanno and Raiteri, 1993). There is also variation in sensitivity to the antagonists phaclofen and CGP 35348. The molecular basis of such heterogeneity awaits the cloning of the GABA_B receptor gene(s).

GABA_B receptors are known to activate at least four different effector mechanisms: (1) inhibition of adenylyl cyclase, (2) stimulation of phospholipase A_2 (which potentiates cAMP formation by other receptor systems), (3) increased K^+ membrane conductance (i.e., activation of a K^+ channel), and (4) inhibition of a voltage-dependent membrane Ca^{2+} conductance (Misgeld, Bijak, and Jarolimek, 1995; Wojcik and Holopainen, 1992). All of these responses appear to be mediated through coupling to pertussis toxin–sensitive G protein(s). Potassium channel activation by GABA_B receptors has been found to underlie the GABA-induced slow hyperpolarization of CA1 and CA3 hippocampal pyramidal neurons, thalamocortical cells, cells of the dorsal raphe nucleus, and dorsal horn spinal cord neurons. Through a complicated mechanism, GABA_B receptor–mediated IPSPs help to prime thalamocortical neurons to engage in burst firing, which is thought to be important in the oscillatory activity of these cells during slow-wave sleep (Crunelli and Leresche, 1991).

As mentioned earlier, some GABA_B receptors appear to be located presynaptically. Activation of these receptors inhibits the release of neurotransmitters at a number of central and peripheral synapses, thereby presynaptically reducing the amplitude of stimulus-evoked postsynaptic potentials in various areas such as the hippocampus (Bowery, 1989; Misgeld, Bijak, and Jarolimek, 1995; Nicoll, Malenka, and Kauer, 1990). GABA_B receptors can also reduce the duration of action potentials in cultured dorsal root ganglion (DRG) cells. This phenomenon has been considered a model of presynaptic inhibition because these same receptors are found on DRG cell axon terminals in the spinal cord (see below). The presynaptic GABA_B receptors of the DRG cell system have no effect on K^+ currents, but instead inhibit Ca^{2+} influx into the cells (Nicoll, Malenka, and Kauer, 1990; Wojcik and Holopainen, 1992).

GABA_C Receptors

There is a growing acceptance among researchers that some cellular effects of GABA are mediated by a third class of receptors, which has been termed GABA_C receptors. The earliest evidence for this subtype came from studies of Johnston and coworkers, who observed that certain unsaturated, partially folded GABA analogs such as *cis*-4-aminocrotonic acid (CACA), produced inhibitory neuronal responses that were insensitive to both bicuculline and baclofen (see Johnston, 1995).

$$NH_2-CH_2 \diagdown \overset{CH=CH}{\diagup} \diagdown CH_2-COOH$$

cis-4-Aminocrotonic acid

GABA_C receptors are activated not only by the relatively selective agonist CACA, but also by the nonselective agonists GABA and muscimol. In fact, GABA_C receptors are more sensitive to GABA than GABA_A receptors, and GABA_C receptors also desensitize more slowly (Bormann and Feigenspan, 1995). GABA_C receptors, however, show no modulation by BDZs, barbiturates, or neurosteroids.

Like GABA_A receptors, GABA_C receptors appear to contain an integral Cl^- channel that is inhibited by picrotoxin or TBPS. But the subunit structure of these two subtypes differs in that GABA_C receptors appear to be formed from novel subunits designated ρ1 and ρ2 (Bormann and Feigenspan, 1995). Both subunits are found in the retina, particularly in the bipolar cells, where both GABA_C and GABA_A receptor–mediated responses can be observed. Also, ρ2 but not ρ1 subunits have also been identified in the brain and may form homooligomeric GABA_C receptors in some cell populations.

The Role of GABA in Physiological and Behavioral Functions

The presence of both GABAergic neurons and synaptic connections at all levels of the neuraxis (Mugnaini and Oertel, 1985; Nagai et al., 1984) suggests that neural inhibition is a critical regulatory process in behavioral organization and control. A major proponent of this view has been Eugene Roberts, one of the original discoverers of GABA. Roberts (1986) argues that structures possessing GABAergic projection neurons, such as the cerebellar cortex, globus pallidus, substantia nigra pars reticulata, and reticular nucleus of the thalamus, act as coordinative command centers that chronically restrain excitatory output systems. A second source of inhibition comes from local GABAergic interneurons that are found in important structures such as the cerebral cortex and hippocampus. With these inhibitory neurons "acting like reins that serve to keep the neuronal 'horses' from running away" (Roberts, 1986, p. 99), behavioral activation requires the release (disinhibition) of excitatory pathways by a reduction of activity in the appropriate GABAergic systems.

Roberts illustrates these principles with the example of a cat encountering a mouse. When the mouse is first seen, processing of sensory input in the cat's corpus striatum leads to a suppression of inhibitory GABAergic activity from the globus pallidus and substantia nigra to the superior colliculus, thereby permitting collicular neurons to help direct visual tracking of the prey. At the same time, neurons in the thalamic motor nuclei and their projection areas are disinhibited so as to allow the movements required for stalking, killing, and ultimately consuming the mouse. The cerebellum also participates in this process by modulating fine motor activity.

From the standpoint of this theoretical framework, it is not surprising to learn that GABA plays an important role in many different behavioral and physiological mechanisms, including locomotor activity, feeding behavior, aggression, sexual behavior, mood, regulation of pain sensitivity, cardiovascular regulation, and thermoregulation (for review, see Matsumoto, 1989; Paredes and Ågmo, 1992). At a cellular level, GABA has been implicated in the phenomenon of presynaptic inhibition and in the dysregulation of brain excitability that occurs in epilepsy. As it is beyond the scope of this chapter to consider all of the above-mentioned functions of GABA, we have chosen to selectively focus on the role of this transmitter in presynaptic inhibition and in epilepsy. The pivotal role of GABA in motor control by the extrapyramidal motor system is discussed in the Parkinson's disease section of Chapter 20.

Presynaptic Inhibition

As first discussed in Chapter 6, presynaptic inhibition is a process in which transmission at an excitatory synapse is suppressed by an effect occurring at a presynaptic site. This phenomenon, which has been observed in the spinal cord, brain, and peripheral nervous system, is accomplished by means of axoaxonic synapses on the presynaptic fiber or terminal. The biochemical and electrophysiological mechanisms underlying presynaptic inhibition have been studied extensively in the spinal cord, in which the transmission of primary afferent input from DRG cells to second-order sensory neurons in the cord is subject to such inhibition.

Excellent evidence exists that GABA is the transmitter involved in presynaptic inhibition in the spinal cord and probably also in other parts of the nervous system. DRG cells express GABA receptors, these receptors are found in the appropriate layers of the spinal cord, presynaptic inhibition can be attenuated by either bicuculline or picrotoxin pretreatment, and electron microscopic immunohistochemical studies have demonstrated the presence of GABAergic axoaxonal synapses on primary afferent terminals in the cord (Barber et al., 1978; Nicoll and Alger, 1979; Nicoll, Malenka, and Kauer, 1990).

The sensitivity of presynaptic inhibition to bicuculline and picrotoxin implicates a $GABA_A$ receptor–mediated effect; however, the way in which the receptors carry out their action is unusual in this case. Electrophysiologists have long known that presynaptic inhibition of primary afferent fibers involves a *depolarization* of the fibers. Yet the increased Cl^- conductance caused by

$GABA_A$ receptor activation normally results in cellular hyperpolarization. What accounts for this discrepancy? It appears that the afferent fibers possess an inward Cl^- pumping mechanism that leads to a high internal Cl^- concentration and a corresponding Cl^- equilibrium potential in the depolarizing direction. Under these conditions, opening of the $GABA_A$ receptor–coupled Cl^- channels causes an efflux of Cl^- ions instead of the usual influx, and the synaptic terminals are consequently depolarized rather than hyperpolarized. This depolarization leads to a reduction in Ca^{2+} influx when the terminals are invaded by incoming action potentials because the amount of Ca^{2+} influx is determined by the difference in voltage between the preexisting membrane potential and the peak of the action potential. In turn, given that exocytosis is dependent on Ca^{2+}, decreased Ca^{2+} flow into the terminal results in less neurotransmitter release.

Although $GABA_A$ receptor–mediated depolarization clearly plays a major role in primary afferent presynaptic inhibition, $GABA_B$ receptors may be involved as well. As mentioned above, DRG cells possess $GABA_B$ receptors, and these sites also reduce Ca^{2+} influx, although by a different mechanism involving a G protein–mediated inhibition of the voltage-gated Ca^{2+} channels. There is now direct evidence for the involvement of $GABA_B$ as well as $GABA_A$ receptors in spinal presynaptic inhibition (Alford and Grillner, 1991).

GABA and Epilepsy

The term "epilepsy" refers to a class of neurological disorders characterized by recurrent convulsive and nonconvulsive seizures. It is estimated that epileptic disorders afflict approximately 1% of the population of the United States, which corresponds to over 2 million individuals (McNamara, 1994). We saw in Part I of this chapter that brain cell loss can occur in epileptic individuals, and that an excitotoxic, NMDA receptor–mediated process may be involved in such loss. In the present section, we will consider the possible role of amino acid transmitters, particularly GABA, in the etiology of epilepsy.

The GABA hypothesis of epilepsy.   Because seizures are associated with heightened neuronal excitability and abnormal firing, researchers have theorized that inhibitory GABAergic systems might be operating improperly in the epileptic brain. Of particular interest in this regard is focal (localized) epilepsy, which is generally centered in the neocortex or limbic cortex. Focal epilepsy is characterized by the appearance of intermittent, high-amplitude electrical discharges at the site of the epileptic focus during interictal periods (i.e., periods between seizure episodes). Such discharges display two phases, the first being a series of synchronous depolarizing events that are presumably evoked by strong excitatory inputs to the cells within the focal region. This massive depolarization is followed by the second phase, which is a period of hyperpolarization reflecting the activation of inhibitory mechanisms impinging on the cells. One of the processes thought to underlie the transition from interictal discharges to the generation of a full-blown seizure is a decrease in the hyperpolarizing phase, and thus a failure of inhibition. If GABA is one of the principal transmitters involved in neuronal inhibition, then it seems possible that GABAergic dysfunction might play a role in the epileptogenic process (Dichter, 1988; Morimoto, 1989).

Studies concerning the role of GABA in the onset and/or maintenance of seizure activity can be divided into three areas: (1) differences in GABAergic function in the brains of epileptics compared with nonepileptic individuals, (2) the ability of GABAergic drugs to suppress or promote seizures, and (3) the involvement of GABA in seizure production in animal models of epilepsy. Each of these areas will be discussed in turn.

GABAergic function in epileptics. The GABA theory of epilepsy leads to the expectation that the activity of this transmitter system might be abnormally low in epileptics. Some investigators have therefore measured GABA concentrations in the CSF of epileptics, under the assumption that this measure reflects brain GABA levels and/or the activity of GABAergic neurons. Two such studies found reduced CSF GABA concentrations in epileptics compared with control subjects (Manyam et al., 1980; Wood et al., 1979), although an earlier study reported no difference in the epileptic patients (Enna, Wood, and Snyder, 1977). Even the positive findings, however, are problematic in two ways. First, almost all patients were receiving anticonvulsant medication, which may have exerted an effect on GABA levels (although anticonvulsant drugs admittedly would not be expected to decrease the activity of GABAergic neurons). Second, the reduction in CSF GABA concentration was in no way specific to epilepsy. Equivalent decreases were found in a variety of other neurological disorders, including multiple sclerosis, Parkinson's disease, Huntington's disease, cerebellar cortical atrophy, and dementia (Manyam et al., 1980). Although some of these conditions are known to involve a loss of GABAergic cells (e.g., Huntington's disease) and therefore would be predicted to produce lowered GABA concentrations, this result is not as readily explained in other instances (e.g., multiple sclerosis).

Surgical removal of the focal area may be performed in cases of intractable epilepsy in which medication alone has proved ineffective in controlling seizures. Although this opportunity was used by two different Swedish groups to measure extracellular levels of amino acids in the epileptic focus by microdialysis, GABA was unfortunately not included in their analyses (Hamberger, Nyström, and Silfvenius, 1992; Ronne-Engström

et al., 1992). Earlier studies examined various GABAergic markers (e.g., GABA concentrations, GAD or GABA-T activity) in the excised epileptogenic tissue and in "normal" tissue from the same patient that was removed during the surgical approach to the damaged area. For example, Lloyd et al. (1986) analyzed samples from a total of 54 patients, 14 of whom had detectable brain tumors associated with the occurrence of their epilepsy. In both tumor and nontumor cases, these investigators found significant overall reductions in GAD, but not GABA-T, activity in the epileptogenic compared with the normal tissue. In a subgroup of patients, [^{3}H]GABA binding to GABA$_A$ receptors was also decreased in the focal area. In contrast, Sherwin and coworkers (1984) found no change in either GAD or GABA-T in spiking versus nonspiking cortical tissue obtained from a different group of epileptics (whereas the epileptic focus showed significant increases in glutamate dehydrogenase and tyrosine hydroxylase). Although the discrepant results from the two studies may have been related to methodological factors (see Sherwin and van Gelder, 1986), the overall results do not clearly support the GABAergic hypothesis of epilepsy.

GABAergic drugs and seizure activity. In earlier sections of this chapter, we saw that seizures can be induced experimentally by inhibiting GABA synthesis or by blocking GABA$_A$ receptors either competitively or noncompetitively at the picrotoxinin binding site. Conversely, inhibiting GABA breakdown or enhancing GABA action with BDZs, barbiturates, or ethanol leads to an anticonvulsant effect. Therefore, there is no doubt that manipulating the GABAergic system can greatly influence brain excitability and seizure-proneness both in animals and humans.

Examining the mechanisms of action of antiepileptic medications is another way to evaluate the GABA hypothesis of epilepsy. The most widely used antiepileptic drugs in the United States are phenytoin (Dilantin), sodium valproate (Depakene), carbamazepine (Tegretol), ethosuximide (Zarontin), trimethadione (Tridione), primidone (Myidone), BDZs, and phenobarbital. Whereas the BDZs and phenobarbital clearly exert their anticonvulsant effects at least partly through a GABAergic mechanism, the other compounds are thought to act largely by inhibition of voltage-dependent Na$^+$ and/or Ca^{2+} channels (Macdonald and Kelly, 1994). On the other hand, a number of novel antiepileptic compounds are currently undergoing clinical testing or have already been approved for clinical use (Fisher, 1993). Among these are two drugs, vigabatrin (Sabril) and tiagabine, that exert their effects by enhancing GABAergic function (Upton, 1994). As mentioned earlier in the chapter, vigabatrin irreversibly inhibits GABA-T activity, thereby producing increased brain levels of GABA. In animal studies, intracerebral administration of vigabatrin has been

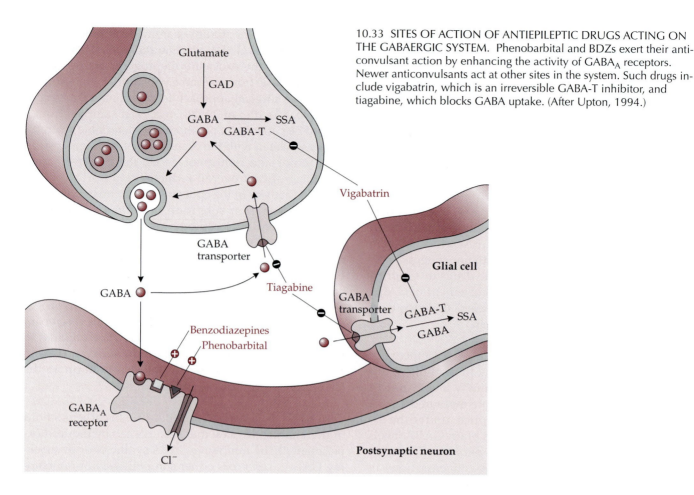

10.33 SITES OF ACTION OF ANTIEPILEPTIC DRUGS ACTING ON THE GABAERGIC SYSTEM. Phenobarbital and BDZs exert their anticonvulsant action by enhancing the activity of GABA$_A$ receptors. Newer anticonvulsants act at other sites in the system. Such drugs include vigabatrin, which is an irreversible GABA-T inhibitor, and tiagabine, which blocks GABA uptake. (After Upton, 1994.)

used to locate specific regions of the brain in which elevated GABA concentrations produce anticonvulsant effects (Gale, 1992). This same compound was found to protect rats from hippocampal cell loss in an animal model of temporal lobe epilepsy (see Part I) (Ylinen et al., 1991). In human clinical trials, vigabatrin has proved efficacious not only in adults, but also in cases of pediatric epilepsy (Gram, Sabers, and Dulae, 1992; Mumford and Cannon, 1994). Tiagabine, which likewise appears to be a promising antiepileptic agent, elevates the concentration of GABA in the synaptic cleft by blocking GABA uptake (Figure 10.33). In considering how these developments bear on the GABA hypothesis of epilepsy, it is important to emphasize that GABAergic agents might suppress seizure activity through a process unrelated to the etiology of those seizures.

GABA and experimental models of epilepsy. Probably the strongest evidence in favor of the GABA hypothesis comes from some of the experimental animal models of epilepsy that have been developed by various investigators. The kindling model, which was first described by Goddard, McIntyre, and Leech (1969), is particularly interesting in this regard. The term "**kindling**" refers to a progressive, more or less permanent epileptogenic process induced by repeated application (typically once per day) of a brief tetanic stimulus to a specific site in the brain. Kindling can be elicited in a variety of areas within the limbic system, cortex, and basal ganglia, although a few structures, such as the cerebellum, have not been found to support kindling (McNamara, Bonhaus, and Shin, 1993). A number of studies have found GABA abnormalities in the kindled brain, including reductions in GAD activity and GABA concentration as well as alterations in GABA-T, GABA receptor binding, and GABA$_A$ receptor–mediated Cl$^-$ flux (reviewed in Burnham, 1989). Although some inconsistent findings have also been reported, the idea that GABAergic function is altered in kindling must be considered seriously.

Like the hyperpolarization observed in the second phase of an interictal discharge in focal epilepsy (see above), the electrophysiological activity elicited by a kindling stimulus entails a period of EEG suppression. As

Tiagabine

the kindling proceeds over a period of several days, the suppression phase comes to be followed by a rhythmic synchronous discharge leading to an epileptiform after-discharge. Morimoto and Goddard (1986) have demonstrated that the duration of EEG suppression in amygdala-kindled rats can be modulated by drugs that act at the GABA$_A$/BDZ receptor complex. That is, diazepam treatment increases the period of poststimulus EEG suppression, whereas bicuculline, picrotoxin, and BDZ inverse agonists all tend to reduce this period. Excitatory amino acids and NMDA receptors may also be involved in the kindling process. Both competitive and noncompetitive NMDA receptor antagonists retard the development of kindling and raise the threshold for seizure induction in previously kindled subjects (Dingledine, McBain, and McNamara, 1990).

A model that encompasses these findings has been proposed by Morimoto (1989). According to this model, repeated NMDA receptor activation is required for the development of kindling, much as these receptors are thought to be involved in the induction of long-term potentiation following tetanic stimulation. Inhibitory GABAergic neurons are also triggered by the kindling stimulus, and are responsible for the suppression phase of the EEG response. Morimoto proposes that the transition from the suppression phase to the onset of the rhythmic synchronous discharge results from a collapse of GABA-mediated inhibition and a concurrent activation of NMDA receptors by excitatory amino acids.

Other models of focal epilepsy that use chemical induction have also been investigated with respect to possible GABA involvement. As summarized by Lloyd et al. (1986), decreases in GABA concentrations, GAD activity, and GABA uptake have been found in the cobalt focus, penicillin focus, and alumina gel models of epilepsy. Furthermore, immunocytochemical and ultrastructural studies have indicated a loss of GABAergic nerve terminals in many of these same preparations (reviewed by Houser, 1991). Evidence for structural damage raises the question of whether reduced GABA functioning preceded seizure onset in the treated animals, or whether recurrent seizure activity subsequently injured or destroyed nearby GABAergic neurons, thus leading to biochemical indices of GABA hypoactivity.

Finally, GABA-related markers have been examined in several genetic models of epilepsy, such as the epilepsy (*E1*) mouse, the genetically epilepsy-prone rat (*GEPR*), and the seizure-sensitive gerbil. Somewhat surprisingly, *increases* in the number of GABA- or GAD-immunoreactive neurons have been reported in all three of these animal strains (see Houser, 1991). Some investigators have explained these findings by suggesting that GABAergic interneurons such as basket cells inhibit one another as well as other (excitatory) neurons. In theory, therefore, increased density (or GAD activity) of basket cells might cause a disinhibition of excitatory circuits through excessive mutual inhibition.

GABA and epilepsy: conclusions. The GABA hypothesis of epilepsy has been tested using a number of different research and clinical approaches. Evidence in favor of the hypothesis may be summarized as follows: (1) GABA is a critical inhibitory transmitter, and seizures can readily be elicited by pharmacological disruption of GABAergic mechanisms; (2) some studies have reported reduced GABA concentrations in the CSF of epileptics as well as decreased levels of GABA markers in focal tissue compared with neighboring tissue that appeared to be electrophysiologically normal; (3) some effective antiepileptic drugs act by enhancing GABAergic activity; and (4) GABA abnormalities have been implicated in various animal models of epilepsy. However, the following contrary findings must also be considered: (1) Although blocking GABA functioning is one way of producing seizure activity, it does not follow that all convulsive syndromes must involve the same underlying mechanism; (2) reductions in CSF GABA are not specific to epilepsy alone, and the alternative approach of studying tissue GABA markers has yielded inconsistent results; (3) some of the most potent and widely prescribed antiepileptic drugs exert their primary effects through non-GABAergic mechanisms; and (4) whereas GABA dysfunction may play a role in the onset of kindling-evoked discharges, reductions in GABA markers in chemically induced focal epilepsy could be a secondary consequence of brain damage produced by recurrent seizure activity. Future research should apply molecular biological techniques to the study of various genetic animal models of epilepsy. Moreover, the use of noninvasive imaging techniques such as positron emission tomography (PET) and magnetic resonance imaging (MRI) should permit investigators to study epilepsy-related neurochemical changes without having to obtain surgical tissue samples from subjects.

Part II Summary

GABA is the most important inhibitory neurotransmitter in the CNS. It is synthesized from glutamate in a single step catalyzed by glutamate decarboxylase (GAD), of which two different isoenzymes have been characterized. GAD uses pyridoxal phosphate as an obligatory cofactor; however, much GAD in the brain exists in the form of an apoenzyme that lacks bound cofactor. This pool of inactive enzyme may serve as a reservoir for increasing GABA synthesis when needed. GABA is catabolized by the successive action of GABA aminotransferase (GABA-T) (with α-ketoglutarate as recipient of the amino group) and succinic semialdehyde dehydrogenase (SSADH) to yield succinate. Because this pathway represents a route from α-KG to succinate that bypasses the citric acid cycle, it is sometimes called the GABA shunt. Tissue GABA concentrations can be elevated by various drugs that inhibit GABA-T.

Most investigators believe that GABA is stored in synaptic vesicles and released by exocytosis; however, this mechanism has not been established unequivocally. Following its release, GABA is taken up into both neurons and astrocytes by plasma membrane transporters. Uptake is dependent on both Na^+ and Cl^- ions. Two different GABA transporter proteins have been cloned, GAT-A (also termed GAT-1), which may be both neuronal and glial, and GAT-B, which appears to be mainly neuronal.

Many brain regions are rich in GABA-containing cells and/or terminals, including the cerebral cortex, hippocampus, striatum, substantia nigra, and cerebellum. Within the cerebellar cortex, GABA is used by the Purkinje cells as well as the locally projecting Golgi, stellate, and basket cells. GABA is also an important transmitter for local inhibitory circuits in the spinal cord and peripheral nervous system. Outside of the nervous system, GABA is synthesized and secreted by the insulin-producing β-cells of the pancreas. There it acts on the nearby α-cells to inhibit their secretion of the hormone glucagon.

GABA receptors can be divided into three main subtypes, $GABA_A$, $GABA_B$, and $GABA_C$. The $GABA_A$ receptors are ligand-gated channels that are permeable to Cl^- ions and mediate fast IPSPs in postsynaptic cells. Blockade of these receptors by bicuculline (a competitive antagonist at the GABA binding site) or picrotoxin (a noncompetitive antagonist that binds to a separate site) leads to powerful convulsant effects. In contrast, a number of sedative–hypnotic drugs positively modulate the influence of GABA on the $GABA_A$ receptor. These drugs include BDZs such as diazepam (Valium), barbiturates such as pentobarbital or phenobarbital, anesthetic steroids, and ethanol. With the possible exception of ethanol, each of these drug classes interacts with a distinct binding site on the $GABA_A$ receptor complex. There is evidence for multiple BDZ receptor subtypes, and researchers have also demonstrated the existence of inverse receptor agonists with pharmacological characteristics opposite to the sedative–hypnotic, anxiolytic, and anticonvulsant profile of classic BDZs. So-called neurosteroids (steroids synthesized in the nervous system) may be the endogenous ligands for the steroid modulatory site on the $GABA_A$ receptor complex; however, the endogenous ligands for the BDZ and barbiturate sites have not yet been identified.

The $GABA_A$ receptor is a glycoprotein made up of several different subunits, each coded for by a distinct gene. The most important subunits are designated α, β, and γ, each of which has three to six isoforms. The $GABA_A$ receptor complex is thought to be made up of five subunits that together form the Cl^- channel and the various modulatory sites described above. Although various experimental approaches have been used to ascertain the possible subunit composition of native receptors,

there is still no definitive information on this issue. It does seem clear, however, that cells assemble certain combinations of subunits more readily than others, suggesting that such combinations may also be formed in vivo. Interestingly, the sensitivity of $GABA_A$ receptors to BDZs and ethanol has been linked to the presence of particular subunits, which may help to explain the regional heterogeneity of these receptors and the differential responsiveness of receptor-bearing cells to such drugs.

The $GABA_B$ receptor appears to be a G protein–coupled receptor, although it has not yet been cloned. These receptors are present not only postsynaptically but also on nerve terminals, where they inhibit neurotransmitter release. $GABA_B$ receptors can act via at least four different effector mechanisms: inhibition of adenylyl cyclase, stimulation of phospholipase A_2, K^+ channel activation, and Ca^{2+} channel inhibition.

$GABA_C$ receptors form Cl^- channels that can be inhibited by picrotoxin and TBPS. These receptors are activated by GABA, muscimol, and the more selective agonist cis-4-aminocrotonic acid. They are insensitive, however, to bicuculline, baclofen, and to $GABA_A$ receptor–modulating compounds such as BDZs, barbiturates, and neurosteroids. $GABA_C$ receptors are made up of the novel subunits ρ1 and ρ2, which are found in the retina and (in the case of ρ2) the brain.

GABA is a critically important transmitter for inhibitory control mechanisms in the brain. At the cellular level, this control is mediated not only by direct postsynaptic inhibition, but also by a phenomenon known as presynaptic inhibition. Presynaptic inhibition has been particularly well characterized in primary sensory neurons, in which activation of axonal $GABA_A$ receptors leads to a membrane depolarization rather than a hyperpolarization. This unusual response is the consequence of a Cl^- equilibrium potential across the membrane of the axon that promotes Cl^- efflux rather than the more typical influx when the ion channel is opened. Moreover, the resulting depolarization causes less transmitter to be released when an action potential invades the nerve terminal because the amount of Ca^{2+} entering the terminal depends on the difference between the preexisting membrane potential and the peak amplitude of the action potential.

GABA has also been implicated in the pathophysiology of epilepsy. Several animal models of epilepsy, including the kindling model, focal seizure-inducing treatments, and genetic seizure-prone strains, all show various alterations in the GABA system. On the other hand, it has proved more difficult to demonstrate consistent defects in GABAergic functioning in the brains of human epileptic patients. Nevertheless, several antiepileptic drugs that are either in current use or under development work by enhancing GABAergic function, and it remains possible that some types of epilepsy may stem from combined abnormalities in GABA and other neurotransmitters such as glutamate.

Part III
Inhibitory Amino Acids: Glycine

The second major inhibitory amino acid neurotransmitter in the CNS is **glycine**. The side chain in glycine is a hydrogen atom, which makes it the simplest amino acid structurally. Glycine is present in all tissues, where it participates in a number of metabolic pathways and is one of the constituents of various tissue proteins. Glycine is particularly enriched in collagen, a fibrous protein found in basement membranes, skin, blood vessels, bones, and tendons.

As discussed in greater detail below, there is a much higher concentration of glycine in some areas of the spinal cord than in others. Based in part on this heterogeneous distribution, Aprison and Werman (1965) proposed a possible neurotransmitter role for glycine. Over the next several years, glycine was shown to be synthesized in nerve cells, released following stimulation, taken up by nerve terminals, and capable of mimicking the action of the natural transmitter used by inhibitory spinal cord interneurons (reviewed in Aprison and Daly, 1978). Consequently, this substance is now well established as an important transmitter in vertebrates as well as many invertebrates.

Synthesis and Metabolism of Glycine

The two major pathways involved in glycine biosynthesis are shown in Figure 10.34. Quantitatively, the most important route for glycine synthesis is conversion from the amino acid serine through the action of the mitochondrial enzyme serine hydroxymethyltransferase. Serine, in turn, is produced largely via a multistep pathway from the glycolytic intermediate 3-phosphoglycerate. Thus, most of the glycine synthesized in the nervous system and in other tissues is ultimately derived from glucose metabolism.

An alternate pathway, shown in Figure 10.34b, involves the transamination of glyoxylate, a compound formed from either glycolytic or citric acid cycle intermediates. This pathway is analogous to the synthesis of glutamate by transamination (see Figure 10.2), except that glyoxylate, rather than α-ketoglutarate, serves as the amino acceptor. Although the glyoxylate pathway is found in the CNS, its role in glycine formation is not as important as that of the serine pathway.

The degradation of glycine may involve a number of different routes. In vitro studies have established the existence of biochemical mechanisms by which glycine can be converted to glutathione or guanidoacetic acid, or back to serine or glyoxylate. Which of these pathways are important for the inactivation of glycine in the neurotransmitter pool is not known.

Storage, Release, and Uptake of Glycine

As in the case of other amino acid transmitters, vesicular uptake and storage of glycine has proved difficult to demonstrate. However, there is now evidence that glycine is taken up into synaptic vesicles by an ATP-dependent transporter that uses the common mechanism of an electrochemical proton gradient as the driving force for transport. There is disagreement, however, as to whether this vesicular uptake system is selective for glycine (Kish, Fisher-Bovenkerk, and Ueda, 1989) or is similar to the uptake system for GABA (Burger et al., 1991).

Synaptic release and reuptake of glycine are carried out by mechanisms similar to those for other amino acid transmitters. Several studies have demonstrated Ca^{2+}-dependent release of glycine in tissue slices or synaptosomal preparations, particularly in tissue obtained from spinal cord or medulla (reviewed in Bradford, 1986).

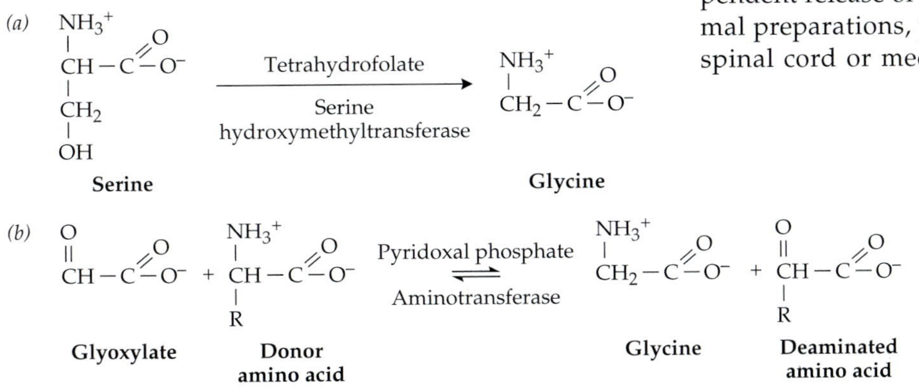

10.34 PATHWAYS OF GLYCINE SYNTHESIS. (*a*) In neural tissues, the major pathway of glycine synthesis is conversion from the amino acid serine. This reaction is catalyzed by the enzyme serine hydroxymethyltransferase and requires tetrahydrofolate and pyridoxal phosphate (not shown) as cofactors. (*b*) An alternate pathway of minor importance in the nervous system involves the transamination of glyoxylate, again using pyridoxal phosphate as a cofactor in the reaction.

Glycine uptake following release occurs by means of a high-affinity, Na$^+$-dependent transport system. Cloning techniques have recently identified three glycine transporter proteins: GLYT-1a (Borowsky, Mezey, and Hoffman, 1993; Guastella et al., 1992), GLYT-1b (Smith et al., 1992), and GLYT-2 (Liu et al., 1993).*

GLYT-1a and GLYT-1b are apparently derived from the same gene by means of either alternative mRNA splicing or alternative promoter usage. Using in situ hybridization histochemistry, Borowsky, Mezey, and Hoffman (1993) found that GLYT-1b mRNA was present almost exclusively in white matter, suggesting a primary localization in glial cells. In contrast, GLYT-1a mRNA was found in the gray matter of many areas within the brain and spinal cord. More recently, rat GLYT-2 mRNA was reported to occur exclusively in the brain stem, cerebellum, and spinal cord (Luque, Nelson, and Richards, 1995). This distribution corresponds well with the location of putative glycinergic neurons in the hindbrain and spinal cord, suggesting that GLYT-2 may be important in glycine uptake within classic glycinergic pathways (see below). The more extensive distribution of GLYT-1a, on the other hand, could reflect either a broader neurotransmitter role for glycine or an involvement of this transporter in regulating glycine concentrations at the glycine modulatory site of NMDA receptors (which are found throughout the CNS).

Anatomy of Glycine Pathways

Glycine has been most conclusively established as a neurotransmitter in inhibitory spinal cord interneurons. Some of these cells, termed Renshaw cells, mediate recurrent inhibition of spinal motor neurons (Eccles, Fatt, and Koketsu, 1954). Although glycine is usually considered the Renshaw cell transmitter, GABA may also play an important role in recurrent inhibition (Schneider and Fyffe, 1992). Moreover, these two inhibitory transmitters may be colocalized in some spinal cord cells, although whether these include the Renshaw cells remains to be determined (Todd and Sullivan, 1990).

Whereas early studies of glycinergic transmission focused almost exclusively on the spinal cord, there is growing evidence for glycine involvement in a number of brain pathways as well. These pathways include the corticohypothalamic tract, brain stem projections to the substantia nigra, spinal afferents from the raphe nuclei and reticular formation, the glossopharyngeal cranial nerve, and a pathway from the ventral cochlear nucleus to the corresponding nucleus on the contralateral side (McGeer and McGeer, 1989; Nieuwenhuys, 1985). In addition, there is evidence for use of glycine by interneu-

rons in the striatum and substantia nigra, certain retinal amacrine cells, and Golgi cells of the cerebellum. As in the case of spinal interneurons, glycine and GABA may be colocalized in some cerebellar Golgi cells (Ottersen, Storm-Mathisen, and Somogyi, 1988). It seems likely that as information concerning central glycine systems continues to grow, this amino acid will be found to play a more important role in behavioral and physiological regulation than previously recognized.

The Glycine Receptor

The glycine receptor functions in much the same way as the GABA$_A$ receptor. It contains an intrinsic Cl$^-$ channel, and glycine-mediated neuronal hyperpolarization is caused by increases in Cl$^-$ conductance across the membrane. Glycine and GABA$_A$ receptor Cl$^-$ channels are similar, though not identical, in their conductance states, apparent pore diameters, and anion permeability sequences (Bormann, Hamill, and Sakmann, 1987).

Biochemical purification of the glycine receptor indicates the presence of a 48-kDa α subunit (which contains the agonist binding site) and a 58-kDa β subunit, with a proposed stoichiometry of 3α:2β (Betz, 1991; Betz and Becker, 1988). An additional 93-kDa protein called gephyrin copurified with the receptor and is thought to play a role in receptor anchoring and clustering (Becker, 1995). The glycine receptor exhibits regional and developmental heterogeneity, which stems from the existence of four isoforms of the α subunit (designated α1–α4). Most glycine receptors in adult animals possess the α1 isoform, which confers a high affinity for the prototypical glycine antagonist strychnine (see below). In contrast, fetal and early neonatal receptors primarily contain the α2 isoform, which results in only a low affinity for strychnine (Becker, 1995).

Glycine Pharmacology and Behavioral Functions

Studies of the functional role of glycine in behavioral processes have been hampered by the relative lack of available pharmacological tools. Several amino acids show agonistic activity at the glycine receptor, including β-alanine, taurine, and β-aminoisobutyric acid. However, these compounds lack both specificity and high affinity for the glycine receptor (Betz and Becker, 1988).

The major drug used to study glycine pharmacology has been the receptor antagonist strychnine, a compound that has a long history in medicine and research. Strychnine is an alkaloid derived from the seeds of a tree native to India, *Strychnos nux vomica*. A related but less potent alkaloid called brucine is also found in these seeds. Nux vomica, as strychnine was known in old pharmacopoeias, has been erroneously translated as "emetic nut"; however, strychnine is not an emetic, and *vomica* means "depression" or "cavity," which is a fea-

---

*At the time of this writing, various investigators have used different systems of glycine transporter numbering. For convenience, we have chosen to use the system of Liu et al. (1993) and Luque, Nelson, and Richards (1995).

Strychnine

ture of the *Strychnos* seed. In the sixteenth century, nux vomica was used as a poison for rats and other pests in Germany, and its use in modern times in "rat biscuits" has been responsible for some accidental poisonings of children (Esplin and Zablocka, 1965).

Early studies showed that strychnine was a potent convulsant and had its greatest effect on the antigravity muscles, causing them to display symmetric extensor thrusts. Such thrusting movements could be elicited by almost any sensory stimulus—tactile, auditory, visual, or otherwise. Strychnine-induced convulsions were also found in spinal animals (i.e., animals with a surgical transection separating the spinal cord from the brain), suggesting that the drug's principal site of action was in the spinal cord. The effects of strychnine on neuronal excitability can be strikingly demonstrated by injecting a subconvulsant dose into a mouse. The mouse seems to act normally in a quiet environment, but a loud clap of the hands will cause it to jump about wildly.

Photoaffinity labeling studies indicate that strychnine binds to the α subunit (mainly the $\alpha1$ isoform) of the glycine receptor, which also contains the agonist recognition site (Betz, 1991; Becker, 1995). Glycine-displaceable binding of [^{3}H]strychnine has been considered a marker for the glycine receptor complex, and [^{3}H]-strychnine autoradiography has accordingly been used to map the distribution of glycine receptors in the spinal cord and brain (Zarbin, Wamsley, and Kuhar, 1981). Within the cord, glycine receptors have been found at particularly high densities in laminae II, III, V, and VII. Significant levels of receptor binding have also been observed in a number of medullary and pontine nuclei, whereas lower levels have been found in midbrain and thalamic structures. One limitation of using [^{3}H]strychnine binding as a glycine receptor marker is that the relatively strychnine-insensitive $\alpha2$ subunit persists into adulthood in a few brain areas (notably the cerebral cortex and hippocampus) (Malosio et al., 1991). Therefore, glycine receptors containing this subunit instead of $\alpha1$ have not been detected in classic [^{3}H]strychnine binding studies.

Despite the limitation just mentioned, the pattern of glycine receptors revealed by [^{3}H]strychnine autoradiography correlates well with the results of electrophysiological studies of glycine sensitivity, and indicates that glycine plays a role in both sensory and motor systems in the CNS. Zarbin, Wamsley, and Kuhar (1981) suggested that the locations of strychnine binding sites can account for many of the clinical symptoms of strychnine intoxication. These hypothesized relationships are presented in Table 10.3.

Further evidence for glycine involvement in sensorimotor function comes from a group of behavioral disor-

Table 10.3 Hypothesized Relationships between Clinical Effects of Strychnine Intoxication and Areas of Labeled Strychnine Binding (Glycine Receptors)

Clinical effect of strychnine	Area of strychnine binding sites
Heightened perceptual acuity	
Visual	Retina (inner plexiform layer)
Auditory	Superior olivary nucleus, nuclei of the lateral lemniscus
Cutaneous	Dorsal horn of spinal cord, cuneate and gracile nuclei, and analogous portions of trigeminal nuclei
Hyperalgesia and pain associated with convulsions	Dorsal horn of spinal cord (esp. laminae II and V) and analogous portions of trigeminal nuclei
Hyperreflexia and muscular stiffness or spasm	
Limb and trunk musculature	Dorsal and ventral horns of spinal cord
Muscles of mastication	Sensory and motor portions of trigeminal nuclei
Muscles of facial expression	Sensory portions of trigeminal nuclei and nucleus of the facial nerve (VII)
Increased respiratory rate, bradycardia, and hypertension	Respiratory and cardiovascular centers in medulla and pons (dorsal parabrachial nucleus; ventral parabrachial nucleus; paramedian reticular nucleus; parvocellular reticular nucleus; gigantocellular reticular nucleus)
Initiation of convulsions by visual and acoustic stimuli	Gray layers of the superior colliculus (superficial, intermediate, and deep)
Disequilibrium	Medial vestibular nucleus

Source: After Zarbin, Wamsley, and Kuhar, 1981.

ders involving abnormal startle responses. In humans, "startle disease" (also called hyperekplexia or Kok's disease) is an inherited disorder characterized by the ability of a sudden loud noise or a touch to trigger sudden muscular rigidity, which results in the victim falling (see Becker, 1995; Rajendra and Schofield, 1995). Startle-induced rigidity is called "myoclonus" in animal species such as dogs, horses, and cows. Two autosomal recessive mouse mutants, *spastic* and *spasmodic*, likewise exhibit exaggerated startle responses characterized by tremor, rigidity, falling, and a retarded righting reflex.

In the case of *spastic* mice, an abnormality in glycinergic function was suggested by the fact that these animals resembled strychnine-intoxicated subjects both behaviorally and in terms of electromyographic responses (Betz and Becker, 1988). Subsequent research has indeed shown that the disorder is caused by a defect in the gene for the glycine receptor β subunit, which leads to a large reduction in subunit expression and receptor assembly (Becker, 1995; Rajendra and Schofield, 1995). In contrast, human startle disease and the *spasmodic* mouse phenotype result from separate missense mutations of the α1 subunit of the glycine receptor. Consequently, affected cells display a markedly reduced sensitivity to glycine

and a large reduction in glycine-activated Cl⁻ currents. These mechanisms are illustrated in Figure 10.35. It is important to note that the behavioral symptoms associated with the *spastic* and *spasmodic* mutations are not manifested until 2 weeks postnatally. Along with other findings, this suggests that glycine receptors may be composed of only α2 subunits (which are unaffected in either disorder) during early development. As immature receptors are subsequently replaced with receptors containing α1 and β subunits, the above-mentioned behavioral abnormalities begin to appear.

Part III Summary

Glycine is an inhibitory amino acid transmitter synthesized primarily from serine. Following release, glycine is taken up by the following membrane transporters: GLYT-1a, GLYT-1b (which may be glial), and GLYT-2 (which is particularly prevalent in the hindbrain and spinal cord). Glycine is best known as a transmitter in the spinal cord, where it is used by Renshaw cells to mediate recurrent inhibition of motor neurons. However, glycinergic pathways are also found in the hindbrain and in other brain areas.

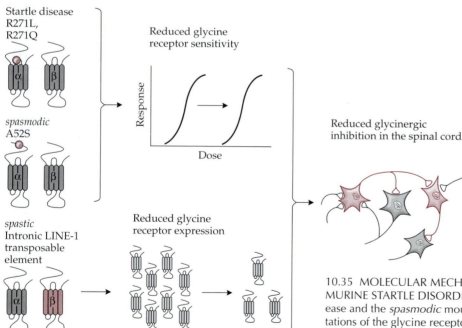

10.35 MOLECULAR MECHANISMS UNDERLYING HUMAN AND MURINE STARTLE DISORDERS. Human familial inherited startle disease and the *spasmodic* mouse disorder are both due to missense mutations of the glycine receptor α1 subunit (mutation sites denoted by colored circles), which in turn cause reduced receptor sensitivity. In startle disease, an arginine (R) residue at position 271 has been replaced by either leucine (L) or glutamine (Q). In the *spasmodic* mutant, an alanine (A) to serine (S) conversion is present at position 52 in the N-terminal extracellular domain of the protein. In the *spastic* mouse mutant, an intronic insertion into the β subunit leads to reduced receptor expression. All three disorders are characterized by impaired glycinergic inhibition in the spinal cord, which is manifested phenotypically by hypertonia (excessive muscle tone) and exaggerated startle responses. (After Rajendra and Schofield, 1995.)

The glycine receptor is similar to the $GABA_A$ receptor. It functions as a ligand-gated channel for Cl^- ions and produces fast IPSPs in postsynaptic cells. The receptor appears to be made up of two subunits, α and β, with a proposed stoichiometry of $3\alpha:2\beta$. There are four known isoforms of the α subunit, $\alpha1$–$\alpha4$. In adulthood, most brain areas express the $\alpha1$ isoform, whereas the $\alpha2$ isoform predominates during early development.

The major drug used to study the glycine system has been strychnine, a glycine receptor antagonist that binds with high affinity to the $\alpha1$ but not the $\alpha2$ subunit. Behaviorally, the drug exerts potent excitatory and convulsant effects. In radiolabeled form, strychnine has also played an important role in mapping the location of glycine receptors in the brain and spinal cord.

The localization of glycine receptors and the effects of strychnine intoxication suggest that the glycinergic system plays an important role in sensorimotor function. This supposition is supported by the existence of inherited disorders in mice, humans, and several other species involving an exaggerated startle response that triggers sudden muscular rigidity and falling. Recent research has shown these disorders to result from genetic errors in either the α or β subunit of the glycine receptor, thereby leading to a loss of normal receptor function.

Part IV
Histamine

The final part of this chapter deals with histamine, a neurotransmitter that is not an amino acid, but which is nevertheless most conveniently presented here. Like serotonin and the catecholamines, histamine is a biogenic amine that is synthesized from an amino acid precursor. Histamine is of interest to neuropharmacologists because of its potential importance in behavioral and physiological regulation as well as its involvement in the actions of some psychotropic drugs.

Histamine is best known for its relationship to respiratory allergies to airborne pollens. Many of the unpleasant symptoms of various allergic and inflammatory reactions can be ascribed to the release of histamine from **mast cells**, a class of connective tissue cells that also contain heparin (a blood-clotting regulator) and, in some species, small amounts of serotonin and dopamine. Histamine released from mast cells produces vascular effects such as local vasodilation and increased vascular permeability, and also influences visceral smooth muscle and exocrine glands. Indeed, the classic pharmacology of histamine was developed using these peripheral systems.

As discussed in more detail below, some mast cells are also found in the brain and contribute to the brain's histamine content. The existence of nonneuronal brain histamine has been one of the complicating factors in determining whether it is used as a neurotransmitter. In addition, the early histofluorescent methods that proved so important in mapping the distribution of catecholaminergic and serotonergic cell bodies and nerve terminals were ineffective for histamine. Nevertheless, early neurochemical studies by Schwartz and his colleagues led to the concept of histamine as a central neurotransmitter (see Schwartz, Pollard, and Quach, 1980). This idea was later strengthened by the immunohistochemical visualization of histamine in neurons (see below). It is now clear that a number of histaminergic pathways are present in the brain, and that this substance has important physiological actions. General reviews of neuronal histamine function may be found in Onodera and coworkers (1994) and Schwartz, Arrang and coworkers (1991).

Histamine Synthesis, Release, and Inactivation

Synthesis and Release

As illustrated in Figure 10.36, histamine is formed by decarboxylation of the amino acid histidine. The reaction is catalyzed by a specific enzyme called histidine decarboxylase, which requires pyridoxal phosphate as a cofactor. The amino acid sequence of the enzyme shows homologies with other pyridoxal phosphate–dependent enzymes such as aromatic L-amino acid decarboxylase (AADC). Although histidine can also be decarboxylated by AADC, it is a poor substrate for this enzyme. Histidine decarboxylase activity is much higher in neurons than in mast cells, which is consistent with the greater rate of histamine turnover in the former cell population.

One major approach to studying the functional significance of histamine has been to deplete this substance by inhibiting its synthesis. The most widely used drug for this purpose is the potent, highly specific, and irreversible histidine decarboxylase inhibitor α-fluoromethylhistidine (α-FMH; Kollonitsch et al., 1978; Watanabe et al., 1990). α-FMH appears to be a suicide substrate, which means that it inactivates the enzyme after being converted to a reactive product by the enzyme's own catalytic reaction. A single injection of α-

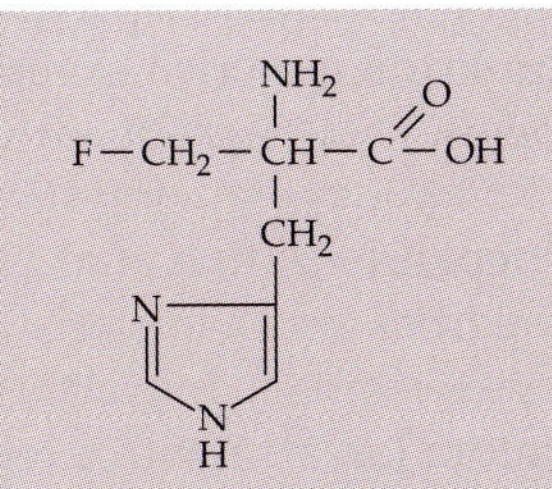

α-Fluoromethylhistidine

FMH only partially depletes brain histamine in normal animals, presumably because of the slower turnover of

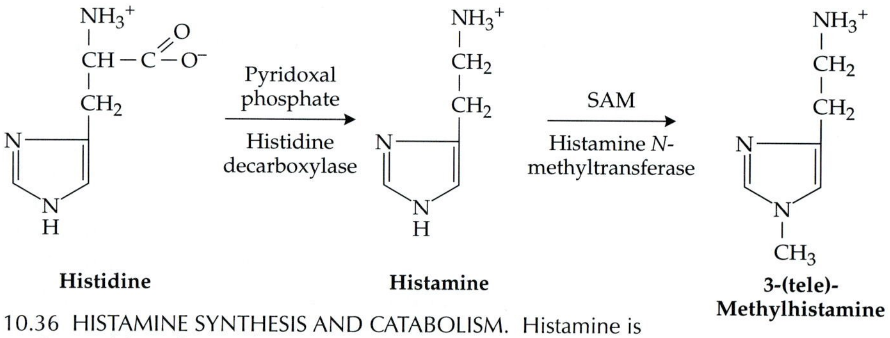

10.36 HISTAMINE SYNTHESIS AND CATABOLISM. Histamine is synthesized from the amino acid histidine by the enzyme histidine decarboxylase. Histamine is converted to its major catabolite, 3-(tele)-methyl-imidazoleacetic acid, by the combined action of histamine N-methyl transferase, monoamine oxidase (MAO), and aldehyde dehydrogenase.

histamine in nonneuronal cell types such as mast cells. This conclusion is supported by the ability of the drug to totally deplete brain histamine in the W/W^V mutant mouse strain, which is deficient in mast cells.

As we have seen in previous chapters, the synthesis rate of a neurotransmitter is governed by multiple factors, including substrate availability, the activity of synthetic enzymes, and so forth. In the case of histamine, histidine availability may be one regulatory factor in its synthesis. Histidine administration leads to increased brain levels and release of histamine (Cumming et al., 1991; Russell et al., 1990; Schwartz, Lampart, and Rose, 1972), indicating that histidine decarboxylase is probably not saturated in vivo with its substrate. Depolarizing stimuli likewise stimulate histamine synthesis in both brain slices and in synaptosomes (Arrang, Garbarg, and Schwartz, 1987), thus providing for a compensatory increase in neurotransmitter availability in response to heightened demand. However, histidine decarboxylase activity in hypothalamic tissue was unchanged following depolarization (Chudomelka and Murrin, 1989), and there is no evidence for stimulation-induced increases in histidine uptake. Thus, although increased impulse flow may be capable of enhancing the rate of histamine formation, the underlying mechanism has not yet been determined.

Several laboratories have examined histamine release in vivo using microdialysis. Histamine overflow in the hypothalamus (an area rich in histamine-containing neurons; see below) was significantly elevated by local application of KCl (a depolarizing stimulus), and this effect was Ca^{2+}-dependent (Itoh et al., 1991; Russell et al., 1990). Such properties are characteristic of transmitter release from nerve terminals. In contrast, histamine overflow in the striatum (an area with a relatively sparse histaminergic innervation) was insensitive to KCl or tetrodotoxin (a drug that blocks voltage-dependent Na^+ channels), and showed only a modest effect of Ca^{2+} removal (Cumming et al., 1991; Russell et al., 1990). These findings raise the possibility that some histamine release in the brain is from nonneuronal cells (e.g., mast cells).

Inactivation

Despite several attempts to demonstrate a high-affinity uptake system for histamine, no such system has been discovered. In this respect, histamine differs from the amino acid neurotransmitters as well as the other neuroactive amines. Histamine in the brain is metabolized by the enzyme histamine N-methyltransferase, using S-adenosylmethionine (SAM) as the methyl donor (Huszti, 1990; see Figure 10.34). This reaction gives rise to an intermediate, 3-(tele)-methylhistamine, which is rapidly metabolized by type B monoamine oxidase (MAO-B) and aldehyde dehydrogenase to yield 3-(tele)-methyl-imidazoleacetic acid. The presence of MAO-B has been reported in histaminergic neurons of the cat hypothalamus (Lin et al., 1991). Histamine in other tissues can be subjected to initial oxidation by diamine oxidase; however, this enzyme appears to be lacking in the mammalian brain.

Sources and Distribution of Histamine in the Brain

Neurons

As mentioned above, immunohistochemical procedures have been important in demonstrating the presence of histamine in nerve cells and in mapping the distribution of these cells and their fibers and terminals. Mapping studies have been performed using antibodies either against histidine decarboxylase or against histamine itself, and the two approaches have yielded similar results (Hough, 1988; Onodera et al., 1994). In the rat brain, histaminergic neurons are found exclusively in a region of the basal posterior hypothalamus called the tuberomammillary nucleus (TM). Wada and coworkers have defined five subgroups of cells within this region, which they have designated E1–E5* (Onodera et al., 1994; Figure

---

*As described in earlier chapters, the dopaminergic and noradrenergic cell groups have designations beginning with the letter "A". Likewise, "B" and "C" are used for serotonin- and epinephrine-containing cells respectively. Finally, Jaeger, Ruggiero, Albert, Joh and colleagues (1984) referred to neurons immunoreactive for tyrosine hydroxylase, but not aromatic L-amino acid decarboxylase, as D1–D14. This left the letter "E" for use for the next monoaminergic system, namely, histamine.

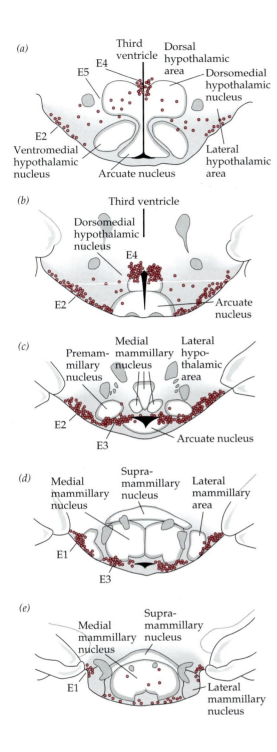

(a)

Third ventricle
Dorsal hypothalamic area
E4
E5
Dorsomedial hypothalamic nucleus
E2
Ventromedial hypothalamic nucleus
Arcuate nucleus
Lateral hypothalamic area

(b)

Third ventricle
Dorsomedial hypothalamic nucleus
E4
E2
Arcuate nucleus

(c)

Medial mammillary nucleus
Premammillary nucleus
Lateral hypothalamic area
E2
E3
Arcuate nucleus

(d)

Supramammillary nucleus
Medial mammillary nucleus
Lateral mammillary area
E1
E3

(e)

Supramammillary nucleus
Medial mammillary nucleus
E1
Lateral mammillary nucleus

10.37 LOCATION OF HISTAMINERGIC CELL GROUPS IN THE RAT BRAIN. Histaminergic neurons are found in a region of the basal posterior hypothalamus that is sometimes called the tuberomammillary nucleus. Within this area, it is possible to delineate five cell clusters, which have been designated E1–E5. The parts of the figure labeled *a–e* represent different levels of the hypothalamus moving from rostral to caudal. (After Yamatodani et al., 1991.)

ascending and (to a lesser extent) descending projections. Figure 10.38 is a schematic illustration of the histamine pathways in the rat brain. Fiber density is highest in the hypothalamus, medial septum, and diagonal band, somewhat lower in the cerebral cortex and amygdala, and lowest in the hippocampus, striatum, olfactory bulbs, brain stem, and cerebellum. The varicose fibers elaborated by histaminergic axons seem to form few synaptic contacts (Takagi et al., 1986), suggesting that histamine may act at a distance from its site of release, perhaps in a neuromodulatory manner. Furthermore, the morphological organization of the histamine system as a small number of cell clusters with diffuse efferent projections resembles the organization of the noradrenergic and serotonergic systems (Steinbusch, 1991). Together, these findings raise the possibility that histamine subserves very basic behavioral and physiological functions, as has been proposed for norepinephrine and serotonin.

Immunohistochemical studies indicate that histamine is colocalized with other neuroactive substances in posterior hypothalamic neurons. In rats, 45% to 100% of TM histamine neurons also exhibit immunoreactivity for GABA (or GAD), adenosine deaminase (a suggested marker for cells that use adenosine as a transmitter), and/or the neuropeptides galanin and methionine-enkephalin-Arg[6]-Phe[7] (see Onodera et al., 1994). There is no information thus far concerning corelease of these substances with histamine or physiological interactions among the transmitters in affecting postsynaptic target cells.

Nonneuronal Cells

Besides neurons, histamine has been detected in at least three other cell types in the brain: mast cells, related cells called neurolipomastocytes (also called type II mast cells), and some capillary endothelial cells (Hough, 1988). Mast cells have been found in the brains of many nonhuman species, although there seems to be wide interspecific as well as intraspecific variation in cell number (Dropp, 1976). Furthermore, the distribution of mast cells within the brain is quite uneven. In rats, one place where these cells are seen is in the leptomeninges (pia and arachnoid membranes), particularly in the vicinity of the cerebral cortex, dorsal thalamus, and median eminence of the hypothalamus (Dropp, 1976; Panula, Yang, and Costa, 1984). Mast cells are also found in the vicinity of blood vessels in some areas of the brain. Rats were found to have the highest concentrations of vascular-associated mast cells in the dorsal thalamus, cerebral cortex, and olfactory peduncles (Dropp, 1976). It is impor-

10.37). The histaminergic neurons receive afferent connections from several structures, including the prefrontal cortex, medial preoptic area, and septum. Electrophysiological studies have shown that these cells are spontaneously active, with a firing rate of approximately 2 Hz. Histamine-containing neurons in the human brain are likewise found in the hypothalamus, although they are spread over a larger area (Airaksinen et al., 1991; Panula et al., 1990).

In contrast to the highly restricted localization of histaminergic cell bodies, the cells give rise to widespread

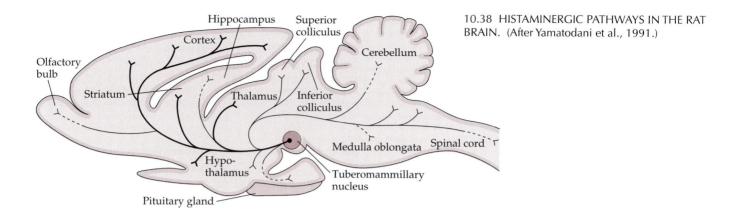

10.38 HISTAMINERGIC PATHWAYS IN THE RAT BRAIN. (After Yamatodani et al., 1991.)

tant to note that most studies have reported an absence of mast cells in the human brain (Hough, 1988). However, human brains apparently do possess neurolipomastocytes, which may perform functions similar to those of traditional mast cells.

The function of mast cell (or neurolipomastocyte) histamine in the brain is still unclear. Hough (1988) has reviewed studies showing that the number of brain mast cells can be altered by environmental manipulations, immune sensitization, and certain types of brain damage, although the significance of these changes has not been established. As peripheral mast cells play a major role in vascular regulation, it is conceivable that mast cells in the brain serve a similar function. Further work, however, is needed to test this hypothesis.

Histamine Receptors

At the present time, histamine receptors are classified into three different subtypes, designated H_1, H_2, and H_3. The following discussion will focus on the H_1 and H_2 subtypes, about which the most is known.

H_1 Receptors

The H_1 receptor subtype mediates the contractile effects of histamine on certain smooth muscle preparations such as the guinea pig trachea, ileum, and uterus. The bovine and guinea pig H_1 receptors have been cloned and shown to possess structures indicative of membership in the G protein–coupled receptor superfamily (Traiffort et al., 1994; Yamashita et al., 1991). Consistent with the receptor's peripheral actions, H_1 receptor mRNA was found in the above-mentioned organs, as well as in spleen and adrenal medulla. In vivo, most H_1 receptor actions have been associated with activation of the phosphoinositide/protein kinase C second messenger system (Hill, 1987). Expression of the cloned guinea pig receptor in Chinese hamster ovary (CHO) or HeLa cells, however, showed that the receptor is also capable of other second messenger effects, including stimulation of cAMP synthesis and arachidonic acid release (presumably via activation of phospholipase A_2) (Traiffort et al., 1993).

The first antihistamines were described by two French researchers approximately 60 years ago (Bovet and Staub, 1937). These and other "classic" antihistamines are all H_1 receptor blockers. Such compounds, many of which are used for the relief of allergy symptoms, include diphenhydramine (Benadryl), chlorpheniramine (Chlor-Trimeton), *trans*-triprolidine, promethazine, and mepyramine (Hill, 1987). The sedative properties of classic antihistamines have been known for many years, and represent an undesirable side effect of these medications for many allergy sufferers. For this reason, several H_1 antagonists have been developed that are nonsedating because they do not readily cross the blood–brain barrier. Astemizole (Hismanal), loratadine (Claritin), and terfenadine (Seldane) are three nonsedating antihistamines that are used clinically.

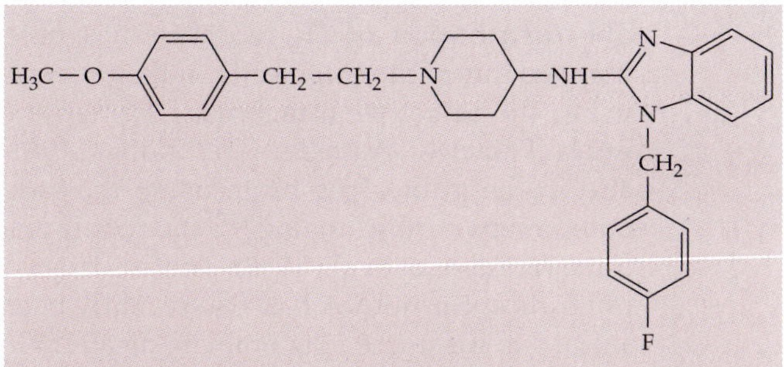

Astemizole

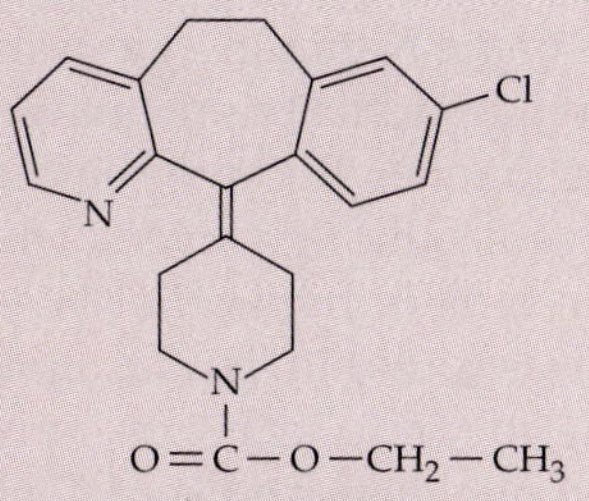

Loratadine

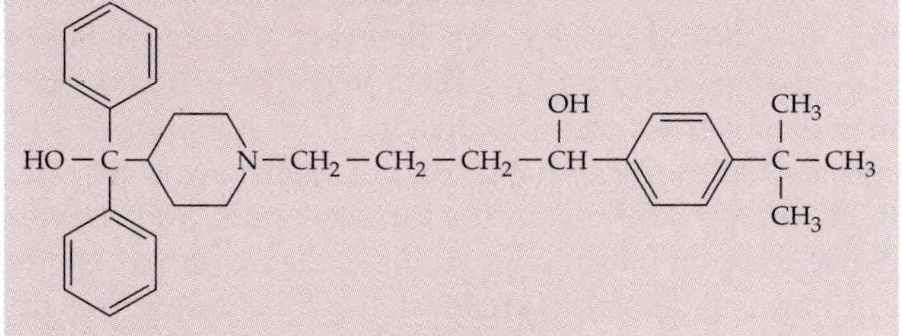

Terfenadine

It is interesting to note that a number of drugs used in the treatment of psychiatric disorders also have significant H_1 receptor blocking ability. These drugs include the antidepressants doxepin, amitryptyline, and mianserin, and the neuroleptic (antipsychotic) drugs chlorpromazine, fluphenazine, thioridazine, and flupenthixol (Hill, 1987). In fact, the development of chlorpromazine came about through the French surgeon Laborit's search for antihistaminergic compounds to use as calming agents in the treatment of shock (Caldwell, 1970). As discussed in Chapter 18, however, the therapeutic efficacy of these psychotropic drugs has been ascribed more to their effects on the catecholaminergic (or in some cases serotonergic) systems than to their interactions with histamine.

In contrast to the situation for H_1 antagonists, it has proved difficult to find specific and potent agonists for this receptor subtype. The major H_1 agonist available at this time is 2-thiazolylethylamine, which has a lower potency than histamine and only about a tenfold selectivity for peripheral H_1 sites versus H_2 sites (Ganellin, 1982; Schwartz, Arrang, and Garbarg, 1986).

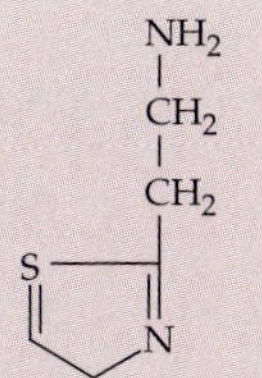

2-Thiazolylethylamine

H_2 Receptors

Although some peripheral actions of histamine are blocked by classic antihistamines, others are not, including the contractile effects on rat uterus and guinea pig atrium as well as histamine-induced stimulation of gastric acid secretion. This finding led to the proposal by Ash and Schild (1966) of an additional class of histamine receptors. This second subtype was subsequently validated pharmacologically and designated the H_2 receptor (Black et al., 1972). The H_2 receptor has been cloned in rats (Ruat et al., 1991), dogs (Gantz, Schäffer et al., 1991), and humans (Gantz, Munzert et al., 1991) and was found to be coupled to G proteins. H_2 receptors are classically associated with stimulation of adenylyl cyclase and cAMP synthesis (Hill, 1987); however, cells transfected with these receptors also respond with an inhibition of arachidonic acid release (opposite to the effect produced by H_1 receptors) (Traiffort et al., 1993).

Specific antagonists of H_2 receptors include cimetidine (Tagamet), ranitidine (Zantac), and tiotidine. Cime-

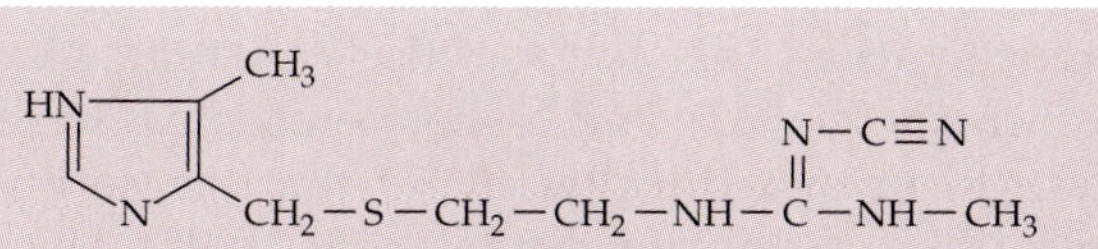

Cimetidine

Ranitidine

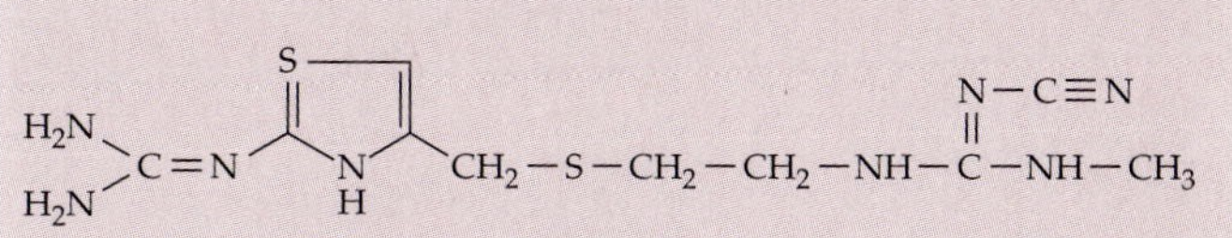

Tiotidine

tidine and ranitidine are widely used clinically to reduce gastric acid secretion in patients with gastric or duodenal ulcers. Another important drug is zolantidine, which is currently the only available H_2 antagonist that readily penetrates the blood–brain barrier. This compound should be useful in future studies of the behavioral and physiological functions of central H_2 receptors.

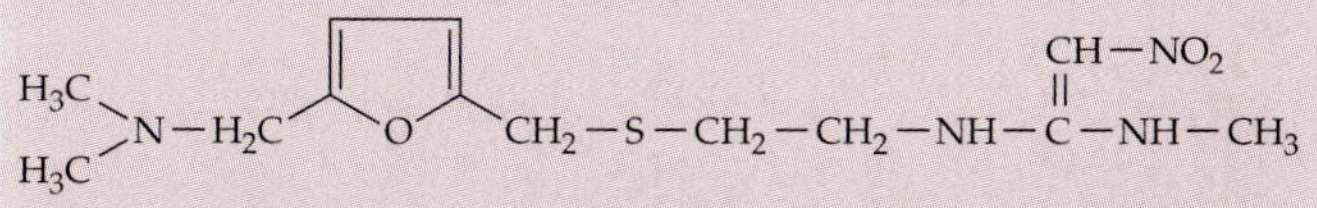

Several useful H_2 receptor agonists are likewise available, including dimaprit, impromidine, and arpromidine. Impromidine and arpromidine, however, lack

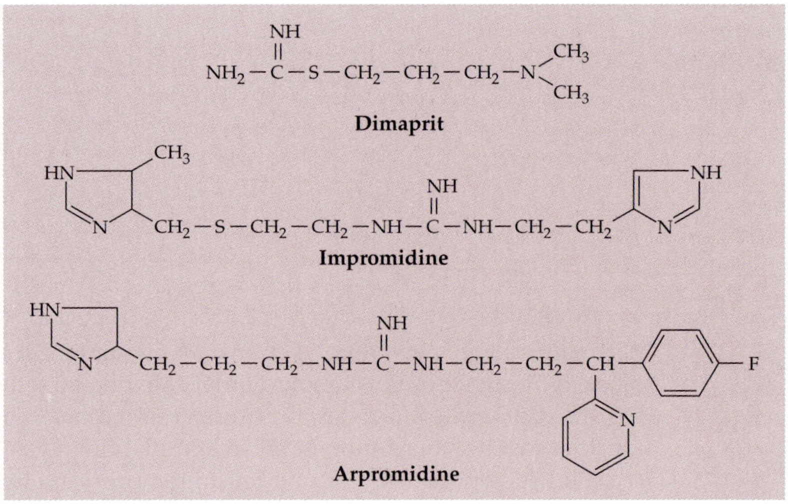

Dimaprit

Impromidine

Arpromidine

selectivity in that they also exhibit H_3 and H_1 antagonist effects, respectively.

H_3 Receptors

A third histamine receptor subtype, H_3, was proposed in 1983 based on the ability of various drugs to influence histamine release from brain slices in vitro (Arrang, Garbarg, and Schwartz, 1983). Briefly, histamine was found to inhibit its own release, presumably through the action of some type of autoreceptor. Moreover, this putative autoreceptor possessed a pharmacology distinct from that of either H_1 or H_2 receptors, and therefore presumably represented a novel receptor subtype. Since this initial work, H_3 autoreceptors have been shown to regulate histamine synthesis as well as release (Arrang, Garbarg, and Schwartz, 1987), and H_3 heteroreceptors have been found to presynaptically inhibit the release of other transmitters (Schwartz, Arrang et al., 1991). The structure of the H_3 receptor is currently unknown, as the gene has not yet been cloned; however, like the other hista-

R-α-Methylhistamine

Thioperamide

mine receptor subtypes, the H_3 receptor appears to belong to the G protein–coupled receptor superfamily. Pharmacological characterization of the H_3 receptor has been facilitated by the development of relatively selective agonists such as R-α-methylhistamine and antagonists such as thioperamide (Arrang et al., 1987).

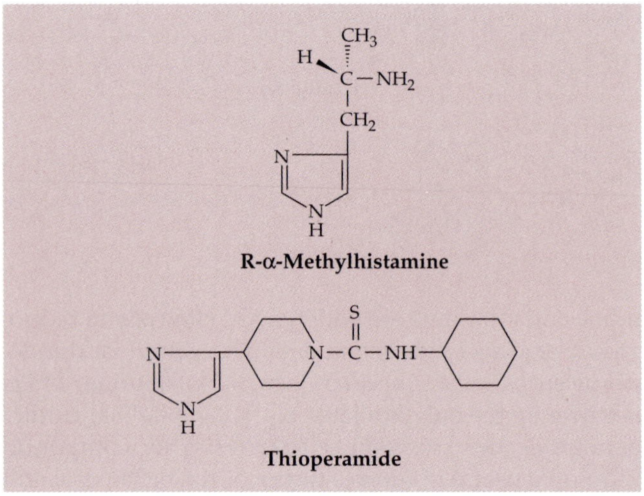

Distribution of Histamine Receptors

The distribution of H_1 receptors has been mapped autoradiographically in the rat brain using the selective antagonist [^{3}H]mepyramine (Palacios, Wamsley, and Kuhar, 1981) and in the guinea pig brain using the iodinated mepyramine analog [^{125}I]iodobolpyramine (Bouthenet et al., 1988). The localization of H_1 receptor mRNA has also recently been studied in the guinea pig brain by means of in situ hybridization histochemistry (Traiffort et al., 1994). As would be expected from the diffuse projections of the histaminergic system, H_1 receptors were found throughout the brain, but were distributed in a heterogeneous manner. Receptor binding was observed in all cortical layers, although layer 4 tended to display a higher receptor density than other layers. Moderate to heavy binding was found in various limbic system structures, including the hippocampus, amygdala (particularly the medial nucleus), and septal area. Many hypothalamic nuclei also showed substantial receptor density in both rats and guinea pigs; however, thalamic labeling was more pronounced in guinea pigs. The caudate–putamen exhibited a fairly low density of H_1 receptors in both species. On the other hand, the cerebellum was very rich in H_1 receptor mRNA in the Purkinje cells, and showed dense receptor binding in the molecular layer (where the Purkinje cell dendrites are located). This finding was unexpected, given that the cerebellum receives only a sparse histaminergic innervation. The reason for this discrepancy is not known; however, it is worth mentioning that such "receptor mismatches" have been described for other neurotransmitters and neuropeptides (for example, see the section on substance P in Chapter 11).

H_2 receptor binding sites have been localized in guinea pig and human brains using the potent and selective antagonist [^{125}I]iodoaminopotentidine. In guinea pigs, high densities of H_2 receptor binding were observed in the striatum, nucleus accumbens, olfactory tubercles, layers 1–3 of the cerebral cortex, and areas of the hippocampal formation (Ruat et al., 1990). The hypothalamus displayed only a low level of H_2 receptors. Similar results were found for the human brain (Traiffort et al., 1992). When the distributions of H_1 and H_2 receptors are compared, it appears that the H_1 subtype is most important in the hypothalamus, the H_2 subtype mediates histaminergic action in the striatum, and both subtypes are present in many other brain areas.

Finally, H_3 receptor distribution in the rat brain has been studied with $[^3H]R$-α-methylhistamine. Moderate to high receptor densities were found in the cerebral cortex (particularly the deep layers 4–6), striatum, globus pallidus, nucleus accumbens, olfactory tubercles, substantia nigra pars reticulata, and certain nuclei within the hypothalamus and amygdala (Pollard et al., 1993). Interestingly, unilateral disruption of ascending histaminergic pathways produced by electrolytic lesions of the medial forebrain bundle caused an *increase* in ipsilateral striatal and cortical H_3 receptor binding, rather than the expected decrease. In addition, striatal infusions of kainic acid (which cause cell loss but spare axons and nerve terminals) led to a decrease in striatal H_3 receptors. These findings, along with significant disparities between H_3 receptor density and abundance of histaminergic fibers, strongly suggest that many H_3 receptors are located postsynaptically rather than on nerve endings (Pollard et al., 1993).

The Role of Histamine in Neural and Behavioral Functions

Electrophysiological Effects

The effects of histamine on neural activity have been studied using a variety of in vivo and in vitro approaches. Iontophoretic application of histamine has generally been found to inhibit the firing of neurons in the cerebral cortex, brain stem, and spinal cord (Haas, 1985). These effects can be blocked by metiamide or cimetidine and mimicked by impromidine, indicating an important role for H_2 receptors. Although H_2-mediated inhibition has also been observed for some neurons in the hypothalamus, many cells in this area are excited by histamine application. Such stimulation can be blocked with mepyramine, and thus appears to involve H_1 receptors.

Histamine was recently reported to exert a novel action on NMDA receptor–mediated excitatory synaptic potentials in cultured rat hippocampal neurons. Application of histamine increased the amplitude of such potentials, while having no effect on non-NMDA glutamate receptor currents, $GABA_A$ receptor currents, or currents carried by voltage-gated Na^+ or K^+ channels (Bekkers, 1993). The potentiating effect of histamine was mimicked by the H_3 receptor agonist R-α-methylhistamine, but not by H_1 or H_2 agonist application. On the other hand, the effect was not blocked by the H_3 antagonist thioperamide. The ability of histamine to enhance NMDA receptor action suggests that this transmitter could modulate processes in which NMDA receptors have been implicated, such as excitotoxicity or long-term potentiation.

Behavioral Functions

Histamine has been implicated in the regulation of a wide range of behavioral and physiological functions in humans and animals, including ingestive behaviors (eating and drinking), sleep and arousal, motor activity, learning, sexual behavior, aggression, pain perception, pituitary gland activity, thermoregulation, and regulation of blood pressure (for review, see Hough, 1988; Onodera et al., 1994; White and Rumbold, 1988). Wada and colleagues have suggested that the diversity of these effects, along with the morphological features of the histaminergic system, indicates that this system plays a widespread and basic role in neural functioning (see Onodera et al., 1994; Wada et al., 1991). Whether or not this view is accurate, it seems clear that histamine is significantly involved in the modulation of arousal. Such involvement has been personally experienced by every individual who has suffered from the drowsiness produced by classic antihistamines (i.e., H_1 antagonists). This effect is recognized in the *Physician's Desk Reference,* where the frequent "adverse reactions" listed for diphenhydramine (Benadryl) include sedation, sleepiness, dizziness, and disturbed coordination. The remainder of this chapter will therefore be devoted to considering the possible functions of histamine in sleep–waking mechanisms and psychomotor performance (since performance on psychomotor tasks is strongly influenced by information processing and level of arousal).

Sleep–waking cycle. In considering how histamine could be involved in the sleep–waking cycle, we might first ask whether the activity of histaminergic neurons follows a circadian rhythm. In rats, histamine overflow in the anterior hypothalamus was shown to be higher during the dark period of the day–night cycle (when the animals are most active) than during the light period (Mochizuki et al., 1992; Figure 10.39). The relationship between histaminergic cell activity and waking was confirmed in a diurnal (daytime-active) species, the rhesus monkey, in which transmitter output was greatest during the light period of the day–night cycle (see Onodera et al., 1994). These neurochemical results are consistent with electrophysiological studies demonstrating that the firing rate of histamine neurons correlates positively with the degree of arousal—that is, it is lower during sleep than during waking (reviewed by Monti, 1993).

Studies on cats have revealed further information concerning the involvement of histamine in sleep and waking. EEG recordings permit the differentiation of four neurobehavioral states in this species: wakefulness (W), light slow-wave sleep (S1), deep slow-wave sleep (S2), and paradoxical or rapid-eye-movement sleep (PS). Intraperitoneal injection of either the histidine decarboxylase inhibitor α-FMH or the H_1 antagonist mepyramine increased S2 and decreased W over the following 22 hours (Lin, Sakai, and Jouvet, 1988; Figure 10.40). Similar effects were observed when the drugs were administered directly into the ventrolateral posterior hypothalamus instead of being given systemically. Further-

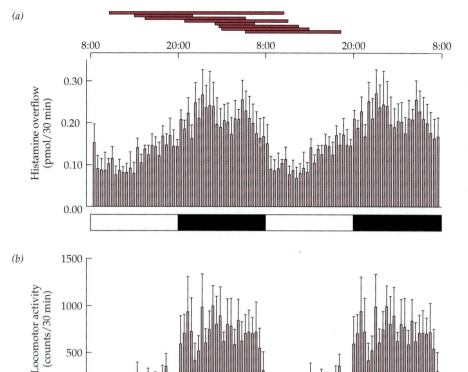

(a)

10.39 CIRCADIAN VARIATION IN ANTE-
RIOR HYPOTHALAMIC HISTAMINE
OVERFLOW AND ITS RELATIONSHIP TO
LOCOMOTOR ACTIVITY IN RATS. Rats
with microdialysis probes in the anterior
hypothalamic area were studied in a behavioral test chamber maintained under a
12:12-hour light–dark cycle. (*a*) Histamine
overflow and (*b*) spontaneous locomotor
activity were recorded for 30-minute time
blocks during various phases of the cycle
(topmost horizontal bars). Histamine overflow and locomotor activity both peaked
during the dark period of the light–dark
cycle (black bars). (After Mochizuki et al.,
1992.)

more, hypothalamic injections of either histamine itself
or SKF-91488, a specific inhibitor of histamine *N*-methyl-
transferase, produced an increase in W but a reduction
in S2 and PS. The effects of histamine were completely
prevented by pretreatment with mepyramine. In a subsequent study, the H_3 agonist R-α-methylhistamine, which
suppresses histamine synthesis and release, led to increased S2 (Lin et al., 1990). In contrast, the H_3 antagonist thioperamide produced an increase in W.

These findings indicate that in cats, histamine acting
through H_1 receptors serves to promote waking (W) and
to suppress deep slow-wave sleep (S2). Research concerning the influence of H_1 histamine antagonists on
sleep patterns in humans has yielded more variable results. Some investigators have reported positive effects in
terms of increased sleep time or decreased sleep latency,
whereas others have found no changes (reviewed by
White and Rumbold, 1988).

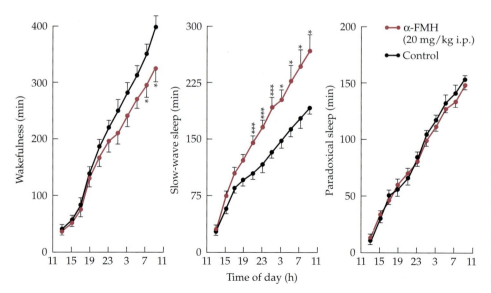

10.40 THE EFFECTS OF INHIBITING
HISTAMINE SYNTHESIS ON SLEEP
AND WAKEFULNESS IN CATS. Subjects were injected with the irreversible
histidine decarboxylase inhibitor α-
FMH at 11:00 A.M., and the cumulative
amounts of wakefulness, deep slow-
wave sleep, and paradoxical sleep
were measured over the next 22 hours.
Compared with the same subjects
given saline instead, inhibition of histamine synthesis led to a significant decline in wakefulness, an increase in
slow-wave sleep, and no change in
paradoxical sleep. (*p < .05,***p < .01
compared with saline). (After Lin,
Sakai, and Jouvet, 1988.)

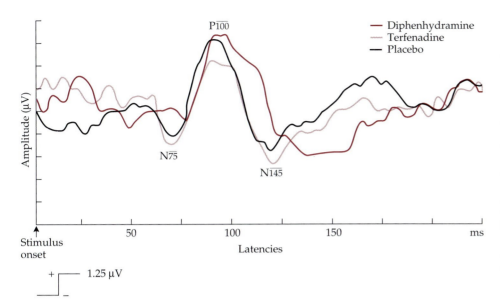

10.41 INCREASED PATTERN REVERSAL EVOKED POTENTIAL (PREP) LATENCIES PRODUCED BY A CLASSIC, BUT NOT A NONSEDATING, ANTIHISTAMINE. Cortical evoked potentials were recorded during reversal of a patterned visual stimulus (black-and-white checkerboard). The figure depicts averaged PREP recorded from a single subject 2.25 hours after administration of either the classic antihistamine diphenhydramine (50 mg), the nonsedating antihistamine terfenadine (60 mg), or placebo. Diphenhydramine produced a significant increase in latencies for the P$\overline{100}$ and P$\overline{145}$ waveforms, which suggests a slowdown in visual information processing. (After Tharion, McMenemy, and Rauch, 1994.)

Psychomotor performance. Patients who take classic (i.e., sedating) antihistamines are warned not to drive or engage in other activities requiring skilled psychomotor performance while under medication. In following these instructions, many individuals evaluate the influence of the drug (in terms of determining when it is safe to drive, for example) by monitoring their state of drowsiness. However, certain experimental findings suggest that impairment in psychomotor performance does not coincide with subjective ratings of drowsiness (reviewed by Manning and Gengo, 1993). Thus, it is important to establish directly whether different antihistamine drugs cause decreased performance on various types of psychomotor tasks.

Researchers have examined the effects of antihistamines on four aspects of psychomotor performance: sensory processing (e.g., vigilance tasks), central integration and processing (e.g., critical flicker fusion and digit symbol substitution tasks), overt motor responses (finger tapping or body sway), and overall sensorimotor coordination (e.g., tasks requiring visual–motor coordination, such as various tracking tasks). In general, classic antihistamines cause impaired performance in all of these domains, whereas few or no effects occur following acute treatment with the newer antihistamines that exhibit poorer penetration across the blood–brain barrier (Manning and Gengo, 1993).

Tharion, McMenemy, and Rauch (1994) recently demonstrated an electrophysiological correlate of the psychomotor impairment produced by sedating, but not nonsedating, antihistamines. These researchers compared the effects of diphenhydramine and terfenadine on the Pattern Reversed Evoked Potential (PREP), an electrophysiological response elicited by a reversing black-and-white checkerboard pattern. As illustrated in Figure 10.41, the PREP involves three major waveforms: negative-going potentials at approximately 75 ms (N$\overline{75}$)

and 145 ms (N$\overline{145}$) following stimulus onset, and a positive-going potential at 100 ms (P$\overline{100}$). Of interest is the finding that diphenhydramine, but not terfenadine, caused a significant increase in latency of the P$\overline{100}$ and N$\overline{145}$ potentials from 1 to 3 hours after drug administration (N$\overline{75}$ latency was increased at 2 hours only). As the PREP is believed to be produced by the visual cortex, these findings suggest that classic antihistamines slow down visual information processing in the cortex, and thus help to explain the deleterious effects of such drugs in many tests of psychomotor performance.

Part IV Summary

Histamine is a biological regulator best known for its participation in various allergic and inflammatory reactions. This role is related to the synthesis and release of histamine from certain connective tissue cells called mast cells, which can produce vascular effects such as local vasodilation and increased vascular permeability. In the brain, histamine is found both in mast cells and in a small population of neurons.

Histamine is synthesized from histidine in a single reaction catalyzed by the enzyme histidine decarboxylase. The drug α-FMH is an important inhibitor of histidine decarboxylase, and has been used experimentally to deplete endogenous histamine stores. Histidine administration leads to increased brain levels and release of histamine, indicating that histidine decarboxylase is probably not saturated in vivo with its substrate.

In contrast to other biogenic amines, no uptake system appears to be present to remove histamine from the synapse following its release. However, histamine can be inactivated enzymatically through a pathway that leads to the major metabolite 3-(tele)-methyl-imidazoleacetic acid. The first step in this pathway is catalyzed by the enzyme histamine *N*-methyltransferase.

Histaminergic neurons are found exclusively in the hypothalamus. In the rat brain, these cells are localized even more specifically to a collection of five clusters (designated E1–E5) within a region of the basal posterior hypothalamus called the tuberomammillary nucleus (TM). In contrast to the highly restricted localization of histaminergic cell bodies, the cells give rise to widespread projections, with a moderate to high density of fibers in the hypothalamus, medial septum, diagonal band, cerebral cortex, and amygdala. Immunohistochemical studies indicate that neuronal histamine is colocalized with other neuroactive substances or their synthetic enzymes. These substances include GABA, adenosine deaminase, and several neuropeptides.

Histamine receptors include three known subtypes, H_1, H_2, and H_3. The first two have been cloned, and belong to the G protein–coupled receptor superfamily. H_1 receptors mediate the contractile effects of histamine on the guinea pig trachea, ileum, and uterus via stimulation of the phosphoinositide/protein kinase C second messenger system. Classic antihistaminergic drugs such as mepyramine and diphenhydramine are all H_1 receptor blockers. Few selective H_1 agonists are available, although the compound 2-thiazolylethylamine has some usefulness in this regard. H_1 receptors exhibit a widespread distribution in the brain, but are particularly enriched in the hypothalamus, cerebellum, and various limbic system structures.

H_2 receptors are known to stimulate adenylyl cyclase activity and hence increase cAMP synthesis. Like the H_1 receptor, this subtype is involved in several peripheral effects of histamine, including stimulation of gastric acid secretion and contraction of the rat uterus and guinea pig atrium. The ability of the selective H_2 antagonists cimetidine and ranitidine to reduce gastric acidity has led to their widespread use in treating gastric and duodenal ulcers. The compound dimaprit is one of several H_2 agonists available for experimental studies.

The central localization of H_2 receptors differs somewhat from that of the H_1 subtype, with high densities in the striatum and other forebrain dopamine terminal areas.

The H_3 receptor was first discovered in the context of its function as a terminal autoreceptor that inhibits histamine synthesis and release. Subsequently, however, evidence has been obtained for H_3 heteroreceptors that presynaptically inhibit the release of other transmitters, and possibly even postsynaptic H_3 receptors. The drugs R-α-methylhistamine and thioperamide function as an H_3 agonist and antagonist respectively. The H_3 subtype exhibits a somewhat different distribution than either H_1 or H_2 receptors.

Local application of histamine generally inhibits cell firing in the cerebral cortex, brain stem, and spinal cord, apparently via an action of H_2 receptors. On the other hand, it excites many hypothalamic cells through stimulation of H_1 receptors. In cultured hippocampal neurons, histamine has also been reported to increase the amplitude of NMDA receptor-mediated excitatory synaptic potentials. This finding suggests that histamine could play a previously unsuspected role in mechanisms involving NMDA receptors and neural plasticity or toxicity.

Finally, classic H_1 receptor-blocking antihistamines have long been known to exert significant sedative effects. This observation has led to various studies, particularly in cats, showing that activation of these receptors promotes wakefulness and suppresses deep slow-wave sleep. In humans, traditional H_1 receptor antagonists produce measurable decrements in psychomotor performance and impair visual information processing as measured by evoked potential recording. However, these effects are lacking in a newer generation of H_1-blocking agents, such as astemizole, terfenadine, and loratadine, that show poorer penetration across the blood–brain barrier. These compounds are now available for allergy sufferers who wish to avoid the drowsiness associated with earlier drug formulations.

Chapter 11

Peptide Neurotransmitters

The Discovery of Peptides in the Nervous System

The generation of neuropharmacologists trained in the 1960s and early 1970s was taught that there were only about half a dozen transmitters in the nervous system, including acetylcholine, norepinephrine, dopamine, serotonin, GABA, and perhaps glutamate. Current estimates would place the number at well over 50, and it is increasing all the time. What has transpired over the past 25 years or so to cause such a massive change in our concept of neurotransmitter diversity? The main answer to this question is that from the 1970s onward, a great variety of peptide transmitters have been discovered in the brain as well as in the peripheral nervous system.

The current era of peptide neurobiology was ushered in by research that proceeded along four different fronts. One of these was the discovery of endorphins and enkephalins, peptides that exert effects similar to those of opiate drugs such as morphine. Opioid peptides are presented in detail in Chapter 12 and therefore will not be covered here. However, the remaining three lines of work will each be discussed briefly from a historical perspective to show their contributions to the birth of modern neuropeptide research. More recent advances in peptide research are summarized in an excellent review by Hökfelt (1991) and are discussed in subsequent sections of this chapter.

Vasopressin, Oxytocin, and the Concept of Neurosecretion

Our first historical theme concerns two peptide hormones, vasopressin and oxytocin, that are found in the posterior lobe of the pituitary gland (also called the neurohypophysis or pars nervosa). Endocrinologists had determined that these substances were clearly secreted from the neurohypophysis, but there were questions about whether the hormones were synthesized there as well. Pioneering work by Bargmann, Scharrer, and their colleagues (Bargmann and Scharrer, 1951) established that vasopressin and oxytocin were actually made by nerve cells in the hypothalamus and then transported to release sites in the pituitary gland. Bargmann and Scharrer used the term *neurosecretion* to refer to the ability of these and other nerve cells to manufacture and secrete physiologically active substances into the circulation. As we shall see, almost all such compounds have since turned out to be peptides and to be used as both transmitters and hormones.

Hypothalamic Releasing Hormones

The second theme in the evolution of neuropeptide research is linked to another major part of the pituitary gland, the anterior lobe (also known as the adenohypophysis or pars distalis). This part of the gland secretes a number of important hormones, including adrenocorticotropin, thyrotropin, growth hormone, luteinizing hormone, follicle-stimulating hormone, and prolactin. Early studies showed that these hormones were under significant CNS control; however, there was little evidence for a direct neural connection between the brain and the pars distalis. As stated by Geoffrey Harris in 1948, "The pars distalis of the pituitary may, in general terms, be described as a gland under nervous control but lacking a nerve supply." The solution to this seeming paradox was provided by the discovery of a system of blood vessels, called the pituitary portal system, linking the adenohypophysis with the hypothalamus. When nerve terminals were later found to come into close proximity with the portal vessels in the median eminence region of the hypothalamus (see the discussion below for more details), Harris brilliantly hypothesized that chemical factors might be secreted from these terminals into the portal circulation and then travel to the pituitary gland, where they could regulate the secretion of the anterior pituitary hormones. Further studies showed that if the pituitary stalk connecting the gland to the brain is severed, relatively normal secretory activity can be restored if the gland is replaced in or near its normal position, but not if it is transplanted to a distant site (Harris, 1955). Because pituitary glands replaced in their normal location are revascularized by portal blood vessels, but do not regrow their neuronal connections, this result provided strong (though still indirect) support for Harris' theory.

Once it was clear that the hypothalamus must contain various substances that serve as "releasing hormones" (so named because they all serve to either stimulate or inhibit the release of an anterior pituitary hormone), several laboratories began striving to identify these factors. The laboratories of Roger Guillemin and of Andrew Schally engaged in a particularly fierce competition to isolate and identify the first hypothalamic releasing hormone (Wade, 1978a,b,c). Their task was extremely difficult because these substances are present in tissues in only nanogram amounts. The researchers had to acquire hypothalami from hundreds of thousands of freshly slaughtered swine and sheep to obtain many kilograms of tissue. From this material, after 20 years of intense work, they isolated a few milligrams of purified thyrotropin-releasing hormone (TRH).*

TRH turned out to be a peptide, as did almost all of the other releasing hormones that were later characterized. The discovery of hypothalamic releasing hormones further supported the concept of neurosecretion as envisioned earlier by Bargmann and Scharrer, and the chemical identity of these substances focused increased attention on peptide communication in the nervous system.

As a final note to this story, the work of Guillemin and Schally was aided by the development of a new method of analysis—radioimmunoassay—that enabled the detection of minute quantities of compounds. Rosalyn Yalow and Solomon Berson were credited with the development of this technique (Yalow, 1978), and in 1977, Yalow, Guillemin, and Schally shared the Nobel Prize in medicine.†

Substance P: The First Gut–Brain Peptide

In 1931, von Euler and Gaddum reported the discovery of a substance in the intestine that exerted powerful contractile effects when applied directly to intestinal smooth muscle and hypotensive effects when injected intravenously. A similar biological activity was detected in brain extracts, suggesting that the same chemical might be present in both the brain and the gut (i.e., the gastrointestinal tract). In their work, von Euler and Gaddum prepared their crude tissue extracts as a dry powder that was abbreviated in their notes simply as "P," and within a few years, the material began to be called substance P (von Euler, 1985). Although subsequent studies suggested that substance P might be a protein or peptide, the compound was not fully characterized until almost 40 years later by Chang and Leeman (1970). Since its original discovery, substance P has been found to play important roles as a sensory transmitter in the peripheral nervous system and as a centrally acting neuropeptide.

The Biochemistry of Peptides

Peptide Structure and Synthesis

Before proceeding with our discussion of peptides and neurotransmission, it is appropriate to summarize the general features of peptide biochemistry. To begin, a peptide is simply a chain of two or more amino acids. Peptides differ from proteins only in that they are smaller (a molecular weight of at least 10 kDa generally qualifies a peptide chain as a protein), and that proteins may be made up of more than one peptide chain. Adjacent amino acids in a peptide or protein are linked to each other by a type of chemical bond called a **peptide bond** (Figure 11.1). As all peptide bonds are assumed to be identical, it is the side chains of the amino acid residues (designated R_1 and R_2 in the figure) that give a particular peptide its chemical identity and biological function. Structurally, a peptide is considered to begin with the amino group at one end (referred to as the amino or N-terminus and conventionally oriented to the left) and to terminate with the carboxyl group at the other end (referred to as the carboxyl or C-terminus and conventionally oriented to the right). Thus, if R_1 happened to represent a tyrosine residue and R_2 a leucine residue, the

---

*Guillemin estimated that the cost of isolating the first milligram of pure thyrotropin-releasing hormone from 300,000 sheep hypothalami was two to five times the cost of transporting a kilogram of moon rock to Earth by the Apollo 13 mission. The cost was borne mainly by the National Institutes of Health and the Veterans Administration (Meites, 1977).

---

†Berson was deceased by that time, and Nobel Prizes are not awarded posthumously.

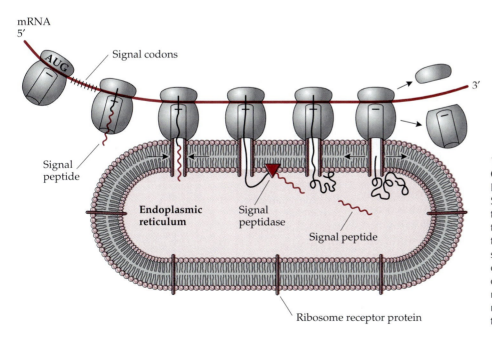

$$H_3\overset{+}{N}-\overset{R_1}{\underset{H}{\overset{|}{C}}}-\overset{O}{\overset{||}{C}}\overset{O}{\underset{O^-}{}} \quad + \quad H-\overset{H}{\underset{H}{\overset{|}{N}}}-\overset{R_2}{\underset{H}{\overset{|}{C}}}-\overset{O}{\overset{||}{C}}\overset{O}{\underset{O^-}{}}$$

Amino acid 1 **Amino acid 2**

$\longrightarrow H_2O$

$$H_3\overset{+}{N}-\overset{R_1}{\underset{H}{\overset{|}{C}}}-\overset{O}{\overset{||}{C}}-\overset{}{\underset{H}{\overset{|}{N}}}-\overset{R_2}{\underset{H}{\overset{|}{C}}}-\overset{O}{\overset{}{C}}\overset{O}{\underset{O^-}{}}$$

Peptide bond

11.1 FORMATION OF A PEPTIDE BOND.

dipeptide (a term for any peptide containing two amino acids) shown in Figure 11.1 would be tyrosine–leucine.

Many years ago, biochemists determined that proteins are synthesized on cellular organelles known as ribosomes (see Chapter 3). The sequence of amino acids constituting a given protein is coded by the messenger RNA (mRNA) transcribed from the gene (DNA) for that protein. This fact is equally applicable to neuropeptides because all neuropeptides appear to come from larger precursor proteins called **propeptides**. The principle that secretory peptides are initially synthesized as larger precursors was first elucidated by Steiner and Dyer (1967) for the peptide hormone insulin. However, there is an additional factor in peptide synthesis that was not appreciated in the earliest studies. The mRNA transcribed from a secretory peptide gene is now known to code for

an even larger molecule than the propeptide mentioned above. Such a precursor to the propeptide is called a **pre-propeptide**. (Fortunately, there is no precursor to the pre-propeptide, because we've probably run out of suitable prefixes!) The difference between a propeptide and its corresponding pre-propeptide is a stretch of hydrophobic amino acids at the N-terminus called a **signal sequence**. When a protein is being synthesized, the presence of this signal sequence causes the associated ribosomes to bind to the membrane of the endoplasmic reticulum (ER) (Figure 11.2) (Blobel et al., 1979), enabling the newly made protein to enter the interior of the ER. This signal is part of a complex process that designates a protein (or peptide) either for eventual insertion into a membrane or for secretion by the cell (as in the case of peptide transmitters and hormones). Inside the ER, the protein can be chemically modified in several ways, such as the attachment of certain sugars that occurs in the formation of glycoproteins. The signal sequence is no longer needed once the protein has entered the ER, and is cleaved off by a specific enzyme called a signal peptidase to yield the propeptide. To summarize, neuropeptides are synthesized in a sequential process, beginning with a pre-propeptide. The presence of a signal sequence allows the newly formed pre-propeptide to enter the ER, where it is converted into a propeptide and subjected to additional chemical modification. Prior to secretion, the active peptide is liberated from the propeptide in a manner to be described below.

Peptide Catabolism

Peptides are broken down into inactive fragments by enzymes called **peptidases**. Peptidases hydrolyze peptide bonds; that is, they cleave the bond with the addition of

11.2 SYNTHESIS AND PROCESSING OF SECRETORY AND MEMBRANE PROTEINS ACCORDING TO THE SIGNAL HYPOTHESIS. Proteins destined for eventual secretion or for insertion into a membrane are initially synthesized with a hydrophobic signal sequence at the N-terminus of the molecule. This signal results in translocation of the protein into the endoplasmic reticulum, where the signal sequence is removed and other chemical modifications are made. (After Stryer, 1981.)

$$\underset{\text{Peptide}}{\overset{\displaystyle R_1 \quad O \qquad R_2 \quad O}{\sim\!\sim\!\sim\!N-C-C-N-C-C\sim\!\sim} + H_2O} \longrightarrow \underset{\substack{\text{Carboxyl}\\\text{component}}}{\sim\!\sim\!\sim\!N-C-C \overset{O}{\underset{O^-}{}}} + \underset{\substack{\text{Amino}\\\text{component}}}{H_3\overset{+}{N}-C-C\sim\!\sim}$$

11.3 HYDROLYSIS OF A PEPTIDE BOND BY A PEPTIDASE.

a molecule of water. Peptide bond hydrolysis is illustrated schematically in Figure 11.3. There are two broad classes of peptidases: exopeptidases and endopeptidases. An exopeptidase cleaves off one amino acid at the very end of the peptide. A given exopeptidase is always specific either for the carboxy (—COOH) terminus of the peptide, in which case it is called a carboxypeptidase, or for the amino (NH$_2$—) terminus, in which case it is called an aminopeptidase. Endopeptidases hydrolyze peptide bonds within the interior of the molecule, thereby cleaving off groups of two or more amino acids from the original peptide. Each type of endopeptidase also is selective in its action, preferring to act on peptide bonds adjacent to specific amino acid residues or on bonds at a particular physical location in the peptide. Peptidases that are thought to be important in terminating the action of peptide transmitters are located on the surface of the plasma membrane, where they can operate effectively on peptides released into the extracellular space (Schwartz et al., 1991).

Features of Peptidergic Transmission

Peptides versus Classical Transmitters

The use of peptides by neurons exhibits several important differences from the so-called "classical" transmitters (e.g., acetylcholine, catecholamines, serotonin, and amino acids) described earlier. A general comparison between peptides and classical transmitters is shown in Figure 11.4. In the case of classical transmitters, the enzyme(s) needed to form the transmitter (e.g., choline acetyltransferase or tyrosine hydroxylase), along with vesicles for storing the transmitter, are synthesized in the cell soma. These elements are then transported down the axon to the nerve terminals by the anterograde transport system described in Chapter 3. Vesicle filling occurs at several different locations, including the soma, the terminals, and possibly also the axon. Exocytotic release of transmitter from the vesicles occurs at specialized regions of the terminal called active zones. Following release, molecules of the transmitter or its breakdown products (such as choline) are taken back up by the presynaptic cell. Finally, replenishment of transmitter stores occurs primarily in the terminal region via a combination of reuptake and resynthesis.

A number of elements in this scenario differ for peptide transmitters. As mentioned above, peptides are initially synthesized as propeptides in the soma and then packaged into vesicles. Converting enzymes (specific endo- and exopeptidases) are necessary to process the precursor appropriately into the active transmitter. Although some processing may occur before packaging, this step is generally thought to occur mainly via the action of peptidases present with the propeptide inside the vesicles (Gainer, Russell, and Loh, 1985). At the nerve terminals, release of the peptide along with the other vesicle contents occurs through exocytosis, as indicated previously for classical transmitters. However, peptide release is not limited to areas of synaptic specialization in the nerve terminals (Morris and Pow, 1991). Furthermore, no formation or packaging of peptides occurs in the nerve terminals because of the lack of mRNA and the necessary cellular organelles. Therefore, neurons can resupply the terminals with peptide transmitters only by synthesizing more propeptide in the soma and shipping it to the terminal area (some cells may cope with this

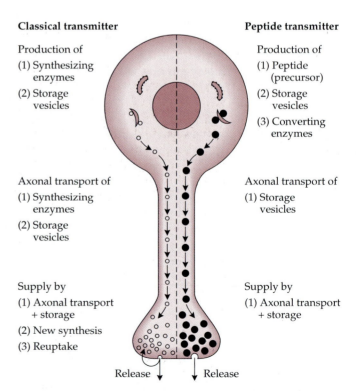

Classical transmitter	Peptide transmitter
Production of (1) Synthesizing enzymes (2) Storage vesicles	Production of (1) Peptide (precursor) (2) Storage vesicles (3) Converting enzymes
Axonal transport of (1) Synthesizing enzymes (2) Storage vesicles	Axonal transport of (1) Storage vesicles
Supply by (1) Axonal transport + storage (2) New synthesis (3) Reuptake	Supply by (1) Axonal transport + storage

Release   Release

11.4 CELLULAR PROCESSES INVOLVED IN THE SYNTHESIS, STORAGE, AND TRANSPORT OF NEUROPEPTIDES VERSUS "CLASSICAL" NEUROTRANSMITTERS. (After Hökfelt et al., 1980.)

problem by storing a large pool of peptide for use when needed; Morgan and Chubb, 1991). With regard to inactivation, the peptidases described above are thought to break down peptides released synaptically. Reuptake is another possible mechanism whereby peptide action could be terminated (McKelvy and Blumberg, 1986); however, this mechanism does not appear to be of major significance.

Coexistence of Peptides with Classical Transmitters

Dale's principle.   Until the early 1970s, it was generally thought that a given neuron utilized only one specific transmitter in communicating with other cells. This idea was often erroneously referred to as "Dale's principle," after the eminent physiologist Sir Henry Dale. Forty years earlier, Dale had in fact said,

> When we are dealing with two different endings of the same sensory neurone, the one peripheral . . . and the other at a central synapse, can we suppose that the discovery and identification of a chemical transmitter [at the peripheral ending] . . . would furnish a hint as to the nature of the transmission process at the central synapse?

(Dale, 1935). Dale's question is basically a speculation that the same transmitter is released at all branches of a particular neuron. When subsequent evidence offered support for this hypothesis, Sir John Eccles codified the hypothesis into a formal statement that he called Dale's principle (Eccles, 1957). Thus, Dale's principle actually concerns the chemical unity of neurons (i.e., different terminals of the same cell behave similarly) rather than the question of how many transmitters a cell might utilize.

Neurotransmitter coexistence.

Neurotransmitter coexistence.   If it was once thought that each neuron synthesized only a single transmitter, the situation has changed so radically that we can hardly find any remaining examples of cell populations containing fewer than two transmitter substances! In fact, up to six different potential transmitters have been found in some neurons (Furness et al., 1989). Several different technical approaches can be used to demonstrate neurotransmitter coexistence, most of which utilize immunohistochemistry (for review, see Hökfelt et al., 1987). Although histochemical techniques are quite useful for determining the localization of a chemical substance, the substance must also be shown to be released from cells under physiological conditions for it to be accorded neurotransmitter status. This additional information is still lacking in many instances of transmitter coexistence, although researchers often assume that release will ultimately be demonstrated when the necessary experiments are finally performed.

Several different patterns of neurotransmitter coexistence are possible, including:

1. One neuropeptide and at least one classical transmitter;
2. Multiple neuropeptides, all derived from the same propeptide, with or without a classical transmitter;
3. Multiple neuropeptides derived from separate propeptides, with or without a classical transmitter;
4. Two or more classical transmitters with no neuropeptides.

All of these possibilities may exist in nature; in practice, however, it is impossible for investigators to be certain that a particular group of cells expresses *only* the peptide(s) and/or classical transmitter(s) currently known to be present in those cells. New peptides as well as new nonpeptide transmitters continue to be discovered, creating additional possibilities for transmitter coexistence that had not been previously considered. Nonetheless, based on our current understanding, a few selected examples of transmitter coexistence can be given (for more examples, see Furness et al., 1989; Hökfelt et al., 1987; O'Donohue et al., 1985). In the peripheral nervous system, some guinea pig primary sensory neurons contain substance P colocalized with other peptides (Morris and Gibbins, 1989), whereas postganglionic cholinergic neurons innervating the cat salivary gland also contain the peptide vasoactive intestinal peptide (VIP) (Lundberg and Hökfelt, 1983). As illustrated in Figure 11.5, a complex array of peptides is present in the noradrenergic sympathetic neurons of the guinea pig superior cervical ganglion (Morris and Gibbins, 1989). Furthermore, enkephalins are found in conjunction with catecholamines in chromaffin granules of the adrenal medulla and are secreted upon stimulation of the chromaffin cells (Viveros and Wilson, 1983).

Peptides also commonly coexist with classical transmitters in the central nervous system. Some notable examples are:

1. The colocalization of either cholecystokinin (CCK) or neurotensin (NT) in some dopaminergic neurons of the mesolimbic and mesocortical pathways;
2. The presence of substance P and/or thyrotropin-releasing hormone (TRH) in certain serotonergic cell groups in the medulla;
3. The presence of the peptide galanin in neurons of the basal forebrain cholinergic system;
4. The colocalization of GABA either with enkephalins or with substance P and dynorphin (another opioid peptide) in output neurons of the caudate–putamen (Hökfelt et al., 1987).

Unfortunately, researchers have not discovered any consistent principles for predicting the coexistence of peptides with specific classical transmitters. CCK, for ex-

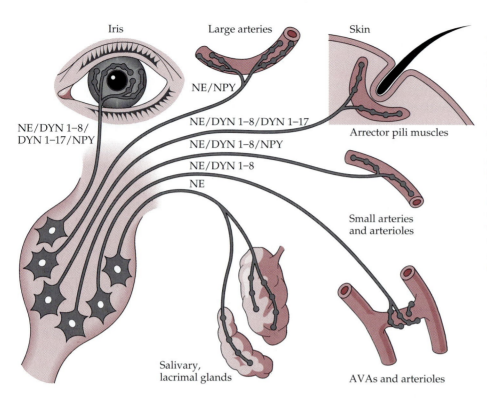

11.5 COEXISTENCE OF PEPTIDES WITH NOREPINEPHRINE in guinea pig sympathetic neurons. Sympathetic fibers from the guinea pig superior cervical ganglion have been found to contain not only norepinephrine (NE) but also a variety of peptides, including neuropeptide Y (NPY) and two different forms of the opioid peptide dynorphin A (DYN 1–8 and DYN 1–17). All of the dynorphin A-containing cells also contain dynorphin B as well as α-neo-endorphin. Different subpopulations of these ganglionic neurons innervate various target organs and contain different combinations of colocalized peptides, except for those innervating the salivary and lacrimal glands AVAs = arteriovenous anastomoses. (After Morris and Gibbins, 1989.)

ample, is found only in a subset of dopaminergic neurons, and is also present in certain nondopaminergic cells.

The concept of neuromodulation.   The discovery of neurotransmitter coexistence has engendered a great deal of excitement among researchers, as aptly stated in a com-

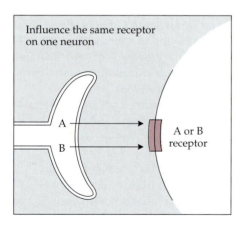

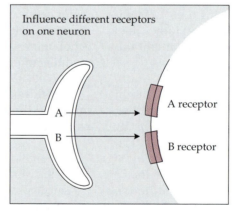

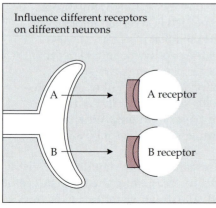

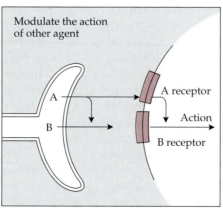

11.6 SOME POSSIBLE INTERACTIONS OF COEXISTING NEUROTRANSMITTERS OR NEUROMODULATORS. (After O'Donohue et al., 1985.)

ment by Bartfai and his coworkers: "The joy of neurobiologists at the discovery of the coexistence of several neuroactive substances within the same neuron terminals can be compared with the delight of a man who has bought a radio he thought would only receive AM broadcasts, but who then discovers that it also gets all the FM stations" (Bartfai et al., 1988). More importantly, the implications of neurotransmitter coexistence for understanding neuronal communication are enormous. Even the simplest case in which just two signaling agents are released by the same cell allows for many functional possibilities, some of which are illustrated in Figure 11.6. Each agent might act independently on the same or different target cells, one substance might alter the sensitivity of target cells to the other substance, or one substance might act presynaptically to influence the release of the other substance (Bartfai et al., 1988; Furness et al., 1989; Kow and Pfaff, 1988). Obviously, these possibilities are multiplied manyfold when more than two different compounds are involved.

Co-storage also plays an important role in determining the nature of neurotransmitter interactions. In some cases, such as adrenal chromaffin cells, peptides are found in the same storage granules or vesicles as the classical transmitter. In many systems, however, nerve terminals contain two populations of vesicles: small vesicles (either clear or dense-core) that contain only the classical transmitter, and large dense-core granules that contain the peptide(s) and perhaps small amounts of the classical transmitter. If only a single population of vesicles exists that stores all of the cell's neurotransmitter substances, those substances are normally co-released upon stimulation. On the other hand, the existence of two different vesicle populations allows for the possibility of selective release of peptides and classical transmitters (Matteoli, Reetz, and De Camilli, 1991). This phenomenon has been observed in some systems in which low-frequency stimulation evokes release of only the classical transmitter, whereas higher frequencies or bursts of impulses lead to release of the coexisting peptide as well (Figure 11.7; Hökfelt, 1991; Hökfelt et al., 1987).

In some cases in which a coexisting peptide interacts with a classical transmitter to alter a cellular response, it has been found that the peptide alone exerts no effect on the cell. In such cases, should the peptide be called a neurotransmitter? The term **neuromodulator** was coined to denote a substance (often a peptide) that modulates the action of a transmitter rather than having a direct physiological effect of its own. A prime example of this kind of neuromodulation was demonstrated by Lundberg and colleagues in their elegant studies of vasoactive intestinal peptide (VIP) and acetylcholine (ACh) in the cat submandibular salivary gland (Lundberg and Hökfelt, 1983). Postganglionic parasympathetic fibers from the submandibular ganglion enter the submandibular salivary gland, where they form endings on both the secretory

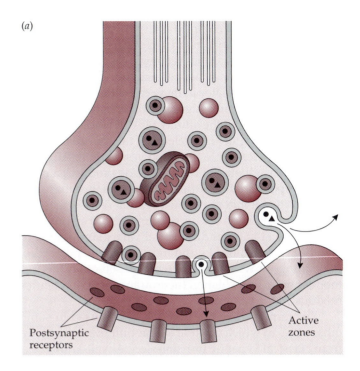

(a)

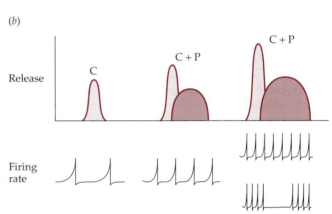

(b)

11.7 FREQUENCY DEPENDENCE OF RELEASE OF A COEXISTING CLASSICAL TRANSMITTER AND A NEUROPEPTIDE (a) When a classical transmitter (solid circles) and a peptide (triangles) coexist in the same nerve terminals, small synaptic vesicles contain only the transmitter whereas large, dense-core vesicles contain both transmitter and neuropeptide. Exocytosis of small vesicles occurs at active zones, whereas large, dense-core vesicles can undergo exocytosis at extrajunctional sites. (b) Release of coexisting transmitters and neuropeptides may be frequency dependent in that the cell releases only the classical transmitter (C) when it fires at a low frequency, whereas high frequency or burst firing causes corelease of the peptide (P). (After Hökfelt, 1991; Lundberg and Hökfelt, 1983.)

cells of the gland (called acinar cells) and blood vessels. Activation of these fibers stimulates salivary secretion while simultaneously causing vasodilation and thus an increase in local blood flow. Work from Lundberg's laboratory showed that ACh and VIP are colocalized in the submandibular parasympathetic fibers and, furthermore, that much more peptide is released at high (10-Hz) than at low (2-Hz) stimulus frequencies. These investigators also demonstrated a complex interplay between the two substances in their effects on secretion and blood flow. ACh acting via muscarinic receptors was found to be the primary stimulus for acinar cell activity. In contrast, VIP acts as a neuromodulator in these cells: it has no effect on secretion by itself, but it significantly enhances the effect of ACh by increasing the affinity of ACh binding to its receptor and by augmenting release of the transmitter (Figure 11.8). With respect to the blood vessels, both ACh and VIP cause vasodilation, but the peptide produces a more potent response. Finally, there is also evidence that ACh may exert an inhibitory control over VIP release, presumably via receptors on the nerve terminals. To summarize, VIP in the cat submandibular salivary gland seems to have both modulator-like and transmitter-like properties, depending on whether its effects on secretion (neuromodulator) or vasodilation (neurotransmitter and neuromodulator) are being considered.

The term "neuromodulation" is also used in some other cases in which peptide action differs substantially from classical synaptic transmission. A well-known example was found in bullfrog sympathetic ganglia by Jan and Jan (1983). As discussed in Chapter 7, bullfrog sympathetic neurons display a number of different synaptic responses following stimulation of the preganglionic fibers. Although most of these responses are clearly cholinergic, a slowly developing and long-lasting EPSP (see Figure 7.13) was observed that could not be blocked by either muscarinic or nicotinic antagonists. From a number of experiments, it became clear that the agent responsible for this late slow EPSP is a peptide with a structure similar to that of mammalian luteinizing hormone-releasing hormone (LHRH). The LHRH-like peptide coexists with ACh in two spinal nerves, the seventh and eighth, that innervate the last two lumbar ganglia. Other preganglionic fibers arising from the third, fourth, and fifth spinal nerves also innervate these ganglia, but contain only ACh. Furthermore, some of the neurons in the ganglia, called B cells, receive synaptic input only from nerves 3, 4, and 5, whereas other neurons, called C cells, are in contact only with terminals from the seventh and eighth nerves. Why is this arrangement of interest? Jan and Jan showed that when nerves 7 and 8 were stimulated, not only did the C cells display the expected LHRH-mediated late slow EPSP, but the B cells responded likewise. It has been estimated that the LHRH-like peptide must have traveled some tens of micrometers from its release sites without being degraded in order to stimulate the B cells. Such "action at a distance" (also termed "volume transmission"; see Chapter 8) represents a form of cellular communication somewhere between classical synaptic transmission, in which the target cell is in extremely close physical proximity to the release site, and hormonal regulation, in which the signaling agent is released into the bloodstream and therefore may affect target cells quite distant from the site of release.

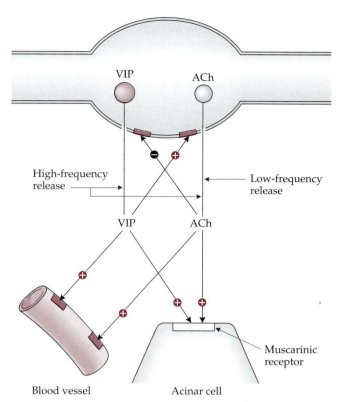

11.8 COEXISTENCE OF ACETYLCHOLINE AND VASOACTIVE INTESTINAL PEPTIDE. Parasympathetic fibers innervating the cat submandibular salivary gland contain ACh and VIP, which are present in two separate populations of vesicles. Low impulse frequencies selectively release ACh, which stimulates salivary secretion by the acinar cells and also increases blood flow somewhat by triggering vasodilation. Higher impulse frequencies lead to the release of VIP as well, which positively modulates the cholinergic effect on secretion and also produces a much more pronounced vasodilatory response. (After Burnstock, 1983.)

The Organizational Framework of Neuropeptide Systems

Because of the large number of peptides already found in the nervous system, it is useful to fit them into some type of organizational scheme. One possible system, which is presented in Table 11.1, classifies neuropeptides into six categories:

1. Opioid peptides, which include compounds that are agonists at opiate receptors (see Chapter 12);
2. Gut–brain peptides, found in both the central nervous system and the gastrointestinal tract;
3. Hypothalamic releasing hormones, which act both as transmitters/modulators and as hypothalamic hormones that regulate the release of other hormones from the anterior pituitary gland;
4. Pituitary hormones, which are found in both the pituitary gland and the nervous system;
5. Other circulating hormones;
6. Miscellaneous peptides.

Table 11.1 Peptides Found in the Vertebrate Nervous System[a]

Opioid peptides
  Met-enkephalin
  Leu-enkephalin
  β-Endorphin
  Dynorphin

Gut–brain peptides
  Substance P (SP)
  Vasoactive intestinal peptide (VIP)
  Cholecystokinin (CCK)
  Neurotensin (NT)
  Neuropeptide Y (NPY)
  Galanin
  Insulin
  Glucagon
  Bombesin
  Gastrin
  Secretin
  Motilin

Hypothalamic releasing hormones
  Thyrotropin-releasing hormone (TRH)
  Luteinizing hormone–releasing hormone (LHRH), also
    known as gonadotropin-releasing hormone (GnRH)
  Corticotropin-releasing factor (CRF)
  Growth hormone–releasing hormone
  Somatostatin

Pituitary hormones
  Vasopressin
  Oxytocin
  Adrenocorticotropic hormone (ACTH)
  Growth hormone (GH)
  Thyrotropin, or thyroid-stimulating hormone (TSH)
  Luteinizing hormone (LH)
  Prolactin
  α-Melanocyte–stimulating hormone (α-MSH)

Other circulating hormones and miscellaneous peptides
  Angiotensin II
  Bradykinin
  Atrial natriuretic factor (ANF)
  Calcitonin gene-related peptide (CGRP)

[a]Although this table presents many of the peptides identified to date in vertebrate nervous systems, it is not meant to be exhaustive.

A number of the compounds mentioned in the table have been identified in the nervous system only by immunochemical criteria (i.e., radioimmunoassay or immunohistochemistry). In such cases, determination of the exact structure of the peptide and its possible physiological role awaits chemical purification and characterization, as well as appropriate synthesis and release studies.

The remainder of this chapter will survey selected peptide systems from several of these categories, al-

though, as mentioned above, the opioid peptides are taken up in detail in Chapter 12 and therefore are not covered here. In most cases, we will consider the peptide's amino acid sequence, localization, and proposed physiological and behavioral functions. To understand the peptide sequences, readers should refer to the list of amino acids and their abbreviations given in Table 3.1.

Vasopressin and Oxytocin

Structure and Synthesis

Vasopressin and oxytocin are small, closely related peptides, as indicated by their amino acid sequences. There are actually two different forms of vasopressin, differing with respect to whether an arginine residue (most mammals) or a lysine (pigs and hippopotami) is found adjacent to the C-terminal glycine. The amino group shown

$$\text{Phe—Tyr—Cys} \\ |\qquad\qquad| \\ \text{Glu—Asn—Cys—Pro—Arg—Gly—NH}_2$$
Arginine vasopressin (AVP)

$$\text{Ile—Tyr—Cys} \\ |\qquad\qquad| \\ \text{Glu—Asn—Cys—Pro—Leu—Gly—NH}_2$$
Oxytocin

on the C-terminal glycine indicates that it is amidated; that is, the free COOH group has been converted to $CONH_2$. Vasopressin and oxytocin, which are synthesized by separate cells (see below), are packaged in secretory granules along with specific carrier proteins called neurophysins. Each neurophysin is formed from the same precursor as the hormone itself.

The structure and processing of the vasopressin precursor, pre-propressophysin, is of interest as a general example of how active peptides are liberated from their precursor proteins. As shown in Figure 11.9, pre-propressophysin contains vasopressin, its corresponding neurophysin, an additional glycopeptide at the C-terminal end, and the expected signal peptide at the N-terminus. Additional amino acids that link vasopressin with neurophysin (—Gly—Lys—Arg—) and neurophysin with the glycopeptide (—Arg—) are involved in the processing of the precursor protein and are ultimately removed.

The conversion process begins within the endoplasmic reticulum, where the signal sequence is removed, a disulfide bond (—S—S—) is formed between the cysteine residues, and a sugar chain (abbreviated CHO) is added to form the glycopeptide. The resulting propeptide, propressophysin, is then packaged into secretory vesicles along with the necessary enzymes for further processing. Within the secretory vesicles, the first step is

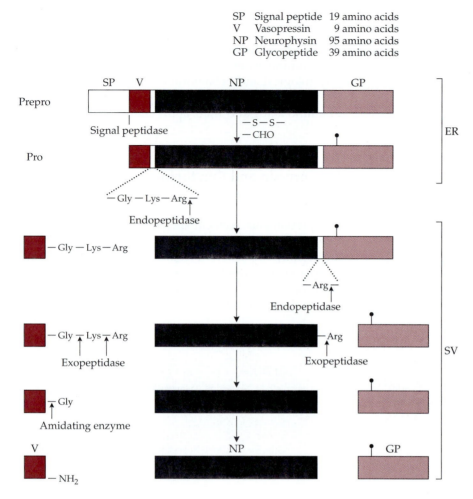

SP   Signal peptide   19 amino acids
V   Vasopressin   9 amino acids
NP   Neurophysin   95 amino acids
GP   Glycopeptide   39 amino acids

11.9 STRUCTURE AND PROCESSING OF THE VASOPRESSIN PRECURSOR (PRE-PROPRESSOPHYSIN). The vasopressin precursor protein contains, in addition to vasopressin itself, a carrier protein called neurophysin, a glycopeptide whose function is still unknown, and a signal peptide. Initial processing occurs in the endoplasmic reticulum (ER), after which the molecule is packaged into secretory vesicles (SV), where the final products are liberated by the action of various peptidases. Note that the exact order of processing steps is somewhat speculative. The solid circles denote the carbohydrate chain (CHO) attached to the glycopeptide. (After Richter, 1988.)

the hydrolysis of the peptide bond on the carboxyl side of each arginine by an endopeptidase (it is actually not yet known whether the same enzyme catalyzes both reactions). Propeptides commonly possess either single arginine or lysine residues or pairs of these amino acids (i.e., —Lys—Lys—, —Arg—Arg—, or —Lys—Arg—) at points where the molecule is to be processed because certain types of proteolytic enzymes specifically cleave the carboxyl peptide bonds formed by these amino acids. The particular endopeptidases involved in propeptide processing are commonly referred to as "converting enzymes" or simply "convertases." After many years of looking for these enzymes in cells that synthesize peptide neurotransmitters or hormones, researchers have finally identified some likely candidates (Lindberg, 1991), although the specific endopeptidase(s) that acts on propressophysin has yet to be identified. Propressophysin processing is completed in several additional steps involving exopeptidase removal of the now unnecessary lysine and arginine residues, followed by a final cleavage of the extra glycine by a so-called "amidating enzyme." Instead of breaking a peptide bond, this enzyme leaves the nitrogen of the glycine residue attached to the preceding amino acid, thus forming the C-terminal amide group.

Localization

Vasopressin and oxytocin were first identified in clusters of large neurons within the paraventricular (PVN) and supraoptic (SON) nuclei of the hypothalamus (Color Plate 2). These so-called **magnocellular neurons** could be stained by a special technique called the Gomori method that was first developed for peripheral secretory glands. The magnocellular system gives rise to the vasopressin and oxytocin projections described above that terminate in the posterior lobe of the pituitary gland (i.e., the neurohypophysis).

Other groups of smaller vasopressin- or oxytocin-containing cells, termed **parvocellular neurons**, are found in several areas of the brain and project to a number of locations in the forebrain, brain stem, and spinal cord (Kozlowski, Nilaver, and Zimmerman, 1983; Sofroniew, 1983). For example, some parvocellular neurons within the PVN contain vasopressin coexpressed with corticotropin-releasing factor. These cells project to the median eminence of the hypothalamus, where they release their secretory products into the pituitary portal vasculature. The anatomical relationships between the PVN, SON, median eminence, and pituitary gland are presented diagrammatically in Figure 11.10. Other vasopressinergic cell groups have been found in the suprachi-

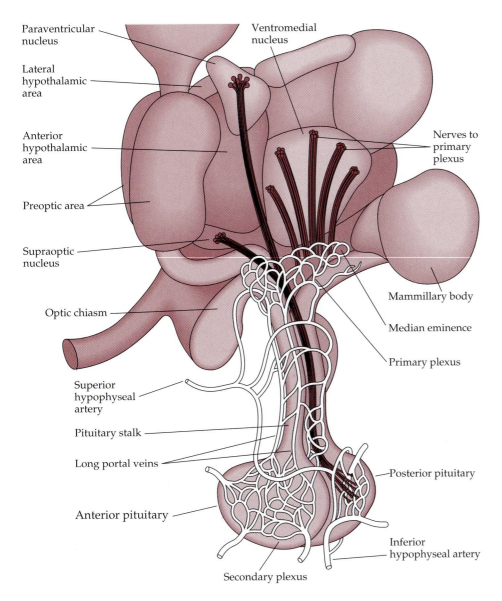

Paraventricular nucleus

Lateral hypothalamic area

Anterior hypothalamic area

Preoptic area

Supraoptic nucleus

Optic chiasm

Superior hypophyseal artery

Pituitary stalk

Long portal veins

Anterior pituitary

Secondary plexus

Ventromedial nucleus

Nerves to primary plexus

Mammillary body

Median eminence

Primary plexus

Posterior pituitary

Inferior hypophyseal artery

11.10 ANATOMICAL RELATIONSHIPS BETWEEN THE HYPOTHALAMUS AND THE PITUITARY GLAND. Magnocellular vasopressin- and oxytocin-containing neurons in the paraventricular nucleus and supraoptic nucleus project to the posterior lobe of the pituitary, where they secrete their respective hormones into the general circulation. Other neurons deliver various hypothalamic releasing hormones to the median eminence, where these substances enter the capillaries of the pituitary portal system ("primary plexus"), travel to the anterior lobe of the pituitary, and regulate the secretion of anterior pituitary hormones. Some parvocellular neurons of the paraventricular nucleus and the supraoptic nucleus also send fibers to the median eminence. (After Frohman, 1980.)

asmatic nucleus (SCN), medial amygdala, bed nucleus of the stria terminalis, and locus coeruleus. In contrast, most of the oxytocin-containing pathways in the brain seem to originate from the PVN (Buijs, 1990). The major vasopressinergic and oxytocinergic pathways in the rat brain are illustrated in Figure 11.11.

Vasopressin Receptors

Vasopressin receptors have been divided into two major subtypes, designated V_1 and V_2, largely on the basis of their actions in nonnervous tissues. V_1 receptors were initially discovered in hepatocytes (liver cells), although their best-known peripheral effect is to stimulate the contraction of vascular smooth muscle. There is pharmacological evidence for two V_1 receptor subtypes, designated V_{1A} and V_{1B}. The V_{1A} receptor gene has recently been cloned (Morel et al., 1992), and the localization of this receptor in the rat brain has been determined autoradiographically (Johnson et al., 1993). Among the areas showing significant V_{1A} receptor density are the lateral septum, dentate gyrus of the hippocampus, nucleus of the solitary tract, and a number of nuclei within the diencephalon. Peripheral V_1 receptors have been shown to stimulate the phosphoinositide second messenger system (Manning and Sawyer, 1989), although a role for this system in the neural actions of vasopressin has not yet been established.

Both the human and rat V_2 receptor genes have also been cloned (Birnbaumer et al., 1992; Lolait et al., 1992). This receptor seems to be expressed only in the kidney, which supports its previously reported involvement in the renal effects of vasopressin (see below). V_2 receptors function by stimulating adenylyl cyclase activity and cyclic AMP formation (Manning and Sawyer, 1989).

Physiological Effects of Vasopressin

The classical physiology of vasopressin is related to its peripheral actions as a hormone secreted from the neu-

(a) Vasopressin

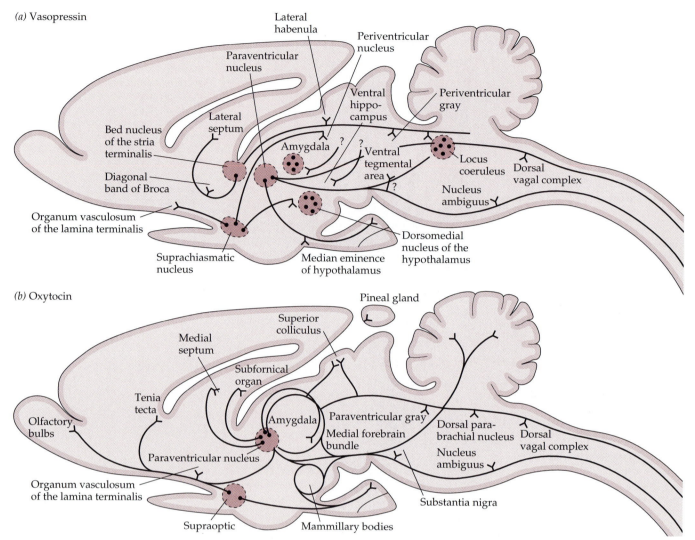

(b) Oxytocin

11.11 MAJOR VASOPRESSINERGIC AND OXYTOCINERGIC PATHWAYS IN THE RAT BRAIN AND THEIR PROBABLE SITES OF ORIGIN. (a) Vasopressin. Pathways from the paraventricular nucleus are indicated by dashed and dotted lines; from the suprachiasmatic nucleus by dotted lines, and from the bed nucleus of the stria terminalis by dashed lines. Triangles depict cell groups that contain sufficient neuropeptide to be stained immunohistochemically in untreated animals. Circles depict cell groups that may possess lower levels of neuropeptide, as they are only stained in animals pretreated with the antimicrotubule agent colchicine (microtubule disassembly prevents axonal transport of neuropeptides, thereby causing them to accumulate in the cell soma and increasing immunohistochemical reactivity). (b) Oxytocin. (After Buijs, 1990.)

rohypophysis. In early studies, circulating vasopressin was found to exert two major effects: (1) a powerful stimulation of water retention by the kidneys at very low doses, and (2) an elevation in blood pressure at higher doses. The name "vasopressin" can obviously be traced to the pressor effect of the peptide; however, its role in diuresis is responsible for the alternative name, "antidiuretic hormone," that is commonly used by endocrinologists. In fact, stimulation of magnocellular vasopressin-containing cells and consequent vasopressin secretion results from dehydration, salt loading, or any other condition (e.g., hemorrhage) that requires conservation of body water (Hatton, 1990).

The pressor and antidiuretic effects of vasopressin are mediated by V_1 and V_2 receptors respectively. Based on this receptor difference, drugs have been developed that act as relatively selective anti-vasopressor or anti-antidiuretic agents (László, László, and De Wied, 1991). However, these agents have generally been peptide analogs of vasopressin or oxytocin, and therefore are relatively ineffective when administered orally due to degradation in the gastrointestinal tract. It is thus noteworthy that an orally effective nonpeptide V_1 antagonist was introduced a few years ago by the Otsuka pharmaceutical company in Japan (Yamamura et al., 1991). This compound, OPC-21268, may eventually prove useful in the treatment of hypertension (high blood pressure) as well as congestive heart failure.

OPC-21268

The importance of circulating vasopressin as an antidiuretic factor is illustrated by considering a disease called diabetes insipidus. Diabetes insipidus differs entirely from the better-known diabetes mellitus in that it is a disorder of water balance rather than sugar metabolism. This disease is not related to insulin, but rather, stems from a deficiency in vasopressin. Without the water-resorbing effects of vasopressin, people lacking this hormone excrete copious amounts of urine each day and consequently must consume enormous quantities of water to survive. An animal model of diabetes insipidus was discovered fortuitously by Henry Schroeder in 1961 (see Valtin, 1982). Although Schroeder was then affiliated with Dartmouth Medical School, he was spending much of his time in his own private laboratory in West Brattleboro, Vermont. One day, Schroeder's assistant noticed that some of the rat pups in one litter from his breeding colony were drinking excessive amounts of water each day. Instead of simply discarding these anomalous animals, Schroeder took an interest in them and performed a simple experiment showing that their drinking behavior could be normalized by administering vasopressin. This result suggested that the subjects had inherited a genetic form of diabetes insipidus. The mutant strain of rats has since been maintained for research purposes, and has come to be known as the Brattleboro strain. As anticipated, Brattleboro rats suffer from a defective vasopressin gene—specifically, a deletion of one nucleotide in the region of DNA that codes for neurophysin. Even though the mutant gene is transcribed, its mRNA is translated, and the resulting precursor contains a correct vasopressin sequence, packaging of the peptide is apparently impaired, and thus little or no detectable vasopressin is transported to or secreted from the neurohypophysis (Richter, 1988). Most humans who suffer from diabetes insipidus likewise exhibit deficient vasopressin secretion; however, there is a rare nephrogenic form of the disorder involving a mutation of the V_2 receptor gene that reduces the kidneys' responsiveness to the peptide (Holtzman et al., 1993).

Virtually all neuropeptides have been found to subserve multiple physiological and/or behavioral functions, and vasopressin is certainly a prime example.

Vasopressin in the various hypothalamic and extra-hypothalamic parvocellular groups seems to exert a multitude of effects unrelated to either water retention or blood pressure regulation. For example, it plays a significant role in activating the hypothalamic–pituitary–adrenocortical system during stress (Gibbs, 1986). This function is probably mediated at least partially by the above-mentioned PVN neurons that contain both vasopressin and corticotropin-releasing factor. In contrast, vasopressin neurons in the SCN may play a role in circadian rhythms, considering that this nucleus has been identified as the site of the "biological clock." Vasopressin in the cerebrospinal fluid, which is thought to be derived in large measure from the SCN, shows a circadian (about 24-hour) rhythm that persists even under conditions of constant light (Reppert et al., 1981). Furthermore, subsequent studies have shown that processing of vasopressin mRNA in the SCN, but not in the PVN or SON, likewise exhibits a circadian rhythm (Robinson et al., 1988). These findings raise the possibility that vasopressin may be one of the transmitters responsible for conveying information concerning circadian rhythmicity from the SCN to other parts of the brain.

The Role of Vasopressin in Learning and Memory

In addition to the above-mentioned physiological actions, vasopressin has been implicated in several behavioral processes. The possible involvement of this peptide in certain social behaviors will be taken up in the discussion of oxytocin below. However, there is also a controversial line of research suggesting a role for vasopressin in learning and memory. This research began in the late 1960s and early 1970s, when David De Wied and his coworkers at the Rudolf Magnus Institute for Pharmacology in the Netherlands set out to investigate the behavioral effects of vasopressin and several other neuropeptides (for reviews, see Kovács and De Wied, 1994; van Wimersma Greidanus, Burbach, and Veldhuis, 1986). In some of their experiments, rats were first tested for the rate at which they acquired a two-way (i.e., shuttle) active avoidance response and then for the rate at which the response was extinguished following discontinuation of the electric shock. Removal of the posterior lobe of the pituitary gland was found to selectively accelerate the rate of extinction. This effect could be blocked by systemic injection of pitressin, a crude vasopressin-containing pituitary extract, and subsequent studies showed that pitressin administration also retarded the rate of extinction in intact animals. Similar results were obtained with purified vasopressin, confirming that this substance was the active agent present in the pitressin mixture. Further experiments showed that even a single dose of vasopressin produced a long-lasting inhibition of response extinction that persisted well after the peptide was presumably cleared from the organism.

Other studies were performed utilizing a simple step-through passive avoidance paradigm. This task involves an apparatus consisting of two connected chambers: a lit chamber with an elevated platform leading to a dark chamber, which is normally preferred by rats and mice. The subject is placed on the platform, allowed to "step through" the opening into the dark chamber, and then immediately given an electric shock to the feet. A single trial of this kind normally produces a lasting avoidance response, as measured by an increased latency to step through the opening on subsequent retention tests. Administration of vasopressin either immediately after the acquisition trial or just prior to the retention test led to enhanced avoidance (i.e., longer latencies) compared with control subjects. Further studies demonstrated similar behavioral effects when small doses of vasopressin were injected directly into the brain rather than being given peripherally. In other experiments, anti-vasopressin antiserum was administered either intravenously or intracerebroventricularly to inactivate the animal's own vasopressin. Intracerebroventricular, but not intravenous, administration led to deficits in passive avoidance retention, suggesting that vasopressin acting centrally as a neurotransmitter or neuromodulator is involved in this behavioral response. Finally, it was shown that vasopressin-deficient Brattleboro rats display significant deficits in some of these same tests of learning and memory.

Together, these findings were interpreted by De Wied's group to mean that vasopressin acts on memory storage and retrieval mechanisms (Kovács and De Wied, 1994; van Wimersma Greidanus, Burbach, and Veldhuis, 1986). Because behavioral extinction was viewed by these researchers as a forgetting phenomenon, vasopressin-induced retardation of active avoidance extinction was thought to represent enhanced memory retention, which had been mediated, perhaps, by facilitation of the consolidation process. Likewise, increased step-through latencies on the passive avoidance task were considered to be indicative of improved memory storage or retrieval, depending on when the peptide was administered relative to the training and test trials. Nevertheless, criticisms have been raised against these interpretations of the results (Martinez, Schulteis, and Weinberger, 1991; Sahgal, 1984; Strupp and Levitsky, 1985). One major point is that learning theorists generally consider extinction to involve "new learning"—that is, learning to withhold the previously trained response—rather than the forgetting of that response. From such an alternative perspective, vasopressin-treated animals that show delayed avoidance extinction are actually manifesting poorer rather than better learning! A second major criticism is that performance of avoidance learning tasks is subject to a number of variables besides those associated with learning or memory per se. Thus, vasopressin treatment might alter the subject's activity, its fearfulness, or simply its general level of arousal. Studies involving peripheral injection may be particularly problematic in this regard. High systemic doses of vasopressin appear to be

aversive to the animals, probably due to the pressor effects of the peptide (Ettenberg et al., 1983). Third, if vasopressin really does play a role in learning or memory processes, it should be possible to demonstrate effects of this substance on appetitive (e.g., food- or water-motivated) as well as aversive (e.g., shock-motivated) tasks. Although some studies have reported a positive influence of vasopressin in appetitive learning situations (van Wimersma Greidanus, Burbach, and Veldhuis, 1986), a number of investigators have found no effects on such tasks (Sahgal, 1984; Strupp and Levitsky, 1985).

Do these criticisms and negative findings mean that vasopressin is definitely not involved in learning or memory? Not necessarily. It is clear that greater care must be taken before applying such an interpretation to the results of the previously described studies, particularly those in which aversive stimuli were used. More extensive behavioral controls would certainly be helpful in attempting to rule out alternative motivational or arousal hypotheses. Nevertheless, those who argue for a learning or memory interpretation of vasopressin action can point to additional evidence to support their case. For example, it has been known for some time that many of the behavioral effects of vasopressin can be mimicked by chemical analogs that are essentially devoid of either the pressor or the antidiuretic effects of the native molecule (van Wimersma Greidanus, Burbach, and Veldhuis, 1986). Moreover, some studies have found improved performance by humans on various cognitive tasks following administration of vasopressin or one of its analogs (for review, see Beckwith et al., 1990; Zager and Black, 1985). Subjects in these studies were either cognitively normal or suffering from a cognitive deficit, most typically some form of dementia. Although some negative findings have been reported, there have been sufficient positive results to support a cognitive interpretation of vasopressin action. It is interesting to note that work on healthy subjects has led to the conclusion that vasopressin does not specifically affect long-term memory storage, but rather enhances selective attention and the efficiency of short-term memory processes (Beckwith et al., 1990). Additionally, the results from cognitively impaired individuals are encouraging in terms of the possibility of using vasopressin therapy in the treatment of cognitive disorders.

To summarize, vasopressin functions as a circulating hormone that stimulates water retention by the kidney, elevates blood pressure, and, when released into the pituitary portal circulation, potentiates the hypothalamic–pituitary–adrenocortical response to stress. This peptide also acts as a neurotransmitter/neuromodulator in the brain, where it has been implicated in circadian rhythms, learning and memory, and other processes not discussed here. The apparent cognitive effects of vasopressin suggest that it or related peptides might eventually be useful in the treatment of dementia or other cognitive disorders.

Physiological Effects of Oxytocin

Like that of vasopressin, the classical physiology of oxytocin involves its actions as a circulating hormone. Despite its close structural similarity to vasopressin, however, oxytocin has a different spectrum of action revolving around female reproductive activities. For example, oxytocin potently stimulates the contraction of uterine smooth muscles and is routinely used by both physicians and veterinarians to enhance uterine contractions in certain types of labor complications. Recent studies with rats indicate that hypothalamic oxytocinergic cells are activated during parturition, and that inhibition of these cells suppresses the normal birth process (Luckman et al., 1993). Other research has shown that oxytocin is also synthesized by the uterus itself, suggesting that locally produced as well as circulating oxytocin may participate in the induction of labor (Lefebvre et al., 1992).

Another vital function of oxytocin involves the triggering of milk ejection (sometimes also called milk "letdown") in lactating females. During lactation, peptide synthesis in oxytocinergic hypothalamic magnocellular neurons is greatly increased, as indicated by in situ hybridization studies of oxytocin gene expression (Lightman and Young, 1987). Suckling stimulation leads to intermittent, synchronized bursts of action potentials in these cells (Hatton, 1990). Consequently, oxytocin is secreted from the neurohypophysis, followed seconds later by milk ejection from the mammary glands. Oxytocin works by stimulating the contraction of mammary gland myoepithelial cells, thereby forcing milk into the ducts and sinuses of the gland, where it can be removed by the suckling offspring. In the absence of this hormone, offspring would obtain far less milk and would presumably die or at least be seriously malnourished. Nursing women have been reported to release oxytocin into the bloodstream several minutes *before* actual suckling begins (McNeilly et al., 1983), suggesting that behavioral conditioning of the secretory process may be possible.

The Role of Oxytocin in Social Behaviors

There is considerable evidence that oxytocin serves not only as a hormone but also as a neurotransmitter or neuromodulator (reviewed by Argiolas and Gessa, 1991; Richard, Moos, and Freund-Mercier, 1991). Various studies have implicated both oxytocin and vasopressin in the control of social behaviors, including reproductive behavior, parenting, and infant attachment (see Pedersen et al., 1992). Let us first consider the possible role of oxytocin in regulating female rodent sexual behaviors. Sexual receptivity in female rodents is manifested by a characteristic mating posture known as lordosis. Lordosis is dependent on the presence of female sex hormones such as estrogen and progesterone, and can normally be elicited in ovariectomized subjects by sequential treatment with these substances. As reviewed by Carter (1992) and Insel (1992b), studies in the 1980s from several laboratories showed that intracerebroventricular administration of oxytocin enhanced lordosis responding in estrogen plus progesterone-primed rats. A similar effect could be obtained with estrogen priming only, but generally required higher doses of oxytocin. The involvement of endogenous oxytocin in sexual receptivity was subsequently demonstrated by the work of Witt and Insel (1991), who showed that intracerebroventricular administration of an oxytocin receptor antagonist called OTA to estrogen and progesterone-primed rats substantially reduced lordosis frequency when OTA was given concurrently with progesterone.

Infusion studies aimed at identifying the site of oxytocin action have demonstrated positive results in both the ventromedial hypothalamus (VMH) and medial preoptic area (MPOA), although these areas may influence different aspects of the lordosis response (Schulze and Gorzalka, 1991). Some investigators have reported that the strongest effect of oxytocin on lordosis is actually elicited from an area lateral to the posterior ventromedial hypothalamic nucleus (VMN) (Schumacher et al., 1993). Moreover, priming of ovariectomized rats with both estradiol and progesterone (but not estradiol alone) was found to increase dramatically the density of oxytocin receptor binding in the VMN and the associated lateral zone, and also to enlarge the area covered by these receptors. The intensity of staining of oxytocin-immunoreactive nerve fibers in the expanded area of receptor binding was likewise enhanced. Consequently, Schumacher and colleagues (1993) hypothesized that the ability of estrogen plus progesterone priming to facilitate oxytocin-induced lordosis may be related to the effect of bringing oxytocin receptors into register with the presumed site of peptide release. A further twist to this story comes from studies showing that the progesterone-mediated changes in oxytocin receptor density and distribution (1) occur relatively rapidly and are independent of protein synthesis, indicating that formation of new receptors is not required, and (2) can even be obtained in dried and frozen tissue sections incubated with the steroid in vitro (Schumacher et al., 1993). Together, these observations argue against mediation by the classical mechanism of steroid action, namely, altered gene transcription and protein synthesis. Perhaps progesterone instead acts within the cell membrane to influence the binding affinity of oxytocin receptors and/or their mobility. These initial results must be confirmed by further studies, but if they are, they will represent an important new mechanism by which neurotransmitter systems can be regulated.

After successful mating, pregnancy, and birth, mammals must care for their young. As we have already seen that oxytocin is critical for milk ejection during lactation, it is interesting to discover that this substance may also be involved in maternal behavior itself. Based on studies of sheep and goats, Klopfer (1971) was the first to speculate that oxytocin might be important in the onset of maternal behavior shortly after delivery of the offspring.

Subsequent work by Keverne, Kendrick, and their co-workers demonstrated increased release of oxytocin in the medial preoptic area, bed nucleus of the stria terminalis, olfactory bulbs, and substantia nigra of sheep during parturition or following vaginocervical stimulation, which is thought to mimic the sensory aspects of the birthing process (Kendrick et al., 1992; Keverne and Kendrick, 1990). Furthermore, maternal behavior in ovariectomized, estrogen-primed ewes can be triggered either by vaginocervical stimulation or by central administration of exogenous oxytocin. Similarly, intracerebroventricular oxytocin administration has been shown to cause a dose-dependent increase in maternal behavior in intact, estrus-cycling rats and in ovariectomized, hormone-primed subjects (Insel, 1990; Pedersen and Prange, 1985; Figure 11.12). Recent experiments have indicated that the stimulatory effect of oxytocin on rat maternal behavior may be mediated by the medial preoptic area and ventral tegmental area (Pedersen, Caldwell et al., 1994).

One of the most intriguing current areas of neuropeptide research concerns a fascinating group of wild rodents called voles (genus *Microtus*). Some members of this group, such as prairie voles (*M. ochrogaster*), exhibit a monogamous mating system (i.e., formation of a pair-bond after mating) and a high level of maternal care for offspring. Others, such as montane voles (*M. montanus*), are polygamous and show a lower level of maternal behavior. Examination of these and other related species allows researchers to perform powerful comparative studies correlating various neural characteristics with these differing social behavioral systems. For example, Insel and Shapiro (1992) found that oxytocin receptor density in the lateral amygdala was substantially higher in virgin female prairie voles than in virgin female montane voles. At the same time, the prairie voles, but not the montane voles, exhibited a high degree of maternal behavior when given pups to care for. After giving birth to their own pups, the montane voles showed a large rise in lateral amygdala oxytocin receptors, and they likewise became almost as maternal as the prairie voles. Other experiments found that central oxytocin administration exerted differing effects on aggressive behavior in male prairie and montane voles (Winslow, Shapiro et al., 1993). Finally, several recent studies have implicated oxytocin and vasopressin in pair-bonding and parental behavior in prairie voles (Insel, Wang, and Ferris, 1994; Wang, Ferris, and De Vries, 1994; Williams et al., 1994; Winslow, Hastings et al., 1993). Thus, both oxytocin and vasopressin may play important roles in many aspects of sociality.

Thyrotropin-Releasing Hormone (TRH)

Structure and Localization

As mentioned in the first part of this chapter, TRH was the first hypothalamic releasing hormone to be identified. Both basic and clinical aspects of TRH have been reviewed by Faglia and Persani (1991). TRH is a small molecule, consisting of only three amino acids: glutamic acid, histidine, and proline. The structure of this tripeptide is unusual in that the N-terminal glutamate residue is modified to form a cyclic arrangement that is designated by the term "pyro." In addition, the C-terminal proline, like the C-terminal glycine in vasopressin and oxytocin, is amidated. Hence, the correct chemical name for TRH is (pyro)glutamylhistidylprolineamide.

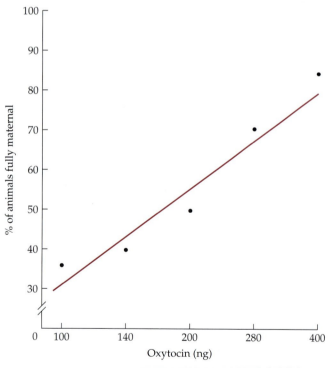

11.12 EFFECT OF INTRACEREBROVENTRICULAR OXYTOCIN ON MATERNAL BEHAVIOR IN VIRGIN FEMALE RATS. Ovariectomized virgin rats were primed with 100 μg/kg estradiol, given oxytocin (100–400 ng into the lateral ventricle) 48 hours later, and then tested for maternal responsiveness to pup exposure. The figure shows the percentage of animals demonstrating full maternal behavior (including grouping of pups, crouching over pups, licking of pups, pup retrieval, and nest building) at 1 hour post-oxytocin injection. Full maternal behavior was exhibited by only 18% of similarly treated females receiving saline instead of oxytocin. (After Pedersen et al., 1982.)

Thyrotropin-releasing hormone (TRH)

Like other neuropeptides, TRH is synthesized from a precursor protein. ProTRH contains within its structure several copies of the TRH sequence, specifically five in the case of the rat protein (Lee et al., 1989). Although we do not yet know how many of these copies are liberated as free TRH molecules during proTRH processing, this example illustrates the general principle that some propeptides contain multiple copies of the same active peptide (see also Chapter 12 for an example of this same phenomenon in the enkephalin precursor family).

The presence of TRH in various brain areas was first demonstrated using biochemical techniques such as radioimmunoassay. Using this approach, TRH was found in the hypothalamus, which accords with its neuroendocrine function, as well as in a number of extrahypothalamic structures. More recent studies have mapped TRH neurons using immunohistochemistry for the peptide itself or in situ hybridization for the pre-proTRH gene. These more sensitive and refined techniques have found TRH cells in a large number of locations, including several hypothalamic nuclei, the olfactory bulbs, hippocampal formation, amygdala, limbic cortex, periaqueductal gray of the midbrain and pons, and the raphe nuclei of the medulla (Hökfelt et al., 1989; Lechan and Segerson, 1989). It has been known for some time that TRH in the medullary raphe coexists with serotonin (5-HT) and substance P in a neural pathway that descends into the spinal cord and innervates ventral horn motor neurons. This has been demonstrated not only immunohistochemically (Johansson et al., 1981), but also by the fact that intracerebroventricular injection of the serotonergic neurotoxin 5,7-dihydroxytryptamine results in a virtual disappearance of spinal 5-HT, TRH, and substance P (Gilbert et al., 1982).

Physiological and Behavioral Effects

In its role as a hypothalamic releasing hormone, TRH is synthesized by cells in the parvocellular part of the paraventricular nucleus (PVN) and transported along the axons of those cells to the median eminence of the hypothalamus (see Figure 11.10). In the median eminence, axons from the various releasing hormone neurons (denoted in the figure as nerves to the primary plexus) give rise to nerve endings in close proximity to the capillaries of the pituitary portal system. These capillaries lack blood–brain barrier characteristics (see Chapter 3 for further details), thus permitting the entry of TRH and the other peptide releasing hormones following their release from the nearby terminals. TRH then travels down the vessels of the pituitary stalk to the anterior pituitary (adenohypophysis), where it stimulates the secretion not only of thyroid-stimulating hormone (TSH, or thyrotropin) but also of another hormone called prolactin.

The neuroendocrine role of TRH is well documented and is extremely important physiologically. However, as in the case of vasopressin, much of the TRH found in the brain seems to function as a neurotransmitter or neuromodulator rather than as a hormone. TRH receptors are widely distributed in the central nervous system (Sharif, 1989), and it is generally assumed that TRH is released from nerve terminals by an exocytotic, calcium-dependent process, as in the case of other neuroactive substances.

If TRH plays a significant transmitter role, what behavioral functions are subserved by this peptide? Early clinical studies reported that TSH (which, as we have just seen, is under the control of TRH), as well as the thyroid hormone triiodothyronine (T_3), potentiated the antidepressant effects of imipramine in depressed patients (Prange et al., 1970; Wilson et al., 1970). Subsequent research has investigated the possible involvement of TRH itself in a number of psychiatric disorders, as well as the possible clinical utility of measuring the TSH response to TRH administration (see Loosen, 1988, for review). The initial clinical reports also prompted an examination of the effects of TRH in animal subjects. Many such studies performed since the early 1970s have convincingly shown that TRH produces stimulant behavioral effects in a variety of test situations. For example, TRH has been found to antagonize the effects of various sedative drugs, including barbiturates, alcohol, chlorpromazine, diazepam, chloral hydrate, and ketamine (see Nemeroff et al., 1984, for review). This analeptic action of TRH, which is manifested by a reduction in sleep time induced by the sedative agent, is not blocked by removal of either the thyroid or the pituitary gland, suggesting that the effect is independent of the neuroendocrine functions of the peptide.

Behavioral effects of TRH have also been observed in the DOPA and 5-HTP potentiation tests. These tests involve treating rats or mice with either the catecholamine precursor L-DOPA or the 5-HT precursor 5-HTP. Pargyline, a potent monoamine oxidase (MAO) inhibitor, is given along with the precursor to induce transmitter "overflow" into the synaptic cleft by blocking intraneuronal metabolism. TRH was found to potentiate the arousing and locomotor-stimulating effects observed in both pharmacological tests, again in a neuroendocrine-independent manner (Nemeroff et al., 1984).

Based in part on the results of the DOPA and 5-HTP potentiation tests, it has been hypothesized that the stimulatory effects of TRH stem from an interaction with catecholaminergic or serotonergic systems. The DA system in particular has been implicated in studies showing that intravenous TRH injections increase extracellular DA concentrations in the corpus striatum (Kreutz et al., 1990), and that administration of TRH directly into the nucleus accumbens enhances locomotor activity, presumably by augmenting DA release from mesolimbic dopaminergic nerve terminals (Nemeroff et al., 1984). However, noradrenergic and serotonergic systems may also be involved in TRH action. Bennett and colleagues (1989) demonstrated that the hyperactivity produced by intraperitoneal injection of either TRH or its more potent synthetic analog CG 3703 (6-methyl-5-oxo-thiomor-pholinyl-3-carbonyl-prolineamide) could be virtually abolished by pretreatment with the α_1-adrenoceptor antagonist prazosin (Figure 11.13). Moreover, TRH also attenuated the hypoactive effect of clonidine, a drug that is thought to inhibit norepinephrine release by stimulating α_2-autoreceptors on noradrenergic nerve terminals. Finally, various studies have demonstrated that wet-dog shakes induced in rats by intrathecal administration (injection into the subarachnoid space of the spinal cord) of TRH analogs may involve both α_1- and 5-HT$_2$ receptors (Bennett et al., 1989; Marsden et al., 1989).

We have seen that TRH has a stimulatory behavioral effect that can be demonstrated in many ways, ranging from antagonism of sedative drugs to the elicitation of wet-dog shakes. Some of the actions of TRH are similar to those of psychomotor stimulants (see Chapter 13). For example, systemically administered TRH can elicit tremors, tail raising (Straub tail), sniffing, grooming, and other excitatory behaviors that resemble the effects of amphetamine. A further comparison of the two drugs showed that they both depress food intake and produce a dose-related decrease in bar pressing on a FR-30 schedule of food reinforcement (Vogel et al., 1979). Neither drug altered shuttle box avoidance learning in the doses tested. However, the drugs' effects were distinct when

bar pressing for low rates of electrical stimulation of the lateral hypothalamus was examined: TRH decreased the rate of responding, whereas amphetamine increased bar pressing for brain stimulation. Moreover, amphetamine has been reported to antagonize, rather than mimic or potentiate, TRH-induced wet-dog shakes (Nemeroff et al., 1984). The similarities and differences of amphetamine and TRH exemplify the danger of classifying psychoactive substances on the basis of a single, presumably dominant, effect. The ability of a drug to act as a "stimulant" is clearly dependent upon the behavior examined, the existing level of arousal of the organism, and previous drug history. We cannot assume a common mechanism of action for all "stimulants," given that various forms of behavioral activation (e.g., enhanced locomotor activity vs. wet-dog shakes vs. seizures) depend at least in part on different underlying neurochemical systems.

Corticotropin-Releasing Factor (CRF)

Structure and Localization

The secretion of adrenocorticotropic hormone (ACTH) from the adenohypophysis is stimulated by a peptide called corticotropin-releasing factor (CRF). CRF was the first of the hypothalamic releasing hormones to be sought. However, its purification and identification lagged behind that of TRH and several other of these compounds for various technical reasons (for a historically oriented review, see Yasuda, Greer, and Aizawa, 1982). In 1981, Vale and colleagues finally reported the characterization of a 41-amino acid peptide from ovine hypothalamus that fulfilled the necessary biological criteria to be considered CRF. Since that time, CRF structure has also been determined in pigs, cattle, rats, and humans. These peptides all contain 41 amino acids and are quite similar in their amino acid sequences (in fact, rat and human CRF are identical).

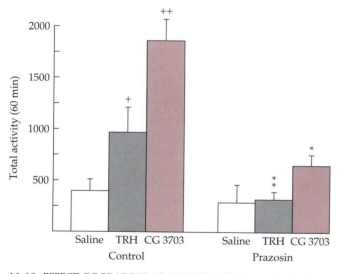

11.13 EFFECT OF PRAZOSIN ON LOCOMOTOR ACTIVITY INDUCED BY TRH OR THE TRH ANALOG CG 3703. Mice were given an intraperitoneal injection of either the α_1-adrenoceptor antagonist prazosin (3 mg/kg) or saline vehicle. Sixty minutes later, subjects received TRH (20 mg/kg), the potent TRH analog CG 3703 (1 mg/kg), or a saline control injection (C) intraperitoneally. Locomotor activity was then measured for a 60-minute period following the second injection. Prazosin significantly inhibited the locomotor activating effects of both TRH agonists (+$p < .02$, ++$p < .01$ compared with saline/saline controls; *$p < .02$, **$p < .01$ comparing prazosin-pretreated vs. saline-pretreated subjects). (After Bennett et al., 1989.)

| Ser—Gln—Glu—Pro—Pro—Ile—Ser—Leu—Asp—Leu—Thr— |
| Phe—His—Leu—Leu—Arg—Glu—Val—Leu—Glu—Met— |
| Thr—Lys—Ala—Asp—Gln—Leu—Ala—Gln—Glu—Ala— |
| His—Ser—Asn—Arg—Lys—Leu—Leu—Asp—Ile—Ala—NH$_2$ |

Ovine corticotropin-releasing factor (CRF)

One interesting feature of CRF is that it shares considerable amino acid homology with two peptides found in lower vertebrates, known as sauvagine and urotensin (Vale et al., 1981). The genes coding for these peptides may all stem from a common ancestral gene that subsequently evolved to serve a variety of physiological roles in different taxonomic orders. Immunohistochemical studies from a number of laboratories have established the existence of widespread CRF-containing cell groups and fiber pathways throughout the brain and in the spinal cord (reviewed by Sawchenko and Swanson, 1989; Sawchenko et al., 1993). Some of the major locations of CRF-containing cells are the parvocellular division of the PVN, the medial and lateral preoptic areas, olfactory bulbs, bed nucleus of the stria terminalis, central amygdaloid nucleus, lateral dorsal tegmental nucleus, parabrachial nucleus, locus coeruleus, dorsovagal complex, regions of the A1 and A5 noradrenergic cell groups, and layers 2 and 3 of the neocortex. CRF-like material has also been observed in peripheral organs such as the pancreas, stomach, small intestine, lung, adrenal gland, and placenta (Petrusz et al., 1985). As the ACTH-stimulating action of CRF is mediated by neurons in the hypothalamus, particularly within the PVN, the extensive extrahypothalamic localization of CRF is fully consistent with an additional nonendocrine role as a neurotransmitter or neuromodulator.

Physiological and Behavioral Effects

The physiological and behavioral actions of CRF are summarized by Müller and von Werder (1991) and by Owens and Nemeroff (1991). CRF is classically associated with regulation of the pituitary–adrenocortical system, an endocrine system first described over 40 years ago as playing a pivotal role in the physiological response to stress (Selye, 1950). More specifically, physical and psychological disturbances experienced by an organism (i.e., "stressors") provoke an increased release of CRF into the pituitary portal capillaries located in the median eminence (see the earlier discussion of TRH). Upon reaching the adenohypophysis, CRF stimulates the release of ACTH, as well as the opioid peptide β-endorphin, from cells called corticotrophs. ACTH and β-endorphin are co-released because they are both liberated from a common precursor, proopiomelanocortin (see Chapter 12 for further details concerning β-endorphin and proopiomelanocortin). The function of circulating ACTH is to stimulate the synthesis and secretion of a class of steroid hormones known as glucocorticoids by the adrenal cortex (hence the name for this system, pituitary–*adrenocortical*). These hormones in turn exert a variety of effects on various target organs. Indeed, persistently elevated glucocorticoid concentrations due to chronic stress can result in hyperglycemia and hyperinsulinemia, increased gastric acid secretion and eventual ulceration, involution (decreased mass) of lymphoid tissues, and a marked suppression of inflammatory and immune responses. Although increased glucocorticoid levels can be pointed to as the *immediate* cause of these effects, we can see that steroid hormone elevations depend on a cascade of events beginning with heightened release of CRF into the pituitary portal vasculature. The neurons responsible for this CRF release are located principally in the PVN, and it is interesting to note that some of these cells also express various coexisting peptides, such as vasopressin, cholecystokinin (see below), or angiotensin II, that may operate together with CRF to enhance the secretory response of the corticotrophs (Sawchenko et al., 1993).

The long-awaited characterization of CRF enabled researchers to begin studying possible functions of this peptide beyond its role in pituitary–adrenocortical regulation. Direct neuronal application of CRF was found to produce potent excitatory effects in the hippocampus, amygdala, locus coeruleus, cortex, and hypothalamus, but it causes an inhibition of cell firing in the thalamus and lateral septum (Owens and Nemeroff, 1991). Moreover, intracerebroventricular administration of CRF led to EEG arousal and behavioral activation. Higher doses even produced seizure activity in the amygdala, hippocampus, and cortex.

Both the endocrine and neurophysiological effects of CRF are mediated by G protein–coupled CRF receptors that stimulate adenylyl cyclase. As recently reviewed by Chalmers and colleagues (1996), there are two major classes of CRF receptors, designated CRF_1 and CRF_2. CRF_2 receptors are also subject to alternative mRNA splicing, thus giving rise to $CRF_{2\alpha}$ and $CRF_{2\beta}$ isoforms. CRF_1 receptors are the dominant form in the pituitary gland, indicating that this subtype mediates the stimulatory effect of CRF on ACTH secretion. Within the brain, both CRF_1 and $CRF_{2\alpha}$ receptors are found in neurons, whereas the $CRF_{2\beta}$ isoform is localized in nonneuronal elements such as the choroid plexus and cerebral blood vessels. Although brain and pituitary CRF receptors share a similar mechanism of action, they are subject to differential regulation in that the pituitary receptors are markedly down-regulated following adrenalectomy (presumably due to increased hypothalamic CRF release), whereas the density of brain receptors is unchanged (Grigoriadis, Heroux, and De Souza, 1993).

CRF_1 receptor mRNA is present in high abundance in the neocortex, the cerebellar cortex, and sensory relay structures (Chalmers et al., 1996). In contrast, highest densities of CRF_2 mRNA are found in the lateral septum, olfactory bulb, and certain amygdaloid and hypothalamic nuclei. Figure 11.14 illustrates the location of CRF-containing cell groups in the rat brain and their projections to CRF_1 and CRF_2 receptor-containing areas.

Going beyond the cellular level, behaviorally and physiologically directed studies have led to a fascinating view of CRF function. Thus far, the only stress response mentioned has been activation of the pituitary–adrenocortical system. However, stressors initiate a much wider range of biological reactions, including stimulation of sympathetic activity and epinephrine secretion from the adrenal medulla, increased heart rate, increased metabolic rate, decreased growth hormone secretion, decreased food intake and sexual behavior, and altered locomotor and grooming behavior. It now appears that

(a)

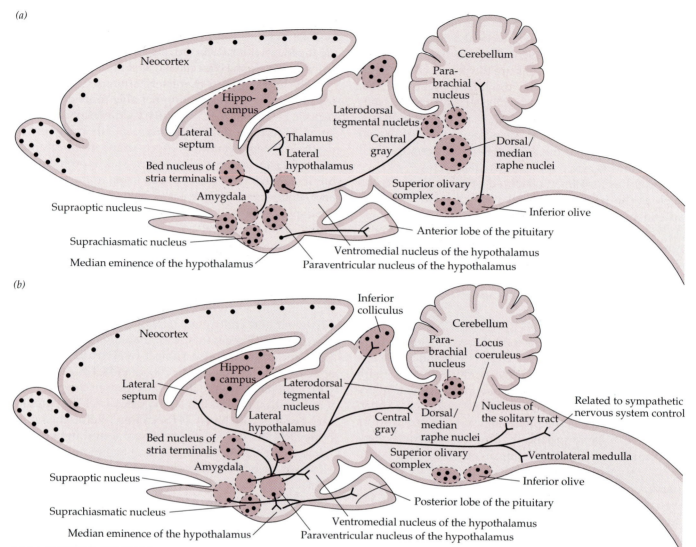

11.14 PUTATIVE CRF PATHWAYS IN RELATION TO CRF$_1$ AND CRF$_2$ RECEPTOR LOCALIZATION. Major CRF-immunoreactive cell groups and fibers are shown by black dots and lines, respectively. Pathways are separated into those that project to brain areas expressing relatively high densities of (*a*) CRF$_1$ or (*b*) CRF$_2$ receptor mRNA. (After Chalmers et al., 1996.)

central CRF systems play a critical role in many, if not all, of these responses (see reviews by Dunn and Berridge, 1990; Fisher, 1993; Koob et al., 1993). If so, then CRF-containing neurons may coordinate a remarkably well integrated mechanism for adapting to the demands of stressful events. Let us now examine the evidence for this hypothesis.

The possible functions of central CRF—that is, CRF that might be released synaptically instead of into the pituitary portal vasculature—have been investigated primarily by administering the peptide either intracerebroventricularly or intracisternally (into the cisterna magna, a large cerebrospinal fluid–filled expansion of the subarachnoid space). Using this approach, a number of studies have shown that CRF acts on the autonomic nervous system to stimulate sympathetic activity and

epinephrine secretion from the adrenal medulla and to inhibit parasympathetic outflow via the vagus nerve (Fisher, 1989, 1993). Among the results of these actions are elevated plasma norepinephrine and epinephrine concentrations, increased heart rate and arterial pressure, and higher circulating levels of the kidney hormone renin (Figure 11.15). The cardiovascular and catecholaminergic consequences of central CRF administration are inhibited by the ganglionic blocker chlorisondamine, but not by hypophysectomy, thus demonstrating mediation by the autonomic nervous system rather than by altered pituitary–adrenocortical function. Other experiments have shown that intracerebroventricular treatment with the CRF antagonist α-helical CRF$_{9-41}$ attenuates the rise in plasma epinephrine provoked by various stressors. These findings are important in implicating endogenous CRF in the regulation of stress responsivity.

CRF also exerts wide-ranging effects on ingestive behavior, gastrointestinal activity, and energy balance. CRF-treated animals show reduced food intake, de-

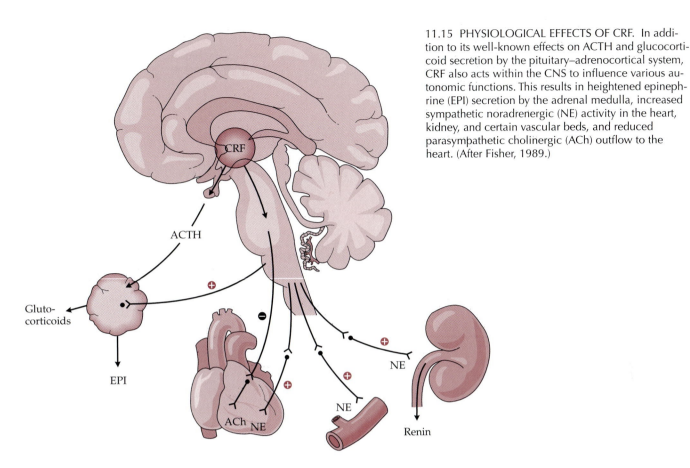

11.15 PHYSIOLOGICAL EFFECTS OF CRF. In addition to its well-known effects on ACTH and glucocorticoid secretion by the pituitary–adrenocortical system, CRF also acts within the CNS to influence various autonomic functions. This results in heightened epinephrine (EPI) secretion by the adrenal medulla, increased sympathetic noradrenergic (NE) activity in the heart, kidney, and certain vascular beds, and reduced parasympathetic cholinergic (ACh) outflow to the heart. (After Fisher, 1989.)

creased gastric acid secretion, decreased gastric emptying and food transit through the small intestine, increased fecal excretion and fecal transit through the large intestine, elevated plasma glucagon levels and hyperglycemia, and increased thermogenesis (heat production) (Dunn and Berridge, 1990; Rothwell, 1990). Most, if not all, of these changes can again be ascribed to increased sympathetic and decreased parasympathetic activity. The effects of CRF on food intake and energy metabolism are noteworthy in several respects. First, stress induces a similar spectrum of behavioral and physiological responses, possibly through the release of central CRF. The result of these reactions seems to be a temporary suppression of nonessential functions with a concurrent mobilization of bodily resources for the purpose of taking immediate physical action (i.e., the "fight-or-flight" response). Second, suppression of appetite by CRF supports the possibility that levels of this neuropeptide could be elevated in certain psychiatric disorders such as depression or anorexia nervosa (see Glowa et al., 1991). Finally, abnormalities in energy metabolism have been found in a number of genetically obese animal strains and may also underlie excessive weight gain in some humans. Given its potentially important role in metabolic regulation, CRF may eventually be implicated in at least some forms of obesity.

In addition to its influence on eating, CRF has been found to influence behavioral activity in a variety of test situations. For rats in a familiar environment, CRF produces dose-dependent increases in locomotor activity, rearing, and grooming (Koob et al., 1993). In contrast, the same doses of CRF cause decreased locomotion and exploratory behavior when subjects are tested in a novel open field or elevated plus maze (situations that are presumed to be more stressful than a familiar environment). CRF has also been reported to decrease responding in conflict tests (such tests are described in Chapter 16 on sedative and anxiolytic drugs) and to decrease interactive behavior in a social interaction test (Dunn and Berridge, 1990; Koob et al., 1993). Together, these findings suggest that CRF may exert an anxiogenic (anxiety-producing) effect that is manifested when subjects are appropriately challenged. Further support for this hypothesis comes from a recent study of transgenic mice that overproduce CRF (Stenzel-Poore et al., 1994). Compared with normal subjects, such mice exhibit signs of increased anxiety in a novel environment and in the elevated plus maze (another standard animal test for screening anxiogenic or anxiolytic treatments).

How might CRF interact with other neurotransmitters or neuromodulators to influence behavior and physiology? One possibility is via the noradrenergic system. The locus coeruleus is innervated by CRF-immunoreactive fibers (Valentino et al., 1992), and neurochemical studies have shown that CRF activates central noradrenergic pathways in both rats (Emoto et al., 1993) and mice

(Dunn and Berridge, 1987). The CRF antagonist α-helical CRF$_{9-41}$ has also been used to demonstrate a role for endogenous CRF in stress-induced activation of the noradrenergic system. Intracerebroventricular injection of this antagonist blocked the induction of tyrosine hydroxylase in the locus coeruleus by a chronic stressor (Melia and Duman, 1991), and it also inhibited stress-induced NE release in the medial prefrontal cortex (Shimizu et al., 1994).

Other studies have suggested that CRF activation of the noradrenergic system might underlie CRF-induced anxiogenesis in rats. In one series of experiments (Butler et al., 1990), CRF was infused either into the ventricular system (i.e., the lateral ventricle or cerebral aqueduct) or directly into the locus coeruleus. Some rats were tested for ambulatory (locomotor) and nonambulatory movement in an activity chamber. Others were subjected to a modified Porsolt test. These animals were fitted with a flotation device and placed in a Plexiglas tank containing 37.5 cm of water at 25°C for 15 minutes. During this period, the amount of time spent either struggling (swimming vigorously) or floating motionless was recorded. Finally, some animals were studied in a "defensive withdrawal" paradigm. This test was performed using a large, brightly lit open field containing an opaque cylindrical chamber that could be entered by the subject. After an initial day of habituation to the apparatus, subjects were tested for defensive withdrawal, as represented by the amount of time spent inside the chamber during a 15-minute period.

Overall, intracerebral CRF administration was found to increase nonambulatory activity, decrease the amount of time spent floating in the Porsolt test, and increase the amount of defensive withdrawal in the open field test. Most importantly, dose–response curves showed that these effects were elicited much more potently by locus coeruleus infusions than by administration into the ventricular system (Figure 11.16). Neurochemical analyses of several forebrain noradrenergic terminal areas further demonstrated CRF-induced increases in the norepinephrine metabolite dihydroxyphenylglycol (DHPG). These findings, coupled with the research cited above demonstrating an excitatory effect of CRF in the locus coeruleus, indicate that the activational and anxiogenic effects of CRF may be mediated at least partially through stimulation of noradrenergic neurons in this area.

Other researchers examined the possible role of norepinephrine in CRF-induced defensive withdrawal by asking whether the behavioral effects could be blocked by selective adrenergic antagonists (Yang and Dunn, 1990). Their results showed that CRF-induced defensive withdrawal could be blocked by central administration of the selective β$_1$-antagonists atenolol or CGP-20712, but not by the β$_2$-antagonist ICI 118,551 or by the peripherally acting, nonselective antagonist CGP-12177. These

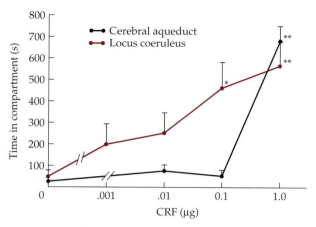

11.16 DEFENSIVE WITHDRAWAL INDUCED BY CENTRAL CRF ADMINISTRATION. Rats were given various doses of CRF infused into either the cerebral aqueduct (the passage connecting the third and fourth ventricles) or the locus coeruleus. Defensive withdrawal was examined 45 minutes later by measuring the amount of time during a 15-minute test period spent in a small, dark compartment located in a brightly lit open field. Note that locus coeruleus infusions were more potent than administration into the ventricular system until a dose of 1 μg was reached (*$p < .025$, **$p < .001$ compared with controls receiving no CRF). (After Butler et al., 1990.)

findings are consistent with the previously described experiments and further suggest that stimulation of β$_1$-adrenergic receptors may play an important role in CRF-induced anxiogenesis.

CRF clearly elicits many behavioral and physiological reactions resembling those observed under conditions of stress. In fact, there are even more stresslike responses to CRF that have not been discussed here due to space limitations, including suppression of reproductive function (Rivier and Vale, 1984b; Rivier, Rivier, and Vale, 1986; Sirinathsinghji et al., 1983), inhibition of growth hormone secretion (Rivier and Vale, 1984a), and alterations in immune function (Irwin, Vale, and Rivier, 1990). Furthermore, as described above and summarized more completely by Dunn and Berridge (1990), α-helical CRF$_{9-41}$ has been found to inhibit many different effects of stress. The combination of CRF administration experiments and studies using CRF antagonist treatment thus provides powerful convergent evidence that this peptide indeed plays a central coordinating role in determining how organisms react physiologically and behaviorally to stressful events in their lives.

Substance P and the Tachykinins

Structure and Localization of the Tachykinins

In the opening section of this chapter, we described how the neuropeptide substance P (SP) was first discovered and characterized. Subsequent research has shown that SP is but one member of a broad family of related peptides known as **tachykinins** (meaning "fast acting"). A number of important tachykinins have been found in various nonmammalian tissues, including eledoisin, which was isolated from octopus salivary glands, and the amphibian peptides physalaemin and kassinin (Maggio, 1988). Besides substance P, other members of the mammalian tachykinin family are neurokinin A (NKA; sometimes also called substance K because of its structural similarity to kassinin), NKA_{3-10}, neurokinin B (NKB; sometimes also called neuromedin K), neuropeptide K (NPK), and neuropeptide γ (NPγ) (Helke et al., 1990; Otsuka and Yoshioka, 1993). All of the mammalian peptides except NKB are derived from a single gene known as the pre-protachykinin (*PPT*) A (or *I*) gene, whereas NKB is derived from a separate gene known as *PPT B* (or *II*).

The processing of the primary transcript (see the section on peptide structure and synthesis above) of the *PPT A* gene is an excellent example of **alternative mRNA splicing**, a phenomenon outlined in Chapter 3. In the 1970s, molecular biologists were surprised to discover that most genes found in higher organisms contain substantial regions of DNA that do not code for any part of the protein products of those genes. These noncoding regions of a gene were found to be interspersed among the coding regions, and hence became known as **introns** (for "*inter*vening sequences"). In contrast, those regions that actually determine the structure of the gene's product were called **exons** (for "*ex*pressed sequences"). To synthesize mRNA molecules that contain the exons, but not the introns, from the primary transcript, a cell must cleave the primary transcript at the exon–intron boundaries and then fuse together the exons by a process called splicing. This is where alternative splicing comes into play. In some instances, different mRNA species are

formed from the same primary transcript because of a failure to splice together all of the available exons. Thus, the same gene can give rise to more than one mRNA and hence more than one set of protein products.

Figure 11.17*a* illustrates the results of alternative mRNA splicing in the case of the *PPT A* gene (which codes for the peptides SP, NKA, and NPγ). Three different mRNA species are formed, which are conventionally called α-, β-, and γ-PPT-A mRNA. Each of these in turn is translated into a slightly different precursor protein (α-, β-, and γ-PPT-A). Exons 2–7 are spliced together in β-PPT-A, whereas exon 6 is lacking in α-PPT-A, and exon 4 is missing from γ-PPT-A (note that exon 1 is not present in any of the mRNAs). This differential splicing is responsible for the different tachykinin peptides processed from each precursor. SP is derived from exon 3 and is therefore produced in each case.

SP is an undecapeptide (11 amino acids) that, like many other neuropeptides, is amidated at the C-terminus. All tachykinins share a C-terminal sequence consisting of —Phe—X—Gly—Leu—Met—NH_2, which is important in conferring similar biological activity on various members of the family. SP is unique among the mammalian tachykinins in possessing a phenylalanine (Phe) residue at position X instead of the valine (Val) residue that is found in all other members of the family (see Figure 11.17*b*).

Determining the distribution of SP in the nervous system has been complicated by the existence of these other peptides, particularly those derived from the same gene (i.e., *PPT A*). This problem has been somewhat overcome in recent work by means of in situ hybridization studies using probes specific for the various *PPT* mRNA species (Helke et al., 1990). Many of the antisera used in immunohistochemical mapping studies,

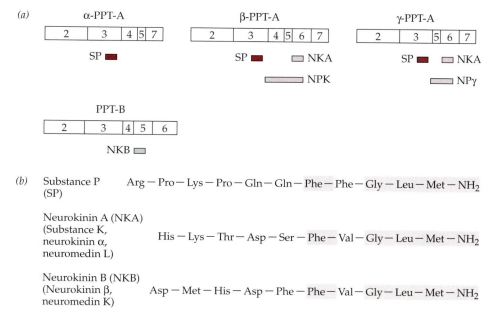

11.17 MAMMALIAN TACHYKININ PEPTIDES AND PRECURSOR PROTEINS. (*a*) The *PPT A* gene gives rise to three precursor proteins (α-PPT-A, β-PPT-A, and γ-PPT-A) through alternative mRNA splicing. Posttranslational processing of these precursors yields the tachykinin peptides substance P (SP), neurokinin A (NKA), neuropeptide K (NPK), and neuropeptide γ (NPγ). A single precursor protein (PPT-B) is derived from the *PPT B* gene and is processed to yield neurokinin B (NKB). (*b*) Amino acid sequences of SP, NKA, and NKB, showing the similar C-terminal region necessary for tachykinin activity (shaded regions). (After Otsuka and Yoshioka, 1993.)

however, have not been selective enough to distinguish between authentic SP and related tachykinins. Use of the term "SP immunoreactivity" in the discussion that follows is therefore not meant to imply that SP is the only tachykinin present in a given cell group or fiber pathway.

There is strong evidence for a neurotransmitter role for SP and other tachykinins in both the central and peripheral nervous systems (see review by Otsuka and Yoshioka, 1993). As shown in Figure 11.18, there is a widespread distribution of presumptive SP-containing cell groups and pathways in the CNS. For example, SP immunoreactivity is found in a subset of the medium spiny neurons that give rise to the output pathways of the corpus striatum. These cells, which also contain GABA and the opioid peptide dynorphin colocalized with SP, project to both the substantia nigra pars reticulata (Gerfen and Young, 1988) and the pars compacta. In the latter area, SP-containing nerve endings appear to synapse directly on dendrites and cell bodies of the nigral dopaminergic neurons (Bolam and Smith, 1990; Chang, 1988). Other SP-immunoreactive cell groups in the forebrain are found in the hypothalamus, amygdaloid complex, and habenula. Serotonin, SP, and in some cases TRH as well have been found to coexist in several cell groups in the brain stem that project to cranial nerve motor nuclei (Tallaksen-Greene, Elde, and Wessendorf, 1993) and also to spinal motor neurons (Wessendorf and Elde, 1987). Yet another descending pathway contains SP

colocalized with the neuropeptide cholecystokinin. This pathway begins in the Edinger–Westphal nucleus and terminates in laminae I and V of the dorsal horn of the spinal cord, where it may be involved in the modulation of somatosensory (especially pain) input (see below) (Maciewicz et al., 1984; Phipps et al., 1983).

Finally, it is important to mention the major functions of SP as a neurotransmitter in the peripheral nervous system. First, there is considerable evidence that SP is one of the transmitters used by primary sensory neurons located in the spinal dorsal root ganglia and the trigeminal ganglion. This topic is covered further in the discussion of SP and pain transmission below. Second, cell bodies and fibers displaying SP immunoreactivity are found in autonomic ganglia, where they are colocalized with various classical transmitters (e.g., acetylcholine or norepinephrine) (Morris and Gibbins, 1989). Both sensory and ganglionic sources of SP contribute to the presence of this compound in the gastrointestinal system and its designation as a "gut–brain" peptide.

Regulation of Substance P Synthesis

The synthesis of most neurotransmitter substances is under complex regulatory control. In some cases, this control is exerted trans-synaptically—that is, by the activity of synaptic inputs to the cells manufacturing the transmitter. Trans-synaptic regulation of SP synthesis has been extensively studied in two different systems: the superior cervical ganglion of the sympathetic nervous

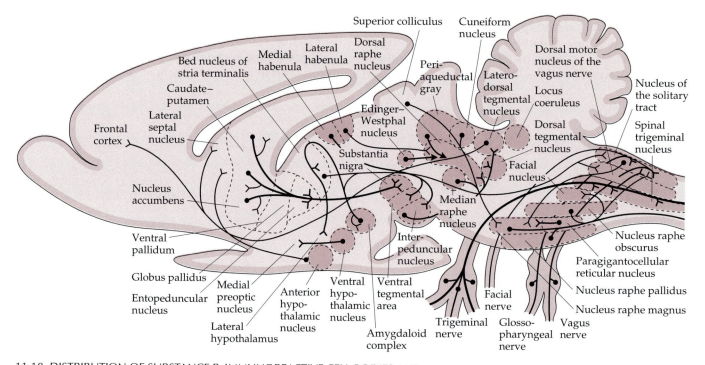

11.18 DISTRIBUTION OF SUBSTANCE P–IMMUNOREACTIVE CELL BODIES AND FIBERS IN THE CENTRAL NERVOUS SYSTEM. Locations of SP-immunoreactive cell bodies and fibers are shown by the dots and solid lines, respectively. Most of the data were obtained from rats. (After Otsuka and Yoshioka, 1993.)

system and the SP-containing neurons of the striatonigral pathway.

Studies of the rat superior cervical ganglion have demonstrated the presence of SP and have elucidated some of the mechanisms regulating its expression (Black et al., 1987). Normal in vivo levels of SP and PPT mRNA in the superior cervical ganglion were found to be quite low. Activation of afferent fibers to the ganglion resulted in a further reduction in SP immunoreactivity, indicating that the normally low level of peptide expression is not due to a lack of ganglionic stimulation. Indeed, SP and PPT mRNA levels in the ganglion rose markedly following pharmacological blockade of synaptic input to the cells, ganglionic denervation in vivo, or removal of the ganglion followed by tissue culture explantation (Black et al., 1987). The mechanism underlying this effect was studied further using explanted (and hence necessarily denervated) ganglia. Veratridine, a drug that depolarizes neurons by increasing sodium influx, blocked the explantation-induced increase in both SP and its mRNA. The effect of veratridine, in turn, could be reversed by the sodium channel blocker tetrodotoxin. These findings suggest that synaptic stimulation of ganglionic neurons suppresses PPT gene expression (or alternatively, decreases the stability of PPT mRNA) by a depolarization-dependent mechanism. Such tonic suppression is alleviated by denervation or by pharmacological blockade of ganglionic transmission, allowing SP levels to rise. It is important to note that markers of noradrenergic function (e.g., tyrosine hydroxylase activity) in these same cells are *increased* rather than decreased by synaptic stimulation. Therefore, different neurotransmitters or neuromodulators in a given cell population can apparently be regulated in different directions by the same set of physiological stimuli.

A different scheme has been found in the regulation of SP in striatonigral neurons. As mentioned earlier, these cells give rise to one of the major output pathways of the striatum. They are also important postsynaptic targets for the massive nigrostriatal dopamine projection (Freund, Powell, and Smith, 1984; Kubota, Inagaki, and Kito, 1986). Evidence from a variety of studies indicates that this dopamine input serves to induce PPT expression and increase SP levels in the striatonigral neurons (reviewed by Angulo and McEwen, 1994). For example, PPT gene expression is markedly increased by the dopamine-releasing drug methamphetamine, whereas striatal SP immunoreactivity and PPT mRNA were significantly decreased by chronic treatment with the dopamine receptor blocker haloperidol or by 6-hydroxydopamine lesions of the substantia nigra. As might be predicted from these lesion results, basal ganglia SP levels also appear to be decreased in human patients with Parkinson's disease (Mauborgne et al., 1983).

Pharmacological studies suggest an interaction between D_1 and D_2 dopamine receptors in the stimulation of striatal tachykinin biosynthesis (Angulo and McEwen, 1994). Elevation of PPT mRNA by methamphetamine can be inhibited by treatment with either a D_1 antagonist (SCH 23390) or a D_2 antagonist (sulpiride). Furthermore, PPT mRNA is increased by treatment with a D_2 agonist (quinpirole), but not a D_1 agonist, yet the D_2 agonist effect is blocked by SCH 23390. This type of interaction between dopamine receptor subtypes has also been found in certain behavioral and electrophysiological assay systems, as discussed previously in Chapter 8.

In summary, the tachykinin system has proved to be extremely valuable for studying trans-synaptic regulation of neurotransmitter gene expression. We have seen that different patterns (and possibly also mechanisms) of control occur in different tissues, and also that the same cell can differentially up- or down-regulate particular transmitter substances in response to the same change in input. Finally, the dopaminergic modulation of tachykinins in the striatum may have important implications for the symptoms of Parkinson's disease, a disorder involving severe damage to the nigrostriatal pathway, and for the appearance of extrapyramidal motor effects in schizophrenics treated chronically with dopamine receptor–blocking drugs.

Tachykinin Receptors

Recognizing the possible roles of the multiple, sometimes colocalized, peptides derived from PPT A and B represents the first step in understanding tachykinin physiology and pharmacology. However, it must also be appreciated that these peptides act on at least three different tachykinin receptor subtypes in the central and peripheral nervous systems (for review, see Gerard et al., 1993; Mussap, Geraghty, and Burcher, 1993). At this time, tachykinin receptors are conventionally designated neurokinin-1 (NK-1; formerly called SP-type), NK-2 (formerly called substance K-type), and NK-3 (formerly neuromedin K-type) receptors. Each receptor subtype has a unique distribution in the brain and periphery, and as illustrated in Table 11.2, each also has a distinctive rank order of potency of the naturally occurring tachykinins. A number of SP analogs have been synthesized that exert relatively selective agonist effects on the various tachykinin receptor classes (Helke et al., 1990; Regoli et al., 1988). Of additional interest is the recent development

Table 11.2	Rank Order of Potency of Tachykinin Peptides at Different Tachykinin Receptor Subtypes
Receptor subtype	**Rank order of potency**
NK-1	SP > NPγ ≥ NKA = NPK > NKB
NK-2	NPK = NPγ ≥ NKA > NKB > SP
NK-3	NKB > NKA > SP

of several nonpeptide tachykinin receptor antagonists, including CP96345 (NK-1) and SR48968 (NK-2) (Watling, 1992; Watling and Krause, 1993). Because of the important central and peripheral effects of SP and the other tachykinins (see below), these novel antagonists may eventually find use in various clinical applications.

CP96345

SR48968

Current information on the binding characteristics and distribution of tachykinin receptors is summarized in Mussap, Geraghty, and Burcher (1993). In determining the localization of tachykinin receptors, investigators noticed certain discrepancies with the anatomy of SP-containing pathways. Similar disparities have been found within some other transmitter systems, thus giving rise to the idea of a "mismatch problem" in receptor mapping research. However, the problem has seemed particularly acute in the case of SP. As noted by Herkenham and McLean (1986), "Immunoreactive substance P fibers and terminals are consistently out of register with substance P receptors" (p. 145). In general, there are a number of possible logical as well as technical reasons for the presence of receptors without an appropriate transmitter nearby, or the presence of high levels of neurotransmitter in the apparent absence of a suitable receptor (Herkenham, 1991; Herkenham and McLean, 1986; Kuhar, 1985). The question is, can such explanations account for the mismatch problem as it pertains to SP?

The tachykinin mismatch problem is observed most clearly in the substantia nigra pars reticulata, which contains perhaps the highest density of SP-immunoreactive fibers and nerve endings in the entire brain. Yet this area is nearly devoid of SP-preferring (NK-1) receptors (Mussap, Geraghty, and Burcher, 1993). One proposed solution to this paradox is related to the fact that NKA is present along with SP in the striatonigral pathway

(Valentino et al., 1986) and, in fact, excites nigral cells with a potency that possibly exceeds that of SP (Collingridge and Davies, 1982; Innis, Andrade, and Aghajanian, 1985). These findings suggest that NKA, rather than SP, might be the physiologically active tachykinin in the substantia nigra (Quirion, 1985). However, the NKA-preferring NK-2 receptor is expressed mainly in peripheral tissues, rather than in the brain. Thus, it may be more appropriate to look for other explanations for the receptor mismatch problem, such as the presence of a previously unidentified receptor subtype or the possibility that SP released in the substantia nigra acts at some distance from its site of origin.

The NK-1, NK-2, and NK-3 receptors have all been cloned, and their putative structures are consistent with membership in the G protein–coupled receptor superfamily (Gerard et al., 1993; Mussap, Geraghty, and Burcher, 1993). Tachykinin receptors are positively coupled to phospholipase C and thus stimulate the phosphoinositide second messenger system. In some tissues and cell types, adenylyl cyclase activation has also been reported (Gerard et al., 1993). At the cellular level, the effect of SP in the brain and spinal cord is mainly excitatory, although neuronal responses to SP are manifested more slowly than responses to excitatory amino acids such as glutamate or aspartate (Piercey, Moon, and Blinn, 1985). The excitatory effects of SP seem to be mediated primarily by a G protein–mediated inhibition of K^+ channel conductance (Nakajima et al., 1993; Nicoll, Malenka, and Kauer, 1990).

Behavioral Effects of Substance P

In the CNS, the tachykinin peptides have been implicated in a number of behavioral functions. For example, intracerebral infusion of SP, NKA, or other tachykinins in rats can lead to behavioral excitation characterized by locomotor activation, stimulation of grooming behavior, and elicitation of wet-dog shakes (Barbeau, Rondeau, and Jolicoeur, 1980; Elliott and Iversen, 1986). Results of both pharmacological and neurochemical studies suggest that these activational effects may be related to stimulation of the nigrostriatal and/or mesolimbic dopamine systems (Barbeau, Rondeau, and Jolicoeur, 1980; Reid et al., 1990). SP may also be involved in the neural pathways underlying female sexual behavior in rodents (Dornan, Malsbury, and Penney, 1987; Dornan, Akesson, and Micevych, 1990). This notion is supported by evidence that in certain hypothalamic areas, many neurons containing estrogen or progestin receptors are also immunoreactive for SP (Akesson and Micevych, 1988; Nielsen and Blaustein, 1990).

The Role of Substance P in Pain Transmission

Although SP undoubtedly is involved in many behavioral systems, by far the greatest attention has been devoted to its role as a sensory transmitter. Based on the discovery that bioassayable SP is much higher in the dorsal than in the ventral roots of the spinal cord, Lembeck (1953) was the first to propose the presence of this peptide in primary afferent fibers. Subsequent studies established the presence of SP-immunoreactive neurons in dorsal root (spinal) and trigeminal ganglia as well as SP-positive fibers in the dorsal horn (Chan-Palay and Palay, 1977; Hökfelt et al., 1975b). The organization of this system is depicted in Figure 11.19. Each neuron gives rise to a bifurcated axon consisting of a short central branch that projects to the dorsal horn of the spinal cord and a longer peripheral branch that innervates the skin (right-hand side), gastrointestinal tract (left-hand side), and other organs (the function of this peripheral branch is discussed in greater detail below). SP can be released from terminals at both branches of the axon.

In addition to the anatomical findings just presented, physiological evidence strongly supports SP as a sensory transmitter (Otsuka and Yanagisawa, 1987; Otsuka and Yoshioka, 1993). First, SP is released in the spinal cord in a Ca^{2+}-dependent manner upon stimulation of sensory nerves. Second, tachykinin receptors are found in the dorsal horn, and neurons in this area exhibit excitatory responses to SP application. Finally, stimulation of the dorsal root leads to a slow EPSP in dorsal horn cells that can be inhibited by a SP antago-

nist or antiserum. However, it is important to note that SP is by no means the sole compound responsible for sensory transmission. This peptide is present in only 10% to 20% of primary afferent fibers and appears to be colocalized with other peptides as well as the excitatory amino acid glutamate (De Biasi and Rustioni, 1988; Holzer, 1988).

The somatosensory system, of course, detects and relays information concerning touch, temperature, and pain. This information is carried by several different classes of fibers that vary in their diameter and degree of myelination (Salt and Hill, 1983). As SP has been implicated particularly in responses to nociceptive (noxious or painful) stimuli, we will concentrate on that modality. Nociceptive input is conveyed by two fiber systems: small, unmyelinated C-fibers and small, myelinated Aδ-fibers. SP is thought to be particularly important in the slowly conducting C-fiber system, which transmits delayed pain information (Otsuka and Yanagisawa, 1987). This idea is consistent with the distribution of SP-containing afferents in the spinal cord. As shown in Figure 11.20, SP is concentrated in laminae I and II (Rexed, 1954) of the dorsal horn gray at levels 5 to 10 times greater than in the ventral gray. These laminae, which consist of the posteromarginal nucleus and the substantia gelatinosa, respectively, are the major termination zones of the C-fiber system.

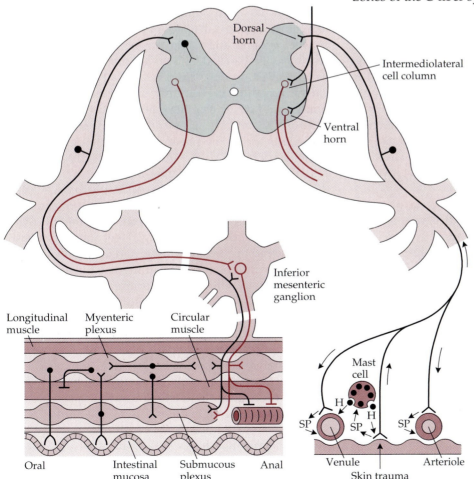

11.19 LOCATION OF SUBSTANCE P–CONTAINING NEURONS AND FIBERS IN THE SPINAL CORD, SKIN, AND INTESTINE. SP-positive cells and fibers are shown as filled circles and solid lines respectively. Non-SP cells and fibers are depicted with open circles and shaded lines. See text for further details. (After Otsuka and Yoshioka, 1993.)

(a)

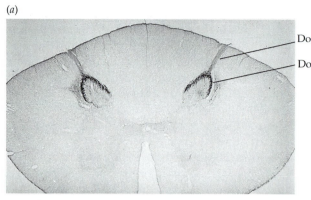

(b)

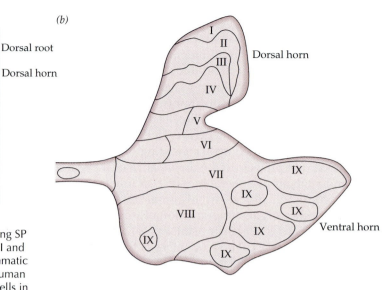

Dorsal root

Dorsal horn

Dorsal horn

Ventral horn

11.20 LOCALIZATION OF SUBSTANCE P IN THE SPINAL CORD. (a) Cross-section through monkey spinal cord showing SP immunoreactivity in the dorsal horn, particularly in laminae I and II, which receive input from nociceptive fibers. (b) A diagrammatic representation of Rexed's laminae in the gray matter of the human cervical spinal cord. Neurons in laminae I and II project to cells in laminae V and VI that form the lateral spinothalamic tract. This pathway then ascends, mostly contralaterally, to higher centers in the brain stem. (a from Iversen, 1979; courtesy of Stephen Hunt.)

Other anatomical, physiological, and pharmacological studies likewise support the participation of SP in transmitting nociceptive information. For example, recent studies with cats demonstrated that dorsal horn neurons that respond to noxious stimuli receive substantial inputs from SP-immunoreactive fibers (Cuello et al., 1993). Such stimuli also increase PPT gene expression in dorsal root ganglion cells and cause a release of SP in the substantia gelatinosa (Duggan et al., 1987; Noguchi et al., 1988). Furthermore, intrathecal injection of exogenous SP or other tachykinins in mice produces a characteristic scratching behavior thought by many researchers to reflect some type of pain sensation. This response can be inhibited by coadministration of various tachykinin antagonists (Vaught, 1988), suggesting a direct involvement of spinal tachykinin receptors.

Perhaps the most compelling evidence favoring SP as a pain transmitter stems from the discovery and exploitation of a substance known as capsaicin. This compound is the pungent principle found in chili peppers (genus *Capsicum*). It produces not only the "hot" sensation experienced upon eating these peppers, but also blistering and pain when applied to the skin. The effects of capsaicin are caused by the stimulation of nociceptive cells that give rise to C-fibers, other cells that serve as C-fiber warmth receptors, and some of the cells associated

with pain-carrying Aδ-fibers (Holzer, 1991). Many of these sensory neurons contain SP, and this peptide is thus believed to play an important role in mediating capsaicin-induced pain sensation.

The activating effects of capsaicin on the above-mentioned sensory neurons are probably mediated by a specific membrane receptor. Support for this hypothesis comes from two major findings: (1) resiniferatoxin, a capsaicin-like compound from the plant genus *Euphorbia*, can be used to label a population of binding sites in sensory ganglia, and (2) the physiological effects of capsaicin can be blocked by a novel antagonist called capsazepine (Dray, 1992; Holzer, 1991). The putative capsaicin receptor is coupled in some manner to a nonselective cation channel that permits the inward passage of Ca^{2+} and Na^+ ions and the outward movement of K^+ ions across the plasma membrane. A net inward positive current results, which accounts for capsaicin's depolarizing effect on its target cells.

Ironically, capsaicin is used medically to treat certain types of painful disorders (Carter, 1991). For example, capsaicin is an active ingredient in some over-the-counter rubs and liniments (e.g., Heet and Capzasin-P) administered to alleviate muscle and joint pain. Because these preparations produce an intense burning sensation, they may alleviate the original pain through a process of counterirritation. At sufficient doses of capsaicin, the initial unpleasant feelings are followed by desensitization, which renders the sensory neurons temporarily unresponsive to painful stimuli. A capsaicin-containing cream (Zostrix) is currently available for the relief of arthritic pain, and this medication has also been tested with painful skin disorders such as psoriasis and postherpetic neuralgia (nerve pain following *Herpes zoster* infection). Although the results suggest some degree of therapeutic efficacy in these disorders, the clinical usefulness of such preparations is limited by the lack of

CH_3O — $CH_2 - NH - \overset{\overset{O}{\|}}{C} - (CH_2)_4 - CH = CH - CH \overset{CH_3}{\underset{CH_3}{<}}$

HO

Capsaicin

tolerance of many patients for the effects of the capsaicin itself (Carter, 1991). Nevertheless, new applications continue to be developed. One of the most recent is a mixture of (capsaicin-containing) cayenne pepper with Betty Crocker taffy, which was formulated by Linda Bartoshuk and Ann Berger at Yale University for treating cancer patients with mouth lesions (see Levenson, 1995).

When high doses of capsaicin are administered systemically rather than locally, a toxic effect is exerted that results in damage to, or even loss of, the capsaicin-sensitive cell population. The greatest degree of neurotoxicity is observed in immature animals. For example, newborn rats treated with 50 mg/kg of capsaicin show a permanent loss of 50% to 90% of all unmyelinated sensory fibers (Holzer, 1988, 1991). A variety of compounds, including SP, are depleted following capsaicin-induced degeneration, a finding that has served as additional support for their putative role in nociceptive transmission. Capsaicin neurotoxicity is probably due to massive sodium and calcium influx, which would lead to cell damage or death by a mechanism similar to that postulated for the excitatory amino acid NMDA receptor (see Chapter 10).

Our final comments concern the interaction of SP and opiates in the control of pain transmission. As we shall see in Chapter 12, opiate drugs and endogenous opioid peptides called enkephalins and endorphins are potent analgesic compounds. Jessell and Iversen (1977) noted a high density of opiate receptors in the superficial laminae of the dorsal horn, where SP is similarly concentrated. These investigators then found evidence that potassium-evoked SP release from slices of spinal trigeminal nucleus was inhibited by opiate drugs as well as by opioid peptides. Consequently, Jessell and Iversen hypothesized that opiate analgesia at the level of the spinal cord involves a presynaptic inhibition of SP release from nociceptive fibers (Figure 11.21).

Subsequent work has supported and extended these initial findings. In several studies, opiate compounds were found to inhibit in vivo SP release evoked by either noxious sensory stimuli or acute capsaicin treatment (Hirota et al., 1985; Yaksh et al., 1980). Moreover, neonatal treatment with a high dose of capsaicin subsequently abolished the effect of opiates on SP release, suggesting that nociceptive fibers, rather than SP-containing descending pathways, are the site of opiate action (Pohl et al., 1989). Although the mechanism by which presynaptic inhibition occurs is not completely established, one possibility is a modulation of voltage-sensitive Ca^{2+} channels, which would lead to decreased Ca^{2+} influx in the nerve terminals and reduced neurotransmitter release (Mudge, Leeman, and Fishbach, 1979). Finally, the identity of the receptors mediating the presynaptic inhibition effect has been investigated by means of receptor-selective agonists and antagonists. Some researchers have suggested that this effect may specifically involve δ

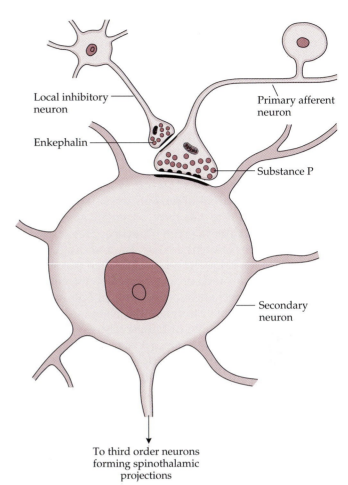

11.21 OPIATE-INDUCED INHIBITION OF SUBSTANCE P RELEASE. According to this model of opiate-mediated analgesia in the spinal cord, opiate receptors are located on the presynaptic terminals of primary afferent (nociceptive) axons containing SP. Local inhibitory neurons release enkephalin onto these terminals, thereby reducing SP release and attenuating the transmission of pain information to the brain.

opiate receptors (Pohl et al., 1989); however, a number of studies have also implicated the other two major opiate receptor subtypes, μ and κ, in spinal analgesia (Collin et al., 1992; Millan, 1990). This apparent discrepancy may be due to the location of opiate receptors not only on primary afferent nerve terminals, but also on the terminals of local enkephalinergic neurons (where they presumably function as autoreceptors), as well as on the cell bodies of spinothalamic neurons. Thus, opiate analgesia probably arises from a combination of pre- and postsynaptic inhibition mediated by several different receptor subtypes.

Substance P and Inflammation

Many types of skin trauma give rise not only to painful sensations, but also to an inflammatory reaction, the so-called "triple response" characterized by (1) erythema (local reddening), (2) flare (a rapidly spreading area of redness), and (3) the gradual development of a wheal (a raised area of the skin). The erythema is caused by local vasodilation, whereas flare stems from expanding arteriolar dilation mediated by axon reflexes. The wheal is produced by increased venular permeability and consequent plasma extravasasion (leakage into the surrounding space). Inflammatory responses to chemical or thermal skin injury are reduced, if not eliminated, by capsaicin treatment, strongly implicating SP-containing C-fibers in these responses (Otsuka and Yoshioka, 1993).

The right-hand side of Figure 11.19 illustrates the role of SP in the inflammatory process. Initially, skin trauma (upward-directed arrow) triggers afferent impulses in the peripheral axon branches. This response rapidly generates efferent activity, leading to a local release of SP in the skin. The released SP then participates in vascular dilation and enhancement of permeability, either through a direct effect on endothelial cells and vascular smooth muscle or through the action of other mediating substances. Finally, histamine released from mast cells (see Chapter 10) also appears to be involved in the flare response by stimulating SP release from sensory terminals. A positive-feedback loop may also occur in which SP provokes histamine secretion from neighboring mast cells. This loop presumably contributes to the expansion and prolongation of inflammation observed in the flare response.

The Role of Substance P in the Gastrointestinal System

Considering that SP was the first peptide to be found in both brain and gut, it is important to discuss the role of this substance in gastrointestinal function. SP is one of a number of transmitters that regulate gut physiology. Its specific actions include a direct contractile effect on intestinal smooth muscle, alteration of ion transport by the intestinal mucosa, and dilation of blood vessels in the intestinal wall (Costa et al., 1985; Otsuka and Yoshioka, 1993). Furthermore, SP may play an important role in triggering or modulating the peristaltic reflex (Barthó and Holzer, 1985). The intestinal actions of SP are mediated by two separate classes of cells: *intrinsic* SP-containing neurons located entirely within the intestinal wall, and dorsal root ganglion SP neurons that provide an *extrinsic* input to the gut. The arrangement of these cells and their fibers is illustrated in the left-hand side of Figure 11.19. The mucosal (glandular) lining of the intestine and the overlying circular muscle layer are served by two parasympathetic ganglia, the myenteric plexus and the submucous plexus. As shown in the figure, the mucosal epithelial cells are thought to receive input from intrinsic SP-immunoreactive neurons located in both plexuses. Cells in the myenteric plexus apparently also innervate the submucous plexus and the circular muscle layer. Finally, the extrinsic SP fibers, which are much sparser than those derived from the intrinsic cells, inner-

vate primarily the submucous plexus and associated blood vessels (although a few are also found in the myenteric plexus). Axon collaterals from the sensory SP-containing cells additionally enter the inferior mesenteric ganglion, thereby providing an afferent pathway from the gut to sympathetic postganglionic neurons.

Cholecystokinin

Structure and Localization

Cholecystokinin (CCK), the last peptide we will discuss in this chapter, is another gut–brain peptide. Cholecystokinin was first discovered in the gastrointestinal system, where it stimulates gallbladder contraction and enhances pancreatic enzyme secretion (Liddle, 1994). Cholecystokinin is actually a family of peptides derived from a common precursor, pre-proCCK. As shown in Figure 11.22, pre-proCCK is made up of four major domains. The first domain, located at the amino terminus, is a 20-amino acid sequence that functions as the signal for entry of the molecule into the endoplasmic reticulum. Next is a 25-amino acid stretch (residues 21–45), termed the "spacer peptide" because it is cleaved off and discarded in the formation of CCK. The third domain is a 58-amino acid region that constitutes the largest form of CCK (i.e., CCK-58) detected in most tissues. The remaining C-terminal peptide (residues 104–115) is also removed and discarded in the process of posttranslational processing of pre-proCCK.

Several other aspects of CCK structure are important to mention. First, the tyrosine (Y) residue at position 97 is almost always sulfated, as shown in the figure. Second, after cleavage of the C-terminal peptide, the phenylalanine (F) at position 103 is amidated. Both of these modifications are absolutely necessary for full bioactivity of CCK. Finally, as mentioned above, other, shorter forms of CCK are present in varying amounts in both the brain and the gut. In fact, biochemical studies have indicated a preponderance of CCK-8 (residues 96–103) in nervous tissue (Rehfeld et al., 1985). Subsequent references to CCK without an accompanying fragment size will refer to this octapeptide form.

The discovery of CCK in the nervous system is credited to Vanderhaeghen, Signeau, and Gepts (1975), who reported the presence of a brain peptide that cross-reacted with antibodies directed against gastrin (a related gut–brain peptide possessing a C-terminal pentapeptide sequence that is identical to that of CCK). CCK-containing neurons have since been found in a widespread distribution throughout the brain, and release of CCK-immunoreactive material has been documented in vivo using microdialysis (Raiteri, Paudice, and Vallebuona, 1993). The localization of CCK-immunoreactive cell bodies and fibers in the rat nervous system has been reviewed by several authors (Fallon

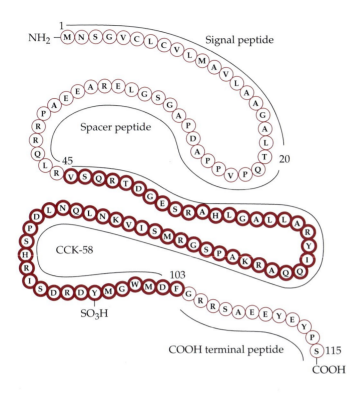

11.22 STRUCTURE OF PRE-PROCHOLECYSTOKININ. In humans and rats, pre-proCCK is made up of 115 amino acids that can be divided into four major domains: the N-terminal signal peptide, a 58-amino acid region that contains the biologically active peptides, a so-called spacer peptide separating the signal peptide from CCK, and a C-terminal peptide. (After Liddle, 1994.)

11.23). Many of these cells are probably local circuit neurons, although CCK-containing fibers are also present in corticofugal pathways as well as in the corpus callosum. Other forebrain structures containing significant numbers of CCK-immunoreactive neurons include the hippocampus, amygdala, claustrum, bed nucleus of the stria terminalis, and a number of thalamic and hypothalamic nuclei. CCK is present in both the paraventricular and supraoptic nuclei and appears to be colocalized with oxytocin in a number of magnocellular neurons. The distribution of CCK in the rat brain as determined immunohistochemically has been confirmed by means of in situ hybridization for pre-proCCK mRNA (Ingram et al., 1989), and this technique has similarly been used to map CCK gene expression in the human brain (Savasta, Palacios, and Mengod, 1990).

CCK-positive perikarya are also found in the midbrain, brain stem, spinal cord, sensory ganglia, autonomic ganglia, and retina (Fallon and Seroogy, 1985). Particular attention has been directed to a group of neurons in the ventral midbrain that possess CCK colocalized with dopamine. These cells are concentrated in the

and Seroogy, 1985; Vanderhaeghen, 1985). To begin, CCK neurons are very prominent in the cerebral cortex (particularly in layers 2 and 3), and indeed, this substance is present at a higher molar concentration in the cortex than any other peptide examined thus far (Figure

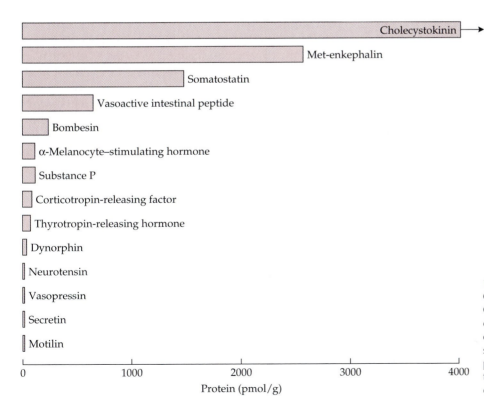

11.23 ESTIMATED CONCENTRATIONS OF NEUROPEPTIDES IN THE CEREBRAL CORTEX. CCK is present in a higher concentration in the cerebral cortex than any other peptide studied to date. The arrow signifies a value greater than 4,000 pmol/g protein. These data are primarily representative of the rat brain and come from references cited by Crawley (1985b).

ventral tegmental area and some parts of the substantia nigra, and their projections have been reported to terminate in the posterior medial regions of the nucleus accumbens and olfactory tubercle, the central nucleus of the amygdala, the bed nucleus of the stria terminalis, and the periventricular zone of the caudate nucleus (Hökfelt et al., 1985). It is interesting to note that although CCK-containing nerve terminals have been found in the main body of the caudate nucleus, the massive dopaminergic nigrostriatal tract does not seem to be the source of these terminals. The main CCK projection to the caudate therefore must arise elsewhere, possibly as a part of the corticostriatal pathway or, alternatively, in subcortical areas other than the ventral mesencephalon.

Cholecystokinin Receptors

As we shall see below, CCK functions not only as a neurotransmitter but also as an important digestive hormone affecting the gallbladder, stomach, and pancreas. When brain and pancreatic CCK binding sites were first compared, evidence was obtained for the existence of a distinct receptor subtype in each tissue (Innis and Snyder, 1980). Moran and colleagues (1986) subsequently proposed a designation of CCK-A for the peripheral site (A = alimentary) and CCK-B for the central site (B = brain). This distinction, however, is an oversimplification, as each receptor subtype has been found in both the periphery and the brain (Woodruff and Hughes, 1991). Researchers have cloned the rat CCK-A and CCK-B receptors, as well as the human CCK-B receptor (Pisegna et al., 1992; Wank et al., 1992, Wank, Pisegna, and De Weerth, 1992). The deduced structures of these receptors indicate that they are members of the G protein–coupled receptor superfamily.

Autoradiographic studies confirm that CCK-B receptors are the predominant subtype in the brain. In rats, moderate to high densities of these receptors have been found in the neocortex (layer 3), olfactory bulbs, nucleus accumbens, ventral striatum, and various regions of the limbic system, diencephalon, and brain stem (Carlberg et al., 1992; Chang et al., 1989; Knapp et al., 1990). In contrast, CCK-A receptors have a much more restricted distribution in the brain, with the highest densities reported in the area postrema, the nucleus of the solitary tract, and the A2 noradrenergic cell group of the medulla (Carlberg et al., 1992; Woodruff et al., 1991).

During the late 1980s, CCK pharmacology was advanced significantly by the development of several nonpeptide, benzodiazepine-based antagonists with high selectivity for the CCK receptor subtypes. The prototypical CCK-A antagonist is MK-329 (originally designated L-364,718 and sometimes also called devazepide), and the corresponding CCK-B antagonist is L-365,260 (Woodruff and Hughes, 1991). Because of their ability to cross the blood–brain barrier and their greater resistance to meta-

bolic breakdown compared with CCK-related peptides, these and other recently developed compounds have already played a prominent role in elucidating the physiological and behavioral actions of CCK in the CNS (see below).

Devazepide

L-365,260

A number of electrophysiological studies have indicated that CCK acts as an excitatory neurotransmitter (Woodruff et al., 1991), although it can also interact with dopamine in an inhibitory manner (see below). The mechanisms underlying these complex actions of CCK in the nervous system are not yet understood. One report suggests that CCK may excite hippocampal neurons by inhibiting an outward K^+ current across the cell membrane (Buckett and Saint, 1989). Based on the mapping studies discussed above, this effect is most likely mediated by CCK-B receptors. In contrast, the mechanism of action of CCK-A receptors in pancreatic acinar cells (cells of the pancreas that secrete digestive enzymes) has been extensively studied. CCK-stimulated enzyme secretion from these cells appears to be mediated principally by stimulation of phospholipase C, intracellular Ca^{2+} mobilization, and activation of protein kinase C and Ca^{2+}/calmodulin-dependent protein kinase (Liddle, 1994). It remains to be determined whether CCK-A receptors in the brain operate by the same mechanism.

Physiological and Behavioral Effects

As would be expected of a peptide with such a widespread distribution in the nervous system, CCK has been implicated in a number of physiological and behavioral processes, including neuroendocrine regulation (Bondy et al., 1989), pain transmission (Baber, Dourish, and Hill, 1989), learning and memory (Itoh and Lal, 1990), and exploratory behavior (Crawley, 1988). The effects of CCK agonists and antagonists on exploratory and "emotional" behavior are particularly interesting because they suggest that central CCK systems might play an important role in anxiety. Indeed, several human studies, as well as a number of experiments using animal models of anxiety, strongly support this contention.

As reviewed by Ravard and Dourish (1990), one line of evidence concerns the possible interactions of CCK with the anxiolytic (anxiety-reducing) drugs called benzodiazepines (see Chapter 16). We have already noted that CCK receptor antagonists can be generated that contain the core benzodiazepine structure. Furthermore, chronic administration of benzodiazepines was found to decrease neuronal responsivity to CCK, whereas CCK receptor density in the hippocampus and frontal cortex was increased following benzodiazepine withdrawal. These findings suggest that the anxiolytic action of benzodiazepines might be related to their effects on central CCK systems.

Human studies are consistent with the hypothesis that CCK can exert an anxiogenic (anxiety-producing) effect in various situations. For example, panic-like attacks have been induced in patients with panic disorder and even in normal individuals by administration of either CCK-4 or pentagastrin, a pentapeptide similar to CCK-5 (Harro, Vasar, and Bradwejn, 1993; Ravard and Dourish, 1990). Although CCK-8 failed to produce the same response, this may have been due to poorer penetration of the larger peptide across the blood–brain barrier.

Animal experiments implicating CCK in the induction of anxiety have used test systems such as the black–white box, elevated plus maze or X maze, holebox, social interaction test, and conditioned suppression of drinking (many of these are also discussed in Chapter 16). In the black-white box test, rats or mice are placed in a chamber containing a black, dimly lit compartment and a white, brightly lit compartment. Subject "anxiety" is determined in part by latency to enter the dark compartment (a shorter latency is considered to indicate greater anxiety) and by the amount of time spent there. Elevated mazes are equipped with open and enclosed arms, and the amount of time spent in the enclosed arms is deemed to reflect the level of anxiety. Holeboxes are enclosed chambers containing several small holes cut in the walls. Nose pokes into the holes are thought to be a kind of exploratory behavior, and would thus be inversely related to the level of anxiety. In the social interaction test, pairs of rats are placed in a novel or brightly lit environment. Anxiolytic agents increase the amount of time the rats spend interacting socially under these conditions. Finally, in the conditioned suppression paradigm, thirsty subjects that are initially allowed to drink freely are then exposed to an auditory stimulus previously paired with electric shock. The degree of suppression of the ongoing drinking behavior serves as a measure of anxiety.

In a number of studies using various combinations of these test systems, CCK antagonists have consistently acted as anxiolytics, whereas CCK agonists have exerted anxiogenic effects (Woodruff and Hughes, 1991). Still to be resolved is the receptor subtype involved in these actions. Experiments with PD134308 and PD135158, two recently developed CCK-B receptor blockers, have suggested an important role for that subtype (Figure 11.24) (Hughes et al., 1990; Singh et al., 1991). Additional support is provided by the above-mentioned human studies showing an anxiogenic effect of the CCK-B selective agonist CCK-4. On the other hand, other studies have implicated the less prevalent CCK-A receptor subtype (Ravard and Dourish, 1990). Particularly provocative are findings indicating a possible involvement of CCK-A receptors in the posterior medial nucleus accumbens (Daugé et al., 1989), a region generally considered devoid of these binding sites on the basis of conventional mapping studies. It is possible that both CCK-A and CCK-B receptors play significant roles in the anxiogenic process, although this remains to be confirmed. In any case, at least some CCK antagonists seem to reduce anxiety without sedative side effects, which makes them interesting candidates for possible therapeutic use in humans (Hughes et al., 1990; Woodruff and Hughes, 1991).

Interactions between CCK and Dopamine

High concentrations of CCK are found in the nucleus accumbens and the caudate nucleus, important projection areas of the mesolimbic and nigrostriatal dopamine pathways, respectively. Furthermore, as discussed above, CCK and dopamine coexist in many of the midbrain neurons that give rise to the mesolimbic system. It is therefore not surprising that the possible interactions of these cotransmitters have been of great interest to many investigators.

In a review of this work, Crawley (1991) noted that CCK–dopamine interactions have been found using various electrophysiological, neurochemical, and behavioral approaches. Electrophysiological experiments have demonstrated that ventral tegmental and nigral neurons exhibit excitatory responses to CCK alone. On the other hand, CCK has been found to potentiate the autoreceptor-mediated inhibitory effects of dopamine and apomorphine on cell firing. The reason for this discrepancy is still unknown, although it could involve differentially acting CCK receptor subtypes.

Studies of functional interactions between CCK and dopamine have focused on locomotor activity and exploration, behaviors known to be regulated by the mesolimbic dopamine system. At low doses, direct administration of CCK alone into the posterior medial nucleus accumbens failed to alter locomotor behavior; however, the peptide did potentiate dopamine-induced hyperactivity. This effect seemed to involve CCK-A receptors (Crawley, 1992), which is noteworthy in view of the fact

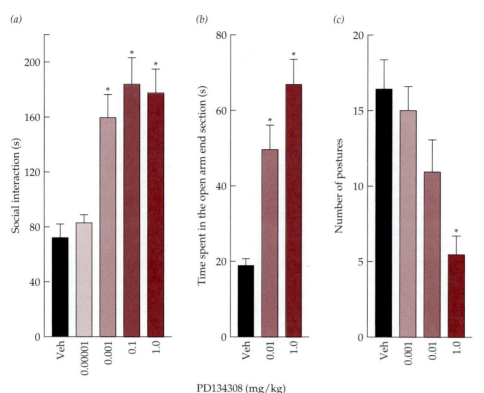

(a)

(b)

(c)

PD134308 (mg/kg)

11.24 EFFECTS OF THE CCK-B AN-TAGONIST PD134308 IN THREE DIFFERENT ANIMAL MODELS OF ANXIETY. PD 134308 was given sub-cutaneously at the indicated doses and then tested for anxiolytic activity in (*a*) the rat social interaction test, (*b*) the rat elevated plus maze, and (*c*) the mar-moset human threat test. The rat mod-els are described in the text. The mar-moset test measures the number of agonistic postures displayed toward a human observer standing near the home cage. *$p < .001$ compared with vehicle (Veh). (After Hughes et al., 1990.)

that some type of "cryptic" CCK-A receptor site in the posterior medial accumbens was also hypothesized to underlie the anxiogenic properties of CCK in this area. In contrast, CCK injected into the anterior nucleus ac-cumbens inhibited dopamine-induced hyperactivity, possibly by an action on CCK-B receptors.

The neurochemical interactions of CCK and do-pamine may shed light on the mechanisms underlying the behavioral phenomena mentioned above. Specifi-cally, CCK has been reported to enhance dopamine re-lease from the posterior nucleus accumbens by a CCK-A receptor–dependent mechanism, but to inhibit release from the anterior part of the nucleus via CCK-B recep-tors (Crawley, 1991). The different effects of CCK on the posterior and anterior nucleus accumbens may be re-lated not only to the receptor subtypes involved, but also to the different sources of CCK in each case. CCK in the posterior region is colocalized with dopamine in the mesolimbic nerve terminals, whereas CCK in the ante-rior accumbens appears to arise from other areas, such as the cerebral cortex.

Finally, evidence has also been presented for receptor interactions between CCK and dopamine. Chronic ad-ministration of the dopamine antagonist haloperidol sig-nificantly increased CCK receptor binding in the nucleus accumbens and cortex, whereas CCK treatment increased dopamine D_2 receptor binding in the accumbens, cortex, and olfactory tubercles (Crawley, 1991). Consequently, re-ceptor changes must be considered when behavioral in-teractions between CCK and dopamine following long-term drug administration are examined.

Considering the critical role of dopamine in Parkin-son's disease, schizophrenia, and possibly other neu-ropathological and psychopathological conditions, the ability of CCK to modulate dopaminergic functioning has important etiologic and therapeutic implications. Al-though definitive results are still lacking, researchers have already begun to examine the possible role of CCK in the genesis of these disorders as well as the selective use of CCK agonists or antagonists as therapeutic agents (Rasmussen, 1994; Wettstein, Buéno, and Junien, 1994). For example, initial reports by Boyce and colleagues in-dicate that the CCK-B antagonist L-365,260 potentiates the therapeutic efficacy of L-DOPA in a monkey model of Parkinsonism, whereas CCK-8 treatment inhibits the oc-currence of dyskinesias, undesirable side effects of chronic L-DOPA administration (Boyce, Rupniak, Steventon et al., 1990; Boyce, Rupniak, Tye et al., 1990).

The Role of CCK in Food Intake and Metabolism

As mentioned earlier, CCK was identified as a hormone in the gastrointestinal system long before its discovery in the brain. Gut CCK is synthesized in a specific type of en-docrine cell found in the duodenum and jejunum regions of the small intestine (Liddle, 1994). When food is present in the lumen of the intestine, these cells are stimulated to release CCK into the bloodstream, through which it trav-els to various target tissues. The first discovered role of CCK was the stimulation of gallbladder contraction, and the term "cholecystokinin" in fact means "that which ex-cites or moves the gallbladder" (Ivy and Oldberg, 1928). Another gut factor, originally called pancreozymin, that enhances the secretion of pancreatic digestive enzymes was later found to be none other than CCK (Mutt and Jorpes, 1971). Other peripheral actions of CCK include stimulation of pancreatic hormone (e.g., insulin) secretion and inhibition of stomach emptying (Liddle, 1994). Thus, we can see that CCK plays a pivotal role in coordinating physiological reactions to food ingestion.

A possible related function involving *behavioral* responses to food was first suggested by the studies of Gibbs, Smith, and their colleagues (Gibbs, Young, and Smith, 1973), who demonstrated an inhibition of food consumption in hungry rats treated intraperitoneally with either a partially purified CCK preparation or synthetic CCK-8. The characteristics of this response, along with the knowledge that CCK is released into the bloodstream when food enters the intestine, prompted these investigators to hypothesize that endogenous CCK might serve as a satiety signal involved in the short-term regulation of food intake. Since then, the ability of CCK treatment to inhibit eating has been demonstrated in a wide variety of species, including mice, hamsters, rabbits, dogs, monkeys, and humans (for review see Morley et al., 1985; Silver and Morley, 1991). Nevertheless, before we can accept the original premise of circulating CCK as a satiety factor, several important issues must be addressed.

One of the challenges posed to the CCK–satiety hypothesis is the possibility that CCK might reduce eating because it makes the organism feel sick or nauseated, or exerts some other type of aversive action. Some investigators have demonstrated that CCK can cause a learned taste aversion, or bait shyness, under certain conditions (Deutsch and Hardy, 1977), whereas others have reported that CCK treatment produces a learned place aversion when tested in a place-conditioning paradigm (Swerdlow et al., 1983). Although these findings must be considered carefully, there are a number of arguments against the aversion hypothesis of CCK action. First, under the experimental conditions used by the Gibbs and Smith group, CCK-treated subjects do not show evidence of bait shyness (Gibbs, Young, and Smith, 1973; Holt et al., 1974). Second, CCK produces not only decreased food intake, but also the complete behavioral sequence of normal satiety in rats, including grooming and exploratory behavior followed by resting or sleeping (Antin et al., 1975). Third, test situations devised to differentiate between satiety and gustatory aversion suggest that CCK acts as a true satiety factor (Billington, Levine, and Morley, 1983; Flood, Silver, and Morley, 1990). Finally, and perhaps most convincingly, human studies, in which self-reports can be obtained, generally do not support the idea that CCK effects are due to feelings of malaise. Although CCK administration did produce mild nausea or stomach sickness in a few individuals, the occurrence of these symptoms was not related to inhibition of food intake in the overall subject population (Smith and Gibbs, 1987; Stacher, 1985).

A second issue concerns the possible sites of CCK action. CCK-8 and larger forms that may also be released from intestinal cells do not seem to pass readily across the blood–brain barrier. Thus, at present, we must assume that the satiating effects of either intestinal CCK or systemically administered CCK are exerted mainly outside of the brain (Crawley, 1985a). The major candidate sites of action are the pyloric sphincter, where CCK is thought to exert its inhibitory effects on gastric emptying, and the abdominal sensory terminals of the vagus nerve (Murphy, Schneider, and Smith, 1988). Both the pyloric sphincter and the vagus nerve possess CCK-A receptors, and both have been implicated in peripherally mediated satiety. The vagus appears to be particularly important in that the effects of CCK on food intake can be inhibited either by subdiaphragmatic vagotomy or by lesions of afferent vagal fibers at the spinal level (Morley, 1990). Indeed, the most recent data suggest that the main satiating action of peripheral CCK is mediated by release from intestinal CCK neurons (rather than the CCK-secreting endocrine cells described earlier), which activates vagal fibers that transmit sensory information to the brain stem (Figure 11.25; Fraser and Davison, 1992; Ritter, Brenner, and Tamura, 1994).

In previous sections of this chapter, we saw that central oxytocin and CRF serve behavioral functions that coordinate exquisitely well with the hormonal actions of those peptides. Somewhat similarly, brain CCK, like CCK from the intestine, seems to participate in the regulation of feeding behavior. Administration of CCK either into the cerebral ventricles or directly into specific brain regions has been reported to decrease food intake in a number of experiments (Della-Fera, Coleman, and Baile, 1990; Schick et al., 1990; Silver and Morley, 1991). The potential relevance of brain CCK is further supported by evidence for an increased density of central CCK receptors following fasting (Saito, Williams, and Goldfine, 1981), as well as for a stimulation of eating behavior in sheep that received CCK antibodies injected intracerebroventricularly (Della-Fera et al., 1981). Furthermore, there is growing evidence that CCK may interact with monoaminergic transmitters such as serotonin to regulate satiety mechanisms (Cooper and Dourish, 1990; Cooper, Dourish, and Clifton, 1992).

The most promising new avenue of CCK satiety research, however, involves some of the nonpeptide, receptor-selective antagonists described earlier. This approach has several advantages over CCK or related agonists. By preventing the action of endogenous CCK, receptor blockers may provide a clearer picture of the physiological role of CCK in satiety. Moreover, because CCK antagonists would be expected to increase rather than decrease food intake, the question of aversion or malaise is not at issue. Finally, the selectivity of these drugs should enable researchers to determine the receptor subtype involved in CCK action and may also provide inferential evidence for either a peripheral or central site of action.

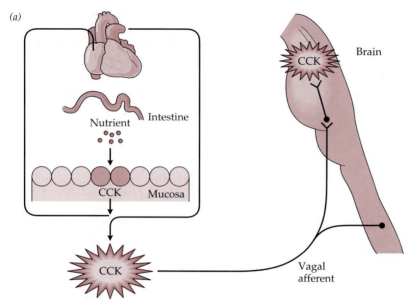

(a)

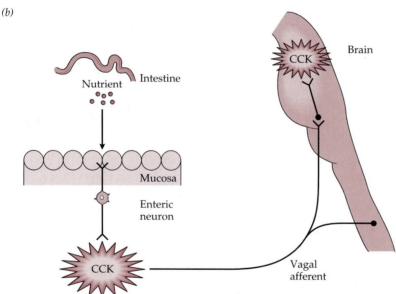

(b)

11.25 HYPOTHESIZED MECHANISMS BY WHICH CHOLECYSTOKININ REGULATES EATING BEHAVIOR IN RESPONSE TO INTESTINAL FOOD STIMULATION. Entry of nutrients into the small intestine stimulates CCK release from both neuronal and nonneuronal (endocrine) cells in the intestinal wall. (*a*) CCK released by the nonneuronal cells could play a role in satiety mechanisms by entering the general circulation (note vascular pathway to and from the heart) and then returning to the gut, where it then activates vagal receptors. (*b*) An alternative (though not mutually exclusive) hypothesis involves the local stimulation of vagal afferents by CCK released from enteric neurons. Note that CCK neurons within the brain may also participate in the regulation of food intake. (After Ritter, Brenner, and Tamura, 1994.)

A number of studies have implicated CCK-A receptors in the regulation of hunger. For example, CCK-A antagonists were reported to inhibit the satiating effect of CCK given either systemically or centrally (Crawley et al., 1991; Laferrere et al., 1991; Melville, Smith, and Gibbs, 1992). Administration of the CCK-A antagonist devazepide (MK-329) alone stimulated food intake in rats and mice (Corwin, Gibbs, and Smith, 1991; Hewson et al., 1988; Silver et al., 1989) and increased self-reported hunger ratings in previously fasted humans (Wolkowitz et al., 1990). The CCK-A receptor agonist L-71623 mimicked CCK in producing a suppression of food intake in mice, dogs, and monkeys (Asin et al., 1992). More recently, Japanese researchers have discovered a mutant strain of rat (named Otsuka Long-Evans Tokushima Fatty; *OLETF*) lacking CCK-A receptors both centrally and peripherally. Cerebroventricular administration of CCK-8 inhibited food intake in control animals, but not in *OLETF* rats (Miyasaka et al., 1994). Although these results strongly implicate CCK-A receptors in the promotion of satiety, at least one study found a much greater potency of the CCK-B antagonist devazepide compared with L-365,260 in stimulating food intake and postponing satiety in rats (Dourish, Rycroft, and Iversen, 1989). Thus, it is premature to conclude that central CCK-B receptors play no role in satiety mechanisms.

In conclusion, many of the actions of CCK revolve around the coordination of ingestive and metabolic processes. In this respect, CCK appears to be yet another example of an integrative peptide. CCK nevertheless has many other behavioral functions, including a possible involvement in anxiety. The importance of CCK as a neurotransmitter is consistent with its widespread distribution in the nervous system.

1 5-HT TRANSPORTER SITES visualized by in vitro autoradiography with [^{3}H]paroxetine in a horizontal section through a 25-day-old rat brain. High concentrations are seen as warm colors, low concentrations as cooler colors. Particularly high transporter densities (red) are seen in the dorsal lateral geniculate nucleus of the thalamus, superior colliculus, periaqueductal gray, caudal striatum, and parts of the cerebral cortex and hippocampus. In contrast to the NE transporter (see cover illustration), the 5-HT transporter shows a laminar distribution in the neocortex and is virtually absent in the cerebellum (blue). (Autoradiogram by Alison McReynolds and Jerrold S. Meyer, University of Massachusetts.)

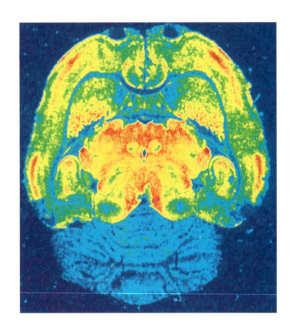

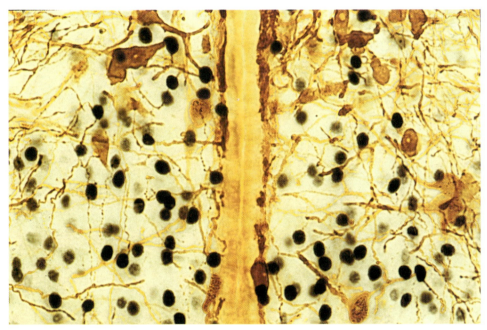

2 OXYTOCIN PEPTIDE AND ANDROGEN RECEPTORS in male rat brain. This coronal section through the hypothalamus at the level of the paraventricular nucleus was double-stained for immunoreactivity to the neuropeptide oxytocin and to receptors for androgen (male sex hormone), which created a brown precipitate for oxytocin immunoreactivity and a black precipitate for androgen receptor immunoreactivity. Oxytocin staining is seen primarily in the cytoplasm of cell bodies and dendrites, whereas staining for androgen receptors is seen mainly in cell nuclei. Note that almost none of the oxytocin-positive neurons show androgen receptor staining. The vertical structure in the center of the photomicrograph is the third cerebral ventricle, which exhibits some nonspecific staining. (Courtesy of Lei Zhou and Geert De Vries, University of Massachusetts.)

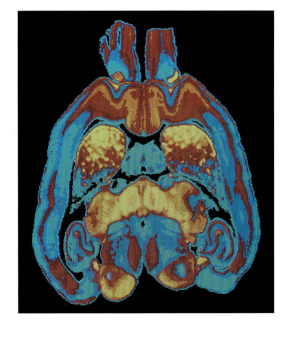

3 OPIATE RECEPTORS are heterogeneously distributed in the rat brain. Areas of high receptor density are shown in this autoradiogram as warmer colors, and are seen in the caudal striatum, medial thalamus, and several brainstem structures, including the locus coeruleus, periaqueductal gray, and the raphe nuclei. Note the laminar binding in the cerebral cortex and hippocampus. (Courtesy of Miles Herkenham, NIMH.)

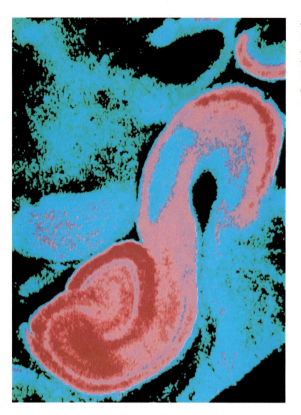

4 CANNABINOID RECEPTORS IN GUINEA PIG HIPPOCAMPUS. As shown in this striking autoradiogram, the hippocampus is one of the brain areas with a high concentration of cannabinoid receptors (red and pink). This localization is thought to be at least partly responsible for cannabinoid-related deficits in cognitive function. Note the very low levels of binding in structures adjacent to the hippocampus (blue and black). (Courtesy of Miles Herkenham, NIMH.)

5 OCCUPANCY OF HUMAN 5-HT$_2$ AND D$_2$ RECEPTORS BY NEUROLEPTIC DRUGS. Positron-emission tomography (PET) scans of a healthy, untreated man (Control) and three schizophrenic patients treated with haloperidol, a "typical" neuroleptic drug, or with an atypical neuroleptic, clozapine or risperidone. In all subjects, striatal D$_2$ receptors were labeled with [^{11}C]raclopride (*top*) and neocortical 5-HT$_2$ receptors were labeled with [^{11}C]N-methylspiperone (NMSP; *bottom*). The scans reveal that both clozapine and risperidone—but not haloperidol—produced substantial reductions in 5-HT$_2$ binding. In contrast, striatal D$_2$ receptors were almost completely blocked by haloperidol and risperidone, but residual binding to these receptors was still present following clozapine treatment. These and other differences in receptor antagonism are thought to underlie the ability of atypical neuroleptics to alleviate schizophrenic symptoms without producing severe parkinsonian side effects. (Courtesy of Svante Nyberg and Anna-Lena Nordström, Karolinska Institute.)

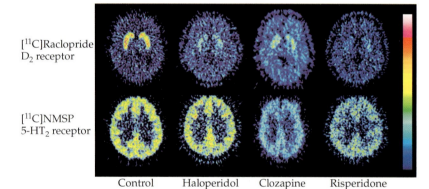

[^{11}C]Raclopride D$_2$ receptor

[^{11}C]NMSP 5-HT$_2$ receptor

Control   Haloperidol   Clozapine   Risperidone

6 SENILE PLAQUES AND NEUROFIBRILLARY TANGLES IN ALZHEIMER'S DISEASE. A 6-μm paraffin-embedded, modified Bielschowsky silver-stained section through the amygdala of a 69-year-old man reveals the neuropathological "plaques and tangles" that are characteristic of the disorder. Two senile plaques are visible: a large one near the center of the photomicrograph and part of a smaller plaque in the lower right-hand corner. The large plaque consists of an extracellular core of amyloid protein surrounded by a halo of swollen, abnormal-appearing ("dystrophic") neurites. (Reactive microglia and astrocytes are also associated with senile plaques, but are not easily visualized in this preparation.) Neurofibrillary tangles are seen here as darkly stained structures that occupy much of the cytoplasm and part of the processes of some of the pyramidal neurons. Other neurons show an unstained cytoplasm and thus appear to be cytologically normal. The man whose brain is depicted here had exhibited progressive Alzheimer's disease-associated dementia for 6 years before his death. (From Selkoe, 1991; courtesy of Dennis Selkoe, Harvard Medical School.)

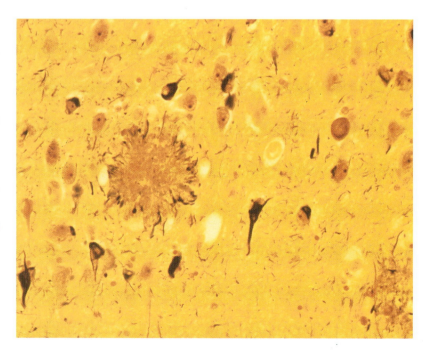

Summary

The neuropeptides constitute an important class of neurotransmitters that pharmacologists have been aware of only since the 1970s. Peptides are chains of amino acids derived from precursor proteins called pre-propeptides. The pre-propeptides are synthesized on ribosomes and then inserted into the lumen of the endoplasmic reticulum, where the signal sequence is removed and the resulting propeptides are further processed. The propeptide and appropriate converting enzymes are packaged into storage granules and transported down the axon, during which time liberation of the active peptide(s) occurs.

Peptides are released synaptically by exocytosis. Termination of the transmission process is thought to occur through peptidase-catalyzed breakdown of the active compound. Although there is little current evidence for peptide reuptake and reutilization mechanisms, this possibility cannot be ruled out.

Peptides have frequently been found to coexist in the same neurons with one another and/or with classical transmitters such as acetylcholine, serotonin, or catecholamines. Transmitter coexistence can give rise to neuromodulation, in which one substance acts primarily to regulate the action of another. The interactions of VIP and acetylcholine in the cat submandibular salivary gland represent one example of this phenomenon. Peptides may also act at some distance from their site of release, as seen in the case of the LHRH-like peptide found in bullfrog sympathetic ganglia.

The peptides selected for detailed coverage in this chapter exemplify the variety of physiological and behavioral roles played by these compounds. Vasopressin and oxytocin are nonapeptides synthesized by nerve cells in the hypothalamus and elsewhere. Some of these cells project from the hypothalamus to the posterior lobe of the pituitary gland, where the peptides are released as hormones into the circulation. Circulating vasopressin has pressor and antidiuretic effects, whereas oxytocin stimulates uterine contraction and triggers milk ejection from the mammary glands. Other vasopressinergic and oxytocinergic pathways are thought to be involved in neurotransmitter-related functions. In this regard, vasopressin may influence learning and memory, and oxytocin may play a role in female sexual and maternal behaviors.

Two of the other peptides described, TRH and CRF, can likewise claim dual status as hormones and neurotransmitters. These peptides serve as hypothalamic releasing hormones that stimulate the secretion of TSH and ACTH, respectively, from the anterior pituitary. In their neurotransmitter capacity, both peptides have excitatory behavioral effects. Moreover, CRF seems to play a special role in regulating physiological and behavioral responses to stressful stimuli.

The last two peptides described, SP and CCK, belong to the category of gut–brain peptides. Both substances were originally discovered in the digestive tract and then later found to be present in the brain as well. SP, which is a member of a larger class of peptides called tachykinins, is believed to be one of the transmitters that regulate gut motility. It is also used by a population of primary afferent neurons involved mainly in nociception. CCK stimulates gallbladder contraction and pancreatic activity, and may also influence food intake by acting as a peripheral satiety factor. CCK-containing neurons are found throughout the brain, and some of these cells may likewise be involved in the control of eating behavior.

The discovery of neuropeptides and the multiple functions they serve has had a major impact on neuropharmacology as well as the other neurosciences. First, we have seen the breakdown of many of the classical distinctions between endocrine and neurally mediated information transmission. Second, we have come to appreciate the existence of complex interactive and regulatory mechanisms unimaginable by previous generations of researchers. Finally, we are witnessing the advent of a new generation of selective nonpeptide antagonists at peptide receptors that exhibit important behavioral and physiological profiles. The entry of these drugs into the clinical realm will signal the beginning of a new era in neuropharmacology in which therapeutic approaches will target the peptides that coexist and interact with the classical neurotransmitters.

Major Drug Classes

Chapter 12

The Opiates

The opiates comprise a class of drugs known as the narcotic analgesics. Their principal effect is pain reduction, and for acute pain, the opiates and their synthetic analogs are vastly superior to all other analgesics. Opiates have a distinctive chemical structure, although even slight structural modifications of the natural substances can cause pronounced changes in their pharmacological effects.

In addition to inducing analgesia, opiates not only have a broad spectrum of side effects but also produce a sense of well-being and euphoria that in some circumstances lead to increased opiate use. Coupled with chronic opiate use is the development of tolerance and of physical dependence, the possibility of fatal overdosing or the transmission of the AIDS virus via contaminated needles, and the social strictures against drug dependence. For these reasons, serious medical, social, and legal problems surround the use of these drugs.

The opiates were once considered unique because their efficacy coincided with a great need for substances to blunt pain. However, this uniqueness rested primarily upon ignorance about the drug's mechanism and site of action. As this ignorance has given way to contemporary research, the opiates have become one of the most exciting and well-studied classes of psychotropic drugs.

The excitement among neuroscientists regarding the opiates is almost universal. Following the identification of specific opiate receptors in the CNS, the discovery of a family of endogenous opioid peptides has led to a large volume of research. Not only does opiate-related research contribute to a more complete understanding of the mechanisms of pain and analgesia, tolerance, reinforcement, and physical dependence, but it also elucidates the function and genetics of a significant neuropeptide transmitter system.

Part I
General Pharmacology: History, Identity, and Use

The opiates, being unsurpassed in reducing pain, have been used for analgesia and other purposes for centuries, and are still widely used in all branches of medicine despite their undesirable side effects and their potential for addiction. Reference to the use of opiates is found in the writings of Theophrastus as early as the third century B.C. For a long time opium was administered as a vapor or given through punctures in the skin. Because of the extreme variability in opium content and its variable rate of absorption, the opiate's effects varied from inadequate analgesia to respiratory depression and death. Fatalities were not uncommon because, lacking our modern narcotic antagonists, futile attempts were made to revive patients from opium-induced unconsciousness by placing a sponge dipped in vinegar under the nose or by dripping the juice of rue (a plant with evergreen leaves that produce an acrid, volatile oil) into the ears.

The administration of opium was greatly improved after 1803 when a German chemist isolated the active ingredient in opium, which he called **morphine**, after the god of dreams, Morpheus. The effects of morphine were

Morphine

more potent and significantly more predictable than those of the parent compound opium, although the problem of accurate administration persisted until 1853, when Pravaz invented the syringe and Alexander Wood developed the hollow needle (Musto, 1991).

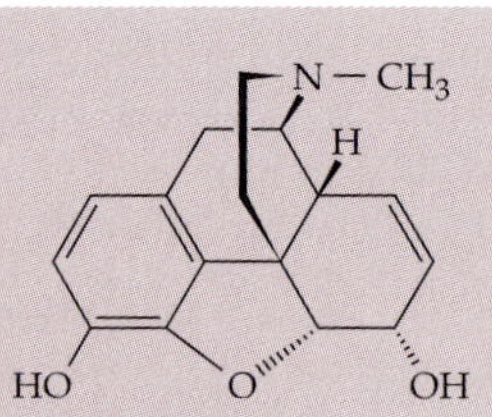

Opium is prepared by drying and powdering the milky juice taken from the seed capsules of the opium poppy, *Papaver somniferum*, just prior to ripening. Experimental cultivation of the opium poppy has been successful in the Temperate Zone as far north as England and Denmark, but the majority of the world's supply comes from Southeast Asia, India, China, Iran, Turkey, Russia, and southeastern Europe.

The active ingredients in opium include over 25 alkaloids, which make up 25% of its content by weight. Although the content varies among different specimens of opium, the percentages of the most important alkaloids include approximately 10% morphine, 0.5% codeine, 0.3% thebaine, 1% papaverine, 6% narcotine, and 0.2% narceine (Reynolds and Randall, 1957). Of these alkaloids, morphine and codeine have the widest clinical use.

In addition to their analgesic effects, the opiates act on the CNS to produce hypnotic effects and drowsiness, mood changes, and mental clouding. Acting on the gastrointestinal tract, opiates produce decreased gastric motility and reduced gastric and intestinal secretion, causing constipation. Autonomic effects include diminished respiration and heart rate, as well as the telltale constriction of pupils.

Structure–Activity Relationships

Although morphine was isolated from opium in the early 1800s, the structure of morphine was not identified until 1925 by Gulland and Robinson. Table 12.1 shows the structure of morphine and lists the structural positions of related compounds. The naturally occurring opiate alkaloid codeine is identical in structure to morphine except for the substitution of a methoxy ($-OCH_3$) for a hydroxyl group ($-OH$), producing a compound that tends to have less pharmacological activity, although codeine is a potent cough suppressant. Despite the fact that codeine's analgesic effects are much less potent than those of morphine, it is adequate for the relief of moderate pain. Its advantage over morphine is that its hypnotic properties are minimal and are not increased significantly by increased dosage. Thus, ordinarily, codeine alleviates moderate pain with fewer side effects.

Of great interest to synthetic chemists and pharmacologists was the discovery that simple modifications of the morphine molecule produce great variations in pharmacological potency. In 1874, a minor chemical modification of the morphine molecule (i.e., the addition of two acetyl groups, $-OCOCH_3$), produced the compound diacetylmorphine, or **heroin**. At the time, the new compound was promoted as a more potent, yet nonaddicting substitute for morphine. Today we know that the pharmacological effects of morphine and heroin are identical because heroin is converted to monoacetylmorphine and then to morphine in the brain. Heroin is, however, faster acting because the diacetylation makes the drug less polar and thus more lipid soluble. Great lipid solubility renders the drug more readily accessible to the brain, where it can act at brain receptors. In more recent years, synthetic narcotics have been developed with the hope of producing more potent analgesic activity accompanied by reduced physical and psychological dependence. Some synthetic compounds, such as etorphine,

Table 12.1 Similarities and Differences in Chemical Structures of the Opiates

	Opiate	Position of change in chemical radical[a]			Other changes
		3	7	17	
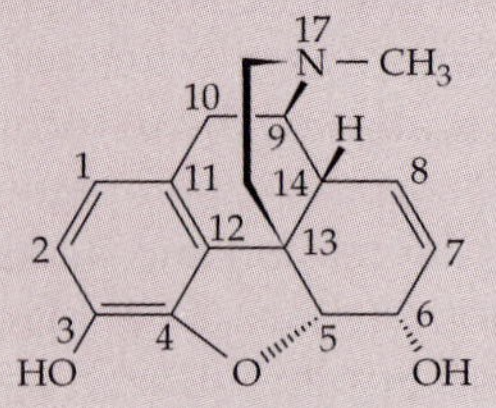 Morphine	Heroin	$-OCOCH_3$	$-OCOCH_3$	$-CH_3$	None
	Codeine	$-OCH_3$	$-OH$	$-CH_3$	None
	Nalorphine	$-OH$	$-OH$	$-CH_2CH=CH_2$	None
	Naloxone	$-OH$	$=O$	$-CH_2CH=CH_2$	Single instead of double bond between C7 and C8
	Naltrexone	$-OH$	$=O$	$-CH_2CH-CH_2$ (with CH_2 bridge)	Single instead of double bond between C7 and C8

[a]Position numbers refer to the morphine molecule shown at left.

are potent analgesics and have many of the same pharmacological effects as morphine, but all of them still possess some potential for addiction.

Several chemical classes of drugs show pharmacological activity in humans similar to that of morphine. They are the 4-phenylpiperidines (e.g., pethidine), the diphenylpropylamines (e.g., methadone), the morphinans (e.g., levorphanol), and the 6,7-benzomorphans (e.g., metazocine). The compounds in these groups share

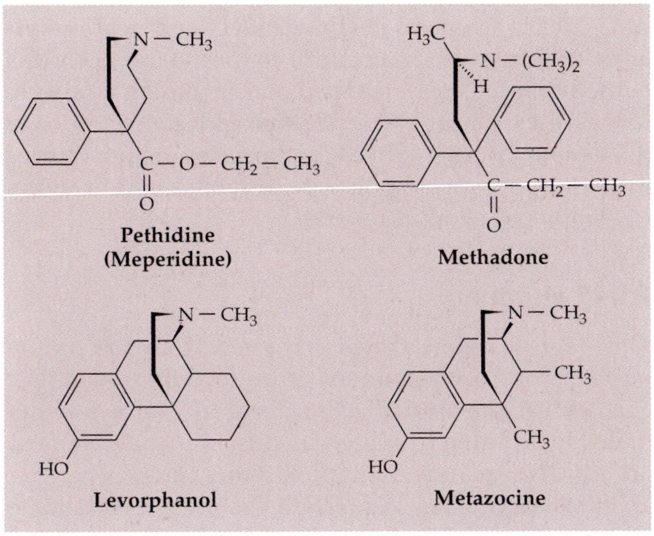

Pethidine
(Meperidine)

Methadone

Levorphanol

Metazocine

the capacity to produce analgesia, respiratory depression, gastrointestinal spasms, and morphine-like physical dependence. If depicted as flat two-dimensional representations, these structurally diverse compounds appear to be quite different, and one may question whether there is indeed a common mechanism of action for these drugs. As shown above, however, the drugs of these different classes all either possess a piperidine ring or contain the critical part of the ring structure. In addition, most have a methyl group attached to the ring as well as a variety of other bulky groups.

Other chemical modifications, such as the substitution of an allyl group (—CH$_2$CH=CH) for the methyl group on the nitrogen atom of morphine, produce the narcotic antagonists, naloxone and nalorphine (see Table 12.1). Opiate antagonists are drugs that have structures similar to those of the opiates but produce no pharmacological activity of their own. These drugs can prevent or reverse the effect of administered opiates because of their ability to occupy opiate receptor sites. As the consequence of receptor occupation is not an all-or-none phenomenon, we can consider most opiates to be mixed agonists–antagonists even though naloxone, for example, has an antagonist–agonist potency ratio that is so large that it is considered to be a "pure" antagonist.

Pharmacodynamics: Absorption and Excretion

Morphine is readily absorbed through most mucous membranes and is administered most commonly by sub-

cutaneous injection. Oral administration, however, is not uncommon; neither is absorption from the nasal mucosa (as when heroin is snorted), nor from the lung (as when opium is smoked). Once absorbed, morphine's distribution is fairly uniform in most tissues. Despite the fact that morphine has its greatest effects in the CNS, the drug does not seem to concentrate there. In fact, only small quantities are capable of passing the blood–brain barrier. It is worthwhile to mention that opiates are capable of passing the placental barrier. Consequently, newborns of opiate-addicted mothers suffer withdrawal symptoms within several hours after birth. Although opiate withdrawal is not considered life-threatening in the adult addict, the syndrome may have severe consequences for the newborn, particularly if his or her nutritional state is poor as a result of inadequate prenatal care.

The kidney is the principal route of excretion. Most of the administered drug is found in the urine within 24 hours of treatment, whereas only 7% to 10% eventually appears in the feces. Some of the morphine is excreted unchanged, but the largest portion is combined with glucuronic acid. The conjugate has an increased filtration rate in the kidney because of the altered ionic charge of the molecule (see Chapter 1). Recent findings suggest that some products of morphine metabolism are in fact active metabolites and are also capable of producing analgesia (Benyhe, 1994). Among these is one of the glucuronide metabolites, morphine-6-glucuronide.

Physiological and Behavioral Effects

CNS Effects

In terms of both pharmacodynamics and physiological effects, the prototypic opiate is morphine. The related opiates have qualitatively similar effects that vary primarily in potency and duration. Morphine has its most pronounced effects in the CNS, and, as we might expect, these drug-induced effects are dose related. At small to moderate doses (5–10 mg), the principal subjective effects are drowsiness, decreased sensitivity to external and internal stimuli, and loss of anxiety and inhibition. At this dose, muscle relaxation occurs, pain is relieved, respiration is somewhat depressed, and pupils are constricted. The ability to concentrate is impaired, and this effect is often followed by a dreamy sleep.

At slightly higher doses, an abnormal state of elation or euphoria may develop that is quite different from the relaxed state obtained with smaller doses. The literature frequently refers to the "kick," "bang," or "rush" that the addict feels immediately after injecting morphine or heroin into a vein. This rush is likened to an "abdominal orgasm." Nonaddicts describe it as a sudden flush of warmth, localized in the pit of the stomach. Individuals who take opiates orally or who smoke, snort, or inject them subcutaneously or intramuscularly do not experience this rush. Because these latter individuals can be just as dependent on opiates as the "mainliners" (i.e., those who inject it intravenously), it is clear that this rush is not the sole basis for abuse. It is interesting to note that the euphoric effect of morphine does not always accompany its intravenous administration. In fact, in well-adjusted, stable individuals who are free of pain, the administration of morphine may produce a dysphoria (restlessness and anxiety). The elation occurs most often in those who are either abnormally depressed or highly excited.

The nausea that often accompanies even small therapeutic doses of morphine is increased with higher doses. The nausea is also a CNS effect of the drug and involves the action of morphine on the chemical trigger zone in the medulla, the area postrema, which ultimately contributes to vagal input to the gut. For the addict, the nauseous episode may become a "good sick" because it has attained secondary reinforcing properties by signaling the onset of euphoria.

At the highest doses of morphine, depression deepens into unconsciousness. Pupils are now quite constricted and respiratory rate is further depressed. At this dose, the respiratory center in the brain stem, which normally responds to high CO_2 levels in the blood by triggering increased rate and depth of respiration, is severely depressed and may be the ultimate cause of death. Of great significance is the fact that even at the highest doses, morphine does not cause slurred speech, significant motor incoordination, or severe mental clouding, unlike other agents (such as nitrous oxide) that cause analgesia only when accompanied by mental confusion or unconsciousness. Analgesia and the mechanism of opiate-induced analgesia is discussed in greater detail in later sections.

Gastrointestinal Effects

Apart from the CNS, effects of morphine are greatest on the gastrointestinal tract. Opium was used for relief of diarrhea and dysentery even before it was used for analgesia. The digestive processes, on the whole, are slowed in most species, and in humans constipation is a common and disturbing side effect of morphine use, even in the addicted person. Morphine also alters the tonus and motility of the stomach and intestines, thereby slowing the passage of the contents and permitting greater absorption of water and increase in fecal viscosity. However, with repeated administration of morphine, most of these pharmacological effects are diminished in magnitude. Demonstrating the phenomenon of "rebound," frequent and copious diarrhea is a prominent part of the syndrome following abrupt withdrawal of morphine after prolonged drug usage.

Although the opiates have been used for centuries, only within the past 25 years have the cellular mechanisms of action for each of morphine's many effects gradually become clear. Researchers have demonstrated

the existence of specific membrane-bound receptors for opiates, and extensive work is underway to identify, characterize, and isolate these receptors. In addition, there is an intense interest in the endogenous opioid substances, which almost certainly represent a class of peptide neurotransmitters involved in modulation of pain transmission as well as in other opiate modified behaviors: eating, social interaction, and mental "set." The discussion of morphine's mechanisms of action will center on opiate receptors and the endogenous opiates because they are among the best understood peptide systems in the nervous system due to the intense interest of neurobiologists. Research methods, including new techniques in molecular biology that provide a description of the genetic coding, mRNA, and precursors for various proteins, provide a model for studying peptide neurotransmitter systems in general.

Part I Summary

The natural opiate drugs extracted from the opium poppy, along with their structurally similar synthetic analogs, are the most effective analgesics known to humans. In addition to analgesia, dose-dependent effects on the CNS include mental clouding, mood changes, and the induction of sleep. Of tremendous importance to modern medicine (particularly in developing countries) is the ability of opiates to slow intestinal motility, causing constipation (or eliminating diarrhea). Despite molecular modifications of the drugs, respiratory and cardiac depression and high abuse potential remain the principal side effects of greatest concern.

Part II
Opiate Receptors

Receptor Characteristics

In-depth analysis of the molecular structures of the opioid drugs provides sufficient information to hypothesize definite structural features of the opiate receptor. Very early it became clear that the piperidine ring was essential to the pharmacological activity of opiates (see Table 12.1). The nitrogen atom of this ring is normally positively charged, so it is likely that one important element of the drug–receptor interaction is the attraction of the drug molecule to a negatively charged site on the receptor surface. It is also evident from the three-dimensional model of morphine that the receptor binding site must have the shape of an irregular pouch into which the morphine molecule can fit, allowing the essential contacts to be made on different walls of the pouch.

The importance of "fit" of the molecule to the receptor is demonstrated by the stereospecificity of the opiates. The D-isomers are identical to the active L-isomers in structure but are mirror images; thus, they are excluded from the receptor site by their "wrong" geometry and have neither agonist nor antagonist activity. The structural requirements of the opiate receptor provide an excellent means to demonstrate the specificity of any opiate pharmacological effect. Thus, if it is suspected that a compound has an opioid effect, that effect should be reduced by a specific opiate receptor antagonist, such as naloxone, and not be produced by D-isomers of the test compound. Such stringent molecular requirements for opiate activity, the great potency of these compounds, and their stereospecificity (i.e., the optical isomers of the analgesic compounds are inactive) all suggest the presence of a specific opiate receptor.

Opiate receptors are proteins embedded in the cell membrane to which morphine and other opiate agonists bind to initiate their pharmacological effects. The methods used for the identification and characterization of the opiate receptors are similar to those used to identify other membrane-localized receptors. Chapter 2 describes these assay procedures in general, as well as the data analysis in some detail.

Receptor Binding Studies

Initial attempts to develop a method for detecting stereospecific receptors in mouse brain were plagued by high levels of nonspecific binding. Opiates apparently will bind to almost any biological or nonbiological membrane. In addition to binding at specific recognition sites (i.e., receptors), the radioactively labeled ligand can also be dissolved nonspecifically in the lipid membrane, or it may nonspecifically bind to anionic groups in the membrane because of the positively charged atoms in the opiate molecule.

The separation of specific binding from nonspecific binding is of great importance because physiological membrane receptors are present in small numbers, while there are many more nonspecific binding sites that may show quite high affinity for the ligand. Binding techniques were greatly improved and used more successfully when radioactive opiates with higher specific radioactivity (e.g., 40 Ci/mM for [³H]naloxone) were developed. Use of the "hotter" ligand means that even a small number of receptors with high affinity can be measured over and above background values.

Biochemical Characterization of Opiate Binding

In addition to stereospecificity, several other criteria have been met to confirm the specificity (see Chapter 2) of opioid binding (see Pasternak, 1987). Although different laboratories used different ligands, their results were quite consistent. Using [³H]naloxone as the primary ligand, Pert and Snyder (1973) found its binding to be saturable, with half saturation occurring at about 1.6×10^{-8} M. Figure 12.1 shows that with increasing amounts of

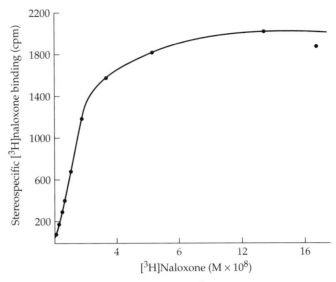

12.1 STEREOSPECIFIC BINDING OF [³H]NALOXONE to rat brain homogenate. By increasing the concentration of the ligand, saturation of the opiate receptors occurs. (After Pert and Snyder, 1973).

[³H]naloxone, stereospecific binding increases and gradually reaches a plateau. The asymptotic curve indicates saturation of the binding sites, which suggests that a finite number of receptors exists. In this case, the concentration of the ligand needed to saturate the receptors is within a concentration range that is meaningfully related to the concentration of agonist necessary to elicit a pharmacological response.

Opiate binding sites have high affinity for narcotic analgesics and their antagonists. Not only do the opioid ligands have affinities in the nanomolar range, but the rate of dissociation of the ligand–receptor complex is consistent with the loss of pharmacological effect observed in a bioassay when the drug is removed from the medium.

Further biochemical studies have shown that stereospecific opiate binding is greatly impaired by proteolytic enzymes such as trypsin and pronase and by sulfhydryl reagents (Pasternak, 1987). This observation strongly supports the idea that the opiate receptor contains a sulfhydryl group occupying a position at or near the binding site. Stereospecific opiate binding is also very sensitive to phospholipase A, which alters the lipid constituents in the membrane or in the receptor itself and thus retards binding. The finding that phospholipase C is less effective than phospholipase A suggests that the more polar groups of the phospholipids that are attacked by phospholipase C are less important to opiate binding.

Ionic Requirements

Sodium (Na⁺), but not other alkali metal ions (except lithium to a limited extent), enhances the binding of opi-

Table 12.2	Effect of Sodium Ions on [³H]Opiate Binding

Radioligand	Change in binding produced by sodium[a]
Agonists	
Dihydromorphine	−70%
Oxymorphone	−44%
Levorphanol	−38%
Antagonists	
Nalorphine	+45%
Naloxone	+145%
Levallorphan	+29%

[a]Binding was determined in the presence and absence of sodium chloride (100 mM).
Source: After Pasternak, 1987.

ate antagonists and greatly reduces the binding of agonists. For example, the binding of the virtually pure antagonist, [³H]naloxone, is increased by 60% by the addition of 1 mM Na^+, and this antagonist binding continues to increase as the sodium ion concentration is raised to 100 mM (Table 12.2). Conversely, binding of the agonists levorphanol, oxymorphone, or dihydromorphine is depressed by the addition of Na^+. The ability of Na^+ to alter the degree to which opiates bind correlates well with the agonist–antagonist properties of these drugs (Pasternak, 1987).

Although the mechanism by which Na^+ acts is not known, its action is likely to be intracellular because the concentration of Na^+ that alters ligand binding is in the range of 10–30 mM (the concentration producing half-maximal inhibition of agonist binding). Extracellular Na^+ concentration is significantly higher than that level, a condition that would put the receptor in a constant inhibitory state if Na^+ were acting extracellularly. Intracellular concentrations are approximately equal to or slightly lower than the Na^+ concentration that inhibits agonist binding, so fluctuations in intracellular Na^+ could have a functional role in altering ligand binding (see Cox, 1993).

Pasternak (1987) summarizes evidence for conformational shifts in the opiate receptor. Apparently, the addition of Na^+ shifts the receptor to an altered conformational state, so antagonists bind effectively whereas agonists show less ability to bind. Removal of Na^+ shifts the receptor back to the agonist form, and antagonists bind less effectively. This "Na^+ shift" is not unique to opiate receptors, but seems to be a general characteristic of G protein–coupled receptors and therefore may be a function of the interaction of the receptors with G proteins in the membrane (see discussion on cellular mechanisms). However, treating cultured hybrid neuronal cells (NG 108-15) with pertussis toxin inactivates the G_i protein and prevents opioid inhibition of adenylyl cyclase, but does not reduce the ability of Na^+ to inhibit agonist binding (Wuster et al., 1984). From that study and others, it seems that Na^+ acts on the receptor itself, rather than on the G proteins. The molecular mechanism is not yet clear.

Opiate Bioassay

The fundamental principle of bioassays is that agonist–receptor interactions lead to a measurable biological response in an isolated tissue that is in its native, functional state. These differ from radioligand assays, which utilize nonphysiological conditions and provide information only on ligand–receptor interactions. Isolated organs have been used for determining structure–activity relationships among opioids, as well as for identifying endogenous opioids isolated from tissue extracts or biological fluids. A discussion of methodological considerations and applications is provided by Smith and Leslie (1993).

The bioassay considered most accurate in measuring opioid activity uses the guinea pig ileum longitudinal muscle–myenteric plexus preparation developed by Kosterlitz, Lydon, and Watt (1970). After dissection, the tissue is maintained in a physiological solution that is aerated with a 95% O_2:5% CO_2 mixture and kept at 37°C. The muscle preparation is fastened at each end to maintain a fixed tension so that when the postganglionic cholinergic neurons are electrically stimulated, the release of acetylcholine (ACh) induces a twitch in the longitudinal smooth muscle that can be recorded on a polygraph. The release of ACh and the resulting twitch is inhibited by opiate drugs. Although a variety of compounds inhibit the twitch response, the specificity of this effect for the opiates is demonstrated by naloxone reversal. Kosterlitz and Waterfield (1975) showed that the naloxone-reversible twitch inhibition is almost perfectly correlated with the potency of the opiates to relieve pain in humans (Figure 12.2).

There is also a very strong correlation between the extent of muscle-twitch inhibition by the opiates tested and their affinities for stereospecific binding sites in the guinea pig intestine (see Snyder, 1986). Furthermore, the affinities of the opioids for intestinal binding sites are also closely correlated with those in brain. Therefore, it is apparent that a correlation exists between analgesic effects in vivo, muscle-twitch inhibition in the bioassay in vitro, and the ability to bind stereospecifically to opiate receptors. These findings were important in demonstrating the functional relevance of the early binding assays.

Opiate Receptor Subtypes

Martin and colleagues (1976) provided the first indication that several subtypes of opiate receptors exist. The authors interpreted the results from classic dose–response curves and agonist–antagonist interactions (see

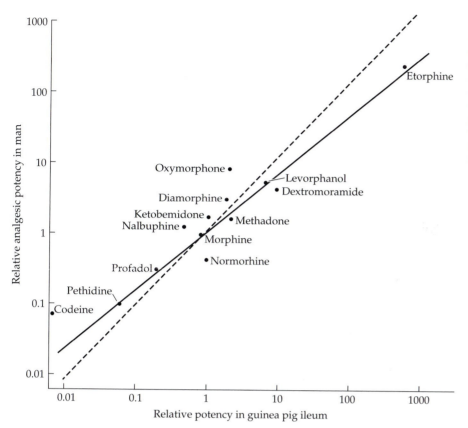

12.2 CORRELATION BETWEEN THE RELATIVE POTENCIES OF OPIOID ANALGESICS in inhibiting guinea pig ileum twitch and producing analgesia in human subjects. The strong positive correlation is represented by the solid line. For purposes of comparison, the dashed line represents a perfect correlation. The values for potency were calculated relative to morphine (morphine = 1). (After Kosterlitz and Waterfield, 1975.)

Chapter 1) as evidence for the existence of multiple receptor subtypes. Using traditional methods in pharmacology, they demonstrated that three distinct syndromes are produced by three different congeners of morphine. Furthermore, they found that while morphine readily suppressed the withdrawal syndrome in morphine-dependent dogs, the morphine analog ketocyclazocine was ineffective. Also, tolerance to one group of opiates did not necessarily produce cross-tolerance to other classes of opiate drugs, as would be expected if all opiates acted at the same receptor. Their results suggested that at least three types of opiate receptors exist: **mu** (μ), which is stimulated by morphine, **kappa** (κ), which binds ketocyclazocine, and **sigma** (σ), for which the experimental compound SKF-10,047 has a high affinity.

With the development of highly selective ligands (both agonists and antagonists), researchers have been able to more directly examine binding to particular receptor subtypes with minimal interference from binding to other subtypes (see Simon, 1991). With these tools, radioligand binding techniques and autoradiography have identified as many as nine receptor subtypes. Three of the nine are now generally accepted, and include the μ, δ, and κ opiate receptors. The σ-receptor described by Martin and colleagues (1976) is no longer considered an opiate receptor. Rather, it binds phencyclidine (PCP) with some affinity, as well as some antipsychotic drugs, such as haloperidol. It is discussed briefly in Chapter 17.

The receptor subtypes bind opiates with different specificities, such that compounds that readily displace a radioligand from the μ-receptor, for example, have very low binding affinity at δ sites. In addition, CNS distribution varies significantly for the different receptors, and some brain regions are more highly enriched in a particular receptor than others. Opiate receptor distribution is also species-specific.

Opiate Receptor Pharmacology and Localization within the CNS

μ-Receptors. The μ-receptor is the morphine receptor and has a high affinity for morphine and related alkaloid opiate drugs. It is present in brain and heavily concentrated in guinea pig ileum. μ-receptors are specifically labeled with the enkephalin analog [3H]DAGO as well as [3H]morphiceptin and its analog, [3H]PL017. Binding to μ-receptors is found in the neocortex, striatum, nucleus accumbens, amygdala, septum, thalamus, hippocampus, substantia nigra, inferior and superior colliculi, locus coeruleus, nucleus tractus solitarius, spinal trigeminal nucleus, and the dorsal horn of the spinal cord. Some μ binding is also found in the periaqueductal gray and the nuclei of the raphe (Color Plate 3).

In addition to qualitative autoradiography, distribution of the receptors has been examined using several other techniques, including quantitative autoradiography (Tempel and Zukin, 1987), grain counting (Moskowitz and Goodman, 1985) and a computerized digital subtraction technique (Goodman and Pasternak, 1985). Postmortem autoradiographic mapping in human brain (Quirion and Pilapil, 1991) and in vivo mapping of opiate receptor subtypes using positron emission tomography (PET) (Mayberg and Frost, 1990) provide additional information on receptor localization and possible roles in pathological conditions such as chronic pain states and psychiatric disorders. Although studies on the concentration of receptor types in discrete areas of rat brain do not always agree between laboratories, in general the localization of the μ-receptor suggests its role in morphine-induced analgesia and positive reinforcement, as well as in sensorimotor integration, cardiovascular and respiratory depression, and neuroendocrine effects (Mansour et al., 1987; Mansour and Watson, 1993).

Similarly, sensory processing roles may be suggested for the μ-receptor in the human brain where concentrated μ binding sites occur in the superficial laminae of the cerebral cortex, the inferior lobe of the temporal cortex, and the visual and auditory cortical areas (Quirion and Pilapil, 1991). Heavy concentrations have also been found in the amygdala and the caudate and putamen, although without the "patchy" characteristic reported for striatal receptors in other species. Despite many similarities, differences in μ- (as well as in σ- and κ-) receptor concentrations between human brain and other species are noteworthy.

μ-Receptor subtypes.   Detailed examination of μ-receptor characteristics has led to the conclusion that several μ-receptor subtypes exist. Pasternak (1987, 1993) has proposed that morphine and the endogenous opioids, the enkephalins, label distinct sites that are not merely conformational changes from one state to another, but are distinct receptors. μ_1-receptors have a high affinity for both morphine and enkephalins, and are blocked by naloxonazine. These receptors are believed to mediate supraspinal analgesia, catalepsy, and prolactin release.

Although μ_1 binding represents only a small part (approximately 30%) of total opioid binding, the concept that the μ_1 binding site is common for morphine and enkephalin has received support from biochemical and competition studies, developmental studies, phylogenetic and regional distribution studies, as well as evaluation by computer analysis (see Pasternak, 1987). Visualization of μ_1-receptor localization suggests high concentrations within the medial thalamus, periaqueductal gray, superior colliculus, median raphe, and clusters within the striatum. Such distribution supports the idea that μ_1-receptors have an important role in mediating analgesia. Furthermore, the CXBK strain of mouse, which is relatively insensitive to morphine analgesia, is apparently deficient in μ_1 sites in brain areas associated with morphine-induced analgesia (Moskowitz and Goodman, 1985). Furthermore, although naloxonazine

was effective in antagonizing the analgesic effects of morphine, suggesting μ_1-receptor function in analgesia, the symptoms of morphine withdrawal were not attenuated by a μ_1-agonist (Ling et al., 1984), indicating that a receptor-specific distinction exists between analgesic effects and drug dependence. Results such as these represent the first step in the search for potent analgesics with low abuse potential.

In contrast to μ_1-receptors, μ_2-receptors have a slightly lower affinity for morphine and have still lower affinity for enkephalins.

δ-Receptors.   The δ-receptor (originally discovered in the mouse) is so named because it is concentrated in the vas deferens, though it is also found in discrete areas of the CNS. When labeled with the enkephalin analogs [^{3}H]DPDPE or [^{3}H]DPDLE, δ-receptors have a distribution similar to that of μ-receptors, but are more restricted. They are predominantly found in forebrain structures such as the neocortex, striatum, olfactory areas, substantia nigra, and the nucleus accumbens. Many of these sites are consistent with a possible role for δ-receptors in olfaction, motor integration, and cognitive function.

δ Subtypes and interaction with μ-receptors.   Subtypes of δ-receptors also have been identified, and a complex relationship with μ-receptors has been proposed and reviewed (Rothman et al., 1988; Rothman, Holaday, and Porreca, 1993; Traynor and Elliott, 1993). Interactions of receptors have been demonstrated in several tissues. For example, Porreca and coworkers (Jiang, Mosberg, and Porreca, 1990) found that the δ-selective agonist DPDPE, at a dose that by itself produces no analgesia, potentiates the analgesic effects of morphine, which presumably acts via μ-receptors. The same group identified a δ-antagonist, DALCE, that attenuates δ-receptor–mediated analgesia without altering the δ-agonist potentiation of morphine. Based on the results of binding studies that showed both competitive and noncompetitive inhibition of δ ligand binding by μ-agonists, Rothman and colleagues (1988) have proposed multiple δ subtypes. The first, called $\delta_{complexed}$, interacts with μ-receptors, while the $\delta_{noncomplexed}$ subtype is not associated with μ-receptors.

Other groups have also identified δ subtypes, called δ_1 and δ_2, based on receptor labeling studies and both in vivo and in vitro pharmacological studies. The results of these groups have been summarized by Traynor and Elliott (1993) and provide evidence for δ ligands that bind differentially to subsets of receptor populations. δ_1-receptors are labeled by DPDPE and δ_2-receptors by deltorphin II and DSLET. A newly developed antagonist, 7-benzylidene naltrexone, is 100 times more potent in competing for [^{3}H]DPDPE than for [^{3}H]DSLET. The antagonist's selectivity in the competitive binding assay is matched by its ability to antagonize analgesia in vivo.

Additionally, the lack of cross-tolerance between DPDPE and deltorphin in analgesia testing suggests multiple δ subtypes. Although multiple δ-receptors certainly exist, a relationship between δ_1 and δ_2 and the receptors called $\delta_{complexed}$ and $\delta_{noncomplexed}$ has not been established, and the matter is complicated by inconsistencies between the studies in binding assays and in vitro experiments where different effector systems may be involved.

While pharmacological interactions between selected μ and δ subtypes have been shown, Simon (1991) provided evidence for specific molecular entities for μ- and δ-receptors by physically separating the binding units of the receptors using affinity cross-linking of labeled ligands to membrane fractions. Gel autoradiography revealed a band at an apparent molecular weight of 65 kDa only in tissues known to have μ-receptors, and an additional band at 53 kDa was correlated with the presence of δ-receptors. Pretreatment of the tissue with DAGO (μ-selective binding) reduced the 65-kDA band without altering the 53-kDa band, whereas DPDPE (δ-selective binding) preferentially suppressed labeling of the 53-kDa band. These results demonstrate that these receptor subtypes are distinct molecular entities, though allosteric interactions between them are not unlikely. The unique nature of the μ- and δ-receptors is discussed further in the section on molecular cloning of receptor subtypes.

κ-Receptors. The κ-receptor is the binding site for ketocyclazocine, an opiate analog that produces hallucination and dysphoria, suggesting a possible role for this receptor in psychosis. The κ-receptors also bind the benzomorphans such as bremazocine, modified dynorphan A (DAKLI or DPRODYN), or nonpeptidergic compounds (U-50,488H or U-69,593.). These receptors may participate in the regulation of water balance, food intake, temperature control, gut motility, pain perception, and neuroendocrine function (Mansour et al., 1988; Wollemann, Benhye, and Simon, 1993). In rat brain, κ-receptors have a distinct distribution pattern compared with μ- and δ-receptors: κ-receptors are found in the preoptic area of the hypothalamus, median eminence, caudate–putamen, amygdala, nucleus accumbens, neural lobe of the pituitary, and nucleus tractus solitarius. These receptors are also present in the periaqueductal gray, nucleus of the raphe, spinal trigeminal nucleus, and the dorsal horn of the spinal cord.

κ-Receptor subtypes. Ligand binding studies and pharmacological evaluation demonstrate the existence of κ-receptor subtypes (Wolleman, Benyhe, and Simon, 1993). Sites sensitive to U-50,488 or U-69,593 are designated κ_1 while those sites sensitive to DADLE, and which have a higher affinity for Met-enkephalin–Arg–Phe than for dynorphin, are considered κ_2. The neuroanatomical distribution in rat revealed the highest concentration of κ_1-receptors in the spinal cord and κ_2-receptors in the brain

stem, though large species differences also exist for κ-receptor distribution. Functional studies of receptor-linked neurochemical and neuroendocrine effects, electrophysiological changes, and analgesic properties support the existence of κ-receptor subtypes, but results of these studies do not correlate well with the classification of κ subtypes based on binding assays. Furthermore, although several authors have possibly identified κ_3- and κ_4-receptor subtypes using selective ligand binding in conjunction with computer analysis, pharmacological and physiological evidence for these additional subtypes is lacking. Cloning and amino acid sequencing of the receptors will ultimately clarify this issue.

It should be clear from the previous discussion that many brain structures have multiple opiate receptor types. For instance, in the rat, both μ and κ subtypes are found in the periaqueductal gray, though their distribution within this region is quite different. Both μ and δ sites are found in the striatum, but the diffuse localization of δ sites is in contrast to the distinct patches of binding of μ-receptors. All three receptor types are found in the temporal cortex with distinct distribution patterns. The μ-receptors are found in layers 1 and 4, δ-receptors in 2, 3, 5, and 6, and κ-receptors in layers 5 and 6. A layered pattern is also found in other structures, such as the olfactory bulb, where μ binding is found in the glomerular layer and δ binding is predominantly in the external plexiform layer. Several recent reports describe the localization of these receptors in more detail, though agreement between them is limited due to differences in radioligand, concentration of ligands used, and method of measurement or visualization (see Akil, Bronstein, and Mansour, 1988; Gouarderes, Cros, and Quirion, 1985; Mansour et al., 1987, 1995; McLean, Rothman, and Herkenham, 1986; Tempel and Zukin, 1987).

Molecular Cloning of Opiate Receptor Subtypes

The biochemical purification and molecular sequencing of the opiate receptor subtypes have been difficult to achieve for many reasons. Among them is the small amount of available protein and its particularly hydrophobic nature (Thompson et al., 1993). Many laboratories have been struggling with the problem, and recently several have met with outstanding success. The recent cloning of the opiate receptor subtypes has immense impact on the study of opioid peptides. The results not only provide crucial information regarding gene and protein structure, but also enhance our understanding of the anatomy, regulation, and function of the opiate receptors (Mansour et al., 1995).

The molecular cloning of opiate receptor subtypes provides several key pieces of information:

1. It tells us about gene structure, that is, the specific nucleic acid sequence that directs the synthesis of each receptor protein.

2. The amino acid sequence of the encoded protein can be deduced and compared with other families of receptor proteins.

3. Other cells can be transfected with receptor-specific DNA so that they can express the particular receptor encoded on the gene.

4. Transfected cells can then be used to perform functional studies on the receptor to clarify its signal-transduction mechanism or second messenger responses, such as accumulation of cyclic AMP (cAMP) or ion channel changes resulting in electrophysiological responses.

5. The recent availability of molecular biological techniques makes it possible to visualize the cells that synthesize the receptor protein and also localize the receptors themselves at a cellular resolution that was previously impossible with standard autoradiographic techniques (see Chapter 2).

δ-Receptor cloning.   The first opiate receptor to be successfully cloned was the δ-receptor. The feat was accomplished almost simultaneously by two independent laboratories (Evans et al., 1992; Kieffer et al., 1992). Each group apparently isolated the same cDNA that encodes a protein of 371 or 372 amino acids. In both cases the protein, when expressed in transfected cells, possesses the properties expected of a δ-receptor. For instance, high specific binding to the cloned receptors occurs with δ-specific radioligands in nanomolar concentrations, similar to values obtained for native δ-receptors. In addition, the protein has structural characteristics similar to

other G protein–coupled δ-receptors, including seven hydrophobic regions thought to be membrane-spanning domains of the receptor. Finally, the cloned δ-receptor is capable of transducing a physiological signal, that is, inhibition of adenylyl cyclase. Selective δ-agonist activation of the receptor in transfected cells decreased cAMP accumulation in a naloxone-sensitive fashion. Figure 12.3 is a schematic drawing of the proposed δ-receptor structure.

Subsequent research (Bzdega et al., 1993) localized the corresponding δ-receptor mRNA in expected brain regions. The unexpected low levels found in the striatum and other disparities with conventional receptor localization may be explained by the fact that mRNA distribution identifies sites of protein synthesis, which may not be identical with receptor localization because the receptor protein can be transported to presynaptic loci. The surprisingly heavy concentration of δ-receptor mRNA in the anterior pituitary and pineal gland suggests that opioid peptides act as classic hormones in these tissues, which are outside the blood–brain barrier.

κ-Receptor cloning.   The cloning of the mouse δ-receptor facilitated the cloning of other opioid receptor subtypes. As in the case for the δ-receptor, a κ-receptor clone was isolated and characterized by two independent laboratories almost simultaneously (Meng et al., 1993; Yasuda et al., 1993). The isolated cDNA encodes a receptor protein having 380 amino acid residues and seven putative transmembrane domains. Much of the protein sequence (59%) is identical to that of the mouse δ-receptor. The homology with δ-receptors is greatest for the trans-

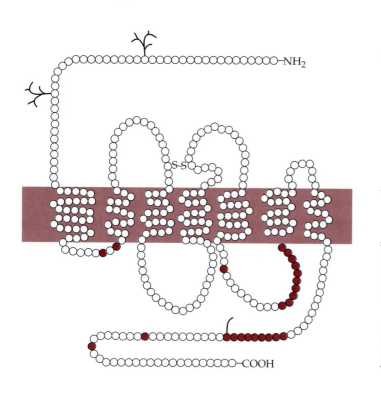

Extracellular

Cell membrane

Intracellular

12.3 PROPOSED STRUCTURE OF THE δ-RECEPTOR PROTEIN. Each circle represents an identified amino acid. The seven regions spanning the membrane are typical for receptors that are coupled to G proteins. Some of the darkened circles on the intracellular portion of the protein are potential sites for phosphorylation by cAMP-dependent protein kinase and protein kinase C. (After Evans et al., 1992.)

membrane domains and the intracellular loops of the receptor, which may be critical for the coupling of these receptors to G proteins, a characteristic typical of all opiate peptide receptor subtypes.

Binding studies using cells transfected with the clone show that κ-selective ligands such as dynorphin and U-50,488 bind selectively with high affinity, while DAGO and DPDPE do not. Sterospecificity is demonstrated by the high affinity for L-naloxone and L-levorphanol but poor affinity for D-naloxone and D-levorphanol. The rank order of κ-receptor–selective ligands in displacement studies suggests that the clone is of the κ₁-subtype.

The expressed receptor is functionally coupled to the cAMP second messenger system, via G protein. Activation of the receptor by κ ligands inhibits forskolin-induced increases in cAMP. Localization of the corresponding mRNA by in situ hybridization shows a distribution similar to that of κ-selective binding sites. The finding that κ-receptor mRNA is high in the ventral tegmentum while κ-receptors are high in the nucleus accumbens suggests that the protein is synthesized in the midbrain nucleus and is transported to presynaptic terminals in the nucleus accumbens. A similar situation exists where high κ-receptor mRNA is seen in the substantia nigra with high receptor localization in the striatum.

μ-Receptor cloning. Simultaneous isolation of a rat cDNA clone (Chen et al., 1993; Thompson et al., 1993) for the μ opioid receptor shows that it is homologous with both mouse δ- and rat κ-receptors. The cDNA encodes a protein of 398 amino acids, which again contains the expected seven hydrophobic domains characteristic of receptors linked to G proteins. Its identification as encoding a selective μ-receptor comes from several characteristics examined in cells transfected with the clone:

1. Classic opioids bind to the cloned receptor with expected affinities and sterospecificity.
2. High-affinity binding in the nanomolar range occurs for the μ-selective agonist DAMGO and the μ-antagonist CTAP but only at micromolar concentrations for κ- or δ-selective agonists.
3. Competition binding studies demonstrate that the rank order of binding to the cloned receptor is consistent with binding of μ-receptor agonists and antagonists.
4. The anatomical distribution of the mRNA generally coincides with the distribution of μ-receptors reported earlier.

A notable exception is in the spinal cord, where the μ-receptor mRNA is most dense in the dorsal root ganglia, while the μ-receptor is localized in layers I and II of the spinal cord, which could indicate that the receptors are manufactured in the ganglia and are transported to presynaptic terminals in the spinal cord (see Mansour et al., 1995). An additional characteristic of the μ-receptor was revealed in transfection studies in which it functionally inhibited adenylyl cyclase in a naloxonazine-sensitive manner.

Localization. Radiolabeled mRNA probes are used to localize the cells that synthesize the opioid receptors using in situ hybridization histochemistry, and antibodies directed to the exact amino acid sequence are used to localize the specific receptor proteins using immunohistochemical techniques. These methods have revealed information about receptor transport and helped to distinguish pre- from postsynaptic receptor sites (see Mansour et al., 1995). When the localization of receptor protein and mRNA are in the same region, local synthesis with no receptor transport is assumed. When a displacement between a receptor and its mRNA exists, it is likely that receptor synthesis occurs in one part of the cell and the receptor is transported to its final location. Mansour and colleagues (1995) provide a detailed map and a discussion of the distribution of μ-, δ-, and κ-receptor mRNAs and their respective binding sites.

Localization studies also provide information regarding the regulatory role of opioids in classical neurotransmitter release. For instance, the high levels of δ-receptor mRNA in the large cholinergic cells of the striatum suggests colocalization with ACh. Such colocalization with ACh is consistent with the inhibitory effect of opiates on ACh release in that brain area, suggesting a presynaptic inhibitory effect. Also μ-receptor mRNA is found in the locus coeruleus, an area that responds to μ-receptor agonists by inhibiting cell firing and reducing subsequent release of norepinephrine in the cerebral cortex (see Mansour et al., 1995).

Cellular Mechanisms of Action

In general, the effects of opiates on nerve cell function include the reduction of membrane excitability with subsequent slowing of cell firing, and the inhibition of neurotransmitter release. The cellular mechanisms responsible for these actions have been thoroughly investigated in isolated tissue preparations.

G Protein Mediation

Biochemical evidence for opiate receptor–G protein coupling has been summarized and reviewed by Cox (1993) and Childers (1993). As is usual for G protein–linked receptors, not only is the effector's function modified by guanine nucleotides (e.g., GTP), but receptor binding affinity is changed. Binding of agonists, but not antagonists, is inhibited by guanine nucleotides (also see Figure 8.21). Guanine nucleotides increase the rate of dissociation of opiate agonists from the opiate receptor, particularly in the presence of Na⁺. Agonist affinity is also reduced by membrane treatments that change G protein function. For example, pertussis toxin, which inhibits G_i (see Chapter 6), significantly reduces binding affinity of agonists to opioid receptors. Opiate agonists also stimulate GTPase activity, thereby enhancing the rate of breakdown of GTP to GDP, which further supports the notion of receptor-mediated G protein activation.

Furthermore, the cloned opiate receptors all contain the characteristic membrane-spanning regions typical of G protein–linked receptors. The receptors are coupled to several of the effector systems that are usually associated with G proteins (Childers, 1993), including adenylyl cyclase activity, phosphoinositide turnover, and direct G protein coupling to K^+ and Ca^{2+} channels. These cellular responses require GTP and are modified by altering G proteins with agents such as pertussis toxin and cholera toxin (which persistently activates G_s). Finally, purified opiate receptor protein and G protein can be reconstituted in prepared membranes for functional studies.

Opiate Receptors Regulate Ion Channels

The effects of opiates on ion channels depend on G protein mediation. Opiate receptor–G protein activation apparently increases K^+ conductance and decreases Ca^{2+} conductance in many different parts of the CNS. Both of these ion channel effects potentially reduce neurotransmitter release and may ultimately be responsible for the analgesic effects of opioids (DiChiara and North, 1992).

Activation of μ- and δ-opiate receptors increases membrane K^+ conductance, causing hyperpolarization and, in most tissues, shortens the duration of the normal action potential. In some tissues, such as the dorsal root ganglion, no membrane hyperpolarization or change in resting membrane potential occurs, but the increase in K^+ conductance speeds up the repolarization phase of the action potential and increases the magnitude of the afterhyperpolarization. Although evidence for κ-receptor regulation of K^+ conductance is lacking, expectations are that in some tissues the κ-receptor will also be found to alter the function of this channel (North, 1993).

Considerable evidence suggests that opiate receptors interact with K^+ channels via G proteins (North, 1993; DiChiara and North, 1992). Pharmacological manipulations interfering with G protein function prevent opiate-induced increases in K^+ conductance. The K^+ conductance can be restored by recoupling the receptor and channel by the further addition of purified G protein to the cells. A role for cAMP in this process has been generally dismissed since no freely diffusible second messenger intervenes between receptor activation and K^+ channel activation.

Opiates suppress a resting Na^+-dependent inward current in cells in the locus coeruleus which reduces their spontaneous firing rate. In this case, mediation by cAMP is likely (see below).

Agonists for the μ-, δ- and κ-receptors are known to close N-type Ca^{2+} channels in various tissues, possibly via direct G protein interactions (Brown and Birnbaumer, 1990). These channels are differentiated from the L and T types by requiring strong depolarization from normal resting potential for activation. These same channels are often closed by agonist occupation of nonopiate receptors (e.g., adenosine A_1, muscarinic M_2, $GABA_B$, $5\text{-}HT_{1A}$, somatostatin, neuropeptide Y, dopamine D_2, and norepinephrine α_2), which, like the opiate receptors, are G protein–coupled and are in some cases associated with the identical channels. Such a multiplicity of receptor regulation of channel function is the likely basis for the overlapping pharmacological effects of agents acting on these receptors.

Inhibition of Adenylyl Cyclase

Of the several G protein–mediated effects of opiate receptor occupation, inhibition of adenylyl cyclase has been most extensively studied. The earliest report of opiate receptor regulation of a second messenger system showed morphine inhibition of PGE_1-stimulated adenylyl cyclase in rat striatal membranes, which was antagonized by naloxone (Collier and Roy, 1974). Subsequent research showed opioid inhibition of adenylyl cyclase activity stimulated by a variety of agonists in a variety of tissues. In addition, the hybrid NG 108-15 cells that have high levels of δ-opiate receptors show opioid inhibition not only of PGE_1-stimulated adenylyl cyclase but also basal activity, adenosine-stimulated, and cholera toxin–stimulated adenylyl cyclase. The requirement for GTP (Law et al., 1981) and importance of Na^+ (Konkoy and Childers, 1989) in adenylyl cyclase inhibition by opiates is clear. Furthermore, pertussis toxin and other treatments that alter G protein function also abolish opioid inhibition of adenylyl cyclase, suggesting once again that inhibitory G proteins are necessary for this action.

All three types of opiate receptors (μ, δ, and κ) can inhibit adenylyl cyclase in various tissues. Within the CNS, for example, μ-inhibited adenylyl cyclase has been identified in rat thalamus, rabbit cerebellum, and rat periaqueductal gray and locus coeruleus. Striatal adenylyl cyclase is readily inhibited by δ-agonists, but evidence for the activity of multiple opioid receptors in that tissue has been reported. κ-receptor–mediated inhibition occurs in rat spinal cord neurons and in guinea pig cerebellum.

Although evidence for opioid inhibition of adenylyl cyclase is clear, its role in cell function is less apparent. In some cases the opioid-induced inhibition of cyclic nucleotide accumulation has been linked to the peptides' modulation of neurotransmitter release, though in most cases inhibition of neurotransmitter release is not mediated by cAMP. Most electrophysiological evidence suggests that changes in cAMP do not play a part in opioid effects on ion channels, although in the spinal cord, inhi-

12.4 THE SUGGESTED MECHANISM OF ACTION OF OPIOIDS ON ENKEPHALIN SYNTHESIS. By binding to the opioid receptor (R_i), the inhibitory G protein (G_i) is activated and in turn inhibits the formation of cAMP by adenylyl cyclase. Since cAMP is required for cAMP-dependent protein kinase phosphorylation, the CREB remains unphosphorylated and proenkephalin mRNA synthesis is inhibited, thus reducing enkephalin levels in the cell. On the other hand, a stimulated receptor (R_s) bound to a stimulatory G protein (G_s) can reverse this process and ultimately increase enkephalin levels in the cell.

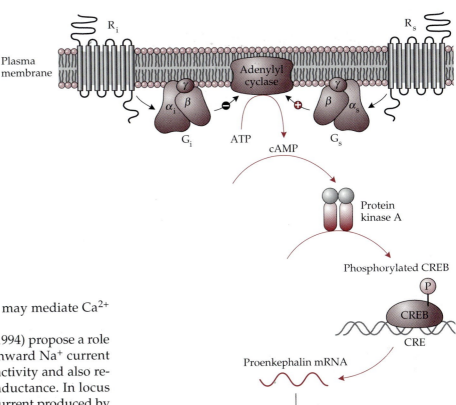

bition of adenylyl cyclase by opiates may mediate Ca^{2+} influx (Chen et al., 1988).

Nestler, Alreja, and Aghajanian (1994) propose a role for cAMP in regulating the resting inward Na^+ current that maintains neuronal pacemaker activity and also reverses the effects of outward K^+ conductance. In locus coeruleus neurons, the net outward current produced by opiates is due to both activation of K^+ conductance and by the inhibition of the Na^+-dependent inward current (Alreja and Aghajanian, 1993). While K^+ conductance is not mediated by cAMP, pacemaker activation of locus coeruleus neurons does seem to be dependent on cAMP-dependent protein kinase. Evidence presented suggests that opiate inhibition of adenylyl cyclase and the subsequently reduced cAMP-dependent kinase activity may be responsible for a decrease in Na^+ channel phosphorylation and subsequent ion conduction.

Opioid-induced inhibition of adenylyl cyclase may also be involved in long-term regulation of opioid neuropeptide synthesis. Childers (1993) describes a model (Figure 12.4) based on evidence that the genes for several neuropeptides, including proenkephalin, contain cAMP-response elements (CRE) and cAMP response element binding protein (CREB). Transcription factors, such as CREB, are proteins that bind to specific DNA sequences in the promoter regions of genes and increase or decrease the rate at which those genes are transcribed (see Chapter 6). When activated by cAMP-dependent protein kinase, the phosphorylated CREB increases mRNA synthesis. This model proposes that opioid inhibition of adenylyl cyclase may represent presynaptic negative feedback in which high concentrations of endogenous opioid neuropeptides released into the synapse may act on presynaptic receptors to inhibit further adenylyl cyclase–induced synthesis of the neuropeptide, thus reducing its availability.

In support of this model, opiate agonists administered in vivo significantly reduce levels of proenkephalin

mRNA in striatum (Uhl, Ryan, and Schwartz, 1988) while chronic antagonist administration increases proenkephalin mRNA levels (Tempel, Kessler, and Zukin, 1990). Childers (1993) found that forskolin-stimulated increases in cAMP and in proenkephalin mRNA were inhibited by opioid agonists. The effect could be antagonized by naloxone and also by pertussis toxin, demonstrating that it is mediated by an opiate receptor coupled to a G protein.

Finally, cAMP-mediated intracellular changes have been implicated in the adaptation of cells to chronic opioid exposure. The up-regulation of the cAMP system may represent a compensatory mechanism to the initial inhibitory effects of the opioids, and could represent the neural basis for tolerance, dependence, and withdrawal. Details of this role for cAMP are described in a subsequent section.

Part II Summary

The binding of specific opioid ligands to distinct receptor subtypes has been thoroughly characterized. Molecular biology has further demonstrated that the cDNAs for μ-, δ-, and κ-receptors each encode a series of amino acids that are strikingly (≥60%) homologous to one another. Each includes within it seven homologous hydrophobic domains that span the neuronal membrane.

These receptors closely resemble others belonging to the large family of receptors that are linked to G proteins and transduce their intracellular signals via G protein–coupled pathways. In addition, by comparing the amino acid sequences of the receptors, structural differences among the subtypes can be identified. These differences provide a basis on which to design highly specific receptor ligands and therapeutic agents that target each receptor subtype more precisely than those currently available.

Transfection studies using the cloned nucleic acid sequence (mRNA or cDNA) for each opiate receptor revealed that the μ-, δ-, and κ-receptors all apparently have an inhibitory effect on the formation of cAMP. This inhibitory action on the second messenger is consistent with previously reported pharmacological studies in vitro (see below).

Moreover, localization studies generally revealed a similar distribution between a specific receptor protein and its mRNA. This suggests that receptor synthesis occurs locally where the receptor functions. However, the discrepancies that do exist between receptor protein location and its mRNA provide important information about receptor transport to presynaptic sites on neuron terminals in selected brain areas.

Opioid receptors clearly reduce Ca^{2+} entry and increase K^+ conductance by G protein–mediated actions on the respective ion channels. There is no clear agreement at this time as to whether one or both of these events is ultimately responsible for diminished neurotransmitter release. The well-documented inhibitory effect of opiates on adenylyl cyclase activity seems to have a modulatory role in Na^+ conductance and the rate of synthesis of endogenous opioid peptides, and may play a large part in the development of tolerance and dependence.

Part III
Endogenous Opioid Peptides

The search for endogenous opioid peptides was prompted by the realization that opiate receptor distribution failed to parallel the regional distribution of any previously known neurotransmitter. Also, since the analgesia produced by electrically stimulating specific areas of the CNS could be partially antagonized by naloxone, it was reasonable to consider the stimulation-induced release of a natural ligand acting on those receptors. The appearance of cross-tolerance between morphine-induced and electrically-induced analgesia also suggested the existence of an endogenous ligand to act on the opiate receptor.

In 1974, two independent laboratories identified a peptide in brain extracts that mimicked opiate activity in its ability to inhibit electrically induced contractions in the guinea pig ileum (Hughes, 1975) and to bind to opiate receptors (Terenius and Wahlstrom, 1974). These studies led to the subsequent identification and characterization of the endogenous opiates, called **endorphins**, from *endo-*, signifying "endogenous," and *-orphin* from the common suffix in the names of opiates. Several peptides of low molecular weight having opiate agonist properties were found in pig brain (Hughes, Smith, Kosterlitz et al., 1975), cow brain (Pasternak, Goodman, and Snyder, 1975), human cerebrospinal fluid (Terenius and Wahlstrom, 1975), and pituitary extracts (Teschmacher et al., 1975). Hughes, Smith, Morgan, and colleagues (1975) sequenced the amino acids of two pentapeptides, Met-enkephalin (H–Tyr–Gly–Gly–Phe–Met–OH) and Leu-enkephalin (H–Tyr–Gly–Gly–Phe–Leu–OH), which differ only in the terminal amino acid. Since these substances were found in the brain they were named *enkephalin*, which is Greek for "from the head."

Within a short time, it was discovered that the amino acid sequence of Met-enkephalin is identical to a peptide sequence within β-lipotropin, a 91-amino acid peptide that was first found in the pituitary (Li and Chung, 1976) and that also has some opioid properties. New purification techniques produced a host of other peptide fragments with varying degrees of opioid activity, such as α-, β-, and γ-endorphin, dynorphin, and peptides E and F. The great similarity in structure among the peptides led researchers to conclude that the larger peptides are prohormones that are broken into smaller active opioids. Whether the smallest of the peptides were the ultimate active synaptic transmitters or were degradation products of the larger active peptides remained to be determined.

Three Families of Peptides

Opioid Peptide Processing

Some of the confusion surrounding the large number of opiate peptides was clarified by techniques in molecular biology showing that three distinct opioid precursors exist (see Uhl, Childers, and Pasternak, 1994). Each of the three large peptide prohormones—**prodynorphin (PDYN)** (Kakidani et al., 1982), **proopiomelanocortin (POMC)** (Nakanishi et al., 1979), and **proenkephalin (PENK)** (Comb et al., 1982)—is coded by a separate gene and separate messenger RNA. The similarities between the three suggests that they may have been derived from a common ancestral gene (Akil, Bronstein, and Mansour, 1988). Each of the precursors must undergo processing by proteolytic enzymes, which are packaged along with the precursor in the Golgi apparatus. The enzymes cleave the prohormone into individual peptide products that are stored in vesicles (Figure 12.5). Further processing occurs within the vesicles. Specific amino acid sequences, or "signals," are embedded within the peptide and direct proteolytic enzymes to cleave the prohor-

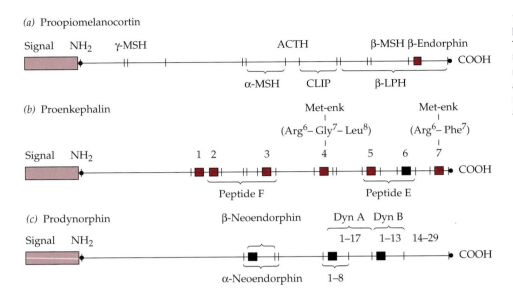

mone between specific amino acids. The cleavage varies depending upon which enzymes are present, resulting in complex cell-specific patterns of prohormone expression. Furthermore, it is suggested that this posttranslational enzyme processing within a particular cell can vary with conditions over time, depending on a wide variety of regulatory events (Akil, Bronstein, and Mansour, 1988; Hollt, 1993; Roberts et al., 1993; Rossier, 1993; Young, Bronstein, and Akil, 1993). In addition, posttranslational processing may include chemical modification (e.g., acetylation) of the peptide to further alter the end product. Clearly, mapping the location of specific peptides within the brain requires more than knowledge of prohormone mRNA expression.

The gene that codes for POMC is transcribed into a mRNA that is translated into a prohormone of 267 amino acids. Posttranslational processing of the large precursor peptide produces several smaller opioid peptides, including β-lipotropin (β-LPH) and β-endorphin (Figure 12.5a). It also contains biologically active peptides that are unrelated to opioid peptides, such as ACTH, α-MSH, β-MSH, and γ-MSH. Since these peptides play an important part in the body's response to stress, POMC could be a link between pain regulation and the stress response.

Complex processing of POMC occurs in the pituitary. Although POMC is found in both the anterior and the intermediate lobes of the pituitary, posttranslational processing differs between the two lobes, resulting in different end products (Eipper and Mains, 1981). In the anterior lobe, POMC is cleaved into three fragments: the β-LPH/β-endorphin domain, the ACTH domain, and the amino-terminal (NH₂) domain (Figure 12.5a). Approximately 30% of the β-LPH/β-endorphin domain is further split into β-LPH and β-endorphin. In the intermediate lobe, POMC is similarly split, but all of the β-LPH/β-endorphin is further broken to form β-LPH and

β-endorphin. Additional cleavage of the peptides also occurs, forming a family of ACTH peptide fragments, as well as α-MSH. POMC processing in brain (Dores et al., 1986; Young, Bronstein, and Akil, 1993) shows further variations in cleavage and processing depending on the brain region.

The PENK gene encodes a protein precursor with 267 amino acids. Within this protein (Figure 12.5b) are four copies of Met-enkephalin and one copy each of Leu-enkephalin, Met-enkephalin–Arg^6–Phe^7, and Met-enkephalin–Arg^6–Gly^7–Leu^8. The PENK precursor can also be processed into larger enkephalin-containing peptides, including peptide E, peptide F, BAM-18P, methorphamide, and amidorphin.

The PDYN gene produces a prohormone of 254 amino acids (Figure 12.5c), which is cleaved into leu-enkephalin and several Leu-enkephalin–containing peptides: dynorphin A, dynorphin B, and α- and β-neoendorphin (Hollt, 1993).

The details of posttranslational processing of proenkephalin (Rossier, 1993) and prodynorphin (Day, Trujillo, and Akil, 1993) are less well understood than is POMC processing. However, there is considerable evidence demonstrating that distinct regional differences in processing exist, yielding varied products. Species variations also exist (Dores and Akil, 1987). The ratio of dynorphin A-(1–17) to its cleavage product, dynorphin A(1–8), in the rat pituitary is 1:2, while it is much higher in the porcine pituitary (10:1) and that of the rhesus monkey (14:1). The relevance of such differences is not immediately evident; however, it is clear that different peptide end products have different receptor subtype selectivity. Dynorphin A-(1–17) binds most avidly to κ-type opiate receptors, while dynorphin A-(1–8) produces a ligand with mixed selectivity for κ- and δ-receptors (see below).

Finally, peptide processing can be modified by cell activity. As demands change, a cell may change the mixture of peptides it produces and subsequently releases. For instance, in the intermediate lobe of the pituitary, *N*-acetylated β-endorphin$_{1-27}$ is normally the most prevalent form of β-endorphin. In contrast, under conditions of foot shock or swim stress, the *N*-acetylated β-endorphin$_{1-31}$ becomes the predominant form stored in the tissue and that which is released (Young, 1990). Prodynorphin peptides are also modified by other pharmacological, physiological, and behavioral manipulations. Changes in prodynorphin processing in the nigrostriatal pathway are produced by treatment with dopamine agonists and other drugs, such as lithium and phencyclidine (Day, Trujillo, and Akil, 1993).

Since many peptides can be formed within the same biosynthetic pathway, many questions still remain. Which of the many peptides formed is the "real" end product? Can the same peptide be a precursor, an end product, and a degradation product in different tissues? Are multiple peptides released to produce varying effects on the target cell receptors? Is the most prevalent product necessarily the most biologically significant? When the ratios of products vary regionally or across species, is release proportional to the stored ratios, or are the various products differentially released? In summary, not only is a large variety of prohormone cleavage patterns possible, but regional differences in peptide concentrations and species-specific processing all suggest a complexity of function that will continue to intrigue researchers for years.

Localization and Regulation

The earliest attempts to localize specific opiate peptides were somewhat problematic because the peptides' amino acid sequences are so similar that they frequently show common immunoreactive characteristics and cross-react with different antisera. Despite these difficulties, early results from anatomical, biochemical, and immunohistochemical studies showed unique distributions of several peptides in the brain (Simantov et al., 1976; Hökfelt et al., 1977; Watson, Barchas, and Li, 1977).

Later, when it became clear that three distinct opioid families with three unique prohormone precursors exist, research became focused on identifying those neuronal perikarya that synthesize each prohormone in hopes of correlating the location of different peptides with opiate receptor subtypes. Mapping was achieved by in situ hybridization to visualize prohormone mRNA or by immunohistochemistry to localize the prohormone itself. In situ hybridization has the potential to identify even minute amounts of mRNA and thereby provides information on the dynamic process of peptide synthesis. With this technique, factors that regulate opioid peptide gene expression can be examined. For instance, chronic morphine administration might be expected to have an effect on the synthesis of endogenous opioids, reflected by a change in the mRNA level for a particular prohor-

mone. These mapping and peptide regulation studies have been summarized in detail elsewhere (Hollt, 1993; Khachaturian, Schaefer, and Lewis, 1993; Kley and Loeffler, 1993; Roberts et al., 1993).

It is also important to realize that opioid peptides are frequently colocalized with other neurotransmitters, including with opioid peptides from other families. At least in some neurons, opioid peptides play a neuromodulatory role that evidently modifies the function of the colocalized neurotransmitter. Table 12.3 provides a partial list of brain areas where colocalization of opioids and other transmitters occurs (see Elde and Hökfelt, 1993, for review).

Proenkephalin.   Proenkephalin (PENK), the precursor to Leu- and Met-enkephalin, as well as peptides E and F and other peptides has extensive distribution throughout the CNS and peripheral autonomic nervous system. It appears to be the most abundant of the three families. While some enkephalin-containing cells have long projections, many are small neurons that contain relatively little PENK and form local circuits. These small neurons are difficult to detect unless colchicine is used to block axonal transport, thereby increasing perikaryon concentration of newly manufactured peptide.

The ability to localize the prohormone and evaluate the factors that regulate prohormone synthesis prompts research into the functional roles of the endogenous opioid. For example, the highest levels of PENK mRNA are found in the medium spiny neurons of the striatum which project to the pallidum. The importance of the dopamine rich striatum to extrapyramidal motor function is well documented. Thus the discovery that dopamine regulates the gene expression for PENK in striatum predicts an important role for the PENK-opioids in motor coordination. (Hollt, 1993).

The ventromedial nucleus of the hypothalamus (VMH) is another brain area with high concentrations of the enkephalin prohormone. In ovariectomized rats, PENK mRNA levels in the VMH are rapidly increased by estrogen treatment. Although removing the estrogen again reduces PENK mRNA, the reduction can be attenuated by progesterone. The differential changes noted in this response in males and females suggest that the enkephalinergic cells may play a role in the hormonal regulation of the estrous cycle (Hollt, 1993; Romano et al., 1990).

Finally, in situ hybridization has shown significant PENK mRNA in the granule cells of the dentate gyrus of the hippocampus. Repeated stimulation of the amygdala, which induces seizures, causes a significant increase in PENK mRNA in the hippocampus. Other techniques for inducing seizures, such as contralateral lesions of the dentate gyrus hilus, direct electrical stimulation, or repeated electroconvulsive shock, also increase PENK gene expression in the hippocampus (Hollt, 1993;

Table 12.3   Selected Examples of Coexistence of Opioids and Other Transmitters in Rat Brain

Brain area	Opioid	Classical neurotransmitter	Peptide neurotransmitter
Caudate	ENK	GAD	SP
Amygdala	ENK		CCK
Supraoptic nucleus	DYN	TH	VP and GAL
Paraventricular	ENK		CRF and VIP
Arcuate	DYN	TH	
Superior colliculus	ENK	GABA	
Raphe nucleus	ENK	5-HT	
Area postrema	ENK	5-HT	
Solitary nucleus	ENK and DYN		SOM
Lateral superior olive	ENK and DYN	ChAT	CGRP
Cerebellum	ENK	GABA	

Abbreviations: 5-HT = serotonin; CCK = cholecystokinin; ChAT = choline acetyltransferase (synthesizing enzyme for ACh that acts as marker for cholinergic neurons); CRF = corticotropin-releasing factor; GAD = glutamate decarboxylase (synthesizing enzyme for GABA that acts as a marker for GABAergic cells); GAL = galanin; SOM = somatostatin; SP = substance P; TH = tyrosine hydroxylase (synthesizing enzyme for catecholamines that acts as a marker for NE and DA cells); VIP = vasoactive intestinal polypeptide; VP = vasopressin.
Source: After Elde and Hökfelt (1993).

Gall et al., 1990). The regulation of peptide synthesis in hippocampus coincides with behavioral evidence of hippocampal μ- and δ- agonist-induced seizure activity and κ-receptor–mediated anticonvulsant effects (see Morris and Johnston, 1995).

Proopiomelanocortin.   Proopiomelanocortin (POMC) is the precursor to β-endorphin, ACTH, and α-MSH and is synthesized in discrete brain areas such as basal ganglia, cortex, and amygdala, as well as in both the anterior and intermediate lobes of the pituitary. Brain sites of most interest include the arcuate nucleus of the hypothalamus with its extensive projections and the nucleus tractus solitarius in the medulla.

The regulation of POMC mRNA synthesis in arcuate nucleus by gonadal steroids implies that these opioid products may play a role in reproductive physiology. In rats, estrogen clearly reduces POMC gene expression, as does castration. The effects of castration can be reversed by testosterone. Other hypothalamic cells (in the medial basal nucleus), however, show castration-induced increases in POMC mRNA. The precise physiological consequences of these hormone-induced changes are not immediately clear. Additional evidence for a relationship between the POMC peptides and hormonal function is shown by the significant increase in POMC mRNA at the onset of puberty in the male rat (Wiemann, Clifton, and Steiner, 1989). The burst of gonadotropin-releasing hormone occurring at that stage of development may be under opioid control.

POMC-containing cells are also found in the nucleus tractus solitarius. Although some of the fibers are short and terminate within the medulla, other cells are the origin of a descending POMC fiber bundle that terminates in the gray matter around the central canal in the spinal cord. These areas are known to contain cells selectively sensitive to noxious stimuli. When the spinal cord is transected, only immunoreactivity below the cut disappears, suggesting that the sources of POMC innervation in the spinal cord must be supraspinal. Since electrical stimulation of the nucleus tractus soliatarius in the medulla produces strong opioid-mediated inhibition of the tail-flick reflex to noxious stimuli, this nucleus is the likely origin of the descending pathway that mediates analgesia (Tsou et al., 1986).

The highest concentration of POMC mRNA is in the pituitary (anterior and intermediate lobes), and regulation of POMC gene expression has been most extensively studied in this tissue (Roberts et al., 1993). In the anterior pituitary, corticosteroids from the adrenal gland provide negative feedback control over POMC gene expression. Thus, removing the adrenal gland increases POMC mRNA levels, while dexamethasone (a corticosteroid drug) reduces them. Corticotropin-releasing factor (CRF) causes a rapid increase in POMC mRNA as do a variety of stressors, such as foot shock, restraint, and swim stress, which also elevate CRF and its mRNA in the paraventricular nucleus of the hypothalamus (Harbuz and Lightman, 1989; Hollt, 1993). The localization of POMC-derived peptides in discrete areas of the CNS related to pain transmission and in the hypothalamic–pituitary–adrenal stress system suggests that these peptides may provide a link between pain regulation and stress regulation (Young, Bronstein, and Akil, 1993).

Prodynorphin.   Prodynorphin (PDYN), the precursor for dynorphin A, dynorphin B, and α- and β-neodynorphin, is found in many areas of the brain and spinal cord as well as in the anterior lobe of the pituitary. Its wide distribution often parallels that of PENK, and they may, in fact, coexist in certain cells. Like PENK-containing neurons, many PDYN neurons are short and form local circuits. Other cells, however, have long projections terminating far from their somata.

High levels of PDYN mRNA are found in magnocellular cells in the hypothalamus, where colocalization with vasopressin occurs. Vasopressin is the antidiuretic hormone (ADH) that is ultimately released from the pituitary to increase water reabsorption by the kidney. This colocalization is paralleled by a close association between the opioid and vasopressin regulation. Osmotic challenges, such as salt loading or dehydration, increase both PDYN products and vasopressin content in those cells.

In the hippocampal formation, both PENK and PDYN mRNAs are expressed in the granule cell layer of the dentate gyrus. Seizure activity in the hippocampus decreases the peptide products of both prohormones, but the levels of PDYN mRNA decrease while PENK mRNA increases significantly (Gall et al., 1990). Other evidence also indicates that, unlike the PENK mRNA, the expression of the PDYN gene is reduced by neuronal firing (Hollt, 1993). Further research into the differences in regulation of these peptides is necessary.

Inactivation

The earliest studies of the newly isolated peptides had difficulty demonstrating biological activity because when even large doses of opioid peptides are injected into the brain, only small and fleeting effects occur. Research soon showed that enkephalin is almost immediately hydrolyzed into constituent amino acids when it contacts brain tissue in vivo or in vitro. Several studies (reviewed by Roques et al., 1993) showed that [³H]Leu-enkephalin disappeared completely within one minute at 37°C when the peptide was incubated with brain tissue, while its principal metabolite, [³H]tyrosine, concomitantly increased.

This rapid degradation of enkephalin is due to the presence of peptidases in the tissue that attack the peptide bond between amino acids and generally cleave a variety of peptides with little specificity. A given peptidase may recognize only one or two amino acids on either side of the bond to be cleaved. The generality of peptidases makes it difficult to determine precisely which one(s) may be involved in breaking down a particular peptide. Detailed analysis of the peptide cleavage pattern, the anatomical and cellular localization of the peptidase, and inhibition of peptide cleavage using specific peptidase inhibitors is necessary (Turner, 1988; Dua, Pinsky, and LaBella, 1985).

Of the peptidases investigated, the two that are likely candidates in the metabolism of enkephalin are endopeptidase-24.11 ("enkephalinase") and aminopeptidase-N. Both of these enzymes are found in the CNS but are also in many other tissues, which means that no specific "neuropeptidase" probably exists (Roques et al., 1993).

The aminopeptidases, which split tyrosine–glycine bonds, were the first enkephalin-metabolizing enzymes to be discovered, since tyrosine is the initial metabolite formed. The majority of brain aminopeptidases are found in the soluble fraction of nerve cells and have an anatomical distribution that does not correlate well with markers for enkephalin neurons. Puromycin inhibits their action but does not enhance opioid activity. On the other hand, the membrane-bound species of aminopeptidase (particularly aminopeptidase-N) is sensitive to inhibition by bestatin, a drug shown to potentiate the analgesic effect of injected Met-enkephalin. Given that enkephalins do not enter cells, the location of this enzyme at the cell surface is particularly significant (Schwartz, 1983a; Roques et al., 1993).

Like aminopeptidase-N, endopeptidase-24.11 (enkephalinase) is an ectoenzyme, which means that it is a protein embedded in the cell membrane with its active site facing the extracellular fluid. Immunohistochemical analysis shows that enkephalinase is distributed heterogeneously in the CNS, with highest concentrations in the caudate, putamen, globus pallidus, olfactory tubercle, substantia nigra, nucleus accumbens, substantia gelatinosa of the spinal cord, amygdala, periaqueductal gray, and hippocampus. Its distribution roughly parallels the areas of enkephalin concentration (Pollard et al., 1989). Additionally, subcellular distribution is closely correlated with opiate receptors in rat and human brain (Roques et al., 1993). For instance, neurotoxic lesions in the striatum cause a decrease both in enkephalinase and opiate receptor binding at terminal sites in the substantia nigra and globus pallidus. Since striatonigral and striatopallidal neurons are well documented, the loss of enzyme activity and receptor binding demonstrates a presynaptic localization for both (Waksman et al., 1987). However, in addition to CNS distribution, enkephalinase is found in a variety of peripheral tissues (Turner, 1988).

Specific inhibition of enkephalinase can be demonstrated by evaluating the recovery of intact enkephalins released by depolarization of brain slices. Depolarization of brain slices normally yields only a small fraction of unmetabolized Met-enkephalin. However, the addition of either the enkephalinase inhibitor thiorphan or the aminopeptidase-N inhibitor, bestatin, increases recovery of intact Met-enkephalin only twofold. The presence of either inhibitor alone apparently shifts the burden of metabolism to the uninhibited peptidase, since the addition of bestatin increases the metabolic products formed by enkephalinase, and thiorphan increases metabolites produced by aminopeptidase-N. When both inhibitors are present, recovery of unmetabolized opioid is virtually complete (Schwartz, 1983a). Figure 12.6 diagrams the re-

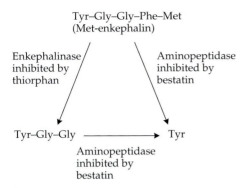

12.6 ALTERNATIVE PATHWAYS FOR METABOLISM OF ENKEPHALINS. Since enkephalin can be metabolized by either enkephalinase or aminopeptidase, inhibiting either one of the enzymes shifts the metabolic load to the other pathway.

lationship between the two peptidases. These results indicate that endogenous enkephalin is likely to be metabolized in vivo by both enkephalinase and aminopeptidase-*N* with little or no effect of other peptidases. In keeping with this finding, new mixed inhibitors of these enzymes have been designed. Kelatorphan and its analogs effectively inhibit both peptidases. However, their high water solubility prevents them from readily penetrating the blood–brain barrier (Roques et al., 1993).

Parallel experiments measuring the effects of peptidase inhibitors on behavioral responses to noxious stimuli confirm the importance of enkephalinase and aminopeptidase-*N* on metabolism of endogenous opioid peptides. In these studies of nociceptive reflexes that are known to be mediated by opioids, tests such as the hot plate and tail flick tests are used. Thiorphan and bestatin each produce analgesia that is significantly increased by dual administration. Since the action of the inhibitors is blocked by naloxone, it is reasonable to assume that the peptidase inhibitors work by increasing the availability of enkephalin. These results and other effects of peptidase inhibitors on analgesia, gastrointestinal function, and behavior are discussed in more detail elsewhere (Roques et al., 1993).

Relationship to Receptor Subtypes

The relationship between the three families of peptides, with their many products, and the principal receptor types is complex. At this time, researchers find no obvious correspondence between any opioid peptide or peptide family and a particular opiate receptor. Rather, each of the peptides can bind to any of the recognized receptors with varying affinities. So rather than being selective, the peptides show a relative preference for a particular receptor type. In general, the natural ligands for the δ site are thought to be those derived from proenkephalin, and products from prodynorphin are likely the natural κ-receptor agonists. No endogenous opioid family has yet been found to bind selectively to the μ site, although several morphine-like molecules found in brain may be en-

dogenous μ-selective compounds (Donnerer et al., 1986). Additionally, enkephalins and perhaps β-endorphin appear to have a very high affinity for the μ_1-receptor.

One way to examine peptide–receptor specificity is to evaluate the localization of peptide-containing neurons in specific brain areas and their corresponding receptor subtype densities. Autoradiographic studies of rat brain show that a strong correlation between receptor density and peptide concentration exists in some brain areas, but not in others (Mansour et al., 1988).

For example, in most of the hypothalamic nuclei there is a good relationship between PDYN and κ-receptors. In cortex, amygdala, and caudate–putamen, correlations exist between δ- and κ-receptor density and PENK and PDYN peptide localization, respectively. In contrast, no apparent relationship exists between POMC peptides and μ-receptors in cortex, hippocampus, caudate, putamen, or thalamus. Although this mismatch is initially disturbing, such disparities are not unique to peptides, and are probably related to distinctions between peptide localization and postsynaptic or presynaptic sites of action.

Several other investigators have also proposed reasons for mismatches, including the lack of sensitivity of the autoradiographic technique to resolve local circuits of opioid neurons, a problem that in situ hybridization may overcome. Also, the existence of "spare" (or nonfunctional) receptors or undetectable low affinity receptors may result in similar disparities (Herkenham, 1987; Khachaturian, Schaefer, and Lewis, 1993). Investigation of the subtypes of μ-, δ-, and κ-receptors (e.g., μ_1 and μ_2), and the possible allosteric interactions between them, is also potentially important when evaluating localization data.

Furthermore, the complexity of the peptide–receptor interaction may also preclude a simple one-to-one relationship. As the cleavage products of a particular prohormone are formed, their affinities for the receptor subtypes change. For example, prodynorphin products are considered to prefer κ-receptors and also bind with somewhat lower affinity at the μ-receptor. However, cleavage into shorter peptides (e.g., dynorphin A-[1–8]) decreases affinity for the κ-receptor, and the order of preference shifts to favor δ-receptors over μ-receptors and lastly, κ-receptors (Akil, Bronstein, and Mansour, 1988).

Khachaturian, Schaefer, and Lewis (1993) propose that evolutionary specialization is the basis for at least some of the disparities. They argue that phylogenetic divergence in the nervous system may be most readily accomplished by an up- or down-regulation of receptor types rather than a restructuring of opioid pathways. Similarly, an up- or down-regulation of precursor processing enzymes is easier to code for genomically than is restructuring neural connections. The great species differences in distribution and concentration of receptor subtypes and in opioid precursor processing support this idea. Further, developmental changes in the expression of opioid peptides and receptors (McDowell and Kitchen, 1987) also reveal mismatches and may provide an optimal physiological way to regulate complex opioid functions.

In summary, it can be said that each peptide family has the ability to bind to every receptor subtype and conversely, each receptor can be occupied by several opioid peptides. Therefore, the ultimate physiological effects of opioid neuron activity are dependent on (1) which peptides are formed and released, (2) in what proportion the peptides are released, (3) which receptors are present at that synapse, and (4) whether allosteric interactions (Rothman, Holaday, and Porreca, 1993) exist between the receptors. Certainly the complexity uncovered thus far predicts a rich and robust function for these natural ligands.

Functional Effects of Opiates and Opioid Peptides

The discovery of the opioid peptides initiated an enormous volume of research into their pharmacological and behavioral properties. The peptides, like the exogenous opiates, produce analgesia (Chang et al., 1976), inhibit electrical stimulation-induced muscle twitch of guinea pig ileum (Hughes, 1975), depress neuronal firing in various areas of the brain and spinal cord (Duggan, Hall, and Headly, 1976; Frederickson and Norris, 1976), and produce physical dependence (Wei and Loh, 1976a).

The large volume of research into the physiological and behavioral effects of the peptides and the functional roles of receptor subtypes continues to expand at an exponential rate. Early studies examined the effects of intracerebral injection of the endogenous peptides on animal behavior and utilized the general opiate antagonist naloxone to demonstrate specific receptor mediation of the measured variable. The recent description and mapping of multiple families of peptides and receptor types suggests the existence of discrete systems serving particular functions. These systems may not be so well defined, however, since exogenous administration of selected agonists or antagonists can act on one or more receptor subtype to produce a variety of effects, making it difficult to pinpoint a specific role for any one agonist. A role for opiates in analgesia and positive reinforcement has been generally assumed, though more recent emphasis has been placed on opiate modification of more complex behaviors, including development and social behavior, motor coordination, feeding and water regulation, and a host of psychiatric disorders.

Methodology

Since the use of opioid peptides themselves is frequently limited by their very short half-lives, the most common way to distinguish between receptor subtypes and biological effects is to use specific receptor agonists

and antagonists (Simon, 1991). Many of the selective ligands are opioid peptide analogs prepared by substituting, deleting, or adding natural or artificial amino acids or by modifying the peptide bonds (Schiller, 1993). These modified peptides are less easily degraded by brain peptidases; however, they often do not easily penetrate the blood–brain barrier and must be administred intracerebrally (Table 12.4). Nonpeptidergic ligands developed for in vivo research have the advantage of easier penetration of the blood–brain barrier so they can be administered peripherally (Portoghese, 1993). In addition, the nonpeptide ligands have been developed to act at specific receptor subtypes and are more stable than the peptides.

The receptor antagonist naloxone is an important tool used to demonstrate opiate function in general. However, it does not readily discriminate between receptor types except at low doses, when specificity for the μ-receptor occurs. Fortunately, selective antagonists have also been developed.

A second approach to studying opioid function is to consider the anatomy of the peptide families. For example, if only one gene family is expressed in a particular brain region that regulates a physiological function, then it increases the likelihood that peptides in that prohormone family modulate the system. For instance, by combining results from several studies (see Akil, Bronstein, and Mansour, 1988), we know that only κ-receptors are found in the posterior lobe of the rat pituitary; prodynorphin, but not proenkephalin, is colocalized with vasopressin, and vasopressin causes antidiuresis, while prodynorphin products or κ-agonists cause diuresis. Thus, prodynorphin products and κ-receptors are implicated in an inhibitory or negative feedback mechanism regulating water balance. Although receptors in the pituitary apparently regulate water balance, other opiates may well modify fluid balance at other sites. While κ-receptors seem to produce diuresis by inhibiting vasopressin secretion, μ-agonists produce antidiuretic effects without the involvement of vasopressin (Leander, Zerbe, and Hart, 1985).

The preceding examples are instances in which receptor localization data, biochemical results, and behavioral experiments provide a relatively consistent pattern of function. There are many more unclear cases in which more experiments are needed to reconcile disparities in the data. For instance, μ-, δ-,and κ- agonists are equipotent in stimulating feeding behavior when injected into the ventral tegmental area (Jenck, Quirion, and Wise, 1987), despite the autoradiographic evidence showing dense μ-receptor concentrations, but few or no κ or δ sites, in this region.

Turnover rate measurements.   Studies measuring regional brain concentrations of specific opiate peptides have found only small changes following physiological

Table 12.4 Advantages and Disadvantages of Ligands Used to Determine Receptor Specificity for Discrete Behaviors and Physiological Functions

Ligands	Advantages	Disadvantages
Opioid peptides	Most similar to endogenous action	Short half-life May need intracranial administration
Modified peptides	Developed for receptor specificity Reduced degradation	May need intracranial administration
Nonpeptide ligands	Developed for receptor specificity Easy penetration of blood brain barrier Reduced degradation	Effects may be very different than endogenous ligands

treatments such as hunger, stress, motor activity, dehydration, addiction, and withdrawal. Despite use of highly sensitive radioimmunoassays to quantify the peptides, measurements of steady state levels do not reflect the dynamic changes that are continually occurring in the system. Turnover studies for the peptides are more difficult than for classical neurotransmitters because mechanisms of peptide regulation are not fully known. In general, the amount of mRNA increases in response to sustained, increased demand for peptide, probably following an increase in transcription. Although the amount of available peptide tends to parallel levels of its mRNA, if demands on the system are sustained and the release of peptide is high, mRNA levels tend to be greatly elevated and stores of peptide low (Akil, Bronstein, and Mansour, 1988).

Regulation of posttranslational cleavage. For short-term events, the measurement of peptide and mRNA is less useful because short-term needs can be met without significant changes in mRNA levels. Many posttranslational events can modulate the rate of formation of peptide fragments by activating the enzymes that determine protein cleavage. Enzymatic activation is coupled to peptide secretion, which provides a feedback mechanism to maintain available peptide stores (Shiomi et al., 1986). If this feedback mechanism is active, it is obvious that neuronal function cannot be determined by merely measuring steady state levels of peptide.

Physiological regulation of product identity, rate of formation, as well as release, is an extraordinarily elegant characteristic of opioid systems. Opioid cells in various brain areas can respond to current environmental conditions with a high degree of flexibility. Their complexity of cleavage in response to environmental events also suggests a possible significance in psychiatric disorders, where errors in gene splicing, transcription, or peptide cleavage may represent a neurochemical basis for abnormal behavior (see below).

Effects on Synaptic Processes

Electrophysiological effects of opioids. In order to examine the opioid characteristics of the endogenous peptides, researchers compared the electrophysiological effects of the endogenous opiates with those of morphine. For example, by making intracellular recordings from myenteric ganglia of the guinea pig ileum, North and Williams (1976) found that those cells that showed normorphine-induced hyperpolarization showed the same hyperpolarization after application of Leu- or Met-enkephalin, which was blocked by naloxone.

At the level of the spinal cord, opiate receptor binding is high in the substantia gelatinosa (Rexed area II; see Figure 11.20b), an area where pain-conducting fibers synapse on their way to higher neural centers. Duggan, Hall, and Headly (1976) recorded an increase in firing rate in cells of the substantia gelatinosa in cats in response to the nonnoxious deflection of hair and a noxious application of heat. The authors found that both morphine and enkephalin inhibited the heat-induced increase in firing, but not the increase in firing due to the nonnoxious hair deflection. This result demonstrates that opioid inhibition of neuronal excitation is selective for pain-conducting, small-diameter afferents (e.g., Aδ and C fibers) rather than generally inhibiting all sensory transmission.

Experiments utilizing ligands with specificity for opiate receptor subtypes also examined inhibition of the spinal neurons. (For review, see Duggan and Fleetwood-Walker, 1993.) For instance, Fleetwood-Walker and co-workers (1988) found that the iontophoretically applied μ-agonist DAGO produced a strong selective, naloxone-reversible inhibition of neurons in the substantia gelati-

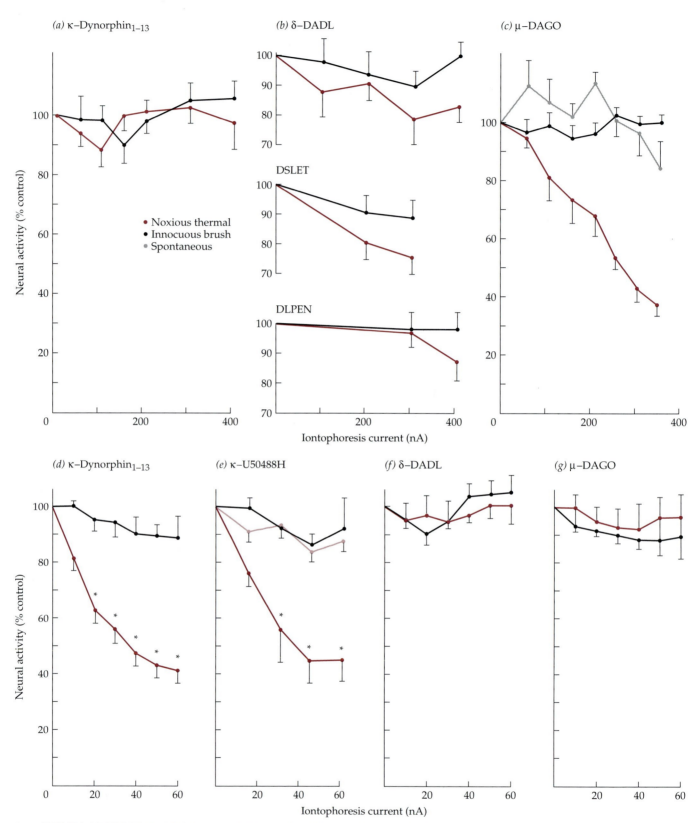

(a) κ–Dynorphin₁₋₁₃

(b) δ–DADL

(c) μ–DAGO

DSLET

DLPEN

Neural activity (% control)

● Noxious thermal
● Innocuous brush
● Spontaneous

Iontophoresis current (nA)

(d) κ–Dynorphin₁₋₁₃

(e) κ–U50488H

(f) δ–DADL

(g) μ–DAGO

Neural activity (% control)

Iontophoresis current (nA)

12.7 EFFECTS OF SELECTIVE OPIOID AGONISTS ON CELL FIRING AFTER EXCITATION BY NOXIOUS OR NON-NOXIOUS STIMULI. The agonists were applied to the receptive field of the neuron by iontophoresis. A dose–response is achieved by increasing the iontophoretic-ejecting current (abscissa) and evaluating the changes in firing rate over background as a percentage of control response (ordinate). (After Duggan and Fleetwood-Walker, 1993; Fleetwood-Walker et al., 1988.)

nosa (Figure 12.7). The μ-agonist inhibited firing following noxious thermal stimulation without changing the cell's spontaneous firing or the response to nonnoxious stimuli. Under the same conditions, the κ-agonist dynorphin (1–13) and the δ-agonists DADL, DSLET, and DLPEN had no effect. In contrast, when the opioids were iontophoresed close to the cell body (laminae IV and V), the κ-preferring agonists were effective in selectively inhibiting the response to noxious stimulation, while the μ- and δ-agonists were not.

These iontophoretic studies show that the receptors are functionally discrete and localized in restricted areas of the spinal cord. These experiments also show how vital it is to evaluate functional results in terms of the location of the relevant receptors: on dendrites, on cell bodies, or on cells innervating the neuron. Opioid modulation of sensory information may take place at the terminals of the primary afferent neurons, at the intrinsic neurons ultimately sending signals to the spinothalamic or spinoreticular cells, or on the terminals of cells originating above the level of the spinal cord.

One example of opioid effects on supraspinal neurons involves the rostroventral region of the medulla (RVM). Its significance to pain modulation is demonstrated by the fact that intact RVM projections to the spinal cord are necessary for systemic opioid analgesia (Azami, Llewelyn, and Roberts, 1982). Single unit recordings of cells within the RVM identify two distinct cell classes: on-cells, which increase firing when peripheral noxious stimuli are applied, and off-cells, which slow their firing under the same conditions. Apparently, on-cell firing in response to noxious stimuli subsequently reduces the inhibitory control normally exerted by the spontaneously active off-cell on spinal cord dorsal horn cells. Systemic opioids reduce the firing of on-cells and increase the firing of off-cells (Fields et al., 1991). On-cell inhibition is due to hyperpolarization following the opening of K^+ channels or reduction of Ca^{2+}-induced release of neurotransmitter.

Pharmacological evidence (Fields, 1993) suggested the model in Figure 12.8, which shows activation of off-cells by opioid-induced inhibition of an inhibitory on-cell. Since the inhibitory on-cell is GABAergic, the off-cell is inhibited by iontophoretic GABA, an effect reversed by $GABA_A$ receptor blockers. Further, microinjection of $GABA_A$ receptor antagonists into the RVM also produces analgesia. Opiate inhibition of GABA cell firing therefore would effectively increase firing of the RVM off-cell, which in turn would increase inhibitory action in the dorsal horn of the spinal cord, producing analgesia. While these and other studies have made great progress in identifying the physiological importance of specific receptor subtypes using selective agonists, the relevance of the endogenous opioids in each of these systems remains to be clarified.

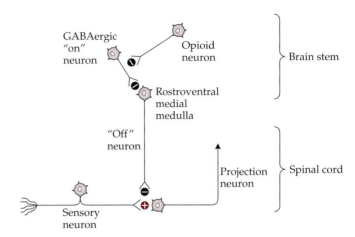

12.8 MODEL OF OPIOID DISINHIBITION OF BRAIN STEM (RVM) NEURONS. Under conditions of noxious stimulation, the GABA-containing "on" cell increases firing and inhibits the spontaneously active "off" cell, thus reducing the inhibitory modulation of pain conduction at the spinal cord. Treatment with opioids inhibits the "on" cell, producing an increase in "off" cell firing and a subsequent inhibition of nociceptive transmission in the spinal cord. (After Fields, 1993).

Effects on neurotransmitter release. Many of the actions of opioids reflect their ability to modulate the processes of neurotransmission by altering the release of other neurotransmitters, especially NE, ACh, DA, and 5-HT. Typical methods involve administering the opioids (systemically, intracerebrally, or locally) and measuring changes in regional brain neurotransmitter steady state levels and turnover. Alternatively, in vivo studies directly measure release of neurotransmitter after opioid administration using push–pull cannulas or microdialysis. In vitro methods using cells in culture, synaptosomes, or brain slices evaluate neurotransmitter release in a simplified system by radioactively labeling neurotransmitter stores and measuring depolarization-induced efflux into the bathing medium. Results from many of these studies indicate a presynaptic inhibition of neurotransmitter release by opiates and opioid peptides.

Opioid effects on release of NE. Opioid effects on NE release have been studied extensively. The results of early studies summarized by Illes (1989) demonstrated the naloxone-reversible inhibition of [³H]NE release from cortical slices by morphine, enkephalin, and β-endorphin. More recent studies using selective receptor subtype ligands show that μ-receptor agonists, but not δ- or κ-agonists, inhibited [³H]NE release from rat cerebral cortex preparations (see Mulder and Schoffelmeer, 1993). β-endorphin was surprisingly selective in its effect on μ-receptors, and an important role for that peptide as an endogenous agonist for presynaptic μ-receptors has been proposed.

The μ-receptor modulation of NE release has been found in many brain areas, including hippocampus, amygdala, periaqueductal gray, cerebellum, and other areas that receive projections from cells within the locus coeruleus. NE cells projecting from regions other than the locus coeruleus tend not to be inhibited by μ- agonists at their terminals. For example, the electrically evoked release of [^{3}H]NE from slices of mediobasal hypothalamus was not inhibited by μ- or κ-agonists (Heijna et al., 1991).

Although the cellular mechanisms responsible for the presynaptic inhibition of NE neurons are not entirely clear, Mulder and Schoffelmeer (1993) have shown that presynaptic opioid effects are distinct from presynaptic α$_2$-adrenergic receptor effects, despite the similarities in their ultimate actions. At the presynaptic terminals of NE neurons, μ-receptor activation results in inhibition of voltage-sensitive Ca^{2+} channels, subsequently reducing the amount of NE released by action potentials. In contrast, at the cell body in the locus coeruleus, μ- and δ-receptors are coupled to K$^+$ channels.

Opioid modulation of DA release.

Opiate receptors can modulate mesolimbic DA release either by altering dopaminergic cell firing or by acting locally within terminal areas. With respect to the first mechanism, infusion of either a selective μ-receptor agonist (DAMGO) or a δ-receptor agonist (DPDPE) into the ventral tegmental area led to a stimulation of DA overflow in the nucleus accumbens, whereas similar infusions of the κ-receptor agonists U-50488H or U-69593 had no effect on accumbens extracellular DA levels (Devine et al., 1993; Spanagel, Herz, and Shippenberg, 1992). The second type of regulatory mechanism can be seen when opioid agonists are administered directly into the nucleus accumbens. In this case, μ-agonists had no effect, whereas DA overflow was stimulated by the δ-agonist (D-Ala2)deltorphin and inhibited by U-69593 (Longoni et al., 1991; Spanagel, Herz, and Shippenberg, 1992). A model emphasizing the role of μ- and κ-receptors in controlling the mesolimbic DA system is presented below in Figure 12.16.

Opioid modification of other transmitters.

In spinal cord preparations, substance P is likely to be a significant neuropeptide transmitter in the unmyelinated primary afferents ending in the substantia gelatinosa. Immunohistochemical localization of opiate receptors on substance P–containing nerve terminals in this area of the spinal cord is one indicator of a presynaptic inhibitory role for opioids (Hökfelt et al., 1977). Stimulation-evoked substance P release from cultured dorsal root ganglia preparations is reduced by μ- and δ-opioids in a dose-dependent fashion. This inhibition is antagonized by naloxone (Chang et al., 1989). Similar results occur using dorsal horn slices stimulated by capsaicin. Substance P release is inhibited by μ- (morphine) and δ- (DPDPE) receptor occupation, but not by κ-agonists (U 50488H or dynorphin) (Aimone and Yaksh, 1989). This same pattern of receptor activity was measured in the in vivo release of substance P from C fibers, which carry nociceptive information, but not from A fibers.

The results in brain stem parallel those found in spinal cord. Hökfelt and colleagues (1977) described a striking immunohistochemical overlap in distribution of Met-enkephalin and substance P cell bodies and nerve terminals in the periaqueductal gray, nucleus raphe magnus, and the caudal trigeminal nucleus. A stable Met-enkephalin analog suppressed the K$^+$-evoked release of substance P from slices of trigeminal nucleus in a naloxone-reversible manner (Jessell and Iversen, 1977). Since enkephalin had no effect on resting efflux, the opioid must be acting at the level of stimulus–secretion coupling.

Evidence for opioid modulation of release of ACh, 5-HT, histamine, GABA, and neuropeptides is accumulating. However, the results are less clear-cut than for the catecholamines, and large regional variations exist. ACh release is inhibited by δ-agonists in striatum, by δ- and μ-agonists in nucleus accumbens and olfactory tubercle, and only by μ-agonists in the hippocampus and amygdala. A more complete discussion of opioid modulation of neurotransmitter release is provided by Mulder and Schoffelmeer (1993).

Analgesia

Of the many pharmacological properties of the opiates, their analgesic effects have received the most attention. However, despite great efforts, the mechanism by which morphine produces analgesia is just beginning to be understood. One key to this problem is the difficulty in identifying and measuring pain.

Pain is considered to be a sensation resulting from any tissue-damaging stimulus and is essential for survival. Pain receptors, unlike the more specialized receptors of the other senses, can be activated by a variety of stimuli, including heat, cold, electrical impulses, pressure or stretching, cuts or tears, and chemical irritants. The quality of pain also varies and may be described as "pricking," "stabbing," "burning," "throbbing," "aching," and so on. Cutaneous or somatic pain comes from the skin or close to the surface of the body and may be intense, but usually involves little emotional reaction. On the other hand, pain that is deeper (visceral) is poorly localized and is accompanied by autonomic responses, such as sweating, fall in blood pressure, or nausea, and has a strong emotional component. This emotional response to pain is one that is not usually found in conjunction with other sensory systems such as audition or taste. The separation of the two components is particularly clear in the patient who, after receiving morphine for protracted pain, maintains that the pain is present and as intense as ever but is no longer aversive. The ability of morphine to modify the emotional component of pain may explain why it is more effective in alleviating chronic or pathological pain than acute pain. Presumably the sensory component of pain is the same for all persons given an identical stimulus, but the reaction process to the initial sensation varies between subjects.

In a classic review of the subject, Beecher (1957) suggested that the reaction process is influenced by the patient's concept of the sensation, by its significance based on past experience, and by its degree of seriousness. A strong emotional reaction may be generated in the patient with a characteristic ache beneath the sternum suggesting heart failure, whereas a pain of the same intensity and duration in the arm is considered trivial and is disregarded. Further evidence of the influence of emotion on pain is the often cited example of the soldier who, during the heat of the battle, is unaware of his mortal wounds. Furthermore, hypnosis, which under some conditions can effectively block the response to pain, reduces the reaction component rather than the sensory component of pain. The effectiveness of analgesics may then be due to (1) reduced sensation, (2) reduced process of recognition, or (3) altered processes of discrimination, memory, or judgment that follow recognition. A summary of the factors that contribute to pain and determine the effectiveness of opioid treatment is discussed in detail by Foley (1993).

Quantification of pain. Although we can get subjective verbal reports of the sensation of pain, quantification is difficult, particularly in the clinical setting. There are a number of factors that may bias a patient's emotional response to pain. For instance, anxiety may result from the anticipation of more pain or the lack of knowledge of the cause of pain, and may affect how a patient responds to drug treatment. This fact is emphasized by the finding that opiates, under certain experimental test situations (such as responding to heat stimuli), do not reliably raise pain thresholds in humans, although they are very effective in the treatment of pathological pain. Tests of analgesia using animal models compare more closely with the tests of human pathological pain than with tests of human experimental pain. This may be due to the fact that the human subject in the experimental setting realizes that the pain stimulus poses no real threat, whereas for the animal subject, all pain is serious and potentially represents a life-threatening situation.

Despite the importance of the emotional response to pain, we must keep in mind that drugs that reduce anxiety (e.g., chlordiazepoxide) do not have significant analgesic properties.

Experimental procedures. In the laboratory the methods used to induce pain at threshold, such as the application of sudden pressure, pinpricks, or stabs, show ineffective or inconsistent analgesic effects in response to opiates, probably because of the low emotional component in that type of pain. More consistent results are obtained with the analgesics when techniques are used that produce slowly developing or sustained pain.

One such technique is the occlusion of blood flow with a tourniquet on an exercising muscle. Using this method, the pain is slow in onset and is directly related to the amount of exercise. Furthermore, cutaneous pain in humans can be produced by the intradermal injection of various chemicals. A reliable method to test this kind of pain uses cantharidin to induce a blister, from which the outer layer of epidermis is removed to expose the blister base, on which small quantities of various agents can be applied for testing. Bathing the area with isotonic solutions enables repeated testing within 10–15 minutes without changing the sensitivity of the nerve endings. Techniques that have been designed to produce more intense or more persistent pain are infrequently used because finding subjects willing to participate in such experiments is more difficult. An alternative and common method to measure analgesic properties uses animal models (see Chapter 2).

Pain Pathways

Spinal cord. The dual nature of the phenomenon we call pain, that is, its sensory and emotional components, is reflected in the anatomy and physiology of pain pathways. At the spinal cord level, pain in humans is carried by several types of sensory neurons. The Aδ fibers are small in diameter and are thinly myelinated. They mediate sharp, pricking types of pain. In contrast, the C fibers are small and unmyelinated and are activated by intense mechanical, chemical, or temperature stimulation. Both types of neurons end on cells in the superficial dorsal horn (lamina I, the marginal zone, and lamina II, substantia gelatinosa). Both types of neurons release an excitatory neurotransmitter that is likely to be glutamate. In addition, C fibers and perhaps Aδ neurons also release excitatory neuropeptide transmitters, including substance P (see Chapter 11). Substance P produces slow excitatory postsynaptic potentials when applied to dorsal horn neurons (see Jessell and Kelly, 1991).

The primary sensory afferents end on three types of cells in the dorsal horn: directly on projection neurons that transmit pain signals to higher brain centers, on small excitatory interneurons, or on inhibitory interneurons that subsequently synapse on the projection neurons. In this way the primary afferents have both direct and indirect influences on the projection neurons (Jessell and Kelly, 1991). It is this multisynaptic pathway for nociception that provides the basis for the theory of spinal opioid analgesia. Not only does the multisynaptic pain pathway provide multiple sites for modulation, but the opioids also are capable of modifying pain transmission via several cellular mechanisms.

Kosterlitz and Hughes (1975) proposed that the opioid peptides could have inhibitory effects on pain pathways in three possible ways, as shown in Figure 12.9. Postsynaptic inhibition occurs by opioid peptides acting directly as inhibitory neurotransmitters by increasing K^+ conductance (Figure 12.9a). The neuron in Figure 12.9b shows opioid-induced presynaptic inhibition that reduces the release of an excitatory neurotransmitter per-

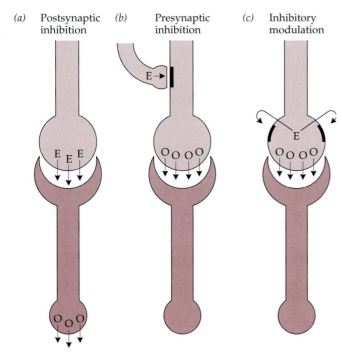

(a) Postsynaptic inhibition *(b)* Presynaptic inhibition *(c)* Inhibitory modulation

12.9 INHIBITORY ACTION OF ENKEPHALIN. Enkephalin (E) may inhibit nerve activity either by postsynaptic inhibition, presynaptic inhibition, or via inhibitory modulation. (0 represents excitatory transmitter.) (After Kosterlitz and Hughes, 1975.)

haps by decreasing Ca²⁺ influx. Finally, inhibitory modulation occurs via opioid autoreceptor activation which inhibits the release of a colocalized neurotransmitter (Figure 12.9c). Evidence exists to support each one of these three models in brain and/or in spinal cord.

The high levels of opiate receptors in spinal cord show localization based on subtype. In general, μ- and κ-receptors are more abundant than δ-receptors and the distribution of the three types shows striking similarity across species. μ-receptor binding is most concentrated in the substantia gelatinosa and in laminae II, V, VI, and VIII. Binding to κ–receptors is highest in the substantia gelatinosa, while δ-receptors are concentrated in lamina I. Experiments of several types have demonstrated that a significant amount of opioid receptor binding occurs on the nerve terminals of afferent nociceptive neurons. This location is consistent with presynaptic inhibitory function, the mechanisms for which are described above. Note that intracellular recordings show a direct postsynaptic action as well (Yoshimura and North, 1983) and opioids may reduce the excitatory effects of glutamate on dorsal horn neurons postsynaptically.

Descending modulatory pathways.   Neurons projecting from supraspinal nuclei also modulate the nociceptive information carried by spinal cord neurons. Many of the supraspinal centers interconnect, forming complex circuits, portions of which have descending modulatory

control over spinal nociceptive pathways. However, it is important to realize that other supraspinal neurons directly inhibit nociceptive transmission at higher centers. Mapping of these antinociceptive pathways is accomplished by focal electrical stimulation or by microinjection of opioids. Figure 12.10 is a flow chart of the relationship of several of the brain stem centers important to antinociception that are discussed in the following section. Fields (1993) and Jessell and Kelly (1991) provide excellent discussions of spinal and supraspinal mechanisms of pain modulation.

Among the descending pain modulating systems, the most extensively investigated is the gray matter adjacent to the third ventricle in the diencephalon (periventricular gray) extending into the midbrain periaqueductal gray (PAG). A second area is the rostroventral region of the medulla (RVM), which includes the serotonergic nuclei of the raphe and the nucleus reticularis paragigantocellularis. Microinjection of opioids into either area produces significant analgesia.

The PAG and RVM have extensive reciprocal connections and provide descending projections to the dorsal horn of the spinal cord. The serotonergic neurons originating in the raphe descend into the spinal cord and synapse on cells in laminae I, II, and V of the dorsal horn. Stimulation of these neurons produces inhibition of cells in the dorsal horn, including spinothalamic tract cells. Lesioning of the fibers connecting the RVM and spinal cord or local microinjection of opioid antagonists prevents systemic opiate-induced analgesia (Azami, Llewelyn, and Roberts, 1982). Thus, opioid analgesia depends on an intact RVM descending projection. The opiates' ability to increase the inhibitory influence on spinal pain pathways is likely due to opiate-induced inhibition

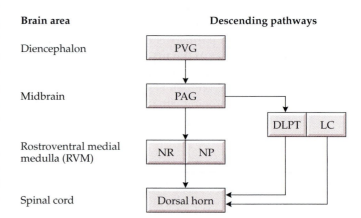

Brain area	Descending pathways
Diencephalon	PVG
Midbrain	PAG
	DLPT | LC
Rostroventral medial medulla (RVM)	NR | NP
Spinal cord	Dorsal horn

12.10 DESCENDING SUPRASPINAL PATHWAYS THAT MODULATE NOCICEPTIVE TRANSMISSION IN THE SPINAL CORD. Neither reciprocal connections between brain structures nor ascending pathways are shown. PVG = periventricular gray; PAG = periaqueductal gray; NR = raphe nuclei; NP = nucleus paragigantocellularis; DLPT = dorsolateral pontomesencephalic tegmentum; LC = locus coeruleus.

of an inhibitory GABAergic input to the 5-HT cells in RVM (see Figure 12.8).

Many of the descending neurons of the RVM have cell bodies in the nucleus of the raphe that utilize 5-HT as their neurotransmitter. Evidence for the serotonergic nature of the RVM descending fibers comes from experiments showing analgesic effects of direct application of 5-HT to spinal cord cells, which in turn may induce release by spinal opioid-containing cells. Also, the effects of opioid microinjection into the PAG or RVM is blocked by applying 5-HT antagonists to spinal cord neurons (Jensen and Yaksh, 1986).

Although the primary projection of the PAG is to the RVM as described above, it also sends input to the dorsolateral pontomesencephalic tegmentum (DLPT), periventricular hypothalamus, and to medial thalamic regions that also receive input from spinothalamic tract neurons carrying nociceptive information from the dorsal horn. Connections to the DLPT are particularly significant, since those cells likely represent the origin of a second major descending pain modulatory system. Its intimate relationship to norepinephrine cell bodies in the locus coeruleus may explain the nociceptive effect of NE agonists applied to the spinal cord (Proudfit, 1988). The importance of locus coeruleus neurons is suggested by the high concentration of endogenous opioids in that area and by the fact that neurotoxic lesions of the descending NE and 5-HT cells prevent systemic morphine-induced analgesia. Further, the excitation of locus coeruleus neurons by noxious stimuli and the opioid-induced hyperpolarization of the cells mediated by μ-opiate receptors is well documented (Aghajanian and Wang, 1987).

The importance of these descending pathways in modulating nociception is well established. However, the inhibition of nociceptive projection neurons in the spinal cord by descending fibers is direct in some cases, while at other times inhibition occurs by acting on intrinsic interneurons. Figure 12.11 summarizes several possible interactions between descending neurons and sensory neurons in the dorsal horn (Fields, 1993). RVM stimulation results in direct inhibition of spinothalamic tract neurons or inhibition of excitatory interneurons in lamina II that synapse on nociceptive projection neurons in lamina I (Figure 12.11a and b, respectively). Finally, evidence for supraspinal excitation of spinal cord inhibitory interneurons containing GABA or enkephalin has also surfaced (Figure 12.11c). Both 5-HT and NE have been shown to excite inhibitory interneurons when applied iontophoretically to the spinal cord.

Ascending pain pathways. The principal ascending projection fiber bundle mediating pain and temperature is the spinothalamic tract. The spinothalamic tract projects from laminae I and V–VII in the dorsal horn neurons contralaterally to several areas in the thalamus, particu-

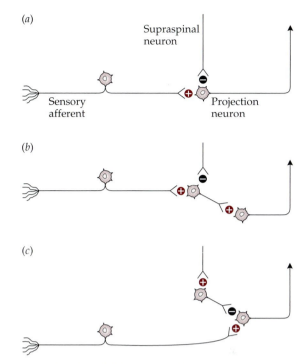

12.11 THE POSSIBLE EFFECTS OF SUPRASPINAL DESCENDING NEURONS ON NOCICEPTIVE TRANSMISSION IN THE SPINAL CORD. (a) Direct inhibition of spinothalamic projection neurons by cells from RVM. (b) RVM cells inhibit excitatory interneurons ending on projection neurons. (c) Supraspinal excitation of spinal cord inhibitory neurons that inhibit the projection neuron.

larly the medial and lateral nuclear groups. In addition, a great many of the spinothalamic fibers synapse at brain stem levels below the thalamus, such as in the tegmental reticular formation (which may have an alerting function). Furthermore, a number of fibers synapse in the central gray of the midbrain, from which neurons project to the hypothalamus and subsequently to limbic structures that may be responsible for the emotional component of pain. Apparently large numbers of nociceptive neurons in the spinal cord project directly to the hypothalamus and telencephalon (Giesler, Katter, and Dado, 1994) and may carry information about noxious stimuli to brain areas that are responsible for affective, autonomic, and neuroendocrine responses to pain.

Opiates may act by blocking signals from the nociceptive pathway to higher sensory areas as well as to limbic structures. The mapping of opiate receptors (Mansour et al., 1995) and the localization of endogenous opioid peptides (Khachaturian, Schaefer, and Lewis, 1993) suggests that significant opioid modulation of pain occurs at the spinal cord level, in limbic structures, as well as in the hypothalamus and medial thalamus which also receive nociceptive input.

In addition, several other tracts relay pain information to the cortex as well as projecting to the reticular formation, thalamus, PAG, and limbic structures. The redundancy and diffuse nature of pain-related pathways probably reflects the evolutionary significance of pain perception (Jessell and Kelly, 1991). Certainly, the anatomical and neurochemical complexity of pain neurotransmission provides ample opportunity for modulatory action by endogenous peptides and explains why a simple relationship between the opioids and analgesia is not forthcoming.

Analgesic Effects of Opioids

Electrically induced analgesia.   The neuroanatomy of pain modulation has been further examined with functional electrophysiological studies. Midbrain areas, most notably the PAG, have been found not only to bind opiates readily but also to produce analgesia when stimulated electrically. In fact, both focal electrical stimulation-induced analgesia and analgesia produced by microinjection of opiates appear to exert maximum effects at sites surrounding the third ventricle, the cerebral aqueduct, and rostral portions of the fourth ventricle (Mayer and Liebeskind, 1974). Clinically, some success has been achieved in treating patients with intractable chronic pain with focal brain stimulation (see Fields, 1987; Young, 1989). Although the subjects do not lose their sense of temperature, touch, or pressure, they do experience less pain. Unfortunately, relief is not always consistent.

Evidence supporting opioid mediation includes the development of cross-tolerance between the analgesic effects of electrical stimulation in the mesencephalic PAG and subcutaneous administration of morphine (Mayer and Hayes, 1975). Akil, Mayer, and Liebeskind (1976) also have shown that naloxone could partially antagonize the analgesia produced by focal electrical stimulation of the PAG in rats without altering responsiveness to other stimuli, and suggested that electrical stimulation might release a morphine-like substance onto naloxone-sensitive postsynaptic receptor sites. However, even large doses of naloxone were no more than 38% effective in blocking the analgesia. Thus, stimulation of the periaqueductal gray almost certainly also activates nonopioid pain mechanisms (Watkins and Mayer, 1982). As discussed above, several nonopioid descending pain-related pathways may be involved.

Acupuncture and endogenous opioids.   The discovery of the endogenous opioids led to a dramatic increase in research into the mechanisms of the ancient Chinese method for pain relief, acupuncture. Acupuncture involves inserting a metallic needle into the skin to reach deep structures, such as muscles and tendons. Rhythmic movement of the needle or application of mild electrical current reduces pain perception.

Mayer, Price, and Rafi (1975) were among the first to demonstrate naloxone antagonism of acupuncture-in-duced analgesia in human dentally evoked pain. Naloxone reversal, however, was not a general phenomenon in this type of analgesia. The ability of naloxone to attenuate acupuncture analgesia is evidently dependent on characteristics of the acupuncture treatment (see Han, 1993). For example, the frequency of the electroacupuncture, the intensity of the stimulation, and the timing of naloxone administration relative to the acupuncture determine whether naloxone is effective as an antagonist. More recent evidence shows that such modifications of the acupuncture technique may be mediated by different opioid peptides. As reviewed by Han (1993), the δ-antagonist ICI 174864 reduced 2-Hz electroacupuncture-in-duced analgesia, but not that induced by 100 Hz. Conversely, the κ-antagonist (MR 2266) blocked the 100-Hz analgesia but not the 2-Hz. In the same study, the authors found that 2-Hz electroacupuncture showed cross-tolerance to morphine, but not to 100-Hz acupuncture. Further investigation showed that 2-Hz acupuncture developes cross-tolerance with δ- but not κ- agonists, while 100-Hz electroacupuncture showed cross-tolerance to the κ-agonist dynorphin, but not the δ-agonist DPDPE.

Several groups have evaluated the levels of opioid peptides in spinal CSF after electroacupuncture (Sjolund, Terenius, and Eriksson, 1977; Han et al., 1991). In studies using both rats and humans, 2-Hz electroacupuncture produced significant elevations in the proenkephalin peptide Met-enkephalin–Arg–Phe, with no change in the prodynorphin peptide dynorphin A. In comparison, 100-Hz acupuncture produced elevated CSF levels of dynorphin A with no change in Met-enkephalin–Arg–Phe levels. Clearly the art of acupuncture has moved into the realm of science and deserves careful evaluation to establish whether or not it has a presence in the field of modern medical science.

Stress-induced analgesia.   Given the intimate relationship between the synthesis and localization of opioids and stress hormones, it is not surprising to find a voluminous literature dealing with the parameters of stress-induced analgesia (SIA). Biologically the phenomenon is adaptive in that suppressing the normal response to pain allows the animal to engage in productive behaviors to cope with potentially life-threatening danger.

A wide variety of stressors induce analgesia, including inescapable electric foot shock, restraint, forced swimming, food deprivation, social isolation, and learned helplessness. Although analgesia produced by some stressors, such as electric shock, is attenuated by naloxone, antagonism is not complete, implying that both opioid and nonopioid mechanisms may contribute to the effect (see Akil et al., 1984). Mediation of SIA by opioids varies depending on the type and parameters of stress involved (see Olson, Olson, and Kastin, 1989), and levels of endogenous opioids in brain and CSF are also paradigm-dependent (see Przewlocki, 1993).

Psychosocial factors. In humans, pain is not only an intense sensory stimulus but is influenced by psychosocial factors such as attention, arousal, anticipation of more pain, coping strategies, and cognitive appraisal of the situation. Evidence shows that CSF levels of opioid peptides are significantly lower in patients experiencing chronic organic pain than in control subjects. In contrast, those suffering from chronic idiopathic (i.e., spontaneous and without organic basis) pain have significantly higher CSF opioid levels than controls (Almay et al., 1985; Simmonet et al., 1986; Terenius, 1982). Pain relief following electrical stimulation of periventricular brain sites and treatment with acupuncture in patients suffering from intractable pain is accompanied by an increase in CSF opioids (Akil et al., 1978; Amano et al., 1982). Almay and coworkers (1985) showed that electrical nerve stimulation that relieved organic pain also increased endorphin in the CSF to normal levels. For those patients with idiopathic pain receiving similar stimulation, no change in CSF opioids was detected.

Cognitive factors also have a role in attenuating pain. Perceived self-efficacy, that is, the individual's confidence in his or her capability to exercise control over events, and placebo medication both have demonstrable analgesic effects. These effects may have opioid components since naloxone reduced subjects' ability to cognitively manage pain (Bandura et al., 1987), suggesting the possibility that placebo medication and coping strategies release pain-attenuating opioids.

Localization of Opioid Analgesia

Spinal cord. Intrathecal administration (within the meninges of the spinal cord) of opiates attenuates the escape response from a wide variety of stimuli including heat, pressure, electric shock, chemical stimulation, and neurogenic stimuli (i.e., chronic nerve compression). Evaluation of intrathecal administration of a large number of opioid agonists (Table 12.5) in several analgesia paradigms clearly shows significant μ- and δ-agonist ac-

Table 12.5 Effects of Intrathecal Opioids on the Response to Noxious Stimuli Using Several Experimental Paradigms[a]

Ligand	Rat			Shock titration (primate)
	Tail flick	Hot plate	Writhing	
μ-Receptor selective				
Morphine	1.0	1.0	1.0	1.0
Dermorphin	2600	4428	1384	—
Lofentanil	99	118.2	—	2100.0
Sufentanil	15	27.7	—	63
DAG	11	15	—	16
Levorphanol	8	10.2	7.8	—
Fentanyl	2	1.7	—	—
Alfentanil	0.9	0.76	—	—
D/L-Methadone	0.1	0.6	—	1.0
Meperidine	0.07	0.05	—	0.2
Codeine	<0.01	<0.01	—	—
δ-Receptor selective				
DADL	1.5	1.0	<0.1	—
DPE	1.3	1.0	<0.06	—
DPLPE	0.7	0.5	<0.1	0.3
Met-enkephalin	0.03	0.02	<0.01	—
Leu-enkephalin	<0.01	<0.01	<0.01	—
DSTLE	—	—	<0.1	—
κ-Receptor selective				
U50488H	<0.01	<0.01	0.03	—
Spiradoline	<0.01	<0.01	0.5	—
Bremazocine	<0.01	0.05	0.09	—
EKG	<0.01	0.03	0.18	—
Dynorphin	<0.1	<0.1	1.1	—

[a]The table provides results accumulated from 16 published studies. The data have been normalized so the figures represent analgesic activity relative to morphine.

Source: After Yaksh, 1993.

tivity, while κ-agonists are minimally effective in these tests. Further, the analgesic effects of δ-agonists are reduced by δ-receptor blockers (e.g., ICI154129) which do not antagonize μ agonist action; while μ-receptor antagonists block μ-induced, but not δ-induced, analgesia (Pasternak, 1993).

Characteristics of the noxious stimuli seem to play a part in determining which receptor agonists mediate analgesia. For instance, μ- and κ-agonists suppress the writhing response to intraperitoneal acetic acid injection, but δ-agonists do not (Schmauss, Doherty, and Yaksh, 1983). The κ-agonists weakly inhibit the writhing response, but have no effect on the tail-flick or hot plate responses. Dirksen (1990) suggests that analgesia for cutaneous thermal stimuli may be modulated by μ- and δ-receptors, whereas modulation of visceral chemical stimuli may depend more on μ- and κ-receptor activation. More detailed discussion of the spinal actions of opiates is provided in several reviews (Dirksen, 1990; Pasternak, 1993; Yaksh, 1993).

Supraspinal effects of opioids.   The modulatory role of supraspinal areas in pain conduction is shown by the loss of analgesia following spinal transection or neurotoxic lesions of the descending pathways (5-HT and NE) described above. Furthermore, μ_1-receptor antagonists, such as naloxonazine, also reduce the antinociceptive effects of intracerebral or systemic morphine without changing spinal cord function (see Pasternak, 1993). A genetic strain of mouse (CXBK) having relatively few μ_1-receptors compared with μ_2-receptors provides a useful tool for determining the relative importance of μ-receptor subtypes (Vaught, Mathiasen, and Raffa, 1988). These animals maintain a normal sensitivity to morphine in the spinal cord but show minimal sensitivity to morphine administered systemically. On the basis of selective antagonism and the high density of μ_1 sites in areas normally associated with processing nociceptive stimuli (Moskowitz and Goodman, 1985), it is suggested that virtually all supraspinal analgesia is mediated via μ_1-receptors (see Porreca and Burks, 1993). This μ_1/μ_2 distinction is expected to have significant clinical impact with the increased use of intrathecal pain management techniques.

κ-receptor subtypes also seem to differentially mediate analgesia at spinal and supraspinal levels. Whereas κ_1-receptors modulate antinociception in spinal neurons, κ_3-receptors mediate supraspinal analgesia, which cannot be blocked by μ-, δ-, or κ_1-receptor antagonists. Moreover, no cross-tolerance develops to the analgesic effects of κ_1- and κ_3-agonists, nor between κ_3-agonists and morphine (Pasternak, 1993). This lack of cross-tolerance further demonstrates unique mechanisms mediated by opioid receptor subtypes.

As is true for κ-receptors, δ-receptor mediation of analgesia is less well established than that for μ-recep-

tors, though they also show subtype distinctions. Selective δ_1-receptor agonists (DPDPE) are relatively specific for modulating spinal analgesia, while δ_2-receptor agonists (deltorphin II) mediate supraspinal analgesia. Detailed discussion of the role of supraspinal receptors in analgesia can be found elsewhere (Pasternak, 1993; Porreca and Burks, 1993).

Opiate Effects on Gastrointestinal Function

An additional clinically useful action of opiates is on the gastrointestinal tract. Therapeutically, the opiates are known for their ability to reduce pain and to stop diarrhea, and in this latter function they are unsurpassed as lifesaving drugs, particularly in developing countries. Details of the gastrointestinal actions of opiates are provided in a review by Kromer (1993).

Opiates delay gastric emptying and inhibit gastric contractions in several species, including humans. The effects on stomach acid secretion are dose dependent, with low doses of morphine enhancing histamine- or feeding-induced acid secretion and higher doses inhibiting it. Opioid action on gastric secretion may be mediated by somatostatin, which inhibits stomach acid secretion, since the same doses of opioids decrease and increase somatostatin. Although this action is antagonized by naloxone, the specific receptor subtype and cellular mechanism is unknown. Significantly, gastric acid secretion is controlled both in the gut and in the CNS. Therefore, the ultimate action of opiates may depend upon the impact of the CNS on the stomach as well as local gastric effects.

The action of opiates on intestinal peristalsis (i.e., the cycle of migrating ring contractions that propels the intestinal contents along its length) is more complex, with opiates showing both excitatory and inhibitory actions. The opiates alter the intestinal motility pattern and cause constipation. Although the circular smooth muscle layer involved has both μ- and κ-opioid receptors, evidence suggests that dynorphin is the endogenous ligand regulating the muscle contraction by acting on κ-receptors. However, species differences exist, and μ-receptors predominate in the rat while μ- and κ-receptors are both involved in other species (see Krevsky et al., 1991). Activation of μ-receptors, which are probably located on neuronal processes that innervate the muscle, reduces excitability by increasing K^+ conductance and shortening action potential duration, thus reducing muscle contraction. κ-receptors, however, reduce the amount of neurotransmitter released at the muscle in response to depolarization by directly inhibiting voltage-dependent Ca^{2+} influx. In that way, both μ- and κ-receptors can work cooperatively to alter intestinal motility.

Opioids alter other autonomic functions, such as respiration, vomiting, temperature, cardiovascular function, as well as endocrine responses. Several reviews are available to those interested in opioid effects on cardiovascular regulation (Faden, 1993), respiration and vomiting (Florez and Hurle, 1993), temperature regulation and neuroendocrine function (Almeida, 1993; Cella, Locatelli, and Muller, 1993).

Opiates and Development

In rats, all three families of opioid peptides appear during embryonic development and generally increase in concentration postnatally (Loughlin et al., 1985). Distinct patterns of development exist for each opiate family depending on the brain region. The mapping and description of the developmental sequence is a complex matter for several reasons. First, the pattern of opioid innervation in the developing organism differs from that of the adult. The peptides and precursor hormones are expressed very early in germinal zones unique to the neonate, preceding cell migration and differentiation. For instance, the first fetal cells to express POMC peptides appear in the diencephalon by embryonic day 12, and these diencephalic cells are the progenitors of arcuate neurons in the mature animal.

Secondly, phasic changes in opioids occur both prenatally and postnatally. In situ hybridization reveals proenkephalin mRNA first on embryonic day 16 in the striatum, where it remains constant until birth; at this time it rapidly increases, reaching a peak at postnatal day 2, after which levels gradually fall back to embryonic levels. A second surge begins at day 14 and reaches adult levels by day 28. Unfortunately, the functional significance of such changes is not clear at the time of this writing.

Finally, significant differences in the developmental pattern occur in various brain areas. The developmental appearance of the opiate receptors is in general correlated with the expression and localization of the peptides and displays a caudal–rostral sequence beginning by embryonic day 15 (Coyle and Pert, 1976). During development, opiate binding increases with no changes in affinity for the ligands, suggesting that the receptors are already in their mature form by embryonic day 15. Labeling studies using specific radioligands show that developmental patterns for μ-, δ-, and κ-receptors vary significantly (Spain, Roth, and Coscia, 1985; Kornblum, Hurlbut, and Leslie, 1987). Details of the ontogenetic pattern of opioids and receptors have been provided by several reviews (McDowell and Kitchen, 1987; Pintar and Scott, 1993).

Although it is premature to ascribe specific functions to the developing opioid systems, temporal modifications of opioid concentrations and receptor densities may be reflected in changes in sensitivity to opiates during development. For example, a significant fluctuation in sensitivity to morphine-induced analgesia occurs during the first few weeks after birth (see Kehoe, 1988). In addition, more recent evidence shows distinct mediation of maternal deprivation–induced analgesia and distress vocaliza-

tion by opioid receptor subtypes (Kehoe and Boylan, 1994).

Another suspected role for opioids in development may involve regulating the formation of brain structures and growth-related processes (Hammer and Hauser, 1992; Zagon, Gibo, and McLaughlin, 1992). Opioid (morphine, β-endorphin, or Met-enkephalin) administration to neonatal rats inhibits DNA synthesis, resulting in a reduced number of cells and reduced cell density in those areas of the brain in which postnatal cell division occurs. Furthermore, endogenous opiates retard dendritic growth and dendritic spine formation in young animals. Because glial cell development is also reduced by opioid treatment, the glial guides that direct the pattern of neuron migration are altered too. In contrast, opiate receptor antagonists administered during the first 3 postnatal weeks stimulate cell proliferation and density of neurons in the cerebellum and hippocampus. In other areas, neuronal differentiation and neuropil development are altered, causing cortical thickening with no accompanying increase in cell number (Zagon and McLaughlin, 1986). Postnatal antagonist administration increases dendritic branching and length of dendrites, particularly in the cortex and cerebellum. The endogenous basis for opioid modulation of growth and elaboration of neurons is presently being investigated.

Zagon and McLaughlin (1991) have identified an opioid growth factor (Met^5-enkephalin) in developing rat brain that exerts tonic inhibitory control over cell proliferation, differentiation, and survival. They propose that the growth factor works through a unique opioid receptor (called *zeta*) that is found in human and rat brain only during development and not at adulthood. At the time of weaning in the rat (around day 21), neurogenesis is complete and binding to the *zeta* receptor is negligible.

The normal inhibition of neuronal growth and changes in glial guides by perinatal opiates may be part of a mechanism for promoting controlled growth and neurite targeting (Savio and Schwab, 1989; Zagon, Gibo, and McLaughlin, 1992). The amount of endogenous opiate control may be critical at specific points in the developmental sequence. Loss of *zeta* receptors or insufficient Met^5-enkephalin may be associated with uncontrolled cell proliferation and overdevelopment of brain circuitry, as may occur in forms of neural cancer common in children. On the other hand, excess *zeta* receptor, overabundance of Met^5-enkephalin, or high levels of exogenous opiate may severely impair cell number and synaptic elaboration, resulting in inadequate information processing and retardation.

Learning and Memory

McGaugh, Introini-Collison, and Castellano (1993) review the extensive evidence supporting the hypothesis that learning and memory are regulated by the endogenous opiate peptides. The complexity of the theoretical constructs involved and the paradigms used to evaluate various aspects of learning and memory (e.g., attention and motivation, acquisition, storage, retrieval, and performance variables) preclude an extensive discussion in this chapter.

In general, opioid agonists impair acquisition and retention of new associations while antagonists enhance them. However, results vary significantly depending upon the agonist, the experimental design, the learning task, and the species. Systemically administered opiates at subanalgesic doses impair acquisition of tasks motivated by either appetitive or aversive stimuli in a naloxone-dependent fashion. For example, γ-endorphin may impair acquisition of an active avoidance response while β-endorphin modulates learning in an inhibitory-avoidance paradigm.

Posttraining treatment with morphine or β-endorphin shows effects of opioids on the retention of learning. Opioids apparently impair consolidation of newly acquired memories in a dose- and time-dependent fashion that can be antagonized by naloxone. Once again the effects of individual peptides on retention are task- and species-specific (see Morris and Johnston, 1995). For example, microinjection of dynorphin into the hippocampus impairs working memory in a radial arm maze, but has no effect on a learned inhibitory-avoidance response.

In summary, evidence from a wide variety of sources using many different experimental designs shows significant modulation of learning by opioids. Their influence on memory is likely to be mediated via other neurotransmitter systems, particularly NE, but ACh, 5-HT, and GABA have also been implicated. Furthermore, interactions between stress, hormones, and learning provide an almost certain role for the opioids in memory.

Opioid Effects on Food Consumption

Food consumption and taste preferences are both significantly altered by opiate treatment (see Cooper and Kirkham, 1993). Naloxone significantly reduces food consumption in food-deprived or nondeprived subjects, as well as reducing eating induced by a stressful tail pinch, 2-deoxyglucose treatment, and stimulation of brain sites that elicit feeding. The assumption is that naloxone acts by blocking endogenous opioid activity, suggesting its role in feeding behavior.

Injection of morphine or β-endorphin into the ventromedial nucleus of the hypothalamus or paraventricular nucleus increases eating in satiated rats, while microinjection of naloxone into the same sites reduces food consumption. Also, naloxone reduces food consumption to a greater extent in genetically obese animals than in normal-weight littermates. Animals that have become obese by eating a palatable high-calorie diet also respond to naloxone treatment by eating less.

A major thrust of current research involves investigation into the importance of endogenous opiates to the palatability or pleasure value of consumed food. Using taste preference tests in which rats normally choose a sweet solution over water, naloxone characteristically reduces preference for either sucrose-sweetened or noncalorically sweetened fluids. Naloxone not only eliminates the established taste preference, but also prevents the establishment of the preference. As anticipated, opiate agonists increase the amount of sweetened solutions consumed by water-deprived rats. The μ- and δ-agonists, but not κ-agonists, increase intake of saccharin solutions without affecting water consumption. Parallel studies show that μ- and δ-agonists also increase preference for isotonic salt (0.9% NaCl) solutions without altering water consumption. The κ-agonists have no effect on these preferences.

The palatability of diet is also modified by endogenous opiates. Opiate antagonists reduce consumption of a highly palatable food (such as chocolate cookies) and reinstate consumption of standard rat food pellets, while systemic morphine administration increases chocolate cookie consumption without increasing standard food consumption (Cooper and Kirkham, 1990). Further evidence supports the idea that opioids modify food preference based on palatability rather than nutritional content. Experiments show that morphine increases fat consumption in fat-preferring rats and carbohydrate consumption in carbohydrate-preferring rats (Evans and Vaccarino, 1990; Gosnell, Krahn, and Majchrzak, 1990).

Kirkham and Cooper (1991) have reviewed evidence for endogenous opioid peptide control of eating in humans with particular emphasis on treatment of obesity and bulimia, and the reader is referred to that source for further detail. Despite some contradictory evidence, endogenous opioids in humans, as in other species, seem to modify the preference or liking of some foods over others. For example, naloxone reduces consumption of tasty fat/sugar mixtures while not altering the intake of less palatable foods. Table 12.6 summarizes results compiled by Cooper and Kirkham (1993) from representative studies which show opioid modulation of the pleasure or palatability associated with food-related stimuli.

Although opiates seem to modulate palatability, some evidence suggests that the degree of palatability may depend on the ability of particular foods to enhance endogenous opioid activity. For example, by increasing the sucrose concentration, the inhibitory effect of naloxone on consumption of that solution is reduced, perhaps because the sucrose solution increases endogenous opioids. Also, infusion of sucrose into rat pups produces analgesia and reduced distress vocalization that is mediated by opioids (Blass, Fitzgerald, and Kehoe, 1987). These studies and others indirectly indicate that sucrose and other palatable foods increase endogenous opioids.

A review (Cooper and Kirkham, 1993) of opioid receptor mediation of food consumption concludes that in

Table 12.6 Summary of Evidence Implicating Endogenous Opioids in the Palatability of Food-Related Stimuli in Rats and Humans

Paradigm	Effects of opioid antagonists	Effects of opioid agonists	General conclusions
Sweet taste preference	Naloxone and naltrexone reduce preference	μ- and δ-receptor agonists increase preference	Endogenous opioid peptides mediate sweet taste preference
Salt taste preference	Naloxone reduces preference	μ- and δ-receptor agonists increase preference	Endogenous opioid peptides mediate salt taste preference
Sucrose sham feeding	Naloxone reduces sham feeding	Not evaluated	Sham feeding is opioid-dependent
Electrical stimulation–induced feeding	Naloxone increases the frequency threshold. Norbinaltorphimine (lateral ventricle) raises the threshold, but given caudally (mesopontine aqueduct) lowers the threshold	Not evaluated	Stimulation-induced feeding is opioid-dependent, but forebrain involvement may differ from lower brain stem involvement
Food preference (rats)	Naloxone and naltrexone reduce intake of preferred food	Morphine increases intake of preferred food	Preference for palatable food is opioid-dependent
Food preference (human)	Naltrexone induces negative alliesthesia. Naloxone and nalfemene reduce palatability of preferred foods	Not evaluated	Human food preference is, in part, opioid-mediated

Source: After Cooper and Kirkham, 1993.

order to identify receptor mechanisms, the characteristics of the feeding model must be considered. In general, κ-receptor agonists increase food consumption, while κ-antagonists tend to reduce consumption of palatable, high-fat diets and decrease eating induced by 2-deoxyglucose. μ_2-receptors have also been implicated in the regulation of those particular eating paradigms. In contrast, μ_1-receptor antagonists decrease overall free feeding as well as consumption due to food deprivation or morphine injection. Specific δ-antagonists also reduce food consumption.

In summary, evidence is clear that opioids modify food consumption and in particular alter the intake of preferred food, suggesting an involvement of reward mechanisms. The microinjection of morphine and selected opioid agonists into the nucleus accumbens elicits increased consumption, particularly of palatable foods. Since the dopaminergic mesolimbic neurons terminating in the nucleus accumbens are considered to be involved in a central reward mechanism, a link has been established between opioids, feeding, and reward mechanisms (see below; Evans and Vaccarino, 1990). Whether such a connection is substantiated by further research and whether the results of that research can be used clinically to treat obesity and eating disorders remains to be seen.

Endogenous Opiates in Social Behavior

Several areas of research demonstrate a role for endogenous opiates in social behavior, and the significance of such investigations is not trivial. Social bonding between adults is vital, not only for reproductive purposes and family formation, but for formation of hunting and defense units. Attachment between infant and parent improves survival of the young.

In contrast, breaking of social bonds following separation of mother and infant or breaking of a pair bond by divorce or death frequently elicits strong, chronic behavioral changes. These changes are characterized by social withdrawal, sadness and despair, decreased food intake, and sleep disturbances. Many forms of mental illness involve difficulties in forming social bonds. Therefore, examination of the biological basis for social attachment is of importance to psychopharmacologists who are interested in social behavior and are concerned with pharmacological intervention in mental disorders.

Panksepp and colleagues found that opiates reduce distress vocalizations and motor agitation in newborn animals of several species following a variety of social and thermal treatments (Panksepp, Siviy, and Normansell, 1985). Further, social stress such as maternal deprivation results in increased endogenous opioid activity, demonstrated by prolonged paw-lift latency after noxious stimulation (Kehoe and Blass, 1986). Demonstration of such early opioid mediation of social behaviors suggests a role for endogenous opiates in the development of affectional relationships.

Opioid modification of other social behaviors, including maternal behavior, play, and aggressive/submissive behaviors, also occurs (see Benton and Brain, 1988). In each case, the neural substrates of the complex behaviors are diverse and opioid interactions with other neurochemical systems are involved.

Endogenous Opiates and Psychiatric Disorders

The importance of endogenous opiates in psychiatric disorders has been suggested by studies of several types: (1) opioid peptide levels in the biological fluids of patients with defined psychiatric disorders are different from controls; (2) the effectiveness of opiate agonist and antagonist treatment on various disorders has been demonstrated; (3) an intimate relationship exists between opiate receptors and brain DA, a neurotransmitter implicated in schizophrenia and in reinforcement; and (4) opiates are well known to produce mood changes (e.g., euphoria, dysphoria, or psychotomimetic effects). For example, cyclazocine and other κ-receptor agonists are particularly effective in eliciting dysphoria. Also, PCP, which induces psychotic symptoms in abusers, alters dopamine function and elevates enkephalin levels in various brain areas. Further, in patients with Parkinson's disease, degeneration of enkephalin-containing neurons may be related to the blunted affect of these patients. These observations lead one to speculate that endogenous opiates have a role in mood disorders or in schizophrenia. Inconsistencies in experimental findings, however, have made it difficult to draw broad conclusions.

The disparities among experimental results may occur for several reasons. When evaluating peptides in biological fluids of the mentally ill, not only are there concerns regarding clinical controls of subjects for age, sex, duration of hospitalization, and so forth, but each of the biological fluids that are sampled (plasma, urine, and CSF) receive peptides from several sources (pituitary and adrenal secretions as well as neuronal sources). At this time, clinical research methods do not provide a means to influence one endogenous system without affecting the others. Therefore, the importance of individual peptide families in the etiology of mental illness remains difficult to determine.

An additional concern is that CSF samples measure only global activity of peptide systems (i.e., steady state levels), which may not be meaningful in light of the known complexity in regulation of peptide cleavage and the vast anatomical differences in regulation. Attempts are being made toward elucidating specific regulatory mechanisms, including gene transcription and the characterization of enzymes regulating the rate-limiting steps in peptide cleavage (Nyberg and Terenius, 1988). However, clinical research still relies on evaluating the amount of opioid at an isolated time point using standard radioimmunoassay or radioreceptor assay techniques (Nyberg, 1993).

It should be mentioned that many of the clinical studies are very difficult to interpret due to methodological flaws, including the lack of control groups, insuffi-

cient subject numbers, lack of diagnostic criteria, and insufficient documentation of biochemical parameters such as binding specificity and characterization of the isolated peptide (Berger and Nemeroff, 1987). Thus, it is not surprising that a consensus among research groups is not readily available. Of great interest is the potential to utilize studies from a variety of research groups that use different methods and patient populations to identify types of mental disorders that vary in endogenous opiate concentrations, responses to physiological challenge, or therapeutic effects.

The following discussion will focus on the possible involvement of endogenous opioids in affective disorders, schizophrenia, and autism. Clinical researchers have also investigated the potential importance of endogenous opioids in other forms of psychopathology, including postpartum psychosis, Gilles de la Tourette's syndrome, anorexia nervosa, Alzheimer's disease, Parkinson's disease, premenstrual syndrome, obsessive–compulsive disorder, and anxiety. Naber (1993) and Nyberg (1993) provide reviews of the more recent literature.

Affective Disorders

A Swedish group led by Terenius provided the earliest measurement of endogenous opiates in patients with affective disorders (Nyberg and Terenius, 1988). They found elevated endogenous opiates in the CSF of patients with major unipolar depression. Furthermore, positive correlations were found between enkephalin levels and the clinical symptoms of suicidal ideation and somatic anxiety. Despite these early encouraging findings, results of subsequent work have been far from unanimous in concluding a significant correlation between affective disorders and endogenous opiate levels.

Differences in the response to pharmacological challenges have also been documented in depressed populations. For example, Risch (1982) found that depressed patients were more sensitive than controls to the physostigmine-induced release of β-endorphin. Since physostigmine (a cholinesterase inhibitor that prolongs ACh action) induces depressive symptoms in normal individuals and has been found to reduce manic symptoms (see Berger and Nemeroff, 1987), the relationship between ACh and opiates may be important. In fact, an earlier study (Janowsky, Khaled, and Davis, 1974) showed that physostigmine-induced mood changes, including increased depression, hostility, and confusion, as well as decreased arousal and mania, were positively correlated with elevations in plasma β-endorphin.

Affective disorders are also associated with abnormalities in circadian rhythms and neuroendocrine function (see Chapter 19). The best established is hypersecretion of cortisol in response to excessive secretion of ACTH by the pituitary. Other neuroendocrine abnormalities include abnormal hormonal responses to pharmacological challenges. Such irregularities occur for vasopressin, growth

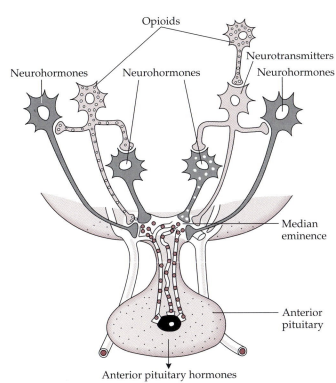

Opioids

Neurotransmitters

Neurohormones   Neurohormones   Neurohormones

Median eminence

Anterior pituitary

Anterior pituitary hormones

12.12 THE RELATIONSHIP BETWEEN OPIOID PEPTIDE NEURONS AND NEURONS UTILIZING CLASSICAL NEUROTRANSMITTERS in the median eminence of the hypothalamus. Opioidergic neurons may also directly influence cells releasing neuro-hormones that ultimately control the release of anterior pituitary hormones. (After Cella et al., 1993)

hormone, thyroid-stimulating hormone, and other pituitary hormones. The median eminence of the hypothalamus is the brain area responsible for the control of anterior pituitary hormones, and it is an area where several classical neurotransmitters and neuropeptide terminals converge to regulate the hypothalamic stimulating and releasing factors that act on the pituitary (Figure 12.12). Although it is not clear precisely where opioids interact with neurons in the median eminence, the high concentration of the opioids in the hypothalamus predicts a significant role for them in neuroendocrine control. Cella, Locatelli, and Muller (1993) provide an excellent summary of the literature.

An additional interaction between opioids and hormones in the pituitary is worth noting. ACTH and β-endorphin are both POMC products in the pituitary and are released under physiological conditions. The well-documented finding that some depressed patients do not show a suppression of cortisol release in response to dexamethasone (see the dexamethasone suppression test in Chapter 19) is paralleled by an inability to suppress β-endorphin secretion. Furthermore, a positive correlation between postdexamethasone levels of β-endorphin and the severity of depression has been reported (Meador-Woodruff et al., 1987; see Naber, 1993). Discussion of the details is beyond the scope of this chapter; however, elucidation of the neuroendocrine correlates of depression,

including patterns of neuropeptide changes, may well provide an important tool for diagnosis and ultimately for treatment.

Early attempts to treat affective disorders with naloxone met with failure, and although mixed agonist–antagonists as well as administration of β-endorphin have been evaluated, no general conclusions can be made regarding the efficacy of opioid treatment for depression. The most consistent results came from therapeutic trials using partial agonists that act on κ opiate receptors. In these cases, significant antidepressant effects were reported with κ-agonists, while μ-receptor agonists (morphine, FK33-824) and mixed μ-/δ-receptor agonists were either ineffective or produced variable results (see Schmauss and Emrich, 1988).

Schizophrenia

Shortly after the discovery of the endogenous opioid peptides, several laboratories showed that intracranial injection of the peptides produced a loss of righting reflex, profound sedation, and prolonged muscular rigidity similar to a catatonic schizophrenic state (Bloom et al., 1976; Jacquet and Marks, 1976). Each of these behavioral effects was antagonized by naloxone. These empirical results were in agreement with the report that CSF levels of endorphin are positively correlated with the severity of symptoms in schizophrenic patients (Gunne, Lindstrom, and Terenius, 1977). The same group reported that naloxone reduced the auditory hallucinations of four chronic schizophrenics in a single-blind test.

Unfortunately, in a series of clinical studies carried out over several years, altered levels of opioid peptides were not consistently documented in the schizophrenic population. While a number of reports have found elevated CSF opioids in acute and/or chronic schizophrenics that are reduced by antipsychotic drug treatment, many others failed to find evidence for abnormal opioid concentrations (see Naber, 1993; Nemeroff, Berger, and Bissette, 1987; Nyberg and Terenius, 1988). Given the recent interest in neurobiological rhythms and their impact on mental function (see Chapter 19), the report by Gil-Ad and coworkers (1986) describing disturbed diurnal rhythms of β-endorphin in schizophrenic patients may generate a new direction of research interest.

Based on some of the preliminary evidence that schizophrenia is associated with excess opioid activity, numerous clinical trials with naloxone have tested the effect of opioid receptor blockade on schizophrenic symptoms. Several studies described in greater detail in other sources (Nemeroff, Berger, and Bissette, 1987; Schmauss and Emrich, 1988) reported a significant reduction in hallucinations, unusual thought content, and other psychotic symptoms in response to naloxone. The time course of effectiveness suggests an intermediate step, such as the naloxone-induced increase in ACTH or β-endorphin release. Clinical trials are suggested (see Naber, 1993).

Endorphins and Autism

If, as discussed earlier, endogenous opioids play a role in mediating the reinforcing effects of social contact, then a potential role in childhood autism might be considered. Autistic children lack the normal social–emotional interest in other people, leading to poor social skills and inappropriate use of language for communication. Whereas perceived loss of emotional support (e.g., maternal separation) normally triggers activation of the neuronal systems involved in social signals such as crying, orienting toward, or following behavior, such a pattern is absent in the autistic child. Additional symptoms of autism include reduced sensitivity to pain as demonstrated by self-abusive behavior, less overt emotional behavior and reduced crying, low desire for social contact and lack of physical expressions of affection, as well as the development of stereotypic behaviors.

Several autistic-like symptoms can be produced in experimental animals using opioids. The naloxone-reversible behavioral effects in animals include reductions in pain sensitivity, decreased crying, diminished desire for social companionship and reduced clinging behavior, and increased learning abnormalities including extreme resistance to extinction (Sahley and Panksepp, 1987).

Additionally, naloxone and other opiate antagonists have been useful to a limited extent in reducing self-injurious and autistic-like stereotypy (Barron and Sandman, 1983; Herman et al., 1989; Richardson and Zaleski, 1983), and in increasing interpersonal behavior (Sandman et al., 1983) in selected populations.

Since opioids retard development (see above) and can induce autistic-like behaviors in animals, it has been suggested that metabolizing enzymes may be absent in the autistic child. Such an absence of enzymes might leave the brain saturated with the opioids, subsequently retarding the development of the child and reducing the normal signal pattern of the peptides (Sahley and Panksepp, 1987). Although the blood levels of β-endorphin in autistic children are lower than those of controls (Weizman et al., 1984), CSF levels of selected opioids (fraction II endorphins) are significantly elevated (Gillberg, Terenius, and Lonnerholm, 1985). Furthermore, elevated fraction II endorphin levels were correlated with decreased sensitivity to pain and increased self-destructiveness. Studies of this type provide some direct support for the hypothesis that excess endorphins may mediate autistic symptoms. Nevertheless, the hypothesis remains highly speculative at this time and needs further evaluation.

Part III Summary

The discovery of natural opioid peptides in neural tissue opened the door to investigations of endogenous modulation of pain, stress, mood, mental illness, reinforcement, dependence, and homeostatic processes such as eating. Three major families of peptides exist with distinct prohormone precursors and cleavage patterns, including proenkephalin, proopiomelanocortin, and prodynorphin. Ca^{2+}-dependent release and inactivation of the neuropeptides by two peptidases support a neuromodulatory function for the endogenous opiates. Localization of the peptides, their biological effects, and receptor subtype mediation are now being intensely investigated.

Application of recent advances in opioid neurophamacology means that highly specific opioid drugs will ultimately provide the long sought-after analgesic effects without dependence liability. Receptor-specific opiate agonists and antagonists or postreceptor probes that target intracellular mechanisms may soon be available for therapeutic intervention in addiction, eating disorders, mental illness, and so forth.

Part IV
Opiate Dependence and Abuse

General Features of Drug Abuse

Drug abuse may be defined as the self-administered use of any drug in a manner that deviates from the approved medical or social patterns within a given culture. According to this definition, misuse of drugs can include agents with profound CNS effects, but might also include laxatives, antibiotics, or vitamins. Exactly what constitutes drug abuse at any one time is determined by society and is variable, not only from culture to culture, but also within a given culture over time. In the United States for much of the nineteenth century, the individual states rather than the federal government had responsibility for health issues, including regulation of medical practice and availability of pharmaceutical products. Most states failed in this regulation, and a condition of free enterprise existed so that drugs such as opium and cocaine were widely available and advertised freely. At the same time, nations having a strong federal government (e.g., Great Britain) had national policies delineating controlled availability of dangerous drugs (Musto, 1991). During times of rapid social change, drug abuse tends to increase within the society. Because adolescents are most vulnerable to rapidly changing mores, drug abuse is highest within this age group. In addition, adolescents' belief in their own invulnerability minimizes their sense of risk and increases their likelihood to experiment.

Diagnostic Criteria

Recent editions of the *Diagnostic and Statistical Manual of Mental Disorders* of the American Psychiatric Association (including the current edition, DSM-IV) use the terms "substance dependence" and "substance abuse" to cate-

Table 12.7 Criteria for Substance Dependence and Substance Abuse According to the *Diagnostic and Statistical Manual of Mental Disorders*, Fourth Edition (DSM-IV)

Substance Dependence

A maladaptive pattern of substance use, leading to clinically significant impairment or distress, as manifested by three (or more) of the following, occurring at any time in the same 12-month period:

(1) Tolerance, as defined by either of the following:
  (a) a need for markedly increased amounts of the substance to achieve intoxication or desired effect,
  (b) markedly diminished effect with continued use of the same amount of the substance.

(2) Withdrawal, as manifested by either of the following:
  (a) the characteristic withdrawal syndrome for the substance,
  (b) the same (or a closely related) substance is taken to relieve or avoid withdrawal symptoms.

(3) The substance is often taken in larger amounts or over a longer period than was intended.

(4) There is a persistent desire or unsuccessful efforts to cut down or control substance use.

(5) A great deal of time is spent in activities necessary to obtain the substance (e.g., visiting multiple doctors or driving long distances), use the substance (e.g., chain-smoking), or recover from its effects.

(6) Important social, occupational, or recreational activities are given up or reduced because of substance use.

(7) The substance use is continued despite knowledge of having a persistent or recurrent physical or psychological problem that is likely to have been caused or exacerbated by the substance (e.g., current cocaine use despite recognition of cocaine-induced depression, or continued drinking despite recognition that an ulcer is made worse by alcohol consumption).

Substance Abuse[a]

A maladaptive pattern of substance use leading to clinically significant impairment or distress, as manifested by one (or more) of the following, occurring with a 12-month period:

(1) Recurrent substance use resulting in a failure to fulfill major role obligations at work, school, or home (e.g., repeated absences or poor work performance related to substance use; substance-related absences, suspensions, or expulsions from school; neglect of children or household).

(2) Recurrent substance use in situations in which it is physically hazardous (e.g., driving an automobile or operating a machine when impaired by substance use).

(3) Recurrent substance-related legal problems (e.g., arrests for substance-related disorderly conduct).

(4) Continued substance use despite having persistent or recurrent social or interpersonal problems caused or exacerbated by the effects of the substance (e.g., arguments with spouse about consequences of intoxication, physical fights).

[a]Substance abuse is diagnosed when an individual meets the above conditions but does not meet the criteria for substance dependence.

Source: American Psychiatric Association (1994). *Diagnostic and Statistical Manual of Mental Disorders* (4th ed.). American Psychiatric Association, Washington, D.C., pp. 181–183.

gorize differing degrees of problematic drug use. This terminology is not ideal, however, because the term "abuse" has historically been used in a more general way in psychopharmacology. The same is also true for the term "dependence" (see below). Nevertheless, the current system does provide a uniform nomenclature for investigators to use in describing the phenomena of compulsive drug-taking in humans and the mechanisms that may underlie these phenomena. DSM-IV does not use the term "addiction" at all, perhaps because of the many negative images, emotions, and associations it evokes. Table 12.7 contains DSM-IV criteria for substance dependence and abuse.

Biopsychosocial Model of Substance Dependence and Abuse

The DSM-IV recognizes that treatment of drug dependence and abuse depends on more than eliminating the drug from the body (detoxification), although detoxification is usually the first step in treatment. Ultimately, a host of behavioral and social factors must be identified and modified for a successful outcome. Figure 12.13 shows the relationship of physiological, behavioral, and social variables that contribute to drug-seeking behavior (see Stolerman, 1992). The model proposes that four main factors determine the strength of the drug-seeking behavior that is the common factor in drug dependence of all types: (1) positive reinforcement by the drug, (2) stimuli conditioned to drug effects, (3) cue effects of the drug, and (4) aversive consequences of taking the drug. Each of these factors in turn reflects a contribution by neural mechanisms, behavioral mechanisms, and modulating variables. Notice that the neural and behavioral mechanisms and modulating variables are shown only for their contribution to the positive reinforcing effects of drugs, but in fact similar mechanisms affect the other

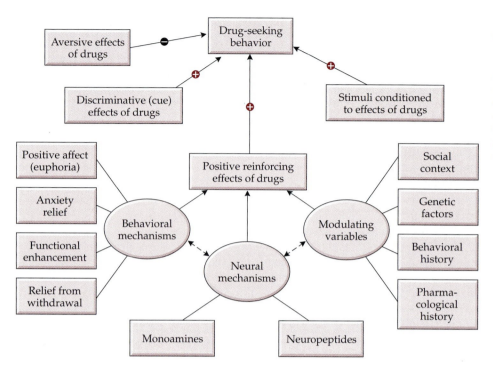

12.13 A BIOPSYCHOSOCIAL MODEL OF DRUG-SEEKING BEHAVIOR. The four principal contributors to drug abuse according to this model are positive reinforcing effects of drugs, cue effects of drugs, stimuli conditioned to drug effects, and aversive effects. The model also shows the nature of the factors that in turn constitute each of the four main components. (After Stolerman, 1992).

major factors in drug-seeking behavior. Much of the remainder of this chapter discusses the factors contributing to opiate abuse and potential treatment modalities for opiate dependence.

Consequences of Opiate Use

Tolerance

Compulsive opiate use involves three independent components: tolerance, psychological dependence, and physical dependence. The three components are not necessary features of substance dependence in general and vary significantly for psychotropic drugs of different classes. Tolerance produces a need to increase the dose of the drug after several administrations in order to achieve the same magnitude of effect. Tolerance occurs for all of the opioids including the endorphins. The extent of tolerance depends on the magnitude and frequency of drug use. After several months of heavy drug use, a user can self-administer 40 to 50 times the normal lethal dose. Tolerance to the opiates develops quite rapidly, although not all the pharmacological effects of morphine undergo tolerance to the same extent or at the same rate. For instance, the euphoria and analgesia show rapid tolerance, but the constipating effects and the pinpoint pupils persist even after prolonged opiate use.

Cross-tolerance for the opiates exists such that when tolerance develops to a particular agent, other substances that are chemically similar also show reduced effectiveness. For the opioids, the degree of cross-tolerance is dependent on receptor subtype. Selective agonists for the μ-receptor show a large degree of cross-tolerance to each other, but only minimal cross-tolerance to κ-receptor agonists. However, κ agonists demonstrate significant cross-tolerance to each other.

Although the development of tolerance is in part due to an increased rate of metabolism (drug disposition tolerance) and to classical and operant conditioning processes, most tolerance is apparently of the pharmacodynamic type; that is, the cells become accustomed to the presence of the drug. The cellular mechanisms of opiate tolerance and dependence are discussed in more detail below (see also Chapter 1).

Physical Dependence

Some drugs also induce a **physical dependence**, which is an adaptive state produced by repeated drug administration and which manifests itself by intense physical disturbance when drug administration is halted. The **withdrawal syndrome** or **abstinence syndrome** comprises a specific array of psychological and physiological symptoms that are characteristic for each drug type. The degree of physical dependence can be measured only by the severity of withdrawal symptoms. For drugs such as alcohol, barbiturates, and the narcotic analgesics, the withdrawal symptoms are so unpleasant that they can be important factors in motivating continued drug-seeking behavior.

The withdrawal symptoms characteristic for the opiates (Table 12.8) are essentially opposite to the acute effects of the opioids and are considered an overshoot rebound to the initial drug-induced state. Opiate withdrawal is not considered life-threatening but the symp-

Table 12.8	Acute Effects of Opioids and Rebound Withdrawal Symptoms	
Acute action	**Withdrawal sign**
Analgesia	Pain and irritability
Respiratory depression	Hyperventilation
Euphoria	Dysphoria and depression
Relaxation and sleep	Restlessness and insomnia
Tranquilization	Fearfulness and hostility
Decreased blood pressure	Increased blood pressure
Constipation	Diarrhea
Pupillary constriction	Pupillary dilation
Hypothermia	Hyperthermia
Drying of secretions	Lacrimation, runny nose
Reduced sex drive	Spontaneous ejaculation
Peripheral vasodilation; flushed and warm skin	Chilliness and "gooseflesh"

toms are extremely unpleasant and flu-like in nature. As for other psychotropic drugs, the symptoms vary in intensity from quite mild to severe. The severity of symptoms, as well as their onset and termination depends on the intensity of the initial drug effects, the dose administered, the frequency and duration of drug use, as well as the health and personality of the addict. The symptoms generally peak at 36–48 hours after the last administration of morphine and disappear within 7–10 days. However, for a drug like methadone, which acutely has a gradual onset of action that is relatively long-lasting, withdrawal symptoms do not abruptly peak but increase to a gradual maximum after several days and decrease gradually over several weeks. Abstinence for the very long acting opiate L-acetylmethadol (LAAM) is even more prolonged, but as is true for all the longer-lasting opiates, the withdrawal signs are milder.

It is assumed that abstinence occurs when the receptors are no longer occupied by the opiate. Due to differences in binding affinities of the opioids for various receptors and differences in bioavailability, particular withdrawal signs may appear gradually and sequentially. The sudden displacement of opiates from all the receptors simultaneously by the administration of an opioid antagonist produces a rapid and dramatic appearance of the withdrawal syndrome that is more severe than that caused by mere abstinence from the drug. At the point when abstinence signs subside, the user is considered to be in a detoxified state. Readministration of the opiate at any point during withdrawal will dramatically suppress all the symptoms. Furthermore, cross-dependence exists among the opiates. Consequently, administration of a sufficient quantity of any opiate will stop or reduce the withdrawal symptoms after cessation of any of the other opiates. However, as was true for the occurrence of cross-tolerance, cross-de-

pendence is also limited within specific receptor subtypes.

Evaluation of selective agonists showed that when compared with morphine, dependence on κ-agonists is both receptor-specific and pharmacologically unique. Evidence for κ-induced physical dependence comes from several types of evidence. First, unique withdrawal symptoms follow the cessation of chronic κ-agonist administration. Secondly, withdrawal signs are selectively suppressed such that only κ-agonists suppress U50,488 withdrawal, and only μ-agonists suppress morphine withdrawal. Finally, μ- and κ-antagonists selectively precipitate withdrawal following chronic μ- and κ-agonist treatment (Gmerek et al., 1987; Woods et al., 1993).

In vivo animal models of opioid dependence involve either multiple injections or pellet implantation of opioid drugs, which maintain significant blood levels of drug over several days up to 2 weeks. Distinctive and quantifiable withdrawal syndromes can be observed in mice, rats, dogs, and monkeys and provide a useful preclinical research tool because of the close species correlation with potencies of agonists and antagonists in humans (see Gmerek et al., 1987; Way, 1993). Withdrawal signs elicited by central antagonist administration include jumping, rearing, wet-dog shakes, and increased locomotor behavior.

Neural substrates of dependence. Just as acute actions of opioids involve multiple sites in the CNS, neural substrates of physical dependence and opiate withdrawal are also widely represented. It is generally assumed that several brain areas are responsible for the physical and motivational signs of opiate withdrawal and that some physical signs may also be mediated by peripheral (gut) receptors (Koob, Maldonado, and Stinus, 1992). Typical experiments investigate the effects of selective lesions on the appearance of opiate withdrawal induced by antagonist administration. Although lesioning the medial forebrain bundle, the ventromedial hypothalamus, or the raphe nuclei blocks portions of opiate-induced withdrawal, even extensive lesions of the thalamus, limbic system, and cortex do not abolish the full withdrawal syndrome. Intracerebral microinjection studies using opiate antagonists also attempt to identify discrete brain areas that produce particular signs of abstinence. Although no brain area has been found to precipitate the entire withdrawal syndrome, brain areas highly sensitive to methylnaloxonium (a potent hydrophilic antagonist that does not readily diffuse from the brain) are the locus coeruleus and PAG. Anterior preoptic area and nucleus raphe magnus are less sensitive to methylnaloxonium, and nucleus accumbens and medial thalamus are the least sensitive of the areas tested (Maldonado et al., 1992).

Although microinjection of opiate antagonists into the nucleus accumbens was not very effective in eliciting somatic signs of withdrawal, Koob, Maldonado, and Stinus (1992) describe experiments showing that the brain area may be important in the aversive stimulus effects of opiate withdrawal. Opiate-dependent rats undergoing antagonist-induced withdrawal in a novel environment tend to develop a place aversion for the novel location (see below). To identify the brain area responsible for the aversive effects of precipitated withdrawal, methylnaloxonium was microinjected into discrete brain areas. High doses of the drug that were introduced into several brain areas, including the ventral tegmental area and medial dorsal thalamus, produced significant place aversion. However, the areas most sensitive to low doses of the antagonist was the nucleus accumbens, followed by the amygdala, and periaqueductal gray. The place aversion occurred despite the fact that little or no sign of abstinence was induced by injection of the low dose into the nucleus accumbens or amygdala. Thus, while the PAG and LC seem to be involved in the physiological signs of abstinence, the nucleus accumbens may be responsible for the motivational aspects of opiate withdrawal.

Psychological Dependence

Psychological dependence is a condition characterized by an intense drive or craving for a drug whose effects the user feels are necessary for a sense of well-being. Psychological dependence varies both with personality characteristics of the individual and with specific drug effects. When the desire to continue taking the drug becomes a "psychic craving" or "compulsion" and the user becomes preoccupied with drug taking, there exists the basis for compulsive drug use. Although it is necessary to distinguish between physical and psychological dependence, keep in mind that neurochemical changes are responsible for psychological dependence just as they are for physical dependence.

Psychological dependence is the most poorly defined of the three factors contributing to compulsive drug use and continues to be the most difficult to identify and quantify. One approach is to examine the reinforcing effects of opiates on behavior.

Opiates as Reinforcers

Opiates have potent effects on motivated—that is, goal-directed—behaviors. Several experimental techniques utilizing both operant and classical conditioning paradigms provide tools to evaluate the rewarding properties of opiates (see Chapter 2, Part II). These methods include drug self-administration, conditioned place preference, and facilitation of intracerebral electrical self-stimulation. The techniques differ in several fundamental aspects. The advantages and disadvantages of each technique are discussed in detail elsewhere (Bozarth, 1987; Carr, Fibinger, and Phillips, 1989; Shippenberg, 1993; Stolerman, 1992; Watson et al., 1989).

Methods of Assessing Drug Reinforcement

Intracerebral electrical self-stimulation.   This operant technique allows subjects to perform a specific task, such as lever pressing, in order to self-administer a weak electric current to discrete brain areas via an indwelling electrode. The underlying assumption is that certain brain areas constitute central reward pathways. When the animal works to stimulate a particular cluster of neurons, it is assumed that the electrical activation causes release of neurotransmitters from the nerve terminals in the region, which in turn mediate a rewarding effect. The fact that morphine and other opioids lower the electric current threshold for intracranial self-stimulation indicates that the drugs enhance the brain reward mechanism (Esposito, Porrino, and Seeger, 1989).

Conditioned place preference.   Place conditioning is another useful technique demonstrating the reinforcement value of psychotropic drugs. This procedure relies on the formation of a classically conditioned association between drug effect and environment. A typical place conditioning apparatus is shown in Figure 12.14. As previously described in Chapter 8, exposure to each chamber of the apparatus is repeatedly paired with either drug or vehicle administration. During these conditioning trials, the sensory cues provided by the drug-paired chamber are thought to become associated with the drug state and to take on reinforcing values themselves (that is, they become secondary reinforcers). An increase in the amount of time spent in the drug-paired chamber is therefore assumed to reflect approach behavior by the subject to these reinforcers (Shippenberg, 1993; Stoler-

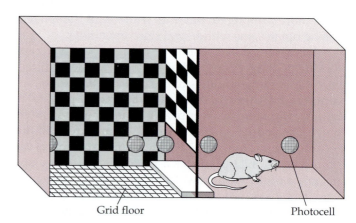

Grid floor   Photocell

12.14 A TYPICAL PLACE CONDITIONING APPARATUS. The apparatus consists of two compartments that vary along several sensory dimensions, including the characteristics of the floor and the pattern or color of the walls. After each compartment has been repeatedly paired with drug or saline administration, the reinforcing or aversive effect of the drug is determined in a test session in which the animal has access to both compartments, and the amount of time spent in each is monitored with photocells or by visual observation. (After Stolerman, 1992.)

man, 1992). Aversive effects of withdrawal symptoms can be evaluated in the same way.

Drug self-administration. Weeks (1964) developed the technique of implanting a catheter into the jugular vein of a rat during brief surgical anesthesia and connecting the catheter's tubing to an injection device (infusion pump). The animal controls the delivery of drug by pressing a lever in the operant chamber (Figure 12.15). The device can be operated without restraining the animal.

Using the self-administration technique, several critical studies were performed that demonstrated its reliability and validity in evaluating the self-administration of drugs from several major classes by both rats and rhesus monkeys. The basic premise of self-administration studies is that psychotropic drugs can control behavior by acting as positive reinforcers. Table 12.9 lists some of the drugs that have been self-administered by rhesus monkeys and are consequently considered to have primary reinforcing effects. It is highly significant that one characteristic common to all the drugs listed as reinforcers is that these drugs are all self-administered by humans and have a significant abuse potential.

The drugs listed in Table 12.9 are not equally reinforcing, nor are the daily patterns of self-administration the same for each. The striking finding is that the reinforcement value and the patterns of drug taking are quite similar to those seen in humans. For example, chlorpromazine, an antipsychotic drug that is not abused in humans, is not self-administered by monkeys. Furthermore, hallucinogens are rarely self-injected by animals, and it is rare to see compulsive self-administration of these drugs in humans. The finding that nearly all monkeys will self-inject particular psychotropic drugs suggests that self-administration of these compounds is

Table 12.9	Drugs Acting as Reinforcers in the Rhesus Monkey
Central stimulants	
Cocaine	
Amphetamine	
Pipradrol	
Methylphenidate	
Nicotine	
Caffeine	
Narcotics	
Morphine	
Methadone	
Meperidine	
Codeine	
Pentazocine	
CNS depressants	
Pentobarbital	
Amobarbital	
Phenobarbital	
Hexobarbital	
Chlordiazepoxide	
Ethanol	

not abnormal behavior, but is normally restrained in humans by social values and customs.

Self-administration experiments in non-physically dependent rhesus monkeys show that self-injection frequency gradually increases over time until the monkeys self-administer a stable and apparently optimal amount of drug. The rate of opiate self-administration is evidently determined by plasma levels of the drug. For example, pretreatment of animals with morphine, codeine, or meperidine reduces intravenous self-administration of morphine. In contrast, pretreatment with naloxone increases the response rate of morphine self-administration to a rate similar to that seen during morphine abstinence. It is evident from these studies that the animals learn to regulate with some accuracy the amount of morphine that they require. Dose–response curves can be used to compare the reinforcing effects and the relative potencies of opiate drugs (Woods et al., 1993).

Comparisons of self-administration patterns across drug classes also reveal some important features. The characteristics of acquisition, patterning of self-infusions, and pattern of extinction (responding after reinforcement is discontinued) are distinct for the opiate drugs and for the stimulant cocaine. Differences between patterns of opiate and cocaine use may provide significant information about the nature of drug reinforcement and dependence.

Of current interest is the discovery that µ-agonists support self-administration responding in a variety of

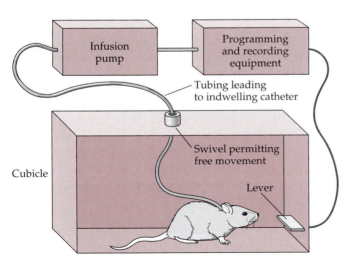

12.15 OPERANT CONTROL OF DRUG SELF-ADMINISTRATION predicts abuse liability of psychotropic drugs. Pressing the lever according to a predetermined schedule of reinforcement provides the delivery of drug into a vein or into discrete brain areas.

experimental designs and species. The potency of opiates such as morphine, fentanyl, heroin, nalbuphine, pentazocine, and others in producing reinforcing effects is correlated with their binding affinity for the μ-receptor (see Shippenberg, 1993). In contrast, κ-agonists (ketazocine, ethylketocyclazocine, and U 50488H) fail to produce self-injection behavior in rhesus monkeys (Woods and Winger, 1987). Although intrahippocampal self-administration of dynorphin has been reported, its reinforcing effects were reduced by specific μ-antagonists rather than κ-antagonists. In addition, others have found κ-agonists to induce aversive states leading to avoidance behavior (see Shippenberg, 1993). Results from these self-administration studies correlate with subjective effects measured with mood rating scales in humans. Human volunteers report aversive effects of the κ-agonist ketazocine.

Studies using intracerebroventricular administration of peptide agonists that do not easily cross the blood–brain barrier showed that δ-receptor agonists also serve as positive reinforcers. The reinforcing effects of several δ-agonists were attenuated by specific δ-antagonists, but not by μ-antagonists, showing receptor specificity. Thus, both μ- and δ-receptors are involved in reward processes. β-endorphin self-administration is antagonized by either μ- or δ-receptor antagonists, demonstrating that both types of receptors may be involved in the reinforcing effect of this peptide (Bals-Kubik, Shippenberg, and Herz, 1990).

Despite their wide variations in experimental design and procedures, drug self-administration studies have provided strikingly consistent results. A description and evaluation of several self-administration techniques, as well as other methods currently used to evaluate dependence, such as drug discriminative stimulus properties, can be found in several sources (Bozarth, 1987; Carr, Fibinger, and Phillips, 1989; Johanson, Woolverton, and Schuster, 1987; Shippenberg, 1993; Stolerman, 1992; Young and Herling, 1986).

Human self-administration studies are important to the understanding of substance abuse, but are much more difficult to accomplish (Preston and Jasinski, 1991). Opiate addicts in a research ward environment may provide answers to some of the many questions about the roles of primary reinforcement, social and environmental components, and the avoidance of pain in chronic drug use in humans. Human research is intended to answer such questions as: What is the role of the subjective emotional state of the individual in drug-taking behavior? How important are interoceptive cues as triggers for the behavior? Are there environmental conditions associated with increased or decreased heroin use? What is the effect of narcotic antagonist administration on the drug-seeking behavior? Can psychological factors predict which individuals will continue to self-administer heroin in the presence of a narcotic antagonist?

None of the answers to the questions posed are simple, and the methodology needed to achieve the answers is complex. The participation of chronic opiate users in research that involves drug self-administration raises several ethical considerations and relies on self-report data, presupposing that addicts have insight into their own motivations and behavior and that they will respond truthfully at all times. Further, appropriate controls are much more difficult to achieve in experiments with human subjects, whose environment and behavior cannot be as rigorously regulated as animal subjects. Nevertheless, the Addiction Research Center (ARC) has developed quantitative methods for assessing subjective effects of drugs in humans that emphasize measures of euphoria, positive mood, or measures of liking (Johanson, Woolverton, and Schuster, 1987). The development of models and measures of drug dependence has increased the understanding of both environmental and biological factors contributing to substance abuse and has aided in the development of treatment strategies (see below).

Drugs as discriminative stimuli.   The animal correlate to the ARC assessment of mood states in humans is the use of drugs as discriminative stimuli (Overton, 1987). In discrimination studies, drugs are used as cues to signal the availability of food reinforcement. For example, in a two-lever operant chamber, rats are trained to press one lever after a drug is administered and to press the alternate lever after saline treatment. Once the discrimination has been learned, the animal begins to press the appropriate lever for food rewards depending on whether it has received the training drug or saline. Trained subjects can be used to determine whether test substances are subjectively experienced as "like" or "unlike" the training drug. Test substances can include drugs in the same class as the training drug, novel compounds with unknown subjective effects, or specific receptor agonists. Pharmacological manipulations with specific antagonists or selective neurotoxic brain lesions can be used to interfere with the learned discriminative behavior.

The significance of discriminative stimuli to drug-seeking behavior is based on the belief that humans use psychoactive drugs to achieve a characteristic subjective effect. Second, following detoxification, drug-seeking behavior is enhanced by cues previously associated with the drug. Finally, abstinence-induced withdrawal can also contribute to drug-associated discriminative stimulus effects (Stolerman, 1992).

Mechanisms of Opiate Reward

Two methods provide information regarding the neural substrates of reinforcement. In one, opioid ligands are microinjected into discrete brain areas and are evaluated for their ability to support self-administration. Second, selective brain lesions are used to identify the neuroanatomical and/or neurochemical basis for drug-induced reinforcement.

Microinjection studies from many laboratories implicate the dopaminergic mesolimbic system (originating with cell bodies in the ventral tegmental area that project to the nucleus accumbens) in opiate reward (see Di-Chara and North, 1992; Koob and Bloom, 1988; Shippenberg, 1993, Watson et al., 1989). Self-administration of morphine or endogenous peptides occurs when the microcannula is implanted near the dopamine cell bodies within the ventral tegmental area (VTA), but not in other brain areas (Bozarth and Wise, 1984). When an opiate antagonist such as nalorphine is injected into the VTA or nucleus accumbens (NA), intravenous self-administration of opiates increases in order to overcome the reduction in reinforcement. In contrast to the VTA, rats do not readily learn to microinject the same dose of morphine into the substantia nigra, caudate–putamen, periventricular gray, or lateral hypothalamus. Intra-VTA microinjection of morphine or selective μ-agonists also induces conditioned place preference (Bozarth, 1987), further substantiating a role for the VTA in opiate reward. Also, microinjection of morphine into the VTA reduces the threshold for intracranial electrical self-stimulation, arguing for a direct action of opiates on central reward mechanisms.

Although animals will learn to press a lever for morphine injection into the NA (Koob and Goeders, 1989), the nucleus is much less sensitive than the VTA and requires significantly greater concentrations to support self-administration. Higher concentrations of morphine are also needed for conditioned place preference, and specific μ-agonists are ineffective in this regard (Bals-Kubik, Shippenberg, and Herz, 1990). The concentration difference may reflect receptor subtype densities: the NA has predominately δ-receptors rather than μ-receptors. Koob and Goeders (1989) showed reinforcing effects for δ-agonists microinjected into the NA. They propose the VTA as the principal site for μ-receptor–mediated reinforcement and the NA as the reward substrate for δ-agonists.

The significance of dopamine (DA) activity in morphine reinforcement is quite clear. First, systemic or intra-VTA opiates increase dopaminergic cell firing in the VTA and increase the release of dopamine and its metabolites in NA. Selective blockade of μ-receptors in the VTA produces a significant decrease in basal DA release (Spanagel, Herz, and Shippenberg, 1992). Intraventricular β-endorphin produces similar enhancements of VTA neuron firing. Interestingly, κ-agonists produce opposite effects on mesolimbic neurons. Selective κ-agonists injected into the NA reduce DA neuronal activity and subsequent DA turnover (release and metabolism). κ-antagonists increase basal dopamine release. Based on these data it is evident that tonic activation of μ- and κ-receptors maintains basal levels of dopamine release in the

NA. The fact that κ-agonists microinjected into either the VTA or NA produce conditioned place aversions suggests that the mesolimbic dopamine system may mediate aversive effects of opiates as well as their reinforcing properties (Shippenberg et al., 1991).

The precise neural mechanism that mediates opioid activation of the mesolimbic cells is not known. However, a model of the dual control suggested above (Spanagel, Herz, and Shippenberg, 1992) provides a basis on which to further investigate the mechanism of opiate dependence (Figure 12.16). The presence of GABA inhibitory neurons in the VTA suggests a mechanism similar to that described earlier for the activation of descending supraspinal neurons (see Figure 12.10). Opioids may inhibit the GABA inhibitory cells via μ-receptors by opening K^+ channels or altering Ca^{2+} flux. The inhibition of inhibitory neurons would lead to subsequent increases in the firing of DA cells in the VTA (Figure 12.16). Dynorphin acting on presynaptic κ-receptors in the NA reduces the release of DA.

Moreover, in rats trained to self-administer heroin intravenously, systemic morphine or injection into the VTA reinitiates responding after the behavior has been extinguished. Morphine is ineffective, however, if injected in the NA. Also, increasing mesolimbic cell activity by systemically administering amphetamine or microinjecting it into the NA reinstates the heroin self-administration. This action of amphetamine strongly suggests that mesolimbic dopamine cell firing is essential for opiate reward. Microinjection of morphine into the VTA also reinstates responding in rats trained to self-administer cocaine. Since opiates increase firing of cells in the VTA and subsequently increase release of DA in the NA, and similar actions are reported for the self-administration of ethanol, nicotine, and psychostimulants, a common link in reinforcement mecha-

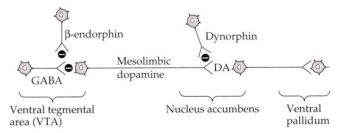

12.16 MODEL OF THE OPPOSING TONIC EFFECTS OF OPIOID NEURONS ON MESOLIMBIC DOPAMINE CELLS. In the VTA, β-endorphin neurons (via μ-receptors) increase mesolimbic activity by inhibiting the inhibitory GABA neurons. The release of dopamine (DA) from mesolimbic nerve terminals is tonically inhibited by dynorphin activity (via κ-receptors). Basal dopamine release is determined by the balance between the two opioid systems. D_1 receptors on cells in nucleus accumbens that go to other brain areas, such as the ventral pallidum, may ultimately be responsible for "motivational" tonus (aversion, neutral state, positive reinforcement).

nisms must involve the VTA–NA pathway (see Shippenberg, 1993; also see Chapter 13).

In addition, DA receptor antagonists block the reinforcing effects of opiates when evaluated by intracranial electrical self-stimulation or conditioned place preference. These results, however, have not been entirely consistent and force us to consider that other brain sites may also be involved. Using specific DA ligands, several groups have concluded that the tonic release of DA and activation of D_1 receptors in the NA are required for maintaining a neutral motivational state, while a reduction in DA activity (as following κ-receptor stimulation in NA) leads to aversion, and an increase (as following μ-receptor stimulation in the VTA) leads to positive reinforcement. D_1 antagonists reduce the primary reinforcing effects of opiates, decrease intracranial electrical self-stimulation, and decrease the self-administration of psychostimulants. D_1 antagonists injected into the NA but not other brain areas produces aversive effects as demonstrated by conditioned place aversions. D_2 antagonists are apparently inactive in these tests.

Finally, the effects of lesions further support a role for the dopaminergic neurons in reinforcement mechanisms. Lesions in the VTA or NA produced by 6-hydroxydopamine (6-OHDA) reduce the conditioned place preference for μ-agonists as well as the conditioned place aversion for κ-agonists, while destruction of other DA pathways (nigrostriatal or mesocortical) has no effect (Shippenberg, 1993). The conditioned place preference for several other abused substances is also attenuated by 6-OHDA lesions of the NA. Self-administration of some abused substances such as cocaine and amphetamine is virtually eliminated by such lesions; however, heroin self-administration is only partially reduced, and a typical response pattern of extinction from heroin is not observed (Pettit et al., 1984).

Why opiate self-administration is only partially reduced by 6-OHDA lesions is not clear at present. However, injecting the neurotoxin kainic acid into the NA does disrupt opiate self-administration. Since kainic acid destroys cell bodies but not fibers of passage, the cells originating in the NA may be a necessary common link for the reinforcing properties of opiates and psychoactive stimulants (see Figure 12.16). The destruction of cells in the ventral pallidum that receive input from NA neurons also abolishes opiate self-administration (Hubner and Koob, 1987), which further substantiates the importance of mechanisms beyond the VTA–NA cells as a final common pathway.

Although the importance of dopamine is clear, involvement of other neurotransmitters is not unlikely. Some evidence suggests a mediating role for serotonin acting at $5-HT_3$ receptors. $5-HT_3$ antagonists also reduce opiate-induced DA release along with reducing the reinforcement value of μ-agonists (see Shippenberg, 1993).

Neurochemical Mechanisms of Opiate Tolerance and Dependence

The classic hypothesis of the mechanism of tolerance to and physical dependence on opiates was formulated by Himmelsbach (1943). This hypothesis suggests that although acute administration of morphine disrupts the organism's homeostasis, repeated administration of the drug induces some undetermined adaptive mechanism that compensates for the acute effects of morphine and restores the original homeostasis. At this point, tolerance to the effects of morphine is said to have occurred, as administration of the same size dose of morphine no longer produces the original physiological disturbance. The abrupt cessation of morphine administration stops all drug effects but leaves the adaptive mechanism active; it then overcompensates and produces a new disturbance in homeostasis, which might be equated with withdrawal.

Himmelsbach's model was entirely theoretical, but in the mid-1970s a physiological correlate was described by Sharma, Klee, and Nirenberg (1975). They developed special hybrid cells (NG108-15) by crossing neuroblastoma cells (cancerous cells from neural tissue) with glial cells and maintained them in cell culture medium (see Chapter 2). The NG108-15 cells have opiate receptors that are coupled to adenylyl cyclase via G protein and regulate the production of the intracellular second messenger cAMP. Studies of these cells have provided a large body of information, not only on cAMP regulation but also on receptors and receptor function (see below).

Down-Regulation of Opioid Peptide Synthesis

Tolerance to administered opiates may occur because exogenous opiates act at the endogenous opioid receptor sites, and by a negative feedback mechanism reduce the synthesis of the endogenous peptides. For example, tolerance to the analgesic effect might develop because the reduction in endogenous peptides means more exogenous opiate is necessary to inhibit transmission in the pain pathway. Abrupt withdrawal of the opiate in conjunction with the already low levels of endogenous opioids would leave the pain fiber uninhibited, producing withdrawal symptoms, such as hyperalgesia. The duration of withdrawal symptoms may depend in part on the subsequent rate of opioid synthesis.

The idea that opiate drugs interact with endogenous opioid peptide systems to bring about tolerance and dependence is not a new one, but empirical support was lacking until the cell biology of the endogenous peptides was clarified and new tools and techniques were developed to investigate these interactions. Numerous studies have documented that chronic administration of opioid drugs alters opioid peptide content in specific brain regions, and that this regulation occurs at the level of gene expression. (For more in-depth reviews, see Kley and Loeffler, 1993; Roberts et al., 1993; Rossier, 1993.)

Childers (1993) described how opioids may regulate the synthesis of proenkephalin by inhibiting adenylyl cyclase (see previous section on cellular mechanisms and Figure 12.4). Briefly, the inhibitory effect of opiate drugs on the production of cAMP by adenylyl cyclase leads to a reduced activation of cAMP-dependent protein kinase and a subsequent reduction in phosphorylation of CREB (cAMP-response element binding protein). As mentioned earlier, CREB is a transcription factor that activates CRE, which is a DNA sequence in the promoter region of genes that regulates the rate at which the genes (e.g., those coding proenkephalin) are transcribed. Thus, increased opioid receptor activation would negatively feed back to reduce synthesis of the endogenous peptide prohormone. Reduction of proenkephalin mRNA does in fact occur in the hypothalamus following chronic morphine treatment. This negative feedback in which exogenous drug reduces the available pool of endogenous ligand is one possible mechanism responsible for the development of tolerance.

Several experiments have found that chronic morphine treatment also leads to a decrease in mRNA encoding for POMC, the prohormone for β-endorphin, in the hypothalamus (Bronstein, Przewlocki, and Akil, 1990) as well as in prodynorphin mRNA in striatum (Trujillo and Akil, 1991). However, the reductions in mRNA are not necessarily reflected in reduced peptide content in these brain areas. Neither β-endorphin nor proenkephalin peptide levels are decreased, despite reduced mRNA, and prodynorphin peptides are actually increased. The basis for these effects is not clear, but may be due to changes in posttranslational processing and release or additional feedback mechanisms that reflect changes in demand (see Trujillo and Akil, 1991).

Role of Receptor Changes

Although the appearance of the withdrawal syndrome is dependent on opioid receptors, the relationship between tolerance and physical dependence and receptor modification is not clear. Although early studies failed to show that chronic treatment with opioid agonists consistently down-regulates opioid receptors, in selected cells opioid receptor changes may be sufficient to account for desensitization to the opiates (Zukin et al., 1993).

Opiate agonists appear to reduce only moderately the number of opiate receptors in vivo. For example, six days of subcutaneous morphine administration in guinea pigs produced a small (approximately 25%) net reduction in μ-receptors without a change in δ- or κ-receptors. More importantly, the chronic treatment induced a change in the relative proportions of the high- and low-affinity forms of the receptor (Cox, 1993). In general, relatively high concentrations of high-efficacy

agonists, rather than partial agonists, may be necessary to produce down-regulation of receptors.

Results of studies using chronic administration of opioid antagonists are much clearer. Chronic, but not acute, naloxone or naltrexone treatment leads to a dramatic increase in receptor number along with an enhanced analgesic response. Specific receptor labeling techniques showed a selective up-regulation of brain μ- and δ-receptors following chronic naltrexone, but no significant change in κ-receptor number or affinity. The brain regions with the largest changes in receptor number include cortical layers 1 and 2, striatum, nucleus accumbens, periaqueductal gray, and ventral tegmental area (see Zukin et al., 1993). In addition, the up-regulated receptors are apparently functional, as demonstrated by an increased coupling to G_i, and an enhanced sensitivity to modulation by GTP.

The effects of chronic opioids appear to be quite different in the developing organism. Exposure to opioids, as well as stress, pain, and a variety of other environmental factors, is known to alter the ontogenesis of brain opioid systems prenatally. In postnatal animals, chronic morphine treatment generally reduces μ-receptors to a greater extent than either δ- or κ-receptors and this degree of down-regulation decreases with age. The significance of the transient effects of morphine on neonatal receptors is not yet clear at the time of this writing (Zukin, et al., 1993).

Desensitization and G protein uncoupling. Since a decrease in receptor number cannot fully account for the development of tolerance to opioids, neurobiologists have considered that agonist action generates nonfunctional receptor forms, a process called receptor desensitization (see Cox, 1993; Trujillo and Akil, 1991). Since each of the three opioid receptor subtypes is linked to a G protein, it is reasonable to assume that chronic agonist activation of the receptor produces a functional decoupling between the receptor and the G protein. In support of this hypothesis, Wuster, Costa, and Gramsch, (1983) found that agonist treatment reduced the number of high-affinity receptors in which the receptor is coupled to the G protein in the absence of guanine nucleotides. Other competition binding studies showed that high-affinity binding sites dropped from 75% of total sites in control membranes to 45% of the total in membranes from cells chronically treated with morphine; low-affinity sites correspondingly increased in opiate-treated cells from control levels of 25% to 55% in treated cells. The assumption is that during the development of tolerance, receptors are shifted into a low-affinity, uncoupled state such that opiate binding to the receptor can no longer induce inhibition of adenylyl cyclase or other second messengers.

Although uncoupling occurs, desensitization does not necessarily mean that changes in the levels of G protein subunits also occur (see Cox, 1993). NG 108-15 cells desensitized by treatment with DADLE did not show reduced concentrations of G protein subunits (Lang and Costa, 1989), despite evidence of altered receptor binding affinities. However, within the CNS, opioid-induced changes in the concentration of G proteins have been found to vary with brain region.

Terwilliger and colleagues (1991) found that 5 days of morphine treatment increased levels of inhibitory G-proteins in the locus coeruleus and amygdala, reduced their levels in the nucleus accumbens and spinal cord dorsal root ganglia, and left G proteins unchanged in frontal cortex, hippocampus, periaqueductal gray, ventral tegmental area, substantia nigra, and dorsal raphe. The authors propose that such regional differences may be the basis for the distinction between homologous and heterologous desensitization. **Homologous desensitization** refers to tolerance developing only to the agonist administered and not to other agonists, which act on different receptors but share receptor-mediated mechanisms. In this case, the functional decoupling between opiate receptor and G protein may produce a compensatory up-regulation of inhibitory G proteins through which other nondesensitized ligands continue to function. This type of desensitization occurs in several brain areas including the locus coeruleus. **Heterologous desensitization** refers to the case in which tolerance develops to the effects of not only the opiate but also other ligands with common receptor-mediated actions. In this case, a decrease in inhibitory G protein subunits would reduce the effectiveness of all inhibitory ligands working via G_i. This type of desensitization occurs in dorsal root ganglia.

Trujillo and Akil (1991) have combined evidence on receptor binding, endogenous opioid biosynthesis, and receptor decoupling from G proteins to develop a model of opiate tolerance and dependence. Acute administration of an opiate increases the number of receptors occupied, and full opiate drug effects occur. With repeated treatment, the receptors become decoupled from G proteins so that opiate actions diminish (i.e., tolerance occurs). Also during chronic administration, the synthesis of the endogenous peptides diminishes although as long as exogenous opiate is present, the consequences are minimal. However, when the exogenous opiate is withdrawn, receptor occupation drops, and demand for endogenous peptides dramatically increases. The abstinence syndrome therefore is due to reduced receptor occupation in combination with decoupling from G proteins, plus an increased but unmet demand for endogenous peptide. Duration of abstinence is determined by rate of recoupling of the receptors to G protein and restoration of peptide biosynthesis.

Role of Adenylyl Cyclase

Using neuroblastoma–glioma hybrid cells (NG 108-15), Sharma, Klee, and Nirenberg (1975; Sharma, Nirenberg,

and Klee, 1975) demonstrated significant changes in the cells' cAMP-generating system during chronic opioid exposure, which provided empirical support for Himmelsbach's original notion of tolerance and dependence. In these cells, acute administration of morphine inhibited prostaglandin E_1-stimulated adenylyl cyclase in a naloxone-reversible manner. However, when the cells were maintained for 2 days in the presence of morphine, they demonstrated tolerance to the acute inhibitory effect of morphine and had levels of cAMP equal to those in control cells. When the opiate was abruptly removed from the cell culture medium or naloxone was added, the concentration of cAMP rose significantly above control levels. This rebound in cAMP levels is considered to correspond to the withdrawal phenomena. Changes in cAMP levels under these conditions can be seen in Figure 12.17.

Collier and Roy (1974) were among the first to investigate opiate action on cAMP using brain cell homogenates. They characterized the enzyme activity and concluded that in response to the chronic inhibition of adenylyl cyclase by morphine, the cAMP generating system within the opioid neuron is up-regulated (Collier, 1984). Further behavioral evidence also implicated cAMP in opioid tolerance and withdrawal. They found that drugs that increase cAMP enhance morphine withdrawal symptoms. Administration of any one of a number of chemically diverse compounds that inhibit cAMP phosphodiesterase, thus increasing cAMP, produced a morphine-like withdrawal syndrome (Collier et al., 1981). The effectiveness of the drugs in producing the syndrome was correlated with their ability to inhibit the phosphodiesterase. Other evidence shows that reduced cAMP degradation by phosphodiesterase occurs in NG 108-15 cells that are chronically treated with opioids and other ligands that inhibit adenylyl cyclase (Thomas, Vagelos, and Hoffman, 1990). This reduction in cAMP breakdown may contribute to the apparent development

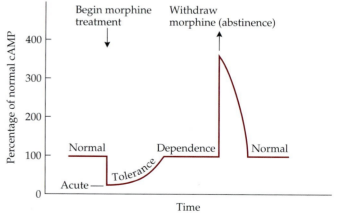

12.17 MORPHINE-INDUCED EFFECTS ON cAMP. Changes in cAMP levels in cultured cells during acute morphine administration, tolerance, and withdrawal of the drug. (After Sharma, Klee, and Nirenberg, 1975.)

of tolerance to the initial inhibitory effects of opioids on cAMP production.

cAMP in the locus coeruleus.

Nestler, Alreja, and Aghajanian (1994) elaborated on earlier results and developed a model of addiction based on biochemical and electrophysiological evidence accumulated from studies in the locus coeruleus (LC). The LC is used as a model system because, as a large cluster of norepinephrine cell bodies, it is a relatively homogeneous brain area that has been well characterized anatomically and electrophysiologically. In addition, the LC has been implicated in the development of physical dependence and withdrawal (see above).

The acute effect of opioids acting at μ-receptors on LC neurons is hyperpolarization and subsequent reduction in rate of firing. This reduced rate of firing is due to both the opening of K^+ channels producing hyperpolarization and the inhibition of slow depolarization due to supressed Na^+ channel opening. These actions both require G protein mediation. However, G proteins can act directly on K^+ channels while inhibition of cAMP and cAMP-dependent protein kinase is required for the opioid action on the Na^+ channels. Repeated exposure to opiates leads to a gradual increase in firing rates of the LC cells as tolerance develops. Administration of an opiate antagonist after chronic opiate treatment induces a significant rise in firing rate to levels well above pretreatment controls, reflecting a rebound withdrawal syndrome.

Many research groups have shown that chronic opioids up-regulate the cAMP system at several points (e.g., increases in adenylyl cyclase, cAMP-dependent protein kinase, and several morphine- and cAMP-regulated phosphoproteins). Since increased cAMP enhances excitability of the cells by activating protein kinase, which increases inward Na^+ current, it was proposed that the second messenger system is responsible for the excitability of LC neurons and is the neurochemical basis for tolerance, dependence, and withdrawal.

The importance of cAMP to neuronal excitation and behavioral manifestations of withdrawal is demonstrated by the parallel time course of changes in the three factors (Rasmussen et al., 1990; Figure 12.18). Naltrexone-induced withdrawal produces behavioral signs (Figure 12.18*a*) and increases in LC neuron firing rates (Figure 12.18*b*), which rise dramatically and peak within 15 to 30 minutes and decrease rapidly over the first 2 to 4 hours, remaining at that level for a 24-hour period before falling gradually to baseline levels by 72 hours. The activities of adenylyl cyclase (Figure 12.18*c*) and cAMP-dependent protein kinase (Figure 12.18*d*) are high before treatment with naltrexone, a characteristic of chronic opiate use. Following antagonist treatment, their increased activity is only temporally related to the first phase of withdrawal, and then decreases over a 6-hour

period and essentially returns to control levels by the end of that time. The authors propose that the increase in the cAMP system occurs during chronic administration of the opiate, but does not manifest itself in behavioral symptoms due to inhibitory actions of exogenous opiate. Upon withdrawal of the drug, the uninhibited cAMP system produces increased electrical activity and behavioral withdrawal signs that diminish with time. This up-regulation of cAMP systems has been noted in several other brain areas in addition to the LC, including dorsal horn of the spinal cord, nucleus accumbens, amygdala, and thalamus, implying that opiate-sensitive neurons in different brain regions may utilize common mechanisms.

Expanding the original hypothesis, Nestler (1992) summarized evidence showing that chronic opiate use may alter gene expression. Altered gene expression would lead to changes in the amounts of both mRNA, and specific proteins that are responsible for the intracellular adaptations described earlier. Testing this idea, Guitart and coworkers (1992) examined the CREB (cAMP-response element binding protein) which is responsible for stimulating the expression of particular genes. They found that both the total amount of CREB and the extent of phosphorylation of the protein changes during chronic drug use. Whereas acute morphine decreases the phosphorylation of CREB protein in LC, tolerance occurs in such a manner that the extent of phosphorylation gradually increases toward control levels while withdrawal significantly enhances phosphorylation of the protein.

Aspects of gene expression other than CREB also have been evaluated in order to find the cell mechanisms responsible for the opioid-induced changes in cAMP-system components. For example, chronic morphine has been shown to increase the mRNAs for cAMP-dependent protein kinase (catalytic subunit), tyrosine hydroxylase, and others. Also under investigation is the family of transcription factors (*c-fos*, *c-jun*, and related immediate–early genes; see Chapter 6) that mediate the effects of extracellular stimulation on neuronal gene expression (see Morgan and Curran, 1991; Nestler, Alreja, and Aghajanian, 1994; Morris and Johnston, 1995). However, specific functional consequences of any changes found in these factors are not yet known.

Mesolimbic adenylyl cyclase.

Opioid-induced changes in the mesolimbic system may also contribute to tolerance, dependence, and withdrawal. Evidence from numerous sources implicates the mesolimbic DA pathway in opioid euphoria and reinforcement (see previous discussion), as well as in reinforcement of other drugs. Since the rebound withdrawal during abstinence from opiates includes dysphoria and feelings of craving, it is reasonable to investigate the chronic changes that occur in the dopaminergic reward pathway.

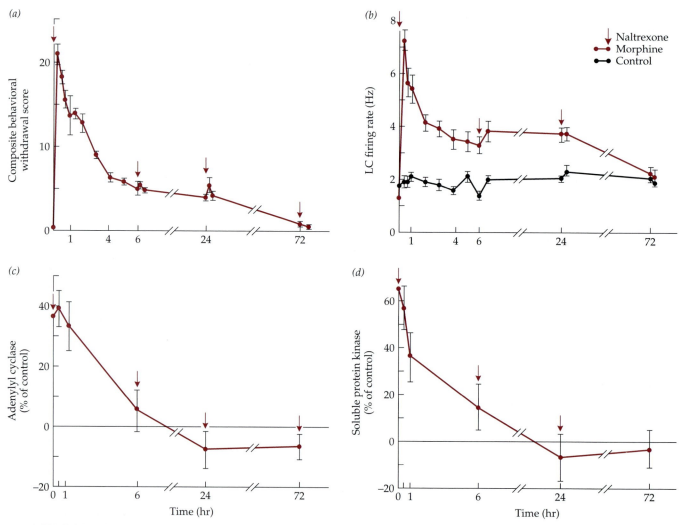

12.18 TIME COURSE OF ABSTINENCE BEHAVIORS, LC FIRING RATE, ADENYLYL CYCLASE ACTIVITY, AND PROTEIN KINASE ACTIVITY DURING OPIATE WITHDRAWAL. After 5 days of morphine treatment, some animals were sacrificed without naltrexone administration (controls) while the remainder received naltrexone at time 0 (see arrows). Behavioral and biochemical measures were made at each time point (0, 20 minutes, 1 hour, or 6 hours). Some animals received a second naltrexone injection at 6 hours and were tested at 24 hours; others received 2 additional naltrexone treatments at 6 and 24 hours and were tested at 72 hours. The withdrawal score is a composite of 14 abstinence behaviors. LC firing rate was evaluated by single-unit recording and presented as mean firing rates of 10 to 40 neurons (taken from 2–4 rats) at each time point. Forskolin-stimulated adenylyl cyclase activity and protein kinase activity were assayed in LC tissue preparations taken from control and naltrexone treated animals. (After Rasmussen et al., 1990.)

Acute opiate administration increases cell firing in the VTA and stimulates DA release in the NA by inhibiting inhibitory GABA influence on the dopaminergic cells (see above). Following chronic drug treatment, opiate withdrawal produces a significant decrease in DA release as measured by microdialysis in the NA (Rossetti, Hmaidan, and Gessa, 1992). Furthermore, Harris and Aston-Jones (1994) report that D_2 dopamine receptor activation within the NA prevents somatic signs of naloxone-induced opiate withdrawal and that blockade of the D_2 receptors in opiate-dependent animals elicits somatic withdrawal symptoms. In addition, firing rate and burst firing of VTA–NA neurons are reduced to about 30% of normal rates during the opiate withdrawal syndrome, an effect readily reversed by administration of morphine (Diana et al., 1995). The prolonged relative refractory periods observed suggest that the membrane machinery controlling ion channel kinetics may be altered by chronic drug treatment. Ion channel function can be regulated by protein phosphorylation under the control of intracellular second messengers.

The changes found in second messenger mechanisms after either chronic morphine or chronic cocaine exposure include a reduction in inhibitory G protein and an increase in adenylyl cyclase and cAMP-dependent protein kinase activity in the NA. Drugs with no reinforcement value do not produce these same changes. It is particularly interesting that one inbred strain of rats (Lewis rats) that demonstrates high levels of self-administration of several abused substances (e.g., morphine, cocaine, and alcohol) also shows a pattern of postreceptor neurochemistry that is similar to that found in animals after chronic drug use. The Lewis rats have low levels of G_i, high adenylyl cyclase and cAMP-dependent protein kinase activity, and low levels of tyrosine hydroxylase when compared with rat strains that show a lower preference for the drugs (Beitner-Johnson, Guitart, and Nestler, 1991). Moreover, these neurochemical differences occurred in drug-naive animals, indicating that naive drug-preferring rats have neurochemical differences that resemble the changes seen in drug-dependent rats, perhaps reflecting a common neuronal substrate for craving or desire.

In summary, increased adenylyl cyclase activity is associated with opioid withdrawal in some CNS neurons. Changes in the coupling between the enzyme and inhibitory G protein may be a significant contributor to this phenomenon. Increased adenylyl cyclase activity enhances the phosphorylation of neuronal proteins by cAMP-dependent protein kinase, and in this way may show adaptation to chronic opioid inhibition and withdrawal once abstinence occurs. The locus coeruleus provides an excellent model system for the investigation of the cellular basis of tolerance and physical dependence, while altered mesolimbic dopamine function may contribute to the dysphoria and cravings that are characteristic of psychological dependence.

Behavioral Mechanisms of Tolerance and Dependence

Despite the present emphasis on the physiological basis for tolerance and dependence, other investigators have identified a behavioral conditioning component of the phenomena. Wikler's (1980) classic model of substance dependence, utilizing principles of both operant and classical conditioning, provides a framework for evaluating the social and behavioral factors that regulate drug-seeking behavior. The initial drug-taking behavior, encouraged by peer pressure and social reinforcement, is soon established by the primary reinforcing effects of the drug (e.g., euphoria and relief of stress). Positive reinforcement following opiate use leads to an increased probability of drug-taking behavior in the future. For the opiates, chronic use leads to a diminished response (tolerance) to the reinforcing psychotropic effects (euphoria), thus encouraging subsequent escalation of dosage or change in route of administration (e.g., intravenous administration) to restore the magnitude of reinforcement.

As opiate use continues on a chronic basis, physical dependence develops. When blood levels of drug fall, withdrawal symptoms provide strong motivation to resume opiate use. Drug-taking to alleviate the withdrawal syndrome becomes a negative reinforcer (i.e., the probability of the behavior occurring increases because an aversive event is terminated by the behavior). This negative reinforcement in combination with the primary reinforcing properties of the drug itself provide a strong motivation for continued opiate use.

Environmental factors classically conditioned to components of the drug experience provide additional strengthening of drug abuse behavior. Features in the drug-taking environment become associated with the cycle of abstinence–withdrawal–drug-taking behavior, so that a detoxified addict experiences drug craving and associated withdrawal symptoms merely by being in the original drug-taking environment. These environmental stimuli become secondary reinforcers (or conditioned reinforcers) and, as such, encourage drug-taking behavior even in the absence of withdrawal symptoms.

Conditioning experiments provide insight into how the drug-using subculture, with its camaraderie, drug-taking rituals, and drug-acquisition procedures, becomes a potent secondary reinforcer to the ongoing drug-taking behavior. As shown for animals pressing a lever for food in an operant chamber, a light previously paired with food reinforcement will significantly slow the rate of extinction when the primary reinforcer is withheld. Many aspects of drug-taking behavior (e.g., membership in a group, peer acceptance, and new status) act like operant chamber lights and are in themselves reinforcing, apart from the primary reinforcement of the drug. Classic animal studies have shown that acute drug effects, withdrawal symptoms, and relief of withdrawal symptoms can each be conditioned to environmental stimuli (Roffman, Reddy, and Lal, 1972; Wikler, 1973).

Roffman, Reddy, and Lal (1972) found that after repeated pairing of morphine injection and the ringing of a bell during the development of physical dependence, the sound of the bell alone was sufficient to prevent withdrawal hypothermia after the cessation of morphine injection. These results may explain why the various rituals and procedures of drug procurement and use may elicit reinforcing effects similar to those of the drug itself. An example of this phenomenon is the "needle freak" who by the act of injection alone or the injection of pharmacologically inert substances derives significant reinforcement.

Abstinence symptoms can likewise be classically conditioned (Figure 12.19). Goldberg and Schuster (1967) trained morphine-dependent monkeys to respond for food reinforcement. During the food reinforcement sessions, a buzzer was presented and was followed by an intravenous injection of nalorphine (an opiate antagonist), which produced withdrawal symptoms. After several pairings, the buzzer alone elicited the signs of withdrawal (salivation, emesis, change in heart rate, and suppression of responding). These conditioned with-

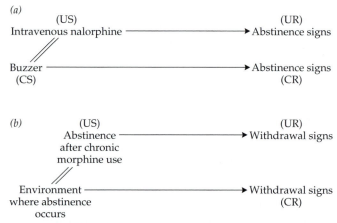

(a)

(US)   (UR)
Intravenous nalorphine ——————————→ Abstinence signs

Buzzer ————————————————————→ Abstinence signs
(CS)   (CR)

(b)   (US)   (UR)
Abstinence ——————————→ Withdrawal signs
after chronic
morphine use

Environment ——————————————→ Withdrawal signs
where abstinence   (CR)
occurs

12.19 CLASSICAL CONDITIONING MODEL to explain conditioned abstinence and the tendency to relapse. In the upper panel, the previously neutral stimulus (buzzer) regularly precedes the administration of intravenous nalorphine (US) which elicits abstinence signs (UR). After several pairings, the neutral stimulus becomes closely associated with the US, and presentation of the buzzer alone (now a CS) without the nalorphine precipitates signs of withdrawal (CR). The lower panel shows how an addict who repeatedly experiences abstinence in a particular environment may show withdrawal signs on returning to that environment, even when he is in a detoxified state.

drawal signs could be elicited for up to 4 months after the withdrawal of morphine.

In other experiments, detoxified rats showed an increase in withdrawal "wet-dog" shakes when returned to a cage where they had undergone morphine withdrawal several months earlier (Wikler, 1973).

In humans, both objective (respiration rate, skin temperature, heart rate) and subjective elements of narcotic withdrawal symptoms can be experimentally conditioned to environmental stimuli (Childress, McLellan, and O'Brien, 1986). This empirical evidence is in direct support of the clinical reports that former addicts experience withdrawal symptoms when they visit areas of prior drug use (O'Brien, 1993). The high relapse rate among detoxified addicts may then in part be due to the conditioned abstinence syndrome in the old environment. The importance of environment to relapse rate among addicts has led to the conclusion that detoxified addicts should not return to their original neighborhoods (Gold, 1989). Because the importance of classical and operant conditioning to drug-seeking behavior has been demonstrated repeatedly, application of these principles to drug treatment programs should be emphasized.

Conditioning theory has also been applied to the development of opiate tolerance. Some aspects of tolerance cannot be fully attributed to drug exposure but involve learning processes. Siegel (1975, 1989) and others (Tiffany, Drobes, and Cepeda-Benito, 1992) propose that narcotic tolerance is the result of the learning of an association between the systemic effects of the drug and those environmental cues that reliably precede the drug effects. Several experiments have shown that the antici-

patory response of the animal, which occurs when it experiences the administration procedure without the active drug, is compensatory in nature (see Chapter 1). Thus, it is argued that tolerance to the analgesic effects of morphine results because environmental cues regularly paired with drug administration begin to elicit the compensatory response (hyperalgesia), which algebraically sums with the stable effects of morphine. With longer drug administration, the association between environment and hyperalgesia become stronger, leading to the appearance of tolerance.

The importance of environment is dramatized in a series of experiments (Siegel, 1976) in which rats were made tolerant to morphine in one of two distinct environments (colony room or experimental room where white noise was a constant background). Tolerance to morphine-induced analgesia was demonstrated by those rats tested in the same environment in which they previously received morphine, but not in the alternate room.

Using the same reasoning, morphine tolerance should be retarded by the administration of the drug in the absence of environmental cues. To test this hypothesis, rats were exposed both to morphine and to an environmental cue (overhead illumination) before analgesia testing with a hot plate (Siegel et al., 1981). Although both groups received the same number of morphine treatments, in the control group, the light and morphine were paired. In the experimental group, the cue signaled a drug-free period. Both groups were subsequently administered morphine in the presence of the cue and the amount of analgesic tolerance was measured. Although both groups demonstrated increasing analgesic tolerance over the test sessions, the rate of development of tolerance was significantly slower in the experimental (unpaired) group. Thus an animal's experiences with environmental cues associated with the drugged state contribute significantly to the appearance of tolerance. Others have shown that drug administration cues themselves may gain associative control over morphine tolerance (Cepeda-Benito and Tiffany, 1992).

Some evidence suggests that both associative and nonassociative processes contribute to the development of morphine tolerance (Tiffany, Drobes, and Cepeda-Benito, 1992). In this series of experiments, the characteristics of associative tolerance (i.e., tolerance that is environment dependent) were examined. The researchers found that tolerance to morphine's analgesic effect develops in animals that have the drug explicitly paired with a distinctive context when the drug is administered with interdose intervals ranging from 12–96 hours. This associative tolerance persisted for more than 30 days after the first test. In contrast, when morphine was administered at 6-hour interdose intervals, association with the environmental cues apparently had no detectable influence on tolerance development. Whether animals received morphine in the distinctive environment or in their home cages during the tolerance development phase, there was a shift in the dose–response curve similar to that seen in saline controls. This type of tolerance was relatively short-lived and was not detected 30 days after the first test. Such research helps to clarify the parameters that lead to the development of tolerance in an organism and define the conditions that identify associative and nonassociative processes relevant to this phenomenon.

Modes of Treatment for Opiate Dependence

Treatment programs are designed with the knowledge that the addict population is a very heterogeneous one and most addicts abuse multiple drugs. Among narcotics users there is a diverse pattern of drug use, and the conditions for initiating drug-taking behavior and reasons for relapse vary widely. Just as there has been no way to predict which individual within a given group will become addicted, there is no reliable way to predict which types of narcotics users will respond to the various modes of treatment. On the whole, it has been found (Meyer, 1972) that older addicts do better in most treatments than do younger addicts. Also, as might be expected, addicts having employment skills and job experience and having little criminal history show more improvement than do other groups.

Detoxification

Unassisted detoxification or "cold turkey" refers to the termination of drug use in an addicted individual without pharmacological intervention to reduce withdrawal symptoms. Drug abusers often experience some portion of the abstinence syndrome on a regular basis because heroin blocks withdrawal for about 4–8 hours and drug availability may not match this schedule of withdrawal.

Alternatively, detoxification may be assisted by the administration of any one of a number of relatively long acting opiate drugs, such as methadone, which reduces the symptoms to a comfortable level. This dose is gradually reduced over the subsequent 5–7 days, depending on the original dose.

Moreover, several nonopioid drugs can be used to partially reduce some of the symptoms of abstinence. One such drug is the antihypertensive medication clonidine. Clonidine is an α_2-adrenergic agonist that acts on norepinephrine autoreceptors to reduce central adrenergic activity. Since the norepinephrine neurons in the locus coeruleus are inhibited by opiates and the cells increase firing during withdrawal, clonidine-induced inhibition of firing reverses this hyperexcitable state to some extent. Clonidine seems most effective at relieving chills, lacrimation, yawning, stomach cramps, sweating, and muscular aches, although some of the symptoms still occur during the peak withdrawal. In addition, clonidine-induced side effects include insomnia, dry mouth, sedation, bone and joint pain, fainting, and hypotension, and so the drug works best in well-motivated opiate users who are willing to tolerate some unpleasant symptoms. However, there is evidence to suggest that addicts may reject clonidine detoxification because of its residual physiological effects and the subjective discomfort and craving that are not ameliorated by the drug (Gold, 1989; O'Brien, 1993).

Treatment Goals

The three principal treatment modalities include (1) psychological treatment, (2) pharmacological support, and (3) enforced treatment. In general, the highly idealistic goals of any treatment program are to help narcotic addicts to become emotionally mature, law-abiding, and productive members of society who require no drugs or medical or social support to maintain such behavior. Clearly, these goals are rarely achieved with any treatment program, so improvement in these areas is used as a measure of success. The particular criteria chosen for improvement and emphasis by a given treatment center play a critical part in measuring the program's success. For example, advocates of incarceration and forced abstinence claim high rates of success because the method is an effective means of detoxifying the addict and reducing criminal activities throughout the duration of "treatment." However, the method by itself does not meet the rehabilitative goals of treatment, such as increased employment, social responsibility, improved self-esteem, and so forth, and relapse rates can be extremely high when such extreme methods are used.

Brill and Lieberman (1969; Lieberman and Brill, 1972), however, have emphasized the need to use "rational authority" in drug addiction programs. Rational authority is authority not intended as a punitive end in itself but as a means to ensure a durable relationship with the addict; that is, to hold unmotivated addicts in a sustained treatment program. Addicts tend to be impulsive and easily frustrated and come from groups that have high delinquency rates. Brill and Lieberman proposed that a graduated series of sanctions be offered to the addict, giving him more responsibility and minimizing the addict's "acting out." Such control helps him to conform to socially acceptable standards and ultimately to internalize the controls he lacks. Most often the rational authority is wielded in conjunction with parole and the threat of a return to prison. Some element of authority has been found necessary in most treatment modalities, although the control may be chemical, custodial, or autocratic, as in the case of the therapeutic community (Meyer, 1972).

Drug Abuse Treatment Programs

Methadone maintenance. Of the pharmacological support methods, the most popular is the methadone maintenance program originally developed by Dole and Nyswander (1965). They propose to make addicts more amenable to rehabilitative efforts by providing pharmacological relief for narcotic craving. By relieving craving, the patient is able to redirect his efforts toward productive activities rather than toward securing drugs to prevent withdrawal. Their program goals include not only elimination of illegal drug use, but also reduction of disease associated with unsterile injection equipment. Furthermore, they aim toward improving socialization and productivity while reducing the need for criminal activity. The underlying philosophy of methadone maintenance programs assumes that protracted and perhaps irreversible metabolic changes exist in opiate addicts and that the use of methadone provides a prolonged maintenance treatment (Langrod et al., 1972).

Methadone is a synthetic narcotic analgesic that has pharmacological effects qualitatively similar to those of morphine. It can substitute for morphine or any other opiate and prevent withdrawal; that is, there is cross-dependence between methadone and the other opiates. The dose of methadone used for maintenance is one that is high enough to relieve craving and prevent withdrawal symptoms, but not high enough to produce euphoria or sedation. Methadone is considered medically safe even with long-term use, and does not interfere with daily activities such as working, attending school, or taking care of a family. However, tolerance to some of its actions is incomplete, so the side effects such as constipation, excessive sweating, decreased sex drive, and sexual dysfunction persist during treatment for some individuals.

Although it is pharmacologically similar to morphine, oral methadone has only mild euphoric actions. Also, in sufficient doses, methadone will prevent or reduce heroin-induced euphoria because of the cross-tolerance between heroin and methadone. The reduced euphoria decreases the probability of repeated heroin use. The euphoria "blockade," however, can be overcome by large doses of heroin because a high concentration of heroin can effectively compete with methadone for the opiate receptors. Furthermore, methadone itself can, if administered intravenously, produce a "rush" of euphoria (Lennard, Epstein, and Rosenthal, 1972), and in those programs in which methadone is self-administered at home, a significant amount of abuse occurs.

Methadone has the advantage of being pharmacologically effective when given orally. Oral administration reduces the use of the needle by the addict and the ritual surrounding its use. In addition, oral administration alleviates the danger of disease due to unsterile injection techniques. The incidence of infectious diseases, including hepatitis B, hepatitis δ, and HIV, among this population is reduced by eliminating the need to share contaminated needles. Furthermore, methadone is longer-lasting than most opiates, so that over a 24-hour period a more constant blood level is achieved. A more stable blood level means that the extremes of drug effect are avoided and greater stability is afforded. Additionally, the stable blood levels of methadone seem to normalize

neuroendocrine function in this population. Particularly important is the restoration of the hypothalamic–pituitary–adrenal function improving the physiological response to stress and the hypothalamic–pituitary–gonadal function central to normal reproductive behavior (Kreek, 1991). Immunological functions are also restored to previous levels. The long half-life also means that the drug needs to be administered only once a day to prevent withdrawal symptoms and craving for 24–36 hours.

One significant problem with methadone use is that methadone, like all opiates, is addictive, and withdrawal symptoms occur with abrupt abstinence. However, because the drug is long acting, withdrawal symptoms are comparatively mild, though longer-lasting, than those following morphine withdrawal. Critics of the methadone program claim that at the high doses of methadone required, abstinence can produce quite intense withdrawal symptoms (Lennard, Epstein, and Rosenthal, 1972).

In contrast, advocates of the program suggest that methadone dependence is actually beneficial because it provides an essential control mechanism, allowing repeated interaction with the clinical staff who can provide many forms of therapy, such as behavioral and occupational therapy, group and family counseling, and individual psychotherapy (O'Brien, 1993). In addition, methadone clinics are prepared to treat medical problems previously left untreated. The daily return to the clinic for methadone may be particularly significant for female addicts who are pregnant and who are provided with the prenatal obstetrical care that they normally would not receive. A methadone program with massive psychological support has been reported to alleviate many of the common maternal problems associated with addiction in pregnancy, such as syphilis and hepatitis. However, neither the high incidence of lower birth weight in infants nor the sometimes severe infant withdrawal signs, including CNS hyperactivity (tremors, irritability, twitching, seizures) and gastrointestinal disturbances (vomiting, diarrhea, poor feeding), is prevented by maintenance on methadone.

Since the establishment of the pilot programs in the 1960s, more methadone centers have opened, although not at a rate that keeps pace with need. Furthermore, demands on the staff have increased over time because of the high incidence of polydrug use and multiple chemical dependency on alcohol and cocaine. A higher percentage of abusers entering the program are more disturbed and less motivated. Nevertheless, benefits seem to outweigh costs. In general, patients show reductions in criminal activity, decreases in drug use, and fewer psychological symptoms such as depression (Jaffee, 1987). The percentage of patients who remain abstinent for 1–3 years after withdrawal of methadone varies dramatically, ranging from 10% to 12% abstinence among those dropped from the program to 80% success among those who elected to terminate with consensus by the clinical staff. One study conducting a 6-year follow-up found 40% of former methadone patients were abstinent from opioids and free of other drug problems (Simpson et al., 1982). Among polydrug abusers, recidivism may be between 70% and 80% within 1–2 years after leaving treatment (Kreek, 1991). For that reason, prolonged (1–2 years) involvement with the program, including counseling and rehabilitation, is advocated, and continued methadone maintenance beyond that time in a general medical setting is suggested (Dole, 1988; Novick et al., 1988).

Of the available treatment methods, methadone maintenance is considered far more acceptable to drug abusers than the alternative therapeutic approaches (Meyer, 1972). Voluntary participation in long-term methadone maintenance treatment ranges from 40% to 60% of eligible addicts, and voluntary retention rates in the program for more than 2 years are estimated to be between 45% and 85% (Ball and Corty, 1988). Since success depends in no small part on the individual's motivation and effort, acceptance of the treatment program is an important factor. However, many have questioned whether the prolonged administration of a potent psychotropic drug is in fact reinforcing the illusion that any drug can be "a fast, cheap, and magical answer to complex human and social problems" (Lennard, Epstein, and Rosenthal, 1972).

Therapy with narcotic antagonists.   An alternative pharmacological therapy is the use of a specific narcotic antagonist like naloxone, naltrexone, or cyclazocine following detoxification. Given to a nondetoxified drug user, the antagonists cause abrupt onset of withdrawal symptoms and discourage further participation in the program. After detoxification, the antagonists block the reinforcing effects of opiates.

The pure antagonist **naloxone** lacks agonist activity and has a short duration of action. These characteristics make it suitable for reversing potentially lethal respiratory depression following opiate overdose. However, its short duration of action makes it less useful for addiction programs, where frequently supervised drug administration becomes unwieldy. **Cyclazocine** is a longer-acting antagonist but produces both analgesia and respiratory depression. Further, the drug may produce irritability, psychotomimetic symptoms including delusions and hallucinations, and motor incoordination. Withdrawal from this drug frequently leads to periods of weakness and loss of environmental contact. For these reasons, despite its ability to block opiate-induced euphoria, cyclazocine has been replaced by naltrexone.

Naltrexone, a μ-receptor antagonist, is most commonly used because of its relatively long duration of action and its minimal side effects. It is considered a medically safe drug with a large therapeutic index. The drug is effective given orally and is almost completely ab-sorbed from the gastrointestinal tract. Steady state plasma levels are rapidly reached, and no increase in dose is required. Once antagonist treatment has begun, use of heroin or other opiate agonists produces few or no effects. The blockade of subjective heroin-induced effects, such as euphoria, is directly correlated with naltrexone plasma levels. Therefore, it is possible to identify the dose needed for 100% blockade in individual patients (see Gold, 1989). Opiate use decreases rapidly under these conditions. However, if antagonist use is stopped, resumption of opiate use often occurs.

Because a good deal of motivation is needed to voluntarily substitute an antagonist for a drug with highly reinforcing properties, this treatment modality is not a preferred method among addicts and perhaps appeals to only 10% of the addicted population (O'Brien, 1993). Compliance is lowest among addicts having minimal occupational skills and poor social support. With this population, external motivation (e.g., threat of prison) is needed to initiate antagonist treatment. For those addicts who are highly motivated, have strong family support, and are involved in careers (e.g., addicted medical personnel), compliance is higher and dropout rates are much lower. As many as 70% remain abstinent 1 year later (Washton, Gold, and Pottash, 1984). Reliable patients have taken naltrexone for 5 to 10 years without relapse to drug-taking behavior and with minimal side effects on appetite, sexual behavior, or endocrine function (O'Brien, 1993).

The use of the narcotic antagonists in the treatment of addiction is based on the rationale that the compulsive drug abuser has acquired a complex set of operantly and classically conditioned responses that both perpetuate his drug-taking behavior and make relapse after detoxification highly probable. The antagonist, by binding to the opiate receptor site but having little or no activity, will block the reinforcing properties of the opiate. Under these conditions, extinction of the response should occur. That is, when reinforcement is stopped, the drug-taking behavior should gradually stop.

To test the operant hypothesis, one study (McLellan and Childress, 1985) attempted to enhance the extinction of conditioned stimuli by having patients who were receiving naltrexone act through the sequence of drug preparation steps and subsequently self-inject saline. Under these conditions the withdrawal response was severe and the craving was so great that the test was discontinued. In a later study a gradual reduction in conditioned craving was achieved in a significant number of addicts by using less potent conditioned stimuli and greater psychological support. Because of the nature of the extinction process, the antagonist administration is best for those addicts with a short drug reinforcement history.

Long-term antagonist use has potential ramifications regarding endogenous opioid systems. Chronic naltrexone elevates plasma and CSF levels of selected endogenous opioids, suggesting an increased release in response to receptor blockade (O'Brien, 1993). Also, long-term, but not acute, antagonist administration increases opiate receptors (particularly μ and δ) and results in enhanced morphine-induced analgesia (see Zukin et al., 1993). Despite these changes, no apparent risk of overdose exists for patients terminating naltrexone and resuming opiate use, perhaps because of rapid restoration of normal physiological function.

Further preclinical evaluation of opiate receptor subtypes and their relationships to reinforcement, subjective effects, tolerance, and dependence may in the future provide highly selective and maximally effective antagonists useful in addiction programs.

Psychological treatment programs.   Among the various psychological treatment programs, traditional psychotherapy is generally considered to be the least successful unless it is teamed with other methods. A second type is "self-help" or "communal" therapy, which includes residence programs like Synanon, Day Top, Horizon House, and others (Brill and Lieberman, 1969; Cherkas, 1965). These programs are run almost entirely by former addicts and are based on the belief that their "extended family" members are able to stay drug-free because of membership in the group. Criticism by the group and banishment from the unit are the primary means of punishment and social control.

The addict must demonstrate sufficient motivation to enter the group by undergoing a sometimes traumatic first interview in which he is confronted with his own weakness by the successful ex-addicts. Once accepted into the group, he must stop all use of drugs "cold turkey" (i.e., without pharmacological aid), but with a large amount of emotional support. Undergoing unassisted withdrawal may be a second test of the abuser's motivation. Such nonmedical treatment programs usually have a philosophical aversion to pharmacological intervention. They believe that all drug use is bad and that drug-assisted detoxification prolongs the addict's reliance on drugs and encourages the erroneous belief that drugs reduce problems. Such an attitude may also prohibit drug treatment for other psychiatric conditions such as depression or bipolar disorder.

The program provides basic living needs, including medical care, and strives to understand the addict and help him find need-satisfying roles in a drug-free community. Intensive group therapy and self-appraisal sessions are held regularly for this purpose. Drug abusers in this setting find that their previous patterns of behavior, their values, and their expectations are vehemently rejected. The reward for conformity is acceptance by the group. The original programs were based on the idea that the addicts would not leave the residence unit permanently, but would provide support and services for others within the group or in a similar group elsewhere. More commonly, a 6-to-12 month treatment program is advocated, with a gradual reintroduction to work and a normal environment. However, the cost of such programs often precludes a lengthy treatment period and a 1-month program is now most common (O'Brien, 1993). Such abstinence-oriented rehabilitation programs have a high recidivism rate but are a viable option for the highly motivated addict who is not suffering from other psychiatric disorders.

Part IV Summary

Opiate dependence and abuse remains a complex biopsychosocial problem that defies simple answers. Opiates clearly have potent reinforcing properties, which are evident in several research paradigms using a variety of species. The reinforcement value of opiates is apparently related to their ability to modify DA function in the VTA–NA pathway, and long-term changes in that system may be responsible for withdrawal-induced dysphoria and craving. The locus coeruleus provides a model system to study the cellular basis for tolerance and dependence, which may exclude changes in opioid peptide synthesis, changes in receptor number, desensitization and G protein uncoupling, or changes in the components of the cAMP second messenger system. Combining our knowledge of the neurochemical characteristics of tolerance and dependence with what we know about contributing behavioral and environmental factors provides the basis for effective drug abuse treatment strategies.

Chapter 13

Stimulants: Amphetamine and Cocaine

Stimulants are drugs that increase alertness, heighten arousal, and cause behavioral excitement. The most potent of these drugs are amphetamine, cocaine, and related compounds, which together are called **psychomotor stimulants**. As discussed in greater detail below, this term refers to the marked sensorimotor activation that occurs in response to drug administration. Considering the widespread illicit use of cocaine, amphetamines, and the legal stimulants discussed in Chapter 14, it is apparent that the effects of stimulant drugs are highly prized in most human cultures. In this chapter, we shall consider the behavioral and physiological effects of amphetamine and cocaine, their mechanisms of action, and their potential for producing abuse and dependence.

Part I
Amphetamine

Amphetamine is the common name for β-phenylisopropylamine (see structure on page 295). Two stereoisomeric forms of amphetamine exist: D-amphetamine (dextroamphetamine; trade name Dexedrine), and L-amphetamine (levoamphetamine). D-amphetamine is more potent than L-amphetamine in producing most of the behavioral effects we will be discussing. The term D,L-amphetamine (trade name Benzedrine) refers to the **racemic mixture**, meaning that the D- and L-isomers are present together in equal amounts. Methamphetamine (trade names Methedrine and Desoxyn) is a potent analog of amphetamine that will also be discussed below. Readers interested in more detailed information concerning structure–activity relationships within the family of amphetamine-like compounds are referred to the review by Biel and Bopp (1978).

Amphetamine is structurally related to several naturally occurring plant compounds, one of which is called cathinone. Cathinone is the principal ac-

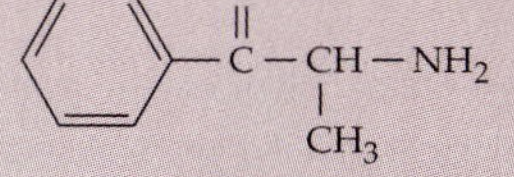

Cathinone

tive ingredient in khat (*Catha edulis;* alternatively spelled qat), an evergreen shrub native to East Africa and the Arabian peninsula (Karch, 1993). Khat was unknown to most Americans until 1992, when the troops sent to provide humanitarian aid to Somalia encountered young Somali soldiers chewing khat leaves for their energizing properties. The psychostimulant effects of cathinone can be readily appreciated by comparing its chemical structure to that of amphetamine. Indeed, recent reports indicate that cathinone is being

549

manufactured illegally in the United States and sold on the street as an alternative to amphetamine or methamphetamine.

A second amphetamine-like compound is ephedrine, which comes from the herb *Ephedra vulgaris*. Chinese

Ephedrine

physicians have used *Ephreda* (known to them as Ma Huang) for over 5,000 years as an herbal remedy. However, the properties of ephedrine were not appreciated in the West until the 1920s, when the drug was found to be useful as an antiasthmatic agent due to its powerful bronchodilator (widening of the airways) action. Many over-the-counter and prescription drugs marketed as decongestants still contain pseudoephedrine (an isomer of ephedrine) as their active ingredient.

As the popularity of ephedrine grew, the medical profession became concerned that demand for the drug might soon exceed its supply. Hence, investigators began to search for an appropriate synthetic substitute. That substitute turned out to be amphetamine, which had first been synthesized in 1887 by Edeleano. In 1932, the infamous Benzedrine inhaler was introduced by the Smith, Kline & French pharmaceutical company as a nasal and bronchial decongestant. The Benzedrine inhaler, which contained 250 mg of D,L-amphetamine sulfate in a cotton plug, proved to be effective in the temporary relief of nasal congestion. When used sparingly, there were relatively few side effects. Unfortunately, repeated dosing caused a rebound swelling, prompting more and more use of the device with an upward spiraling of symptoms. One of the authors (R.S.F.) recalls using a Benzedrine inhaler during insufferable bouts of pollen allergies before the advent of modern antihistamines. Due to the rebound effect described above, he escalated to a pattern of continuous dosing and began to experience hallucinatory episodes and other bizarre visual phenomena. The family physician had no explanation for these effects, nor did the author connect them with the trusted inhaler that he carried with him all the time.

The availability and use of amphetamine rapidly increased following the introduction of the Benzedrine inhaler (see Grinspoon and Hedblom, 1975). Inhalers were not only overused (many varieties could be purchased without prescription), but people soon learned to open the container and remove the drug-containing plug. Some individuals extracted the cotton to recover the amphetamine for injection purposes, while others simply chewed the cotton or even swallowed it whole! Amphetamine in tablet form was first marketed in 1935 as a treatment for the sleep disorder narcolepsy (see below). By the 1940s, amphetamine had become so widely embraced

by the medical profession that one author documented 39 supposed clinical uses for the drug (Bett, 1946). In addition, many American military personnel were given amphetamine to forestall sleep and maintain a heightened level of alertness during prolonged periods on duty. At the same time, methamphetamine was serving a similar purpose in the Japanese armed forces, and Japan consequently suffered a serious methamphetamine problem during the early postwar years (Suwaki, 1991).

After World War II, the United States likewise experienced a surge in the street use of amphetamine (Rawlin, 1968). During the 1950s and 1960s, students were casually using amphetamines to remain awake during preexam "all-nighters." Use of amphetamines was so common among long-haul truck drivers that the trucker subculture developed its own terminology for different drug preparations: a supply of "St. Louies" could get you halfway across the continent, whereas "West Coast turnabouts" were good for an entire transcontinental run. A further indication of amphetamine's acceptance by the general culture was the appearance of popular songs such as "Who Put the Benzedrine in Mrs. Murphy's Ovaltine." The peak of amphetamine use in the United States occurred during the early 1970s, when the legal production of amphetamine exceeded 10 billion tablets (Grinspoon and Hedblom, 1975), and at least one survey estimated that approximately 25% of young men had used stimulant drugs (mainly amphetamine or related compounds) on one or more occasions (Newmeyer, 1979). Since that time, amphetamine has lost popularity while being supplanted to a major degree by cocaine (see below). One exception to this trend has been a recent upsurge in methamphetamine use, primarily through smoking.

Basic Pharmacology of Amphetamine

Amphetamine is typically administered either orally or by intravenous or subcutaneous injection (the latter is sometimes called "skin popping"). Street names for amphetamine include "uppers," "bennies," "dexies," "black beauties," or "diet pills." Amphetamine is a weak base with a pK_a of approximately 9.9 (Mack and Bönisch, 1979). Consequently, absorption following oral consumption is slow because almost all of the drug is positively charged in the acidic environment of the stomach and is therefore prevented from passing across the membranes of the gastric mucosa. Nevertheless, effects are generally experienced within 30 minutes after a typical oral dose of 5–15 mg.

As would be expected, intravenous injection provides a much more rapid and more intense subjective reaction ("high") than oral consumption. Some amphetamine or methamphetamine users (called "speed freaks") go on binges of repeated intravenous injections to experience recurrent highs. Such "speed runs" can last many hours or even days. Yet another approach is to moderate the extreme stimulatory effect of intravenous amphetamine or methamphetamine by combining it with heroin to yield a so-called "speedball."

Methamphetamine is more potent than amphetamine in its CNS effects, and is therefore favored by substance abusers when available. Typical street names for

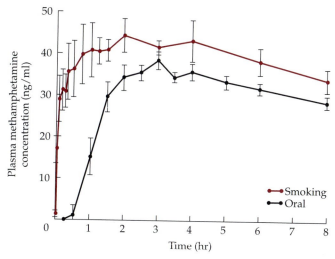

methamphetamine are "speed," "crystal," "crank," and "go." Besides being taken orally or by injection, methamphetamine can be smoked in either its hydrochloride or freebase form. Smoking can be accomplished either by using a glass pipe or by heating the methamphetamine on a piece of aluminum foil (a practice sometimes called "chasing the dragon"). As shown in Figure 13.1, plasma levels of methamphetamine peak much more rapidly following smoking than following oral administration. Methamphetamine hydrochloride in a crystalline form particularly suitable for smoking began showing up in Hawaii in the 1980s. This material, which is called

13.1 TIME COURSE OF PLASMA DRUG CONCENTRATIONS FOLLOWING METHAMPHETAMINE ADMINISTRATION BY SMOKING OR ORAL CONSUMPTION. Human subjects received methamphetamine at a dose of 0.25 mg/kg (oral) or 21 mg total (smoking). Data represent the mean ± *SEM* for six subjects per group. (After Cook, 1991.)

"ice" on the street, has since spread to California and other parts of the United States (Cho, 1990). Because "ice" is inexpensive to make and highly addictive, it poses a serious challenge to society's attempts to control and reduce the incidence of stimulant abuse.

Amphetamine and its congeners are metabolized by the liver, albeit at a slow rate. The principal metabolic pathways in humans are shown in Figure 13.2. Metabolites (as well as some unmetabolized amphetamine) are

Amphetamine (26%)

p-Hydroxylation β-Hydroxylation Deamination

4-Hydroxyamphetamine (3%) **Norephedrine (2%)** **Phenylacetone (1%)**

4-Hydroxynorephedrine (0.4%) **Benzoic acid (24%)**

Hippuric acid (16%)

13.2 PATHWAYS OF AMPHETAMINE METABOLISM. Hepatic metabolism of amphetamine occurs mainly by *p*-hydroxylation, β-hydroxylation, and deamination. To determine the relative proportion of each metabolite excreted, subjects were given 5 or 20 mg of amphetamine sulfate, and urine was then collected over the following 24 hours. The average percentage of the original dose represented by each metabolite is shown in parentheses. The percentages do not add up to 100 because amphetamine elimination continues for several days following a single dose. (Data combined from Dring, Smith, and Williams, 1970, and Caldwell, Dring, and Williams, 1972; figure after Morgan, 1979.)

excreted primarily in the urine. The elimination half-life ($t_\frac{1}{2}$) can range from 7 to over 30 hours depending on urinary pH (Creasey, 1979). Acidification of the urine decreases the half-life and increases the proportion of amphetamine that is excreted unchanged. A significant portion of methamphetamine is also excreted intact in the urine (Caldwell, Dring, and Williams, 1972). As in the case of amphetamine, p-hydroxylation occurs on the phenyl ring. There is also a small amount of demethylation to yield the parent compound.

Mechanisms of Amphetamine Action

Amphetamine is an indirect agonist of the catecholaminergic systems. This agonist activity stems from the combined ability of the drug to release catecholamines from presynaptic endings, to block catecholamine reuptake, and (at high doses) to inhibit catecholamine metabolism by monoamine oxidase (MAO). The releasing and reuptake blocking effects are most important for understanding amphetamine action, and these effects will therefore be emphasized in the discussion below. Extensive reviews of amphetamine mechanisms may be found in Kuczenski (1983), Seiden, Sabol, and Ricaurte (1993), and Kuczenski and Segal (1994).

Neurochemical Effects on Catecholamine Systems

Catecholamine release and reuptake. Because of amphetamine's behavioral stimulant properties, researchers hypothesized that the drug might interact with catecholaminergic neurons. Early studies using synaptosomal or slice preparations soon showed that amphetamine competitively inhibited uptake of dopamine (DA) in the corpus striatum and of norepinephrine (NE) in the cerebral cortex (Azzaro, Ziance, and Rutledge, 1974; Harris and Baldessarini, 1973). Serotonin (5-HT) uptake could also be inhibited, but only at much higher amphetamine concentrations (Taylor and Ho, 1978). At about the same time, other investigators were demonstrating that amphetamine is a potent DA releasing agent (Arnold, Molinoff, and Rutledge, 1977; Azzaro, Ziance, and Rutledge, 1974; Raiteri et al., 1975). The extent to which amphetamine also releases NE is less clear. Studies using static incubations, in which the synaptosomes or slices are maintained in an unchanging medium during the experiment, seemed to indicate a clear NE releasing effect (Arnold, Molinoff, and Rutledge, 1977; Azzaro, Ziance, and Rutledge, 1974); however, release can be difficult to distinguish from reuptake inhibition under these conditions. Procedures have since been developed to differentiate these processes, including the double-labeling method of Bonnet, Lemasson, and Costentin (1984) and the superfusion system of Raiteri, Angelini, and Levi (1974). In the superfusion system, synaptosomes are exposed to a continuously moving stream of incubation medium to minimize reuptake of released neurotransmitters by the nerve terminals. Using this approach, Raiteri's group found relatively little stimulation of NE release (Raiteri, Levi, and Federico, 1974; Raiteri et al., 1975). On the other hand, amphetamine markedly elevates extracellular NE concentrations in vivo (Kuczenski and Segal, 1992b), which may reflect NE release in addition to uptake inhibition.

The mechanism underlying amphetamine-induced release of catecholamines, particularly DA, has generated considerable interest. To appreciate this work, it is useful first to review what we know about the general phenomenon of DA release (also see Chapter 8). In dopaminergic nerve terminals, DA is synthesized in the cytoplasmic compartment and then transported into synaptic vesicles. Electrically evoked release is blocked by removal of Ca^{2+} from the extracellular fluid, which is consistent with an exocytotic process involving the vesicular pool. Reserpine, a drug that inhibits vesicular uptake and thus depletes vesicular catecholamines, similarly blocks stimulus-evoked release. However, DA is also continuously released in a spontaneous manner from nerve endings. This spontaneous release is Ca^{2+}-independent and insensitive to reserpine; however, it is sensitive to the tyrosine hydroxylase inhibitor α-methyl-p-tyrosine (AMPT). These observations indicate that spontaneous DA release occurs mainly from a cytoplasmic pool of DA that is maintained by ongoing transmitter synthesis.

The same characteristics of Ca^{2+} independence, sensitivity to AMPT, and relative insensitivity to reserpine have been shown for DA release elicited by amphetamine in vitro (Arnold, Molinoff, and Rutledge, 1977; Parker and Cubeddu, 1986a), and for amphetamine-stimulated DA overflow measured by in vivo microdialysis (Butcher et al., 1988) (Figure 13.3). Microdialysis experiments have further shown that prevention of nerve impulses by administration of tetrodotoxin fails to eliminate the effect of amphetamine on striatal DA release (Nomikos et al., 1990; Westerink et al., 1987). Finally, amphetamine enhances spontaneous release not only from dopaminergic nerve terminals in areas such as the striatum, but also from the dendrites of nigral DA neurons (Robertson, Damsma, and Fibiger, 1991). Somatodendritic DA release does not emanate from synaptic vesicles, nor does it require generation of action potentials by the cells. Thus, one major effect of amphetamine is to provoke DA release from the cytoplasmic compartment in an activity-independent manner. Amphetamine has also been reported to enhance stimulation-evoked DA overflow under some conditions (Parker and Cubeddu, 1986b), although the significance of this finding is not entirely clear.

What is the mechanism underlying the DA-releasing effect of amphetamine? First, it is important to note that amphetamine enters nerve terminals by two distinct

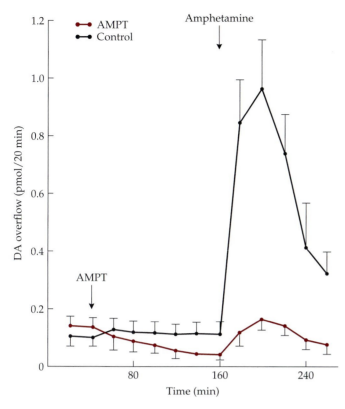

13.3 EFFECT OF α-METHYL-*p*-TYROSINE (AMPT) ON AMPHET-AMINE-STIMULATED DOPAMINE OVERFLOW IN THE STRIA-TUM. Rats were treated intraperitoneally with 250 mg/kg of AMPT or vehicle 120 minutes before intraperitoneal administration of 4 mg/kg of amphetamine. DA overflow in the striatum was measured by in vivo microdialysis. (After Butcher et al., 1988.)

processes. The first process, which is energy-independent and which presumably occurs throughout the brain, is passive diffusion across the plasma membrane. The second is an active process that occurs specifically in dopaminergic nerve terminals and is mediated by the DA transport system. Amphetamine interacts with a site on the DA transporter, as indicated by the drug's DA uptake-inhibiting properties as well as its ability to displace the binding of [³H]mazindol (a drug that labels catecholamine transporters) to striatal membranes (Parker and Cubeddu, 1988). However, unlike many other uptake inhibitors that simply block the action of the transporter, amphetamine appears to be a substrate for transport. Transporter-mediated uptake of amphetamine was actually first demonstrated in PC-12 cells (Bönisch, 1984), which are a clonal line of adrenal chromaffin-like cells that synthesize and take up catecholamines via an NE transporter. These initial experiments were followed by the work of Zaczek, Culp, and De Souza (1991), who found that [³H]amphetamine transport into striatal synaptosomes was saturable, temperature-dependent, and stereoselective (exhibiting an eightfold preference for D- over L-amphetamine). Moreover, transport was in-

hibited by ouabain (which eliminates the transmembrane sodium gradient by blocking Na^+–K^+ ATPase), reduced by 6-hydroxydopamine (6-OHDA) lesions of the striatum, and exhibited a pharmacology consistent with mediation by the DA transporter. The apparent K_m for [³H]amphetamine transport was approximately 100 nM, supporting the possible involvement of this process both in DA release and in the behavioral responses to low-dose amphetamine administration (see below).

There is additional evidence that the effects of amphetamine depend on the DA transporter. For example, amphetamine-stimulated DA release is inhibited by drugs that block DA uptake (Fischer and Cho, 1979; Liang and Rutledge, 1982; Raiteri et al., 1979). Furthermore, DA transporter knockout mice mentioned previously in Chapter 8 exhibit neither DA release nor locomotor activation in response to amphetamine treatment (Giros et al., 1996). Taken together, these findings have led to an **exchange diffusion model** of amphetamine-stimulated DA release (Fischer and Cho, 1979; Liang and Rutledge, 1982). The idea of exchange diffusion had previously been developed from studies of glucose efflux from human erythrocytes (red blood cells) (Stein, 1967). As applied to the phenomenon of DA release by amphetamine, the model proposes that extracellular amphetamine binds to the DA transporter, is taken up into the terminal, and is released into the cytoplasm. The transporter binding site is now facing inward, where it can bind an intracellular DA molecule. Once this has occurred, the DA molecule is transported in the opposite direction from normal reuptake and released into the extracellular fluid. There are precedents for such "reverse transport" of DA and other monoamines under appropriate conditions (see Seiden, Sabol, and Ricaurte, 1993).

Two other factors must be considered in relation to amphetamine stimulation of DA release. First, although exchange diffusion is thought to be the principal mechanism operating at low amphetamine concentrations, high concentrations (which would saturate the transporter) probably result in substantial amphetamine accumulation by passive diffusion across the plasma membrane. Second, amphetamine increases cytoplasmic catecholamine concentrations at the expense of the vesicular pool. This occurs in part because the drug is a weak inhibitor of the vesicular uptake process (Knepper, Grunewald, and Rutledge, 1988; Philippu and Beyer, 1973). Perhaps even more importantly, amphetamine evokes release of catecholamines from their vesicular storage sites due to its previously mentioned properties as a weak base (Sulzer and Rayport, 1990; Sulzer, Maidment, and Rayport, 1993). The lipophilicity of amphetamine in its uncharged form allows it to penetrate catecholamine vesicles. However, because the interior of these vesicles is quite acidic compared with the cytoplasmic compartment (see Chapter 8), the amine group on the amphetamine molecule will tend to become protonated (i.e., to pick up a H$^+$ ion). One consequence of amphetamine protonation is that the drug becomes sequestered within the vesicles because it does not readily cross the vesicular membrane when carrying an electric charge. Second, a reduction in the concentration of free H$^+$ ions means that the vesicle interior has become less acidic. This change reduces the pH gradient across the vesicle membrane, thereby inhibiting uptake and promoting efflux of catecholamines from the vesicle. Based on these findings, Sulzer and his colleagues have developed a **weak base model** of amphetamine action (Sulzer and Rayport, 1990; Sulzer, Maidment, and Rayport, 1993). This model proposes that amphetamine and other lipophilic weak bases promote catecholamine release from vesicular stores, followed by reverse transport of the transmitter across the cell membrane. Because the large increase in cytoplasmic catecholamine levels is thought to shift the concentration gradient across the plasma membrane, the weak base model (unlike the exchange diffusion model) does not rely on transporter-mediated uptake of the drug.

The weak base model appears to adequately explain the catecholamine-releasing effects of lipophilic bases that are not substrates for the plasma membrane trans-

porter. However, because the evidence indicates that amphetamine is carried by the transporter, we may conclude that both exchange diffusion and vesicular release/reverse transport contribute to the DA-releasing effects of amphetamine. The potential mechanisms by which amphetamine might release DA from dopaminergic nerve terminals are summarized in Figure 13.4. Possible relationships between the dose of amphetamine and the relative importance of different releasing mechanisms remain to be determined.

Catecholamine synthesis and metabolism.   The influence of amphetamine on catecholamine synthesis has also been studied primarily with respect to the DA system. In the striatum (caudate nucleus), low concentrations or doses of amphetamine tend to enhance DA synthesis (Connor and Kuczenski, 1986; Elverfors and Nissbrandt, 1992; Nielsen, Chapin, and Moore, 1983; Uretsky, Kamal, and Snodgrass, 1979). Because this effect can be blocked by DA uptake inhibitors (Connor and Kuczenski, 1986), it may result from a reduction in end-product inhibition of tyrosine hydroxylase due to amphetamine-stimulated DA release. On the other hand, high concentrations or doses of amphetamine either inhibit striatal DA synthe-

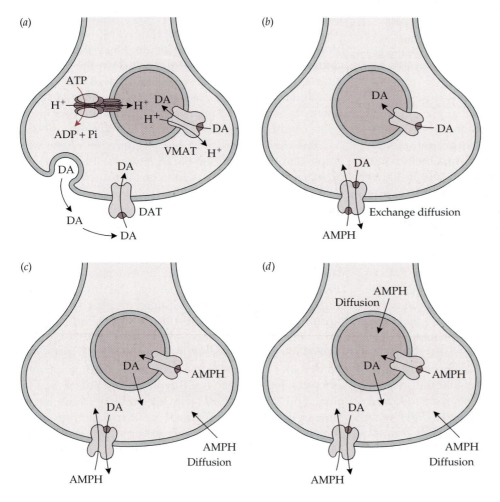

13.4 POSSIBLE MECHANISMS OF AMPHETAMINE-INDUCED DOPAMINE RELEASE. (a) Some of the normal processes occurring in a dopaminergic nerve terminal, including exocytotic DA release, DA uptake into the terminal via the plasma membrane transporter (DAT), and DA uptake into synaptic vesicles via the vesicular monoamine transporter (VMAT). Possible mechanisms of amphetamine action: plasma membrane transport-mediated amphetamine uptake coupled to cytoplasmic DA release (exchange diffusion) (b–d); amphetamine entry into the terminal by passive diffusion (c–d); amphetamine entry into the vesicles mediated by the vesicular transporter and/or by passive diffusion (c–d); and release of vesicular DA (c–d). Seiden and colleagues have postulated that the processes shown in b–d occur in sequential order as the dose of amphetamine is raised (for example, at low doses, only exchange diffusion would take place); however, this hypothesis remains to be validated. (After Seiden, Sabol, and Ricaurte, 1993.)

sis (Connor and Kuczenski, 1986; Uretsky, Kamal, and Snodgrass, 1979) or have no effect (Elverfors and Nissbrandt, 1992; Nielsen, Chapin, and Moore, 1983). Decreased DA synthesis could be related to two processes: progressive displacement of vesicular DA, which would increase cytoplasmic DA concentrations and facilitate end-product inhibition, and DA reuptake inhibition, which would activate synthesis-inhibiting presynaptic autoreceptors or postsynaptically mediated negative feedback loops that suppress dopaminergic cell firing.

In contrast to the striatum, other dopaminergic terminal areas such as the nucleus accumbens, olfactory tubercle, and prefrontal cortex show little or no stimulation of DA synthesis following amphetamine administration (Nielsen, Chapin, and Moore, 1983; Tyler and Galloway, 1992; Westerink and Van Putten, 1987). Moreover, doses of amphetamine that enhance DA synthesis in the striatum cause a reduction in synthesis rate in the substantia nigra, the location of the cell bodies of the nigrostriatal tract (Elverfors and Nissbrandt, 1992). These different responses are thought to result from differences in the mechanisms regulating DA synthesis in particular projection areas and in the cell bodies versus the nerve terminals.

Early work demonstrated that amphetamine is an inhibitor of monoamine oxidase (MAO) activity in vitro (Mann and Quastel, 1940). Inhibition is reversible, and is preferential for type A MAO compared with type B (Mantle, Tipton, and Garrett, 1976) (see Chapter 8). Although inhibition of catecholamine metabolism by MAO could contribute to the indirect agonist effects of amphetamine, this mechanism generally has not been considered important in vivo. Yet Miller, Shore, and Clarke (1980) showed that pretreatment of rats with 10 mg/kg amphetamine significantly reduced subsequent inactivation of striatal MAO by the irreversible inhibitor phenelzine. This effect was specific to the D-isomer, occurred only with MAO-A, and was presumed to result from interaction of amphetamine with the enzyme in vivo. Thus, MAO inhibition might play at least a modest role in the response to amphetamine, particularly at high doses.

Other Neurochemical Effects

As we have seen, most studies on the neurochemical actions of amphetamine have focused on the presynaptic side of the dopaminergic system. More recently, however, investigators have begun to turn their attention to postsynaptic events, particularly in the striatum. For example, striatal output neurons, which receive direct synaptic connections from nigrostriatal DA terminals, respond to acute amphetamine treatment by increasing transcription of the pre-protachykinin gene, which codes for substance P (Hurd and Herkenham, 1992), and the *c-fos* immediate–early gene (Graybiel, Moratalla, and Robertson, 1990). Induction of *c-fos* by amphetamine was

recently shown to depend on phosphorylation of the transcription factor known as cAMP response element binding protein (CREB) (Konradi et al., 1994; see Chapter 6 for a discussion of immediate–early genes and transcription factors). A single amphetamine injection also leads to a transient dose-dependent desensitization of DA D_1 receptor-stimulated adenylyl cyclase activity in the striatum (Barnett and Kuczenski, 1986; Roberts-Lewis et al., 1986) (Figure 13.5). This effect was not observed in mesolimbic terminal areas (nucleus accumbens and olfactory tubercle), demonstrating another difference between the mesolimbic and nigrostriatal systems in responsivity to amphetamine. Finally, the 2-deoxyglucose method has been used to examine changes in cerebral glucose utilization following amphetamine injection (Porrino et al., 1984). A low dose of amphetamine (0.2 mg/kg i.v.) that elicited increased locomotor behavior but no focused stereotypies (see below) selectively stimulated glucose utilization in the nucleus accumbens. Higher doses (1–5 mg/kg) that gave rise to stereotyped sniffing and oral behaviors increased glucose utilization throughout the extrapyramidal motor system and neocortex, as well as in selected limbic and thalamic structures. The association of heightened locomotor activity with enhanced glucose utilization in the nucleus accumbens is consistent with other findings discussed below that link the nucleus accumbens to this behavioral effect of amphetamine. On the other hand, it is clear that high doses of amphetamine produce a much more widespread, though not universal, stimulation of brain metabolic activity.

Electrophysiological Effects

Another approach to studying the mechanism of amphetamine action has been to examine electrophysiological changes in various brain regions. Researchers have found consistent evidence that amphetamine administration depresses the firing of dopaminergic, noradrenergic, and (at higher doses) serotonergic neurons (Bunney et al., 1973; Engberg and Svensson, 1979; Graham and Aghajanian, 1971; Rebec, Curtis, and Zimmerman, 1982). These effects seem to be mediated by activation of somatodendritic autoreceptors or stimulation of a negative feedback loop, particularly in the case of the dopaminergic system (Bunney and Aghajanian, 1978a). It is interesting to note that autoreceptor-mediated inhibition of A_{10} DA neurons is desensitized in response to chronic amphetamine treatment (White and Wang, 1984a) or even following a short period of continuous exposure in vitro (Seutin et al., 1991).

Amphetamine also leads to complex electrophysiological effects in the striatum. Terminal excitability is decreased due to activation of presynaptic autoreceptors (Groves et al., 1989). Furthermore, systemic administration of amphetamine to awake, freely moving animals tends to stimulate striatal neurons previously character-

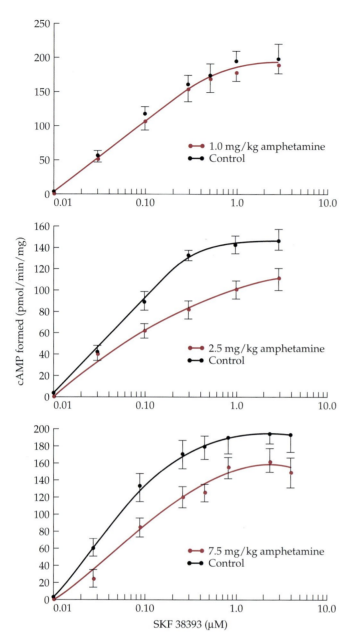

13.5 DESENSITIZATION OF STRIATAL DOPAMINE D₁ RECEPTOR–STIMULATED ADENYLYL CYCLASE BY A SINGLE AMPHETAMINE TREATMENT. Rats received either 1, 2.5, or 7.5 mg/kg amphetamine intraperitoneally and were sacrificed 30 minutes later. Striatal membranes were analyzed for adenylyl cyclase activity in the presence of varying concentrations of the D_1 agonist SKF 38393. Note the reduction in maximal D_1-stimulated cAMP formation following treatment with the two higher doses of amphetamine. (After Roberts-Lewis et al., 1986.)

ized as having a relatively high baseline firing rate along with movement-associated excitatory responses (Haracz et al., 1993). In contrast, cells exhibiting a low rate of spontaneous firing have been reported to be further inhibited by amphetamine treatment (Groves et al., 1989). Assuming that a low level of baseline activity represents background "noise," Haracz and colleagues (1993) have

interpreted these findings to mean that amphetamine enhances the signal-to-noise ratio of information transmission in the striatum.

Acute Behavioral and Physiological Effects of Amphetamine in Humans

Effects on Mood and Behavior

In humans, amphetamine causes heightened alertness, increased confidence, feelings of exhilaration, lowered fatigue, a decrease in boredom, and a generalized sense of well-being (for review, see Grinspoon and Hedblom, 1975). The mood-enhancing and subjectively positive effects of amphetamine were first described in the medical literature in the mid-1930s (Myerson, 1936; Nathanson, 1937; Peoples and Guttmann, 1936), and were subsequently confirmed using questionnaires such as the Addiction Research Center Inventory (ARCI) (Martin et al., 1971) and the Profile of Mood States (POMS) (Johanson and Uhlenhuth, 1980).* A brief report some years ago indicated that the euphoric effects of amphetamine could be antagonized by AMPT or by DA receptor–blocking neuroleptic drugs (Gunne, Änggård, and Jönsson, 1972). Although these results are consistent with a dopaminergic mediation of amphetamine's euphoric effects, more research clearly needs to be performed in this area.

Various studies have demonstrated that amphetamine improves performance on simple, repetitive psychomotor tasks, presumably due to the drug's ability to enhance confidence, increase interest in the task, and reduce fatigue (Grinspoon and Hedblom, 1975; Weiss and Laties, 1962). The drug causes a delay in sleep onset and a reduction in sleep time, particularly with respect to rapid eye movement (REM) sleep. Indeed, amphetamine administration permits sustained physical effort without rest or sleep, which accounts for its use by soldiers and aviators during World War II as well as by truck drivers and other workers desirous of foregoing sleep for extended periods of time. It can also enhance athletic performance (Laties and Weiss, 1981), and is therefore one of the many substances banned from athletic competitions.

Physiological Effects

Amphetamine is classified as a sympathomimetic compound (i.e., it mimics the effects of sympathetic stimulation). The physiological consequences of acute amphetamine administration include elevated systolic and diastolic blood pressure, relaxation of bronchial and in-

---

*As currently used, the ARCI is a questionnaire containing 49 items organized into five scales. These scales reflect the mood states typically produced by specific classes of abused drugs (e.g., opiates, amphetamines and other psychostimulants, barbiturates and other sedative–hypnotic drugs). The POMS is a more general psychological instrument that is widely used to assess emotional states.

testinal smooth muscle, tachypnea (increased respiration rate), heightened metabolic rate and oxygen consumption, and hyperthermia (elevated body temperature) (Martin et al., 1971; Morgan, 1979). The effect on heart rate is complex, but mainly involves tachycardia (increased heart rate). These effects could be related to amphetamine's NE-releasing and reuptake-blocking effects at sympathetic nerve endings, or to a central activation of sympathetic outflow (see the discussion below on the physiological effects of cocaine).

Therapeutic Uses of Amphetamine

Amphetamine and related psychostimulants are used therapeutically for three major purposes: treatment of narcolepsy, promotion of weight loss, and treatment of attention deficit hyperactivity disorder.

Narcolepsy. Narcolepsy is a disorder characterized by one or more of the following symptoms: recurring and irresistible attacks of sleepiness during the daytime hours; cataplexy, which refers to a sudden loss of muscle tone while the patient remains conscious; sleep paralysis, which occurs during the transition between the waking state and sleep; and hypnagogic hallucinations, which are vivid hallucinations that also take place during the sleep–waking transition. Both amphetamine and the nonamphetamine stimulant methylphenidate (Ritalin) have been used successfully in the treatment of narcolepsy (Soldatos, Kales, and Cadieux, 1979). Unfortunately, high doses may be needed to achieve therapeutic efficacy, and patients thus face the risk of becoming dependent on the drugs. Moreover, chronic stimulant treatment can lead to unwanted side effects such as anorexia and weight loss, hypertension, irritability, and disruption of normal sleep patterns.

The etiology of narcolepsy and the mechanism underlying the therapeutic efficacy of CNS stimulants remain to be determined. However, it is interesting to note that a narcolepsy-like syndrome has been found in certain genetic strains of Labrador retrievers and Doberman pinschers. The brains of these narcoleptic dogs were found to possess elevated levels of DA and the DA metabolite dihydroxyphenylacetic acid (Mefford et al., 1983). These findings suggested that the animals had lower levels of DA utilization and higher levels of intraneuronal DA degradation than normal dogs.

Obesity. A second medical use of amphetamine is in the treatment of obesity. Many clinical studies have shown that amphetamine is an anorectic agent, which means that it suppresses appetite and food intake (Grinspoon and Bakalar, 1979; Silverstone, 1981) (Figure 13.6). Amphetamine and methamphetamine have therefore been very popular historically in the treatment of obese patients. However, serious problems arose in the course of amphetamine use for weight loss. First, the abuse po-

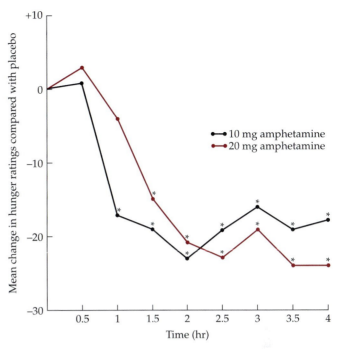

13.6 ANORECTIC EFFECT OF AMPHETAMINE. Normal male subjects were given a single dose of 10 or 20 mg D-amphetamine and then asked to rate their subjective feelings of hunger using a visual analog scale. Over a 4-hour period, the two doses produced approximately equivalent reductions in self-reported hunger compared with placebo administration (*, significantly different from placebo rating). (After Silverstone, 1981.)

tential of these compounds is very high (see below), which led to many individuals becoming psychologically and physically dependent on their "diet pills." Second, anorectic efficacy diminishes with chronic administration (Cawthorne, 1981; Grinspoon and Bakalar, 1979), which can lead either to a potentially dangerous escalation in dose or to dropping out of the weight loss program. Although amphetamines are still sometimes prescribed for the treatment of obesity, they have been largely replaced by nonamphetamine anorectic compounds such as diethylpropion (trade name Tenuate), phenmetrazine (trade name Preludin), mazindol (trade names Sanorex and Mazanor), or the serotonergic drug dexfenfluramine (trade name Redux; see Chapter 9).

Attention deficit hyperactivity disorder. A third clinical use for stimulants, particularly methylphenidate, is in the treatment of a developmental disorder once known as minimal brain dysfunction, but more recently called attention deficit hyperactivity disorder (ADHD) (Towbin and Leckman, 1992). Children diagnosed as suffering from ADHD exhibit extreme degrees of inattentiveness, impulsivity, and hyperkinesis (excessive motor activity). They have an extremely short attention span and impulsively turn their attention to almost anything in the environment. Other behavioral characteristics include low frustration tolerance, obstinacy, bullying, obtuseness to the needs of other, and lack of response to discipline. In graver cases, there may be destructiveness, stealing, lying, fire-setting, and sexual "acting out." The child is frequently disruptive in the classroom, and has trouble learning. Problems likewise occur in the child's interactions with parents and other family members in the home.

For many years ADHD was thought to be restricted to childhood and adolescence; however, subsequent observations have shown that in some cases symptoms persist into adulthood. This discovery led to the proposal of a diagnostic category termed attention deficit disorder, residual type (ADD-RT) (Wender, 1978). Adults considered to be suffering from ADD-RT show symptoms of distractibility, impulsivity, restlessness, hyperemotionality, and problems both at work and in interpersonal relationships (Gualtieri, Ondrusek, and Finley, 1985). Moreover, such individuals are at heightened risk for developing conduct disorder, antisocial personality disorder, or substance abuse problems (Gittleman-Klein et al., 1985).

The relevance of stimulants for the treatment of ADHD is that these drugs paradoxically produce a calming effect in affected children. This phenomenon was first reported by Bradley in 1937 and has since been observed in many other studies (see Brown and Cooke, 1994; Oades, 1987). Amphetamine, methylphenidate, and a third stimulant, pemoline (trade name Cylert), are the medications usually prescribed for ADHD. For the best results, concomitant psychotherapy and parental counseling are also required. More than 50% of ADHD patients show a positive response to drug treatment. In most cases, all three drugs are equally effective, although there are rare selective responders to one or the other (Zametkin and Rapoport, 1987). Side effects may occur, as described above in the treatment of narcolepsy. A recent review by Wilens and coworkers (1995) indicates that many, though not all, adults diagnosed with ADD-RT are likewise helped by psychostimulant treatment.

Although methylphenidate is an indirect catecholamine agonist like amphetamine, it differs from the latter in several important ways: methylphenidate is more potent as a DA uptake inhibitor than as a releasing agent (Ferris, Tang, and Maxwell, 1972); methylphenidate only weakly blocks vesicular uptake of DA (Ferris and Tang, 1979); and methylphenidate-evoked DA overflow depends on neuronal activity (Nomikos et al., 1990) as well as on the integrity of the vesicular compartment (Chiueh and Moore, 1975). From these findings, we may conclude that methylphenidate blocks reuptake and to a lesser extent promotes release of DA from the vesicular (but not the cytoplasmic) pool. As such, it belongs in a group of other nonamphetamine stimulants (e.g., cocaine, mazindol, nomifensine, and amfonelic acid) that share similar properties (McMillen, 1983).

The ability of psychomotor stimulants to alleviate the symptoms of ADHD implies that the disorder might arise from an underlying pathology of the catecholaminergic system. Support for this hypothesis comes from the work of Porrino and Lucignani (1987), who showed that treatment of rats with a low dose of methylphenidate stimulated glucose utilization in the nucleus accumbens and olfactory tubercle, two target areas of the mesolimbic DA pathway. Furthermore, several clinical studies found abnormally low urinary levels of either the DA metabolite homovanillic acid (HVA) or the NE metabolite 3,4,-methoxy-hydroxy-phenylglycol (MHPG) in subpopulations of ADHD children (Oades, 1987). However, in some cases the already low metabolite concentrations fell even further following stimulant treatment. It thus remains unclear whether there are neurochemically distinct subtypes of ADHD (dopaminergic vs. noradrenergic mediation), why some patients show normal catecholaminergic activity, what differentiates treatment responders from nonresponders, and what neurochemical processes are responsible for the therapeutic efficacy of stimulant drugs in this disorder. Because of the side effects mentioned earlier, it would be desirable to minimize the drug doses used in ADHD treatment. Animal studies by Woods and Meyer (1991) raise the possibility that coadministration of the catecholamine precursor tyrosine might augment the therapeutic effectiveness of methylphenidate, thereby allowing lower doses to be given.

Acute Behavioral Effects of Amphetamine in Animals

Locomotor and Stereotyped Behaviors

Purely motor stimulants such as strychnine and pentylenetetrazol (Metrazol) cause undirected running, jumping, crashing into obstacles, and so forth. In contrast, psychomotor stimulants such as amphetamine produce a more organized sensorimotor activation. In rodents and other animal subjects, this activation is manifested by increased locomotor behavior, various stereotyped activities, and altered rates of reinforced lever pressing (reviewed by Segal and Kuczenski, 1994). A single low dose of amphetamine (0.25–1.0 mg/kg i.p.) administered to rats leads to a characteristic response pattern consisting of locomotor activity, rearing, mild sniffing, and head bobbing. Gradually increasing the dose to 10 mg/kg results in a decrease in locomotion and rearing, which are replaced by focused stereotypies (repetitive, seemingly aimless behaviors performed in a relatively invariant manner) confined to a small area of the cage floor. After a single large dose given subcutaneously to retard absorption, the animal's behavior goes through the same stages that occur with increasing intraperitoneal doses.

Amphetamine-induced stereotypies take many forms, depending on the species, dose, time after injection, environmental conditions, and previous experience. In rats, mice, and guinea pigs, one observes intense sniffing, repetitive head and limb movements, and licking and biting. Amphetamine-treated cats show sniffing if tested in a cage, but in the open they show rapid head movements and changes in visual fixation between near and far objects. Such movements cease if the subjects are blindfolded, confirming that the behavior is sensorimotor in nature and not merely motorically driven. Stereotypies in monkeys consist of staring, chewing, tongue protrusions, jerking of the neck and shoulders, rocking behavior, repetitive grooming, snatching at the air, or seizing the cage bars (Randrup and Munkvad, 1967; Ridley and Baker, 1982; Wallach, 1974).

It is common in the literature to assume a major distinction between enhanced locomotion, which is the predominant response in rodents to low doses of amphetamine, and the elicitation of focused stereotypies by high doses of the drug. However, Rebec and Bashore (1984) have pointed out that amphetamine-induced locomotor behavior is likewise stereotyped in nature. Whereas untreated subjects ambulate around the entire test apparatus, amphetamine administration leads to repetitive back-and-forth movements along the side of the enclosure. The dose-related effects of amphetamine can be further understood in terms of the theory proposed by Lyon and Robbins (Lyon and Robbins, 1975; Robbins and Sahakian, 1983). These investigators argue that the fundamental behavioral effect of amphetamine is to stimulate all responses that have some minimal likelihood of occurrence under nondrugged conditions. Consequently, as the dose is increased, pauses between or within behavioral sequences become shorter and shorter. Moreover, competition begins to occur between different responses, leading to truncation of some behavior patterns and virtual elimination of others. Ultimately, the subject is rapidly switching between a few simple and repetitive behavioral elements, all of which are performed at a high rate. This hypothesis thus explains why stereotyped sniffing, head movements, and oral behaviors predominate at high doses of amphetamine, whereas longer-duration ambulatory behaviors are truncated under such conditions (Rebec and Bashore, 1984).

Schedule-Controlled Behavior

The influence of amphetamine and other psychomotor stimulants on schedule-controlled (operant) behavior has been extensively studied. Overall, this work indicates that the effect of amphetamine depends heavily on the baseline rate of responding. Amphetamine tends to increase response rates under conditions of low baseline responding, but to depress responding when the baseline rate is already high (Dews and Wenger, 1977). These effects can be readily demonstrated by training animals on a fixed interval (FI) schedule. As described in Chapter 2, FI schedules give rise to a characteristic scalloped pattern of responses in which responding is low early in the interval but dramatically accelerates as the end of the interval approaches. Administration of amphetamine increases responding early in the interval, but either decreases or has no effect on responding late in the interval. When animals are working under a DRL (differential reinforcement of low rates of responding) schedule, amphetamine increases the rate of responding even though the animals consequently receive fewer reinforcements. Yet another interesting reinforcement schedule that has been tested with amphetamine is the progressive ratio (PR) schedule. In this paradigm, rats start out pressing a lever for food under conditions of continuous reinforcement. Every 2 minutes, however, the number of presses required per reinforcer doubles (that is, from 1 to 2 to 4 to 8 and so forth). Nondrugged subjects typically begin to show marked declines in response rate within 12–14 minutes after the beginning of testing. However, administration of 0.5 or 1.0 mg/kg amphetamine or appropriate doses of other stimulants led to a high and consistent response rate despite the decreasing frequency of reinforcement (Poncelet et al., 1983).

Several factors may contribute to the complex influence of amphetamine on operant responding. First, amphetamine appears to enhance the effectiveness of conditioned reinforcers (Robbins, 1978), which may include various cues associated with lever pressing in a Skinner box. This could help to account for the activating effects of amphetamine under low baseline levels of responding. Second, as discussed by Seiden, Sabol, and Ricaurte (1993), the suppressant effects of amphetamine on operant behavior at high levels of responding and at high drug doses can be understood at least partially in terms of Lyon's and Robbins' hypothesis. Under such conditions, amphetamine tends to reduce response rates by eliciting competing behaviors that are incompatible with performing the operant reponse or by truncating the pattern of behavior required to perform the response (that is, approaching the lever, placing a paw above the lever, and pressing down) before it reaches completion.

Discriminative Stimulus Properties of Amphetamine

One of the most powerful techniques used to study the behavioral effects of drugs is drug discrimination testing (see Stolerman, 1992). Although this technique was discussed in Chapter 2, we will briefly recapitulate here. Just as exteroceptive stimuli (e.g., sounds or lights) can serve as discriminative stimuli controlling operant behavior, many psychoactive drugs produce interoceptive cues that can be used in the same way. Thus, animals can be trained to perform one response (e.g., entering the left arm of a shock escape apparatus or pressing the right-hand lever in a two-lever Skinner box) when given a drug injection and to perform a different response (e.g., entering the right arm of the apparatus or pressing the left-hand lever) when given the drug vehicle instead.

Amphetamine has been shown to serve as a discriminative stimulus in a number of species (see Fischman, 1987). Figure 13.7 shows the results from a typical experiment that was carried out by Kuhn, Appel, and Greenburg (1974). In this study, water-deprived rats were trained to respond on two levers for water reinforcement under a tandem VI 1/FR 10 schedule (i.e., to obtain reinforcement, the subject was required to make 10 responses on the correct lever after an interval averaging 1 minute had elapsed). On different days, subjects received either saline or 1 mg/kg D-amphetamine 30 minutes before the onset of testing. The animals began to reliably discriminate amphetamine from saline by session 13, finally reaching a plateau at approximately 90% correct responding (Figure 13.7*a*). The animals were then given various test doses of amphetamine below and above the training dose. A dose of 0.50 mg/kg effectively substituted for the training dose, 0.25 mg/kg yielded essentially random responding, and the lowest test dose (0.0625 mg/kg) elicited responding mainly on the saline lever (Figure 13.7*b*). When generalization studies have been performed using this paradigm to determine whether other compounds will substitute for the amphetamine cue, full substitution has been found using appropriate doses of methamphetamine, several other N-substituted amphetamine analogs, cocaine, and methylphenidate (Huang and Ho, 1974; Kuhn, Appel, and Greenburg, 1974; Young and Glennon, 1986). However, a number of other compounds, including mescaline, LSD-25, Δ^9-tetrahydrocannabinol, the amphetamine analog and 5-HT releasing agent fenfluramine, nicotine, and caffeine (Kuhn, Appel, and Greenburg, 1974; Schechter and Rosecrans, 1983; Young and Glennon, 1986), failed to show stimulus generalization at the doses tested. The fact that nicotine and caffeine failed to substitute for amphetamine indicates that the amphetamine cue is not due to a simple stimulant effect.

Chait, Uhlenhuth, and Johanson (1984) have developed a procedure for testing the discriminative stimulus effects of drugs in humans. Application of this technique to amphetamine showed that subjects reliably discriminated a 10 mg oral dose of the drug from placebo (Chait, Uhlenhuth, and Johanson, 1986).

Reinforcing Effects of Amphetamine

As discussed in Chapter 12, the willingness of animals to self-administer various drugs has proved, in most cases, to be an excellent predictor of their abuse liability in humans. This is certainly true of amphetamine, methamphetamine, and cocaine, which are among the most powerfully reinforcing drugs in this paradigm. As reviewed by Yokel (1987), intravenous self-administration of amphetamine and/or methamphetamine has thus far been demonstrated in rats, dogs, cats, squirrel monkeys, rhesus monkeys, and baboons. Animals given unlimited

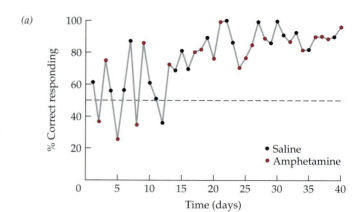

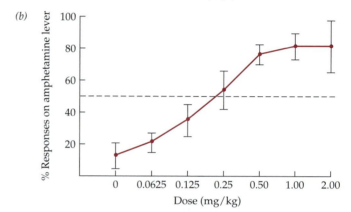

13.7 DISCRIMINATIVE STIMULUS PROPERTIES OF AMPHETAMINE IN RATS. (*a*) Acquisition of the discriminative response. Subjects were first trained to press a lever for water reinforcement under a tandem VI 1/FR 10 schedule. Amphetamine discrimination was then instituted by starting daily intraperitoneal injections of either 1 mg/kg *d*-amphetamine or saline vehicle. Within 3–4 weeks, the animals were reliably discriminating amphetamine from saline with an accuracy approaching 90%. (*b*) Amphetamine discrimination as a function of dose. After the acquisition phase was completed, the subjects were tested for their generalization to differing doses of amphetamine. Doses near the training dose of 1 mg/kg elicited amphetamine-appropriate responding, whereas low doses elicited responding mainly on the saline-appropriate lever. Data represent the mean ± *SEM*. (After Kuhn, Appel, and Greenburg, 1974.)

access to these and other stimulants typically exhibit alternating periods of drug intake and abstinence. Intervals of drug responding are characterized by an appearance of stereotyped behaviors, reduced food and water consumption, and little or no sleep. Consummatory behaviors and sleep occur during the periods of nonresponding. Despite the fact that drug intake is discontinuous, unlimited access to amphetamine leads to a high fatality rate due to severe weight loss, convulsions, and other toxic effects (Pickens, Miesch, and Thompson, 1978; Yokel, 1987). On the other hand, animals will generally maintain their health if access to the drug is limited to only part of the day.

Piazza and colleagues (1989) noted that individual rats differ in their propensity to self-administer amphetamine at low doses. To determine whether vulnerability to amphetamine self-administration could be related to any preexisting behavioral tendencies, these investigators first tested a group of rats for the rapidity with which they habituated to placement in a novel environment. Animals that habituated slowly to the novel environment (called "high responders") were found to acquire low-dose amphetamine self-administration (10 µg per injection), whereas the rapidly habituating subjects ("low responders") failed to self-administer the drug under these conditions (Figure 13.8*a*). Further experiments showed that four injections of amphetamine (1.5 mg/kg i.p.) at 3-day intervals prior to the beginning of self-administration testing abolished the difference between the groups (Figure 13.8*b*). These interesting results suggest that preexisting behavioral reactivity and prior drug exposure may both contribute to an individual's potential for abusing a particular substance.

Another method of studying the reinforcing or aversive effects of drugs is place conditioning, which was discussed earlier in Chapters 8 and 12. Many studies have demonstrated conditioned place preferences with amphetamine and other psychomotor stimulants (reviewed by Hoffman, 1989). These findings are consistent with the reinforcing properties of these drugs in the self-administration paradigm. However, amphetamine has been shown to induce a conditioned place avoidance when a large number of drug injections and training trials were used (Wall et al., 1990). Because intermittent amphetamine administration sensitizes animals to the activating effects of the drug (see further discussion below), these results provide some indication that such sensitization is aversive to the subject.

Mechanisms Underlying Behavioral Effects of Amphetamine

Since the earliest descriptions of amphetamine's behavioral effects in animals, there has been great interest in the neural mechanisms underlying these effects. Some of

the many reviews of this topic may be found in Cole (1978), Swerdlow and colleagues (1986), Fischman (1987), Evenden and Ryan (1990), and Seiden, Sabol, and Ricaurte (1993). In the discussion below, we will focus on the mechanisms thought to be involved in amphetamine-induced locomotor and stereotyped behaviors, the discriminative properties of amphetamine, and its reinforcing effects in the self-administration and place conditioning paradigms.

Locomotor and stereotyped behaviors. The DA system has traditionally been considered crucial to the ability of amphetamine to stimulate locomotor activity and stereotyped behaviors. Which DA receptors mediate the activational effects of amphetamine is not yet fully understood, although recent work suggests that both D_1 and D_2 receptors may be involved (Petry et al., 1993). Inhibition of tyrosine hydroxylase by AMPT antagonizes the elicitation of stereotyped behaviors by amphetamine (Weissman, Koe, and Tenen, 1966). On the other hand, several laboratories have demonstrated that reserpine pretreatment fails to block the amphetamine-induced stereotypies, and may even enhance the occurrence of such behaviors (Callaway, Kuczenski, and Segal, 1989; Hong, Jenner, and Marsden, 1987). This phenomenon is not due to increased DA release (Callaway, Kuczenski, and Segal, 1989) and hence must be caused by some other factor, such as receptor supersensitivity following reserpine treatment.

With respect to the anatomic substrates of amphetamine action, a view has developed over the past 15 to 20 years that stimulation of DA activity in the nucleus accumbens is responsible for amphetamine-induced locomotor activity, whereas DA in the caudate–putamen (dorsal striatum) is linked to the focused stereotypies produced by high doses of the drug. Some of the early evidence in support of this hypothesis is as follows: First, both amphetamine and DA itself evoked locomotor ac-

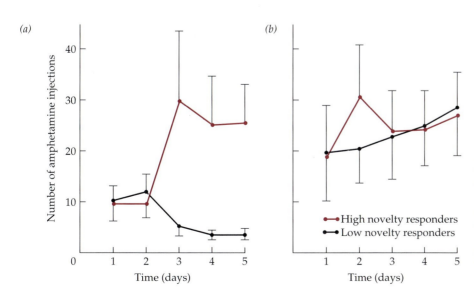

(*a*)

(*b*)

●—● High novelty responders
●—● Low novelty responders

13.8 FACTORS INFLUENCING LOW-DOSE AMPHETAMINE SELF-ADMINISTRATION. (*a*) Rats that were high responders to novelty self-administered amphetamine at a low dose (10 mg per infusion), whereas low responders showed little self-administration. (*b*) After subjects were sensitized by four injections of 1.5 mg/kg amphetamine, both groups showed equivalent amphetamine self-administration. (After Piazza et al., 1989.)

tivity when microinjected directly into the nucleus accumbens, but not the caudate (Elkhawad and Woodruff, 1976; Pijnenburg et al., 1976; Staton and Solomon, 1984). Second, amphetamine microinjected into the caudate, but not the nucleus accumbens, elicited stereotyped behaviors (Kelley, Lang, and Gauthier, 1988; Staton and Solomon, 1984). Third, locomotor stimulation by a low dose of amphetamine was blocked by 6-OHDA lesions of the nucleus accumbens, but not the caudate nucleus (Kelly, Seviour, and Iversen, 1975; although see also Fink and Smith, 1980). Fourth, amphetamine-stimulated locomotor behavior was also antagonized by injection of the DA receptor blocker haloperidol into the nucleus accumbens, but not the caudate (Pijnenburg, Honig, and van Rossum, 1975b). Finally, amphetamine-induced stereotypies were abolished by 6-OHDA lesions of the caudate, but not the nucleus accumbens (Creese and Iversen, 1974; Joyce and Iversen, 1984; Kelly, Seviour, and Iversen, 1975).

More recent studies have focused on correlations between behavioral responsivity to amphetamine and regional changes in DA overflow measured by microdialysis. Using this approach, Sharp and colleagues (1987) observed increases in extracellular DA concentrations in both the caudate and the nucleus accumbens following subcutaneous amphetamine doses of 0.5, 2.0, or 5.0 mg/kg (Figure 13.9). However, locomotor activity in response to the 0.5 and 2.0 mg/kg doses was significantly correlated only with accumbens DA overflow, whereas the intensity of stereotyped head and forepaw movements at all amphetamine doses was significantly correlated with DA overflow in the caudate. Although these findings are basically consistent with the microinjection and lesion studies described above, they must still be interpreted cautiously because other studies have failed to demonstrate a clear relationship between amphetamine-induced behaviors and DA changes in any brain area (reviewed by Segal and Kuczenski, 1994).

Discriminative stimulus effects.   As in the case of locomotor and stereotyped behaviors, the discriminative stimulus effects of amphetamine have been linked to its influence on central DA systems. The cue produced by systemic amphetamine (usually at a dose of 1 mg/kg) was found to be antagonized by AMPT, by intraventricular administration of 6-OHDA in conjunction with intraperitoneal desipramine to protect noradrenergic neurons, and by D_1 or D_2 receptor blocking drugs (Nielsen and Jepsen, 1985; Schechter and Cook, 1975; West, Van Groll, and Appel, 1995; Woolverton and Cervo, 1986). In contrast, amphetamine's discriminative stimulus properties were not affected by the dopamine β-hydroxylase inhibitor disulfiram, the tryptophan hydroxylase inhibitor *p*-chlorophenylalanine, or various adrenergic or serotonergic receptor antagonists (Schechter and Cook, 1975; West, Van Groll, and Appel, 1995).

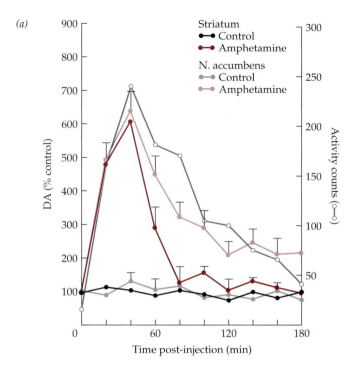

(a)

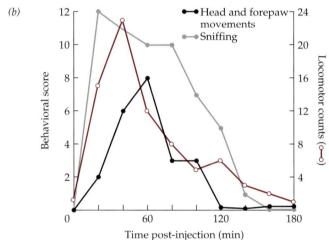

(b)

13.9 RELATIONSHIP BETWEEN REGIONAL DOPAMINE OVERFLOW AND BEHAVIOR FOLLOWING AMPHETAMINE TREATMENT. Rats were implanted with microdialysis probes in either the anterior striatum (caudate–putamen) or the nucleus accumbens and then were allowed to recover. DA overflow and behavioral responses were monitored for 180 minutes following subcutaneous injection of 0.5 mg/kg amphetamine or saline. (a) Time course of regional DA overflow and general activity counts measured in a circular photobeam apparatus. (b) Time course of locomotor activity measured by the photobeams as well as stereotyped sniffing and head and forepaw movements scored by an observer. (After Sharp et al., 1987.)

Nielsen and Scheel-Krüger (1986) performed a particularly interesting experiment aimed at localizing the neural site mediating the amphetamine discriminative stimulus. Rats previously trained to discriminate systemic amphetamine (1 mg/kg i.p.) from saline were tested for stimulus generalization following microinjec-

(a) Intracerebral amphetamine

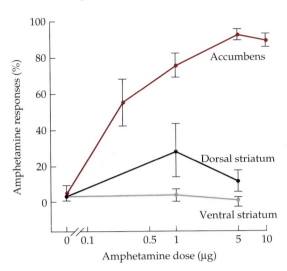

(b) Intraaccumbens amphetamine (1 µg) + sulpiride

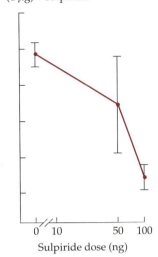

13.10 DISCRIMINATIVE STIMULUS PROPERTIES OF AMPHETAMINE ADMINISTERED DIRECTLY INTO THE BRAIN. Rats were trained to discriminate systemically administered amphetamine (1 mg/kg i.p.) from saline. They were then tested to determine whether intracerebral amphetamine administration generalized to the systemically produced cue. (a) Microinjection of amphetamine into the nucleus accumbens, but not into the dorsal or ventral caudate (striatum), led to a dose-dependent generalization as indicated by responding on the amphetamine-appropriate lever. (b) This effect was blocked by coadministration of the D$_2$ receptor antagonist sulpiride. (After Nielsen and Scheel-Krüger, 1986.)

tion of 0.25–10 µg of amphetamine directly into either the nucleus accumbens or the dorsomedial or ventrolateral caudate. As shown in Figure 13.10, generalization, as indicated by responding on the amphetamine-appropriate lever, occurred only following the accumbens injections. Also shown are additional results demonstrating antagonism of the intra-accumbens stimulus generalization by coinjection of the D$_2$ receptor blocker sulpiride. These results provide intriguing evidence that dopaminergic synapses involving D$_2$ receptors (although not necessarily excluding the additional participation of other receptor subtypes) play an important role in the discriminative stimulus properties of amphetamine.

Reinforcing effects. Studies aimed at determining the neurochemical mechanisms of drug self-administration have generally examined the influence of various pharmacological challenges on drug responding in previously trained subjects. In this situation, low doses of an appropriate antagonist usually increase response rate as the animal attempts to overcome the reduced reinforcement value by consuming more of the drug. Once a sufficiently high antagonist dose has been reached, however, this strategy becomes ineffective and the response rate drops off. With respect to amphetamine, this pattern has been observed following treatment with AMPT or with various DA receptor antagonists (reviewed by McGregor and Roberts, 1994; Yokel, 1987) (Figure 13.11). As no such effect was observed with either α- or β-adrenoreceptor blockade, it appears that DA again underlies the reinforcing effects of amphetamine in the self-administration paradigm. Similar conclusions have been reached in the case of amphetamine-induced conditioned place preferences (Hiroi and White, 1990, 1991; Hoffman, 1989).

A different approach was taken by Ritz and Kuhar (1989), who were interested in whether the monoamine

reuptake blocking effects of amphetamine could be related to its reinforcing properties. These investigators attempted to correlate the potency of amphetamine and various analogs in self-administration with the drugs' binding potencies to the DA, NE, and 5-HT transporters. No significant positive correlations were obtained for any of the transporters, although a modest trend was found with respect to DA transporter binding. The authors noted that amphetamine was more potent behaviorally than would be predicted from its DA uptake blocking effects alone. Thus, the DA-releasing effect of amphetamine may be quite important in its ability to support self-administration.

The principal neural locus of amphetamine's reinforcing effects appears to be the nucleus accumbens. Rats will self-administer amphetamine directly into this structure (Hoebel et al., 1983), but not into other DA terminal areas such as the caudate nucleus or medial prefrontal cortex (Carr and White, 1986). Di Chiara's group has carried this idea further by arguing that amphetamine treatment preferentially increases DA overflow in the nucleus accumbens compared with the caudate (Carboni et al., 1989). Although other laboratories have failed to confirm these findings (Kuczenski and Segal, 1992a; Robinson and Camp, 1990), the mesolimbic DA system is nevertheless thought to play an important role in amphetamine reinforcement. Mechanisms of psychostimulant reward will be discussed further in the section on cocaine below.

Role of transmitters other than dopamine. A recurring theme in this section has been the central role of DA in almost all of the behavioral effects of amphetamine. However, there are hints in the literature of some involvement of NE and 5-HT as well. For example, several reviews provide evidence that the noradrenergic system may contribute to the locomotor-stimulating effect of

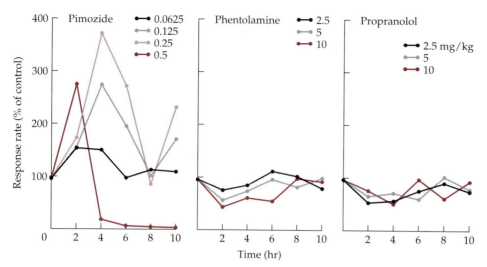

13.11 EFFECTS OF CATECHOLAMIN-ERGIC ANTAGONISTS ON AMPHETA-MINE SELF-ADMINISTRATION. Rats were trained to self-administer amphetamine intravenously (0.25 mg/kg per infusion). The roles of DA and NE in amphetamine's reinforcing properties were assessed by injecting subjects intraperitoneally with varying doses of pimozide (D_2 receptor antagonist), phentolamine (α-receptor antagonist), or propranolol (β-receptor antagonist). Whereas the adrenergic receptor blockers had no effect on the rate of amphetamine self-administration, a moderate dose of pimozide caused an increase in response rate, and the highest dose led to a cessation of responding. (After Yokel and Wise, 1975.)

amphetamine (Cole, 1978; Tessel, 1990). On the other hand, pharmacological manipulations of the serotonergic system suggest that 5-HT antagonizes amphetamine-induced locomotion (Lucki and Harvey, 1979; Segal, 1976) as well as amphetamine self-administration (Leccese and Lyness, 1984; Ritz and Kuhar, 1989; Yu et al., 1986). It remains unclear how the serotonergic and catecholaminergic systems interact to modulate behavior in amphetamine-treated subjects. This question is of particular importance in the case of drug reinforcement, because appropriate serotonergic agonists (for example, reuptake inhibitors like fluoxetine) might have therapeutic value in treating individuals who abuse amphetamine or other drugs (Yu et al., 1986).

Amphetamine Abuse and the Effects of Chronic Amphetamine Exposure

Initiation and Progression of Amphetamine Abuse

This section deals with amphetamine abuse, which will be taken to mean any instance of uncontrolled, compulsive use that continues to occur despite significant adverse consequences for the user. Even though amphetamine abuse is not as widespread as it was 20 or 30 years ago, it is important to understand this drug in the broader context of psychostimulant abuse. The development and course of amphetamine abuse has been described by Kramer, Fischman, and Littlefield (1967) and by Grinspoon and Hedblom (1975). Different patterns of initiation may occur: some individuals first obtain amphetamine through a prescription, whereas many others immediately begin with illicitly obtained material. Furthermore, initial drug consumption may be either oral or via intravenous injection. Regardless of the route of administration, if drug usage continues, the development of tolerance leads to a large escalation in the dose (see below). Moreover, even if the individual has previously taken amphetamine only orally, he or she may be

tempted to switch to intravenous administration (or possibly smoking in the case of methamphetamine) in order to obtain a more powerful "rush." The resulting chronic, high-dose intravenous (or smoking) pattern of consumption represents the most serious form of amphetamine or methamphetamine abuse.

Habitual intravenous amphetamine users commonly take the drug in patterns called "runs." During a run, the drug is typically injected approximately every 2 hours for a period of up to 3–6 days or longer (Kramer, Fischman, and Littlefield, 1967). Little sleep or eating occurs during a run. The user finally becomes exhausted, ends the run, and goes to sleep for many hours. Barbiturates or other depressant drugs are sometimes used either to "take the edge off" during a run or to assist in sleeping following the run.

Amphetamine Tolerance and Sensitization

For many years, the development of tolerance was considered one of the hallmarks of drug addiction. However, the occurrence of tolerance varies widely across different drugs, species, patterns of administration, and dependent variables. Therefore, many researchers now focus instead on the compulsivity of drug use and other aspects of drug-seeking behavior as crucial to defining drug abuse or addiction (Stolerman, 1992).

Despite this change in emphasis, tolerance is still important to consider in any discussion of chronic drug effects. Tolerance has been reported to the anorexic, hyperthermic, cardiovascular, and reinforcing effects of amphetamine (Lewander, 1971; Miller and Gold, 1989; Perez-Reyes et al., 1991), as well as to its disruptive influence on operant responding for food reinforcement (Fischman and Schuster, 1977; Schuster, Dockens, and Woods, 1966). Amphetamine tolerance is usually not a consequence of heightened drug metabolism or clearance (Kuhn and Schanberg, 1978; Perez-Reyes et al., 1991), although a possible exception may occur in humans in cases of extreme drug-induced anorexia, in which the resulting acidification of the urine hastens the excretion of unmetabolized amphetamine. We must turn, therefore, to cellular and behavioral mechanisms instead. Research to date has not yielded a consensus as to how amphetamine tolerance develops at the cellular level. However, Demellweek and Goudie (1983) have argued that behaviorally, amphetamine tolerance might be understandable as an adaptive reaction to behavioral disruption and the resulting loss of reinforcement.

Particularly important for understanding amphetamine abuse is the question of tolerance to its euphoric effects in humans. A recent laboratory study found no significant change in the subjective response to methamphetamine following 14 daily doses of 10 mg of the drug in a slow-release preparation (Perez-Reyes et al., 1991). In contrast, reports from chronic street users have consistently affirmed the occurrence of tolerance to amphetamine's euphoric effects (Grinspoon and Hedblom, 1975; Kramer, Fischman, and Littlefield, 1967). This often results in tremendous dose escalation, even during the course of a single run, as the user attempts to overcome the tolerance and achieve a satisfactory high. Such exposure to extremely high doses of amphetamine can lead to the development of psychotic reactions, which will be discussed further below.

One of the most interesting features of chronic psychostimulant administration is the development, in some cases, of reverse tolerance, or sensitization. A number of animal studies over the past 25 years have demonstrated that when amphetamine is given in a repeated, intermittent pattern, subjects become sensitized rather than tolerant to the locomotor-stimulating and stereotypy-inducing effects of the drug. Some of the main features of amphetamine sensitization are as follows: first, not all stereotyped behaviors become sensitized (Figure 13.12); second, the degree of sensitization may grow over time following the last drug administration; third, behavioral hyperresponsiveness can be extremely long-lasting (up to 1 year or more); fourth, a single low-dose injection can sensitize animals to a second drug exposure given at a later time; and finally, repeated amphetamine treatments and repeated exposures to stress can lead to cross-sensitization (that is, amphetamine-sensitized subjects are hyperresponsive to stress, and vice versa) (Robinson and Becker, 1986). Possible mechanisms of psychostimulant sensitization will be considered below in the section on cocaine.

Sensitization of amphetamine-induced stereotypies occurs not only in animals, but in humans as well. Some of the reported stereotyped behaviors in chronic amphetamine users include bizarre limb movements, continuous chewing or licking of the lips, nail biting, and aimless walking (Schiørring, 1981). Other behaviors may fall under the category of "punding,"* a term coined by

*According to Schiørring (1981), "punding" is derived from the Swedish word *pund-huvud*, which translates to the English "blockhead." "Punding" therefore connotes foolish or stupid behavior.

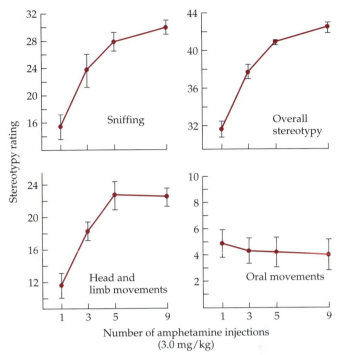

13.12 SENSITIZATION OF STEREOTYPED BEHAVIORAL RESPONSES TO REPEATED INTERMITTENT ADMINISTRATION OF AMPHETAMINE. Rats received 3 mg/kg amphetamine intraperitoneally once every 3–4 days for a total of 9 treatments. Using standard rating scales, observers assessed stereotyped behaviors at several intervals following the first, third, fifth, and ninth injections. Stereotyped sniffing and head and limb movements increased significantly with repeated amphetamine administration, whereas oral movements did not change over the course of treatment. (After Robinson and Becker, 1986.)

the Swedish psychiatrist Rylander (1972) to subsume a variety of stereotyped examination and manipulative behaviors shown by chronic amphetamine users. Punding may be manifested as persistent manipulation of a single small object, compulsive sorting of many small objects such as pebbles, or even the dismantling and reassembling of complicated equipment such as radios or television sets (Ellinwood, Sudilovsky, and Nelson, 1973; Ridley and Baker, 1982). In many instances, the appearance of these behavior patterns seems to be related to the development of an amphetamine psychosis (see below).

Amphetamine Dependence

In addition to tolerance, the other classic criterion for determining addiction was drug dependence. This typically meant the presence of somatic withdrawal symptoms following abrupt termination of drug use (abstinence syndrome), particularly autonomic symptoms like those observed during opiate withdrawal (see Chapter 12). With this criterion in mind, the initial view was that amphetamines and other psychostimulants did not produce dependence and hence were not addictive. However, as we saw in the case of tolerance, physical dependence is no longer considered synonymous with addiction. Moreover, interviews with chronic amphetamine users have revealed that both somatic and psychological reactions occur in the course of drug withdrawal. The symptoms of amphetamine withdrawal consist of extreme lethargy, difficulty in concentrating, lack of motivation, anxiety, increased sleep time along with excessive dreaming due to REM rebound, and craving for the drug (Grinspoon and Hedblom, 1975; Kramer, Fischman, and Littlefield, 1967). As would be expected, the degree of withdrawal symptomatology varies with the length of drug use and the doses taken. In severe cases, the symptoms may be sufficient to warrant a diagnosis of clinical depression. There is some evidence that the depression, dysphoria (unpleasant mood), and craving associated with withdrawal from a variety of abused substances (including amphetamine and cocaine) may be related to reduced DA release from mesolimbic neurons (Rossetti, Hmaidan, and Gessa, 1992).

Amphetamine Psychosis

Connell (1958), and later Ellinwood (1967) and Kramer, Fischman, and Littlefield (1967), described a type of psychotic reaction that occurs in a substantial number of high-dose amphetamine users. This reaction typically consists of visual or auditory hallucinations, behavioral disorganization, and the development of a paranoid state with delusions of persecution. In severe cases, the user may perceive that he or she is infested with parasites under the skin (colloquially termed "crank bugs"). Such parasitotic hallucinations lead to frantic picking and gouging at the skin in a futile attempt to rid oneself of the imagined scourge.

The users studied by Kramer, Fischman, and Littlefield (1967) reported that paranoia and hallucinations did not usually begin until the second or third day of a "speed run." Furthermore, these reactions to amphetamine generally did not occur upon first exposure to the drug, but only after a chronic abuse pattern had developed. Nevertheless, users who previously experienced a psychotic reaction were more susceptible to a recurrence if they used the drug again, even following a long period of abstinence (Sato et al., 1983). This phenonenon is suggestive of long-term amphetamine sensitization in humans.

Many of the symptoms of amphetamine psychosis are remarkably similar to those of paranoid schizophrenia, and amphetamine abusers have sometimes been misdiagnosed as schizophrenics. Moreover, the symptoms are ameliorated by neuroleptic (antipsychotic) drugs. Consequently, amphetamine (or cocaine) psychosis is commonly regarded as one of the best available models for schizophrenia, even though it only poorly resembles nonparanoid forms of the disorder (see Chapter 18). To study the possible etiology of schizophrenia, several laboratories have developed animal models involving either intermittent amphetamine injections or contin-

uous exposure via subcutaneously implanted osmotic minipumps or drug-filled silicone tubing. The contrasting reviews of Robinson and Becker (1986) and Ellison (1991) show that debate persists over which is the better model for eliciting schizophrenia-like neurological and behavioral effects.

Neurotoxic Effects of Amphetamine

Beginning in the 1970s, animal studies involving repeated administration of methamphetamine found persistently reduced DA concentrations and tyrosine hydroxylase activity in the caudate nucleus (Koda and Gibb, 1973; Seiden, Fischman, and Schuster, 1975, 1976). Subsequent work by Ellison and his colleagues (1978) showed that continuous amphetamine exposure led to the appearance of many swollen, catecholamine-containing axons in the caudate. Because administration of the catecholamine neurotoxin 6-OHDA causes a similar effect, the investigators hypothesized that the amphetamine treatment resulted in damage to the dopaminergic fibers of the nigrostriatal tract.

The neurotoxicity of amphetamine, methamphetamine, and certain of their congeners is now well established (for reviews see Axt, Mamounas, and Molliver, 1994; Gibb et al., 1989; Seiden and Kleven, 1989). Here we will focus closely on amphetamine and particularly methamphetamine, which is more toxic than its parent compound. The neurotoxicity of amphetamine congeners such as 3,4-methylenedioxymethamphetamine (MDMA), which has potent effects on the serotonergic system, is covered in Chapter 9.

In addition to the findings mentioned above, other evidence for the DA neurotoxicity of amphetamine and methamphetamine includes reduced density of DA transporter sites (Wagner et al., 1980) and histological signs of nerve terminal degeneration using the Fink-Heimer silver stain (Ricaurte et al., 1982; Ricaurte, Seiden, and Schuster, 1984). Indices of neurotoxicity are greatest in the caudate nucleus, whereas the mesolimbic and mesocortical pathways are less affected, and the hypothalamic DA neurons seem to be completely spared (Ellison et al., 1978; Morgan and Gibb, 1980; Ricaurte, Schuster, and Seiden, 1980; Ricaurte et al., 1982). Despite the severe damage to the DA terminals of the nigrostriatal tract, the cell bodies in the substantia nigra appear to remain intact (Ricaurte et al., 1982). However, recent results using cultured fetal mesencephalic neurons indicate that cell damage can occur at very high concentrations of methamphetamine (Bennett et al., 1993).

In addition to the dopaminergic system, several other neurotransmitter systems and brain regions have been examined for evidence of amphetamine neurotoxicity. These studies indicate that the serotonergic system is also severely damaged by methamphetamine (though less so by amphetamine) (Hotchkiss and Gibb, 1980; Morgan and Gibb, 1980; Ricaurte, Schuster, and Seiden,

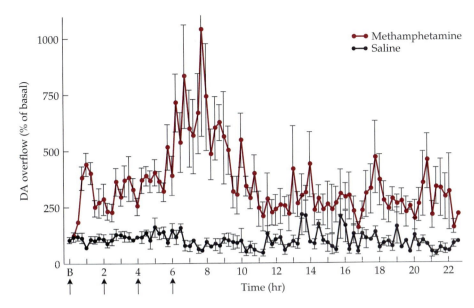

13.13 DOPAMINE OVERFLOW IN THE CAUDATE–PUTAMEN FOLLOWING A NEUROTOXIC DOSING REGIMEN OF METHAMPHETAMINE. Rats were implanted with microdialysis probes in the anterior caudate–putamen. After several days of recovery, the subjects were given four subcutaneous injections of either 4 mg/kg methamphetamine or saline at 2-hour intervals (arrows). Note that each of the first three drug injections caused a small to moderate increase in DA overflow, whereas the fourth injection at 6 hours led to a massive increase in extracellular DA. Moreover, DA overflow continued to be elevated above baseline for at least 22 hours following the first treatment. Basal DA overflow values were 14.0 ± 4.7 and 13.0 ± 4.0 pg/30 µl sample for the saline-and methamphetamine-treated subjects, respectively. (After O'Dell, Weihmuller, and Marshall, 1991.)

1980), whereas noradrenergic, cholinergic, and GABAergic neurons are thought to be relatively unaffected (Hotchkiss, Morgan, and Gibb, 1979; Morgan and Gibb, 1980; Wagner et al., 1980). It is also interesting to note that continuous amphetamine treatment has been reported to induce axonal and even cellular degeneration in certain areas of the rat neocortex (Ryan et al., 1990).

The possible mechanisms underlying amphetamine and methamphetamine neurotoxicity have been studied mainly with respect to the dopaminergic system. Methamphetamine-induced degeneration of caudate DA terminals can be prevented by AMPT pretreatment or by DA uptake inhibitors (Fuller and Hemrick-Luecke, 1980; Hotchkiss and Gibb, 1980; Ricaurte, Seiden, and Schuster, 1984), which is consistent with the notion that the neurotoxic effect requires DA release via exchange diffusion. Indeed, recent results suggest that damaging treatment regimens of amphetamine or methamphetamine produce their neurotoxic effects by triggering particularly large elevations in extracellular DA concentration (O'Dell, Weihmuller, and Marshall, 1991) (Figure 13.13). Less easily explained are the findings that antagonists of either DA or N-methyl-D-aspartate (NMDA) receptors block methamphetamine toxicity in the caudate nucleus (Marshall, O'Dell, and Weihmuller, 1993; O'Dell, Weihmuller, and Marshall, 1993; Sonsalla, Riordan, and Heikkila, 1991). However, Marshall's group has proposed that these agents exert their neuroprotective action by attenuating the DA-releasing effects of multiple methamphetamine injections (Marshall, O'Dell, and Weihmuller, 1993; O'Dell, Weihmuller, and Marshall, 1993). The proximate causes of DA terminal degeneration have not yet been elucidated; however, recent theories have centered around the possible roles of oxygen free radical formation (Cadet et al., 1994; Cubells et al., 1994) and disruption of energy metabolism (Chan et al., 1994).

Finally, animal studies of amphetamine and methamphetamine neurotoxicity raise the crucial question of whether human abusers of these drugs may be susceptible to brain damage, particularly in the extrapyramidal motor system. At present, there is no clinical evidence (i.e., parkinsonian symptoms) of nigrostriatal system deficits in chronic amphetamine or methamphetamine users (Seiden and Ricaurte, 1987). However, because the drug-induced damage to this system is only partial, even methamphetamine-treated animals do not exhibit behavioral deficits unless they are pharmacologically challenged (Seiden and Kleven, 1989). It thus remains possible that some human users suffer from latent neurotoxic effects that are manifested later in life as a heightened vulnerability to or an earlier onset of Parkinson's disease. Just as in vitro autoradiography can be used to demonstrate the loss of dopaminergic transport sites (and hence DA nerve terminals) in amphetamine-treated animals, the technique of positron emission tomography (PET) could be applied to determine whether nigrostriatal damage is present in human users. We hope that such studies will be performed to resolve this important question.

Part I Summary

Amphetamine and methamphetamine are synthetic drugs that belong to a group of compounds known as psychomotor stimulants. They are closely related structurally to two plant compounds, cathinone and ephedrine, which possess similar behavioral and physiological properties. Amphetamine was first introduced in the United States in 1932 in the form of a nasal inhaler. People soon realized that they could achieve powerful stimulatory and euphoric effects by consuming the drug orally or by injecting it intravenously or subcutaneously.

The incidence of amphetamine use and abuse grew until a peak was attained in the 1970s. Since that time, the drug has been largely supplanted by cocaine, except for a recent upsurge in the smoking of a crystalline form of methamphetamine known as "ice."

Amphetamine exerts complex effects on the catecholaminergic, particularly dopaminergic, systems. The drug releases DA from the cytoplasm of nerve terminals by a process called exchange diffusion. It also seems to enter synaptic vesicles and displace DA from its storage sites. Other effects include the blocking of DA uptake and (at high doses) the inhibition of DA degradation by MAO. From these findings, it is clear that amphetamine is a potent indirect agonist at dopaminergic synapses. At least some of these effects have also been demonstrated for the noradrenergic system.

Acute administration of amphetamine in humans leads to a well-known constellation of behavioral reactions, including increased arousal, reduced fatigue, and feelings of exhilaration. Sleep is delayed, and performance of simple, repetitive tasks is improved. Physiologically, amphetamine acts as a typical sympathomimetic agent, causing elevated blood pressure, heart rate, respiration rate, and energy metabolism. Despite these and other "side effects," amphetamine and other stimulants such as methylphenidate are used therapeutically in the treatment of narcolepsy, attention deficit hyperactivity disorder, and obesity.

Amphetamine also causes a spectrum of behavioral changes in animal subjects. At low doses, locomotor activity is stimulated. As the dose is increased, locomotor activation is replaced by increasing levels of focused stereotyped behaviors, the components of which depend on the species. Amphetamine also exerts rate-dependent effects on operant responding, produces a discriminative stimulus that generalizes to other psychomotor stimulants, and is strongly reinforcing, as demonstrated by self-administration and place-conditioning studies. The behavioral effects of amphetamine can be attributed primarily to its actions on the DA system. The nucleus accumbens in particular has been associated with amphetamine's locomotor-stimulating and reinforcing effects, whereas the caudate nucleus appears to mediate amphetamine-induced stereotypic behaviors.

As would be predicted from its reinforcing properties in animal models, amphetamine has severe abuse potential in humans. Some individuals develop a binge pattern of use, during which the drug dose may be increased tremendously due to the development of tolerance. This pattern can also lead to the development of a psychotic state that closely resembles paranoid schizophrenia. In both animal subjects and human users, intermittent regimens of amphetamine administration can lead to sensitization of certain stereotyped behaviors. Finally, animal studies have demonstrated that high doses of amphetamine or, particularly, methamphetamine can be neurotoxic to the dopaminergic and serotonergic systems. In the case of DA, the nigrostriatal tract is most vulnerable to amphetamine neurotoxicity. Whether this effect also occurs in human high-dose users remains an open question at the present time.

Part II
Cocaine

The history of cocaine is detailed in several excellent reviews (Johanson and Fischman, 1989; Van Dyke and Byck, 1982); hence we will present only a brief summary here. Cocaine is an alkaloid found in the leaves of the shrub *Erythroxylon coca*. The coca shrub grows in the eastern highlands of the Andes mountains in Bolivia, Peru, Ecuador, and Colombia. The inhabitants of these regions consume cocaine by chewing the leaves, a practice that may have begun over 5,000 years ago according to some archeological evidence (Van Dyke and Byck, 1982). Like amphetamine, cocaine is a weak base ($pK_a = 8.6$). Hence, coca chewers take some lime or ash with the leaves to make the pH of the saliva more alkaline, thereby decreasing ionization of the cocaine and promoting absorption across the mucous membranes of the oral cavity. Because the Incas thought of coca as a gift from the Sun God, use of the drug was initially restricted to ceremonial or religious occasions. However, coca chewing later became more widespread and commonplace until the practice was banned by the Spanish conquerers in the 1500s. The Spaniards subsequently lifted the ban when they discovered that Incan slaves worked harder and longer when allowed to chew their coca.

Although coca leaves were brought back to Europe, coca chewing never caught on, possibly due to degradation of the active ingredient during the long sea voyage. The situation changed, however, when Niemann isolated and characterized the pure alkaloid in 1859. Over the next 30 years, cocaine became tremendously popular as many notable scientists and physicians lauded its properties. A chemist named Mariani concocted an infamous mixture of cocaine and wine ("Vin Mariani"), while the Italian neurologist Mantegazza wrote, "I would rather have a life span of ten years with coca than one of 1,000,000 centuries without coca" (Petersen, 1977). The most famous cocaine user was Sigmund Freud. In 1884, Freud published the monograph *Uber Coca* ("On Coca"), which extolled the drug's virtues and recommended its use in the treatment of alcoholism, morphine addiction, depression, and a variety of other ailments. Freud also performed the first recorded psychopharmacological experiments on cocaine and published the results in an 1885 paper entitled "A Contribution to the Knowledge of the Effect of Cocaine" (see Rosecran and Spitz, 1987).

In the late nineteenth and early twentieth centuries, cocaine's popularity also grew in the United States (Das and Laddu, 1993; Musto, 1991). By 1885, Parke Davis & Co. was manufacturing 15 different forms of cocaine and coca, including cigarettes, cheroots (a type of cigar), and inhalants. One year later, a Georgia pharmacist named John Pemberton introduced a new beverage, "Coca Cola," that contained cocaine from coca leaves and caffeine from cola nuts.* Coca Cola and similar concoctions with names like "Koca Nola" and "Nerv Ola" were marketed as alternatives to alcoholic drinks because of the growing strength of the alcohol temperance movement at that time. Cocaine-containing tooth drops were even given to infants to relieve the discomfort of teething (the local anesthetic effects of cocaine are discussed further below). Not surprisingly, widespread cocaine abuse started to appear across the United States. Finally, President Taft declared cocaine to be "public enemy number one" in 1910. Congress then passed the 1914 Harrison Narcotic Act, prohibiting the inclusion of cocaine (as well as opium) in patent medicines and specifying other restrictions on its importation and sale. Subsequent state and federal laws, of course, placed even tighter regulations on cocaine distribution and use.

From the 1920s to the 1960s, cocaine use continued primarily among a relatively small group of "avant garde" artists, musicians, and other performers (Petersen, 1977). Beginning in the 1970s, however, we have seen two successive waves of increasing cocaine use in the United States. The first involved an escalation of cocaine use by snorting or intravenous injection, whereas the most recent epidemic of cocaine use has been driven by the smoking of "crack" cocaine.

According to the 1990 National Household Survey on Drug Abuse conducted by the National Institute on Drug Abuse (NIDA), approximately 1.6 million people (less than 1% of the U.S. population) were current users of cocaine at that time (National Institute on Drug Abuse, 1991). By "current user," we mean an individual who had used cocaine at least once during the previous month. A larger number of individuals (6 million) had used cocaine during the previous year, whereas the lifetime prevalence rate (use at least once during one's lifetime) was reported to be nearly 23 million (about 11% of the population). The highest rates of use were found in adults between the ages of 18 and 34.

When these data were compared with comparable surveys conducted from 1974 to 1988, it appeared that cocaine use peaked during the late 1970s and early 1980s, and that the prevalence of use was subsequently declining. However, two limitations of these data are important to consider. First, the study sample did not include some important segments of the population, such as students living in college dormitories, hospitalized patients (including those currently hospitalized for drug-related problems), jail inmates, and homeless people. Second, the data were based on personal interviews with the respondents and therefore depended on both the memory and honesty of the subjects. These aspects of the survey are likely to lead to an underestimation of overall cocaine (or other drug) use in our society, although the degree of underestimation is impossible to determine.

Basic Pharmacology of Cocaine

Coca leaves contain between 0.6% and 1.8% alkaloidal cocaine. Initial extraction from the leaves results in a coca paste containing about 80% cocaine. The alkaloid is then converted to the hydrochloride (HCl) salt and crystallized. Cocaine HCl is readily water soluble and thus can be taken orally (as in Vin Mariani), intranasally ("snorting"), or by intravenous injection. One disadvantage of cocaine HCl is its vulnerability to pyrolysis (heat-induced breakdown), which prevents it from being smoked effectively. However, the hydrochloride salt can be transformed back into cocaine freebase by dissolving it in an alkaline solution, followed by precipitation. The resulting material resists pyrolysis and thus can be smoked (hence the term "freebasing"). "Crack" or "rock" cocaine are street terms for chunks of cocaine freebase generally sold in small amounts sufficient for only a single dose.

Different routes of consumption yield somewhat different patterns and levels of plasma cocaine concentration. Extremely rapid absorption occurs with both intravenous injection and smoking. Hence, typical single doses taken by these routes yield rather high concentrations of circulating cocaine (500–1,000 ng/ml) (Jatlow, 1988; Johanson and Fischman, 1989), although even higher values can be attained with multiple doses that mimic the pattern of a cocaine "binge" (Isenschmid et al., 1992; see below). Absorption is somewhat slower following oral administration or snorting; consequently, these routes yield lower cocaine levels in the range of 100–500 ng/ml. Figure 13.14 depicts the time course of plasma cocaine concentration as a function of route of administration. It is also interesting to note that a few hours of coca leaf chewing delivers enough drug to mimic the plasma concentrations produced by a modest dose taken either orally or intranasally (Jatlow, 1988).

The two primary metabolites of cocaine are ecgonine methyl ester and benzoylecgonine, both of which are excreted in the urine. Together, ecgonine methyl ester and benzoylecgonine account for 75% to 90% of cocaine metabolism (Jatlow, 1988). Smaller amounts of ecgonine and the biologically active metabolite norcocaine are also formed. Breakdown of cocaine to ecgonine methyl ester

---

*In case any readers are wondering, whereas the caffeine still persists in regular Coca Cola, the cocaine was eliminated in 1906.

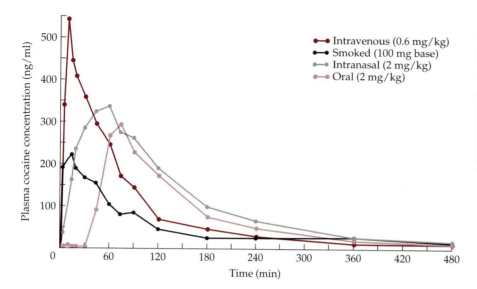

13.14 TIME COURSE OF PLASMA CO-CAINE CONCENTRATIONS FOLLOWING DIFFERENT ROUTES OF ADMINISTRATION. Each curve shows the mean for ten human subjects. For the cocaine freebase smoking, subjects were allowed only 1–3 puffs of the vapor from 100 mg of drug heated in a flask; the peak plasma concentrations produced under these conditions probably underestimate the levels occurring from recreational use. (After Jones, 1990.)

is rapidly catalyzed by cholinesterases found in serum and liver. In contrast, hydrolysis of the other ester linkage to form benzoylecgonine may be nonenzymatic (Shuster, 1992). Finally, the demethylation of cocaine to form norcocaine occurs through the hepatic mixed function oxidase system.

Considerable individual variability has been observed in the rate at which cocaine is cleared from the circulation. This can be seen in studies using intravenous injections, which theoretically should give the most valid results because the entire dose is administered over a short time and absorption is rapid. Yet even under these seemingly ideal conditions, estimates of the elimination half-life range from 16 to 90 minutes across different individuals and studies (Shuster, 1992). Despite this interindividual variability, it is clear that cocaine is eliminated much more rapidly than amphetamine. For this reason, the subjective "high" produced by a single intra-venous or smoked dose of cocaine may last only about 30 minutes (Jones, 1990), compared with the longer effect produced by a typical dose of amphetamine.

Mechanisms of Cocaine Action

Neurochemical Effects on Monoamine Systems

The pharmacology of cocaine and its mechanisms of action are reviewed in Woolverton and Johnson (1992). In contrast to amphetamine, cocaine appears to have little effect on catecholamine release (Heikkila, Orlansky, and Cohen, 1975; Nicolaysen and Justice, 1988). However, it interacts with the plasma membrane transporters for DA, NE, and 5-HT, thereby blocking cellular uptake of all three monoamines. The influence of cocaine on monoamine systems has been investigated using several different approaches, beginning with early studies of transmitter uptake in synaptosomal or tissue slice preparations (Harris and Baldessarini, 1973; Taylor and Ho, 1978). These experiments demonstrated that cocaine acts on all three uptake systems with a similar, though not identical, potency. Later microdialysis studies demonstrated that acute cocaine treatment causes increases in extracellular DA levels (Carboni et al., 1989; Nomikos et al., 1990), and that the time course of such increases is correlated with changes in extracellular cocaine concentration (Figure 13.15; Hurd, Kehr, and Ungerstedt, 1988; Nicolaysen, Pan, and Justice, 1988). These findings confirmed that the reuptake blockade observed in vitro likewise occurs in vivo, and they further suggested that such blockade enhances monoaminergic synaptic activity by increasing transmitter availability within the synaptic cleft.

Investigators have recently begun to study the interaction of cocainelike drugs with monoamine trans-

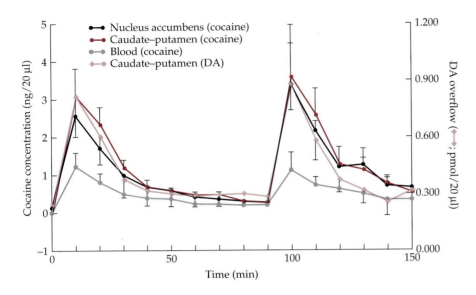

13.15 RELATIONSHIP BETWEEN BLOOD AND BRAIN COCAINE CONCENTRATIONS AND COCAINE-INDUCED DOPAMINE OVERFLOW IN THE CAUDATE–PUTAMEN. Rats were implanted with microdialysis probes and then, while still under anaesthesia, injected intravenously with 1.5 mg/kg of cocaine at time 0 and again at 90 minutes. In some subjects, cocaine concentrations were determined in blood and in dialysate samples from the anterior caudate–putamen and nucleus accumbens (left-hand scale). DA overflow was measured in the anterior caudate–putamen in a separate group of subjects treated in the same manner (right-hand scale). Note that changes in striatal DA overflow closely parallel the time course of blood and tissue cocaine levels. (After Hurd, Kehr, and Ungerstedt, 1988.)

porters using membrane binding and autoradiographic techniques. To date, most of these experiments have used either of two compounds, 2β-carbomethoxy-3β-(4-fluorophenyl)tropane (referred to either as WIN 35,428 or CFT) and 2β-carbomethoxy-3β-(4-iodophenyl)-tropane (referred to as RTI-55 or β-CIT). These compounds belong to a series of potent phenyltropane cocaine congeners originally synthesized by chemists at the Sterling-Winthrop company (Clarke et al., 1973). It can be seen that both substances lack cocaine's ester linkage between the two rings, and that both also possess a halogen substituent at the *para* position on the phenyl ring. These structural changes give rise to certain pharmacological differences from cocaine itself. For example, WIN 35,428 blocks DA uptake somewhat more selectively than cocaine, and radiolabeled forms of the drug bind mainly to the DA transporter (Kaufman, Spealman, and Madras, 1991; Madras et al., 1989). On the other hand, RTI-55 binds with high affinity to both the DA and 5-HT transporters in vivo and in vitro (Boja et al., 1992; Cline, Scheffel et al., 1992; Scheffel et al., 1992). When labeled with an appropriate photon- or positron-emitting isotope, RTI-55 should be useful for SPECT (single photon emission computed tomography) or PET (positron emission tomography) imaging of the human brain to study the transporter changes associated with degenerative disorders such as Parkinson's disease (Brücke et al., 1993; Farde et al., 1994; see Chapter 20).

Although cocaine produces a net enhancement of monoaminergic transmission due to its uptake-blocking effects, Galloway (1990) showed that DA and 5-HT synthesis are transiently inhibited by acute cocaine administration. This result is understandable when one considers that elevated extracellular neurotransmitter levels may stimulate both synthesis-inhibiting presynaptic autoreceptors and somatodendritic autoreceptors that slow the frequency of cell firing (as discussed in previous chapters, the rate of neurotransmitter formation is often correlated with neuronal activity). Consequently, dopaminergic and serotonergic neurons exhibit a compensatory response to cocaine by reducing their neurotransmitter synthesis.

Other Neurochemical Effects

At high concentrations, cocaine interacts with several membrane proteins in addition to the monoamine transporters. These proteins include σ sites (Sharkey, Glen et al., 1988; see Chapter 17), 5-HT$_3$ receptors (Kilpatrick, Jones, and Tyers, 1987), muscarinic cholinergic receptors (Sharkey, Ritz et al., 1988), and most importantly, voltage-gated Na$^+$ channels (Matthews and Collins, 1983). Because of its ability to block axonal Na$^+$ channels, cocaine is a potent local anesthetic. Indeed, two synthetic local anesthetics that are widely used in medical and dental practice, procaine (Novocain) and lidocaine (Xylo-

Procaine

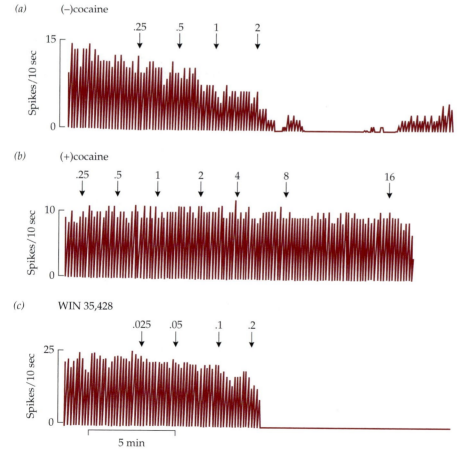

C_2H_5
C_2H_5
N — CH_2 — C — NH
O
H_3C
H_3C

Lidocaine

caine), were developed from the structure of cocaine, although they lack cocaine's tropane ring.

Like amphetamine, cocaine induces expression of the immediate–early gene *c-fos* in the rat striatum. However, the pattern of expression within the striatum differs between the two drugs (Graybiel, Moratalla, and Robertson, 1990). Recent work has shown that cocaine induction of striatal *c-fos* occurs primarily in neurons that project to the substantia nigra (i.e., neurons that form the striatonigral pathway) (Cenci et al., 1992). Such induction has generally been attributed to activation of D_1 receptors (Young, Porrino, and Iadarola, 1991); however, D_2 receptor activation also seems to be required (Ruskin and Marshall, 1994).

We saw earlier that low doses of amphetamine preferentially stimulated cerebral glucose utilization in the nucleus accumbens. Porrino and her coworkers (1988) found similar results with cocaine, except that the me-

dial prefrontal cortex was activated as well. At high doses, cocaine, like amphetamine, produced more widespread increases in glucose utilization.

Electrophysiological Effects

Cocaine has important effects on the electrophysiological activity of monoaminergic cell groups and also on the activity of neurons that receive monoaminergic input. Various studies have demonstrated cocaine-induced inhibition of dopaminergic cell firing in the substantia nigra and ventral tegmental area (Einhorn, Johansen, and White, 1988; Lacey, Mercuri, and North, 1990), noradrenergic cell firing in the locus coeruleus (Pitts and Marwah, 1987), and serotonergic cell firing in the dorsal raphe nucleus (Cunningham and Lakoski, 1990). Some of these findings are illustrated in Figure 13.16, which shows extracellular recordings of single dorsal raphe units in anesthetized rats. Repeated intravenous doses of (−)cocaine (the active isomer) led to a progressive reduction in firing rate until the cells were completely silenced following a cumulative dose of 2.0 mg/kg. The inactive isomer (+)cocaine had no effect on raphe single unit activity, whereas the cocaine congener WIN 35,428 was ten times more potent than cocaine in terms of the dose required for 100% inhibition of cell firing (WIN 35,428 is thus less selective for DA in this sys-

13.16 EFFECTS OF COCAINE STEREOISO-MERS AND THE COCAINE ANALOG WIN 35,428 ON THE SPONTANEOUS ACTIVITY OF SEROTONERGIC NEURONS. Rats were anesthetized with chloral hydrate and electrodes were acutely implanted for extracellular recording of serotonergic neurons in the dorsal raphe nucleus (DRN). Test drugs were administered intravenously in a cumulative dosing paradigm (arrows indicate when a particular dose infusion was completed), and the effect on DRN single-unit activity was observed. (*a*) The active stereoisomer of cocaine [(−)cocaine] produced a dose-dependent suppression of DRN neuron firing. Within several minutes after the cumulative cocaine dose had reached 2 mg/kg, the cells were completely silenced. (*b*) The inactive stereoisomer [(+)cocaine] had no effect on neuronal activity. (*c*) The phenyltropane cocaine analog WIN 35,428 was approximately tenfold more potent than cocaine itself in suppressing neuronal firing in the DRN. (After Cunningham and Lakoski, 1990.)

tem than it is in radioligand binding studies). Other experiments of Cunningham and Lakoski (1990) demonstrated that the influence of cocaine and WIN 35,428 on single-unit activity was mimicked by the selective 5-HT uptake inhibitor fluoxetine (Prozac; see Chapter 9), but not by the DA uptake inhibitor GBR 12909, the NE uptake inhibitor desipramine, or the local anesthetics lidocaine or procaine.

The inhibitory effects of cocaine on monoaminergic neurons appear to be mediated at least partly by stimulation of the somatodendritic autoreceptors described in previous chapters. Cocaine-induced blockade of the cell membrane transporter presumably increases transmitter activation of these autoreceptors, thereby reducing impulse flow. Activation of negative feedback pathways from target neurons (e.g., in the nucleus accumbens) represents another potential mechanism whereby cocaine may inhibit monoaminergic cell firing (Einhorn, Johansen, and White, 1988).

Because of its reuptake-blocking action at nerve terminal transporters, cocaine would be expected to enhance the electrophysiological effects of DA, NE, and 5-HT on postsynaptic neurons that receive input from these transmitters. One example of this phenomenon was reported by Uchimura and North (1990), who made intracellular recordings in vitro from slices of rat nucleus accumbens. Application of DA tended to produce a hyperpolarizing effect mediated by D_1 receptors, whereas D_2 receptors mediated a depolarizing effect in some cells. 5-HT caused depolarization in most neurons examined. As anticipated, all three effects were enhanced by cocaine. Interestingly, however, low concentrations of the drug had a greater potentiating effect on 5-HT than on DA. This finding is consistent with evidence that cocaine has a somewhat greater affinity for the 5-HT than for the DA transporter (Ritz et al., 1987).

Finally, it should be noted that monoamine uptake inhibition by cocaine increases extracellular transmitter concentrations in the vicinity of presynaptic as well as somatodendritic autoreceptors. This reduces the amount of neurotransmitter released when an action potential invades the nerve terminal. Consequently, even though cocaine administration produces a net enhancement of monoaminergic transmission, the effect of the drug is to some extent self-limiting due to autoreceptor stimulation and the resulting inhibition of cell firing and transmitter release.

Acute Behavioral and Physiological Effects of Cocaine in Humans

Effects on Mood and Behavior

Not surprisingly, cocaine yields a classic amphetamine-like psychostimulant profile on the ARCI and POMS when administered to subjects under controlled laboratory conditions (see Johanson and Fischman, 1989). More subjective accounts of cocaine's acute behavioral effects are presented in Grinspoon and Bakalar (1985) and in Spotts and Shontz (1980). Typical aspects of the cocaine "high" are feelings of exhilaration and euphoria, a sense of well-being, and great self-confidence. Taken by intravenous injection or by smoking, cocaine also produces a brief "rush" that is sometimes described as being like an orgasm but even more intense. At low and moderate doses, cocaine often increases sociability and talkativeness. There are also reports of heightened sexual interest and performance under the influence of cocaine, although the drug's legendary ability to enhance sexual prowess is highly exaggerated. Finally, Licata and colleagues (1993) recently found that cocaine increased aggressiveness under controlled laboratory conditions. This important finding suggests that some of the street violence associated with cocaine might be attributable to a direct effect of the drug.

The major subjective and behavioral effects of cocaine and other psychostimulants are summarized in Table 13.1. The effects listed in the "mild–moderate" category are generally produced by single, low to moderate doses of cocaine in naive subjects or in users who have not yet progressed to heavy, chronic patterns of drug intake. "Severe" effects are most likely to be seen with high-dose use, particularly in individuals with long-standing patterns of chronic intake. It is easy to see that many of the positive effects of cocaine that may contribute to its powerful reinforcing properties become negative or aversive with escalation of dose and duration. Some of these aversive effects (e.g., irritability) are present in most high-dose users, whereas others occur mainly in cases of cocaine-induced psychosis (e.g., incoherence or delusions; see below). Like amphetamine, cocaine may lead to stereotyped motor responses when taken chronically (see Brady et al., 1991; Johanson and Fischman, 1989); however, cocaine stereotypies seem to be less common than amphetamine stereotypies. For example, Spotts and Shontz (1980) never observed this phenomenon in their extensive case studies of nine cocaine-using men, some of whom ingested up to 11 g of cocaine per day for several days.

The mechanisms underlying the mood-altering effects of cocaine in humans have not yet been elucidated. DA probably plays some role, as Sherer and coworkers found that pretreatment with the D_2 antagonist haloperidol attenuated the "high" produced by intravenous cocaine administration, but had no effect on the self-reported "rush" (Sherer, 1988; Sherer, Kumor, and Jaffe, 1989). Recent work suggests that 5-HT may also be involved, as acute depletion of tryptophan (a procedure that decreases brain 5-HT levels) reduced the subjective "high" obtained from intranasal cocaine administration (Aronson et al., 1995).

Table 13.1   Mild to Moderate versus Severe Behavioral and Subjective Effects of Cocaine and Other Psychostimulants in Humans[a]

Mild–moderate effects	Severe effects
Mood amplification; both euphoria and dysphoria	Irritability, hostility, anxiety, fear, withdrawal
Heightened energy	Extreme energy or exhaustion
Sleep disturbance, insomnia	Total insomnia
Motor excitement, restlessness	Compulsive motor stereotypies
Talkativeness, pressure of speech	Rambling, incoherent speech
Hyperactive ideation	Disjointed flight of ideas
Increased sexual interest	Decreased sexual interest
Anger, verbal aggression	Possible extreme violence
Mild to moderate anorexia	Total anorexia
Inflated self-esteem	Delusions of grandiosity

[a]The actual effects observed show individual variability and depend on the dose, route of administration, pattern and duration of use, and environmental context.
Source: After Post and Contel, 1983.

Several research groups have investigated the influence of cocaine on psychomotor performance. Fischman and Schuster (1980) found no statistically reliable effect of cocaine on the reaction time of rested subjects. However, Higgins and colleagues (1990) subsequently reported that intranasal cocaine administration produced a modest but significant improvement in performance on the Digit Symbol Substitution Test.

Physiological Effects

Cocaine produces a spectrum of sympathomimetic effects similar to that described earlier for amphetamine (reviewed by Pitts and Marwah, 1989). It might be assumed that these effects of cocaine are mediated by a blockade of NE reuptake at peripheral sympathetic neuroeffector junctions. However, evidence obtained in rats indicates that the cardiovascular actions of cocaine are mainly due to stimulation of central sympathetic outflow (Kiritsy-Roy et al., 1990; Tella, Schindler, and Goldberg, 1992, 1993). Cocaine-induced catecholamine release then causes a pressor response (i.e., increased blood pressure) through α_1-adrenergic receptor–mediated vasoconstriction (Branch and Knuepfer, 1992).

Acute Behavioral Effects of Cocaine in Animals

As summarized by Johanson and Fischman (1989), cocaine is similar to amphetamine in its acute behavioral effects on various animal species. Like amphetamine, cocaine produces locomotor activation and, at higher doses, stereotyped motor behaviors. Interestingly, Scheel-Krüger and colleagues (1977) reported that cocaine and amphetamine stereotypies were similar when the drugs were administered subcutaneously, but that cocaine stereotypies were less pronounced than those following

amphetamine administration when the intraperitoneal route was used.

We saw earlier that the influence of amphetamine on schedule-controlled behavior is largely rate-dependent; that is, responding is typically increased under conditions (schedules) that yield low baseline rates, whereas responding is decreased when the baseline rate is high. Most studies with cocaine have yielded comparable rate-dependent changes (Johanson and Fischman, 1989).

Animals can readily learn to discriminate cocaine from vehicle treatment. Cocaine's discriminative stimulus properties were first shown in rats by Colpaert, Niemegeers, and Janssen (1976), and were subsequently demonstrated in other species such as pigeons, rhesus monkeys, and squirrel monkeys (Johanson and Fischman, 1989). Animals initially trained on cocaine readily generalize to amphetamine, indicating a fundamental similarity in the cue properties of the two drugs. Generalization also occurs to potent phenyltropane congeners such as WIN 35,428 and RTI-55 (Cline, Terry et al., 1992), which further supports the cocainelike characteristics of these compounds.

Reinforcing Effects of Cocaine

Three major approaches have been used to demonstrate the reinforcing effects of cocaine in animals: self-administration, enhancement of brain stimulation reward, and place conditioning. Animals readily learn to self-administer cocaine intravenously. Within the appropriate dose range, response rate varies inversely with dose per infusion; that is, relatively low doses lead to high response rates, and vice versa. Although most cocaine self-administration studies have used the intravenous route, Carroll, Krattiger and colleagues (1990) have been able to demonstrate cocaine freebase smoking in rhesus monkeys.

As in the case of amphetamine, unlimited access to cocaine leads to gradual weight loss, the appearance of convulsions, and eventual death in a high percentage of subjects (Johanson, Balster, and Bonese, 1976). Interestingly, somewhat less toxicity has been reported for long-term unlimited access to heroin compared with cocaine (Bozarth and Wise, 1985).

The seemingly compulsive nature of cocaine and amphetamine self-administration when access is unlimited seems to accurately reflect the high abuse potential of these compounds. On the other hand, it is important to recognize that such compulsivity is not observed under all conditions. For example, Nader and Woolverton (1992) trained mildly food-deprived rhesus monkeys on a discrete-trials choice procedure involving intravenous cocaine injections versus 1-g banana-flavored food pellets. The subjects chose between the two reinforcers under varying fixed ratio (FR) schedules. The results indicated that cocaine was not uniformly preferred over food, but rather, that the animals' preference depended on the relative magnitude of each reinforcer as well as the response requirements as determined by the FR schedule (Figure 13.17). Thus, the group mean data show that a four-pellet reinforcement under an FR 30 schedule (i.e., 30 lever presses were required to obtain the pellets) was chosen about 50% of the time when matched with a cocaine dose of 0.1 mg/kg under either an FR 30 or an FR 120 schedule.

Humans show similar behavior, at least under some conditions. Four young adults who had occasionally snorted cocaine in the past were each given 20 trials in which they were allowed to choose between snorting a small but reinforcing amount of cocaine (10 mg) or receiving a small amount of money ($0.50 to $2.00). Whereas most of the subjects chose cocaine over the $0.50 reinforcement, they all consistently preferred $2.00 rather than the drug (Higgins, Bickel, and Hughes, 1994).

One theoretical approach to understanding the behavior of organisms when multiple reinforcers (including drugs) are available under varying response requirements is known as **behavioral economics**. The central tenet of this theory is that demand for a drug (measured as drug consumption) will decrease in a predictable manner as unit price (UP) increases (UP is measured in terms of responses required per dose, that is, the responses/mg/kg) (Bickel et al., 1990). Although behavioral economics represents an interesting new way of examining drug consumption, it may not be the best approach in all circumstances (see Nader, Hedeker, and Woolverton, 1993). With humans, for example, the choice of money over cocaine in a laboratory setting by someone who occasionally snorts the drug is probably not predictive of what a heavy crack smoker will do when experiencing intense craving during withdrawal from a binge in a "crack house."

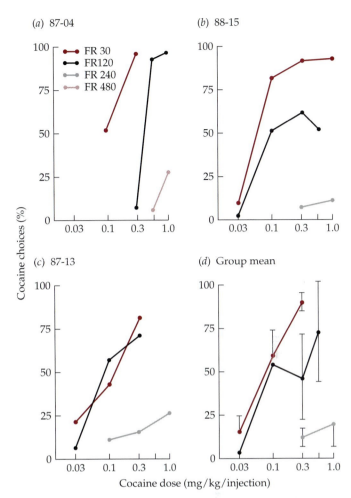

13.17 CHOICE BETWEEN COCAINE AND FOOD REINFORCEMENT IN RHESUS MONKEYS. Monkeys were mildly food-deprived and trained in a two-lever operant chamber to press one of the levers for food. The reinforcer was four 1-g banana-flavored pellets delivered under an FR 30 schedule. Each subject was then equipped with an indwelling venous catheter and trained to select either the food or an infusion of cocaine (obtained by pressing the second lever in the chamber) using a discrete-trials choice procedure. In separate sessions, cocaine was available at various doses (0.03–1.0 mg/kg per infusion) and under differing schedules of reinforcement (see key). (a–c) Results from individual monkeys. (d) Group mean data, which show that food reinforcement was chosen equally or more often than cocaine at low drug doses (0.03–0.1 mg/kg) and at a very high cocaine response requirement (the FR 480 schedule). (After Nader and Woolverton, 1992.)

A second method of studying the reinforcing properties of cocaine and other drugs of abuse is to examine their effects on brain stimulation reward. In Chapter 8, we discussed the neural circuits that mediate intracranial self-stimulation (ICSS) and the role of DA in this phenomenon. Cocaine enhances ICSS in both the medial forebrain bundle (Wise et al., 1992) and the prefrontal cortex (McGregor, Atrens, and Jackson, 1992). Figure 13.18 illustrates the influence of cocaine on ICSS in an individual rat using the curve-shift procedure described in Chapter 8. The baseline (no cocaine) curve shows that re-

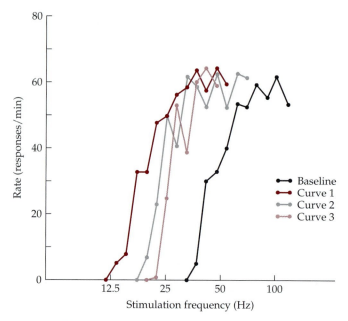

13.18 THE REINFORCING EFFECT OF COCAINE AS DEMON-STRATED BY ENHANCEMENT OF INTRACRANIAL SELF-STIMU-LATION. Data are shown from a single rat in which successive frequency–rate self-stimulation curves were generated at 30-minute intervals before and after cocaine administration (15 mg/kg i.p.). Drug treatment led to a leftward shift in the frequency–rate curve compared with baseline, indicating an enhancement of the reinforcing effect of the electrical stimulus. The rightward shift of curves 2 and 3 compared with curve 1 could be due to several factors, including rapid tolerance to the cocaine or a gradual diminution of the reinforcing effect due to clearance of the drug from the animal's circulation. (After Wise et al., 1992.)

sponding was first elicited at a stimulation frequency between 25 and 50 Hz, and that the response rate reached a plateau between 50 and 100 Hz. Following a single intraperitoneal injection of cocaine, subsequent stimulus frequency–response rate curves retained the same basic shape, but were significantly shifted to the left. This effect, which is reminiscent of shifts in drug dose–response curves, indicates that cocaine enhanced the reinforcing effect of the electrical stimulus and suggests that psychostimulants may operate on the same neurochemical mechanisms that underlie ICSS.

The reinforcing effects of cocaine have also been investigated using place conditioning procedures. The strength of cocaine-induced place conditioning depends heavily on the dose, route of administration, and other experimental variables. In general, the strongest place preferences are produced by intravenous injections, followed by intraperitoneal administration (Nomikos and Spyraki, 1988). The subcutaneous route has yielded the most variable results, with some investigators reporting a place preference (Durazzo et al., 1994) and others reporting no conditioning (Mayer and Parker, 1993).

Finally, it is important to note that aversive effects of cocaine can be observed in animals under certain condi-

tions. This has been demonstrated by experiments in which cocaine treatment paired with consumption of a novel flavored solution elicited a subsequent avoidance of that flavor (i.e., a conditioned taste aversion) (Ferrari, O'Connor, and Riley, 1991; Mayer and Parker, 1993). Cocaine's aversive properties may stem from its ability to increase anxiety, both in human self-reports (see Table 13.1) and in animal behavioral tests (Ettenberg and Geist, 1991; Yang et al., 1992). Although we have just seen that subcutaneous injections of cocaine are less reinforcing than intravenous or intraperitoneal injections in place conditioning procedures, the subcutaneous route of administration seems to yield the most robust aversive conditioning. This difference could be related to the different pharmacokinetic characteristics of each injection route. Intravenous injections (which are the most reinforcing) produce rapid peaking of blood and brain cocaine concentrations, whereas intraperitoneal injections require some time for absorption to occur, and subcutaneous injections lead to even slower absorption due to local vasoconstriction. Slow absorption probably reduces the reinforcing properties of the drug, which may permit the accompanying aversive effects to be seen more readily than in the case of intravenous or even intraperitoneal injections.

Mechanisms Underlying the Behavioral Effects of Cocaine

Locomotor behavior. There is substantial evidence linking cocaine-induced locomotor activation to blockade of DA reuptake. The most recent and compelling evidence for this hypothesis comes from studies of the DA transporter knockout mice mentioned in the amphetamine section of this chapter. In contrast to wild-type (i.e., genetically normal) subjects, the mutant mice showed no change in locomotor activity when administered a high dose of cocaine (Giros et al., 1996). This presumably occurred because in the absence of the transporter cocaine had no effect on extracellular DA concentrations.

As in the case of amphetamine, the locomotor stimulating effects of cocaine have been ascribed largely to enhancement of dopaminergic transmission in the nucleus accumbens. This was first suggested by Kelly and Iversen (1976), who demonstrated reductions in cocaine-induced locomotor behavior following 6-OHDA lesions of the mesolimbic DA pathway. Further supporting this hypothesis are more recent studies showing that locomotor activity can be elicited by direct microinjection of cocaine into the nucleus accumbens (Figure 13.19; Delfs, Schreiber, and Kelley, 1990) and that the locomotor effect of systemically administered cocaine is significantly attenuated by the injection of sulpiride (a D_2-like antagonist) into the accumbens (Neisewander, O'Dell, and Redmond, 1995). Dopaminergic activation of the *c-fos* immediate–early gene may also play a role in this

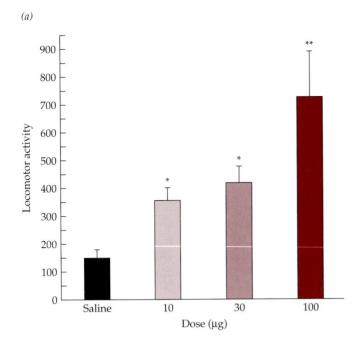

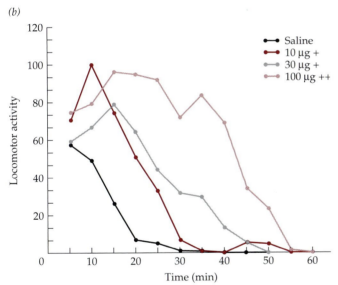

13.19 STIMULATION OF LOCOMOTOR ACTIVITY BY COCAINE MICROINJECTION INTO THE NUCLEUS ACCUMBENS. (a) Total activity (measured as photocell beam breaks over a 60-minute period) as a function of dose of cocaine microinjected into the nucleus accumbens. (*$p < 0.05$, **$p < 0.01$ compared with saline treatment.) (b) Time course of activity (measured as beam breaks in 5-minute time blocks) as a function of cocaine dose. (+$p < 0.05$, +++$p < 0.001$ for the dose × time interaction compared with saline.) (After Delfs, Schreiber, and Kelley, 1990.)

the relationship between neurochemical activity in this system and behavioral stimulation does not seem to be a simple one. For example, Kuczenski, Segal, and Aizenstein (1991) showed that 10 mg/kg cocaine given intraperitoneally stimulated locomotor behavior more than 0.5 mg/kg amphetamine given subcutaneously; however, the amphetamine treatment caused a greater increase in DA overflow in the nucleus accumbens as measured by in vivo microdialysis. Moreover, a variety of drugs besides DA antagonists have been reported to inhibit the locomotor stimulant effects of cocaine. These drugs include NMDA receptor blockers (Karler and Calder, 1992), non-NMDA glutamate receptor blockers (Kaddis, Wallace, and Uretsky, 1993; Witkin, 1993), the α_1-adrenoreceptor antagonist prazosin (Berthold, Gonzales, and Moerschbaecher, 1992), 5-HT$_3$ receptor antagonists (Reith, 1990), σ-receptor ligands (Menkel et al., 1991), and antagonists of corticotropin-releasing factor (CRF) (Sarnyai et al., 1992). Such results suggest that the psychostimulant properties of cocaine are mediated by a complex neurochemical circuit involving many transmitters and presumably a number of different brain areas.

Discriminative stimulus effects. DA appears to play a prominent role in the discriminative stimulus properties of cocaine. DA uptake–inhibiting drugs such as GBR 12909, mazindol, nomifensine, and bupropion readily substituted for cocaine in rats (Baker et al., 1993; Cunningham and Callahan, 1991) and monkeys (Kleven, Anthony, and Woolverton, 1990; Spealman, 1993) previously trained to discriminate cocaine from saline. Such drugs also induced a leftward shift in the dose–response curve (i.e., percentage of responses on the cocaine-appropriate lever as a function of cocaine dose) when administered together with cocaine. These findings indicate a potentiation of cocaine's stimulus properties by DA uptake inhibition. In contrast, NE and 5-HT uptake inhibitors did not induce responding on the cocaine-appropriate lever by themselves, nor did they potentiate the cocaine cue. 5-HT may actually antagonize the cocaine cue in some way, because squirrel monkeys showed a rightward shift in the dose–response curve when the selective 5-HT uptake inhibitor citalopram was given along with cocaine (Spealman, 1993).

Current evidence suggests that both D$_1$ and D$_2$ receptors are involved in the discriminative stimulus effects of cocaine. In rats, full D$_2$ agonists such as quinpirole and bromocriptine completely substituted for cocaine, and also enhanced responding on the cocaine-appropriate lever when administered with cocaine (Callahan, Appel, and Cunningham, 1991; Callahan and Cunningham, 1993). The D$_1$ agonist SKF 38393 mimicked the cocaine cue less effectively than the above-mentioned D$_2$ agonists (Barrett and Appel, 1989; Callahan, Appel, and Cunningham, 1991), although it is

process. Blockade of *c-fos* gene expression in the nucleus accumbens by local application of a *c-fos* antisense oligonucleotide was recently reported to virtually abolish the locomotor stimulant effect of cocaine given intraperitoneally (Heilig, Engel, and Söderpalm, 1993).

Although nucleus accumbens DA undoubtedly plays an important role in cocaine-induced locomotion,

important to note that this compound is only a partial agonist in many assay systems (see Chapter 8).

Antagonist experiments further support a role for DA receptors in the discriminative stimulus effects of cocaine. Studies in both rats and monkeys have shown that responding on the cocaine lever is reduced by treatment with either a D_1 or a D_2 receptor blocker (Baker et al., 1993; Barrett and Appel, 1989; Callahan, Appel, and Cunningham, 1991; Kleven, Anthony, and Woolverton, 1990). Of particular interest is a recent study by Callahan, De La Garza, and Cunningham (1994) investigating the possible role of nucleus accumbens D_1 receptors in cocaine's discriminative stimulus properties. Rats were first trained to discriminate intraperitoneal cocaine from saline in the usual manner. The investigators then showed that microinjection of cocaine directly into the nucleus accumbens fully substituted for systemically administered cocaine. Finally, intra-accumbens administration of the D_1 antagonist SCH 23390 blocked the stimulus effects of intraperitoneal cocaine. Taken together, the receptor agonist and antagonist studies indicate that D_2 receptors are most important for the discriminative stimulus properties of cocaine, although concurrent D_1 receptor activation is probably also required (see Chapter 8 for a discussion of D_1–D_2 receptor interactions). Moreover, the work of Callahan and coworkers suggests that the nucleus accumbens may be a critical site for DA receptor stimulation.

As a final point, the discriminative stimulus effects of cocaine in squirrel monkeys can be modulated by certain opioid receptor subtypes (see Chapter 12). Several μ-receptor agonists were found to potentiate the cocaine cue, whereas κ-agonists antagonized the cue, and a δ-agonist had no effect (Spealman and Bergman, 1992, 1994). The mechanism by which opiate drugs influence the discriminative stimulus properties of cocaine is not yet known.

Reinforcing effects.   In discussing the neural mechanisms of cocaine reinforcement, we will focus on the self-administration paradigm. Early studies showed that low doses of DA antagonists increased the rate of cocaine self-administration, whereas high doses of the same compounds led to a cessation of responding (De Wit and Wise, 1977; Ettenberg et al., 1982). More recent experiments have investigated the influence of dopaminergic drugs on cocaine self-administration using not only the standard fixed ratio (FR) schedules, but also progressive ratio (PR) schedules. In the typical PR schedule used for cocaine self-administration, the first lever press at the beginning of a test session delivers a drug infusion. However, each successive drug delivery requires a greater number of operant responses (e.g., 2, 4, 6, 9, and so forth). The animal eventually stops responding when the response requirement is too great for the amount of reinforcement provided at a given drug dose. This point

in the progressive ratio schedule, called the "break point," is a sensitive index of the animal's motivation to self-administer the drug. DA antagonists were found to decrease the average break point, indicating a reduction in cocaine reinforcement (reviewed by Roberts and Ranaldi, 1995).

Ritz and colleagues (1987) used a correlative approach to determine the relative importance of DA versus 5-HT and NE uptake blockade in cocaine reinforcement. The potencies of various cocainelike drugs in self-administration experiments correlated well with their relative affinities for the DA transporter, but not with their affinities for either of the other two monoamine transporters. Serotonin may actually antagonize the reward value of cocaine, as also suggested earlier for cocaine's discriminative stimulus properties. This conclusion stems from several studies demonstrating reductions in cocaine self-administration following administration of the 5-HT uptake inhibitor fluoxetine (Carroll, Lac et al., 1990a; Richardson and Roberts, 1991) or the 5-HT precursor L-tryptophan (Carroll, Lac et al., 1990b; McGregor, Lacosta, and Roberts, 1993).

In general, both D_1 and D_2 receptors have been implicated in cocaine self-administration (Britton et al., 1991; Caine and Koob, 1994; Hubner and Moreton, 1991). Moreover, the putative D_3 agonist 7-hydroxy-N,N-di-*n*-propyl-2-aminotetralin (7-OH-DPAT) was recently found to decrease the rate of cocaine self-administration (interpreted as an increase in reinforcing efficacy) and was also self-administered when substituted for cocaine (Caine and Koob, 1993). Hence, multiple DA receptors seem to participate in cocaine reinforcement.

In light of its presumed role in the reinforcing effects of amphetamine, the nucleus accumbens is also likely to be important in the reinforcing effects of cocaine. Indeed, cocaine self-administration is attenuated by 6-OHDA lesions of either the nucleus accumbens (Roberts, Corcoran, and Fibiger, 1977) or the ventral tegmental area (VTA), the site of the dopaminergic neurons that project to the accumbens (Roberts and Koob, 1982). Furthermore, intra-accumbens administration of a D_1 or D_2 antagonist increases cocaine self-administration rates, just as in the case of systemic administration of such drugs (Maldonado et al., 1993; Robledo, Maldonado-Lopez, and Koob, 1992).

Consistent with the above findings, in vivo microdialysis experiments have shown that cocaine self-administration leads to increased extracellular DA concentrations in the nucleus accumbens (Pettit and Justice, 1991). However, the relationship between accumbens DA and cocaine reinforcement may not be a simple one. Although a particular unit dose of cocaine was found to produce a relatively consistent rise in DA overflow, the degree of rise was greater at higher doses (Figure 13.20). This occurred despite the the fact that self-administration rates decreased as unit dose increased. Conse-

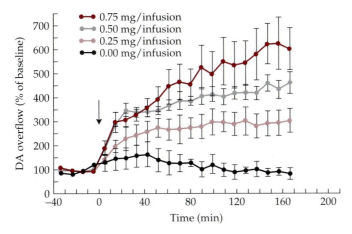

13.20 EFFECT OF COCAINE DOSE ON NUCLEUS ACCUMBENS DOPAMINE OVERFLOW DURING COCAINE SELF-ADMINISTRATION. Rats self-administered various doses of cocaine (0.25, 0.50, or 0.75 mg/infusion) while nucleus accumbens DA overflow was monitored by in vivo microdialysis. After the beginning of the self-administration session, DA overflow significantly increased at all doses compared with the 0.0 group, which represents subjects responding under extinction conditions in which no cocaine was available. However, the plateau of DA overflow was not the same at each dose, but rather increased with higher doses. (After Pettit and Justice, 1991.)

quently, rats do not appear to regulate accumbens DA concentrations at some optimal level regardless of the dosing conditions. Rather, it is possible that self-administration of higher cocaine doses is more reinforcing due to the greater increases in extracellular DA. Alternatively, there might be a "ceiling" effect (i.e., reinforcement is maximized) once the DA concentration reaches a certain level, either because of saturation or desensitization of the postsynaptic receptors.

We saw earlier that animals will self-administer amphetamine directly into the nucleus accumbens. However, attempts to demonstrate cocaine self-administration into this area have, surprisingly, not been successful (Goeders and Smith, 1983). Combined with the other findings presented in this section, such results seem to imply that increased DA transmission in the nucleus accumbens is a necessary, but not a sufficient, condition for cocaine reinforcement. Interestingly, rats have been found to self-administer cocaine into the medial prefrontal cortex (Goeders and Smith, 1983; Goeders, Dworkin, and Smith, 1986). Furthermore, cocaine self-administration into the medial prefrontal cortex was recently reported to enhance DA turnover in the ipsilateral nucleus accumbens (Goeders and Smith, 1993). This interaction may be mediated by excitatory synaptic connections from the prefrontal cortex to dopaminergic neurons in the VTA (Sesack and Pickel, 1992). In any case, the reinforcing effects of cocaine may involve a complex interaction between the medial prefrontal cortex, VTA, and nucleus accumbens. Finally, anatomic structures

that receive outflow from the accumbens can also be expected to participate in cocaine reinforcement (see, for example, Robledo and Koob, 1993).

Is There a Common Neural Mechanism Underlying the Reinforcing Effects of All Abused Drugs?

In comparing opiates (Chapter 12) with psychomotor stimulants and also the various abused drugs discussed in succeeding chapters, we can see that these compounds differ markedly in their molecular and anatomical sites of action. Nevertheless, it might the case that most, if not all, such drugs eventually converge on a final common pathway. Wise and Bozarth (1987) have argued that the ability to elicit psychomotor activation is common to all abused drugs, and that such activation is intimately involved in the reinforcing properties of such drugs. Even drugs typically considered to be CNS depressants, such as opiates, alcohol, barbiturates, and benzodiazepines, stimulate locomotor activity at low doses (whereas higher doses lead to behavioral depression). Wise and Bozarth further hypothesized that the psychomotor and reinforcing effects of abused drugs are due to increased DA transmission in the nucleus accumbens. This hypothesis was subsequently supported by in vivo microdialysis studies showing increased DA overflow in the accumbens and locomotor activation following administration of amphetamine, cocaine, morphine, nicotine, and alcohol (Di Chiara and Imperato, 1988). Drugs that are not abused by humans or self-administered by animals failed to produce these effects.

The notion that enhanced dopaminergic transmission is common to most abused drugs has received widespread attention; however, some important findings are inconsistent with this hypothesis. For example, Hemby and coworkers (1995) found no change in accumbens DA overflow in rats self-administering heroin. An alternative theory proposed by Koob and his colleagues posits the existence of a midbrain–forebrain–extrapyramidal drug reward circuit activated by the major classes of abused drugs (i.e., psychostimulants, opiates, and sedative–hypnotics) (Koob, 1992; Koob and Bloom, 1988). In this model, the nucleus accumbens plays a key role in receiving motivational information from various limbic structures and then activating behavioral responses through its efferent connections to the extrapyramidal motor system (Figure 13.21). DA is critical to the reinforcing effects of amphetamine and cocaine; however, other transmitters may be equally or more important for other classes of abused drugs. This circuit-based (rather than neurotransmitter-based) model is attractive because of its ability to integrate a broader range of experimental findings than other models that require the participation of the DA system.

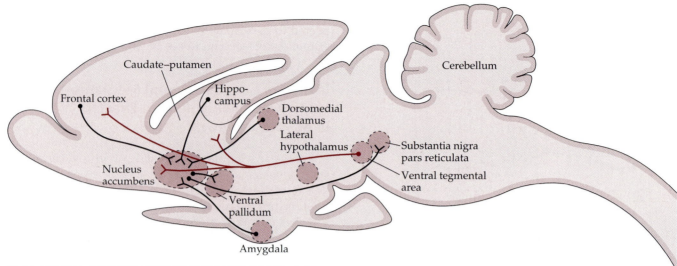

13.21 NEURAL CIRCUITS MEDIATING THE REINFORCING EFFECTS OF PSYCHOSTIMULANT DRUGS. A sagittal rat brain section showing the limbic–extrapyramidal circuit believed to underlie the reinforcing properties of psychostimulants. A critical part of this circuit involves DA pathways from the VTA to the nucleus accumbens, ventral caudate–putamen, and frontal cortex. The accumbens is additionally regulated by limbic system afferents from the frontal cortex, amygdala, hippocampus, and dorsomedial thalamus. The behavioral output of this circuit is thought to be mediated by efferent pathways from the accumbens to the ventral pallidum and substantia nigra pars reticulata, which are components of the extrapyramidal motor system. (After Koob, 1992.)

Cocaine Abuse and the Effects of Chronic Cocaine Exposure

Initiation and Progression of Cocaine Abuse

There is no common pattern to the initiation of cocaine use, nor to the personalities and backgrounds of cocaine users. This variation is exemplified in the work of Spotts and Shontz (1980), who conducted detailed case studies of nine male cocaine users. The men included a burglar and armed robber who was the son of a poor Arkansas sharecropper, a musician in a rock band who grew up in an upper-middle-class family, a successful young salesman, a street hustler, a gas station attendant, a pimp, and several drug dealers. Despite this diversity, when the subjects were asked their reasons for using cocaine, two frequent responses were (1) to provoke feelings of strength and self-confidence, and (2) to escape from feelings of depression, frustration, and/or anger. Furthermore, all of the subjects described early experimentation with both legal (e.g., alcohol) and illegal drugs, often beginning by 13 or 14 years of age. Early use of other substances may therefore be an important risk factor for the initiation of cocaine use.

Most individuals who try cocaine, particularly via the intranasal route, do not progress to a pattern of abuse. Some report a strong anxiety response as their initial reaction to cocaine, and are thereby dissuaded from further experimentation. Other factors may likewise mitigate against the development of a long-term abuse pattern, including unavailability of the drug, the cost of maintaining a steady supply, the social and legal consequences of illicit drug use, and the very real fear of losing control over one's drug-taking behavior.

Nevertheless, surveys performed by NIDA suggest that approximately 10% to 15% of initial intranasal users do eventually become abusers. The details of this transition process certainly vary among individuals, yet a few factors that may generally be important have been summarized by Gawin and his colleagues (Gawin and Ellinwood, 1988; Gawin, 1991). The stimulating, euphoric, and confidence-enhancing effects described above provide a powerful reinforcing effect during the early stages of cocaine use. Furthermore, these aspects of cocaine reinforcement may be augmented by social responses from friends and acquaintances who react positively to the user's newfound energy and enthusiasm. Over time, cocaine use escalates as the individual discovers that higher doses produce a more powerful euphoric effect. Even more importantly, the user may switch from intranasal administration to smoking or intravenous injection. For many, this is a significant event in their drug history because of the greater abuse potential of these latter routes of administration.

Psychiatric evaluation of heavy cocaine users has shown that the majority of such individuals suffer from concurrent mental disorders, including major depression, anxiety disorders, and personality disorders such as antisocial personality (Kleinman et al., 1990; Rounsaville et al., 1991). Many also have a childhood history of attention deficit hyperactivity disorder (ADHD). The onset of ADHD and/or the development of anxiety disorders or antisocial personality typically precede the beginning of cocaine abuse. The high rate of occurrence of other psychiatric disorders in this population raises the possibility that for many people, "self-medication" is an underlying factor in the onset and maintenance of their drug abuse pattern (Khantzian, 1985).

Relatively low-dose, occasional cocaine use can persist for long periods of time (see, for example, Kaplan, Bieleman, and TenHouten, 1992). However, individuals who progress to a compulsive use pattern may exhibit daily or near-daily use, or they may develop a binge pattern of abuse (Gawin and Ellinwood, 1988). Like the amphetamine "runs" described earlier in this chapter, cocaine binges are episodic bouts of repeated use lasting from hours to days, during which the user gets little or no sleep. During these periods, nothing is important to the user except maintaining the "high," and all available supplies of cocaine are consumed in this pursuit. A 3-day freebasing binge can involve the consumption of as much as 150 g of cocaine, which is an enormous amount (Grinspoon and Bakalar, 1985).

Cocaine Tolerance and Sensitization

Human laboratory studies have demonstrated tolerance to the subjective and cardiovascular effects of cocaine over repeated doses taken within a single session (Fischman et al., 1985; Foltin, Fischman, and Levin, 1995). Habitual users similarly report tolerance to cocaine's euphoric effects, both within a binge and over longer time periods as drug use gradually escalates (Grinspoon and Bakalar, 1985). Emmett-Oglesby and coworkers (1993) recently described a possible animal model of this phenomenon in which rats self-administering cocaine increased their operant response rate (and hence their amount of cocaine consumption) across test sessions.

As in the case of amphetamine, the behavioral effects of chronic cocaine administration in animals depend on the pattern of administration. Continuous drug infusion by means of subcutaneously implanted osmotic minipumps or intravenous infusion causes the development of tolerance (Figure 13.22*a*; Inada et al., 1992; Reith, Benuck, and Lajtha, 1987). This tolerance appears to be primarily of a cellular type, although an increased rate of drug metabolism apparently can also occur over time (Johansson et al., 1992). In contrast, intermittent cocaine administration (e.g., by daily injection) typically leads to

(a)

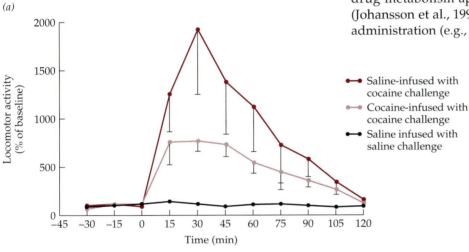

(b)

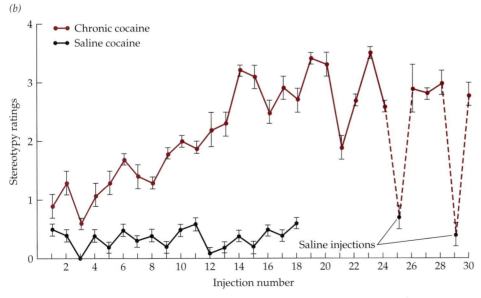

13.22 CHRONIC COCAINE ADMINISTRATION CAN PRODUCE TOLERANCE OR SENSITIZATION DEPENDING ON THE PATTERN OF ADMINISTRATION. (*a*) Rats were given a continuous intravenous infusion of either saline or 60 mg/kg of cocaine per day for 11 or 12 days. One day after the end of the infusion, subjects were given a saline injection or challenged with cocaine (20 mg/kg i.p.), and were then tested for locomotor activity. The previously cocaine-exposed animals showed tolerance as indicated by a decreased locomotor response to the challenge dose. (*b*) Rats given once-daily cocaine injections (10 mg/kg i.p.) showed a progressive increase in stereotyped behavior (sensitization) compared with saline-treated controls. The behavior patterns observed in these animals consisted of repetitive corner-to-corner locomotion, vertical rearing and nose poking, and head bobbing. Saline test injections on days 25 and 29 showed that the high levels of stereotypy seen on the other days were due to the cocaine injections on those days and were not a residual effect of the prior treatments. (*a* after Inada et al., 1992; *b* after Post and Contel, 1983.)

sensitization of cocaine's psychostimulant (Figure 13.22b) (Kilbey and Ellinwood, 1977; Post and Contel, 1983) and reinforcing (Horger, Shelton, and Schenk, 1990) effects. As previously mentioned for amphetamine, there is a cross-sensitization between stress and cocaine (Sorg and Kalivas, 1991).

The mechanisms underlying cocaine and amphetamine sensitization have been intensively studied but are still not completely understood. As stated in a review by Kalivas, Sorg, and Hooks (1993), it is useful to distinguish between the initiation and the expression of sensitization. *Initiation* refers to early processes that are necessary for the development of heightened reactivity but that may not persist for very long after the period of drug administration. In contrast, the *expression* of sensitization is related to enduring changes in the nervous system that are directly manifested as altered behavioral responses when the organism is given a drug challenge. Given that these mechanisms may be different, it is particularly important to determine the temporal pattern of neurochemical changes that accompanies chronic psychostimulant treatment.

Because of the central role of DA in the acute effects of psychostimulants, researchers have focused on the dopaminergic system in their search for the underlying mechanisms of sensitization. Indeed, sensitizing treatments have been reported to alter basal extracellular DA levels in the nucleus accumbens, DA reuptake, D_1 or D_2 receptor density, and D_2 autoreceptor sensitivity at various times following the end of the treatment regimen (Kalivas, Sorg, and Hooks, 1993). However, such changes have not been consistently observed, and hence may not be critical to the sensitization process. Instead, Kalivas and colleagues argue that the most important and consistent correlates of psychostimulant sensitization are (1) elevated accumbens DA release in response to stimulant challenge, stress, or even electrically induced depolarization, and (2) increased electrophysiological sensitivity of accumbens D_1 receptors. According to this model, the expression of sensitization involves enhanced dopaminergic transmission in the nucleus accumbens, mediated both pre- and postsynaptically.

Even though the nucleus accumbens is probably a critical site for the expression of psychostimulant sensitization, it may not be the neural locus of initiation. This conclusion follows from the observation that sensitization to amphetamine or cocaine can be produced by amphetamine microinjection directly into the VTA, but not the accumbens (Dougherty and Ellinwood, 1981; Kalivas and Weber, 1988). Systemic as well as local administration of psychostimulants causes increased somatodendritic DA release in the VTA (Bradberry and Roth, 1989). This may play an important role in the initiation process, as intra-VTA administration of the D_1 antagonist SCH 23390 prevents the initiation of amphetamine sensitization (Stewart and Vezina, 1989).

Finally, it should be noted that in addition to DA, excitatory amino acids seem to be a necessary component of psychostimulant sensitization. NMDA receptor antagonists have been reported to block the initiation of sensitization (Karler et al., 1989; Stewart and Druhan, 1993), and non-NMDA receptor antagonists prevented both initiation and expression (Karler, Calder, and Turkanis, 1991). Consequently, Kalivas (1995) recently proposed a model in which (1) psychostimulants enhance somatodendritic DA release in the VTA, (2) DA stimulates D_1 receptors on nerve terminals of cortical afferents projecting to the VTA, (3) D_1 receptor activation produces increased release of excitatory amino acids from the terminals, (4) the amino acids stimulate NMDA receptors on the dopaminergic cells, and (5) the resulting increase in intracellular Ca^{2+} concentrations leads to persistent alterations in gene expression and cellular functioning. Although this model is still hypothetical, it represents a further step in elucidating the complex mechanisms of cocaine and amphetamine sensitization.

Cocaine Dependence

Until the early 1980s, cocaine was not believed to produce a syndrome of dependence and withdrawal, and hence the drug was not considered addictive by classic criteria. For example, cocaine dependence was not listed as a substance abuse disorder in the 1980 version of the Diagnostic and Statistical Manual of Mental Disorders (DSM-III). This situation began to change, however, when Frank Gawin and Herbert Kleber (then at Yale University School of Medicine) described a pattern of abstinence symptomatology occurring in chronic cocaine bingers withdrawing from a binge (Gawin and Kleber, 1986, 1988). Based on a combination of clinical observations and patient interviews, Gawin and Kleber concluded that the cocaine abstinence syndrome occurs in three phases, which they called "crash," "withdrawal," and "extinction" (Figure 13.23). Early in the crash phase (i.e., within 15–30 minutes following the final dose), users experience extreme dysphoria manifested as feelings of agitation and anxiety, depression, and intense cocaine craving. Within a few hours, however, cocaine craving subsides, and the individual feels increasing fatigue and a desire for sleep. At this time, sleep induction may be aided by taking drugs such as alcohol, sedatives, anxiolytics, opiates, or marijuana. Finally, the user becomes exhausted and sleeps for many hours or even days (hypersomnolence). Sleep may be interrupted by periodic awakenings accompanied by strong feelings of hunger and eating (hyperphagia), which are presumably related in part to the absence of food consumption during the binge. There is no desire or craving for cocaine during this late part of the crash phase.

The second (withdrawal) phase of the cocaine abstinence syndrome begins with a period of several hours or

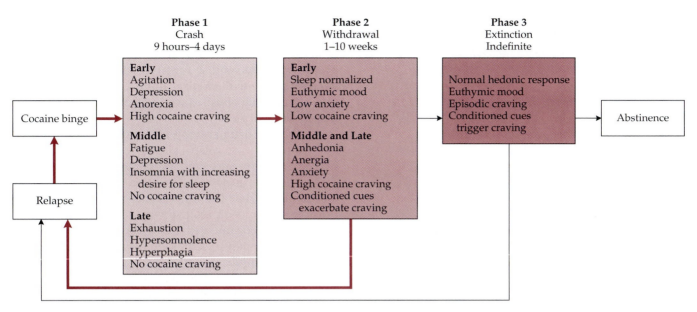

13.23 PHASES OF ABSTINENCE SYMPTOMATOLOGY FOLLOWING A COCAINE BINGE. Cocaine binges reportedly last for varying periods of time, ranging from several hours to 6 days or longer. The figure illustrates the typical pattern of post-binge symptomatology observed in experienced users, although the duration and intensity of symptoms are somewhat variable depending on the binge characteristics and other factors. (After Gawin and Kleber, 1986.)

days characterized by a relatively normal mood state (euthymic mood), normal sleep–waking cycles, and little anxiety or cocaine craving.* Over the next few days, however, there is a gradual onset of a dysphoric syndrome manifested by intense boredom, anergia (lack of energy), anhedonia (the inability to experience normal pleasure from the environment), and anxiety. Cocaine craving increases, particularly when triggered by environmental stimuli (cues) previously associated with cocaine-induced euphoria (Ehrman et al., 1992). Along with the other symptoms just mentioned, such conditioned craving places the user at extreme risk of relapse. Indeed, at this point, most chronic bingers obtain a new batch of cocaine and embark on their next binge. Consequently, most of the subjects studied by Gawin and Kleber reported regular 3–10-day cycles of cocaine use: typically 6–36 hours of cocaine bingeing, 1–2 days of "crash," 1–2 days of normalization, 1–2 days of resistance while cocaine craving grew, and then relapse.

Users who maintain abstinence through the crash and withdrawal phases enter a third phase (extinction) characterized by normal mood and feelings of pleasure. Intermittent episodes of cocaine craving may persist for a long time, however, particularly in response to condi-

tioned cues. Many users thus suffer eventual relapse even if they manage to reach this phase.

As mentioned earlier, some heavy cocaine users exhibit a daily rather than a binge pattern of consumption. It is important to note, therefore, that a multiphasic model of cocaine withdrawal may not apply to non-bingers. This conclusion can be drawn from the work of Weddington and coworkers (1990), who studied withdrawal symptomatology in a group of long-term daily intravenous users admitted to a treatment facility. The subjects exhibited severe dysphoria (consisting of depression, fatigue, anxiety, and anger) and cocaine craving at the time of admission. But instead of passing through several distinct phases of withdrawal, they experienced a gradual normalization of mood and a reduction in self-reported craving over the next 4 weeks.

As drug craving is such an important factor in cocaine relapse, understanding its neurobiological determinants might prove very useful in developing effective strategies for treating cocaine abuse. One of the most influential theories of cocaine withdrawal symptomatology (including craving) has been the "dopamine depletion" hypothesis of Dackis and Gold (1985). According to these investigators, increased synaptic levels of DA occur during cocaine use and are critical for the euphoric effects experienced by the user. Dackis and Gold further hypothesize that termination of drug use leads to abnormally low DA availability, which in turn causes dysphoria and cocaine craving (e.g., as during the early part of the "crash" and perhaps also during the middle to late

---

*Although subjects seemed normal during the early withdrawal phase according to the findings of Gawin and Kleber, preliminary results from a more recent study suggest that cocaine abusers may suffer from cognitive impairment during this time (Berry et al., 1993).

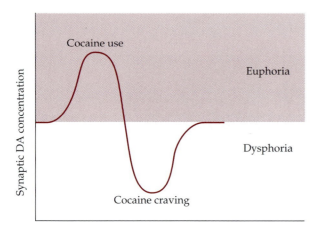

13.24 HYPOTHETICAL RELATIONSHIP BETWEEN COCAINE USE, SYNAPTIC DOPAMINE LEVELS, AND MOOD. Cocaine use acutely elevates synaptic DA concentrations, which is thought to play a critical role in the euphoric effects of the drug. After use has ended, synaptic DA concentrations may decrease below normal levels, thus leading to cocaine craving and a dysphoric mood. (After Dackis and Gold, 1985.)

stages of the withdrawal phase) (Figure 13.24). Direct human studies to test the dopamine depletion hypothesis are difficult to carry out and thus far have been inconclusive. In fact, two small studies found that craving during cocaine abstinence was associated with increased rather than decreased concentrations of the DA metabolite homovanillic acid (HVA) in the cerebrospinal fluid or plasma (Knoblich et al., 1992; Martin et al., 1989). The results of animal studies have likewise been inconsistent; however, a few experiments do seem to support the hypothesis. In one case, rats withdrawing from 3 weeks of cocaine self-administration exhibited decreased tissue DA concentrations in the VTA and nucleus accumbens (Bozarth, 1989). A subsequent microdialysis study found that withdrawal from chronic experimenter-administered cocaine was associated with reduced DA overflow in the nucleus accumbens (Rossetti, Hmaidan, and Gessa, 1992).

Robinson and Berridge (1993) recently proposed a different theory of drug craving based on the concept of "incentive-sensitization." This theory distinguishes between the motivational process of "liking" (i.e., pleasure) and the process of "wanting" (which Robinson and Berridge formally refer to as "attribution of incentive salience"). The latter process, which is not consciously experienced, causes the perception or psychological representation of an object to become desirable and to be pursued. Most importantly, repeated exposure to an addictive drug such as cocaine in the presence of various drug-related stimuli is hypothesized to produce a conditioned sensitization of the neural mechanisms that mediate attribution of incentive salience. Consequently, the user becomes driven by an ever-increasing "wanting" of

the drug, even though he may actually "like" the drug less and less (e.g., he may derive less pleasure from drug consumption due to tolerance, development of dysphoric reactions, and so forth). It will be interesting to see how this new theoretical approach influences future research on drug abuse as well as the search for effective treatment strategies.

Although drug craving is obviously an extremely important factor in relapse, other variables are also involved. McKay and coworkers (1995) subjected 95 chronic cocaine users to a structured interview designed to elucidate what the individuals were experiencing prior to a relapse (a relapse was defined here as 1 or more days of cocaine use following at least 2 weeks of voluntary abstinence). Common factors associated with relapse were unpleasant affect (including loneliness, depression, anxiety, and anger), social pressure to use drugs, desire to get "high," boredom and need for excitement, and, of course, cocaine craving. Users who relapsed also typically reported that they had a lot of free time, had money available to buy drugs, and did not avail themselves of the self-help treatment program in which they were enrolled. It seems clear that relapse must be seen as a multidimensional problem requiring a comprehensive treatment approach that accounts for the above factors.

Cocaine Psychosis

Cocaine-induced psychosis has not been as well characterized as the psychotic reactions associated with high-dose amphetamine use. However, several studies indicate that a transient paranoid psychosis with delusions and hallucinations is a common feature of chronic high-dose cocaine abuse (Brady et al., 1991; Satel, Southwick, and Gawin, 1991). As in the case of amphetamine psychosis, cocaine psychosis occurs more frequently over time, which is consistent with an underlying sensitization or kindling mechanism. Psychotic reactions are usually restricted temporally to the period of drug use. Nevertheless, Manschreck and colleagues (1988) reported that in the mid-1980s in the Bahamas, a sudden upsurge in freebase cocaine smoking was associated with the appearance of psychotic reactions that, in some cases, persisted for many days or even weeks.

Cocaine Toxicity

Cocaine can exert toxic effects on the CNS as well as on other organ systems. Brown and colleagues (1992) have reviewed the major CNS complications associated with cocaine abuse, which range from seizures to vascular disorders such as stroke and intracerebral hemorrhage. Although such events obviously lead to the death of brain cells, cocaine differs from amphetamine and methamphetamine in that it apparently does not directly damage neurons except at extremely high doses (Bennett et al., 1993). Measurements of DA, 5-HT, NE, and their metabolites indicate that the systems using these transmitters remain intact in animals subjected to long-term cocaine administration (Kleven, Woolverton, and Seiden, 1988; Yeh and De Souza, 1991). Histological examination of cocaine-treated animals has similarly revealed no evidence of neuronal damage (Goodman and Sloviter, 1993; Ryan et al., 1988), except for one study by Ellison (1992), which found that several days of continuous exposure to either cocaine or amphetamine produced signs of degeneration in the lateral habenula and fasciculus retroflexus.

Effects of Prenatal Cocaine Exposure

Women who are heavily dependent on cocaine may not curtail or terminate their drug habit even when they become pregnant. Hence, the upsurge in cocaine (particularly "crack") use in the inner cities that began in the 1980s has led to a large increase in cocaine consumption during pregnancy. By the late 1980s and early 1990s, researchers at urban public hospitals were reporting that at least 10% to 15% of newborn infants had been exposed to cocaine prenatally (Frank et al., 1988; Matera et al., 1990; Streissguth et al., 1991). Because individuals are not always honest about their drug-taking behavior, it is generally important to use some type of clinical testing to determine the presence of cocaine or its metabolites (e.g., see Zuckerman et al., 1989). One approach is to assay for the presence of cocaine metabolites such as benzoylecgonine in the mother's or infant's urine. Such metabolites usually persist for several days after the mother's last usage, thus allowing investigators to detect recent exposure. However, women who have used cocaine earlier in pregnancy, but not during the last week before giving birth, cannot be identified by this method. Recent studies have shown that cocaine metabolites are also deposited in the hair of the fetus and in a fecal material called meconium that is excreted during the first few days following birth. Thus, detection of cocaine metabolites in the newborn's meconium or hair allows investigators to verify cocaine exposure during earlier periods of prenatal development (Callahan et al., 1992).

The influence of maternal cocaine use on pregnancy outcome and offspring development has been reviewed by Frank, Bresnahan, and Zuckerman (1993) and Meyer and colleagues (1996). Cocaine-exposed neonates (newborns) are frequently reported to exhibit reductions in average birth weight and head circumference (which is an indirect measure of brain size). Although these reductions are sometimes associated with premature delivery, even full-term infants may be small for their gestational age. Furthermore, there are some indications that prenatal cocaine exposure might increase the risk for certain kinds of structural malformations. However, these findings are controversial, and more research is needed on this issue.

A popular misconception is the notion that offspring of cocaine-using women are born addicted to the drug.

As mentioned in Part I of this chapter, drug craving and a pattern of compulsive use are currently considered to be the defining characteristics of addiction (Stolerman, 1992). Although newborn infants are obviously incapable of exhibiting organized drug-seeking behavior, we can look for signs of pharmacological dependence (i.e., withdrawal symptoms) that might be construed as including some element of drug craving. Some cocaine-exposed neonates do exhibit behaviors that could be related to drug withdrawal (see below); however, as a group, they do not show a consistent withdrawal syndrome such as that observed in the offspring of opiate (i.e., heroin or morphine) users (see Neuspiel and Hamel, 1991). Thus, there is little evidence at this time indicating that prenatal cocaine exposure causes infant addiction to the drug.

Other potential behavioral abnormalities in cocaine-exposed newborns have been investigated using a well-known battery of tests called the Neonatal Behavioral Assessment Scale (NBAS) (Brazelton, 1984). The various components of the NBAS are typically grouped into the following clusters: sensory orientation, habituation, motor function, range of state, regulation of state, autonomic regulation, and presence of abnormal reflexes. Cocaine-exposed infants have exhibited various abnormalities on the NBAS, although the effects have not been consistent across studies (Frank et al., 1993; Neuspiel and Hamel, 1991). Furthermore, some of the most recent and best-controlled studies have found few or no cocaine-associated deficits on the NBAS (see Meyer et al., 1996).

Considering the overall findings summarized above, many researchers now believe that the risks of prenatal cocaine exposure have been seriously overestimated, not only by the communications media but by the scientific community itself (e.g., see Day and Richardson, 1993; Hutchings, 1993). Nevertheless, long-term studies are still needed to determine whether behavioral abnormalities will emerge as the offspring of cocaine-abusing women develop further. This is particularly important considering that follow-up studies over the first several years of life have begun to indicate that cocaine-exposed children may be at risk for deficits in language development and other cognitive functions (Azuma and Chasnoff, 1993; Nulman et al., 1994; van Baar, 1990).

Another criticism of this research area concerns the lack of adequate controls for confounding factors (Frank et al., 1993; Neuspiel and Hamel, 1991). For example, women abusing cocaine may be malnourished and may have received little or no prenatal care. These factors alone increase the risk of pregnancy complications and intrauterine growth retardation. In addition, it is rare to find individuals who use cocaine exclusively. Consequently, cocaine abuse is usually accompanied by a consumption of alcohol, tobacco, or illicit drugs (such as marijuana, opiates, or sedatives) greater than that of non-cocaine-abusing subjects.

Because these and other maternal variables will presumably continue to pose a problem for clinical investigators, it is important to consider the results of controlled studies on laboratory animals. This work, most of which has been performed with rats, has clearly shown that prenatal cocaine exposure can produce later learning deficits (Heyser et al., 1990; Heyser, Spear, and Spear, 1992) and other behavioral changes (Meyer, Robinson, and Todtenkopf, 1994; Moody, Frambes, and Spear, 1992). Animal studies have also identified several mechanisms by which cocaine's effects might be mediated. First, the vasoconstrictive action of cocaine reduces blood flow to the uterus and placenta, thereby leading to fetal hypoxia (Plessinger and Woods, 1991). This hypoxia may be responsible for cocaine-induced intrauterine growth retardation, and it has also been hypothesized to cause depressive symptomatology in a subset of cocaine-exposed infants (Lester et al., 1991). Another likely mechanism of prenatal cocaine action is the blocking of monoamine uptake in the fetal brain. Cocaine readily crosses the placenta into the fetus (Schenker et al., 1993), and cocaine interaction with monoamine transporters has been demonstrated in the fetal rat brain (Figure 13.25; Meyer et al., 1993; Shearman, Collins, and Meyer, 1996). Interference with reuptake during some critical period could perturb monoamine system development, with later consequences for the many behaviors regulated by these neurotransmitters.

In summary, prenatal cocaine exposure has been associated with intrauterine growth retardation and behavioral deficits in human infants. However, its effects overall are not as severe as was once thought. It has been difficult to ascribe these effects specifically to cocaine due to the presence of various confounding factors. Nevertheless, animal studies have confirmed that cocaine administered under controlled conditions can alter later offspring behavior, perhaps through the drug's ability to produce fetal hypoxia and/or its monoamine uptake blocking actions.

Treatment of Cocaine Abuse

Pharmacotherapies.   High rates of cocaine abuse in the United States have spurred a great deal of interest in developing effective therapies for this problem. As summarized by Kleber (1995) and Witkin (1994), NIDA is currently directing an active program to identify and test pharmacological agents that might facilitate abstinence and prevent relapse by reducing the reinforcing effects of cocaine or the craving that ensues during cocaine withdrawal. Table 13.2 presents some of the major candidate drugs either being considered for cocaine pharmacotherapy or actually undergoing clinical testing. As space considerations do not permit discussion of all of these compounds, we will focus on bromocriptine, fluoxetine, desipramine, buprenorphine, and ibogaine.

Several different strategies could be useful in the development of dopaminergic drugs for treating cocaine abuse. For example, if cocaine craving and other withdrawal symptoms stem from DA depletion, as hypothesized by Dackis and Gold, then direct or indirect DA agonists might reduce such symptoms by enhancing dopaminergic transmission. Bromocriptine is a D_2 receptor agonist that has already undergone preliminary clinical trials in cocaine users. Although some reduction in cocaine craving has been reported, the long-term prospects for this compound are probably not good because of its high incidence of adverse side effects (Kleber, 1995). The 5-HT uptake inhibitor and antidepressant drug fluoxetine (Prozac) is another potential therapeutic agent for cocaine abuse. The rationale for its use is based on preclinical results described earlier indicating serotonergic antagonism of cocaine's reinforcing effects, as well as the observation that many cocaine-abusing patients suffer from varying degrees of depression. Research with fluoxetine is still ongoing; however, recent results from a large double-blind study do not support the efficacy of this compound in reducing cocaine use (Grabowski et al., 1995). Desipramine, which is a tricyclic antidepressant that mainly inhibits NE uptake, has been used for a number of years as an adjunct to psychotherapy in cocaine abuse treatment. Levin and Lehman (1991) performed a meta-analysis of previous randomized trials of desipramine efficacy. They concluded that this drug is somewhat effective in maintaining abstinence, but not in promoting patient retention in treatment programs.

Buprenorphine is an opiate partial agonist originally developed as a pharmacotherapeutic agent for opiate (i.e., heroin) addiction; however, it was unexpectedly

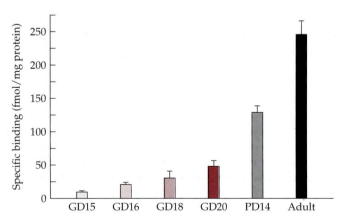

13.25 NORMAL PRE- AND POSTNATAL ONTOGENY OF [³H]-COCAINE BINDING SITES IN THE RAT BRAIN. Whole-brain membrane preparations were incubated with 10 nM [³H]cocaine to label high-affinity binding sites. Such sites, which represent cocaine interaction with plasma membrane monoamine transporters, were detected as early as gestational day (GD) 15 and gradually increased in density through postnatal day (PD) 14 and up to adulthood. (After Meyer et al., 1993.)

Table 13.2 Drugs under Consideration or Already in Clinical Testing for the Treatment of Cocaine Abuse

Drug	Pharmacological activity
Dopaminergics	
Bromocriptine	D$_2$ receptor agonist
Flupenthixol	DA receptor antagonist
Amantadine	DA releaser
Methylphenidate	DA uptake inhibitor
Mazindol	DA uptake inhibitor
Antidepressants	
Fluoxetine	5-HT uptake inhibitor
Sertraline	5-HT uptake inhibitor
Desipramine	NE uptake inhibitor
Imipramine	Mixed 5-HT and NE uptake inhibitor
Miscellaneous	
Buprenorphine	Opiate receptor partial agonist
Ibogaine	Unknown
Buspirone	5-HT$_{1A}$ receptor partial agonist
Ritanserin	5-HT$_2$ receptor antagonist
Nimodipine	Calcium channel blocker
Carbamazepine	Antiepileptic agent

Sources: After Johnson and Vocci, 1993; Kleber, 1995.

found to suppress cocaine self-administration by rhesus monkeys (Mello et al., 1989). This compound is currently being evaluated for the treatment of patients with a dual cocaine and opiate dependency. However, buprenorphine in conjunction with cocaine may actually mimic the effect of a cocaine–heroin "speedball" (Foltin and Fischman, 1994), and it is not yet clear that buprenorphine actually reduces cocaine consumption in cocaine–opiate users (Kosten et al., 1992).

Perhaps the most unusual drug under consideration for treating cocaine abusers is an indole alkaloid called ibogaine, which comes from the root bark of the African shrub *Tabernanthe iboga*. As noted in Table 13.2, this com-

Ibogaine

pound has not yet been adequately characterized neuropharmacologically, although effects on various neurotransmitter systems have been reported (reviewed by Popik, Layer, and Skolnick, 1995). According to Cappendijk and Dzolijc (1993), the drug has been used in West Central Africa for many years as a stimulant and (at higher doses) a hallucinogenic agent. In the United

States, a businessman named Lotsof has claimed that ibogaine enables addicts to achieve abstinence from a variety of addictive agents, including cocaine, and he has patented specific treatment methods using this drug (e.g., Lotsof, 1986). Several studies have found that ibogaine administration can suppress cocaine self-administration in rats (Cappendijk and Dzolijc, 1993; Glick et al., 1994), although in one case this occurred only with a very high dose that caused motor impairment (Dworkin et al., 1995). It remains to be seen whether ibogaine is effective in promoting abstinence in human cocaine abusers under controlled study conditions.

Behavioral therapies. It should be apparent that researchers have not yet discovered any compound that is broadly effective in treating cocaine abuse. Although this situation could change with the development of newer medications, it is necessary to consider the potential role of behavioral and social therapies in dealing with this problem. Indeed, Tims and Leukefeld (1993a) point out that while pharmacotherapy may aid in patient stabilization (e.g., by reducing craving or other abstinence symptoms), equally important are counseling and support structures enabling the patient to learn new coping responses, avoid triggers for relapse, and function effectively in a drug-free lifestyle. Readers who are interested in more information are referred to recent NIDA monographs edited by Tims and Leukefeld (1993b) and Onken, Blaine, and Boren (1993), both of which present a variety of approaches to cocaine abuse treatment. Here we will briefly discuss two such approaches: treatments to reduce conditioned craving, and a multicomponent behavioral program that includes the Community Reinforcement Approach.

In his classic work with opiate addicts, Wikler (1973) was the first to document withdrawal-like symptoms in previously detoxified individuals who were exposed to stimuli (cues) previously paired with drug acquisition or use. This "conditioned withdrawal" was hypothesized to play an important role in the high risk of relapse among users of opiates, cocaine, and other drugs with strong abuse potential. Conditioned withdrawal has since been demonstrated in laboratory studies of both humans and animals (reviewed by O'Brien et al., 1993); some of the specific research on conditioned craving in cocaine addicts was mentioned above. The apparent power of this phenomenon to precipitate a relapse argues that methods of reducing or counteracting such conditioning may prove critical to the long-term success of any treatment program. Childress, O'Brien, and their colleagues at the University of Pennsylvania Addiction Research Center have been investigating the use of both cue extinction techniques (exposing subjects to drug-related cues without allowing consumption of cocaine) and active response techniques designed to counteract conditioned craving responses to cocaine (Childress et al., 1993; O'Brien et al., 1993). They have achieved some success with these techniques; however, further work is needed to refine the methodology and to assess long-term efficacy in maintaining drug abstinence.

Another recently introduced therapeutic approach was developed by Higgins and his coworkers at the University of Vermont. This 24-week, outpatient, multicomponent behavioral treatment program is based on the premise that drug taking is an operant response that persists mainly due to the reinforcing properties of the drug (Higgins, Budney, and Bickel, 1994). Hence, altering reinforcement contingencies to reduce drug-associated reinforcement and increase the availability of nondrug reinforcers should help to promote abstinence and the adoption of a drug-free lifestyle. The treatment program accordingly has four interrelated aims: (1) to detect drug use and abstinence by means of frequent urinalyses (three or four times weekly), (2) to positively reinforce abstinence through contingency management proce-

dures, (3) to penalize drug use by the loss of earned reinforcers, and (4) to further increase the availability of nondrug reinforcement using a Community Reinforcement Approach (CRA). The contingency management procedure used in this program involves the awarding of vouchers for each negative urine test. Although the vouchers cannot be redeemed for money (to avoid patients accumulating funds for drug purchases), they can be exchanged for items approved by the individual's counselor, particularly things that promote a healthy lifestyle, such as YMCA passes and educational materials. The CRA, which was first developed by Hunt and Azrin (1973) for the treatment of alcoholism, is aimed at improving the patient's social (including family) relationships, recreational activities, and job opportunities. In the University of Vermont program, these goals are implemented through extensive counseling sessions with the participation of nondrug-abusing family members and friends, instruction in how to recognize the fac-

(a)

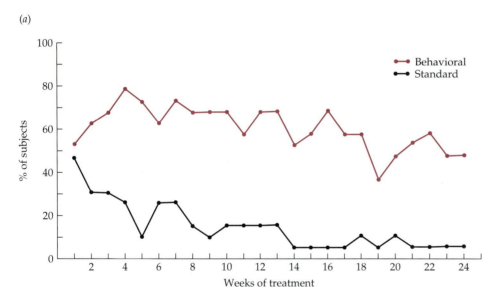

(b)

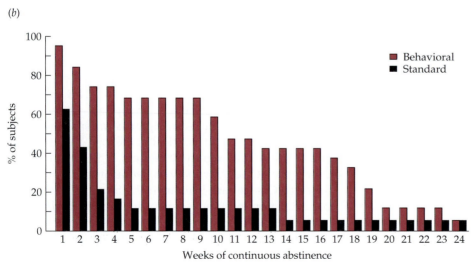

13.26 RESULTS OF A MULTICOMPONENT BEHAVIORAL TREATMENT PROGRAM VERSUS STANDARD DRUG ABUSE COUNSELING FOR COCAINE DEPENDENCE. Cocaine-dependent subjects volunteered for enrollment in an outpatient treatment program. Approximately half of the subjects used cocaine intranasally, while the remainder mainly used the intravenous injection or freebase smoking routes of administration. Subjects were assigned to one of two programs: the multicomponent treatment program described in the text, or a standard twelve-step counseling program (*n* = 19 per group). Urine samples were collected either thrice weekly (weeks 1–12) or twice weekly (weeks 13–24) for toxicological analysis. (*a*) By the second week of treatment, subjects in the behavioral treatment program exhibited much higher abstinence rates (as shown by negative urinalyses) than subjects given the standard treatment. (*b*) The percentage of subjects in each program who achieved a duration of abstinence equal to or greater than the number of weeks shown (e.g., 20% of the subjects in the behavioral treatment program achieved at least 19 weeks of continuous abstinence, compared with approximately 5% of subjects in the standard program.) (After Higgins et al., 1993.)

tors involved in the patient's drug use and how to minimize such use, educational and employment counseling as well as help with housing and social services, and finally, the identification of recreational activities that could take the place of drug use.

Cocaine-dependent patients enrolled in the multicomponent behavioral treatment program exhibited substantially greater levels of abstinence than other patients treated with standard drug abuse counseling (Figure 13.26; Higgins et al., 1993). At a 1-year follow-up, 80% of the subjects in the behavioral treatment program had negative urinalyses for cocaine, compared with approximately 40% of the subjects given counseling alone (Higgins, Budney et al., 1995). One possible criticism of this program is that it was developed and initially tested only on white males in Vermont, a mostly rural state. However, Silverman and colleagues (1995) recently reported the successful use of a voucher-based program in promoting cocaine abstinence in urban cocaine- and methadone-dependent patients. Much more research obviously needs to be performed; however, current findings suggest that voucher-based programs are among the best new strategies available for dealing with the problem of cocaine abuse.

Part II Summary

Cocaine is an alkaloid derived from the leaves of the shrub *Erythroxylon coca*, which is indigenous to the eastern highlands of the Andes mountains in South America. Although the peoples of that region have been chewing coca leaves for perhaps 5,000 years, cocaine use did not become popular in Western cultures until after the pure compound was isolated in 1859. In the United States, cocaine was a constituent of many popular beverages and over-the-counter pharmaceutical products in the late nineteenth and early twentieth centuries until its nonprescription use was banned by the Harrison Narcotic Act of 1914. Cocaine then went "underground" until the 1970s, at which time the first of two waves of increased cocaine use began. Household survey data indicate that over 10% of the U.S. population has used cocaine at least once, whereas fewer than 1% are current users.

Cocaine HCl is water soluble and therefore can be taken orally, intranasally, or by intravenous injection. Cocaine freebase (including "crack" cocaine) is the chemical form most suitable for smoking. The most rapid absorption and distribution of cocaine occurs following intravenous injection and smoking, which may account for the highly addictive properties of these routes of administration. Cocaine is metabolized by several biochemical pathways, yielding benzoylecgonine, ecgonine methyl ester, and several other metabolites.

At low to moderate doses, cocaine acts mainly to block synaptic uptake of DA, 5-HT, and NE by binding to their plasma membrane transporters. This action enhances transmission at the monoaminergic synapses by increasing the synaptic concentrations of these transmitters. Concurrent stimulation of the autoreceptors on monoaminergic nerve terminals and cell bodies, however, causes acute reductions in both cell firing and transmitter synthesis. At higher concentrations, cocaine also blocks several other membrane proteins, including voltage-gated Na^+ channels, σ sites, 5-HT_3 receptors, and muscarinic cholinergic receptors.

Cocaine exerts amphetamine-like psychostimulant effects on mood and behavior. The cocaine "high" is characterized by feelings of exhilaration, euphoria, well-being, and self-confidence. Other acute effects of cocaine include heightened energy, motor excitement, and sleep disturbances. At high doses or with prolonged use, cocaine can give rise to a number of negative effects such as irritability, anxiety, exhaustion, total insomnia, and even psychotic symptomatology. Cocaine produces sympathomimetic effects like those of amphetamine. The cocaine "high" is probably mediated at least partially by stimulation of the DA system, whereas the sympathomimetic effects involve peripheral adrenergic receptors.

In animal studies, cocaine is again amphetamine-like in eliciting locomotor activity, stereotyped behaviors, and rate-dependent changes in operant responding. Cocaine can function as a discriminative stimulus, and it exhibits powerful reinforcing effects in standard experimental paradigms involving drug self-administration, brain stimulation reward, and place conditioning. It is noteworthy, however, that cocaine also seems to be aversive under some conditions, which may be related to the drug's apparent anxiogenic (anxiety-provoking) properties.

Most of the behavioral effects of cocaine in animals have been attributed to activation of dopaminergic transmission, particularly in the nucleus accumbens. Both D_1 and D_2 receptors are involved in these mechanisms. However, some of cocaine's effects are modulated by other transmitters, such as 5-HT, excitatory amino acids, and opioids. Moreover, the role of the nucleus accumbens in cocaine reinforcement must not be emphasized to the exclusion of other brain areas. Current evidence suggests that this structure is part of a broader midbrain–forebrain–extrapyramidal drug reward circuit that is activated by several classes of abused drugs. DA is critical to the reinforcing effects of cocaine and amphetamine; however, other transmitters may be equally or more important for other drug classes.

Continuous exposure to cocaine or repeated dosing over a short time can cause behavioral and physiological tolerance. In contrast, intermittent treatment leads primarily to sensitization. In animals, the VTA is thought to be the site of initiation of cocaine's locomotor-sensitizing effects, whereas sensitization is expressed mainly in the nucleus accumbens.

Cocaine use occurs in individuals from all walks of life, although a common feature seems to be early use of other substances (legal or illegal). Some users quickly stop taking cocaine for various reasons, others maintain controlled use for long periods of time, and still others progress to a pattern of uncontrolled use (i.e., abuse). Such progression may come about through dose escalation or switching from intranasal use to smoking or intravenous injection, routes of administration with greater abuse potential. Cocaine abuse may be manifested by daily or near-daily use, or by a pattern of bingeing similar to the amphetamine "runs" described in the previous section. The end of a cocaine binge is followed by a complex abstinence syndrome, some of the symptoms of which (e.g., cocaine craving, anhedonia, anergia) place the user at high risk for relapse. These symptoms have been hypothesized to result from a temporary reduction in synaptic DA availability.

The adverse effects of cocaine use include the development of a psychotic state, cerebral vascular disorders such as stroke and intracerebral hemorrhage, and growth retardation and neurobehavioral deficits in offspring exposed to cocaine prenatally. Recent studies suggest that although certain infants may be severely affected, prenatal cocaine exposure is generally not as damaging as once thought. Nevertheless, animal research has demonstrated that cocaine does interact with the developing nervous system and that prenatal exposure can lead to later behavioral abnormalities.

Much effort in the area of treating cocaine abuse has been focused on the development of medications that might reduce craving and promote abstinence among users. Some of the compounds being tested are bromocriptine, fluoxetine, desipramine, buprenorphine, and ibogaine. Medications alone, however, will probably not be successful in dealing with our society's cocaine abuse problem. Effective behavioral treatment programs must therefore also be developed. Two new behavioral programs currently under consideration are treatments designed to extinguish or counteract conditioned drug craving and voucher-based treatment programs aimed at reinforcing abstinence and helping patients to develop and maintain a drug-free lifestyle. Over time, these and other novel methods, along with new pharmacotherapies, may help to reverse the devastating effects of cocaine on our society.

Chapter 14

Stimulants: Nicotine and Caffeine

In the previous chapter, we saw the powerful stimulant and reinforcing properties of amphetamine and cocaine. Nevertheless, the use of these drugs is relatively limited because of their illegality except for limited medical purposes. Many more individuals are users of the legal stimulants nicotine and caffeine. The present chapter is concerned with the properties of these substances, their mechanisms of action, and their potential for abuse.

Part I
Nicotine

Nicotine (1-methyl-2-[3-pyridyl]pyrrolidine) is one of the several alkaloids that can be extracted from tobacco leaves. When nicotine was first isolated in

Nicotine

1828 by Posselt and Reimann, it was found to constitute about 5% of the total weight of the dry plant leaves. However, this relatively minor fraction imbues tobacco with many physiological and psychological effects when the leaves are smoked, chewed, or snorted (as snuff) and the nicotine is absorbed into the human bloodstream. Without nicotine, it is quite likely that tobacco would be regarded as a useless weed.

In 1988, the U.S. Surgeon General reported that evidence had been accumulating for a long time showing that using tobacco products has unfavorable consequences for human health (see below). Because nicotine consumption is a critical aspect of smoking-related reinforcement, the Surgeon General proposed that nicotine be included with alcohol, the opiates, amphetamines, and cocaine in the category of addictive or dependency-producing drugs. Indeed, the widespread use of tobacco makes it the prime source of preventable premature death among Americans and members of many other societies where smoking is commonplace.

The widespread use of tobacco began after Europeans learned about it from crew members of the Columbus voyages in the latter part of the fifteenth century who saw the indigenous Americans smoking tobacco leaves for hedonistic, ritual, or magical purposes. These effects were later traced to the action of nicotine, which is one of many cholinomimetics that have been used for these purposes, such as lobeline, arecoline, hyoscine, muscarine, physostigmine, pilocarpine, and morphine (Rand, 1989; see Chapter 7). When tobacco plants were brought to Europe they were given the name *Nicotiana tabacum* in honor of Jean Nicot (1530–1600). Nicot had introduced tobacco chewing to Catherine de Medici and had promoted the importation and cultivation of the plant, believing it to have medicinal value. As one of the several plant substances mentioned above, nicotine became far better known than most other cholinotropic substances because it confers an interoceptive "pleasurable effect" (Di Chiara and Imperato, 1988) or euphoria that has instigated and sustained tobacco use by large proportions of human populations virtually the world over.

Basic Pharmacology of Nicotine

Tobacco: A Vehicle for Delivering Nicotine

Inhaled tobacco smoke contains a complex mixture of substances including carbon monoxide (CO) and thousands of different particulate substances such as carcinogenic hydrocarbons that are generated by the tobacco combustion process. These inhalants make up tobacco "tar," which provides the principal taste and smell of the

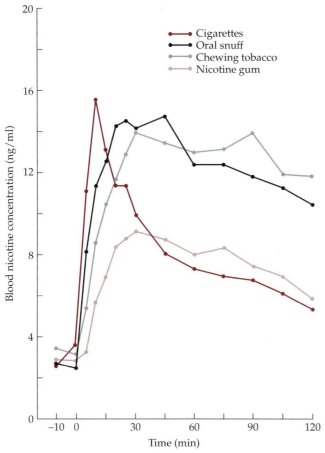

14.1 NICOTINE INGESTION AND PLASMA CONCENTRATION. Blood concentrations during and after cigarette smoking (one and one-third cigarettes) for 9 minutes and use of oral snuff (2.5 g), chewing tobacco (average 7.9 g), and nicotine gum (two 2-mg pieces) for 30 minutes. The points represent average values for 10 subjects. (After Benowitz, 1990b.)

smoke. Unfortunately, tobacco tar and CO are responsible for most of the diseases associated with long-term tobacco use. This subject is discussed below.

The major psychoactive ingredient in tobacco is nicotine. A typical American cigarette contains approximately 9 mg of nicotine, and the yield to the smoker is about 1 mg (Benowitz, 1990b). When tobacco smoke is inhaled, nicotine readily passes through the absorbent surface of the lungs, whose total area has been estimated to be about equal to the surface of a tennis court. Nicotine is absorbed to a lesser degree through the membranes of the mouth and nostrils when tobacco is chewed or snorted. Figure 14.1 illustrates these differences, showing that the most rapid absorption and elimination of nicotine occurs with cigarette smoking compared with other routes of ingestion.

When tobacco smoke is inhaled, 25% of the nicotine reaches the brain in about 7 seconds, about twice as fast as when the drug is administered intravenously. Thus, for nicotine, tobacco smoke inhalation via the modern cigarette is the fastest and the most efficient method of drug delivery to the brain. In general, reinforcement of a conditioned response is strongest when there is a short time interval between performing the response (e.g., pressing a lever for food or smoking a cigarette for nicotine) and obtaining the reinforcement. Consequently, the rapid transit time of nicotine to the brain—a few seconds—makes the drug a powerful reinforcer of smoking behavior (Oldendorf, 1992). The rapidly repeated, puff-by-puff intake of nicotine that occurs during smoking is unmatched by any other form of drug-taking. Moreover, the relatively short half-life of nicotine in blood and brain (see next section) allows frequent use without loss of effect (Russell, 1977).

Metabolism of Nicotine

Though some inhaled nicotine is metabolized in the lungs, about 80% to 90% of it is metabolized in the liver, with small amounts in the kidneys. The elimination half-life of nicotine varies among individuals but is typically around 2 hours (Jones, 1987b). Consequently, circulating nicotine levels are lowest upon waking and gradually increase through the day with repeated cigarette smoking. The major metabolites of nicotine are cotinine and nicotine-N-oxide. These compounds are eliminated mainly

Cotinine

in the urine, leaving trace amounts in other body fluids, such as saliva. Nicotine is also excreted in the milk of nursing mothers who smoke.

Acute Behavioral and Physiological Effects of Nicotine

Reinforcing Effects

What is the evidence that nicotine reinforces and maintains tobacco use? In the U.S. Surgeon General's report in 1988, drug dependence was defined as substance-seeking behavior involving a psychoactive agent that acts on the central nervous system. Drugs of abuse are usually euphoriants whose effects are dose-dependent and centrally mediated. This was shown in an experiment with human subjects who pressed a lever for intravenous nicotine administration. This self-administration of nicotine elicited dose-related euphoric effects similar to those resulting from cocaine and morphine, and when saline was substituted for nicotine, the subjects discontinued lever pressing. Further, when the subjects could choose between a placebo or nicotine, they preferentially chose to self-administer nicotine, showing that nicotine was a positive reinforcer (Pomerleau, 1992).

Moreover, there seem to be many instigators and secondary reinforcers of smoking behavior. For example, the taste and smell of cigarettes become conditioned stimuli associated with nicotine-induced euphoria and the satisfaction of the smoking process. The reinforcing effects of these stimuli thus enhance the desirability of tobacco and contribute further to tobacco dependence. Another consequence of this process is the craving that may occur from observing another smoker "lighting up" and sensing the smell of tobacco smoke. Environmental context can also be strongly conditioned to smoking behavior, which is exemplified by habitual smoking after a meal, when drinking coffee or alcoholic beverages, while watching sporting events, or while using the telephone.

Such considerations raise questions as to the exact role of nicotine in eliciting and maintaining cigarette smoking. However, the role of nicotine becomes clear from the demonstration that nicotine can initiate and support drug-seeking behavior by animals. Specifically, animals will self-administer nicotine intravenously, although the phenomenon is not as robust as that seen with amphetamine or cocaine. Figure 14.2 illustrates the results of one study involving rats that had learned to self-administer nicotine solutions of various concentrations. In this case, the experimental chamber contained two levers—one activating the infusions, the other inactive. The data show significantly more dose-related responses with the active than with the inactive lever. The decline in responding at the highest dose (0.06 mg/kg per infusion) probably represents a longer-lasting nicotinic effect, since that dose provided the most nicotine intake per response and thus longer interresponse intervals. Self-administration methods have shown clear patterns of nicotine seeking by rats, dogs, and primates

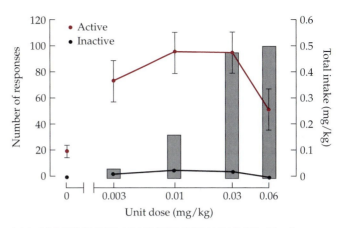

14.2 NICOTINE SELF-ADMINISTRATION IN RATS. The line graph shows the average number of responses leading to an infusion of a unit dose of nicotine via an implanted intravenous cannula. The superimposed bar graph shows the total intake of nicotine at each unit dose during a 60-minute session. Learning to self-administer nicotine is shown because an active lever (color circles) that supplies nicotine was pressed significantly more often than an inactive lever (black circles). (After Corrigal and Coen, 1989.)

(Stolerman and Shoaib, 1991; also see Swedberg, Henningfield, and Goldberg, 1990 for more details).

These and other experiments performed since the mid-1970s, as well as additional findings from human studies, provide strong evidence that nicotine induces drug-seeking behavior and dependency. In turn, this leads to the conclusion that nicotine should be designated as an addictive drug despite persistent denials by representatives of the tobacco industry (some of which have come as recently as mid-1995; see Corrigall and Coen, 1989; Robinson and Pritchard, 1995; Stolerman and Jarvis, 1995).

Tar and nicotine content are usually closely correlated among different brands of cigarettes. After smoking thousands of cigarettes (a pack a day is 7,300 cigarettes a year), individuals have readily learned the relationship between a cigarette's flavor and its nicotine content. Sensing public concern about the health dangers of smoking, the tobacco industry experimented with the marketing of nicotine-free cigarettes, but these were rejected by smokers. Moreover, cigarettes with low concentrations of nicotine that fail to supply the expected effect are puffed strongly and more often to optimize the ingestion of whatever nicotine they do contain (Schelling, 1992). Small wonder, then, that cigarette advertising emphasizes "flavor" (which to practiced smokers immediately indicates the nicotine content) as its catchword rather than "nicotine," which sounds ominous and is best left unmentioned.

Plasma levels and nicotine reinforcement.   One way to understand the compulsive use of tobacco products is to establish the relationships between the plasma level of the suspected euphoriant, nicotine, its physiological and psychological effects, and the mechanisms by which drug dependence develops and is sustained (for reviews, see Rand, 1989; Sherwood, 1993). In one of several experiments performed by Pomerleau and Pomerleau (1992), evidence was sought for euphoriant sensations that might serve as reinforcers during cigarette smoking. Groups of smokers were carefully monitored for subjective feelings of euphoria while smoking cigarettes with different nicotine contents.

On each of three separate test days, the subjects smoked a single cigarette after an overnight abstinence. Three types of special research cigarettes were used: ultralow nicotine (0.2-mg yield), medium nicotine (1.3-mg yield), and high nicotine (2.4-mg yield). The subjects were instructed to depress a button at any time while they were smoking when they experienced "pleasurable sensations . . . which may be described as a 'rush,' a 'buzz,' or a 'high,' and to hold the button down for the duration of the sensation." Blood samples were also collected for the measurement of plasma nicotine concentrations.

Examination of the blood plasma concentrations revealed that some of the subjects given the medium and high nicotine cigarettes had apparently adjusted their smoking behavior to compensate for the varying nicotine content. Hence, the data were analyzed by regrouping the subjects according to plasma nicotine level: low dose (mean nicotine concentration = 4.5 ng/ml), medium dose (mean nicotine concentration = 13.4 ng/ml), and high dose (mean nicotine concentration = 22.8 ng/ml). The behavioral findings from this analysis are shown in Figure 14.3. The number of button presses for both the medium- and high-dose groups differed significantly from the number of presses for the low-dose subjects. There was also a trend toward a dose-related increase in button press duration, but it was not statistically significant.

In subjects smoking a high-nicotine cigarette as the first cigarette of the day, there was a positive correlation between the number of years the subjects had smoked and the number of button presses ($r = 0.48$, $p < 0.05$). This suggests that more experienced smokers obtained greater subjective pleasure from smoking and may be more tobacco-dependent. Furthermore, a correlation was found between the number of puffs and total duration of button presses ($r = 0.43$, $p < 0.05$), indicating a relationship between the parameters of smoking behavior and the subjective effects of smoking.

These data support and extend earlier findings that nicotine produces euphoric sensations in a dose-related manner. It should be noted, however, that it is difficult to assess the unanimity of what constitutes a "rush," a "buzz," or a "high," which presumably are the indicators of euphoria. The authors therefore acknowledged uncertainty as to whether the pleasurable effects re-

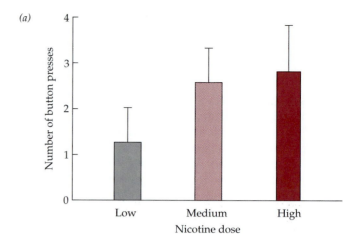

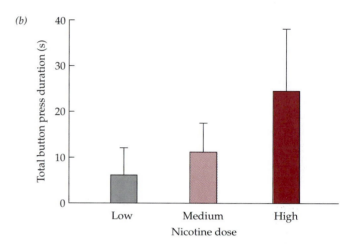

14.3 INFLUENCE OF NICOTINE DOSE ON SELF-REPORTED EUPHORIA IN SMOKERS. In smokers smoking a single cigarette following an overnight abstinence, higher nicotine doses (as determined by plasma nicotine concentration) were associated with a significant increase in the number of euphoria-associated button presses (a) and a trend toward an increased button-press duration (b). (After Pomerleau and Pomerleau, 1992.)

ported by the subjects indeed constituted euphoria. Rather, the subjects may have confused euphoria with the avoidance of withdrawal symptoms, which might be somewhat pronounced after a relatively long sleep-time abstinence (see below).

Psychomotor Performance

As mentioned in Chapter 7 and discussed in more detail below, nicotine acts as an agonist at nicotinic cholinergic receptors in the brain and peripheral nervous system. Because of the hypothesis that acetylcholine (ACh) plays an important role in certain aspects of cognitive functioning, nicotine obtained from smoking cigarettes might conceivably facilitate psychomotor performance and enhance cognition. Animal studies on nicotine have focused on learning and memory using a variety of tasks. Many of these studies have found that nicotine administration enhances learning and/or memory, whereas treatment with a nicotinic antagonist, such as mecamyl-amine, causes learning deficits (reviewed by Levin, 1992). The human literature encompasses a broader array of nicotine effects, including attentional processes and sensorimotor function. Recent reviews by Heishman, Taylor, and Henningfield (1994) and Sherwood (1993) have summarized and critically evaluated the current status of nicotine effects on human psychomotor performance. We will therefore not attempt to cover this topic exhaustively, but rather, we will discuss some of the methodological aspects of the field, highlight a few representative studies and some general research findings, and conclude with an overall assessment of the literature.

Methodological issues.   The most widely used paradigm for investigating nicotine effects on human psychomotor performance involves the study of regular smokers who are asked to abstain from tobacco for some period of time in order to reduce circulating nicotine levels. In one type of experimental approach, all the subjects are smokers, and comparisons are made between still-abstinent smokers and smokers who are tested after being allowed to self-administer nicotine by smoking. In a second type of approach (a within-subject design), the same subjects (all of whom are smokers) are tested repeatedly, sometimes after abstinence and other times after having access to cigarettes. Yet a third variation involves comparing smokers (who are allowed to smoke before testing) and nonsmokers, who serve as control subjects.

It can readily be seen that all of these experimental approaches suffer from various methodological problems (Heishman, Taylor, and Henningfield, 1994; Sherwood, 1993). First, smoking subjects may have widely disparate preexperimental histories in terms of cigarette brand, smoking frequency, smoking duration, and so forth. These factors could influence both the amount of residual nicotine in the circulation after the abstinence period and sensitivity to the nicotine administered during the experimental test. Second, different studies have used abstinence periods ranging from 3 hours to 5 days, which makes comparisons between studies somewhat problematic. Third, because many studies do not use any placebo control procedures, both the subject and experimenter know whether or not nicotine is being administered in a given test trial. Even when they are used, placebo (i.e., nicotine-free) cigarettes may be ineffective as a control if subjects sense the lack of subjective effects normally produced by nicotine ingestion. Fourth, experiments in which smokers are compared with nonsmokers can be criticized on the basis that these groups may have inherently different levels of "normal" performance. Finally, we shall see later that nicotine abstinence produces a variety of withdrawal symptoms, including increases in irritability, anxiety, and depression, as well as restless-ness and difficulty in concentrating. Some abstinent smokers are virtually free of such effects, whereas others are significantly affected even after an overnight sleep abstinence. Consequently, it is very problematic to assess behavioral effects of nicotine under abstinence conditions because any positive effects that are observed may be due to the amelioration of withdrawal-related behavioral deficits rather than enhancement of function above baseline levels.

Experimental findings.   Roth and colleagues (1992) used the within-subject design to assess the influence of smoking on performance in remembering a maze and in a word recognition task. The subjects were tested either while smoking normally or after an 8-hour abstinence period. The general result was that the subjects did equally as well on both tests under both conditions, although there was some evidence that smokers who normally smoked early in the day were helped by smoking, whereas those who smoked later in the day performed better when not smoking. If this experiment was meant to assess the effects of abstinence on memory, a range of abstinence times should have been tested in both smoking and nonsmoking subjects.

Spilich and colleagues (1992) performed a study comparing abstinent smokers with nonsmokers on several tasks. These investigators found that smokers who were abstinent for 3 hours prior to tasks of continuous attention, memory scanning, or text comprehension performed significantly more poorly than did control subjects. On the other hand, scores on a simulated driving test and a simple visual search task were not different. An earlier study showed that task complexity is a significant factor in smoking-related performance (Kleinman, Vaughn, and Christ, 1973). Smokers abstinent for 24 hours learned lists of paired nonsense syllables. In this task, the subjects learn a list of syllable pairs by being presented with the pairs one at a time for a few trials; they are then given the first syllable and must supply the second. The lists are presented over and over again, and the subject's score is the number of repetitions needed to reach a certain criterion of correct responses. In a difficult task in which the syllable pairs had low associative value (e.g., MJZ–RDP), the abstinent smokers did poorly compared with nonsmokers. But in an easy task in which the syllable pairs had high associative value (e.g., TAB–DOT), the abstinent smokers learned the list more quickly. The reason for these findings is open to conjecture.

A number of studies have investigated the effects of nicotine on critical flicker–fusion (CFF) frequency. This task, which requires subjects to distinguish fusion from flicker of an intermittent light source, has often been used to assess overall CNS activity or arousal. The frequency threshold (in Hertz) at which flicker turns to fusion (i.e., a steady light) is presumed to represent the highest number of discrete "bits" of information that the retino-cortical system can process in a unit of time, and thus is an index of the functional state of the CNS. As expected, therefore, stimulant drugs raise the CFF (i.e., the fusion threshold occurs at higher frequencies, indicating an elevated sensory processing), while sedative drugs reduce the threshold. A large number of CFF studies have been reported utilizing differing conditions of abstinence, routes of nicotine administration (cigarettes, nicotine gum, or subcutaneous injection), types of control groups, and so forth, and the general conclusion drawn from this work is that nicotine does elevate CFF threshold in abstinent smokers, but has a less clear effect in nonsmokers. This would seem to indicate that the major influence of nicotine is to reverse withdrawal-induced deficits in function (Heishman, Taylor, and Henningfield, 1994). Nevertheless, Sherwood (1993) argues that nicotine may produce an absolute enhancement of performance on this measure regardless of prior experience.

The influence of nicotine has also been evaluated with respect to motor function, focused attention, selective attention, sustained attention, divided attention, learning, and memory. Some of the tasks used to evaluate these parameters include finger tapping and hand steadiness (motor function), reaction time (focused attention), the Stroop test (selective attention), a rapid visual information processing (RVIP) task (sustained attention), and various types of verbal learning tasks (learning and memory). In the RVIP task, subjects are presented visually with a series of digits at a rate of 100 per minute (600 ms between stimuli) and are asked to detect sequences of three consecutive even or odd numbers. As in the case of CFF, many studies found that nicotine enhanced performance in abstinent smokers, but fewer instances were reported of similar enhancement in nonsmoking subjects (Heishman, Taylor, and Henningfield, 1994). One exception is simple motor function (e.g., finger tapping), in which nicotine administration has consistently been shown to enhance performance regardless of previous smoking experience.

Finally, it is of interest to consider the possible influence of nicotine on complex performance in which two or more tasks must be performed simultaneously. A common example of a complex task is automobile driving, which requires sustained divided attention to multiple stimuli as well as continuous psychomotor performance. Studies on the influence of nicotine on simulated driving have yielded variable results, with no consistent pattern of effects having been observed (Sherwood, 1993).

Conclusion.   We have seen that the study of nicotine effects on psychomotor performance has been plagued by methodological weakness and inconsistent findings. The typical use of cigarettes as a delivery vehicle raises many concerns, such as limiting the subject population to smokers, administering nicotine by a route that produces highly variable drug intake, and invoking problems associated with abstinence. Both Sherwood (1993) and Heishman, Taylor, and Henningfield (1994) thus conclude that studies on abstinent smokers can be taken to show only that nicotine reverses deficits in psychomotor performance that are produced by drug abstinence. This effect may contribute to nicotine dependence in regular smokers.

A more contentious issue is whether nicotine can increase performance above normal baseline levels in nonsmokers or in nonabstinent smokers. Heishman, Taylor, and Henningfield (1994) argue that very few measures are reliably enhanced by nicotine without prior abstinence. In contrast, Sherwood (1993) concluded that nicotine exerts small but noticeable improvement on several aspects of psychomotor performance, including simple motor responses, CFF threshold, sustained attention, and memory. These results are consistent with a possible role for ACh and nicotinic cholinergic receptors in attentional or memory processes. Furthermore, because memory impairment in Alzheimer's disease is correlated with a decrease in cerebral cortical ACh activity, it is possible that nicotinic receptor activation might have an ameliorative effect on this disorder (see Chapter 20).

Peripheral Physiological Effects

Small doses of nicotine have an excitatory effect upon the nicotinic cholinergic receptors at neuromuscular junctions and in autonomic ganglia (Taylor, 1985c). At a given dose, the autonomic effects are more pronounced than the neuromuscular effects. However, though larger doses stimulate neuromuscular junctions, the postsynaptic membranes may undergo a prolonged depolarization and desensitization leading to muscle weakness and paralysis. In contrast, by stimulating autonomic ganglia, nicotine can cause a wide spectrum of physiological and behavioral manifestations. For example, even the small amount of nicotine absorbed when smoking cigarettes increases heart rate and blood pressure by stimulating the sympathetic ganglia and the adrenal glands to release norepinephrine and epinephrine. Furthermore, nicotine stimulates chemoreceptors in the aorta and carotid arteries that also cause vasoconstriction, tachycardia, and increased blood pressure. It can thus be understood why smokers, especially those who have high blood pressure to begin with, are at greater risk than nonsmokers for cardiovascular disease and cerebrovascular accidents.

The nicotinic action on parasympathetic autonomic ganglia increases hydrochloric acid secretion in the stomach, which exacerbates or contributes to the formation of stomach ulcers (Taylor, 1985c). It also increases motor activity in the bowel, which sometimes leads to chronic diarrhea that is especially harmful to individuals who are vulnerable to colitis, a chronic irritability of the colon. These and other nicotine-induced effects produce the deleterious consequences of heavy and prolonged use of tobacco products. This subject is discussed in more detail below.

Physiological Effects on the CNS

Systemic doses of nicotine obtained during tobacco smoking exert profound pharmacological effects on the human CNS. Circulating nicotine readily passes the blood–brain barrier and enters the brain, where it activates nicotinic cholinergic receptors (see below). In addition to influencing the motivational and cognitive processes described earlier, nicotine can produce tremors and convulsions at high doses. At lower doses, it increases respiration rate, it acts upon vasomotor centers in the medulla to induce cardiovascular changes, and it causes the release of antidiuretic hormone from the pituitary gland (Volle and Koelle, 1975).

A number of studies have investigated the effects of tobacco-derived nicotine on cortical activity. At doses absorbed by a typical smoker, nicotine induces an alerting neocortical electroencephalogram (EEG) (a 13–30 Hz low-voltage pattern) and increases theta wave activity in the hippocampus (a 4–7-Hz high-voltage pattern). Simultaneous occurrence of both EEG patterns is associated with heightened arousal. Further, subcutaneous administration of nicotine can produce dose-dependent increases in cerebral glucose uptake, indicating elevated brain metabolic activity and brain energy utilization, which is also associated with states of arousal. Similar effects have been found with cocaine (Pomerleau, 1992).

Toxic Effects of Nicotine

Nicotine is very toxic; as little as 60 mg can be fatal to an adult. It may be surprising to learn that an ordinary cigar contains enough nicotine to provide about two lethal doses. However, the burning of tobacco destroys much of the nicotine so that only the amount contained in the smoke drawn through the cigar is available to the smoker. When tobacco is chewed, nicotine is poorly absorbed through the oral membranes, but other ingredients in the tobacco are harmful to the teeth, gums, and buccal mucosa.

When tobacco is accidentally swallowed, for example by children, the nicotine is less toxic than would be expected. The low toxicity occurs because nicotine is slowly absorbed from the stomach owing to the fact that the drug is a weak base and is therefore mostly ionized in the acidic environment of the stomach. If nicotine passes into the duodenum, it can be absorbed more rapidly; however, even then, the amount absorbed into the bloodstream is rapidly metabolized during its first passage through the liver.

In cases of nicotine overdose (e.g., due to cigarette swallowing), the amount absorbed may be sufficient to activate the chemical trigger zone (vomiting center) in the medulla and cause the expulsion of the remaining tobacco in the stomach. The onset of vomiting is rapid and vigorous because nicotine has an excitatory effect on the sensory nerves of the vomiting reflex pathways. Smokers may remember that when they began to smoke, even slightly inhaling the smoke often caused symptoms of nicotine toxicity: nausea, vomiting, pallor, abdominal pain, headache, dizziness, and weakness (Volle and Koelle, 1975). Continued smoking usually leads to tolerance and the absence of these signs, but the serious diseases associated with chronic tobacco use, such as lung cancer, respiratory diseases, coronary artery disease, tobacco amblyopia (dimness of vision), and complications of pregnancy, testify to the fact that tolerance does not occur to the toxic effects of other tobacco ingredients (Gritz and Jarvik, 1978).

Most cases of severe nicotine poisoning are the result of accidental exposure to nicotine-based insecticides, which may be sprayed over large agricultural areas. If not adequately protected from the spray, a person applying such an insecticide can readily absorb nicotine through the skin. Nicotine is toxic to insects because the high dose causes nicotinic receptor blockade, leading to paralysis; thus the insects die either of asphyxiation or because they cannot feed. In humans and animals, excessive doses of nicotine produce a continuous depolarization of the postsynaptic membrane at neuromuscular synapses, resulting in receptor desensitization. The block of synaptic transmission in the excitatory innervation of the respiratory muscles, diaphragm, and intercostal muscles can cause severe respiratory distress. In acute toxicity, the sympathetic ganglia are affected as shown by severe autonomic symptoms that occur very rapidly. These symptoms include nausea, excessive salivation, abdominal pain, vomiting, diarrhea, cold sweat, headache, dizziness, disturbed hearing and vision, mental confusion, and marked weakness. This is quickly followed by falling blood pressure, difficulty in breathing, weakening of the pulse, which becomes rapid and irregular, and collapse. The end result may be terminal convulsions, with death following in a minute or two due to respiratory failure. The treatment of nicotine poisoning, if the poison has been swallowed, involves the induction of vomiting, placing adsorptive charcoal in the stomach, giving artificial respiration, and treating for shock (see Taylor, 1985c).

Carbon Monoxide Toxicity

As mentioned above, CO is a component in the tobacco smoke inhaled during smoking. Its presence in the lungs and bloodstream is scarcely noticed by smokers, but heavy smoking can cause enough CO accumulation to have deleterious effects on respiration. The affinity of CO for hemoglobin (Hb) to form carboxyhemoglobin (COHb) is 220 times greater than the affinity of oxygen for hemoglobin to form oxyhemoglobin (O_2Hb). COHb cannot transport oxygen and has a half-life of 3–4 hours. In addition, COHb interferes with the release of oxygen from O_2Hb, so that a relatively small amount of COHb in the blood severely reduces the availability of O_2 for respiration. Furthermore, COHb has a direct toxic effect upon other O_2-dependent enzymes. Over the long term, tolerance to CO in the blood occurs through increased production of Hb and red blood corpuscles, and these changes partially compensate for the presence of COHb. Nevertheless, it should be emphasized that the compensations described above do not diminish the harmful effects of these substances in the body (Jarvik, 1979; Klaassen, 1985).

Mechanisms of Nicotine Action

Nicotinic Receptors

The primary sites of action of nicotine are the nicotinic cholinergic receptors (nAChRs). These receptors are ligand-gated channels that represent one of the major ACh receptor subtypes (see Chapter 7). Central nicotinic receptors have been identified in the midbrain tegmentum, in subcortical forebrain nuclei such as the striatum and nucleus accumbens, in the substantia nigra pars compacta and ventral tegmental area (VTA), and in various cortical areas. In the brain, many nAChRs appear to be presynaptic and to be associated with cholinergic, dopaminergic, and glutamatergic nerve terminals. This contrasts with the classic neuronal muscarinic receptors that are located mainly postsynaptically.

In accordance with their presynaptic localization, stimulation of central nAChRs is thought to enhance presynaptic Ca^{2+} influx and thereby enhance the amount of neurotransmitter (cholinergic or noncholinergic) liberated from nerve endings. Nicotine particularly affects nerve endings in the terminal fields in limbic and cortical areas, which are implicated in cognition and other functions that are altered by nicotine administration (McGehee et al., 1995; Ochoa, 1994).

Furthermore, iontophoretic application of nicotinic agonists in the rat hippocampus and in the prefrontal cortex increased the amplitude of excitatory postsynaptic potentials (EPSPs) mediated by NMDA glutamatergic receptors. Thus, a cholinergic system may control the excitation of pyramidal cells in the prefrontal cortex by modifying their responsiveness to glutamate (Vidal, 1994). Given that NMDA receptors are important in learning and memory (see Chapter 10), this phenomenon may account for the enhancing effects of nicotinic agonists on cognitive functioning. Interactions between nicotine and glutamate may also be relevant to cognitive deficits in the offspring of mothers who smoked during pregnancy and in whom nicotine perturbed the development of nicotinic receptors in the fetus (Vandekamp and Collins, 1994).

Neural Mechanisms of Nicotine-Induced Behavioral Effects

As shown in Figure 14.4, several different brain areas have been implicated in the behavioral effects of nicotine. Among these are the nucleus accumbens, striatum, VTA, and substantia nigra pars compacta, all of which possess high densities of nAChRs (Clarke and Pert, 1985). As discussed above as well as in Chapter 8, the nucleus accumbens and VTA comprise an important part of the mesolimbic DA system and play a significant role in regulating locomotor activity and drug reinforcement. Current evidence indicates that the stimulant and reinforcing effects of nicotine are mediated by activation of this system and consequent release of DA in the accumbens. For example, in vivo microdialysis studies by Di Chiara and Imperato (1988) found that nicotine was similar to other abused drugs (amphetamine, cocaine, morphine, and alcohol) in causing enhanced accumbens DA overflow, which is correlated with the drug's locomotor activating effect.

Because nAChRs are found in both the VTA and nucleus accumbens, there has been some controversy as to the anatomical (VTA vs. accumbens) and subcellular (pre- vs. postsynaptic) localization of the receptors involved in the stimulant and reinforcing effects of nicotine (reviewed by Clarke, 1990). However, the majority of evidence at this time seems to favor a predominant action of nicotine on postsynaptic receptors located directly on the VTA mesolimbic DA neurons. For example, Corrigall and colleagues (1994) demonstrated a disruption of nicotine self-administration following infusion of the nicotine antagonist dihydro-β-erythroidine into the VTA, but not when the antagonist was infused into the accumbens. This suggests that a nicotine-mediated increase in VTA neuron firing is necessary for nicotine reinforcement, whereas activation of nicotinic receptors on the dopaminergic nerve terminals in the accumbens is less important. Reavill and Stolerman (1990) also found that stimulation of locomotor activity was produced by injection of nicotinic agonists specifically into the VTA. Finally, the role of VTA and accumbens nicotinic receptors in regulating DA release was investigated in a recent microdialysis study of nicotine-induced DA overflow in the accumbens (Nisell, Nomikos, and Svensson, 1994). As previously observed by other investigators, systemic administration of nicotine by subcutaneous injection led to significantly increased DA overflow in the accumbens. However, prior infusion of the nicotinic antagonist mecamylamine directly into the VTA, but not the accumbens, blocked the nicotine-induced increase in extracellular DA levels. On the other hand, it should be noted that when nicotine was administered directly into the VTA or accumbens instead of being given systemically, both areas yielded significant enhancement of accumbens DA overflow at a high concentration of nicotine (1 mM), but not at lower concentrations. Thus, stimulation

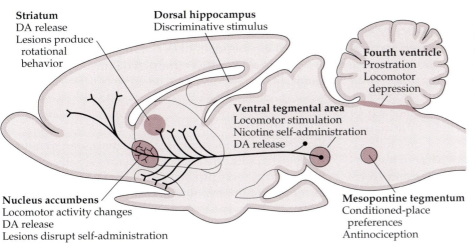

Striatum
DA release
Lesions produce rotational behavior

Dorsal hippocampus
Discriminative stimulus

Fourth ventricle
Prostration
Locomotor depression

Ventral tegmental area
Locomotor stimulation
Nicotine self-administration
DA release

Nucleus accumbens
Locomotor activity changes
DA release
Lesions disrupt self-administration

Mesopontine tegmentum
Conditioned-place preferences
Antinociception

14.4 BRAIN REGIONS AND PATHWAYS IMPLICATED IN THE BEHAVIORAL AND NEUROCHEMICAL EFFECTS OF NICOTINE. The mesolimbic dopamine (DA) pathway projecting from the VTA to the nucleus accumbens plays an important role in the stimulant and reinforcing properties of nicotine. Other brain areas shown are thought to be involved in additional effects of nicotine. (After Stolerman and Shoaib, 1991.)

of VTA nicotinic receptors seems to be a necessary condition for enhancement of nucleus accumbens DA release by systemic nicotine (because the effect can be inhibited by local nicotinic receptor blockade in the VTA). However, stimulation of these receptors alone is not sufficient to induce DA release, since intra-VTA nicotine had only a weak releasing effect in the accumbens.

In an effort to establish the role of DA in the reinforcing properties of nicotine, Corrigall and Coen (1991) trained rats to self-administer nicotine and then examined the effects of pretreating the animals with the D_1-receptor antagonist SCH23390 or the D_2-receptor antagonists spiperone or haloperidol. The results showed that pretreatment with either SCH23390 or spiperone significantly reduced self-administration of nicotine in a dose-dependent manner, although the effect of spiperone was not as robust as that of SCH23390. In contrast, no significant changes occurred following haloperidol pretreatment within the selected dose range. These findings suggest that DA D_1 receptors play the most prominent role in nicotine self-administration. In general, the notion of DA involvement in nicotine's reinforcing properties is consistent with the previous discussions of reinforcement mechanisms above and in Chapters 8 and 13.

Who Are the Smokers and Why Do They Smoke?

In this section, we will turn our attention away from nicotine and focus on the wider problem of tobacco smoking. To understand smoking behavior more fully, we must consider not only the pharmacology of nicotine but also demographic variables, subjective reasons for smoking, and the commercial promotion of tobacco use.

Characteristics of Smokers

Socioeconomic factors and gender. With respect to socioeconomic status, a report by Reeder (1977) stated that

better-educated groups had a lower proportion of smokers, particularly in the case of men. Further, upwardly mobile men whose socioeconomic status was above that of their parents were less likely to smoke, whereas men who moved down the social order tended to be heavy smokers. With respect to occupations, white-collar males were less likely to be smokers than workers in all other classes. In contrast, white-collar women workers were more likely to smoke than women in all other occupations, though women were overall less likely to smoke than men. Similarly, men in upper to middle income categories were less likely to smoke, whereas women in this category were more likely to be smokers than women in lower income categories. This apparent inverse relationship between smoking tendencies and gender was considered to be the result of the changing gender roles of women in the 1970s. At that time, 46% of women who were 16 and over were in the labor force, and this number was increasing year by year. There was also a greater number of women in colleges and in the professional world, and an ongoing general trend toward equality in virtually all aspects of social and economic life. Thus, the change in smoking behavior of women at that time may have reflected their increased social power and independence. Surgeon General Koop's 1989 report stated that young women were going against the trend of quitting smoking (U.S. Department of Health and Human Services, 1989), a finding of some concern because of evidence showing that smoking by pregnant women is injurious to the fetus.

A number of studies examining the determinants of smoking in children in the United States, Canada and Great Britain showed that schoolchildren, especially girls, were smoking at younger ages, and that peer pressure was instrumental in the initiation of smoking. The children reported that they smoked because their "best friend" or group of friends smoked, and one investigator found that the most significant variable in explaining smoking behavior in English and Welsh schoolboys was the number of their friends that smoked (Evans et al., 1979). Among teenagers, those less academically successful and inclined to choose vocational programs were more likely to smoke than their peers who were more academically oriented toward college preparatory programs and who were high in their need for recognition. However, with the increasing implementation of school health education programs that include information about unhealthy practices of drug, alcohol, and tobacco use, familial and peer influences have become less important as smoking determinants (see Kolbe and Newman, 1984; Severson, 1984).

Moreover, a survey in Canada among 4,828 men in the Quebec area, age 35–64, revealed that 62.5% were smokers, and that smoking was significantly less prevalent among those completing at least 13 years of school than among those completing 12 years or less (Robitaille, Dagenais, and Christe, 1984). A 1978 survey in the former West Germany correlated smoking with 125 different occupations (Borgers and Menzel, 1984). The results indicated that the highest percentages of smokers and heavy smokers were found among blue-collar workers, and in many jobs the number of female smokers and male smokers were equal. Among traditional female occupations such as waitress, supermarket cashier, and typist, 60% to 70% were smokers. The lowest percentages of smokers were found among professionals and academics. Thus, there appears to be a definite inverse relationship in Western societies between the likelihood of tobacco smoking and educational, occupational, and socioeconomic status. This relationship was identified over 20 years ago and was still found to exist in the United States according to Surgeon General Koop's 1989 report.

Familial factors.   Smoking among family members is a significant determinant of smoking behavior: teenagers are most likely to be smokers if both parents smoke, less likely if only one parent smokes, and least likely if neither parent smokes. Teenagers in single-parent homes are more likely to smoke than teenagers in two-parent homes. Both boys and girls are more likely to smoke if an older sibling smokes and less likely if siblings do not smoke. Both boys and girls are more likely to smoke if only the mother smokes than if only the father smokes, and if both parents and a sibling smoke the likelihood of a teenager becoming a smoker increases fourfold (Reeder, 1977; Evans et al., 1979). For more details on parental influences on teenage smoking see Oechsli and Seltzer (1984).

Higgins, Whitley, and Dunn (1984) studied smoking within families involved in tobacco production. Children in these families had more favorable attitudes toward smoking than children whose families were in other occupations. Also, a larger proportion of children from tobacco families smoked, and they smoked more than their peers from non-tobacco families. Tobacco-family children, therefore, appear to be at greater risk for smoking-related diseases, and they may be more resistant to antismoking messages unless more persuasive messages are designed for this group (Higgins, Whitley, and Dunn, 1984).

Determinants of Smoking Behavior

Smokers smoke for nicotine.   We have seen in animal studies that nicotine delivery provides significant reinforcement of lever pressing. There are also human data in support of the hypothesis that nicotine reinforces tobacco smoking. For example, administration of the central nicotinic antagonist mecamylamine to cigarette smokers was found to increase smoking behavior (presumably in an attempt to overcome the nicotinic receptor blockade), whereas the peripheral nicotinic blocker pentolinium had no effect on smoking (see Jarvik, 1979).

Other pertinent findings are related to the use of low-nicotine cigarettes by smokers who are attempting to curb their habit. Surveys show that 80% to 90% of smokers express the desire to quit smoking (mostly for health reasons), but admit that they can't. As an alternative, many smokers smoke filtered cigarettes or cigarettes low in nicotine and tar that have been made commercially available, purportedly to serve the health of smokers. However, smokers change their behavior when smoking such cigarettes: they puff harder and more often, they inhale more deeply and smoke more cigarettes, and they smoke more of each cigarette before it is discarded. To assess whether or not smokers of low-nicotine cigarettes actually do have lower intakes of nicotine, their blood and urine concentrations of nicotine and tar were compared with those of smokers of regular cigarettes. The results showed that the differences were very small, and certainly did not reflect the difference in yields between the two types of cigarettes. This powerful biochemical evidence shows that smokers have ways to compensate for reduced nicotine delivery and negates the claim that low-yield cigarettes are significantly safer than regular cigarettes (Benowitz et al., 1983).

Further indication of the smoker's compelling need for nicotine is the fact that cigarettes with less than a 0.3-mg yield of nicotine are not very popular, and sales of nicotine-free lettuce cigarettes were so poor that the two companies that made them quickly went bankrupt. The low-nicotine and nicotine-free cigarettes had most of the attributes that are deemed part of the cigarette habit; that is, they gave the smoker the opportunity to handle, light, and puff the cigarettes, see the smoke, and obtain olfactory and oral gratifications. Nevertheless, these cigarettes were quickly given up for the usual high-nicotine varieties. Clearly, the correlation between nicotine content and the preference for and satisfaction obtained from cigarettes leads to the conclusion that nicotine is the major desired and reinforcing agent, though not necessarily the only one, that maintains smoking behavior.

Subjective reasons for smoking. Smoking is a complex behavior that involves not only nicotine delivery but also a host of other sensorimotor experiences. These all contribute to the subjective experience of smoking and thus to the acquisition and maintenance of this behavior. Individuals smoke in situations that vary widely in arousal value. Some examples include when relaxing after a meal, when trying to "get yourself together" before a possibly stressful confrontation or before taking an examination, or when just doing something to fill up time while waiting for the car pool driver. The variety of contexts in which smoking occurs suggests that it may be used in different ways to modulate an individual's state of arousal. Smoking obviously serves as a mild stimulant due to the psychoactive properties of nicotine. This effect is manifested by increases in EEG signals that are indicative of behavioral arousal and sustained attention. On the other hand, for some individuals smoking acts as a sedative to diminish stress and anxiety.

To gain a better understanding of the subjective reasons for smoking, Jaffe and Jarvik (1978) interviewed smokers about the characteristics of their smoking behavior and their reasons for smoking. Responses to a questionnaire showed that smoking had a calming effect on many subjects. In some cases, smoking seemed to provide a pleasurable state of relaxation after an initial period of alertness and tension had passed. Smoking sometimes helped the smoker cope with feelings of tension, anxiety, or anger that occurred in difficult life situations. Other respondents experienced a stimulating effect of smoking and/or an enhancing effect on social interactions. Other reasons given for smoking included the enjoyment of handling and lighting cigarettes, avoidance of an unpleasant state of craving produced by not smoking (i.e., withdrawal symptoms), or that smoking was simply a habit that did not make the smoker feel any different. The results further indicated that some smokers had one predominant reason for smoking, whereas most had multiple reasons. These and other findings (see Spielberger, 1986) indicate that there is no consistent relationship between smoking and arousal among individuals, and that we cannot explain smoking behavior or nicotine intake by this variable alone.

Given that different individuals report smoking to be either calming or stimulating, it is important to determine the influence of these subjective reactions on smoking-related changes in performance. This issue was examined in a study involving two groups of light smokers (fewer than 15 cigarettes per day) selected using a smoking questionnaire (Myrsten et al., 1975). One group indicated that they usually smoked during boring, monotonous situations (the low arousal group), whereas the other group smoked mostly during tense, stressful situa-

tions (the high arousal group). Half of the members of each group were then given either a difficult task (requiring high arousal) or a simple task (easily managed with low arousal). Subjects were allowed to smoke if they wished. The results showed that smoking improved performance if there was concordance between the arousal level of the task and the arousal level that elicited smoking (boredom vs. stress), but impaired performance if there was discordance between the arousal level of the task and the arousal level of the subjects. In a nonsmoking situation, there were no differences in performance for either group in either task. Thus, the effect of smoking on task performance (and the likelihood of an individual smoking during task execution) seems to depend on a complex interaction between prior arousal level, task difficulty, and the subjective reasons for smoking for that individual.

Social factors. In the last two decades there has been a progressive change in public attitude toward tobacco use. Cigarette smoking was once widely accepted. Smoking was found frequently in feature films and advertising, and was promoted by sports figures and attractive models. The aim was to connect cigarette smoking with good looks, healthy activity, and affluence, an approach that snared millions upon millions of habitual smokers.

Currently, though, millions of nonsmokers and former smokers see cigarette smoking as an unhealthful and annoying habit. This change in attitude was fostered by local and federal antismoking campaigns that aggressively publicized the deleterious health effects of smoking. These antismoking efforts have resulted in a tightening of laws regulating where smoking is permitted, and they have also reduced the social acceptance of smoking (Goldstein, 1994). This is reflected in historical data showing per capita cigarette consumption in the United States from 1900 to 1985 (Figure 14.5). In fact, millions of adult smokers in the United States have given up the habit despite continued commercial promotion of tobacco products (see below). Thus, although as long as tobacco is available there will inevitably be smokers, the number of smokers can be influenced by educational campaigns, changing cultural norms, legal proscriptions, and taxation to increase the cost of tobacco products.

Commercial Promotion of Smoking and Tobacco Products

While some governmental agencies and private groups are attempting to reduce the incidence of smoking, commercial tobacco interests continue to advertise their products in the mass media. Indeed, high school children and even preschoolers (age 3–6 years) showed high recognition of Camel's Old Joe cartoon character (DiFranza et al., 1991; Fischer et al., 1991). Despite arguments to the contrary by the tobacco industry, these find-

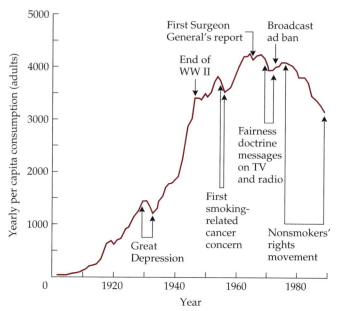

14.5 PER CAPITA CIGARETTE CONSUMPTION IN THE UNITED STATES FROM 1900 TO 1985. (After Goldstein, 1994; original data from Slade, 1989.)

ings suggest that one function of cigarette advertising is to attract new smokers from young age groups (also see Pierce et al., 1991).

Hanson (1984) describes a 10-year period during which the tobacco industry attempted to circumvent the fear of respiratory disease associated with smoking. They suggested the use of smokeless tobacco in the form of snuff, including small drip-through packets of snuff that were to be placed between the cheek and gums. In order to reshape the negative attitudes toward this practice, the tobacco industry initiated a high-pressure media campaign, including endorsements by professional athletes, that was directed toward impressionable elementary through college-age students. The result was an 11% annual increase in sales from 1974 to 1984, which translated to about 1 boy in 5 becoming a habitual user of smokeless tobacco (see Warner, 1986).

During this campaign, the industry promoted the use of snuff in place of cigarettes because the incidence of oropharyngeal cancer was lower than that of lung cancer. It did not point out that this difference would soon disappear as more and more people used snuff. It has been known for a long time that the use of chewing tobacco and snuff leads to its own variety of pathologies such as gum recession, periodontal disease, leukoplakia (precancerous lesions in the mouth), and cancer of the gums and cheeks, bladder, and stomach (Negin, 1985). After a while, direct television advertising of smokeless tobacco products disappeared from the air, partly due to a spirited attack by health authorities, who fortified their arguments with gruesome pictures of a young man who had chewed tobacco and had since developed terminal cancer of the mouth and jaw.

The Brown and Williamson documents. The most recent criticisms of the tobacco industry are based largely upon several thousand pages of memoranda on research findings, conference presentations, and discussions that comprised 1,384 internal documents from the Brown and Williamson (B&W) Tobacco Corporation and its parent company, the British American Tobacco Company (BAT Industries). BAT is the second largest private cigarette manufacturer in the world, and the third largest in the United States. The documents, which surfaced publicly in May 1994, ultimately came into the possession of the American Medical Association. Some of the documents were anonymously donated to Stanton A. Glantz, professor of medicine at the School of Medicine, University of California at San Francisco. Some were obtained by Congress from B&W, and some came from private papers of a deceased former BAT officer. These documents, which covered a 30-year period, were examined by the editors of the *Journal of the American Medical Association* (*JAMA*), who published reviews that provided a highly detailed and candid look into the company's internal workings with respect to the smoking and health controversy of the last 50 years (see Barnes et al.,1995; Bero et al., 1995; Glantz et al., 1995; Hanauer et al., 1995; Slade et al., 1995).

The B&W documents revealed that both B&W and BAT clearly recognized that their own sponsored research showed that nicotine is pharmacologically active, that it is addictive, and that cigarettes are, in essence, nicotine delivery devices. Some of the documents pertained to a research institute, The Council of Tobacco Research-U.S.A. (CTR), which had been established by the tobacco industry. CTR claimed to award research grants to independent researchers who were assured complete scientific freedom in conducting their studies on the health effects of smoking. However, some representatives later admitted that the institute was created more for public relations purposes, and that there were special projects designed to find scientists and medical doctors who would serve as industry witnesses in lawsuits against the industry. In addition, there was abundant evidence in the documents showing that adverse findings against nicotine and smoking were withheld from publication and outside scrutiny.

B&W was very concerned about the threat of product liability lawsuits, and lawyers were therefore called upon to avoid the discovery of documents that could be useful to plaintiffs in such lawsuits and to control the language of scientific discourse on issues related to smoking and health. The company also arranged to bring potentially damaging internal scientific documents under attorney–client privilege to maintain the secrecy of damaging scientific information and insulate B&W from similar information from other BAT companies (Hanauer et al., 1995). For example, CTR research supported the conclusions of other scientists that smoking is causally related to lung cancer and heart disease, yet these research findings were never published, and CTR publicly denied that such links had been proven. Furthermore, throughout the 1970s B&W and BAT privately engaged in a massive research program to identify and remove any toxic compounds found in tobacco smoke. Their goal was to create a "safe" cigarette, but their research showed that there were so many different toxic compounds in tobacco smoke that it would be very difficult to remove them all. Yet, publicly, the industry continued to deny that smoking had been proven harmful to health (Glantz et al., 1995).

A concluding editorial in *JAMA* at the end of the article series stated that the documents provide massive, detailed, and damning evidence of the tactics of the tobacco industry. They show how the industry has spread confusion by suppressing, manipulating, and distorting the scientific record. They show in a stark way that some who speak for the industry dissemble, distort, and deceive, despite the fact that the industry's own research was consistent with the scientific community's conclusion that continued use of their product will endanger the lives and health of the public at home and abroad. With the staggering estimation that 3 million deaths occur worldwide each year due to tobacco use, the importance of bringing this hazard under control is correspondingly great (*JAMA* Editorial, 1995).

Effects of Chronic Tobacco Use

Chronic use of tobacco products leads to a number of unhealthy consequences. Smokers become partially tolerant to nicotine, and they also develop nicotine dependence. Repeated exposure to nicotine, tar, and CO also has important effects on health, as mentioned above and discussed in detail below.

Nicotine Tolerance

Animal studies have shown that repeated nicotine treatment causes tolerance to at least some of the drug's behavioral effects (reviewed by Balfour, 1990). There is also considerable evidence for tolerance to the cardiovascular effects of nicotine in humans. One example was shown in an experiment by Pomerleau and Pomerleau (1992) similar to the one described above. In this case the subjects smoked two cigarettes, 30 minutes apart, after an overnight abstinence. The cigarettes used in this study included the same ultralow- and high-nicotine cigarettes described previously, but the third type of cigarette used was the usual brand that each subject smoked (average nicotine yield was approximately 1 mg). In addition to the euphoria measurements mentioned previously, heart rate data were collected before and during smoking of each cigarette by means of electrocardiography.

As shown in Figure 14.6, cigarette smoking induced tachycardia, and the effect was significantly greater after an overnight abstinence than after the 30-minute abstinence prior to the second cigarette of the day. The differ-

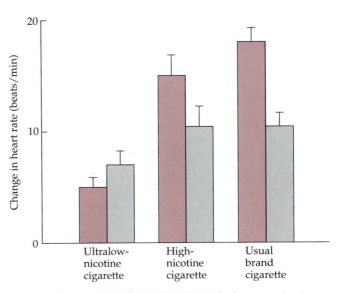

14.6 NICOTINE: STIMULANT EFFECTS. The heart rate is stimulated by nicotine in a dose-dependent way. Also, the nicotine effect is stronger after overnight abstinence (color bars) than after the one-hour abstinence between the first and the second cigarettes of the day (gray bars). (After Pomerleau and Pomerleau, 1992.)

ence in the increases in heart rate between the two smoking episodes suggested tachyphylaxis (a rapid tolerance) for the tachycardiac effect. Tolerance typically develops very quickly when the drug effect has a rapid onset and a short duration, which is true of the nicotine effects. Also, the degree of increase was related to the nicotine content of the cigarettes. That is, the high-nicotine cigarettes had a significantly greater influence on heart rate than the ultralow-nicotine cigarettes. There was also some evidence for tolerance to the euphoric effects of the high-nicotine cigarettes; however, this was not as clear as the cardiovascular results.

A more recent study examined the possibility of detecting tolerance to the subjective effects of nicotine after repeated smoking (Parrott, 1994). In this experiment, a brief feeling-state questionnaire, the Smoking Motivation Questionnaire (SMQ), was used to separate the subjects into two groups: (1) a "sedation" group comprised of subjects who were prone to stress and who experienced calming and sedative effects from smoking; and (2) a "stimulation" group comprised of subjects who tended to be at low arousal levels and who became activated or stimulated by smoking (see Mackay et al., 1978). The SMQ was thus used to assess two psychological effects of nicotine: a decrease in stress (sedation) or an increase in arousal (stimulation) over a whole day of smoking. The subjects chose their own brand of cigarettes and completed the questionnaire immediately before and after smoking each cigarette of the day.

For the "sedation" group, stress factors were found to be significantly affected by smoking. Stress was higher presmoking than postsmoking for each cigarette, with stress values increasing between cigarettes. Overall, the nicotine effects on stress were gradually reduced over the day, although the drug × time interaction was not significant. Self-rated feelings of arousal for the "stimulation" group were likewise influenced by nicotine. Arousal was higher postsmoking than presmoking and decreased during the interval between cigarettes. The greatest increase in arousal occurred after the first cigarette of the day. In general, arousal followed an inverted-U function across the day, with low arousal in the morning, peak arousal at midday, and reduced arousal in the evening.

The observation that the degree of nicotine-induced arousal was lower during the day than following the first cigarette is similar to the findings of Pomerleau and Pomerleau (1992) and might reflect an acute tolerance to the stimulant effects of nicotine. Alternatively, the large nicotine-induced increase in arousal caused by the first cigarette might be a consequence of the previously low plasma nicotine level associated with overnight abstinence. Thus, the first cigarette of the day produces a relatively greater increase in plasma nicotine than later cigarettes. For this reason, the first cigarette of the day could lead to a larger perceived enhancement of arousal. In contrast, subjects in the "sedation" group reported little or no arousal under any condition, even after the first cigarette of the day. This lack of smoking-induced change in arousal generally reflected high levels of arousal prior to smoking.

In summary, although some of these results of Parrott (1994) could have been due to acute pharmacodynamic (cellular) tolerance, the author concluded that this was not a major determining factor in the subjective effects of repeated smoking. The greater effects produced by the day's first cigarette may be explicable in terms of the low nicotine level present in the blood at this time. Furthermore, subjects exhibited mood changes throughout the day, not just after the first cigarette. The general pattern observed was of vacillating mood/cognitive states, with deleterious moods developing between cigarettes and mood normalization after cigarettes.

Nicotine Abstinence and Withdrawal Symptoms

Compulsive drug use can often be traced to positive subjective feelings such as the onset of analgesia, sleep, anxiolysis, or general euphoria. Such feelings serve to reinforce the acquisition and use of licit or illicit drugs. In the case of nicotine, smoking in many instances is associated with an enhancement of cognition and alertness, easing of tensions and muscular relaxation, and a better response to stress. On the other hand, abstinence after sustained use of a euphoriant may precipitate unpleasant and even life-threatening symptoms, as seen in cases of sudden withdrawal during severe alcoholism (see Chapter 15).

Abrupt abstinence from regular tobacco use can result in withdrawal effects that are usually not life-threat-

ening, but that are still severe enough to make abstinence extremely uncomfortable. Abstinence symptoms consist of severe craving for nicotine, irritability, anxiety, difficulty concentrating, restlessness, decreased heart rate, dysphoria, impatience and insomnia, and increased appetite and weight gain (Hughes et al., 1991; Pomerleau, 1992). A return to smoking will forestall these symptoms and thus increase its reinforcing properties, which contribute to further dependence. Among self-quitters who were considered to have been strongly motivated to quit smoking cigarettes, 60% to 65% relapsed in the first month after cessation.

Some of the typical characteristics of smoking withdrawal can be seen in a series of studies performed by Hatsukami, Hughes, and Pickens (1984). These investigators initially performed a 1-week inpatient study of 27 smokers. For the first 3 days, the subjects were allowed to smoke ad lib while a battery of tests was administered once or twice a day. For the next 4 days, 20 subjects were required to abstain from smoking while the remainder continued smoking as a control condition. The results of this study, however, revealed fewer withdrawal symptoms during abstinence than expected from earlier reports.

Although previous research may have overestimated the severity of tobacco withdrawal due to methodological flaws, these investigators were nevertheless concerned that abstinence symptomatology may have been minimized in their study because the test environment (the hospital) lacked many of the stimuli usually associated with (and hence conditioned to) smoking. Therefore, a second experiment was conducted using outpatients who returned to the smoking clinic in the evening to measure the effects of smoking cessation. Comparing the inpatient with the outpatient group showed many similarities as well as a few differences in the effects of smoking deprivation. Symptoms found in both groups were decreased heart rate, increased craving for tobacco, difficulty concentrating, increased eating behavior, increased awakening during sleep, and feelings of confusion, depression, and dejection as measured by the scores on the Profile of Mood States (POMS) questionnaire. In the outpatient, but not in the inpatient group, there was a decrease in tremulousness, an increase in anger–hostility and tension–anxiety scores, and a decrease in the vigor score on the POMS. Increased craving for tobacco was reported by up to 90% of deprived smokers, and increased irritability and anger were frequently reported. Most withdrawal symptoms began about 24 hours after the beginning of deprivation, peaked within 36–72 hours, and then gradually declined.

Despite these and other findings, abstinence symptomatology may not be always a critical factor in preventing smoking cessation because the severity of tobacco withdrawal varies widely among smokers. Indeed, abstinence symptoms do not always follow smoking cessation, for it has been found that some people can smoke for many years and stop abruptly without showing such effects. Moreover, some investigators in withdrawal clinics have reported that most relapses occur well after withdrawal symptoms have abated.

Determinants of withdrawal symptoms. It is not yet clear why the profile of withdrawal symptoms varies so greatly among smokers who quit. It is possible, for example, that the severity of withdrawal effects is related to the frequency of smoking. However, unlike the positive correlation between these variables in morphine and heroin abuse, the connection with respect to smoking is unclear (Shiffman, 1979). In an effort to establish the causes or determinants of the various self-reported withdrawal symptoms, Fagerström (1978) investigated the value of several precessation variables as symptom predictors. The variables investigated were age, sex, marital status, education, occupation, income, number of cigarettes per day, nicotine yield of cigarette choice, self-reported severity of past withdrawal symptoms, and duration of smoking. The analysis showed that there was virtually no relationship between any of these factors and the magnitude of any self-reported or observed withdrawal symptoms. Consequently, the causes of individual variability in tobacco abstinence symptomatology remain poorly understood.

Health Effects of Smoking

As mentioned earlier, the tar in tobacco is mainly responsible for the diseases that are associated with long-term tobacco use. In 1990, a total of 420,000 deaths (about 20% of all deaths) in the United States were attributed to smoking (see Bartecchi, MacKenzie, and Shrier, 1994), and Henningfield (1992) stated that smoking tobacco contributes to four of the five major causes of death in the world today: cardiovascular diseases, lung and other cancers, stroke, and chronic obstructive pulmonary diseases (see Ochoa, 1994). Although there has been a substantial (approximately 50%) drop in the number of smokers since the mid-1980s, a recent report indicated that 25.7% of adults (46.3 million, roughly half men and half women) in the United States still smoke (Bartecchi, MacKenzie, and Shrier, 1994). In industrialized countries, tobacco will cause approximately 30% of all deaths among those 35 to 69 years of age, making it the largest single cause of premature deaths in the industrialized world. Further, it has been estimated that by the next century, one in five deaths worldwide will be caused by tobacco, many of them in developing as well as industrialized nations (Peto, 1986).

Many young people are unfortunately being recruited to cigarettes and becoming dependent on them, despite warnings on tobacco packages and public advertising concerning the adverse health consequences of smoking. Young smokers tend to feel immune to the harmful consequences of smoking because, after initial autonomic dysfunction is overcome through adaptation or tolerance, smoking does not impair performance (Russell, 1977). Unlike alcohol and many other drugs of dependence, nicotine from smoking is perceived as enhancing rather than impairing the capacity of young people to work and socialize, and there are no immediate negative consequences. Consequently, because all the grave health consequences are remote in time for the young smoker, they are of weaker influence.

Figure 14.7 presents some of the classic findings demonstrating a powerful relationship between the number of cigarettes smoked daily and the mortality rate from lung cancer. The figure also shows that the likelihood of dying from lung cancer diminishes over time after an individual stops smoking. The tobacco industry has repeatedly argued that the data showing a relationship between smoking and serious illnesses such as lung cancer are only correlational and therefore do not prove a cause-and-effect relationship between these variables. However, research in epidemiology is always statistical, and in some circumstances correlation can be interpreted as causation. The necessary conditions are: (1) the consistency of the association; (2) the strength of the association; (3) the specificity of the association; (4) the temporal relationship of the association; and (5) the coherence of the association. Rarely have these conditions been met as well as in the case of smoking and respiratory disease (Warner, 1986). In addition there is voluminous laboratory evidence that supports the epidemiological findings. For example, laboratory studies have shown what happens to the lungs of smokers and what happens when they quit, that tars in cigarette smoke induce skin cancers in mice, and that dogs living in a tobacco-smoke environment develop lung cancer.

A relatively new area of health concern is that of exposure to environmental (i.e., "secondhand") smoke. Based on an analysis of various studies, the U.S. Environmental Protection Agency (EPA) issued a report in 1992 asserting that environmental smoke is a demonstrated risk factor for lung cancer and other respiratory disorders (U.S. EPA, 1992). However, Witschi and colleagues (1995) recently argued that the experimental and epidemiological data upon which the report was based are weak at best. Because of the potentially important implications of so-called passive smoking, it is important that further studies carefully address this issue.

The health costs of tobacco use. In 1985, Owen estimated that tobacco-related illness was responsible for 145 million extra days of hospitalization and 80 million lost workdays. Monetarily, these effects translated to more than $65 billion per year in medical bills, Medicaid and Medicare, and reduced productivity. As the cost of medical care has increased, the current total may approach or even exceed $100 billion. This is a staggering societal price to pay for the use of just one psychoactive agent.

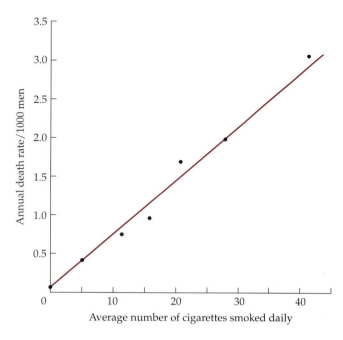

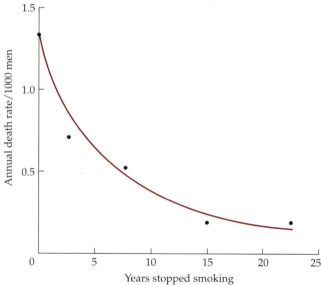

14.7 RELATIONSHIP BETWEEN CIGARETTE SMOKING AND DEATH FROM LUNG CANCER. Early epidemiological studies on male smokers demonstrated a strong relationship between the number of cigarettes smoked daily and annual death rate from lung cancer (*top*). However, the lung cancer death rate of former smokers falls over time after smoking cessation (*bottom*). (After Goldstein, 1994; original data from Doll and Hill, 1964.)

Treatment Strategies for Nicotine Dependence

Characteristics of Nicotine Dependence

Nicotine can produce a powerful dependence, as indicated by the finding that 90% of people who smoke say they would like to quit but can't, and of those that do quit by their own efforts, only 10% to 27% remain abstinent for 1 to 5 years (Grabowski and Hall, 1985b). In general, drug dependence may be defined as a behavioral pattern of compulsive drug use characterized by overwhelming involvement with the use of a drug, the securing of its supply, and a high tendency to relapse after withdrawal (Jaffe, 1985). Specific nicotine dependence is characterized by continuous use of tobacco for at least 1 month, and by at least one of the following being true:

1. Serious attempts to stop or significantly reduce the amount of tobacco use on a permanent basis have been unsuccessful.
2. Attempts to stop smoking led to the development of tobacco withdrawal; i.e., craving for tobacco, irritability, anxiety, difficulty concentrating, restlessness, headache, drowsiness, and gastrointestinal disturbances.
3. The individual continues to use tobacco despite a serious physical disorder (e.g., respiratory or cardiovascular disease) that he or she knows is exacerbated by tobacco use.

Nicotine ingestion by smoking tobacco is thus compulsive, difficult to give up, and involves tolerance and withdrawal effects (see U.S. Department of Health and Human Services, 1988). The *Diagnostic and Statistical Manual of Mental Disorders*, Fourth Edition (DSM-IV; American Psychiatric Association, 1994), recognizes both nicotine dependence and nicotine withdrawal as substance-related disorders.

Treatment Goals

The contemporary search for optimal techniques for treating tobacco dependence is directed not only toward smoking cessation, but also toward the maintenance of abstinence. Attaining this goal appears to be possible with combinations of behavioral intervention, group support, and use of pharmacological adjuncts (Grabowski and Hall, 1985a). However, the success rate of any treatment approach will be influenced by numerous variables, including the intensity of the abstinence syndrome, the differing subjective factors involved in smoking, the duration of smoking behavior, the intellectually based insight as to why quitting would be desirable, the motivation to quit, whether or not the smoker lives and/or works in a smoking environment, and so on. Furthermore, even if a given therapeutic program claims a high success rate for its clients, such claims are meaningless unless there is careful follow-up for months and years to ascertain permanent abstinence.

Behavioral Interventions

There are a number of strategies directed toward discouraging young people from beginning tobacco use or encouraging them to give it up if it is already habitually being used. For example, there are antismoking appeals in the media by the Surgeon General's office, National Cancer Institute, National Heart, Blood, and Lung Institute, Office on Smoking and Health, and the National Institute on Drug Abuse (NIDA). The laws mandating the display of health warnings on cigarette packages and advertisements are examples of the efforts of these institutions. Also, state legislatures have found that increasing cigarette taxes significantly reduces the beginning of smoking or its continuation among young people. Further, the increased revenue to the state from increased cigarette taxes is frequently used for educational antismoking programs.

There are self-help programs provided through books and manuals, and while such programs are generally inexpensive, the success of self-help "bibliotherapy" is not considered to be very substantial. There are treatment entities such as group and social support programs run by nonprofit organizations, health maintenance organizations (HMOs), and for-profit groups (e.g., Smokenders). These programs emphasize social pressure and reinforcement to help smokers analyze why and when they smoke, and plan a cessation program to be completed by a certain date. Unfortunately, there are few data on the permanent effectiveness of these programs. Individual programs are undertaken with psychologists, psychoanalysts, hypnotists, and even acupuncturists and herbalists. The evaluations of these efforts are hampered by the lack of data on how many smokers attempt these routes or how effective they are. (For references on behavioral cessation methods, see Bibliography on Smoking and Health, 1985).

Pharmacological Interventions

Early strategies. Over the years, a number of chemical agents have been tried as possible pharmacological treatments for tobacco dependence. One approach was to administer a drug that would block nicotine action, thereby promoting extinction of the smoking response. Alternatively, because some smokers report that cigarettes have a calming effect while others report a stimulating effect, sedative or antianxiety agents were thought to be appropriate for the former group and psychostimulants for the latter group.

None of these strategies has been proven effective in fostering tobacco abstinence. The nicotinic antagonist mecamylamine did block nicotine action at doses that were free of side effects, but there were other consequences that made the drug unpopular among those treated with it. In addition, blocking the sympathetic activation of heart rate and blood pressure with the drug propranolol (Inderal) had no effect on smoking. When amphetamine was tested to determine whether it might serve as a nicotine substitute for those reporting stimu-lating effects of smoking, the treatment caused an acute increase rather than a decrease in smoking. Finally, sedative and antianxiety drugs given in acute or long-term programs were likewise ineffective as cigarette substitutes for those who seek the calming effects of smoking (Shuster, Lucchesi, and Emley, 1979; Kozlowski, 1984).

Nicotine chewing gum. In contrast to the disappointing results described in the above studies using stimulants and sedatives, more success was found by direct administration of nicotine without the tobacco delivery system. This was first accomplished by formulating a special nicotine-containing chewing gum, which has the advantage that nicotine can be absorbed by the buccal mucosa rather than the gastrointestinal tract where absorption is minimal and there is substantial first-pass metabolism in the liver. This approach is based on several premises: (1) the difficulty associated with smoking cessation is significantly related to nicotine withdrawal symptoms; (2) blocking these symptoms by maintaining a certain circulating level of nicotine can assist in terminating smoking; and (3) gum chewing is a much safer way for individuals to obtain nicotine than by smoking.

Although Ferno and coworkers reported the experimental use of nicotine gum in 1973, its approval by the U.S. Food and Drug Administration as a phamacotherapeutic aid in the treatment of cigarette dependence did not occur until 1984. The gum (polacrilex) is marketed under the trade name Nicorette and is usually dispensed with 2 mg or 4 mg of nicotine bound to an ion-exchange resin in the gum that releases the nicotine upon chewing. Patients are instructed to chew the piece of gum 12 to 15 times until a peppery taste is felt, then park the gum between the teeth and cheek until the taste fades, and repeat the procedure until there is no more peppery taste. This "chew and park" procedure maximizes the absorption of nicotine through the buccal mucosa.

Although the patients chew the nicotine gum on an ad lib basis, they are advised to take no more than 20 pieces per day of 4-mg gum or 30 pieces per day of 2-mg gum. Chewing 2-mg or 4-mg gum produces a plasma nicotine concentration of approximately 11.8 µg/L and 23.2 µg/L, respectively. These compare well with the lower range of plasma nicotine concentrations that occur during cigarette smoking (see the review by Jorenby, Keehn, and Flore, 1995).

Nicotine gum should be prescribed only after the physician first ascertains that the patient is free of heart disease or high blood pressure. Generally, the gum is taken with few side effects, but dizziness and vomiting are occasionally reported. The 4-mg doses are more effective for more highly dependent smokers.

Blocking of withdrawal effects and abstinence In one of the early nicotine gum experiments by Russell, Raw, and Jarvis (1980), 100 smokers were enlisted who had a history of tobacco withdrawal syndrome as defined by the DSM. The subjects smoked ad lib for 2 days, after which they submitted to 4 days of tobacco deprivation during which half the smokers received 2-mg nicotine gum and the other half received placebo gum. The subjects chewed the gum as often as they wished.

Self-rating of abstinence symptomatology using a checklist showed that after smoking cessation, the nicotine gum group experienced significantly less irritability, anxiety, difficulty concentrating, restlessness, impatience, and somatic complaints than did the placebo gum group. However, there was little or no effect of nicotine replacement on craving for tobacco. These results were confirmed by observer ratings and by lower scores on feelings of confusion, depression, and dejection on the POMS questionnaire. Group differences were evident on the first day and lasted throughout the 4 days of smoking deprivation. Almost identical findings were reported by Hughes and colleagues (1984) and West and colleagues (1984).

In a later study, Hughes and colleagues (1991) assessed the effect of nicotine gum on withdrawal symptoms and abstinence in 315 subjects selected from a larger group of smokers who wanted to quit smoking and who answered an advertisement for an outpatient abstinence program. The subjects started the program with 10 minutes of counseling and a prescription for a chewing gum to be taken as needed. Two-thirds of the subjects were given nicotine-containing gum, while the remaining one-third received placebo gum with the same taste. Individuals were told not to smoke and were randomly assigned to the nicotine or placebo group in a double-blind manner; that is, neither the subjects nor their therapists knew which gum the subjects were receiving until the end of the experiment. After smoking cessation, the subjects recorded the daily nature and intensity of their withdrawal symptoms, and these observations were verified by an observer such as a friend, spouse, or relative. There were additional visits to the clinic after 1 and 2 weeks, and there were queries by mail after 1 and 6 months asking the subjects if they had smoked and how much, and requesting a description of any withdrawal symptoms. One year after the start of the study, subjects were again queried by mail to report their abstinence status.

In this study, nicotine replacement was found to relieve some withdrawal symptoms such as anger, anxiety, and impatience. However, there was only marginal relief of difficulty in concentrating and restlessness, and no evidence for reductions in drowsiness, insomnia, or physical symptoms. In contrast to earlier findings, subjects in this study reported a robust decrease in cigarette craving and hunger. This effect was noted only after 1 to 2 weeks of treatment, which may explain why it was not observed in the previous study that lasted only 4 days.

Thus, nicotine replacement during tobacco abstinence relieves some, but not all, of the symptoms of tobacco deprivation. This may be due to the nicotine dose, or to the difference between oral administration (which leads to slow continuous absorption from the mouth) and smoking (which produces an intermittent dosing pattern with rapid absorption from the lungs). There is also the possibility of the presence of psychoactive substances other than nicotine in tobacco smoke. However, it is more likely that withdrawal symptoms are influenced by behavioral and psychological as well as pharmacological factors. For example, tobacco craving and hunger may be governed mainly by expectancy during the early abstinence period (which explains why nicotine replacement initially fails to diminish these symptoms), whereas later these feelings are determined more by the level of circulating nicotine.

Nicotine gum also showed some effectiveness in promoting smoking abstinence, although the improvement was modest. For the 105 placebo subjects, 80% were still abstinent at the 2-week time point; however this figure dropped to 41% by 1 month and only to 19% at 6 months. Comparable figures for the 210 subjects receiving nicotine gum were 75%, 54%, and 29%. Therefore, even with nicotine gum treatment, many subjects relapsed or dropped out of the study, presumably because of a return to smoking. It is interesting to note that the effectiveness of nicotine gum in different subjects during the early stages of the Hughes and coworkers (1991) study did not predict which subjects would maintain abstinence for 6 months or longer. This indicates that smokers should be encouraged to persist in their attempts at smoking cessation, even if they meet with early failure.

As in the case of other drugs such as cocaine or opiates, a combination of counseling with pharmacotherapy may be more effective than either alone. This hypothesis was tested by Schneider and Jarvik (1985) in a 1-year study of 96 heavy smokers (30–35 cigarettes per day) who had previously tried repeatedly to quit smoking without success. Subjects were assigned to 1 of 4 groups: (1) nicotine gum plus counseling; (2) placebo gum plus counseling; (3) nicotine gum only; and (4) placebo gum only. The first two groups received clinical support and guidance at various intervals during the study, whereas the latter two groups were given little instruction or support.

The results showed that the nicotine-treated subjects reported milder abstinence symptoms and selected more positive states and fewer negative states on the POMS questionnaire than did their placebo-treated counterparts. Figure 14.8a clearly shows that receiving clinical support along with nicotine gum led to the best abstinence rates, whereas those subjects receiving little or no clinical support (Figure 14.8b) exhibited virtually the same low abstinence rates regardless of whether they received nicotine replacement. Unfortunately, however, the tendency to relapse is so strong that only 30% of the sub-

(a) Groups receiving counseling and gum

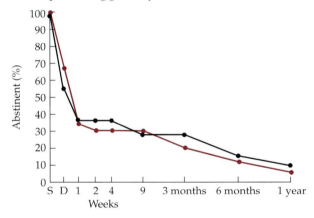

(b) Groups receiving gum only

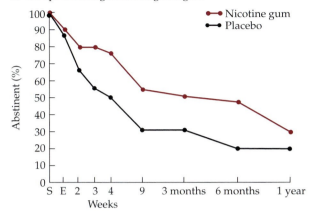

14.8 INFLUENCE OF CLINICAL GUIDANCE ON NICOTINE GUM EFFECTIVENESS (a) Subjects who received counseling along with nicotine gum were more likely to remain abstinent than those who received counseling along with a placebo gum, and had far better abstinence rates than either group that received no counseling (b). However, only 30% of the group remained abstinent after 1 year. S = start of treatment; E = end of daily treatment; D = days 1–3. (After Schneider and Jarvik, 1985.)

jects were still abstinent at 1 year even under the best conditions.

In support of these findings, a meta-analysis of data from 17,000 individuals that participated in many experiments concluded that the use of any kind of nicotine replacement therapy increased the odds ratio (OR) of abstinence to 1.7 relative to placebo (Silagy et al., 1994). This means patients receiving replacement nicotine have a 70% better chance of achieving abstinence than those who are given placebos. For example, if 10 smokers out of 100 became abstinent while treated with placebos, nicotine replacement would likely result in 17 cases of abstinence. Other meta-analyses (Cepeda-Benito, 1993; Lam et al., 1987) have confirmed that nicotine gum is superior to placebo in promoting abstinence, particularly when accompanied by intense behavioral treatment. However, the overall success rate remains disappointingly low.

Side effects of nicotine replacement. Because the user of nicotine gum can titrate the doses if the gum has adverse effects, the occurrence of significant side effects can be minimized. Nevertheless, 37% of users complain about soreness in the mouth and throat, and 10% report gastrointestinal distress (which, however, may be due to incorrect chewing or swallowing the gum) (Jorenby, Keehn, and Flore, 1995). Hiccups and heart palpitations have also been reported.

The other major problem associated with nicotine gum is the possibility of dependence. There is evidence that some smoking-abstinent users become dependent on nicotine gum (estimates range from 17% to 25% of abstinent users), suggesting that nicotine dependence has transferred from tobacco to the replacement vehicle (Jorenby, Keehn, and Flore, 1995). Although nicotine gum chewing is not as toxic as smoking, the stimulant effects of the drug can still be a source of many symptoms, particularly for individuals already at risk for cardiovascular disease. The gum is often taken without medical supervision after being obtained over the counter in some foreign countries and recently in the United States. Indeed, sales of nicotine gum are increasing despite its relatively high cost (about $30 per box of 96 doses). Close control over this product may therefore be necessary to prevent the rise of another source of substance abuse.

Despite these problems, comparisons between the health risks of long-term tobacco use and those of nicotine gum reveal that tobacco use is the much greater health hazard. Thus, prolonged use of nicotine gum is an acceptable risk if it prevents relapse to tobacco use. Nevertheless, it is important that physicians carefully instruct patients concerning the parameters of gum use and strictly advise against using gum in conjunction with cigarette smoking.

Transdermal nicotine systems. The transdermal method of nicotine replacement consists of multilayered adhesive patches made of a variety of binding substances saturated with a lipid-soluble nicotine solution. These skin patches are sold under a number of brand names (Habitrol, Nicoderm, Nicorette, Nicotrol, and Prostep), and each is available in two or three doses depending on the size of the patch and the duration of wear (from 16 to 24 hours). Delivered doses range from a total of 5 mg to 22 mg per application period, resulting in average plasma nicotine concentrations of 9.4 to 17 µg/L, which are slightly lower than the concentrations produced by chewing nicotine gum.

This delivery mode was meant for those who are highly motivated to quit cigarette smoking and who are willing to engage in intensive behavioral therapy to enhance the possibilities of achieving permanent abstinence. A prospective patient must also meet one of three criteria: (1) smokes 20 or more cigarettes per day; (2) smokes his or her first cigarette within 30 minutes of awakening; or (3) has experienced strong cravings for cigarettes during the first week of previous attempts to quit. Skin patch therapy was also designed to avoid some of the difficulties encountered with nicotine gum. Wearing nicotine skin patches is probably the easiest nicotine delivery system currently available. During treatment the patches are normally applied once per day and are worn for either 16 or 24 hours, depending upon the prescribed patch. Thus, the patch is akin to one dose per day, and there is nothing more to attend to. In contrast, using nicotine gum requires continued attention all day to know when and how to chew the gum.

Meta-analysis of experimental studies showed that nicotine patches are a highly effective form of nicotine-replacement, producing two or three times the number of abstainers as placebo treatments (see Jorenby, Keehn, and Flore, 1995). The patches reduce cigarette craving more consistently than nicotine gum, and they also decrease other withdrawal symptoms such as anger, anxiety, difficulty concentrating, and impatience. Moreover, compliance with medical directives not to smoke is more easily obtained with nicotine patches than when patients use nicotine gum. There is only one dose administration per day, and smoking can occur only after the patch has been removed for between 1 to 3 hours to allow plasma nicotine concentrations to decline to safe levels. (Patients are warned about the importance of abstaining from smoking while wearing a nicotine patch because in some cases smoking when a patch was in place has resulted in nicotine overdose and adverse cardiovascular events.) In contrast, the shorter duration of nicotine delivery from each gum dose and the possibility of gum avoidance provide more opportunities for treatment evasion, and thus more safe opportunities to smoke. Consequently, superior treatment outcomes in smoking cessation and withdrawal suppression using transdermal nicotine patches as compared with nicotine gum can be attributed at least partly to better patient compliance with the treatment program (Jorenby, Keehn, and Flore, 1995).

There are modest aversive characteristics of patch use and a low abuse liability. For example, some users report local skin irritation from the patch, but the effect in most cases disappears within a few days. About 7% to 22% report more severe skin reactions that may intensify with further patch use, but fewer than 5% of users require immediate cessation of patch therapy (Jorenby, Keehn, and Flore, 1995). Further, in contrast to the 17% to 25% of nicotine gum users who become dependent, the virtual absence of abuse of nicotine patches is presumed to be due to the steady flow of transdermal nicotine, which does not create a surge in circulating nicotine levels as in the case of smoking and, to some extent, nicotine gum chewing. Clinical findings indicate that few abstinent smokers wear prescribed patches for a long time and that many voluntarily discontinue their use before completing the prescribed treatment regimen,

suggesting that the patches are not euphoriant or reinforcing. Therefore, nicotine patches may now be obtained over the counter.

Nicotine nasal spray and inhalers.   A relatively new mode of nicotine replacement utilizes an aerosol spray that delivers into each nostril 50 µl of a solution containing 0.5 mg of nicotine, thus yielding a total dose of 1 mg. The suggested maximum use is 5 mg/hr and 40 mg/day, which will produce approximately 50% of the plasma nicotine concentration achieved by smoking. Efficacy of this treatment approach was assessed in a double-blind, placebo-controlled study of 227 patients who also received six group counseling sessions (Sutherland et al., 1992). The results showed that the spray treatment reduced cigarette craving and overall severity of withdrawal symptoms. Furthermore, 32% of the treated patients were abstinent at 6 months postcessation compared with 12% of placebo subjects (OR = 2.7). At 1 year postcessation, the respective abstinence rates were 26% for nicotine-treated and 10% for control subjects (OR = 2.6). These results suggest that the nasal spray may be a promising method for nicotine-replacement therapy, but further research is necessary.

The newest delivery system is a nicotine inhaler, which consists of a perforated plastic plug containing nicotine and through which a puff of air can be drawn containing 0.016 mg of nicotine. Each inhaler contains about 300 puffs, and the recommended dosage is 2 to 10 inhalations per day. This usage is estimated to produce plasma nicotine concentrations of about 38% of those achieved by smoking. Current findings indicate an excellent degree of efficacy for the inhaler system (Jorenby, Keehn, and Flore, 1995). This may be due, in part, to the inhaler's functional similarities to cigarettes as something to handle and something to inhale. As of this writing, the nicotine inhaler is still in development and is not yet approved for use in the United States.

Evaluation of nicotine pharmacotherapies.   At the time of this writing, transdermal nicotine replacement appears to be the best method for withdrawal suppression and smoking cessation due to its relative efficacy, modest adverse effects, and low abuse potential. It has been found to be two to three times more effective than placebo treatments regardless of what concurrent behavioral therapy is used. Further, this treatment mode generates high rates of "no smoking" compliance, so that nicotine patches may be the treatment of choice in primary care settings.

At present, an abstinence rate of about 30% appears to be the best attainable long-term outcome with the available pharmacotherapies combined with behavioral therapy or counseling. However, future methodological improvements may permit an increase in this success rate. For example, one recent study showed that a combination of nicotine patches and nicotine gum was superior to either treatment alone in suppressing withdrawal (Fagerstrom et al., 1993). It is possible that the quick rise in circulating nicotine produced by the gum can counteract acute craving or other symptoms that are not blocked by the steady state levels produced by the skin patch. Thus, a combination of patches with a rapid self-administered treatment (such as gum, nasal spray, or inhaler) would theoretically assist the patient in maintaining abstinence in high-risk situations that elicit a strong craving response.

Part I Summary

Nicotine is one of many substances found in tobacco leaves. Smoking tobacco was probably practiced for centuries by native Americans for hedonistic, ritual, or magical purposes. In the fifteenth century, voyagers to the New World introduced tobacco use to Europe, and tobacco is now used by many individuals in countries all over the world. The presence of nicotine in tobacco is the overriding reason for tobacco use and dependence.

Nicotine is easily extracted from tobacco smoke when the smoke is drawn into the lungs, and within a few seconds it stimulates nicotinic cholinergic receptors in the brain and the autonomic nervous system. These receptors are found on postsynaptic cells and also presynaptically where they modulate the release of various neurotransmitters. Nicotinic receptors concentrated in the VTA and nucleus accumbens activate the mesolimbic DA system, which is thought to be responsible for nicotine's reinforcing and euphoric effects. In this way, nicotine is similar to other abused drugs such as amphetamine, cocaine, morphine, and alcohol. Nicotine also enhances certain aspects of learning and performance, although these effects are most pronounced in smokers who have been abstinent from tobacco for some period of hours or days.

Smoking is a complex behavior that is governed by a variety of factors. For example, some smokers report that smoking provides a stimulating effect, whereas others report that they are calmed by smoking. Regardless of the subjective reasons given for smoking, however, it is clear that the delivery of nicotine plays a critical role in the acquisition and maintenance of smoking behavior. Because of the rapid absorption of nicotine from tobacco smoke in the lungs and its rapid transit to the brain, the act of smoking is ideally suited to maximize the reinforcing and dependence-producing effects of nicotine.

Chronic use of tobacco results not only in nicotine dependence, but also in tolerance (particularly to the drug's cardiovascular effects) and in many adverse health consequences. Tobacco tar, which results from the combustion of the tobacco and which contains a number of toxic substances, is drawn into the lungs along with nicotine and is the major cause of smoking-related illnesses. These illnesses constitute four of the five major causes of death in the world today: lung and other cancers, stroke, and severe cardiovascular and pulmonary diseases. The prevalence of cigarette smoking consequently makes it one of the most important sources of premature mortality in the United States.

Abstinence from nicotine after chronic use causes well-defined withdrawal symptoms such as tobacco craving, anxiety, irritability, difficulty concentrating, restlessness, headache, drowsiness, and gastrointestinal disturbances. Because abstinence symptomatology is a major contributor to relapse in individuals who are attempting to quit smoking, several nicotine replacement methods have been developed as therapeutic adjuncts in smoking-cessation treatment programs. These replacement vehicles include nicotine-containing gum, nicotine patches for transdermal delivery, and most recently, nicotine sprays and inhalers. Research clearly indicates that nicotine replacement is helpful in achieving abstinence from tobacco, although overall success rates are still low and more effective treatment programs must continue to be sought.

Part II
Caffeine

If you are like most people living in Western societies, you probably had at least one cup of coffee (or perhaps tea) this morning, possibly followed up by additional cups as the day progressed. Whether you like the taste of coffee (which is bitter when taken black) or not, you are probably consuming it at least partly for its pharmacological properties as a stimulant. This, of course, brings us to the subject of caffeine, the principal psychoactive ingredient in coffee.

Caffeine and the closely related drug theophylline are methyl derivatives of the compound xanthine. The

Caffeine   **Theophylline**

major source of caffeine is coffee beans, which are the seeds of the plant *Coffea arabica*. Tea leaves contain significant amounts of both caffeine and theophylline (which means "divine leaf"). Caffeine is one of the most widely consumed drugs in the world. In the United States, for example, it is estimated that approximately 80% of adults drink coffee or tea on a daily basis. The typical caffeine content of various foodstuffs and over-the-counter drugs is shown in Table 14.1. Calculated from

Table 14.1 Typical Caffeine Content of Common Food Items and Drugs

Source	Caffeine content
Beverages	
Brewed coffee	85 mg/5-oz. cup
Decaffeinated coffee	3 mg/5-oz. cup
Tea (brewed 3 minutes)	28 mg/5-oz. cup
Cocoa or hot chocolate	30 mg/5-oz. cup
Cola drinks	30–46 mg/12-oz. can
Chocolates	
Baking chocolate	35 mg/oz.
Milk chocolate	6 mg/oz.
Analgesic drugs	
Anacin, maximum strength	32 mg/tablet
Excedrin	64.8 mg/tablet
Over-the-counter stimulants	
No Doz	100 mg/tablet
Vivarin	200 mg/tablet

Source: After Somani and Gupta, 1988.

these various sources, the average adult caffeine intake in the United States has been estimated to be approximately 400 mg per day (Weidner and Istvan, 1985). As discussed below, individuals who are compulsive users can greatly exceed even this rather high dose. Furthermore, even children may ingest considerable amounts of caffeine, mainly through consumption of caffeinated soft drinks and chocolate (Benowitz, 1990a).

Basic Pharmacology of Caffeine

The basic pharmacology of caffeine has been reviewed by Arnaud (1993). When caffeine is consumed orally, as in a beverage, virtually complete absorption occurs from the gastrointestinal tract within approximately 45 minutes. Although caffeine absorption begins in the stomach, this process takes place mainly within the small intestine. Caffeine has a plasma half-life in humans that ranges from about 2.5 to 4.5 hours. Consequently, people who drink coffee repeatedly over the course of a day experience gradually rising plasma caffeine concentrations, but most of the caffeine is cleared from the circulation during sleep. The rate of plasma clearance is stimulated by smoking and reduced when smoking is terminated. The resulting increase in plasma caffeine levels could contribute to cigarette withdrawal symptoms in heavy coffee drinkers, particularly since caffeine is anxiogenic at high doses (see below).

Caffeine is converted to a variety of metabolites by the liver microsomal enzyme system (Arnaud, 1993). These metabolites account for almost all caffeine excretion, as only 1% to 2% of an administered dose is ex-

creted unchanged. In humans, approximately 95% of caffeine metabolites are eliminated through the urine, 2% to 5% through the feces, and the remainder through other bodily fluids such as saliva. The majority of urinary caffeine excretion can be accounted for by a combination of the metabolites 1-methyluric acid, 1,7-dimethyluric acid, 1-methylxanthine, paraxanthine, and 5-acetylamino-6-formylamino-3-methyluracil (AFMU).

1-Methyluric Acid   1,7-Dimethyluric Acid

1-Methylxanthine   Paraxanthine

AFMU

Acute Behavioral and Physiological Effects of Caffeine

In laboratory animals such as rats and mice, caffeine increases locomotor activity and may also be anxiogenic, particularly in the social interaction test (see Chapter 16; Bättig and Welzl, 1993). Like other stimulants, caffeine exerts complex effects on operant responding that vary as a function of dosage, schedule of reinforcement, and other methodological factors.

The effects of caffeine on humans are well known to any student who needs to "pull an all-nighter" before an exam. At typical doses (100–500 mg), caffeine has been found to increase arousal, reduce fatigue, and depress sleep (reviewed by Bättig and Welzl, 1993; Benowitz, 1990a; Snel, 1993). At higher doses, it can also produce feelings of tension and anxiety. Interestingly, patients suffering from panic disorder appear to be hypersensitive to caffeine's anxiogenic effects and may even suffer panic attacks in response to caffeine administration (Boulanger et al., 1984; Charney, Heninger, and Jatlow, 1985).

A number of studies have found that caffeine improves performance on various psychomotor tasks (Bättig and Welzl, 1993). However, James (1994b) has questioned whether caffeine actually enhances attention or performance over baseline levels, or whether it merely reverses the deleterious effects of caffeine withdrawal on these measures. This issue arose because the subjects in most caffeine studies drink at least moderate amounts of coffee, and those individuals selected for the control (i.e., no caffeine) condition may therefore exhibit reduced attention and psychomotor performance as part of an abstinence syndrome (see below). On the other hand, a large survey study conducted in Great Britain found significant correlations between amount of caffeine consumption (coffee and tea drinking) and performance on several cognitive tasks (Figure 14.9; Jarvis, 1993). These data provide additional, though still not conclusive, support for an ability of caffeine to enhance performance above baseline levels.

Studies with both animals and humans have demonstrated that caffeine can serve as a discriminative stimulus (Bättig and Welzl, 1993; Heishman and Henningfield, 1992). Rats trained to discriminate caffeine from saline showed partial generalization to other stimulants, including amphetamine, cocaine, and methylxanthine derivatives such as theophylline and theobromine. An interesting study of low-dose caffeine discrimination in humans was conducted by Griffiths and colleagues (1990a). These investigators showed that in subjects whose baseline caffeine consumption was low (approximately 1 cup of coffee per day) and who abstained from all dietary sources of caffeine during the study, reliable discrimination of a caffeine-containing capsule from a placebo capsule could eventually be achieved at doses of 56 mg or lower.

Some of the subjective effects of caffeine may be related to its peripheral physiological effects. These include increased blood pressure and respiration rate, enhanced water excretion (diuresis), and stimulation of catecholamine, particularly epinephrine release (Benowitz, 1990a). Caffeine was also reported to decrease whole brain cerebral blood flow in humans (Cameron,

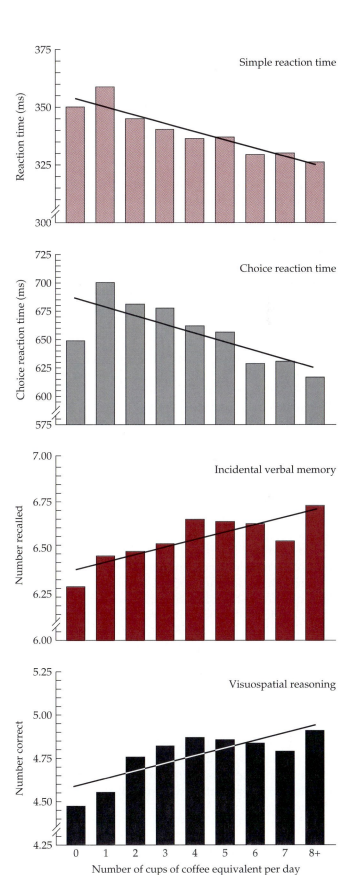

14.9 COGNITIVE AND PSYCHOMOTOR PERFORMANCE AS A FUNCTION OF AVERAGE DAILY CAFFEINE CONSUMPTION. Over 7,000 men and women in Great Britain were surveyed for information on their coffee- and tea-drinking habits and for other potentially relevant lifestyle variables. They were subsequently tested for their performance on four tasks: simple reaction time, choice reaction time, incidental verbal memory, and visuospatial reasoning. Average daily self-reported caffeine intake from both coffee and tea was converted to coffee equivalents (assuming that coffee contains twice the caffeine content of tea). Caffeine intake was then related to task performance by multiple linear regression, which permitted statistical correction for the influence of potential confounding factors such as educational level and other demographic variables, health, and use of other legal drugs including tobacco and alcohol. The results indicate a significant relationship between overall daily caffeine intake and improved performance on every task. (From Jarvis, 1993.)

Modell, and Hariharan, 1990), although the behavioral significance of this finding is not yet clear.

Therapeutic Uses of Caffeine

Although caffeine is not usually regarded as a medicinal agent, it does have several therapeutic uses. As shown in Table 14.1, caffeine is a constituent of several over-the-counter analgesic agents. This use is based on studies suggesting that caffeine is mildly effective in the treatment of nonmigraine headaches, either alone or acting synergistically with aspirin or acetaminophen (see Bättig and Welzl, 1993; Benowitz, 1990a). Caffeine has also been combined with ergotamine in a medication (Cafergot) for migraine headaches. However, this approach creates a risk that caffeine withdrawal following the treatment could actually precipitate another migraine. Probably the most important clinical use of caffeine is in the treatment of newborn infants who show apneic episodes (periodic cessation of breathing) (Benowitz, 1990a). Caffeine can be lifesaving in these patients by regularizing their breathing.

Effects of Chronic Caffeine Exposure

Caffeine Tolerance and Sensitization

As we have seen previously with amphetamine and cocaine, repeated treatment of animals with caffeine can lead to either tolerance or sensitization, depending on the pattern of administration. Thus, continuous treatment of rats by the addition of caffeine to their drinking water produced tolerance to the drug's locomotor activating effects (File et al., 1988; Finn and Holtzman, 1986). In contrast, locomotor sensitization was found to occur following intermittent intraperitoneal injection or oral administration (Meliska, Landrom, and Loke, 1985; Meliska, Landrom, and Landrom, 1990).

In humans, tolerance occurs to the cardiovascular effects of caffeine (Heishman and Henningfield, 1992), although such tolerance may not be complete (James, 1994a). Less clear is whether tolerance also occurs to the drug's psychological and behavioral effects. Studies on the activating influence of caffeine during the daytime have demonstrated only a weak tolerance (Heishman and Henningfield, 1992). In contrast, caffeine administration produces less sleep disruption in heavy coffee drinkers than in light coffee drinkers (Snel, 1993). Unfortunately, however, it is impossible to determine whether these results are due to tolerance or to preexisting differences in caffeine sensitivity (which would also explain the disparity in voluntary caffeine consumption between the groups).

Caffeine Dependence

Caffeine withdrawal syndrome.   Readers who are regular caffeine users may have experienced various psychological and physical symptoms either when they attempted to reduce their caffeine intake voluntarily, or when they were forced to terminate their consumption abruptly (e.g., during a hospital stay). In recent years, these anecdotal reports have been confirmed in controlled studies by several research groups. The main withdrawal symptoms were found to be headaches, drowsiness, fatigue, impaired concentration and psychomotor performance, and in some cases mild anxiety or depression (Hughes et al., 1991; Silverman et al., 1992). An intense craving for coffee may also be experienced. It is important to note that caffeine withdrawal symptoms can be severe enough to cause occupational and/or social dysfunction in heavy users who are physically dependent on the drug (Strain et al., 1994).

Although caffeine withdrawal symptoms were first observed in high-dose consumers (>600 mg/day), they can occur in individuals who are consuming as little as 100 mg/day, which is the equivalent of one 6-oz. cup of regular coffee or three cans of caffeinated soft drink (Griffiths et al., 1990b). As shown in Figure 14.10, the caffeine withdrawal syndrome begins on the first day of abstinence and lasts for several more days. Researchers now believe that relief from withdrawal is a major factor in chronic coffee drinking, particularly with regard to the first cup in the morning.

Caffeine abuse.   Although caffeine is not normally associated with the compulsive drug-taking patterns seen in severe alcoholics or individuals dependent on cocaine or opiates, physicians occasionally encounter patients who persist in consuming large amounts of coffee or other caffeinated beverages despite strong medical advice to the contrary. Chronic ingestion of excessive amounts of caffeine can lead to a syndrome called "caffeinism," which is characterized by restlessness, nervousness, insomnia, and physiological disturbances including tachycardia (Benowitz, 1990a). At extremely high doses (>1,000 mg/day), even more severe psychiatric effects may be observed. Due to the similar symptomatology, caffeinism is sometimes difficult to distinguish from a primary anxiety disorder (Greden, 1974). Although the origins of caffeinism are not yet known, it may be that individuals suffering from this disorder experience particularly strong withdrawal symptoms and craving when they attempt to curtail their usage.

We have seen that caffeine consumption causes physical dependence and can also lead to a compulsive use pattern. Moreover, caffeine is reinforcing to regular users (Evans, Critchfield, and Griffiths, 1994; Heishman and Henningfield, 1992). Caffeine therefore possesses some of the characteristics of an abused substance. On the other hand, most caffeine use is noncompulsive and does not impair the user's daily functioning. Furthermore, the reinforcing effects of caffeine are not due to an intense drug-induced euphoria as in the case of cocaine, opiates, and certain other heavily abused substances.

Headache

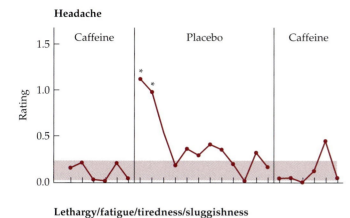

Lethargy/fatigue/tiredness/sluggishness

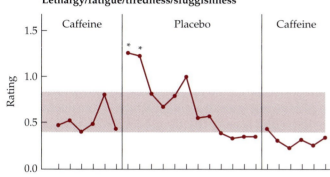

Energy/activity

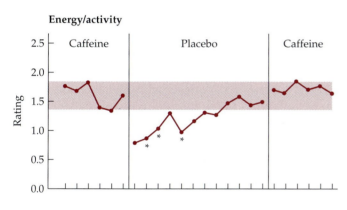

Ablity to concentrate

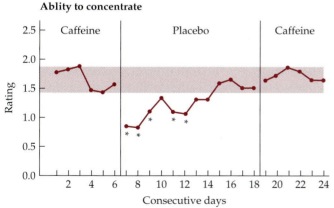

14.10 TIME COURSE OF CAFFEINE WITHDRAWAL SYMPTOMS. The subjects of this study were seven men and women, all of whom were regular caffeine users (mean prestudy consumption was estimated to be 384 mg/day). During the study, the subjects refrained from all dietary caffeine intake. In the first phase (Caffeine), subjects were given 10 capsules/day, each containing 10 mg caffeine, for a total of 100 mg/day. In the second phase (Placebo), the caffeine capsules were replaced with identical-looking placebo capsules. Subjects were aware that one or more placebo conditions would occur in the course of the study, but they were not informed when drug replacement would be instituted. The final phase (Caffeine) involved reexposure of subjects to 100 mg/day of caffeine. Throughout all phases, the subjects completed a questionnaire four times daily in which they rated 33 variables related to their mood and behavior. Substitution of placebo for this low dose of caffeine produced a rapid appearance of withdrawal symptoms followed by a gradual return to normalcy over the next several days. *$p \geq 0.05$ compared to the mean of the initial caffeine period. (From Griffiths et al., 1990b.)

1986). Animal self-administration studies have likewise found little evidence for caffeine reinforcement compared with the powerful reinforcing effects reported for cocaine, amphetamine, and opiates (Heishman and Henningfield, 1992). Together, these findings lead to the conclusion that caffeine has only a limited dependence potential, which is reflected in the lack of either a caffeine dependence or abuse syndrome in the DSM-IV. However, it is worth noting that DSM-IV does list several caffeine-related disorders, including caffeine intoxication (caffeinism), caffeine-induced anxiety disorder, and caffeine-induced sleep disorder. Moreover, one group of investigators has recently suggested that a caffeine-dependence syndrome can be demonstrated in some users, and they argue that the prevalence and characteristics of this syndrome deserve further study (Strain et al., 1994).

Adverse Physiological Effects of Chronic Caffeine Consumption

In addition to the previously mentioned psychological and behavioral consequences of chronic caffeine consumption, caffeine may act as a risk factor for certain physiological disorders. For example, Benowitz (1990a) reviewed evidence linking heavy coffee drinking with an increased incidence of coronary heart disease. There have also been several reports of an association between amount of caffeine consumption by pregnant women and low infant birth weight (Fortier, Marcoux, and Beaulac-Baillargeon, 1993; Martin and Bracken, 1987). It is therefore reasonable to conclude that all individuals, and especially pregnant women, should moderate their caffeine intake.

Mechanisms of Caffeine Action

Although the mechanism by which caffeine exerts its stimulant effects is not yet completely understood, substantial progress has been made over the past 15–20 years (reviewed by Daly, 1993). It is clear that caffeine

Rather, caffeine reinforcement seems to be related to a combination of functional enhancement (i.e., improved attention and psychomotor performance) (Silverman, Mumford, and Griffiths, 1994) and relief from withdrawal symptoms (Griffiths, Bigelow, and Liebson,

does not directly influence catecholamine systems like the psychomotor stimulants amphetamine and cocaine. How else might it work? When the biochemistry of cAMP was first being investigated, the discovery was made that caffeine and theophylline are inhibitors of cAMP phosphodiesterase. This led to the theory that caffeine- or theophylline-induced behavioral stimulation resulted from an accumulation of brain cAMP. Subsequent research, however, demonstrated that behavioral activation by these drugs can occur at brain concentrations that are insufficient to inhibit phosphodiesterase. In addition, nonxanthine phosphodiesterase inhibitors are behavioral depressants rather than stimulants, thus casting serious doubt on the relevance of this biochemical action for the behavioral properties of caffeine and theophylline (Daly, 1993).

An intriguing alternative hypothesis was advanced by Snyder and coworkers in 1981. This hypothesis proposed that the stimulant effects of methylxanthines such as caffeine are due to a blockade of receptors for the neurotransmitter/neuromodulator adenosine. Because of the importance of adenosine for understanding caffeine pharmacology, we will present a summary of adenosine biochemistry and pharmacology before proceeding with our discussion of caffeine's mechanism of action.

Adenosine

Adenosine is a purine nucleoside, which means that the compound consists of a ribose sugar linked to the purine base adenine. The majority of cellular adenine is found in the nucleotide (phosphorylated) forms, particularly 5'-adenosine monophosphate (5'-AMP) and adenosine triphosphate (ATP). As we have noted earlier in this volume, ATP is critically involved in cellular energy metabolism. However, adenine nucleotides are also constituents of DNA, RNA, and many enzyme cofactors, including nicotinamide adenine dinucleotide (NAD), flavin adenine dinucleotide (FAD), and coenzyme A.

Adenosine as a neuroregulator.   Adenosine is known to exert a variety of important effects on peripheral physiology, including coronary vasodilation, relaxation of gastrointestinal smooth muscle, inhibition of blood platelet aggregation, and stimulation of triglyceride formation in adipose cells (Daly, 1993; Ohisalo, 1987). Interest in the possibility that adenosine might have neuroregulatory properties, in addition to its other cellular functions, began to emerge following Sattin and Rall's (1970) discovery that this compound could stimulate cAMP formation in cerebral cortical slices. Since that time, a number of studies have examined the electrophysiological effects of adenosine, investigated its release and uptake by nerve cells, demonstrated the presence of adenosine receptors in the brain, and attempted to explain the actions of certain psychoactive and neuroactive drugs by means of interactions with adenosinergic systems. It is clear

from this extensive body of research that adenosine plays some type of regulatory role in the nervous system. As we shall see, however, the exact nature of this role remains something of an enigma at the time of this writing.

Adenosine synthesis and release.   Adenosine can be formed in a biochemical pathway involving de novo synthesis of the purine nucleoside inosine 5'-monophosphate. However, this pathway is thought to be of only minor significance in the brain (Geiger and Nagy, 1990). The most important source of brain adenosine seems to be adenosine 5'-monophosphate (AMP), which yields adenosine upon hydrolysis by the enzyme 5'-nucleotidase (Figure 14.11a). Intracellular adenosine synthesis is catalyzed by a cytoplasmic form of 5'-nucleotidase. Alternatively, it can be formed on the outside of the cell membrane by an ecto-5'-nucleotidase. An ectoenzyme is embedded in the membrane with its catalytic site oriented toward the extracellular space. Extracellular AMP is derived at least partly from ATP, which is colocalized and co-released with several classical neurotransmitters (e.g., acetylcholine and NE) in the peripheral nervous system and possibly also the brain (Burnstock, 1990a; Salter, De Koninck, and Henry, 1993). Following its release, ATP activates specialized membrane receptors (not discussed here due to space limitations) and is then rapidly dephosphorylated to 5'-AMP by several ectonucleotidases. Consequently, conditions that cause enhanced release of ATP presumably also increase adenosine availability in the extracellular space (Geiger and Nagy, 1990).

A second and entirely different source of adenosine stems from its role as a by-product of transmethylation reactions. Transmethylations are important in a number of biochemical pathways, including the catabolism of catecholamines and histamine (via catecholamine O-methyltransferase and histamine N-methyltransferase). The methyl donor for these reactions is S-adenosylmethionine (SAM), which in the process is converted to S-adenosylhomocysteine. The relevance of this fact is that adenosine can be liberated from S-adenosylhomocysteine by the enzyme S-adenosylhomocysteine hydrolase (Figure 14.11b). This pathway is thus another potential source of adenosine in neural tissues.

Adenosine has been detected in the brain extracellular fluid by means of in vivo microdialysis (Ballarín et al., 1991). A number of studies have also shown stimulation-evoked release of adenosine from neural tissues, although the source of adenosine has been difficult to ascertain (Meghji and Newby, 1990; Nagy, Geiger, and Staines, 1990). One possibility, of course, is that stimulation causes release of ATP, which is followed by extracellular production of adenosine as described above. Alternatively, under some conditions adenosine itself might be released from the cytoplasm by reversal of the mem-

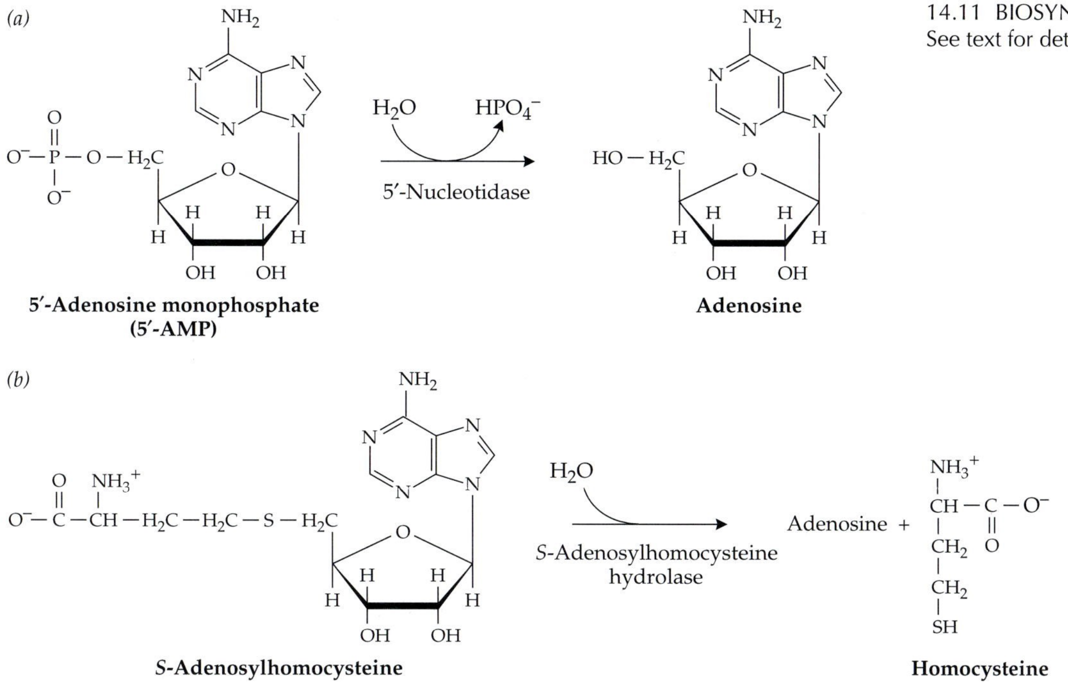

(a)

5'-Adenosine monophosphate
(5'-AMP)

5'-Nucleotidase

Adenosine

14.11 BIOSYNTHESIS OF ADENOSINE.
See text for details.

(b)

S-Adenosylhomocysteine

S-Adenosylhomocysteine
hydrolase

Adenosine +

Homocysteine

brane nucleoside transporter normally responsible for adenosine uptake (see next section). There is currently no evidence indicating vesicular storage of adenosine, although such a possibility has not been ruled out experimentally.

Adenosine release from both neural and nonneural tissues is enhanced by conditions of metabolic stress and oxygen deprivation (e.g., hypoxia or ischemia) (Hagberg et al., 1987; Zetterström et al., 1982). This is an adaptive response because adenosine has a vasodilatory action that helps restore blood flow and oxygen to the affected area. On the other hand, the clarification of adenosine's role in normal behavioral and physiological regulation has been hampered by a lack of information concerning the characteristics of its release under nonstressful conditions

Adenosine inactivation. The immediate mode of inactivation of extracellular adenosine is believed to be uptake into nerve terminals and glial cells carried out by a plasma membrane transporter (Snyder, 1985). Relatively selective adenosine-uptake blockers have been developed, including nitrobenzylthioinosine (NBI) and dipyridamole (DPR). Moreover, [³H]NBI and [³H]DPR have been used to study the distribution of adenosine transporters in the brain (Deckert, Morgan, and Marangos, 1988). It is interesting to note that a number of psychoactive drugs also block adenosine uptake with respectable potencies, including neuroleptics of the phenothiazine and butyrophenone classes and benzodiazepines. However, at present there is no clear evidence that such an effect is important for the clinical actions of these compounds.

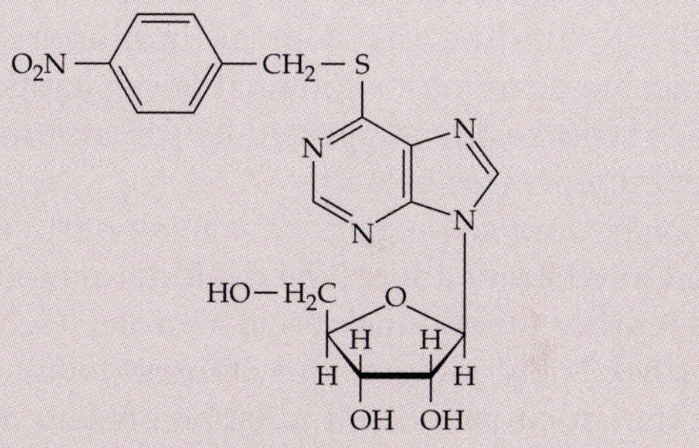

Nitrobenzylthioinosine
(NBI)

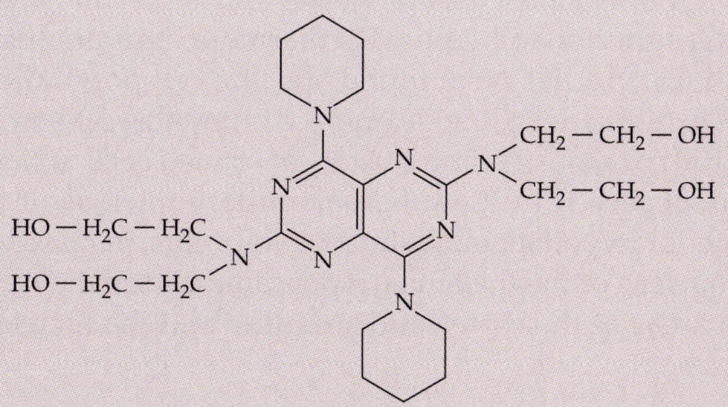

Dipyridamole (DPR)

Intracellular adenosine in the brain is inactivated by two main pathways illustrated in Figure 14.12. One pathway involves oxidative deamination to inosine, which is catalyzed by the cytoplasmic enzyme adenosine deaminase. This enzyme is potently inhibited by the drug 2'-deoxycoformycin (Padua et al., 1990). Inosine is converted to hypoxanthine, which is then either cleared from the cell, oxidized to xanthine and then the waste product uric acid (reactions not shown), or phosphoribosylated by the enzyme hypoxanthine phosphoribosyltransferase (HPRT). The latter reaction is a salvage pathway that may be important in recycling adenosine for the synthesis of new 5'-AMP. Alternatively, adenosine can be metabolized to 5'-AMP directly through phosphorylation by adenosine kinase. Formed in this manner, 5'-AMP may then be phosphorylated further to form ATP. The relative importance of these pathways in neural tissues is still a matter of conjecture (Geiger and Nagy, 1990).

Distribution of putative adenosinergic neurons. As with the excitatory amino acid transmitters glutamate and aspartate, we can expect to find significant concentrations of adenosine in all cells in the brain. Consequently, determining (1) whether certain neurons synthesize and release a specific pool of adenosine for neurotransmitter/neuromodulator purposes, and (2) where these certain neurons might be located, has proved to be a daunting task. Nevertheless, several markers have been proposed for the identification of putative adenosinergic neurons or nerve terminals, including the presence of adenosine uptake sites as indicated by [³H]NBI or [³H]DPR binding, as well as immunoreactivity for adenosine deaminase. Potential postsynaptic sites of action, of course, are suggested by the location of adenosine receptors (see below).

Nagy and coworkers have been particularly interested in whether adenosine deaminase might be useful as a marker for adenosinergic neurons (Geiger and Nagy, 1990; Nagy, Geiger, and Staines, 1990). Despite the fact that adenosine itself must be present in all cells in the brain, adenosine deaminase activity varies widely across different regions, with highest levels in the posterior hypothalamus, olfactory bulb, and superficial layers of the superior colliculus. Furthermore, immunohistochemical studies have found specific cell populations that exhibit adenosine deaminase immunoreactivity. In rat and/or mouse brain, clusters of stained cells or fibers were observed in the tuberomamillary nucleus of the posterior hypothalamus, superior colliculus, parafascicular nucleus of the thalamus, hippocampal formation, certain areas of the cortex and striatum, and the olfactory

nerve (Staines, Daddona, and Nagy, 1987; Yamamoto et al., 1987). The apparent high level of adenosine deaminase in restricted groups of neurons has led to the hypothesis that cells using adenosine in a neurotransmitter/neuromodulator role might require an enhanced capacity to metabolize the compound (Nagy, Geiger, and Staines, 1990).

Thus, both biochemical and immunohistochemical studies of adenosine deaminase are consistent with the notion that specific adenosinergic neurons are present in the brain, and that this enzyme may serve as a marker for such cells. Nevertheless, a number of questions remain. First, it has not yet been established whether adenosine deaminase–immunoreactive cells contain a releasable pool of adenosine, which would be expected of true adenosinergic neurons. Second, in mouse, though not rat brain, many glial cells were observed to stain with an adenosine deaminase antibody (Yamamoto et al., 1987). How this relates to the usefulness of adenosine deaminase as a marker in neuronal populations is unclear, although staining of glial cells could be clearly distinguished from neuronal staining. Third, whereas there is some concordance between the distribution of adenosine deaminase activity/immunoreactivity and the location of adenosine uptake sites as measured by [³H]NBI binding (Deckert, Morgan, and Marangos, 1988), the distribution of adenosine receptors in the brain does not correspond well with these other measures. Admittedly, receptor mismatches of this sort have been found with a number of well-established transmitters, so this fact alone is insufficient to cast serious doubt on the use of adenosine deaminase as a neurotransmitter/neuron marker. However, this apparent discrepancy indicates that new approaches may be needed to confirm the location of adenosinergic pathways in the brain.

Adenosine receptors. There are three main subtypes of adenosine receptors, designated A_1, A_2, and A_3 (reviewed by Collis and Hourani, 1993; Van Galen et al., 1992). There is also evidence that the A_2 subtype can be further subdivided into A_{2A} and A_{2B} receptors (Bruns, Lu, and Pugsley, 1987). Although this classification system was initially developed primarily on the basis of pharmacological criteria, over the past several years researchers from several laboratories have succeeded in

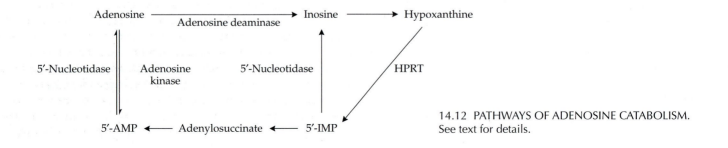

14.12 PATHWAYS OF ADENOSINE CATABOLISM. See text for details.

cloning all three receptor subtypes (reviewed in Collis and Hourani, 1993; Linden, 1994). The cloned receptors exhibit substantial sequence homology with one another, and they all belong to the G protein–coupled receptor superfamily.

The pharmacological differentiation of A_1 and A_2 receptors is based partly on the relative potencies of the agonists 5'-N-ethylcarboxamide adenosine (NECA), N^6-cyclohexyladenosine (CHA), N^6-cyclopentyladenosine (CPA), 2-chloroadenosine (2-CA), R-N^6-phenylisopropyladenosine (R-PIA), and the stereoisomer S-N^6-phenylisopropyladenosine (S-PIA) for each subtype. The rank order of potency of these agonists at A_1 sites is CPA > R-PIA = CHA ≥ NECA > 2-CA > S-PIA, whereas the potency order for A_2 sites is NECA > 2-CA > R-PIA = CHA = CPA > S-PIA (Collis and Hourani, 1993). In radioligand studies, cloned A_3 receptors exhibit approximately equal affinities for R-PIA and NECA and thus differ from both the A_1 and A_2 subtypes in their agonist specificity (Linden, 1994).

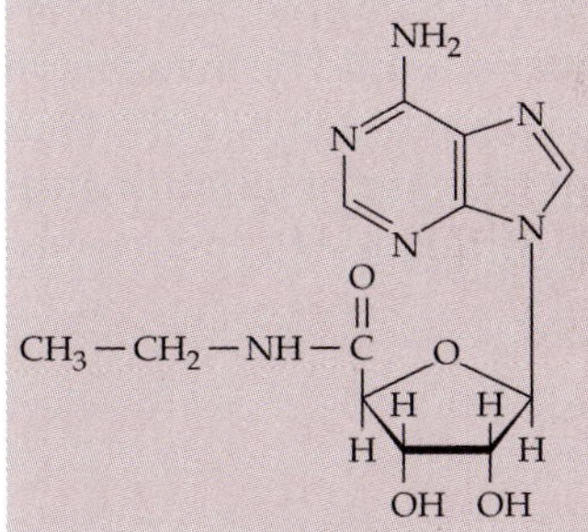

A number of adenosine receptor antagonists have also been identified, most of which are xanthine derivatives. Caffeine and theophylline are relatively weak, nonselective adenosine antagonists in that they block both A_1 and A_2 receptors with roughly equal potencies (van Galen et al., 1992). However, other compounds have been developed with greater selectivity and potency. For example, 1,3-dipropyl-8-cyclopentylxanthine (DPCPX) is a useful A_1-selective antagonist, whereas the quinazoline CP66713 is rel-

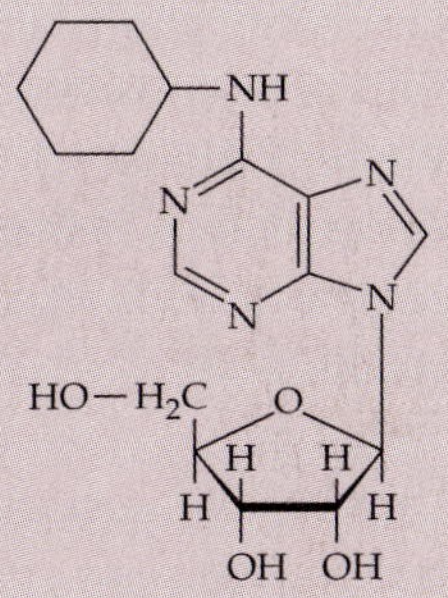

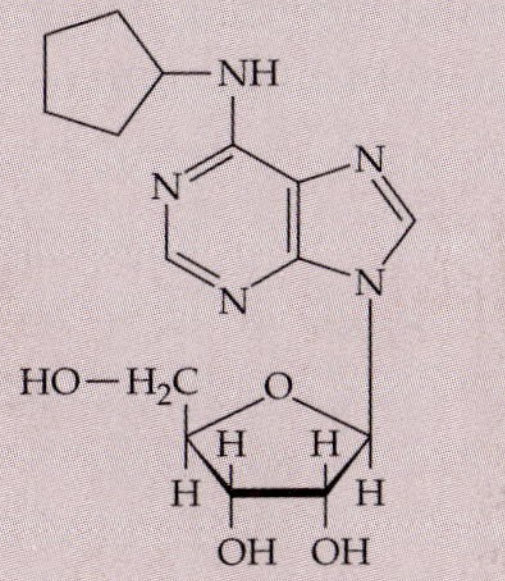

DPCPX

CP66713

atively selective for the A_2 receptor subtype (Collis and Hourani, 1993). The rat A_3 receptor is relatively insensitive to inhibition by xanthine derivatives; however, human and sheep A_3 receptors are potently blocked by certain xanthines such as 1-propyl-3-(3-iodo-4-aminobenzyl)-8-(4-oxyacetate)-phenylxanthine (I-ABOPX) (Linden, 1994).

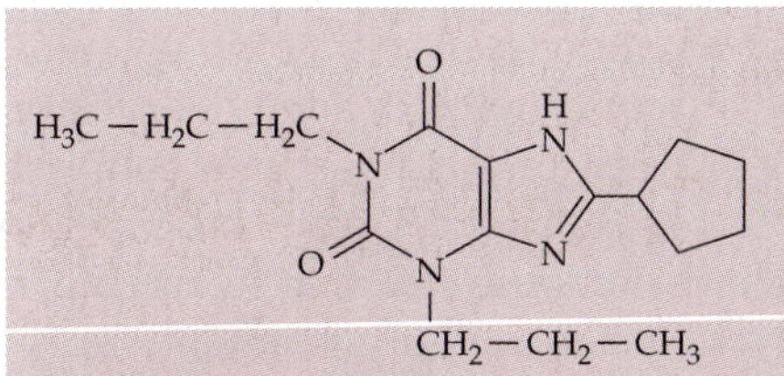

NECA

CHA

CPA

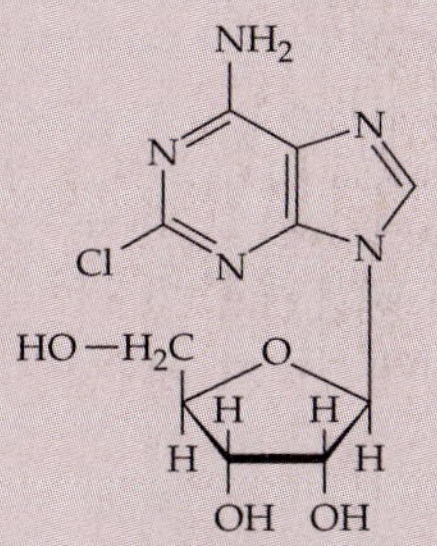

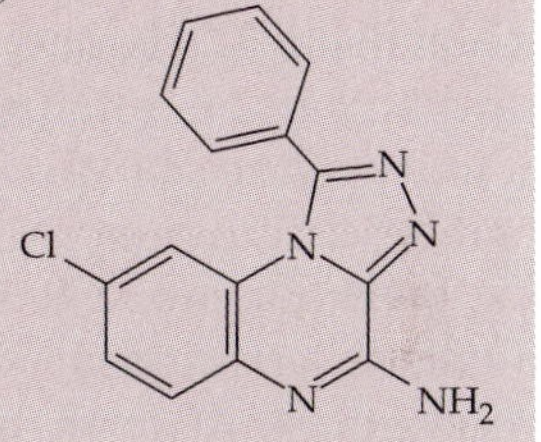

2-CA

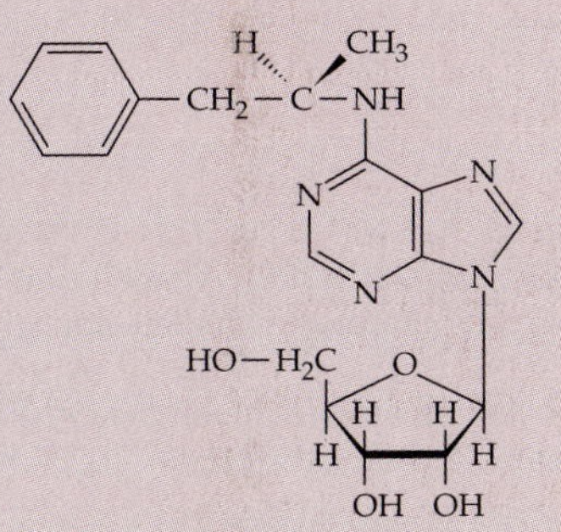

R-PIA

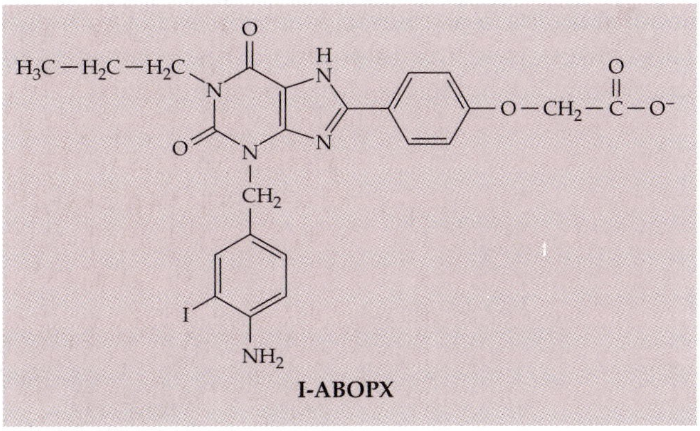

I-ABOPX

Autoradiographic studies in the rat brain found the highest densities of A_1 receptors in the hippocampal formation, molecular layer of the cerebellar cortex, and diencephalon, with lower but measurable levels in the cerebral cortex and striatum (Jarvis and Williams, 1989; Weber et al., 1990). A_2 receptors showed a strikingly different distribution, with highest levels of binding in the striatum, nucleus accumbens, and olfactory tubercle, somewhat lower levels in the globus pallidus, and essentially no specific binding in any other brain area (Jarvis and Williams, 1989). Subsequent experiments using in situ hybridization histochemistry for A_{2A} receptor mRNA found essentially the same localization as determined by autoradiographic studies and further demonstrated a cellular coexpression of A_{2A} receptor mRNA with DA D_2 but not D_1 receptor mRNA (Fink et al., 1992). The presence of A_2 receptors in the basal ganglia may well be related to the ability of adenosine agonists and antagonists to modulate locomotor behavior (see below).

Like other G protein–coupled receptors, adenosine receptors operate through multiple signal transduction mechanisms. Early work showed that A_2 (both A_{2A} and A_{2B}) receptors are positively coupled to adenylyl cyclase through G_s, whereas A_1 receptors are negatively coupled through G_i (Figure 14.13) (Stiles, 1991; Van Galen et al., 1992). Other studies have demonstrated that A_1 receptors also stimulate guanylyl cyclase activity in smooth muscle, activate K^+ channel opening in hippocampus and in cardiac muscle, inhibit neuronal Ca^{2+} influx, and alter activity of the phosphoinositide second messenger system in various tissues. Relatively little is known about the mechanisms of action of the A_3 receptor, although initial observations indicate that it inhibits adenylyl cyclase and cAMP formation (Linden, 1994).

Cellular effects of adenosine.   Electrophysiological studies have demonstrated that adenosine inhibits the firing of neurons throughout the brain. This effect is mediated in part by the above-mentioned K^+ channel activation, which has the effect of hyperpolarizing the nerve cell membrane (Greene and Haas, 1991). Another postsynaptic electrophysiological action of adenosine is to enhance neuronal accommodation and the after-hyperpolarization that occurs in reaction to persistent excitatory input. This causes a selective inhibition of responsiveness to long-lasting but not to brief synaptic stimulation.

It is well known that adenosine inhibits the release of many neurotransmitters, including ACh, NE, DA, 5-HT, GABA, and glutamate (Fredholm and Dunwiddie, 1988), probably by adenosine inhibition of Ca^{2+} influx into nerve terminals. Prince and Stevens (1992) investigated the influence of adenosine on synaptic transmission at perforant path synapses on dentate granule cells in a hippocampal slice preparation, and found that adenosine selectively inhibited excitatory, but not inhibitory, transmission at these junctions. This effect appeared to be mediated entirely by a presynaptic effect on neurotransmitter release. Finally, the adenosine antagonist 3-isobutyl-1-methylxanthine (IBMX) enhanced excitatory synaptic currents when applied in the absence of exogenous adenosine. This suggests that endogenous adenosine is present at sufficient concentrations at these synapses to produce a tonic inhibition of excitatory transmission.

The widespread effectiveness of adenosine in damping neuronal firing raises the possibility that extracellular adenosine may exert a tonic inhibitory effect on neural excitability throughout the brain. In this way, adenosine might be considered an endogenous anticonvulsant compound. It is further conceivable that abnormalities of adenosinergic regulation could be involved in the etiology of some forms of epilepsy (Chin, 1989; Dragunow, 1988). However, as in the case of another anticonvulsant transmitter, GABA, this idea remains unproven at the present time.

Adenosine Antagonism as the Mechanism of Caffeine Action

Behavioral effects of adenosine agonists and antagonists. There is some physiological evidence that caffeine and theophylline are adenosine antagonists in humans (Biag-

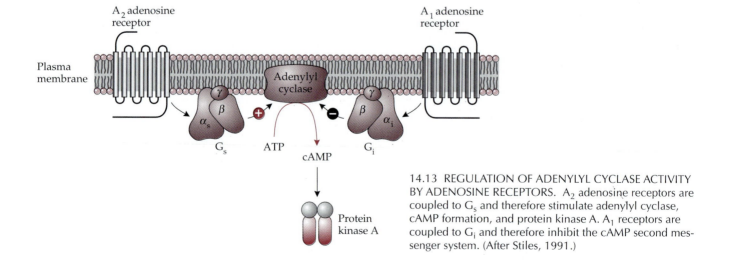

14.13 REGULATION OF ADENYLYL CYCLASE ACTIVITY BY ADENOSINE RECEPTORS. A_2 adenosine receptors are coupled to G_s and therefore stimulate adenylyl cyclase, cAMP formation, and protein kinase A. A_1 receptors are coupled to G_i and therefore inhibit the cAMP second messenger system. (After Stiles, 1991.)

gioni et al., 1991). However, this concept is based mainly on animal studies, beginning with the classic experiments of Snyder and coworkers (1981). These investigators showed that various methylxanthines bound to adenosine receptors with a potency that correlated with their ability to stimulate locomotor activity in mice. Moreover, the adenosine agonist R-PIA was found to be a potent behavioral depressant, an effect that was reversed by concurrent treatment with caffeine or theophylline. Based on these findings, it was argued that the stimulant effects of caffeine and theophylline are due to a blockade of adenosine receptors. A further implication of this hypothesis is that endogenous adenosine exerts a tonic suppressive effect on activity and arousal.

Our earlier discussion on adenosine receptors indicated that R-PIA is relatively selective for A_1 receptors. Also, Snyder and coworkers (1981) used [^{3}H]CHA, which likewise prefers the A_1 subtype, for their receptor binding experiments. These and other findings (Kaplan et al., 1992) seem to implicate A_1 receptors in the locomotor effects of adenosinergic drugs in rodents. On the other hand, several studies have indicated an equal, if not more important, role for the A_2 receptor subtype (Durcan and Morgan, 1989; Ferré, Rubio, and Fuxe, 1991; Nikodijević, Daly, and Jacobson, 1990). Particularly noteworthy is recent work of Barraco and colleagues (1993) in which the A_1 selective agonist CPA and the A_2 selective agonists NECA and 2-(carboxyethylphenylethylamino)adenosine-5′-carboxamide (CGS 21680) were microinjected directly into the nucleus accumbens of mice. As illustrated in Figure 14.14, CPA had little or no effect on locomotor activity, whereas a profound depression of activity was produced by both CGS 21680 and NECA. Moreover, this activity-suppressing effect was significantly attenuated by the A_2 receptor antagonist 3,7-dimethyl-1-propargylxanthine (DMPX), particularly in the case of CGS 21680. Therefore, at least in the nucleus accumbens, A_2 rather than A_1 receptors appear to be responsible for adenosine-mediated locomotor depression.

The neural mechanisms underlying adenosine's behavioral effects are still being explored; however, at least two plausible hypotheses have been advanced. First, Rainnie and colleagues (1994) recently presented evidence that adenosine exerts a tonic inhibitory effect on the firing of cholinergic neurons in the laterodorsal tegmental nucleus (LDT), pedunculopontine tegmental nucleus (PPT), and the diagonal band of Broca (DBB). LDT and PPT cholinergic neurons project to the thalamus and forebrain, and they are thought to play an important role in waking and behavioral arousal (see Chapter 7). Cells of the DBB are part of the basal forebrain cholinergic system that projects heavily to the neocortex and is involved in attentional and possibly other cognitive processes. If these cell groups are normally inhibited to some extent by adenosine, then this provides an important means by which adenosine antagonists such as caffeine could stimulate arousal at both the electrophysiological and behavioral levels.

A second possible mechanism (which does not exclude the first) involves interactions between adenosine and DA. In one experiment, for example, the D_2 receptor agonist BHT-920 attenuated the cataleptic effect of CGS 21680 in rats (Ferré, Rubio, and Fuxe, 1991). Several other studies have found that DA receptor blockers inhibit the behavioral effects of caffeine (Garrett and Holtzman, 1994; Josselyn and Beninger, 1991). Figure 14.15 shows that the stimulatory effect of caffeine in rats was suppressed by both D_1 and D_2 receptor antagonists. Together these findings suggest that adenosine antagonizes the functioning of DA (i.e., it acts like a neuroleptic drug), whereas adenosine antagonists (e.g., caffeine) enhance dopaminergic activity. This interaction may occur, in part, at the level of adenosinergic inhibition of DA release (Fredholm and Dunwiddie, 1988). An additional intriguing possibility involves an interaction between A_{2A} and D_2 receptors in the membrane of striatal neurons. We have already seen that these two receptor populations are coexpressed in cells of the rat striatum (Fink et al., 1992). In vitro receptor binding experiments further demonstrated that CGS 21680 stimulation of A_{2A} receptors reduced the affinity of D_2 agonist binding sites in striatal membranes (Ferré, Rubio, and Fuxe, 1991). Finally, this adenosine–DA interaction was shown to have

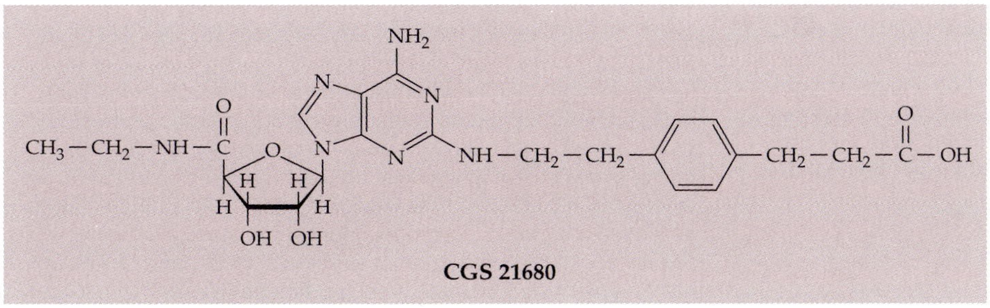

CGS 21680

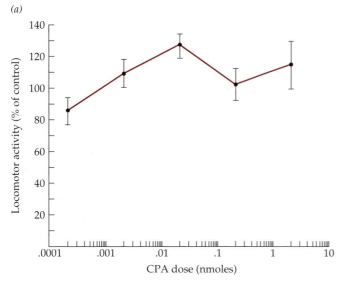

(a)

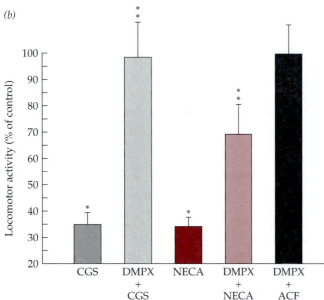

(b)

14.14 INFLUENCE OF ADENOSINE RECEPTOR AGONISTS MICROINJECTED INTO THE NUCLEUS ACCUMBENS ON LOCOMOTOR ACTIVITY. (*a*) Microinjection of varying doses of the A_1 adenosine receptor agonist CPA into the nucleus accumbens of mice had no significant effect on locomotor activity measured over a 40-minute test period. Results are expressed as percentage of the activity displayed by control mice given artificial cerebrospinal fluid (ACF) vehicle. (*b*) In contrast to the results obtained with CPA, intra-accumbens injection of the A_2 agonists CGS 21680 or NECA greatly suppressed locomotor activity. This effect was significantly attenuated by prior intraperitoneal injection of the A_2 antagonist DMPX, which had no effect on activity in vehicle-treated (ACF) animals. (*, significantly different from ACF vehicle controls [$p < 0.01$]; **, significantly different from the respective agonist-only group [$p < 0.01$], but not from the DMPX + ACF group.) (From Barraco et al., 1993.)

functional consequences in that intrastriatal infusion of CGS 21680 blocked the inhibitory effect of the D_2 agonist pergolide on GABA release by striatopallidal neurons (Ferré et al., 1993).

Role of adenosine in caffeine tolerance.   Based on the apparent role of adenosine in the acute behavioral effects of caffeine, an up-regulation of adenosine receptors has often been assumed to underlie the tolerance produced by continuous caffeine administration. However, this hypothesis suffers from at least two major problems. First, although modest up-regulation has been observed for cortical or hippocampal A_1 receptors, the potentially more important A_{2A} receptors in the striatum appear to be unaffected by chronic caffeine treatment (Johansson et al., 1993; Shi et al., 1993). Second, tolerance to chronic caffeine is frequently unsurmountable, meaning that the subjects still do not respond even when the caffeine dose is increased. This pattern is inconsistent with mediation by elevated receptor density (Holtzman, Mante, and Minneman, 1991). It is therefore important to look for

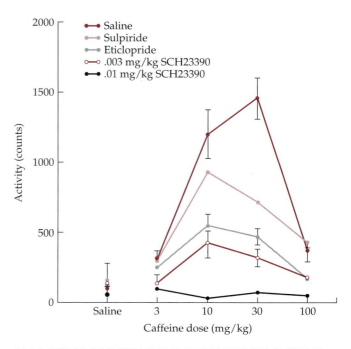

14.15 EFFECT OF DOPAMINE ANTAGONISTS ON CAFFEINE-STIMULATED MOTOR ACTIVITY Rats (*n* = 9/group) were tested for motor activity after administration of either saline or 3–100 mg/kg caffeine i.p. Some subjects were additionally pretreated with 30 mg/kg of the dopamine D_2 antagonist sulpiride, 0.03 mg/kg of the D_2 antagonist eticlopride, 0.003 mg/kg of the D_1 antagonist SCH23390, or 0.01 mg/kg of SCH23390. Caffeine alone produced a biphasic dose-dependent stimulation of activity, which has also been reported in other studies. Both D_1- and D_2-antagonist treatment significantly attenuated the response to at least one dose of caffeine. (From Garrett and Holtzman, 1994.)

other factors that might be responsible for caffeine tolerance. Possible candidates include other transmitter systems that are modulated by adenosine, particularly since Shi and colleagues (1993) reported alterations in the cholinergic, adrenergic, serotonergic, and GABAergic systems in response to only 4 days of continuous caffeine treatment in mice.

Other effects of caffeine.   Adenosine antagonism remains the best current explanation for the behaviorally activating effects of caffeine and related methylxanthines. As mentioned earlier, these compounds also inhibit cyclic nucleotide phosphodiesterase and mobilize Ca^{2+} from intracellular storage sites. Such effects require very high caffeine concentrations and therefore may not contribute to the behavioral changes seen at normal doses (Daly, 1993). Nevertheless, it is premature to conclude that all effects of caffeine can be explained by antagonism of adenosine receptors.

Part II Summary

Caffeine is a xanthine derivative contained in a number of foods, especially coffee and tea. It exerts a stimulant action in humans and laboratory animals, although this effect is not as extreme as that produced by amphetamine or cocaine. At typical doses, human subjects experience heightened arousal, reduced fatigue, reduced sleep, and improved psychomotor performance. Higher doses can lead to feelings of anxiety and dysphoria. Caffeine can act as a discriminative stimulus, even at relatively low doses. Various physiological effects are also produced, such as increased blood pressure and respiration rate, diuresis, and enhanced catecholamine secretion.

Laboratory animals show tolerance to the behavioral effects of caffeine, particularly when the compound is administered continuously (as in the drinking water). Humans exhibit tolerance to caffeine's cardiovascular effects; however, psychological and behavioral tolerance appear to be weak under typical experimental conditions.

A number of studies have shown that regular caffeine use leads to physical dependence. Symptoms of caffeine withdrawal include headache, drowsiness, fatigue, impaired concentration, and reduced psychomotor performance. The ability of caffeine to produce dependence and withdrawal accounts for the anecdotal observations of those who insist that they cannot "get started" in the morning without a cup of coffee. Although most users consume caffeine at low to moderate doses, a small number of individuals consume extremely high amounts that can lead to adverse psychological and physiological consequences (caffeinism). The existence of this syndrome, along with the evidence for caffeine

withdrawal symptoms, support the notion that caffeine possesses some of the characteristics of an abused substance. In addition to the obvious problems associated with caffeinism, even more modest caffeine consumption has been associated with a heightened risk for coronary heart disease and low infant birth weight (when the drug is taken by pregnant women).

Caffeine has a number of effects on neural and other tissues. It inhibits cyclic nucleotide phosphodiesterase and mobilizes Ca^{2+} from certain intracellular stores. However, the best explanation for caffeine's behavioral and physiological properties is that it competitively blocks receptors for the neuromodulatory substance adenosine.

Adenosine is a purine nucleoside that is formed from ATP in the extracellular fluid by a series of plasma membrane ectoenzymes. Its formation/release is enhanced by metabolic stress and oxygen deprivation. Adenosine is cleared from the extracellular space through uptake by a plasma membrane transporter that can be blocked by the compounds NBI and DPR. Once inside the cell, adenosine is metabolized to either inosine or 5'-AMP. Based on immunohistochemical staining for adenosine deaminase (the enzyme that converts adenosine to inosine), putative adenosinergic neurons are particularly concentrated in the posterior hypothalamus, superior colliculus, parafascicular nucleus of the thalamus, hippocampal formation, certain areas of the cortex and striatum, and the olfactory nerve.

Adenosine receptors are members of the G protein–coupled receptor superfamily. They can be divided into A_1, A_{2A}, A_{2B}, and A_3 subtypes. CPA is a relatively selective A_1 agonist, whereas NECA and CGS 21680 are selective agonists for the A_{2A} receptors. DPCPX and CP66713 are antagonists with selectivity for A_1 and A_2 receptors, respectively. Highly selective agonists or antagonists have not yet been developed for the A_3 subtype, although the compound I-ABOPX has some usefulness as an antagonist at human and sheep A_3 receptors. A_1 receptors inhibit cAMP synthesis, stimulate cGMP formation, activate K^+ channels, inhibit Ca^{2+} channels, and also affect the phosphoinositide second messenger system. In contrast, A_2 receptors have thus far only been found to stimulate cAMP. At the cellular level, adenosine can act postsynaptically to hyperpolarize neurons and inhibit their firing. It also exerts widespread presynaptic effects to inhibit neurotransmitter release from nerve terminals. The net effect of these actions is to dampen neuronal firing throughout the brain.

The concept that caffeine and related compounds exert their behavioral effects via adenosine antagonism arose from early studies showing that the behavioral potency of a series of methylxanthines correlated with their adenosine receptor–blocking potency. Moreover, adenosine agonists cause a profound depression in activity that is prevented by caffeine. Recent studies suggest that the A_2 receptor subtype is most important for these actions of adenosine agonists and antagonists, although A_1 receptors may also be involved. There are two major hypotheses concerning how adenosinergic compounds exert their psychological and behavioral effects. One hypothesis is based on evidence that adenosine tonically inhibits mesopontine and basal forebrain cholinergic neurons that play a critical role in electrophysiological and behavioral arousal. The second hypothesis proposes that adenosine antagonizes the actions of DA in the striatum and nucleus accumbens. Such antagonism may occur through adenosine inhibition of DA release and/or modulation of D_2 receptors by A_{2A} receptors in the membranes of striatal output neurons. Despite this substantial evidence for adenosine mediation of the acute effects of caffeine, attempts to demonstrate that caffeine tolerance is due to up-regulation of adenosine receptors have thus far not been convincing.

Chapter 15

Alcohol

No doubt the earliest drug in common use as an anodyne (something that calms, soothes, or comforts) was ethanol or ethyl alcohol, commonly referred to as alcohol. There is evidence that alcoholic beverages came into being in prehistoric times, probably by accidental fermentation of honey, grains steeped in water, or fruit juices, and that the consumption of these products found favor in human societies in most parts of the world. Even on remote islands, the native cultures had their beers made by the fermentation of substances rich in sugar or starch. Mead (meed), a fermentation product of honey, is regarded as the oldest alcoholic beverage, having existed in the paleolithic age, about 8000 B.C.E. (Blum and Associates, 1969). Archaeological records show that beer and wine were made by the fermentation of carbohydrates in what may have been the first brewery, dating back to 3700 B.C.E. in Egypt. The process of distillation to obtain higher alcohol concentrations was discovered in the Arab world around A.D. 800, and the word "alcohol" is of Arabian origin, from the word that is transliterated as *alkuhl* or *al-koh'l* ("something subtle") (Roueché, 1966).

$$CH_3 — CH_2 — OH$$
Ethanol

Alcohol is a fermentation product of yeast. Yeasts are quite common in the air where plants are grown, and contain enzymes that catalyze the conversion of sugars to alcohol and CO_2. It is small wonder that alcoholic beverages were produced when yeast acted upon solutions of fruit and grain that were left standing in a warm place. In fact, any carbohydrate that can be converted to sugar, such as potato starch, can be a source of alcohol through the fermentation process.

Although it would be hard to prove, it is unlikely that human use of alcoholic beverages can be explained by thirst, taste, or nutritional factors. Rather, it was the psychoactive sedative, anxiolytic, and euphoriant properties of alcohol beverages that made them so desirable. The social organization of early societies determined what the role of alcohol would be in those societies. (See Segal, 1987, for an extensive review of this subject.)

In the Middle Ages, the distillation process introduced by the Arabs enabled alcohol to be concentrated at high levels. Normally, the accumulation of alcohol above 12% to 15% during fermentation kills the alcohol-producing yeast, thus limiting the fermentation process. By means of distillation, the alcohol can be drawn off and consumed by itself, or it can be added to other mixtures and consumed in concentrations of about 40% to 50%. In this way, alcoholic beverages distilled from fermented grain mixtures gained common use, one variant coming to be known as whiskey (from the Gaelic *usquebaugh*, meaning "water of life"). Alcohol in this form came to be used in almost every country in the world, with the exception of those embracing the Moslem religion and culture.

Used in moderation, alcoholic beverages produce relaxation, elevation of mood, increased appetite, and release from inhibition by social constraints. Recently, it was found that older persons in good health obtain significant benefits from daily consumption of an ounce or two of alcohol, especially that found in wines. In contrast, total abstinence is associated with increased mortality compared with light or moderate drinking. It has been suggested that this effect occurs because light drinking increases plasma concentrations of high-density lipoprotein, which confers protection from coronary artery disease (see Ritchie, 1985).

It is easy to imagine that if alcohol were discovered today, it would be hailed as a wonder drug for its anxiolytic, soporific, hypnotic, analgesic, astringent, antibacterial, and solvent properties. Even as a food, although deficient in amino acids, vitamins, and minerals, it has the shortest possible metabolic pathway and hence provides the fastest source of calories among known foods. Were it not for its abuse potential, its toxicity at high doses, and its relatively short duration of effect, it would truly deserve the high esteem connoted by the name "whiskey." Yet, despite heroic research efforts, the mechanisms of action and the causes of alcohol's toxic effects on the CNS and other organs are just beginning to be understood.

In the late nineteenth and early twentieth centuries in America, alcohol was a prime ingredient in a wide assortment of nostrums such as nerve tonics, vegetable compounds, and elixirs. With a proof equal to that of a fairly good sherry, these compounds conferred their euphoric benefits even upon the ladies of the Women's Christian Temperance Union. At high doses, alcohol was also used as a general anesthetic in the nineteenth century, before the advent of chloroform and ether. However, the short duration of the effect required speedy action on the part of surgeons, many of whom were renowned for this aspect of their skill. Unfortunately, the low therapeutic index of the anesthetic—that is, the small difference between a lethal dose and that required for anesthesia, the absence of resuscitative devices and skills, and the haste of the surgeon contributed to the peril of patients so treated.

Alcohol Pharmacokinetics

Alcohol Absorption and Distribution

Alcohol is rarely consumed in its pure state; rather, it is found in 10% to 12% concentrations in wines, 3% to 5% in beers, and 40% to 50% in liquors; in the case of vodka, the alcohol is simply diluted with water. (The concentration is usually expressed as the alcoholic "proof," which is twice the percentage of concentration; e.g., 80 proof whiskey is 40% alcohol.) Thus, when we discuss alcohol consumption by humans, the reader can assume that it is consumed in one of the usual types of alcoholic beverages.

Alcohol differs significantly from other drugs in that a comparatively huge amount is required for the desired effects. The partition coefficient of alcohol between water and oil is about 30:1, indicating low lipid solubility. Thus, the diffusion of alcohol throughout the body very closely approximates that of water. Comparing alcohol with other sedatives, the effects of 1.5 ounces of liquor containing 18.7 grams of 95% alcohol can be obtained from just 5 milligrams of diazepam (Valium), a potency ratio of 1:3,740; and the effects of diazepam would last for at least 4 hours, while the effects of alcohol would dissipate in about an hour. The relative potency of diazepam and the duration of its effects are largely due to its high lipid solubility and slow dissociation from its receptor, whereas the low lipid solubility and high dissociation rate of alcohol explain the short duration of its effects and their rapid reversal in vivo (see Samson and Harris, 1992).

The reaction to alcohol intake depends upon many factors and thus is quite variable. One factor is the rate of alcohol absorption from the stomach and intestine into the bloodstream. Alcohol is a simple molecule that is completely miscible in water and can be almost completely absorbed into the bloodstream after oral ingestion. The mode of alcohol transport into or out of cells or tissues is passive diffusion, which is governed principally by the concentration gradient across cell membranes. Consequently, the rate of entrance of alcohol into the tissues of the body depends upon the blood supply to the tissues. Therefore, the alcohol concentration in the highly vascularized CNS rapidly comes into equilibrium with that in the systemic arterial blood, whereas relatively poorly perfused tissues, such as resting skeletal muscle and depot fat, accumulate alcohol more slowly. Further, as the alcohol slowly diffuses into the large mass of skeletal muscle, the blood level of alcohol falls, reversing the concentration gradient between the blood and the brain so that alcohol diffuses out of this organ. Thus, the psychological effects of an ounce or two of whiskey or a few bottles of beer are dissipated in a relatively short time, although there are many factors that determine the precise duration of that interval (see below).

One factor in determining the effects of alcohol after ingestion is the rate of alcohol absorption into the bloodstream. Under normal conditions, only about 10% of alcohol is absorbed from the stomach; most of the rest is absorbed at a higher rate when the stomach contents are emptied into the duodenum, the upper part of the small intestine. The high rate of absorption from the duodenum was demonstrated in patients that had undergone a massive gastrectomy (removal of the stomach). These patients experienced severe effects from even a small amount of alcohol, which after ingestion was immediately carried to the small intestine.

The overall rate of absorption is most rapid when alcohol is ingested in a 15% to 30% solution, and less rapid when the concentration is below 10% or above 30%. Higher concentrations may delay absorption by inhibiting gastric peristalsis and producing spasm of the pylorus, the valve between the stomach and the duodenum. These effects slow or prevent emptying of the stomach.

The rate of alcohol diffusion depends partly upon the volume of intake and the alcohol concentration of the beverage. The intrinsic properties of the beverage may also affect absorption; for example, beer is absorbed more slowly than whiskey or brandy, even if the alcohol concentrations are equated among the three beverages. The stomach contents also influence diffusion: the presence of food in the stomach slows the diffusion of alcohol out of the stomach and this effect is more pronounced when the stomach contents are proteins and carbohydrates rather than fats (see Pohorecky and Brick, 1990).

Body size and gender are additional factors in alcohol diffusion. Men tend to be larger than women and have a higher ratio of muscle to fat; thus, men have a proportionately greater vascular capacity because fat is not vascularized. Therefore, drink for drink, alcohol will be more diluted in the bloodstream of a man than in that of a woman. Furthermore, compared with men, women have proportionally more body fat, which does not absorb alcohol; therefore, even more alcohol, drink for drink, will be concentrated in the bloodstream of a woman.

Another factor is the rate of intake. Some alcohol abusers drink alcohol steadily in small doses from early morning to late at night, but they may not show signs of intoxication because the rate of alcohol metabolism keeps pace with their intake (see below). In contrast, some habitually drink rapidly until they become intoxicated, and some go on sporadic binges of heavy drinking over a few days that lead to gross intoxication over the entire period.

Alcohol Metabolism

The rate of alcohol metabolism and elimination also has a bearing on the drug's effects. The metabolism of alcohol occurs at a steady rate immediately after the drug is absorbed into the bloodstream and begins to pass through the liver. It is the balance between the absorption rate and the metabolic rate that largely determines the effect of alcohol consumption. Ninety percent of al-

cohol metabolism occurs in the liver, while the remaining 10% is exhaled through the lungs, excreted in the urine, or lost in perspiration.

Liver metabolism occurs in three steps. The first is oxidation via alcohol dehydrogenase (ADH) to form acetaldehyde (Figure 15.1a). ADH is a zinc-containing enzyme located in the cytoplasm of liver cells that utilizes the coenzyme nicotinamide adenine dinucleotide (NAD) as a hydrogen acceptor. Two other types of enzymes, catalase and mixed-function oxidases, are able to oxidize alcohol to acetaldehyde, but normally their effect is small. However, their activity may come into play during heavy and sustained drinking (see Israel and Mardones, 1971). Further, small amounts of ADH have been found in the mucosa of the stomach and small intestine, so a small amount of metabolism occurs there as well.

Acetaldehyde is a highly reactive and toxic substance, but normally its concentration is small and insignificant because it is rapidly converted by a second oxidative step, mediated by the cytoplasmic enzyme aldehyde dehydrogenase (ALDH) and NAD, into acetate (Figure 15.1b). Acetate is then released into the hepatic venous blood, where it combines with coenzyme A to form acetyl CoA, which enters the citric acid cycle. There it is oxidized to CO_2 and H_2O while yielding 7 calories per gram of alcohol.

The average person metabolizes 6–8 grams (7.5–10 ml) of alcohol per hour, and the rate is fairly constant for a given individual. Smaller amounts of alcohol are metabolized more slowly, but greater amounts are metabolized at a rate independent of the quantity present in the bloodstream. The maximal amount of alcohol that can be metabolized in 24 hours is 170 grams, and the rate-limiting factor is the availability of NAD, which requires the oxidation of the reduced form NADH. In the interest of obtaining a quick route from intoxication to sobriety, many attempts have been made to increase the rate of alcohol metabolism, but no practical method has been found. In some cases, however, some increase in metabolism after an increase in alcohol concentration has been shown, and this effect is presumed to be the result of the involvement of the other metabolizing pathways utilizing catalase and mixed-function alcohol hydroxylases. Early experiments by Gordon (1966, 1968) showed that perfusing rat livers with highly oxygenated blood (95%) markedly increased metabolism of high alcohol concen-

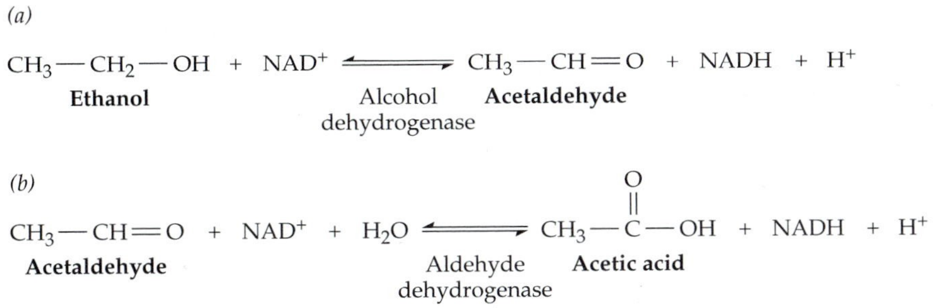

(a)

$$CH_3-CH_2-OH + NAD^+ \rightleftharpoons CH_3-CH=O + NADH + H^+$$
Ethanol   Alcohol **Acetaldehyde** dehydrogenase

(b)

$$CH_3-CH=O + NAD^+ + H_2O \rightleftharpoons CH_3-\overset{O}{\underset{||}{C}}-OH + NADH + H^+$$
Acetaldehyde   Aldehyde **Acetic acid** dehydrogenase

15.1 ALCOHOL METABOLISM. (a) Ethanol is oxidized by alcohol dehydrogenase to form acetaldehyde; (b) a second oxidative step converts acetaldehyde to acetate. See text for details.

trations, but the effect was not considered to be the result of direct aerobic oxidation of NADH in the cytoplasm.

There is an important gender difference in alcohol metabolism. It has been established that after ingestion of equivalent alcohol doses, there is substantially less alcohol dehydrogenase (ADH) activity in the gastric mucosa of women than in men, and the little gastric oxidation that does occur in women is virtually abolished in alcoholic women. Specifically, when ethanol equivalent to a few drinks was introduced into the stomachs of patients, ADH activity in the stomachs of nonalcoholic men was 70% to 80% higher than in nonalcoholic women; among alcoholics, the rate was reduced by 37% to 46% in men and 11% to 20% in women. These findings were buttressed by data showing that oxidation rates, after intravenous ethanol administration that bypassed the "first-pass" oxidative metabolism in the stomach, were no different between men and women and between alcoholics and nonalcoholics (Figure 15.2).

Despite the known toxicity of acetaldehyde, the ingestion of small or moderate amounts of alcohol does not present a threat of acetaldehyde toxicity, because of the rapidity of the second oxidative step (as mentioned above). Even in cases of intoxication, it is not likely that the symptoms are related to blood acetaldehyde levels. Evidence in support of this view was found by comparing the severity of alcohol-induced impairment with the time scale of the rise and fall of blood alcohol concentration (BAC) and that of acetaldehyde. As shown in Figure 15.3a, after rats received alcohol (2 g/kg) by gavage,

blood levels of acetaldehyde remained stable over time because the rate of alcohol oxidation and acetaldehyde formation was constant (due to enzyme saturation) while the BAC rose and fell. Figure 15.3b compares the course of behavioral impairment and the BAC, showing that the severity of behavioral symptoms correlates with the BAC rather than with the blood concentration of acetaldehyde. Further evidence comes from the use of pyrazole, which inhibits alcohol dehydrogenase and acetaldehyde formation.

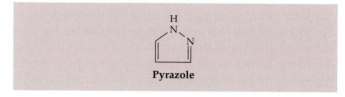

Rats treated with pyrazole were more impaired at a given BAC than control rats with the same BAC without pyrazole. Thus, blocking alcohol metabolism increased impairment, whereas if acetaldehyde were the cause of intoxication, the pyrazole-treated animals should have been symptom-free (see Goldstein, 1983). This finding is consistent with the difficulty of detecting acetaldehyde in the brain even when the BAC is high (see Deitrich et al., 1989). Nonetheless, though acetaldehyde itself may not be directly responsible for the symptoms of intoxication, it could contribute to the formation of biogenic aldehydes and other products that may be related to alcohol dependence (see below).

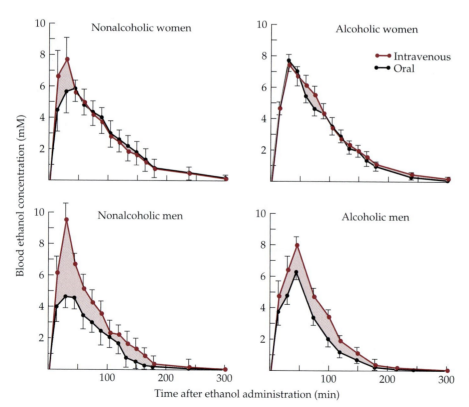

15.2 EFFECTS OF GENDER AND CHRONIC ALCOHOL ABUSE ON BLOOD ETHANOL CONCENTRATIONS. Ethanol was administered orally or intravenously in a dose of 0.3 g/kg body weight. The higher blood ethanol levels after oral ethanol intake by women compared to men, and the smaller shaded areas between their blood ethanol curves, show that first-pass metabolism (in the stomach) is lower in women than in men, and especially so in alcoholic women. (After Frezza et al., 1990.)

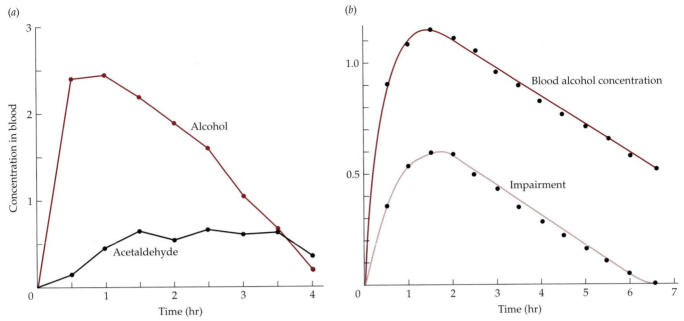

15.3 ALCOHOL-INDUCED IMPAIRMENT IS RELATED TO BLOOD ALCOHOL CONCEN-TRATION. (*a*) Blood acetaldehyde concentration remains stable while blood alcohol concentration rises and falls over time. (Blood levels of alcohol are in mg/ml; those of acetaldehyde are in μg/ml.) (*b*) The degree of behavioral impairment over time, as indicated by arbitrary units of motor incoordination, is a function of the blood alcohol concentration, not that of acetaldehyde as shown in (*a*). (After Goldstein, 1983; data from Goldberg, 1943 and Kalant et al., 1972.)

Another factor in determining the effects of alcohol ingestion is the acquired alcohol tolerance that results from chronic use. The subject of alcohol tolerance is discussed in greater detail later in this chapter.

Alcohol Use and Abuse

The Prevalence and Cost of Alcoholism

In the United States, nearly 75% of all adults drink alcohol occasionally. Most of these individuals have a drink or two to relieve the tensions of the working day. These drinking habits, along with occasional drinking at cocktail parties, weddings, and yes, funerals, are practiced by most alcohol users without deleterious effects.

For some drinkers, however, alcohol becomes a fast-acting anodyne that is easily available for reducing tension and anxiety brought on by serious problems with far-reaching consequences over which the drinker may have little or no control, such as a divorce, the loss of employment, the threat of a lawsuit, or a financial loss. In a culture that has few strictures on the use of alcohol, and in which it is readily available, its use as an anxiolytic for self-treatment can become a habit, albeit an expensive one.

Moreover, habitual drinking itself may become a source of conflict and anxiety in that time and money are wasted during drinking behavior, social relationships are lost or compromised, trustworthiness is diminished, little illegalities such as too many parking tickets grow into bigger ones such as auto accidents, health problems develop, and so on, so that relatively small anxieties begin to assume major proportions and threaten the drinker's career and family. The 15% of alcohol users in the United States that fit this description are considered to be heavy drinkers or subject to alcoholism. Other estimates are that 100 million Americans drink, and 10 million of those are classed as alcoholics.

What, then, defines an alcoholic? As defined by the American Medical Association in its *Manual on Alcoholism,*

> Alcoholism is an illness characterized by preoccupation with alcohol and loss of control over its consumption such as to lead usually to intoxication if drinking is begun; the condition is chronic, progressive, and has a tendency toward relapse. It is typically associated with physical disability and impaired emotional, occupational, and/or social adjustments as a direct consequence of persistent and excessive use of alcohol.

Among the problems of substance abuse in the United States, alcoholism is by far the most severe. More people become dependent on alcohol, become psychotic through excessive use of it, and are killed or disabled by it than by all other abused drugs (excluding tobacco) put together. For example, alcohol abuse accounts for 11 million accidents each year; in one year, 24,000 alcohol-related highway fatalities occurred. Also, 40% of admissions to mental hospitals and 50% of arrests are alcohol-related. Alcohol is a significant factor in the battered child syndrome, desertion, divorce, and impoverishment of families (see Miller, 1990). In 1990 alone, alcohol abuse was responsible for a drain of $136 billion from the U.S. economy due to lost production, health and welfare services, property damage, and medical expenses (Buck and Harris, 1991). In 1991 the Secretary of Health and Human Services, Louis Sullivan, reported that 18% of Americans had grown up living with an alcoholic or problem drinker, 10% of adults had been married to an alcoholic or problem drinker, and about 38% of adults had at least one blood relative who was an alcoholic.

Anxiety and Alcoholism

It has long been known that people suffering from chronic anxiety have an affinity for alcohol that is self-perpetuating because of alcohol's anxiolytic effects, which reinforce drinking. Alcohol ingestion rapidly diminishes anxiety, tension, and the perception of stress. Consistent with this view is the often-reported finding that persistent anxiety expressed as phobias, panic disorders, or obsessive–compulsive disorders frequently antedates the misuse of alcohol. The coprevalence of alcoholism and the anxiety disorders has been reviewed by Kushner, Sher, and Beitman (1990). Surveys of outpatients being treated for alcoholism show that a quarter of them manifest comorbid anxiety. In other studies it has been found that the coprevalence of alcoholism is 20% with the phobias, 10% with general anxiety disorders, 1.2% with panic disorder, and is 24% among those diagnosed as obsessive–compulsive, which is twice the rate of alcoholism in non-obsessive–compulsive controls (see Tollefson, 1991).

We may conclude that alcoholism is generated by cultural acceptance of the regular use of alcohol, its easy availability, the amount of stress that bears upon an individual, and one's sensitivity to that stress and to the reinforcing quality of an anxiolytic. It is also proposed that within the set of vectors converging on the individual leading to alcoholism, there is a genetically determined vulnerability that must also be taken into account (see below).

Alcohol-Related Fatalities

With so many individuals prone to alcoholism, it is not surprising that a significant number of dangerous alcohol overdoses occur. Alcohol is second only to carbon monoxide as an immediate cause of death by poisoning, and these two agents cause more deaths than all other lethal poisons put together. Acute alcohol poisoning results in death by causing edema (swelling) in the base of the brain, which contains the medullary centers of respiratory and cardiovascular regulation. Inexperienced young people are especially at risk when they rapidly consume large amounts of alcohol on a dare, or when they participate in an ill-advised drinking competition among peers. Also, because many substance abusers are multidrug users, fatal synergies are not uncommon. For example, if a person, after a heavy bout of drinking, takes a few capsules of a barbiturate hypnotic before going to bed, the effect of the two drugs will be additive and could be lethal. Ingesting this drug combination leads to competition between the two drugs for the metabolizing liver enzymes, which results in high blood levels of both drugs. Such an event may occur when a semi-stuporous person forgets about a previous dose of a barbiturate and takes another dose, which is enough to be fatal. This subject is discussed further in the section on barbiturates in Chapter 16.

Alcohol may also be a strong contributor to dangerous risks frequently taken by young people who become fatalities in auto and other accidents. Alcohol is also a factor in the deaths of intoxicated pedestrians killed in falls or while crossing busy streets and highways, people killed in fires set by smoking in bed, and people who die from exposure when they lose consciousness on deserted streets on a wintry night. Finally, a certain number of alcohol-related injuries and fatalities occur when alcoholics drink, by accident or out of desperation, alcohol that has been denatured with methyl (wood) alcohol (methanol). Methanol, as well as acetone, phenol, iodine, and other hydrocarbons, is added to ethanol when it is to be used in paint removers and thinners, antifreeze fluids, and canned fuels. Whereas the ultimate metabolites of ethanol are acetate, CO_2, and H_2O, methanol, which is not toxic in itself, when oxidized by the same enzymes is converted to formic acid and formaldehyde, which are especially toxic to the optic nerves. Fractional distillation may be attempted to separate the methyl from the ethyl alcohol, but the difference in the boiling points between the two alcohols is so small that complete separation is almost impossible, and chronic ingestion of even small amounts of the contaminated mixture can lead to blindness. The lethal dose of methanol is between 100 and 250 milliliters. If methyl alcohol poisoning is suspected, one mode of treatment is giving the patient ethyl alcohol, which competes favorably for the metabolizing enzymes until the methyl alcohol leaves the bloodstream via the kidneys, breath, and perspiration.

With respect to statistics on deaths related to alcohol, death certificates may not provide accurate data because the involvement of alcohol may not be known, and when it is known, it is often not reported in an attempt to protect the sensibilities of family survivors (Hofmann, 1983).

Adverse Systemic Effects of Alcoholism

When alcohol is used to excess, it can be damaging to almost all the tissues of the body, directly or indirectly.

This is partly due to the relatively large amounts that need to be ingested to obtain the desired effects, and partly due to the fact that alcohol is completely miscible in water and thus is rapidly distributed to virtually all tissues and organs. Moreover, high concentrations of alcohol are inherently toxic to biological tissue.

Some indirect effects are the result of alcohol metabolism involving the interaction of enzymes that become unbalanced, leading to kidney and liver dysfunction. Further, alcohol has no nutritional value outside of its caloric content. In contrast to the appetite-stimulating effect of a drink before dinner, excessive drinking depresses appetite and prevents an adequate absorption of amino acids, vitamins, and other nutrients, leading to the malnourished and debilitated state of the problem drinker. Further, although alcohol is not known to be a carcinogen, it is an effective solvent for known carcinogens, and thereby may enhance their circulation and metastases (the formation of new tumor sites). This effect may account for the epidemiologic finding of a linkage between alcoholism and certain cancers (see below) (Noble, 1984).

Table 15.1 lists most of the organic sites that are vulnerable to the toxic effects of alcoholism and other signs that may be present in alcoholism. Obviously, not all of these signs are seen in all alcoholics; after persistent alcohol abuse, there is a wide range in the occurrence and the severity of organ damage and other indirect effects. We shall describe the causes and the nature of specific alcohol-induced injuries below.

Effects on the Gastrointestinal System

Excessive use of alcohol can induce a wide range of injuries to the gastrointestinal (GI) system and associated organs. Frequent drinking of undiluted whiskey causes

---

Table 15.1   Signs of Alcoholism[a]

Bodily site or system affected	Sign
Skin	Pellagra; signs of trauma; infestation
Head	Fracture; subdural hematoma; other trauma
Mouth	Nutritional stomatitis; cheilosis; increased cancer incidence
Eyes	"Tobacco–alcohol" amblyopia; ophthalamoplegia (Wernicke–Korsakoff syndrome)
Gastrointestinal system	
Esophagus	Esophagitis; diffuse esophageal spasm; esophageal rupture; increased cancer incidence
Stomach and duodenum	Acute erosive gastritis; chronic hypertropic gastritis; peptic ulcer; hematemesis (bloody vomit); increased cancer incidence
Bowel	Malabsorption; "alcoholic diarrhea"
Liver	Steatosis (fatty degeneration); alcoholic hepatitis; cirrhosis
Pancreas	Acute pancreatitis; chronic recurrent pancreatitis
Respiratory system	Susceptibility to infection; fractured ribs; complications from smoking
Cardiovascular system	Cardiomyopathy
Genito-urinary tract	Hypogonadism (in men); impotence (in men); infertility (in women)
Endocrine and metabolic disorders	Decreased testosterone; hypoglycemia; hyperglycemia; protein malnutrition; vitamin B deficiencies
Neurological disorders	Acute withdrawal syndromes; amblyopia (optic neuropathy); Wernicke–Korsakoff syndrome; cerebellar degeneration; polyneuropathy; pellagra; Marchiafava–Bignami disease; central pontine myelinolysis; cerebral atrophy with dementia
Muscles	Myopathy

[a]Signs include direct and indirect physiological effects of chronic excessive alcohol intake, as well as indirect consequences of alcohol-impaired behavior.
Source: After Solomon, 1984.

irritation and blood engorgement of the tongue, erosion of the mucous membranes, ulceration inside the mouth, and cheilosis (bleeding of the lips and corners of the mouth). Similar effects occur in the esophagus, stomach, and small intestine.

One of the worst consequences of alcoholism is the increased risk of cancer of the tongue, mouth, oropharynx, esophagus, stomach, and liver. In North America, epidemiological studies have revealed that these cancers constitute 6.1% to 9.1% of all cancers in the white population, and 11.3 to 12.5% of cancers among blacks. Liver cancer is rarely a primary cancer in North America and Europe, but its presence is associated with cirrhosis, which is almost always associated with alcoholism. Also, there is a synergistic effect when alcohol and tobacco are used together. A study by Noble (1984) showed that heavy drinkers who smoked had risks of head and neck cancers that were 6 to 15 times greater than the risk to abstainers from both substances, and that the risk of esophageal cancer was 44 times greater among heavy users of both, whereas the risk was 18 times greater for users of alcohol and 5 times greater for users of tobacco alone (Figure 15.4). Finally, alcoholics with various cancers have poorer chances of survival and greater chances of developing another primary tumor than do nonalcoholic patients with the same cancer (see Noble, 1984).

Alcohol also causes a derangement in fat synthesis in the liver that leads to fat accumulation, a condition known as "fatty liver." This condition may be a precursor to cirrhosis, wherein damaged liver cells are replaced with connective tissue. Cirrhosis is the eighth leading cause of death in the U.S., and is the fourth leading cause of death in males between the ages of 35–54 (about 30,000 deaths per year; Noble, 1984; Sultatos and Soranno, 1991). A secondary consequence of alcohol-induced liver disease is damage to the brain. Known as hepato-encephalopathy, it is a result of malnutrition and the decreased ability of the liver to cleanse the blood of toxic substances that adversely affect the brain. If liver damage reaches this state, the chances of a reversal of the liver disease are remote.

Effects on the Cardiovascular System

Alcohol causes a vasodilation that produces a warm, flushed skin; thus, alcohol is frequently used to "warm up" the body in cold weather. However, the dilated peripheral blood vessels cause a greater heat loss, so that after the brief "warm-up," the person is colder than before. Furthermore, alcohol prevents reflexive cold-induced peripheral vasoconstriction, so that an intoxicated person will rapidly succumb to the cold. Bringing alcohol to sufferers from cold should be avoided in favor of hot soups and beverages. Frequent episodes of alcohol-induced vasodilation lead to the display of broken blood vessels in the upper cheeks adjacent to the nose, as well as an overall flushing of the face, which may become permanent.

With respect to the heart itself, some heavy drinkers develop alcohol cardiomyopathy (heart muscle damage), rhythm disturbances, and congestive heart failure. Some of these symptoms are due to thiamine deficiencies and are reversible by thiamine therapy, but others are not, and are probably due to the direct action of alcohol or its metabolites. Damage to the heart muscles is due to damage to the mitochondria, which results in impaired energy metabolism and respiration within the muscle cells. There are indications that protein synthesis is also impaired by acetaldehyde, thereby inhibiting the action of the enzymes within the heart muscles. These conditions are exacerbated by alcohol-induced hypertension. Some individuals who drank as much as three drinks per day had higher systolic and diastolic pressures than abstainers and those who drank fewer than three drinks daily. This relationship was independent of coffee and salt intake, cigarette smoking, adiposity, blood group, and educational attainment (see Noble, 1984).

15.4 RELATIVE RISK OF ESOPHAGEAL CANCER in relation to the daily consumption of alcohol and cigarette smoking. Compared with nonsmokers and moderate or nondrinkers (*lower left*), the risk is 44.4 times greater for individuals who daily smoke 20 or more cigarettes and drink 81 or more grams of alcohol, about six or more drinks (*upper right*). (After U.S. Congress on Alcohol and Health, June 1978.)

Effects on Reproductive Functions

Alcohol abuse is known to affect male and female reproductive organs and sexual function. In males it may cause impotence, testicular atrophy, a decrease in the size of the prostate and seminal vesicles, a decrease of facial and body hair, gynecomastia (enlargement of male breasts), and loss of sexual interest. Chronic alcoholism also diminishes testosterone levels, and even nonalcoholic men show a transient drop in testosterone levels after a drinking bout. Among alcoholic women ovarian functions are disrupted, leading to anovulation, luteal phase dysfunction, and amenorrhea. An extensive investigation of the effects of alcohol on a nonclinical sample of 917 women revealed an alcohol-related incidence of menstrual disorders such as dysmenorrhea (painful menstruation), heavy menstrual flow, and premenstrual discomfort. Women who consumed six or more drinks per day at least five times per week had a higher incidence of gynecological surgery (other than hysterectomy) and obstetric disorders.

Effects on the CNS

Behavioral manifestations.

Whereas alcohol has substantial effects on many organ systems, the central nervous system is most obviously affected by this drug, judging by its almost immediate elicitation of change in subjective feelings and motor effects. The rapidity of these effects is due to the complete solubility of alcohol in water, which results in its rapid absorption into the blood and distribution throughout the highly vascularized brain.

Although alcohol is often thought of as a stimulant, it is foremost a CNS depressant, and the perception of its stimulating effects reflects unrestrained activity in some parts of the brain because of the alcohol-induced suppression of inhibitory control mechanisms. Alcohol depresses both excitatory and inhibitory postsynaptic potentials, but the centers mediating the most highly integrated functions of the brain are especially sensitive to alcohol effects. Among these centers are the polysynaptic linkages of the reticular activating system and certain cortical sites. Hence, under the influence of high doses of alcohol, the cortex is released from a major part of its integrated control. Consequently, the processes that are related to thought, sobriety, and self-restraint are among the first to be disorganized, and the smooth operation of psychomotor activities such as speech, locomotion, and fine motor coordination are disrupted.

The physical and psychological effects of alcohol can be related to the BAC, which is given as grams of alcohol per 100 milliliters of blood. For example, a person having 0.1 grams of alcohol per 100 milliliters of blood (100 mg/dl) would have a BAC of 0.1%. This level can be reached by consuming one drink (1.5 oz of 80 proof liquor, 5 oz of wine, or 12 oz of beer) for every 35 pounds of body weight in an hour (5 drinks for a 175-lb person). In most of the United States, such a person would be considered legally drunk, and he or she would be staggering, drowsy, and incoherent.

Neuropathology.

Chronic alcoholics are subject to a variety of neuropathologies caused by the direct or indirect effects of alcohol. An indirect effect of alcoholism is evidence of brain lacerations or subdural hematomas (blood clots) that may have resulted from blows to the head from falls or other accidents while intoxicated. Another indirect effect is the alcohol-induced nutritional deficiencies described above that adversely affect normal brain function. Most of the early data were supplied from brain autopsies of known alcoholics, which showed that 50% to 100% of them (depending upon the selectivity of the referring alcohol treatment centers) had significant brain pathologies.

Later studies by Carlen and coworkers (1978) examined the brains of heavy drinkers and alcoholics using noninvasive brain scanning techniques. Their data confirmed early autopsy findings of brain shrinkage, increased ventricle size, and a widening of the sulci that is related to a reduction in the volume of white matter in the cerebral hemispheres. Brain scanning techniques have also revealed Marchiafava-Bignami disease, a rare disorder formerly identified only by autopsy. This disorder is characterized by necrosis of the corpus callosum and the adjacent subcortical white matter. This condition, predominantly found in malnourished alcoholics, is marked by dementia, spasticity, dysarthria (poor speech articulation), and locomotor difficulties. The course of this syndrome is variable—some patients recover, some survive for many years in a demented condition, and some lapse into a coma and die (Charness, Simon, and Greenberg, 1989). Another study using scanning methods showed that thinning of the corpus callosum appeared even among some heavy social drinkers (Bergman et al., 1980).

With respect to the gray matter in the brains of alcoholics, there was a specific loss and shrinkage of neurons, as well as supporting glia and vasculature, in the superior frontal cortex, suggesting that this area is more susceptible to alcohol brain damage than other cortical areas. Although there were no neuron losses in other areas, there was neuron shrinkage in the cingulate and motor areas that was related to reduction of the dendritic arborizations and the diameter of the cell bodies. Autopsies showed similar shrinkage effects and loss of synapses in the Purkinje cells of the cerebellum and the hippocampal pyramidal cells. Thus, excessive alcohol intake may detrimentally affect behavioral and mental processes. Among the elderly, alcohol-induced peripheral and CNS neural degeneration may be superimposed upon the normal attrition of nerve cells that occurs characteristically with aging.

How does alcohol damage the brain? Studies with animals have shown that alcohol depresses the synthesis of brain protein and RNA, substances that are necessary for neuronal maintenance and function. These deficiencies have been related to defects in human cognitive functions such as memory and learning. Fortunately, alcoholics who curtailed their alcohol intake or abstained altogether showed significant reversals of brain shrinkage as early as 1 month after the start of abstinence. These studies suggested that the effect of abstinence is the remyelination of axons in the white matter and the regrowth of the axonal and dendritic neuropil as well as the supporting glia and vasculature. These changes presumably underlie the reversible aspects of alcohol-induced brain atrophy and functional brain impairment (see Carlen et al., 1978).

Nevertheless, there are some changes in the brain that are irreversible. This is especially true in the cerebellum, where atrophy occurs among 27% to 42% of alcoholics, compared with an overall incidence of 1.7%. Cerebellar atrophy typically occurs only after about 10 years of excessive alcohol use. It is characterized by cell losses variously estimated at between 11% and 36%, and is clinically manifested by ataxia and incoordination, particularly in the lower limbs (Harper and Kril, 1990). It is not known whether these effects are directly related to alcohol, as the cerebellar ataxia does not correlate with the daily, annual, or lifetime consumption of alcohol.

Another condition, the Wernicke–Korsakoff syndrome (WKS), is a two-stage pathology associated with heavy drinking, alcoholism, and a thiamine deficiency. In the Wernicke stage, there is a widespread polyneuropathy characterized by peripheral neuritis, leading to sensory disturbances in the extremities, including localized areas of hyperesthesia (excessive skin sensitivity) or anesthesia, numbness and pain in the lower legs, and signs of impaired motor and sensory innervation and reduced reflexes. These signs may ultimately progress to the upper extremities, along with contractures and paralysis. In some cases there are visual abnormalities, such as nystagmus, which are due to weakness of the oculomotor muscles, alcohol amblyopia (blurred vision for near and far objects), central scotomata (black areas in the visual fields), which may be related to inflammation of the optic papilla (the blind spot), and damage to the optic nerve where it passes through the papilla. There are also states of delirium representing acute toxic episodes.

In the later Korsakoff stage, there are amnestic–confabulatory states (loss of memory leading to fictitious descriptions of past events). These memory deficits were described by Sergei Korsakoff in 1889; hence the disorder was known as Korsakoff's psychosis. The amnesia is anterograde, meaning that there is an inability to learn anything new, although there is fairly good recall for events that occurred prior to the brain damage.

With respect to the role of thiamine in WKS, it has long been known that thiamine deficits produce polyneuropathy including the sensory and motor deficits described above. In addition to the thiamine deficit brought about by alcohol-related malnutrition, alcohol may also block intestinal thiamine absorption. Finally, the symptoms of peripheral neuritis and confusional states can be reversed by thiamine therapy if it is initiated promptly, although the amnestic symptoms may not be completely reversed.

Gender and Alcohol-Related Pathology

Neuropsychological and neuroradiological studies, as reported by Harper and Kril (1990), have suggested that females are more susceptible to alcohol-related brain damage than males. First of all, as mentioned earlier, for a given amount of ingested alcohol, women attain higher peak levels of blood alcohol concentration per unit of body weight than men because the lower muscle/fat ratio in women results in lower vascular volumes. At the same time, because alcohol is soluble in water and there is little water in fat, there will be proportionately more alcohol in the blood of females, who generally have more body fat than males. Furthermore, as described earlier, gastric metabolism of alcohol is slower in women than in men.

All of these gender-related factors—muscle/fat ratio, water and vascular volume, and first-pass alcohol oxidation by the stomach mucosa—contribute to the higher bioavailability of, and consequent higher vulnerability to, given amounts of alcohol in women than in men. The greater bioavailability of alcohol in women may account for the occurrence of liver damage in women after shorter drinking histories and at lower levels of alcohol intake than for men. Also, neuropsychological studies have shown that after similar drinking histories, women performed worse during psychological testing than men; and neuroradiological studies have shown that women alcoholics experienced brain shrinkage and ventricular enlargements equal to those in men, even though the women had shorter drinking histories and lower peak alcohol consumption (Jacobson, 1986). However, in this same study, it was shown that the women who became abstinent had a faster and more complete return to normalcy than the men (see Harper and Kril, 1990; and Frezza et al., 1990).

Neuromolecular Effects of Alcohol

The development of microanalytic methods has provided information about the direct effects of alcohol upon neural tissue (Fleurel-Balter et al., 1983; Goldstein and Chin, 1981; Klemm and Foster, 1986). Here, it should be noted that, for the most part, these microanalytic methods have been used on animal tissue, and the question has been raised whether the effects are similar to those in humans. For example, rats may be subjected to forced intake of alcohol, or some species may have a predisposition for preferring alcohol solutions over tap water, but these are hardly the same patterns of alcohol intake as that of a human alcoholic; and using human volunteers for various patterns of chronic alcohol intake and then asking them to supply tissue samples for analysis is difficult to justify. Nonetheless, there are sufficient morphological and physiological similarities among mammalian nervous systems so that studying the biochemical reaction of animal neural tissue to alcohol can be justified. However, the interpretation of animal data must carefully take into account the precise goal of the experiments, as well as the species used and the conditions under which the experiments were performed (see McClearn, 1988; Ollat, Parvez, and Parvez, 1988; Tipton, 1988).

Among researchers hoping to understand alcohol-induced changes in the CNS, attention has been drawn to the binding affinity of neural membranes for various drugs and to patterns of ion transport. Many investigations have revealed that alcohol affects some structures and functions of neuronal membranes in a general way, but the influences can also be highly specific. Alcohol readily penetrates cell membranes and alters the fatty acid interaction of the lipid layers, thereby increasing membrane "fluidity" and permeability (see Chapter 3). This effect is common to virtually all anesthetics, whose potency is directly related to lipid solubility, and the sedative effect of alcohol has been at least partly traced to this effect. For example, comparisons between brain membranes taken from long-sleep (LS) and short-sleep (SS) mice showed that the LS mice, which are more sensitive to the sedative effects of alcohol, also had membranes that were more sensitive to the lipid-fluidizing effects of alcohol added in vitro. However, after prolonged consumption, alcohol increased the cholesterol/phospholipid ratio in membranes, thereby altering the lipid layers to increase membrane rigidity. This change reduced the effects of alcohol and is presumed to be a factor underlying the development of tolerance and dependence (Buck and Harris, 1991; Deitrich et al., 1989; Johnson et al., 1979).

In another study, Rottenberg, Waring, and Rubin (1981) used an electron paramagnetic resonance (EPR) technique to examine the effects of chronic alcohol treatment on liver mitochondrial and brain synaptosomal membranes of rats and mice. They found that in animals chronically fed with alcohol, both types of membranes became resistant to the fluidizing effects of alcohol and showed a reduction in alcohol binding. Moreover, the membranes of these animals were also resistant to the disordering effect of the inhalation anesthetic halothane, even though halothane is about 50 times more potent

than alcohol in disordering membranes. Similar effects were found for the binding of the sedative drug phenobarbital; hence, these mechanisms are presumed to underlie not only tolerance and dependence, but cross-tolerance as well. However, later studies suggested that whereas the precise mechanisms underlying the cross-tolerance between alcohol and barbiturates may be similar with respect to the drug-induced changes in the cell membrane lipid processes, they may not be identical with respect to the receptors, ionophores, and enzymes that are affected by these two substances (Tabakoff, Cornell, and Hoffman, 1986; see also the section on tolerance below).

Ion channels are among the membrane elements influenced by alcohol. For example, Cl^- flux through the ionophore associated with the $GABA_A$ receptor is inhibited in the presence of alcohol. (This subject is discussed in greater detail in the following section on alcohol–GABA interactions.) Various cation channels can also be affected by alcohol. For example, studies have shown that alcohol decreases voltage-dependent Na^+ and Ca^{2+} influx into synaptosomal preparations. These effects contribute to the inhibitory influence of alcohol on neural excitability and neurotransmitter release. Alcohol also seems to suppress ion currents associated with the NMDA and kainate receptor subtypes for excitatory amino acids (see Chapter 10 for further details). In contrast, the action of acetylcholine at nicotinic receptors and of 5-HT at $5-HT_3$ receptors is enhanced by acute alcohol treatment (Figure 15.5; Buck and Harris, 1991; Ollat, Parvez, and Parvez, 1988; Samson and Harris, 1992).

Many of the effects of acute alcohol exposure on ion channels are reversed when the drug is administered

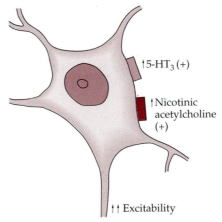

15.5 EFFECTS OF ACUTE ALCOHOL EXPOSURE ON $5-HT_3$ AND NICOTINIC CHOLINERGIC RECEPTORS. Alcohol (ethanol) has been reported to facilitate (up arrow) the action of two ligand-gated channels, the $5-HT_3$ receptor and the nicotinic cholinergic receptor. Because both receptors gate cation channels and thus lead to depolarization (+), the influence of alcohol would be to increase the excitability of the cells expressing these channels. (After Samson and Harris, 1992.)

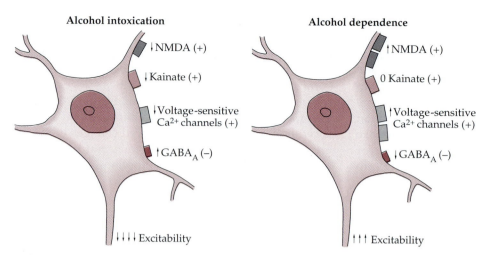

15.6 EFFECTS OF ACUTE AND CHRONIC ALCOHOL EXPOSURE ON AMINO ACID NEUROTRANSMITTER RECEPTORS AND CALCIUM CHANNELS. Acute alcohol intoxication has been reported to facilitate (up arrow) the action of some $GABA_A$ receptors and to inhibit (down arrow) NMDA and kainate receptors as well as voltage-sensitive Ca^{2+} channels. These effects would be expected to reduce cell excitability. However, chronic alcohol treatment causes increases in the density of NMDA receptors and voltage-sensitive Ca^{2+} channels, as well as a decrease in $GABA_A$ receptor function. Such changes should lead to increased excitability when alcohol is abruptly withdrawn, thus contributing to the phenomena associated with dependence; 0 indicates no change. (After Samson and Harris, 1992.)

chronically. Chronic alcohol administration leads to reduced $GABA_A$ receptor function and an increased density of NMDA receptors (Figure 15.6). Another potentially important effect concerns L-type Ca^{2+} channels, which are located on neuronal cell bodies and dendrites and are thought to mediate many Ca^{2+}-activated second messenger functions. The density of these channels is thought to increase as a result of repeated alcohol treatment. Moreover, this change may play a significant role in alcohol tolerance and dependence. When L-type channel antagonists such as nitrendipine or PN 200-100 were repeatedly coadministered with alcohol, tolerance to alcohol's ataxic effects was either prevented or delayed. Furthermore, these same drugs have been reported to reduce convulsions following withdrawal from chronic alcohol treatment (Buck and Harris, 1991; Ollat, Parvez, and Parvez, 1988; Samson and Harris, 1992).

In addition to ion channels, certain second messenger systems are targets of alcohol action. The cAMP system is particularly noteworthy in this regard, since alcohol has been shown to stimulate adenylyl cyclase activity in both neural and nonneural tissues. Although an elevation of basal activity has sometimes been reported, the greatest effects found have generally been on cAMP formation in response to hormones or neurotransmitters. For example, alcohol enhances dopamine-stimulated adenylyl cyclase activity in the striatum and β-adrenergic receptor–mediated activity in the cerebral cortex (Buck and Harris, 1991; Hoffman and Tabakoff, 1990; Ollat, Parvez, and Parvez, 1988). It was also found that the brain concentration of cGMP undergoes a sharp

decrease, especially in the cerebellum, after a single alcohol dose, and that this effect is dose related. However, the effect is quickly reversed once alcohol is eliminated. Furthermore, these same effects are seen after treatment with anxiolytic drugs such as barbiturates and benzodiazepines, and may be related to the ataxia seen after the drug treatment (see Goldstein, 1983; and Ollat, Parvez, and Parvez, 1988).

One site at which alcohol influences second messenger systems is the stimulatory G protein G_s (see Chapter 6 for further information on G proteins). In both the cortex and striatum, alcohol increased the rate of G_s activation. Depending on the area being examined, other effects included enhancement of the interaction of α_s (the α-subunit of G_s) with either guanine nucleotides or the catalytic unit of adenylyl cyclase. The inhibitory G protein G_i shows little response to alcohol, indicating at least some specificity concerning the interaction of alcohol with G_s. Furthermore, various lipid fluidizing substances, such as halothane or the organic solvent chloroform, differed at least somewhat from alcohol in their effects on G proteins and adenylyl cyclase activity. Hence, this aspect of alcohol action may not result entirely from its perturbing influence on membrane lipids (Buck and Harris, 1991; Hoffman and Tabakoff, 1990).

The cAMP system appears to undergo an adaptive response to repeated alcohol administration in that receptor-stimulated adenylyl cyclase activity in many tissues is reduced rather than elevated. This finding has been obtained not only in animal models in which neural changes can be studied, but also in blood lymphocytes and platelets obtained from human alcoholics. Alterations in G_s again are intimately involved in the response to chronic alcohol exposure, although the exact nature of these alterations is still being investigated. The important point is that second messenger systems and G proteins are likely participants in the neural mechanisms underlying the reinforcing effects of alcohol, as well as in the development of alcohol tolerance and dependence (Buck and Harris, 1991; Hoffman and Tabakoff, 1990).

We have seen that alcohol exerts a number of effects on cell membrane constituents. Alcohol has an inhibitory influence on voltage-dependent Na^+ and Ca^{2+} channels, which results in reduced excitability and neurotransmitter release. Such effects are rather diffuse, reflecting the involvement of virtually all areas of the CNS. On the other hand, alcohol also influences several ligand-gated channels, and acutely stimulates G_s activation and receptor-mediated cAMP formation. These effects are, of course, more specific with respect to brain region and cell type. Finally, many of the elements that respond to acute alcohol exposure show compensatory changes following chronic treatment, and at least some of these changes may play important roles in the phenomena of alcohol tolerance and dependence.

Alcohol–GABA Interactions

Although alcohol–GABA interactions are described in some detail in Chapter 10 as well as in earlier sections of this chapter, a brief review of those discussions will serve as an introduction here. Alcohol–GABA interactions are significantly and directly involved in the central effects of alcohol. On the molecular level, Cl^- ionophores are more reactive to alcohol than the Na^+ and the K^+ channels. In particular, alcohol activates the $GABA_A$ receptor–coupled Cl^- channel, thereby increasing Cl^- conductance and postsynaptic inhibition by means of a transient decrease in the postsynaptic membrane potential. This is in keeping with the finding that alcohol at concentrations of 5 mM or lower potentiates $GABA_A$ receptor–coupled Cl^- uptake to effect postsynaptic inhibition in neocortical, cerebellar, and spinal cord neurons. At 50 mM, alcohol acts in a GABA-mimetic fashion to directly activate Cl^- channels.

Moreover, the wide distribution of the $GABA_A$ receptors is indicative of the multiple effects they have on CNS functions, and seems to explain many of the effects of alcohol on the CNS. For example, activating $GABA_A$ receptors results in sedation and a decrease of muscle tone, whereas blocking these receptors with bicuculline or picrotoxin results in excitation and generalized seizures. Further, the $GABA_A$ receptor is presumed to mediate tonic inhibition within the CNS, as it affects cognition, motor activity, and sensory functions. Thus, the effect of alcohol on the $GABA_A$ complex may be involved in the impaired cognition and incoordination caused by mild intoxication, or with the ataxia and seda-

tion caused by moderate alcohol intake (Buck and Harris, 1991).

In an early experiment, Nestoros (1980) demonstrated this alcohol–GABA interaction by using multi-barreled micropipettes to release alcohol, GABA, and other substances, alone or successively, on cortical cells of cats. When GABA was released from one barrel followed by alcohol from another, the GABA-induced inhibition of postsynaptic cell firing was potentiated. All the effects of alcohol occurred within 10 seconds after its release, and were fully reversible within 1–3 minutes. Similar effects were obtained when alcohol was administered intravenously while cortical cells were electrically stimulated or iontophoretically stimulated with GABA. These findings raised questions as to whether the effect was caused by blockade of GABA uptake, induction of GABA release, or a direct effect on postsynaptic receptors. In one attempt to answer these questions, glycine was released from one barrel followed by alcohol from another. Though glycine inhibited postsynaptic cell firing, alcohol neither enhanced nor antagonized glycine-induced inhibition. Thus, it is unlikely that alcohol was acting directly upon Cl^- channels. This conclusion was supported by the finding that alcohol could potentiate the effects of GABA at alcohol doses that were ineffective by themselves at opening Cl^- channels. Therefore, rather than being a direct GABA receptor agonist, it is more likely that alcohol potentiates GABA by acting upon a regulatory site located on or near the GABA receptor binding site. There is evidence that GABA mediates the sedative and antianxiety effects of alcohol, as shown by the effect of the GABA antagonist bicuculline, which diminished the behavioral effects of alcohol intoxication, and that of GABA agonists such as aminooxyacetic acid (AAOA), which potentiated them.

These findings were later supported by evidence that GABA receptors, at least to some degree, are associated with other receptor sites for anxiolytic drugs such as the benzodiazepines (see Chapter 10). It is within these receptor complexes that alcohol exerts its influence. This was dramatically shown when the benzodiazepine derivative Ro 15-4513, which binds to the complex, was found to block the intoxicating and anxiolytic effects of alcohol by antagonizing the alcohol-stimulated Cl^- ion transport. The Ro 15-4513 effect on alcohol was itself blocked by benzodiazepine receptor antagonists, which block the binding of Ro 15-4513. These findings provided additional evidence that alcohol exerts these effects within the GABA–benzodiazepine receptor complex.

Interactions between Alcohol and Other Neurotransmitters

Many investigators have attempted to establish the possible connection between neurotransmitter action and alcohol effects: intoxication, tolerance, dependence, craving, and withdrawal. These attempts have been reviewed by Ollat, Parvez, and Parvez (1988) and Deitrich and colleagues (1989). We have already mentioned the involvement of GABA activity as it relates to activation of Cl⁻ ionophores. With respect to the other known transmitters, the interdependence among them must be taken into account in the sense that alteration in the activity of one transmitter nearly always induces changes in the others. However, one can examine the role of one transmitter at a time in the expression of a given effect that is associated with alcohol ingestion.

Alcohol–dopamine interactions.   One obvious question concerns the role of dopamine (DA) in alcohol-induced craving because such craving may reflect the activity of a DA-mediated reward system (see Chapter 8). In a review of animal studies by Wise and Bozarth (1987), it was reported that depressing central DA function by a variety of means reduced voluntary alcohol consumption in alcohol-craving rats. That finding suggested that DA may mediate alcohol reinforcement and craving. In related work, low doses (0.5–2.0 g/kg) of alcohol stimulated the activity of DA pathways and enhanced spontaneous as well as experimentally induced synaptic release of DA. Alcohol also stimulated DA synthesis, accelerated DA turnover, and increased cerebral DA concentrations. These effects were due to direct effects of alcohol and were not due to a compensatory rebound from blockade of DA receptors. These effects might be related to the euphoriant effects in humans of low alcohol doses. Behaviorally consistent effects were shown when low doses stimulated rodent motor activity, an effect that was DA-dependent and was blocked by pretreatment with catecholamine synthesis blockers. Also, low doses of alcohol increased the firing rate of DA neurons in the ventral tegmental area (VTA) and the substantia nigra, whereas high doses had the opposite effect, presumably because at high doses alcohol directly stimulated the GABAergic striatonigral inhibitory feedback pathway, which projects from the striatum to the DA cells in the substantia nigra (see Di Chiara and Imperato, 1985, 1986, 1988).

Using an in vivo microdialysis technique in the brains of awake and freely moving rats, Di Chiara and Imperato (1985) found that low doses (0.5 g/kg) of alcohol increased the release of DA from the nucleus accumbens, but had no effect on the striatum. Larger doses (2.5–5 g/kg) also caused an increase; however, still higher doses decreased DA release in the nucleus accumbens but caused a release in the striatum. This finding suggested that rats having a preference for alcohol might be more sensitive to the stimulatory effects of alcohol upon the DA cells of the VTA.

Experiments on the effect of chronic alcohol intoxication showed that it produced DA hypofunction by diminishing DA release by 80% compared with controls. Alcohol reduced the stimulant effect of the DA agonist apomorphine, reduced the hypothermic effect of the DA receptor agonist piribedil, and reduced DA-sensitive adenylyl cyclase activity. In other words, chronic alcohol intoxication tends to down-regulate DA systems. This conclusion is borne out further by the finding that chronically intoxicated animals, when temporarily abstinent, are insensitive to the stimulant activity of low alcohol doses. They also show reduced DA turnover and reduced DA release in the striatum. They display decreased withdrawal signs with L-DOPA and an aggravation of symptoms after receiving doses of the DA receptor blocker haloperidol (see Wise and Bozarth, 1987). Finally, recent studies by Diana and colleagues (1993) showed a marked reduction in VTA cell firing and nucleus accumbens DA overflow during alcohol withdrawal in rats. If similar effects occur in humans, they could play an important role in the dysphoria associated with alcohol abstinence in alcoholics.

Alcohol and biogenic amine metabolites.   In the 1970s there was considerable interest in the interactions among the metabolites of alcohol and the biogenic amines (norepinephrine, dopamine, serotonin, etc.). It was proposed that such interactions might lead to the synthesis of alkaloids and other biotransformation products that are toxic to the nervous system as well as to other organs (see Goldstein, 1983). It was also thought that those products could play a role in the autonomic and behavioral side effects of alcohol and might underlie the mechanism of alcohol dependence. This approach, known as the "biogenic aldehyde hypothesis" (Deitrich and Erwin, 1975), developed from earlier findings about the toxicology of the alcohol metabolite acetaldehyde. For example, acetaldehyde is 10 to 30 times more toxic than alcohol. It releases catecholamines, an effect that has been implicated in alcohol cardiomyopathy. Acetaldehyde is believed to be the basis of the disulfiram–alcohol reaction (see the section below on this subject). Acetaldehyde can form condensation products with catecholamines and indoleamines to form biogenic aldehydes such as tetrahydro-β-carbolines (THBCs) and tetrahydroisoquinolines (TIQs), which are precursors to morphine alkaloids in plants. TIQs and related products have been postulated to play an etiologic role in various pathologies such as Parkinson's disease, schizophrenia, and phenylketonuria.

In the course of alcohol intoxication, biogenic aldehydes are found both in animals and humans, and in excess probably participate in the effects of alcohol on the CNS. (For more details and references, see Ollat, Parvez, and Parvez, 1988; Rahwan, 1975.) Normally after high rates of alcohol ingestion, the activity of ALDH to metabolize acetaldehyde is accelerated, and therefore less of the enzyme is available to oxidize the aldehyde intermediates of catecholamine metabolism. For example, it was found that alcohol administration to human subjects resulted in impaired ALDH activity on exogenously administered [14C]norepinephrine (NE). Specifically, alcohol diminished the oxidative metabolism of 3,4-dihydroxyphenylglycoaldehyde (DHPGA) to form 3,4-dihydroxymandelic acid (DHMA) and elevated reductive metabolism to form 3,4-dihydroxyphenylglycol (DHPG) (see Figure 8.18). A similar response occurs during serotonin metabolism; that is, after alcohol ingestion, the reductive metabolic path for the intermediate 5-hydroxyindoleacetaldehyde to form 5-hydroxytryptophol is preferred to the usual oxidative path to form 5-hydroxyindoleacetic acid (5-HIAA) (see Figure 9.8). These findings imply an alcohol-induced impairment of ALDH activity and an increase of aldehyde reductase activity.

When DA is metabolized within axon terminals, it is first oxidized and deaminated by MAO to form the intermediate 3,4-dihydroxyphenylacetaldehyde (DHPA) (see Figure 8.17). In the next step DHPA is further oxidized by ALDH to form the corresponding acid 3,4-dihydroxyphenylacetic acid (DOPAC). However, a substantial intake of alcohol and its metabolism to high concentrations of acetaldehyde would saturate the small amount of ALDH in the brain, leaving little or no ALDH to oxidize DHPA, thus causing a buildup of DHPA. It is to be noted, however, that because alcohol dehydrogenase is virtually absent in the brain, very little alcohol is metabolized there. Consequently, any appreciable amount of brain acetaldehyde would have to come from the liver via the bloodstream, but if the blood level of acetaldehyde were high enough, it could affect brain DA metabolism.

An early study by Davis and Walsh (1970) examined the possibility that an acetaldehyde-induced impairment of ALDH-mediated DA metabolism could lead to a buildup of DHPA, which could form condensation products with dopamine. One such product is tetrahydropapaveroline (THP), which turns out to be an intermediate in the biosynthesis of morphine in the opium poppy.

Such reactions could readily occur at high rates in brain areas rich in DA, such as the substantia nigra and the VTA and the target sites of the mesostriatal and the mesolimbocortical projections. Furthermore, because these areas are relatively low in aldehyde-oxidizing activity, they are inordinately sensitive to inhibitors of ALDH. In turn, morphinelike derivatives of these products could be the basis for the addictive property of alcohol.

To test their hypothesis, Davis and Walsh incubated rat brain stem homogenates with dopamine and acetaldehyde or alcohol. They found significant increases of THP levels among the catechol metabolites. Moreover, they also found that in rats, THP can undergo biotransformation to morphinelike compounds. Specifically, intravenous administration of [14C]THP resulted in radioactive excretions, 50% of which indicated the presence of normorphine, morphine, norcodeine, and codeine. Figure 15.7 shows the steps in the condensation of dopamine and DHPA to form THP, as well as the nonenzymatic condensation of acetaldehyde and dopamine to form the biogenic aldehyde salsolinol. Based on this demonstration of alcohol-induced enhanced biosynthesis of THP and opiate derivatives in neural tissue, Davis and Walsh (1970) proposed that endogenous THP formation might be the basis of alcohol addiction (see Rahwan, 1975). However, this hypothesis has been largely unsupported by subsequent research (see Ollat, Parvez, and Parvez, 1988).

Alcohol and the opioid system. In line with the above discussion, we will mention some experimental research on direct alcohol interactions with opiates and with opioids, which are endogenous peptides with opiatelike characteristics (see Chapter 12). The importance of this subject rests upon the knowledge that these three substances—alcohol, opiates, and opioids—produce many similar neuropharmacological responses—namely, hy-

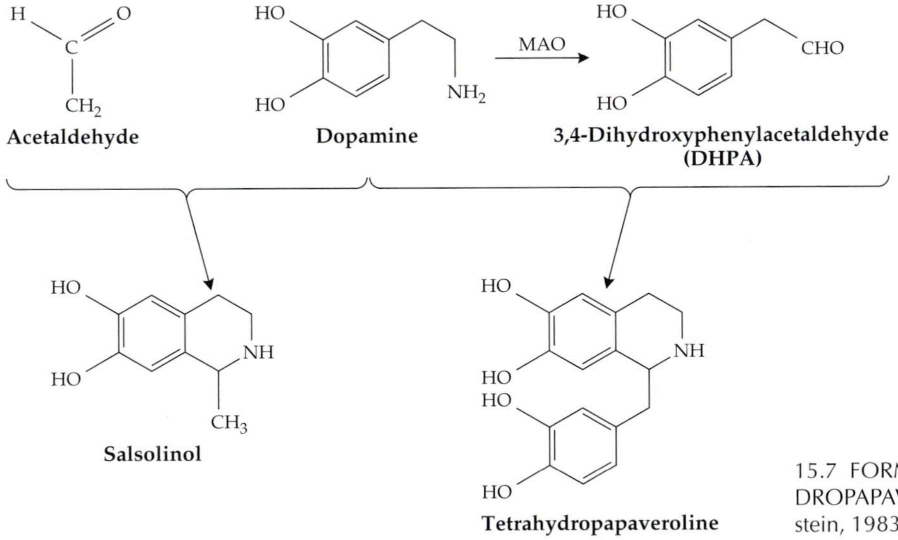

15.7 FORMATION OF SALSOLINOL AND TETRAHYDROPAPAVEROLINE FROM DOPAMINE. (After Goldstein, 1983.)

pothermia, euphoria, analgesia, and motor activation, as well as tolerance and dependence. First, it was reported that acute alcohol administration increased plasma levels of the opioid β-endorphin in humans and increased Met-enkephalin levels in the rat brain (hypothalamus, striatum, and midbrain) and pituitary gland. Whether the alcohol-induced alterations in Met-enkephalin were due to changes in the release, synthesis, or degradation of the opioid was not known. It has been found, however, that drugs that block the degradation of enkephalins increase voluntary alcohol consumption in rats (Froehlich et al., 1990, 1991). Other studies have shown that alcohol-preferring strains of mice and rats had higher levels of basal β-endorphin and met-enkephalin in the pituitary gland and in some brain areas compared with alcohol-nonpreferring rodents.

Another way of demonstrating a relationship between alcohol and opiates is by the use of opioid receptor antagonists. For example, it was shown that the opiate antagonists naloxone suppressed alcohol consumption without altering water intake in rats that were bred for high voluntary alcohol drinking (Froehlich et al., 1990, 1991), and that naloxone and naltrexone partially reversed alcohol-induced analgesia as measured by the tail-flick test (see Chapter 2). Analgesics markedly increased the time of tail exposure, and naloxone blocked this effect. Naloxone also partially protected rats from alcohol-induced hypothermia, and protected rats from alcohol-induced conditioned taste aversion. In the taste-aversion tests, rats drank alcohol that included lithium carbonate, which later caused a gastrointestinal (GI) upset. Normal rats then showed an aversion to drinking alcohol, presumably because the taste of alcohol had been associated with the GI upset. Naloxone attenuated the taste aversion—that is, the naloxone-treated rats drank alcohol despite the prior aversive experience. Thus, it is clear that opioid receptors and/or their endogenous ligands play a role in mediating alcohol effects.

A number of other experiments have investigated the effect of chronic administration of alcohol on the binding characteristics of opiate receptors. In general, binding to opiate receptors is diminished by alcohol treatment, but the effect is not easily explained. It has been suggested that alcohol influences the interaction of specific opiate receptor complexes with G proteins, or that the effect of alcohol on ligand binding may be mediated by conformational changes in the ligand rather than in the receptor. However, these effects occurred under relatively high alcohol concentrations (e.g., 1.0% which is ten times 0.1%, the criterion for legal drunkeness).

We may conclude that although there is evidence that alcohol interacts with opiates and opioids in certain ways, it may simply reflect the ever-present finding that alcohol is capable of altering virtually every tissue with which it comes in contact. With respect to the possibility that alcohol may induce the formation of opioid condensation products such as THP and TIQs, little light on that subject has been generated by experiments on the direct effects of alcohol on opiate systems.

Alcohol–norepinephrine interactions.   Alcohol–norepinephrine interactions have been reviewed and summarized by Goldstein (1983) and Ollat, Parvez, and Parvez (1988). A single dose of alcohol was found to stimulate the synthesis and turnover of NE in the CNS, and after prolonged administration of alcohol, NE turnover remained accelerated for as long as 3 days during the withdrawal period. Alcohol also accelerated the decline of NE levels when NE synthesis was blocked by tyrosine hydroxylase inhibitors.

In mice, blocking NE synthesis with α-methyltyrosine or blocking β-receptors with propranolol during alcohol withdrawal briefly intensified withdrawal convulsions. Reserpine treatment (which depletes NE and serotonin) during withdrawal had a severe and prolonged effect that was sometimes fatal. In humans, propranolol aggravates several acute effects of alcohol. Because both D- and L-propranolol have this effect, this enhancement was not attributable to β-blockade, but rather to another property of the drug: its ability to inhibit alcohol dehydrogenase, thus potentiating the effects of alcohol. On the other hand, patients undergoing alcohol withdrawal may obtain beneficial effects from propranolol because it decreases heart rate, tremor, and blood pressure, and its potentiation of alcohol effects provides a "tapering off" effect after an alcoholic binge. Also, by potentiating alcohol effects and slowing the withdrawal process, propanolol diminishes the possibility of convulsions and delirium tremens (see Goldstein, 1983).

In other experiments, chronic intoxication had little effect on the binding and the sensitivity of α-adrenergic receptors, whereas β-receptors were altered. In intoxicated animals the number of β-receptors was reduced, and in in vitro studies alcohol reduced the affinity of high-affinity isoproterenol binding sites. During withdrawal, the number of β-receptors suddenly increased, together with their sensitivity. Also, the adenylyl cyclase associated with β-receptors was activated by alcohol, and this effect underwent tolerance during chronic intoxication.

In summary, alcohol intoxication stimulates NE turnover and function in the CNS, with probable involvement of cAMP. The effect may be directly alcohol-induced or may be mediated by alcohol's effects as a general stressor. In the long term, chronic intoxication leads to NE hypofunction due to postsynaptic adaptation of β-receptors and their associated adenylyl cyclase. Also, NE hypoactivity is associated with alcohol craving, whereas NE hyperactivity is revealed during withdrawal, and these effects differ depending upon the brain loci being studied.

Alcohol–acetylcholine interactions.   Neuromuscular junctions were studied for the effects of alcohol on acetylcholine (ACh) synapses because of their accessibility and the absence of other neurotransmitters at those synapses. Acting presynaptically, alcohol increased the rate of spontaneous release of ACh and the frequency of miniature end-plate potentials (MEPPs). In stimulated preparations, alcohol increased the amplitude of end-plate potentials, indicating that an increased number of quanta were released in response to the stimulation. Tolerance to the above effects develops so that nerve–muscle preparations from rats that were chronically treated with alcohol were resistant to the action of alcohol in vitro. The postsynaptic response to alcohol is an increased amplitude and duration of the MEPPs brought about by a slow rate of decay of the potentials, probably because of the perturbation of membrane lipids by alcohol.

In the brain, alcohol decreases ACh release, thereby elevating the amount of ACh in neural tissue. When alcohol is applied to electrically stimulated brain slices in vivo or in vitro, the release of ACh declines. However, within a half hour, tolerance to these effects develops despite the continued presence of alcohol in the blood or perfusion fluid. Tolerance in mice is accompanied by an increase in muscarinic receptors in some brain areas, but this effect disappears within a day. Further, whereas alcohol increases brain levels of ACh, there is disagreement about its effects on choline acetyltransferase: some investigators found an alcohol-induced increase in enzyme activity in vitro and in vivo, but others did not. These discrepancies may be due to genetic differences among the species used and differences among the brain areas tested. Some reports describe an alcohol-induced increase of ACh receptors, but the effect may have been due to unusually high alcohol levels. Also, in animals, acute intoxication increased the excitatory responses of the pyramidal cells of the hippocampus following iontophoretic administration of ACh. These alcohol-related perturbations in the hippocampus may be related to the amnesias that sometimes occur after bouts of intoxication (see Goldstein, 1983).

On the other hand, a review of studies on the neurobehavioral effects of alcohol on cholinergic-mediated systems by Deitrich and colleagues (1989) did not present a coherent picture with respect to alcohol–acetylcholine interactions. Thus, no significant effect of alcohol upon cholinergic cells, synapses, or systems has been found that contributes to a better understanding of the effects of alcohol on behavior. Whereas some alcohol effects on ACh may occur, such findings are difficult to replicate because, as we mentioned above, the effects are diffuse and variable with respect to the dosages used, the species studied, and the brain area under investigation. (For more details, see the review by O'Brien, 1994.)

Alcohol–serotonin interactions. Until recently, the sizable literature on the possible role of serotonin (5-HT) in alcoholism was at considerable variance. Some studies found alcohol-induced changes in 5-HT levels and turnover rates (Roy and Linnoila, 1989), whereas other studies could not confirm them (see Ollat, Parvez, and Parvez, 1988). On the other hand, there is consistent evidence that 5-HT is a factor in alcohol consumption. In rats, low blood levels of 5-HT coincided with an enhanced preference for alcohol, whereas stimulation of 5-HT production or intravenous infusions of 5-HT attenuated alcohol consumption. Similar attenuating effects were obtained by bilateral microinfusions of 5-HT into the nucleus accumbens, and by postsynaptic 5-HT agonists such as MK 212, quipazine, and buspirone. Voluntary alcohol consumption was also diminished by the 5-HT uptake blocker fluoxetine (later known as Prozac). In contrast, selective destruction of 5-HT cells with 5,7-dihydroxytryptamine increased alcohol consumption.

5-HT hypofunction likewise accompanies alcohol consumption by spontaneously alcohol-craving rats, whereas stimulation of central 5-HT function reduces alcohol craving. For example, 8-OH-DPAT, a potent selective 5-HT_{1A} receptor agonist (see Chapter 9), reduced alcohol consumption in alcohol-craving rats, but not in low-alcohol-consuming rats. Further, rats that were treated with zimelidine, a 5-HT uptake blocker, showed a diminished alcohol intake when they had a choice between tap water and increasing concentrations of alcohol. Zimelidine presumably reduced alcohol intake by increasing 5-HT availability at synapses. In humans, zimelidine reduced alcohol intake among heavy drinkers; alcoholics treated with this drug were abstinent for more days, and when they were drinking, they decreased the number of daily drinks (Naranjo et al., 1984; Naranjo, Sellers, and Wu, 1985). However, central 5-HT stimulation is known to have anoretic effects, which may account for the fact that zimelidine reduced not only alcohol consumption but the consumption of any flavored drink. Thus, zimelidine probably is not a specific inhibitor of alcohol intake.

There is more substantial evidence that 5-HT plays a role in the development of tolerance to alcohol. For example, central stimulation of 5-HT nuclei of the median raphe (MR) accelerates alcohol tolerance, whereas 5-HT depression (after lesions in the MR) delays it or hastens its disappearance (Le et al., 1981a,b). Similar effects were obtained with specific lesions of the 5-HT pathway from the median raphe to the hippocampus; that is, the lesions slowed the development of tolerance for alcohol-induced hypothermia and motor deficits. Also, whereas depletion of brain NE in rats did not affect the development of alcohol tolerance, combined destruction of the NE and 5-HT pathways completely blocked tolerance development.

The effect of 5-HT on tolerance was demonstrated in another way by Frankel and colleagues (Frankel et al., 1975; Frankel, Khana, and LeBlanc, 1978), who examined the effect of 5-HT depletion in rats on the acquisition of tolerance to ethanol-induced ataxia. Serotonin depletion was obtained by daily treatments with the 5-HT synthesis-blocking drug *p*-chlorophenylalanine (PCPA) (100 mg/kg, p.o.), which lowered and maintained brain 5-HT levels at 5% of normal. The degree of ethanol-induced ataxia was measured during 2-minute tests of running on a motor-driven circular belt. This miniature treadmill, devised by Gibbins, Kalant, and Le Blanc (1968), was mounted over an electrified grid that delivered an annoying foot shock to the rat if a foot left the belt during the test. The circuitry of the grid also recorded the number of contacts with the grid and their duration. After being pretreated with PCPA for 5 days, the rats were tested on the treadmill 20 minutes after an acute injection of one of four doses of ethanol (1.6, 1.9, 2.2, or 2.5 g/kg) given in an 8% saline solution. As shown in Figure 15.8*a*, the PCPA treatment had no effect on dose-related ethanol-induced motor impairment.

To examine the effect of PCPA on tolerance acquisition, PCPA was given with ethanol for 25 days, and on every fifth day the rats were given a challenge dose of ethanol just before a treadmill test. A control group was given ethanol alone. Also, after the last three tests, blood

samples were taken from the tip of the tail 20 minutes after the ethanol administration to establish the blood ethanol concentration for both groups. As shown in Figure 15.8*b*, PCPA did retard tolerance acquisition during chronic ethanol intake, but there was no significant difference in blood ethanol levels on the 4th, 5th, and 6th test days or between the groups or days.

In a third test, rats that had developed tolerance were returned to the treadmill to determine the effect of PCPA on the loss of tolerance. In order to maintain low brain 5-HT in the PCPA animals, the drug was given for 5 days prior to the withdrawal of ethanol and throughout the abstinence period up to the time of treadmill testing. The controls received H_2O injections. As in the previous experiments, the tests of tolerance were based on locomotor performance on the treadmill following the ethanol test dose (2.2 g/kg). Four tests were given, on the 4th, 6th, 10th, and 14th day post–alcohol withdrawal. As shown in Figure 15.8*c*, the ethanol-tolerant rats showed a progressive return to locomotor impairment as a function of the duration of abstinence, but the animals that received the prior PCPA treatment lost tol-

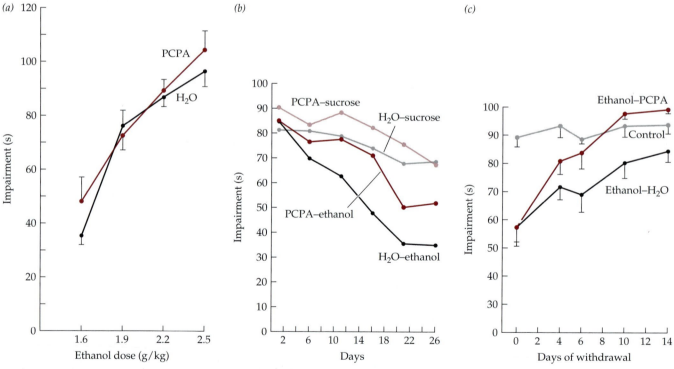

15.8 EFFECT OF 5-HT DEPLETION ON ETHANOL TOLERANCE. (*a*) The effect of PCPA on acute ethanol-induced motor impairment expressed as the time (s) off the treadmill. Pretreatment for 5 days with PCPA had little or no effect on acute ethanol-induced motor impairment compared with controls. (*b*) Effect of PCPA on the acquisition of tolerance to ethanol. Ethanol tolerance is indicated by the decrease in ethanol-induced impairment with repeated testing. Pretreatment with PCPA diminished the acquisition of tolerance. (*c*) Ethanol tolerance declined over time of alcohol withdrawal, as indicated by the return of alcohol impairment during withdrawal. Controls with no prior alcohol treatment showed no tolerance at all, but among ethanol-tolerant animals, pretreatment with PCPA hastened the loss of tolerance and the return to ethanol-induced motor impairment. (After Frankel et al., 1975; Frankel, Khana, and LeBlanc, 1978.)

erance at a faster rate than those that received the water placebo. Taken together, these experiments demonstrated that depressing brain levels of 5-HT with PCPA slowed the acquisition and accelerated the loss of tolerance to the locomotor effects of alcohol in rats (Frankel et al., 1975; Frankel, Khana, and LeBlanc, 1978).

From the results of the experiments described above, we may conclude that chronic alcohol consumption leads to complex changes in 5-HT metabolism that have been generally interpreted as a stimulation of serotonergic activity. Repeated alcohol administration to rats led to a depletion of the 5-HT metabolite 5-HIAA in the corpus striatum, hypothalamus, and hippocampus, presumably because 5-HT synthesis could not keep pace with the chronic activation of the serotonergic system. Although studies on human alcoholics have reported both high and low levels of CSF 5-HIAA (Ollat, Parvez, and Parvez, 1988; Roy and Linnoila, 1989), Ballenger and coworkers (1979) have proposed a unifying theory to explain the relationship between alcohol and serotonergic function. These investigators argue that at least some alcoholics suffer from a preexisting, possibly inherited, deficit in central serotonergic activity that is reflected in low 5-HIAA concentrations. Consequently, such individuals would be selectively vulnerable to alcoholism, and might begin drinking chronically in an attempt to ameliorate the deficiency by stimulating 5-HT release. Although this idea remains speculative at present, it is consistent with a considerable number of findings from both human and animal research.

Alcohol Tolerance

Drug tolerance is a decreased physiological response to a particular drug dose, generally because of prolonged, frequent, or excessive use; the greater the tolerance-inducing doses, the greater is the tolerance effect. In some individuals, chronic use of alcohol contributes to tolerance and ever-increasing rates of consumption, with the result that the alcoholic can remain sober while having a BAC that may be many times higher than the level that would be associated with intoxication in a nontolerant individual.

Acute Tolerance

There are two types of tolerance to alcohol: acute and chronic. Acute tolerance is apparent within the time in which a single dose is cleared from the bloodstream. This was demonstrated in early experiments showing that shortly after alcohol ingestion by humans, when the blood alcohol concentration (BAC) is increasing, signs of intoxication appear at a certain point on the rising slope of a curve representing the BAC over time. As shown in Figure 15.9, signs of intoxication appeared when the BAC was about 200 mg/dl. During the declining slope, however, the subjects appeared to be sober when the BAC was about 265 mg/dl (Mirsky et al., 1941). Thus, it

was held that whereas the effect of alcohol on the CNS is proportional to the BAC, the behavioral effect is more pronounced when the BAC is rising than when it is falling, illustrating an acute tolerance effect (Charness, Simon, and Greenberg, 1989; Tabakoff, Cornell, and Hoffman, 1986; Ritchie, 1985).

However, this interpretation has been questioned on the following grounds. It is known that after alcohol ingestion, the brain alcohol concentration rises rapidly because a large proportion of the circulating arterial blood perfuses the highly vascularized brain. In contrast, blood circulation through less vascularized tissues such as muscles is slower; consequently, the alcohol concentration in such tissues rises considerably more slowly (Harger, Hulpieu, and Lamb, 1937). Within 10 minutes after oral administration of alcohol, the brain/arterial blood alcohol ratio is virtually at equilibrium (1.00:1.18), whereas in muscle tissue there is a lag of about an hour before equilibrium is reached (Forney and Harger, 1971). In the Mirsky study and similar experiments, the BAC levels were ascertained from venous blood samples taken from the cubital vein in the forearm (which contains venous drainage from the forearm muscles), whereas in later experiments, blood drawn from the radial artery of the forearm was used. This arterial blood had alcohol levels significantly higher than those determined from venous blood at the same time after alcohol comsumption (Forney et al., 1964). Given that the arterial BAC more closely approximates the brain alcohol concentration, and that the degree of intoxication pre-

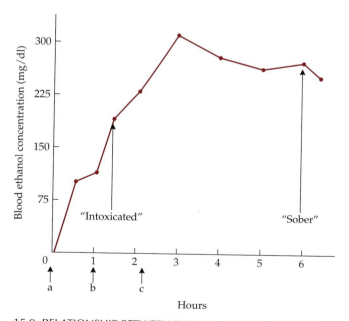

15.9 RELATIONSHIP BETWEEN BLOOD ALCOHOL CONCENTRATION AND SIGNS OF INTOXICATION. After three doses of alcohol (1.0 g/kg at time *a*, and 0.25 g/kg at times *b* and *c*), signs of intoxication appeared during the rising phase of the BAC curve when the BAC was about 200 mg/dl. However, when the BAC was declining, the subject became sober even though the BAC was about 265 mg/dl. (After Mirsky et al., 1941.)

sumably is a function of the brain alcohol concentration, venous samples taken during the rising slope of the curve would underestimate brain alcohol concentrations and make it appear that intoxication occurred at lower brain alcohol levels than it really did (Forney and Harger, 1971; Hofmann, 1983).

Goldstein (1983) tested this hypothesis by giving ethanol (2 g/kg i.p.) to groups of mice and alternately measuring tail and brain ethanol levels after varying time intervals. That is, each animal provided a venous tail blood sample at one time interval, and at the next interval it was sacrificed to provide a brain blood sample. As Figure 15.10 shows, brain ethanol reached a peak in about 15 minutes and did not equate with the ethanol level in tail blood until 60 minutes after the alcohol injection. Thus, the ethanol concentration in venous blood did not represent brain ethanol levels during ethanol absorption when intoxication became apparent. However, the ethanol concentration for venous blood on the declining slope reasonably approximated cranial ethanol BAC levels. Here it is worth noting that some recent reports describe alcohol-related phenomena in rats that are dependent upon the rising slope of BAC curves obtained from tail-vein samples (Lewis and June, 1990). According to the data shown in Figure 15.10, it appears that such reports may be in error by relying on venous BAC measurement to infer brain alcohol concentrations.

It must be conceded, however, that evidence of acute tolerance has been found even when brain alcohol concentration was correlated with the behavioral effects of the drug. In one experiment, three groups of rats were given various intraperitoneal doses of alcohol and, after a delay of 10, 30, or 60 minutes, were given a 2-minute test on Gibbins' miniature treadmill, described above. Immediately after the test, each animal was sacrificed

and its brain alcohol concentration measured. The three separate and parallel dose–response lines in Figure 15.11 indicate that rats that were tested 30 or 60 minutes after alcohol treatment had significantly higher brain alcohol levels than, but performed as well as, the rats tested after a 10-minute delay. For example, one rat, which was tested after 10 minutes, was off the belt for about 88 seconds and had a brain alcohol level of 1.80 mg/g, whereas one of the rats that was tested after 60 minutes was off the belt for only 10 seconds and had a brain alcohol level of about 2.50 mg/g. In general, there was a twofold tolerance that developed over an hour (LeBlanc, Lalant, and Gibbins, 1975). Another study found that acute alcohol tolerance is dose-related: intoxicated dogs sobered up at higher BAC levels after high doses of alcohol than after low doses. In this case the behavioral tests were performed and the blood samples taken from the jugular vein at a time when blood and brain alcohol concentrations were the same (Maynert and Klingman, 1960; see also Goldstein, 1983).

From the foregoing we are led to the conclusion that acute alcohol tolerance is a demonstrable phenomenon, but in many cases it appears that faulty procedures may point to the phenomenon when its presence is questionable. Moreover, in human subjects, a number of important factors limit the value of quantitative assessments of any kind of tolerance. Because alcohol and other drugs are metabolized in the liver and/or cleared from the bloodstream by the kidneys, the ages of the subjects and the status of their hepatic and renal functions are critical factors in any experimental results. Furthermore, measures of drug absorption, metabolism, and clearance are contaminated by tobacco smoking, drug interactions, and drug abuse and dependence, along with the limits imposed by small numbers of subjects, extremely vari-

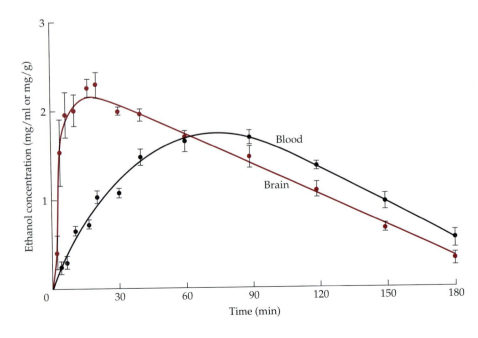

15.10 TIME COURSE OF BRAIN AND VENOUS ETHANOL CONCENTRATIONS. After administration of ethanol (2 g/kg i.p.) to mice, the brain ethanol concentration reached its peak in about 15 minutes, and did not equate with ethanol levels in venous blood taken from the tip of the tail until 60 minutes had passed. (After Goldstein, 1983.)

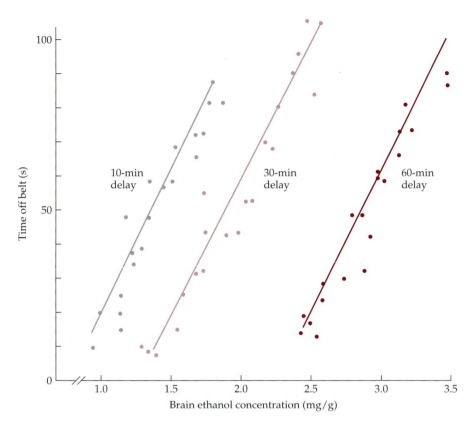

15.11 ACUTE ALCOHOL TOLERANCE IN RATS. Each point represents the relationship between brain alcohol concentration and the degree of alcohol-induced motor impairment for an individual rat in one of three groups. The rats were tested on the treadmill after various delays (10, 30, or 60 minutes) following alcohol administration. The shift of the concentration–response line from the 10-minute to the 60-minute position represents a substantial tolerance effect, that is, animals tested 30 or 60 minutes after high ethanol doses had higher BACs but similar degrees of intoxication compared with rats tested after a 10-minute interval. (After LeBlanc, Lalant, and Gibbins, 1975.)

able and poorly described clinical conditions, and failure to adequately describe and control for diet, weight, body composition, concurrent medication, and racial and genetic background. Also, individual differences, even among "healthy normal volunteers," are such that four- to sixfold variations in drug half-life and clearance are common. Consequently, even if a change in a single variable is detected in a carefully controlled study, it is questionable that the result can be generalized to a less selected population (see Sellers and Bendayan, 1987). Nonetheless, with the help of animal studies, some general principles of alcohol tolerance can be described.

Chronic Tolerance

Chronic tolerance develops after repeated dosing with alcohol, and is manifested by a lower effectiveness of the same doses that were given earlier. This effect occurs because of one or two kinds of alcohol-induced physiological changes: metabolic (pharmacokinetic) tolerance and tissue (pharmacodynamic) tolerance.

Metabolic tolerance. Metabolic tolerance results from alcohol-induced changes in the absorption, distribution, degradation, and excretion of alcohol, and is characterized by a diminished peak BAC, faster clearance from the bloodstream, and diminished or absent alcohol effects. In one experiment to assess the degree of tolerance that can occur in humans, subjects were given increasing hourly doses of alcohol solutions until they were consuming in

excess of the equivalent of 400 ml of 95% alcohol daily and were judged to be markedly intoxicated. However, within 10 days, though this alcohol intake was maintained, BACs in this group fell to nearly zero and signs of intoxication disappeared. At this point these subjects were metabolizing alcohol at a rate of about 455 ml/day, in comparison to 346 ml/day during a control period. This appeared to be about the maximum tolerance that could be achieved, because when total daily alcohol was increased by only 3–65 ml, BACs rose sharply and signs of intoxication reappeared (see Hofmann, 1983). Limits to the degree of metabolic tolerance were also found in animal studies. Maximum tolerance amounted to about 30% to 50%, which means that among tolerant animals, alcohol intake could be maximally increased 30% to 50% without signs of intoxication. Tolerance in humans was found to be transitory in that the effect was lost after 3 weeks of abstinence, and the same effect was found even among individuals who had been severe alcoholics for 5 years or more (Mendelson, 1968).

The basis of metabolic tolerance was presumed to be an alcohol-induced increase in alcohol dehydrogenase (ADH) activity (see Figure 15.1a). However, there are limits to the degree of ADH activity because the rate of regeneration of the ADH coenzyme nicotinamide adenine dinucleotide (NAD^+) may be insufficient to keep pace with the extra enzyme that is produced. Rather, it is more likely that the increase in the rate of alcohol inactivation is brought about by a proliferation of the smooth endoplasmic reticulum in liver cells and a concomitant enhancement of the hepatic mixed function oxidase system, which handles a variety of exogenous substances. (See Goldstein, 1983; Kalant et al., 1976; Lundquist, 1971.)

There are related findings suggesting that hepatomegaly (enlargement of the liver) may occur after prolonged alcohol abuse, and that this could be a factor in increased rates of alcohol metabolism. Evidence shows that after chronic alcohol ingestion, increases in alcohol metabolism were congruent almost exactly with increases in the ratio of liver weight to body weight. Furthermore, the rate of ADH activity per gram of liver was not increased, but because liver weight was greater, total ADH activity was higher (see Tabakoff, Cornell, and Hoffman, 1986). Nonetheless, whether or not tolerance occurs, a lethal dose of alcohol is still possible because tolerance does not extend equally to all of alcohol's effects.

Metabolic tolerance and cross-tolerance.   In the simplest case, cross-tolerance refers to the loss of effectiveness of a drug due to tolerance to another drug similar in its chemical composition to the first drug. However, cross-tolerance between chemically unrelated substances may also occur. Metabolic cross-tolerance in alcoholics is presumed to occur because the increased rate of metabolism of alcohol is extended to the metabolism of other substances. Consequently, excessive alcohol use leads to reduced plasma drug concentration, a shorter drug elimination half-life, and an increased rate of clearance of CNS depressants, anxiolytics, and antidepressants, as shown

in Table 15.2. Alcohol-induced activity of pentobarbital hydroxylase was found to be increased twofold in both rats and human subjects, which may account for the known resistance of alcoholics to barbiturates. Similarly, if the anticonvulsant phenytoin is taken while a chronic alcoholic is sober, it is metabolized at an exaggerated rate that severely reduces its blood concentration, thereby rendering the drug ineffective (Ritchie, 1985). This effect has been traced to the proliferation of the smooth endoplasmic reticulum in liver cells and the augmentation of the microsomal mixed-function oxidase system.

Cross-tolerance can be quite variable across animal species because of the induction of different metabolizing isoenzymes among various animals, only some of which are appropriate for metabolism of a certain drug. Thus, alcohol-induced increases in a variety of drug-metabolizing enzymes may account for cross-tolerance between chemically unrelated substances. Moreover, it has also been found that in vitro, 50 mM alcohol significantly *inhibited* some drug-metabolizing enzymes, which may account for the increased sensitivity to certain drugs found in intoxicated nonalcoholics (Lundquist, 1971). Finally, cross-tolerance can be a manifestation of a different form of tolerance that has nothing to do with drug metabolism.

Cellular tolerance.   Cellular tolerance differs from metabolic tolerance in that it has a different mechanism and site of action, a different time course, and different dose relationships. Cellular tolerance is demonstrated by a shift

---

Table 15.2   Pharmacokinetic Interactions of Chronic Ethanol Ingestion and Psychotropic Drug Administration

Drug (route of administration)	Effect of ethanol on drug pharmacokinetics[a]
CNS depressants	
Pentobarbital (p.o.)	Decreased $t_{\frac{1}{2}}$ (25%)
Meprobamate (p.o.)	Decreased $t_{\frac{1}{2}}$ (50%)
Phenytoin	Decreased $t_{\frac{1}{2}}$ (40%); Cl increased (50%)
Benzodiazepines	
Chlordiazepoxide (p.o.)	Decreased plasma concentrations of chlordiazepoxide and desmethylchlordiazepoxide
Chlordiazepoxide (p.o.)	Decreased chlordiazepoxide AUC
Chlordiazepoxide (p.o.)	Increased $t_{\frac{1}{2}}$
Diazepam (i.v.)	Decreased AUC up to 24 hrs
Diazepam (i.v.)	$t_{\frac{1}{2}}$ shorter on day 1 than after withdrawal; Cl and V_d unchanged
Antidepressants	
Imipramine	Decreased concentrations of imipramine and 2-hydroxyimipramine; decreased bioavailability (?)

[a]Abbreviations: $t_{\frac{1}{2}}$, elimination half-life; Cl, clearance; AUC, area under the drug concentration–time curve; V_d, volume of distribution.
Source: After Sellers and Bendayan, 1987.

to the right in the BAC response curve after repeated drug use, or, stated another way, it is identified by diminished or absent drug effects despite the constancy of BAC levels during repeated alcohol doses. Achieving a given alcohol effect therefore requires a higher BAC, made possible by a greater alcohol intake. Such tolerance indicates that the brain and other organ systems have become less sensitive to a given dose of alcohol. A number of theories have been proposed to explain this phenomenon, but none of them is completely satisfactory.

Cellular tolerance is illustrated in an experiment in which dogs were tested for the relationship between blood alcohol and behavior before and after a 3-month period of chronic intoxication. The dogs were given alcohol in their drinking water, which was available for only an hour once in the morning and once in the evening. In this way the dogs were made noticeably intoxicated twice a day. Their degree of intoxication was measured by trained observers using a rating system devised by Newman (see Newman and Lehman, 1938). The results shown in Figure 15.12 clearly indicate that after the 3-month period of chronic intoxication, a given degree of intoxication required a significantly higher blood alcohol level in the dogs.

After tolerance to alcohol has been established, cross-tolerance is conferred upon other drugs such as anesthetics, barbiturates, and benzodiazepines that have pharmacological profiles similar to those of alcohol, but are chemically dissimilar. Furthermore, cross-tolerance between these substances, to a significant degree, may be due to a combination of metabolic and tissue elements. (See Tabakoff, Cornell, and Hoffman, 1986; and the section on barbiturates in Chapter 16.)

Earlier in this chapter we described some molecular mechanisms that may be instrumental in alcohol cellular tolerance. In this section we will discuss some hypothetical mechanisms that may be involved in the way the molecular mechanisms are expressed. Explanations for cellular tolerance are somewhat tentative, but there are some reasonable possibilities.

It has been proposed that when drugs depress neural activity in some systems, there is a counteradaptation that results in a "latent hyperexcitability" in the system. This counteradaptation becomes manifest by rebound or overshoot phenomena when the drug is withheld or blocked by an antagonist. It may be effected by changes in the drug receptors themselves—by an alteration in their numbers or in their sensitivity to the drug.

Another possibility is that if a drug effect is due to the diminished action of an enzyme necessary for transmitter synthesis, then the pharmacological effect of the drug is due to a diminished supply of the transmitter. However, if the activity of the enzyme is regulated by end-product inhibition, the product being the transmitter, the diminished supply of the transmitter could cause an acceleration of enzyme synthesis and activity

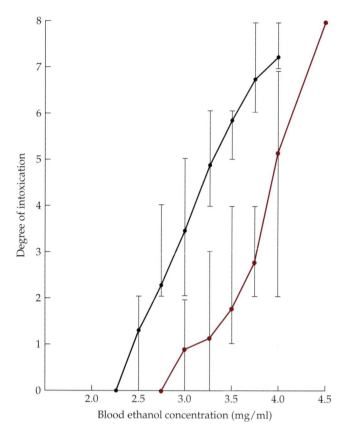

15.12 BAC RESPONSE CURVES FOR NORMAL AND ALCOHOL-TOLERANT DOGS. Using the Newman rating scale, dogs were rated for alcohol effects before (black plot) and after (color plot) a 3-month period of chronic intoxication. The shift of the concentration–response curve to the right represents tissue or functional tolerance. (After Goldstein, 1983; Newman and Lehman, 1938.)

that restores the transmitter, thereby resulting in tolerance. After drug withdrawal, there is an excess of enzyme and thus increased transmitter synthesis and rebound until the enzyme is restored to its original concentration.

Another proposal holds that one action of a drug could be the opening of redundant pathways in the CNS when the primary pathway is blocked by the drug. With drug withdrawal, the primary pathway is reactivated, which, when added to the activity in the redundant pathway, results in rebound hyperexcitability. Finally, there is the suggestion that the drug–receptor interaction induces effects that are antagonized or compensated by changes that occur in other biochemical pathways, which account for tolerance, and that rebound is the result of continued activity in the compensating systems (see Jaffe, 1985; and Chapter 12).

Alcohol Interactions with Other Drugs

First, it should be noted that alcohol is consumed in doses, measured in grams, that are far in excess of the doses of other drugs, usually measured in milligrams. A 1.5 oz (45 ml) drink of 80 proof whiskey, for example, contains about 18 grams of pure alcohol. In a tolerance study that was described above, human subjects were given over 400 ml of suitably diluted 95% alcohol a day to induce intoxication, whereas a similar effect could be attained with a few 100 mg pentobarbital tablets. Consequently, during significant alcohol consumption, many normal liver processes come to a halt while the liver deals with alcohol metabolism. During a fairly heavy evening of drinking during which six strong drinks are consumed, about 100 g of alcohol would be ingested. This is about 2 M of alcohol, which requires 2 M of NAD to oxidize it via the ADH pathway. This amount of NAD would weigh about 1.5 kg; therefore, the liver must continuously regenerate its much smaller supply of NAD (Goldstein, 1983). Thus, it is obvious that alcohol–drug interactions can be of major significance to a chronic alcoholic, especially when liver-based oxidative metabolism is involved.

Three types of alcohol–drug interactions can take place: (1) concurrent ingestion of alcohol and another psychotropic drug; (2) ingestion of a single dose of a psychotropic by an intoxicated or recently abstinent alcoholic; and (3) ingestion of an acute single dose of alcohol by a chronic user of therapeutic psychotropics.

Acute Alcohol–Drug Interactions

If a related drug is taken shortly after the ingestion of alcohol that has not been cleared from the bloodstream, both substances may compete for the available metabolizing enzymes, thereby increasing the half-life and plasma concentration of both substances. In such instances, the side effects of both drugs may become prominent. The degree of the interaction, as one would expect, depends upon the bioavailability of each substance, which is determined by its rate of absorption into the bloodstream, its rate of hepatic extraction from the blood, and the biotransformation process, which in this case is mostly oxidation.

Thus, a drug with high bioavailability (i.e., easily absorbed into the bloodstream and taken up at the target sites) and low hepatic clearance would be less susceptible to the effects of concurrent ingestion of alcohol than a drug with low bioavailability and a high rate of hepatic clearance. In humans, acute alcohol administration caused a 96% increase in blood diazepam concentration 18 minutes after intravenous administration of diazepam and a 100% increase after an oral dose compared to subjects receiving diazepam alone. This effect may be related to the finding in animals that acute administration of alcohol inhibits the mixed-function oxidase enzymes. Depending upon the doses of diazepam and alcohol and the time factors of their administration, the degree of the resulting CNS depression in humans could lead to respiratory arrest, severe brain damage, and irreversible coma (see Sellers and Bendayan, 1987).

Chronic Alcohol–Drug Interactions

Chronic use of alcohol, on the other hand, causes proliferation of the smooth endoplasmic reticulum and an increase in microsomal protein content in the liver, thereby augmenting the drug metabolizing activity of the microsomes. Consequently, the biotransformation and clearance of benzodiazepines, barbiturates, and phenytoin is increased and the clinical benefit of these drugs is diminished, but at the same time a dangerous potentiation of drug effects is avoided. On the other hand, the proliferation of the hepatic smooth endoplasmic reticulum may lead to the enhanced biotransformation and the more efficient production of toxic metabolites of other drugs, such as acetaminophen, cocaine, and vitamin A (see Tabakoff, Cornell, and Hoffman, 1986).

Acute Alcohol–Chronic Drug Interactions

The effects of an acute dose of alcohol on a chronic user of psychotropic drugs have been the least studied; theoretically at least, because of the rapid elimination of alcohol and the long half-life of psychotropic drugs, it is less likely that a deleterious kinetic interaction will occur. Alcohol ingestion would probably be safe if the regimen of chronic drug use is therapeutically sound and the acute alcohol intake is moderate. It is further assumed that liver and kidney functions are within normal limits. Under these circumstances a chronic user of Valium, for example, would not be at risk were he or she to have a small glass of wine at dinner.

From the foregoing discussion, it can be seen that alcohol–drug interactions can occur under many different circumstances. When a psychotropic or any other drug is ingested during an alcohol intoxication episode and both substances must compete for finite sources of metabolizing enzymes, there may be exaggerated drug effects, especially if the drugs rapidly enter the bloodstream and are competitively dependent on hepatic biotransformation for their metabolism and elimination. In cases in which chronic alcoholism has led to increased growth of the endoplasmic reticulum and increased levels of oxidizing enzymes, the increased rates of hepatic clearance could easily render the accompanying drug ineffective, or toxic metabolites of some drugs might materialize. Alcohol–drug interactions also depend upon the plasma half-life of the accompanying drug and its bioavailability, and whether there is cross-tolerance between alcohol and the coingested substance. Therefore, because so many factors can influence the outcome of alcohol–drug interactions, inconclusive and or contradictory results can be the result of multiplying or offsetting combinations of actions (see Sellars and Bendayan, 1987).

Alcohol Withdrawal Syndrome

Withdrawal symptoms are associated with alcohol dependence, which becomes evident when alcohol is precipitously withheld from a tolerant person. Hence, the alcohol-dependent individual frequently requires alcohol to forestall withdrawal effects in order to function normally. This phenomenon is seen when alcoholics desperately seek alcohol to quiet "the jitters" after they have been abstinent for many hours. However, it should not be assumed that the compulsive use of a drug such as alcohol depends solely on its negative reinforcing effect of forestalling withdrawal symptoms. Other factors may be equally important.

The alcohol withdrawal syndrome (AWS) is among the most serious consequences of alcoholism. The appearance of the withdrawal symptoms defines the extent of alcohol dependence. The intensity of these symptoms is, for the most part, dependent on the daily amount of alcohol consumed and the duration of use. However, it has been proposed that many signs and reactions characteristic of withdrawal effects can be observed after a single exposure to a high dose of alcohol. Such signs are hyperactivity, agitation, sleeplessness, and dysphoria; in fact, some observers suggest that the common "hangover" has many similarities to withdrawal symptoms. More serious symptoms occur after prolonged periods of heavy drinking, and they can be protracted, extremely unpleasant, and even life-threatening. An average-sized individual metabolizes about 30 ml, or 7–10 grams, of alcohol per hour, which corresponds roughly to the alcohol in an ounce of 90-proof whiskey or 12 ounces of beer. If this rate of consumption occurs over the day, it is unlikely that there will be an inordinate rise in the BAC. However, if larger amounts are consumed, or if the intake is at shorter intervals so as to exceed the rate of metabolism, there will be a buildup of the BAC over time, leading to a clinically significant physical dependence within a few days. If there should then be a change in the pattern of drinking, or a marked decline or sudden cessation of alcohol intake with a corresponding drop in the BAC, withdrawal symptoms may appear within 12 to 72 hours. Thus, the pattern of drinking as well as the total intake can influence the BAC in ways that precipitate the AWS. Even though there is considerable overlap between stages of dependence and AWS, we can reasonably describe different levels of dependence and withdrawal symptoms.

Low levels of dependence are associated with chronic intoxication at BACs of about 0.1%. After abstinence, the first stage of withdrawal symptoms may appear within a few hours after the last drink. The earliest symptoms are tremulousness (the "shakes"), headache, disturbed sleep, weakness, and anxiety (the "jitters"), which may last for less than a day. At a somewhat higher level of dependence, the tremulousness is more pronounced, and there is profuse sweating, which is accompanied by anxiety, anorexia, and nausea and abdominal cramps, followed by retching and vomiting. The patient has a flushed face, bloodshot eyes, is restless, agitated, hyperreflexive, and easily startled, but is usually alert and persistently expresses a desire for alcohol. At these levels of dependence the symptoms gradually disappear in a few days.

The second stage of withdrawal is sometimes referred to as acute alcoholic hallucinosis, although hallucinosis is not necessarily the indicator of the severity of the condition. At this stage the tremors may be so severe that the subject is unable to drink out of a glass; the other symptoms, such as nausea, weakness, anxiety, sweating, cramps, and vomiting, are also more severe. The patient may be desperate to obtain alcohol, and some alcoholics will drink flavorings such as vanilla extract, medicines such as cough syrups that contain alcohol, or denatured alcohol such as rubbing alcohol or highly toxic mixtures of ethyl and methyl alcohol. One of the authors (R.S.F.) is familiar with the case of a temporary laboratory assistant who worked at night cleaning equipment. He was discovered to be an alcoholic and was fired because his craving was so great that he drank alcohol after removing animal brain tissue that was being dehydrated by soaking in it.

At this stage abstinence-induced convulsive seizures develop in some alcoholics, but the necessary antecedents of this symptom are unknown. EEG recordings taken during withdrawal may show abnormalities such as mild dysrhythmias, random spikes, and brief episodes of high-voltage slow waves, but these signs are not prognostic of whether convulsions will appear. At first, hallucinatory images are seen with the eyes closed and later when the eyes are open, but the patient retains insight and remains oriented; that is, he knows that the images are imaginary and he knows his whereabouts. At this stage the patient may have seizures within the first 24 hours after withdrawal. In a study of 272 alcoholics undergoing withdrawal, 13% had seizures resembling the grand mal type, and the number of seizures ran from just one per day to status epilepticus, a state of continuous epileptic activity that can be fatal unless stopped by intravenous perfusion of antiepileptic drugs (Buck and Harris, 1991).

The third stage, known as delirium tremens (DT) (from the Latin *de lira*, "off the track," + "trembling"), occurs in 1% to 15% of alcoholics. These effects occur within a week after the cessation or reduction of heavy drinking and a few days after the early symptoms have diminished. As the syndrome progresses further into the third day of withdrawal, the patient becomes weaker, more confused, disoriented, and agitated, and may become terrified by his persecutory hallucinations, which are so vivid that even after recovery the patient cannot believe they were unreal. This syndrome is further characterized by hyperthermia, exhaustion, fever, sweating, tachycardia, elevated blood pressure and respiratory rates, and insomnia. These symptoms dissipate within 24 hours for 15% of patients, and 80% are in remission in less than 3 days. In the past, DT was fatal for about 15% of alcoholics because of cardiovascular collapse, but improvement in hospital management of the syndrome has brought the fatality rate to less than 1%. Unless the patient dies, he or she recovers within 5 to 7 days without treatment (Jaffe, 1985). It should be noted that if there are repeated cycles of continuous alcohol consumption separated by 2-week abstinent periods, the severity of AWS increases after each cycle (Buck and Harris, 1991).

The peak incidence of DT is between the ages of 30 and 50, with a decline in frequency after age 60. On average, blacks who are admitted to hospitals for DT are 8 years younger than whites, and men are at higher risk for DT than women. Both differences are suspected of being due to a higher incidence of alcoholism and particular drinking patterns among the respective high-risk groups (see Nathan, 1990).

In conclusion, we may reiterate that the precise antecedents of particular patterns of withdrawal symptoms are unknown. Furthermore, even severely addicted alcoholics may undergo withdrawal without exhibiting these signs and symptoms. Nonetheless, it can be said that the nature and intensity of the AWS seem to depend upon the degree and duration of chronic intoxication before drinking cessation or a sharp reduction in intake (Hofmann, 1983). Consequently, the detoxification of an alcoholic must be undertaken under careful supervision to avoid epileptiform or delirious states that can be fatal.

In considering pharmacological management of AWS, theoretically, alcohol itself should be an effective agent for suppressing AWS, but because of its short duration of action and narrow safety range, it gives way to longer-acting benzodiazepines such as chlordiazepoxide (Librium), diazepam (Valium), and flurazepam (Dalmane) that show cross-dependence with alcohol. These drugs are effective in preventing AWS or suppressing the symptoms once they develop. Other drugs are effective, but the benzodiazepines seem to be the drugs of choice in the United States (Jaffe, 1985). The use of these drugs is consistent with the hypothesis that alcohol tolerance and dependence are due to a compensatory decrease in GABAergic neurotransmission, and the benzodiazepines counteract these effects by increasing GABAergic transmission. Similar effects are found with GABA agonists such as GABA itself, the GABA mimetics such as muscimol, GABA aminotransferase inhibitors such as ethanolamine-O-sulfate and di-N-propylacetate, which block GABA metabolism, and GABA uptake inhibitors such as 2,4-diaminobutyric acid. Withdrawal signs are not suppressed by pharmacologically unre-

lated drugs such as opiates and antipsychotic drugs. Finally, AWS is exacerbated by agents such as picrotoxin that reduce GABA-mediated transmission (Buck and Harris, 1991).

Alcohol Abuse and Alcoholism

Models of Alcoholism

Throughout this chapter, we have presented evidence of the serious behavioral and health-related consequences of chronic alcohol intake. Yet we have not yet addressed the question of how alcoholism develops. What are the factors that can lead to a pattern of alcohol abuse, and why do so many people fall prey to the destructive influence of this drug?

Before considering the specific factors that may underlie alcoholism, it is useful to review some of the important models that have been proposed to explain this disorder. Until about 35 years ago, ideas about the nature of alcoholism were dominated by what we now call the **moral model**. In this view, alcoholics suffer from a lack of normal self-control over alcohol consumption that results in excessive drinking. Because such lack of control was thought to be a character defect, alcoholics were subjected to punishment rather than treatment. The first significant departure from the moral model was the **disease model** (sometimes also called the **medical model**), which was initially proposed by E. M. Jellinek in his 1960 book *The Disease Concept of Alcoholism*. The disease model has undergone some revision and elaboration since Jellinek's time, but it has remained a widely held theoretical perspective. Contemporary versions of this model generally hold that (1) although there may be stages in the development of alcoholism-related behaviors, the disorder itself is a unitary, definable entity (one is either alcoholic or not); (2) alcoholics are endowed with a constitutional factor (e.g., an "allergy" to alcohol, abnormally low or high sensitivity to alcohol, or some other type of pathology) that is present prior to any alcohol exposure and that ultimately manifests itself in uncontrolled drinking after exposure does take place; (3) because of the innate nature of this putative factor, alcoholics are not responsible for the loss of control that occurs when drinking; (4) the alcoholism-inducing factor is permanent and untreatable (i.e., there is no such thing as a "former alcoholic" in this model); and (5) total abstinence from alcohol therefore must be maintained over the individual's lifetime. The evidence presented below for a genetic contribution to alcoholism might be considered supportive of at least some features of the disease model. It must be emphasized, however, that no pathophysiological state has yet been *clearly and consistently* associated with alcohol abuse. Moreover, the disease model fails to acknowledge the variety of patterns of alcohol abuse, and places little, if any, importance on environmental factors. Hence, this model suffers from a number of serious problems.

A more recent view is encompassed by the so-called **behavioral model**. This model proposes that (1) alcohol consumption ranges from complete abstention to levels that induce chronic intoxication, and individuals can move up or down this continuum as a function of varying circumstances; (2) for those persons who do consume alcohol, the consequences of ingestion (at least in the short term) are positively reinforcing; (3) alcohol drinking is subject to the same control mechanisms that govern other reinforced behaviors; (4) excessive drinking (i.e., alcoholism) is therefore a learned, but maladaptive, behavior pattern; and (5) this behavior pattern can presumably be altered by the appropriate reinforcement contingencies, allowing for the possibility of controlled drinking in former alcoholics. The reader may wonder at this point how reinforcement mechanisms could ever engender a behavior pattern as self-destructive as chronic excessive alcohol intake. The important point here is that the *immediate* consequences of a response generally exert far greater control over the response than consequences that are delayed. Thus, in the early stages of development of an alcohol abuse problem, the punishing effects of a drinking bout, which are usually delayed (e.g., the next day's hangover), are easily outweighed by the drug's rapid reinforcing effects in terms of anxiety reduction, euphoria, social facilitation, and so forth. Even though the deleterious effects of drinking may increase greatly as the abuse problem progresses, the individual now faces an increased need for alcohol to quell his or her growing anxiety and to prevent or alleviate the unpleasant psychological and physiological symptoms of withdrawal. The development of tolerance, of course, exacerbates the problem as more alcohol than before is required to accomplish these effects.

One additional and important aspect of the behavioral approach is that it does not preclude the possibility of biological (for example, genetic) factors that confer heightened vulnerability to alcoholism in some individuals. Postulating the existence of such factors does not make alcoholism a disease, but rather, recognizes the fact that behavioral mechanisms alone are unlikely to account completely for individual differences in the response to alcohol. The notion of genetic–environmental interactions and the implications of the behavioral model for the treatment of alcoholism can now be considered.

Genetic and Environmental Factors in Alcoholism

There is substantial evidence of a genetic basis for alcoholism, as shown by selective breeding experiments that have produced strains of rats with tendencies to self-administer alcohol. Rats in free-choice situations could drink either tap water or a 10% alcohol solution from similar dispensing bottles. Based on their preferences, rat strains were developed that were alcohol preferring (P) or alcohol nonpreferring (NP). This preference was not simply a taste preference because P rats also self-administered alcohol intragastrically (Waller et al., 1984). These results suggest that there is a genetic basis for the predilection to ingest alcohol (Li, 1986; Meisch and George, 1988).

Data from human studies also support the hypothesis that genetic factors are at work in alcoholism. For example, it has been ascertained that 20% to 50% of the sons of alcoholics and about 3% to 8% of daughters become alcoholics. Also, the rates of alcoholism among first-degree relatives of alcoholics are severalfold higher than most general population estimates. In addition, compared with probands (alcoholic subjects) without alcoholic family members and those with alcoholism on only one side of the family, probands with alcoholism on both sides of the family experienced significantly more impaired control over their drinking behavior, more physical symptoms, and more pathological symptoms associated with chronic alcohol use (Stabenau, 1988). These findings, however, do not rule out environmental contributing factors.

With respect to gender, 46% of male siblings of male alcoholics become alcoholics, as do about 5% of their female siblings (see Fialkov, 1985). This gender differential appears to have existed throughout history and in many cultures, and it is presumed to be related, at least in part, to a gender-based physiological sensitivity and intolerance to alcohol. As many as 50% of Caucasian women develop a cutaneous flush following alcohol ingestion, while others feel dizzy and have headaches. These unpleasant consequences contribute to a disinclination to drink and a diminished alcoholism rate among women (Goodwin, 1991). On the other hand, recent surveys have shown females "catching up" to male subjects in heavy drinking patterns over the last two decades, owing, perhaps, to diminished differences in gender roles.

Pickens and coworkers (1991) studied 169 same-sex pairs of human twins raised together with respect to their concordance for two aspects of alcoholism: alcohol abuse (i.e., acute alcohol effects) and alcohol dependence (i.e., withdrawal effects). Specifically, the investigators compared groups of male and female monozygotic (identical) twins with groups of same-sex male and female dizygotic (fraternal) twins. There was a significantly higher concordance in the risk for alcoholism among monozygotic than among dizygotic male twins for both alcohol abuse and dependence, separately or together (Table 15.3). Again, it was found that the male concordance rates were two to three times higher than corresponding female concordances. For the female twins, whereas there was a significant difference in concordance between monozygotic and dizygotic twins with respect to alcohol dependence, the difference was not significant for alcohol abuse, alone or combined with

Table 15.3   Concordance Rates for Alcohol Abuse and/or Dependence in Twins[a]

	Male subjects			Female subjects		
	Monozygotic ($n = 50$)	Dizygotic ($n = 64$)	p-value[b]	Monozygotic ($n = 31$)	Dizygotic ($n = 24$)	p-value[b]
Alcohol abuse and/or dependence	0.760	0.609	.04	0.355	0.250	NS
No. of probands	50	64		31	24	
Alcohol abuse	0.740	0.578	.04	0.267	0.273	NS
No. of probands	50	64		30	22	
Alcohol dependence	0.590	0.362	.02	0.250	0.050	.04
No. of probands	39	47		24	20	

[a]Alcohol abuse and dependence were defined according to *DSM-III* criteria.
[b]p-values correspond to a one-tailed test and are reported as not significant (NS) if greater than .05.
Source: After Pickens et al., 1991.

dependence. Most importantly, these findings showed that if one twin is an alcoholic, there is a greater probability that an identical twin, compared with a fraternal twin, will also be an alcoholic. These findings support earlier reports of higher concordance for alcoholism among identical twins than among fraternal twins raised together, and strengthen the hypothesis that heredity is a significant etiologic factor in alcoholism. The finding that monozygotic male and female twins both showed higher concordance for alcohol dependence than fraternal twins suggests that the pattern of genetic factors has a greater effect upon alcohol dependence than upon alcohol abuse. Thus, there are commonalities in the inheritance of alcoholism in the two sexes, and it is proposed that shared environmental factors are more closely related to alcohol abuse than to alcohol dependence (see Pickens et al., 1991).

Furthermore, the increase in risk found among sons of alcoholics still applies when these children are adopted and raised by nonalcoholics. Similar findings have been reported for adopted daughters of alcoholics, but with the same lower vulnerability. On the other hand, adoptees from nonalcoholic parents, when raised by alcoholics, seem to incur little, if any, increased risk (for references, see Goodwin, 1991; Pickens et al., 1991; and Schuckit, 1986, 1987).

Schuckit (1987) has compared the biobehavioral phenotype displayed by sons of alcoholics (high risk) with that of sons of nonalcoholics (lower risk). Members of the former group (family history positive, or FHP men) were matched with members of the latter group (family history negative, or FHN men) with respect to age, sex, race, religion, educational level, drinking history, drug use history, and smoking history. The subjects were university students and nonacademic staff members of a university. The subjects were given, in random order, a placebo, a low dose (0.75 ml/kg), and a high dose (1.1 ml/kg) of alcohol (the equivalent of three and five drinks, respec-

tively) as a 20% solution in a carbonated beverage consumed over 10 minutes. Following the ingestion of the drinks, the subjects were observed over a 5-hour period during which they rated themselves for feelings of intoxication in terms of dizziness, nausea, and level of "high." The subjects were also objectively rated for performance in cognitive and motor skills, and for changes in hormones known to react to alcohol intake.

The results established, first, that following equivalent alcohol consumption, the FHP and the FHN subjects had the same blood alcohol concentrations over time. However, after the low-dose challenge, the FHP men rated themselves as significantly less intoxicated than the FHN subjects, though there was no significant difference between the groups after the high-dose challenge. These differences between the groups were buttressed by the finding that the FHP subjects had a smaller decrement in cognitive and psychomotor performance associated with the low dose of alcohol. For example, while both groups were similar for the level of body sway at baseline and after placebo, the FHN subjects had a significantly greater increase in body sway after the low-dose drink than the FHP subjects. Also, the FHP subjects showed less change in two hormones affected by drinking, namely, cortisol and prolactin. Thus, among the high-risk subjects, there were consistent reports of less intense subjective feelings of intoxication after relatively low alcohol doses, and these self-evaluations were supported by the objective physiological and cognitive–psychomotor measures.

Schuckit (1987) proposed that these particular findings relate to future vulnerability to alcoholism among FHP subjects in the following way. Hypothetically, an FHP person having a decreased sensitivity to low doses of alcohol, but a "normal" sensitivity to high doses, would be disadvantaged in a heavy-drinking environment. It is presumed that most young men and women "learn" how to control their alcohol consumption by occasionally overimbibing and then using this experience to recognize when to stop drinking to avoid severe intoxication. In contrast, a relative insensitivity to the effects of moderate levels of alcohol could impair an FHP person's ability to learn to stop drinking when control of behavior is still intact. Whereas this factor by itself may not be a sufficient cause of alcoholism, it may be instrumental in an environment in which drinking is a popular pastime, and it exemplifies how biological and environmental factors may interact and contribute to the probability of alcohol abuse (see Schuckit, 1987).

Other biological processes have been investigated as possible phenotypes relating to alcoholism. As mentioned earlier, alcohol is metabolized in two oxidizing steps: first, via the action of alcohol dehydrogenase (ADH) to form acetaldehyde, and second, via the action of aldehyde dehydrogenase (ALDH) to form acetate and then CO_2 and H_2O. Although ADH and ALDH exist in different forms that are quite varied in their activity with regard to biochemical factors such as substrate specificity, sensitivity to inhibitors, and quantity, none of these characteristics reliably predicts high or low risk. There are reports that the congenital absence of a particular ALDH isoenzyme may reduce vulnerability to alcoholism. The gene for this form of ALDH is altered in up to 85% of Asians, who cannot efficiently metabolize acetaldehyde to acetate. Consequently, within several minutes after alcohol ingestion, acetaldehyde levels rise considerably, causing a quite pronounced vasodilation or "flushing" of the face that resembles measles or the hives, heart palpitations or tachycardia, and nausea—symptoms similar to a mild ethanol–disulfiram reaction (see below). This effect, known as the alcohol-flush syndrome, serves as an aversive consequence of drinking and is a protective factor against alcoholism in this population (Fialkov, 1985).

Is There a Gene for Alcoholism?

In their attempts to identify genes that may confer susceptibility to various psychiatric disorders (including substance abuse), molecular biologists have used a powerful approach based on the phenomenon of **restriction fragment length polymorphism** (**RFLP**). This approach relies on several principles, the first being that DNA strands can be broken down into relatively small fragments by enzymes called restriction endonucleases. A restriction endonuclease recognizes a specific sequence of bases (usually 4–8 bases long) in the DNA molecule, and cleaves the molecule at a precise site within that sequence. The resulting collection of fragments can then be separated on the basis of size using the technique of gel electrophoresis. Now consider that the DNA that is being digested encodes a number of genes, some (or all) of which may exist in variable forms (known as alleles) that produce differing phenotypic outcomes (for example, alleles for eye color that result in brown vs. blue eyes). When two or more alleles exist for a given gene, digestion of that gene by an appropriate restriction endonuclease may produce fragments of differing sizes that will generate a RFLP when the fragments are run on a gel (Figure 15.13). Researchers can then attempt to determine whether there is a consistent relationship between the presence of a particular DNA fragment, which presumably indicates a specific allele for the gene, and the presence of the disorder under investigation.

RFLP has been used in recent years to search for an identifiable gene that might result in (or at least predict) vulnerability to alcohol abuse. One focus of this search has been the gene for the dopamine D_2 receptor. This gene has been localized to the q22–q23 region of chromosome 11, a chromosome that carries other genes previously associated with a variety of medical disorders (Figure 15.14). The D_2 receptor gene story began in 1990,

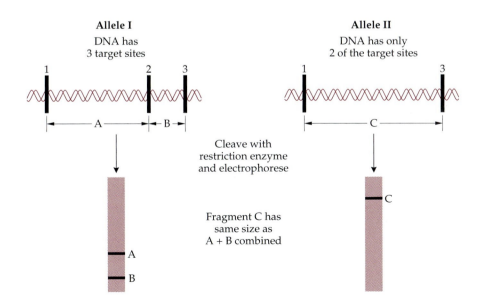

Allele I
DNA has
3 target sites

Allele II
DNA has only
2 of the target sites

Cleave with restriction enzyme and electrophorese

Fragment C has same size as A + B combined

15.13 RESTRICTION FRAGMENT LENGTH POLYMORPHISM. Two different alleles of the same gene may vary with respect to cleavage sites for particular restriction endonucleases. Consequently, the application of an appropriate restriction enzyme to DNA from individuals bearing these alleles will generate two related patterns of fragments, as shown by gel electrophoresis. This phenomenon, which is called restriction fragment length polymorphism (RFLP), has been used extensively to study possible genetic factors in psychopathology and drug abuse. (After Voet and Voet, 1990.)

when a research team at the University of Texas Health Science Center headed by Kenneth Blum generated considerable excitement by reporting a strong association between a particular allele of the D_2 gene and the presence of alcohol abuse (Blum et al., 1990; Roberts, 1990). In this study, postmortem brain tissue was obtained from 35 alcoholics and 35 nonalcoholic controls. Assignment of subjects to groups was made on the basis of alcohol consumption data, examination of medical records, and interviews with family members and treatment center staff. A sample of frontal cortex from each subject was then analyzed using four different restriction endonucleases. The results indicated that one allele (designated A_1) was present in 69% of the alcoholics, but only 20% of the nonalcoholics. Furthermore, a follow-up study found that the density of D_2 binding sites in the caudate nuclei of A_1^+ individuals was significantly lower than that observed in A_1^- subjects (Noble et al., 1991), suggesting that the polymorphic variants may differ in their dopamine binding characteristics.

The significance of these findings is obvious in light of the fact that the dopaminergic system has been shown to play a major role in neural reinforcement mechanisms and in the rewarding and euphoric properties of such drugs as alcohol, cocaine, nicotine, and opiates. Moreover, abnormalities in this system have been strongly implicated in a number of neurological and psychiatric disorders, some of which have been associated with alcoholism. Consequently, the notion that a specific form of the D_2 receptor gene might be selectively associated with alcoholism commanded a great deal of attention when first proposed. However, subsequent studies by several research groups produced inconsistent results with respect to A_1 allele frequency and alcoholism (see review by Uhl et al., 1993). Particularly disappointing was a failure to link this genetic marker with either the presence or the severity of alcohol abuse in families with multigenerational pedigrees of alcoholism. This finding is consistent with the existence of multiple vulnerability-enhancing genes, only one of which is the A_1 allele of the D_2 receptor gene. The follow-up research also provided important evidence for an elevated A_1 allele frequency in many patients with neural disorders such as Tourette's syndrome, attention deficit hyperactivity disorder, postraumatic stress disorder, and autism, as well as in a variety of substance abusers, not just alcoholics.

The fact that the A_1 allele is prevalent in neural disorders as well as in alcoholism and drug abuse, is consistent with the view that these are part of a spectrum of disorders with a common substrate of impulsive–compulsive–addictive behaviors that are mediated by dopaminergic systems through the action, at least in part, of the D_2 gene. Furthermore, others have noted the wide diversity of alcoholism in terms of pattern of drinking, age of onset, the rate of development of alcoholism, drinking associated with psychiatric and child-

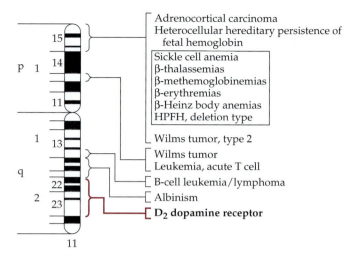

15.14 THE D_2 DOPAMINE RECEPTOR GENE. In humans, the gene for the D_2 receptor is located on chromosome 11 in the q21–q22 region. (The boxed disorders are allelic mutations of the same gene.) (After Roberts, 1990.)

hood conduct disorder which is seen in close to 50% of alcoholics, and alcoholism associated with multidrug abuse. Thus, coupled to the extensive variety of the antecedents and the patterns of alcoholism, and the widespread and easy availability of alcoholic beverages, and the implicit acceptance of their use in numerous social occasions, it is doubtful there is a single gene for the expression of alcoholism. Rather, it appears that substance abuse (including alcoholism) and perhaps also compulsive gambling, certain eating disorders, and other disorders of impulse control all derive from a complex interplay between environmental variables and a number of genotypes that confer increased vulnerability (Cloninger, 1991).

Serotonin, Personality Disorders, and Alcohol Abuse

In support of the animal research described earlier, a number of investigators have found diminished 5-HT activity among individuals with personality disorders. For example, correlations have been found between low CSF levels of the 5-HT metabolite 5-HIAA and histories of aggressive behavior, as well as scores on the psychopathic deviate scale of the Minnesota Multiphasic Personality Inventory (MMPI). Similar correlations have been found between low CSF 5-HIAA levels and self-rated childhood problems, as well as psychotism (i.e., aggressiveness, nonconformity) as measured by the Eysenck Personality Questionnaire (EPQ). Using a variety of other personality inventories, other investigators have found similar correlations with high scores for monotony avoidance and impulsivity and low scores for socialization. It was also reported that depressives with low 5-HIAA levels, compared with depressives with normal levels, had significantly more contact with the police, had more arguments with relatives, spouses, colleagues, and friends, were more hostile in interviews, and had impaired employment histories because of arguments. Low CSF levels of 5-HIAA were also found among individuals who attempted suicide and who were violent offenders and arsonists, the majority of whom were also alcohol abusers (see Chapter 9; for references see Roy and Linnoila, 1989).

With respect to alcohol abuse, diminished 5-HT activity may not be a factor for all alcoholics; rather, it is probably most characteristic of those known as Type II cases. According to Goodwin (1979), Cloninger (1987a,b), and Cloninger and colleagues (1988), Type I alcoholism is characterized by an indeterminate genetic predisposition, late onset, anxious personality traits, and a rapid development of tolerance to and dependence on the antianxiety effects of alcohol. In contrast, Type II alcoholism is generally limited to males and is characterized by early onset, high genetic predisposition, antisocial personality traits (as described above), and persistent seeking of alcohol for its euphoriant effect. Its results include an early inability to abstain from alcohol, and fighting when arrested for drunkenness. Consequently, it was proposed that Type II alcoholism, which is probably associated with diminished 5-HT activity, be regarded as a distinctly different clinical entity than Type I alcoholism.

These views are supported by the results of an extensive study by Cloninger (1987), who was able to obtain extensive personality ratings on 431 Danish early adolescents, then follow them as independent records became available of alcohol abuse among these subjects as young adults. The prediction that early onset of alcohol abuse would be correlated with Type II alcoholism was confirmed. Earlier studies had also found that people who became alcoholics as adults had demonstrated aggressive and antisocial traits in their youth. When tested on the Karolinska Scales of Personality, Type II alcoholics had significantly higher scores than Type I alcoholics on the Verbal Aggression and the Impulsive Sensation-Seeking Psycopathy scales, as well as significant lower scores on the Inhibition of Aggression scale. Moreover, comparisons were made between 19 alcoholics and 21 nonalcoholics who committed suicide while in psychiatric treament. More of the alcoholic than nonalcoholic suicide victims had been rated as showing "markedly outwardly directed aggressiveness" (32% vs. 5%) or "violent behavior toward others" (26% vs. 10%.) Also, among alcoholics who were admitted to a clinic, the ratings on the first admission of those who subsequently committed suicide, as compared with those who did not, showed significantly more irritability, dysphoria, or aggressiveness, lability of affect, explosiveness, or affective incontinence, or brittleness and hypersensitivity (see Roy and Linnoila, 1989).

Thus it was proposed that a 5-HT deficiency may be associated with violent and suicidal behavior (see Chapter 9) and with Type II alcohol abuse. Alcohol is presumed to promote synaptic release of 5-HT acutely and chronically to further reduce presynaptic stores. The effects of a functional 5-HT deficit include poor impulse control and violent outbursts, which may be the forerunners of suicide attempts. These findings initiated attempts at treatment of alcoholism with 5-HT-enhancing medications, and as mentioned earlier, some benefits have been reported by Naranjo and colleagues (1984, 1985).

It has also been reported that human subjects with alcoholic fathers had lower mean cerebrospinal 5-HIAA concentrations and more impulse-oriented behavior than matched subjects with nonalcoholic fathers (see Tollefson, 1991). Related to these findings are those of Ballenger and colleagues (1979), who found that human alcoholics had lower baseline levels of 5-HIAA, which were transiently elevated by alcohol consumption. These findings may mean that those who are vulnerable to alcoholism have a relatively low level of 5-HT activity that can be increased by alcohol consumption. All in all, these findings suggest that a low level of brain 5-HT activity, perhaps genetically mediated, characterizes those who are vulnerable to alcohol abuse, and enhances the preference for alcohol. We may further hypothesize that the craving for alcohol by alcoholics represents an attempt to modify this relative 5-HT deficiency.

Gender-Specific Drinking Styles

Earlier in this chapter, we showed that there are different biological consequences of alcohol consumption in men and women; these differences may be responsible for the higher incidence of aversive consequences that many women experience, drink for drink, as compared with men. On the one hand, these aversive consequences may explain the lower incidence of alcoholism among women. On the other hand, women who do abuse alcohol are more vulnerable to the adverse physical and psychological consequences. From another standpoint, some investigators have suggested that because relatively few empirical studies have compared male and female alcoholics, it may be inappropriate to generalize the data from predominantly male studies to the epidemiology and treatment of female alcoholics. This problem has been rectified to some extent by a study by Olenick and Chalmers (1991), who examined the drinking styles and self-evaluations of those styles by male and female alcoholics and nonalcoholics.

Among the findings of this study was support for the popular notion that alcoholic and nonalcoholic men use alcohol more often than similar groups of women to increase their congeniality in social gatherings. But among these four groups, alcoholic women were the least gregarious in their drinking styles. This may indicate that alcoholic women are more self-conscious about their drinking. It was also found, as expected, that men consumed more alcohol at greater frequencies than women and were more likely to incur alcohol-related social and legal difficulties. Moreover, both alcoholic and nonalcoholic men drank in a more sustained pattern (without periods of abstinence) than their female counterparts, which is contrary to the idea that women drink more continuously and surreptitiously than men. Alcoholic women were also found to use alcohol more often than men to manage stress and anxiety and to relieve depression, and they used alcohol just prior to the onset of their monthly menses, which may indicate attempts to manage the mood changes that frequently occur at that time. In a similar vein, other studies reported "escapist drinking," heavy drinking during stressful events in women's lives.

Among alcoholics, females reported drinking in response to marital difficulties more often than than their male counterparts, whereas there was no difference between nonalcoholic men and women. This is in agreement with other findings that women cite marital difficulties as the cause of drinking more often than men do; but the women were less likely to see drinking as the cause of their marital problems than the men were. Further, alcoholic women were more likely to have alcoholic spouses than were alcoholic men, and the alcoholic husbands tended to be instrumental in maintaining the heavy drinking of their spouses. It was concluded that alcohol impacts uniquely on the sexes in two areas, mood changes and marital problems, which may have implications for the treatment or prevention of alcoholism in women.

Treatment of Alcoholism

In the United States in the early years of the twentieth century, the cure for alcohol abuse and dependence was based on the simple premise that alcoholic beverages put any user at risk for drunkenness and degradation. Thus, to prevent this calamitous condition, there had to be a total ban on alcohol availability. These ideas led to the Eighteenth "Prohibition" Amendment to the Constitution of the United States, which made it illegal to manufacture and sell alcohol beverages in any form, except when made and used for medicinal purposes. However, in 1933, the Eighteenth Amendment was declared null and void by the Twenty-First Amendment, which was heavily favored during the severe ongoing economic depression due to the promise of many jobs in the reconstituted alcoholic beverage industry.

Because of the influence of the moral model of alcoholism, up until the last few decades, public drunkenness (sometimes combined with vagrancy) was considered a crime and led to arrests, jail sentences, and/or fines and other punitive measures. This "treatment" had little, if any, effect on the incidence of alcohol abuse. Rather, jails had merely become revolving doors for public drunkards. Finally, in 1970, the U.S. Congress passed

a law known as the Comprehensive Alcohol Abuse and Alcoholism Prevention, Treatment, and Rehabilitation Act, which recognized the alcoholic not as morally corrupt, but rather as a physically sick person with a disease requiring health rehabilitation services. Following this law, most states repealed their punitive laws regarding public intoxication and instituted services for detoxifying and rehabilitating alcoholics. This brought into being the professional treatment centers that were needed to deal with the problem.

Except for emergency cases involving severe alcohol poisoning, most therapeutic efforts took place on an outpatient basis in private or hospital-associated clinics utilizing medical, psychological, and social work specialists. In addition, a group known as the Fellowship of Alcoholics Anonymous (AA) began to play a rapidly increasing role in helping alcoholics. This organization, which was founded in 1935, promotes the concept that alcoholism is a disease, an incurable "allergy" to alcohol. The implication is that alcoholics can never drink safely and that total and lifelong abstinence is the only solution. The AA program has been characterized as a "quasi-religious" pragmatic approach to the problem of alcoholism. We will return to this subject later.

The chronic alcoholic has always presented, and still presents, a formidable challenge to treatment facilities, which out of necessity have developed a variety of pharmacological and psychotherapeutic approaches to deal with alcoholism. The long-term treatment of the persistent craving for alcohol and the prevention of relapse into alcoholism are not easily handled.

By the mid-1980s, among patients in designated clinics and treatment programs with well-integrated modern medical, psychiatric, and psychosocial treatment, short-term (6 months) improvement rates had reached 80%, and there was a significant drop in death rates from complications such as delirium tremens. However, long-term improvement rates (defined as abstinence for 1 year) were only 50%, and the national average was estimated to be closer to 25% (West, 1984). This assessment was echoed by Enoch Gordis, director of the National Institute on Alcohol Abuse and Alcoholism and the director of an extensive hospital program, when he wrote in 1987 (see Peele, 1991) that

> contemporary alcoholism treatment is, at best, of limited effectiveness . . . and our whole treatment system, with its innumerable therapies, armies of therapists, large and expensive programs, endless conferences, and public relations activities is founded on a hunch, not on evidence, and not on science.

Further, Dr. George Vaillant, a psychiatrist and researcher who worked in what he called "the most exciting alcoholism program in the world ... consisting of hospital detoxification, compulsory AA attendance, and a counseling program based on the disease concept" had to admit that his patients fared no better after 8 years than alcoholics who were left to their own devices. He reflected, "Perhaps the best that can be said . . . is that we were certainly not interfering with the natural recovery process." Moreover, Dr. Forrest Tennant, in an editorial in the *Journal of the American Medical Association,* wrote that any sophisticated critic using statistical analysis to measure treatment effectiveness would be appalled by affidavits from media and sports personalities supporting claims by specific treatment centers of cure rates of 80% to 90% (see Peele, 1991). Because of the tremendous variability of treatment methods and providers, it is beyond the scope of this volume to evaluate each one in detail. However, the interested reader is referred to Heather (1990) for an analysis of this subject and an extensive reference list dealing with various treatment methods.

Pharmacotherapy for Alcoholism

The pharmacological approach has been directed toward counteracting the acute effects of alcohol, reducing the craving for it, reducing the severity of withdrawal symptoms, and ameliorating the sharp discomfort of abstinence. Consistent with the idea that alcoholism is a manifestation of a psychological or psychiatric dysfunction, the advent of psychotherapeutic drugs in the 1950s brought about initial drug trials for the treatment of this disorder. Clinical experiments were conducted in which anxiolytics, antidepressants, antipsychotics, and lithium were used alone and in combination to treat various aspects of alcoholism. However, none of these medications were found to be effective for alcohol problems per se, although they may have been helpful in alleviating some psychological disorders associated with alcoholism, such as anxiety or depression. Also, during the 1960s and early 1970s, there was some enthusiasm for trying the so-called "hallucinogens" such as LSD and related substances as adjuvants toward finding the "inner" part of the personality at fault for alcoholic compulsion. But controlled trials revealed nothing of any benefit from that method (see Heather, 1990).

Drugs for the acute effects of alcohol. One of the earliest and still widely used treatments for the ataxia, dysarthria, and semi-stupor characteristic of acute alcohol intoxication is coffee, presumably because of its stimulating ingredient, caffeine. However, there is no evidence that coffee has a true sobering effect, and the fact that it is usually recommended to be served black and hot adds to the folk-remedy status of its use. However, coffee may be beneficial to overcome drowsiness for the drive home after a wine-embellished dinner. CNS-stimulating drugs such as pentylentetrazol (Metrazol) were also found to be ineffective in treating acute alcoholism, and dangerous as well.

The strategy in later attempts at reversing acute alcohol intoxication was to hasten its metabolism. Substances such D-glyceraldehyde, methylene blue, fructose, and pyruvate, which are NADH oxidizing compounds, were found to be effective in some cases, but not consistently so (see Pohorecky and Brick, 1990). There is no specific antidote for acute alcohol poisoning; thus, the treatment of this condition is similar to that used for other drug poisoning and is directed toward maintaining the patient's vital functions, emptying the stomach of residual alcohol, and clearing the blood of alcohol by hemodialysis (Ritchie, 1985).

Recently, a benzodiazepine compound, Ro 15-4513, was found to block the neurochemical, behavioral, and intoxicating effects of alcohol. Investigations into its mechanism of action revealed that alone, it produced no overt behavioral activity at doses as high as 10 mg/kg body weight, although there was some evidence that it caused seizures in nonhuman primates (see Britton, Ehlers, and Koob, 1988). Also, the drug effect was not due to an induced reduction of blood alcohol concentration because there was no change in peak BAC levels in Ro 15-4513-treated rats. However, the antialcoholic effects of Ro 15-4513 were reversed by the selective benzodiazepine receptor antagonist Ro 15-1788. This suggested that Ro 15-4513 acts upon the $GABA_A$ receptor complex by inhibiting the alcohol-induced potentiation of GABA-mediated Cl^- uptake. Ro 15-1788 presumably is able to reverse the effect of Ro 15-4513 by blocking its binding to the GABA receptor complex (Suzdak et al., 1986). These findings caused a flurry of suggestions that Ro 15-4513 could be taken before or during alcohol intake to prevent intoxication. But it was soon realized that the effects that could lead to some level of intoxication are precisely what one wants when drinking; thus, Ro 15-4513 would probably be unpopular among drinkers, or if taken, there might be attempts to overcome its effect by heavier alcohol intake, with its deleterious systemic effects. Moreover, the drug does not alter the lethal threshold, so increasing alcohol intake to override the effects of Ro 15-4513 could be fatal.

Other drugs that diminish alcohol effects as well as alcohol craving are 5-HT reuptake blockers. One such drug mentioned earlier in this chapter is zimelidine, which seemed to reduce the memory-impairing effects of acute intoxication and to reduce alcohol craving. This drug was also found to decrease alcohol use in nondepressed alcoholic men, with a corresponding increase in abstinent days (Naranjo, Sellers, and Larwin, 1986). However, it was later found that zimelidine aggravated the performance-impairing effect of alcohol and its effect on mood. Because of these and other effects, the drug was withdrawn from clinical use by the manufacturer (Jaffe, 1987).

Drugs for withdrawal symptoms. The symptoms of alcohol withdrawal were described in detail earlier in this chapter; the ways these symptoms can be avoided or subdued was also discussed. Here we may point out that mild withdrawal effects can be managed with sedatives and antianxiety agents, or simply with nutritional supplements and good nursing care. If seizures occur, diazepam or phenytoin should be given, and the antipsychotic drug haloperidol can be used to control hallucinations after the risk of seizures has passed (usually after the first 48 hours of withdrawal).

Most patients undergoing withdrawal report depression and anxiety, but while most improve fairly quickly, 15% to 30% report high levels of these symptoms. For this latter group, there may be some relationship between these postwithdrawal symptoms and preexisting conditions such as major or minor depression, bipolar depression, antisocial personality, drug dependence, agoraphobia with panic episodes, or Attention Deficit Disorder, Residual Type. In any case, these symptoms can be treated with appropriate antidepressants, anxiolytics, and antipsychotic drugs. However, for alcoholism per se, these drugs are not generally useful. For postwithdrawal anxiety states and sleep disturbances, the benzodiazepine anxiolytics have superseded the previously used sedatives and have been generally effective, but there is a growing tendency to restrict the use of these agents in order to avoid a combined alcohol–benzodiazepine dependence. Other related drugs have been used with some success in recently detoxified alcoholics, but in some studies placebo groups did better with respect to work and activity.

Aversion therapy.   Several pharmacological strategies have been attempted to prevent or delay relapse to uncontrolled drinking so that patients can remain accessible to counseling with better probabilities for success. After Pavlov's studies of conditioning became known in the 1920s, there were attempts to treat alcoholism by creating negative conditioned responses to alcohol through the pairing of stimuli associated with drinking (i.e., the sight, taste, or smell of alcohol) with powerfully unpleasant unconditioned stimuli such as nausea or electric shock (Kantorovich, 1930). Later, an extensive program was carried out using emetine, which induces nausea, as the unconditioned stimulus (Voegtlin et al., 1941a,b). The investigators reported abstinence rates as high as 60% to 70% after a 1-year follow-up, but they admitted that the success of the program may have rested upon the selection of alcoholic subjects with a good prognosis—those having an intact marriage, high occupational status, and high motivation demonstrated by their willingness to pay fees (Voegtlin and Broz, 1949). It is likely that these characteristics would contribute to the success of these alcoholics with almost any form of treatment.

Similar studies by West (1984) used other emetics such as lithium and apomorphine. In one study, pairing lithium with alcohol intake resulted in a clinically relevant aversion to alcohol, as indicated by abstinence in 36% of the drug-treated subjects versus 12% of controls at 6 months posttreatment. Further follow-up data were not reported. Some investigators used electric shock as the unconditioned stimulus, feeling that it was more controllable in terms of intensity and onset. However, shock was found to be less effective than chemically induced nausea, apparently because it failed to create a strong aversion to the taste of alcohol. Efforts were also made to deter drinking by pairing with alcohol a number of drugs or compounds that result in disagreeable odors or tastes. The antidepressant MAO inhibitor isoniazid, for example, when given before or during alcohol intake, alters the taste of alcohol in an unpleasant way. When tested for its ability to inhibit drinking (West, 1984), however, this treatment was not significantly beneficial (see Pohorecky and Brick, 1990).

Disulfiram therapy.   Disulfiram (Antabuse) has been used to promote abstinence in patients who have been detoxified and want to avoid a relapse into alcoholism. In this case, the drug negatively reinforces abstinence, given that alcohol consumption along with disulfiram use would lead to an extremely disagreeable consequence. It may be recalled that disulfiram irreversibly inhibits the action of aldehyde dehydrogenase (ALDH) (as well as other enzymes), which metabolizes acetaldehyde to acetate. Consequently, in the absence of ALDH activity, the consumption of alcohol results in highly toxic levels of acetaldehyde in the bloodstream. Because ALDH inhibition is irreversible, the disulfiram effect will be expressed if drinking occurs within 6 to 14 days after the last dose of the drug, the time it takes for synthesis to restore normal levels of ALDH.

If a disulfiram-treated patient drinks as little as 7 ml of alcohol (about 0.24 fl oz, or the amount in a few doses of cough medicine), the resultant sharp rise of blood acetaldehyde causes an unpleasant syndrome characterized by facial flushing, tachycardia, pounding in the chest, decreased blood pressure, nausea, vomiting, shortness of breath, sweating, dizziness, and confusion. In severe cases that follow substantial alcohol intake by disulfiram-treated individuals with coronary disease, there may be myocardial infarction, cerebrovascular hemorrhage, cardiovascular collapse, and congestive seizures. An antidote to the development of these symptoms is the drug 4-methylpyrazol, which inhibits the metabolism of alcohol to acetaldehyde. However, the availability of this treatment does not justify the risk of disulfiram treatment with such patients.

It is obvious that disulfiram does not cure alcoholism. Rather, it serves to fortify the desire to stop drinking with the knowledge that any drinking within a week or two after taking the drug will be followed by the extremely unpleasant experience of the "acetaldehyde syndrome." Early research on disulfiram produced results that were not very promising, largely because of lack of compliance with taking the drug at home and a high rate of dropout from treatment. In one experiment, subjects receiving either low or high doses of disulfiram showed modest improvement over placebo controls; that is, they were a little more likely to remain abstinent, especially in the early months of treatment. Yet there were no significant clinical differences between the drug and control groups with respect to days worked, days drinking, or family stability. Again, those clients that did benefit from disulfiram treatment were said to be volunteers or selected individuals with a good prognosis for any form of treatment (Ritchie, 1985; Jaffe, 1987). Other studies have shown that compliance with the disulfiram dose schedule can be improved and dropout rates reduced by recruiting relatives to supervise and record the daily ingestion of the drug, and by contracts drawn up by the client, a relative, and a counselor.

A variety of side effects of disulfiram have been reported, including drowsiness, lethargy, tremor, dizziness, headache, and GI disturbances. The severity of these side effects has sometimes been overrated. On the other hand, because of these side effects, alcoholics with severe physical or psychiatric problems and those taking psychotropic drugs, or other drugs for organ dysfunctions, are not good candidates for disulfiram treatment. There are other substances, such as calcium carbamide (cyanamide or Abstem), that reversibly inhibit ALDH for shorter durations (less than a day) and are more selective in their action. Such compounds have fewer side effects, are better tolerated than disulfiram, and have approximately equivalent efficacy in preventing relapse into alcoholism for as long as treatment continues. Unfortunately, the pharmacokinetics of cyanamide make it easier for the patient to stop treatment and resume drinking.

Further considerations must be noted for disulfiram therapy. Disulfiram treatment should begin in a hospital because the patient must be alcohol-free for at least 12 hours before the first dose, and the maximal dose without undue side effects must be established. Also, clinicians recommend extensive mental, physical, and laboratory examinations followed by monthly or quarterly test repetitions. Thus, large-scale disulfiram treatment programs present major logistical problems with respect to implementation and maintenance.

Naltrexone treatment. Naltrexone, like naloxone, is a morphine derivative that is often used to treat individuals with opiate dependence. The mechanism of action of these drugs, as mentioned earlier in this chapter, is their ability to block μ and δ opiate receptors, thereby diminishing the positively reinforcing euphoria that opiates generate (see Chapter 12). Naltrexone is superior to naloxone in that it is orally effective, relatively free of side effects, and depending upon the dose, can produce receptor blockade for more than 24 hours. Given orally three times per week in doses of 100–150 mg, it provides almost continuous blockade (Jaffe, 1985).

Evidence from animal experiments, described above, has been found to link the endogenous opioid system to the reinforcement of alcohol drinking. Also, naltrexone reduced alcohol drinking in monkeys, as well as in strains of rodents that were selected for alcohol preference (Froehlich et al., 1991). There may be a similar relationship in humans. Studies compared nonalcoholic volunteers from families having a strong history of alcoholism (high risk) with volunteers with no family history of alcoholism (low risk). Baseline levels of plasma β-endorphin were lower in the high risk subjects, and a test dose of alcohol given to both groups produced a significantly greater increase in plasma β-endorphin in the high risk group. Thus, the opioid system may be more sensitive to alcohol in those at high risk of becoming alcoholics (Gianoulakis et al., 1990). Further, since opioid reinforcement has been linked to limbic dopamine activation, the opioid effects of alcohol consumption are consistent with the data implicating dopamine in the alcohol reinforcement mechanism.

These findings led to the hypothesis that naltrexone would diminish the rewarding effects of alcohol and reduce the urge to continue drinking. Clinical trials were begun with a double-blind experiment using naltrexone versus placebo in male chronic alcoholic volunteers who were patients applying for treatment at the Philadelphia Veterans Administration Medical Center (Volpicelli et al., 1992). All patients were first detoxified and then placed in a counseling program that extended over 3 months. Fifty percent of the patients received 50 mg of naltrexone daily, and the others received a placebo. During the 3 months of the study, the naltrexone-treated patients reported significantly less craving for alcohol, and they reported significantly fewer days of alcohol use. The overall rates of relapse for the two groups during the 3-month study are shown in Figure 15.15a. As is typical in rehabilitation programs, 54% of the placebo patients met the criterion for uncontrolled drinking for relapse to alcoholism, whereas only 23% in the naltrexone-treated group met that criterion. Further, in the placebo group, among those patients that "slipped" and resumed drinking, 95% met the criterion for relapse; whereas in the naltrexone group, only 50% of those who resumed drinking showed uncontrolled alcohol consumption. Thus, among alcoholics after detoxification, the consumption of even small amounts of alcohol usually leads to loss of control and relapse. In contrast, the chances of relapse were significantly less if the patient that drank happened to be on naltrexone.

When asked about the effects of alcohol, the placebo subjects reported nothing different, whereas those receiving naltrexone reported less euphoria from their drinking than expected based on prior experience. It was also found that patients can drink while on naltrexone with no noxious consequences, and can stop the medication without withdrawal symptoms.

A similar study on the efficacy of naltrexone utilized a different psychotherapy program with 97 alcohol-dependent subjects. Those randomly assigned to naltrexone treatment drank on half as many days and con-

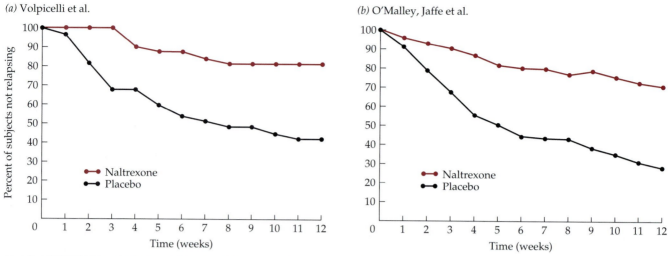

15.15. NALTREXONE ENHANCES PSYCHOTHERAPY FOR ALCOHOL DEPENDENCE. (a) In the Volpicelli et al. clinical trials, the naltrexone-treated subjects were significantly less likely to relapse to uncontrolled drinking. (b) Similar results were found in the O'Malley, Jaffe et al. study. (After O'Brien, 1994.)

sumed one-third the number of standard drinks as did subjects in the placebo group. Further, the naltrexone-treated subjects that had at least one drink had one-fourth the risk of relapse compared with subjects receiving placebo. In a follow-up evaluation 6 months after the end of the study, it was found that the naltrexone-treated subjects showed significantly less return to symptomatic drinking than those who had received placebo (O'Malley, Jaffe et al., 1992) (Figure 15.15b).

The aims of these treatment programs were to obtain total abstinence, not to use naltrexone to teach controlled drinking. However, by reducing the immediate reward produced by alcohol, the drug may support the efforts of rehabilitation programs by enabling patients to remain in treatment and receive the benefits of long-term behavior change (O'Brien, 1994).

In summary, while there have been reports of some drug-assisted improvements in the rate and degree of abstinence, as well as diminished withdrawal and post-withdrawal symptoms, there seems to be no generally approved pharmacotherapy for alcoholism and its after-effects (see Jaffe, 1987). This unfortunate situation again attests to the heterogeneous nature of alcoholism and the consequent difficulty of having to treat the condition practically on an individual basis. Nevertheless, the findings obtained thus far with naltrexone offer some hope that effective pharmacotherapies can be developed for the treatment of alcoholics.

Nondrug Approaches to the Treatment of Alcoholism

Individual and clinic-oriented psychotherapy. Some individuals who recognize that they have an alcohol problem will seek out a psychotherapist for one-on-one treat-

ment. Such therapy can be provided by psychiatrists, psychoanalysts, psychologists, or social workers. Psychoanalytically oriented treatment may be based on the notion that the patient has an "oral personality" characterized by lack of self-control, passive dependence on others, self-destructive impulses, and a tendency to use the mouth as a primary means of gratification. Psychoanalysts and psychiatrists (who are often Freudian in their approach) charge high rates, and the treatment usually goes on for a long period of time. Even though other treatment professionals may charge lower fees than psychiatrists or psychoanalysts, a course of individual therapy can still be prohibitively expensive unless covered by medical insurance.

A major alternative to individual psychotherapy by a private practitioner is treatment in a clinic setting. Most individuals seeking therapy for alcoholism are probably referred for treatment by family physicians, clergy, business organizations, or by the courts following a drunk-driving incident. In such cases, referral is often to a clinic that specializes in alcohol abuse, or more generally, substance abuse problems. Several steps occur upon acceptance into a clinic treatment program. If the patient is acutely alcoholic, then detoxification (clearance of alcohol from the system) must be accomplished first. During this time, withdrawal symptoms may be minimized by pharmacological interventions such as those described above. The next step is a thorough assessment of the patient as to his or her general health, intellectual status, social skills and attitudes, family relations, work status, possible legal problems, and so on. The patient is then assigned to a therapeutic team, and a treatment plan is outlined that may initially involve individual psychotherapy followed later by group sessions. Within the group, patients interact with one another to clarify their thoughts about their drinking problems and to verbalize ways of dealing with these problems.

Alcoholics Anonymous.

Some of the basic features of Alcoholics Anonymous (AA) were presented above. AA is an organization in which the membership (all alcoholics) directs its own affairs, and the participants are free to come and go as they please. As mentioned, AA subscribes to a variation of the disease model of alcoholism in which members must place themselves in the hands of a "higher power" that will help them remain sober. Emphasis is placed on educating individuals about the consequences of alcoholism through the testimonials of other group members. Continuing total abstinence is each member's goal, and support is provided any time someone needs help in maintaining this state. An important underlying assumption of AA is that only a peer group is able to understand and respond to the denials and rationalizations that prevent alcoholics from accepting the fact of their disorder.

Analysis has shown that the typical AA member is a middle-aged person with a severe degree of alcohol dependence and alcohol-related problems. AA is frequently sought out by the problem drinker who is headed toward or has reached "rock bottom," with major disintegration of health, job, and family life. Evidence further suggests that individuals best suited for AA have a particular psychological, social, and ethnic profile. Psychologically, they tend to have an authoritarian personality and a strong need for affiliation, and they are also likely to be overtly religious (Heather, 1990; Ogborne and Glaser, 1981). With respect to social and ethnic variables, AA seems to appeal more to middle- and upper-class whites from socially stable backgrounds than to individuals from other socioeconomic and/or ethnic groups.

Behavioral therapy.

The various models of alcoholism discussed earlier clearly lead to different types of therapeutic approaches. In contrast to the disease model, the behavioral model predicts the possibility of achieving either abstinence or controlled drinking (if desired) through the use of an instrumental conditioning approach. Such an approach is aimed at reducing or eliminating alcohol consumption by modifying the reinforcement contingencies associated with this behavior.

One of the earliest attempts at applying this method was carried out by Hunt and Azrin (1973), who developed the Community Reinforcement Approach (CRA). CRA was a systematic arrangement worked out with the client's spouse, employer, friends, and participating community agencies. Contingencies were carefully planned so that positive reinforcements predictably occurred only when the client was abstinent, and not when he was drinking. Clients were also provided with family counseling, vocational and financial assistance, and a social club serving exclusively nonalcoholic beverages to facilitate recreational activities without alcohol. Subsequent improvements to the CRA program added disulfiram treatment to discourage impulsive drinking as well as other techniques to improve long-term outcome (see Azrin, 1976).

A more recent type of behavioral therapy is known as cue exposure. This approach is based on experimental findings indicating that tolerance and withdrawal are partly conditioned responses (see MacCrae, Scoles, and Siegel, 1987), and the assumption that it should therefore be possible to extinguish the craving that is associated with alcohol withdrawal in dependent individuals. This approach generally consists of exposing alcoholics to cues for drinking (to elicit craving), then discouraging or preventing subsequent alcohol consumption. An interesting variation on this theme involves the interoceptive cues associated with a rising blood alcohol concentration. Through conditioning processes, these internal stimuli may become cues for further drinking, thus accounting for the loss of control typically associated with chronic alcoholism. Rankin, Hodgson, and Stockwell (1983) reported some success in extinguishing this learned association by repeatedly giving subjects moderate priming doses of alcohol, each of which was followed by a period during which the subjects were exposed to the sight and smell of alcohol but were not allowed to actually drink.

The Effectiveness of Different Treatment Approaches

In evaluating any treatment program for alcoholism, it is important to consider the rate of spontaneous remission of this disorder. Knowledge concerning the factors that contribute to spontaneous remission is also desirable for the purpose of incorporating such information into existing intervention strategies. Remission rates may vary considerably depending on what criteria are used. Perhaps the best available estimates come from long-term (15-year) follow-up studies in Sweden and the United States that reported spontaneous abstinence rates of 30% and 35%, respectively (Ojesjo, 1981; Vaillant, 1983). These figures suggest that substantial numbers of alcohol abusers are able to cope with their problem without professional assistance. For some, changes in drinking pattern may be triggered by an event in the person's life such as an alcohol-associated injury, marital separation or divorce, or alcohol-related financial and legal problems. Nevertheless, statistics on spontaneous remission rates must be viewed cautiously because of the difficulties inherent in selecting the sampling population as well as in defining and demonstrating remission.

According to most outcome research, the effectiveness of either individual or clinic-oriented psychotherapy for treating alcoholism is questionable at best. With respect to long-term outcome, several studies found no advantage for more intensive over less intensive treatment programs (e.g., inpatient vs. outpatient programs, extensive therapy vs. brief counseling) (for reviews, see Drummond, 1991; Heather, 1990). Moreover, some investigators have concluded that professional treatment does not even lead to higher long-term remission rates than are observed spontaneously (for example, Vaillant, 1983). This conclusion may be an oversimplification, however. Because of their differing personality characteristics, educational status, motivation, problem severity, and treatment goals (i.e., complete abstinence vs. achievement of controlled social drinking), alcohol abusers may need to be matched up with the appropriate treatment approach (Glaser, 1980). This so-called "matching hypothesis" predicts that client matching should lead to increased compliance and better long-term treatment outcome. Some studies appear to support this hypothesis (reviewed by McLellan and Alterman, 1991), but further research is needed to refine assessment methodology as well as the matching process itself.

Relatively few studies have been conducted to assess the outcome of behavioral therapies for alcohol abuse. The most controversial work comes from Sobell and Sobell (1973, 1976), who reported impressive results using individualized behavior therapy to achieve controlled drinking in a group of subjects who had been physically dependent on alcohol. Almost 10 years later, questions were raised about the integrity of this work, and the matter remains unresolved despite exoneration of the Sobells by several investigative committees (the interested reader is referred to Heather, 1990; Heather and Robertson, 1983). Despite the potential value of behavioral therapy, the long-term efficacy of this approach remains largely unknown. Thus, additional follow-up studies are clearly needed, as well as continuing research on the feasibility of controlled drinking versus abstinence as realistic treatment goals.

The effectiveness of AA has likewise been a matter of contention for many years. The organization has made extravagant assertions in this regard, claiming success rates as high as 75% (Alcoholics Anonymous, 1955). However, it has been extremely difficult to verify such claims because the anonymity of the membership precludes record keeping, and because AA itself has not been especially cooperative with researchers. Nevertheless, it is interesting to note the outcome of one study in which alcohol abusers facing legal sanctions were randomly assigned to AA, individual psychotherapy, two different types of behavioral therapy, or to a control group that received no intervention. When follow-up was conducted 1 year later, all of the treatments generally produced better outcomes than no treatment; however, AA was inferior to the other approaches used (Brandsma, Maultsby, and Welsh, 1981). In accordance with the matching hypothesis, it may have been the case that the subjects assigned to AA were not well suited to that organization's theory and methods. We may reasonably conclude that AA does work well for many individuals, but is inappropriate for many others. Advantages of AA include its lack of cost, ready accessibility, and continuing support for clients as they struggle with their drinking problems. On the other hand, the model of alcoholism promoted by AA may impede progress in certain areas, such as early intervention and secondary prevention (Heather, 1990).

The Relapse Prevention Approach

Almost any treatment approach can claim success in reducing or eliminating alcohol consumption by the end of the treatment period. The problem, of course, is that most patients have relapsed when they are studied again months or years later. Attention has therefore been focused on the possible causes of relapse and the means by which treatment goals can be maintained over the long term. An underlying assumption of the behavioral model is that the habits associated with drinking have become so deeply ingrained over the years that the relatively short period of time allocated to treatment is insufficient to extinguish these behaviors fully or to modify them in the desired way. Rather, months or even years may be necessary for new habits and coping strategies to become firmly incorporated into the individual's behavioral repertoire. Whether better results are achievable by the supplementary use of opiate receptor blocking agents such as naltrexone may be revealed by more experience with this promising method (see above).

Marlatt and his colleagues have developed a useful model of relapse and relapse prevention (Marlatt and George, 1984). Their approach is based in part on interviews with problem drinkers indicating that the most common precipitating factors (i.e., high-risk situations) in relapse are (1) negative emotional states such as anger, anxiety, frustration, and depression, (2) social conflicts involving spouses, other family members, friends, or work associates, and (3) social pressures, including direct pressure to drink. The relapse prevention strategy of Marlatt is based on social learning theory and aims to help clients anticipate high-risk situations and develop coping strategies for such situations, learn how to deal with an initial lapse to avoid a full-blown relapse, and cope with a serious relapse without collapsing or dropping out of treatment. To achieve these goals, clients receive training in a variety of self-management skills. Cognitive restructuring is also used, for example, to alter client attitudes toward a lapse. Lapses are thus regarded as errors in the learning process underlying recovery, rather than a reaffirmation of the individual's belief that he is unable to prevent further drinking (dubbed by Marlatt the "abstinence violation effect"). It seems clear that the relapse prevention approach can be a powerful adjunct, or perhaps even an alternative, to more traditional treatment strategies. Indeed, Heather (1990) views it as the most influential recent development in the treatment of alcoholism.

Fetal Alcohol Syndrome

In the section above on the systemic effects of alcohol, we mentioned that a number of structures and functions of the female reproductive system are adversely affected by chronic alcohol use. Further, it has been found that the adverse effect of alcohol on the menstrual cycle is frequently associated with infertility and spontaneous abortion. In many cases, however, alcohol-abusing women who become pregnant come to term with offspring, and these infants are sometimes born with congenital anomalies. This unfortunate result comes about because alcohol freely passes the placental barrier, causing the fetus to be exposed to the same effective dose as the mother. However, whereas it takes the mother about 1 hour to metabolize the alcohol in one drink, the alcohol remains in the fetal system for 6–12 hours. In addition, alcohol causes a number of placental abnormalities, one of which is the constriction of the umbilical blood vessels that connect the placenta to the fetus. The result may be a diminished placental blood flow that reduces the supply of oxygen and nutrients to the fetus and the removal of CO_2. The resulting fetal hypoxia may be an indirect factor in the toxicity of alcohol. Recent reviews of the subject have concluded that evidence about the effects of alcohol on the growth, maturation, and survival of cells is rapidly accumulating, even though present proposals about the mechanism of cell damage associated with fetal alcohol exposure are based on weak and circumstantial evidence (Michaelis, 1990; Randall, Ekblad, and Anton, 1990; Schenker et al., 1990).

Frequency and Antecedents of Fetal Alcohol Syndrome

The term "Fetal Alcohol Syndrome" (FAS) was coined by Jones and colleagues (1973) to describe a pattern of physical malformations and mental retardation that they encountered among 11 children born to alcoholic mothers; Clarren and Smith (1973) added a working definition of FAS after collating information on 245 subsequent case reports.

Full FAS cases occur in the offspring of approximately 6% of alcoholic mothers and in 0.1% to 0.3% of live births (Charness, Simon, and Greenberg, 1989). These numbers suggest that there will be approximately 1,200 new cases in the United States each year, which will account for 10% of all persons born with mental retardation. These individuals will generate an annual medical and special education cost of $74.6 million, and an estimated $1.4 million lifetime expenditure per FAS child (Abel and Sokol, 1991; Clarren, 1990; Streissguth et al., 1991). Other studies have reported that FAS occurs in one-third of the infants born to mothers who consume 150 g or more alcohol per day during pregnancy, and that another third show some degree of mental retardation without the other overt features of the syndrome

that are described below. Finally, it is important to note that ethnic groups with high rates of alcoholism may show extremely high incidences of FAS. For example, whereas the proportion of FAS cases to live births in Seattle, Washington, is 1:700, the proportion on one southwestern Native American reservation is 1:97; the highest reported proportions were 1:8 on one Canadian reservation and about 1:4 in an interior Alaskan area (Backover, 1991; Conry, 1990; Streissguth et al., 1991).

Knowing that there is a direct relationship between habitual and excessive maternal alcohol use and the occurrence of FAS, various public health agencies in the United States set about acquainting women of childbearing age with the health risks to their offspring that are associated with alcohol use. Similar programs focused on the risks of cigarette smoking and the illicit use of cocaine, "crack," heroin, barbiturates, and other drugs. Despite these educational programs, however, continued alcohol use and a heightened risk for poor pregnancy outcome remains a significant problem, especially for young, unmarried women who have a high school education or less, and who smoke.

Alcohol Effects on Fetal Development and Postnatal Behavior

Effects of alcohol on the fetal nervous system. As shown by animal studies, alcohol and acetaldehyde are directly toxic to fetal nervous tissue and cause brain growth deficits and neuron loss (Randall and Taylor, 1979; O'Shea and Kaufman, 1979). The fetus is subject to alcohol-induced disruption of neuronal cell membrane integrity and cytoskeletal elements, and to inhibition of RNA and protein synthesis, which are crucial to cell multiplication. Also, alcohol causes interference with transmembrane signaling, which is crucial for neuron division, migration, differentiation, and synaptogenesis (see Schenker et al., 1990, Michaelis, 1990; West et al., 1990). Autopsies on aborted and nonsurviving FAS infants revealed numerous instances of neuronal and glial pathology in the cerebrum, hippocampus, and cerebellum, displacement of neurons and glia into the brain membranes (the pia mater and the arachnoid), and agenesis of the corpus callosum (Figure 15.16).

Alcohol, organogenesis, and FAS. In humans, organogenesis (the laying down of the body organs in the fetus) occurs during the first 10 weeks of embryonic life, which corresponds to the major part of the first trimester. During this period the developing organs, including the CNS, may be especially vulnerable to the toxic effects of alcohol because of its depressant effect upon the rapid rate of cell division and protein synthesis that occurs at this time (West et al., 1990).

Unfortunately, many women with a pattern of persistent drinking may be unaware they are pregnant dur-

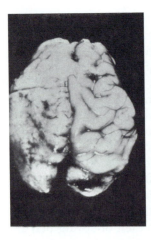 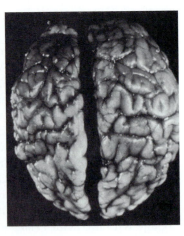

15.16 ABNORMAL BRAIN DEVELOPMENT ASSOCIATED WITH FETAL ALCOHOL SYNDROME A brain from an FAS infant (*left*) compared to a brain from a normal infant of the same age (*right*). The FAS brain shows microcephaly, cerebral cortical gyri, and the presence of a sheet of ectopic (abnormally migrated) glia over the surface of the left hemisphere. (Courtesy of S. Clarren.)

ing the early stages and may unknowingly inflict significant, irreversible damage on the developing embryo. Maternal drinking during the first trimester may contribute to the deficient pre- and postnatal growth and congenital injury to organ systems that characterize FAS (Maxwell, 1984).

Moreover, whereas the brain is one of the first organs to begin development, it is also the last to become fully mature, as its development is not complete until 2 years postnatally, or even later. Consequently, because the brain is vulnerable to various insults throughout the course of pregnancy, alcohol-induced neural and mental anomalies are encountered most frequently, even when other teratogenic effects are barely detectable (Michaelis, 1990). (See also Abel, 1985; Aronson and Olegård, 1985; Charness, Simon, and Greenberg, 1989; Maxwell, 1984; Streissguth et al., 1991; Thomson et al., 1988.)

Systemic signs of FAS/FAE. As established by the Research Society on Alcoholism, an FAS diagnosis is confirmed by a history of maternal alcohol abuse and the fulfillment of three criteria by the child: prenatal or postnatal growth retardation (height and weight below the 10th percentile), CNS dysfunction (neurological, developmental, or intellectual impairment), and at least two of the craniofacial abnormalities described below. In cases in which the symptoms are fewer and less severe, such as when a child shows two, but not all three, of the above indicators for FAS, the diagnosis is that of Fetal Alcohol Effects (FAE) (see Rosett, 1980; and Conry, 1990).

The overt signs of FAS include prenatal and postnatal growth retardation, mild to moderate microcephaly (small head circumference), and irritability and jitteriness in infancy. Other common features of FAS are facial

dysmorphology consisting of craniofacial abnormalities that correlate with the amount of alcohol taken during the first trimester, a time when pregnancy is frequently unrecognized. Typical craniofacial signs include a narrow upper lip, a small nose, and the absence of the philtrum (the groove between the nose and the upper lip). There are also short palpebral fissures (the openings between the eyelids), folds over the upper lid, and abnormally small eyeballs; there is sometimes an inordinate amount of hair on the face at birth, along with an underdeveloped jaw, cleft palate, misaligned teeth, and malformations of the middle ear. One investigator reported that more than 50% of FAS infants had retinal malformations such as hypoplasia (abnormal or incomplete development) of the optic disc and tortuosity (multiple twists and turns) of retinal blood vessels, such that 50% of these infants later showed moderately reduced vision and 25% of them had severely reduced visual acuity. (See Abel and Sokol, 1991, for a breakdown of the frequencies of occurrence of these and other FAS-related effects, and the costs of their medical management.)

There are additional systemic findings of congenital injuries to the genitourinary system and cardiac malformations, and there are reports of musculoskeletal anomalies such as joint dysplasias and postnatal muscular weakness. Consequently, many of these infants are late in beginning to walk and show persistent balance difficulties and clumsiness. Shortly after birth, neonates of severely alcoholic mothers show signs of alcohol withdrawal symptoms, including seizures. They are also irritable, jittery, tremulous, and difficult to feed, and they gain weight slowly. At this point the caregiving by the alcoholic mother often breaks down, and the child is frequently given over to foster care. (See Aronson and Olegård, 1985; Clarren, 1990; Streissguth et al., 1991.)

Later in life there may be isolated brain dysfunctions such as mental retardation, learning disabilities, and attention deficit hyperactivity disorder (ADHD) (see below). Generally, these findings are included in the category of Fetal Alcohol Effects, but some individuals who have not been exposed to alcohol in utero may have the same isolated malformations or brain dysfunctions, possibly caused by other toxic substances in the uterine environment. One such situation may occur when the mother has phenylketonuria and does not sufficiently restrict phenylalanine from her diet (see Chapter 8). Although the mother may tolerate high phenylalanine levels in adulthood, the fetus may be significantly affected by this condition in utero, with severe mental retardation being the consequence (Prensky, 1975). Thus, the isolated appearance of many of these symptoms is not reliably diagnostic of FAS.

Reversible and irreversible characteristics. In a longitudinal study of 36 FAS and 11 FAE patients as adolescents and adults, Streissguth and coworkers (1991) found that some of the overt symptoms, such as the facial dysmorphologies, became less noticeable as the child grew through adolescence to adulthood, but the retarded postnatal growth in body length and head circumference persisted. With respect to intellectual functioning, the average IQ scores (Wechsler Intelligence Scales-Revised for adults and children where appropriate) for the FAS and FAE groups were 66 and 73, respectively, which represented significantly subaverage intellectual function. The IQ range was wide, from 20 (severely retarded) to 105 (normal), but 58% of the patients had IQs below 70, which is a commonly used cutoff point for the classification of the developmentally disabled. The average reading, spelling, and arithmetic grade levels for these individuals were fourth, third, and second grade, respectively, showing that arithmetic ability was most severely compromised. The older patients did not, in general, function better academically than the younger patients, thus testifying to the permanent nature of the mental deficits. In an earlier study, Streissguth (1988) compared 58 FAS patients with 34 FAE patients in young adulthood with respect to their intellectual and social functioning. Although the FAS adults were intellectually more impaired, there were no differences between the groups in terms of academic and social functioning. Thus the long-term consequences of FAE can be as severe as those of FAS.

Considering adaptive functioning, patients with FAS and FAE functioned at about the 7-year level, even though they averaged 17 years chronologically. Most of them were lacking in age-appropriate social and communication skills, and they characteristically failed to consider the consequences of their actions. Further, they showed a lack of appropriate initiative, were unresponsive to subtle social cues, and lacked reciprocal friendships.

With respect to maladaptive behaviors, as measured by objective tests, 62% of the patients had "significant" levels of maladaptive behaviors and 38% had "intermediate" levels, but no patient was in the "insignificant" range. The most frequent findings were poor concentration and attention, dependence, stubbornness and sullenness, social withdrawal, teasing or bullying, crying or laughing too easily, impulsivity, and periods of high anxiety. In addition, some of the patients were found to lie, cheat, or steal, and exhibited excessive unhappiness.

Behavior problems are an expected concomitant of mental retardation, but compared with patients with Down's syndrome, of which 15% to 32% were labeled as having severe behavior problems, 62% of FAS patients were so designated (see Streissguth et al., 1991). Contributing to the unfortunate status of these patients was their unstable early environment. On average, the FAS patients had lived in five different receiving homes in their lifetimes, and only a few were still with both biological parents or their biological mothers. It was found that 69% of the biological mothers of the FAS group were dead of alcohol-related illness or from other alcohol-related causes such as suicide, homicide, falls, and automobile accidents. Nearly one-third of the patients had never been raised by their biological mothers; they were either given up for adoption at birth or abandoned in the hospital.

Judging from these limited data, the outlook for these patients in adulthood was bleak indeed. Their limited intellectual resources and severe behavioral problems made these individuals unsuitable for training programs, even those that have been devised for patients with Down's syndrome. Furthermore, there was a predictable long-term progression of the disorder into adulthood, leading to severe difficulties in living independently and avoiding criminal activity. These findings point out the need for facilities to provide more favorable remedial experiences for FAS patients, and to serve as shelters to prevent their victimization. (See Streissguth et al., 1991, for more details.)

Prenatal alcohol exposure and ADHD.   A number of reports describing manifestations of FAS and FAE have mentioned that these children are hyperactive, destructive, impulsive, and have short attention spans. Some mothers reporting alcohol consumption in "social" amounts during pregnancy have also described their children as being inattentive, fidgety, and restless. These behavior patterns frequently resembled those of children that were diagnosed as suffering from the Attention Deficit Hyperactivity Disorder (ADHD) (see Chapter 13).

Nanson and Hiscock (1990) compared FAS/FAE children with ADHD and normal children, all within the ages of 5–12 years, using questionnaires, intelligence tests, and attention-demanding tasks to measure attention and impulsivity. The attention test was the Delay Reaction Time Task (DRTT), which requires that the subject respond to a tone by pressing a button and maintain that response until a visual signal appears.

Test results showed that the FAS/FAE children were significantly more impaired intellectually than the normal and the ADHD groups, but the signs of behavioral problems were about the same for the FAS/FAE and the ADHD children. Even their parents described the social behavior of the FAS/FAE and ADHD children in similar terms as being inattentive and hyperactive, despite the differences in the intellectual abilities between the two groups, and these ratings were in direct contrast to the parental ratings of the normal children.

On the DRTT measures of attention, the FAS/FAE children made significantly more impulsive errors (presses before the tone signal was presented) and also responded more slowly than the normal children. The ADHD subjects likewise displayed excessive impulsivity; however, they responded as rapidly as the normal children. Thus, both groups were marked by impulsivity, but motor deficiencies were characteristic only among the FAS/FAE subjects.

In summary, comparisons of FAS/FAE and ADHD children showed that FAS/FAE children were more intellectually impaired than were ADHD children, but that the behavioral characteristics of fidgety inattention and restlessness were characteristic of both groups. Moreover, based on the observation that preschool children of social drinkers display behavior similar to that of preschoolers who are later diagnosed as having ADHD, it can be concluded that children diagnosed as having ADHD may include a number of children who may have been exposed in utero even to relatively small amounts of alcohol at inopportune times during their fetal development (Nanson and Hiscock, 1990).

Factors Contributing to FAS

In epidemiological FAS studies it has been noted that many, if not most, women who reported substantial alcohol consumption during pregnancy gave birth to infants who were quite free of obvious birth defects, whereas other women reporting similar rates of alcohol consumption had infants with FAS with considerable CNS damage (Sokol, Miller, and Reed, 1980). It had been proposed that these differences were due to genetically determined degrees of alcohol sensitivity on the part of the mother and/or her fetus. The more valid explanation may be that the likelihood of fetal teratogenesis depends mainly on the peak blood alcohol levels attained, the pattern of consumption, and the period and duration of fetal exposure to alcohol during the pregnancy.

Peak blood alcohol levels and FAS.   It is now established that the peak blood alcohol levels in the mother and the fetus, rather than the overall amount consumed, is the critical factor in causing organ damage. For example, it is very likely that the effects on a fetus of 30 grams of alcohol per day for a week would be far different from those of a binge episode of 210 grams once per week, even though the weekly average of alcohol intake was the same.

This view was supported by evidence concerning the effect of alcohol on neonatal rats undergoing their peak brain growth spurt, which corresponds to that occurring during the third trimester in the human fetus. Among these rats, brain growth was severely retarded after condensed alcohol administration leading to high peak blood alcohol levels (270 mg/dl). In contrast, there were minimal brain effects when the same dose was administered over an extended time period, resulting in stable maximum blood alcohol levels of 46 mg/dl. These BAC-dependent effects were also observed when alcohol-induced neuronal loss and behavioral deficits were measured. For example, alcohol-induced cell loss in the hippocampus and the cerebellum was greater in neona-

tal rats that received a condensed dose of 4.5 g/kg than in those that received distributed doses totaling 6.6 g/kg, with the lower dose causing higher peak blood levels (Schenker et al., 1990; West et al., 1990.)

In another experiment by West and colleagues (1990), a daily total of 6.6 g/kg of alcohol was given in a milk formula to rat pups on postnatal days 4 through 9. One group received a dose of a 2.5% alcohol solution during each of 12 daily feedings (1 every 2 hours) over a 6-day period. Another group received doses of a 7.5% solution during 4 of the 12 daily feedings, and a third group received doses of a 15% solution during 2 of the daily feedings. On postnatal day 6, the mean peak BACs for the three groups were 53, 383, and 523 mg/dl, respectively. On postnatal day 10, the pups were sacrificed and their brains weighed. There were no differences between a group of nonalcohol controls and the rats exposed to the multiple 2.5% doses, but the brain weights of the rats receiving 4 daily condensed 7.5% doses or 2 daily condensed 15% doses were diminished by 19% and 31%, respectively. Moreover, in subsequent experiments on cell loss in the rat cerebellum, the correlation between cell loss and the BAC was maintained: when the BAC was maintained at 85 mg/dl there was virtually no cell loss, but when the dose was condensed and there were peaks at 480 mg/dl, cell loss was considerable. This strong correlation between peak BAC and microencephaly supports the hypothesis that the pattern of exposure determines the severity of alcohol-induced neuronal injury. In addition, there were differences in alcohol vulnerability among the various lobules of the cerebellum: some lobes in the cerebellum showed cell loss, whereas others appeared to be normal.

Regional CNS and organ vulnerability.   The course of human fetal development is not a steadily progressive one; rather, growth occurs with spurts of activity from time to time. For example, the first trimester is considered to be the period of organogenesis and neuronal multiplication. During this period exposure to alcohol results in a variety of neuronal, skeletal, and visceral anomalies in the fetus. In the second and third trimesters there are significant spurts in brain growth and weight when neurons and glia grow to establish their branches and connections and axon myelinization occurs. It is in these latter stages that an initial alcohol exposure can lead to neuronal and behavioral deficits in the absence of overt physical defects. As we pointed out earlier, chronic alcohol consumption throughout pregnancy results in a wide variety of effects ranging from CNS injury and structural anomalies to the growth retardation that is characteristic of FAS. On the other hand, episodic binge drinking at high levels of alcohol consumption is more likely to yield abnormalities in organ systems or parts of the brain that are in a phase of intense development. Consequently, alcohol-induced injury may appear selective when, in fact, the areas undergoing critical development coincide with binge episodes to produce localized anomalies. Similar changes occur in the growth rates of various subcellular components such as DNA and RNA. For example, in the human fetus, there is a rapid increase of DNA content during two periods: the first occurs during the 15th and 20th weeks of gestation, and the second begins after the 25th week and continues into the second year of postnatal life. Also, there are changes in the free pool concentrations of various amino acids, some of which are rising while others are falling. In addition, changes occur in the concentrations of gangliosides, proteins, phospholipids, and neurotransmitters, which are different in the various brain regions (see Alling, 1985; Michaelis, 1990).

Clarren and colleagues carefully studied the impact of binge alcohol ingestion on pregnant pigtailed macaque monkeys while monitoring the pregnancies to maximize physical health and minimize stress. They were interested in the teratogenicity of binge drinking, and whether behavioral effects can occur without overt physical effects. The alcohol regimen in this experiment modeled the most common drinking schedule of nonalcoholic-dependent women, the binge at the Saturday night party. Thus the animals were given alcohol doses at various concentrations (0.3–1.8 g/kg) diluted in four parts water once per week for 24 weeks. The highest dose was 1.8 g/kg because preliminary tests showed that fetuses were aborted at higher doses. Also, some animals were not dosed until after 5 weeks of gestation; after that, they were given higher doses (2.5–4.1 g/kg).

The results showed that none of the macaque infants had the full constellation of anomalies characteristic of human FAS patients, but each component was found in at least one animal. The data suggested that certain anomalies, such as facial dysmorphologies, occured after fetal alcohol exposure during specific focal periods of gestation, and that growth deficiencies and microcephaly appeared when the mothers received the highest doses. Concerning developmental and cognitive effects, there were significant deficits in animals whose mothers' mean peak plasma ethanol concentrations were above 140 mg/dl and who were dosed from the beginning of pregnancy. Among the animals receiving alcohol after a 5-week gestational delay, there was a marked diminution of symptoms despite the high doses they received. These findings strongly suggest that the brain is especially vulnerable to alcohol during the early period of gestation. Further, they suggest that binge-type exposure to alcohol can alter brain function without necessarily producing concomitant physical malformations, and that prolonged exposure to higher doses is most likely to produce developmental and cognitive deficits. (For more details and references see Clarren, 1990.)

The role of maternal nutrition. Because malnutrition is a common adjunct of alcohol abuse, its role in FAS has been thoroughly investigated. Many alcoholic mothers may be malnourished before giving birth to FAS children, but investigation has shown that although the dietary intake of such mothers showed some deficiencies, their diets were not obviously inferior to those of mothers in the same setting with normal children. Though the fetus depends upon a maternal supply of some key nutrients such as certain amino acids and vitamins, and though maternal dietary deficiencies can result in impaired fetal growth, it is thought that malnutrition is not obligatory for the development of alcohol-induced fetal damage. Further, there is no clear indication that fetal damage results from aberrations of glucose metabolism as it may be related to maternal alcohol intake; nor does it seem to be related to specific deficiencies in vitamin intake, absorption, utilization, and excretion.

Effects of multiple drug use. Estimating the precise relationship between the degree of alcohol abuse and fetal damage is sometimes difficult because in utero exposure to other drugs and other conditions may be factors in the presenting case. Among alcohol abusers there is a prevalence of multiple drug use. Alcohol abuse is frequently accompanied by the use of opiates, cocaine, cigarettes, and marijuana, which may further exacerbate fetal injury. It is informative to note that a 1990 survey of emergency rooms in the United States by the National Institute for Drug Abuse (NIDA) showed that alcohol combined with other drugs was the most frequently mentioned cause of problems necessitating acute medical care. The same report stated that among emergency room visits for drug-related problems, heroin combined with alcohol and, in some cases, one or more other drugs accounted for 30% of heroin abuse cases, and cocaine combined with alcohol and sometimes other drugs accounted for 42% of the cocaine abuse cases. Other data indicate that alcohol combined with cocaine and alcohol combined with heroin were among the eight drug combinations most frequently cited by medical examiners in the United States in postmortem reports of causes of death or related to death in drug-related cases (Kreek, 1987).

Moreover, alcoholics tend to be heavy cigarette smokers, a habit that investigations show is intensified during concurrent drinking (see Mello, 1987). It has long been known that cigarette smoking by pregnant women contributes to retarded fetal growth, which may be due to nicotine-induced constriction of placental blood vessels that deprives the fetus of well-oxygenated blood and nutrients. Alcohol has a similar effect, and the two effects are additive (Leichter, 1989; Meyer and Tonascia, 1977). Marijuana smoking has been reported to exert adverse effects upon reproductive hormones in women, which increases the risk of failure to maintain pregnancy and contributes to uterine dysfunction and possibly fetal abnormalities (Braude and Ludford, 1984; Mendelson,

and contributes to uterine dysfunction and possibly fetal abnormalities (Braude and Ludford, 1984; Mendelson, 1987). Thus, whereas the more severe FAS cases seem to be among the children of mothers who drank heavily throughout pregnancy, the possibility exists that multiple drug use may be an important contributing factor.

Is There a No-Risk Level of Alcohol Use for Pregnant Women?

Until recently, it had been held that there was no precise dose–response curve for alcohol-induced fetal pathology, but evidence suggested that a mother's consumption of more than three drinks per day tripled the risk of her offspring having a subnormal IQ (<85) at the age of 4. Despite the fact that the ingestion of less than three drinks per day has not been found to correlate with fetal damage, some studies suggest that a linear relationship exists between the dose of alcohol and behavioral and morphological measurements, and thus reject the notion that there is a threshold for adverse alcohol effects (Mello, 1987).

This view was buttressed by the results of an extensive longitudinal study by Streissguth, Barr, and Sampson (1990) of 500 infants born to 1,529 pregnant women who were receiving prenatal care in two hospitals in Seattle, Washington. These women were primarily white, middle class, and at low risk for adverse pregnancy outcomes. They were queried about their age and education and their family history of learning disabilities. The amount and frequency of their drinking of beer, wine, and liquor during midpregnancy and during the 4–5 weeks before pregnancy recognition was assessed in fine detail. They were also interviewed regarding their use of caffeine, tobacco, and drugs, their nutrition, and the course of their pregnancy. Their use of the above substances ranged from heavy drinking and smoking to infrequent drinking and abstinence.

The offspring of these mothers were carefully studied on their first and second days of life, at approximately 8 and 18 months, and at approximately 4 and 7 years. Other covariates among the infants and children that might bear upon the data were considered, such as illnesses, accidents, hospitalizations, minor illnesses on the day of an examination, preschool attendance, and major life changes in the household at 8 and 18 months and 4 and 7 years. Other factors, such as the sex of the child and the grade and age in days at time of testing, were also taken into account. The children were tested with the Wechsler Intelligence Scale for Children-Revised (WISC-R), the Wide Range Achievement Test, and the Connors' Parent Rating Scale, and the children's teachers filled out the Myklebust Pupil Rating Scale (MPRS) on the child's classroom behavior. Other behavior ratings and computerized vigilance tests were also performed. At no time were the examiners aware of any prior test result.

The results showed that the mean WISC IQ of the full cohort of 482 children was 107.6 ± 14.4. However, the IQs for the full scale, the verbal scale, and the performance scale were all significantly lower for children exposed, on average, to more than 1 ounce of alcohol per day in midpregnancy, even after adjustment for the many covariates listed above. With respect to academic achievement, women who reported ever drinking five or more drinks on any occasion during the month or so prior to pregnancy recognition had children who were, on average, 1–3 months behind their peers in reading and arithmetic by the end of the first grade in school. Among the 154 children of mothers reporting binge drinking before or after pregnancy recognition, 24% were in remedial programs at school, compared with 15% of the 328 children of nonbingers. Furthermore, on the basis of their MPRS scores, 17% of the first group (vs. 10% of the second group) were judged at risk for learning disabilities. The results of the other tests showed similar differences in the signs of fetal alcohol effects. It should be noted that the mothers who admitted to binge drinking were, on average, younger, less educated, and less likely to be married. In the analysis of the effect of alcohol on the results of subtests, such as Arithmetic and Digit Span, Comprehension of Words, and Cooperation/Impulsivity, there were uniformly negative correlations with possible fetal alcohol exposure; that is, the more often the mothers drank, the lower the test scores.

It was concluded that two alcohol consumption patterns stand out as being related to the deficits described above: over two drinks per day during midpregnancy, and binge patterns of five or more drinks per occasion, especially before pregnancy recognition. The data also showed that even 1 ounce of alcohol per day during pregnancy can lead to almost half of a standard deviation (almost 7 points) decrement in IQ score, which in this population would increase by 3.5-fold the number of IQ scores below 85.

These effects are of basic organic etiology rather than stemming from factors in the postnatal environment, as shown by the appearance of alcohol-induced effects shortly after birth. On postnatal day 1, the affected infants showed manifestations of attentional deficits as measured by habituation (the ability to withhold responses to redundant and irrelevant stimuli): the more alcohol use reported by the mothers, the more poorly the infants habituated to repetitive light, rattle, and bell stimuli. Alcohol-related decrements of attention were also observed at ages 4 and 7 years in a laboratory vigilance paradigm that was sensitive to sustained attention. The children who had experienced prenatal alcohol exposure showed "errors of commission" by impulsively pressing the response key. The apparent permanence of prenatal alcohol effects was demonstrated in children of moderately drinking mothers by the finding of decrements of attention and speed of central process-to attach to the nipple by the newborn, the longer the latency to self-correct errors on a fine motor maze task at the age of 4, and the longer the reaction time on vigilance tasks at ages 4 and 7.

These findings have been buttressed by the results of animal studies showing that prenatal alcohol exposure can lead to behavioral deficits similar to those found in humans, including problems of response inhibition, suckling, gait, and spatial memory. Thus, learning problems in school-age children can be linked to maternal social drinking during pregnancy. Because 10% of schoolchildren are designated as having learning disabilities, it is imperative to isolate the biological antecedents of these problems. Consequently, the American Medical Association and the Surgeon General have advised that women attempting to conceive should abstain from alcohol (Charness, Simon, and Greenberg, 1989; Mello, 1987). This measure may be the first step in the prediction, prevention, and treatment of a major proportion of learning disabilities (Streissguth, Barr, and Sampson, 1990).

Summary

Alcohol is a drug of worldwide distribution, use, and concern. A large majority of humans (75% of American adults, for example) enjoy the consumption of alcoholic beverages. At small doses, alcohol rapidly bestows upon the consumer a warm, relaxed feeling of tranquility that contributes to conviviality in social situations. However, consumption of larger amounts frequently leads to disinhibition by social constraints, so that conviviality turns to boisterousness and irresponsibility, or social tension and conflict. As consumption continues, motor control is compromised so that the drinker is inarticulate and ataxic to the point at which he may be a danger to himself or to others. Under these conditions the judgement of the drinker may be diminished so that even more alcohol is consumed, leading to severe intoxication characterized by stupor, insensibility, and blackouts (a loss of memory for episodes that occurred prior to the developing intoxication). Thus, what was initially a relaxant and a mood elevator becomes a toxic substance with dangerous consequences.

These events in varying degrees occur occasionally to almost all steady users of alcohol. However, for a considerable number of individuals (15% of alcohol users, with men outnumbering women 6 to 1), intoxication occurs with regularity. The resultant health consequences and other adverse effects have caused alcohol to be considered the foremost drug of abuse, doing damage far exceeding that done by the abuse of all other known substances put together (except tobacco). Alcohol abuse is frequently associated with personality and affective disorders such as anxiety and depression, and it can lead to physical pathology of the gastrointestinal, cardiovascular, and the central nervous systems. It also results in psy-

chosocial pathology exemplified by severe accident proneness, child and spouse abuse, divorce, economic incompetence, suicide and homicide, and dementia. In addition to these consequences to the alcoholic, there is serious danger to others who come into contact with alcoholics, such as those in families that are disrupted by alcoholic parents, and those who are injured or killed by drunken drivers. Also, there is the danger of damage done by some alcoholic pregnant women to their fetuses, who are injured by the transplacental invasion of alcohol into their rapidly developing bodies. Such offspring are designated as having fetal alcohol syndrome. They enter life with physical handicaps and mental retardation, and suffer from lifelong disadvantage, social incompetence, and dependence upon civic support.

Investigations into the biochemistry of alcohol have shown that alcohol potentiates GABA-mediated postsynaptic inhibition by enhancing the uptake of chloride ions. These findings, together with the unique character of the $GABA_A$ benzodiazepine receptor–chloride ionophore complex indicate that this particular receptor system plays a central role in the actions of alcohol. Also, there has been considerable attention to serotonergic (5-HT) mechanisms that are related to alcoholism. It was found that serotonin hypofunction accompanies increased alcohol consumption in alcohol-craving rats, whereas the stimulation of the 5-HT raphe or zimelidine-induced blockade of 5-HT uptake (which facilitates 5-HT synaptic action) diminishes alcohol consumption. Further, zimelidine reduced alcohol consumption among human alcoholics. With respect to tolerance, 5-HT stimulation facilitated the acquisition of alcohol tolerance, whereas 5-HT lesions or drug-induced 5-HT depletion delayed tolerance acquisition and hastened its disappearance during abstinence.

Two key characteristics of alcoholism are tolerance and dependence. Chronic consumption of relatively large amounts of alcohol induces tolerance for many of the drug's behavioral effects. Thus, heavier consumption is needed for the desired or rewarding effects of the drug. However, because tolerance for many of the effects of alcohol is uneven, high alcohol intake can occur without ataxia or garbled speech, but the heavy intake can still cause severe damage to organ systems and increase the susceptibility to acute alcohol toxicity, because the toxic threshhold does not undergo tolerance and remains the same.

Alcohol dependence is associated with the rebound that occurs with abstinence after cellular tolerance has been established. For example, the synaptic inhibition following alcohol intake may reduce the occurrence of epileptic seizures in a seizure-prone individual. But sudden abstinence may exacerbate the release of neural discharge from epileptic foci, and the seizures, if undetected, may have lethal consequences. Even if an alcohol abuser is not prone to epilepsy, higher alcohol intake provokes more severe withdrawal symptoms, which can ultimately become life-threatening.

The phenomenon of cross-tolerance exists for both metabolic and cellular tolerance. The consequence of metabolic cross-tolerance is that in the presence of alcohol, another drug for an unrelated illness could compete for the metabolizing enzymes, thereby exaggerating the effect of both drugs. On the other hand, if a required drug is administered to a sober alcoholic with an exaggerated enzyme activity, the drug may be broken down so rapidly that its therapeutic effect would be diminished or lost altogether.

In epidemiological studies of alcoholism, the role of inheritance is being extensively investigated. There is substantial evidence that children of alcoholics raised as adoptees of nonalcoholics have the same vulnerability for alcoholism as nonadopted children of alcoholics. But, children of nonalcoholics that are raised by alcoholics are not adversely affected. Also, twin studies have shown that there is a greater concordance of alcoholism among identical than among fraternal twins. Women make up a significantly smaller proportion of alcohol abusers than men, and these smaller numbers are also reflected in a smaller percentage of risk of inheriting alcoholism. In searching for the inherited trait that is responsible for vulnerability, some investigators have proposed that the principal defect is a decreased sensitivity to the effects of alcohol, so that the subject fails to sense the cues of overindulgence soon enough to curtail drinking. Thus, in a drinking milieu, such individuals are more prone to heavy drinking.

The crucial factor that would establish the genetic basis of alcoholism is the identification of the gene that expresses the significant trait. A search led to the discovery of an allele (A_1) for the gene that codes for the D_2 dopamine receptor. The A_1 allele was consistently found with greater frequency in alcoholics than in nonalcoholics. These and other findings led to the suggestion that the genetically disturbed dopamine activity at D_2 receptors conferred susceptibility to severe alcoholism. However, the presence of the allele was not concordant with alcoholism in the pedigrees of family members with alcoholism; that is, many alcoholics in the family cohort were free of the allele while many nonalcoholics had it. Also, a significant percentage of patients with neural disorders such as Tourette's syndrome, attention deficit hyperactivity disorder, posttraumatic stress disorder, and autism, also had the allele, suggesting that it was not specific to alcoholism. Therefore, the most parsimonious explanation for these findings is that the A_1 allele is a modifying agent that intensifies the symptoms of these disorders, and is neither necessary nor sufficient to cause alcoholism, and that other genes, yet unknown, are more directly responsible for alcoholism.

Pharmacological approaches to relieve the effects of alcohol abuse aim to counteract the acute effects of overindulgence of alcohol, to ameliorate the withdrawal symptoms, and to reduce the cravings for alcohol. The acute effects of rapid sustained alcohol intake are ataxia, dysarthria, and semi-stupor. One pharmacological strategy to reverse these effects might be to hasten the metabolism of alcohol. If that were possible, it could also apply to the reversal of acute life-threatening alcohol poisoning, but no such reliable antidote exists at the present time. Therefore, current practice involves preventing the intoxicated person from injury to himself and others, while waiting for alcohol metabolism to run its course. In severe cases, such as alcohol poisoning, hospital care is required to maintain the patient's vital functions by emptying the stomach of residual alcohol, and clearing the blood of alcohol by hemodialysis. If withdrawal symptoms are mild they can be managed with sedatives and antianxiety agents. However, if seizures occur, the person is at risk and should be treated with antiepileptic agents.

The most difficult aspect of pharmacological treatment of alcoholism is controlling craving. Different strategies involved using conditioning procedures to create disagreeable associations (such as unpleasant odors or induced nausea) with alcohol intake or even with the thought of it. These techniques were, by and large, poorly predictive of long-term sobriety. For those who are detoxified and highly motivated to maintain sobriety, the drug disulfiram and similar compounds have been used with some success in certain patients. These drugs block the complete metabolism of alcohol so that if the patient drinks as little as 0.24 oz of alcohol within 6 to 14 days after the last dose of the drug, there will be a sharp rise of the alcohol metabolite acetaldehyde in the blood. This causes a hyperactivity of the autonomic nervous system characterized by facial flushing, tachycardia, pounding in the chest, decreased blood pressure, nausea, vomiting, shortness of breath, sweating, dizziness and confusion. The severity of these reactions will motivate drinking abstinence provided that the patient accepts supervision, usually by family members, who insure that long-term treatment with disulfiram is taken on schedule. It is obvious that disulfiram does not cure alcoholism. Rather, it serves to fortify the desire to stop drinking. However, there are sometimes significant side effects from disulfiram treatment such that alcoholics taking drugs for organ dysfunctions or those taking psychotropic drugs are not good candidates for disulfiram treatment.

A more recent pharmacological candidate for treating alcoholism is naltrexone, which is an opiate antagonist that blocks μ and δ opiate receptors. The use of this drug is based upon the hypothesis that alcohol ingestion stimulates the release of endogenous opioids such as β-endorphin and Met-enkephalin, which increase the rewarding effects of alcohol. Naltrexone, by blocking the opioid receptors, also blocks the rewarding effects of alcohol. This hypothesis is supported by the finding that the opioid effect of alcohol ingestion is fully consistent with the evidence implicating dopamine in the alcohol reinforcement mechanism. The use of this agent has additional positive features: naltrexone is relatively free of side effects and needs only 3 doses per week to provide continuous receptor blockade. Clinical studies have shown that naltrexone-treated patients may drink alcohol without adverse effects, and stopping the naltrexone treatment is free of withdrawal symptoms. A follow-up 6 months after a 12-week program of naltrexone treatment showed significantly fewer relapses into symptomatic drinking than patients receiving placebos. The overall benefit to alcoholic patients undergoing rehabilitation in this way is achieved by reducing the immediate rewards produced by alcohol, thus enabling the patient to receive the benefits of long-term psychotherapy to bring about behavior change.

With respect to psychotherapy for alcoholism, it is known that because environmental factors are highly significant in determining the course and the persistence of alcoholism, the concept of alcoholism as a disease that will ultimately yield to a medicinal magic bullet is rapidly going out of favor. This leaves alcoholism—or better, alcohol-related problems—to be treated as a socio-psychological phenomenon that requires behavioral redirection. The fact that drugs to subdue alcohol craving are still in the developmental stage makes this alternative approach all the more important.

This behavioral approach has led to an explosion of clinics and therapists of unimaginable variety, making it extremely difficult to assess their effectiveness. If the criteria for successful treatment were expressed as abstinence from alcohol or use with sobriety at 4-year follow-ups, one would find that the rate of effectiveness would be no better than the rate of spontaneous remissions, which is estimated at 30% to 35%. Though, admittedly, there are problems in specifying what spontaneous remissions are, the estimated rate of effectiveness for all legitimate therapies are in the same range.

The explanation offered by treatment providers is that the critics suffer from "therapeutic nihilism" and fail to acknowledge that treatment failures are the inevitable result of the poor operating conditions of many clinics, which suffer from low morale, ill-defined goals, poor working relationships, low funding, staff insecurity, and other aspects of "organizational melancholia." It is also claimed that too often clients and their therapists are poorly matched, and that treatments fare better when they take into account the particular kind of alcohol problem presented.

On the other hand, sometimes the fault is attributed to the traditional views of conventional therapists whose methods are not empirically based and who are unwilling to give up traditional methods of therapy irrespective of their lack of success, and who are not able to adapt their strategies of treatment to those which have the potential to integrate theory, research, and practice (Heather, 1990). These new treatments are based on well-established laws of behavior change under the rubric of operant conditioning as practiced in the Community Reinforcement Approach. When they are utilized, significantly higher success rates emerge, although there must be a commitment from the family and the community to ensure that behaviors that are consonant with sobriety are positively reinforced, and those that are deemed unacceptable are not. Whereas it may be prohibitively expensive to set up and supervise the therapeutic environment, the program may have its greatest value in directing attention to the behavior-changing strategies that can be adapted in significant ways to more commonly used techniques of therapy. In addition, when the elements of the strategy are recognized, research on what works best in this context can be assessed more reliably. Further, it is proposed that in dealing with alcohol problems a strong effort should be directed to prevention and early intervention when the alcohol abuse is in its early phases.

Chapter 16

Sedative–Hypnotic and Anxiolytic Drugs

Part I
The History and the Study of Anxiolytic Drugs

During all of human history there have been searches for antidotes for the symptoms of anxiety, with alcohol among the earliest to be discovered, as described in the preceding chapter. In the late nineteenth and the early twentieth century, a number of sedative drugs were formulated and used, but most of them were found to promote tolerance and dependence, as well as severe intoxication upon overdosage. In the late 1950s, the benzodiazepines were discovered, and became widely used because of their efficacy and relative safety. Because of the widespread need for drugs to ameliorate the symptoms of anxiety, these drugs are the front runners, judging by the number of prescriptions written, among all other drugs used in medical practice (see Baldessarini, 1985). Furthermore, because of their predictable effects, the benzodiazepines are useful tools for investigating the mechanisms of anxiety and identifying the drug receptor sites and neural circuits that mediate the anxiety response.

Early Sedative–Anxiolytic Drugs

The principal action of early sedatives and anxiolytics was CNS depression, and even today this is a major feature of drugs in this class. In addition to their sedative and anxiolytic properties, the early drugs had euphoric and soporific, or **hypnotic** (sleep-inducing), effects. The fact that these same properties are characteristic of contemporary sedative–anxiolytic compounds justifies the argument against referring to these compounds as anxiolytics or tranquilizers, because none of them are that specific. Nevertheless, with this caveat in mind, we shall frequently refer to these compounds as anxiolytics and hypnotics, only because that is our major interest.

Bromides

Bromide compounds were very popular a century ago as CNS depressants and sedatives that were effective against some forms of epilepsy (Sharpless, 1970). In the latter half of the nineteenth century, bromides were used on an enormous scale, and in the 1870s it was reported that in London, a single hospital dispensed several tons annually as sedatives and anticonvulsants. Bromides were also found in nostrums, nerve tonics, and headache remedies (e.g., Bromo Seltzer), but since bromides were found to be toxic, their use has been largely discontinued. Whereas bromides in low doses do act as sedatives, bromide intoxication can occur because these drugs are excreted slowly by the kidneys (their plasma half-life is about 12 days). Thus, when bromides were taken on a regular basis for a few weeks, dangerous blood levels were attained that resulted in bromism: impaired thought and memory, drowsiness, dizziness, irritability, and emotional disturbances. These symptoms frequently induced the user to increase the dose, with dire consequences: a bromide psychosis characterized by delirium, delusions, vivid hallucinations, mania, and ultimately, lethargy and coma. Bromism was also accompanied by a repulsive skin eruption and gastrointestinal disturbances. The intoxication occurs because the kidney preferentially reabsorbs bromide and excretes chloride, thus causing an increasing buildup of bromide in the blood. Fortunately, bromides are no longer produced or sold, so bromide poisoning is now a rare occurrence.

Belladonna Alkaloids

The belladonna alkaloids have been used over many centuries and are still used today. The most familiar drugs in this class are atropine and scopolamine; a variety of their applications are described in Chapter 7. These compounds block cholinergic muscarinic receptors, and of the two, scopolamine is the more potent CNS depressant. It has not been used as a sedative or anxiolytic drug by itself in modern times, but it continues to be used in preanesthetic medication to block secretions in the nasopharynx that might be induced by anesthetic inhalants. It also promotes drowsiness, euphoria, and amnesia. When scopolamine is administered, alone or supplemented with barbiturates or opiates, the patient tolerates surgical procedures under local anesthesia, sometimes appearing fully awake but in a state of quiet repose. When the procedures are complete, the patient hardly remembers that they ever started, and hours are condensed into minutes. These effects are difficult to explain physiologically. Scopolamine is also used to combat motion sickness and is sometimes administered via a small skin patch on the neck behind the lower part of the ear. However, drowsiness is sometimes an unwelcome side effect.

Narcotic Analgesics (Opiates)

Narcotic drugs are derived from the alkaloid constituents of the exudate from the seed pod of the poppy plant, and were well known before recorded history. As far back as 4000 B.C.E., the Sumerians had an ideograph for the poppy plant that was composed of the characters *hul* ("joy") and *gil* ("plant") (Jaffe, 1975). Opiates in their various forms are associated with strong psychological effects such as euphoria, drowsiness, changes in mood, and mental clouding. Individuals suffering from pain, discomfort, tension, and worry may experience euphoria with as little as 5–10 mg of morphine. However, frequent use leads to drug tolerance and increasing doses. It is easy to appreciate how easily one can become dependent upon a drug that seems to alleviate psychological stress and to replace boredom, frustration, worry, anxiety, and fear with feelings of peace, repose, and surcease of all cares (see Chapter 12).

The Development of Modern Anxiolytics

For the most part, bromides, ethanol, belladonna alkaloids, and opiates were the prominent drugs in use for the relief of fear and tension until about the 1930s (see Caldwell, 1970, for a review). At about that time, there was a developing awareness of concepts of anxiety, probably initiated by Freud's book *The Problem of Anxiety* (1936), which was first published in the 1920s but was not translated into English until approximately 10 years later. Before that there were no formalized concepts of the role of fear and anxiety in behavior, nor of their consequences of maladaptation, psychosomatic manifestations, and compulsive, phobic, and hysterical symptoms. Even in World War I, soldiers who were psychologically incapacitated by their battlefield experiences were diagnosed as being shell-shocked or as suffering from battle fatigue. In 1935, a paper by Thorner entitled "The Psycho-Pharmacology of Sodium-Amytal" described the use of this barbiturate psychosedative in psychiatric practice to reduce tension and anxiety. This may have been the first use of the term "psychopharmacology" in the psychiatric literature (Caldwell, 1970, p. 10). During World War II and the Korean War, American psychiatrists turned to barbiturates for pharmacological treatment of soldiers who were overcome by the rigors of combat in an effort to hasten the return of those soldiers to duty. These treatments with barbiturate psychosedatives such as amobarbital (Amytal) and thiopental (Pentothal) seemed to facilitate psychotherapy. These developments were described in the notable book *Men Under Stress* by Grinker and Spiegel (1945). In retrospect, it seems that these were the beginnings of specific treatment of recognized anxiety states by the use of drugs.

Experimental Methods for the Assessment of Anxiolytic Drugs

As described in Chapter 2, certain techniques have been developed for the study of behavioral pharmacology. In the search for medicinal drugs, preclinical experiments with animals are obviously necessary to assess the safety and effectiveness of the compounds that are developed. Although it is virtually impossible to assess the subjective feelings and mental states of animals that are treated with drugs, animal research has clearly shown that the physiological effects of psychoactive drugs are almost always identical in animals and humans. Indeed, a drug's distribution in the CNS, its binding sites and receptors, its metabolism and elimination, the mechanisms of tolerance, and even the proportional effective dose are highly correlated between animals and humans. These findings provide a face validity that permits the results of animal tests to be applied to the understanding of the results of tests on humans.

With respect to the behavioral effects of a drug, the human response may not seem to resemble the behavioral response in animals, but if there is a correlated quantifiable measure of the human and the animal responses; the animal response may be predictive of a clinical effect in humans. As the following discussion of anxiolytic drug research will show, behavioral psychopharmacology will have impressive heuristic credits (see Chapter 2).

As mentioned above, therapeutic psychopharmacology began in the 1930s with the use of the barbiturates amobarbital and thiopental. These and related compounds were the dominant anxiolytic and hypnotic agents at the time, and continued in popularity for three or four more decades until they were gradually superseded in the 1960s and 1970s by the benzodiazepines, such as Librium and Valium (see below). Nonetheless, many of the behavioral effects of the drugs were discovered using operant conditioning techniques that were largely developed in the laboratory of B. F. Skinner at Harvard University, several of which were described in Chapter 2 (see Dews, 1955).

Classical Paradigms for Assessing Anxiolytic Effects

Conditioned suppression. The conditioned suppression paradigm is very similar to the one that evokes a conditioned emotional response (CER), described in Chapter 2, but conditioned suppression is a more objective term because the focus is on the animal's behavior rather than its internal states of fear and anxiety. Early experiments showed that barbiturates had marked effects in conditioned suppression paradigms. In these experiments, warning cues signify that if responses are made, shocks will occur, which, as expected, causes animals to refrain from responding. However, if animals are pretreated with barbiturates, the response suppression is diminished. Kelleher and Morse (1964), for example, trained pigeons to peck an orange transilluminated disk for food rewards. They were on an FR-30 schedule, meaning that food rewards were given after every 30th response. After 5 reinforcements (150 responses), the color of the disk was changed to white. During this segment, the FR-30 schedule was still in effect, but after the 10th, the 20th, and the 30th response (in each 30-response section), the birds received a brief (35 ms) shock applied by a gold wire implanted in the tail region. This segment continued until there had been 5 food reinforcements or until 3 minutes had elapsed. As shown in Figure 16.1*a*, after a few tests, the birds pecked vigorously at the orange light (nonpunishment segment) and completely suppressed responses to the white light (punishment segment), thus demonstrating conditioned suppression. Pentobarbital (10 mg/kg) increased the response rate during the punishment segment so that it was almost equal to the response rate during the nonpunishment segment, but the drug had no appreciable effect on the nonpunishment segment.

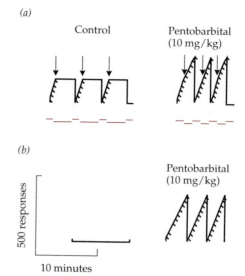

16.1 PENTOBARBITAL INCREASES RESPONDING IN THE CONDITIONED SUPPRESSION TEST. (*a*) The upward displacement of the bottom record indicates a nonpunishment segment with an FR-30 schedule of reinforcement accompanied by an orange light. During the punishment segments (downward displacement of the bottom record), an FR-30 schedule was accompanied by white light. Each of the first 10 responses in each 30-response section produced a brief (35 ms) 6-mA electric shock. Pecking was suppressed during the punishment segment in the controls. With pentobarbital treatment, pecking responses occurred during both the nonpunished and the punished components. The termination of each punishment component is indicated by the resetting of the recording pen to the bottom of the record. (*b*) The punishment procedure was in effect throughout each session in the presence of the white light stimulus. The control condition shows no response. With pentobarbital, pecking was continuous during the session. (After Kelleher and Morse, 1964.)

In another part of the experiment (Figure 16.1*b*), the white-light condition was maintained continuously, during which time the birds responded hardly at all, but under the influence of pentobarbital, high pecking rates were restored. This finding indicated that behavior suppressed by punishment is disinhibited by low or moderate doses of pentobarbital. As we shall see below, the ability to disinhibit behavior under aversive control is a strong marker for clinically useful anxiolytic drugs of high efficacy.

The Geller–Seifter paradigm. Geller and Seifter (1960) developed a refinement of the methods used to identify anxiolytic drugs (see Chapter 2). Their method was described as an experimentally induced conflict paradigm and had its origin in work done in Pavlov's laboratory (see Maier, 1949; Pavlov, 1928; Yates, 1962). But Geller and Seifter's method had the added ability to produce quantifiable data from highly controlled procedures.

The experimental design utilized a multiple VI-2/continuous reinforcement (CRF) schedule. Rats were trained to press a lever on a VI-2 minute schedule for liquid food rewards. After 15 minutes, a tone of 3 minutes' duration signaled a change to a CRF schedule during which every lever press was followed by food reinforcement, but the food reinforcements were accompanied by foot shocks that were sufficiently annoying to suppress responding to very low levels. When the trained animals were given pentobarbital (5.0 mg/kg), the response rate during the VI segment was decreased slightly, but the average number of responses during the 3-minute CRF segment increased from 4 to 18, a 350% increase (Geller, 1962). An identical effect occurred when another anxiolytic drug, oxazepam, was substituted for pentobarbital (Figure 16.2). (It should be noted that the rate of responding during the CRF segment is low partly because each response is rewarded and the rat takes time to lick up the sweetened milk reward that is offered.)

The water-lick suppression test.   The water-lick suppression test, developed by Vogel, Beer, and Clody (1971), was another reliable method for identifying anxiolytic drugs, and it had the significant advantage of requiring little training of the animals (usually rats). The animals were trained for the experiments by being deprived of water and then learning to lick the tip of a small metal spout for water when the spout was inserted into the cage. During the experiments, the thirsty rats were given the spout for 3 minutes, but after every 20th lick, the rats received a mild tongue shock (0.4 mA, 0.5 s duration), which caused a marked suppression of drinking behavior. When rats were pretreated with anxiolytic drugs before the tongue shock tests, the drinking suppression was significantly diminished. The minimally effective dose (MED) of the drug was determined as the average dose that produced a significant increase in licking rates during the tests: that is, the smaller the MED, the more potent the drug. This method of drug assessment turned out to be extremely sensitive (see below).

Drug discrimination tests.   The testing of drugs as discriminative stimuli was also described in Chapter 2. As developed by Lal (1977), this method has the unusual ability to discriminate interoceptive differences between drugs. That is, animals, especially rats, can readily be trained to make a response for food rewards by pressing one of a pair of levers when a drug has been administered and the other lever when given saline. Drug discrimination refers to the subjective awareness by a person or animal of interoceptive cues of the presence of a drug in the body. For example, most persons would be able to detect the presence of amphetamine or morphine after injection, as compared with penicillin or aspirin, because the first two drugs provide discriminative cues while the latter two do not.

The method of training for the drug discrimination test is as follows: First, food-deprived animals (usually rats) are trained to press one of a pair of levers placed

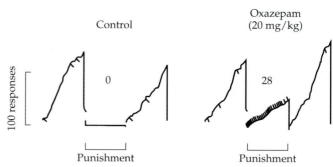

16.2 PERFORMANCE RECORDS FROM THE GELLER–SEIFTER CONFLICT TEST. Lever-press responses are cumulated over time; the slope of the tracings at any point gives the response rate. When there is no lever pressing, the trace is horizontal. Punishment periods of 3 minutes duration, signaled by a tone, are flanked by equivalent periods of nonpunished responding. Punished responses are numbered and indicated by upward strokes of the pen; presentations of the milk rewards in the nonpunished schedule are indicated by downward strokes of the pen. Oxazepam causes a marked disinhibition of punishment-suppressed behavior, but does not importantly influence nonpunished behavior. (After Stein, Wise, and Berger, 1973.)

side by side for food rewards. Drug days and saline days are randomly alternated, and testing occurs 30 minutes after drug or saline is injected intraperitoneally. For example, on drug days, pressing the lever on the right is rewarded with food on an FR-10 schedule (i.e., a fixed ratio schedule in which every tenth press of that lever is rewarded). Pressing the lever on the left has no effect. On saline days, pressing the left-hand lever is rewarded under the same contingency (FR-10). On drug days, a rat's daily score is the percentage of responses made on the drug lever up to the first reinforcement. On saline days, the animal is scored by the percentage of responses made on the saline lever up to the first reinforcement. For instance, on a drug day, a well-trained rat that discriminated the benzodiazepine chlordiazepoxide (CDP) from saline might make 2 responses on the saline lever and 10 responses on the CDP lever, the last response being followed by an automatic presentation of a dipper with a few drops of a highly preferred milk mixture. In this case, the rat's score would be 10/12, or 83.3%. On a saline day, the rat might make 3 responses on the drug lever and 10 responses on the saline lever for the first reward, and its score would be 10/13, or 77%. An animal is assumed to be reliably discriminating between the drug and saline after it reaches a certain criterion, such as three consecutive daily tests without more than one inappropriate response per day (10/11, or 91%).

After criterion is reached, animals can be given threshold, generalization, and antagonist tests. In threshold tests, varying doses of the drug are given to find the dose that yields discrimination accuracy of at least 75%. The dose obtained may then serve as a baseline dose for a variety of other procedures, such as the generalization test, in which a new compound is substituted for the training compound to see whether the animal responds to the drug lever, and at what dose. It is generally accepted that generalization has occurred if the rats press the drug lever with 80% consistency when the new drug has been injected. This procedure can also establish relationships among drugs and their potencies; that is, if a different drug can be substituted at about the same dose as the training drug, it is assumed that the two drugs share similar properties. If a larger dose is required for the substitution, it is a sign that the substituted drug is less potent than the training drug. (See Figure 10.27 for the results of other tests of comparative potency.) Antagonist testing can establish the effect and the potency of a compound that diminishes or blocks responding to the training drug when the two drugs are given together. Such data may help in formulating the mechanisms of action of both drugs.

Corticosterone assessment. The steroid corticosterone is released from the adrenal gland along with epinephrine and norepinephrine in response to stress. Thus, the level of plasma corticosterone can indicate the level of stress that is induced in an animal. Stress can be induced by a variety of behavioral manipulations or by anxiogenic drugs, which will be described below. Further, the effectiveness of anxiolytic drugs can be assessed by their ability to block behavioral or chemically induced steroid release.

Alternative Testing Procedures

It is obvious that some of the procedures described above, especially the conditioned suppression, Geller-Seifter, and water-lick suppression tests, are characterized by animal conflict and stress. Further, some of these tests require a substantial amount of training in unnatural environments using unnatural stimuli (e.g., foot shocks). To be sure, these tests were designed to induce anxiety and fear, and the procedures were designed to produce data that could be objectively evaluated. Nonetheless, there have been frequent instances in which the results of replicated studies were at variance (see Gardner, 1986; Johnston and File, 1986; and Treit, 1985). Because most of these discrepancies occurred between different laboratories rather than within the same laboratories, it followed that the differences might be due to differences in the training procedures, the animal environments, the magnitude of the shocks, and the introduction of sensory, motor, or associative phenomena that complicate the interpretation of experimental results.

It was therefore proposed that the research designs of the last two or three decades should give way to simpler procedures utilizing responses for which the animals are biologically prepared, and that this might result in more consistent results. Operationally, such "prepared" responses may range from reflexive reactions, as in the tail-flick test (see Chapter 2), to the extremely rapid response in a test for ataxia in which the animal simply has to cling to an inclined plane.

It follows that researchers screening for anxiolytic compounds may be able to obtain data more rapidly, and that the data may be more reliable, with a prepared learning paradigm than with one that depends upon lengthy training to respond to novel stimuli coupled with aversive consequences. Also, the neural substrates of biologically prepared fear reactions may be less complex and more directly related to anxiety than the neural substrates of more difficult learned adaptations. Some examples of these simpler learning paradigms are described below. It will be seen that studying models based upon prepared fear reactions may have advantages for understanding the neural mechanisms underlying antianxiety drug action (Treit, 1991).

The light–dark crossing test. The light–dark crossing test (described in Chapter 2) was put forward as an alternative to the Geller–Seifter procedures, in which animals have to be trained (prepared) for a considerable period of time to make the appropriate responses, such as pressing a lever for food in a strange environment. The crossing test uses techniques that are more in keeping with the natural tendencies of animals. Rodents, for example, have an almost reflexive tendency to avoid brightly lit areas. Mice placed in the brightly lit side of a two-compartment test chamber quickly cross to the dark side and make few transitions in the opposite direction. Tests showed that anxiolytics increased the number of light–dark transitions, whereas nonanxiolytic agents had no effect. Moreover, the relative potencies of the anxiolytic compounds that increased the number of transitions correlated positively with their clinical potency. As a control procedure to test for a possible motoric stimulation by the anxiolytics, mice were tested with two undifferentiated compartments—that is, both compartments had the same illumination. Mice treated with anxiolytics behaved in the same way as vehicle-treated subjects. Thus, in the light–dark crossing test, the animals give an avoidance response that they are biologically "prepared" to make in what may be an aversive situation, and drugs may be quickly assessed for anxiolysis, which is expressed as diminished avoidance behavior.

The social interaction test. The social interaction test (see Chapter 2) was also designed as a more sensitive predictor of the efficacy of psychotropic drugs than the so-called artificially contrived conflict tests. This test, like the light–dark crossing test, takes advantage of the rodent proclivity to avoid bright lights and unfamiliar surroundings. In the social interaction test, pairs of rats are introduced into an experimental arena, and the time spent in active social interactions (e.g., sniffing, nipping, grooming, following, kicking, boxing, crawling over each other, and so on) is recorded. In one such test, the overall level of social interactions was suppressed in unfamiliar or brightly lit environments, and periodic injections of chlordiazepoxide counteracted this suppression at doses that did not significantly affect ambulation (Treit, 1985).

The distress vocalization test.   Another test for anxiolysis utilizes the ultrasonic "distress" vocalization of rat pups as the reflexive response. As described by Winslow and Insel (1991), when rat pups are removed from their nest, they emit ultrasonic vocalizations that are monotonic whistlelike sounds with a frequency range of about 35–45 kHz, which is within the region of high auditory sensitivity for adult rats. From the first day of postnatal life, these calls, known as "distress vocalizations" or "isolation calls," are extremely potent stimuli for maternal retrieval of the pups. The calls increase in number and intensity during the second week and decrease abruptly around day 14, about the time of eye opening. The particular stimuli that elicit these calls remain unclear, but lowering the ambient temperature stimulates their production, whereas exposure to littermates as well as to the mother terminates them. Also, sensory inputs from social contact indicate that texture, contour, warmth, and odor have additive effects toward reducing isolation calls.

When isolated rat pups were treated with benzodiazepines, their distress vocalizations were significantly decreased at doses that did not alter locomotor activity. Also, the drugs decreased the average peak frequency of the calls from 38.8–36.7 kHz, as well as the loudness of the calls (Gardner, 1985; Insel, Hill, and Mayor, 1986).

The fear-potentiated startle test.   In the fear-potentiated startle test, rats are tested for the magnitude of their startle response to a sudden loud sound. The response is measured by the activity of the rat in a cage that is lightly balanced on a movement sensor. The animals are then conditioned to associate a cue (a brief light) with a shock, and if the sound is paired with the cue, the startle response to the sound is potentiated. This conditioned effect is readily established in most animals. When rats so trained were treated with a benzodiazepine compound, there was a selective dose-related reduction of the fear-potentiated startle compared with the magnitude of the startle on the noise-alone trials (see Treit, 1991).

The elevated plus-maze.   The elevated plus-maze is described in Chapter 2 and is yet another device that presumes to exploit the natural avoidance tendencies of rodents and thus avoids the possible complicating effects of intensive training and punishment in evaluating anxiolytic drugs.

Thus, we see that these simple behavioral tests for drug-induced anxiolysis are more akin to natural reactions to aversive conditions and less dependent upon lengthy training procedures such as conflict/punishment paradigms. These tests have thus proved useful in efforts to assess the mechanisms by which anxiolytic drugs influence anxiety.

Part I Summary

For humans, anxiety, at one level or another, is a pervasive aspect of life. If anxiety exists at relatively high levels, the discovery and use of anxiolytic substances is highly rewarded and reinforced. Alcoholic beverages may have been the first anxiolytic drug in common use; opiates and belladonna alkaloids came close behind. In the nineteenth century bromides and the early barbiturates were recognized or synthesized and became part of the physicians' armamentarium. World War II gave impetus to find substances to treat anxiety-induced casualties, and after the war the search for effective sedatives and anxiolytics became a high priority. This led to the development of therapeutic psychopharmacology, which sought to supplement the pharmacologists' preclinical assessment of safe and efficacious new products. Psychopharmacology's highest achievement was in providing methods to obtain behavioral data from animal studies, which were significantly predictive of human responses to the newly developed psychoactive products.

Part II
The Barbiturates

Although the therapeutic use of barbiturates has significantly diminished during the last three decades, these drugs are reviewed here in some detail because their biochemistry and pharmacology provide a strong background for the study of the drugs that have superseded them, the benzodiazepines.

The History of Barbiturates

In 1864 Adolph von Baeyer (or Bayer), who was later instrumental in forming the great Bayer chemical firm in Germany, synthesized, for unknown reasons, barbituric acid (malonylurea) by combining malonic acid (from apples) and urea (Figure 16.3). The name of the compound

Malonylurea
(Barbituric acid)

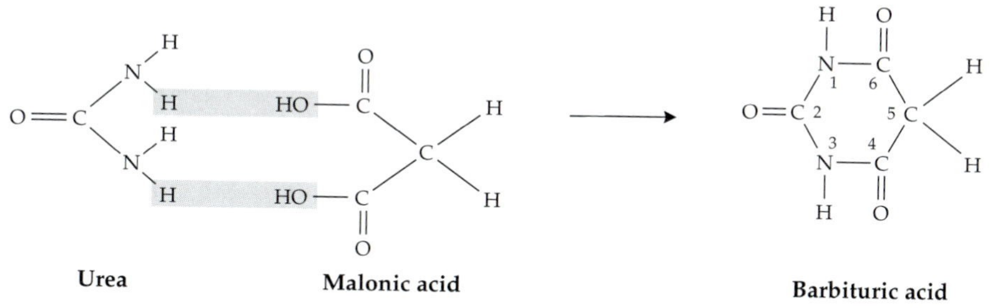

Urea   **Malonic acid**   **Barbituric acid**

16.3 BARBITURIC ACID is made by combining urea with malonic acid with the elimination of water. The barbiturate families arise from substitutions of other chemical groups for hydrogen at position 5 in the basic barbiturate structure.

is said to be derived from von Baeyer's presence, on the day of the experiment, at a tavern frequented by artillery officers who were celebrating the Day of St. Barbara, their patron saint (Sharpless, 1970).

Barbituric acid itself had no clinical value, but in 1903, Fischer and von Mering synthesized diethylbarbituric acid by substituting ethyl groups for hydrogens at position 5 in Figure 16.3. This compound was given the generic name of barbital and was found to have soporific or hypnotic (sleep-inducing) potency. The compound

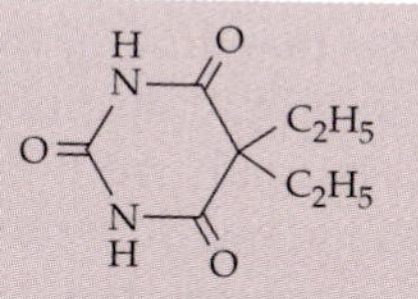

Barbital
(Veronal)

was given the trade name Veronal, presumably because of von Mering's presence in Verona when he first heard that Fischer had synthesized the compound. (Another version of the story claims that the drug was named after Verona because of the peace and solace that is associated with that Italian town.) Barbital became medically popular as a drug that facilitated sleep and had relaxing properties when taken during the daytime. However, barbital is low in lipid solubility, and therefore it is distributed to and penetrates the brain slowly. It is also metabolized slowly, thereby conferring drowsiness that may extend over a day and a half. Although it was regarded as an excellent hypnotic, barbital has been supplanted by compounds with a shorter duration of action.

In 1912 two independent teams of researchers introduced phenobarbital (Luminal) to therapeutics. This

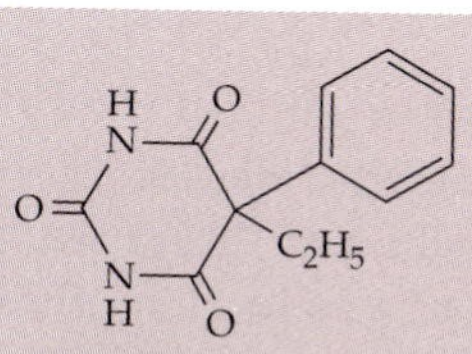

Phenobarbital
(Luminal)

drug had excellent sedative and anticonvulsant properties; given orally twice a day, it served, in mild or moderate cases, to keep chronic seizure activity in abeyance. Interestingly, the sedative and the anticonvulsive effects seemed to be independent of each other because the sedative effect could be reversed with amphetamine without disturbing the anticonvulsant activity. Later developments led to barbiturates with shorter durations of action, such as amobarbital (Amytal), pentobarbital (Nembutal), and secobarbital (Seconal). All three of these

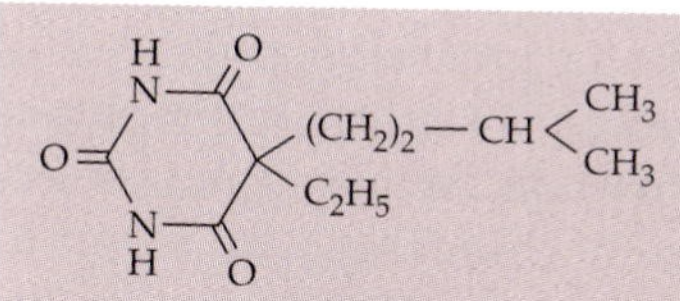

Amobarbital
(Amytal)

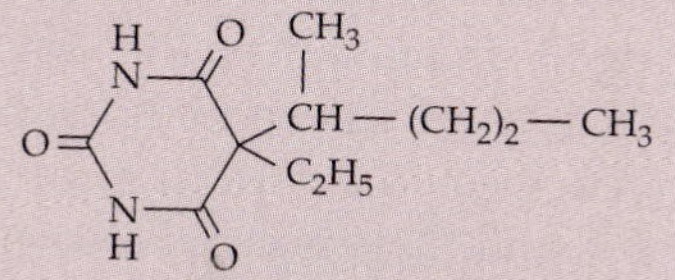

Pentobarbital
(Nembutal)

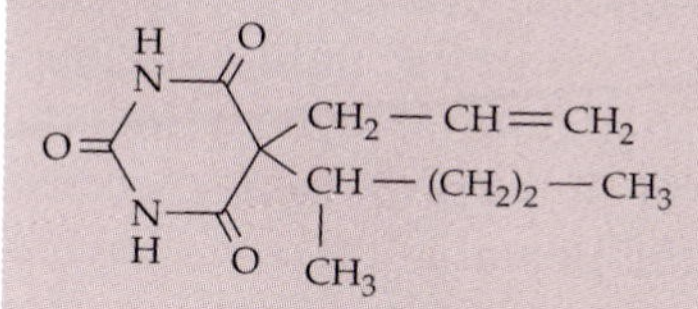

Secobarbital
(Seconal)

compounds were found to be useful for inducing sleep and, in smaller doses, providing relief from mental stress. Because of their rapid onset and short duration of action, these drugs can be given intravenously to terminate acutely generated convulsions (e.g., caused by drugs such as strychnine or by brain injury). In cases of chronic seizure episodes, other more specific anticonvulsants have been introduced to supplement or replace barbiturates (some anticonvulsant drugs and their mechanisms of action are described in Chapter 10). Over the years, 2,500 different barbiturates were synthesized, many of which were tested for their clinical usefulness. About 50 barbiturates were marketed, but five seemed to fulfill most clinical needs.

In the 1930s the ultrashort-acting barbiturates, such as hexobarbital (Evipal), thiopental (Pentothal, not to be confused with pentobarbital), and methohexital (Brevital), were introduced as intravenous anaesthetics. Thiopental is one of a few barbiturates in which a sulfur

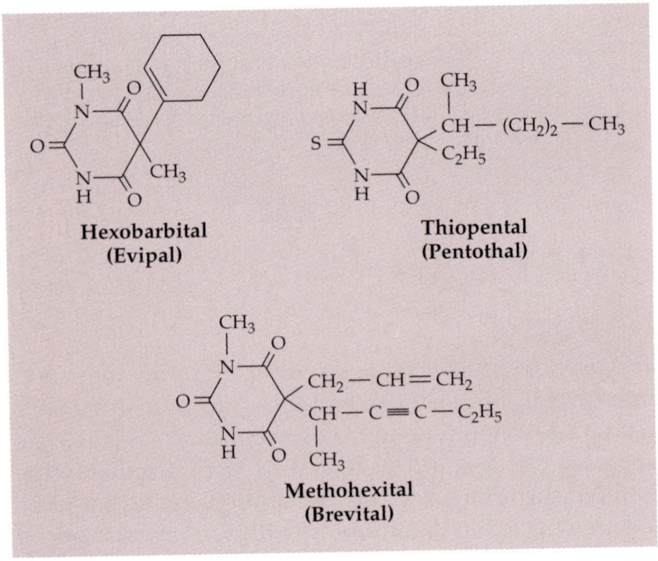

Hexobarbital
(Evipal)

Thiopental
(Pentothal)

Methohexital
(Brevital)

atom replaces oxygen at position 2 in Figure 16.3, and this is the only difference between it and pentobarbital. Currently, thiopental enjoys the greatest popularity, followed by methohexital, which is slightly more potent and has effects of shorter duration. An intravenous injection of a single small dose of thiopental can result in anesthesia within 10–20 seconds, the time it takes for the drug to circulate from the arm to the brain. A talking patient may fall asleep in the middle of a sentence. There is no excitement, vomiting, or salivation, respiration is quiet, and there is rapid recovery after small doses. After infusion, the depth of anesthesia increases for up to 40 seconds, then begins to slowly decrease until consciousness returns in about 20–30 minutes, at which time the plasma concentration is 10% of the peak value. Because the duration of action of thiopental is short, prolonged surgical procedures require supplementation by inhalant anesthetics (Marshall and Wollman, 1985).

Barbiturate Pharmacology

We have seen that the important differences among the barbiturates are in their time of onset and duration of action. These differences can be explained in terms of the lipid solubility, rates of ionization, plasma protein binding, metabolism, and excretion of the various barbiturate compounds. (The mechanisms of these factors are described in Chapter 1). These factors can be illustrated in a comparison of the actions of thiopental and pentobarbital, whose chemical structures are very similar but whose onset duration characteristics are very different.

Pentobarbital is about equal in potency to thiopental in that the same brain concentration of each drug is necessary for anesthesia. But no dose of pentobarbital will mimic the fast onset and ultrashort duration of anesthesia brought on by thiopental. An injected dose of pentobarbital equal to an anesthetic dose of thiopental will result in no anesthesia. The explanation for these differences became clear when it was discovered that thiopental was

rapidly redistributed to fat and muscle; virtually the whole dose was found there after a few hours. This finding led to the suggestion that the high lipid solubility of thiopental was the basis of the rapid onset and the short duration of anesthesia. Indeed, studies have shown that the brain reaches its peak thiopental concentration within 30 seconds after intravenous administration of the drug, whereas muscle and skin require from 15–30 minutes and fat requires about 2 hours to become saturated. After 30 minutes, the brain may give up as much as 90% of its peak concentration (Marshall and Wollman, 1985). In contrast, pentobarbital, being much less lipid soluble, enters the brain very slowly—so slowly, in fact, that by the time the drug in the brain has reached equilibrium with the plasma level, the plasma level is already falling because of the drug's metabolism and excretion. Thus, at equal doses, no anesthesia occurs. With respect to metabolism, thiopental is metabolized slowly in the liver: 10–15% per hour, a rate which is much too slow to account for its short duration of action.

Finally, comparisons among thiopental, pentobarbital, and barbital showed that barbital has a partition coefficient of 0.002 (less than that of thiopental by a factor of 1,650) and thus is so lipid insoluble that even after an intravenous injection, many minutes elapse before any effects appear. Consequently, barbital is not an effective anesthetic or hypnotic agent, but serves well as a long-acting sedative.

Synaptic Effects of Barbiturates

Barbiturates depress the actions of skeletal muscles, smooth muscles of the viscera, and cardiac muscle as well as the actions of neurons. They also depress kidney function and the nonneurogenic aspects of respiration. However, the CNS is much more sensitive to barbiturates than other tissues, and when given at sedative or hypnotic doses, barbiturates have virtually no effect upon tissues other than those of the CNS. Even at anesthetic doses, the direct effect upon peripheral excitable tissue is weak as long as the duration of anesthesia is not prolonged. In cases of acute barbiturate-induced intoxication, however, there may be serious compromise of cardiovascular and other peripheral functions such as the protective reflexes (coughing and sneezing) (Harvey, 1985) (see the section on barbiturate toxicity below.)

The Site of Barbiturate Action

Within the CNS, barbiturates exert a membrane effect that has been described as "electrical membrane stabilization," referring to a reduction of the membrane conductance that usually occurs after physiological or artificial stimuli. Under the influence of barbiturates, such stimulation is immediately followed by little or no alteration of membrane resting potentials (Haefely, 1977).

Barker and Gainer (1973) investigated the question of whether barbiturate-induced neuronal depression was due to a decrease in excitatory or an increase in inhibitory synaptic events. They studied the effects of barbiturates on nerve–muscle preparations from several molluscan and crustacean species in which EPSPs and IPSPs could be readily recorded and measured. They found that the depressant action of pentobarbital is related to the selective depression of transmitter-coupled Na^+ conductances, with preservation of transmitter-coupled Cl^- and K^+ conductances. Furthermore, there was a close correspondence between the pentobarbital concentrations that produced the experimental membrane effects and pentobarbital plasma concentrations found during anesthesia and anticonvulsive therapy. This finding suggested that EPSP suppression, anesthesia, and anticonvulsive effects are related in significant ways.

Once it had been established that pentobarbital suppressed Na^+-dependent EPSPs, the next step was to identify which step in synaptic events was altered. Nicoll and Iwamoto (1978) investigated this question by examining the effects of barbiturates on synaptic transmission through the ganglia of the sympathetic trunk of bullfrogs. The preganglionic fibers were electrically stimulated and recordings were made of membrane changes in the postsynaptic ganglion cells. The experiment demonstrated that the fast EPSP, which reflects a change in Na^+ conductance, was preferentially depressed by 50% at pentobarbital concentrations significantly lower than those required to reduce the slow IPSP, which reflects the influx of Cl^- (Figure 16.4). Thus, it was reasonable to assume that barbiturates exert their neurodepressant action by rendering postsynaptic membranes less responsive to Na^+-dependent excitatory transmitter action, and it was later found that this effect combines with a dose-dependent enhancement of Cl^--dependent postsynaptic

inhibitory effects (Haefely, 1978, 1983; Nicoll, 1978). However, while these conclusions seemed to fit the experimental results, further developments in the understanding of GABA receptor morphology were required to better explain these phenomena.

The Role of GABA in Barbiturate Effects

As described in Chapter 10, GABA-mediated inhibitory transmission is found in virtually every brain region and every functional circuit. The most commonly occurring GABA receptor is the $GABA_A$ type, which is associated with postsynaptic membrane Cl^- channels and regulates Cl^- permeability. Because the Cl^- equilibrium potential is near the resting membrane potential (see Chapter 3), the opening of channels to a Cl^- influx firmly stabilizes the membrane potential near resting, thereby preventing depolarizing responses to excitatory transmitters and inhibiting the tonic firing that is typical of many neurons in the CNS (Olsen, 1987). Thus, $GABA_A$ receptors are seen as the major molecular sites whereby GABA mediates neuronal inhibition.

GABAergic function is sensitive to a wide variety of agonist and antagonist drugs (Fonnum, 1987), of which two classes are especially important: the barbiturates and the benzodiazepines. These drugs are Cl^--dependent ligands for allosteric sites on the GABA receptor, such that these substances interact with GABA and with one another to modulate inhibition of the GABAergic target cells via $GABA_A$ receptors.

Barbiturate Effects on the $GABA_A$ Receptor Complex

Pentobarbital (PBT) potentiates GABA-induced increases in Cl^- conductance by increasing the affinity of the $GABA_A$ receptors for GABA and increasing the duration of the opening of GABA-activated Cl^- channels (see

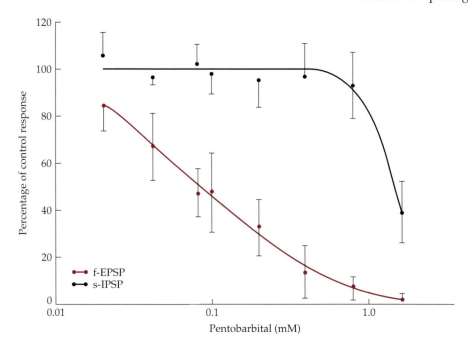

16.4 PENTOBARBITAL-INDUCED DE-PRESSION of fast (f-) EPSP and slow (s-) IPSP synaptic potentials in the sympathetic trunk ganglia of bullfrogs. Group data show that 0.1 mM pentobarbital reduced the fast EPSP 50%, whereas the concentration of pentobarbital had to be increased tenfold to block the slow potential. Each point represents the average ± *SD* of 3 to 11 preparations. Responses were recorded after their amplitude had reached a stable value (20–45 minutes). (After Nicoll and Iwamoto, 1978.)

Figure 10.25). Furthermore, at high doses, pentobarbital has a direct GABA-mimetic effect of opening the Cl^- channels in the absence of GABA (Barker et al., 1984; Haefely, 1983; see Chapter 10). The benzodiazepines have similar effects on the $GABA_A$ receptors, but they bind at a different site on the receptor. Furthermore, barbiturates do not displace BDZs from their binding sites, but rather enhance BDZ binding. These and other findings have established that GABAergic dysfunction plays a role in human neurological disorders such as epilepsy and Huntington's chorea, and there are suspicions that it is involved in psychiatric disorders such as profound anxiety reactions, depression, and schizophrenia (Lloyd and Morselli, 1987). For example, any serious loss or blockade of GABA function may cause epileptic seizures, whereas any enhancement of GABA-mediated inhibition by barbiturates and BDZs has anticonvulsant effects. Paradoxically, phenobarbital is only a weak competitor of the GABA antagonist picrotoxin and a weak enhancer of GABA and BDZ binding, yet it is relatively potent as an anticonvulsant in certain forms of epilepsy (Harvey, 1985; Rall and Schleifer, 1985).

Barbiturate Effects on the CNS

With this knowledge about the synaptic effects of barbiturates, we can now examine the general effects that barbiturates exert on the CNS. Because excitatory synaptic events are suppressed and inhibitory effects are either unaffected or enhanced, it is not surprising that the overall effect of these drugs is one of depression of neuronal excitability, which, of course, is directly responsible for their anticonvulsant effects. Nevertheless, the barbiturates, as well as the benzodiazepines, have a variety of effects—hypnotic, anesthetic, anticonvulsant, anxiolytic, euphoric—and some barbiturates are even convulsants (Nicoll, 1978a). Regional effects of the drugs within the brain may account for their different pharmacological effects.

The consensus among early investigators was that barbiturates do not exert selective neurochemical actions on specific parts of the CNS such as the "sleep center" or on the hypothalamus or cerebral cortex. On the other hand, there is evidence of a selective effect upon the neurons of the brain stem reticular formation, which subserves modulating effects on many aspects of psychomotor activity, and this could account in large part for the most prominent effects of these drugs (see the discussion of the reticular formation in Chapter 4). It is now held that the pontine region of the reticular formation serves to activate cortical centers, whereas the medullary area suppresses them, and that the equilibrium between these two areas can be altered even by small doses of barbiturates. If the medullary system is affected first, there will be activation and euphoria; if the pontine system is affected, the result will be relaxation, drowsiness, or sleep. Thus, although the direct effects of barbiturates on

neural tissues are roughly the same throughout the nervous system, their special effects on the reticular activating system are due to its unique characteristics and its location in the central core of the brain stem, where it modulates the level of attention and alertness and provides a gating function for sensory input consistent with needs. Barbiturates also influence the descending reticular pathways that modulate spinal reflexes and the activities of the sympathetic nervous system.

Barbiturate Abuse and Toxicology

Barbiturate Abuse

It is almost a truism that any substance that induces euphoria, allays anxiety, and promotes sleep will have a high abuse potential, and barbiturates certainly have these characteristics. To satisfy the phenomenal demand for them two decades ago, 500 tons of barbiturates were produced annually in the United States. Fort (1970) and Cohen (1969) then estimated that at least 10 billion doses were produced annually, enough for 40–50 doses for every man, woman, and child. A significant percentage of this production was diverted into black market channels, where it found its way into the hands of drug abusers. The consequence of this problem has been a severe reduction of the supply of sedative barbiturates over the last two decades, and the subsequent unavailability of barbiturates has nearly eliminated their abuse. However, we shall discuss the dynamics of barbiturates as prototypical drugs of abuse.

Assessment Methods

Which drugs are most subject to abuse? Animal and human studies have relied on comparative rates of self-administration to answer this question, assuming that self-administration rates reflect the magnitude of the reinforcing effect. In studies with rats and nonhuman primates, animals self-administered drugs such as barbiturates and benzodiazepines (BDZs) by intravenous, oral, and intragastric routes via implanted catheters that were connected to infusion pumps. The pumps were activated briefly whenever the animals pressed a lever that was continuously available 24 hours a day. In general, the barbiturates with intermediate half-lives, such as pentobarbital, amobarbital, and secobarbital, were more efficacious as reinforcers than were the BDZs. The validity of these studies was supported by the good correspondence between those drugs that are vigorously self-administered by laboratory animals and those that are self-administered and abused by humans (see Griffiths and Ator, 1980).

Human studies were done with well-validated, double-blind, placebo-controlled methodologies on subjects with histories of drug abuse. Comparisons were made among a number of BDZs and barbiturates having different pharmacokinetic profiles (fast vs. slow onset, fast vs. slow elimination, or drugs that were primarily hypnotics vs. anxiolytics). The results showed that pentobarbital was superior to the BDZs in maintaining self-administration, thereby indicating that it had the greater liability for abuse. However, written comments by the subjects stated that among the BDZs, diazepam (Valium) was more like pentobarbital than the other BDZs, that it produced recognizable euphoria, and that its rapid onset of effects was a desirable feature of the drug. It was also judged by the subjects as having a greater monetary street value than the other BDZs (Griffiths and Sannerud, 1987).

Barbiturate Toxicity

When barbiturates were in common use, it was estimated that there were 1,500 deaths annually and six or seven times as many sublethal poisonings in the United States directly involving barbiturates, taken alone or in combination with other CNS depressants such as alcohol. Most fatalities were the result of suicide attempts; some were due to accidental poisoning of children and drug abusers. In the early stages of acute intoxication, the symptoms are similar to those of alcoholic inebriation; the later signs are characterized by depressed reflexes, depressed cardiovascular, respiratory, and renal functions leading to shock, and coma. Similar symptoms are encountered with opiate intoxication, but the effects of opiate overdoses can be readily reversed by opiate antagonists such as naloxone. Unfortunately, there are no fast-acting antidotes to the toxic effects of barbiturates.

Parameters of Barbiturate Dependence

Barbiturate Tolerance

We have discussed drug tolerance in considerable detail as it pertains to alcohol in the preceding chapter, and the same principles apply to barbiturate tolerance. As mentioned earlier, chronic use of barbiturates leads to increasing drug tolerance and dependence and to an upward spiral of higher and higher doses to obtain the desired effects. When the intake of the barbiturate reaches 400 mg/day over several weeks, a pronounced withdrawal syndrome becomes evident when the drug is suddenly and completely withheld.

Like tolerance to alcohol, tolerance to barbiturates is of two principal types: metabolic (pharmacokinetic) tolerance and tissue (pharmacodynamic) tolerance. Metabolic tolerance results from the induction of metabolizing enzymes in the liver by the drug. When more enzymes are available, the drug is metabolized at higher rates, and a higher drug intake is required to maintain sufficient plasma and tissue levels for effective drug activity. This effect was demonstrated when animals were pretreated with low doses of pentobarbital or secobarbital for a few days and then injected with a hypnotic dose

of the drug. The pretreated animals slept for a shorter period than animals that were tested with the same dose but were not pretreated, yet the blood plasma levels at the time of awakening were the same for both groups. The fact that the waking plasma level occurred earlier in the pretreated animals showed that the drug was metabolized faster in those animals.

Cellular tolerance, which also occurs with barbiturates, is indicated by lower or absent drug effects despite the constancy of blood plasma levels during repeated doses of the same strength. This suggests that the tissue of the CNS undergoes changes so that it is less reactive to the drug. In addition, as the required dose increases as a result of metabolic tolerance, so too will cellular tolerance increase. Moreover, whereas metabolic tolerance may reach its maximal value in a few days, cellular tolerance may continue to increase over weeks and months depending upon the dose schedule. Thus, by the time overall tolerance becomes maximal, the effective dose of the barbiturate may be increased sixfold, and this increase is two- or threefold greater than can be accounted for by enhanced metabolic disposition (Jaffe, 1985).

Here it should be noted that, as with alcohol, metabolic and cellular tolerance lead to reduced barbiturate effects, but the size of the lethal dose is not altered (Jaffe, 1985; Sharpless, 1970). Thus, tolerance is not evenly conferred to all effects of barbiturates. Whereas tolerance to the sedative effect does increase, this tolerance is not conferred upon depression of the respiratory centers. Hence, if a person increases barbiturate doses to maintain a wanted state of sedation, he or she increases the risk that the blood levels of the drug may reach the lethal level as far as the respiratory centers are concerned. Similar effects can occur if BDZs and alcohol are taken together, although the margin of safety is significantly greater for BDZ–alcohol effects.

Withdrawal effects. The study of the barbiturate withdrawal syndrome, first begun in 1950, has been intensively conducted with animal and human subjects (Essig, 1970; Okamoto, 1984) and has been extended to many other drugs that were regarded as having a significant abuse potential. A number of effective behavioral and physiological tests have been developed for this endeavor. (See Brady and Lukas, 1984, for a review.)

Barbiturate Tolerance and Dependence in Animals

Tolerance and dependence are more likely to occur with some barbiturate agents than with others. Differences in pharmacokinetics may be related to differences in abuse potential, but differences in the target sites for the various agents have not been ruled out.

Okamoto (1984) reviewed recent techniques for assessing the abuse potential of sedative–hypnotic and anxiolytic drugs in animals. He described a number of experiments from his laboratory in which rating scales were developed for quantifying the induction of tolerance and the effects of sudden drug withdrawal after repeated dosing with barbiturates. In one experiment he made quantitative comparisons between the effects of the prototypical sedatives pentobarbital (PBT) and barbital (BBT) using numerical scales for induced depth of anesthesia, level of ataxia, and the loss of fine motor coordination. First, it should be recalled that PBT and BBT differ in their onset and duration times: PBT has a rather short onset time, an intermediate to short duration of action, and is rapidly metabolized by liver enzymes. In contrast, BBT has a slower onset time, a long duration of action, and is slowly eliminated via the kidneys.

The tolerance induction phase.   In the first phase of the experiment, cats were treated with PBT (twice daily) or BBT (once in 3 days) for 5 weeks, with doses just great enough to induce a light surgical anesthesia. (These doses will be referred to as the effective doses, EDs.) Over the course of treatment, the EDs of PBT and BBT had to be increased to obtain the adverse effects, but the rate of increase was greater for PBT than for BBT. Also, weekly tests showed that the half-life of PBT rapidly declined over days, but for BBT it remained constant. These results showed that a rapid induction of drug-metabolizing enzymes and metabolic tolerance had occurred with PBT. But, in keeping with renal clearance of BBT, this tolerance did not occur with that drug. However, weekly measures of the plasma drug concentration at the peak of the adverse effects following the administration of the EDs showed a gradual increase over the 5-week period for both drugs. This finding showed that a slow-developing cellular tolerance had occurred for both drugs.

The withdrawal phase.   After 5 weeks, the drugs were withdrawn and the PBT-treated animals were challenged with the drug every 3rd day for 2 weeks; in other words, the animals were treated as they were during the induction phase, but less often. This rate of administration would not add tolerance to that which already existed. During this period the EDs of PBT gradually declined and the half-life of the drug gradually increased, showing that metabolic tolerance was declining. However, the plasma drug concentration at the peak of the adverse effects declined very slowly, and it did not return to normal in the 2-week withdrawal period. This finding showed the typically slow pace of the dissipation of cellular tolerance.

Dose frequency.   In investigations of the frequency of barbiturate administration as a factor in tolerance and dependence, the most important dependent variable was found to be the plasma concentration of the drug, which is directly related to dose frequency and drug elimination. If a drug with a long half-life is repeatedly given at short intervals, the plasma drug level will rise; if the half-life is short, the plasma level will fall sharply after administration and no drug accumulation will occur.

Barbiturate metabolism and elimination.   It has long been known that after heavy usage, the long-acting barbiturates such as phenobarbital and barbital are less likely to lead to drug dependence than the short-acting drugs such as pentobarbital and secobarbital. Also, when comparing the time parameters of dependencies on BBT and PBT, one finds that the onset of withdrawal symptoms is slower and their intensity is less severe in BBT dependence than in PBT dependence. The average elimination half-lives of the two drugs are 30 and 5 hours respectively. Thus, researchers wanted to know whether the slow rate of metabolism and elimination of BBT was responsible for the slow onset of mild withdrawal symptoms, and whether the fast metabolism and elimination of PBT was related to its high incidence of dependence and withdrawal symptoms.

To answer these questions, the short half-life of PBT was experimentally lengthened and the long half-life of BBT was shortened. The half-life of PBT was lengthened by administering proportionally smaller doses intravenously at computer-generated intervals based upon PBT elimination kinetics. The effect of this manipulation was to lengthen the PBT half-life from 5 to 27 hours. This procedure slowed the onset of withdrawal symptoms and reduced their severity. With BBT, the long half-life was shortened by peritoneal dialysis after the last dose, which reduced the half-life from 30 to 7 hours. In this case withdrawal signs appeared much sooner, with markedly intensified symptoms. Thus, the signs of drug withdrawal were slower to appear and were less severe when the rate of drug metabolism and elimination was low. And in contrast, a high blood level and rapid drug elimination contributed to a stronger rebound after abstinence. These data support the idea that the rate of drug metabolism is a factor in the onset and severity of the withdrawal syndrome.

It is generally accepted that barbiturates having short onset times and half-lives, such as secobarbital, are more likely to be abused and to be associated with severe withdrawal syndromes than compounds with long onset times and half-lives. Because secobarbital's effects occur soon after ingestion, the drug is presumably very rewarding. In contrast, drugs whose effects have a long, gradual onset are probably less reinforcing because of the time delay between ingestion and the drug consequences, which probably explains why such drugs are less desirable to drug abusers. For example, phenobarbital, used to control epilepsy, has a long onset time and is long-acting; this drug is rarely abused, and termination of the drug after prolonged treatment has few consequences. Moreover, drugs with long half-lives allow the CNS time to adjust to the absence of the drug, which also lessens the severity of withdrawal symptoms. Thus, it is more likely that strong dependence on barbiturates and severe withdrawal symptoms will follow the frequent ingestion of high doses of fast-acting compounds with comparatively short half-lives. It will be seen that these principles apply to drugs other than barbiturates as well.

Barbiturate Tolerance and Dependence in Humans

There is an extensive literature on human tolerance and dependence on barbiturates (see Fraser et al., 1958; Isbell, 1950; Isbell et al., 1950). The research on humans was accomplished at the U.S. Public Health Service hospital for drug addicts in Lexington, Kentucky. It involved giving human subjects, who were long-term prisoners, large doses of sedative barbiturates for extended periods and then abruptly withdrawing the drugs. Even though the subjects gave their consent to participate in these studies, it is questionable whether such procedures would be acceptable today.

At first, the general procedure was to induce barbiturate intoxication by giving drugs such as secobarbital, pentobarbital, and amobarbital at doses that were 4 to 12 times greater than normal therapeutic doses. The researchers found that the peak sedative effects occurred after 30–90 minutes, depending on the drug used, that after 2 hours the sedative effects declined, and that after 4 hours the subjects were fully awake. But this period was followed by difficulty in thinking, dysarthria (poorly articulated speech), coarse tremor of the hands, and depressed superficial reflexes. Some subjects became boisterous and silly; others became quiet and depressed.

In other tests, the volunteers were given one of the three drugs in gradually increasing doses every 12 hours over a period of 92–140 days. These doses caused a continuous mild intoxication in most instances; the men were confused and unable to do ordinary tasks, they were unkempt, their living quarters were untidy, and they were irritable, quarrelsome, and aggressive. They staggered, frequently fell, and occasionally injured themselves. During this period their pulse rates increased about 10 beats per minute, but most vital signs and blood chemistry appeared normal.

After the last dose of the drug, there was an interval of 12–16 hours when the subjects seemed to "sober up." Then they became anxious and weak with increasing severity until at 24–36 hours, they could hardly stand or walk unassisted. Their blood pressure dropped, causing them to feel faint on standing. They showed tremulousness, muscular fasciculations, anorexia, vomiting, abdominal distress, mydriasis, hyperreflexia, insomnia, weight loss, and increased startle responses to auditory and visual stimuli.

What was more significant was the appearance of generalized convulsions and/or the onset of a reversible psychosis. The time course for the onset of convulsions was quite variable: some occurred between the 30th and 39th hour after withdrawal, and the latest convulsion occurred as late as the 115th hour of abstinence. The psychotic episodes began between the 3rd and 5th day and lasted as long as 9 days. These episodes were similar to alcohol-induced delirium tremens and were characterized by agitation, insomnia, confusion, disorientation of time and place, delusions, and auditory and visual hallucinations. Body temperature was elevated, pulse rates were rapid, and the appearance of exhaustion was evident. The delirium tended to occur after the convulsions, but the two symptoms could occur alone or together. These were the life-threatening aspects of the withdrawal syndrome. In general, the more severe signs and symptoms were observed only following prolonged exposure to high doses (Griffiths and Sannerud, 1987).

Thus, we have seen that the withdrawal syndrome becomes evident when the drug in question is suddenly and completely withheld. This is not to say that drug dependence and the withdrawal syndrome define the presence of drug abuse, for there are drugs that can produce physical dependence without eliciting substantial drug-seeking behavior, and vice versa. For example, cocaine is a drug with a high abuse potential, but there are virtually no serious physical withdrawal symptoms; on the other hand, phenobarbital taken over a long period of time can produce dependence, but at the same time the drug has a low incidence of abuse.

Diagnosis and Treatment of Barbiturate Abuse

If a therapist's patient is suspected of being an abuser of barbiturates, his or her dependence can be assessed by the patient's reaction to a barbiturate test dose. The patient is given an oral dose (60 mg) of phenobarbital, and the reaction to the drug indicates the degree of barbiturate tolerance that has developed. If the patient, 1 hour after ingestion, is asleep or grossly intoxicated, the tolerance level is minimal and withdrawal symptoms will be mild. If the patient is comfortable, has normal speech, has no ataxia, and shows only a fine lateral nystagmus, the tolerance level is moderate, and withdrawal symptoms can be prevented with 200–300 mg of phenobarbital per day. With high levels of tolerance, there is no response to the 60-mg test dose, and the patient may even show withdrawal effects. In such cases daily doses of 300–500 mg of phenobarbital may be required to prevent withdrawal symptoms. After establishing the level of tolerance that has developed, the phenobarbital dose is gradually reduced by approximately 30 mg every other day until the patient is drug free. This treatment should be supplemented by psychotherapy to help forestall a return to drug abuse.

Part II Summary

The barbiturates are a class of chemical agents having a long history of use for the treatment of anxiety, insomnia, and epilepsy, with some forms being used for surgical anesthesia. The differences between their modes of action can be traced to their lipid solubility and to the mode and time course of deactivation. The effects of barbiturates are related to their ability to enhance GABA-mediated neuronal depression. Numerous animal experiments have demonstrated the anxiety-reducing effects of these drugs and support the results found in clinical data. Also, as we have seen, barbiturates are excellent tools for studying the mechanisms of the tolerance and dependence syndromes that are instrumental in drug abuse. Unfortunately, because of these characteristics, some barbiturates have a high abuse potential, and were once frequent instruments of suicide, unintentional self-poisoning, and drug addiction, with its consequent dangers of injury or death following abrupt withdrawal. Consequently, these drugs, although clinically useful in many instances, have given way to other drugs that are considerably safer.

Part III
The Benzodiazepines and Other Nonbarbiturate Anxiolytics

Early Nonbarbiturate Anxiolytics

In the 1940s, chemists at Wallace Laboratories came upon the compound mephenesin carbamate (2-hydroxy-3-[tolyloxy] propyl carbamate), a compound that had been known since 1908. When tested in animals, mephenesin produced profound muscle relaxation and a sleep-like condition from which the animals could easily be aroused. After clinical studies, there were reports that mephenesin allayed anxiety without clouding consciousness. However, in practice, the drug was found to be impractical because it was rapidly metabolized in the liver and thus required frequent administration or high doses. The Wallace researchers attempted to alter the mephenesin molecule to correct these shortcomings, with the result that meprobamate (MPB) was developed by Ludwig and Piech (1951; Berger and Ludwig, 1964).

Meprobamate (MPB) (11-methyl-2-propyl-1,3-propanediol dicarbamate) was given the trade name Miltown after Milltown, New Jersey, a town near Wallace Laboratories. This compound, like mephenesin, had muscle relaxant qualities, but had a slower induction period and a longer sustained effect. It was also found that MPB had a marked tranquilizing action when tested on monkeys, which, while fully in touch with their environment, lost their fear, hostility, and aggressiveness and became friendly. Further research showed that MPB, like the barbiturates, was effective in disinhibiting behavior suppressed by punishment (Geller, 1962).

In clinical studies it was found that MPB could induce a tranquil state without the suppression of the reticular formation that occurred with barbiturates. This finding suggested that MPB had a uniquely selective action on the CNS in suppressing anxiety states without the impairment of intellectual performance, coordination, and perception, all of which were characteristic of barbiturates at doses that had anxiolytic effects. Consequently, after licensing, MPB was widely prescribed and sold for virtually all the conditions for which the barbiturates were formerly recommended. Miltown became a household word, and in the 1950s and 1960s MPB became one of the most widely used drugs in the world.

Before long, however, studies revealed that the uniqueness and safety of MPB were more imagined than real: there were numerous reports of lethal overdoses, and reports that ingesting MPB with alcohol could be fatal. After further study of the drug, a consensus developed that the mode of action of MPB was not significantly different from that of the barbiturates (Jarvik, 1970), and that MPB carried an unacceptable risk of addiction and fatality on overdosage. The result was a rapid disappearance of MPB as a therapeutic drug.

The Development of the Benzodiazepines

It is obvious that the commercial success of a drug can inspire competing members of the pharmaceutical industry to design a similar drug, if not a better one. When MBP became a commercial success in the 1950s, the drive to find a competing drug was certainly there, and was no doubt accelerated when the shortcomings of MPB became known. What was needed was an agent that was effective in allaying anxiety at doses that were benign in most other respects. In other words, the drug should have a high therapeutic index so that fatal accidental or intentional overdoses would be unlikely, and it should be free of physiological side effects and properties contributing to dependence and withdrawal symptoms.

A team at Hoffman–La Roche led by Leo Sternbach (1973), which started work in 1955, elected to study some compounds that Sternbach had synthesized at the University of Cracow in Poland as a postdoctoral research assistant in the 1930s. These compounds were selected because they were easily available and were expected to lend themselves to many variations and transformations. The hope was to find reaction products to which side chains could be added that were known to impart biological activity. According to Tinklenberg (1977), the sequence of events went something like this: Sternbach, now a medicinal chemist at Roche Laboratories, decided to screen the drugs he had synthesized in Poland for biological activity. He first discovered that the compounds were not heptoxdiazines as he had thought, but quinazolone 3-oxides. Sternbach then synthesized 40 derivatives and found that all but one of these were pharmacologically inert. The last one was not tested; instead, it was labeled Ro 5-0690 and shelved because of other research priorities. In May 1957, during a cleanup of the laboratory, one of Sternbach's chemists turned up the compound and suggested that it be tested. It was given to the Roche pharmacology team headed by Lowell O. Randall, which subjected the compound to a battery of tests and discovered that it had a number of clinically important properties. Ro 5-0690 turned out to be what was first called methaminodiazepoxide and, shortly after, chlordiazepoxide (CDP).

Randall and his colleagues (1960) first announced that CDP had potent sedative, muscle relaxant, taming, and anticonvulsant activity. Soon afterward it was reported that the drug, now given the trade name Librium (from "equilibrium"), had potent antianxiety effects in humans. Others showed that CDP acted almost as a psychostimulant by conferring feelings of well-being that led to an increase in social activity, verbal productivity, and appetite and a reduction of anxious depression. The drug's anticonvulsant properties were demonstrated by its ability to increase the threshold to pentylenetetrazol-induced convulsions (Randall and Kapell, 1973).

Within a year, a more potent congener, diazepam (Valium), was developed (Randall et al., 1961). This was followed in 1965 by oxazepam (Serax), which is a metabolite of diazepam and differs from it essentially by having a shorter plasma half-life than either chlordiazepox-

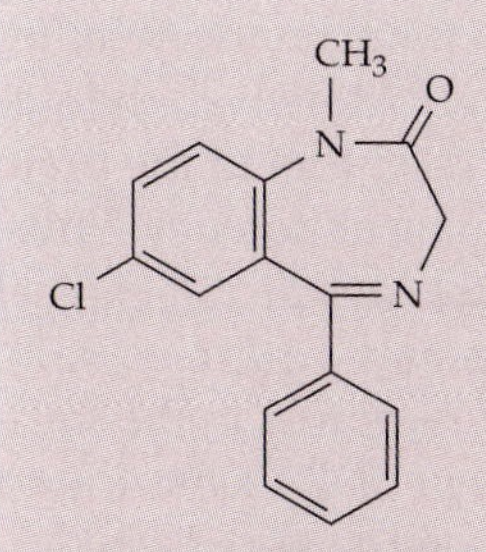

Diazepam (Valium)

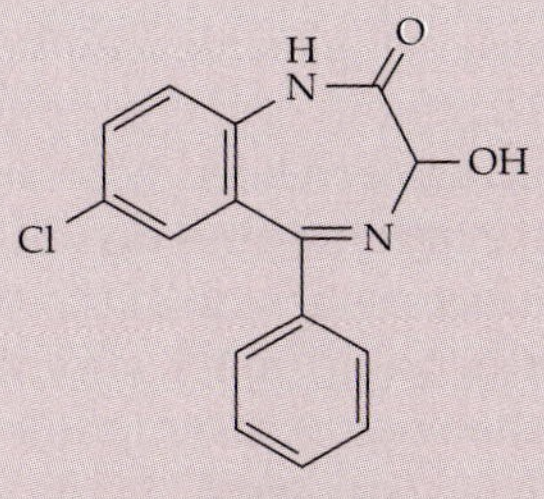

Oxazepam (Serax)

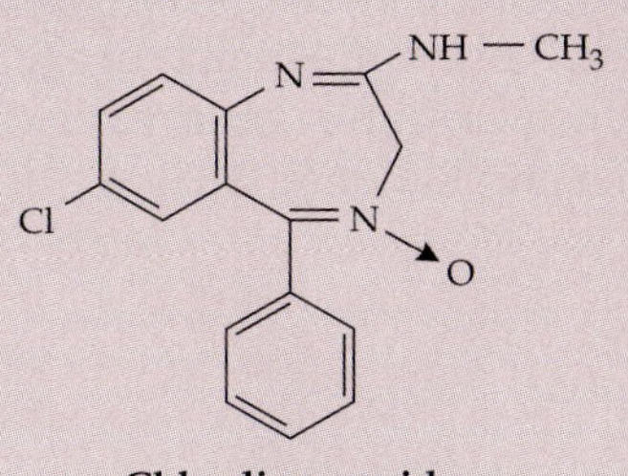

Chlordiazepoxide (Librium)

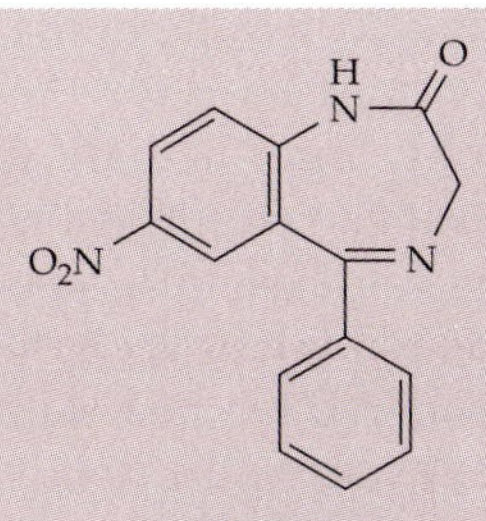

Nitrazepam (Mogodon)

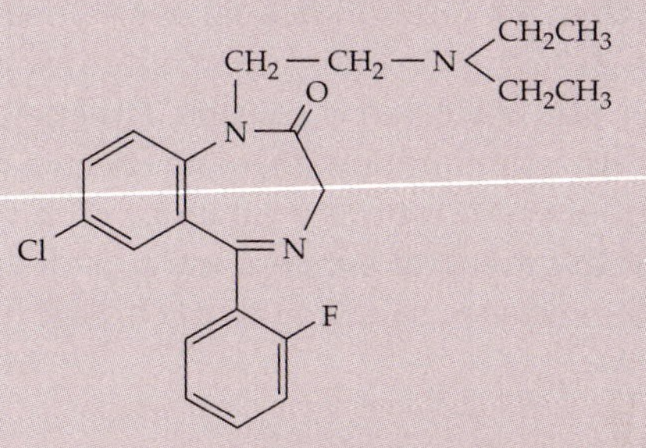

Flurazepam (Dalmane)

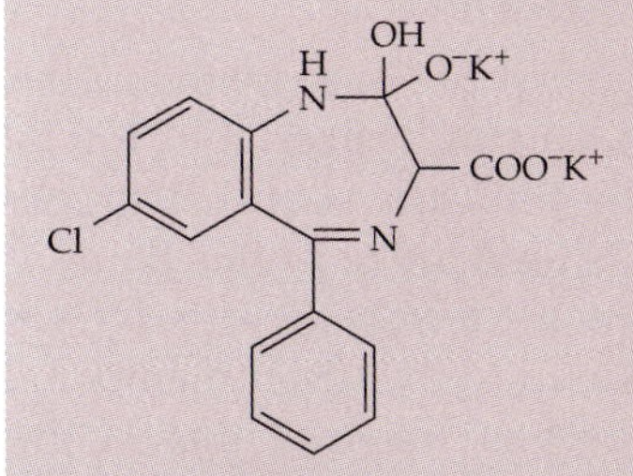

Clorazepate (Tranxene)

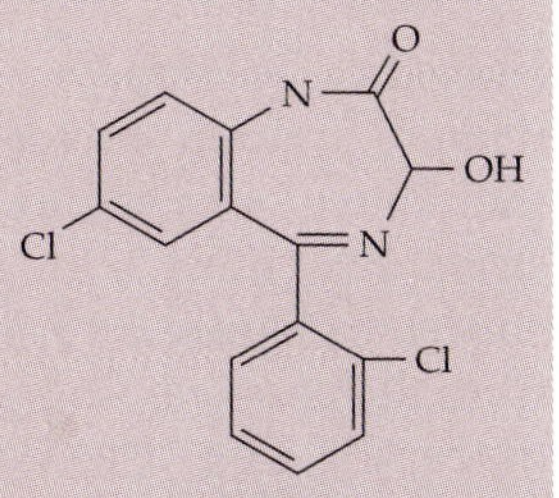

Lorazepam (Ativan)

ide or diazepam. Nitrazepam (Mogodon), which also appeared in 1965, and flurazepam (Dalmane), which appeared in 1970, were found to have marked hypnotic properties. In 1972 clorazepate (Tranxene) was added to the list of commercially successful antianxiety agents, and was followed by lorazepam (Ativan) in 1975. In 1985, the seventh edition of Goodman and Gilman's *Pharmacological Basis of Therapeutics* listed 17 BDZ compounds, most of which are used clinically in the United States (Gilman et al., 1985).

When Librium and Valium became known to physicians, their popularity was almost instantaneous and their commercial success was assured. In 1972 these two substances together accounted for an estimated 49% of all psychoactive drug prescriptions in the United States, virtually displacing all other known sedative–hypnotic and anxiolytic agents in the United States pharmacopeia (Blackwell, 1973). Over 100 million prescriptions for these two drugs were filled annually, at a cost of over $500 million; this figure includes 3 million refills written for Valium each month. In 1977 the newest BDZ, clorazepate, reputed to equal diazepam in effectiveness but with fewer side effects, was reported to be selling in the United States at a rate of about 188,000 prescriptions per month (Shader and Greenblatt, 1977).

The popularity of these drugs peaked in 1973; then, because of adverse publicity (see below), there was a drop of about 20 million prescriptions per annum over the next 5 years, partly due to a drop in prescription refills (Rickels, 1980). In 1981 the United States Food and Drug Administration (FDA) reported that the annual BDZ prescription rate was down to 65 million and was holding steady at that level. Even at that rate, household surveys showed that 11% to 13% of the adult population had taken an anxiolytic drug one or more times during the last year, and that 2.3% to 2.5% of the population had taken anxiolytics on a daily basis for 4 months or longer. This rate of use is only intermediate when compared with the rates in European countries, where the prevalence of use was as high as 18%, and steady use (4 months or more) was as high as 7.2%. Nonetheless, this level of use was considered by the health care system to be within an appropriate, and possibly conservative, range, although some inappropriate prescribing could not be ruled out. Although a recent estimate ascertained that more than 500 million people over the last 30 years have taken BDZ medications for anxiety, insomnia, muscle spasms, stress-related disorders, epilepsy, or as part of preoperative preparation, there has been a decrease in the number of prescriptions written for BDZ compounds because of the medical concern about side effects and physical dependence resulting from chronic use.

Molecular Studies

Chemistry of the Benzodiazepines

Since the development of the first BDZs, more than 2,000 related compounds have been synthesized, but few of them have been found to be clinically useful. The core structure of most of the BDZs used in the United States is shown in Figure 16.5. The name *benzodiazepine* derives from the benzene ring (A) fused to the seven-membered diazepine ring (B). Also, because most of these compounds contain a 5-aryl substituent ring (C) and a 1,4-diazepine ring (N atoms at positions 1 and 4), the complete generic name is 5-aryl-1,4-BDZs. Furthermore, other substituent rings have been fused at positions 1 and 2, such as triazolo and imidazo rings. Other substituent electron-withdrawing atoms or groups, when added at position 7 in ring A or 2′ in ring C, markedly enhance potency, whereas electron-releasing groups at position 7 or elsewhere on ring A reduce activity. The replacment of ring C with a keto function at position 5 and a methyl substituent at position 4 are important structural features of

BDZ antagonists such as the imidazobenzodiazepine Ro 15-1788, which came to be known as flumazenil. (For more details, see Haefely, 1983; Harvey, 1985.)

Benzodiazepine Binding Characteristics

The central binding of BDZs has already been described in Chapter 10, but a few additional comments may be appropriate here. First, the brain distribution of BDZ receptors in humans and rats is remarkably similar (Young and Kuhar, 1980; Zezula et al., 1988). It was also found that displacement of [^{3}H]diazepam binding in vitro occurred only with other BDZs, whose potencies in this regard correlated well with their potencies in the muscle relaxant tests mentioned earlier. It was later found that their displacement potencies were also correlated with their clinically demonstrated anxiolytic potencies, and with the potencies of their anticonflict and muscle relaxant effects in animals (see Figure 10.26).

It was also mentioned in Chapter 10 that there are some peripheral-type binding sites in the liver, adrenal glands, and testes, as well in as some cortical neurons and glia. There have also been reports of peripheral binding in the kidney and lung, but there is virtually no diazepam binding in skeletal or visceral muscle. Moreover, the peripheral binding, where it did exist, was of significantly lower affinity than that for the usual receptors in the brain, and was associated with a mitochondrial rather than a cytoplasmic membrane fraction. Moreover, the low BDZ affinity of the peripheral-type receptors in the brain was not correlated with any neuroclinical potency. Thus, these binding sites do not mediate the significant clinical characteristics of BDZs (Braestrup and Squires, 1977). Furthermore, in the absence of BDZ receptors in the sympathetic or parasympathetic systems, BDZs were found to have only weak, if any, effects upon the peripheral autonomic nervous system. Consequently, BDZ-mediated difficulties involving cholinergic or adrenergic effects on cardiovascular, gastrointestinal, urogenital, and pulmonary systems were rarely observed in BDZ-treated patients (Zbinden and Randall, 1967).

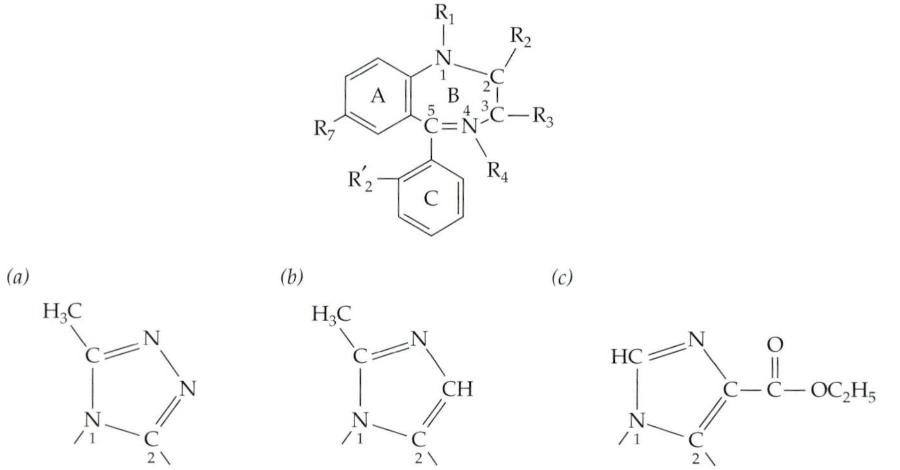

16.5 CHEMICAL STRUCTURE OF THE BENZODIAZEPINES. Shown at the top is the core structure made up of the benzene ring (A), the seven-membered diazepine ring (B), and the aryl substituent ring (C). Below the core structure are the triazolo ring (*a*) and two imidazo rings (*b* and *c*) that are fused to the diazepine ring at positions 1 and 2.

Mechanisms of Action

Neurophysiological Studies

The BDZs have significant effects on the limbic structures of the CNS. Chlordiazepoxide (CDP) was found to inhibit after-discharges induced by electrical stimulation of the septum, hippocampus, and amygdala. In these experiments the brain structures were electrically stimulated for a few seconds; when the stimulus was terminated, the neurons of these structures continued to fire in unison. Systemic administration of CNS-depressant drugs shortened the duration or prevented the occurrence of electrically induced after-discharges. Suppressant effects with CDP occurred at a dose of 10 mg/kg, but the effective doses for meprobamate and phenobarbital were twice as great.

CDP blocked convulsions induced by pentylenetetrazol and electroshock. After 30 mg/kg of CDP, the dose of the convulsant drug had to be increased sixfold to elicit convulsant patterns in the EEG. In the brains of cats sensitized by pentylenetetrazol, CDP at the same dose blocked the induction and spread of convulsant activity induced by flashing lights. These findings formed the basis for the clinical use of some BDZs as antiepileptic agents.

Biochemical Studies: The Interaction with GABA

The ultimate clarification of the mechanism of action of most drugs comes from the identification of the cellular binding sites that are either activated or blocked by the drugs, thereby inducing or preventing changes in subcellular components such as enzymes or ionophores in the cell membrane. In order to establish the mechanism of action of the BDZs, researchers investigated the ability of these compounds to enhance or diminish the activity of neurotransmitters in the CNS. For the most part, the early reports of changes in neurotransmitter turnover were inconclusive except for a growing accumulation of evidence showing consistent patterns of GABA involvement in BDZ-induced effects, as well as probable interactions with serotonergic mechanisms (Gardner, 1986; Thiebot, 1986).

The precise way in which BDZs interact with GABA synapses is discussed in Chapter 10, but here we reiterate that BDZs do not produce the same effects as the GABA mimetic muscimol, nor do they interfere with high-affinity binding of the GABA antagonist [^{3}H]bicuculline or with neuronal or glial uptake of GABA. Rather, BDZs act on the GABA$_A$ receptor to increase its affinity for GABA. Consistent with this finding, the BDZs exert their effects only during the activity of GABAergic neurons. Thus, BDZ potency is limited by the availability of GABA, and this property, plus the absence of GABA–BDZ receptors associated with the autonomic nervous system, may account for the safety of BDZ compounds. Investigations into the BDZ–GABA relationship ultimately led to the discovery of BDZ receptors that were part of an unusual

molecular structure, the GABA–BDZ–Cl$^-$ ionophore receptor complex (see Chapter 10).

Pharmacological Studies

Studies of the pharmacokinetics of BDZ compounds were directed toward establishing such parameters as lipid solubility, absorption, protein binding, receptor affinity, potency, tissue distribution, toxicity, compatibility with other compounds, plasma concentration half-life, metabolism and clearance half-lives, and tolerance. Most of these factors are related to the onset time and duration of effects in human recipients of the drugs. These pharmacokinetic factors may determine the appropriate therapeutic choice, as illustrated by the following comparison between diazepam and lorazepam. The elimination half-life of diazepam is between 20 and 70 hours, whereas that of lorazepam is 10–20 hours, yet the duration of effective action of lorazepam (8 hours) is much greater than that of diazepam (1–2 hours) (Figure 16.6). This apparent paradox is explained by the fact that diazepam is twice as lipid soluble as lorazepam, so

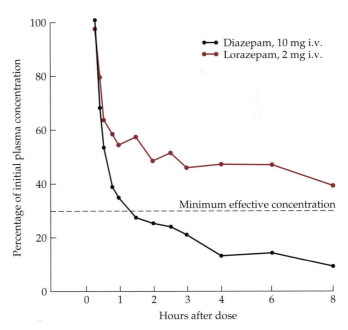

16.6 COMPARATIVE PHARMACOKINETICS OF DIAZEPAM VERSUS LORAZEPAM. A normal individual received diazepam (10 mg i.v.) on one occasion, and lorazepam (2 mg i.v.) on another occasion. Blood plasma concentrations were sampled after drug administration at half-hour intervals for 4 hours, then once every 2 hours for a total of 8 hours. The plasma concentrations measured are shown as the percentage of the initial peak concentration. It was assumed that there was a drug effect as long as the plasma concentration was at least 30% of the peak. Because diazepam is more lipophilic than lorazepam, it has a larger volume of distribution, leading to a rapid fall in plasma concentration and drug effectiveness. Lorazepam is less lipophilic and has a smaller volume of distribution, and therefore maintains an effective plasma concentration longer, even though lorazepam has a shorter elimination half-life. (After Greenblatt and Shader, 1987.)

that it is rapidly taken up by the brain, but it also rapidly exits the brain and blood plasma as it diffuses to peripheral storage sites such as adipose tissue, skeletal muscle, and the liver. With lorazepam, the exit from the brain is slower and the extent of peripheral distribution is smaller. Moreover, because diazepam readily binds to plasma protein (albumin), the free fraction of the plasma concentration is very small (1.6%) compared with that of lorazepam (9.7%). Thus, the kinetics of diazepam are characterized by a large volume of distribution, a small proportion of free drug in the blood plasma, and a rapid exit from the brain. The effective plasma concentration falls below the minimum effective

level between 1 and 2 hours after dosage, whereas a smaller dose of lorazepam, due to its different kinetics of availability, is effective for 8 hours after dosing, even though its elimination half-life is shorter than that of diazepam.

It is beyond the scope of this book to supply detailed pharmacokinetic data on each and every BDZ and related drug mentioned in these pages, but BDZ kinetics will be mentioned in specific instances. Table 16.1 will serve as a quick reference to assist the reader in identifying most of the BDZs and their principal characteristics. (For a brief survey of BDZ kinetics and an extensive reference list, see Greenblatt and Shader, 1987.)

Table 16.1   Pharmacokinetic Summary of the Benzodiazepines

Administered drug	Most common indication	Initial biotransformation pathway	Substances present in blood (with usual range of elimination half-life [hr])[a]
Diazepam	Anxiolytic	Oxidation	Diazepam (20–70)
			Desmethyldiazepam (36–96)
			Oxazepam*
			Temazepam*
Clorazepate[b]	Anxiolytic	Oxidation	Desmethyldiazepam (36–96)
Prazepam[b]	Anxiolytic	Oxidation	Desmethyldiazepam (36–96)
Oxazolam[b]	Anxiolytic	Oxidation	Desmethyldiazepam (36–96)
Alprazolam	Anxiolytic	Oxidation	Alprazolam (8–15)
Lorazepam	Anxiolytic	Conjugation	Lorazepam (10–20)
Oxazepam	Anxiolytic	Conjugation	Oxazepam (5–15)
Bromazepam	Anxiolytic	Oxidation	Bromazepam (20–30)
Clobazam	Anxiolytic	Oxidation	Clobazam (20–30)
			Desmethylclobazam
Flurazepam	Hypnotic	Oxidation	Desalkylflurazepam (36–120)
			Hydroxyethyl flurazepam (1–4)
			Flurazepam aldehyde
			Flurazepam*
Temazepam	Hypnotic	Conjugation	Temazepam (8–20)
Lormetazepam	Hypnotic	Conjugation	Lormetazepam (8–20)
Triazolam	Hypnotic	Oxidation	Triazolam (1.5–5)
Nitrazepam	Hypnotic	Nitroreduction	Nitrazepam (20–30)
Flunitrazepam	Hypnotic; perioperative	Oxidation; nitroreduction	Flunitrazepam (10–40)
			Desmethylflunitrazepam
Quazepam	Hypnotic	Oxidation	Quazepam (15–35)
			Oxoquazepam (25–35)
			Desalkylflurazepam (36–120)
Estazolam	Hypnotic	Oxidation	Estazolam (20–30)
Midazolam	Perioperative; hypnotic	Oxidation	Midazolam (1–4)
			1-Hydroxymethyl midazolam*
			4-Hydroxy midazolam*
Clonazepam	Antiseizure	Nitroreduction	Clonazepam (30–60)

[a]Asterisk (*) indicates compounds present in quantitatively minor amounts, and/or those that have reduced pharmacological activity.
[b]Clorazepate, prazepam, and oxazolam all serve as desmethyldiazepam precursors.
Source: After Greenblatt and Shader, 1987.

Benzodiazepine Receptors and Their Ligands

As noted in Chapter 10, there are two types of GABA receptors, $GABA_A$ and $GABA_B$, and the $GABA_A$ receptors are the ones involved in BDZ binding. These receptors were first described in Chapter 10. Although these findings are presented in detail in Chapter 10, the major conclusions will be reiterated here.

As mentioned above, the binding of GABA, barbiturates, or BDZs is allosterically regulated by the other ligands. For example, a BDZ such as diazepam will bind more tightly when GABA is bound to the receptor, and vice versa: GABA will bind more tightly if a BDZ is bound to the receptor. Finally, there is an additional site within the supramolecular complex that is associated with, and regulates, the opening of the Cl^- channel. This site binds picrotoxinin and other convulsants, such as some barbiturates and t-butylbicyclophosphorothionate (TBPS) (see below).

$GABA_A$ receptors can be subdivided into subgroups that differ in their affinity for GABA agonists and antagonists. The $GABA_A$ agonist muscimol recognizes both high- and low-affinity $GABA_A$ receptors (subunits of the $GABA_A$ complex); however, BDZ binding sites have primarily been associated with the low-affinity subgroup of $GABA_A$ receptors. This has been demonstrated by the use of autoradiographic techniques to localize the individual components of the $GABA_A$ receptor complex. BDZ binding sites can be labeled with [^{3}H]flunitrazepam; high-affinity GABA binding sites can be labeled with [^{3}H]muscimol; the barbiturate-sensitive anticonvulsant sites can be labeled with the convulsant [^{3}H]TBPS; and the low-affinity GABA site can be labeled with [^{3}H]bicuculline in the presence of thiocyanate. By labeling serial brain sections with different ligands, the distribution and density of these components of the macromolecular complex can be individually examined in the same regions of the brain. The results of this approach showed that high-affinity $GABA_A$ receptor sites exist in many brain regions where BDZ receptors could not be localized to any great extent, and vice versa (Wamsley, Gehlert, and Olsen, 1986). In contrast, low-affinity GABA sites are correlated with the presence of BDZ receptors.

Recordings from single isolated Cl^- channels revealed that in the presence of diazepam, the GABA-mediated response was enhanced by an increased frequency of Cl^- channel opening, an effect that was identical to the response that occurred after increasing the concentration of GABA in the absence of the drug. (In contrast, barbiturates prolonged the mean channel opening time by a factor of five compared with GABA alone.) Thus, the general effect of the anxiolytic, anticonvulsant, and sedative–hypnotic BDZs is presumably to alter the conformational state of the receptors so that they are more effectively coupled to the Cl^- channels, the consequence of which is the enhancement of Cl^- conductance and hyperpolarization of the target cells, which renders them less excitable to depolarizing transmitters.

The β-Carbolines and Other BDZ Receptor Ligands

As described in Chapter 10, searchers for endogenous BDZ receptor ligands identified the β-carbolines (e.g., β-CCE, β-CCM, and DMCM), which were potent displacers of radiolabeled BDZs from their receptor sites and had in vitro receptor binding affinities equal to those of some of the most potent BDZs. Some of these ligands exerted effects opposite to those of BDZ anxiolytics and came to be known as "inverse agonists" whose common feature was an antagonism to pharmacological, electrophysiological, and all other BDZ effects. These inverse agonists are presumed to uncouple the receptors from the Cl^- channels, thereby reducing the frequency of channel opening, diminishing Cl^- conductance, and increasing membrane excitability. Not all β-carbolines were inverse agonists: some actually were BDZ agonists, such as ZK 93-423, which in a number of experimental tests had all the earmarks of a regular BDZ agonist (see below). Another agonist, ZK 95 962, had muscle-relaxing properties without sedation, and also had anticonvulsant effects on a few photoepileptic patients without sedative effects. (Photoepileptics show epileptiform EEG signs when they are exposed to flashing lights.) Other BDZ receptor ligands were chemically related BDZ receptor blockers, such as Ro 15-1788 (flumazenil), as well as the related BDZ receptor blockers CGS 8216, CGS 9896, and the β-carboline ZK 93 426, which bind to the receptor complex but have no effect of their own other than blocking the binding and activity of the agonists and inverse agonists. Figure 16.7 is a schematic view of a BDZ receptor showing different binding sites for a variety of ligands. (For additional discussions of Ro 15-1788, see below.)

In addition to the BDZ ligands described above, there are partial agonists and partial inverse agonists that are intermediates between full BDZ agonists and inverse agonists. These compounds have less efficacy than typical BDZ agonists in that they require a significantly greater degree of receptor occupancy for given levels of anxiolytic or anxiogenic effects. For example, a congener of the BDZ antagonist flumazenil is the imidazoBDZ Ro 15-3505 (sarmazenil). This compound is a partial inverse agonist that is also a potent antagonist of BDZ anxiolytics, yet it has a very low inverse (negative) intrinsic efficacy at BDZ receptors. The degree of positive or negative effect of these compounds can be ascertained in terms of their ability to modulate GABA-induced Cl^- flux in membrane preparations from rat cerebral cortex. Figure 16.8 shows comparisons among some full and partial agonists and inverse agonists, with flumazenil occupying the midpoint of the scale.

Another substance with effects similar to those of the β-carbolines is the diazepam binding inhibitor (DBI) (this substance is described in Chapter 10). With respect

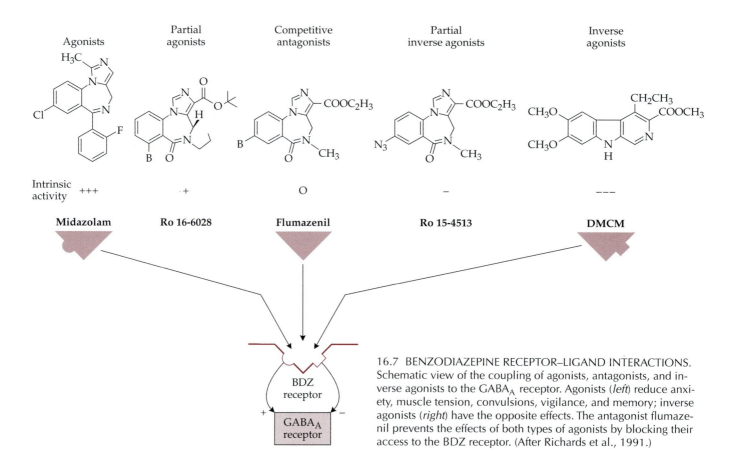

16.7 BENZODIAZEPINE RECEPTOR–LIGAND INTERACTIONS. Schematic view of the coupling of agonists, antagonists, and inverse agonists to the GABA_A receptor. Agonists (*left*) reduce anxiety, muscle tension, convulsions, vigilance, and memory; inverse agonists (*right*) have the opposite effects. The antagonist flumazenil prevents the effects of both types of agonists by blocking their access to the BDZ receptor. (After Richards et al., 1991.)

to its behavioral effects, intraventricular injection of DBI has proconflict effects, which means that animals treated with DBI are affected more adversely in stressful conflict situations. For example, when rats were given noncontingent foot shocks prior to a drinking conflict test, drinking behavior was suppressed more than it was in nonshocked rats, and perfusing DBI into the brains of shocked rats suppressed drinking behavior even more. It will be seen below that the proconflict characteristics of the β-carbolines and related compounds can serve as valuable tools in the assessment of anxiety and the efficacy of BDZs.

Endogenous Benzodiazepines in Mammalian Brains

During the search for peptides with BDZ-like actions, there were reports of the isolation of a number of endogenous substances from mammalian brains that not only bound to BDZ receptor sites, but also had remarkable similarities to BDZs themselves (de Blas et al., 1987; de Blas and Sotelo, 1987; Sangameswaran et al., 1986). Like other brain extracts, these compounds were also found in kidney, liver, spleen, and testes, although the concentration was highest in brain tissue. Among the compounds that were first extracted from rat brains and purified using monoclonal anti-BDZ antibodies (mAb 21-7F9) and immunoaffinity chromatography, one was found to possess the same characteristics as N-desmethyldiazepam,

which is the active metabolite of BDZs such as diazepam, clorazepate, and prazepam (see Table 16.1). A number of

N-desmethyldiazepam

Prazepam (Verstran)

chemical tests validated this identity: the absorption spectrum of this new ligand, designated endogenous BDZ (EBDZ), from bovine cerebellum and cerebral cortex was very similar to the spectra of N-desmethyldiazepam (DDZ) and diazepam (DZ), but different from those of chlordiazepoxide, medazepam, oxazepam, flunitrazepam, Ro 5-4864, Ro 15-1788, the β-carbolines, and other previously proposed endogenous BDZ ligands. Further, the mass spectra of DDZ and EBDZ were virtually identical, and EBDZ from bovine brains and DDZ had similar affinities for mAb 21-7F9 and for neuronal BDZ receptors—that is, both EBDZ and DDZ inhibited [3H]flunitrazepam binding to neuronal BDZ receptors, but they

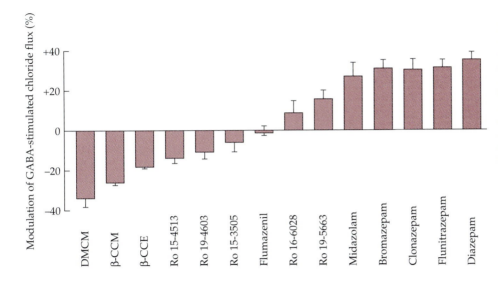

16.8 BENZODIAZEPINE RECEPTOR LIGAND POTENCY. Benzodiazepine receptor ligands modulate Cl⁻ flux in rat cortical membranes. Agonists enhance, whereas inverse agonists reduce, the GABA-mediated Cl⁻ influx. Increased Cl⁻ influx lowers the excitability of neurons; reduced influx increases excitability. Benzodiazepine antagonists do not alter the effect of GABA on Cl⁻ influx, although they block the changes produced by BDZ agonists and inverse agonists. (After Richards et al., 1991.)

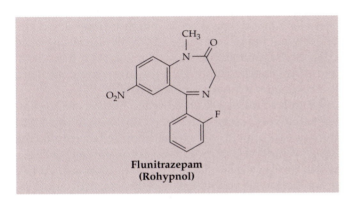

Flunitrazepam (Rohypnol)

did not inhibit [³H]Ro 5-4864 binding to peripheral-type BDZ receptors. Further, GABA potentiated the affinity of EBDZ and DDZ for neuronal BDZ receptors to a similar extent. Thus, in nearly all respects, EBDZ and DDZ are the same, and will be so treated in this discussion.

To support the notion that DDZ was truly an endogenous substance, human cerebella from one infant and four adults that had been stored in paraffin blocks since 1940 were tested for immunoreactivity and compared with fresh rat cerebella. The cellular distribution of the immunoreactivity in the human cerebella was identical to that observed in the rats (see below). Further, the immunoreactivity could be blocked by diazepam, flunitrazepam, and Ro 5-4864, but not by β-CCE or Ro 15-1788. As to the source of the endogenous BDZs, it was argued that because the first synthetic BDZ, chlordiazepoxide, was not synthesized until 1955 and not marketed until 1960, the human brains used could not have been subjected to exogenous BDZs before they were preserved. Moreover, in other studies wherein DDZ was isolated from human sera by a method that did not involve antibodies, it was found in the sera of some of the researchers who had never taken BDZs. Thus, it was presumed that the DDZ molecules were of biological rather than chemical origin.

As expected, these findings prompted further questions about where the purportedly endogenous BDZs came from. For example, was the laboratory equipment contaminated by BDZs from previous experiments, or was DDZ a contaminant introduced during the purification procedures? These questions were answered negatively because DDZ and its precursors (diazepam, etc.) were seldom used in the laboratory before the isolation of DDZ had taken place, and those BDZs that were used, such as flunitrazepam and clonazepam, are not converted to DDZ. Also, control purification procedures without brain tissue did not yield any recoverable DDZ.

Another possibility was that BDZs could be biosynthesized by microorganisms or plants and thus become diet components (like vitamins) that modulate GABA-mediated neurotransmission. This notion could explain the finding of BDZ-like molecules in human brains that had been preserved since 1940. Moreover, Medina and coworkers (1988) even found several extracts from powdered and fresh milk that had chemical characteristics and binding affinities to mAb 21-7F9 similar to those of diazepam. Further support for endogenous sources of BDZs in plants and animals was reported by Wildmann and coworkers (1987) and by Unseld and Klotz (1989), who detected DZ and DDZ in rat cortex, cerebellum, hypophysis (pituitary), and adrenals at concentrations that inhibited the binding of [³H]Ro 15-1788 to BDZ receptors in brain membranes. These results were the same for normal rats and those that lived in pathogen-free environments. Similarly, substances having BDZ-binding inhibitory (BBI) activity were extracted from the contents of the bowel tract and stomach from normal and pathogen-free rats. DZ and DDZ were also detected in human food plants such as wheat grains, soya, corn, and potatoes, in all the constituent cereals in standardized rat diets, and in a fish powder supplement. Similar results were found among grains that were not treated with herbicides or fungicides. But DZ and DDZ were undetectable in the daily quantities of tap water given to rats as well as in other water supplies.

In the sera of drug-free humans, maximal BBI levels of 0.01 ng/ml were measured. In the daily diet of humans, about 3–7 µg/kg BBI was found in wheat grains, whereas after BDZ treatments in humans, serum levels amount to about 1–20 ng/ml. From these data it was estimated that human brain concentrations of BDZs derived solely from ingestion of plantfoods would be about two orders of magnitude below pharmacological relevance. It was suggested that the discrepancy between dietary intake, the amounts of BDZ-like ligands that have been isolated in animal and human brains, and the amounts needed for pharmacological efficacy may be explained by a particular compartmentalization of these agents after chronic intake or by additional biosynthesis in the animals, although it is unlikely that mammals can synthesize a chlorinated heterocycle such as N-desmethyldiazepam (de Blas, 1988; Wildmann et al., 1987).

DZ and DDZ have been found in the brains of animals at different evolutionary stages, including salmon, frogs, lizards, rats, cats, dogs, deer, bovines, chickens, and humans, in concentrations ranging from 0.005 to 0.02 ng/g. They have also been detected in the whites of chicken eggs, showing that these BDZs appear very early in ontogenesis. It remains to be seen whether animals can synthesize them or whether exogenous sources, such as microorganisms or plants, are responsible for the minute amounts that are found in the bodies of animals. A variety of other BDZs have been identified in animal brain and liver, and in wheat grains and potatoes.

Wildmann and colleagues (1987) concluded that diazepam and its major biologically active metabolite, N-desmethyldiazepam, are natural products. It is noteworthy that the fungus *Penicillium cyclopium* can synthesize BDZs, and that a bacterial product of *Streptomyces refuineus*, called antramycin, contains the basic 1,4-BDZ structure. Further, it appears that BDZs are naturally present in plants and plant products and find their way to the brain via the bloodstream when they are consumed. Depending on the nature and the amount of consumption, indirect administration of BDZs via such foods could have some effect on receptor regulation or modification of vigilance and anxiety. But the biological significance of endogenous BDZs is still uncertain.

Anxiety and the Inverse Agonists

In a series of experiments on the intrinsic pharmacological activity of β-CCE, the behavior of adult male rhesus monkeys was rated before and after β-CCE administration. As mentioned above, the effects of β-CCE were virtually opposite to those of the BDZs. Whereas the monkeys were placid and unperturbed when the experimenter approached their cage after a vehicle administration, after an intravenous injection of β-CCE, their behavior was marked by agitation, struggling in a restraining

chair, piloerection, distress vocalizations, and aggressive postures and grimacing. This activity was accompanied by increases in heart rate, blood pressure, and the release of the stress hormone corticosterone as well as the transmitters epinephrine and norepinephrine. All of these responses were blocked by pretreatment with diazepam or the selective BDZ receptor blocker flumazenil, neither of which had any effect by themselves on behavior or autonomic activity. These findings suggested that the BDZ receptor not only mediates the anxiolytic effect of the BDZs, but also mediates the anxiogenic effects of β-CCE in specific ways (Insel et al., 1984; Ninan et al., 1982).

Further, it was found that after a low dose of β-CCE, behavioral effects occurred that were similar to reactions to threats and provocations. Also, there was considerable variability among animals in their response to the drug, and the intensity of the drug-induced response was a good predictor of an individual animal's response to a variety of stressful or fear-provoking stimuli. For instance, if an animal had a robust response to β-CCE, it was likely that it would become highly aroused and agitated when being confronted by a human stranger; in contrast, an animal that showed a low overt behavioral and physiological response to the drug would also be a low responder to environmental stress.

Similar findings resulted when humans were challenged by inverse agonists. When it was established that human experimentation would not be hazardous, the drug N'-methyl-β-carboline-3-carboxamide (FG 7142), which is closely related to β-CCE, was administered to a group of human volunteers. Shortly after drug administration, the subjects experienced muscle tension, autonomic hyperactivity, and extreme apprehension. Subjectively, the subjects interpreted their experience as being similar to anxiety. In one volunteer, the drug effects were so severe that an intravenous dose of the BDZ lormetazepam was administered, which dissipated the symptoms within a few minutes (see Hommer, Skolnick, and Paul, 1987). The fact that a low pharmacologically relevant dose of a BDZ completely blocked the anxiety-related behaviors caused by FG 7142 in this case supports the hypothesis that the reaction to FG 7142 is a reliable pharmacological model of human fear and anxiety.

Additional experiments showed that the antihypertension drug clonidine, an α-adrenergic agonist that is known to have anxiolytic effects in humans, also blocked the β-CCE-induced syndrome, especially the symptoms mediated by the autonomic nervous system. It was also found that serotonin antagonists partially blocked β-CCE effects, which supports the notion that serotonin has a significant role in anxiety production and suppression (see below).

What Is the Natural Role of BDZ Receptors?

Up to this point, our tacit assumption has been that BDZs should be designated as agonists for BDZ receptor

sites. However, if the inverse agonists are indeed the endogenous ligands for those receptors, then perhaps they should be designated as agonists and the BDZs should be designated as inverse agonists. This idea could be extended to include the notion that the BDZ receptors naturally serve an anxiogenic rather than an anxiolytic function (Guidotti, Corda, and Costa, 1983). As we mentioned early in this chapter, anxiety is a natural response to conflict and fear that may be instrumental in modifying behavior in beneficial ways. It may at least alert the animal to behaviors associated with nonreward or punishment, and may be a deterrent to repeating those behaviors. Also, the anxiogenic response may serve a learning function when it leads to corrective action. It follows that if a person is not alert, attentive, and sensitive to well-deserved rebukes and the denial of reinforcements, he or she may be well served to be motivated by the reaction to inverse agonists (see the section on attention deficit disorder in Chapter 13.)

The β-Carbolines: Pharmacological Assessment

In the decade following the discovery of the BDZ receptor ligand β-CCE, a dozen or more related compounds were found and evaluated for their pharmacological properties. These BDZ ligands were then compared in a number of tests to determine their potency for behavioral effects (see Stephens et al., 1987).

Binding Potency

The binding potency of BDZ ligands was assessed in rat brains by giving intraperitoneal ligand injections 30 minutes before sacrifice. The measure of potency was the ligand dose that would inhibit binding by 50% of [^{3}H] lormetazepam that was injected into the tail vein 2 minutes before sacrifice. Further, the allosteric properties of the ligands were evaluated by comparing the ability of the GABA agonist muscimol to enhance the binding of the ligand to BDZ binding sites. Each compound was given a value, the GABA ratio, which expressed the difference between binding in the presence and binding in the absence of muscimol. It was assumed that because the affinity of inverse agonists is decreased in the presence of muscimol, their GABA ratios would be less than 1.0; whereas because the binding of anxiolytic BDZs is enhanced by muscimol, their GABA ratios would be greater than 1.0. The inverse agonist DMCM, for example, had a GABA ratio of 0.46; the BDZ agonist ZK 93-423 had a GABA ratio of 2.17 (Table 16.2).

To estimate the ability of the BDZ receptor ligands to influence the Cl⁻ channels, tests similar to those establishing the GABA ratio were designed to measure each ligand's effect on [^{35}S]TBPS binding. TBPS is a convulsant that, like picrotoxinin, modulates BDZ ligand binding to the GABA$_A$ receptor complex (Wamsley, Gehlert, and Olsen, 1986). In general, inverse agonists and convulsants tend to diminish TBPS binding, whereas anxiolytic anticonvulsants enhance it. Thus, a

---

Table 16.2   TBPS and GABA Ratios, and Direction of Effect in Four Pharmacological Tests

	TBPS ratio	GABA ratio	CDP cue[a]	PTZ cue[b]	Plasma CS[c]	Lick suppression[d]
DMCM	0.58	0.46	A	G	S	PC
FG 7142	0.79	0.87	A	G	S	PC
CGS 8216	0.88	1.15	A	G	S	PC
ZK 90 886	0.86	1.18	A	(G)	S	PC
ZK 93 426	0.89	1.37	A	O	(S)	PC
Ro 15-1788	1.05	1.22	A	O	(S)	0
ZK 95 962	1.08	1.40	G	(A)	(S)	0
ZK 91 296	1.20	1.23	G	(A)	AS	0
CGS 9896	1.03	—	G	(A)	—	AC
CL 218 872	0.98	1.98	G	A	—	AC
Diazepam	1.24	2.3	G	A	AS	AC
Clonazepam	1.38	2.1	G	A	AS	AC
Lorazepam	1.46	1.75	G	A	—	AC
Lormetazepam	1.43	1.71	G	A	AS	AC
Triazolam	1.56	1.00	G	A	—	—
ZK 93 423	1.58	2.17	G	A	AS	AC

[a]Drug discrimination tests with chlordiazepoxide as training drug. A, antagonism of cue; G, generalization.
[b]Drug discrimination tests with pentylenetetrazol as training drug. A, antagonism; (A), partial antagonism; 0, no effect; (G), partial generalization; G, generalization.
[c]Changes in plasma corticosterone. S, stresslike effect; (S), stresslike effect at high dose; AS, antistress (stress-protective) effect.
[d]Activity in water-lick suppression test. PC, proconflict; 0, no effect; AC, anticonflict.
Source: After Stephens et al., 1987.

TBPS ratio was established by comparing TBPS binding in the presence and absence of each ligand. As shown in Table 16.2, GABA ratios correlated highly with TBPS ratios, suggesting a mutual relationship between the two variables.

Comparative Anxiolysis

To assess the comparative anxiolytic properties of the BDZ receptor ligands, they were compared for their efficacy in disinhibiting behavior suppressed by punishment. Petersen and Buus Lassen (1981) used a variant of the water-lick suppression test originally developed by Vogel, Beer, and Clody (1971) (see above). In this procedure, water-deprived rats were given brief, mild tongue shocks (0.4 mA, 0.5 s) after every 20th lick of a water spout during a 3-minute test period. At that shock level, some of the rats showed a high degree of drinking suppression, whereas others showed a low degree of suppression. The high-suppression group was given agonist β-carbolines to test for *antipunishment* effects, and the low-suppression group was given inverse agonists to test for *propunishment* effects. Thirty minutes later, the rats were tested in a second (postdrug) punished drinking period, and finally, the animals were given a no-punishment drinking period.

The results are summarized in Figure 16.9. Going from left to right, the first two groups were high-suppression groups, as identified by the low rate of predrug licking. It can be seen that the BDZ agonist ZK 93-423 increased punished drinking in the first group, whereas the partial agonist ZK 91 296 had only a slight effect on the second group, even at the high dose of 60 mg/kg. In contrast, the third group, with a higher level of predrug drinking, showed a suppression of drinking when they were treated with the receptor antagonist ZK 93 426. Similarly, the inverse agonists FG 7142 and DMCM significantly depressed the relatively high drinking rates of

the last two groups. Because the rate of postdrug (nonpunished) drinking behavior was uniformly high for all groups, it was unlikely that drinking suppression was the result of drug-induced lethargy or motor inadequacy. Comparing the results of this test with other tests of drug effects illustrates the reliability of the water-lick suppression test (see Table 16.2). Thus, this test can stand as a screening device for the anxiolytic or anxiogenic potency of psychoactive drugs.

Drug Discrimination Tests

The β-carbolines were also examined with drug discrimination tests (see Chapter 2 and the discussion earlier in this chapter for the details of this procedure.) In one such experiment performed by Stephens and colleagues (1987), rats were trained to discriminate between a subconvulsant dose (15 mg/kg) of pentylenetetrazol (PTZ) and saline. After training, antagonism and generalization tests were done with a number of BDZ receptor ligands. Antagonism tests showed that PTZ combined with BDZ agonists (e.g., lormetazepam) caused the rats to ignore the PTZ lever and respond to the saline lever in proportion to the dose of the BDZ agonist (Figure 16.10*a*), whereas substituting doses of a convulsant (DMCM) caused a dose-related increase of responses on the PTZ lever and fewer on the saline lever (Figure 16.10*b*). These and other agonists and inverse agonists were tested for their antagonism to or generalization with BDZ and PTZ cues, and these results are also summarized in Table 16.2.

Generalization tests were also done with chlordiazepoxide (CDP). After training to discriminate CDP (5 mg/kg) from vehicle, increasing doses of the BDZ agonist lormetazepam and several partial agonists were substituted for CDP. As shown in Figure 16.11 and Table 16.2, lormetazepam was more potent than the partial agonists in eliciting responding on the drug lever.

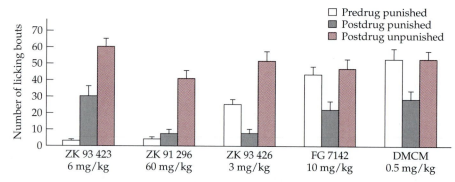

16.9 β-CARBOLINE EFFECTS ON THE WATER-LICK SUPPRESSION TEST. The effects of minimally effective doses of five β-carbolines on licking when it was accompanied by weak tongue shocks. The agonists ZK 93 423 and ZK 91 296 increased licking in high-suppression rats, whereas the inverse agonists ZK 93 426, FG 7142, and DMCM diminished licking in low-suppression rats. The rate of nonpunished licking was approximately the same for all groups. (After Stephens et al., 1987.)

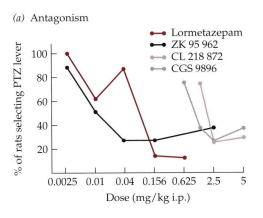

(a) Antagonism

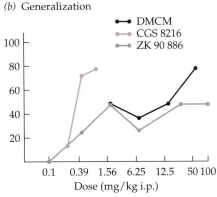

(b) Generalization

16.10 THE PENTYLENETETRAZOL (PTZ) DISCRIMINATIVE STIMULUS: ANTAGONISM AND GENERALIZATION. (*a*) Combining PTZ with a BDZ receptor agonist such as lormetazepam, ZK 95 962, CL 218 872, or CGS 9896 shows a dose-related rejection of the PTZ lever. (*b*) Substituting inverse agonists DMCM, CGS, 8216 or ZK 90 886 shows a dose-related generalization by selection of the PTZ lever. (After Stephens et al., 1987.)

Corticosterone Reactions

As mentioned above, plasma corticosterone levels are indicative of stress endured by animals. The potency of an anxiolytic drug can be ascertained by finding the dose given before the stress episode that will block or significantly diminish the corticosterone response. Further, as might be expected, the administration of anxiogenic drugs (e.g., β-carboline inverse agonists) can induce corticosterone stress responses by themselves.

In one such experiment, rats were subjected to a swim stress test after being pretreated with BDZ receptor agonists. The rats were placed in a large glass cylinder of water about 5 inches deep for 5 minutes, a procedure that usually results in significant increases in plasma corticosterone. As shown in Table 16.2, diazepam, clonazepam, and lormetazepam, as well as ZK 91 296 and ZK 93-423, reduced stress-induced increases in plasma corticosterone. The BDZ receptor antagonist ZK 93 426, however, showed no stress-protective effect; note that it also antagonized the CDP cue in drug discrimination tests.

To assess the effect of inverse agonists on plasma corticosterone levels in unstressed rats, the animals were habituated to handling and drug injection, and then injected with one of the following: DMCM, FG 7142, ZK 90 886, or CGS 8216. After a waiting period, it was found that all of the drugs had a stresslike effect and caused significant increases in corticosterone levels (see Table 16.2). Further, when these anxiogenic drugs were combined with anxiolytic drugs, the corticosterone response was significantly diminished.

In summary, as Table 16.2 indicates, there are strong relationships among GABA and TBPS ratios and the results of the four pharmacological tests on the BDZs and β-carboline agonists, partial agonists, inverse agonists, and BDZ receptor blockers. In general, the inverse agonists in the upper part of the table have low TBPS and GABA ratios, antagonize the BDZ (chlordiazepoxide) cue, generalize with the convulsant PTZ cue, cause stresslike induction of plasma corticosterone, and have proconflict effects in the water-lick suppression test. In contrast, the BDZ agonists at the lower part of the table have high TBPS and GABA ratios, generalize with the CDP cue, antagonize the PTZ cue, have antistress effects on plasma corticosterone, and have anticonflict effects in the lick suppression test. The partial agonists and the receptor blockers align themselves between the other two groups.

Effects of Stress on GABA and BDZ Receptors

One way of measuring emotionality and fearfulness is to evaluate animals' responses in a conflict situation such as the water-lick suppression test described earlier. When substantial numbers of rats were exposed to this procedure, some animals became acclimated to the tongue shock and drank almost as much as nonshocked controls, whereas others drank little despite their considerable thirst, and therefore were assumed to be more fearful than the animals that drank almost normally. Consequently, researchers examined the possibility that a relationship exists between GABA receptor kinetics

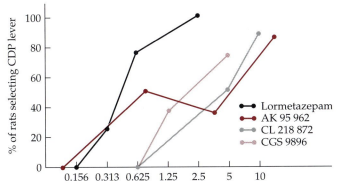

16.11 THE CHLORDIAZEPOXIDE (CDP) DISCRIMINATIVE CUE: GENERALIZATION. Rats trained to discriminate CDP from saline selected the CDP lever when lormetazepam, ZK 95962, CL-218 872, or CGS 9896 was substituted for CDP. The effects were dose-related. (After Stephens et al., 1987.)

with respect to BDZ binding and the manifestations of emotionality and fearfulness.

Comparisons were made between BDZ binding properties in strains of rats and mice that differed in behavioral dimensions of emotionality or fearfulness as indicated in the water-lick suppression test. It was found that the presumably more emotional animals with fewer drinking responses had a lower density of BDZ receptors than the less emotional ones with more drinking responses. It was further found that when less emotional rats were subjected to more intense tongue shocks in the water-lick suppression test, there was a 14% to 24% decrease in specific [^{3}H]diazepam binding (see Sepinwall and Cook, 1980). This finding suggested that anxiety or stress, or anxiolytic or anxiogenic drugs, can induce changes in the GABA$_A$ receptor complex that are related to an organism's response to stress.

Stress-Induced Proconflict and Proconvulsant Effects

In other experiments, stressed and nonstressed rats were tested to see whether one stressful episode would influence behavior in a succeeding one. Specifically, water-deprived rats were first tested for 3 minutes for drinking rates without tongue shock. Then half the animals were given 5 minutes of noncontingent foot shocks, after which drinking without tongue shock was measured again. Next, the animals underwent the water-lick suppression test (with tongue shock). Compared with non-foot-shocked controls, the foot-shocked rats showed only slightly fewer 3-second water-lick periods during the 3-minute control drinking test (i.e., without tongue shocks). But when these animals received tongue shocks, the rats with prior foot shock averaged only about 7 lick periods during a 3-minute test, compared with about 24 lick periods among the non-foot-shocked controls. Thus, it was proposed that the noncontingent foot shock had a proconflict effect that was caused by a stress-induced decrease in GABA receptors, which was manifested as a hypersensitivity to tongue shocks in the water-lick suppression test.

Other experiments provided corroborative evidence for the effect of stress on BDZ receptor binding. For example, Weizman and colleagues (1989) reported that subjecting mice to prolonged swim stress caused a marked suppression of Ro 15-1788 binding in some brain areas, but not in others. In these experiments, mice were placed in a water-containing cylinder in which they were forced to swim for 2 or 10 minutes on 7 consecutive days. Additional tests demonstrated a relationship between the swim stress–induced changes in BDZ receptor binding and their effect on the function of the BDZ receptors. This was done by comparing the effective doses of the anticonvulsant BDZ clonazepam that would protect stressed and nonstressed mice from drug-induced seizures. After various doses of clonazepam (0.04–0.50

mg/kg i.p.), pentylenetetrazol (PTZ) was tail-infused in stressed and nonstressed mice at an ED$_{100}$ dose (150 mg/kg). (An ED$_{100}$ dose implies that the dose would normally have a convulsant effect—sustained contractions of the forelimbs and neck—on 100% of mice tested.) The results indicated that the stressed mice required significantly greater protective doses of clonazepam than nonstressed controls. Further, mice treated with clonazepam before daily swim stress tests and then challenged with PTZ showed a significantly elevated convulsant threshold; that is, more PTZ was needed for convulsive effects. Thus, environmental stress appears to reduce the number and effectiveness of BDZ receptors in discrete brain regions of mice, and such changes lower the convulsant threshold. On the other hand, pretreatment with an anxiolytic drug such as clonazepam seems to diminish the effects of stress and/or raise the convulsant threshold. These findings suggest that BDZ receptor agonists can diminish the effects of chronic or acute stress, as measured by the status of convulsant thresholds, and that these effects are mediated by the GABA$_A$ receptor complex.

Benzodiazepine Effects on Transmitter Systems

In studies investigating the neurochemical action of anxiolytic drugs, many investigators have found that barbiturates, meprobamate, and the BDZs decrease the turnover of norepinephrine (NE), serotonin (5-HT), and other biogenic amines in the brain. These findings suggest that the anxiolytic effects of the drugs are the result of changes in neurotransmitter activity.

The Limited Role of GABA

Polc, Mohler, and Haefely (1974) had shown that the GABA agonist aminooxyacetic acid (AOAA), which blocks GABA metabolism and raises brain GABA levels as much as 500%, not only mimicked diazepam's enhancement of presynaptic inhibition in the spinal cord, but also enhanced the action of diazepam when both drugs were given together. Conversely, the GABA synthesis inhibitor thiosemicarbazide (TSC) blocked the action of diazepam, and the GABA antagonist bicuculline competitively reduced the action of diazepam, in the spinal cord. Thus, with respect to presynaptic inhibition in the spinal cord, GABA agonists mimicked the actions of BDZs, whereas GABA antagonists blocked them.

However, these alterations of GABA synthesis and metabolism are not reflected in antianxiety effects. To assess the role of GABAergic mechanisms in antianxiety effects, Cook and Sepinwall (1975) examined the effect of AOAA on punished behavior in a modified Geller–Seifter (1960) multiple schedule procedure in which rats were rewarded on a VI schedule, but received rewards plus foot shocks during an alternating CRF schedule.

Treatment of these animals with AAOA at various doses had no appreciable effect on nonpunished or punished responses, nor did it enhance the effect of diazepam when the two drugs were given together. Thus, no synergistic anticonflict effect was found, in contrast to the synergistic effects found by Polc, Mohler, and Haefely (1974) in their spinal cord experiments. These experiments showed that increasing brain levels of GABA with AOAA neither resulted in anticonflict activity, nor did it synergize with diazepam in that respect.

Similar negative findings were reported when the GABA agonist muscimol was given to rats in the Vogel water-lick suppression test: there were no signs of an anxiolytic effect. Also, when GABA metabolism was blocked, there were some signs of antipunishment activity, but they were not correlated with the elevation of GABA levels (Lloyd and Morselli, 1987). Further, in clinical trials with anxious patients, treatment with the GABA-mimetic anticonvulsants progabide and THIP produced only weak beneficial effects, much less than those observed with BDZs. These negative and marginal findings further support the hypothesis that BDZs enhance the affinity of GABA for its receptors, especially when GABA activity is submaximal, and that raising brain GABA concentration by itself does not ensure that the transmitter will be synaptically utilized.

Benzodiazepine–Catecholamine Interactions

There is substantial evidence that BDZs reduce the turnover of dopamine (DA) in the olfactory tubercles, the nucleus accumbens, the caudate nucleus, and the cerebral cortex, and these effects seem to be due to enhanced GABA-mediated inhibition of the DA cell bodies that give rise to the ascending mesolimbic DA pathway. Similarly, BDZs diminish NE effects by inhibiting CA cells of the locus coeruleus (LC) (Fuxe et al., 1975). Therefore, the LC was examined for a possible role in anxiety expression and the anxiolytic effect of BDZs.

The extensive outputs from the LC provide the neural substrates for the behaviors that are under its influence. The receptors within the LC respond to a number of excitatory and inhibitory neurotransmitters, including GABA acting on GABA$_A$ receptors. There are also self-modulating feedback mechanisms within the LC that are expressed via NE autoreceptors.

Recent studies revealed that neurons within the LC are activated by novel sensory input and respond with increased bursts of activity. In the LC of an awake monkey, there is rapid habituation to novel benign stimuli and marked activation in response to fear-associated stimuli. These responses suggest that these neurons have a role in orienting and attending to sudden contrasting or aversive sensory input. Electrical stimulation of the LC of macaque monkeys induced a wide range of behaviors such as yawning, chewing, scratching, startling, wringing of the hands, pulling of the hair or skin,

tongue movements, grasping of the restraining chair, struggling, self-mouthing, and self clasping. These effects were accompanied by pupillary dilatation, piloerection, alerting, and increases in heart rate, blood pressure, and respiratory rate. These effects appeared in different patterns on repeated tests, suggesting a progression of adaptation. There were no responses to the electrical stimulation that were indicative of pain; rather, the signs were similar to those seen under circumstances of anxiety, uncertainty, and fear, and were also similar to some drug withdrawal states. These effects could be blocked by BDZs and morphine.

In contrast, bilateral electrothermal lesions of the LC in monkeys resulted in diminished emotional responses to threats. The monkeys withdrew during persistent and vigorous threats and from mildly painful stimuli, but they were without apparent fear of approaching humans or dominant monkeys. They were also more aggressive in social situations, and moved around in their cages more frequently than they did prior to the lesions.

The general picture of locus coeruleus function that emerges from these findings is that of an "alarm" system that filters and discriminates between potentially noxious and irrelevant stimuli. High LC activity produces effects on nearly every major brain and autonomic function that is activated by fear, with profound effects upon behavior. At moderate levels, LC activity is correlated with attentiveness and vigilance to physiologically relevant stimuli. Progressive subnormal functioning of the system is best characterized by inattentiveness, impulsivity, carelessness, recklessness, and fearlessness (Redmond, 1987; Role and Kelly, 1991). It follows that the LC/NE system is regarded as a neural substrate for alarm or fear that might be involved in pathological anxiety, panic, and the effects of antianxiety drugs and rebound withdrawal following their chronic use. However, it should be noted that the locus coeruleus, with its manifold diversity of inputs and outputs, is but one of the contributors to organized arousal and emotion, and is described here simply to explain its possible role in responses to BDZ treatment.

Stress, β-carbolines, and DA activity. More recent experiments examined the role of the dopaminergic mesoprefrontal pathway that emanates from the ventral tegmental area (VTA) of the midbrain and projects to the mesoprefrontal cortex (MPFC) (see Chapters 4 and 8). In rats, this system has been shown to respond to footshock stress by activation and increased DA turnover in the MPFC. Further, the anxiogenic β-carboline FG 7142 produced a dose-dependent increase in DA metabolism in the prefrontal cortex without causing any significant increase in DA metabolism in other terminal areas of the mesocortical, mesolimbic, or nigrostriatal pathways. These FG 7142 anxiogenic effects were prevented by pretreatment with anxiolytic BDZs such as diazepam and lorazepam, or with the BDZ antagonist Ro 15-1788 (Roth et al., 1988; Tam and Roth, 1985). Consequently, anxiogenic β-carboline inverse agonists mimic the effects of stress on the dopaminergic system.

In another experiment, rats were "psychologically" stressed by being placed in cages with transparent plastic walls that separated them from other rats that were receiving stressful foot shocks (3.0 mA, 5-s duration at 30-s intervals) for up to 30 minutes. Though the shocks could be anticipated after a few presentations, the stress among the shocked rats was readily apparent to the observing rats. The shocked rats displayed several somatic and visceral responses, including vocal screeching, struggling to escape, running and jumping, and urinating and defecating. The observing rats received no shocks themselves. After the stress session, the observer rats were sacrificed for blood serum and brain tissue assays, which showed increased DA turnover in the VTA and the MPFC as well as increased blood serum corticosterone. Moreover, these effects were antagonized by pre-stress treatments of diazepam (5 mg/kg), and the attenuating effects of diazepam were antagonized by a 15 mg/kg dose of Ro 15-1788 that preceded the diazepam treatment by 10 minutes.

These data show that the mesoprefrontal DA system is activated by environmental stress, inverse agonists, and "psychological" stress, and that BDZ/GABA recognition sites have a selective influence on mesoprefrontal DA neurons. In other words, certain DA neurons in the VTA are influenced by a GABAergic input that regulates their activity. It is also clear that diazepam exerts inhibitory effects on the mesoprefrontal DA neurons, as well as on the hypothalamic–pituitary axis, which mediates the adrenal release of corticosterone; and that these effects are closely implicated in the anxiolytic action of BDZs (Kaneyuki et al., 1991).

Benzodiazepine–Acetylcholine Interactions

Cholinergic systems within the CNS are also affected by BDZs. At the cellular level, BDZs increase ACh levels in synaptosomes in the guinea pig, mouse, and rat brain, and they decrease ACh turnover without affecting choline, choline acetytransferase, or cholinesterase activity. All of this evidence suggests a blockade of ACh release. There also exists a parallel between increases in striatal acetylcholine levels and the duration of the muscle-relaxant action of diazepam in rats. Diazepam (17 μmol/kg i.v. or higher) increased ACh levels in hemispheric structures, the striatum, and the hippocampus in rats, mice, and guinea pigs. These effects were also attributed to blockade of ACh release. Blockade of ACh release in the hippocampus may be related to the amnestic effects of some BDZs, and to the memory difficulties that can occur when BDZs are overused by the elderly. Also, the reduced turnover of ACh in the cortex and midbrain caused by diazepam was mimicked by the GABA receptor agonist muscimol. This finding suggests that a GABAergic mechanism intervenes in the effects of BDZs on ACh turnover (Guidotti, 1978).

Benzodiazepine–Serotonin Interactions

An extensive literature suggests that a decrease in serotonin turnover is involved in the anxiolytic effects of the BDZs. This hypothesis was strengthened by the finding that direct alteration of 5-HT activity by an assortment of 5-HT agonists and antagonists affected behavior in conflict paradigms, as shown in the following experiments. Pigeons that pecked at an illuminated disc for food rewards showed marked reductions in pecking rates when the food rewards were occasionally accompanied by shocks in the tail region. However, the rate of responding with the shocks increased dramatically after intramuscular injections of 5-HT antagonists such as methysergide and D-2-bromolysergic acid diethylamide (BOL), and the effect was of the same magnitude as that produced by chlordiazepoxide, diazepam, and nitrazepam. In contrast, the 5-HT receptor agonist α-methyltryptamine (α-MTA) suppressed both punished and nonpunished behavior in rat and pigeon conflict experiments.

Similar increases in punished behavior were obtained in rat conflict tests with the 5-HT antagonists methysergide and cinanserin and with the 5-HT synthesis inhibitor p-chlorophenylalanine (PCPA). Also, after PCPA injections, the time course of serotonin depletion coincided closely with the increase in punished behavior, and when serotonin was replenished by administration of the 5-HT precursor 5-HTP, the rate of punished responding again declined (Robichaud and Sledge, 1969; Wise, Berger, and Stein, 1973). Furthermore, a profound, but transitory, increase in punished behavior was found in a rat conflict test after a single intraventricular administration of 5,6-dihydroxytryptamine (5,6-DHT), an agent toxic to 5-HT terminals that presumably blocked 5-HT release (Baumgarten et al., 1971; Stein, Wise, and Belluzzi, 1975). In another procedure, Stein, Wise, and Berger (1973), using rats with stable punished and nonpunished response rates in a conflict test, applied minute amounts (about 5 μg) of crystalline carbachol via permanently indwelling cannulas whose tips were placed in the dorsal raphe region. (Carbachol has an excitatory effect upon many neuron types.) Within 1–2 minutes of this treatment there was a marked suppression of both punished and nonpunished behavior. A subsequent dose of oxazepam (10 mg/kg i.p.) reversed the suppression of both types of behavior. These data support the hypothesis that 5-HT-mediated systems are instrumental in behavior suppression, and that the blockade of the system favors a release of behavior that has been suppressed by punishment (Cook and Sepinwall, 1975; Geller et al., 1974; Graeff and Schoenfeld, 1970; Stein, Wise, and Berger, 1973).

16.12 EFFECTS OF FLUOXETINE AND CHLORDIAZEPOXIDE ON PUNISHED AND NONPUNISHED BEHAVIOR. Each daily session consisted of six alternations of 5-minute VI-40 second and 5-minute CRF schedules. Each interval ended with a pen reset. Reinforcements are indicated by small diagonal pen deflections. When reinforcements occurred close together (as in some CRF sessions), the pen tracings were blurred together. The drug(s) and their doses (in parentheses) and the responses per minute are shown at the left of each record. (*a*) A typical rat on the last control (no drug) day and in 4 additional drug tests with increasing doses of fluoxetine (FXT). The drug selectively decreased responding during the CRF (punishment) component. (*b*) Records of a different rat receiving FXT and chlordiazepoxide (CDP) alone or in combination. CDP increased VI and especially CRF responding, FXT decreased this responding, and the drugs given together cancelled each other's effects. (After Feldman and Quenzer, 1984.)

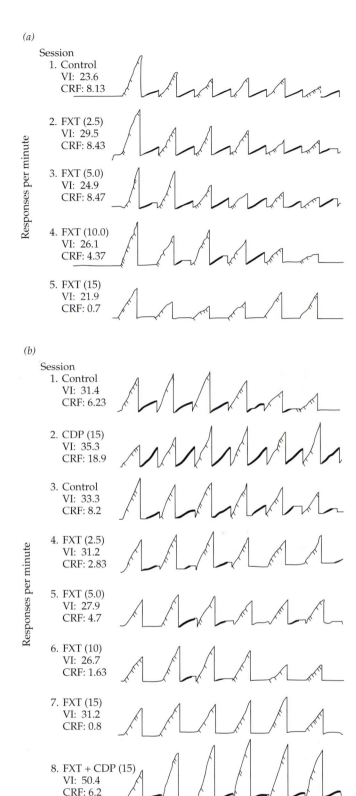

To determine whether the reversal of 5-HT-induced behavior suppression by oxazepam was specific for the antagonism of the effects of punishment or was due to a general disinhibitory action, Margules and Stein (1967) examined the properties of oxazepam using a variety of methods for inducing response suppression. They found that oxazepam markedly reversed behavior suppression caused by foot shock, nonreward (extinction), punishing brain stimulation, or suppression of feeding behavior by tainting food with bitter-tasting quinine. The drug also disinhibited feeding behavior in satiated rats. Because of these and similar findings from a large assortment of BDZs and 5-HT antagonists among a wide variety of animals, it was proposed that the BDZs act on a final common pathway mediated by 5-HT for the suppression of behavior.

Effects of Serotonin Agonists and Antagonists in the Geller–Seifter Paradigm

An early experiment examined the effects of a 5-HT agonist, fluoxetine, alone and in combination with chlordiazepoxide (CDP) in the Geller–Seifter paradigm. Fluoxetine (FXT; now commonly known by its trade name, Prozac) is a serotonin reuptake inhibitor that increases serotonin concentration within synapses and enhances synaptic events. In this experiment, rats received liquid food rewards on a VI 40-second schedule that was alternated every 5 minutes with a CRF schedule for food accompanied by foot shock. The change from the VI to the CRF schedule was signaled by a light that stayed on during the CRF interval. The shock intensity was adjusted to a level that allowed for sufficient responding so that drug-induced response rates could be increased or decreased. Each test session lasted 1 hour (12 5-minute sessions, 6 VI, 6 CRF).

In the first series of drug tests, FXT at increasing doses was given 30 minutes before testing. Figure 16.12*a* shows cumulative response records for one rat during one control (no drug) session and four drug sessions with increasing doses of FXT. It can be seen that the re-

sponse rate (responses per minute) during the VI schedule is much higher than the CRF rate, although the lower rate during the CRF schedule was at least partly due to frequent pauses to consume the food rewards. But, more importantly, at the higher FXT doses, response suppression was proportionally greater for punished (CRF) than for nonpunished (VI) responding—that is, the greater the dose, the more selectively the punished responses were suppressed.

In Figure 16.12b, response records are shown for a different rat that was treated with CDP and FXT alone and in combination. In session 2, CDP (15 mg/kg) elicited only a small increase in VI responding, but a threefold increase in CRF responding. During sessions 4 and 5 with FXT, at 2.5 or 5.0 mg/kg, there were marked reductions in the CRF rates (65% and 47% respectively), but there was little change in the VI rates (6% and 16%). Sessions 6 and 7, with higher FXT doses, showed further selective suppression of CRF rates, whereas combining CDP and FXT in session 8 caused a marked increase in the VI rate and a restoration of the CRF rate to near control levels. With respect to the FXT-induced suppression of CRF responding, the data suggest that this drug enhanced serotonergic synaptic activity, which increased the aversiveness of the shocks, as shown by the virtual disappearance of CRF responses after the higher doses (Feldman and Quenzer, 1984).

In addition, these procedures have the ability to provide quantitative estimates of relative clinical potency. Figure 16.13 shows the relationship between the effectiveness of various anxiolytic drugs in the Geller–Seifter conflict test and the potency of the drugs in clinical tests with human patients (Cook and Davidson, 1973). For the anxiolytic drugs shown, there was a correlation coefficient of +.98 between the minimum effective anticonflict dose in rats and the average daily dose used for clinical treatment of psychoneurotic disorders.

The above findings support the concept, as proposed by Stein, Wise, and Belluzzi (1977), that blocking of serotonergic activity in the brain is associated with the disinhibition of responses suppressed by punishment, possibly by diminishing the effect of aversive consequences of the behavior, whereas enhancing serotonergic activity is associated with increased response inhibition by aversive consequences. Further support for this hypothesis was found by Feldman and Quenzer (1984) when behavior that was suppressed by punishment was further suppressed when 5-HT activity was enhanced by 5-HT uptake inhibitors such as fluoxetine, which also competitively diminished the behavior-disinhibiting effect of chlordiazepoxide. Furthermore, if it is assumed that disinhibition of behavior under aversive control is indicative of anxiolysis, then serotonin is presumed to play a significant role in anxiety and anxiolysis.

Alternative Testing Procedures

Jones, Paterson, and Roberts (1986) used the social interaction test (briefly described above) to investigate the role of 5-HT systems in modulating anxiogenesis and anxiolysis. In this test, pairs of animals (rats) were placed in a small arena and records of the time they spent in active social interaction were kept, as described above. In some of the rats, fine cannulae implanted in the brain

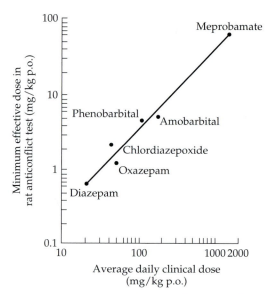

16.13 CORRELATION OF RAT ANTICONFLICT POTENCY WITH CLINICAL POTENCY. The rat minimum effective dose represents the lowest dose producing significant anticonflict effects. The average clinical daily dose represents the dose found effective in treating psychoneurotic disorders, as estimated from over 100 studies. Pearson correlation coefficient $r = 0.987$; $p < .01$. (After Cook and Sepinwall, 1975.)

stem permitted microinjections (0.1–10 ng) of the inverse agonist β-carboline β-CCM into the serotonergic dorsal raphe nucleus (DRN). It was presumed that β-CCM would diminish Cl⁻ flux in the DRN, making the cells hypersensitive to depolarizing transmitters and thereby increasing 5-HT activity. The sites of the cannula tips were verified histologically after completion of the behavioral experiments. In the tests, one cannulated rat and one control partner were placed in a dimly lit arena with which the animals were familiar. The cannulated rats were tested twice, once with β-CCM and once (at least 4 hours later) with vehicle. In addition to the assessment of social interaction, locomotor activity was assessed by counting light beam crossings within the arena. The effects of the microinjections were also compared with the effects of intraperitoneal β-CCM injections (1, 2, and 4 mg/kg).

The results revealed that the microinjections of β-CCM consistently reduced social interaction without significant depression of locomotor activity (Figure 16.14a), whereas the highest intraperitoneal dose (4 mg/kg) of β-CCM suppressed both social interaction and locomotion (Figure 16.14b). However, the lower intraperitoneal doses (1 or 2 mg/kg) suppressed only social interaction. Furthermore, in the histological examinations, the microinjection sites were found to be within the DRN when microinjection diminished social interactions, and ineffective microinjections were found to be outside the DRN. Also, some of the misplaced microinjections produced *increases* in social interaction, which could not be explained. Further, microinjections were as

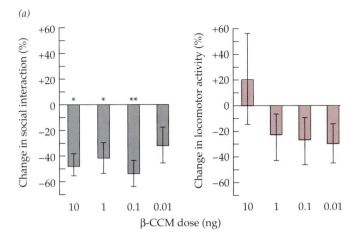

(a)

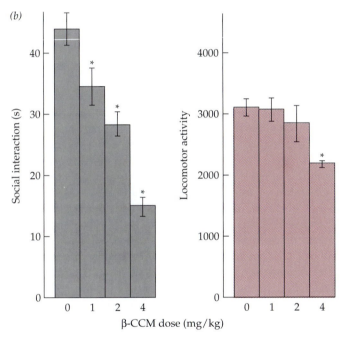

(b)

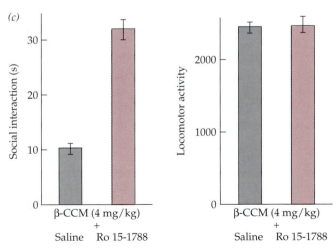

(c)

16.14 EFFECTS OF AN INVERSE AGONIST ON RAT SOCIAL INTERACTION. (a) The effects of β-CCM microinjected into the dorsal raphe nucleus (DRN). The changes in the degree of social interaction are shown as the difference between measurements from the same rats—once after β-CCM and once after vehicle treatment. β-CCM reduced social interaction without significant reduction of locomotor activity. (b) β-CCM injected intraperitoneally had the same effect, but at the highest dose (4 mg/kg), locomotor activity was also reduced. (c) Microinjecting 1.0 ng of Ro 15-1788 into the DRN blocked the effect of the high dose (4 mg/kg) of β-CCM on reduction of social activity but locomotor activity was unaffected ($^*p < .05$; $^{**}p < .01$). (After Jones, Peterson, and Roberts, 1986.)

CCM, and the reversal was the same regardless of the route of β-CCM administration (see Figure 16.14c). Finally, the lack of locomotor effects did not support an alternative hypothesis that the loss of social interaction was due to general motor depression. These findings added support for the role of BDZ receptors in the DRN in the mediation of anxiogenic and anxiolytic effects, and strengthened the hypothesis that 5-HT pathways emanating from the DRN have a major involvement in BDZ-mediated activities.

Serotonergic Drugs and Anxiety

Other approaches to the problem of the role of 5-HT in anxiolysis and anxiogenesis became possible when the variability of 5-HT binding sites became known and different 5-HT systems were implicated in various functional processes. (The varieties of 5-HT receptors and their pharmacological significance are described in Chapter 9.) Coincident with the identification of a variety of 5-HT receptors, a number of 5-HT ligands with specific binding characteristics were developed for these 5-HT receptor subtypes, and some of them were found to have anxiolytic properties. Among these compounds were the arylpiperazines, including buspirone and its congeners, which have been significant additions to the clinical anxiolytic pharmacopeia as well as valuable assets in the study of anxiety disorders. It was these discoveries that provided the impetus to examine further the role of 5-HT in anxiety and anxiolysis.

Among the numerous subtypes of 5-HT receptors that have been described in the research literature (Glennon, 1990), there is substantial evidence for at least two subtypes that are related to anxiolytic effects, the 5-HT$_{1A}$ and the 5-HT$_3$ receptors. The 5-HT$_{1A}$ receptors are found in high density in the hippocampus, and they are richly distributed in the septum, parts of the amygdala, and the dorsal raphe nucleus. These neural regions are related to or are among the neural components of the limbic system, which serves to modulate emotions. Principally, the postsynaptic excitation of 5-HT$_{1A}$ receptors leads to a diminished neuronal effect at the target site. Thus, because the general effect of this serotonergic system is inhibitory, diminished serotonergic activity could lead to the release

effective as intraperitoneal β-CCM administration with respect to anxiogenic effects. It was also found that microinjection (1 ng) of the BDZ receptor blocker Ro 15-1788 into the DRN reversed the anxiogenic effects of β-

or enhancement of some excitatory neuronal activity or behavior that might be suppressed by punishment.

The 5-HT$_3$ receptors are known to be ligand-gated channels and are widely distributed in the brain as well as in the periphery, where they mediate a depolarizing action on peripheral nerves and contractile action of the gut. Studies have revealed a single site of high affinity for this receptor in the entorhinal cortex in rodents, a characteristic that has been confirmed in other species, including humans.

5-HT$_{1A}$ Receptor Ligands

Neuropharmacology of buspirone.   Since the clinical efficacy of buspirone, an anxiolytic that binds to 5-HT$_{1A}$ receptors, was demonstrated, intensive study of this compound has contributed to our understanding of the role of 5-HT in anxiety. Buspirone is a nonBDZ anxiolytic of the arylpiperazine class. It was initially researched as a potential antipsychotic agent because it, like many other antipsychotics, has an affinity for D$_2$ dopamine receptors; however, clinical studies revealed that it was of limited value for psychotic patients, although it did have an antidepressant effect. Subsequent animal studies revealed that it had anxiolytic properties. At first, research on the anxiolytic action of buspirone centered on dopamine as the mediating transmitter, but the finding that buspirone was potent in displacing the radioactive 5-HT agonist [^{3}H]8-OH-DPAT from 5-HT$_{1A}$ binding sites in the hippocampus led to the conclusion that the anxiolytic action of buspirone was mediated via that receptor.

In 1979, Goldberg and Finnerty published the results of controlled comparisons among buspirone, diazepam, and placebo in 54 anxious outpatients. The study revealed that though the onset of anxiolysis took 1 to 3 weeks, the efficacy of buspirone compared favorably with that of diazepam, as well as with clorazepate, lorazepam, alprazolam, clobazepam, and oxazepam in later comparisons. The drug was favorably regarded because it was free of sedating properties, did not add to the sedative effects of ethanol, and did not lead to dependence. However, buspirone was similar to the BDZs with respect to its side-effect profile, producing dizziness, headache, and nausea in about 10% of buspirone-treated patients. Shortly after the original clinical trials of buspirone, two related derivatives, gepirone and ipsapirone, also demonstrated anxiolytic activity. These arylpiperazine 5-HT$_{1A}$ agonists are known collectively as **second generation anxiolytics (SGAs)**.

Binding of buspirone.   Binding experiments revealed that buspirone and its congeners have no significant binding affinity for BDZ receptors; rather, they bind to 5-HT$_{1A}$ and to D$_2$ sites. Further, the main metabolite of these compounds, 1-pyrimidylpiperazine (1-PP), has no affinity for the 5-HT$_{1A}$ site, but it has an affinity for α_2-adrenoreceptors, where it acts as an antagonist. By this antagonist action, 1-PP blocks the negative feedback for NE synthesis, thus increasing NE synthesis and turnover. This effect may account for the antidepressant action of these drugs.

In the brain, buspirone has a more marked effect in reducing 5-HT turnover in the hippocampus and the striatum, and to a lesser extent in the cortex. These findings suggest that the anxiolytic action of buspirone and its congeners is related to the reduction of 5-HT turnover in the limbic regions of the brain, while the antidepressant action could be attributed to the role of 1-PP in selective enhancement of NE turnover in that area. Furthermore, the abdominal discomfort occasionally associated with initial treatments with buspirone could be due to the stimulation of 5-HT receptors in the gastrointestinal tract (Glennon, 1990b; Olivier, Tulp, and Mos, 1991).

Drug discrimination experiments.   A number of drug discrimination experiments compared the SGAs with BDZs to see whether they produced similar interoceptive stimuli (Barrett and Gleeson, 1991). When rats were trained to discriminate the 5-HT$_{1A}$ agonist 8-OH-DPAT from saline, stimulus generalization occurred with the SGAs, and vice versa; that is, animals trained to discriminate SGAs from saline also generalized the discrimination to 8-OH-DPAT. However, neither the SGAs nor 8-OH-DPAT were recognized by animals trained to discriminate diazepam or other BDZs from saline, nor were animals able to recognize diazepam when they were trained to discriminate 8-OH-DPAT or the SGA ipsapirone from saline. All in all, these findings show that there is no stimulus generalization between SGAs and BDZs, providing additional confirmation for the pharmacological separation of these two types of anxiolytics. (For an extended discussion of drug discrimination of SGAs and its implications, see Barrett and Gleeson, 1991.)

5-HT$_{1A}$ ligands in conflict procedures.   In experiments using classic conflict procedures, such as the Geller–Seifter paradigm or the Vogel water-lick suppression test, it was clear that these procedures could discriminate anxiolytic drugs such as the barbiturates and BDZs from nonanxiolytic compounds. However, in experiments using SGAs with rats, mice, or nonhuman primates in these classic conflict models, the results were not altogether convincing in implicating a role for serotonin in anxiolysis, nor was buspirone particularly active in those models that were normally predictive of anxiolytic properties. For example, in an experiment in which BDZ (midazolam)-treated squirrel monkeys were tested in the Geller–Seifter conflict procedure, punished responding was increased 350% over control levels, whereas buspirone, 8-OH-DPAT, and related compounds produced no effect or decreased responding (Gleeson and Barrett, 1990).

In another study using the Geller–Seifter conflict procedure, buspirone-treated rats were examined in a series of manipulations involving the schedules of reinforcement, pharmacological experience (i.e., drug-naive vs. previous drug treatment), strain of rats, route of drug administration (subcutaneous vs. orally), and time course. At no time did buspirone affect the rate of punished responding (Howard and Pollard, 1990). Among 8 Geller–Seifter–type experiments with buspirone, 2 showed buspirone-induced increases of punished responding, and 6 showed decreased responding or no effect. Among 15 Vogel-type experiments with buspirone, 11 showed more drinking with tongue shocks, and 4 showed less drinking or no effect (see Barrett and Gleeson, 1991).

In contrast, buspirone given to pigeons significantly increased pecking under aversive control, as shown when pigeons were trained to peck at a colored key for food rewards under an FR-30 schedule (i.e., after every 30th peck, the bird was rewarded with food). When the key color changed, the bird was on the same FR-30 schedule, but it received a mild shock along with the food reward. As shown in Figure 16.15, buspirone increased punished responding in a dose-dependent manner over a wide range of doses (0.03–3.0 mg/kg), an effect that was also demonstrated with CDP, although at significantly higher doses. It is also interesting to note that when buspirone-treated rats and squirrel monkeys did show an increase in punished responding, the effect was typically smaller than those produced by BDZs. The species difference with regard to which drug is more effective or more potent is presumed to depend on differences in the presence and distribution of 5-HT receptor subtypes (Barrett and Gleeson, 1991).

Buspirone is thought to diminish excessively active 5-HT transmission during anxiety by stimulating 5-HT$_{1A}$ somatodendritic autoreceptors, thereby inhibiting serotonergic neuronal firing. This proposal led to clinical trials of buspirone on alcoholic outpatients with dual diagnoses of chronic anxiety and substance dependence according to DSM-IV criteria. Following buspirone treatment, subjects displayed significantly reduced scores on anxiety rating scales, and alcohol craving was significantly lower for the buspirone treatment group than for controls. Further, 16 of the 22 buspirone-treated subjects, but only 6 of the 20 placebo subjects, achieved a full response to the treatment, and significantly more placebo-treated subjects left treatment because they felt their condition had worsened during the experiment. Thus, considering that 5-HT is a common denominator in anxiety and alcoholism, subjects with a codiagnosis of anxiety and alcoholism may be dually benefited by the anxiolytic buspirone (Cloninger, 1987b). Whether the anxiolytic effect is directly related to diminished craving for alcohol is not yet known.

Other effects of BDZ and 5-HT$_{1A}$ agonists. In the light–dark crossing test (see above), BDZ-treated mice showed dose-dependent increases in dark–bright transitions in their home environments. In tests examining the effect of buspirone (0.1 mg/kg), increases in dark–bright transitions also occurred, but compared with the effect of diazepam, the effect was small and the active dose range was extremely narrow. However, some researchers reported that buspirone at high doses (1.0–10.0 mg/kg) was as effective as diazepam treatment in these tests,

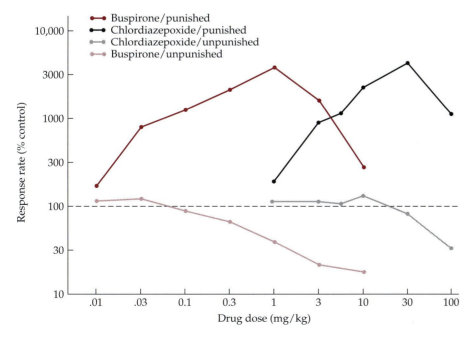

16.15 COMPARISONS BETWEEN THE EFFECTS OF CHLORDIAZEPOXIDE AND BUSPIRONE ON PIGEON BEHAVIOR. Dose–response functions for the effects of chlordiazepoxide and buspirone on punished and nonpunished behavior in a conflict paradigm. Buspirone is more potent in this procedure. The horizontal dashed line represents control measures. (After Barrett and Gleeson, 1991.)

whereas others reported that it was not, and that in a few cases, especially at high doses, there were decrements in locomotor activity. It was concluded that the dark–bright test was sensitive to 5-HT$_{1A}$ agonists such as buspirone and 8-OH-DPAT, but only in a few cases were their effects comparable to those of BDZs.

On the other hand, when the social interaction test was used, it was seen that BDZs were highly effective in promoting social interaction under unfavorable conditions, as when the illumination was bright and the arenas and partners were unfamiliar. In social interaction tests with buspirone, gepirone, ipsapirone, and 8-OH-DPAT, the anxiolytic effects of these compounds were similar to those of diazepam treatment, usually without changes in motor activity. BDZs were also effective in suppressing ultrasonic "distress" vocalizations (see above), and tests with SGAs (buspirone and ipsapirone) and 8-OH-DPAT had similar effects on preweanling rat and mouse pups, as well as on shock-elicited vocalizations in adult rats. Furthermore, shock-enhanced acoustic startle reflexes were subdued by BDZs compared with startle elicited by sound alone. Similar effects were obtained with SGAs, but not with 8-OH-DPAT, a result that was possibly compromised because of a difference of methodology (Treit, 1991). Thus, we see that there are some inconsistencies between species and between methodologies, making it difficult sometimes to select the proper instruments to establish the presence or the effectiveness of putative anxiolytics.

5-HT$_3$ Receptor Ligands

Neuropharmacology. As mentioned earlier, there is a significant presence of 5-HT receptors on peripheral nerves and smooth muscle of the viscera. These receptors were first known as 5-HT-M receptors, then later redesignated 5-HT$_3$ receptors. Their identification led to the development of 5-HT$_3$ receptor antagonists because of their possible utility in controlling visceromotor dysfunctions such as migraine, excessive gastric secretions, or nausea and vomiting associated with chemotherapy. A number of these compounds were examined for anxiolytic activity even though, at that time, there was no evidence that 5-HT$_3$ receptors were present in the brain or had a central functional role in the expression of anxiety. One of the compounds, GR 38032F (ondansetron), was found to modify limbic dopamine hyperactivity, and it compared favorably with buspirone and diazepam in antianxiety activity in a number of animal models. Many experiments with this compound were reviewed by Costall and Naylor (1991), some of which are described below.

Compared with diazepam, ondansetron has no affinity for BDZ receptors; it has no anticonflict effect in the Vogel water-lick suppression test; it does not antagonize pentylenetetrazol-induced convulsions; nor does it induce sedation, locomotor depression, or muscle relaxation. Further, in drug discrimination experiments, animals trained to discriminate anxiolytic 5-HT$_{1A}$ ligands from saline showed no generalization or antagonism to substituted 5-HT$_3$ receptor antagonists, indicating that the two receptors are distinctly different (Barrett and Gleeson, 1991). However, in one experiment, ondansetron was highly potent in increasing social interaction in paired rats under bright light and unfamiliar conditions. In that experiment, ondansetron was 100 times more potent than diazepam and caused no significant change in locomotor activity over an extensive dose range. Further, under dim light and familiar conditions, the drug had no effect on rat social interaction, thereby demonstrating the specificity of the drug effect in diminishing anxiety.

Anxiolytic effects were also demonstrated in the light–dark crossing test with mice, wherein ondansetron, again, was 100 times more potent than diazepam in increasing the exploration of the brightly lit box and decreasing the time spent in the poorly illuminated box. And in the shock-enhanced startle paradigm (which was described earlier), ondansetron significantly reduced the startle amplitude. In contrast, the startle amplitude was significantly increased by the 5-HT precursor 5-HTP, which in turn was antagonized by ondansetron. In additional experiments with marmosets and cynomolgus monkeys that showed emotionality and agitation in confrontations with human observers, ondansetron diminished the marmosets' retreats to the rear of their cage and aggressive posturing, and diminished 10 of 33 behavioral parameters of emotionality in the monkeys. Similar tests with diazepam showed, yet again, that ondansetron was more potent in these effects than diazepam.

Additionally, the possible consequences of chronic treatment with ondansetron—namely, tolerance and withdrawal effects—were examined in a variety of behavioral tests. For example, the behavior of mice in the light–dark exploration test was observed while ondansetron (0.01 μg/kg) was administered twice daily (b.i.d.) for 14 days, after which the drug was withdrawn and observations continued during 10 additional days. Similar tests were made with buspirone and diazepam. As shown in Figure 16.16, ondansetron maintained its anxiolytic effects during the 14-day drug series with no evidence of tolerance or sensitization, and during the withdrawal period, time in the bright box slowly declined to the control level. Similar effects were found with the 5-HT$_{1A}$ agonist buspirone, whereas after similar treatment with diazepam, there was an abrupt anxiogenic effect (within 8 hours) marked by suppression below control values of time in the bright box during the withdrawal period. There were no signs of anxiogenesis at any time after withdrawal from high-dose repeated treatments with ondansetron or other 5-HT$_3$ antagonists such as granisetron and zacopride. Furthermore, almost identical results were found when the drugs were used in the social interaction test. The finding that 5-HT$_{1A}$ agonists and 5-HT$_3$ antagonists maintain their anxiolytic effects

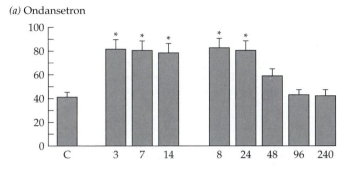

(a) Ondansetron

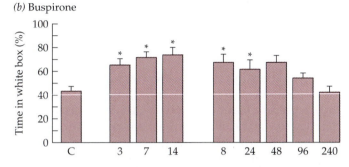

(b) Buspirone

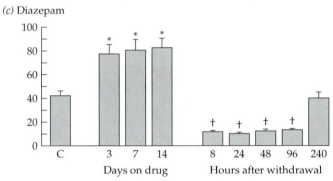

(c) Diazepam

Days on drug   Hours after withdrawal

16.16 CHRONIC TREATMENT WITH ONDANSETRON OR BUS-PIRONE, FOLLOWED BY DRUG WITHDRAWAL, PRODUCES NO TOLERANCE OR ABSTINENCE EFFECT. Mice were treated with ondansetron, buspirone, and diazepam for 14 consecutive days and underwent a light–dark exploration test on days 3, 7, and 14. All three drugs increased bright box explorations without any tolerance effect. The tests continued after 8, 24, 48, 96, and 240 hours of drug abstinence. Mice that had been treated with ondansetron or buspirone showed a slow, gradual return to control values of bright box exploration, whereas diazepam-treated mice showed an abstinence-induced rebound to less than control levels and did not reach control levels until sometime between the 4th and 10th day. ($^*p$ < .01–.001 compared with control values; $^†p$ < .01–.001 [one-way ANOVA followed by Dunnett's *t* test]). (After Costall and Naylor, 1991.)

during chronic treatment with no apparent withdrawal symptoms has important clinical implications.

Further tests investigated the possibility that ondansetron or buspirone could mitigate withdrawal effects after chronic diazepam treatments. Mice were treated with diazepam (10 mg/kg i.p., b.i.d.) for 7 days. After the first dose on day 7, they were tested with the light–dark crossing test, and showed a significant increase in time spent in the bright box. After 8 or 24 hours of diazepam abstinence, additional tests revealed a with-

drawal effect of suppression of time spent in the bright box below control values. Other groups of mice, 24 hours after the same diazepam treatment, received ondansetron (10 µg/kg i.p., b.i.d.) or buspirone (1 mg/kg i.p., b.i.d.), and the effects of the drugs were observed after 48, 96, and 240 hours of diazepam withdrawal. The treatment with ondansetron restored control values within 48 hours, and the time in the bright box increased significantly thereafter; whereas with vehicle (control) or buspirone treatment, it was 10 days (240 hours) before control values returned (Figure 16.17). The same effect was found when buspirone failed to attenuate BDZ withdrawal symptoms in a clinical study (Schweizer and Rickels, 1986). Also, when the same experiment was done using the social interaction paradigm with rats, the ondansetron inhibition of the withdrawal effects was even more marked, whereas the buspirone-treated rats were hardly distinguishable from no-drug controls. Thus, it appears that the drug profiles of 5-HT$_{1A}$ agonists and 5-HT$_3$ antagonists with respect to the attenuation of BDZ-induced withdrawal symptoms are distinctly different.

The fact that ondansetron counteracts BDZ withdrawal symptoms was also thought to have important clinical implications. It is generally held that such symptoms following withdrawal from alcohol, nicotine, or cocaine fall under the rubric of anxiogenic phenomena, and these symptoms have been adequately identified among animal species without overt changes in motor performance. Also, the finding that ondansetron reduced alcohol consumption in marmosets and rats suggests that it may influence craving. Thus, the study of 5-HT$_3$ receptor antagonists may lead to new therapies that support drug withdrawal programs (Costall and Naylor, 1991).

Neural mechanisms of 5-HT$_3$ receptor antagonists. In earlier experiments on the role of 5-HT in anxiety and anxiolysis, the evidence suggested that the anxiolytic action of BDZs is mediated, at least in part, by an inhibitory projection of the dorsal raphe nucleus (Stein, 1981). It was also found recently that microinjections of BDZs into the DRN, as well as into the amygdala, have anticonflict effects, suggesting that there are forebrain sites of action as well. Further, there is evidence that these sites are sensitive to 5-HT$_3$ antagonists, which serve as anxiolytics even though their effects are not mediated via BDZ receptors. For example, in recent light–dark crossing tests, injection of ondansetron into the DRN and the amygdala, whose cells project to the forebrain, attenuated the aversion of mice to the bright box, and the profile of the ondansetron-induced change was virtually the same as that for injected diazepam. Thus, anxiolytics such as BDZs and 5-HT$_3$ antagonists, when injected into the DRN and the amygdala, have their appropriate effects: the BDZs supposedly by enhancing GABA-mediated inhibition of cells in the DRN or amygdala, and the 5-HT$_3$ antagonists

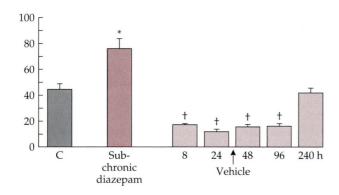

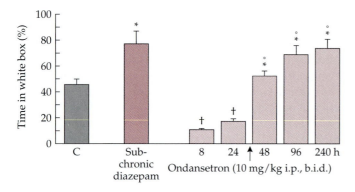

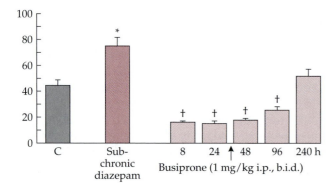

16.17 ONDANSETRON BLOCKS REBOUND EFFECTS OF DIAZEPAM ABSTINENCE. Mice were treated with diazepam (10 mg/kg i.p., b.i.d.) for 7 days. A light–dark exploration test after the first dose on the 7th day showed a significant increase in time spent in the bright box. Abstinence resulted in a rebound of time-in-bright levels to below control values (first two columns on the right). After the 24-hour exploration test, groups of mice were repeatedly treated with vehicle, ondansetron, or buspirone (arrows) and tested again at 48, 96, and 240 hours after diazepam withdrawal. Ondansetron immediately increased time-in-bright to control and higher levels, but buspirone was no better than vehicle treatments. Thus, ondensetron blocks rebound effects (*p < .001 for increased exploration; †p < .001 for decreased exploration; °p < .001 for inhibition of the decreased exploration in the light). (After Costall and Naylor, 1991.)

anxiety and anxiolysis. However, we have seen that experimental models may differ in the degree to which they represent fear or anxiety in different species, and that discrepancies among animal species in drug effects may be due to differences in the concentration and distribution of appropriate 5-HT receptors in the brains of different animals.

Part III Summary

The BDZs, developed by Hoffman-LaRoche, started with the discovery of chlordiazepoxide (CDP) (Librium). This substance had potent anxiolytic, sedative–hypnotic, and anticonvulsant activity. Its action resembled a psychostimulant, eliciting feelings of well being, increasing social activity and appetite, and reducing anxious depression. Many congeners were developed while searching for compounds that were more selective in expressing their effects in terms of onset time and duration. Moreover, the absence of receptors of the BDZs in the ANS resulted in the absence of side effects that could be generated from BDZ effects on autonomic systems.

The principal role of BDZ receptors and their ligands is the modulation of GABA binding within the GABA$_A$ receptor complex, which influences Cl$^-$ conductance in the target neurons. Experimental studies of the interactions between GABA$_A$ receptors and stress have shown that BDZ receptor ligands may have either anxiolytic or anxiogenic effects that are related to the binding properties and changes in the conformation of GABA$_A$ receptors. The anxiolytic ligands, such as the BDZs, enhance GABA binding, increase Cl$^-$ conductance in postsynaptic membranes, and decrease membrane sensitivity to depolarizing neurotransmitters. These effects lead to increased inhibition of neuromuscular reflexes, induction of sleep, anticonvulsant effects, and diminished fear and anxiety.

In contrast, anxiogenic ligands, such as some of the β-carbolines, diminish GABA binding, decrease Cl$^-$ conductance, and increase postsynaptic membrane sensitiv-

probably by acting more directly on presynaptic or postsynaptic 5-HT receptors.

The discovery of the heterogeneity of 5-HT receptors, and the development of specific anxiolytic ligands for some of them, has cast new light on the substrates of anxiety. The hypothesis that there is a role for 5-HT in anxiety and anxiolysis is marked by much supportive data, and recent endeavors have contributed even more. One implication of these findings is that serotonergic systems may either be parallel partners or serve as sequential stages with the GABA$_A$ receptor complex in the manifestation and control of anxiety, and it follows that there is a place for 5-HT pharmacology when anxiety has clinical consequences.

Nonetheless, there have been many reports of inconsistent data that have led some investigators to express considerable doubt about the role of serotonin in

ity. These effects lower convulsant thresholds, sensitize animals to adverse stimuli, further diminish punishment-suppressed behavior, and elicit fear and anxiety reactions in animals and humans that parallel the effects of environmental stress. All of these anxiogenic effects are prevented or reversed by anxiolytic ligands.

There are also "neutral" ligands, such as Ro 15-1788, that have strong competitive affinities for blocking the binding of anxiolytic and anxiogenic ligands, but they have few or no postsynaptic effects except under special circumstances. Thus, the BDZ receptors are unique in that their activation serves to modulate the activity of another neurotransmitter, GABA, without themselves being able to affect neuronal membranes. Further, from the findings described above, BDZ receptors seem to assume three different conformational states: one for an unoccupied receptor; a second for binding BDZ ligands that enhance GABAergic transmission to produce muscle relaxation, anxiolysis, and so on; and a third for reducing GABAergic transmission, resulting in anxiogenesis and seizures, or at lower concentrations, wakefulness, alertness, and the milder aspects of anxiety. Further, there is evidence for the presence of two types of BDZ receptors, BZ_1 and BZ_2, each with its own CNS distribution and BDZ affinity, which may account for some of the variation in effects among different ligands (Guidotti, Corda, and Costa, 1983). BZ_1 receptors are widespread in the CNS, but are found in particularly high levels in the cerebellum. BZ_2 receptors occur in high density notably in the hippocampus, striatum, and spinal cord. It has been proposed that stimulating the BZ_1 sites would induce anxiolytic effects with less sedation than ocurs with a nonselective agent (Handley, 1994; Squires et al., 1979).

These findings support the concept of a macromolecular receptor complex in particular parts of the brain wherein these ligands bind and interact allosterically to modulate the effects described above by increasing or decreasing inhibitory influences upon the target sites. Thus, we may imagine that in the neutral state, the $GABA_A$ complex is relatively quiescent, but when the animal or human is stressed, the complex is shut down or blocked by inverse agonists, leading to decreased inhibition and increased postsynaptic sensitivity resulting in muscular tension, high levels of alertness, and fear and anxiety. In contrast, when the complex is activated by endogenous agonists or anxiolytic drugs, the result is postsynaptic inhibition, leading to relaxation, anxiolysis, and sleep. In the following sections of this chapter, more evidence will be presented to justify the widespread confidence in these conclusions. These findings have contributed greatly to a better understanding of the substrates of emotion, anxiety, and fear, which can be addressed pharmacologically when they become dysfunctional in humans.

Part IV
Benzodiazepine Therapeutics

Pharmacological Considerations

The Efficacy of Benzodiazepines

A large number of BDZs have been formulated, and though some of these drugs are sufficiently specific for clinical treatments, a significant overlap of effects is usually present. Clinically, BDZs have been used as hypnotics (sleep inducers) and preanesthetic sedatives, and some BDZs can be used alone as light anesthetic infusions. But unlike barbiturates, which induce deep sleep and anesthesia, BDZs by themselves are not true anesthetics. One of the newer BDZ hypnotics, midazolam (Versed), is used for rapid induction of tranquility and deep sleep during brief surgical procedures done with local anesthetics. The drug is water- and lipid-soluble, so

**Midazolam
(Versed)**

it is rapidly transported into brain tissue after intravenous infusion. Thus, the drug induces a hypnotic effect within a few minutes, and because it has a short effective half-life, there is a recovery time of only a few hours without hangover. It also induces an anterograde amnesia that creates an illusion of anesthesia in some patients (Doenicke, 1984; Marshall and Wollman, 1985).

BDZs have been used with good effect to promote tranquility in dental patients who are fearful as they approach dental treatments. BDZs have also been prescribed to reduce anxiety and fear in patients with cancer, stroke, and cardiovascular diseases. They have been effective in psychosomatic disorders and those organic diseases with a heavy psychological overlay such as asthma, angina pectoris, irritable colon, gastric ulcers, and skin diseases. The BDZs have also been used to treat neuromuscular disorders associated with cerebral palsy, multiple sclerosis, hemiplegia, paraplegia, and bone fractures. Some of them are anticonvulsants and thus have been useful in managing some forms of epilepsy, especially *status epilepticus*, a period of severe and persistent convulsions for which intravenous infusion of diazepam is the treatment of choice (Gastaut et al., 1965). Acute alcohol withdrawal symptoms and neurotic sleep disorders have also been controlled with these drugs (Zbinden and Randall, 1967). These early clinical uses were well justified, and most of them are still valid today. On the other hand, not every patient improves with BDZ treatments, but moderate to marked improvement occurs in about 65% to 75% of those treated (Rickels and Schweizer, 1987).

The Safety of Benzodiazepines

BDZs are prescribed for the most part as hypnotics and anxiolytics, and it is in these modes that the question of safety is of greatest importance. Safety in these instances refers to the absence of risk of severe side effects when the prescribed dosages are adhered to, as well as when intentional or accidental overdoses or multidrug interactions occur. Also, the abuse potential and the risk of drug dependence has to be considered.

Throughout the history of BDZ treatment, there have been frequent criticisms of these drugs and their use. Part of this concern was due to their immense popularity and the resulting possibility of inappropriate prescribing, and part was based on reports of drug toxicity, dependence, and bizarre idiosyncratic reactions. To illuminate this controversy, we will examine the molecular attributes of BDZs and some experimental and clinical findings regarding BDZ safety and appropriateness.

BDZs interact with the $GABA_A$ receptor complex to enhance GABA binding and GABA-mediated inhibition. However, this effect is limited by the availability of GABA, thus providing a built-in limiting factor in GABA utilization and BDZ effects. Further contributing to BDZ safety is the virtual absence of BDZ receptors in visceral organs, or receptors that could directly activate catecholamine- and acetylcholine-mediated inputs to the sympathetic and parasympathetic nervous systems. Consequently, the BDZs, unlike the barbiturates and other nonBDZ compounds, have little effect upon cardiovascular, respiratory, gastrointestinal, or genitourinary systems, through which the most severe symptoms of overdose or withdrawal are expressed. Because of these factors, BDZs, taken by themselves in large doses as in a suicidal gesture, virtually cannot be taken in lethal amounts. With respect to cases of reactions to BDZ overdose or sudden abstinence, the reports of life-threatening effects are rare and usually attributed to multidrug intoxication.

In contrast, pentobarbital and possibly alcohol also enhance GABA-mediated inhibition, but in addition, they may produce an increment of sedative–hypnotic effects by acting directly upon Cl^- channels without the intervention of GABA–BDZ receptors. Moreover, pentobarbital and other barbiturates also block Na^+-dependent channels, thereby depressing excitatory as well

as enhancing inhibitory effects upon the target cells. Therefore, alcohol and the barbiturates serve as ligands for a greater range of receptor sites, thereby raising the possibility of unrestrained physiological depression of central systems controlling psychomotor stability, sleep, consciousness, and cardiovascular and respiratory activity. Further, the pharmacodynamics of alcohol and barbiturates promote tolerance, dependence, and life-threatening withdrawal effects. In contrast, because long-term use of BDZs does not cause hepatic enzyme induction, there is no metabolic tolerance. A 1977 study showed that among scores of cases of intoxication involving BDZs, the only patients requiring respiratory assistance were those that had also taken another CNS-depressant drug, usually alcohol.

In tests comparing the safety of BDZs with that of other sedative–relaxants, the superior margin of safety of diazepam and related agents against inducing locomotor side effects was especially significant. This superiority was illustrated in rotarod tests of motor coordination in mice (Randall and Kapell, 1973). In this test mice were compared in their ability to maintain their hold on a horizontal rotating cylinder after receiving various doses of barbiturates and BDZs. The drugs were scored by the dose at which 50% of the mice fell off the cylinder within a certain time (ED_{50}). Comparing chlordiazepoxide (CDP) and phenobarbital showed them about equal at 31 mg/kg p. o., but the animals could sustain doses of diazepam and flurazepam 5 times higher than that before falling off the cylinder, and the ED_{50} of flunitrazepam was 310 times higher. The **certain safety factor**, which is the ratio of the LD_{50} (the lethal dose for 50% of the mice tested) to the ED_{50}, ranged from 17:1 for CDP to 20,000:1 for flunitrazepam, whereas the ratio was only 7.8:1 for phenobarbital. These data illustrate the greater margin of safety against inducing muscle relaxation and ataxia with the BDZs compared with that of even as safe a drug as phenobarbital.

Tolerance and Dependence

BDZ effects in the Geller–Seifter paradigm.   In an early series of classic experiments, Margules and Stein (1968) assessed the effects of the BDZ oxazepam on conflict-induced behavior suppression using the Geller–Seifter paradigm described earlier. In this experiment, rats were treated over 22 days to assess the effects of continuous treatment. The animals were first trained to press a lever on a variable interval schedule (average interval 2 min) for milk rewards for 15 minutes. This segment was followed by a continuous tone for 3 minutes, during which a CRF schedule was in place. During this segment, each lever press led to a mild and brief (0.25 s) foot shock, which was immediately followed by a brief presentation of a dipper with a few drops of a milk mixture. On the first day after training, the animals were given a control session following an intraperitoneal saline injection. This session consisted of four 18-minute VI/CRF sequences and lasted 72 minutes (four 18-minute sequences). This was followed by 22 consecutive daily drug tests wherein oxazepam (20 mg/kg i.p.) was given immediately before each test session. Thus, the records would show the changes in behavior as the drug was being absorbed.

Figure 16.18 shows cumulative records for a typical rat in the control test with saline: the first 4 drug tests, and the 12th and 22nd drug tests. On the control (saline) day, nonpunished VI responding was persistent and vigorous, but during the punished CRF segments, there was virtually no responding at all. During the first oxazepam test, there was a rapid decline in the VI response rate as the drug took effect, but ten responses appeared during the first CRF segment. Thereafter, on that day, responding during both segments was minimal. On successive days, however, the rates for both nonpunished and punished responding increased markedly, until on the 4th day, nonpunished responding throughout the session had almost returned to normal, and there was a 350% increase in punished responding compared with the first drug test. By the 22nd day, there was an above normal rate for nonpunished responses, while punished responses had increased from two to over a hundred in a daily session, which was about as many as possible within the allowed time (four 3-minute segments per day).

It was concluded that during the early drug tests, oxazepam caused a transient sedative effect, marked by

diminished response rates, which masked the anxiolytic effect—the increased rate of punished responding. But with repeated testing, the rats developed a tolerance for the sedative effect of the drug, so that the anxiolytic effect was unmasked and punished response rates increased. Nonpunished response rates also increased, but proportionately less than punished response rates did.

To validate the interpretation that tolerance had occurred for the sedative effect, Margules and Stein (1968) did a second experiment in which rats were given a dose of diazepam or chlordiazepoxide (CDP) once a week for several months prior to being tested with oxazepam in the conflict test described above. With these drug-experienced animals, the first test with oxazepam produced a high rate of punished and nonpunished responding, and these responses persisted for 11 more daily tests. Thus, it was clear that in the first experiment, the initial response to oxazepam was sedation and response suppression, but as tolerance developed for the sedative effect, the disinhibition of punished responses became evident. It has also been found that in humans, initial treatments with many BDZs are accompanied by sedative effects, which undergo tolerance within 5–7 days.

Other studies. The pharmacokinetics of anxiolytic BDZs that might give rise to tolerance and severe withdrawal effects were made clear in an experiment by Lucas and Griffiths (1982). This experiment utilized the BDZ receptor blocker Ro 15-1788 to examine the effects of a simulated abrupt drug withdrawal. Four male baboons were implanted with intragastric catheters, and placed in a harness–tether restraint system. A diazepam suspension (10 mg/kg) was administered intragastrically twice daily, at 9:00 A.M. and at 5:00 P.M., for 45 consecutive days. During the first 7 diazepam days, the subjects were sedated, ataxic, and hypokinetic, but remained ambulatory, and over the course of drug treatment they developed virtually complete tolerance to these sedative and ataxic effects.

On days 7 and 35, the BDZ receptor blocker Ro 15-1788 (5.0 mg/kg) was administered intramuscularly at 11:00 A.M. This treatment produced an artificially abrupt BDZ withdrawal with signs of bruxism (grinding of the teeth), retching, vomiting, abnormal postures suggesting nausea, lethargy, and withdrawal depression. One animal also had body and foot tremors. The symptoms peaked 10 minutes after the Ro 15-1788 injection and lasted about 2 hours. After the Ro 15-1788 injection on the 35th diazepam day, the same symptoms appeared, but they persisted for 4–6 hours. Two of the animals had body, limb, and head tremors, and one had grand mal convulsions.

After 45 diazepam days the drug was withdrawn and the animals were observed for spontaneous withdrawal effects. No clear effects were observed until about a week later, when withdrawal signs progressively

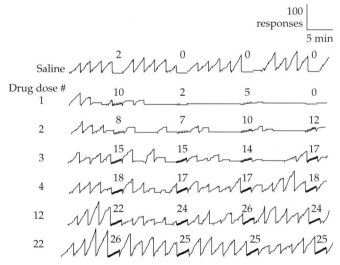

16.18 OXAZEPAM EFFECTS ON PUNISHED AND NONPUNISHED BEHAVIOR. Cumulative records are shown for the last control day and the drug days as indicated. The slopes of the tracings indicate the response rates. The recording pen reset after every 3 minutes. The numbers indicate the frequency of punished responses that occurred during 3-minute tone periods, and these responses are indicated by the short upward strokes of the pen. Downward pen strokes indicate rewarded responses during the nonpunished periods. (After Margules and Stein, 1968.)

developed, peaked during the following few days, and subsided thereafter. During this period there was a 25% reduction of food intake that persisted for 15 days of postdrug observation. Eight weeks after the last diazepam day, three of the subjects were injected with one double diazepam dose (20 mg/kg), followed 1 hour later by an Ro 15-1788 injection. During the interdrug interval the animals showed no signs of BDZ tolerance, since they displayed a marked ataxia and sedation that was completely reversed by the Ro 15-1788 dose, and no other withdrawal signs appeared during a 4-hour postinjection period.

These experiments demonstrated that withdrawal effects similar to those seen after barbiturate withdrawal can occur after long-term BDZ use, but the severity of the effect depends upon the doses used, the duration of continuous use, and most importantly, the suddenness of drug withdrawal, which is, in turn, dependent on the effective half-life and the elimination half-life of the drug as well as the suddenness of drug cessation. It was seen that sudden withdrawal, as effected by Ro 15-1788, has especially severe consequences, and it will be seen below that when hypnotic BDZ drugs with short effective and elimination half-lives are suddenly withdrawn during the treatment of insomnia, similar symptoms can occur.

When BDZs are administered to humans on a daily basis at anxiolytic or hypnotic doses, there may be sedation and muscle relaxation to the point of muscle weakness and ataxia, but in most cases tolerance to these effects occurs after a few days of treatment. On the other hand, these effects may be quite severe in the elderly, or when exacerbated by alcohol intake (see below). In elderly persons with diminished liver function, oxidative biotransformation of compounds such as diazepam, desmethyldiazepam, and alprazolam (Xanax) may be severely impaired. This impairment could result in a prolonged plasma half-life, and with continuous treatment there could be a plasma drug accumulation three to four times greater than normal and a potency factor contributing to falls and vehicular accidents. These effects are less likely to occur with drugs that are metabolized in the liver by conjugation, such as oxazepam and lorazepam, or metabolized by nitroreduction, such as nitrazepam and clonazepam (Sellers and Bendayan, 1987). Thus, for the compromised patient receiving prolonged BDZ treatment, the choice of drug should be one of the compounds with intermediate half-lives prescribed at wide dosing intervals, or one of the drugs that do not depend upon oxidation for metabolism and clearance (see Ellinwood and Nikaido, 1987; Greenblatt, 1990).

Whereas we have shown that under most circumstances, BDZs are comparatively safe, some conditions may lead to contrary effects. Fortunately, the discovery of the BDZ receptor blocker Ro 15-1788 (flumazenil) has provided an antidote for BDZ overdose or cases in which BDZs are combined with other sedative–hypnotic agents. In animals and humans this drug blocks the anxiolytic, muscle relaxant, sedative, anticonvulsant, amnestic, and anesthetic effects of BDZs. For example, BDZ-overdosed patients in coma were rapidly aroused by an intravenous injection of 2.5 mg of flumazenil without any side effects such as rebound epileptic phenomena. This treatment also rapidly reversed respiratory depression, which sometimes occurs when BDZs are used as anesthetics. Further, the effects of flumazenil are highly specific for agents acting through the BDZ receptors. Thus, the effects of barbiturates, ethanol, meprobamate, GABA mimetics, and other agents are unaffected, but non-BDZ agonists of BDZ receptors, such as zopiclone and triazolopyridazines, are blocked (Haefely, 1983).

However, because the effective half-life of flumazenil is rather short, it may have to be administered more than once to block the effects of BDZs still circulating in the blood and affecting the brain. In some cases adverse effects of flumazenil treatment, such as dizziness, nausea, fatigue, hot flashes, and sweating, have been reported, but these effects may be due to the reversal of the therapeutic effects of BDZs. Further, there have been reports of seizures following flumazenil treatment, but this effect may have occurred in patients who were chronically using BDZs to manage a seizure disorder, or in individuals who were polydrug users, especially those using tricyclic antidepressants, which have a mild convulsant potential (Krisanda, 1993).

With respect to concerns about drug dependence in patients under long-term BDZ treatment, it has been estimated that no more that 5% of patients in family practice receive BDZ treatment for more than 4 months, and patients, especially those treated by psychiatrists, who are seriously and chronically anxious can be effectively maintained on diazepam for 1 year or longer without developing tolerance for the therapeutic effects. Further, many such patients taking diazepam tend to lower their dosage voluntarily over time. With respect to the small number of patients who cannot function adequately without BDZs, it is inappropriate to conclude that they are addicted or dependent. Rather, because of their personality structure or the underlying cause of their disease, long-term pharmacotherapy may be required. Drug withdrawal from such individuals may lead to misery in their lives and possibly self-medication with other substances such as alcohol. Nonetheless, there are a sufficiently large number of dependent BDZ users to be cause for concern (see below). But, unlike the incidence of barbiturate dependence, the number of these cases is minuscule when considering the numbers of patients that are treated with BDZs (Greenblatt, 1990).

The termination of treatment among dependent patients is usually without abstinence effects because most of the BDZs used in this way, such as diazepam, chlordiazepoxide, and clorazepate, have long half-lives as well as active metabolites that are slowly cleared from the body even when the parent drugs are abruptly withdrawn. However, even though these pharmacokinetics are unlikely to induce drug dependence, tapering the daily dose by 25% per week is frequently recommended to further reduce the chances of withdrawal symptoms. In the case of continued use of BDZs with short half-lives, such as the hypnotic triazolam (Halcion), rebound insomnia and anxiety may follow abrupt discontinuance, so long-term tapering is required (see below).

In summary, it is probably fair to say that the discovery of the BDZs signified, for the first time in the twentieth century, the development of a class of comparatively safe and effective sedative–hypnotics and anxiolytic drugs. This is not to say that indiscriminate use of these substances is without adverse consequences, but the safety record of these agents, when taken as properly prescribed, has been a major pharmaceutical achievement.

Alcohol–Benzodiazepine Interactions

One of the more frequent factors compromising the safety of BDZs is the combination of BDZs and alcohol. Because of the widespread availability and use of alcohol, it should not be surprising that BDZs will be prescribed for one reason or another for an alcohol user. This is not to say that an alcoholic drink once or twice a day would have a disastrous effect on a patient taking a BDZ hypnotic at bedtime, or a sedative during the day. On the other hand, persons being treated with BDZs should not partake of one of these substances while under the influence of the other, especially if they are elderly persons or persons with limited liver function. This is due to the synergistic effects of alcohol and BDZs, in which simultaneous ingestion of even normal BDZ doses along with excessive amounts of alcohol can induce CNS depression of lethal proportions.

Benzodiazepine Treatment of the Anxiety Disorders

Parameters of Anxiety Disorders

It is fair to say that anxiety is a normal emotion which, in a mild form, contributes to physical and social adaptation and survival. In excess, however, anxiety may result in behavioral disorganization or unremitting expression of the autonomic symptoms of anxiety, which often lead to multiple psychosomatic sequelae that are physically debilitating as well. Among humans, the social environment provides ample opportunities for conflict and frustration that contribute to sometimes almost intolerable levels of anxiety, such as a failing marriage, pressures in the workplace, or the threat of a job loss in combination with an elaborate lifestyle that is supported by heavy spending. In some of these cases an environmental change, such as a new job, might have a significant ben-

efit, but such changes generate their own anxieties, such as separation from family and friends and radical changes in lifestyle. The prevalence of anxiety disorders in the United States (8.3%) exceeds that of all other psychiatrically diagnosed disorders (Rickels and Schweizer, 1987). How BDZs can aid in the restoration of a more balanced emotional life is the subject of this section.

First of all, we will define anxiety disorders as they are described in the *Diagnostic and Statistical Manual of Mental Disorders,* Fourth Edition, (DSM-IV, 1994). Anxiety disorders are divided into eight subtypes:

1. Panic disorder with or without agoraphobia
2. Agoraphobia without history of panic disorder
3. Social phobia
4. Simple phobia
5. Obsessive–compulsive disorder (OCD)
6. Posttraumatic stress disorder
7. Generalized anxiety disorder
8. Unspecified anxiety disorder

These eight subtypes have important differences in symptom profiles, pathogenesis, course, and treatment. (See Fyer et al., 1987, for detailed descriptions and differential diagnoses of these subtypes of anxiety disorders.) Moreover, anxiety may be primary and be expressed as a hypersensitivity to the omnipresent vicissitudes of life; or secondary in that it accompanies serious physical or psychiatric illness. The symptoms may be acute, intermittent, or chronic, and they may be mild, moderate, or severe. The anxiety disorders most often seen by physicians are panic disorder and generalized anxiety disorder (Bowden, 1990; Rickels and Schweizer, 1987).

Panic Disorder

Panic disorder is characterized by recurrent attacks of intense fear or discomfort that usually last for a number of minutes, or more rarely, hours. The disorder usually begins in late adolescence and may extend into the midlife period. The incidence of attacks after age 50 is about a third of that for people in their 20s. The syndrome affects women disproportionately at a ratio of two or three to one. There is evidence of a hereditary predisposition for this disorder. Some patients will endure the debilitating symptoms for as much as 7 years before seeking psychiatric treatment (Fyer et al., 1987; Rickels and Schweizer, 1987).

A frequent accompaniment of panic disorder is agoraphobia (Gk. *agora*, "marketplace"), which is a fear and/or avoidance of certain places by patients who perceive them as places in which they could not function, escape from, or get help if they had a panic attack. As required by the DSM-IV criteria, the avoidance and/or fear must be severe enough so that the patient's life is progressively restricted (Fyer et al., 1987). The principal panic symptoms are palpitations, trembling, shortness of breath, dizziness, sweating, choking, nausea, numbness and tingling, chest pain, fear of dying or going crazy, and feelings of depersonalization or derealization. These symptoms are frequently perceived as an impending heart attack, which fuels the panic even more. There is a sudden onset of symptoms, which become more intense within a few minutes after the start of the attack. The initial attack may be brought on by a stressful event, but later attacks may be unexpected or unrelated to a precipitating event. The combination of panic attacks and anticipatory anxiety between attacks may lead to phobic avoidance behavior resulting in an inability to work, drive a car, or engage in social behavior, symptoms that frequently lead to self-confinement in the home.

The role of catecholamines.   Based on the assumption that panic attacks are an expression of adrenergic hyperactivity, β-adrenergic blocking agents such as propranolol (Inderal) were tried in the early 1980s for treatment of the symptoms of acute stress, which might be considered mild panic symptoms. For example, propranolol was effective in controlling acute stress symptoms such as tachycardia and tremor in actors and musicians who were required to perform in public and in managers who, for instance, had to present progress reports at meetings of the executives of the corporation. Such persons were considerably calmed by a prophylactic administration of the drug, and their performances were said to be improved (see Weiner, 1985b).

However, it was generally found that except for some amelioration of tachycardia and palpitations, propranolol was ineffective for the management of panic disorders. Thus, it was proposed that the exclusive focus on adrenergic symptoms as the sole manifestation of panic was unwarranted (Rickels and Schweizer, 1987). This conclusion was supported by research findings described in a recent review stating that, with one exception, there were no studies demonstrating that β-blockers were superior to placebos in treating panic disorders. Moreover, the role of catecholamines is probably different in stress and panic. For example, during stressful emergencies, norepinephrine and cortisol are released from the adrenal glands, but the release of these substances frequently fails to occur during chemically provoked panic attacks (i.e., with sodium lactate), the mechanism of which has not been explained. Researchers were mystified by the finding that such panic attacks can produce all the symptoms of stress without the release of all the classic stress hormones, and the question of why some drugs or situations produce an attack with the release of stress hormones and others do not remains unanswered (Johnston, 1991). (See Gorman et al., 1987 for a discussion of sodium lactate–induced panic.) Thus, the manifestations of panic do not seem to be catecholamine dependent.

When propranolol and other β-blockers were compared with BDZs such as CDP, diazepam, and alprazo-lam, the BDZs were found to be superior in alleviating panic attacks, and there were no appreciable differences in antipanic effect among the various β-blockers. On the other hand, when stress led to moderate autonomic and somatic symptoms not normally amounting to panic, the effect of β-blockers was somewhat beneficial, but the effect of an appropriate BDZ was more pronounced. Nonetheless, propranolol may be preferred in some instances because the action of β-blockers is not accompanied by sensorimotor or cognitive impairment, and if the treatment is for chronic symptoms, the risk of dependence is even lower than it would be with BDZ treatment. For these reasons, the use of β-blockers may be superior to most other treatments for reducing mild symptoms of stress.

Antidepressant drugs such as imipramine and MAO inhibitors (MAOI), particularly phenelzine, were among the first agents that proved to be effective in curtailing panic attacks, but because of the unpleasant side effects of imipramine and the diet restrictions associated with MAOIs, many patients were reluctant to continue drug therapy with these agents. Thus, in the early 1980s, the drugs of choice for panic disorder were chlordiazepoxide (Librium), a low-potency BDZ, and diazepam, which were both reported as providing moderate to marked improvement of panic symptoms.

Alprazolam and clonazepam.   First marketed in 1981 as a treatment for generalized anxiety disorder, the use of alprazolam (Xanax) in the treatment of panic disorder was established in several controlled studies involving over 700 patients. Alprazolam was promoted as an antipanic

**Alprazolam
(Xanax)**

remedy because of its rapidity of action, its high benefit–risk ratio, and its generally minimal and well-tolerated side effects. Its principal drawbacks were interdose anxiety and its potential for withdrawal symptoms and physical dependence after discontinuation of long-term therapy. These effects were due to the high lipid solubility of alprazolam and its fast rate of redistribution into inactive tissue, which rapidly reduces drug plasma concentration and shortens the duration of action. These factors contribute to the risk of withdrawal effects and dependence.

In the meantime, another BDZ, clonazepam (Klonopin), originally used as an antiepileptic, was found to be twice as potent as alprazolam for blocking panic attacks as well as for blocking background and anticipatory anxiety. The difference between the two drugs is

**Clonazepam
(Rivotril)**

due to the lower lipid solubility of clonazepam. Clonazepam is absorbed more slowly from the GI tract, thereby extending the onset time of its maximum effect to as much as 2 hours after administration, whereas the peak effect of alprazolam occurs within 30 minutes. In addition, the low lipid solubility of clonazepam increases the duration of its effects. The duration of action of clonazepam is further increased because its effective elimination half-life is 3 to 4 times longer than that of alprazolam. Whereas the usual dose for alprazolam is between 2 and 6 mg, given in four daily doses to minimize interdose anxiety, the dose for clonazepam is 1–3 mg given in morning and evening doses, and initial doses can be as little as 0.25 mg once a day. On the other hand, because of the sudden nature of panic attacks, clonazepam's very gradual latency to peak effect can be disadvantageous to a person with panic disorder who is taking clonazepam "as needed," because by the time the drug reached its peak effect, the attack probably would be over. Consequently, drugs with shorter onset times such as alprazolam, diazepam, and lorazepam would be a better choice for "as needed" use. Further, if there is a need for a more sustained drug effect, a person with agoraphobia could take extra clonazepam about an hour before visiting a shopping area (see Rosenbaum, 1990).

Generalized Anxiety Disorder

In contrast to the rather sudden appearance and episodic nature of panic disorder, generalized anxiety disorder (GAD) has a more gradual development. Its symptoms are chronically manifested because of unrealistic and excessive worry that never seems to be fully resolved. GAD is characterized by combinations of the symptoms listed in Table 16.3. Unlike patients with panic disorder, individuals with GAD retain some ability to cope with the anxiety even when it is at its most severe level. The awareness of the symptoms and attempts to control them are indicative of a syndrome less malignant than schizophrenia or the affective disorders.

Obviously, a diagnosis of generalized anxiety disorder does not automatically call for pharmacotherapy, because many of the causes can be effectively treated by other means, such as advice, psychotherapy, and situational intervention. Further, if medication is indicated after a thorough investigation of the cause and nature of the anxiety disorder, it may be prescribed for a short period to overcome the effects of a nonrecurring stress, or for longer periods during persistent states of stress such as those induced by a terminal illness. With respect to drug choice, a BDZ with a long half-life is prescribed for most patients because of the safety of these compounds and because their dosing frequency is no more than three times a day. Diazepam, clorazepate, and prazepam are recommended because they undergo primary metabolism to desmethyldiazepam, which has an elimination half-life of 36–200 hours (see Table 16.1). Many variables must be considered to determine what antianxiety medication is appropriate in a particular case (Bowden, 1990), but the details of such considerations are beyond the scope of this volume.

Paradoxical Benzodiazepine Effects

A potentially serious consequence of BDZ treatment is the infrequent paradoxical increase of excessive assertiveness and aggression. A number of clinical reports revealed that such adverse behavior was released in some subjects being treated with diazepam. For example, some patients, after less than 30 days of diazepam treatment, demonstrated such symptoms as tremulousness, apprehension, confusion, insomnia, depression, and suicidal ideation (i.e., feeling like killing themselves but not really wanting to die). Once these responses were recognized, they were resolved within a week of discontinuation of medication. Six drug-discontinued patients were followed up for 1 year with a report of no recurrence of symptoms.

Greenblatt and Shader (1974) suggested that BDZs could produce a paradoxical increase in aggression if fear or anxiety were serving to inhibit aggression or hostility, and that individuals with such proclivities might express these behaviors when disinhibited by anxiolytics such as the BDZs. In animal studies, low doses of CDP induced aggression after aggression was previously suppressed by punishment. Other researchers reported that patients receiving diazepam showed a progressive development of dislikes or hates; and when taken by some parents, such drugs were linked to actual or threatened child abuse. It was not implied that the drug by itself caused child abuse; rather, the drug disinhibited aggressive impulses that were implicated in child abuse (see Cormack, Owens, and Dewey, 1989).

It is logical to assume that fear and anxiety may serve to suppress obnoxious or antisocial behavior, and it is not uncommon to observe that alcohol can serve as a disinhibiting agent and produce inappropriate boister-

Table 16.3   Diagnostic Criteria for Generalized Anxiety Disorder

Unrealistic or excessive anxiety and worry about two or more life circumstances for a period of six months or longer.

Focus of anxiety and worry not related to another disorder such as anxiety or worry about having a panic attack.

Disturbance does not occur only during the course of a mood disorder or a psychotic disorder.

At least six of the following 18 symptoms are often present when anxious (does not include symptoms present only during panic attacks):

Motor tension
  Trembling, twitching, or feeling shaky
  Muscle tension, aches, or soreness
  Restlessness
  Easy fatigability

Autonomic hyperactivity
  Shortness of breath or smothering sensations
  Palpitations or accelerated heart rate (tachycardia)
  Sweating or cold clammy hands
  Dry mouth
  Dizziness or light-headedness
  Nausea, diarrhea, or other abdominal distress
  Hot flushes or chills
  Frequent urination
  Trouble swallowing or "lump in throat"

Vigilance and scanning
  Feeling keyed up or on edge
  Exaggerated startle response
  Difficulty concentrating or "mind going blank" because of anxiety
  Trouble falling or staying asleep
  Irritability

Lack of evidence that an organic factor initiated and maintained the disturbance, e.g., hyperthyroidism, caffeine intoxication.

Source: After Bowden, 1990; adapted from *DSM-III-R*, 1987, pp 235–253.

---

ousness and dangerous pranks as well as scapegoating, violence, and aggression. It is unlikely that special neurochemical events are responsible for such paradoxical effects during the intake of alcohol or BDZ treatment; rather, in some individuals, the drugs reduce the fear of disapproval that usually inhibits such expressions, and during the disinhibition some element of antisocial or psychopathic behavior emerges. However, compared with the number of persons being treated in one way or another with BDZs, such occurrences are extremely rare, and are likely to be found in greater proportions among alcohol abusers (Baldessarini, 1985; Bowden, 1990; Harvey, 1985).

Abuse Liability of Benzodiazepines

There has been enough concern about the abuse liability of long-term treatment with BDZs to identify actual or potential drug-dependent users and to design programs to reduce the chronic use of these agents (see Cormack, Owens, and Dewey, 1989). On the other hand, there is some question as to how many patients on long-term anxiolytic treatment are truly drug dependent. Investigations to assess the magnitude of problems associated with long-term BDZ use have revealed that in many instances in which adverse effects of psychotherapeutic drugs have occurred, there were findings, or at least suspicions, that the drugs were misused because of inappropriate prescriptions, doses, or treatment schedules; or that the drugs were used without medical approval and oversight. For example, physiological dependence (as shown by withdrawal symptoms of increased anxiety and insomnia) can develop in patients taking high doses of BDZs for prolonged periods, but less severe symptoms were found when the doses were within the therapeutic range.

In two double-bind placebo-controlled experiments on the effects of long-term treatment with therapeutic doses of BDZs, it was found that the risk of developing dependence with therapeutic doses of BDZs was virtually nonexistent for the first 6 weeks of treatment, but there was a slightly increased risk between 3 and 8 months of treatment, and a considerably greater risk beyond that point. However, among patients who had been taking BDZs daily for 1 year, the termination of the short half-life BDZ lorazepam produced a markedly more intense withdrawal syndrome than the termination of long-acting BDZs such as diazepam or clorazepate.

To deal with the problem of BDZ dependence, the abuse potential of BDZ compounds had to be assessed. Thus, self-reports were employed to obtain an appraisal of the degree of euphoria or other positive subjective responses to various drugs. After drug-naive volunteers were given drugs or placebos in color-coded capsules, subjects receiving low doses showed no preference for BDZs over placebos, and even at moderate doses of diazepam, they generally exhibited a preference for the placebo. Similar effects occurred with low doses of flurazepam, lorazepam, and placebo: the subjects chose the drug and placebo capsules equally, and at the higher doses they again generally chose the placebo over the medication. Thus, for drug-naive subjects, the drugs were devoid of significant reinforcing effects, and may even have been aversive. Similar findings were obtained from subjects who were sedative abusers and from highly anxious individuals. In general, at low and therapeutic doses there were no preferences for BDZs except for high doses by sedative abusers, and barbiturates were preferred when the choice was between them and BDZs. These studies suggested that self-administration of BDZs among drug-naive subjects is quite meager, even among anxious subjects. Among sedative abusers, barbiturates were the usual choice when compared with BDZs. (See Katz, Winger, and Woods, 1991, and Woods, Katz, and Winger, 1992, for extensive reviews.)

The Parameters of BDZ Abuse

Survey research has revealed that nonmedical or recreational use of BDZs among adults and youths in the general population is trivial, and where it was found to any degree, it was among subjects with histories of drug abuse, including alcoholics and patients receiving methadone. These groups made up the greater part of the 4.8% of the U.S. population who reported in 1988 ever having used tranquilizers nonmedically, with a 1-year prevalence of 2.2% and a 1-month prevalence of 0.6%. A similar survey in Sweden reported that 15 (0.06%) of 2,566 BDZ users developed regular purchase patterns, and 4 (0.15%) had patterns indicative of abuse or overuse, but most users decreased their purchases over time. Thus, nonmedical or recreational use of BDZs does not reflect a high abuse potential.

In considering whether a drug or drug class has abuse liabilities, surveys show that the lack of significant

reinforcement by BDZs is such that the extent of such use is trivial, even among abusers of other drugs, and that among patients who have been prescribed BDZs, only a small percentage have developed a pattern of consumption indicative of drug abuse. Further, it has been proposed that just as it is unjustifiable to withhold opiates for the relief of pain because of the risk of physiological dependence, it is likewise unjustifiable to withhold appropriate anxiolytic or hypnotic therapy because of the risk of BDZ dependence. Evidence suggests that anxiety can be a chronic illness that requires chronic treatment, and that the fact that only a small proportion of such patients seek treatment indicates that long-term antianxiety medication is underutilized, rather than unnecessarily widespread.

Serotonergic Anxiolytics

Partly because of the adverse effects of BDZs described earlier, there has been an aggressive search for alternatives to BDZs despite their record for efficacy and safety; quite possibly this search is also motivated by the huge potential market for such alternatives. The search was accelerated by the discovery of multiple central 5-HT binding sites and site-selective ligands by Peroutka and Snyder (1979). Given that 5-HT probably plays a significant role in BDZ-induced anxiolysis, finding a 5-HT receptor ligand with anxiolytic properties was a good possibility. The result of 10 years of research activity has been the production of an abundance of such ligands with varying affinities, potencies, and specificities. Glennon, Naiman, and coworkers (1989), in reviewing the progress of these endeavors, described an almost bewildering scene of effects that appeared to be consistent at one time and paradoxical shortly thereafter, of ligands that have agonistic effects at one site and antagonistic effects at another, of agonists that are inhibitory and others that are excitatory, and so on. Nonetheless, a few ligands have emerged that seem to have desirable clinical properties without undesirable side effects.

Buspirone Characterization and Therapeutics

The 5-HT ligands that are most relevant to the subject of the pharmacotherapy of generalized anxiety disorder are buspirone and its congeners gepirone and ipsapirone, which are members of the arylpiperazine family of compounds. Buspirone has been heavily researched and is already widespread in clinical use. Accordingly, we shall describe the characteristics and efficacy of this compound as an alternative non-BDZ anxiolytic (see Schweizer and Rickels, 1991).

Buspirone (Buspar) was thoroughly tested and was found to have anxiolytic actions that compared favorably with those of diazepam, but it did not bind to BDZ receptors or modulate GABA activity. It had a slower onset of action and produced fewer adverse psychomotor effects than diazepam, but unfortunately, it could take 5–10 days, or as much as 2–4 weeks of treatment, before clinical anxiolytic improvement was felt. Moreover, some patients who had been taking BDZs experienced a dysphoria (a feeling of restlessness and malaise) when switched to buspirone, and requested that they be returned to BDZ treatment. This may have been partly due to the slow onset of anxiolysis with buspirone and the return of anxiety with the cessation of BDZ treatment. Accordingly, it was suggested that the two drugs be combined to obtain the positive characteristics of each by gradually tapering diazepam off and tapering buspirone on. Because of its slow onset, buspirone would be inappropriate for the treatment of transient anxiety, or as a drug to be used on an "as-needed" basis; in these cases, most BDZs would be preferable (Bowden, 1990; Rickels and Schweizer, 1987).

Buspirone differs from BDZ anxiolytics in several important ways: it does not cause drowsiness; it does not impair psychomotor function or cause muscle weakness and ataxia; and it does not cause the typical muscle relaxation that is sometimes a desired effect of BDZ treatment for patients experiencing muscle tension as part of their anxiety syndrome. Further, buspirone does not impair vigilance or attention, nor does it have adverse effects on memory or cognition, as is sometimes observed during BDZ treatment. Buspirone has no antiepileptic characteristics, nor does abrupt termination after long-term buspirone treatment pose the risk of seizures. It has no demonstrable abuse potential, and coadministration with other sedatives or alcohol has no additive effect on psychomotor impairment. Finally, in contrast to the occasional induction of paradoxical aggression by BDZs, buspirone may reduce aggression (Schweizer and Rickels, 1991). Whether these differences are due to the absence of buspirone binding to the GABA$_A$ receptor complex is not known.

Buspirone Side Effects and Overdoses

As favorable as the above report might seem, buspirone is not free of side effects. As with almost all anxiolytics, about 10% of patients report certain complaints with buspirone, namely, dizziness, headache, and nausea, and with BDZs, drowsiness and fatigue. Still, severe side effects are rare with buspirone, and its therapeutic index is high. There have been no fatalities related to buspirone overdoses; when overdoses have occurred, the symptoms were only exacerbated side effects—nausea, vomiting, headache, and dizziness. For significant overdoses there is no special treatment other than induced emesis, gastric lavage, supportive measures, and careful monitoring. When buspirone is coadministered with other commonly used drugs, no serious reactions occur, except that hypertensive episodes have been reported when buspirone was given with MAO inhibitor antidepressants. Therefore, to avoid double dosing, buspirone

should be discontinued 24 hours before MAOI therapy is begun, and MAOI therapy should be discontinued 10–14 days before buspirone therapy begins.

Buspirone versus BDZ Treatment

Several studies have examined the effects of substituting buspirone for BDZs on chronic users of BDZ anxiolytics. One study on the long-term use of buspirone in the treatment of GAD reported efficacy comparable to that of BDZs after 4 weeks, but not after 1 or 2 weeks of treatment, thereby illustrating the delayed efficacy of buspirone. Buspirone is also known to have antidepressant characteristics, and there is evidence that supports the recommendation of buspirone for treating mixed anxiety–depressive states. Similar effects have been reported for gepirone and ipsapirone. There are some indications that buspirone is more effective for reducing the cognitive aspects of anxiety (i.e., interpersonal sensitivity and irritability), whereas the BDZs may have more effect on the somatic symptoms of anxiety.

Finally, the treatment with buspirone eliminates the psychomotor, attentional, and memory impairments that can be induced by BDZs. Buspirone may therefore be an appropriate treatment for elderly patients, who are particularly sensitive to these BDZ effects. Buspirone may also be appropriate for patients being treated on a long-term basis for chronic GAD if they work in environments where BDZ-induced psychomotor or attention impairment would be hazardous. Such patients should be informed that improvement might be slow in developing. Other patients for whom buspirone might be a more appropriate choice than BDZs are those who consume alcoholic beverages daily, because there are no buspirone–alcohol interactions.

Discontinuation of long-term GAD treatment with BDZs after 4–6 weeks of treatment, especially with the short half-life BDZs, led to rebound anxiety, and after 6 months of treatment, the majority of patients exhibited a withdrawal state. In contrast, no withdrawal state has been demonstrated in buspirone-treated patients. Further, there seems to be no tendency for buspirone abuse, or for its use as a recreational substance. These characteristics favor buspirone for use on a long-term basis with patients who are at risk for substance abuse or when there is limited supervision of the drug regimen. With these advantages, buspirone and the other azapirones could become adequate substitutes for BDZs in some instances, as well as therapeutic agents alongside the BDZs to expand their reach. (See Schweizer and Rickels, 1991, for an extensive bibliography on this subject.)

The Treatment of Insomnia

By definition, hypnotics are drugs that promote sleep and are used as adjunctive treatments for insomnia. In other words, hypnotics are not a cure, but rather an aid in the treatment of insomnia. Before the barbiturates were in common use, a number of other sedative–hypnotics, such as chloral hydrate and paraldehyde, were used in hospital settings to sedate patients and to ensure restful sleep. They were considered to be effective, safe, and inexpensive, but they were not generally prescribed for outpatients. As mentioned earlier, the barbiturates, some of which were the most commonly used hypnotics until the 1960s, were often misused and abused because frequent use induced tolerance, increased dosage, dependence, and serious withdrawal effects. The BDZs, even with chronic use, are less likely to do so. Nevertheless, with continued use, most of the sedative–hypnotic effects of BDZs undergo cellular tolerance, which limits their utility for treating persistent insomnia.

Other products have appeared in the last few decades, such as ethchlorvynal (Placidyl), ethinamate (Valmid), glutethimide (Doriden), methaqualone (Quaalude, Sopor), and methyprylon (Noludar). Many of these compounds, particularly Placidyl, were promoted as alternatives to barbiturates, but they were chemically related to barbiturates, and the "product information" for them contained warnings that were virtually identical to those for barbiturates with respect to dependence and severe withdrawal symptoms. Thus, most of these drugs, like the barbiturates, had characteristics that led to their abuse, and when used in conjunction with alcohol they were especially dangerous. Consequently, most of them were withdrawn from the market, especially when the effectiveness and relative safety of the BDZs was established (Harvey, 1985). A recent report estimated that approximately 20 million prescriptions for hypnotic BDZs such as flurazepam and triazolam are being written each year (D. D. Kelly, 1991a).

The Nature of Sleep

A brief review of the nature of sleep will add to our understanding of insomnia. In most living mammals daily alternations between sleep and waking occur because of endogenous circadian rhythms that are essentially linked to environmental cues, especially light and darkness. Moreover, the need for sleep is coupled to restorative processes such as cellular proliferation, which occur at peak rates during sleep. These processes contribute to bone and skin growth in children and the repair and replacement of tissues that perpetually break down and require renewal in adults. The entire lining of the gut, for example, is sloughed off and replaced every 24 hours. This process requires the synthesis of considerable amounts of new protein, and it proceeds faster during sleep, and is diminished in individuals that are denied sleep. Also, the brain is especially sensitive to sleep deprivation, and the longer the time without sleep, the greater the impairment of physical and mental performance, the poorer the mood, and the greater the need and motivational pressure to sleep. Recovery can be ac-

complished only by sleep; bed rest will not substitute for sleep in rejuvenating physical status and mental performance (see Adam, 1984).

Sleep is not a unidimensional state. Sleep proceeds from wakefulness through four or five stages of sleep that are described in various ways (Figure 16.19; see also Chapter 7). Simply stated, the stages and the rough percentages of total sleep time (in parentheses) spent in the various stages are as follows:

1. Descending sleep or dozing (3% to 6%)
2. Unequivocal sleep (40% to 52%)
3. Deep sleep transition (5% to 8%)
4. Deep sleep (also known as cerebral or slow-wave sleep or SWS) (10% to 19%)

The depth of sleep increases through the various stages, with the deepest sleep in the slow-wave stage. Each of these stages is defined on the basis of a particular electroencephalographic pattern, as shown in Figure 16.19.

In general, the waking state is characterized by a low-voltage, high-frequency wave pattern that gradually progresses to high-voltage, low-frequency patterns as the depth of sleep increases. It takes about 30–45 minutes for sleep to progress to the slow-wave stage (stage 4), and after a short interval there is a reversal of sleep stages that takes an equal amount of time. Usually, when sleep returns to stage 1, another type of sleep appears, known as rapid eye movement (REM) sleep. REM sleep is accompanied by rapid eyeball movement, active middle ear muscles, a loss of skeletal muscle tone, and recallable dreams, especially just before waking. Dreams that occur at other times are only vaguely recalled with few details. During REM sleep the threshold for arousal by environmental stimuli is increased, and by this criterion , REM is the deepest stage of sleep. On the other hand, animals and humans are more likely to awaken spontaneously from REM sleep than from any other sleep stage. Thus, the depth of sleep is not a unitary parameter. The sleep cycles repeat four or five times during the night with an elongation of REM sleep periods and a gradual loss of sleep stages 3 and 4.

In children and young adults, the repetition of the stages occurs in rather uniform sequences, with deeper sleep than is found among adults and especially among the elderly, who sleep for shorter periods with frequent alternations of the sleep stages and frequent awakenings. Further, there are wide differences among individuals in sleep latency (the time it takes to fall asleep) and total sleep duration. Some adults fall asleep within a few minutes, whereas others take a half hour or more. Some adults need at least 8–10 hours of sleep per night, whereas others, especially older persons, need only 5 or 6 hours, and in rare cases 2 or 3 hours of sleep seem to be enough. Moreover, objective observations of sleep among normal sleepers and professed insomniacs reveal

(a)   *(b)*

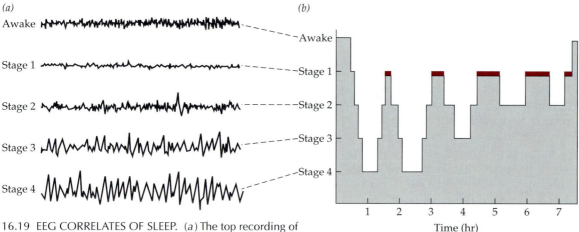

16.19 EEG CORRELATES OF SLEEP. (*a*) The top recording of low-voltage and high-frequency activity is that of an awake brain. Stages 1 through 4 represent the successively deeper stages of slow-wave sleep. In stage 2 there are short (1–2 seconds) bursts of sleep spindles. Stage 1 rapid eye movement (REM) sleep is distinguished from stage 1 non-REM sleep only by electrooculographic (EOG) and electromyographic (EMG) criteria. (*b*) A typical pattern of sleep in a young adult. The time spent in REM sleep is represented by colored bars. The first REM period is usually short (5–10 minutes), but these periods lengthen in successive cycles. Conversely, stages 3 and 4, which together are referred to as "delta sleep," dominate the slow-wave sleep periods in the first third of the night, but are often completely absent during the later, early morning cycles. The amount of stage 2 slow-wave sleep increases progressively until it completely occupies the slow-wave periods toward the end of the sleep period. In this example, morning awakening interrupted the last REM period, which increased the likelihood of good dream recall. Had the last REM period been completed and the awakening occurred during the next stage 2 period, dream recall would have been greatly reduced. (After D. D. Kelly, 1991b.)

that the variation in sleep latency and the duration and consistency of sleep does not provide agreed upon measures of normal or abnormal sleep patterns (Dement, Seidel, and Carskadon, 1984). (See Chapter 7 for a discussion of the biochemistry of sleep, and D. D. Kelly, 1991a,b for reviews of sleep phenomena.)

The Nature of Insomnia

Insomnia is a periodic complaint of about 40% of the population, but only about 4% seek a medical explanation and treatment. It is estimated that the greater part of the adult population will experience transient insomnia at some time in their lives because of travel, time zone shifts, time changes in work schedules, and acute emotional disturbances; and that 15% of people living in industrialized countries have serious or chronic insomnia.

Like sleep, insomnia is not a unidimensional state. It may refer to long sleep latency (an inability to fall asleep quickly), multiple awakenings, or early awakenings and difficulty in returning to sleep. In some cases daytime sleepiness is prevalent, with dozing and short naps that may contribute to insomnia at normal bedtime. Thus, insomnia is a dissatisfaction with the quality of sleep, which largely refers to "lightness" of sleep marked with frequent arousals.

The prevalence of insomnia is age- and sex-related, with 12% of adolescents, 20% of 18–30-year-olds, and 40% of those aged 51 and older complaining about poor sleep, and with more women complaining about it than men (see Adam, 1984). For some, insomnia may be transient, lasting for a few days to a few weeks, suggesting that insomnia in most cases is probably self-limiting in that sleep deprivation leads to sleepiness and motivation to get more sleep. For others it may be chronic, usually measured in months or years, and in some cases insomnia is a lifelong burden. The insomniac usually describes his or her perceptions of disturbed or inadequate sleep in terms of the quality of sleep experiences and how he or she feels during the day in terms of fatigue, drowsiness, and loss of initiative. Other daytime consequences of sleep loss are nervousness, irritability, vague dysphoria, feelings of depression, and impairment of performance. On the other hand, some insomniacs do not mention sleepiness and generally feel fine during the day, and some report that if the day's events are exciting or associated with vigorous physical activity, sleepiness attributed to insomnia can be overcome. The validity of these observations has been buttressed experimentally: many volunteers that are sleep-deprived report no ill effects during subsequent waking hours.

Although the onset and duration of sleep can be measured objectively, the important dimension, the quality of sleep, has no objective measure or criterion. When EEG records of sleep from large groups of normal and insomniac adults were compared for sleep latency, sleep duration, and number of arousals, there was a wide overlap of these sleep parameters between the normal sleepers and the insomniacs, despite a significant difference between the means. This finding shows that there is no consensus about the subjective and objective boundaries between disturbed and undisturbed sleep.

The tenuous nature of insomnia notwithstanding, there are a number of objective deterrents to sleep that may be the root cause of insomnia in many cases. Sleeplessness may be due to grief over one's own or family misfortunes, or chronic pain or other physical discomforts (indigestion, nausea, nasal congestion, coughing). There may be indoor or outdoor environmental noise, excessive heat or cold, drug-induced stimulation such as by caffeine or adrenergic drugs for cold symptoms, or rebound symptoms following the use of antidepressant drugs or alcohol. Also, sleep may be deterred because of residual anxiety related to job stress or other forms of interpersonally induced anxiety. Furthermore, insomniacs sometimes become anxious even about falling asleep because of their past experiences with long sleep latencies. Periods of sleeplessness are also associated with endogenous depression, some forms of psychotic behavior, paroxysmal muscle contractions, and nightmares.

Another frequent deterrent to sleep is the rebound insomnia that results from chronic use of barbiturate hypnotics such as secobarbital or pentobarbital. These drugs, when first used, may be very effective in shortening sleep latency and maintaining sleep, but with chronic use there is tolerance and overdosing. Further, because the metabolizing enzymes for these drugs are nonspecific, a broad cross-tolerance to other hypnotics develops at the same time. The result is rebound insomnia with frequent awakenings during the night. The effect on a typical patient is shown in Figure 16.20.

One form of insomnia, known as pseudoinsomnia, is characterized by dreams of being awake and trying to fall asleep. This condition is discovered when EEG monitoring indicates normal duration and depth of sleep, but upon awakening the patient claims to have been awake all night. In diagnostic laboratory situations only 1 patient in 70 lies awake all night, although many patients make this unfounded claim.

A serious form of insomnia is caused by sleep apnea, characterized by loud snoring and transient cessations of breathing (apnea) during sleep due to the collapse of the pharynx and other muscular tissues in the upper airway, leading to frequent awakenings. Thus, the patient sleeps poorly, and during the day exhibits sleepiness, poor concentration, irritability, memory difficulties, and depres-

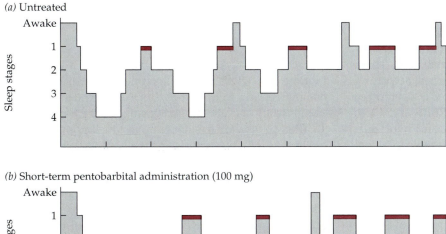

(a) Untreated

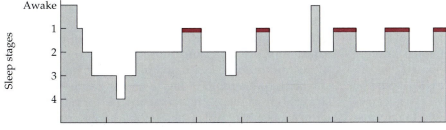

(b) Short-term pentobarbital administration (100 mg)

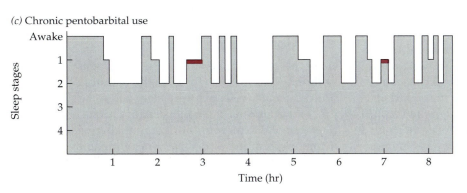

(c) Chronic pentobarbital use

Time (hr)

16.20 PENTOBARBITAL EFFECTS ON SLEEP CYCLES. (*a*) The sleep cycles of an untreated young adult who complained of early morning awakenings, with REM sleep represented by colored bars. (*b*) Pentobarbital (100 mg) initially lengthened the first REM period and decreased spontaneous awakenings. (*c*) With chronic nightly use of pentobarbital and increased dosage, drug tolerance is manifested by the lengthening of sleep latency (1 hour) and 12 awakenings during the night. Also, both REM sleep and stages 3 and 4 slow-wave sleep are suppressed. (After Kales and Kales, 1973.)

sive symptoms. Patients with sleep apnea are frequently middle-aged or older, overweight, and hypertensive. No drugs have been found for ameliorating these symptoms. Treatment includes loss of weight as well as the surgical removal of the uvula and the trimming away of mucous and lymphoid tissue from the oropharynx. These measures are successful in eliminating sleep apnea in 50% to 60% of cases. In milder cases, relief is obtained when patients learn to sleep on the side instead of the back. One way to accomplish this is to have the patient wear a small sack containing a tennis ball at the small of the back.

When insomnia is related to an unfavorable environment for sleep, psychiatric problems, physical impairment, or anxiety, the treatment should be directed at changes in the environment, treatment of the psychiatric and physical infirmities, and psychotherapy for the social dysfunction that is responsible for the sleep-preventing anxieties. On the other hand, during such ongoing therapeutic procedures, persistent insomnia may require an adjunctive hypnotic on a short-term basis (see below.)

The Assessment and Diagnosis of Insomnia

The objective signs of sleep can be obtained during an all-night polysomnographic evaluation, which includes an electroencephalogram (EEG), electrooculogram (EOG), electromyogram (EMG), electrocardiogram (EKG), measures of respiratory airflow, and records of leg movements from electrodes placed over the tibialis muscles of both legs. In addition, patients are diagnosed according to standard procedures established by the Association of Sleep Disorders Centers (ASDC). (See Roffwarg, 1979, and D. D. Kelly, 1991a; also see DSM-IV and see Hindmarch, 1984 for procedures in evaluating psychological performance during treatment with hypnotic drugs.)

Objective measures of the daytime effects of insomnia can be made with the Multiple Sleep Latency Test (MSLT), which measures sleepiness or the tendency to fall asleep during the day. Specifically, at five or six times during the day, measures are taken of sleep latency when the subject is offered a nap. It is assumed that the sooner the subject falls asleep, the more drowsy he or she was. This technique can also be used to assess carryover daytime sleepiness after drug treatment to improve sleep (for details, see Mitler, 1982; Richardson et al., 1978). Some experimental results of this test are illustrated in Figure 16.21, showing the effect of restricted sleep on daytime sleepiness. The subjects were 10 normal young adult males whose sleep duration was restricted from about 9 hours to 5 hours for 7 consecutive nights. After waking, sleep latency was measured at 2-hour intervals beginning at 9:30 A.M. and ending at 7:30 P.M. The test results on days 1, 3, 5, and 7 clearly show a shortening of daytime sleep latency over days, demonstrating that a relatively small reduction of sleep produces a substantial and highly significant increase in

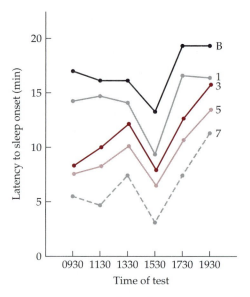

16.21 ASSESSMENT OF THE EFFECTS OF SLEEP DEPRIVATION. The Multiple Sleep Latency Test measures the time taken to fall asleep at 2-hour intervals during the day. The sleep period of normal subjects was reduced from 9 hours to 5 hours for 7 nights. Their sleep latency during the daytime decreased as a function of the number of nights of restricted sleep; that is, the longer the sleep deprivation, the greater the degree of drowsiness during the daytime. B = baseline sleep tendency averaged after 3 nights of approximately 9 hours of sleep. Days 1, 3, 5, and 7 represent day of sleep restriction (SR). (After Dement et al., 1984.)

daytime sleepiness (Carskadon and Dement, 1981). It is also interesting to note that there is a consistent dip in sleep latency at 3:30 P.M. (1530), suggesting a natural inclination toward drowsiness at that time of day.

In addition, many mental, psychophysiological, psychomotor, and performance tasks, as well as questionnaires about the quality of sleep and perceptions following sleep, have been devised for the evaluation of insomnia. These tests, when properly applied with adequate controls, can reveal whether hypnotics significantly improve sleep and subsequent daytime activity. Efficacy should be evaluated in terms of the patient's subjective perception of improvement of the quality of sleep, improvements in mental and performance scores upon awakening, and an absence of carryover sleepiness and weariness (D. D. Kelly, 1991a).

Pharmacological Treatment of Insomnia

Over-the-counter sleep aids.   In the United States, $30 million a year is spent for over-the-counter (OTC) hypnotics (usually referred to as sleep aids). The active ingredient in most of these preparations is one or more antihistamine (H_1 receptor blocker) antiallergenics such as diphenhydramine or doxylamine, which have drowsiness as a side effect. Sodium salicyclamide, an aspirin-related substance that has some sedative properties, is another hypnotic ingredient. Diphenhydramine is found in Sominex, doxylamine is used in Unisom, and sodium salicyclamide is used in many other brands that differ only in packaging and cost. It is interesting to note that the OTC hypnotics sell for 25¢ to 30¢ per tablet dose, whereas the OTC antihistamines sell for as little as 6 cents per tablet dose for use as antiallergenics.

Sleep laboratory tests of OTC hypnotics showed that they did not, at their recommended doses, have an appreciable effect on inducing or sustaining sleep, and sodium salicyclamide was devoid of any hypnotic efficacy. Contributory factors may be the rapid development of tolerance and the inadequacy of doses currently approved (Douglas, 1985; Harvey, 1985).

With respect to side effects, even when used at recommended doses, the OTC hypnotics may precipitate acute glaucoma in vulnerable elderly persons. When users become tolerant to OTC hypnotics, they frequently take more than the recommended dose. Ingesting two or three times the regular dose may result in transient disorientation and hallucinations, especially in emotionally unstable individuals. Further, marked overdoses (15 to 30 tablets) taken accidentally by children may result in stupor, confusion, and extreme psychiatric disturbance; coma and even death have been reported (Goth, 1984).

Benzodiazepine treatment of insomnia. There are some clinical conditions that call for periods of adjunctive use of hypnotics. For example, drugs may be given to manage chronic insomnia that is unrelated to physical or environmental deterrents to sleep, or transitory insomnia brought on by stressors of one sort or another. They can also be useful for persons traveling across many time zones in a short period of time, or for persons experiencing a shift in working hours. Each of these conditions may call for different types of hypnotic medication.

A hypnotic used for insomnia during a brief hospital stay should have a long duration that leads to restful nights, and if some of the hypnotic effects last into the normal waking hours, the additional sleep time is of little consequence and may even be beneficial. In this instance flurazepam, with its gradual onset and long duration of action due to the prolonged half-life of its active metabolite, desalkylflurazepam (40–250 hours), would normally be appropriate. Also suitable would be diazepam, with its long-lasting metabolite desmethyldiazepam (36–200 hours). Further, when treatment is terminated, these drugs disappear from the body as slowly as they accumulate, thereby minimizing the development of withdrawal effects.

When prescribed for outpatient insomniacs, flurazepam (30 mg) or nitrazepam (5 mg) also can be effective, at least for a while. In a 1-month trial in a sleep laboratory, polysomnographic studies revealed that flurazepam increased total sleep time by only 6% to 8%, with a modest shortening of sleep latency and an increase in stage 2 slow-wave sleep. Nevertheless, the patients subjectively reported marked sleep improvement. It was also found that these BDZs sharply curtailed the number of microawakenings, which, though lasting but a few seconds, each severely reduce the restorative aspects of sleep. Thus, the drug benefits may reside in the ability to enhance the continuity of sleep, if not its duration.

However, these drugs may not be appropriate for the long-term treatment of insomnia in elderly patients in hospitals or nursing homes. Patients with diminished metabolic efficiency can develop high plasma drug and metabolite accumulations, leading to daytime drowsiness, sedation, and impaired psychomotor and intellectual performance. In more serious instances, there were reports of light-headedness, increased reaction time, motor incoordination, confusion, dysarthria (slurred speech), and anterograde amnesia. Higher than recommended doses may also cause weakness, headache, blurred vision, vertigo, nausea and vomiting, epigastric distress, diarrhea, joint or chest pains, and incontinence. There may also be adverse psychological effects; for example, hypnotics can sometimes increase the incidence of nightmares, and flurazepam may cause garrulousness, anxiety, irritability, tachycardia, sweating, euphoria, restlessness, hallucinations, and manic behavior. These symptoms are frequently misdiagnosed as symptoms of senility, especially when elderly patients in nursing homes are routinely dosed with hypnotics at bedtime to minimize nocturnal awakenings. In the past flurazepam was prescribed for as many as 94% of nursing home patients, mostly, as it turned out, as a convenience to the nursing staffs, who believed that a sleeping patient is a good patient. If flurazepam is taken routinely, after the seventh night a patient may have 4 to 6 times the plasma level of the metabolite that was measured after the first night. Similar but less severe effects occur with chronic administration of nitrazepam. Even though some of these effects are partly offset by adaptation and tolerance, the resulting impairments were frequently confused with irreversible senility or dementia, which led to other inappropriate medication. For the elderly, hypnotics that do not undergo hepatic oxidation, such as oxazepam and lorazepam, would be better alternatives, but vigilance and caution within the medical staff would be just as important (Smith, 1979).

In the case of elderly outpatients, nightly use of flurazepam could also lead to a cumulative buildup in the blood plasma and brain, resulting in exaggerated hypnotic effects. Taken just before bedtime these effects of flurazepam would hardly be noticed, but if the effects persisted to the waking hours and the patient attempted to drive a motor vehicle, there might be serious consequences. Some serious accidents, particularly in elderly patients, have been directly attributed to the residual effects of BDZ hypnotics, and interactions with alcohol can be especially dangerous (Harvey, 1985; Hindmarch and

Ott, 1984). On the other hand, extensive studies in North America, Western Europe, and Australia on the possible role of anxiolytic and hypnotic BDZs in auto accidents, industrial accidents, and falls among the elderly have not shown that BDZ use, by itself, is a major contributor to those events, since the frequency of finding blood BDZs in the victims of nonfatal and fatal accidents alike is no greater than the frequency of their use in the general population. Moreover, insomniacs have frequently shown improvements of psychomotor control after use of hypnotics to improve sleep (see Woods, Katz, and Winger, 1992, pp. 229 ff.). Nonetheless, the possibility of severe drug buildup or hangover effects suggests cautionary measures for elderly BDZ users. One strategy to prevent drug buildup is the imposition of "drug holidays"; that is, the patient is advised not to take the drug for more than 2 or 3 nights in a row.

Lormetazepam, a drug that was designed to eliminate hangover effects, was investigated by Vogel (1984).

Lormetazepam

The drug has an intermediate to short elimination half-life, in the range of 5 to 15 hours, and thus is less likely to cause a cumulative plasma buildup and a hangover effect during daytime in elderly patients. Vogel tested the drug with otherwise healthy insomniac subjects aged 55 years and older (mean age 60) who were carefully screened to eliminate cases with obvious physical and psychiatric factors that might cause insomnia.

Comparing baseline sleep time with drug sleep time showed that lormetazepam increased the average total sleep time by about 25 minutes per night, and sleep latency and the number of awakenings were significantly reduced. Further, there was no evidence of drug tolerance over the 7 consecutive nights of drug treatment, nor any carryover of hypnotic effects or rebound insomnia upon drug withdrawal. Also, the subjects reported that they fell asleep sooner. Physical examination of the subjects every morning after drug treatment revealed a few reports of drowsiness or headache, but nothing more of any consequence. Hence, drugs with intermediate half-lives were deemed to be safe and efficacious and free of the consequences of hypnotics with longer elimination half-lives for this age group of patients.

Treatment of transient insomnia.   Some drugs are more appropriate than others for the complaint of delayed onset of sleep. The ideal drug would produce a short onset time for sleep, a 6–8 hour duration of sleep, and a prompt clearance to avoid carryover effects. Triazolam (Halcion) evolved from a search for such a drug. It is re-

Triazolam
(Halcion)

garded as being suitable for younger adult insomniacs who want to get to sleep more promptly, but do not want any daytime carryover of sleepiness. Triazolam is also appropriate when sudden shifts in the sleep–waking cycle have to be made. It is well known that intercontinental travelers require a few days to overcome jet lag, the daytime sleepiness and nighttime insomnia that results from traveling rapidly through several time zones. Jet lag may be a mere inconvenience during a vacation trip, but for a traveling diplomat, it may contribute to significant reductions in alertness, efficiency, and mood. For workers who undergo shift changes, the more often the switches occur, the worse are the effects, which may lead to accidents, impaired judgement, and loss of productivity in the workplace, as well as disturbances in family and interpersonal relationships. When these factors affect airplane pilots, truck drivers, and nuclear power plant personnel, the results of shift changes can have catastrophic consequences.

According to the U.S. Bureau of Labor Statistics, 20 million Americans (1 in 5) work other than daytime hours either consistently or on a rotating basis, and 80% of them have trouble sleeping. The number of night workers is increasing as telecommunications and transportation bind the U.S. economy to markets in different time zones. The *Wall Street Journal* reported that shift work costs companies $70 billion a year in lost productivity, medical bills, and industrial accidents, and there are reports that shift workers are more likely to suffer from digestive disorders, heart disease, and emotional problems, and are prone to accidents from falling asleep while driving home from work. Further, labor union studies have reported that shift work contributes to a higher incidence of divorce and juvenile delinquency. Presumably the juvenile problems were with the shift workers' children, who did not have the benefit of adequate parental supervision (see Levin, 1992).

Assuming that loss of sleep was a major factor in these circumstances, it seemed appropriate for physicians to prescribe hypnotics to promote rapid onset of sleep and to overcome the consequences of changes in sleep–waking cycles, with triazolam often being the drug of choice. Triazolam is rapidly absorbed and highly lipid soluble, which insures rapid uptake in the brain. It also has a short elimination half-life (2.7–4.5 hours), and is highly potent—the usual effective dose can be as low as 0.25 mg. When taken just before bedtime, the drug is usually cleared by oxidation before breakfast, thereby minimizing the possibility of work-time sleepiness.

The effectiveness of triazolam was investigated by Seidel and colleagues (1984), who compared it with flurazepam. Human subjects underwent drug treatment during 180° shifts in their sleep–waking schedules. After two placebo baseline nights of sleeping from midnight to 8:00 A.M., the subjects were switched to sleeping from noon to 8:00 P.M. During the double-blind drug tests, the subjects received either 0.5 mg triazolam, 30 mg flurazepam, or placebo 30 minutes before each sleep period, and upon awakening, completed a questionnaire about mood states. Also, a total of seven sleep latency tests (MSLT) were given to each subject at 2-hour intervals during waking time, along with other standard performance tests beginning at 10:00 P.M.

The results showed that during the first phase-reversal session (i.e., sleeping noon to 8:00 P.M.), there was a significant disruption in the sleep of the placebo-treated subjects, and somewhat less disruption during the second and third session, whereas the flurazepam and the triazolam groups did not differ significantly from baseline (Figure 16.22*a*). However, the results of the MSLT (Figure 16.22*b*) showed that the triazolam group did not

experience significant sleepiness, but the flurazepam-treated subjects, despite sufficient sleep, had a decidedly significant shorter average sleep latency when they were tested for sleepiness during the waking hours. The placebo-treated subjects also demonstrated significant sleepiness, although of a lesser severity than that of the flurazepam group. With respect to performance measures during waking time (data not shown), the same relationship held: the flurazepam group was impaired, the placebo group was less so, and the triazolam subjects either maintained or improved their performance over baseline.

However, in contrast to the differences among treatment groups on objective measures of waking-time functions, the subjective appraisals were the same for all three groups; that is, all subjects, including those who showed little waking-time sleepiness on the MSLT, reported an overall increase in sleepiness and mood disturbance during waking hours. This finding might be related to a retarded readjustment of circadian rhythms in these subjects, which may account for the mood disturbances that accompany changes in sleep–waking schedules.

In conclusion, the behavior of the placebo group confirmed that sleep and subsequent alertness is seriously impaired by sudden 12-hour shifts of sleep–waking schedules, and taking flurazepam or triazolam just prior to bedtime reversed the insomnia and sleep loss. Moreover, by promoting good sleep, the short half-life hypnotic triazolam contributed to normal, if not better, waking-time performance despite the 12-hour shift of bedtime. On the other hand, treating insomnia with flu-

(a)

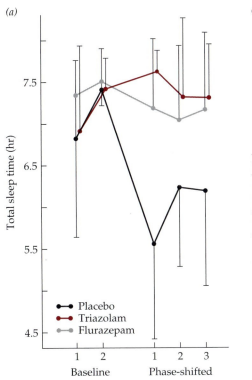

(b)

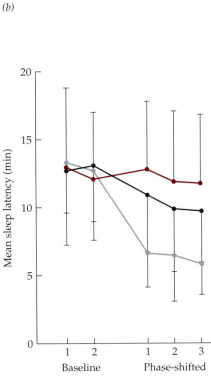

16.22 DRUG TREATMENT OF SLEEP–WAKE PHASE SHIFT INSOMNIA. (*a*) During two baseline nights (no drug), all subjects slept during the allotted sleep time (from midnight to 8:00 A.M.). Sleep time was then shifted to noon to 8:00 P.M., and the subjects received either triazolam, flurazepam, or placebo 30 minutes before bedtime. Placebo-treated subjects showed a statistically significant ($p < .05$) loss of sleep on the first phase-shifted night with partial recovery during the next two nights. The drug-treated groups slept normally during all three phase-shifted nights. (*b*) After phase-shifted sleep time, the subjects were given sleep latency tests (MSLT) beginning at 10:00 P.M. The placebo-treated subjects showed a significant decline in sleep latency, the triazolam-treated subjects showed no sign of sleepiness, and the flurazepam-treated subjects showed the most sleepiness. Each data point represents the mean sleep latency of seven tests (After Seidel et al., 1984.)

razepam, with its long half-life, can result in carryover hypnotic effects and decrements in alertness and performance even exceeding the effects of the 12-hour shift in bedtime without hypnotic treatment. Thus, flurazepam and drugs with similar kinetics are considered inappropriate in these situations, and BDZs with short half-lives seem to be a fair solution to the problem of sleep-time insomnia and waking-time sleepiness for workers who must undergo shift changes.

Adverse Effects of Triazolam

Within the last few years, there have been a number of stories of unusual and criminal behavior by users of triazolam. At the time of this writing, triazolam is the most widely prescribed hypnotic in the world, with about 7 million users in the United States using about half a million prescriptions per month. The drug is sold in more than 90 countries, and has annual sales of $250 million ($100 million in the United States alone). With such a large pool of users, there is a strong probability that there will be some reports of adverse effects that occur for a variety of reasons. Drug abusers and multidrug users will make a share of the claims of adverse effects. There will be mistaken recommendations for long-term use, and precipitous drug cessation will produce severe withdrawal effects. Also, the large population of insomniacs will include some social deviants and persons with psychiatric or behavioral disorders whose aberrant behavior may be released by the disinhibitory effects of BDZs. Finally, the drug may act in an inexplicable way in patients with an idiosyncratic hypersensitivity to BDZs.

The legal indictment of a drug and its manufacturer often depends upon a pattern of complaints related to the drug in question, but to be valid, the indictment should show that the drug had serious side effects even when it was appropriately prescribed and used. Also, when bizarre effects are traced to a licit drug like triazolam, adequate evidence to indict the drug is usually unavailable. For example, in a case in which overdose or multidrug usage may have been present, a replication of such events to prove or disprove the point is unlikely to be performed. During drug development, preclinical and clinical trials establish drug dosage and frequency and time of administration. However, these procedures do not apply when a drug is blamed for criminal acts; that is to say, the offender is not brought to a laboratory to have his or her pharmacokinetic reactions to the drug evaluated. Instead, the offender, through an expensive attorney, will claim immunity from prosecution and sue the drug company for all the trouble he has encountered. The court decision no doubt will depend somewhat upon the testimony of expert witnesses, whose views usually depend on whether the witness is testifying for the defending drug company or the plaintiff.

A few examples from an article in *Newsweek* (Cowley et al., 1991) will illustrate the controversy over the safety of Halcion:

1. A 57-year-old woman who had been taking Halcion for over a year shot her 83-year-old mother eight times, fatally wounding her. While taking Halcion, she became increasingly agitated and paranoid. After she had been taking the drug for months at a time, her doctor raised the dose when the usual drug effect dwindled. The charge of second-degree murder was dismissed, and she sued Upjohn Pharmaceutical Company, the manufacturer, for $21 million. Upjohn made an undisclosed settlement.

2. A physician, who was a director of a sleep disorder clinic, thought his mother was developing Alzheimer's disease or some other rapidly progressing dementia until he discovered that she was using Halcion and martinis to help her sleep. When she became anxious and confused, her husband gave her more Halcion during the day to help her. When the doctor discovered all the pill bottles and stopped the drug, she recovered uneventfully.

3. At 11:00 P.M. one night in Kalamazoo, Michigan (coincidentally, where Upjohn manufactures Halcion), a police officer with no criminal record took two 0.5 mg Halcion tablets, which was twice the already high dose his doctor recommended. At 2:00 A.M., he drove 30 miles to Battle Creek, where his ex-wife was staying. He broke down the door with a tire iron and found her with another man. He then stabbed her in the chest, almost killing her. At his trial he said he had no recollection of breaking down the door and the assault. He was convicted for assault with intent to commit murder. While in prison he saw an item on a television program about the dangers of Halcion. He hired a lawyer, got a retrial, and after two and a half years in prison, won his freedom. He now works as an electrician.

4. A California novelist received a prescription for Halcion and took it for the next 6 months. She became depressed and anxious and ended up "convinced that the world was on the brink of nuclear war or invasion from space." She also reported that after 2 weeks on Halcion, "my heart pounded and I was on the verge of tears much of the time. The slightest danger, such as having to make a left turn in traffic, put me in a sweat." Her therapist, instead of taking her off the drug, added alprazolam (Xanax), Halcion's close chemical cousin.

The "experts" cited in the *Newsweek* article disagreed over Halcion's safety. For example, Dr. Anthony Kales wrote,

This is a very dangerous drug. No other BDZ has such a narrow margin of safety. The only justification for keeping it on the market is to ensure the company's profitability. From the public health standpoint, there is no reason at all.

Dr. Thomas Roth wrote, "If used properly, this is a very, very safe hypnotic." Studies by Dr. David Greenblatt led to the conclusion that age has a lot to do with a patient's sensitivity to Halcion. He said he sees no special risks to older patients as long as the drug is properly prescribed. And Dr. Stuart Yudofsky, a neuropsychiatrist who studies aggression at the University of Chicago, said,

> I do believe that BDZs can be dangerous drugs. They can affect memory. They can affect concentration. They can affect attention. They can affect mood. They can affect spatial discrimination and perception. But, I don't believe they can cause people to murder other people. Far more people become violent on alcohol than on Halcion, but we don't excuse their behavior and sue the distilleries.

In response to a large number of spontaneous adverse reports over a 6-year period, the Food and Drug Administration's Psychopharmacological Drug Advisory Committee met to consider the evidence. Except for their recommendation that the warning label should mention that amnesia occurs at a higher rate with Halcion than with any other BDZ hypnotics, the committee members voted not to require any special measures. The committee chairman stated, "Given the limitations of the information we had, we did not sense [Halcion] had a special problem of side effects."

The cases and opinions cited above are not presented here to make a case for or against triazolam or any other drug. They are presented as a sample of the kind of controversy that sometimes develops with the appearance and use of any kind of drug.

Rebound insomnia. Unfortunately, drugs such as triazolam with short elimination half-lives have features that make their chronic use counterproductive. Kales, Scharf, and Kales (1978) found that after 2 weeks of nightly administration, triazolam markedly improved the induction and maintenance of sleep among insomniacs, but after the drug was withdrawn, sleep was markedly worsened: there were significant increases in sleep latency, time awake after the onset of sleep, and total time awake. The researchers designated these phenomena as components of rebound insomnia. In fact, after drug withdrawal, the total time awake was as much as three times over the predrug baseline level (Figure 16.23). Similar results were found after even 1 week of triazolam or nitrazepam (10 mg) treatment (half-life 18–34 hours); and although a small dose (1 mg) of flunitrazepam (half-life 10–20 hours) was ineffective for inducing or maintaining sleep during this period, sleep worsened significantly after drug withdrawal. Moreover, after 2 weeks of treatment, triazolam lost its effectiveness

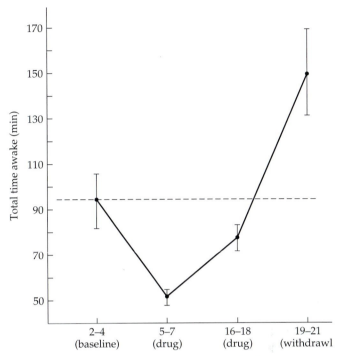

16.23 EFFICACY AND WITHDRAWAL EFFECTS OF TRIAZOLAM. Subjects were scored for the last 3 of 4 nights for time awake during sleeping hours to establish baseline. This was followed by 2 weeks of treatment with triazolam (0.5 mg) before bedtime (nights 5–18). The subjects were evaluated for wake time on nights 5–7 and 16–18. The subjects then underwent drug withdrawal and were observed for 3 additional nights (19–21). During the first 3 nights of drug treatment, there was an improvement of sleep, but by the last 3 nights, some drug tolerance had occurred. When triazolam was withdrawn, there was a marked rebound of sleeplessness (insomnia) above baseline. (After Goth, 1984; Kales et al., 1983.)

for improving sleep, but still worsened sleep after withdrawal. These effects are in contrast to the lack of withdrawal symptoms following treatments with flurazepam, diazepam, and lormetazepam, as well as other non-BDZ hypnotics whose elimination half-lives are considerably longer. Thus, the merits of BDZs with short half-lives are compromised by their tendency to cause rebound phenomena after sudden abstinence.

Early morning insomnia. It has long been known that although alcohol has sedative properties, its usefulness as a hypnotic is limited because its short elimination half-life increases wakefulness during the second half of the night. In an experiment using single nightly doses of hypnotic drugs with short elimination half-lives, induction of sleep was improved and sleep was maintained for about 6 hours, but thorough awakening occurred during the final hours of sleep, a phenomenon designated as early morning insomnia (Kales et al., 1983). In this experiment, which used subjects being treated for chronic insomnia, 20 mg of midazolam (half-life 1–4 hours) or 0.5 mg of triazolam (half-life 1.5–5 hours) were compared with 30 mg of flurazepam or quazepam, which are BDZs with long elimination half-lives (36–120 and 15–35 hours, respectively). Midazolam was administered for 7 nights, and the other drugs were administered for 14 nights.

The results showed that during nights 1 through 3, all the drugs significantly reduced time awake during the first 6 hours of sleep, but during the last 2 hours, the short half-life drugs (midazolam and triazolam) produced only slight, insignificant decreases in time awake, whereas flurazepam (Dalmane) and quazepam produced decreases in time awake equal to or greater than those in the first 6 hours. Further, during nights 5 through 7, the time awake for the midazolam subjects was reduced during the first 6 hours, but was increased by 103.3% during the last 2 hours. For the triazolam subjects during nights 12 through 14, time awake was decreased during the first 6 hours, but by the last 2 hours the drug efficacy was lost. In contrast, during nights 12 through 14, flurazepam and quazepam subjects maintained significant reductions in time awake during the last 2 hours just as they had during the first 6 hours.

Hence, hypnotics with short elimination half-lives rapidly induce sound sleep for about 6 hours, at which time the plasma concentration decreases below the efficacy threshold, and a rebound awakening occurs that shortens sleep time by about 2 hours (25%). In contrast, hypnotics with long elimination half-lives do not cause early morning awakening, nor do they cause rebound effects when the drugs are withdrawn. The differences between the drugs with short versus long half-lives becomes more pronounced the longer the drugs are taken. Thus, drugs that are rapidly eliminated produce the most frequent and intense worsening of sleep—either rebound insomnia or early morning insomnia. These effects are not unique to BDZs, as shown by the severe withdrawal effects that occur after long-term use of barbiturates with short half-lives.

The early morning insomnia, daytime anxiety, and rebound insomnia that accompany the use of triazolam and related compounds could reinforce drug-taking behavior and thus contribute to drug dependence. However, these findings should not automatically condemn such compounds as dangerous, because appropriate prescribing and treatment management can control the emergence of undesirable side effects.

BDZ Hypnotics: Management of Treatment

The adverse effects of BDZ hypnotics described above may well be the consequences of tolerance and withdrawal effects. Consequently, in clinical cases, the drugs should be administered intermittently and eventually withdrawn in a stepwise reduction of dose. If a patient uses the drug on an "as needed" basis over a considerable period, he or she should be advised to reduce the doses over time rather than abruptly discontinuing

them. If patients are not advised of this, and they abruptly stop using such hypnotics, they may sleep poorly on the first posttreatment night, and may therefore conclude that they can no longer sleep without the drug, thus embarking on a course of continued drug use while sleep worsens, doses increase, and the ultimate rebound effects become severe (Greenblatt, 1990).

The consequences of unsupervised long-term drug use and abrupt cessation of such use may be related to reports in the United States, as well as in Europe, of serious triazolam-related behavioral side effects such as confusional states, depersonalization, severe anxiety, or hallucinations. In 1990, the U.S. Food and Drug Administration reported that Halcion ranked first among 329 prescription drugs for the number of violent acts associated with those drugs in the United States. Media reports of cases such as those described above led to accusations of improper testing and a cover-up of adverse findings on the part of drug manufacturers. These cases caused enough concern that some countries banned the sale of triazolam until tablets of more than 0.25 mg were removed from sale. (In 1988 Upjohn even stopped manufacturing 0.5-mg tablets. Only 0.25-mg and 0.125-mg tablets are now available.)

Whereas the clinical consensus is that triazolam can be useful and safe and that the proportion of serious adverse effects is extremely small, some attention must be paid to these adverse effects. But first, it must be considered that the number of annual Halcion prescriptions (over 7 million) is several times higher than the number of prescriptions for other hypnotics such as flurazepam (Dalmane) or temazepam (Restoril). Hence, one would expect a greater incidence of adverse reactions even if all drugs are equally safe.

Second, Halcion, as a fast-onset, short-duration hypnotic, has a built-in proclivity toward adverse reactions if it is not prescribed and used appropriately. In particular, patients with a history of substance abuse, especially with alcohol and barbiturates, are at extreme risk after Halcion overdoses even if they took only two or three times the recommended dose. Further, the risk is greater after long-term use. This means that the drug should be prescribed only for otherwise healthy individuals, at low doses, for short-term intermittent use, and not when drug abuse or multidrug reactions are possibilities. Further, attention has to be paid to other factors that affect drug responses, even when a patient seems to be at low risk. Such factors are the nature and causes of the insomnia complaint, the emotional stability of the patient, and his or her relationship to the physician in charge of the case. Ignoring these factors and allowing unsupervised long-term use of drugs with short half-lives followed by precipitous cessation creates a scenario with possibly dire consequences.

Above all, sedative–hypnotic and anxiolytic drugs may be categorized as a special group of drugs that are subject to abuse primarily because they directly affect consciously perceived feelings of well-being. Because these drugs promptly reduce anxiety, tension, and insomnia, taking them is highly reinforcing, which may contribute to persistent use. Thus, they need to be dispensed with great care.

Part IV Summary

Anxiety is a constant presence that can at times be severe and disabling. Until the advent of the BDZs, there were no anxiolytic drugs that were as safe and effective and had a low abuse potential. The magnitude of any possible danger in the use of BDZs is sharply lower than that of their pharmacological predecessors. Moreover, molecular studies have provided a rational basis for BDZ treatment of anxiety and some sleep disorders. Newer compounds, particularly the serotonergic anxiolytics, such as buspirone, also seem to be appropriate treatments in some cases.

However, the popularity of the BDZs has also become a source of concern. This concern applies mainly to the relatively small number of of long-term users of BDZ anxiolytics or hypnotics. Many of these cases have been found to have links with past or current use of alcohol or other hypnotics, and some users have become tolerant to the BDZs and have escalated their doses. Most of these rare cases have occurred where there was a history of substance abuse, or among persons with a history of emotional instability. Such individuals tend to select a pattern of drug use for short-term relief of anxiety or insomnia, but come to perpetuate their use, which leads to an increase of dosages to dangerous levels and withdrawal effects.

In conclusion, the consensus seems to be that the need for anxiolytic drugs is real and that the BDZs are superior to most other drugs in their efficacy, their range of applicability, and their therapeutic indices. Compared with alcohol, which is a daily alternative anxiolytic drug for many people, the benefits of the BDZs are even more pronounced. But it goes almost without saying that drugs by themselves do not solve personal problems, even though they can interrupt the production of anxiety or suppress its symptoms so that problems become more amenable to psychotherapy when it is needed. Nonetheless, though some patients may legitimately require long-term assistance with BDZs, some members of the medical profession are concerned about the chronic use of BDZs as anxiolytics, sedatives, and hypnotics. Whereas BDZs have a relatively low abuse potential, in some instances misuse, abuse, or dependence can have serious consequences, especially when their use is combined with other drugs and alcohol.

Chapter 17

Mind-Altering Drugs

This chapter covers a collection of chemically disparate substances: marijuana, phencyclidine (PCP), and LSD. These substances do not fit readily into either of the classic categories of CNS stimulants or depressants. They all share an ability to profoundly alter mood state and perceptual–motor functioning; nevertheless, a reading of the individual sections below will quickly reveal that the grouping together of these substances is primarily a matter of convenience, and in no way is meant to imply a common mechanism of action.

Part I
Marijuana and the Cannabinoids

In this section we focus on the flowering hemp, a weedlike plant given the botanical name of *Cannabis sativa* by Linnaeus in 1753. Historically, hemp has served an important function in many cultures as a source of fiber for making rope, cloth, and even paper. At times, its seeds have also been used for their oil content and as bird feed. More importantly for neuropharmacologists, cannabis plants contain over 60 compounds collectively known as **cannabinoids** (Turner, 1984). The psychoactive properties of some of these compounds account for the use of cannabis as a drug. Although cannabinoids can be found to some extent in all parts of the plant, they are concentrated in a sticky yellowish resin that is secreted in particularly large amounts by the flowering tops of female plants.

Cannabis can be consumed in a number of different forms. The form that is most familiar to Americans, of course, is **marijuana** (from the Mexican word *maraguanquo*, meaning "an intoxicating plant"), a crude mixture of dried and crumbled leaves, small stems, and flowering tops. It is usually smoked, although an alternative approach is to bake it in cookies or brownies for oral consumption. Marijuana potency (in terms of active cannabinoid content) varies widely, depending on the genetic strain of the plant as well as its growing conditions. One method of significantly increasing potency is to prevent pollination of, and hence seed production by, the female plants. Marijuana produced by this method is called sinsemilla (meaning "without seeds"). In general, marijuana potency is higher now than it was some years ago, and regular users indeed have been found to prefer the stronger drug (Chait and Burke, 1994).

Another type of cannabis derivative is **hashish**, which also may be smoked or eaten. The potency of hashish depends greatly on how it has been prepared. In the Middle and Far East, "hashish" generally refers to a relatively pure resin preparation that is quite high in cannabinoid content. Alternatively, the term may be used to describe solvent extracts of leaves or resin that are more variable in their potency. A particularly potent form of hashish is "hash oil," an alcoholic extract that has been reduced to an oily, viscous liquid ranging in color from amber to black. A single drop of hash oil may be placed on a standard tobacco cigarette and smoked, or a drop may be added to a marijuana cigarette to effectively double the dose.

The History of Cannabis Use

Cannabis is believed to have originated in central Asia, probably in China. The earliest historical reference to cannabis dates back over 4,000 years to a legendary Chinese emperor named Chen Nung (Li, 1975). However, Western interest in this substance did not begin until the early to middle 19th century, when some of Napoleon's soldiers reportedly brought hashish from Egypt back with them to France (Mickel, 1969). At about the same time, a French physician named Jacques-Joseph Moreau encountered the intoxicating effects of hashish in the course of several trips to the Middle East. After returning to Paris, Moreau helped to found a notorious association of French writers and artists known as "Le Club des Haschischins" ("Club of the Hashish Eaters"), which included such notables as Victor Hugo, Alexander Dumas, Théophile Gautier, and Charles Baudelaire.

The history of cannabis in the United States dates back to the colonial era, when hemp was an important agricultural commodity. George Washington himself was a hemp farmer (Grinspoon, 1977), which is ironic in view of the patriotic fervor associated with the contemporary "War on Drugs." Yet domestic hemp growers of the 17th and 18th centuries apparently had little awareness of the plant's intoxicating properties. Rather, historians believe that the social practice of consuming cannabis (mainly marijuana smoking) was brought into the United States in the early 1900s by Mexican immigrants crossing the Mexican–American border, and by the Caribbean sailors and West Indian immigrants entering the country by way of New Orleans and other ports on the Gulf of Mexico (Bonnie and Whitebread, 1974).

Marijuana use spread rapidly outward from these points of origin. By the 1920s and 1930s, the popular press was filled with lurid accounts attesting to the violent and criminal propensities of marijuana smokers. Finally, in 1937, the federal government passed the Marijuana Tax Act, which instituted a national registration and taxation system aimed at discouraging all use of cannabis for commercial, recreational, and medical purposes. Although this legislation was overturned as unconstitutional by the U.S. Supreme Court in 1969, cannabis remains tightly regulated by state laws and by the federal Controlled Substances Act of 1970. As the reader is undoubtedly aware, the issues surrounding the legal status of marijuana and the penalties associated with marijuana use continue to be controversial in many societies, including our own (see Kleiman, 1989).

Cannabinoid Pharmacology: Chemical Structures, Pharmacokinetics, and Metabolism

The basic structure common to most cannabinoids is shown in Figure 17.1. Historically, cannabinoid nomenclature has been plagued by the use of two different

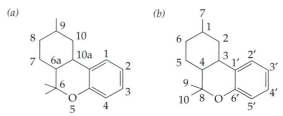

17.1 BASIC CANNABINOID STRUCTURE AND NUMBERING SYSTEMS. Naturally occurring cannabinoids possess a three-membered ring structure that can be numbered using two different systems: (*a*) the dibenzopyran numbering system and (*b*) the monoterpenoid numbering system. (After Nahas, 1975.)

numbering systems by different investigators. One system treats cannabinoids as dibenzopyrans, whereas the second system is based on conventions used for monoterpenoids. The dibenzopyran numbering system favored by most American investigators will be used in this chapter, although figures from other sources may use the monoterpenoid system.

Cannabinoid Structure and Activity

An early review by Todd (1946) describes chemical studies of cannabis dating back to the mid-nineteenth century. Modern cannabinoid pharmacology really began in 1964, however, when Gaoni and Mechoulam identified Δ^9- (alternatively Δ^1-) tetrahydrocannabinol (THC) as the major active ingredient of *C. sativa*. Another cannabinoid

Δ^9-**Tetrahydrocannabinol**

found in *C. sativa*, Δ^8-THC, is about three-fourths as potent as THC, yet it contributes little to the psychoactive effects of marijuana because it is found in only small amounts in the plant. Cannabinol (CBN) and cannabid-

Δ^8-**Tetrahydrocannabinol**

iol (CBD) are major constituents of the plant quantitatively and are active in some cellular systems in vitro (Martin, 1986). However, CBN and CBD are relatively inactive in several animal models of cannabimimetic activity, and neither compound is psychoactive in humans when administered orally (Hollister, 1974; Pertwee, 1990). These cannabinoids are therefore not of major importance to neuropsychopharmacologists.

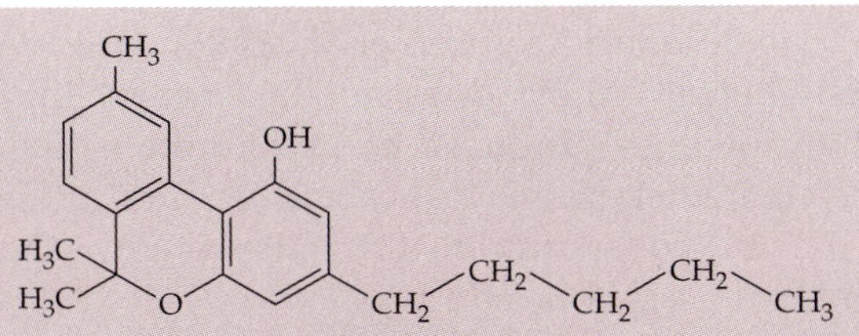

Cannabinol

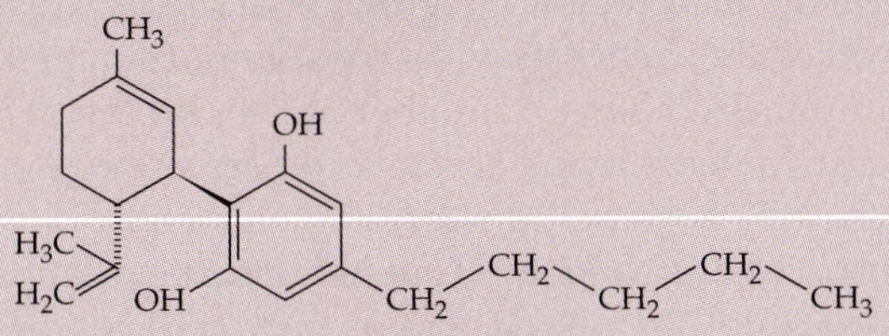

Cannabidiol

Since the discovery of THC over 25 years ago, much has been learned about the structural requirements for cannabinoid activity. The study of cannabinoid structure–activity relationships has given rise to a variety of potent synthetic cannabinoids, including levonantradol, nabilone, dimethylheptyl derivatives of Δ^9- and Δ^8-THC, such as 9-nor-9-β-hydroxyhexahydrocannabinol and 11-OH-Δ^8-tetrahydrocannabinol-dimethylheptyl, the bicyclic compounds CP 55,940 and CP 55,244, and a group of novel aminoalkylindole compounds including WIN 55212. These drugs have proved highly useful in canna-

Levonantradol

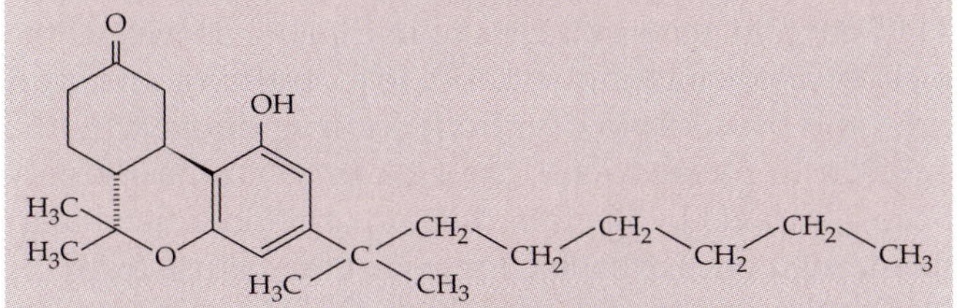

Nabilone

9-Nor-9-β-Hydroxyhexahydrocannabinol

11-OH-Δ^8-Tetrahydrocannabinol-dimethylheptyl

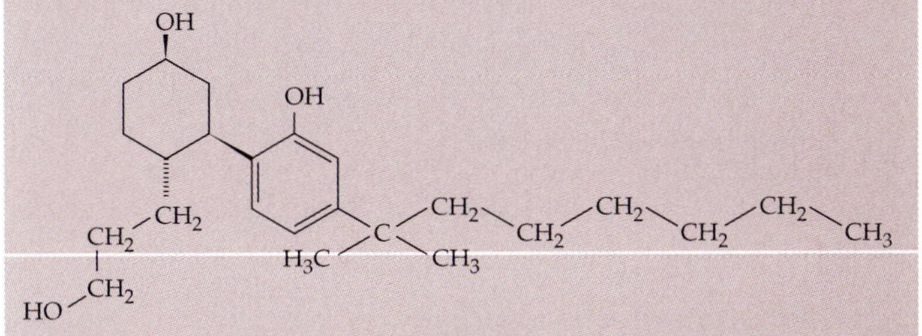

CP 55,940

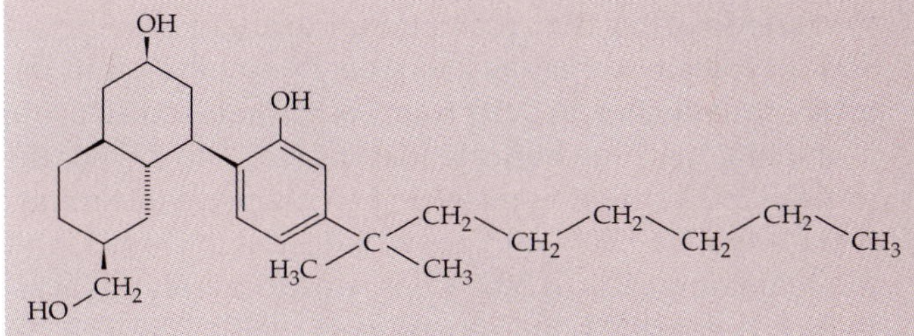

CP 55,244

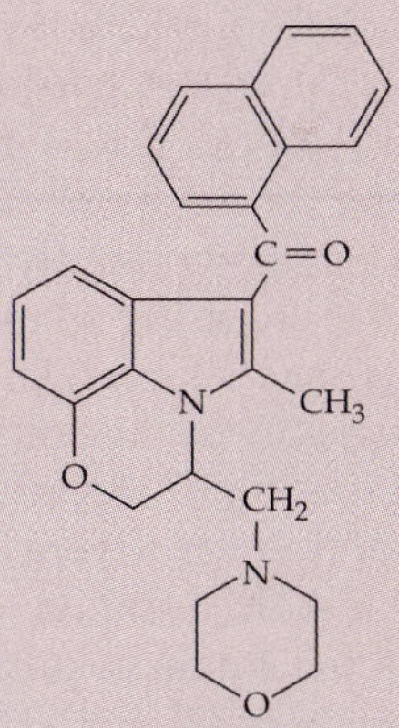

WIN 55212

binoid research and, in some cases, in the clinical realm as well. Readers who want further information on cannabinoid structure–activity relationships are referred to excellent reviews by Makriyannis and Rapaka (1990), Martin and coworkers (1991), Mechoulam and Feigenbaum (1987), and Razdan (1986).

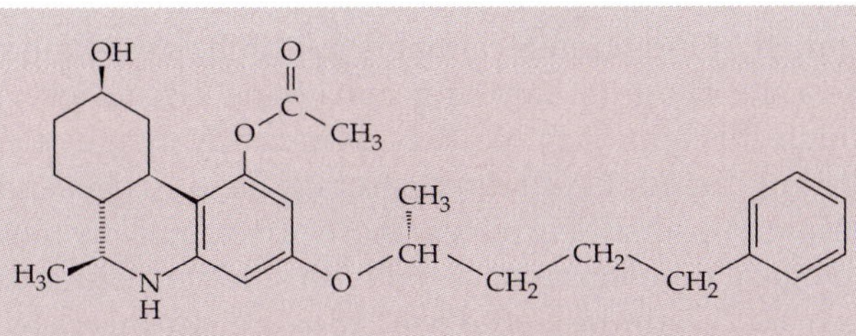

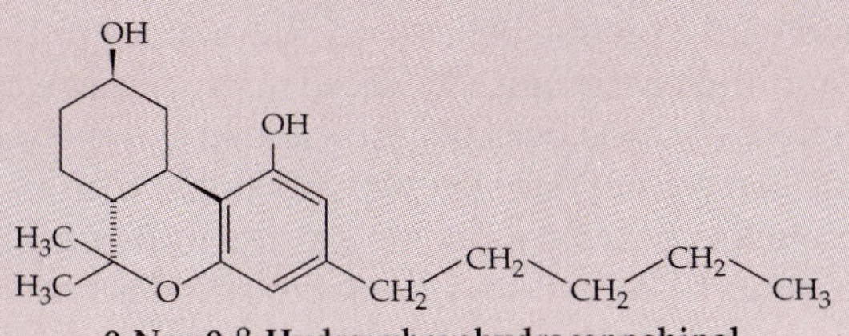

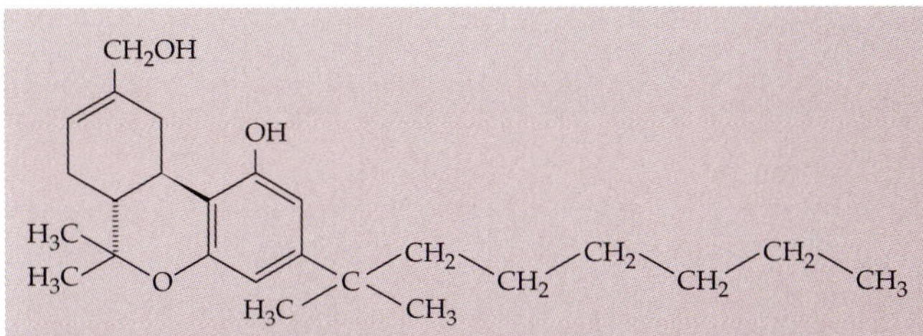

Few, if any, selective cannabinoid antagonists were available prior to the cloning and characterization of CNS cannabinoid receptors in the late 1980s (see below); however, several useful antagonists are now available. These antagonists include bromopravadoline, iodopravadoline (AM630), and SR 141716A (Pertwee et al., 1995; Rinaldi-Carmona et al., 1995).

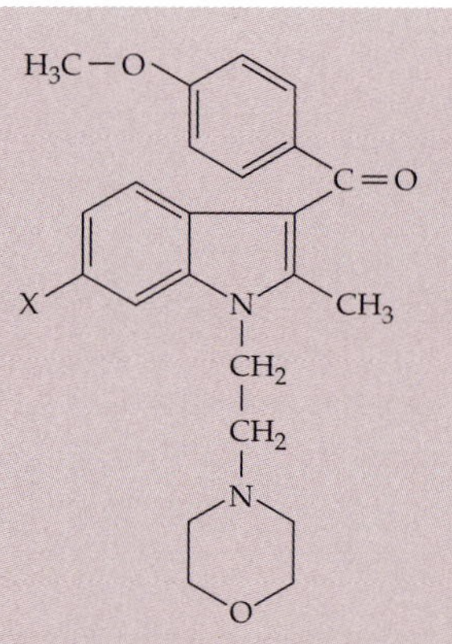

Bromopravadoline (X=Br)
Iodopravadoline (AM630) (X=I)   SR 141716A

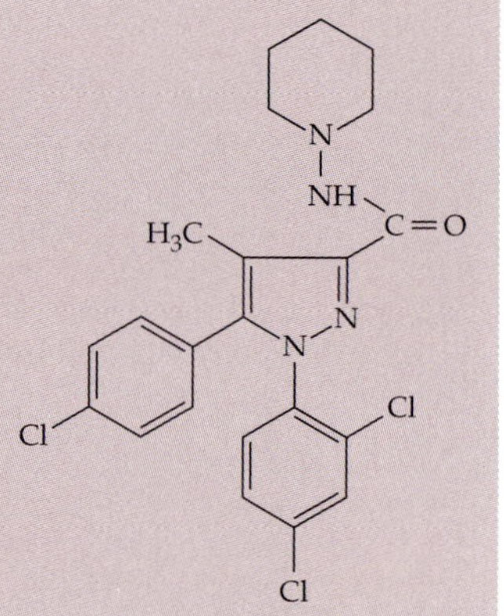

Cannabinoid Absorption, Metabolism, and Clearance

We noted earlier that recreational users in the United States typically consume cannabis by smoking it in the form of marijuana. Results from controlled studies using a smoking machine indicate that only 20% to 37% of the initial THC content is recovered in mainstream smoke, whereas 40% to 50% escapes in sidestream smoke, and the remaining 23% to 30% is lost due to pyrolytic (heat-induced) degradation (Perez-Reyes, 1990). The THC in the mainstream smoke is rapidly absorbed through the lungs into the circulation, where it is almost completely bound to plasma proteins. According to the studies of Perez-Reyes (1990), plasma THC concentrations peak at the time of smoking termination when marijuana cigarettes are smoked relatively rapidly; however, peak levels may be reached even earlier when the smoking rate is slower. Other experiments found that increasing the puff volume caused significant elevations in plasma THC concentration and the "high" reported by subjects (Azorlosa, Greenwald, and Stitzer, 1995). On the other hand, increasing the breathhold duration (which is widely believed to enhance marijuana's subjective effects) produced smaller changes in plasma THC and had virtually no effect on the marijuana "high."

Once the plasma peak has been attained, the rate of clearance of THC from smoked marijuana is similar to that observed for pure THC given by intravenous injection (Figure 17.2). In contrast, oral consumption of marijuana leads to prolonged but poor absorption of THC, resulting in low and variable plasma concentrations. The reduced bioavailability of THC following oral consumption compared with smoking probably results from a combination of degradation in the stomach and "first-pass" hepatic metabolism (Agurell et al., 1986; Chiang and Barnett, 1989). That is, once orally ingested THC has been absorbed from the gastrointestinal tract, it must pass through the liver, where it undergoes extensive transformation before entering the systemic circulation.

By performing clearance studies over periods of 48 hours or longer, researchers have been able to calculate the final elimination rate (expressed as terminal half-life; $t_{\frac{1}{2}}$) of THC. Most such studies have found the $t_{\frac{1}{2}}$ to average 20 to 30 hours (Agurell et al., 1986). However, the psychological "high" does not last nearly this long. Rather, the high produced by smoking a single marijuana cigarette typically lasts about 3 hours, after which the plasma concentration has fallen below the level needed for a euphoric effect.

THC metabolism and excretion have been covered in several detailed reviews (Agurell et al., 1986; Chiang and Barnett, 1989); hence only the most important points will be summarized here. A number of sites on the THC molecule are subject to metabolic transformation. As shown in Figure 17.3, these transformations include allylic and aliphatic hydroxylations, double-bond epoxidation or reduction, and glucuronic acid or fatty acid condensation reactions. THC metabolites are excreted mainly in the feces (about two-thirds of an administered dose), with the remainder appearing in the urine. More than 24 THC metabolites have been identified in human excreta thus far, some of which are biologically active. Even after intravenous injection of a single THC dose, the metabolites have not been fully cleared within 5 days. Slow clearance of THC and its metabolites is due to sequestration of these compounds in adipose (fat) tissue followed by their gradual release back into the circulation.

Acute Behavioral and Physiological Effects in Humans

In much of the human cannabis research, subjects have taken the drug by smoking marijuana cigarettes. Although this approach has the obvious advantage of duplicating the route of administration usually chosen by marijuana users themselves, there are numerous methodological problems associated with studying drugs that are usually administered via smoking. In the case of cannabis, these problems include wide variations in THC content across batches of marijuana as well as the influence of smoking patterns (e.g., puff volume, puff rate, and breathhold duration) on drug delivery to the subject. In recent years, the first problem has largely been alleviated by the introduction of standardized marijuana cigarettes available for experimental use from the National Institute on Drug Abuse (NIDA). With respect to the parameters of smoking behavior, investigators routinely give precise behavioral instructions to the subjects and then ascertain that these instructions were followed as closely as possible. In summary, contemporary cannabis research has successfully dealt with many of the problems posed by smoking as the route of drug administration. These issues must nevertheless be kept in mind, particularly when evaluating earlier studies in which these control procedures were not in use.

(a)

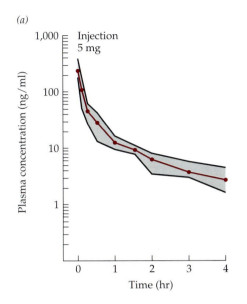

(b)

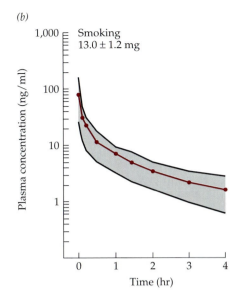

17.2 PLASMA THC CONCENTRATIONS VARY WITH THE ROUTE OF ADMINISTRATION. Plasma THC concentrations (mean ± range) were measured for 4 hours following administration of the indicated dose of Δ^9-THC by (a) intravenous injection, (b) smoking, or (c) oral ingestion in a chocolate cookie. Note the lower concentrations, broader peak, and greater variability produced by oral administration. (After Agurell et al., 1986.)

(c)

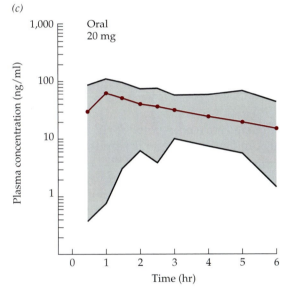

reported profound personality changes and perceptual distortions, even frank hallucinations. Indeed, administration of high doses of pure THC can produce hallucinogenic effects in human subjects (Isbell et al., 1967).

The lower cannabis doses associated with smoking one or two marijuana cigarettes produce a somewhat more modest reaction, although many of the same *kinds* of effects are found across the dose–response curve. The subjective and behavioral effects commonly associated with marijuana intoxication are summarized in Tart (1971) and in Grinspoon (1977). These effects include feelings of euphoria and exhilaration, a sense of disinhibition manifested as increased laughter, volubility (talkativeness), and/or hyperactivity, and heightened hunger and thirst. Users often feel calm, relaxed, perhaps even in a dreamlike state, although opposing reactions of restlessness, agitation, and even anxiety can also be experi-

Cannabis Intoxication

The earliest recorded clinical studies on the intoxicating properties of cannabis were performed by Moreau, the French physician mentioned earlier who introduced hashish to nineteenth-century Parisian literary society. As a result of his experiences with hashish, Moreau (who is sometimes called the "Father of Psychopharmacology") became interested in the possible relationship between the state of intoxication produced by this substance and the characteristics of mental illness. Consequently, Moreau and his students meticulously recorded their subjective experiences after consuming varying amounts of hashish.* Due to the potency of their preparation, these individuals

---

*Moreau's work culminated in a book entitled *Du Hachich et de l'aliénation mentale* (*Hashish and Mental Alienation*), major excerpts of which can be found in Nahas (1975).

17.3 MAJOR SITES OF THC METABOLISM. (After Halldin et al., 1984.)

enced. A number of sensory effects have been reported, such as feelings of lightheadedness, floating sensations, enhanced visual and auditory perception, visual illusions, and a tremendous slowing of time passage. Cognitive effects are varied. Some individuals report feeling more childlike and open to new experiences. On the other hand, cognitive decrements are noticeable in terms of poorer problem solving, illogical thinking, impaired short-term memory, and a tendency to be sidetracked more easily (see the section below on performance measures). Sociability can also undergo different types of changes in that the user may experience either an increased desire to be with others or a desire to be alone. As with most psychoactive drugs, the characteristics of marijuana intoxication vary greatly with the dose, the setting, the subject's mental set, and his or her past exposure to the drug.

Hollister (1986) noted that marijuana use can evoke several types of psychopathological reactions, including strong feelings of anxiety or panic, paranoid reactions, and (at high doses) a state of delirium. Flashbacks, which are widely known to occur in LSD users, have occasionally been reported for marijuana as well. Although some authors have suggested the existence of a specific cannabis-induced psychosis, this concept remains questionable (Thomas, 1993).

In accordance with the previously discussed time course of THC absorption and appearance in the circulation (see Figure 17.2), the peak "high" is reached much more rapidly with smoking or intravenous injection than with oral administration (Figure 17.4). Nevertheless, users who are smoking marijuana do not reach this peak until sometime after the cigarette has been finished. This delay means that the maximum level of intoxication occurs when plasma THC concentrations are already declining (Agurell et al., 1986; Chiang and Barnett, 1984), suggesting that the brain and plasma THC concentrations are not yet equilibrated at the time when the plasma level is peaking. Another possible factor is the contribution of active THC metabolites (whose peak does not coincide with that of THC itself) to the psychoactive properties of marijuana.

Learning, Memory, and Other Cognitive Functions

Clinical accounts of marijuana intoxication have commonly noted deficits in thought processes and in verbal behavior. These deficits may include illogical or disordered thinking, fragmented speech, and difficulty in remaining focused on a given topic of conversation (see Tart, 1971). The early descriptive work subsequently gave rise to quantitative experimental assessments of marijuana's effects on learning, memory, and other cognitive processes. Marijuana administration does not seem to impair subjects' ability to recall simple, "real-world" information (Block and Wittenborn, 1986; Darley et al., 1977). On the other hand, drug-induced perfor-

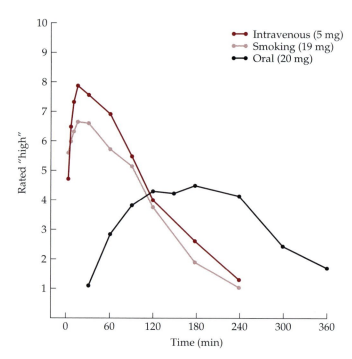

17.4 TIME COURSE OF SUBJECTIVE "HIGH" RATINGS AS A FUNCTION OF ROUTE OF THC ADMINISTRATION. (After Agurell et al., 1986.)

mance decrements have been noted for a variety of verbal, spatial, time estimation, and reaction time tasks (Block, Farinpour, and Braverman, 1992; Ferraro, 1980). Many of these results can be explained by postulating some type of drug-induced memory impairment, although other possibilities exist as well. One factor accounting for diminished performance in verbal free recall tasks is the occurrence of memory intrusions, extraneous items not on the original stimulus list but seemingly "remembered" by the subject (Hooker and Jones, 1987). It is also interesting to note that significant prior marijuana usage may reduce the adverse cognitive effects of acute marijuana exposure. Some investigators have accordingly proposed that behavioral ("cognitive") tolerance develops in heavy marijuana smokers (Cohen and Rickles, 1974).

Psychomotor Performance

Marijuana not only can impair cognitive functioning, but also has deleterious effects on psychomotor performance (Manno et al., 1974; Tinklenberg and Darley, 1975). When low doses of marijuana and relatively simple tasks are used, drug-induced performance deficits may show up only in previously naive subjects (Weil, Zinberg, and Nelsen, 1968). However, it is clear that even experienced users display impaired psychomotor functioning when difficult tasks are used and when the marijuana dose is moderate or high (Barnett, Licko, and Thompson, 1985).

Psychomotor deficits caused by marijuana can have very real social consequences if the user attempts to drive an automobile, operate heavy machinery, or even fly an airplane before the effects of the drug have fully dissipated. Klonoff (1974) investigated the performance-altering effects of marijuana on an off-street driving course as well as on the streets of Vancouver during varied traffic conditions.* Smoking a single 700-mg marijuana cigarette with a THC content of 1.2% led to a decline in driving performance by most subjects, although performance actually improved in a few cases. In laboratory experiments conducted by Barnett, Licko, and Thompson (1985), the effects of smoking a single standardized marijuana cigarette were examined using several different tasks thought to reflect skills important for driving. Not only were substantial decrements found on all measures, but performance generally was not restored to normal levels until 10 to 12 hours after smoking (Figure 17.5). Because of such marijuana-induced psychomotor deficits, it is prudent for users to avoid heavy machine operation for a substantial period of time after smoking. Nevertheless, a consideration of all available evidence suggests that marijuana is not a major risk factor for automobile accidents, particularly in comparison to alcohol (Jones, 1987a; Gieringer, 1988).

Acute Physiological Effects of Cannabis

Marijuana smoking typically produces tachycardia (increased pulse rate) (Dewey, 1986; Hollister, 1986), an effect that is thought to be due to reduced activity of the vagus nerve. Blood pressure is either unchanged or may drop slightly. Other common physiological changes include reddening of the conjunctiva (sometimes called "red-eye"), decreased muscle strength, and increased hunger. Acute effects on the endocrine system have been reported by several investigators (Cone et al., 1986). Finally, marijuana smoking or pure THC administration has an analgesic action under some conditions (Segal, 1986), although the literature in this area is far from consistent.

Therapeutic Uses of Cannabinoids

Medicinal use of cannabis in various cultures can be traced back for many hundreds, perhaps thousands, of years (see Mechoulam, 1986). During the late nineteenth and early twentieth centuries, crude cannabis extracts were accepted pharmaceuticals in Europe and the United States (six different types of preparations were listed in the 1896 Merck Index), although they tended to be unstable and had inconsistent potency. Although the medicinal use of cannabis later declined, interest in the possible therapeutic benefits of cannabinoids was revived following the discovery of THC and the subsequent manufacture and testing of various synthetic

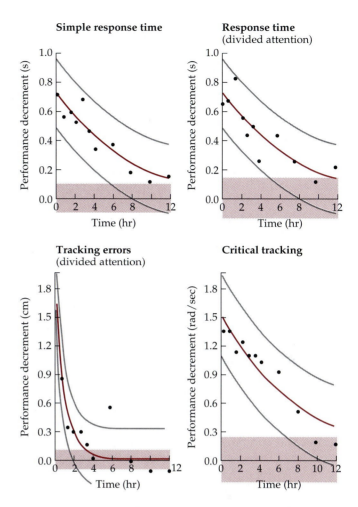

17.5 TIME COURSE OF PERFORMANCE DECREMENTS FOLLOWING MARIJUANA SMOKING. Subjects smoked one marijuana cigarette containing 250 μg THC per kg body weight. Over the next 12 hours, psychomotor performance was assessed using four different tasks. The shaded area at the bottom of each graph indicates the standard error of baseline performance (0 decrement) on that task. The curves represent the mean (middle curves) ± *SE* performance decrement as a function of time. (After Barnett, Licko, and Thompson, 1985.)

analogs. At present, both THC (under the trade name Marinol) and the synthetic analog nabilone (trade name Cesamet) are prescribed in oral form for the treatment of nausea and vomiting (emesis) in cancer patients undergoing chemotherapy who are not helped by other antiemetics. Marinol is also approved for use as an appetite stimulant in AIDS patients suffering from anorexia. One disadvantage of orally administered cannabinoids is the variable absorption described earlier. With this in mind, a THC-containing rectal suppository was recently developed that avoids first-pass hepatic metabolism and produces higher, more sustained circulating drug concentrations (Mattes et al., 1993).

Beyond the limited uses of THC in cancer chemotherapy and AIDS, researchers have been interested in

---

*Lest the reader fear that safety concerns were overlooked, it should be noted that the on-street driving tests were performed using a dually controlled automobile with an expert driver at the auxiliary controls.

possible cannabinoid applications in analgesia, bronchodilation (antiasthma), anticonvulsant/antispasmodic action, and the reduction of intraocular pressure (in glaucoma patients) (Hollister, 1986; Lemberger, 1980; Mechoulam and Feigenbaum, 1987). For cannabinoid drugs to achieve significant acceptance as clinical agents, psychoactivity (with its associated performance decrements and abuse potential) must be minimized or eliminated while therapeutic efficacy is retained. Although this goal has not yet been reached, neuropharmacologists are continuing to search for novel cannabinoids with selective (and hence therapeutically useful) biological actions. The identification and cloning of the cannabinoid receptor several years ago (see below) should help tremendously in this quest.

Acute Behavioral Effects in Animals

With the exception of some primate studies involving inhalation of marijuana smoke, most of the cannabis research on animals has involved injection of purified THC or other naturally occurring or synthetic cannabinoids. Using this approach, investigators have made great strides in elucidating the mechanisms of cannabinoid action, understanding structure–activity relationships within the cannabinoid family, and developing new experimental compounds. Some of these topics will be taken up in later sections.

Unconditioned Behavior

Following the identification in 1964 of THC as the major biologically active constituent of cannabis, researchers began to examine the effects of this drug on unconditioned behaviors in various animal species. These early studies quickly showed that THC produced motor impairment, catalepsy, hypothermia, and analgesia in mice and rats (Gill, Paton, and Pertwee, 1970; Grunfeld and Edery, 1969). At low doses, THC actually elicits a mixture of excitatory and depressant effects. At higher doses, the drug produces a more uniform motor depression and catalepsy, although hyperactivity may be seen initially as the plasma drug concentration rises. The neural pathways mediating these responses include the nucleus accumbens (Conti and Musty, 1984) and the corpus striatum (Gough and Olley, 1978), structures known to be involved in the motoric effects of dopaminergic drugs.

Other effects of cannabinoids on rodent behavior include decreased food intake, anticonvulsant or proconvulsant activity (depending on the dose and test system), and increased aggressive behavior (Dewey, 1986). THC has been observed either to enhance aggressiveness by itself (typically following chronic administration) or to potentiate aggressive behavior elicited by other stimuli.

The effects of THC on spontaneous behavior have been used to devise several screening tests for cannabi-

mimetic activity (Mechoulam and Feigenbaum, 1987). One such procedure, the "ring immobility test," is a means of quantifying cannabinoid-induced cataleptic behavior in mice (Pertwee, 1972). The subject is placed across a horizontal wire ring and its activity monitored for 5 minutes. The proportion of time spent immobile ("immobility index") is dose-dependent and is taken as a measure of catalepsy. Other useful procedures are based on the behavior of dogs and monkeys. THC-treated dogs exhibit a characteristic static ataxia, typically accompanied by a tucking of the tail. Administering larger amounts leads to a stuporous state that may last for over an hour. The effects in monkeys are likewise dose dependent. Low doses of THC elicit partial motor impairment and an apparent taming effect, whereas high doses cause ptosis (drooping eyelids), severe ataxia, stupor, and assumption of a crouched posture sometimes termed the "thinker position" (Grunfeld and Edery, 1969; Mechoulam and Feigenbaum, 1987).

Operant Behavior

The influence of THC on animals has also been assessed by examining changes in stimulus-controlled operant behavior. Such changes can be taken as indices of potential drug effects on human cognitive and motivational functioning. Early studies showed that THC administration reduced the rate of operant responding in both rats and pigeons (see Dewey, 1986). Accuracy of performance was also affected in some cases. Subsequent experiments have obtained similar findings using rhesus monkeys (Schulze et al., 1988, 1989).

Discriminative Stimulus Properties of THC

Although the behavioral measures described in the previous two sections have proved useful in screening for cannabinoid activity, they do not have a high level of specificity. Neuroleptic drugs such as chlorpromazine and haloperidol, for example, produce a cataleptic state indistinguishable from that produced by THC in the above-mentioned ring test. Moreover, the ability of various cannabinoids to produce an intoxicating state in humans is not always correlated with the drugs' effects on spontaneous behaviors or operant response rates in nonhuman subjects.

Fortunately, application of the drug discrimination learning paradigm has been able to surmount these problems to a significant degree. THC has been known for a number of years to produce internal stimulus effects that can direct responding in standard drug discrimination paradigms. Indeed, the stimulus properties of cannabinoids thus far seem to be unique in that no other drugs (including LSD and PCP) have yet been shown to substitute for the THC cue (Balster and Prescott, 1992). Moreover, with only minor exceptions, there is a good correspondence between the ability of various drugs to produce a THC-like discriminative stimulus and their effectiveness in producing a cannabis-like intoxicated state in humans. Thus, the drug discrimination paradigm probably provides the best animal model at this time for studying the mechanisms of human cannabinoid intoxication. A verbal response form of this technique has even been used to demonstrate that marijuana produces discriminable subjective effects in humans (Chait et al., 1988).

Reinforcing Effects of Cannabinoids

As we have seen in previous chapters, many drugs that are abused by humans are self-administered by laboratory animals. The self-administration paradigm has thus come to serve as an important measure of drug-induced reinforcement and a useful predictor of abuse liability. Several exceptions to this generalization have been found, however, including cannabis. Although a few early studies reported some limited success in producing THC self-administration in rats and monkeys (reviewed by Kaymakçalan, 1981), other laboratories have not been able to induce self-administration of either THC (Carney, Uwaydah, and Balster, 1977; Harris, Waters, and McLendon, 1974; Mansbach et al., 1994) or the potent synthetic cannabinoids nantradol, levonantradol, or CP 55,940 (Mansbach et al., 1994; Young, Katz, and Woods, 1981). Moreover, place conditioning and taste aversion studies in rats have even provided evidence that THC administration is aversive (Elsmore and Fletcher, 1972; Parker and Gillies, 1995). From these results, it appears that cannabinoids do not have strong reinforcing properties in animal subjects, at least under the conditions that have been used to demonstrate powerful reinforcing effects of cocaine, opiates, and many other compounds that are abused by humans.

Cannabis Abuse and the Effects of Chronic Cannabis Exposure

Marijuana is the most widely used illicit drug in the United States. According to the 1990 National Household Survey on Drug Abuse conducted by NIDA (National Institute on Drug Abuse, 1991), over 66 million Americans (about 37 million males and 29 million females) report having used marijuana at least once. Current users, defined as those who used the drug during the past month, number approximately 10 million. As shown in Figure 17.6, the percentage of individuals reporting marijuana use has been declining steadily since a peak in 1979. Although this finding may be valid and may reflect changing societal attitudes toward cannabis, such self-report data must be interpreted cautiously. It is further important to recall, as previously mentioned in Chapter 13, that this is specifically a *household* survey. Hence, it does not include homeless individuals or people living in group settings such as college dormitories, military bases, or prisons.

Initiation and Progression of Cannabis Use

Dedicated cannabis users may smoke marijuana on a near-daily basis for years; hence, questions related to chronic cannabis use are of considerable interest to pharmacologists as well as to medical practitioners. Such questions include the factors associated with the initiation of marijuana use and with progression (in some individuals) to regular usage, as well as the relationships between marijuana and other drugs. Initial marijuana use generally occurs during adolescence (Kandel and Logan, 1984). If an individual has not yet tried marijuana by the mid-20s, he or she probably will never do so. As we can see from the 1990 NIDA survey (see Figure 17.6), peak usage occurs during young adulthood. Older adults (defined here as those aged 35 years or older) show a much lower rate of current usage than adults in the younger age brackets.

Most adolescents have prior experience with alcohol or cigarettes before trying marijuana (Kandel and Faust, 1975). For this reason, it has been suggested that alcohol and tobacco serve as "gateway" drugs to marijuana use. Some evidence exists that marijuana, in turn, may serve as a gateway to the use of other illicit drugs (e.g., cocaine) or prescribed psychoactive drugs such as sedatives (Golub and Johnson, 1994; Kandel, Yamaguchi, and Chen, 1992). However, it is rather difficult to determine whether marijuana actually facilitates the progression to "hard" drugs or whether certain users are already predisposed to seek out these more dangerous substances due to some combination of personality traits, life circumstances, or other factors independent of their exposure to marijuana.

A further issue to consider is the progression from occasional to regular (i.e., daily or near-daily) marijuana use. Risk factors for the development of a marijuana abuse problem in adolescents include emotional problems in the family, heavy drug use in the household or by peers, poor school performance, and an early age of onset of marijuana use (Hawkins, Catalano, and Miller, 1992; Kandel and Davies, 1992). Ultimately, heavy marijuana use by adolescents may come to serve a number of psychological functions, including defiance of authority, escape from competitive pressures and the expectations of others, and the engendering of positive mood changes while dissipating anger and hostility (Hendin et al., 1981).

Tolerance

In differentiating between marijuana use and abuse, one possible criterion for abuse might be a pattern of near-daily consumption over prolonged periods of time. However, we would expect to see other characteristics as well, including significant drug craving (psychological dependence) and possibly tolerance and physical dependence. Considering tolerance first, reduced sensitivity has indeed been demonstrated following repeated expo-

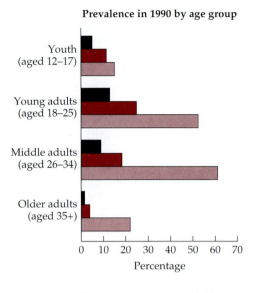

Prevalence in 1990 by age group

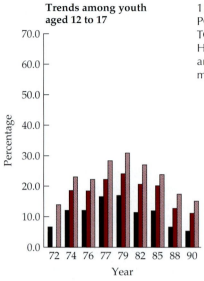

Trends among youth
aged 12 to 17

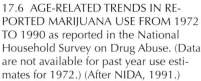

17.6 AGE-RELATED TRENDS IN RE-
PORTED MARIJUANA USE FROM 1972
TO 1990 as reported in the National
Household Survey on Drug Abuse. (Data
are not available for past year use esti-
mates for 1972.) (After NIDA, 1991.)

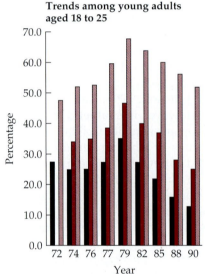

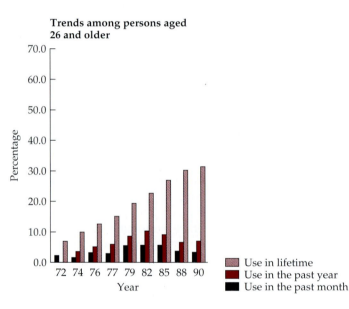

sure to either marijuana or pure THC, although the rate of tolerance development depends on the behavior being studied (Compton, Dewey, and Martin, 1990; Dewey, 1986). Table 17.1 presents data on the effect of THC on key-pecking responses in pigeons under a mixed fixed-ratio (FR)/fixed-interval (FI) schedule of reinforcement (McMillan, Dewey, and Harris, 1971). Consistent with our earlier discussion of its operant effects, THC caused a marked reduction in response rate upon first administration; in fact, the dose chosen for the first drug session (1.8 mg/kg) completely abolished responding in the subjects. Note that some tolerance was already present by the second drug session and that nearly complete tolerance to a 100-fold higher dose (180 mg/kg) was present by session 66. This is a considerable degree of tolerance, particularly considering that such a dose is lethal in previously untreated birds. Cannabinoid tolerance appears to be largely pharmacodynamic in nature and to depend at least partly on receptor changes (see below). Differ-

ences between tolerant and nontolerant animals are generally not attributable to changes in drug absorption, metabolism, or clearance.

In reviewing the literature on human cannabis tolerance, Hollister (1986) concluded that tolerance can develop to both the psychological and physiological (e.g., heart rate elevating) effects of marijuana or pure THC. However, most studies reporting the acquisition of tolerance used high doses and/or extended exposure periods characteristic of heavy users. To determine whether more modest usage also leads to tolerance, Perez-Reyes and colleagues (1991) examined the subjective and cardioacceleratory effects of smoking a single 1% THC marijuana cigarette on 13 consecutive days. At the end of this interval, significant tolerance had developed to the cardioacceleratory influence of the drug, but not to the "high" reported by the subjects. If the psychological effects of cannabis in humans show tolerance only following a pattern of high and/or prolonged dosage, then occasional

Table 17.1 Development of Tolerance to the Behavioral Effects of THC in Pigeons[a]

Session	Dose of THC (mg/kg i.m.)	FI component	FR component
0	0	81–120	85–119
1	1.8	0	0
2	1.8	45	49
6	1.8	90	107
14	3.6	144	104
18	5.6	101	95
21	10	138	94
25	36	125	97
57	60	55	106
61	100	61	93
66	180	77	101

[a]Two pigeons were trained to peck a key under a mixed fixed ratio 30-response, fixed interval 5-minute schedule (discriminative light stimuli in the apparatus served to designate presence of the FR and FI schedules, which alternated during a 1-hour session). Data for session 0 represent the range of response rates (pecks/minute) for the two birds under each reinforcement schedule prior to drug administration. For subsequent sessions, THC was injected intramuscularly at the indicated doses, and the mean response rates at 2 hours post-injection were recorded. Subjects with no prior THC exposure were also tested at the indicated doses on days 18, 25, 61, and 66. In all cases, the response rates were reduced to 0.
Source: After McMillan, Dewey, and Harris, 1971.

users may not be required to increase their intake in order to experience the same intoxicating effects.

Dependence and Withdrawal

A number of early animal studies failed to show abstinence symptomatology with a regimen of repeated THC administration followed by withdrawal. Compton, Dewey, and Martin (1990), however, suggested that the slow rate of THC clearance, along with the previous lack of a selective antagonist (to abruptly block its effects), contributed to the apparent difficulty in demonstrating cannabinoid dependence. Indeed, use of the recently developed antagonist SR 141716A enabled two research groups to finally demonstrate a clear cannabinoid abstinence syndrome in rats. The withdrawal symptoms, which are similar to those found in antagonist-precipitated opiate withdrawal, include "wet-dog shakes," facial rubbing, head shakes, ptosis, ear twitching, biting, and chewing (Aceto et al., 1995; Tsou, Patrick, and Walker, 1995).

Earlier studies of THC-induced physical dependence used rhesus monkeys given frequent intravenous injections or continuous intravenous infusions of this compound (Beardsley, Balster, and Harris, 1986; Fredericks and Benowitz, 1980; Kaymakçalan, 1972). Reported symptoms include irritability, tremors, yawning, piloerection, tooth-baring, anorexia, and disruption of operant responding. It must be noted, however, that continuous infusions of THC or repeated daily intravenous injections of high doses over several weeks may lead to significantly more severe neurochemical effects than seen with other treatment regimens. This fact raises important

questions about the relevance of such an approach for modeling dependence in marijuana-smoking humans.

The issue of cannabis dependence in humans has been a contentious one. Jones (1992) notes that at least some marijuana smokers experience sufficient craving for the drug that they have serious difficulty terminating their use even when faced with possible job loss or other sanctions. In recognition of this fact, the idea of a marijuana dependence syndrome has become increasingly accepted in the clinical realm (Miller and Gold, 1989; Tennant, 1986). Clinicians have also begun to propose specific intervention strategies for the treatment of this problem (Miller, Gold, and Pottash, 1989; Schnoll and Daghestani, 1986; Zweben and O'Connell, 1988). Although it has generally been difficult to demonstrate clear marijuana or THC withdrawal symptoms in the laboratory, Jones, Benowitz, and Bachman (1976) were able to produce an abstinence syndrome by abruptly withdrawing subjects from an intensive six-dose-per-day treatment regimen with oral THC. Interestingly, the symptoms observed by Jones and colleagues, which included sweating, mood disturbances, sleep disruption, and gastrointestinal upset, have also been noted anecdotally in former heavy users undergoing abstinence in the course of professional therapy (Tennant, 1986).

Thus, indices of dependence, including craving and difficulty in voluntarily terminating the drug habit, appear to be present in some marijuana smokers; however, their likelihood of occurrence and their severity are strongly dependent on the amount and pattern of prior usage. The cultural context surrounding drug consumption may also be important. Ethnopharmacological studies were carried out in Jamaica (Rubin and Comitas, 1975) and in Costa Rica (Carter, 1980), two countries in which heavy, daily cannabis smoking occurs within a large male subculture. In neither study did researchers observe, nor did the subjects report, withdrawal symptoms when smoking was abruptly stopped. Given the apparent complexities associated with the issue of cannabis dependence, it will be important to continue both laboratory and field research on this question.

Psychological and Neurological Effects of Long-Term Exposure

It is not unusual for dedicated cannabis users to consume the drug on a regular, even daily, basis for many years. Concern naturally has arisen over whether such lengthy periods of chronic drug exposure might lead to adverse psychological effects. For example, in light of the previously described cognitive deficits that occur during acute marijuana intoxication, it is possible that chronic use might produce residual effects on learning, memory, or attentional processes.

Unfortunately, research on this issue has not yet provided a clear answer. According to two careful literature reviews, there is relatively little evidence for cannabis-associated cognitive impairment in well-controlled studies (Pope, Gruber, and Yurgelun-Todd, 1995; Wert and Raulin, 1986b). Nevertheless, a few recent positive findings should be given some consideration. Researchers at the University of Iowa reported that heavy marijuana use (defined as seven or more times per week for an average of 6 years) in young adults was associated with modest but significant deficits in memory retrieval, verbal expression, and mathematical performance as compared with nonusers (Block and Ghoneim, 1993). A noteworthy aspect of this study was that the subjects were matched on the basis of school achievement tests given in the fourth grade and hence had a comparable level of intellectual functioning (as measured by this instrument) prior to the onset of drug use. Other studies performed by Solowij and her coworkers (Solowij, Michie, and Fox, 1991, 1995) in Australia have assessed selective attention in long-term cannabis users by means of brain event-related potentials (ERPs) and performance on an auditory selective attention task. The cannabis users performed significantly worse than controls on the attentional task. Furthermore, ERP data from the cannabis users suggested that duration of drug use (number of years) was significantly correlated with deficits in focusing attention and filtering out irrelevant information, whereas frequency of use (number of days per month) was correlated with deficits in speed of information processing.

One possible criticism of the studies described above, as well as many others in this field, is that users were required to be abstinent for only 1 day prior to testing. Consequently, any observed cognitive impairments might have been due to an effect of residual THC still in the subject's system (see Pope, Gruber, and Yurgelun-Todd, 1995). To address this issue, Solowij (1995) compared attentional performance and ERP responses in ex-cannabis users (abstinence periods in the study ranged from 3 months to 6 years, with a mean duration of approximately 2 years), current users, and controls. Both the performance and the ERP results indicated a partial, but not complete, recovery of attentional function in the ex-user group. These findings raise the possibility that long-term cannabis use produces lingering deficits in selective attention, although additional research is needed to confirm this hypothesis.

The most extensive studies of chronic cannabis effects on learning and memory in laboratory animals were carried out by Kalant and his colleagues. Rats were treated for 90 or 180 days with a daily oral dose of a marijuana extract containing 20 mg/kg of THC. When the subjects were tested 30 days or more after the last treatment (to allow for washout of the drug), they showed impaired performance in a radial arm maze, poor learning of a DRL operant schedule, hyperactivity in an open field, and enhanced learning of a two-way (shuttle) avoidance task (Stiglick and Kalant, 1982a, 1982b; Stiglick, Llewellyn, and Kalant, 1984; Figure 17.7 shows some of the radial maze results). A remarkable feature of the syndrome identified by Kalant's group is that it very closely resembles the pattern of changes produced by hippocampal damage. Indeed, Drew and Miller (1974) had previously pointed out similarities between cannabinoid-treated and hippocampectomized animals, and had hypothesized that the effects of cannabinoids on learning and memory might be related to a disruption of hippocampal functioning.

The deleterious effects of long-term cannabis exposure on learning and cognitive performance raise the possibility that drug-induced neurotoxicity might mediate these behavioral effects. At the present time, we are not aware of any published histological comparisons of the brains of human users and nonusers. Neurological approaches, including electroencephalography (EEG), computerized axial tomography (CAT scanning), echoencephalography, pneumoencephalography, and standard neurological examination, have generally found no evidence of brain abnormalities in cannabis users compared with controls (see Wert and Raulin, 1986a, for review). On the other hand, histological studies in rats have found that chronic treatment with THC for many months is associated with decreased dendritic branching of hippocampal CA3 neurons (Scallet et al., 1987) and a dose-dependent reduction in neuronal density in the CA1 pyramidal layer (Landfield, Cadwallader, and Vinsant, 1988). Although these findings must still be considered preliminary, they could provide a cellular basis for the behavioral alterations reported in cannabis-treated

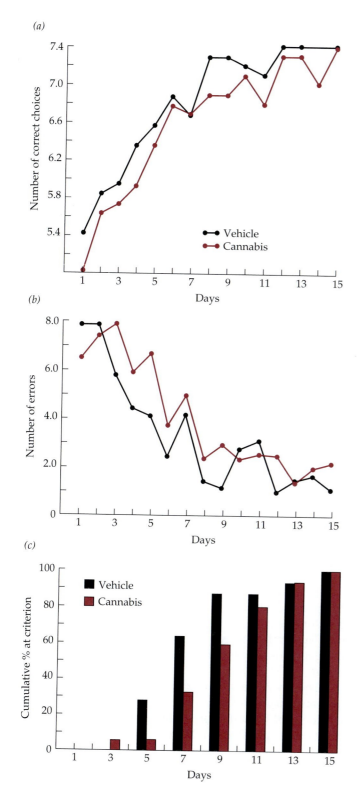

(a)

(b)

(c)

17.7 RADIAL MAZE PERFORMANCE IN CANNABIS-TREATED AND CONTROL RATS. Rats were given a cannabis extract (containing 20 mg/kg THC) orally each day for 6 months. Following a 30-day drug-free period, the cannabis-treated rats and vehicle-treated control subjects were tested for 15 days on an eight-arm radial maze. The figures show (a) the cumulative number of correct choices, (b) the number of incorrect arm entries (errors), and (c) the cumulative percentage of animals reaching a criterion of at least one perfect trial. The cannabis-treated group differed from the controls on all three measures. (After Stiglick and Kalant, 1982a.)

and decreased productivity. These symptoms, which have collectively been termed the "amotivational syndrome" (McGlothlin and West, 1968), are of particular concern in relation to the academic success of high school and college students and the job performance and employment history of older individuals. Some authors have reported an apparent relationship between heavy marijuana use and poor academic performance (e.g., Campbell, 1976). Others, however, stress that psychological and sociological factors associated with the adolescent drug-using subculture are much more important contributors to poor academic achievement and rejection of conventional work-related values than are the direct effects of drugs themselves (Mellinger et al., 1976). We do not rule out the possibility that some human marijuana users might experience a loss of drive and achievement motivation after heavy, chronic exposure. Nevertheless, even when these characteristics are present, it is possible that they are a cause, rather than a consequence, of adopting a marijuana-centered lifestyle (Weil, 1972).

Physiological Effects of Long-Term Exposure

Because cannabis is almost always consumed by smoking, the possibility of lung damage is one area of physiological concern. Hashish smoking has been associated with chronic coughing, bronchitis, and other respiratory symptoms (Henderson, Tennant, and Guerney, 1972). Rhesus monkey studies have confirmed the presence of pulmonary pathology following 12 months of daily marijuana smoking (Fligiel et al., 1991). On the other hand, Hollister (1986) has noted that even heavy marijuana users smoke far fewer cigarettes per day than heavy tobacco smokers. Hence, tobacco use generally poses a much greater health risk to the respiratory system than does marijuana use (see Chapter 14).

Another major concern that has been raised with respect to cannabis is its purported effects on reproductive function. Various adverse effects of chronic marijuana or THC exposure on the male reproductive system have been reported, ranging from reduced sperm counts to decreased circulating levels of testosterone and other reproductive hormones (Ehrenkranz and Hembree, 1986; Hollister, 1986; Vescovi et al., 1992); however, these findings have not been consistently replicated (e.g., Block, Farinpour, and Schlechte, 1991). Consequently, the influ-

animals as well as for the cognitive impairment that may occur in some very heavy human users.

In addition to the purported effects of long-term cannabinoid use on cognitive functioning, many clinicians have suggested the occurrence of undesirable motivational changes including apathy, aimlessness, loss of achievement motivation, lack of long-range planning,

ence of marijuana on the endocrine system remains a subject of controversy.

Mechanisms of Action of Cannabinoids

In this section, we will examine the mechanisms of action of cannabinoids at the neurochemical and neurophysiological levels. Where appropriate, these mechanisms will be related to some of the behavioral and other functional effects discussed above. A good review of cannabinoid mechanisms may be found in Abood and Martin (1992).

Cannabinoid Receptors

Discovery and characterization.   Until recently, our understanding of the neurochemical substrates of cannabinoid action was severely hampered by the lack of an identified cellular receptor for these compounds. Not long ago, some researchers hypothesized that cannabinoids did not interact with a specific receptor at all, but instead worked by perturbing cell membranes due to their extreme lipophilicity. By the mid-1980s, however, the existence of a putative cannabinoid receptor had been inferred from the demonstration of enantioselectivity* for various physiological and behavioral effects of cannabinoid compounds, and also from the observation that cannabinoids appeared to inhibit adenylyl cyclase activity via a G protein–mediated mechanism (see below). In 1988, pharmacological characterization of a CNS cannabinoid receptor was announced by a group of researchers that included William Devane and Allyn Howlett at St. Louis University and Lawrence Melvin and M. Ross Johnson at the Pfizer pharmaceutical company (Devane et al., 1988).

Several reviews have summarized the properties of the central cannabinoid receptor (Howlett, 1995; Howlett et al., 1990; Mechoulam, Hanuš, and Martin, 1994). The critical tool that made the identification of this receptor possible was a potent synthetic bicyclic cannabinoid, CP-55,940, developed at Pfizer (structure shown above; see Johnson and Melvin, 1986, for a historical account of the discovery of this compound). CP-55,940 has THC-like behavioral effects in rats and rhesus monkeys (Gold et al., 1992), which is important in validating its use as a probe for the cannabinoid receptor. When [^{3}H]CP-55,940 was incubated with rat cortical membranes, saturable high-affinity binding occurred to a single site according to Scatchard analysis. [^{3}H]CP-55,940 binding was reduced in the presence of a guanine nucleotide (which is indicative of a G protein–coupled receptor), and the

binding was displaced by THC and other cannabinoids with a rank order of potency consistent with the biological activity of these compounds (Devane et al., 1988). Subsequent studies of a large number of cannabinoid drugs found high correlations ($r \geq 0.81$) between in vitro affinity for the [^{3}H]CP-55,940-labeled cannabinoid receptor and in vivo potency in rat drug discrimination tests, human psychoactivity measures, and several of the previously discussed indices of cannabinoid action in mice (locomotor depression, catalepsy, analgesia, and hypothermia) (Compton et al., 1993). These results powerfully support the hypothesis that most, if not all, of the pharmacological effects of cannabinoids are mediated by interaction with the binding site identified by [^{3}H]CP-55,940.

The initial characterization of the cannabinoid receptor was quickly followed by other studies concerned with its neuroanatomical localization. Herkenham and coworkers (Herkenham et al., 1990; Herkenham, Lynn, Johnson et al., 1991) found the highest levels of [^{3}H]CP-55,940 binding in rat brain in the substantia nigra pars reticulata, globus pallidus, entopeduncular nucleus, molecular layers of the cerebellum and the dentate gyrus, the caudate–putamen, the ependymal and the subependymal layers of the olfactory bulbs, and the CA1 and CA3 areas of the hippocampal formation (Figure 17.8). Moderate binding was found in many other forebrain areas, including the cerebral cortex. Similar, though not identical, patterns were found in rhesus monkey and human brains (Herkenham et al., 1990). The distribution of cells in the rat brain that synthesize the cannabinoid receptor was recently examined by means of in situ hybridization histochemistry for the receptor mRNA (Mailleux and Vanderhaeghen, 1992; Matsuda, Bonner, and Lolait, 1993). Some of the areas with heavy receptor binding, such as the substantia nigra, globus pallidus, entopeduncular nucleus, and the innermost layers of the olfactory bulbs, showed at best a weak hybridization signal. This finding suggests that many of the receptors in these regions may be located on the terminals of afferent fibers.

The presence of cannabinoid receptors in the hippocampus and neocortex helps to explain the profound influence of cannabis on memory and other cognitive functions (Color Plate 4). Moreover, high levels of receptors in the basal ganglia and cerebellum may be responsible for the motoric and coordination-impairing effects of marijuana or THC. Receptor densities in the corpus striatum and in the areas to which it projects (the globus pallidus, substantia nigra, and entopeduncular nucleus) were greatly diminished following intrastriatal lesions with the cellular neurotoxin ibotenic acid (Herkenham, Lynn, de Costa et al., 1991). This finding suggests that cannabinoid receptors are localized on the dendrites and cell bodies as well as on the terminals of striatal projection neurons, which is consistent with the in situ hy-

---

*Enantiomers are structural isomers of a molecule that constitute nonsuperimposable mirror images of each other. When enantiomers of a drug exist, one of the enantiomers usually acts much more potently on that drug's receptor than the other enantiomer.

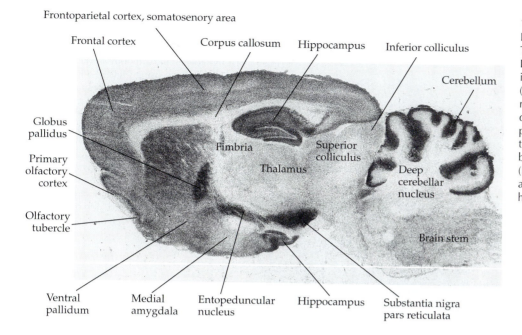

Frontoparietal cortex, somatosenory area
Frontal cortex
Corpus callosum
Hippocampus
Inferior colliculus
Cerebellum
Globus pallidus
Fimbria
Superior colliculus
Deep cerebellar nucleus
Primary olfactory cortex
Thalamus
Olfactory tubercle
Brain stem
Ventral pallidum
Medial amygdala
Entopeduncular nucleus
Hippocampus
Substantia nigra pars reticulata

17.8 LOCALIZATION OF RAT BRAIN CANNABINOID RECEPTORS BY [³H]CP-55,940 AUTORADIOGRAPHY. High levels of binding are seen in the basal ganglia (including the substantia nigra pars reticulata, globus pallidus, entopeduncular nucleus, and caudate–putamen), the hippocampal formation, the molecular layer of the cerebellum, and the olfactory bulbs. (From Herkenham, Lynn, Johnson et al., 1991; courtesy of Miles Herkenham, NIMH.)

bridization results mentioned above. Finally, Herkenham, Lynn, Johnson, and colleagues (1991) have pointed out that the well-known safety of cannabis (as indicated by an absence of lethal overdose in humans) can be related to the extremely low density of receptors in the cardiovascular and respiratory control centers of the medulla.

At about the same time that the St. Louis University and Pfizer researchers were first characterizing the cannabinoid receptor pharmacologically, a group of investigators at NIMH, including Lisa Matsuda and Tom Bonner, cloned a novel cDNA from rat cerebral cortex that predicted a membrane protein with the characteristics of a G protein–coupled receptor. Further studies revealed that these investigators, who were working on an unrelated problem, had actually cloned the gene for the rat brain cannabinoid receptor (Matsuda et al., 1990). This is a good example of an approach that is sometimes called "reverse pharmacology," namely, the cloning of a novel receptor or transporter gene, the identity of which must then be determined by more traditional pharmacological methods. The CNS cannabinoid receptor is currently designated CB_1. A second cannabinoid receptor (CB_2) was cloned several years later from a human leukemia cell line and was found to be moderately homologous with CB_1 (68% sequence identity within the putative transmembrane domains) (Munro, Thomas, and Abu-Shaar, 1993). This receptor was observed in spleen and macrophages, but does not appear to be present in brain. Our discussion of cannabinoid receptors will therefore focus on CB_1.

Receptor mechanisms. The signal transduction mechanisms identified thus far for cannabinoids are consistent with those of a G protein–coupled receptor. Thus, a variety of naturally occurring and synthetic cannabinoids produced a consistent inhibition of adenylyl cyclase activity in rat brain and in cultured N18TG2 mouse neuroblastoma cells (Bidaut-Russell, Devane, and Howlett, 1990; Howlett et al., 1990). The effect of these compounds on cyclic AMP (cAMP) accumulation rapidly desensitized when the cells were continuously exposed to the drug. Moreover, the inhibitory action of cannabinoids on adenylyl cyclase could be reversed by the addition of pertussis toxin, which implicates the G protein G_i in this process. As Self and Stein (1992) have pointed out, μ- and δ-opioid receptors and D_2 dopamine receptors also couple to G_i. This G protein may therefore be part of a common mechanism underlying the reinforcing properties of cannabis, opiate drugs, and dopaminergic drugs such as cocaine and amphetamine. In the cerebellum, adenylyl cyclase-inhibiting cannabinoid and opioid receptors appear to coexist in many granule cells, where they presumably mediate convergent effects of these drug classes on motor function and coordination (Childers et al., 1992).

Other receptor-mediated effects of cannabinoid drugs include stimulation of phospholipase activity in a number of different cell types (Pertwee, 1990) and an inhibition of voltage-dependent Ca^{2+} influx that was found in the NG108-15 neuroblastoma × glioma hybrid cell line (Mackie and Hille, 1992). Phospholipase activation releases arachidonic acid, which can lead to several different biochemical cascades including the synthesis of prostaglandins. The effect of cannabinoids on voltage-regulated Ca^{2+} channels could underlie the inhibition of acetylcholine or monoamine release reported in some studies (see below).

Receptor regulation. Several laboratories have recently begun to investigate the regulation of cannabinoid re-

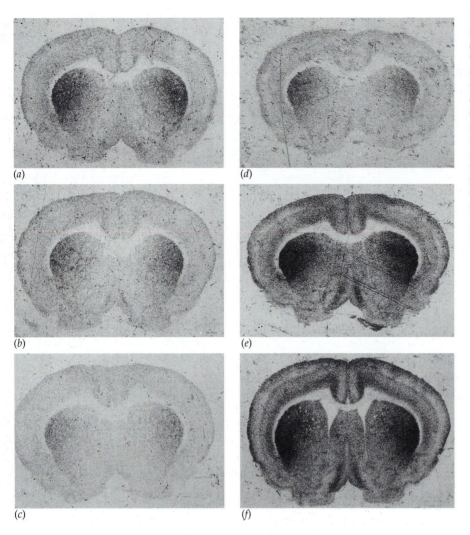

17.9 DOWN-REGULATION OF CANNA-BINOID RECEPTORS FOLLOWING CHRONIC CANNABINOID ADMINISTRATION. Rat brain cannabinoid binding sites were visualized using [^{3}H]CP-55,940 autoradiography following 14 daily injections of (a) 1 mg/kg CP-55,940; (b) 3 mg/kg CP-55,940; (c) 10 mg/kg CP-55,940; (d) 10 mg/kg Δ^9-THC; (e) 10 mg/kg cannabidiol; and (f) vehicle. Note the marked down-regulation of binding sites in the subjects treated with CP-55,940 or THC compared with subjects receiving vehicle or the relatively inactive compound cannabidiol. (From Oviedo, Glowa, and Herkenham, 1993; courtesy of Miles Herkenham, NIMH.)

ceptors. Mailleux and Vanderhaeghen (1993), for example, found that rat striatal CB_1 mRNA levels were significantly elevated following either 6-hydroxydopamine lesion of the ascending DA fibers to the striatum or chronic administration of DA receptor antagonists. These findings indicate that cannabinoid receptor gene expression in the striatum is negatively modulated by normal DA transmission, which is similar to the dopaminergic control of preproenkephalin gene expression demonstrated in other studies (see Chapter 8).

Chronic administration of THC or CP-55,940 to rats has also been shown to dramatically down-regulate cannabinoid receptor binding sites in the striatum, nucleus accumbens, olfactory tubercle, and septum (Oviedo, Glowa, and Herkenham, 1993; Rodríguez de Fonseca et al., 1994; Figure 17.9). This reduction in receptor density was accompanied by substantial behavioral tolerance and presumably plays an important mechanistic role in the development of such tolerance.

Endogenous cannabinoids.   The recent history of neuropharmacology has seen several important cases—namely, opiates, benzodiazepines, and PCP (see below for more details)—in which receptors were discovered

for compounds that are not endogenous to the nervous system. The identification of these receptors as valid entities led to the subsequent discovery of the opioid peptides and to the ongoing search for benzodiazepine-like and PCP-like substances in the brain. Most recently, the cannabinoid receptor has been added to this group. In fact, the density of cannabinoid receptors in the brain is higher than that of any other G protein–coupled receptor, suggesting that these receptors and their endogenous ligand(s) must constitute a novel and important neural system. Proof that any new factor is an endogenous ligand for the cannabinoid receptor minimally requires demonstrating that the factor is synthesized and released by cells in the nervous system, that it binds to the receptor with appropriate specificity and affinity, that it mimics the biological effects of cannabinoids in various physiological and behavioral assays, and that antagonists to the factor are physiologically and behaviorally active in the expected ways. Although several research groups had been searching for endogenous cannabinoids, little progress was made in this area until the appearance of an exciting report by Devane, Mechoulam, and their colleagues (Devane et al., 1992). These investigators isolated an arachidonic acid derivative from pig brain that was identified chemically as arachidonylethanolamide. The compound was given the trivial name "anandamide," from *ananda*, the Sanskrit word for "bliss." In vitro studies have demonstrated anandamide binding to cells expressing cloned cannabinoid receptors and the activation of appropriate signal transduction mechanisms such as inhibition of adenylyl cyclase activity (Felder et al., 1993; Vogel et al., 1993). When administered to mice and rats, anandamide was found to produce classic cannabinoid effects such as hypothermia, analgesia, hypomotility, and catalepsy (Crawley et al., 1993; Fride and Mechoulam, 1993; Smith et al., 1994). Finally, several reports have appeared describing the synthesis of anandamide in brain tissue (Deutsch and Chin, 1993; Devane and Axelrod, 1994). Synthetic activity was particularly high in the hippocampus (one of the brain regions rich in cannabinoid receptors) and low in the cerebellum and medulla.

Together, these findings suggest that anandamide may be an endogenous ligand for brain cannabinoid receptors. To confirm this hypothesis, however, researchers still must demonstrate anandamide release in response to physiological or behavioral stimuli as well as a convincing role for this compound in neural regulation. Because of its lipid solubility, anandamide presumably diffuses rapidly through membranes and therefore may not be stored in vesicles or granules like classical neurotransmitters and neuropeptides. Like other diffusional messengers such as arachidonic acid and nitric oxide (see Chapter 6), anandamide is probably synthesized and released upon demand.

It is important to note that the endogenous cannabinoid story did not necessarily end with the discovery of anandamide. Research groups are still looking for compounds that might either replace anandamide as the major candidate substance or that might serve as cannabinoid agonists in addition to anandamide (the possibility of multiple endogenous cannabinoids is not so strange when one considers that both norepinephrine and epinephrine are endogenous agonists for adrenergic receptors, and that several different endogenous peptides activate opiate receptors). Indeed, the discovery of anandamide was followed closely by the identification of two similar compounds in the brain that likewise bind to cannabinoid receptors (Hanuš et al., 1993). Researchers have suggested that a family of anandamides may exist in the brain and have additionally proposed that each anandamide-like compound be named according to standard fatty acid shorthand nomenclature* (Me-

choulam, Hanuš, and Martin, 1994). It will be interesting to see how the question of endogenous cannabinoids is resolved as further information is collected.

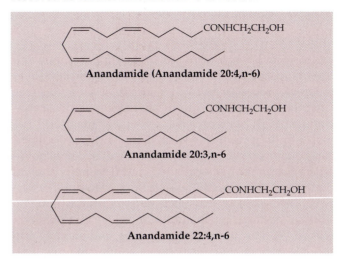

Anandamide (Anandamide 20:4,n-6)

Anandamide 20:3,n-6

Anandamide 22:4,n-6

Electrophysiological Effects

Cannabinoid electrophysiology has been studied using several different model systems, including electrically stimulated smooth or striated muscle preparations, monosynaptic and polysynaptic spinal reflexes, and evoked potentials measured in various brain areas (for review, see Dewey, 1986; Pertwee, 1990). Stimulated muscle contraction and spinal reflex amplitude are generally inhibited by THC and other biologically active cannabinoids. The effects of these compounds on evoked potentials in the brain are more complex, however, and depend on the dose, the type of stimulus, and the pathway being studied. Thalamocortical projections are among those influenced by cannabinoids, a fact that may underlie some of the sensory disturbances produced by marijuana smoking (Pertwee, 1990). Dewey (1986) has suggested that low cannabinoid doses tend to enhance CNS excitability, whereas higher doses tend to reduce excitability. Such dose-dependent electrophysiological changes could be related to the biphasic effects of cannabinoids on locomotor activity and on seizure susceptibility described above.

Electrophysiological studies aimed at understanding the cognitive impairments produced by cannabinoids have focused on the hippocampus. One model system, for example, is the evoked potential waveform that can be recorded in the outer molecular layer of the rat hippocampal dentate gyrus during performance of a two-tone auditory discrimination task. Administration of 1.0 to 2.0 mg/kg of THC disrupted behavioral performance on this task, and at the same time altered specific components of the potential waveform that was evoked (Deadwyler et al., 1990; Hampson, Foster, and Deadwyler, 1989). As mentioned earlier, human studies comparing long-term cannabis users with nonusing control subjects likewise found changes in evoked potentials associated

---

*The fatty acid shorthand naming system specifies the number of carbons in the backbone, the number of unsaturated bonds, and the position of the first double bond. Thus, anandamide 20:4, n-6, the originally described anandamide, possesses a 20-carbon backbone with 4 unsaturated bonds, and the first double bond begins at the sixth carbon from the nonacidic end of the molecule. The two subsequently discovered compounds are called anandamide 20:3, n-6 and anandamide 22: 4, n-6.

with an auditory selective attention task (Solowij, Michie, and Fox, 1991, 1995). Thus, it is possible to demonstrate electrophysiological correlates of cannabis-induced cognitive impairments.

Effects on Neurotransmitter Systems

Because cholinergic afferents to the hippocampus and cerebral cortex are thought to play a significant role in memory processes and other cognitive functions (see Chapter 7), the influence of cannabinoids on acetylcholine (ACh) has received considerable attention.* The major finding from this work is that THC and related compounds exert a presynaptically mediated anticholinergic effect in the hippocampus, as well as in the cerebral cortex and striatum (Miller and Branconnier, 1983; Pertwee, 1990). This conclusion is derived from various results suggesting cannabinoid-induced decreases in ACh release, ACh turnover, choline uptake, and possibly also firing rates of cholinergic neurons. Inhibition of ACh release or choline uptake could be mediated by cannabinoid receptors on the axon terminals of some cholinergic neurons. The involvement of the hippocampus in these effects is consistent with previously discussed evidence that this structure is one of the primary targets of cannabinoid action.

Acute THC administration has been reported to stimulate norepinephrine (NE) synthesis and turnover in rat and mouse brain. THC also exerts complex biphasic effects on synaptosomal NE uptake and release in vitro. Relatively low concentrations (0.1–0.2 μM) were found to increase uptake but decrease release, whereas the opposite effects were produced by higher concentrations (over 10 μM). Studies using several different cannabinoids found that the low-concentration neurochemical responses (i.e., increased uptake and decreased release) were associated only with compounds possessing behavioral potency, whereas the presence of the high-concentration response pattern was independent of behavioral activity (Pertwee, 1990).

Synaptosomal and turnover studies investigating the dopaminergic effects of THC have found many of the same kinds of changes as reported for NE (Pertwee, 1990). However, researchers have recently proceeded beyond these older methods by using microdialysis to examine the influence of THC on dopaminergic functioning in vivo. Such experiments have demonstrated increased extracellular DA levels in the nucleus accumbens and medial prefrontal cortex following intraperi-

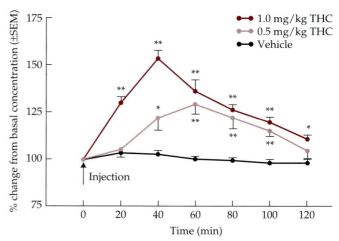

17.10 THC-INDUCED ENHANCEMENT OF DOPAMINE EFFLUX IN THE NUCLEUS ACCUMBENS. Rats were implanted with microdialysis probes in the nucleus accumbens. The next day, extracellular dopamine concentrations were measured in the freely moving animals following intraperitoneal injection of either 0.5 mg/kg THC, 1.0 mg/kg THC, or vehicle. Asterisks denote a statistically significant difference from the vehicle condition (*$p < 0.05$; **$p < 0.01$). (After Chen, Paredes, Li et al., 1990.)

toneal administration of 0.5 to 2.0 mg/kg THC (Chen, Paredes, Li et al., 1990; Chen, Paredes, Lowinson et al., 1990; Figure 17.10). This effect could reflect an inhibition of DA uptake and/or a stimulation of DA release. An interesting aspect of these results is that the influence of THC in the nucleus accumbens was significantly attenuated by naloxone, indicating possible mediation by opioid receptors (Chen, Paredes, Li et al., 1990). Naloxone was not tested in the prefrontal cortex, so we do not yet know whether opioid involvement is specific to the nucleus accumbens.

The stimulation of DA efflux in dopaminergic terminal areas may be related to several behavioral effects of cannabinoids. THC administration into the nucleus accumbens has been shown to mimic the locomotor activating effect of low systemic doses of cannabinoids (Conti and Musty, 1984). Sakurai and colleagues (1985) further observed that in rats previously given unilateral lesions of the substantia nigra, THC produced ipsilateral circling, just like the indirect DA agonist methamphetamine. THC-induced circling was blocked by haloperidol, indicating a dopaminergic involvement in this response. Finally, Gardner and Lowinson (1991) have proposed a model whereby cannabinoids influence the central reward system by interacting with opioid peptide neurons to modulate dopaminergic transmission in the nucleus accumbens and possibly also in other parts of the mesotelencephalic DA system.

DA, NE, ACh, opioid peptides, and other transmitters not discussed here probably play important roles in the mechanisms of cannabinoid action. However, it is

---

*Pertwee (1990) has summarized the literature concerning cannabinoid effects on neurotransmitter biochemistry. Due to space limitations, we will focus on the cholinergic, noradrenergic, and dopaminergic systems. It is important to note that some of the studies summarized below used relatively high (micromolar) concentrations of THC, which raises questions about their physiological relevance in vivo.

clear that much more work must be done before a precise understanding of these mechanisms is achieved.

Part I Summary

Cannabis sativa, the flowering hemp plant, exudes a resin containing a number of intoxicating compounds known as cannabinoids. Cannabis can be obtained in several different types of preparations, including marijuana and hashish, both of which may be smoked or taken orally. The consumption of cannabis for its intoxicating effects is thought to date back thousands of years in Eastern cultures. The practice of marijuana smoking was introduced into the United States in the early 1900s by Mexican and West Indian immigrants.

The major naturally occurring cannabinoid is Δ^9-tetrahydrocannabinol (THC). Inhaled THC is rapidly absorbed from the lungs into the circulation, where it is almost completely bound to plasma proteins. Oral THC consumption yields slower absorption and lower plasma peaks than either smoking or intravenous injection. THC is extensively metabolized in the liver, and the metabolites are excreted mainly in the feces and urine. Following a single dose of THC, total clearance of the drug and its metabolites may take days because of sequestration of these compounds in adipose tissue.

The subjective characteristics of cannabis intoxication include feelings of euphoria, disinhibition, volubility, altered sensations, and memory impairment. Psychopathological reactions can occur, particularly at high doses or in inexperienced users. Cannabis adversely affects memory, psychomotor performance, and other cognitive functions. The impairment produced by smoking a single marijuana cigarette may persist for many hours, even after the subjective "high" has worn off.

In rodents, THC produces changes in motor activity (which may involve both excitatory and depressant components), catalepsy, hypothermia, and analgesia. Anticonvulsant and proconvulsant effects are also observed, depending on the dose and the test system used. THC has also been shown to reduce operant response rates and to act as a discriminative stimulus in a standard drug discrimination learning paradigm. The cannabinoid drug cue appears to be unique to this class of compounds and to correlate well with the intoxicating potency of different cannabinoids in human subjects. On the other hand, cannabinoids do not seem to support self-administration by laboratory animals as readily as most other abused drugs.

According to the 1990 National Household Survey on Drug Abuse, marijuana use in the United States has been declining since 1979. Nevertheless, marijuana remains the most heavily used illegal drug by far. Initial exposure to marijuana usually occurs during adolescence, after the individual has already had experience with alcohol or cigarettes. Some investigators have hypothesized that alcohol and tobacco are "gateway" drugs to marijuana, which then serves as a potential gateway to other illicit substances. As the cannabis user progresses to more frequent consumption, tolerance to at least some of the drug's effects may occur. Whether chronic cannabis exposure produces physical or psychological dependence (as evidenced by withdrawal symptomatology) has been controversial, although it appears that prolonged heavy use can lead to an abstinence syndrome.

Concerns have been raised over the possible adverse consequences of long-term cannabis consumption. Animal experiments using high doses and long exposure periods have demonstrated persistent deficits in various learning tasks, particularly those involving hippocampal function. On the other hand, most of the human studies have found little or no evidence of neuropsychological abnormalities in regular marijuana users, although recent work indicates a possible drug-related impairment of selective attention. Some clinicians have also suggested that heavy cannabis use can produce an "amotivational syndrome" characterized by apathy, loss of achievement motivation, and decreased productivity. However, even if such a syndrome exists (which is controversial), it may precede, rather than result from, the adoption of a marijuana-centered lifestyle.

Significant progress has recently been made in our understanding of the mechanisms of cannabinoid action. A specific cannabinoid receptor has been identified using the potent synthetic cannabinoid [^{3}H]CP-55,940, and the gene for this receptor has been cloned. The cannabinoid receptor is found throughout the forebrain, but is particularly concentrated in the output nuclei of the basal ganglia, the cerebellum, and parts of the hippocampal formation. Localization of the receptor in these areas is consonant with the influence of cannabinoids on locomotor activity, coordination, and memory. At the cellular level, the cannabinoid receptor inhibits adenylyl cyclase via coupling to the G protein G_i. Continual administration of cannabinoids leads to receptor down-regulation, which appears to be an important mechanism in cannabinoid tolerance. Although the endogenous ligand for the cannabinoid receptor has not yet been conclusively identified, the best current candidate is an arachidonic acid derivative called anandamide.

Cannabinoids exert complex effects on electrophysiological and neurochemical functioning. Muscle contraction and spinal reflexes are generally inhibited, and evoked potentials in the hippocampus and other areas are also altered. ACh, NE, and DA are some of the neurotransmitters influenced by THC and other cannabinoids. In vitro studies have found that THC may either stimulate or inhibit the release of these transmitters, whereas in vivo microdialysis experiments have shown THC-induced increases in extracellular DA concentrations in the nucleus accumbens and prefrontal cortex. Further work is needed to characterize the precise pathways and neurotransmitter systems by which cannabinoids exert their behavioral and physiological effects.

Part II
Phencyclidine

Phencyclidine, which is short for 1-(1-*p*henyl*c*yclo-hexyl)*p*iperidine (PCP), belongs to a class of compounds known chemically as arylcyclohexylamines. PCP (trade name Sernyl) was first synthesized in the mid-1950s by Parke, Davis, and Company (see Maddox, 1981, for a historical account of the development of PCP). The level of

Phencyclidine (PCP)

PCP abuse is relatively low at the time of this writing, and no human clinical studies on this compound are currently being performed. Hence, information concerning the effects of PCP in humans was obtained almost entirely from studies beginning in the late 1950s and ending around 1980, a time span encompassing the peak period of PCP abuse during the late 1970s. Early PCP studies revealed that the drug possessed unusual anesthetic properties. Patients given 0.25 mg/kg intravenously of either PCP or the related compound *N*-ethyl-1-phenylcyclohexylamine (PCE; formerly called cyclohexamine) seemed to be anesthetized in that they showed no responsiveness to nociceptive (painful) stimuli. However, these patients differed in other respects from individuals

PCE

given traditional anesthetics, such as barbiturates. They exhibited a catatonic-like state characterized by a vacant facial expression with fixed and staring eyes, and by a lack of true muscle relaxation (Collins, Gorospe, and Rovenstine, 1960; Greifenstein et al., 1958; Johnstone, Evans, and Baigel, 1959). Indeed, it was not unusual for these individuals to develop either rigidity or waxy flexibility (motor symptoms often observed in catatonic schizophrenics). Because patients treated with PCP, PCE, or a third drug called ketamine seemed to be dissociated from

their environment without completely losing consciousness, these compounds came to be known as "dissociative anesthetics" (Corssen and Domino, 1966).

Ketamine

In some respects, the dissociative anesthetics showed initial clinical promise because they did not produce the respiratory depression typically associated with barbiturate anesthesia, and were thus considered to have a high therapeutic index (see Chapter 1). Early enthusiasm was soon tempered, however, by reports of problematic reactions in many patients. In a few cases, this took the form of marked agitation rather than calmness during the drug-induced state. In other instances, the drugs induced postoperative reactions ranging from blurred vision, dizziness, and mild disorientation to much more serious reactions involving hallucinations, severe agitation, and even violence (Collins, Gorospe, and Rovenstine, 1960; Greifenstein et al., 1958; Johnstone, Evans, and Baigel, 1959). PCP was therefore withdrawn from clinical use by 1965, although ketamine continues to be used today in both medical and veterinary practice. The latter agent still occasionally causes adverse emergence reactions, although a number of techniques have been developed to minimize the frequency of such occurrences (Albin, Bunegin, and Garcia, 1990).

In 1967, PCP found its way onto the streets of several cities, including San Francisco, where it was dubbed the "PeaCe Pill" by the drug culture protesting the Vietnam war. After some initial reports of negative drug experiences, publicity regarding PCP use declined for the next few years. By the mid-1970s, however, it was clear that PCP abuse was widespread across the United States and that the drug had become a significant health problem. The popularity of PCP can be gauged, in part, by the profusion of its different street names, such as "angel dust" and "hog," which are included in a list of over 100 names compiled by Linder, Lerner, and Burns (1981). Regional names for PCP-containing drug combinations are also of interest. For example, Californians refer to a PCP–marijuana mixture as "lovely," whereas Chicagoans speak of PCP combined with cocaine as "rocket fuel" or "space base" (Linder, Lerner, and Burns, 1981).

Basic Pharmacology of PCP

One of the factors contributing to PCP's popularity is that it can be ingested by virtually any common route. It can be taken orally, administered intranasally (i.e., snorted), or injected intravenously or intramuscularly.

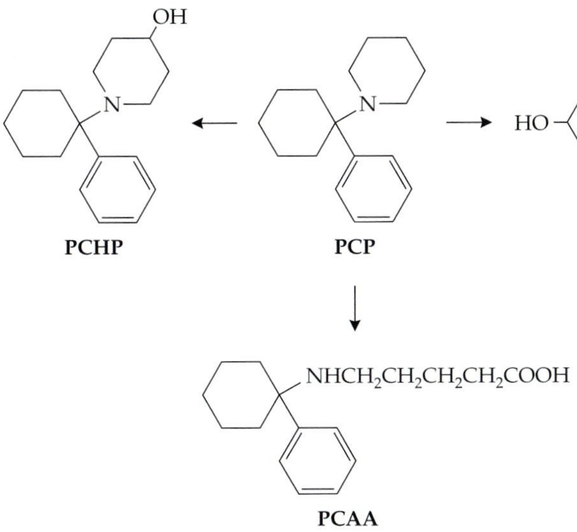

17.11 METABOLISM OF PHENCYCLIDINE. Phencyclidine (PCP) is metabolized by several different pathways. Major metabolites include the hydroxylated compounds 1-(1-phenylcyclohexyl)-4-hydroxypiperidine (PCHP) and 4-phenyl-4-(1-piperidinyl)cyclohexanol (PPC), as well as the compound 5-[*N*-(1-phenylcyclohexyl)]-aminopentanoic acid (PCAA).

Many PCP abusers apply the drug to parsley or marijuana cigarettes for purposes of smoking. Burns and Lerner (1976) reported the following time course of drug action in chronic PCP smokers: 2–5 minutes for the onset of action, 15 to 30 minutes duration of the peak response (the "high"), 4 to 6 hours of continuing effects (the individual remains "loaded"), and 24–48 hours to return to normalcy. Due to its low cost, ease of synthesis, ready availability in various forms, and wide-ranging effects (see below), PCP has frequently been sold on the street under the guise of other abused substances. According to Giannini (1989), PCP has been "marketed" by drug dealers as amphetamine, cocaine, heroin, morphine, barbiturate, LSD, mescaline, psilocybin, marijuana, and amyl nitrate.

The pharmacokinetics, tissue distribution, and metabolism of PCP have been studied in a number of controlled experiments on humans and animals. A 1-mg dose of PCP was found to produce average peak plasma concentrations of 2.7–2.9 ng/ml in human subjects (Cook et al., 1982). A similar peak concentration was produced whether the drug was given intravenously or orally, although in the latter case the peak was not reached until 1–2 hours after treatment. Pharmacokinetic studies have demonstrated that the terminal half-life ($t_{\frac{1}{2}}$) of PCP is approximately 16 hours when given intravenously, but 27 hours when taken orally (Cook et al., 1982; Wall et al., 1981). Giles and coworkers (1982) re-

ported that only about 20% to 25% of total plasma PCP is free, with the remainder bound to various plasma proteins. When Martin (1982) administered either single or repeated doses of PCP to mice, the drug appeared to be stored in adipose tissue where it was slowly released back into the plasma compartment. These findings may account for reports of prolonged or delayed behavioral symptomatology in some PCP abusers.

Clearance of PCP and its metabolites is accomplished mainly via the urine, although a small amount of excretion also occurs through the feces and sweat. When 1 mg of [^{3}H]PCP was administered intravenously or orally to human subjects, 16% of the radioactive material excreted in the urine was found to be nonmetabolized PCP (Cook et al., 1982). The remaining radioactivity was excreted in the form of various metabolites, including PPC (20%), PCAA (15%), PCHP (8%), and several unidentified compounds (Figure 17.11). Most of the hydroxylated metabolites were present in conjugated form, possibly bound with glucuronic acid.

Special considerations apply when PCP is smoked. Because the drug is not stable at the temperature of a burning cigarette, some of it is pyrolyzed to yield PC and piperidine (Martin and Boni, 1990) (Figure 17.12). Much of the piperidine is further modified to form *N*-acetylpiperidine and other compounds. Due to both pyrolysis and loss of material in sidestream smoke, PCP smokers have been estimated to ingest only about 40% of the initial dose present in the drug-laced cigarette (Cook and Jeffcoat, 1990).

Acute Behavioral Effects of PCP in Humans

Results From Controlled Studies

Following early reports by anesthesiologists of potent psychological effects of PCP, psychiatric researchers began to show a great interest in the drug. One of the first studies detailing the subjective experience produced by PCP was performed by Luby and coworkers (1959), who administered a subanesthetic dose (0.1 mg/kg i.v.) to nine normal subjects and nine psychiatric patients (the majority of whom had been diagnosed as schizophrenic).

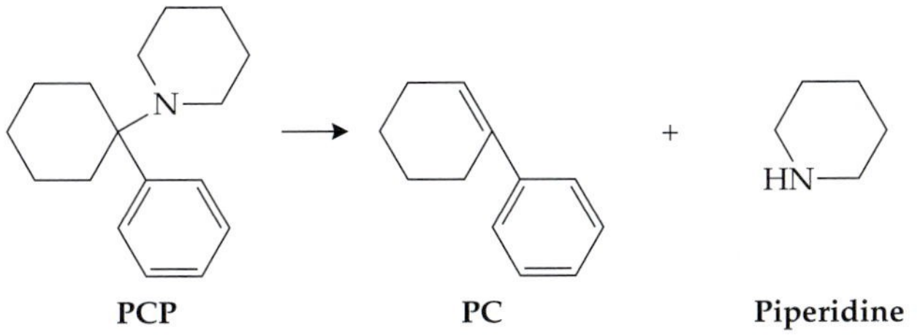

17.12 PYROLYSIS OF PCP. When PCP is smoked, some of the drug is broken down by heat to form 1-(1-phenyl)-1-cyclohexene (PC) and piperidine.

Reactions to the drug generally began within 3 minutes and persisted up to 1 hour following PCP injection.

Interviews during the period of drug intoxication revealed a variety of common responses in both the normal and psychiatric subjects (Table 17.2). One of the most profound effects was an altered body image, as revealed by such characteristic statements as "I feel far away . . . my arms and legs feel distant." This phenomenon was accompanied by a disappearance of normal "ego boundaries." In other words, subjects under the influence of PCP experienced a reduced ability to differentiate between self and nonself. Other sensory effects included feelings of vertigo or floating. Another common reaction to PCP was a strong feeling of isolation and aloneness, which was unpleasant for some subjects but not others. Moreover, all PCP-treated subjects exhibited a marked cognitive disorganization manifested by difficulty in maintaining concentration or focus, deficiency in abstract thinking, and halting speech. Various affective reactions were also observed in many subjects, including drowsiness, apathy, negativism or hostility toward the experimenters, or feelings of euphoria and inebriation. The latter sensation was conveyed by such statements as "I feel half-plastered" or "this is a cheap hangover." In addition, several of the subjects reported experiencing a dreamlike state while under the influence of the drug. The results from the subject interviews were supplemented by neurological tests that demonstrated the presence of ataxia (muscular incoordination, particularly in walking), rotary nystagmus (oscillating movements of the eyeballs), reduced sensitivity of the somatosensory system, and in some cases diplopia (double vision).

Later studies confirmed and extended these initial findings (Bakker and Amini, 1961; Davies and Beech, 1960; Rosenbaum et al., 1959). Experiments using standard cognitive and motor tasks clearly demonstrated PCP-induced impairment, particularly when task difficulty was high. Some of these same studies also reported that PCP exacerbated the symptoms of psychotic patients (see below). Obviously, PCP is a complex drug capable of eliciting a wide range of responses. Nevertheless, the type of reaction that occurs in any given instance is not arbitrary, but rather depends on the dose, the physical and social setting, the personality of the user, previous experience with the drug, and other aspects of the individual's mental set.

PCP Intoxication in Drug Abusers

Information concerning the behavioral and physiological effects of PCP can also be gleaned from clinical reports of drug abuse cases, although such findings are limited by the uncertainty of dose, variability in the interval between drug ingestion and arrival at the hospital, and so forth. Burns and Lerner (1976) described 18 emergency room cases of acute PCP intoxication between 1972 and 1975 in San Francisco. At the time of presentation, the

Table 17.2   Self-Reported and Observed Effects of PCP in Controlled Studies
Altered body image
Feelings of isolation/aloneness
Cognitive disorganization
Drowsiness and apathy
Negativism and/or hostility
Feelings of euphoria and inebriation
Hypnagogic (dreamlike) states

patients were either in a stuporous/comatose state or were confused or delirious. Instances of bizarre or (in one case) violent behavior were also noted. Based on a major survey of 1,000 clinical cases involving PCP abuse, either alone or in combination with other drugs, McCarron and coworkers (1981) proposed the following four major syndromes of PCP intoxication: (1) acute brain syndrome, (2) catatonic syndrome, (3) toxic psychosis, and (4) coma. The acute brain syndrome referred to the presence of marked disorientation, often accompanied by confusion, poor judgment, inappropriate emotional responses, and/or amnesia for recent events. Agitation, bizarre behavior, or violence were also seen in some of these patients. Patients diagnosed as having the catatonic syndrome displayed various combinations of symptoms such as rigidity or catalepsy, psychosocial withdrawal (negativism, mutism), excitement (agitation, violence), and/or lethargy or stupor. The term toxic psychosis was used to denote the presence of drug-induced hallucinations and/or delusions, with or without accompanying acute brain syndrome, but without significant symptoms of the catatonic syndrome. Finally, severe PCP intoxication was associated with varying periods of coma that occasionally persisted for more than a day. Although emergency room observations can aid in our understanding of PCP intoxication, it is important to recognize that some of the responses observed during the recovery period may represent acute withdrawal reactions rather than primary effects of the drug.

PCP and Psychopathology

During the late 1950s, many researchers favored LSD as producing the best available drug-induced model of schizophrenia. However, when Luby and colleagues observed the effects of PCP on normal volunteers, they proposed that this drug was superior to LSD in mimicking the primary deficits found in schizophrenia (Cohen et al., 1962; Luby et al., 1959; Rosenbaum et al., 1959). As discussed by Javitt and Zukin (1991), the effects of PCP on body image, thought processes, and affect closely resemble the primary symptoms of schizophrenia proposed many years ago by Bleuler (1950). A further link between PCP and psychopathology came from several reports of schizophrenia-like psychotic episodes that occurred either immediately following heavy PCP use or after a delay of a few days (Allen and Young, 1978; Luisada, 1978; Rainey and Crowder, 1975). The process by which PCP produces psychopathological effects is still unclear; however, knowledge of its underlying mechanisms of action may eventually help in the elucidation of schizophrenic pathophysiology, as well as in the development of novel pharmacological approaches for treating psychoses (Javitt and Zukin, 1991; also see Chapter 18).

Acute Behavioral Effects of PCP in Animals

Many different experimental paradigms have been used to study the influence of PCP on the behavior of animals. Here we will selectively focus on the complex activational and depressant effects produced by PCP, its ability to alter learning and memory processes, the properties of PCP as a discriminative stimulus, and its reinforcing effects in several experimental paradigms.

Excitatory and Depressant Effects

PCP can have either excitatory or depressant properties when given to animal subjects, depending on the dose, species, and test situation. As reviewed by Balster (1986), some of the stimulatory effects of PCP are amphetamine-like, whereas its depressant effects are reminiscent of those produced by barbiturates and other sedative–hypnotic agents. We shall see that these varied consequences of PCP administration are probably related to modulation of different neurotransmitter systems and ion channels. Nevertheless, because of the complexity of PCP-induced behavioral responses, this unusual drug continues to defy simple classification as either a psychomotor stimulant, a CNS depressant, or a hallucinogen.

Chen and coworkers (1959) first reported the effects of various PCP doses on unconditioned motor behavior in rats and mice. Rats injected subcutaneously with as little as 2 mg/kg of PCP displayed elevated locomotor activity in a jiggle cage apparatus. Stronger behavioral excitation along with ataxia was elicited by 10 mg/kg of PCP injected intraperitoneally, whereas a 50 mg/kg intraperitoneal dose caused a "cataleptoid" state with severe tremors. Mice given 2–4 mg/kg intraperitoneally dose of PCP, were highly excited, but showed deficient performance on the rotarod test of neuromuscular coordination. This neuromuscular deficiency reported in mice, together with the ataxic effects of PCP in rats, reflect a depressant influence of the drug manifested simultaneously with its locomotor activating effects.

Chen and coworkers (1959) further observed that PCP produced primarily a calming or "taming" effect in a wide variety of other species, including guinea pigs, hamsters, rabbits, pigeons, dogs, cats, and rhesus monkeys. Why PCP is predominantly excitatory in some animals yet calming in others is still not known, although the answer is presumably related to species differences in neurotransmitter responsivity to the drug.

In rats, PCP can also elicit a variety of stereotyped behaviors, including persistent sniffing, grooming, gagging, head weaving, turning, backpedaling, and reciprocal forepaw treading. Whereas general locomotor activation was the principal response to 5 mg/kg or less of PCP, stereotyped behaviors and ataxia predominated at higher doses (Sturgeon, Fessler, and Meltzer, 1979; Figure 17.13).

Another important measure of PCP-related excitation or depression is its ability either to promote or inhibit seizure activity. Very high doses of PCP induce seizures in both humans and animals. On the other hand, lower doses of the drug have potent anticonvulsant effects in several standard animal models. For example, PCP antagonized tonic-extensor seizures in mice, whether they were audiogenic, pentylenetetrazol-induced, or electroshock-induced (Chen et al., 1959; Chen and Bohner, 1961). The drug also inhibited hippocampal kindled seizures in rats (Buterbaugh and Michelson, 1986). The anticonvulsant effects of PCP and similar drugs appear to be related to their ability to block N-methyl-D-aspartate (NMDA) receptors (Leander, Rathbun, and Zimmerman, 1988; see below).

Finally, researchers have investigated the influence of PCP on schedule-controlled operant behavior. In several different species, certain doses of PCP were found to promote food-reinforced lever pressing, particularly when given under conditions in which baseline rates of responding were low (see Balster, 1986). Such effects are similar to those produced by amphetamine, and therefore reflect the stimulatory aspects of PCP.

Effects on Learning and Memory

PCP has been tested in a variety of tasks to determine its effects on acquisition and retention of learned behaviors. Although early studies indicated a disruptive effect of PCP on conditioning (for review, see Balster and Chait, 1976), a number of these experiments suffered from design problems that precluded differentiating between *learning and memory* deficits and *motor* deficits induced by the drug. Later studies using spatial or avoidance learning tasks were able to minimize these problems by introducing better control procedures, and generally confirmed that PCP can interfere with learning and/or memory mechanisms (Handelmann, Contreras, and O'Donohue, 1987; Kesner, Hardy, and Novak, 1983; Kesner, Dakis, and Bolland, 1993; Tang and Franklin, 1983). For example, Tang and Franklin (1983) examined the effects of PCP, ketamine, and the related dioxolane derivative dexoxadrol [(+)-2-(2,2-diphenyl-1,3-dioxolan-4-yl) piperidine] on performance in a discrimination shock-avoidance task. In this paradigm, rats were trained to escape/avoid foot shock by running to the dark arm of an automated Y-maze. The

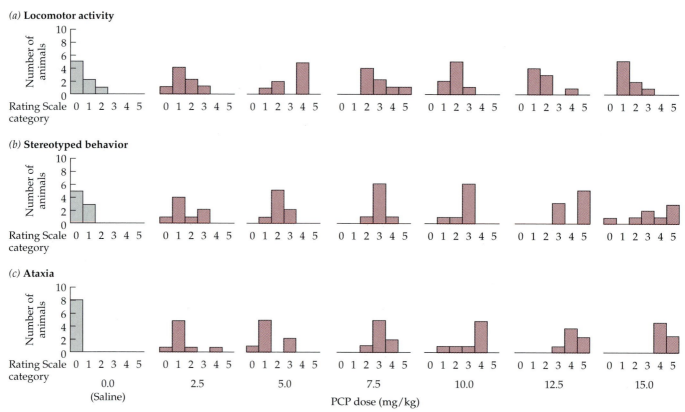

(a) **Locomotor activity**

(b) **Stereotyped behavior**

(c) **Ataxia**

17.13 DOSE-DEPENDENT BEHAVIORAL EFFECTS OF PCP IN RATS. Rats were administered saline or PCP (2.5–15.0 mg/kg i.p.) and then rated 15 minutes later for intensity of *(a)* locomotor activity, *(b)* stereotyped behavior, and *(c)* ataxia. The bars show the number of animals (out of 8 per group) receiving each rating for a given dose of PCP. (After Sturgeon, Fessler, and Meltzer, 1979.)

subjects were thus required to learn a brightness discrimination in addition to the avoidance response, allowing the investigators to assess changes in discrimination behavior independently of altered avoidance responding (which can be confounded by the motor effects of drugs). All three drugs produced a dose-dependent inhibition of discrimination accuracy in animals trained to a preestablished performance criterion. A second experiment examined the influence of repeated injections of PCP in animals given only five initial training sessions. Whereas avoidance responding was unchanged by the drug treatment, 3 mg/kg of PCP consistently reduced discrimination accuracy down to chance levels (i.e., 50% response accuracy) (Figure 17.14). This dose also produced locomotor stimulation, as indicated by a significant increase in movement during the intertrial interval. Finally, several α-adrenergic receptor antagonists were able to reverse the above-mentioned deficit in discrimination behavior, suggesting a possible role for these receptors in some of PCP's behavioral effects.

Discriminative Stimulus Properties of PCP

Like THC, PCP has marked discriminative stimulus properties. Moreover, certain drugs have been found to generalize to the PCP cue, and in one study in which several drug stereoisomers were tested (i.e., dexoxadrol vs. levoxadrol and (–)2-MDP vs. (+)2-MDP), this generalization effect showed stereospecificity (Figure 17.15; Browne, 1986). This result is consistent with the hypothesis that the PCP discriminative cue is mediated by a specific receptor (see below). Other studies by Shannon (1981) found that PCE and another PCP analog, 1-[1-(2-thienyl)cyclohexyl]piperidine (TCP), are more potent than PCP itself in producing a PCP-like discriminative stimulus.

TCP

One of the most interesting drugs that generalized to the PCP cue was SKF 10,047 (N-allylnormetazocine). This compound is a benzomorphan opiate with psy-

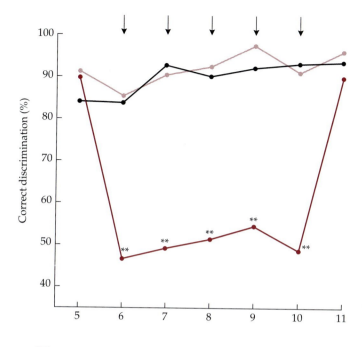

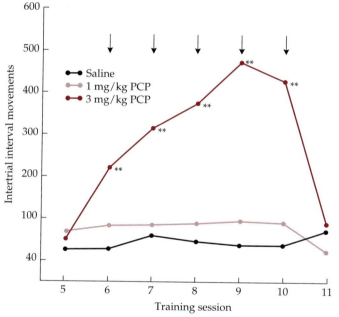

17.14 EFFECTS OF PCP ON BEHAVIOR IN A DISCRIMINATED Y-MAZE ESCAPE–AVOIDANCE TASK. Rats were given five initial training sessions in an escape–avoidance task that required a simultaneous brightness discrimination (see text for details). For sessions 6 through 10, saline or PCP were administered subcutaneously 30 minutes prior to testing (arrows). The higher dose of PCP completely eliminated the learned discrimination while simultaneously eliciting hyperactivity as indicated by increased intertrial interval (ITI) movements. (After Tang and Franklin, 1983.)

chotomimetic properties in humans. In dogs, it exerts a range of physiological and behavioral effects that have been called "canine delirium" (see Walker et al., 1990). PCP–SKF 10,047 cross-generalization in the drug discrim-

ination paradigm is probably mediated by the so-called PCP receptor, which will be discussed later. However, SKF 10,047 also interacts with a second site termed the "σ-receptor." The σ-receptor was first proposed by Martin and his colleagues (1976) as a novel type of opiate receptor that mediated the unique effects of SKF 10,047 in dogs. Although the σ-receptor is no longer considered to be a member of the opiate receptor class, it does appear to be a distinct entity with physiological relevance (London, 1993; Walker et al., 1990). Sigma receptors can be la-

beled with either (+)-[³H]3-3(hydroxyphenyl)-N-(1-propyl)piperidine (3-PPP) or [³H] di-*o*-tolylguanidine (DTG) (Walker et al., 1990), and they probably consist of multiple subtypes (Quirion et al., 1987, 1992). Sigma receptors also have a high affinity for the neuroleptic drug haloperidol, and some investigators have been developing novel sigma ligands to be screened as potential antipsychotic agents (Taylor and Schlemmer, 1992).

Reinforcing Effects of PCP

Researchers have found that PCP is highly reinforcing to animals in the self-administration paradigm. Thus far, PCP self-administration has been demonstrated in rats (Carroll, France, and Meisch, 1981; Marquis and Moreton, 1987), dogs (Risner, 1982), rhesus monkeys (Balster and Woolverton, 1980; Carroll, 1987), and baboons (Lukas et al., 1984). In most cases, the drug was self-administered intravenously; however, rhesus monkeys can also be trained to ingest PCP orally (Carroll, 1987). As in the case of cocaine (see Chapter 13), PCP self-administration is subject to modulation by factors such as unit price (i.e., number of responses required per dose unit) and availability of other reinforcers (Carroll, 1993).

Work on laboratory primates has shown that PCP will support self-administration at doses that are behaviorally toxic to the animal. Indeed, rhesus monkeys self-administering high doses of PCP were intoxicated almost continuously (Balster and Woolverton, 1980, 1981). Under the influence of PCP, the subjects could not support themselves on four legs, but instead were typically found near the response lever either in an awkward sitting position or lying on the cage floor. The ability to elicit self-intoxication in animals is not unique to PCP, but has also been observed with cocaine, amphetamine, opiates, and in some cases alcohol.

Compound	Structure	ED$_{50}$ PCP cueing
PCP		0.55
(±)Ketamine	Cl, NHCH$_3$, O	2.20
Tiletamine	S, NHCH$_2$CH$_3$, O	0.46
Dexoxadrol Levoxadrol	N H O O	1.68 >100
(−)2-MDP (+)2-MDP	HO—C—C—CH$_2$NH$_2$, H, CH$_3$	2.13 >10
± SKF 10047	—NCH$_2$CH=CH$_2$, HO, CH$_3$, CH$_3$	2.74

17.15 POTENCY OF VARIOUS COMPOUNDS IN GENERALIZING TO A PCP-INDUCED DISCRIMINATIVE STIMULUS. Rats were trained to discriminate PCP (1.78 mg/kg s.c.) from vehicle as described in the text. Other drugs were then tested for their potency (ED$_{50}$) in generalizing to the PCP cue. MDP, 2-methyl-3,3-diphenyl-3-propanolamine. (After Browne, 1986.)

A few studies have examined the reinforcing effects of PCP using the place conditioning paradigm. In one case, 0.45 mg/kg of PCP elicited a modest place preference in rats, whereas lower doses had no effect (Marglin et al., 1989). In contrast, a high dose of 4 mg/kg PCP was found to produce a conditioned place aversion (Barr, Paredes, and Bridger, 1985). Consequently, it appears that in the place conditioning paradigm, PCP is at best weakly reinforcing at low doses and aversive at high doses.

PCP Abuse and the Effects of Chronic PCP Exposure

Why Is PCP Abused?

The 1990 National Household Survey on Drug Abuse estimated that about 300,000 Americans had used PCP during the past year, and that approximately 6 million individuals had used the drug at least once during their lifetime (National Institute on Drug Abuse, 1991). Compared to marijuana and even cocaine, these numbers are rather modest. Yet PCP seems to be the drug of choice for a small segment of the population. Why is this so?

Psychoactive drugs can produce many different kinds of subjective reactions. Intuitively, we would expect that the positive effects of a drug reinforce drug-taking behavior, whereas the negative effects discourage further use of the drug. The situation is far from this simple, however. We have seen that PCP can lead to many negative reactions, including agitation, confusion, heightened anxiety, dysphoria, and lethargy. Indeed, the accounts of acute PCP intoxication discussed above might seem so peculiar and disturbing as to preclude anyone from knowingly using the drug more than once.

This seeming paradox may be explained by considering the characteristics of "typical" PCP users and the type of experience sought when using PCP. Detailed information concerning PCP users during the 1970s (when the popularity of the drug first surged) was obtained in a major ethnographic study carried out simultaneously in Philadelphia, Chicago, Miami, and Seattle/Tacoma. According to a summary of this research (Feldman, 1980), groups that experimented with PCP consisted primarily of working- and middle-class white adolescents. These individuals commonly expressed feelings of boredom and a lack of interest in conventional lifestyles. They took drugs in order to achieve a sense of excitement, challenge, and risk that was otherwise lacking in their lives. In fact, most users took PCP to some extent *because of* rather than despite the attendant risks. Moreover, careful planning of the social and environmental setting surrounding the drug experience, along with attempts to control dosage, allowed users to avoid "bad trips" most of the time. Indeed, sharing of the strange experiences induced by PCP seemed to forge a strong sense of solidarity among group members.

Finally, other studies found that chronic PCP users described their first experience with the drug in terms such as "exhilarating," "fun," "happy," "euphoric," "a dream world," "the perfect escape" (Linder, Lerner, and Burns, 1981). A positive experience with PCP in one's initial encounter is reinforcing and likely to increase the probability of subsequent use.

Tolerance and Dependence

Both tolerance to and dependence on PCP have been investigated in studies examining the effects of chronic drug treatment and withdrawal on animals performing an operant task. Other measures included effects on motor and ingestive behaviors. In the development of tolerance to PCP, researchers have generally observed no more than two- to fourfold shifts in its dose–response curve (Balster, 1986), which represents only a modest tolerance compared with that obtained with many other abused drugs. Tolerance to PCP may result at least partially from alterations in drug disposition, although functional tolerance (i.e., the ability to perform the response while intoxicated) may also develop under some conditions (Spain and Klingman, 1985). Balster (1986) noted a somewhat greater tolerance to the behaviorally disruptive effects of PCP in monkeys self-administering very high doses. Since these subjects were continuously intoxicated, as described above (see Balster and Woolverton, 1981), the relevance of these findings to human PCP abusers is uncertain.

PCP dependence has been demonstrated in animals abruptly withdrawn from the drug following a period of chronic administration. For example, withdrawal from PCP significantly suppressed food-reinforced operant responding in both monkeys (Slifer, Balster, and Woolverton, 1984; Carroll and Carmona, 1991) and rats (Wessinger and Owens, 1991) (Figure 17.16). The severity of this effect was dependent upon the number of responses required for each reinforcement, suggesting that PCP

withdrawal may alter motivational processes (Carroll and Carmona, 1991). In general, animals shown to be behaviorally dependent on PCP exhibited few if any physical signs of drug abstinence. One exception, however, was the study by Slifer, Balster, and Woolverton (1984), in which some of the monkeys withdrawn from PCP showed mild abstinence symptoms such as oculomotor hyperactivity, tremors and/or twitches, and hyperaggressiveness.

These results demonstrate that chronic administration of low to moderate doses of PCP produces a behavioral dependence without a significant physical dependence. On the other hand, withdrawal from high doses of PCP can lead to more severe symptomatology. For example, rats infused with 45 mg/kg/day of PCP for 7 days displayed an abstinence syndrome consisting of piloerection, bruxism (teeth grinding), decreased exploratory activity, and extremely impaired rotarod performance (Spain and Klingman, 1985). Additionally, the monkeys of Balster and Woolverton (1980, 1981) that were self-administering intoxicating doses of PCP (4–7 mg/kg per day) showed severe symptoms upon drug withdrawal, including excessive vocalizations, fearfulness, bruxism, diarrhea, piloerection, oculomotor hyperactivity, twitches, and in one case convulsions.

Does chronic PCP use lead to physical and/or psychological dependence in humans? Surprisingly little has been published concerning this issue. The little research available seems to indicate that PCP abusers do not usually develop a strong physical dependence on the

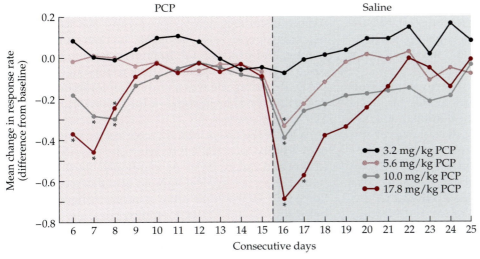

17.16 DISRUPTION OF OPERANT RESPONDING DURING WITHDRAWAL FROM PCP. Rats were first trained to lever-press for food reinforcement. Response rates were then monitored while the subjects were infused intravenously with saline for 5 days (data not shown); PCP for 10 days at a dose of 3.2, 5.6, 10.0, or 17.8 mg/kg/day; and then saline again for the final 10 days. The data displayed are mean changes in response rate compared with the baseline rates measured during the first saline infusion period. Note the disruption of operant behavior during initial administration of high doses of PCP and during withdrawal from all but the lowest PCP dose. Asterisks denote a statistically significant difference ($p < 0.05$) from the baseline response rate. (After Wessinger and Owens, 1991.)

drug, perhaps because PCP's dysphoric effects preclude taking extremely high doses for prolonged periods of time. Whether a psychological dependence can develop to PCP is less clear. Withdrawal from chronic PCP use may entail some abstinence symptomatology. An open clinical study by Tennant, Rawson, and McCann (1981) found that cessation of PCP by a group of chronic users led to feelings of anergia, restlessness, depression, and drug craving. These symptoms could be alleviated by treatment with the antidepressant desipramine. On the other hand, Feldman (1980) reported that individuals often voluntarily reduced or even terminated their use of PCP when faced with the prospect of impaired pyschological functioning due to long-term use (see next section). Furthermore, in many cases users seemed to lose their desire for PCP as they approached adulthood. From these various findings, we may surmise that long-term PCP abuse leads to psychological dependence in some individuals, but that this dependence syndrome is not a common phenomenon that inevitably develops in all chronic PCP users.

Psychological and Neurological Effects of Chronic PCP Use

The psychological effects of chronic PCP use have been described by Feldman (1980) and Linder, Lerner, and Burns (1981). According to Feldman, heavy PCP use over a long period of time can lead to significant cognitive impairment characterized by confusion, disjointed thought, and severe memory loss. This state is referred to on the street as "burnout" and is a matter of concern for many users. Chronic PCP also causes severe emotional disturbances, including depression and even suicidal thoughts. When persistent feelings of depression are periodically interrupted by states of drug-induced euphoria, the individual may feel as if he or she is on an "emotional roller coaster."

Does prolonged PCP use lead to permanent tissue damage? Although chronic exposure to PCP has been reported to reduce frontal lobe glucose utilization (Wu, Buchsbaum, and Bunney, 1991), which could adversely affect certain cognitive abilities, neuropsychological tests performed on heavy users demonstrated a recovery of behavioral and cognitive function when the subjects significantly reduced or eliminated their PCP intake during a 4-week period (Cosgrove and Newell, 1991). Furthermore, rhesus monkeys that self-administered PCP daily for up to 8 years did not appear to suffer any adverse physical reactions to the drug (Carroll, 1990). On the other hand, research with rats indicated that PCP may exert neurotoxic effects under some conditions. Olney and coworkers (Olney, Labruyere, and Price, 1989; Olney et al., 1991) initially described a transient cytopathological reaction to PCP and related drugs in a population of neurons in the cingulate and retrosplenial cortices. More recently, Ellison (1995) found that

5 days of continuous PCP treatment led to neuronal degeneration in a number of limbic system and limbic-related structures, including the posteroventral entorhinal cortex, ventral hippocampus and dentate gyrus, olfactory tubercle and anterior olfactory nuclei, and retrosplenial cortex. These structures have also been shown to be sites of cytological and/or metabolic abnormalities in the brains of many schizophrenic patients. If, as many researchers now believe, structural and metabolic deficits play a critical role in producing the negative symptoms of schizophrenia (see Chapter 18), then chronic PCP use may be a valuable model for studying these aspects of the disorder.

Mechanisms of PCP Action

The PCP Receptor

Characterization of binding sites.   We have seen that PCP produces a wide variety of behavioral effects, which has complicated the task of determining the mechanism of action of this compound. However, a major step toward understanding PCP mechanisms came with the discovery in 1979 of specific binding sites for radiolabeled PCP. The first studies were performed by two groups of researchers, both of which reported that [^{3}H]PCP bound with submicromolar affinity to a single class of sites in rat brain membranes (Vincent et al., 1979; Zukin and Zukin, 1979). Binding could be displaced by various PCP analogs with potencies that correlated well with their potencies in the mouse rotarod test and in the rat discriminative stimulus paradigm. In contrast, a variety of neurotransmitters, neuropeptides, and classical receptor blocking agents (e.g., atropine, haloperidol, phentolamine, and propranolol, to name a few) failed to displace PCP receptor binding. These results suggested that the PCP binding site was a novel receptor in the brain responsible for at least some of the behavioral effects of PCP administration.

One of the drugs initially reported to possess significant affinity for [^{3}H]PCP binding sites was SKF 10,047 (Zukin and Zukin, 1979). As mentioned above, this compound is a prototypical agonist of the σ-receptor site. Since SKF 10,047 (and other σ-receptor ligands) competes strongly for [^{3}H]PCP binding sites, and since PCP likewise has respectable affinity for sites labeled with [^{3}H]SKF 10,047, many investigators initially postulated that PCP receptors and σ-receptors were one and the same (publications from this period of uncertainty commonly refer to the "PCP/σ-receptor"). However, by the mid-1980s, studies from several laboratories provided convincing evidence that there were two separate sites in the brain to which both PCP and SKF 10,047 could bind (Figure 17.17). The non-σ-receptor site, which is now simply called the PCP receptor, can also be labeled selec-

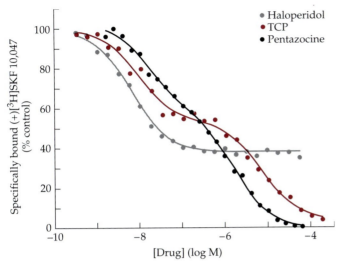

[Drug] (log M)

• Haloperidol
• TCP
• Pentazocine

17.17 EVIDENCE FOR MULTIPLE BINDING SITES FOR (+)-[³H]-SKF 10,047. Haloperidol, TCP, and pentazocine were tested for their ability to inhibit specific binding of 8 nM (+)-[³H]SKF 10,047 to rat whole-brain membranes. Haloperidol displacement was consistent with a one-site model of binding; however, the TCP and pentazocine competition curves were fit best with a two-site model. The (+)-SKF 10,047-labeled site displaced by all three drugs is considered to be the σ-receptor, whereas the additional site recognized only by TCP and pentazocine is currently called the PCP receptor. (After Largent, Gundlach, and Snyder, 1986.)

tively with [³H]TCP, [¹²⁵I]TCP, or the tricyclic compound [³H]MK-801 (5-methyl-10,11-dihydro-5H-dibenzo[a,d]-cyclohepten-5,10-imine; also called dizocilpine) (Price et al., 1988; Reynolds et al., 1992; Vignon et al., 1983). The PCP receptor has a high affinity for PCP and dexoxadrol, but a very low affinity for haloperidol and the sigma ligands 3-PPP and DTG.

(+)-MK-801

Autoradiographic studies of the rat brain have found high densities of PCP receptors in the hippocampal formation (particularly in the strata radiatum and oriens of CA1 and in the dentate gyrus), striate cortex, and layers 1 and 2 of the somatosensory and motor cortices (Johnson and Jones, 1990; Maragos, Penney, and Young, 1988). Intermediate receptor densities were observed in the amygdala, caudate–putamen, nucleus accumbens, olfactory tubercle, lateral septum, parts of the olfactory system, and certain nuclei of the thalamus. A different distribution has been reported for the σ-receptor (Walker et al., 1990), which further discriminates this receptor from the PCP receptor.

PCP and the NMDA receptor. The PCP receptor has been identified as a part of the N-methyl-D-aspartate (NMDA) receptor complex (see Chapter 10). To review briefly, the NMDA receptor is one of the major receptor subtypes for excitatory amino acids such as glutamate and aspartate. The receptor complex gates a cation channel with permeability to Na⁺, K⁺, and Ca²⁺, and possesses multiple regulatory sites that bind not only PCP and related drugs but also glycine, polyamines, Mg²⁺, and Zn²⁺.

The idea of a link between PCP and NMDA receptors stems from several lines of research.

1. Electrophysiological studies carried out in the early and mid-1980s by Lodge and coworkers showed that activation of NMDA receptors could be selectively and noncompetitively blocked by a variety of chemical agents, including initially PCP and related arylcyclohexylamines (see Chapter 10). The list was then expanded to include the sigma benzomorphan cyclazocine, 1,3-substituted dioxolanes such as dexoxadrol, benz-(f)-isoquinolines, and diphenylpropanolamines (reviewed by Johnson et al., 1989).

2. Binding studies performed by other investigators showed that these same compounds possess affinities for the PCP receptor that correlate well with their potencies in behavioral assays of PCP action (Johnson et al., 1993; see below for further discussion).

3. When *Xenopus* oocytes were injected with rat brain mRNA, PCP receptors were coexpressed with NMDA receptors, as indicated by the ability of PCP ligands to effectively modulate the electrophysiological effects of NMDA on these cells (Kushner et al., 1988).

4. In almost all brain areas examined, an excellent correlation was found between the anatomical distribution of PCP receptors labeled with [³H]-TCP and the distribution of NMDA receptors labeled with either [³H]glutamate or [³H]3-([±]-2-carboxypiperazin-4-yl)-propyl-1-phosphonic acid (CPP) (Jarvis, Murphy, and Williams, 1987; Maragos, Penney, and Young, 1988).

One notable exception was the cerebellar granule layer, which displayed a much higher relative density of NMDA receptors than PCP receptors. This raises the possibility that certain NMDA receptors may not possess a PCP modulatory site.

PCP receptor binding is influenced by substances that interact with other regulatory sites on the NMDA receptor complex. Thus, addition of an NMDA agonist stimulates binding of both [³H]TCP and [³H]MK-801 (Johnson et al., 1989, 1993). Activation of the NMDA receptor complex may induce a conformational change in the associated PCP receptor that increases its affinity for its ligands. Because the PCP recognition site is thought to be located within the channel of the NMDA receptor complex (see Chapter 10), receptor activation could also increase ligand accessibility merely by opening the channel. Glycine, Mg^{2+}, and Zn^{2+} also modulate ligand binding at the PCP site, further illustrating the complex interactions within the NMDA receptor complex.

Endogenous ligand for the PCP receptor.   In the previous section on marijuana, we discussed the recent discovery of a putative endogenous ligand for the cannabinoid receptor. Existence of a PCP receptor likewise implies that: (1) there must be one or more endogenous ligands for this site that play a significant role in regulating excitatory amino acid transmission; and (2) insofar as this substance may mimic the behavioral effects of PCP, it might have an important influence on locomotor behavior, brain excitability, learning and memory, reinforcement mechanisms, and even the etiology of certain psychotic states. Although researchers have begun to search for endogenous PCP-like substances (Contreras et al., 1993; Zukin et al., 1987), at the time of this writing no group has yet announced the isolation and characterization of any candidate compound.

Other Neurochemical Actions of PCP

Ion channels.   Considering that the PCP recognition site on the NMDA receptor complex seems to be associated with the receptor's ion channel, it is not surprising that PCP can additionally block several other types of channels. These include voltage-sensitive Na^+ and K^+ channels (Aguayo and Albuquerque, 1987; Allaoua and Chicheportiche, 1989; ffrench-Mullen and Rogawski, 1989) and the cation channel gated by the nicotinic cholinergic receptor (Albuquerque et al., 1983). Since the affinity of PCP for these ion channels is significantly lower than its affinity for the PCP binding site on the NMDA receptor, low doses of the drug should preferentially inhibit NMDA receptor-gated currents without having effects on these other channels. At higher doses of PCP, K^+ channel blockade might prolong action potential duration, enhance activity-dependent neurotransmitter release (see below), and even mediate the proconvulsant effects seen at high drug concentrations. In contrast, inhibition of nerve conduction following Na^+ channel blockade might be responsible for the PCP-induced anesthesia observed in some species (Allaoua and Chicheportiche, 1989).

Acetylcholine.   In addition to blocking nicotinic receptor channels, PCP also blocks muscarinic receptors and inhibits acetylcholinesterase (Kloog et al., 1977; Weinstein, Maayani, and Pazhenchevsky, 1983). However, these direct interactions with the cholinergic system occur only at extremely high PCP concentrations, and are thought to have little or no relationship to the drug's behavioral effects (Johnson, 1982; Johnson and Hillman, 1982; Vincent et al., 1983). In contrast, PCP, ketamine, and other drugs with PCP-like behavioral effects (e.g., etoxadrol and SKF 10,047) have been shown to inhibit NMDA-stimulated ACh release from rat cerebral cortical and striatal slices at nanomolar to low micromolar concentrations (Lodge and Johnston, 1985; Snell and Johnson, 1985, 1986). Potency correlation studies suggest that this indirect anticholinergic effect is due to action at the NMDA receptor-linked PCP binding site.

Norepinephrine and serotonin.   PCP interacts in a complex manner with the noradrenergic and serotonergic systems. It competitively inhibits the uptake of NE by cortical, hypothalamic, and hippocampal synaptosomes (Garey and Heath, 1976; Smith et al., 1977; Snell, Yi, and Johnson, 1988), and also reduces NMDA-induced NE release from hippocampal slices (Jones, Snell, and Johnson, 1987; Snell, Yi, and Johnson, 1988). Systemically administered PCP was reported to decrease the firing rate of noradrenergic neurons in the locus coeruleus (LC) under baseline conditions (Raja and Guyenet, 1980; Murase et al., 1992), and to inhibit responsivity of LC neurons to sensory stimulation (Murase et al., 1992). In contrast, locally applied PCP seemed to enhance the synaptic effects of NE in the hippocampus and cerebellum (Bickford et al., 1981; Marwaha et al., 1980). It is possible that the former action is due to antagonism of NMDA receptor-mediated excitatory input to the LC cells, whereas the latter effect is related to the direct NE uptake-blocking properties of PCP.

With respect to serotonin (5-HT), PCP was found to inhibit 5-HT uptake (Smith et al., 1977), enhance the conversion of [^{3}H]tryptophan to [^{3}H]5-HT in the rat forebrain (Johnson, 1982), and increase 5-HT overflow in the nucleus accumbens (Hernandez, Auerbach, and Hoebel, 1988). The firing rate of serotonergic neurons, however, was less influenced by PCP than was the firing of noradrenergic cells (Raja and Guyenet, 1980).

Dopamine.   As in the case of ACh, low concentrations of PCP have been shown to inhibit NMDA-evoked DA release from striatal slices (Snell and Johnson, 1986). The potency of various PCP-like drugs to inhibit DA release correlates well with their affinity for the PCP binding site on the NMDA receptor complex. This indirect antidopaminergic effect observed in vitro is probably mediated by PCP receptors located directly on the nigrostriatal dopaminergic nerve endings (Johnson and Jeng, 1991). On the other hand, the role of endogenous glutamate (acting via either NMDA or non-NMDA receptors) in regulating striatal DA release in vivo is still subject to considerable debate and uncertainty (see, for example,

Imperato, Honoré, and Jensen, 1990; Leviel, Gobert, and Guibert, 1990; Moghaddam and Gruen, 1991), which makes the interpretation of PCP effects on DA release even more difficult.

Although the ability of PCP to antagonize NMDA-stimulated DA release in the striatum may contribute to some of its behavioral actions, there has been even greater interest in the DA agonist-like properties of this compound. Many of the behavioral properties of PCP resemble those of a DA agonist, including its psychotogenic effects in humans and its ability to stimulate locomotor and stereotyped behaviors in rodents. PCP has been reported to stimulate locomotor activity when infused directly into the nucleus accumbens of rats (McCullough and Salamone, 1992). The drug is also active in the circling-behavior model produced by a unilateral lesion of the nigrostriatal DA pathway. Like amphetamine, an indirect DA agonist, PCP elicits ipsilateral turning when administered to lesioned rats (Johnson, 1983).

Various studies have provided evidence for an enhancement of dopaminergic transmission by PCP. Intravenously administered PCP increased the firing rate of cells in both the substantia nigra pars compacta and the ventral tegmental area (Freeman and Bunney, 1984; French and Ceci, 1990; French, Mura, and Wang, 1993). French and coworkers (French and Ceci, 1990; French, Mura, and Wang, 1993) showed similar effects for other PCP-like drugs such as TCP, MK-801, ketamine, and SKF 10,047, but not for the selective σ-receptor ligand DTG or the κ-opioid agonist U50,488H (Figure 17.18). Systemic PCP, MK-801, and other PCP-related drugs likewise stimulated DA turnover measured by increased formation of the DA metabolites dihydroxyphenylacetic acid and homovanillic acid (Rao et al., 1990a,b; Tanii et al., 1990). This activation, however, is probably not due to a direct effect of PCP on the dopaminergic neurons, since iontophoretically applied PCP or MK-801 either inhibited or had no effect on the firing of midbrain dopaminergic cells (Freeman and Bunney, 1984; Zhang, Chiodo, and Freeman, 1992). In addition, the stimulatory effect of intravenous MK-801 was reduced by an acute hemitransection between the forebrain and midbrain (Zhang, Chiodo, and Freeman, 1992). The latter finding suggests that descending glutamatergic projections may mediate the influence of PCP and related drugs on dopaminergic cell activity.

Although electrophysiological activation of the dopaminergic system may occur indirectly, PCP does interact directly with these cells in at least two ways. First, PCP can release DA from striatal slices (Vickroy and Johnson, 1982; Snell et al., 1984) and from fetal rat mesencephalic cell cultures (Mount et al., 1990). This property seems to be inconsistent with the DA release-inhibiting effect described above. However, relatively high concentrations (at least 10–100 mM) of PCP are needed for the DA-releasing effect, which probably rules out

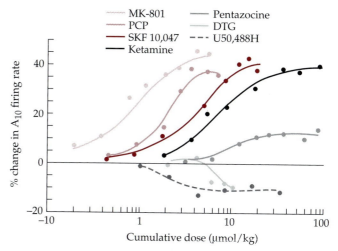

17.18 PCP-LIKE DRUGS STIMULATE FIRING OF VENTRAL TEGMENTAL AREA (A_{10}) DOPAMINERGIC NEURONS. Single-unit activity of A_{10} dopaminergic neurons was recorded in chloral hydrate-anesthetized rats during intravenous infusion of various drugs. PCP, MK-801, ketamine, SKF 10,047, and pentazocine increased the firing rate with a rank order identical to their potency ranking at the PCP receptor. No increase in cell activity was produced by either the selective σ-receptor ligand DTG or the κ-opioid agonist U50,488H. Basal firing rate across all groups was 3.7 ± 0.2 spikes/second. (After French and Ceci, 1990.)

mediation by the NMDA receptor-linked PCP binding site. The K^+ channel blocker 4-aminopyridine was found to exert a DA-releasing effect similar to that of PCP in mesencephalic cell cultures, suggesting that PCP-induced DA release might be related to blockade of membrane K^+ channels (Mount et al., 1990).

An additional means by which PCP interacts with dopaminergic neurons is to block DA uptake. In contrast to amphetamine, PCP is much more potent as a DA uptake inhibitor than as a DA releasing agent (Bowyer, Spuhler, and Weiner, 1984). PCP competitively inhibits synaptic DA uptake with IC_{50} or K_i values below 1 μM (Garey and Heath, 1976; Smith et al., 1977; Vignon and Lazdunski, 1984), and it has a similar potency in displacing [³H]mazindol binding to the rat striatal DA transporter (Kuhar, Boja, and Cone, 1990). These in vitro findings are supported by in vivo microdialysis studies showing increased DA overflow in both the nucleus accumbens and striatum following either systemic or local administration of PCP (Carboni et al., 1989; Hernandez, Auerbach, and Hoebel, 1988; McCullough and Salamone, 1992). Increased extracellular DA following local application of PCP is presumably due to the direct inhibition of DA uptake by these neurons, whereas systemic PCP administration could also induce heightened DA release by stimulating firing of the dopaminergic neurons.

DA uptake inhibition is unlikely to be mediated by the NMDA receptor-linked PCP binding site. This was shown by the finding that MK-801, which has greater potency than does PCP as a noncompetitive NMDA receptor antagonist, was about 250-fold *less* potent than PCP ($IC_{50} > 100 \mu M$) in blocking synaptosomal DA uptake (Snell, Yi, and Johnson, 1988). A possible alternative mechanism by which PCP inhibits DA uptake is that it directly binds to a site on the DA transporter. This idea has been advanced by Rothman and his colleagues, who have provided evidence that the PCP ligand [³H]TCP labels a site on the DA transporter in addition to its acknowledged interaction with the PCP receptor (Akunne et al., 1991, 1992; Rothman et al., 1989).

Other interesting evidence comes from studies of a novel PCP analog, BTCP (*N*-[1-(2-benzo(b)thiophenyl)cyclohexyl]piperidine). This compound was found to ex-

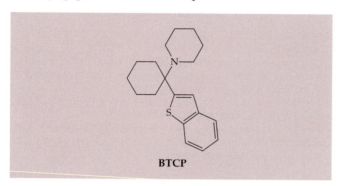

BTCP

hibit behavioral properties more similar to those of cocaine (a potent DA uptake blocking drug; see Chapter 13) than PCP (French, 1994; Koek et al., 1989). Biochemical studies further indicated that [³H]BTCP also has a high affinity for the DA transporter (Maurice et al., 1991; Vignon et al., 1988). Altogether, these results suggest that direct inhibition of DA uptake may contribute to some of the behavioral effects elicited by PCP.

Role of the NMDA Receptor and Other Neurochemical Systems in the Behavioral Effects of PCP

As researchers have begun to understand how PCP influences neurochemical and electrophysiological functioning, a number of questions have arisen concerning how these cellular changes might underlie PCP's complex psychological and behavioral properties. For example, can the various effects of PCP all be attributed to action at the NMDA receptor-linked PCP binding site? Furthermore, in those cases in which the PCP binding site is involved, can similar effects be produced by non-PCP-like (i.e., competitive) NMDA receptor antagonists? Finally, what roles may be played by other neurotransmitter systems?

Discriminative stimulus properties of PCP. The discriminative stimulus properties of PCP have provided fertile ground for studying its neurochemical–functional relationships (see Willetts, Balster, and Leander, 1990, for review). One important outcome from this work is that

MK-801 readily generalizes to either a PCP or a ketamine cue in rats, monkeys, and pigeons. Similarly, PCP and related drugs can substitute for MK-801 in subjects trained to discriminate the latter drug from saline. These findings confirm the importance of the PCP receptor in the discriminative stimulus properties of this compound. However, experiments testing the ability of *competitive* NMDA receptor antagonists (compounds blocking the agonist binding site rather than the *noncompetitive* PCP site) to generalize to a discriminative stimulus produced by PCP or ketamine have yielded complicated results. Some of the competitive NMDA antagonists that were examined in this paradigm include AP5 (2-amino-5-phosphonovalerate), AP7 (2-amino-7-phosphonoheptanoate), NPC 12626 (2-amino-4,5-(1,2-cyclohexyl)-7-phosphonoheptanoic acid), CPP (3-([±]-2-carboxypiperazin-4-yl)-propyl-1-phosphonic acid), and CGS 19755 (1-(cis)-2-carboxypiperidine-4-yl)-methyl-1-phosphonic acid). The degree to which these compounds generalize to a PCP, ketamine, or MK-801 cue seems to depend on the species tested, the route of drug administration, and the dose of the training compound (France, Woods, and Ornstein, 1989; Jackson and Sanger, 1988; Koek et al., 1987, Koek, Woods, and Colpaert, 1990; Willetts and Balster, 1988). For instance, in one study, generalization of CPP to PCP was greatest when low PCP doses were used in training (i.e., where the drug cue is less specific and also less intense (Figure 17.19); Mansbach and Balster, 1991). Consequently, it seems possible either that unique interoceptive effects are produced by noncompetitive NMDA receptor blockade, or that the stimulus properties of PCP-like drugs depend not only on interaction with the PCP receptor but also on one or more other mechanisms involving different neurotransmitter systems.

Locomotion, stereotypy, and ataxia. The underlying mechanisms for the activational and, at higher doses, ataxic effects of PCP in rats and mice have also been examined. Since MK-801 has been shown to exert similar effects (Koek, Woods, and Winger, 1988; Löscher and Hönak, 1992; Tricklebank et al., 1989), stimulation of locomotor and stereotyped behaviors by PCP probably depends more on interactions with the NMDA receptor rather than the drug's cocaine-like ability to block DA uptake. Other studies found that metaphit, a drug that acylates and hence irreversibly inactivates PCP receptors (Rafferty et al., 1985), specifically antagonized PCP-induced ataxia and stereotyped behavior, but not similar behaviors induced by the σ-preferring compounds (+)-SKF 10,047 and (−)-cyclazocine (Contreras et al., 1986). These results indicate that the similar behavioral effects observed with PCP-like drugs and σ-receptor drugs (at least in terms of ataxia and stereotyped behavior) are mediated largely, though perhaps not exclusively, by selective activation of their respective receptor systems.

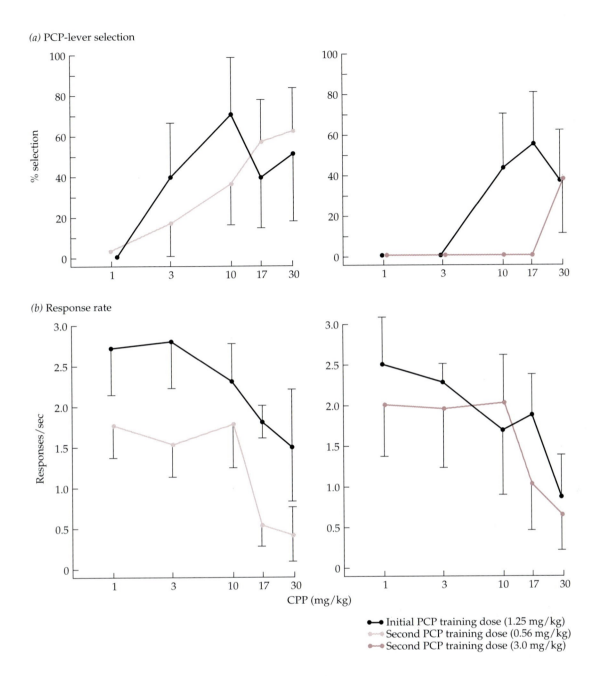

(a) PCP-lever selection

(b) Response rate

CPP (mg/kg)

●—● Initial PCP training dose (1.25 mg/kg)
○—○ Second PCP training dose (0.56 mg/kg)
●—● Second PCP training dose (3.0 mg/kg)

17.19 PCP LEVER SELECTION AND RESPONSE RATE IN PCP-TRAINED RATS TESTED WITH CPP. Rats were trained to discriminate PCP from saline using a two-lever, food-reinforced operant schedule. Subjects were initially trained at a PCP dose of 1.25 mg/kg i.p. and then switched either to 0.56 mg/kg (left panels) or to 3.0 mg/kg (right panels). The graphs illustrate percent PCP lever selection (upper panels) and response rate (lower panels) when the subjects were tested with varying doses of the competitive NMDA antagonist CPP. The unconnected points at the left side of each graph represent the results following administration of either the saline control solution (C) or the PCP training dose (P). CPP produced only a partial generalization to PCP, particularly at the highest PCP training dose. Also note the decrements in response rate associated with high doses of either PCP or CPP. (After Mansbach and Balster, 1991.)

Competitive NMDA receptor antagonists exert PCP-like activational and ataxic effects, albeit typically with a lower potency (Compton et al., 1987; Koek, Woods, and Ornstein, 1987; Tricklebank et al., 1989). This supports the hypothesis that these behaviors are mediated via NMDA receptors, though other neurotransmitter systems must also be considered. For example, DA receptor-blocking neuroleptic drugs generally antagonize PCP-induced stereotypic behavior (see Johnson, 1983, for review). Moreover, PCP-induced hyperactivity is reversed by 6-hydroxydopamine (6-OHDA) lesions of either the nucleus accumbens or the A_{10} region of the ventral tegmental area (French and Vantini, 1984; French, Pilapil, and Quirion, 1985). Although locomotor stimulation produced by the indirect DA agonist amphetamine was also attenuated by 6-OHDA pretreatment, these lesions failed to influence the activating effects of caffeine (Figure 17.20). It is also interesting to note that some of the PCP-elicited stereotypic behaviors in rats resemble those found in the "5-HT syndrome" produced by certain serotonergic agonists (see Chapter 9). Indeed, several studies suggest that the serotonergic system may contribute to the hyperlocomotion and the stereotyped behaviors observed following PCP or MK-801 administration (Löscher and Hönack, 1992; Nabeshima et al., 1987). Considering these various findings, it appears that NMDA receptor antagonism, together with DA and 5-HT stimulation, all contribute to the activational effects of PCP and related compounds.

PCP self-administration and abuse.   It may be possible in the future to control PCP abuse by means of drugs that quell the craving for PCP (in chronic users) without producing a state of psychological dependence. Achieving this goal, however, requires knowledge of how PCP exerts its reinforcing and dependence-producing effects. Too little attention has been paid to this issue, although a few clues are available for consideration. For example, Risner (1982) found that many PCP-related drugs, such as ketamine, TCP, PCE, and the PCP metabolites PPC and PCHP, will support self-administration in dogs. The

potency rank-ordering of these compounds was TCP ≥ PCP > PCE > PPC ≈ PCHP ≥ ketamine. The potencies of these compounds, and others not mentioned here, in the self-administration paradigm were highly correlated with their relative potencies in displacing [^{3}H]PCP binding to rat brain membranes. However, there was a much lower correlation between self-administration potency and potency in generalizing to the PCP cue in drug discrimination studies. Consequently, the neurochemical mechanisms underlying the reinforcing effects of PCP-like compounds may not be identical to the mechanisms responsible for their discriminative stimulus properties. In other studies, rhesus monkeys initially trained to self-administer either PCP or ketamine were shown to continue their pattern of drug administration when MK-801 was substituted for the original compound (Beardsley, Hayes, and Balster, 1990; Koek, Woods, and Winger, 1988). In contrast, when the subjects were first trained to self-administer cocaine, PCP but not MK-801 could be effectively substituted. Recent theories of drug reinforcement and dependence have focused on the mesolimbic and mesocortical DA pathways (Koob and Bloom, 1988; Wise and Bozarth, 1987; see also Chapters 4, 8, and 13). The potential involvement of these systems in PCP self-administration and abuse is a topic for further study.

Part II Summary

PCP was the first identified compound of a group of novel anesthetic agents known as dissociative anesthetics. It was subsequently found to have adverse side effects and abuse potential in humans, and it was withdrawn from clinical use. The acute effects of PCP include alterations in body image, feelings of isolation, cognitive impairment, and various affective changes. At high doses, PCP produces severe intoxication and even coma. Chronic abuse can give rise to a schizophreniform psychosis lasting for days or weeks.

Animal studies have revealed complex behavioral properties of PCP. Whereas many species will show a predominantly sedative or "taming" response to PCP, rodents display locomotor activation, stereotyped behavior, and ataxia. PCP and related drugs have anticonvulsant properties at low to moderate doses, but can themselves elicit seizures at very high dose levels. PCP also disrupts learning and/or memory processes, possesses discriminative stimulus properties, and supports self-administration in a range of species. At moderate doses, chronic PCP exposure does not produce observable signs of physical dependence in either animals or humans, although behavioral disruptions have been demonstrated during PCP abstinence in animal subjects.

Most of the functional effects of PCP can be attributed to action at the so-called PCP receptor. This receptor is a modulatory binding site in the NMDA receptor

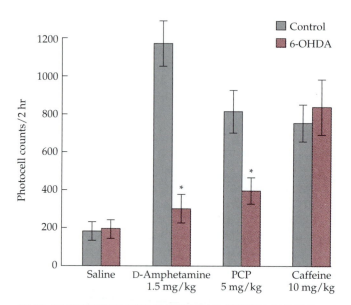

17.20 6-HYDROXYDOPAMINE LESIONS OF THE NUCLEUS AC-CUMBENS BLOCK PCP-INDUCED LOCOMOTOR ACTIVATION. Rats were injected bilaterally in the nucleus accumbens either with the catecholamine neurotoxin 6-hydroxydopamine (6-OHDA) or with vehicle. At least 14 days later, the animals were given saline, PCP, D-amphetamine, or caffeine intraperitoneally (doses are shown under each drug). 6-OHDA lesions of the nucleus accumbens significantly antagonized the locomotor activating effects of PCP and amphetamine, but not that of caffeine. Asterisks denote a significant treatment effect. (After French and Vantini, 1984.)

complex that, when occupied, produces a noncompetitive antagonism of NMDA receptor activity. The highest densities of PCP receptors are found in the hippocampal formation and regions of the neocortex. PCP also exerts a number of other neurochemical effects, including inhibition of DA uptake and, at high doses, blockade of voltage-sensitive K^+ and Na^+ channels. PCP-like drugs stimulate the firing of A_{10} dopamine neurons and increase extracellular DA concentrations in the nucleus accumbens. The dopaminergic effects of PCP may contribute to its reinforcing properties, although this hypothesis remains to be confirmed. Finally, since PCP is a synthetic compound, we must assume the existence of an endogenous ligand for the PCP receptor. Although the search for this endogenous substance has begun, definitive results have not yet been obtained.

Part III
LSD

Synthesis and Characteristic Effects of LSD

LSD, D-lysergic acid diethylamide (also known as LSD-25*), is a semisynthetic compound that was first prepared in 1938 by the Swiss chemist Albert Hofmann (1970) while working in the pharmaceutical research laboratories of Sandoz in Basel. He combined lysergic acid,

LSD-25

an alkaloid obtained from ergot (*Claviceps purpurea*), with diethylamide, a synthetic compound. The molecular structure of lysergic acid contains the indole nucleus, and thus LSD and its congener 2-bromo-LSD (BOL) are related to the neurotransmitter serotonin (5-HT). Ergot is a parasitic fungus found on rye and wheat that manufactures a number of alkaloids, some of which are extremely toxic and responsible for epidemic outbreaks of ergotism, a disease caused by consuming ergot-infested grains. This disease was quite common in the Middle

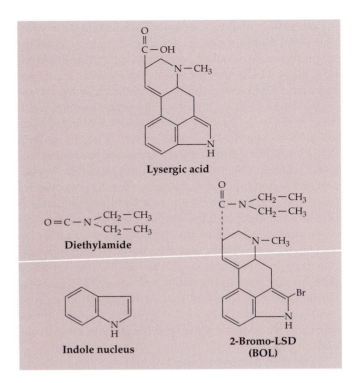

Lysergic acid

Diethylamide

Indole nucleus

2-Bromo-LSD (BOL)

Ages. Forty thousand deaths in Europe in the year A.D. 944 were later attributed to ergotism. Anthropologists who found evidence of the use of hallucinogens in religious practices in many areas of the world as early as 3,500 years ago attributed many of the hallucinogenic effects to the ingestion of plants that were infected with ergot, although many other plant substances (e.g., those derived from certain mushrooms) were implicated as well. One type of ergotism was characterized not only by vivid visual hallucinations, but also by dry gangrene of the extremities due to extreme vasoconstriction. The symptoms of another type, convulsive ergotism, included distorted sensory perceptions, delirium, psychosis, hallucinations, painful muscular contractions, and convulsions. While these hallucinatory effects were ultimately attributed to ergot in the middle of the eighteenth century, the term "hallucinogen" was not introduced until 1954, when it was used by A. Hoffer and H. Osmond to describe a substance that in small doses can alter perception, thought, and mood to create illusions in the mind of the user (Liska, 1986).

Hofmann and his associates were studying ergot compounds, which are vasoconstrictors and, in appropriate doses, are useful in controlling migraine headaches and postpartum hemorrhage. The synthesis of LSD was planned during their search for a circulatory and respiratory stimulant within a drug class known as analeptics (CNS stimulants). LSD, however, was not noteworthy in early experimental tests with animals, so the compound was shelved. Five years later, while still searching for a suitable analeptic, Hofmann either accidentally ingested a small amount of LSD, or possibly absorbed it through his skin. He experienced a very unusual reaction consist-

---

*LSD was the twenty-fifth compound synthesized in a series of experiments; hence, LSD-25.

ing of vertigo, restlessness, optical distortions, a dream-like state, feelings similar to drunkenness, a kaleido-scope-like play of colors, and an exaggerated imagination, all of which he regarded as rather pleasant. Three days later he investigated his suspicion that he had in-gested some LSD by intentionally ingesting 0.25 µg, a dose based on hallucinogenic doses of other ergot alka-loids. However, this dose was several times more than the later-determined adequate dose for the hallucino-genic reaction (50/100 µg). This time Hofmann's reac-tions were quite spectacular, with an extremely powerful physiological response that included autonomic stimula-tion as well as dissociative feelings, hallucinations, and other mental aberrations that lasted 6 hours or more. He also found it significant that after the sleep that followed this drug-induced episode, he awoke feeling refreshed without any trace of the drug experience. Furthermore, Hofmann was astonished that such a small dose could have such a powerful effect, suggesting that LSD must specifically stimulate some kind of a trigger zone in the brain.

The first printed account of these phenomena ap-peared in 1947 after Hofmann's colleague Stoll (1947) sampled the drug and did some studies on human sub-jects at a psychiatric clinic in Zurich. His report con-firmed Hofmann's original observations. Sandoz then began to synthesize the compound, which was marketed as Delysid, a drug available at no cost to medical re-searchers. (For a detailed and interesting history of the discovery and use of LSD, see Ulrich and Patten, 1991.)

Basic Pharmacology of LSD

Though LSD is the most potent psychoactive drug known, it has an extremely high safety margin; it can have effects at doses of 10–15 µg, yet doses hundreds of times higher are unlikely to be fatal. In fact, one estimate of the LD_{50} in humans was 14,000 µg (see Moreines, 1989). On the other hand, an effective dose can be so small that its presence in the blood or urine is barely de-tectable, even when the drug user is clinically intoxi-cated. Because of its high potency, LSD solutions are di-luted many times in order to measure doses more con-veniently. When prepared for illicit distribution, small drops of the diluted solution are distributed on blotting paper, and once dried, the paper is cut so that each piece contains one drop, making up one dose. The user chews the paper to obtain the drug.

After ingestion, LSD is distributed to all parts of the body including the brain, though surprisingly, only a small part of the dose (about 1%) is found in the brain. The greatest concentration is found in the liver, where it is degraded before being excreted in the bile and feces. LSD is degraded rather rapidly in humans with a plasma half-life between 2 and 3 hours. The small amount in the brain is distributed to receptors that are widely scattered

throughout the CNS, which may account for the variety of effects caused by the drug.

Psychological and Physiological Effects

Oral ingestion of 100 µg of LSD is usually sufficient for a significant hallucinatory effect in humans, and as little as 0.3 µg/kg can subjectively detected. Sympathomimetic effects are felt within a few minutes after ingestion, with mydriasis (dilated pupils) being a reliable sign of LSD activity in animals and humans. Psychological effects follow within 30 to 90 minutes, with peak effects occur-ring at 2–4 hours. This is followed by a gradual return to the pre-drug state within about 6–12 hours.

Experienced users of LSD report visual and auditory illusions and synesthesias, which are mixed sensations such as "seeing" smells or "hearing" colors after a small dose. The sense of touch is magnified and the sense of time is distorted. Thoughts are visualized, and thinking does not proceed in logical sequences, but jumps irra-tionally to conclusions that appear to the subject to be more valid than those that are obtained by more normal thought processes. Such experiences are usually judged as desirable or as "having a good trip."

Previous good trips do not guarantee that the next trip will be a good one. A negative response to these LSD-induced episodes (i.e., a "bad trip") consists of acute panicky feelings in which one's personality seems to be falling apart, with paranoia, depression, and feel-ings of confusion and fragmentation. Chronic adverse reactions include flashbacks (reliving an earlier drug ex-perience), psychoses, depression, and chronic personal-ity changes. Flashbacks, with time, decrease in number, intensity, and duration, whether the subject is undergo-ing treatment for drug abuse or not. It is unclear whether LSD itself causes these major psychological ef-fects, or whether it merely unmasks existing emotional problems. (For descriptions of the wide range of LSD-in-duced effects, see Hofmann, 1983; Brown and Braden, 1987; Moreines, 1989.)

At relatively high doses, LSD has strong sympatho-mimetic effects, which probably result from a distur-bance in the balance between the cholinergic and the catecholaminergic systems. LSD induces tachycardia, increased blood pressure, mydriasis, piloerection, in-creased body temperature, sweating and chills, in-creased blood glucose levels, and sometimes headache, nausea, and vomiting. However, these effects are slight with small doses and do not interfere with the percep-tual effects described above. In fact, patients presented at an emergency center due to a drug overdose are not there because of the autonomic effects, but rather, they are usually reacting to the fear and panic generally felt by novice drug users.

Tolerance to LSD develops rapidly so that after a few consecutive daily doses, the initial dose becomes in-effective. However, after 3 or 4 days of abstinence (which does not lead to withdrawal symptoms), the tolerance is lost. There is cross-tolerance of LSD to other hallucinogens such as psilocin, mescaline, DOM, and DMT (see below), which suggests that all of these substances have a common mode of action. It has been shown that if a person has a full-blown hallucinatory experience following a dose of LSD, the normal hallucinatory response to mescaline taken the next day will be dramatically blunted or abolished. Moreover, though marijuana and PCP are sometimes classified as hallucinogens, they do not belong to the class of LSD-like drugs since they show no evidence of cross-tolerance with them (Jacobs, 1987).

Does LSD Cause Hallucinations?

Despite the persistence of referring to LSD and related substances as hallucinogens, it is considered to be a misnomer to label these drugs as such because their effects are not truly hallucinogenic. Genuine hallucinations are characterized as perceptions that are superimposed upon the environment, are usually auditory and threatening, and the subjects tend to think of them as real. The perceptual perturbations caused by LSD and related substances, however, are more likely to be visual and interesting, with the subjects being *aware* that they are experiencing these strange perceptions, as though they were watching a private television show. Thus, the perceptual changes occur in the presence of a clear sensorium (i.e., without toxic delirium). Some investigators suggest that LSD and related drugs produce a distortion of perceived reality rather than genuine hallucinations, which involve perceived experiences that do not truly occur. Therefore, the drugs may be better described as "phantasticants" (derived from the word *phantasmagoria*) (Shulgin, 1978) or as "illusogens" (see Brown and Braden, 1987). On the other hand, though the term may be misleading, "hallucinogen" is still commonly used in the neuroscience literature, and consequently, it will be used here to describe LSD and related substances. (For a variety of suggested alternatives see Cohen, 1985b.)

LSD and Schizophrenia

LSD and related compounds are also sometimes referred to as psychotogenic or psychotomimetic, implying that their induced effects are similar to psychotic states. This characterization is also misleading, since the resemblance to psychotic states is only superficial, and well-trained observers can easily discriminate between drug-induced effects and those of schizophrenia (Hollister, 1978). Furthermore, reports from schizophrenics who were in remission and had taken LSD indicated that they could distinguish between psychotic states and LSD-induced reactions. This, however, is not true of the psychotic states induced by PCP, cocaine, amphetamine, and some of their derivatives; that is to say that the latter substances seem to produce genuine hallucinations in some circumstances.

Though there are now reservations about the similarities of LSD-induced effects and symptoms of schizophrenia, early findings regarding the hallucinogenic-like effects of LSD provided the impetus for pharmacological studies investigating a possible relationship between them. In fact, the LSD response gave some credence to the notion that schizophrenia is caused by some kind of an endogenous catabolic "mistake" that produces a substance that is toxic to the brain, and that substance might be chemically related to LSD. Moreover, it was assumed that this toxic substance must exist in infinitesimal amounts and be extremely potent, since it remained almost undetectable in the blood. It was also thought that LSD might provide a means to experimentally induce schizophrenia, thereby aiding research leading to the treatment and/or the prevention of this disease.

After Stoll's report in 1947, efforts were made to identify this putative connection between LSD and schizophrenia. One proposal was that adrenaline, the release of which is increased during stress, can be degraded into a substance called adrenochrome, which is further converted to adrenolutin, both of which are psychoactive. In normal subjects these hormones would be further converted into neutral substances, but in schizophrenics the conversion of adrenochrome was thought to be blocked, leading to its buildup in the blood and the manifestation of schizophrenic symptoms. This hypothesis suggested that LSD may be the blocking agent resulting in an accumulation of adrenochrome (Hoffer and Osmond, 1959). However, even though Osmond dosed himself with adrenochrome and personally reported that he experienced psychotomimetic effects, later research revealed that adrenochrome was not present in the blood of schizophrenics, nor did it have any psychological effects (Snyder, 1974b).

Wooley and Shaw (1954) found that LSD inhibited serotonergic activity in peripheral organs, and perhaps acted centrally to inhibit 5-HT in the brain. However, brominated LSD (BOL), which had even greater antagonistic effects on 5-HT than did LSD, had absolutely no psychoactivity. Ultimately, a consensus was reached that LSD effects did not serve as a reasonable model for schizophrenia. Nevertheless, LSD came to serve for a time as an adjunct to the treatment of schizophrenia, purportedly by inducing dreamlike states to promote the release of childhood memories and important life events in attempts to shorten the course of psychoanalysis (Frederking, 1955). These activities will be discussed in a later section.

Psychedelic Properties of LSD

At about the time that LSD was being tested as an adjunct to psychotherapy for schizophrenia, one of its proponents saw another possible place for its use. In an address to the prestigious New York Academy of Sciences, Osmond (1957) claimed that LSD possessed more than just psychotomimetic properties because many volunteers who had sampled the drug had reported insightful and pleasurable experiences that enabled them to better understand themselves and their relationships with the world. Consequently he advocated the use of LSD not only to aid in psychotherapy, but also to educate psychiatrists and psychologists in the strange ways in which the mind can operate, and to explore the social, religious, and philosophical applications of this drug. He also proposed that the drug be "recategorized as a psychedelic, meaning mind-manifesting—a name that implies concepts of enriching the mind and enlarging its vision." This view was challenged on many grounds, including the difficulty in defining the parameters of the mind, let alone how one determines whether it has been enriched and enlarged.

Nonetheless, these and other pronouncements served as a catalyst to a psychology professor at Harvard University, Timothy Leary, who had experimented on himself with psilocybin mushrooms and experienced a "profound religious ecstasy, a vitalizing transaction that he believed would revolutionize psychology." Leary recruited a colleague, Richard Alpert, who conducted experiments in their Center for Research in Personality and gave approximately 3,500 doses of psilocybin to 400 volunteers, reporting that 95% of them said afterwards that their lives were changed for the better.

After Leary became acquainted with LSD, his experiments with psilocybin subsided in favor of studies investigating the incredible power of LSD. After a few trips to Mexico, he and others formed the International Federation for Internal Freedom, whose position was that psychedelics were "educational instruments" and whose stated purpose was "to work to increase the individual's knowledge and control of his/her own nervous system." Their LSD experiments, especially those with undergraduate students, drew criticism that their research was being conducted irresponsibly and that psychedelic drugs were too dangerous for nonmedical research. Consequently, they were asked to terminate their enterprise or leave Harvard. They left in 1953 and moved to Mexico, from which they were later expelled. Returning to the United States, they continued their promulgation of LSD and psilocybin, encouraging young people to use psychedelics to produce heightened emotional feelings and increased awareness with the ultimate goal of an "exalted spiritual experience."

These activities gained the attention of the news media, and the publicity helped to create an underground movement that included intellectuals, students, and hippie groups who wanted to experiment with the drugs. The fear that LSD use was becoming a public health problem caused the federal government to outlaw the use, sale, and possession of psychedelic drugs in 1965. As a consequence, in 1966 Sandoz, the last U.S. supplier of legal LSD, stopped all distribution and sent their remaining stocks to the National Institute of Mental Health (NIMH) in the United States. This led to the virtual demise of research on LSD except that which was permitted and supervised by the NIMH. The desire for LSD among members of the drug cults was satisfied, however, by illicit manufacturers who profited greatly since a dose of LSD that was estimated to cost 10 cents to manufacture was frequently sold for $10.00. This illegal source of LSD is still active at the time of this writing (see Ulrich and Patten, 1991). An additional discussion of illicit LSD use appears below.

Other hallucinogenic drugs.   A number of other compounds elicit similar physiological and behavioral effects and are chemically related to LSD.

The first group, the indolealkylamines, includes, along with LSD, psilocybin, which is obtained from the mushroom *Psilocybe mexicana*, with psilocin being the active ingredient. These mushrooms have been used for

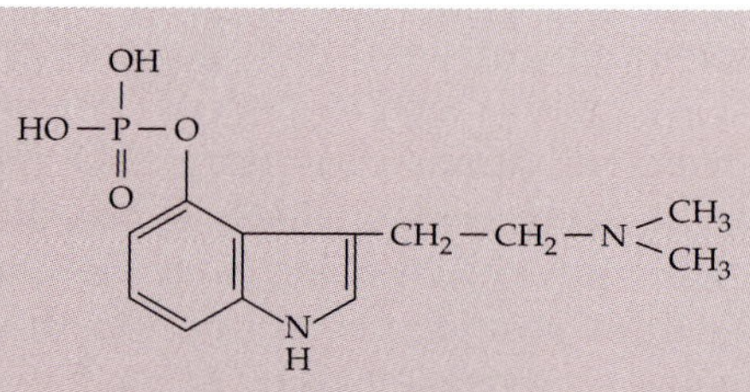

Psilocybin
(*N,N*-Dimethyl-4-phosphoryltryptamine)

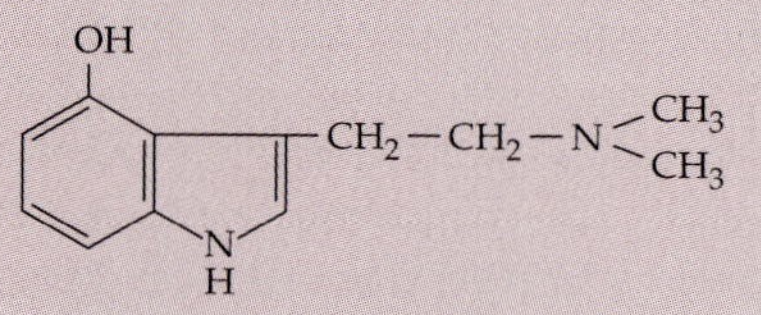

Psilocin
(*N,N*-Dimethyl-4-hydroxytryptamine)

centuries by the native inhabitants of Central America in their religious ceremonies. Bufotenine, a related substance, is derived from the mushroom *Amanita muscaria*, and is also found on the skin and in the poison glands of some toads. There was some evidence that bufotenine

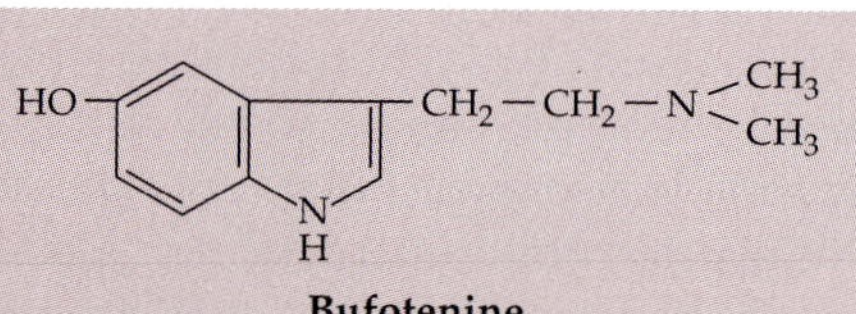

Bufotenine
(*N,N*-Dimethyl-5-hydroxytryptamine)

was found in the urine of some schizophrenics, but other investigators found less of it in schizophrenics than in normal subjects (Gillin, Stoff, and Wyatt, 1978). DMT (N,N-dimethyltryptamine) is derived from the plant *Mimosa hostilis* and is an ingredient of cohoba snuff, used by American and Caribbean Indians. DMT becomes inactive when taken orally, hence it must be taken as a snuff or injected. It and its *O*-methyl derivative 5-OMe-

DMT
(*N,N*-Dimethyltryptamine)

DMT are substituted tryptamines and are thus among the indolealkylamine hallucinogens. On the other hand, the active ingredient of marijuana, Δ^9-tetrahydrocannabi-

5-Methoxy-*N,N*-dimethyltryptamine

nol, can produce some LSD-like effects in high doses, but it is not related to the indolealkylamine group and shows no cross-tolerance with LSD. Other hallucinogens, such as atropine, scopolamine, and ditran, are anticholinergics and are not related to the substances described above. There is no cross-tolerance between the anticholinergics and LSD, mescaline, or psilocybin (Cohen, 1970).

The second group of hallucinogens is the phenethylamines, which include mescaline. Mescaline is derived

Mescaline
(3,4,5-Trimethoxyphenethylamine)

from the peyote cactus plant and has been used in religious ceremonies by the Mexican Indians since pre-Columbian times. Its name is derived from the mescal bean, which was used in ceremonies prior to the peyote plant but, being somewhat toxic, was supplanted by peyote as it became more popular among the various tribes. (See Weinswig 1973 for a brief history of the use of mescaline in the Americas.) The phenethylamines also include the methoxylated amphetamines TMA, (3,4,5-trimethoxyamphetamine), DOET (2, 5- dimethoxy-4-ethylamphetamine), and DOM (2, 5-dimethoxy-4-methylamphetamine). The latter compound was given the street name of STP, which is also the trade name of an oil additive presumed to increase the efficiency of auto engines, but in this case the letters stand for "serenity, tranquility, and peace." (For relative hallucinogenic potencies of many of these compounds, see Glennon, Titeler, and McKenney, 1984, and Shulgin, 1978.) Because of their structural simi-

TMA
(3,4,5-Trimethoxyamphetamine)

DOET
(2,5-Dimethoxy-4-ethylamphetamine)

larities to amphetamines, some of these compounds may have stimulating and/or hallucinogenic characteristics. For example, whereas MDA (3,4-methylenedioxyamphetamine) has more LSD-like stimulus properties, MDMA (3,4-methylenedioxymethamphetamine) induces more amphetamine-like effects.

MDA
(3,4-Methylenedioxyamphetamine)

MDMA
(3,4-Methylenedioxymethamphetamine)

Pharmacological similarities among hallucinogens. The interrelationships among all of these compounds have been established in a number of ways. One of the initial findings was that the tolerance that develops to LSD after only a few doses in animals and humans shares a cross-tolerance with many of the other compounds (Isbell, Miner, and Logan, 1959; Isbell, Wolbach, and Miner, 1961; Isbell, Wolbach, and Rosenberg, 1962). For example, mescaline, though it is chemically similar to catecholamines rather than to serotonin, has effects similar to those of LSD and shares a cross-tolerance with LSD (Appel and Freedman, 1968). The major pharmacological difference between mescaline and LSD seems to be that of potency—the hallucinogenic effect from 5 mg/kg of mescaline is equivalent to that from 1.5 µg/kg of LSD, a ratio of about 3,300:1. Moreover, a greater cross-tolerance between mescaline and psilocin is revealed by an equivalence ratio of about 150–200:1.

A second method for examining potential relationships among these drugs is to compare the relative similarities between their interoceptive cues that allow for drug substitutions in drug discrimination experiments. Here we shall merely mention, with respect to those cues, that there are substantial similarities among these agents, and the degree of similarity even correlates with hallucinogenic potency in humans. This is further discussed below.

LSD–5-HT Interactions

At the time of LSD discovery and characterization, 5-HT was also being studied, and it was soon noticed that LSD and 5-HT were chemically related, at least insofar as they both contained the indole nucleus shown above. As mentioned above, these early studies showed that LSD blocked the effects of 5-HT in peripheral organs; for example, it blocked the stimulating effect of 5-HT on smooth muscle of the rat intestine and uterus. Thus, it was proposed that LSD might have similar 5-HT blocking effects in the brain. However, the related compound, 2-bromo-LSD (BOL) also is a 5-HT antagonist in peripheral tissues, though it produces none of the subjective experiences of LSD, even though it freely passes the blood–brain barrier. This finding created doubt about the hypothesis that LSD might block 5-HT systems in the brain, but it did not rule out the possibility that central receptors sensitive to LSD may not be responsive to BOL. Nevertheless, these findings supported the hypothesis that 5-HT and LSD, might be related in significant ways.

About a decade later, histochemical fluorescence studies of Dahlström and Fuxe (1964, 1965) revealed the location of 5-HT cells in the raphe nuclei of the brain stem. Thus, it became possible to study the direct effects of LSD on serotonergic cells in the brain. These experiments have been reviewed by Aghajanian and coworkers (1974, 1975), Heym and Jacobs (1987), and Vandermaelen (1985). Early studies showed that systemic administration of LSD produced a slight increase in brain 5-HT, a decrease in brain 5-HIAA, and a decrease in brain 5-HT synthesis. These results led to the conclusion that LSD suppressed the activity of 5-HT neurons in the raphe and slowed the turnover of 5-HT. This conclusion was supported by the finding that electrical stimulation of the raphe had the opposite effects (i.e., lower brain 5-HT and increased brain 5-HIAA). Also, when 5-HT synthesis was inhibited, LSD slowed the rate of 5-HT depletion that normally occurred. This finding also supported the idea that LSD slows the firing rate of 5-HT neurons in the raphe nuclei.

To account for the LSD-induced serotonergic suppression in the brain, more recent studies showed that, in the dorsal raphe nucleus, LSD and other indoleamine hallucinogens mimic the action of 5-HT by acting as powerful agonists on somatodendritic autoreceptors. Stimulation of these autoreceptors results in inhibition of

the neurons and diminishes their firing rate. This type of self-inhibition is mediated by the cells' own recurrent axon collaterals which normally release 5-HT to activate autoreceptors either on their own somata or dendrites or those on adjacent cells. This leads to hyperpolarization of the cell membranes along with an increase in ionic conductance. Studies with rats showed that the autoreceptors in the dorsal raphe are of the $5-HT_{1A}$ type. This was demonstrated by the suppression of the firing rate of these cells using the highly selective $5-HT_{1A}$ receptor agonist 8-OH-DPAT administered either intravenously or microiontophoretically. This inhibitory effect was comparable to that observed with LSD. Similarly, the nonbenzodiazepine anxiolytic buspirone, which displays a high affinity for $5-HT_{1A}$ receptors, also suppressed the firing rate of 5-HT neurons in the dorsal raphe when administered systemically, microiontophoretically, or when added to brain slices in vitro. Studies in brain slice preparations have shown that the ionic basis for this inhibitory effect is the opening of the potassium (K^+) channels to facilitate K^+ efflux. These studies revealed that LSD is a much more potent 5-HT agonist at the 5-HT autoreceptor than at postsynaptic inhibitory receptors (Vandermaelen, 1985). Such inhibition provides negative feedback upon the modulation of calcium-dependent electrically released 5-HT.

Another type of 5-HT autoreceptor is present on 5-HT axon terminals. This receptor is comprised of two subtypes, $5-HT_{1B}$ or $5-HT_{1D}$, which also modulate 5-HT release. LSD can act as an agonist at these autoreceptors as well, providing additional negative feedback on the cells of the raphe nuclei, thereby further inhibiting the synthesis and release of 5-HT (Aghajanian, Sprouse, and Rasmussen, 1987; Langer, 1987).

It is of additional interest to note that systemic administration of LSD induces a decrease in spontaneous activity of noradrenergic cells in the locus coeruleus (LC). The effect appears to be mediated by LSD binding to $5-HT_2$ receptors because the effect is reversed by selective $5-HT_2$ antagonists, such as ritanserin and LY-53857. However, this LSD effect is not direct because the effect is not mimicked by iontophoretic application of LSD upon LC cell bodies. Consequently, the implication is that LSD acts either directly or indirectly upon $5-HT_2$ receptors that affect afferent inputs to the LC (Aghajanian, Sprouse, and Rasmussen, 1987).

Receptor Binding of LSD

Early studies by Bennett and Snyder (1975) determined how LSD binding sites were distributed in mammalian brains. Using radioactively labeled LSD and related compounds, they found highly specific LSD binding sites in rat brain, with D-LSD having a binding affinity 1,000 times stronger than that of the psychotropically inactive L-LSD. It was also found that total binding was unaffected by the destruction of the 5-HT neurons in the raphe nuclei, indicating that the preponderance of [³H]LSD binding sites are on postsynaptic nonserotonergic neurons rather than on serotonergic presynaptic sites. Configurational changes in the LSD molecule that reduce psychotropic potency also reduce binding affinity in the brain, except in the case of BOL, which equals *d*-LSD in binding affinity although it is psychotropically inactive.

A wide range of tryptaminergic compounds, 5-HT antagonists, and other hallucinogenic indolealkylamines were tested for their ability to displace [³H]LSD from cortical binding sites. Again, in general, psychotropic potency correlated positively with potency for displacing [³H]LSD binding. Furthermore, Bennett and Snyder (1975) also found that tissue samples from various monkey brain areas that showed high degrees of LSD binding also showed high levels of 5-HT uptake. The highest binding of LSD was found in cerebral cortical regions; diencephalic (midbrain) areas showed intermediate binding; and the lowest binding was seen in the white matter and in the cerebellum. Later studies also showed that there was a heterogeneous distribution of [³H]LSD binding that could be displaced by 5-HT in the choroid plexus, hippocampus, septal nuclei, and cortex (see Heym and Jacobs, 1987). Thus, having established that the postsynaptic cortical LSD binding sites in rat brains also bound 5-HT and its ligands, it remained to be determined which of the 5-HT receptor subtypes(s) are involved, and what role these receptors play in hallucinogenesis.

Single-Cell Studies

Further investigations on the effects of LSD were done on single serotonergic neurons (Aghajanian and Haigler, 1974). This was feasible because the histochemical mapping by Dahlström and Fuxe (1965) made accurate placement of microelectrodes possible. With single-cell recording microelectrodes in the raphe of rat brains, experiments showed that small intravenous doses of LSD (10–20 µg/kg) produced brief, but total, inhibition of firing of 5-HT neurons in the dorsal and median raphe nuclei (Figure 17.21*a*). However, larger doses (more than 100 µg/kg) that increased the duration of inhibition were required to alter the brain levels of 5-HT and 5-HIAA significantly. In these studies it was also found that BOL (the nonpsychoactive analog of LSD) displayed less than 1% of the activity that LSD had on raphe neurons. These findings support the hypothesis that LSD leads to decreased 5-HT turnover by reducing neuronal firing of 5-HT neurons.

Microiontophoretic LSD was also directly applied to raphe neurons using multibarreled micropipettes, which allowed for controlled ejection of the drug directly onto a neuron while simultaneously recording its neural activity. The results showed that raphe neurons, which have a slow rhythmic firing rate, were extremely sensitive to LSD

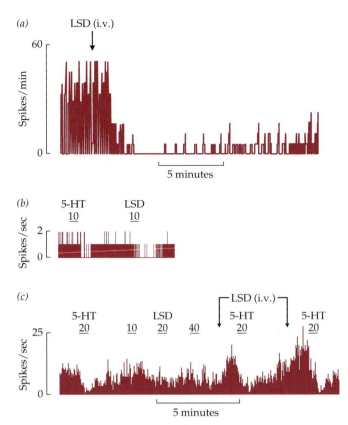

17.21 LSD EFFECTS ON DORSAL RAPHE NEURONS. (*a*) The baseline rate of discharge of a raphe cell during a slow intravenous infusion of LSD (20 µg/kg) which began where indicated by the arrow. An almost total inhibition of the firing for about two minutes was followed by a gradual recovery. Each deflection is the integrated firing rate during a 10-second sampling period. (*b*) The effect of iontophoretic administration of 5-HT and LSD. The numbers above the bars are the ejection currents in nA. Recovery was more rapid after 5-HT than after LSD treatment. (*c*) The effect of iontophoretically applied 5-HT and LSD on a cell in the ventro-lateral geniculate nucleus. An intravenous dose of LSD (10 µg/kg) accelerated the firing in this cell. The inhibition by iontophoretic 5-HT during the intravenous infusion was not blocked. Each inflection in this trace was the integrated firing rate during a 1-second sample time. (After Aghajanian and Haigler, 1974.)

in that their firing rate was clearly inhibited in both anesthetized and unanesthetized rats. It was also found that 5-HT itself inhibited raphe neurons, but LSD was much more potent in this respect (Figure 17.21*b*). When LSD and 5-HT were combined, the inhibitory effect was cumulative, and there was no evidence that LSD even partially blocked the action of 5-HT or vice versa. Therefore, the evidence supported the view that LSD has direct effects on raphe neurons, but it still did not rule out the possibility that feedback effects from higher brain centers could also be involved. However, this possibility became unlikely when it was discovered that LSD still inhibited the firing rate of dorsal raphe neurons even after the brain stem was transected above the midbrain, thereby separating it from the forebrain and other cortical regions.

The next step was the assessment of the effect of LSD on postsynaptic receptors. Again, with the aid of histochemical fluorescence techniques, it was possible to localize accurately terminals of raphe neurons in forebrain areas such as the ventrolateral geniculate nuclei, the basolateral and cortical amygdala, and the optic tectum. Assuming that the cell bodies juxtaposed to the 5-HT terminals received a serotonergic input, microiontophoretic studies assessed the sensitivity of these postsynaptic elements to 5-HT and to LSD. The postsynaptic cells were inhibited by 5-HT but were quite insensitive to LSD at ejection currents that were highly effective in raphe neurons (Figure 17.21c). However, the postsynaptic cells could be inhibited by very high concentrations of LSD. When LSD (10 µg/kg) was administered intravenously, the postsynaptic neurons appeared to be *stimulated*, though LSD-induced stimulation did not interfere with the inhibitory effects of 5-HT applied iontophoretically (Figure 17.21c). Thus, while high iontophoretic doses of LSD did not inhibit the postsynaptic neurons, intravenous doses appeared to stimulate them.

In order to explain this apparent discrepancy, it is necessary to consider which receptors are the primary locus of action of LSD in the brain, the presynaptic receptors on the raphe cell bodies or those on the postsynaptic target cells. Given that raphe neurons exert an inhibitory effect on postsynaptic cells, and that low doses of LSD inhibit raphe neurons, one would expect LSD-induced inhibition of raphe neurons to result in a disinhibition of the target cells, causing an acceleration of their firing rates. As just mentioned, the experiments showed just that: intravenous administration of LSD at a dose sufficient to inhibit raphe neurons caused an acceleration of firing in postsynaptic cells in the geniculate nuclei. Thus, these data supported the notion that LSD inhibition of 5-HT neurons in the raphe caused a disinhibition of serotonergic target cells, resulting in increased postsynaptic activity in many areas in the brain, which could explain the wide variety of LSD effects.

It is interesting to note that many of the postsynaptic neurons under the influence of neurons in the raphe are in structures of the visual system, such as the lateral geniculate nucleus and the optic tectum, as well as in limbic structures. Excitation of these areas as a result of their release from 5-HT inhibitory influences is thought to account at least in part for the distortions of visual perceptions that are characteristic of LSD effects.

Parenthetically, it was found that BOL, even at iontophoretic currents ten times greater than that for LSD, had no effect on raphe neurons, nor did BOL interfere with the effects of 5-HT in the brain. This evidence showed that LSD and BOL act differently from one another on central 5-HT receptors. That is, only LSD mimics the inhibitory action of 5-HT at central receptors, even though both it and BOL block the action of 5-HT on peripheral receptors. This distinction between these re-

lated compounds may explain the inability of BOL to elicit LSD-like hallucinations.

LSD-Induced Raphe Activity and Behavior

Though the studies described above supported the hypothesis that LSD has a suppressant effect on 5-HT neurons in the raphe, it was not known whether this effect is in fact related to hallucinogenesis. Moreover, the electrophysiological data presented above were obtained from anesthetized or immobilized animals, while the behavioral data were taken from freely moving animals or obtained from human reports after drug ingestion. To overcome potential confounds caused by anesthesia, Trulson and Jacobs (1979) and Trulson, Heym, and Jacobs (1981) developed a technique for recording via microelectrodes the activity of cells in the raphe nuclei of freely moving animals. Thus, after an LSD treatment they were able to measure the activity of single neurons in the dorsal raphe nucleus as well as the behavioral effects of LSD.

Even though it is conjectural whether "hallucinations" in animals can be measured, one can monitor the constellation of identifiable behavioral effects in animals resulting from LSD or 5-HT treatment known as the "5-HT syndrome" (see Chapter 9). For example, LSD given to cats causes limb flicking, abortive grooming, head shaking, staring, investigatory and play behavior, and constant eye movements. These effects develop tolerance with repeated dosing, and cross-tolerance occurs with related compounds. Thus, the profile of these LSD effects strongly suggests that they are related to hallucinatory effects in humans. Earlier studies had suggested that these effects are exclusive to 5-HT or drugs that mimic its action, but it was later found that some aspects of the 5-HT syndrome, such as head twitching and shaking, may be mediated by mechanisms other than those involving 5-HT (Glennon, 1990a). Nonetheless, the 5-HT syndrome is a reliable indicator of LSD-induced activity.

After LSD was given to cats (50 µg/kg i.p.) raphe unit activity was significantly decreased (by as much as 48%), with the maximal decrease occurring 1 hour after drug administration, and the peak level of behavioral effects occurring at about the same time. Unit activity remained depressed for about 3 hours after the injection, yet some of the behavioral effects, especially limb flicking, were significantly elevated over baseline levels for as long as 8 hours after drug injection.

There were no changes in neuronal firing rates that were correlated with limb flicks, but some neural units were completely suppressed during staring, and there was increased firing during digging or grooming behavior. A lower LSD dose (10 µg/kg) produced a smaller decrement of raphe unit activity (18%) that lasted for about 2 hours, but again limb flicks lasted up to 4 hours, further suggesting a disassociation of this behavior with neuronal discharge. Neither saline nor BOL had any effect on raphe unit activity or behavior; nor did LSD affect nonserotonergic cells outside the raphe nucleus.

Twenty-four hours after the first injection, a second 50 μg/kg injection of LSD was given, but this dose was virtually without any behavioral effects, even though there was an even greater suppression of raphe unit activity (62.4%). This finding showed that tolerance developed for the behavioral effects elicited by LSD, but not for the LSD-induced suppression of unit activity.

In addition, other phenylethylamine hallucinogens, such as mescaline and DOM, produced robust behavioral effects similar to those in the 5-HT syndrome, despite the absence of significant suppression of 5-HT neuronal activity. Moreover, the 5-HT syndrome could be elicited by LSD from animals whose brains were depleted of 5-HT. In fact, the behavioral effects were *enhanced* in animals whose serotonergic nerve terminals were destroyed by neurotoxic drugs such as 5,6-DHT. These increased LSD-induced effects were probably due to denervation supersensitivity of postsynaptic 5-HT receptors. Thus, these studies showed that the suppression of serotonergic unit activity in the raphe was not necessary to produce the behavioral effects elicited by hallucinogens. These findings cast doubt on the role of presynaptic serotonergic inhibition in hallucinogenesis. On the other hand, these results did not necessarily invalidate a serotonergic basis in central LSD effects as proposed by Aghajanian and Haigler (1974). Rather, they only pointed to the possibly greater importance of LSD effects on raphe target neurons rather than the raphe neurons themselves. Consequently, the next step was the identification of the postsynaptic 5-HT receptor(s) that might be related to LSD-mediated hallucinogenic phenomena.

The Role of the 5-HT Receptor in Hallucinogenesis

An important step in determining which receptors may be involved in hallucinogenesis is to identify which receptors selectively bind a number of compounds that have hallucinatory effects. This was studied by using the two-lever drug discrimination technique that was described in Chapters 2 and 16. Using this technique, many investigators found that rats trained on this procedure invariably perceive all of the major hallucinogens as LSD-like, and drugs from other classes as not LSD-like.

For example, Glennon, Titeler, and McKenny (1984) found that rats trained to discriminate 5-OMe-DMT from saline generalized this discrimination to DOM, DMT, and mescaline. Schechter and Rosecrans (1972) reported that rats trained on LSD generalized their response to mescaline and psilocin, but not to amphetamine, although later experiments showed that some of the phenethylamines will generalize to amphetamine. For example, 3,4-MDA is a stimulant hallucinogen that has one isomer, D(+)3,4-MDA, that generalizes from amphetamine, and another, L(-)3,4-MDA, that generalizes

from DOM, a hallucinogen (see Moreines, 1989). Moreover, it was found that nonselective 5-HT receptor blockers such as cinanserin, cyproheptadine, and methysergide were effective in blocking the discriminative stimulus properties of the hallucinogens DOM, mescaline, and LSD, but not the discriminative properties of the adrenergic drugs amphetamine and methylphenidate. Corroborative data were obtained when the dopamine antagonist haloperidol did not antagonize the discriminative properties of DOM (see Heym and Jacobs, 1987).

Although the above results showed that many hallucinogenic drugs behave similarly in fundamentally physiological ways, there was one feature of the drug discrimination tests that raised an important question. Surprisingly, no drug tolerance was observed in these procedures that involved frequent hallucinogenic drug administrations. This finding was noteworthy because the development of tolerance and cross-tolerance after repeated administration of hallucinogens is the general rule for these drugs.

Of further significance was the finding that drugs such as pirenperone and ritanserin, which are full receptor antagonists and have a high specific affinity for the 5-HT$_{2A}$ postsynaptic receptor subtype, are highly effective in blocking the discriminative cues of LSD in rats. Thus, the discriminative properties of LSD and perhaps other hallucinogens require an agonist action at brain postsynaptic 5-HT$_{2A}$ receptors.

Jacobs (1987) reported using 5-HT$_{2A}$ receptor antagonists to extend his findings that LSD-induced behavior is not dependent upon neuronal depression in the raphe nuclei (see Heym, Rasmussen, and Jacobs, 1984). Cats were first pretreated with 5-HT$_{2A}$ antagonists, then treated with LSD while cellular activity in the raphe nuclei was monitored. Consistent with previous results described above, there was an almost complete blockade of the LSD-induced behavioral effects by 5-HT$_{2A}$ antagonists, though suppression of activity in the raphe remained regardless of antagonist pretreatment. This was added evidence that LSD-induced hallucinogenesis is independent of suppression of activity in the raphe, and instead is the result of agonist effects on postsynaptic 5-HT$_{2A}$ receptors.

These findings were further supported by other experiments. For example, Appel and Rosecrans (1984) proposed that if hallucinogens act by suppressing raphe neurons and reducing 5-HT activity, then prior destruction of the raphe nuclei or depletion of 5-HT from its terminal sites should diminish or abolish the behavioral effects of subsequent LSD, since the system would already have been maximally suppressed. Contrarily, these manipulations enhanced LSD effects rather than diminished them, an effect that was attributed to the loss of 5-HT input to the target cells, resulting in a postsynaptic denervation supersensitivity because of a compensatory proliferation of postsynaptic receptors. This same effect has been seen in human patients treated with reserpine; that is, reserpine-induced depletion of 5-HT led to increases in postsynaptic 5-HT receptors and an increased sensitivity to LSD.

An additional approach in support of these findings used monoamine oxidase inhibitors (MAOIs), compounds that are used to treat psychological depression. Chronic treatment with MAOIs causes a down-regulation of postsynaptic 5-HT receptors, and when rats were chronically treated with MAOIs and later received a dose of LSD, the rats showed almost no behavioral response to the drug. The same effect was also seen in human patients treated with MAOIs; they showed very weak or no effects at all even when given LSD doses four to eight times the effective adult dose (Lucki and Frazer, 1981).

Similar effects occurred with chronic LSD treatments. That is, repeated LSD treatments led to the development of a tolerance to LSD effects that corresponded to a specific loss of 5-HT_{2A} receptor binding, though binding to 5-HT_1 receptors was unchanged. In an experiment by Buckholtz and coworkers (1990), daily intraperitoneal administration of LSD (130 μg/kg) for 5 days led to a selective decrease in 5-HT_{2A} receptor binding in the rat cortex, as measured 24 hours after the last LSD administration. This decrease was evident after three doses but not after the first dose of LSD. The effect was still present 48 hours, but not 96 hours after the last dose. Psilocin (1.0 mg/kg) had a similar effect, but neither BOL (1.3 mg/kg) nor mescaline (10 mg/kg) affected 5-HT_{2A} binding, even with treatments lasting 5 or 10 days. Furthermore, the time course of decreased binding paralleled the development and the loss of behavioral tolerance to LSD (i.e., as binding declined, tolerance increased, and as binding increased during drug abstinence, tolerance was lost). These findings further support the role of postsynaptic LSD receptors in hallucinosis, though some aspects of the cross-tolerance phenomena and loss of 5-HT_{2A} receptor binding remain unclear.

In other highly significant experiments, Glennon, Titeler, and McKenny (1984) examined the relationship between 5-HT receptor affinity, the generalization of a cue from the phenethylamine hallucinogen DOM in drug-discrimination tests, and hallucinogenic potency in humans. First, 22 psychoactive agents taken from the indolealkylamines and the phenethylamines including LSD, 5-OMe-DMT, and DOM, were examined for their binding potency to 5-HT_1 and 5-HT_{2A} receptors in tissue from rat prefrontal and parietofrontal cortex. It was found that there was a greater affinity for 5-HT_{2A} than 5-HT_1 sites, and stereoselectivity was high for the 5-HT_{2A} receptor but was not as evident for the 5-HT_1 site.

The compounds were also evaluated for their relative potencies in generalization tests with DOM. Generalization potency was expressed as the ED_{50} value of the test dose that displayed generalization to the training drug. The smaller the dose, the more potently the drug generalized to the DOM-induced cue. When the relative binding potency to the 5-HT_{2A} receptor was compared to the relative generalization potency there was a highly significant correlation between these two variables, but there was no correlation when comparing binding potency to the 5-HT_1 receptor. More importantly, for the 15 drugs for which human data were available, human hallucinogenic potency was found to be significantly correlated with both 5-HT_{2A} receptor affinity ($r = 0.924$) and ED_{50} values for compounds that generalize to the DOM cue in trained rats. Similarly, in a later experiment, a significant correlation was found between the discrimination-derived potency of 33 agents and human hallucinogenic potency (see Glennon, 1990a).

Thus, the binding affinity of a drug for the 5-HT_{2A} receptor site predicts its potency for evoking hallucinations in humans. How this receptor may trigger the LSD effects of perceptual distortions and mood alterations rests upon the recently discovered significant presence of 5-HT_{2A} receptors in neocortical, limbic, and brain stem areas that are concerned with sensory–perceptual processes and affect. With respect to the clinical significance to these findings, it was suggested that if hallucinogenic effects can be blocked by 5-HT antagonists, then to the extent that hallucinogenic experiences parallel certain psychiatric symptoms, these antagonists might be of psychotherapeutic value. In fact, ritanserin, which was developed as a selective 5-HT_{2A} receptor antagonist and blocks LSD discrimination, demonstrated usefulness in clinical tests compared with haloperidol in the treatment of schizophrenia (see Heym and Jacobs, 1987; and Glennon, 1990a, b). Furthermore, several atypical antipsychotic drugs, such as clozapine and risperidone, exhibit substantial 5-HT_{2A} antagonist activity which may play an important role in their therapeutic efficacy.

Although there are slight differences among the effects of the various hallucinogens, all seem to possess high affinity for the 5-HT_{2A} site. On the other hand, the 5-HT_{2A} receptor is not the sole domain of the indolealkylamines (including LSD). These agents are somewhat nonselective and display a high affinity for other populations of 5-HT sites in the brain, such as the 5-HT_{1A} and the 5-HT_{2C} sites; although the affinity is about 100 times less than for the 5-HT_{2A} site. Nevertheless, there is a correlation between hallucinogenic potency and 5-HT_{2C} affinity ($r = 0.78$), as well as with 5-HT_{2A} binding affinity ($r = 0.90$).

It should also be noted that a functional relationship seems to exist between 5-HT_{1A} and 5-HT_{2A} mediated behaviors. This is illustrated by the induction of head twitching in mice treated with DOI, which is mediated by 5-HT_{2A} receptors, an effect that is attenuated by the 5-HT_{1A} agonist 8-OH-DPAT. This suggests that 5-HT_{1A} agonists can functionally antagonize a 5-HT_{2A}–mediated behavioral effect. This may also explain the biphasic effects of LSD on head twitching, in which low doses elicit head twitching and high doses do not. This suggests that the low doses selectively stimulate the 5-HT$_{2A}$ receptor, whereas high doses also stimulate the 5-HT$_{1A}$ receptor, thus modulating the effects of 5-HT$_{2A}$ stimulation. This interaction may also explain the biphasic nature of many other effects of LSD and other indolealkylamine hallucinogens (Glennon, 1990a).

Despite the findings discussed above, this explanation for the central mechanisms involved in the production of hallucinogenic responses remains tentative. It is doubtful, for example, that the 5-HT$_{1A}$ receptor has a critical role in hallucinogenesis because the anxiolytic agonist, buspirone, has a high affinity for this receptor and binds with no signs of hallucinogenesis. Furthermore, the exact role of 5-HT$_{2A}$ receptors is still unclear. In different test systems, LSD may act at this site either as a full receptor agonist, a partial agonist, or an antagonist (Frazer, Maayani, and Wolfe, 1990; Glennon, 1990b). It should also be noted that not all substances that have a high affinity for 5-HT$_{2A}$ receptors are hallucinogenic. For example, BOL has a high affinity for the 5-HT$_{2A}$ receptor, but it has no hallucinogenic properties and even antagonizes some of the effects of LSD. The LSD nonhallucinogenic analog lisuride has the same affinity for the 5-HT$_{2A}$ receptor as does LSD, but has no known behavioral effects. Also, the 5-HT$_{2A}$ antagonists, pirenperone and ritanserin have a high affinity for the receptor, but they also block LSD activity, perhaps by interfering with LSD binding to and/or stimulation of the receptor. Further, *l*-DOM and *d*-DOM, as well as LSD, also behave as 5-HT$_{2C}$ agonists, so a possible role for this receptor subtype in hallucinogenesis cannot yet be excluded (Frazer, Maayani, and Wolfe, 1990; Glennon, Naiman et al., 1989).

LSD and 5-HT in Review

The foregoing discussion has described the characteristics of LSD as determined by subjective reports of its psychological effects, and by a considerable amount of biochemical and pharmacological research on its mode of action. Due to the limited techniques of early studies, satisfactory answers to questions about its mode of action were not forthcoming, but greater steps were made in the 1980s. For example, LSD was found to suppress the activity of serotonergic neurons in the nuclei of the raphe, though these effects did not correlate well with the behavioral effects of the drug. This was clearly established when measurements of raphe activity in freely moving LSD-treated rats and cats showed that the behavioral effects of LSD were independent of raphe activity. Moreover, with repeated testing, behavioral tolerance developed to LSD, in spite of maintained suppressant effects on the raphe nuclei. This prompted the search for the role of 5-HT postsynaptic receptors in hallucinogenesis.

Studies revealed that chronic administration of monoamine inhibitors (MAOIs), which down-regulate postsynaptic 5-HT receptors, causes both animals and humans to have no behavioral reaction to LSD. Similar effects were also found when other means were used to reduce postsynaptic receptor density. Also, 5-HT receptors are heterogeneously distributed in the brain, and are the major binding sites in the brain for a wide variety of hallucinogenic drugs. Moreover, 5-HT receptor antagonists block the effects of LSD, the most potent of which (pirenperone and ritanserin) selectively block the 5-HT$_{2A}$ receptor subtype.

The paramount importance of this receptor in the effects of LSD was further enhanced when it was found that tolerance to LSD was associated quite specifically with a loss of 5-HT$_{2A}$ binding in the cortex. Lastly, it was established that the relative binding potencies of 22 hallucinogens on 5-HT$_{2A}$ receptors were highly correlated with their relative potencies in generalizing to the interoceptive cues provided by DOM in a two-choice discrimination paradigm. These relationships also correlated highly with the potency of these agents in evoking hallucinatory events in humans, thereby bridging the gap between the animal and human responses to these compounds.

Isoergine (Lysergic Acid Amide)

An interesting account of the possible role of another hallucinogen in an important historical event is presented by Caporael (1976). This author sought a rational basis for the accusations that were made and acted upon during the Salem witchcraft crisis of 1692. She examined numerous historical narratives and documents that might explain the strange events of that time. For the most part, the episode at Salem started in December 1691, when an affliction of "distempers" was suffered by eight girls in Salem. The distempers were characterized by disorderly speech, odd postures and gestures, and convulsive fits. Because there was no logical explanation for their behavior, the New England Puritans looked upon them as the work of Satan brought about by the practice of witchcraft by some women of ill repute as well as by some respected members of the community. By the end of September 1692, 19 men and women were sent to the gallows, one man was pressed to death (a procedure designed to force him to enter a plea to the court so that he could be tried), and two of the accused died in prison.

During the trials, the girls described the activities of invisible specters and "agents of the devil in animal form." They often had violent fits that were attributed to torture by apparitions, and they complained of being choked, pinched, pricked with pins, and bitten by the accused. One man volunteered that he also had been choked and strangled by an apparition of a witch sitting on his chest, and that a black thing came through the window and stood before his face; he claimed that "the body of it looked like a monkey, only the feet were like cock's feet, with claws, and the face somewhat more like a man's than a monkey. . . ." (Caporael, 1976, p. 25.)

After discounting fraud and hysteria, Caporael proposed that there were physiological bases for these behaviors stemming from ergot contamination of the food grains used in the area. Ergot, the parasitic fungus that grows on cereal grains, contains a number of pharmacological agents, one of the most potent being isoergine (lysergic acid amide), an alkaloid having 10% of the potency of LSD-25.

Isoergine

From written records it was established that weather conditions were favorable in the 1691 growing season for an ergot infestation (i.e., a warm, rainy spring and summer), and that other factors favored the ingestion of contaminated cereal products by the residents of the town. It was the practice to harvest grain in August and store it in barns until cold weather began. Usually in November it was threshed and then used as food. Until the mid-nineteenth century, ergot was not known to be a parasitic fungus; rather, ergot-infested grain was regarded as sunbaked kernels.

The children's symptoms appeared in December of that year. It is noted that these events were strictly localized within the village of Salem, and there was no support from neighboring areas for what had transpired. It is not known how far the ergot-infested grain was distributed; however, in Salem most of the food was grown locally, and it was there that the accusations, convictions, and executions occurred.

In the summer of 1692 there was a drought, which did not favor another ergot infestation. In late 1692 the accusations and trials ceased as suddenly as they had begun. In the following years nearly all who were responsible for the accusations and sentences publicly admitted to their errors in judgment. Thus it was proposed that ergotism and the ingestion of isoergine, coupled with the ignorance and superstitions of the times, were responsible for the Salem affair.

However, Spanos and Gottlieb (1976), after careful examination of early descriptions of ergotism and the records of Salem witchcraft, took exception to Caporael's conclusions. They failed to find support for Caporael's assertion that the accusers had symptoms of ergotism, and suggested instead that the behavior of the accusers had been faked in order to mimic the symptoms of "demonic possession," the stereotypes of which were well known to them. These authors contend that their hypothesis is supported by many instances of sixteenth century demoniacs, who displayed all of the symptoms of the Salem girls and who later confessed that they had faked their displays and confirmed their confessions by publicly enacting their supposedly involuntary symptoms. This method does not prove that the Salem girls were totally guilty of conscious faking, but it does suggest that this behavior could be accounted for without recourse to explanations based on an unusual disease.

Therapeutic Use of Hallucinogens

In the 1960s, LSD-related compounds were tested in what was known as psychedelic therapies. As mentioned earlier, the term "psychedelic" was invented by Humphrey Osmond, who with Abram Hoffer published a number of papers on LSD as a therapeutic agent (see Aaronson and Hoffer, 1970). The term "psychedelic" is associated with a number of meanings, such as "mind-manifesting," " mind-revealing," or "mind-expanding," and such meanings, whether accurate or not, were deemed more appropriate for a therapeutic agent than the narrower definition hallucinogen, or the more pejorative term psychotomimetic.

With respect to using psychedelic drugs in the treatment of schizophrenia and other disorders, Masters and Houston (1970) wrote:

> Reports of therapeutic success have come from hundreds of psychotherapists working in many of the countries and cultures of the world . . . describing treatment of thirty to forty thousand patients . . . Types of conditions repeatedly stated to respond favorably to treatment with psychedelics include chronic alcoholism, criminal psychopathy, sexual deviations and neuroses, depressive states, phobias, anxiety neuroses, compulsive syndromes, and puberty neuroses. In addition, psychedelics have been used with autistic children to make them more responsive, . . . with terminal cancer patients, with adult schizophrenics, to condense the psychosis temporarily and to help predict its course of development . . . The drugs have been used as "adjuncts" or "facilitating agents" to a variety of existing psychotherapeutic procedures. (p. 323–325)

These statements were followed by detailed accounts of many case studies in which psychedelic drugs were used primarily with psychoanalysis.

Hoffer (1970) described the use of psychedelics, particularly LSD, for treating alcoholism. LSD supposedly provided the necessary setting that allowed for proper psychotherapy in the treatment of alcoholism . That is to say, the drug itself did not produce the cure, but rather served as an adjunct that allowed psychotherapy to proceed faster. This psychedelic therapy worked best when it was used to prepare the patient for treatment by Alcoholics Anonymous, which Hoffer regarded as "the only established treatment for alcoholics."

Further, it was asserted that the psychedelic therapist is supposed to work with the material that the LSD-treated patient experiences and discusses during therapy, and to help the patient "resynthesize a new model of life or a new personal philosophy." With the aid of the therapist, the patients evaluate themselves more objectively, and become more aware of their own responsibility for their situation, and more importantly, for doing something about it. These patients presumably become more aware of their inner strengths and qualities, which help them in the long and difficult struggle toward sobriety.

The basis for this approach by Hoffer and Osmond rested upon their perception that there were similarities among the psychotomimetic effects of LSD, schizophrenia, and delirium tremens (DTs), the toxic psychosis stemming from persistent alcohol abuse.

> It occurred to us that LSD might be used to produce a model of DTs. Many alcoholics ascribed the beginning of their recovery to "hitting bottom," and often "hitting bottom" meant having had a particularly memorable attack of DTs. We thought that LSD could be used to induce a psychotomimetic state that would lead to something like a religious conversion with no risk to the patient. We treated two alcoholics in a hospital setting and one recovered. (Hoffer, 1970, p. 360)

They reported other "encouraging" results, and raised the tempo of their research to the point where they had treated one thousand alcoholics. They found that a large proportion of their patients did not report having psychotomimetic experiences; rather, their experiences were pleasant and exciting and yielded insight into their drinking problems. Osmond (1957) reported these findings at the meeting of the New York Academy of Sciences that was mentioned above. Hoffer later concluded that after 10 years of major studies of psychedelic therapy, the same proportion of recoveries was always found. "Whether the experiments were considered controlled or not", he wrote, "about 50 percent were able to remain sober or to drink much less. This seems to be a universal statistic for LSD therapy." (Hoffer, 1970, p. 361)

In the treatment of schizophrenia, Hoffer seemed to differ with Osmond by suggesting that psychedelic drugs were countraindicated in these cases because these patients were more likely to have psychotic rather than psychedelic reactions to the drugs, which could lead to severe anxiety or panic, to suicide, and, very rarely, to other violent acts. However, he proposed that psychedelic treatment would not harm these patients if treatment was conducted in a hospital so that if any resurgence of schizophrenia occurred, the patient could be treated promptly and vigorously (e.g., with mega-vitamin B_3 [nicotinic acid]).

Assessment of LSD Therapies

From one point of view, it seems needless to assess LSD therapies since such therapies have virtually disappeared from the psychological and psychiatric scenes. This may be due in part to the results of a 10-year follow-up of 250 persons who had participated in psychedelic treatment, and who displayed no characteristic changes in behavior, attitude, or values as a result of their previous therapy. And, even though many patients in the experimental group eloquently reported a profound experience at the time of therapy, it had little value in predicting the ultimate outcome (McGlothlin and Arnold, 1971). An important reason for the demise of psychedelic therapy was the declaration by the United States Federal Bureau of Narcotics and Dangerous Drugs that LSD be placed in Schedule I, the most restrictive class of substances with no medical value. Hence, LSD was banned from importation, which was followed by Sandoz's decision to stop production. These events for all practical purposes brought LSD treatment to an end, although LSD could be made and sold to be used in biochemical research that was permitted and overseen by appropriate federal agencies.

Even if the supply and use of LSD had not been banned, there was mounting public criticism concerning its therapeutic value that could not be ignored. First of all, the psychedelic studies were said to have frequently included poorly defined patient samples, vague goals of treatment, lack of control groups, and unorthodox investigators. Most of the claims that these drugs were beneficial could not be substantiated in replicated studies, and many favorable outcomes were deemed to be no better than placebo effects. In an evaluation of a study claiming success in treating depression with a single dose of ditran (an anticholinergic drug having severe autonomic side effects), it was proposed that the reported beneficial response might just as well have been based on the patient's fear that he might receive a second dose (Hollister, 1978). Bowers (1987) cited a number of investigators who found that for most psychotic patients who had not shown signs of illness for long periods, hallucinogens such as LSD and mescaline intensified their psychosis. Furthermore, he reported that when LSD was used as an adjunct to psychotherapy by means of the intense emotional experience that the drug produced, there were other precautionary notes that the procedure aggravated psychotic reactions. And, as mentioned previously, in some cases of casual LSD use, there were accounts of psychotic sequelae that were similar to schizophrenic symptoms. This finding was buttressed by the results of epidemiological studies in Connecticut, which revealed that in the late 1960s there was a large increase in drug-abuse patients as first admissions to state hospitals, and 3–5 years later there was a substantial increase in first admissions of former drug users that were diagnosed with schizophrenia and paranoid disorders. Further, this increase was age specific, that is, it occurred in psychotic patients 15–34 years old, but not in older psychotic patients. It was concluded that hallucinogen use had created new cases of bona fide schizophreniform psychosis and related disorders during the 1960s and 1970s.

Misuse and Abuse of LSD

At the same time that psychedelic therapy was being tested, normal volunteers offered themselves as subjects in experiments to assess the effects of LSD. These subjects and those willing to experiment on themselves frequently reported interesting and pleasurable effects of the drug. Ultimately, LSD and other phantasticants were embraced in the 1960s by hundreds of thousands of American and European youths. These substances were taken for an occasional thrill experience or because the users thought that the drugs were "consciousness expanders" and would open up their minds and provide insight into religious, sensual, aesthetic, artistic, and creative endeavors of all sorts, as well as provide a profound understanding of one's place in society and the world.

Because the primary effects of the drug act upon the central nervous system, the mental content of which, for all intents and purposes, is derived from each individual's experience, there are as many drug-induced experiences as there are drug takers. Thus, those seeking religious insights will see a deity in altered perceptions, the writer will see his experiences and hopes rearranged, the artist will see new geometric and color arrangements, and the disenchanted, the alienated, and the lonely will experience what they think is love, gentleness, innocence, and freedom. Theodore Roszak (1969), who wrote in defense of the youth of the counterculture (those expressing opposition to the forms and goals of the current "materialistic" society), and yet decried their commitment to drug use, expressed his view as follows:

> Perhaps the drug experience bears significant fruit when rooted in the soil of a mature and cultivated mind. But the experience has, all of a sudden, been laid hold of by a generation of youngsters who are pathetically a-cultural and who often bring nothing to the experience but a vacuous yearning. They have, in adolescent rebellion, thrown off the corrupted culture of their elders and, along with that soiled bath water, the very body of the Western heritage—at best, in favor of exotic traditions they only marginally understand; at worst, in favor of an introspective chaos in which the seventeen or eighteen years of their unformed lives float like atoms in a void. (p. 159)

Not surprisingly, the anticipated promise of the phantasticant drugs could not be fulfilled; and because unique experiences were no longer unique when frequently repeated, the use of these substances markedly declined within a relatively short time. The drugs did not evoke a physiological dependence. Instead, there was a rapid development of tolerance and a psychological satiation of the intense emotional effects of the drugs. Moreover, there was a lack of dependability in these drugs to produce a desirable effect in mood alteration, as well as decreased gratification as the "trips" became commonplace (McGlothlin and Arnold, 1971).

Furthermore, there were many reports of "bad trips" characterized by being taken over by the drug and losing control of one's psychological experience. These "trips" included such illusions as spiders crawling over one's body, being on the verge of falling into a black and bottomless pit, or of one's hand being purple and remaining so.

The most common nonpsychotic adverse reaction was a state of acute panic, accompanied by fear of imminent insanity. Careful analyses of such "bad trips" have concluded that there was no single factor that could guarantee immunity from an adverse LSD reaction, and psychiatrists and psychologists were not able to find any significant or useful criteria by which experienced users of LSD who had "bad trips" could be distinguished from similar users who did not.

It was difficult to establish the incidence of such adverse reactions because of the reluctance of users to come forward for treatment. But starting with a marked increase in illicit use of LSD in September 1965, several large hospitals in Los Angeles reported that their psychiatric emergency services, which previously had seen only 6 LSD cases per year, were beginning to see patients at a rate of 60 to 180 per year. Whereas unpleasant acute reactions in those hospital cases were not uncommon, more often there were instances of more pervasive effects such as mental confusion, perceptual distortions, and poor concentration that lasted for days or even weeks. In rare cases, individuals complained of mental and emotional disturbances for several years after exposure to LSD.

For these and other reasons, interest in experimenting with LSD markedly declined, but interest in the drug obviously did not end, because new thrillseekers can always be found. In the 1990s, there was an apparent upsurge in LSD use. From 1988 to 1992 LSD use by high school seniors rose from 4.8% to 5.6%. Thus in this group of survey respondents, use of LSD was almost twice as high as that of cocaine, and 7 to 8 times higher than heroin use. Further, in 1991, the National Institute on Drug Abuse (NIDA) reported that a household survey on drug use revealed that between 13 and 17 million individuals in the United States had used a hallucinogen at least once that year (see NIDA, 1991). Also, televised news programs at that time even resurrected old films of reports given by former psychedelic therapists, and some spoken affidavits from individuals who claimed that their long-standing alcoholism was completely eliminated after one LSD treatment. However, aside from the scientific interest in the physiological basis of the psychotomimetic effects of these drugs, their potential therapeutic use for restructuring the sick or dissatisfied personality is virtually over for now.

However, notwithstanding the negative findings described above, a grant from NIDA was recently awarded to the Department of Psychiatry at the University of New Mexico to support new investigations in psychiatric research with hallucinogenic drugs (see Strassman, 1995, for review). The aims of this research project are to probe into the mind–brain interfaces between these drugs and their effects on characteristics of the human mind, such as affect (emotions), cognition, volition, interoception, and perception. The proposed investigations are to proceed with better controlled studies, newly developed Hallucinogen Rating Scales (HRS), and advanced in vivo brain-imaging techniques to better characterize hallucinogen effects and their mechanisms of action. Also, topographic pharmacoelectroencephalography, positron emission tomography, and magnetic resonance imaging will be used to assess the metabolic effects of psychoactive doses of these drugs, as well as their functional distribution within the brains of human subjects. This new approach should yield some interesting data, but because of the recent upsurge of hallucinogen abuse, there will likely be a spate of adverse psychiatric sequelae such as those seen during the illicit use of hallucinogens in the 1960s. Thus, this research is needed to provide safe, selective, and efficacious treatment for acute and chronic negative effects of these drugs.

Part III Summary

The hallucinogenic properties of LSD were serendipitously discovered in 1943 during research with ergot alkaloids, some of which have beneficial therapeutic vascular effects. Attention was drawn to this event because of the uncommonly powerful potency of LSD in producing a bizarre constellation of psychological effects. During this period, many laboratories were searching for a biological basis for schizophrenia, a disease notable for its malignant effects on the human personality, which at that time was virtually uncontrollable by existing pharmacological or psychotherapeutic means. LSD was thought to produce psychological phenomena similar to the symptoms of schizophrenia, so the drug was studied as a possible probe into the mental compartments where thought distortions and perceptual misinterpretations of schizophrenia may have their origin.

LSD and related hallucinogens have significant inhibitory effects upon the serotonergic cells of the raphe, and widely distributed agonistic effects on serotonergic postsynaptic receptors in the brain. Normally the raphe neurons exert a tonic inhibition on most of their target cells in the diencephalon and forebrain. However, the LSD inhibitory effects on the raphe neurons do not seem to be related to the behavioral effects of these drugs. With the discovery of the subtypes of serotonergic receptors, the behavioral effects, including the so-called hallucinogenic response, seem to be mediated via agonistic effects upon postsynaptic 5-HT$_{2A}$ receptors in the forebrain. However, LSD and other hallucinogens bind to other serotonergic receptor subtypes as well, and though their binding potencies to these other sites correlate with their hallucinogenic potencies, this correlation is not nearly as high as when comparing binding to the 5-HT$_{2A}$ site.

Although LSD and related indolealkylamines, as well as a number of phenethylamines, have been and remain valuable tools for studying brain function, the behavioral research on hallucinogens as adjunctive aids to psychotherapy was difficult to interpret because of the wide gamut of physiological and psychological effects that are characteristic for these drugs. Nonetheless, reviews of past controlled studies show little or no evidence for either acute or long-term differences in clinical outcomes as a result of psychedelic therapy, and thus provide little support for the continuation of such treatment. In its defense, there was little evidence of harmfulness of psychedelic therapy when carefully performed in a supervised setting with selected patient groups.

In the 1960s the use of the indolealkylamines was promoted in attempts to expand awareness or consciousness for the purpose of self-realization. At the urging of some professionals, who in retrospect should have known better, large numbers of young people used the drugs in what was deemed a "recreational" way. This was also abetted by the participants of the counterculture, who proposed that the use of these drugs would increase awareness and facilitate solutions to the inconsistencies and conflicts in daily life. Though the drug was declared illegal to possess, the profit motive insured the manufacture and the availability of the drug. Furthermore, the use of an illicit drug that was lacking in the control of its quality, dose, and purity, predictably resulted in many mishaps, some of which were exaggerated and others fabricated. A crackdown ensued, and the illegal manufacturers and purveyors were heavily fined and jailed. Nonetheless, use of LSD and other hallucinogens continues into the 1990s, though at a significantly slower pace than when they were first introduced. (For a detailed discussion of the harmful effects of LSD and other related substances, see Hofmann, 1983, and Moreines, 1989.)

More should be said about the persistent adverse reactions associated with LSD use and their potential modes of treatment, not to mention the possible dangers to the fetuses of pregnant women who are drug users. However, because these drugs are manufactured in secret, purchased illegally, and used in an unregulated manner, there is little hard evidence from which to draw any conclusions. It can be said, however, that as an adjunct to psychotherapy, or as a proactive agent of happiness, self-improvement, creativity, enlightenment, and religious intensification, the benefit–risk ratio is quite small, if not nonexistent. Nonetheless, there is new support for fresh attempts in using improved methods and techniques to better understand the intriguing effects of these drugs upon the central nervous system, and to determine how their adverse effects may be suppressed so that these drugs might be used therapeutically.

Clinical Applications

Chapter 18

Schizophrenia

Despite enormous strides in the advancement of our knowledge of the neurochemical bases of behavior and emotion, our understanding of neural mechanisms mediating abnormal behavior is still in its infancy. Many answers to our questions will be forthcoming as more sophisticated biochemical, physiological and behavioral measurement techniques are developed. Each techniques will further increase accessibility of the CNS to experimental manipulation and measurement. Presently, the bulk of information we possess comes from examining drug effects on animal neurochemistry and from a variety of animal models of psychiatric illness. An alternate approach is to sample the accessible biological fluids (e.g., blood, urine, CSF) of patients with mental disorders or to measure brain amines and metabolites in human brains postmortem. Since it is unlikely that distinct mental illnesses stem from a common neurochemical entity, research results will be highly dependent on the test populations chosen. Thus, increased validity and reliability in diagnosis of psychiatric conditions is critical in determining the biological correlates of specific disorders (see below). In addition, many factors related to hospitalization, drug treatment, and duration of illness must be controlled for in the clinical research design.

Although a genetic factor has been identified in the etiology of psychosis, psychological, biological, and sociological factors combine in a unique manner to contribute significantly to the development of mental disorders. For instance, increased emotional stress is related not only to the appearance of psychotic symptoms but also to widespread physiological effects on circulating hormone levels and CNS neurochemistry. Thus, neurochemistry, which we now assume regulates behavioral responses to environmental stimuli, is in turn regulated by external influences and behavior. The dynamic state of the individual explains why steady state neurochemistry may not be a reflection of ongoing CNS function.

This chapter describes the major hypotheses regarding the etiology and pathogenesis of schizophrenia. The hypotheses presented here are constantly changing as new data accumulate and old ideas are modified. In this chapter perhaps more than any other, critical evaluation of the ideas presented is urged. Only through diligent questioning and carefully controlled experiments will the frontiers of neuropsychopharmacology be extended.

Diagnosis, Etiology, and Pathology

The psychoses are characterized by marked distortions of reality and disturbances in perception, intellectual functioning, affect (mood), motivation, and motor behavior. The psychotic individual's incapacity is often so complete that voluntary or involuntary hospitalization is required. One class of psychoses includes the affective disorders (major depressive disorder, mania, bipolar disorder) and is discussed in Chapter 19. A second class is schizophrenia, which poses a very great social problem and is responsible for filling a majority of mental hospital beds.

Symptoms

Schizophrenia is very clearly a thought disorder, and is characterized by both disturbed form and content of thought. Bizarre delusions having no basis in fact are common. Particularly prevalent are persecutory delusions involving the belief that others are spying on or planning harm to the individual. Also quite common is the delusion that one's thoughts are broadcast from one's head to the world or that thoughts and feelings are not one's own but imposed by an external source. The form of thought is disturbed, leading to confused and illogical communication patterns that frequently do not follow conventional rules of semantics. Speech may be vague or repetitive and characterized by loosening of associations such that ideas shift from one subject to another completely unrelated subject.

Disturbances in perception are also a frequent occurrence in schizophrenia. The major disturbance is hallucination, most often auditory in nature. Generally the hallucinations consist of voices, which are insulting or commanding. Tactile hallucinations, usually electrical, tingling, or burning sensations, also occur.

In many schizophrenics, emotions are either absent or inappropriate to the situation. Inappropriate emotion is demonstrated by the individual who smiles or laughs while describing electrical tortures, for instance. Individuals with blunted emotions show no sign of expression, speak in a monotone, and frequently report a lack of feeling. Sudden and unpredictable changes of emotion are also common.

Schizophrenics are frequently withdrawn, preoccupied with their own thoughts and delusions. They are often withdrawn both physically and emotionally. Motor activity is generally reduced and characterized by inappropriate and bizarre postures, by rigidity that resists efforts to be moved, or by purposeless and stereotyped movements, for example, rocking or pacing.

The combination of symptoms varies significantly in schizophrenia, and the disorder has been divided into more distinct categories, including catatonic, paranoid, and disorganized type. For a further account of clinical symptoms, see any standard text in psychiatry or the Diagnostic and Statistical Manual of Mental Disorders (DSM-IV; American Psychiatric Association [APA], 1994).

The onset of schizophrenia is most often between the late teens and early twenties and episodes recur throughout life, disrupting the individual's most productive years. On that basis, the direct (e.g., hospitalization and medication costs) and indirect (loss of productive employment and participation in society) costs of schizophrenia have been estimated to be between $30 and $40 billion a year in the United States (Rupp and Keith, 1993).

Diagnosis

Estimates of the incidence of schizophrenia are handicapped by differences in diagnostic criteria, which depend to a large extent on the training of the clinicians making the diagnoses as well as their experience, theoretical beliefs, types of practice, and other biases (Haier, 1980). For example, studies in Europe and Asia, using a relatively narrow concept of schizophrenia, found a lifetime prevalence rate from 0.2% to 1%. Studies that were done in the United States which used broader criteria suggested significantly higher rates, at least for urban populations (DSM-III-R, p. 186). Because diagnosis is a summary of subjectively evaluated symptoms at a given time, it is easy to see that diagnostic criteria may vary from society to society, institution to institution, or clinician to clinician.

Diagnosis classically has two principal problems: (1) Not everyone uses the same criteria in making diagnoses; and (2) many criteria are unreliable. Nevertheless, a significant attempt to provide standard criteria for several discrete categories of mental illness and to test them for reliability is represented by the most recent version of the DSM-IV. The DSM-IV includes a set of official definitions of mental illnesses and specifies descriptive criteria for distinguishing among them. The manual was designed by a task force of the APA, who debated what information was to be included and the symptoms to be used to diagnose specific illnesses. Field trials using thousands of patients and several hundred clinical psychiatrists resulted in a manual that reduces diagnostic confusion and provides more reliable criteria for diagnoses than did earlier attempts. However, critics of the modified criteria exist, and many of the DSM-IV revisions have been controversial.

Despite the difficulties, the importance of accurate and reliable diagnosis is fourfold. First, diagnosis improves communication among mental health professionals and between psychiatrist and patient regarding the symptoms, course of the illness, and prognosis. Second, accurate diagnosis precedes the prescription of appropriate treatment. As more specific neurochemical correlates are identified and pharmacological intervention becomes more precise, specific diagnosis will take on further importance. Third, reliable diagnostic categories are vital for accurate estimates of incidence and for demographic research. In addition, diagnosis helps to establish criteria for clinical evaluation of and improvement in treatment. Also, standard criteria are vital in identifying homogeneous populations on which to assess particular treatment modes or to evaluate neurochemical correlates. Fourth, it has been argued (Heinrichs, 1993) that it is insufficient to identify abnormalities in brain structure and neurochemistry without demonstrating a direct relationship to specific behavioral and neuropsychological diagnostic symptoms. With advances in techniques available to neuropsychopharmacologists, an integrated biobehavioral approach to understanding this complex disorder will ultimately provide a comprehensive picture.

The heterogeneity of symptoms among those patients diagnosed as schizophrenic is enormous. No specific characteristics or symptoms are focal to a diagnosis of schizophrenia; that is, no single symptom is consistently present in all schizophrenics. Further, different patients with the same disorder frequently exhibit a very different constellation of symptoms, and schizophrenic patients inevitably exhibit symptoms of more than one diagnostic category. Moreover, within even a short time span, some symptoms tend to become more prominent while others recede. It is apparently not uncommon to find that a patient admitted with catatonic manifestations of schizophrenia may be diagnosed as a paranoid schizophrenic several years later. The question of whether schizophrenia is a single disorder or a collection of disorders has not been resolved, but the issue is discussed in several sources (Cardno and Farmer, 1995; Tsuang and Farrone, 1995).

Historically, the heterogeneous character of schizophrenia has been recognized and the study of the disease has been organized based on a subtype strategy (Kraepelin, 1913). The schizophrenia subtypes, classified as catatonic, paranoid, hebephrenic, and simple, were intended to organize diagnoses, but discrete symptom clusters do not exist to validate these categories. Nor are there consistent differences among the subtypes in terms of abnormalities in information processing, psychophysical measures, regional cerebral blood flow, or neuroanatomical or neurochemical changes. However, modifications of the original subtypes are still used in DSM-IV diagnoses and represent one of several viable approaches for understanding the disorder.

In an attempt to simplify the diagnostic categories, the symptoms are conceptually divided into **positive and negative symptoms**. Stemming from the early work of Kraepelin (1913) and Bleuler (1950), a two-syndrome hypothesis was synthesized by Crow (1980). Crow's distinction between Type I (positive) and Type II (negative) symptoms, although an oversimplification, has had a major impact on biological theorizing in schizophrenia research. Andreasen (1990) summarizes the symptom categories and provides a detailed historical perspective. Positive schizophrenia is characterized by the more florid symptoms of the disorder, including delusions and hallucinations, disorganized speech, and bizarre or disorganized behavior. Patients who demonstrate predominately positive symptoms tend to have had an acute onset of the disorder and had relatively normal premorbid functions. When their symptoms are in remission, their social functioning tends to be relatively good. Rather than finding structural brain abnormalities in these individuals, current thinking suggests that neurochemical abnormalities are a significant cause of the symptoms. These patients respond well to antipsychotic medications that block dopamine (DA) receptors while their symptoms are exacerbated by drugs that enhance dopamine function.

Negative symptoms represent a loss or decrease of normal functions and include poverty of speech and content of speech, blunting of emotions, loss of energy and drive, and loss of sociability and the ability to derive pleasure from normally pleasurable activities. These symptoms are among those that are most resistant to treatment with currently available antipsychotic drugs and may actually be exacerbated by drug treatment. Unlike patients with prominent positive symptoms, patients with negative symptoms tend to show a long course of progressive deterioration, perhaps reflecting long-term brain degenerative changes. Among the most consistent findings is that ventricular enlargement is related to negative symptom schizophrenia (Andreasen, 1987; Meltzer, 1987).

The positive–negative symptom typing of schizophrenics has continued to be challenged and modified to enhance reliability and validity of classification (Flaum and Andreasen, 1995; Peralta, deLeon, and Cuestra, 1992). It is clear, for example, that both positive and negative symptoms occur in other major mental disorders, including mania and depression. Figure 18.1 shows the results when global ratings of positive symptoms, negative symptoms, and mood symptoms were made for acutely ill schizophrenics, manic patients, and individuals with major depressive disorder (Andreasen, 1990). Notice that the schizophrenic group has the highest scores of the three on both positive and negative symptoms, although manic patients have relatively high scores on positive symptoms and depressed patients have high scores on negative symptoms. The greatest difference among the groups, however, occurs on the mood scale. Clearly, manics score high on euphoria, depressed individuals score high on dysphoria, and schizophrenic patients have low ratings on both. Therefore, though no single symptom is specific for any one disorder, their specific patterns of symptoms are significant to diagnosis. It is important to note that although depressed individuals score relatively high on negative symptoms, those symptoms are apparently part of the depressive disorder because antidepressant treatment that effectively reduces depression in these individuals, reduces their negative symptoms in parallel. In contrast, antidepressant drugs have very little or no effect on negative symptoms in a schizophrenic patient.

In addition to the subtype strategy, the other methods used to put order into the heterogeneity of schizophrenia include the symptom strategy, the dimensional strategy, and the unitary strategy (Andreasen, Arndt, Alliger et al., 1995; Andreasen, Arndt, O'Leary et al., 1995). The utilization of one organizing strategy does not preclude the usefulness of the others, and Andreasen and colleagues have explored and utilized each of them. The

(a)

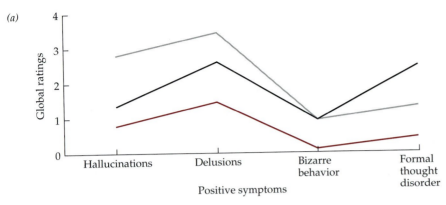

Positive symptoms

18.1 GLOBAL RATING SCORES ON POSITIVE, NEGATIVE, AND MOOD SYMPTOMS for schizophrenic, depressed, and manic individuals. Schizophrenics score significantly higher on most categories for both positive and negative symptoms, but show relatively few abnormalites in mood. Depressed individuals score high on negative symptoms and dysphoric mood. Manic patients have prominent positive symptoms along with striking euphoria. (After Andreasen, 1990.)

(b)

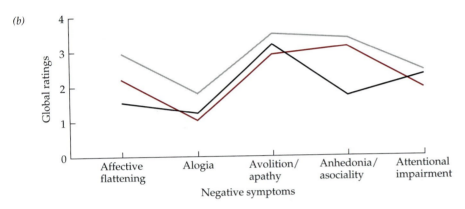

Negative symptoms

(c)

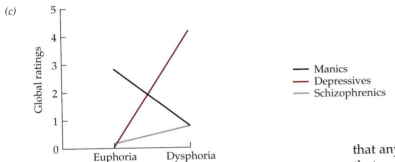

Mood symptoms

symptom approach involves an attempt to identify the neural mechanisms responsible for individual symptoms. Lesion studies and brain imaging techniques are important tools for understanding the neural substrates of normal cognitive processes, as well as abnormal ones. Examples of this approach in studies of schizophrenia include investigations into the relationship between auditory hallucinations and the superior temporal gyrus or between disorganized speech and the perisylvian language areas of the brain (see Andreasen, Arndt, Alliger et al., 1995; Flaum et al., 1995). The nature of this research strategy examines the neural correlates of isolated symptoms and does not attempt to understand the multiple symptoms that constitute the global syndrome.

While the subtype strategy is based on medical models that describe a disease based on discrete categories that do not overlap, dimensional analysis assumes that any symptom can be described as a continuum and that symptoms often do overlap. An important part of dimensional analysis is the use of factor analysis, which identifies groups of symptoms that are correlated with one another. Researchers assume that symptoms that frequently occur together have a clinical or neurochemical relationship. A number of studies using factor analysis have identified three dimensions called psychoticism, disorganization, and negative symptoms (see Andreasen, Arndt, O'Leary et al., 1995). In order to know whether the three groups represent functional clusters, Andreasen and coworkers have evaluated the relationship between the three dimensions and neuropsychological deficits (see Andreasen, Arndt, Alliger et al., 1995). They found that the negative dimension was associated with general dysfunction on a broad range of tests, including those of verbal learning and memory, verbal fluency, visual memory, and motor sequencing. The disorganized dimension was correlated with abnormal higher-order verbal processing, lower IQ, and low scores on the Wisconsin Card Sorting Test. The psychotic dimension was apparently not correlated with performance deficits on any of the tests used. Finding such correlations provides empirical validation for the three dimension strategy. The same group (Flaum et al., 1995) also evaluated the relationship between each of the three dimensions and specific brain regions, visualized with MRI. Their results are discussed below in the section on pathology.

The unitary strategy is based on the idea that schizophrenic symptoms are a consequence of an error or a series of misconnections in the neuronal wiring of the brain. The model assumes that such misconnections, which probably occur during development, could produce multiple symptoms depending on the nature of the miswiring. For example, Andreasen and coworkers (1994) have investigated possible miswiring in the circuits running from the reticular activating system to the thalamus and basal ganglia and on to the prefrontal cortex. The rationale for a unitary strategy is that miswiring in the reticular formation and thalamus, which normally filter most sensory information before relaying it to the cortex for further action, could be responsible for an overload of information reaching the cortex, leading to disturbed perceptions (hallucinations), disturbed beliefs (delusions), and withdrawal from overwhelming sensory input. Goldberg and Weinberger (1995) review some of the relevant data that argue for a unitary pathogenesis in which patients vary along a dimension of severity, but one that has many etiologies.

Prognosis

Figure 18.2 shows a steady increase in the number of hospitalized psychiatric patients from 1900 to 1956, when the number of patients began a gradual decline. This reduction in the number of hospitalized mental patients has been attributed to a large increase in hospital discharges despite the steady increase in new cases admitted yearly. The increased discharge rate correlates temporally with the initiation of psychotropic drug therapy.

We must remember that most patients released from the hospital are not considered "cured," but are in some stage of remission. Thirty percent may be considered to be completely recovered while approximately 10% of schizophrenic patients fail to respond to treatment and remain hospitalized. The remaining 60% experience varying degrees of recovery characterized by social isolation, erratic employment or reduced occupational level, and/or the need for help in daily functioning. Relapse rates for psychiatric disorders are high, but drug treatment has greatly improved the condition of a large number of patients and enabled them to reenter the community, where they may avoid the general deterioration that occurs with prolonged institutionalization. A secondary benefit of community living may be that the mentally ill are now more visible to the community, thus dramatizing the need for greater social concern for mental health and removing a small portion of the social stigma connected with the disorder.

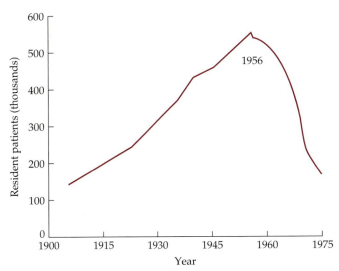

18.2 PATIENT POPULATIONS in public mental institutions, 1900 to 1975. (After Bassuk and Gerson, 1978.)

Although a return to the community is generally believed to provide mental patients with the opportunity to reestablish family ties, social responsibility, and useful employment, many patients live with poor or marginal adjustment to their environment. In addition, because many discharged patients are atypical in their dress, inept in social functioning, and marginal in their economic productivity, there is frequent community resistance to the establishment of community residences for the mentally ill. The establishment of such residences usually occurs in areas populated by the poor, where there is less resistance. The outcome is increased social segregation of the patients. In addition, Arnhoff (1975) and others have suggested that the impact on the families of psychiatric patients may be very great. Among potential problems are increased stress on family members and exposure of children to a distorted model (parental or sibling) further increasing emotional turmoil. Concern has also been expressed about the increase in reproduction rate among severely mentally ill individuals who reside in the community as compared with hospitalized patients. Because a genetic factor has been identified for both schizophrenia and affective disorders, the increased reproduction rate foreshadows an increase in incidence of mental disorders in the future.

Etiology

Epidemiology. Although the question of who is likely to develop schizophrenia has been examined repeatedly, few consistent answers have been found. One of the epidemiological findings is the inverse relationship between socioeconomic status and the incidence of schizophrenia (Dohrenwend and Dohrenwend, 1974). Despite the fact that the relationship has been found repeatedly, it has not held true in all cases. For instance, the relationship is apparently quite strong in metropolitan centers but weak or absent in smaller cities. In addition, if one excludes the lowest socioeconomic group, the relationship is not so strong. Two traditional hypotheses have been suggested to explain the phenomenon. The first suggests that the social and economic stresses experienced by the poor are a possible basis for the higher incidence of schizophrenia. The second hypothesis suggests that poverty is secondary to schizophrenia because schizophrenic patients, who frequently maintain bizarre behavior and are unemployed, are downwardly mobile on the socioeconomic scale.

A third hypothesis has evolved, which suggests that the reduced social network and social communication typical of the lowest socioeconomic group may be an explanation for the elevated numbers of schizophrenics (Hammer, Makiesky-Barrow, and Gutwirth, 1978). These investigators suggest that the poor have a higher risk of severed connections among individuals because of death, forced change of residence, or migration. Such disruption in the social network of an individual and its associated loss of social reinforcement and feedback may be the link to the prevalence of schizophrenia. Such disruption occurs most often in the "disorganized" parts of society, that is, where people experience excessive mobility, ethnic conflict, overcrowding, and social isolation. The advantage in identifying such factors is the possibility of developing preventive action for those individuals with the highest risk.

The hereditary nature of schizophrenia.   The search for a neurochemical pathology responsible for the disease state or for a vulnerability to the disease has been encouraged by genetic studies that demonstrate the importance of heredity to the etiology of the disorder. Classic family and adoption studies have been conducted by American–Danish teams of investigators, who have taken advantage of the excellent record-keeping system of Denmark to explore the relative contribution of heredity and environment to the development of schizophrenia (Kety et al., 1975; Wender et al., 1974). In more recent years, these studies have been reevaluated in light of newer and more uniform diagnostic categories. Despite numerous criticisms of the early work, including the lack of structured interviews, the lack of blind diagnoses, and inappropriate control groups, the interpretation of these results strongly suggests that relatives of schizophrenics are afflicted with the disease much more frequently than members of the general population. Indeed, the closer the genetic relationship, the greater the probability of schizophrenia in the relative.

Demonstrating this relationship, Gottesman and colleagues (Gottesman, McGuffin, and Farmer 1987; Gottesman, 1991; Prescott and Gottesman, 1993) have summarized a large number of family and twin studies of schizophrenics completed between 1920 and 1987 (Figure 18.3). Compared with the general population lifetime risk of about 1%, first-degree relatives have a lifetime risk of about 12%, while second-degree relatives have a 4% risk. The 6% rate among parents of schizophrenic children appears unexpectedly low, although the rate may reflect the selection process in marriage, which tends to exclude schizophrenics. These data also show a higher concordance for monozygotic twins (48%)

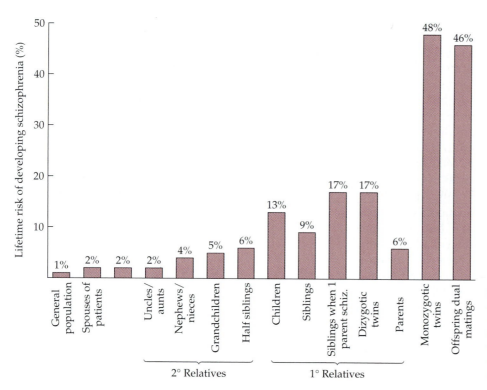

18.3 LIFETIME RISKS OF DEVELOPING SCHIZOPHRENIA among relatives of an affected individual. Data are summarized from about 40 European family and twin studies conducted between 1920 and 1987. (After Gottesman, 1991; Prescott and Gottesman, 1993.)

compared with dizygotic twins (17%). Furthermore, monozygotic twins, even when reared apart (i.e., in different environments), have a severalfold higher probability of concordance for schizophrenia than do dizygotic twins. The operation of genetic factors is strongly suggested by the finding that the offspring of a schizophrenic parent have essentially the same risk for the disorder whether or not they are raised by that parent.

A review of ongoing research in Finland and Denmark using the newest techniques to evaluate relatives of schizophrenic and control adoptees shows a distinct pattern of schizophrenic symptoms in the biological families of schizophrenic adoptees (see Tienari and Wynne, 1994). This might suggest a genetic influence to some component of the disorder. However, in addition to the genetic component, evaluation of the rearing families is used to assess significant environmental effects or environmental-genetic interactions.

The significance of the intrauterine environment has also been suggested by twin studies (Davis, Phelps, and Bracha, 1995). This work suggested that concordant monozygotic twins were more likely to have a shared chorionic membrane (a membrane that surrounds the embryo from the time of implantation) and a shared single placenta, while discordant monozygotic twins were generally dichorionic with separate placentas. Thus, simple monozygotic concordance rates may overestimate schizophrenic heritability because prenatal factors may be a significant contributing factor. The sharing of fetal blood circulation may mean that fetal infection plays a role in the etiology of schizophrenia.

Current molecular genetic research is attempting to uncover a linkage between schizophrenia and specific genomic sites (see Baron, 1995; Cardno and McGuffin, 1994). One area of interest is a portion of the sex chromosomes, called the pseudoautosomal region. Although several types of research have pointed to a linkage between this chromosomal region and the occurrence of schizophrenia, the conclusion has not been universally supported. As for neurobiological research in general, failure to replicate experimental results in molecular genetics may be due to several factors, including statistical artifacts, procedural problems, and misinterpretation of data. Other gene loci, particularly on chromosome 22, have also been found to be associated with the disorder and occur in close proximity to chromosomal aberrations responsible for other syndromes that frequently occur with psychosis (e.g., particular cardiac malfunction). The search for genetic links to schizophrenia is in its early stages, and new findings must be evaluated conservatively. Since the manifestation of the disease is heterogeneous, linkage studies may be enhanced by further clarification of diagnostic criteria.

Developmental errors. Several pieces of evidence have suggested that schizophrenia is due to a pathological process during neurodevelopment (see Nasrallah, 1993;

Weinberger, 1995; Wyatt, 1996). First, a higher incidence of perinatal complications occurs among schizophrenics than in the general population. Brain insult during pregnancy and delivery due to hypoxia, drugs, infections, endocrine disorders, or other events occurs with higher frequency in schizophrenics. Several groups have shown that exposure to the influenza A virus during the second trimester of pregnancy significantly increases the risk for schizophrenia in the child (see Yakeley and Murray, 1995). The virus evidently interferes with the normal neuronal migration that occurs during development. This neuronal abnormality, caused by the virus, may mimic gene-induced defects that lead to the same final outcome. Thus schizophrenia is considered to have phenocopies—forms of the illness caused by environmental agents that are clinically indistinguishable from schizophrenia.

Second, not only have gross morphological abnormalities been found in the brains of schizophrenic patients (see below), but more subtle histoarchitectural abnormalities also occur. These cellular irregularities are likely to be due to disruption in programmed developmental processes, such as neuronal proliferation, migration, differentiation, and elimination. Table 18.1 provides a partial list of postmortem histopathological abnormalities found in schizophrenic brains. Particularly interesting is the fact that little gliosis (mulitplication of astrocytes and microglia) occurs. Since gliosis is a response to neuronal damage that occurs in the mature brain, but not in the immature brain, it is likely that the histological cell damage found in schizophrenic brains occurred during the developmental process. Keshavan, Anderson, and Pettegrew (1994) discuss evidence for neurobiological abnormalities of schizophrenics in the normal synaptic pruning that occurs during adolescence. Excessive pruning of connections in the prefrontal cortex and reciprocal failure of pruning in certain subcortical structures, such as the lenticular nuclei, occur with greater frequency in schizophrenics. Whether such postnatal developmental differences are due to genetic programming errors, early brain insults, or environmental factors is not clear. The initial hypothesis proposed by Feinberg (1982) attempted to explain why, if a neurological abnormality is present at birth, the symptoms do not appear until early adulthood. He argued for a second pathological process in synaptic elimination occurring independently of the initial pathology. Other possible mechanisms for delayed onset include abnormalities in myelination, neuronal sprouting, or stress-induced modifications in neural transmission. Weinberger (1995) provides a review of the physical, neurological, and cytoarchitectural abnormalities that occur coincident with schizophrenia. In addition, possible neural mechanisms of delayed onset of symptoms is also discussed.

The biopsychosocial model. Further research into psychosocial aspects of schizophrenia has been proposed by

---

Table 18.1   Postmortem Histoarchitectural Abnormalities in Schizophrenic Brains[a]

1. Reduction (20% to 40%) in the granule layer of the dentate gyrus in the hippocampal formation consistent with a failure of proliferation of the granule cells.

2. Lower neuronal density in layer 6 of the prefrontal cortex, layer 5 of the cingulate gyrus, and layer 3 of the motor cortex, and reduced number of glia per unit volume in the cingulate cortex.

3. Poorly developed upper layers in the parahippocampal gyrus, with heterotopic displacement of single Pre-α groups without the presence of gliosis (suggestive of a disruption of neuronal migration during brain development).

4. Reductions in the absolute number of nerve cells in the granule cell layer of the dentate gyrus by 10% to 30% without a difference in the number and density of glial cells.

5. Reduction in the volume and neuron number without increased glial cell numbers in the entorhinal cortex.

6. Increased distance (23% to 30%) between the pial surface of the entorhinal cortex and the center of Pre-α cell clusters in some patients (suggestive of a disruption of cell migration during fetal neurodevelopment).

7. Decreased cell density in all areas of the hippocampus with the greatest difference in the left CA4 region.

8. Reduced numbers of neurons and glial cells in the mediodorsal thalamic nucleus and nucleus accumbens.

9. Disruption of cortical layers, heterotopic displacement of neurons, and paucity of neurons in superficial layers in the entorhinal cortex.

10. Reduced numbers of interneurons (possibly inhibitory) in most layers of the cingulate cortex, but mostly in layer 2. Also, lower interneuron density in layer 2 of the prefrontal area but a higher density of pyramidal neurons in layer 5 of the pre-frontal area.

[a]Compiled from numerous studies.
Source: After Nasrallah, 1993.

---

the biopsychosocial medical model of Engel (1980). This model emphasizes the interaction among numerous factors that impinge on the individual, leading to his disturbed behavior. Just as the memory (psycho) of an embarrassing event (social) can produce autonomic nervous system arousal (bio), the argument has been made that environmental stresses (social) can be associated with changes in neurochemistry (bio) that lead to schizophrenia (psycho) in the vulnerable individual (genetic) (Carpenter, 1987). This approach utilizes evidence for both genetic predisposition and the structural brain changes and biochemical abnormalities sometimes observed in patients with schizophrenia. The relative importance of physiological changes that are a consequence of stressful experiences or pathological changes in the CNS leading to alterations changes in subjective experience is not clear at present.

Vulnerability–stress model. Evidence strongly suggests that schizophrenia occurs following the interaction of genetic susceptibility and some as yet unidentified environmental stress. The adoption studies show us that the environmental stress does not have to include the presence of a schizophrenic individual, since children of a schizophrenic parent adopted into a nonschizophrenic family have the same probability of developing schizophrenia.

The vulnerability–stress model (Figure 18.4) developed by Nuechterlein and Liberman (see Goldstein, 1987) specifies the variables contributing to the onset of schizophrenia (vulnerability markers and environmental stressors) and the "protectors" that may reduce the probability of onset of psychiatric symptoms. The contributing factors described are those that have an effect both on the onset of schizophrenic symptoms (premorbid) and on relapse after an episode has occurred. Such a model suggests intervention strategies to modify negative affective climate within the family along with antipsychotic medication.

In Figure 18.4 the vulnerability factors in the uppermost boxes include some of the abnormalities identified by studies of schizophrenics or those who are "at risk," including altered brain neurochemistry, hyperreactivity of the autonomic nervous system, difficulties in attentional and information processing tasks, and particular personality traits. The personal protectors that diminish

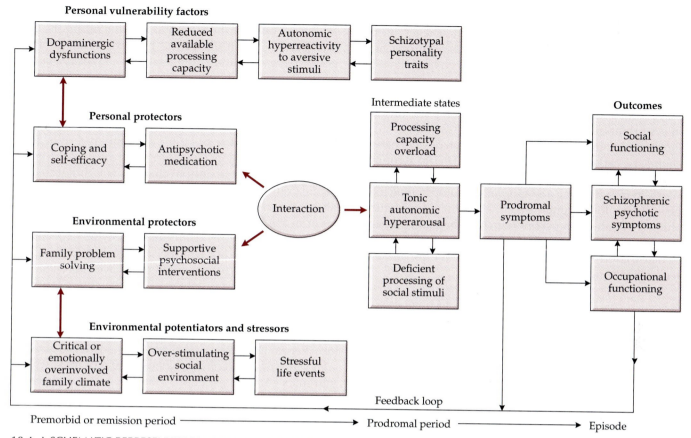

18.4 A SCHEMATIC REPRESENTATION OF THE VULNERABILITY–STRESS MODEL developed by Nuechterlein and Liberman. The variables shown alter the probability of the onset and course of development of schizophrenia in a given individual. (After Goldstein, 1987.)

the damaging effects of the vulnerability factors include the individual's own coping strategies and confidence in problem solving as well as antipsychotic medication for those with a history of schizophrenia.

The environmental stressors include stressful life events, such as a series of adverse events that are beyond the individual's control. Some evidence also suggests that the family climate may contribute to stress when it is critical and emotionally turbulent and when communication patterns are distorted. Excessive social stimulation may be a factor particularly for those individuals who do not live with their families. Countering the environmental stressors are the protectors, which include effective problem-solving strategies within the family and psychosocial therapies that help family members to modify the stress-producing, negative emotional climate. All of these factors interact, producing "intermediate states" that may develop further toward schizophrenic symptoms as the stressors and protectors change. (For a more detailed discussion, see Goldstein 1987.)

The vulnerability–stress model as described by Goldstein (1987) suggests a developmental approach to identify the "high-risk" individual. Evidence suggests that some children who are at risk for schizophrenia show unusual patterns of development in early infancy. Although a single deviant factor was not consistent across studies, some of the factors identified were passivity and apathy, less responsiveness to verbal commands, more difficult temperaments, and poor sensorimotor performance. In the later childhood years, unusual performance on attentional and information-processing tasks, along with impairments in fine motor coordination, were the best predictors of psychiatric disorders in adolescence. In addition, children of a schizophrenic parent are more impaired in social role functioning than children of nonschizophrenic parents. As one might expect, the signs of psychiatric dysfunction that are present in infancy become more pronounced by later childhood and adolescence, but only a subsample of children of schizophrenics show these signs. Thus their usefulness as screening devices is limited at best.

Neuropathology

Until recently, little gross or cellular pathology had been found in the brains of schizophrenics. While significant anatomical and biochemical abnormalities have been identified with the newest techniques, many of the differences discovered may be effects of the disorder rather than causes. Biochemical differences have been attributed to long-term and multiple drug use by psychiatric patients, institutional diet and vitamin deficiency, differences in physical activity, or other effects of chronic hospitalization. It is important to use objective diagnostic criteria to identify the pathology underlying the various forms of schizophrenic behavior. Errors involved in sampling from a heterogeneous population explain the lack of confirmation of results by different research groups. Furthermore, in postmortem examination of CNS neurochemistry, experimental results must take into account a variety of enzymatic changes following death. Both death-to-morgue time and morgue-to-autopsy time have been shown to be significant variables in neurochemical studies. Variations in postmortem handling and preparation of tissue for morphological or histological examination also contribute to difficulties in the interpretation of research findings.

Structural abnormalities.   Brain imaging techniques such as CT scans and MRI (see Chapter 2) provide a rapidly accumulating body of evidence demonstrating structural abnormalities in the brains of schizophrenics. The majority of studies (see Raz and Raz, 1990; Weinberger, 1995) provide evidence for diffuse cerebral atrophy and ventricular enlargement, results which have been confirmed by postmortem examination (Brown et al., 1986; Crow, Ball, and Bloom, 1989). The enlarged ventricles seem to be the result of cell loss, particularly in the temporal lobe, although this conclusion is far from universal (Pfefferbaum et al., 1990).

Although gross degenerative changes are of significance, quantitative neuropathology studies have examined the size, the number, and the organization of neurons in discrete brain areas. Most research focuses on changes in brain structures that may be associated with the unique symptoms of schizophrenia: disturbances in emotion, attention, planning, information processing, and thought disorders. Since DA has been implicated in the etiology of schizophrenia (see below), those brain areas heavily innervated by DA-containing neurons are also of special interest. Hence, emphasis has been placed on the examination of the limbic system, frontal cortex, and basal ganglia. The most consistent results, as summarized by Meltzer (1987) and Weinberger (1995), show reduced volume of the basal ganglia, temporal lobe, and limbic regions, disorganization of the pyramidal cell layer of the hippocampus, and atrophy of discrete cortical layers.

In a series of neuropathology studies (Bogerts, Meertz, and Schonfeldt-Bausch, 1985), quantitative evaluation of Nissl-stained sections of brain from schizophrenics showed significant decreases in volume of the nigrostriatal area without an increase in glial cells. Also, the mean volume of nerve cells in the substantia nigra was decreased when compared with sections from normal age-matched brains and brains from Parkinson's patients. Subsequent experiments showed 20% to 40% re-

ductions in the size of the internal pallidum along with limbic portions of the temporal lobe including the dentate gyrus, subiculum of the hippocampus, parahippocampal gyrus, and amygdala. The temporal lobe and hippocampal changes in chronic schizophrenics compared with controls are among the most consistent MRI findings (DeLisi et al., 1991). Structural differences in these areas have also been reported in monozygotic twins who have the disorder as compared with their healthy twin siblings (Suddath et al., 1990). Additional importance of hippocampal changes was suggested by replicated studies (Kovelman and Scheibel, 1984) that showed marked disorganization of the pyramidal cell layer in the hippocampus of schizophrenics. These limbic-related structures could reasonably be expected to play a role in schizophrenic behavioral dysfunction.

A number of cortical differences have also been documented. Reduced numbers of neurons were found in the prefrontal, anterior cingulate, and primary motor cortices of ten schizophrenics, although most distinct was the cell loss in layers 2, 3, and 6 of the prefrontal cortex (Benes, Davidson, and Bird, 1986). MRI also showed abnormalities in the frontal lobes of 40% of male schizophrenics (Andreasen et al., 1986). Unfortunately these structural differences did not correlate with scores on the Wisconsin Card Sort test, a measurement of frontal lobe functioning. Although the differences reported are modest, corroboration by PET scan studies showing brain metabolic changes (see below) and electrophysiological differences in the frontal lobes of schizophrenics (above) enhances the significance of the structural differences found.

More recent MRI results replicated earlier findings (DeLisi et al., 1991) that increased ventricular size occurs in first-episode schizophrenic patients, before treatment has begun. Increased ventricular size was not correlated with either the duration of time since the onset of symptoms or the duration of time since the first hospitalization. However, a significant correlation exists between ventricular size and age of illness onset, such that the earlier the age of onset of symptoms, the larger the ventricles. Based on these results, the researchers conclude that ventricular enlargement is not due to a progressive deterioration of brain cells, but may represent an insult to the brain occurring during a time of brain growth and development. In contrast, additional brain changes reported by the same group and others, such as the reduction in size of the temporal lobe and hippocampus in chronic schizophrenics, were not apparent in acute schizophrenics. Thus, some of the structural brain changes may represent progressive deterioration or effects of antipsychotic medication. Unfortunately, there were very few correlations between scores of neuropsychological functioning and regional brain volumes.

Heinrichs (1993) recommends caution in interpreting evidence of neurodegeneration. He has pointed out that even massive cerebral atrophy may or may not have an effect on behavior and that the neuroanatomical differences reported are often not reflected in neuropsychological assessment. For example, hippocampal damage might be expected to produce amnesia-like effects in the schizophrenic, such that the individual would forget new information and events rapidly. Although schizophrenics do show memory impairment (Saykin et al., 1991), along with other impaired neuropsychological functions such as ineffective cognitive strategies, they rarely show amnesia-like forgetting. Frontal lobe abnormalities have some relationship to the negative symptoms of schizophrenia, such as the inability to shift strategies as shown with neuropsychological testing, loss of motivation, defective attention, and emotional blunting. However, since frontal lobe lesions do not produce distinctive positive symptoms, damage to that brain area may explain only part of the symptomology. Finally, interest in the basal ganglia stems from its high concentration of DA, which is believed to play an important role in schizophrenic symptomatology (see below). The basal ganglia were traditionally thought only to modulate motor function; however, more recent studies have demonstrated additional involvement in sensory processing and cognition (see Chapter 20). Overall there is a need for more biobehavioral research that will utilize methods from several fields to evaluate the relationship between brain pathology and behavioral consequences of that pathology.

One such attempt to correlate anatomical abnormalities and psychiatric symptoms measured the volumes of specific brain regions using MRI. The study correlated brain volume changes with symptom severity using the dimensional analysis: psychoticism, disorganization, and negative symptoms (Flaum et al., 1995). They found that overall symptom severity was correlated with enlarged ventricles and reduced volume of temporal lobe, hippocampus, and superior temporal gyrus, while symptoms of psychoticism and negative symptoms were associated with increased size of the third ventricle. The severity of psychotic symptoms alone was associated with significant reductions in the superior temporal gyrus and increases in temporal horn volume. Hallucinations (one part of the psychotic dimension) were correlated with decreases in the left superior temporal gyrus. Disorganized symptoms seemed to be unrelated to changes in regional brain volume.

Positive- and negative-symptom neuropathology. Since structural abnormalities are found in only a portion of schizophrenic brains, attempts have been made to correlate the cerebral changes with positive–negative subtypes of schizophrenia. Among the most promising hypotheses is the possibility that ventricular enlargement is related to negative symptom schizophrenia (Andreasen, 1987; Meltzer, 1987). Schizophrenics suffering predominantly from negative symptoms often have had a prolonged history of maladjustment, suggesting long-term

degenerative changes. Also, if structural abnormalities are responsible for negative symptoms, it would explain their relative resistance to pharmacological treatment. Additionally, patients with negative symptoms tend to have lower educational achievement than do patients with positive symptoms, suggesting once again that cognitive impairment begins early and continues over a prolonged period (see Andreasen, 1990). Unfortunately, ventricular enlargement is not found in all patients with negative symptom schizophrenia. Furthermore, ventricular enlargement is not specific to negative symptom schizophrenia and can occur under a variety of conditions, including following environmental stresses and neurological insults (DeLisi et al., 1991). In addition, enlarged ventricles have been found in patients suffering from affective disorders and dementia of the Alzheimer's type and in alcoholics. Thus, although neurodegeneration has potential importance in negative symptom schizophrenia, continued refinement of this hypothesis is required before substantive conclusions can be drawn.

Functional abnormalities. In addition to gross and microscopic structural differences in the brains of schizophrenics, studies of regional brain function, including rate of metabolism, blood flow, electrical activity, and chemistry, have identified significant differences between schizophrenic brains and normal controls. The neuropathological results (described above) showing frontal lobe abnormalities are of particular interest because regional cerebral blood flow measured by means of xenon inhalation (Weinberger, Berman, and Zec, 1986) showed a reduction in the ratio of frontal lobe to whole brain surface blood flow. In addition, schizophrenic patients showed less increase in cerebral blood flow than normal subjects while they were performing a cognitive task requiring use of the frontal lobes. Cerebral blood flow is closely associated with glucose utilization, an accepted indicator of cell metabolic rate. Several recent studies using PET mapping of glucose utilization have shown reduced metabolic activity in the frontal lobes of schizophrenics compared with controls. Buchsbaum and Haier (1987) performed a meta-analysis of eight PET studies from several laboratories by transforming data into comparable ratios. It is evident that despite the heterogeneity of sensory conditions, analytical methods, and patient medication, seven out of the eight studies showed relatively lower frontal cortex metabolism in schizophrenic patients, although the differences were not always statistically significant. Unfortunately, a review of PET results several years later showed less consistent findings (Buchsbaum, 1990), suggesting again that brain dysfunction is heterogenous in the schizophrenic population.

The hypofrontality of schizophrenic brains—the reduced metabolic activity in the dorsolateral prefrontal cortex (Buchsbaum, 1990)—is particularly interesting because the negative symptoms of schizophrenia have some resemblance to deficits seen following surgical disconnection of the frontal lobes. Loss of the dorsal prefrontal cortex produces patients who are poorly motivated, plan poorly, and have a flat affect. They also perform poorly on neuropsychological tests that require shifting mental sets or strategies to solve problems (see Gur, 1995; Heinrichs, 1993). In addition, research with nonhuman primates has shown that monkeys with frontal lobe lesions are unable to suppress irrelevant stimuli, have poor concentration, and perform poorly in tasks requiring a delayed response. In addition, the lesioned animals begin to show poor social functioning during the equivalent of monkey adolescence, a parallel with the onset of schizophrenia in humans during that developmental period. In fact, social functioning was so poor in some cases that the lesioned monkeys were ostracized from their groups (see Davis et al., 1991; Kandel, 1991d).

A majority of studies also found significantly lower glucose metabolic rates in the basal ganglia of nonmedicated schizophrenics compared with normal controls (see Buchsbaum and Haier, 1987). The withdrawal–retardation factor (emotional withdrawal, blunted affect, and motor retardation) of the Brief Psychiatric Rating Scale is negatively correlated with metabolic activity in the basal ganglia (Wolkin et al., 1985). Also, neuroleptic treatment tends to increase metabolic rates in the basal ganglia. However, a similar reduction has been reported for patients with affective disorders (Buchsbaum et al., 1986) and for patients with Huntington's disease (Kuhl et al., 1985), indicating a lack of specificity for the effect. Nevertheless, the altered basal ganglia activity deserves further evaluation because there is evidence of a potential interrelationship between basal ganglia function and frontal lobe activity in these patients, which may distinguish schizophrenics from those with affective disorders or Huntington's disease. For example, not only is blood flow to the dorsolateral prefrontal cortex in response to the Wisconsin Card Sorting Test lower in schizophrenics than in controls, but unlike control subjects, schizophrenics do not show a reciprocal decrease in basal ganglia flow as prefrontal flow increases (Rubin et al., 1991). Furthermore, various studies examined glucose activity in cortical–striatal–thalamic circuits in nonmedicated schizophrenics in an attempt to correlate regional metabolic changes with various treatment stategies (see Gur, 1995).

Psychophysiological irregularities. Several identifiable physiological irregularities have been found in schizophrenics that may aid in diagnosis and evaluation of behavioral symptomatology. Eye movement dysfunctions characterized by an interruption of normal visual tracking of an object by fast saccadic eye movements or by an absence of slow pursuit movements have been found in a majority of schizophrenic patients (see Siever, Kalus,

and Keefe, 1993). The genetic nature of the abnormality has been shown in family and twin studies. Matsushima (1991) reviewed a series of experiments designed to evaluate the eye movements of schizophrenics as they look at horizontal S-shaped figures for 15 seconds. The data include the number of eye movements and the scanning length of eye movements, as well as the "responsive" eye movements (called responsive search score, RSS) that occur in the 5 seconds immediately following the question, "Are there any other differences?" Schizophrenics' eye movements rather consistently were fewer in number and limited to a smaller area of the figure. Further, the RSS as compared with nonschizophrenics was lower not only in chronic schizophrenics but also in acute and remitted schizophrenics. Patients with methamphetamine-induced psychosis also showed the reduced scanning, but they could be distinguished from the schizophrenic group because they did not have the low RSS. In a similar fashion, patients with right frontal lobe lesions, who often show psychiatric symptoms resembling the negative symptoms of schizophrenia, also showed the low number of eye movements and short scanning length, but their RSS resembled that of normal subjects. When a statistical discriminant analysis was done on 41 acute and chronic schizophrenics and over 70 normal controls, methamphetamine-induced psychotics, epileptics, depressed patients, alcoholics, and patients with obsessive–compulsive disorder, the schizophrenic and nonschizophrenic groups could be distinguished by their RSS and number of eye fixations. These psychophysical measures are suggested as a potential aid in the clinical diagnosis of schizophrenia. Although it is likely that these eye movements depend on the integrated functioning of several brain areas, such as the frontal lobe, basal ganglia, superior colliculus, and other regions, imaging of the brain with PET may localize the area of abnormality associated with low RSS scores.

A second neurophysiological abnormality involves event-related brain electrical potentials as measured with EEG. The EEG records neural activity associated with the perception of an event and related cognitive processes. Schizophrenic EEGs differ from those of control subjects in a variety of ways, some of which correlate with the extent and type of psychiatric symptoms. In contrast to the normal individual who shows localized stimulus-induced electrical activity in a specific area of the brain, schizophrenics respond to specific stimuli with diffuse electrical activity in the brain. These studies, along with the eye movement studies, suggest an impairment of information processing at a very preliminary stage. Schizophrenics apparently have a deficit in stimulus perception and subsequent psychological processing. Details of the psychophysiological research in schizophrenics can be found in several sources (Baribeau and Laurent, 1991; Holzman, 1987; Nuechterlein and Dawson, 1995).

Models of Schizophrenia

The development of an animal model of schizophrenia has been difficult because the primary symptom is thought disorder, an obviously cortical process that we would not expect to find in lower mammals. During the 1950s, LSD-induced hallucinations in humans were compared with schizophrenic episodes and extensive research was initiated into the mechanism of the drug's action. However, the differences between the drug state and endogenous schizophrenia were found to be more pronounced than were the few similarities. Of the greatest significance is the fact that the LSD-induced state is rarely confused with an endogenous schizophrenic episode by trained clinicians. In addition, drug-induced hallucinations are visual and usually pleasant, whereas in endogenous schizophrenia, hallucinations are usually auditory and threatening. Furthermore, LSD-induced hallucinations are perceived by schizophrenic patients as different from their existing disorder. Also, it has been noted that schizophrenics are highly resistant to suggestion and withdraw from interpersonal contacts. Withdrawal from personal interaction is much less frequent during drug-induced psychoses, and subjects that have been administered LSD are highly suggestible.

In contrast with the LSD-induced state, the toxic psychosis following frequent high doses of amphetamine consists of well-formed paranoid delusions, various forms of stereotyped, compulsive behavior, and either visual or auditory hallucinations (see Chapter 13). These toxic effects of amphetamine are apparently not due to lack of sleep, overexcitement, or precipitation of an underlying disorder (Snyder et al., 1974). Amphetamine-induced psychotic symptoms can be alleviated by those agents that are also most effective in treating endogenous psychosis. Also, amphetamine exacerbates the existing symptoms of schizophrenia rather than superimposing new symptoms over the old (Janowsky and Davis, 1976). However, low doses of amphetamine do not affect the symptoms of manic, depressed, or neurotic patients. These similarities have led to the conclusion that the toxic reaction after high doses of amphetamine is almost indistinguishable from paranoid schizophrenia.

In animals, high doses of amphetamine produce a characteristic stereotyped sniffing, licking, and gnawing that was first identified by Randrup and Munkvad (1967). Because stereotyped behavior also occurs in response to high doses of amphetamine in humans and is similar to the compulsive repetitions of meaningless behavior seen in schizophrenia, the amphetamine-induced stereotypy is used in the laboratory as an animal model for schizophrenia. The amphetamine model is appealing because it mimics both behavioral and neurochemical abnormalities found in some schizophrenics.

A second significant human model of schizophrenia is the syndrome induced by high doses of phencyclidine (PCP). At low doses PCP produces symptoms of inebriation and mild stimulation, while the symptoms of severe PCP intoxication include disorientation, muteness, cognitive impairments, various motor symptoms (e.g., agitation, grimacing, rigidity, catalepsy, or tremors) and occasionally paranoid delusions (see Chapter 17). PCP-induced psychosis in normal individuals is apparently indistinguishable from an acute episode of schizophrenia (Erard, Luisada, and Peele, 1980). Furthermore PCP intensifies the primary symptoms of schizophrenia, as does the structural analog ketamine (Lahti et al., 1995). The usefulness of the PCP model stems from its ability to produce both positive and negative symptoms of schizophrenia (Javitt and Zukin, 1991), unlike toxic doses of amphetamine, which produce the more florid positive symptoms of paranoid schizophrenia. Note that both amphetamine and PCP enhance DA release and block reuptake, while PCP and ketamine in addition antagonize NMDA-sensitive glutamatergic transmission (Lahti et al., 1995). The PCP model of schizophrenia plays an important role in the DA–glutamate interaction hypothesis of schizophrenia (see Bunney, Bunney, and Carlsson, 1995; Freed, 1988; Grace, 1992; Nishikawa et al., 1991).

A third type of model (sensory gating) is based on the evidence that schizophrenics fail to filter or gate most of the sensory stimuli they receive. Such a defect may lead to sensory overload and fragmented thinking. Both animal and human subjects can be used to evaluate habituation to novel stimuli as well as sensory gating with measures such as the prepulse inhibition of startle response or the gating of acoustic event-related electrical potentials. The clinical validity of these measures as well as several others is discussed by Geyer and Markou (1995).

Pharmacotherapy: Phenothiazines and Butyrophenones

The phenothiazines are currently the largest and most commonly used class of antipsychotic drugs. Drugs of this class are also called "neuroleptics," which is an older term referring to their ability to selectively reduce emotionality and psychomotor activity. They were originally synthesized in 1883 in the course of investigating two chemically related dyes, but were not used medicinally until much later (1940s).

Structure–Activity Relationships of Neuroleptics

The phenothiazine nucleus (Figure 18.5) is a three-ring structure: two benzene rings joined by sulfur and nitrogen atoms. Various substituents at R_1 and R_2 change the potency, pharmacological activity, and side effects of the different phenothiazines. Figure 18.5 shows the structural relationships of several phenothiazines. The structural substituent at R_1 determines the three major subgroups of the phenothiazines: the aliphatic (e.g.,

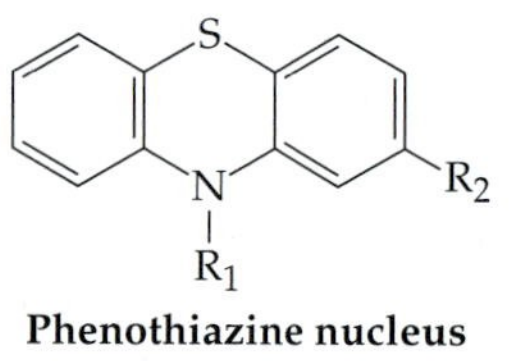

Phenothiazine nucleus

18.5 PHENOTHIAZINE NUCLEUS AND RELATED COMPOUNDS. Minor molecular modifications determine the three major subgroups of phenothiazines and change drug potency, pharmacological activity, and side effects.

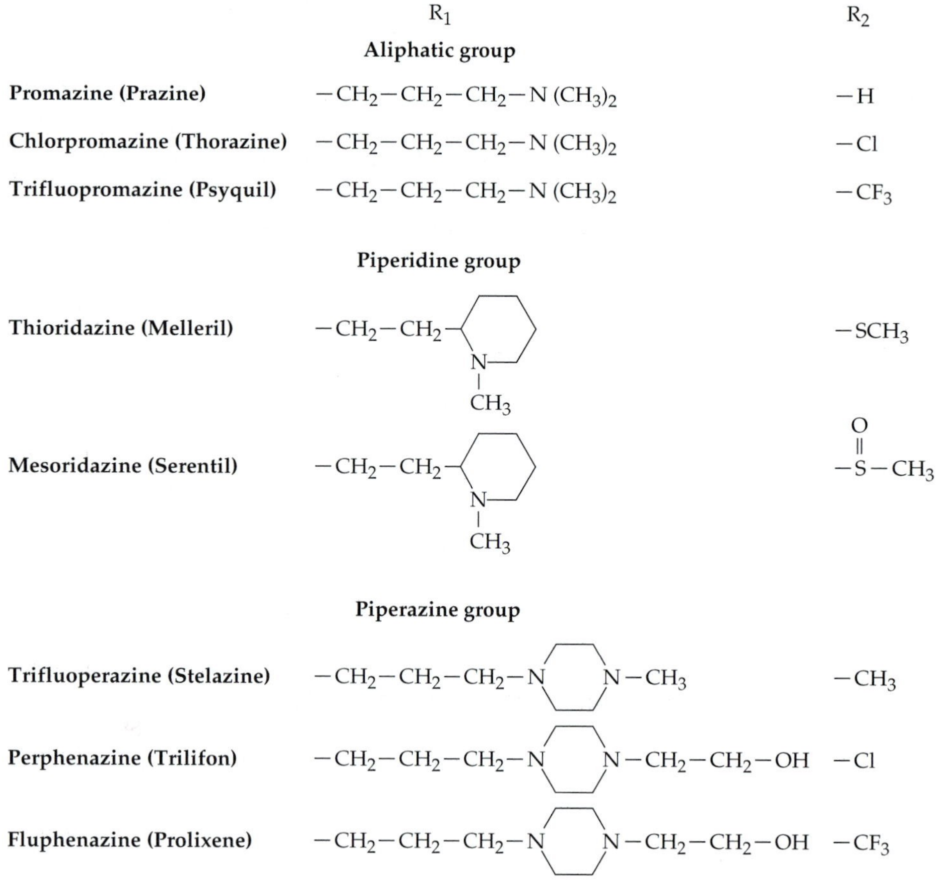

	R_1	R_2
Aliphatic group		
Promazine (Prazine)	$-CH_2-CH_2-CH_2-N(CH_3)_2$	$-H$
Chlorpromazine (Thorazine)	$-CH_2-CH_2-CH_2-N(CH_3)_2$	$-Cl$
Trifluopromazine (Psyquil)	$-CH_2-CH_2-CH_2-N(CH_3)_2$	$-CF_3$

Piperidine group

| **Thioridazine (Melleril)** | $-CH_2-CH_2-$ (piperidine, N-CH₃) | $-SCH_3$ |
| **Mesoridazine (Serentil)** | $-CH_2-CH_2-$ (piperidine, N-CH₃) | $-\overset{O}{\overset{\|}{S}}-CH_3$ |

Piperazine group

Trifluoperazine (Stelazine)	$-CH_2-CH_2-CH_2-N$ (piperazine) $N-CH_3$	$-CH_3$
Perphenazine (Trilifon)	$-CH_2-CH_2-CH_2-N$ (piperazine) $N-CH_2-CH_2-OH$	$-Cl$
Fluphenazine (Prolixene)	$-CH_2-CH_2-CH_2-N$ (piperazine) $N-CH_2-CH_2-OH$	$-CF_3$

chlorpromazine [Thorazine]), piperidine (e.g., thioridazine [Mellaril]), and piperazine (e.g., trifluoperazine [Stelazine]) groups. Additional substitutions at R_2 further alter potency. For example, within the aliphatic group, chlorpromazine (which has a chlorine at R_2) is much more potent pharmacologically than is promazine (which has no R_2 substituent). A CF_3 radical at R_2 (trifluopromazine [Psyquil]) further increases potency for depressing motor activity as well as alleviating psychotic symptoms.

The second group contains a piperidine moiety in the side chain and includes thioridazine and mesoridazine. This substitution is apparently responsible for a lower incidence of extrapyramidal side effects.

In the third group, the replacement of the propyldimethylamino side chain of the aliphatic group by a propylpiperazine side chain (e.g., the change from trifluopromazine to trifluoperazine) greatly augments the potency of the neuroleptic drugs. Within this third group,

the replacement of the terminal $-CH_3$ on the piperazine ring (as on trifluoperazine) with $-CH_2CH_2OH$ (e.g., fluphenazine [Prolixin]) further increases antipsychotic potency as well as antiemetic effects and extrapyramidal side effects.

An explanation for the structure–activity relationship has been provided by the use of X-ray crystallography. The three-dimensional configurations of the phenothiazines, as determined by X-ray crystallography, can be superimposed on the three-dimensional structure of DA (Feinberg and Snyder, 1975). From that work it is apparent that a change in substituents, such as the lack of a substituent at R_2, alters the ability of the phenothiazine to conform to the structure of DA and thus reduces the pharmacological activity at the receptor.

In addition to the classic phenothiazines, several other classes of antipsychotic drugs exist. The thioxanthene derivatives (e.g., chlorprothixene [Taractan]) are very similar in structure to the phenothiazines. The

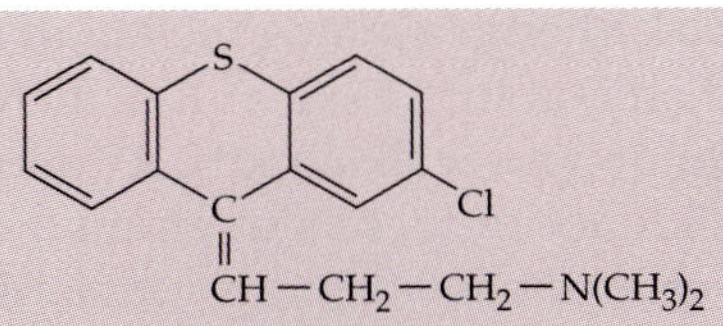

Chlorprothixene
(Taractan)

thioxanthenes, along with the butyrophenone derivative haloperidol (Haldol) are among the traditional drugs used to treat schizophrenia and have pharmacological effects very similar to those of the phenothiazines. Other antipsychotic drugs are atypical in their structures and effects. These include the benzamides (e.g., sulpiride) and several miscellaneous agents such as loxapine (Loxitane) which is a dibenzoxapine, molindone (Moban) which is an indole structurally similar to serotonin, pimozide (Orap) from the diphenylbutylpiperidines, and clozapine (Clozaril), the dibenzodiazepine that has received a lot of popular attention recently because of its unusual spectrum of effects. Our discussion will refer primarily to the phenothiazines because they are most often used. Atypical neuroleptics will be described briefly at the end of this section.

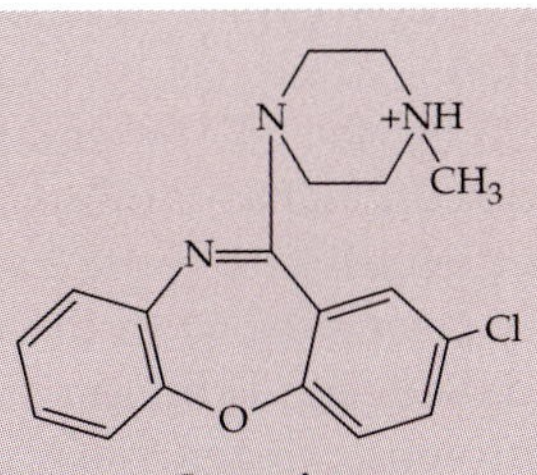

Loxapine
(Loxitane)

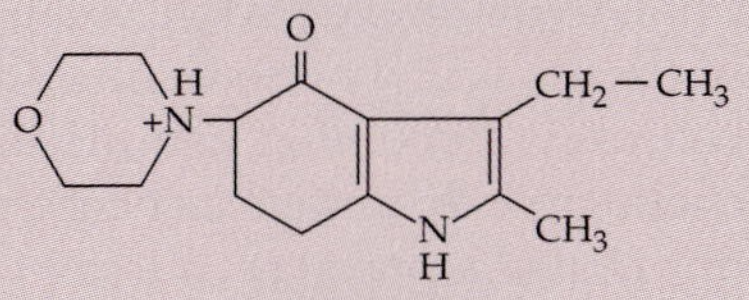

Molindone
(Moban)

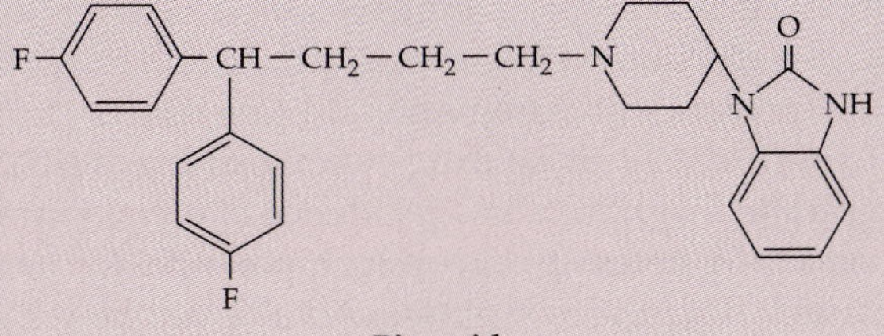

Pimozide

Effectiveness

The introduction of antipsychotic drugs during the 1950s dramatically improved the treatment of schizophrenic patients. Not only do they calm agitated and excited pa-

tients, but they also modify the positive symptoms of schizophrenia including delusions, hallucinations, and disordered thinking. The effectiveness of drugs of this class has been demonstrated hundreds of times in double-blind, placebo-controlled trials. When adequate doses are used, the effectiveness of antipsychotics over placebo has been demonstrated by a significant reduction in symptoms and/or reduction in the average length of hospitalization. However, determining the "adequate" dose is not trivial since full therapeutic effectiveness frequently takes 4–6 weeks or longer (Kane, 1987). Thus, determining the appropriate dose of a neuroleptic for a particular patient is not a simple adjustment. For example, if after 2 weeks a moderate dose of a given drug is ineffective and the dose is raised, resulting in subsequent improvement, it is unclear whether increased drug concentration was required or simply increased duration of treatment.

Second, in general, very high doses do not seem to be more effective than moderate doses, except for selected patients. Attempts to correlate therapeutic effect with blood drug level have produced mixed results due to methodological flaws such as heterogeneity of diagnoses and duration of treatment (see Kane, 1987). However, for haloperidol, a curvilinear relationship has been reported (Van Putten et al., 1985) that suggests the existence of a "therapeutic window" of effectiveness. Doses below or above the therapeutic optimum produce less than maximum clinical effectiveness. It is also possible that behavioral side effects at the high doses mask the therapeutic effects of the drug.

Although a large number of antipsychotic drugs have been developed, none have been found to be consistently more effective than others. However, several of the newest atypical antipsychotics may be more effective in reducing negative as well as positive symptoms. Also, a given individual may respond preferentially to a particular drug. The drugs do vary widely in potency, that is, they are equally effective but differ in the dose required to achieve the same effects. Thus a consideration of "dose equivalents" is necessary when comparing clinical assessments of the effectiveness of different drugs. Chlorpromazine is usually the standard drug against which potency is compared. The equivalent to an oral dose of chlorpromazine (low potency) at 300 mg is 10 mg of a high-potency drug, such as trifluoperazine. Caution should be taken when comparing experimental results testing multiple drugs at widely different "equivalent doses."

What role does psychotherapy play in acute or long-term recovery? Apparently individual psychotherapy, group therapy, or milieu therapy have minimal beneficial effects on long-term recovery of schizophrenics (Klerman, 1984; Kane, 1987), and are not considered substitutes for pharmacotherapy. Social skills training may lead to improvement in some targeted social behaviors, although the individual skills may not generalize to broader social situations and durability of the skills following termination of training may be limited. The limited number of controlled studies available suggest an interactive as well as additive effect of medication and psychosocial treatment. In addition to social skills training, the use of family therapy may diminish relapse rates as well as improve medication compliance and social functioning (Goldstein, 1995). Both psychosocial therapy and family therapy emphasize education about the illness, techniques to improve communication, and coping with stress and real life issues as opposed to insight therapy, which is relatively ineffective (Schooler and Hogarty, 1987).

Following the initial recovery, antipsychotic drugs may be prescribed as maintenance therapy to prevent relapse. Numerous double-blind placebo-controlled studies have shown that continued treatment significantly reduces the probability of reappearance of psychotic symptoms and rehospitalization (Kane and Lieberman, 1987), although the drug treatment does not improve social adjustment. Hogarty and colleagues (Hogarty et al., 1974) found that patients maintained on placebo for 2 years after hospitalization had a 20% chance of remaining in the community, while those patients maintained on antipsychotic drugs had a 55% chance of avoiding rehospitalization.

One summary (Kane and Lieberman, 1987) of double-blind studies aimed at evaluating the effectiveness of antipsychotics in preventing relapse reports a relapse rate that varies between 7% and 86%. Several variables may contribute to the large differences in reported relapse rates. Among these variables are high rates of noncompliance, incidence of side effects leading to variable dropout rate, interaction with other types of psychological support modalities, diagnostic subtype of schizophrenia and individual personality variables, investigators' definition of relapse, and methodological differences among clinical trials. Unfortunately there is no available method to identify those schizophrenics who will relapse without drug treatment. At present only by withdrawing the drug and watching for relapse can the need for continued drug treatment be determined. Since side effects of drug treatment can appear at any time, it is considered optimum to identify the minimum dose required to prevent relapse before beginning long-term maintenance.

Side Effects of Neuroleptics

Parkinsonism

The most common and troublesome side effects are the appearance of extrapyramidal disorders such as parkinsonian symptoms. Extrapyramidal refers to the involvement of the basal ganglia, which are part of an auxiliary system to the pyramidal system for controlling voluntary movement. The symptoms, which undergo remission after drug treatment stops, include tremors, akinesia (a slowing of voluntary movements), spasticity and

rigidity, and akathesia (a strong feeling of discomfort in the legs and an inability to sit still, which compels the patient to get up and walk about). Although estimates vary, the incidence of these symptoms was as high as 90% of patients treated with antipsychotic drugs in some studies. We know that Parkinson's disease is caused by a deficiency of DA in the basal ganglia, which leads to less restrained cholinergic neural activity. Experiments using PET and selective DA receptor ligands showed that phenothiazine-treated patients with acute extrapyramidal symptoms had higher D_2 receptor occupancy in the basal ganglia than those who did not experience those side effects (Farde et al., 1992). The receptor up-regulation is likely to occur subsequent to reduced DA transmission. Thus, the phenothiazine-induced tremors and rigidity are almost certainly due to the blockade of DA receptors in the basal ganglia, the projection region of the nigrostriatal DA neurons. However, despite the fact that DA receptor blockade is responsible for the side effects as well as the antipsychotic effects, the two are not necessarily correlated.

Snyder and colleagues (1974) found that neuroleptic drugs also bind to muscarinic cholinergic receptors in the brain and that their affinity for the acetylcholine receptors is inversely correlated with their ability to produce extrapyramidal effects. Therefore, it may be possible to produce neuroleptic drugs that have high affinity for the DA receptors (and therefore effective antipsychotic action) and at the same time have strong anticholinergic action to minimize parkinsonian side effects. One example that is widely used clinically is thioridazine. Alternatively, combining neuroleptic treatment with an anticholinergic drug such as benztropine mesylate (Cogentin) is also a popular course of action. The risk of anticholinergic side effects is real, however, and for patients who do not require the antiparkinsonian drug, prophylactic use is controversial (Kane, 1987). In addition, several atypical antipsychotics, such as clozapine and risperidone (Risperdal), produce a lower than normal incidence of extrapyramidal side effects.

Unfortunately, those drugs with a strong anticholinergic profile that have a low incidence of extrapyramidal side effects by necessity have a high potential for peripheral anticholinergic symptoms. An alternative is to develop drugs that block specific DA receptor subtypes. Such drugs would have the potential to maximize clinical effectiveness by acting on DA receptors associated with the psychopathology without interfering with nigrostriatal function associated with parkinsonian side effects (see below for further discussion of this issue).

Tardive Dyskinesias

A second group of neurological syndromes associated with the prolonged use of antipsychotic drugs is the tardive dyskinesias (TD). Tardive dyskinesias are characterized by stereotyped involuntary movements particularly of the face and jaw, such as sucking and lip smacking, lateral jaw movements, and "fly-catching" darting of the tongue. There may also be purposeless, quick, and uncontrolled movements of the arms and legs or slow squirming movements of the trunk, extremities, and neck. These spontaneous movements are increased during high vigilance and agitation, whereas drowsiness and sleep have the opposite effect. Voluntary use of the muscle groups that ordinarily exhibit dyskinesia reduces the symptoms, but abnormal movements are enhanced in other muscle groups. For instance, during conversation the oral manifestations of TD are diminished, but the dyskinesia of the hands and pelvis become more conspicuous. On the other hand, writing or the performance of a manual task abolishes spontaneous dyskinesia of the hands, but seems to release oral movements. More recently, attention has been directed to several atypical forms of TD. Tardive dystonia involves sustained abnormal positions with torticollis (neck muscle spasm causing the head to be held abnormally tilted), grimacing, and truncal torsion. Tardive akathesia is persistent restlessness with continuous motions of the trunk.

Although it has been assumed that the dose of neuroleptic and duration of treatment are implicated in the appearance of TD, not all clinical investigations support this view. The conflicting results may be explained in part by methodological differences regarding controls for the complex interaction between increasing age and duration of treatment (Casey, 1987). A conservative estimate suggests that TD appears in about 10% to 20% of patients treated with neuroleptics overall. While TD may appear in any age group, its prevalence increases to 50% in patients over 60. Most often affected are geriatric patients who are especially vulnerable to the toxic effects of drugs due to impaired liver and kidney function. Prevalence may exceed 70% in such high-risk populations. Because most patients have been treated with a variety of neuroleptics, it is not possible to single out any one agent as being more toxic than any of the others for a given individual. Extrapyramidal symptoms seem to be the most important factor affecting compliance with medication schedules and for that reason, they represent a significant treatment concern.

Despite reports of the irreversible nature of TD, improvement has been demonstrated even in some patients continuing drug treatment. Reports of improvement vary from 0% to 92% depending on patient variables such as age, sex, and diagnosis, and on treatment variables such as dose and duration of treatment (see below). The most significant factor is age, with younger patients experiencing a better recovery (Casey, 1985). In addition, early detection and duration of treatment seem to be correlated with the likelihood of reversibility. A review of the epidemiology and clinical presentation of TD can be found in Kane (1995).

Neuropathology of tardive dyskinesia. There have been many attempts to establish the neuropathology of TD, however, autopsy material is scarce and contradictory. Christensen, Moller, and Faurbye (1970) attributed the "irreversible" nature of TD to their finding of gliosis in the substantia nigra and other parts of the brain, which usually denotes neuron degeneration. However, other investigators failed to confirm their findings. Experiments have shown that lesions in the head of the caudate nucleus of the cat brain will cause a vast array of abnormal movements with some features in common with human TD. Since the caudate and other parts of the striatum are central components of extrapyramidal motor control, injury to these areas of the brain or abnormal neuronal function may be responsible for TD.

Although chronic neuroleptic treatment leads to TD in some patients, terminating neuroleptic treatment or lowering the dose aggravates the symptoms. Reinstating treatment or raising the dose temporarily alleviates the disorder. Further, DA agonists increase the severity, and, in contrast to parkinsonian symptoms, anticholinergics further aggravate the syndrome. Such observations suggest that the neuroleptics, by blocking DA receptors, induce a DA receptor supersensitivity, and that this state could be the basis for TD. Such hypersensitivity could be reversed functionally only by returning to drug treatment or by raising the drug dose.

Snyder, Creese, and Burt (1977) tested the hypersensitivity hypothesis by investigating changes in DA receptor binding in rats after chronic treatment with the neuroleptics haloperidol, fluphenazine, and reserpine, as well as the nonantipsychotics phenothiazine, promethazine, and amphetamine. One week after 21 days of treatment with the neuroleptics there was a 20% to 30% increase in DA receptor binding, as reflected by an increase in the number of [^{3}H]haloperidol binding sites (B_{max}) rather than a change in their binding affinity (K_d). Chronic treatment with the nonneuroleptic drugs did not increase binding. Subsequent studies showed a selective increase in the D_2 receptor subtype in rat brain following prolonged neuroleptic treatment (Porceddu et al., 1986; see also Chapter 8).

Further evidence suggests that the supersensitivity in rats after chronic treatment with haloperidol is accompanied by alterations in the ultrastructure and number of synapses in the caudate nucleus (Uranova et al., 1991). Electron microscopic examination revealed changes in both axodendritic and axospinous synapses. Synaptic density on dendritic shafts increased by 83% and on spines by 53%. The area of postsynaptic density and length of the active zone were also increased. Such morphological changes may well be indicative of more efficient neural transmission and enhanced D_2 receptor binding. Thus, behavioral supersensitivity and tardive dyskinesia following chronic treatment with neuroleptics may be due to an increase in DA receptors. The receptor changes found in animals, however, do not explain the varied vulnerability of individuals treated with the drug.

The results of the binding experiments are consistent with behavioral evidence in animals. Chronic neuroleptic treatment induces DA receptor hypersensitivity in rats as measured by the enhanced response (motor activity and stereotypy) to apomorphine after withdrawal of the neuroleptics (Halperin, Guerin, and Davis, 1989). Interestingly, clozapine, a neuroleptic with low incidence of parkinsonian side affects and TD, failed to induce hypersensitivity using the same measures. Long-term exposure to antipsychotic drugs also induces hypersensitivity as measured by electrophysiology and a variety of biochemical events (Blaha and Lane, 1987; Chiodo and Bunney, 1983; Hu and Wang, 1989; Uranova et al., 1991).

As appealing as the hypersensitivity theory is, human postmortem measurement of DA receptor sites showed no difference in D_1 or D_2 receptors in neuroleptic-treated schizophrenics with and without TD (Crow et al., 1982). That is, although neuroleptic treatment does commonly lead to increased D_2 receptor density (see Davis et al., 1991), the extent of receptor increase is not correlated with the occurrence of TD. Nor is there a difference in prolactin release in patients with TD and those lacking TD symptoms, as would be expected if DA receptor hypersensitivity were responsible for TD (Casey, 1987). Since prolactin release from the pituitary is under inhibitory control by DA from the tuberoinfundibular tract, if DA receptors in that system were supersensitive, levels of circulating prolactin should be reduced. However, it must be kept in mind that subtypes of DA receptors vary from one brain region to another and that functional compensatory changes in distinct DA pathways are likely to vary. For example, the atypical antipsychotic clozapine, which has a reputation for a low incidence of extrapyramidal side effects, demonstrates selective action on mesolimbic DA cells that is consistent with its high binding affinity for D_3 (Sokoloff et al., 1990) and D_4 (Van Tol et al., 1991) subtypes of DA receptors in the limbic regions. Nevertheless, attempts to desensitize the DA receptors have also met with failure (Gerlach, Casey, and Korsgaard, 1986). Clearly, a simple neurochemical explanation for TD and a clear-cut method of dealing with the disorder are not yet available.

Treatment for tardive dyskinesia.   No treatment for TD has been consistently successful and found safe over a prolonged period. If the DA receptor hypersensitivity hypothesis is correct, one would assume that reducing DA transmission by depleting the store of transmitter or producing false transmitters would alleviate symptoms. In fact, treatment with reserpine, tetrabenazine, α-methyltyrosine, or α-methyl-dopa does seem to suppress symptoms in a significant number of cases, although others report only a minimal change in symptoms (Jeste and Wyatt, 1982). Unfortunately, since DA transmission blockade may be responsible for the pathophysiology of

TD, further reduction in DA function may well exacerbate the underlying disorder while reducing the symptoms. In harmony with the DA hypersensitivity model, anticholinergic drugs usually aggravate the symptoms. Since striatal DA hyperpolarizes ACh follower cells, further anticholinergic action would further diminish the effectiveness of ACh neurotransmission. A logical therapeutic step might be to enhance ACh activity with physostigmine, the acetylcholinesterase inhibitor, or increase ACh synthesis by precursor loading with choline or deanol. The former drug treatment is complicated by frequently unacceptable side effects, while the latter pharmacological approach has produced both highly encouraging results and reports of limited success (Casey, 1987; Jeste and Wyatt, 1982).

An alternative treatment approach involves manipulation of GABA neurotransmission. Evidence exists to show that GABA in the substantia nigra modulates DA function in the basal ganglia and may mediate hyperkinetic involuntary movements in animals (Scheel-Krüger, 1986). Reduced CSF levels of GABA in patients with TD have also been reported (Thaker et al., 1987). Thus treatment strategies utilizing GABA-mimetic agents such as direct and indirect GABA agonists or GABA-T inhibitors have been suggested. While results have been variable, those agents that act on $GABA_A$ receptors have been the most promising (Casey, 1987). Since benzodiazepines (BDZs) enhance GABA-induced chloride channel opening by binding to the $GABA_A$–BDZ complex, their usefulness in treating TD has been investigated by several groups, with predictably mixed results. Thaker and colleagues (1990) present a summary of such attempts, and although most of these studies report some antidyskinetic effect with or without sedation, it is very clear that more placebo-controlled, double-blind studies are needed before any conclusions can be drawn.

Using the BDZ clonazepam, Thaker and colleagues (1990) have shown a significant improvement in TD in chronically ill patients receiving neuroleptics. Their evaluation was based on the results of a 12-week, double-blind, randomized crossover trial with placebo control in 19 patients. Dramatic improvement was limited to those patients with predominantly dystonic as opposed to choreoathetotic symptoms. Since there was no significant increase in reaction time in the patients and the dose was raised gradually to minimize drowsiness, the improvement in TD symptoms is evidently distinct from sedation. Unfortunately, in the 5 patients studied for prolonged periods, tolerance developed to treatment over a 5–8 month period. However, gradual withdrawal of the BDZ and a 2-week, drug-free "holiday" restored the antidyskinesia effects.

Other Effects of Neuroleptics

In addition to their use as antipsychotics, the phenothiazines are used clinically to reduce nausea and vomiting, to delay ejaculation, for preanesthetic sedation, and to relieve severe itching. These drugs not only have DA-blocking effects but also anticholinergic and antiadrenergic actions, as well as antihistaminic and antiserotonergic actions. These complex interactions produce widespread effects on the autonomic nervous system, endocrine system, and renal–urinary system. For example, blockade of cholinergic synapses produces effects such as dry mouth, blurred vision, constipation, difficulty in urination, and decreased gastric secretion and motility. Orthostatic hypotension from the antiadrenergic action of the antipsychotics leads to dizziness, faintness, or blacking out. Several of the antipsychotics have significant sedative effects that may be unacceptable to some patients.

Other CNS effects of the phenothiazines include inhibition of nausea and vomiting as a result of their actions on the medullary chemical trigger zone. In addition, the neuroleptic drugs may produce neuroendocrine side effects following DA receptor blockade of the tuberoinfundibular neurons. Most common are breast enlargement and tenderness, decreased sex drive, lack of menstruation, increased release of prolactin frequently leading to lactation, and inhibition of the release of growth hormone. Clinical trials have demonstrated reduction of the neuroendocrine and extrapyramidal side effects with the DA agonist amantadine (Correa et al., 1987). Since amantadine does not diminish antipsychotic efficacy, it has been suggested that it may selectively attenuate the neuroleptic-induced blockade in the tuberoinfundibular pathway and the nigrostriatal pathway but not at mesolimbic sites.

Of the side effects occurring following the use of high-potency neuroleptics such as haloperidol, the most serious is the life-threatening occurrence of neuroleptic malignant syndrome (NMS). NMS is characterized by fever, rigidity, altered consciousness, and autonomic nervous system instability (including tachycardia and labile hypertension), which is correlated with the drug's ability to block DA D_2 receptors. Although potentially lethal, rapid diagnosis and intervention have significantly reduced the risk of fatalities (Caroff and Mann, 1988). See Kaufmann and Wyatt (1987) for a detailed discussion of the syndrome and its neurochemical correlates.

In general, the drug selected for a particular patient usually depends upon minimizing side effects. For instance, chlorpromazine or thioridazine may be used because they tend to minimize the extrapyramidal side effects, although their sedative effects may be undesirable and the probability of autonomic side effects is relatively high. Haloperidol, in contrast, tends to produce less sedation and fewer autonomic side effects, but greater probability of movement disorders. For patients who are not compliant regarding self-medication, a high-potency phenothiazine with a very long duration of action may be prescribed and injected subcutaneously.

Clozapine, an unusual antipsychotic, has several unique characteristics including low incidence of extrapyramidal side effects and TD (Small et al., 1987). While it appears to be effective for a portion of those patients who are nonresponsive to classic antipsychotics (Kane et al., 1988), it is not a potent blocker of D_1 and D_2 receptors (see below). Unfortunately, clozapine has the potential for a lethal suppression of bone marrow function. Thus, regular monitoring of patients is necessary.*

Tolerance and Dependence

Clinically, tolerance to the sedative effect of neuroleptics develops gradually, while the antipsychotic effect may take weeks to fully develop. The difference in the time courses of these pharmacological effects is useful in identifying adequate drug screening methods, because any behavioral or neurochemical effect of the phenothiazines that undergoes tolerance is probably related to the sedative rather than to the antipsychotic action of the drug.

The phenothiazines do not produce euphoria and are often considered to have unpleasant effects, particularly in individuals who are not psychotic. For these reasons, the neuroleptic drugs are a class of drugs that are rarely, if ever, abused. Animal studies also demonstrate low incidence of self-administration, confirming low abuse potential.

Effects on Conditioned Avoidance in Animals

Acute administration of the neuroleptic drugs produces reduced motor activity and indifference to environmental stimuli in humans and animals. In animals the indifference to environmental stimuli is demonstrated in conditioned avoidance experiments. In such experiments, a rat is trained to escape electric foot shock by climbing a pole. If the shock onset is signaled by a buzzer, the rat will learn in a few trials to climb the pole whenever it hears the buzzer. After small doses of chlorpromazine, the rat ignores the buzzer even though it is able to climb the pole when the shock is applied. The ability of chlorpromazine to block the conditioned avoidance response (CAR) is a relatively specific characteristic of antipsychotic drugs and has been used as a screening device to identify new efficacious agents. A good correlation between antipsychotic potency and suppression of CAR has been demonstrated.

To evaluate the effect of a drug on the CAR, however, the contribution of nonspecific sedation to the suppression of the CAR must be considered. That is, the animal may merely be responding more slowly to the warning signal because of sedation. By lengthening the

---

*Although typical neuroleptics are discussed briefly in subsequent sections, it is not within the scope of this chapter to describe in detail the intricate effects of these drugs on physiology or to assess therapeutic concerns. For further discussion, refer to a standard text in medical pharmacology.

interval between signal and shock, the two effects can usually be separated. Under these conditions, neuroleptic drugs still produce a decrement in the CAR (Lipper and Kornetsky, 1971). A second method to avoid the contaminating contribution of general sedation is to use passive avoidance procedures such as the step-down platform. In this test, the animal is placed on a platform suspended above an electrified grid floor. After several trials, a normal animal avoids the shock by remaining on the platform. Animals treated with neuroleptic drugs continue to make the step-down response, indicating that the drugs produce an indifference to environmental stimuli without significant sedation.

Mechanisms of Neuroleptic Action

It is well known that neuroleptic drugs modify several neurotransmitter systems; however, the efficacy of the drugs in alleviating psychotic symptoms is best correlated to their effects on DA. Effective antipsychotics interfere with DA transmission by blocking DA receptors or by inhibiting DA release. Evidence comes from several sources, including the drugs' three-dimensional structures, their side effects, receptor binding studies, and subsequent DA turnover, second messenger function, and neuroendocrine changes.

First, the three-dimensional configurations of the phenothiazines, as determined by X-ray crystallography, can be superimposed on the three-dimensional structure of DA (Feinberg and Snyder, 1975). From that work it is apparent that a change in substituents, such as the lack of a substituent at R_2 (see Figure 18.5), alters the ability of the phenothiazine to conform to the structure of DA and thus reduces its pharmacological activity. Second, the common occurrence of parkinsonian symptoms indirectly suggests that neuroleptics reduce the normal DA-mediated inhibition of cholinergic and GABAergic cells in striatum, which play a significant role in the extrapyramidal side effects of neuroleptic treatment (see above).

Receptor binding. Third, early in vitro biochemical studies showed that phenothiazines and butyrophenones inhibit the binding of [^{3}H]haloperidol to the DA receptor in caudate homogenates (Creese, Burt, and Snyder, 1976). Ability to displace the labeled ligand was closely correlated with both the clinical efficacy of the various drugs tested and their ability to inhibit DA-sensitive adenylyl cyclase. Furthermore, an excellent correlation exists between the neuroleptics' inhibition of [^{3}H]haloperidol binding and their ability to inhibit amphetamine-induced sterotypy.

Since the identification and cloning of DA receptor subtypes, neuropharmacological research has been directed toward elucidating the specific receptor-mediated mechanism responsible for both therapeutic and side effects of the neuroleptics. At least six types of DA receptors have been identified and classified into two main groups. D_1-like receptors include D_1 and D_5 while D_2-like receptors include D_{2L}, D_{2S}, D_3, and D_4 (see Chapter 8 for details). The D_2 receptors, located in the basal ganglia, nucleus accumbens, amygdala, hippocampus, and cerebral cortex, have a high affinity for neuroleptics, including the phenothiazines, butyrophenones, and thioxanthenes. Both D_2 subtypes are linked to an inhibitory G protein, through which they inhibit adenylyl cyclase activity. These receptors may also increase phosphoinositide turnover in some cells (Jackson and Danielsson, 1994). Antipsychotics readily bind to presynaptic DA autoreceptors of the D_{2L} type that are located on their cell bodies, dendrites, and nerve terminals. These inhibitory sites are responsible for controlling the rate of firing of the cell as well as the rate of synthesis and release of neurotransmitter. Acute application of DA or a DA agonist (apomorphine) to DA cell bodies in the substantia nigra or ventral tegmentum stimulates the autoreceptors and decreases the rate of firing of the DA neurons (Aghajanian and Bunney, 1977). This inhibition can be antagonized by systemic administration of an effective neuroleptic drug such as chlorpromazine, but not by an inactive phenothiazine. In addition, the antipsychotic drugs block the effects of iontophoretic DA on the firing of striatal neurons (Siggins, Hoffer, and Ungerstedt, 1974) and block the effects of amphetamine on DA neurons in midbrain (Bunney and Aghajanian, 1975a).

The binding selectivity of agonists and antagonists to the various DA receptor subtypes is currently being evaluated, but some important examples are clear. In all cases, the affinities of dopaminergic drugs are relative; that is, receptor occupancy depends on both affinity and concentration, and at high concentrations the relative selectivity is lost. Table 18.2 shows the dissociation constants for the binding of selected agonists and antagonists to the DA receptor subtypes. Recall that low values for dissociation constants represent higher affinities for the receptor. For example, the agonist bromocriptine and the antagonist raclopride are about two orders of magnitude more potent in binding to D_2 and D_3 receptors compared to D_4 binding. Of particular interest is that chlorpromazine is ten times less effective in binding at D_4 receptors compared with D_2 or D_3 binding, while clozapine is ten times more potent at D_4 receptors than at D_2 or D_3 receptors. Since the clinical potencies of effective antipsychotic drugs are positively correlated with their abilities to block D_2 receptors, the low binding of the novel antipsychotic clozapine has complicated the neurochemical interpretation. Figure 18.6 shows that the therapeutic concentration (free neuroleptic in patients' plasma) of antipsychotic drugs is directly related to their dissociation constants for binding to D_2 receptors, except for clozapine. However, when the plasma level of clozapine is compared with its dissociation constant for binding to the D_4 receptor, the correlation is restored, arguing

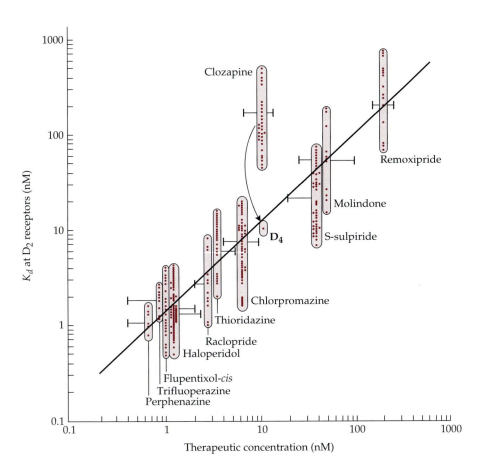

18.6 NEUROLEPTIC DISSOCIATION CONSTANTS (K_d) REPRESENTING AFFINITY FOR THE D_2 RECEPTOR are correlated with the plasma or CSF drug concentrations that are clinically effective in schizophrenic patients. Each individual point indicates a K_d value calculated by a different laboratory. The large ovals demonstrate the range of K_d values for each drug binding to D_2 receptors. The K_d values for clozapine binding to D_2 receptors are distinct from the others (large oval), but its affinity for D_4 receptors (small oval indicated by arrow) falls closely to the calculated correlation. (After Seeman, 1995; Seeman, 1992).

that the D_4 receptor is the primary target of clozapine and the likely mediator for its antipsychotic effect (Seeman, 1995). Although clozapine also blocks muscarinic receptors, 5-HT_2 receptors and D_1 receptors, Seeman (1995) argues against a significant role for these in the neuroleptic action of the drug.

PET studies of receptor occupancy have been used by a Swedish group at the Karolinska Institute to examine the relationship between pharmacological effects and DA receptor subtypes. Several studies have shown that chemically different categories of antipsychotic drugs occupied 70% to 89% of the D_2 receptors at therapeutic doses used in the clinic, suggesting that antipsychotic effects of classical neuroleptics are related to a blockade of D_2 receptors (Nordstrom, Farde, and Halldin, 1992). However, although the effect is dose dependent and fully reversible, the binding appears much earlier than does the antipsychotic effect, and it also occurs in treatment-resistant patients (Sedvall, 1992). Binding occurred within 3 hours after administration, long before antipsychotic efficacy occurs. Although some effects, such as emotional quieting, occur rapidly, the antipsychotic effects apparently require some time-dependent process to occur, subsequent to DA receptor blockade. Bunney (1992) has suggested that depolarization blockade is one possible explanation, since 3 weeks or more of drug treatment are needed to see that particular effect (see below).

Further PET studies (Farde et al., 1992) showed that patients with acute extrapyramidal effects had a higher D_2 receptor occupancy (82%) in the basal ganglia than those without side effects (74%). In contrast, clozapine-treated subjects showed no extrapyramidal symptoms and a lower D_2 occupancy (38% to 63%), suggesting that a therapeutic effect can be achieved at a substantially lower receptor occupancy. However, clozapine also produced a significant (38% to 52%) D_1 receptor occupancy, which they suggest may supplement the antipsychotic effects induced by D_2 occupation. Classical neuroleptics, however, do not occupy D_1 receptors to a significant extent (Color Plate 5).

DA turnover. The ability of phenothiazines to block inhibitory DA autoreceptors and increase cell firing is responsible for the increase in DA turnover suggested first by Carlsson and Lindqvist (1963). They originally speculated that phenothiazines block DA receptor sites and by a feedback mechanism increase the synthesis and release (i.e., the turnover) of DA. In support of this idea, they found a large increase in *O*-methylated DA metabolites after administration of phenothiazines, indicating increased extraneuronal metabolism. They also found that the neuroleptic drugs increased the formation and disappearance of [^{14}C]DA from its precursor [^{14}C]tyrosine, demonstrating more rapid DA turnover.

Table 18.2   Agonist and Antagonist Dissociation Constants for Dopamine Receptor Subtypes

		D_1-like group			D_2-like group			
Agonist	Affinity state of receptor	D_1 native[a] (nM)	D_1 clones (nM)	D_5 clones (nM)	D_2 native[b] (nM)	D_2 clones (nM)	D_3 clones (nM)	D_4 clones (nM)
Apomorphine-(−)	High	0.7	—	—	0.7	39	—	—
	Low[c]	206	417	252	127	86	32	—
Bromocriptine	High and low[d]	439	672	454	4.8	12	4.8	285
Dopamine	High	0.9	~250	~18	7.5	~33	~4	~30
	Low	383	~2,000	228	4,300	924	31	50–150
Fenoldopam-R	High	0.8	—	~0.6	2.8	—	—	—
	Low	45	~33	~18	1,000	—	—	—
Pergolide	High	0.8	0.8	—	~0.8	—	—	—
	Low	322	1,363	918	60	~20	~1.5	—
Antagonist								
Chlorpromazine		94	73	133	3	1.4	4.4	35
Clozapine (no Na⁺)		—	—	—	86	—	—	6
Clozapine (with Na⁺)		172	141	331	229	216	174	21
Emonapride		55–102	26	98	0.06	0.06	0.3	0.09
Haloperidol		—	—	—	1.2	1	~4–10	2.3
Melperone		—	—	—	240	182	—	~460
Olanzapine		18,000	—	—	45	—	—	27
Raclopride		—	—	—	1.8	1.8	3.5	1500
Remoxipride		—	—	—	~300	178	2,300	~2,000
Risperidone		—	—	—	5.6	—	—	7
SCH 23390		0.17	0.37	0.3	1,690	634	780	~3,000
Spiperone		212	~350	~3,500	0.06	0.07	0.6	0.08
Sulpiride-S-(−)		57,000	34,500	77,270	15	18	~13	1,005
Sulpiride-R-(+)		12,000	25,800	28,636	868	347	422	965

[a]Calf brain striatum and/or calf parathyroid used.
[b]Pig anterior pituitary and/or canine brain striatum used.
[c]Low-affinity state of receptor, or dissociation constant from IC_{50}.
[d]High- and low-affinity states for bromocriptine are identical.
Source: After Seeman, 1995.

It is now generally agreed that clinical response to neuroleptic treatment is associated with an initial increase in plasma HVA concentration followed by its decrease. Improvement in symptoms is associated with higher initial plasma HVA levels (i.e., good responders have higher mean levels of plasma HVA than do nonresponders) and greater drug-induced reductions of the metabolite over time (see Siever, Kalus, and Keefe, 1993). Interestingly, negative symptom patients do not show the initial increase in HVA, nor do they show the decline in HVA with continued neuroleptic treatment (Davila, Manero, and Zumarraga 1988). The proposed mechanism of HVA changes involves the acute block of pre- and postsynaptic D_2 receptors. The presynaptic D_2 receptor blockade increases the amount of DA released on subsequent action potentials, but because D_2 postsynaptic receptors are competitively blocked with a high affinity antipsychotic, acute DA transmission is attenuated. However, chronic antipsychotic treatment leads to up-regulation of postsynaptic D_2 sites as well as depolarization blockade (see below), which is ultimately responsible for the gradual return of DA release to normal or below baseline levels. The mechanism for depolarization block is not clear, but it is associated with a reduction in tyrosine hydroxylase activity, subsequent reduction in synthesis of DA, and parallel changes in plasma HVA. When initial neuroleptic-induced DA release is high, plasma HVA is elevated. As the postsynaptic receptors increase and depolarization block occurs, DA synthesis and subsequent release decrease as reflected in low plasma levels of HVA (see Friedhoff and Silva, 1995).

Depolarization block.   In order to understand the mechanism responsible for the gradual decline in HVA after the initial neuroleptic-induced increase, a series of electophysiological studies examined changes in cell firing in the dopaminergic cell bodies of the substantia nigra (origin of nigrostriatal cells) and the ventral tegmental area (origin of fiber projections through the mesolimbic and mesocortical tracts) (Bunney, 1992; Grace, 1992). Using an extracellular recording technique that passed the electrode through this region in a defined pattern, data were obtained on the number of DA cells firing, their average firing rate, and their firing pattern. As an example, haloperidol acutely activated DA neurons by increasing average firing rates, altering cell firing from a single-spike mode to burst-firing with a subsequent increase in DA release, and increasing the number of spontaneously firing cells. Chronic treatment, on the other hand, not only reduced cell firing but also made the cells unresponsive to normally excitatory substances. Since the iontophoretic application of hyperpolarizing GABA concentrations antagonized the reduced responsiveness of DA cells, it is assumed that the chronic antipsychotic drug effects were due to overexcitation of the cells (due to inactivation of their spike-generating mechanism), which could be reversed by hyperpolarization. Although the cellular mechanism for this phenomenon is unclear, feedback pathways from projection areas must be intact in order to induce depolarization blockade. The phenomenon of depolarization block was first described for spinal cord cells exposed to excitatory amino acids (Curtis, Phillis, and Watkins, 1960).

Of particular interest is the evidence that shows that drugs with both antipsychotic and extrapyramidal effects cause depolarization block in both mesolimbic and nigrostriatal neurons, while clozapine, which has a low incidence of extrapyramidal effects, causes depolarization block only in mesolimbic cells. Further, the ineffective antipsychotic drug that causes extrapyramidal symptoms (metoclopramide) produces depolarization block only in nigrostriatal cells (see Grace, 1992; Bunney, 1992). Dopamine cells that project to the frontal cortex do not demonstrate depolarization block, nor are the hypofrontal lobe symptoms attenuated by neuroleptic treatment. Based on these results, one might argue that the clinical effectiveness, at least for positive symptoms, is due to depolarization block in mesolimbic neurons. The hypothesis has further appeal because like the appearance of depolarization block, the time course of effectiveness shows continuing improvement over several weeks.

Although the idea of depolarization block as the basis for antipsychotic efficacy is appealing, alternative explanations are possible. Several experimental designs do not support the requirement of altered cell firing to produce neuroleptic-induced changes in HVA. For example, neuroleptics are able to increase DA metabolites in striatal slices even when nigrostriatal neurons have been eliminated or when the development of DA cell depolarization block is prevented by kainic acid treatment (Biggio et al., 1980). Also, developmental studies show a temporal correlation between the timing of autoreceptor development and tolerance in DA turnover following chronic antipsychotic treatment, but a disparity between receptor development and behavioral tolerance to neu-

roleptics (Coyle, Napier, and Breese, 1985). Furthermore, the importance of presynaptic autoreceptor function and their DA synthesis modulating effects must be considered. Autoreceptors on DA terminals that are blocked by neuroleptics acutely increase synthesis of DA with subsequent increased release and metabolism. Chronic blockade with neuroleptics leads to supersensitivity of the autoreceptors, allowing them to respond appropriately to elevated synaptic DA by reducing DA synthesis, subsequent release, and metabolism (see Cooper, Bloom, and Roth, 1991). The relative importance of depolarization block and presynaptic autoreceptors to the neuroleptic-induced changes in DA turnover is not clear. Resolution of the issue may reside in the realization that neuronal response mechanisms may be quite different in normal cells, which maintain stable levels of activity through a variety of means, compared with those operating under conditions showing abnormal responsivity, as in the schizophrenic brain (see Grace and Bunney, 1995).

Adenylyl cyclase. Early reports showed that DA-stimulated adenylyl cyclase is effectively inhibited in a competitive manner by the addition of low concentrations of neuroleptic drugs (Clement-Cormier et al., 1974). Since destroying the presynaptic cell did not prevent the effect, it is likely that the drug-induced inhibition is a postsynaptic phenomenon (Iversen, 1975a). When various phenothiazine drugs were compared, their individual potencies as inhibitors of DA-sensitive adenylyl cyclase correlated to some degree with their in vivo potencies as antipsychotics (Karobath and Leitich, 1974). How these early intriguing results reconcile with the latest binding evidence is unclear. More recent results suggest that neuroleptics bind to D_2 receptors, which are linked to a G protein that inhibits adenylyl cyclase. D_1 receptors that activate adenylyl cyclase have only a low affinity for most antipsychotic drugs (Kebabian and Calne, 1979).

Prolactin release. Further evidence for DA blockade comes from neuroendocrine measures of prolactin. Neuroleptics, by blocking D_2 receptors in the pituitary gland, stimulate the secretion of prolactin because under normal conditions, DA inhibits prolactin release. Thus an estimate of the extent of D_2 receptor blockade can be made by measuring serum prolactin in patients. The measure of serum prolactin provides an accessible window into the CNS and is frequently used clincally to evaluate CNS D_2 receptor function. The increase in prolactin release produced by the neuroleptics is responsible for excess lactation, a sometimes disturbing side effect of antipsychotic drug use.

Correlates to discrete DA pathways. The neuroendocrine effects of the antipsychotics are almost certainly due to receptor blockade of the tuberoinfundibular DA pathway, which originates in the arcuate and periventricular nuclei of the hypothalamus and projects into the median eminence and the intermediate lobe of the pituitary. Since it is well known that Parkinson's disease is due to destruction of cells in the Nigrostriatal pathway, it is assumed that the parkinsonian-like side effects of the neuroleptics are due to blockade of DA receptors in that neuronal pathway.

Since limbic structures are closely associated with emotions and cognitive processes, it is tempting to speculate that the mesolimbic DA system may be responsible for the drug's antipsychotic action. The DA mesolimbic system projects from the ventral tegmental area to limbic structures, such as the septum, olfactory tubercle, nucleus accumbens, amygdala, and piriform cortex. Most evidence in support of a unique role for the mesolimbic pathway is indirect. For example, Crow and coworkers (1978) tested the effects of three neuroleptic drugs (chlorpromazine, fluphenazine, and thioridazine) on DA turnover in the striatum and the nucleus accumbens. The drugs are all effective antipsychotics, but produce different amounts of extrapyramidal side effects. Their results demonstrated that the drugs' potencies were quite different in striatal DA turnover but were very similar in the nucleus accumbens. Hence, they suggested that the neuroleptic effect on striatal DA is more likely to be responsible for the extrapyramidal side effects than is DA turnover in the nucleus accumbens. More recently, Grace (1992) suggested that neuroleptic efficacy is related to reduced firing of the cells in the ventral tegmental area that project to limbic structures. In contrast, extrapyramidal effects are correlated with depolarization block of the cells in the substantia nigra that project to the striatum.

Further evidence to support a central role for mesolimbic cells comes from studies of the relatively new antipsychotic, clozapine. Clozapine has a strong action on DA turnover in the limbic system and a relatively weak one in the striatum. Coincidentally, clozapine has antipsychotic efficacy but very few extrapyramidal side effects. Furthermore, Bunney and Aghajanian (1975a) demonstrated that clozapine is capable of reversing amphetamine-induced depression of neuronal firing in DA cell bodies in the ventral tegmentum. Clozapine was not effective in blocking amphetamine-induced depression of neuronal firing in the substantia nigra. Because antipsychotic drugs that also have extrapyramidal effects inhibit amphetamine's effects on both cell groups, it is more likely that the antipsychotic effects of the neuroleptic drugs are due to action on the mesolimbic DA system. These findings demonstrate one potential problem in screening methods: correlations must be examined to determine whether they are related to the desired pharmacological effect or to one of the many side effects. Without such care, a screening test developed to identify potent antipsychotic drugs may in reality select compounds with strong extrapyramidal side effects that have some antipsychotic action.

Although a clear anatomical distinction for antipsychotic drug effects is appealing, not all evidence supports this hypothesis. Lidsky (1995) makes the argument that nigrostriatal cells may play a significant role in the appearance of psychotic symptoms and in their relief by neuroleptics. For example, although mesolimbic cells have been implicated in motivational behavior as measured by response to addictive drugs, others find that DA neurons in the ventral tegmentum and substantia nigra both respond to reward and to stimuli that predict reward in a learning task (Ljungberg, Apicella, and Schultz, 1992). In addition, bizarre movements, abnormal postures and irregularities in eye tracking movements suggest basal ganglia involvement in psychotic symptoms. Furthermore, visualization techniques rather consistently report morphological as well as functional abnormalities in basal ganglia. Metabolic activity in the basal ganglia is inversely related to several withdrawal symptom factors in psychiatric scales (see Gur, 1995). Evidence also exists to demonstrate that the caudate receives significant input from frontal association cortex and is involved in complex functions regarding mnemonic processes and cognitive strategies (Evarts et al., 1984; Lidsky, 1995). Finally, O'Dowd (1993) reports significant colocalization of D_4 receptor mRNA along with D_2 mRNA in the caudate and putamen and the substantia nigra. Thus, although it is tempting to speculate about a possible anatomical distinction of neuroleptic drug effects, the hypothesis remains tentative. A more productive approach to selective treatment may be to further elucidate receptor subtype involvement.

Investigations of the role of the mesocortical DA bundle also suggest a role in neuroleptic efficacy. The mesocortical tract originates in the ventral tegmentum and projects to the limbic cortex, including the medial prefrontal, cingulate, and entorhinal areas. In fact, these fibers may have to be considered as three separate groups, since those cells terminating in the prefrontal and cingulate cortices demonstrate properties distinct from the mesoentorhinal cells. Detailed analysis of these fibers has become possible with development of the highly sensitive techniques needed to evaluate this relatively diffuse system. Of principal interest is the realization that while the nigrostriatal and the mesolimbic tracts respond similarly to drug treatment, the fibers in the mesocortical bundle demonstrate unique characteristics. For instance, acute treatment with neuroleptics increases nigrostriatal cell activity determined by increased DA turnover, increased DA synthesis, and increased HVA levels. Mesocortical cells have a higher baseline rate of physiological activity and are much less sensitive to the acute effects of antipsychotic drugs. However, while nigrostriatal cells demonstrate tolerance with repeated exposure to neuroleptics, no such tolerance occurs for those DA cells in the mesoprefrontal and mesocingulate pathways. Many of these characteristics are consistent with the low incidence of autoreceptors on mesocortical neurons (Cooper, Bloom, and Roth, 1991).

Of further interest is the finding that only the meso-prefrontal DA neurons are activated by stressors such as foot shock, swim stress, conditioned fear, or treatment with natural anxiogenic agents. The metabolic activation of the DA neurons can be antagonized by the anxiety-reducing BDZs. It is enticing to suggest that the mesoprefrontal pathway is critical for the severe anxiety experienced by many schizophrenics and is the site of action for the reduction of symptoms following neuroleptic treatment. However, at this point, such a suggestion is entirely speculative. Nevertheless, the role of these neurons has been considered an integral part of at least one model developed to explain the neuropathology underlying positive and negative symptoms of schizophrenia characterized by hypofrontality of brain function (see below).

Atypical Neuroleptics

The conclusion that schizophrenia is not a unitary disorder but comprises multiple subtypes with heterogeneous symptom patterns and varied pathologies, both structural and neurochemical, prompts research toward the development of novel, symptom-specific neuroleptics. One direction taken is investigation into more selective D_2 receptor antagonists, such as sulpiride. A second trend in psychopharmacology is to evaluate more broad-spectrum antipsychotics, such as clozapine, that block 5-HT, NE, and/or histamine receptors. Several reviews have summarized some current developments in antipsychotic drugs (Casey, 1992; Gerlach, 1991; Meltzer, 1995).

The designation of "atypical" antipsychotics is usually based on the drugs' abilities to reduce symptoms of schizophrenia without causing significant extrapyramidal side effects. Other considerations include failure to increase serum prolactin, effectiveness for positive, negative, and disorganized symptoms, enhanced efficacy in treatment-resistant patients, selective improvement of some aspects of cognitive function, and lack of development of tardive dyskinesia. Still other considerations are the different profiles demonstrated in behavioral screening (see Casey, 1992). Not all atypical neuroleptics meet all the criteria, and their different clinical profiles reflect different underlying neurochemical mechanisms. There seems to be no single neurochemical characteristic that identifies those neuroleptics that produce atypical effects. The best current explanation is that the drugs block D_2 receptors incompletely or they also block other receptors to prevent the undesirable side effects (Seeman, 1990).

Specific D_2 receptor antagonists.
Based on the assumption that the efficacy of neuroleptics is related to DA (particularly D_2) receptor blockade, the first attempt to develop antipsychotic drugs with fewer side effects evaluated selective D_2 receptor antagonists. The drugs in this category, in addition to sulpiride (which has been available in Europe and Asia for some years), are raclopride and remoxipride. All three are substituted benzamides that bind specifically to D_2 receptors along with some affinity for the D_3 receptors, which may explain the fact that their behavioral effects differ from those of traditional neuroleptics. For example, these drugs inhibit apomorphine-induced locomotion at relatively low doses, while high concentrations are needed to produce catalepsy. The assumption is that D_2/D_3 receptor antagonists more selectively alter apomorphine-induced locomotion, an animal analog to psychosis. The same dual receptor blockade is less effective on those apomorphine-sensitive receptors that induce catalepsy, the animal analog to extrapyramidal symptoms. Figure 18.7 shows that for the classical antipsychotic haloperidol, the dose–response curves for inhibiting apomorphine-induced locomotion and producing catalepsy are very similar, suggesting that doses that are effective in reducing the locomotion (psychosis) are almost identical to those that induce catalepsy (extrapyramidal symptoms). In contrast, the dose–response curves for remoxipride and sulpiride show a much larger difference in potency between the hyperactivity inhibition and catalepsy effects.

Clinically, the dual D_2/D_3 receptor antagonists do produce fewer extrapyramidal effects than conventional neuroleptics that act primarily on D_2 receptors in different regions of the brain (Seeman, 1990). The receptor selectivity also means that autonomic and cardiovascular reactions are minimal and sedation is mild. Hormonal effects, however, tend to be common because of increased prolactin levels and other tuberoinfundibular tract endocrine effects (see Gerlach, 1991).

Sulpiride.
Sulpiride is an example of a D_2-specific neuroleptic in binding studies, and it increases DA turnover in DA projection areas, as is typical for DA receptor blockers. Sulpiride is equal to chlorpromazine and haloperidol in antipsychotic effectiveness, although it is significantly less potent. The median dose for sulpiride (2,000 mg/day) as compared with haloperidol (12 mg/day) is very high, probably due to its low lipid solubility and slow access to the CNS.

Long-term use of sulpiride does not lead to supersensitivity of D_2 receptors, although an increase in D_1 receptors has been reported (Jenner, Rupniak, and Marsden, 1985). If TD is caused by hypersensitivity of DA receptors, chronic sulpiride might be expected to have a low incidence of tardive dyskinesia. Uncontrolled clinical reports suggest a very low incidence of TD in patients treated with sulpiride. Furthermore, sulpiride suppresses TD in humans and in monkeys without a rebound aggravation when treatment is halted. Suppression with conventional neuroleptics frequently leads to a

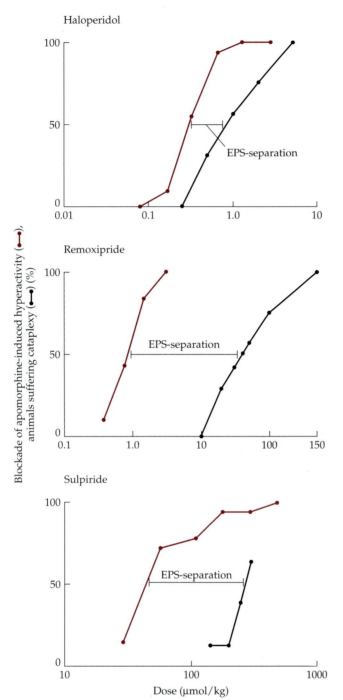

18.7 DOSE–RESPONSE CURVES FOR HALOPERIDOL, SULPIR-IDE, AND REMOXIPRIDE on blocking apomorphine-induced hyperactivity and producing catalepsy in rats. The horizontal distance between the curves on each graph represents the difference in potency of each drug to produce each of the effects. The neuroleptics were injected intraperitoneally 60 minutes before the apomorphine injection. (After Gerlach, 1991.)

the idea that TD is caused by blockade of a special subtype of D_2 receptor not altered by the highly selective drug. Alternatively, sulpiride-induced increases in D_1 receptors may protect against TD by regulating D_2 receptor function. Finally, the hypothesis that TD is not related to DA mechanisms but is a result of nondopaminergic function may be supported by further studies of sulpiride and other D_2 receptor–specific neuroleptics (Tamminga and Gerlach, 1987).

Remoxipride. Remoxipride is the first of this class of drugs to be developed for use in North America. Clinical studies show that remoxipride is as effective as classical neuroleptics in short- and long-term treatment of schizophrenia. Some reports suggest its usefulness in treating the negative symptoms of schizophrenia that are normally resistant to conventional antipsychotics, but others show no difference between remoxipride and haloperidol. Remoxipride has a low extrapyramidal syndrome profile and is well tolerated by patients, who report improvement in cognitive, motivational, and emotional functions. However, there is no evidence to suggest that the drug will not produce TD with long-term use. Also, after a cumulative worldwide collection of data on remoxipride's side effects, eight cases of fatal aplastic anemia were reported with the likely outcome that the drug will not be used in a general clinical population (Wirshing et al., 1995). Certainly further chemical modifications of the drug will be developed and tested. Lewander (1994) and Meltzer (1995) provide further detail.

Multiple receptor antagonists. While some atypical neuroleptics are being developed to target a single receptor type, others have been developed to block both D_2 receptors and one or more other receptors, most often $5\text{-}HT_2$, α_1-adrenergic, or D_1 receptors. The rationale for this work is the clinical efficacy of clozapine, a drug used in Europe prior to being approved in the United States. Clozapine is a broad-spectrum neuroleptic with relatively weak D_1 and D_2 affinities, and substantial serotonergic, α-adrenergic, muscarinic, and histaminergic affinities (Figure 18.8), as well as a high affinity for the recently cloned D_4 receptor. Since the drug is known for its ability to attenuate both positive symptoms and negative symptoms, and has a low incidence of extrapyramidal symptoms and TD, its mechanism of action is being thoroughly investigated.

While there is general agreement that D_2 receptors are important for antipsychotic effects, some laboratories hypothesize that typical and atypical neuroleptics can be differentiated by the ratio of antagonism for various receptors. For instance, some evidence suggests the importance of $5\text{-}HT_2$ antagonism in combination with D_2 blockade (Meltzer, Matsubara, and Lee, 1989). Others consider muscarinic receptor antagonism as a significant factor in defining atypical neuroleptics (Richelson, 1995),

severe rebound of symptoms when treatment is discontinued. The unique characteristics of sulpiride suggest that it may provide new neurochemical evidence of pathology in TD. Hypotheses to be investigated include

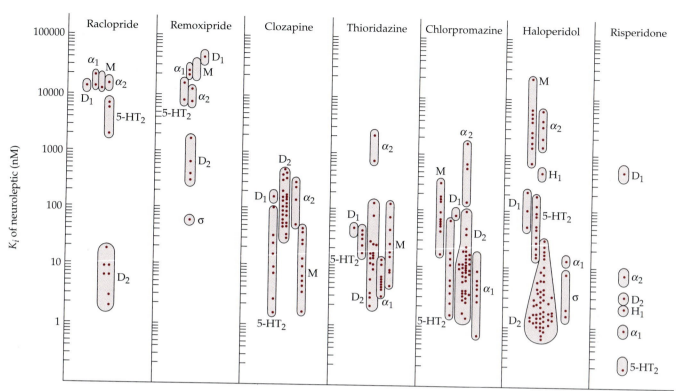

18.8 DISSOCIATION CONSTANTS FOR SEVERAL NEUROLEPTICS AT VARIOUS RECEPTORS summarized from reports in the literature. The K_i represents the estimated affinity of the neuroleptic for each receptor determined from radioligand displacement studies. Each point indicates the K_i from a different publication. D_1 and D_2 = dopamine receptors; $5\text{-}HT_2$ = serotonin receptor; M = muscarinic ACh receptor; α_1 and α_2 = adrenergic receptors; H_1 = histamine receptor; σ = σ opiate receptor. (After Seeman, 1990.)

while some reports support the idea that the ratio of D_1 to D_2 receptor occupation is a defining characteristic of antipsychotic action without extrapyramidal side effects.

PET results suggest that the antipsychotic effect of clozapine may be augmented by effective binding to $5\text{-}HT_2$ receptors along with low D_2 binding. The Karolinska group found that typical antipsychotics produce very little or no in vivo binding to $5\text{-}HT_2$ receptors, while clozapine produces between 80% and 90% receptor occupancy at therapeutic doses (Nordstrom, Farde, and Halldin, 1993). A related atypical multireceptor neuroleptic, risperidone, also binds avidly to the $5\text{-}HT_2$ receptors, but additionally binds to D_2 receptors (80%) as readily as do the conventional antipsychotics. One possibility is that the elevated serotonergic binding might reduce the extrapyramidal symptoms associated with high D_2 binding (see Color Plate 5).

The $5\text{-}HT_2$ receptor occupancy may also be related to the reduction in negative symptoms (see Lieberman, 1994) or to the reduction in symptoms by atypical antipsychotics in patients who are not responsive to classical neuroleptics. When the serotonin agonist *m*-chloro-

phenylpiperazine (*m*-CPP) is given to drug-free individuals, it elevates plasma cortisol, ACTH, and prolactin, an effect that can be blocked by clozapine, but not by fluphenazine or haloperidol. Patients who have greater *m*-CPP–induced increases in plasma hormones have predictably greater responses to clozapine (see Lieberman, 1994). Others found that when treatment-resistant patients were administered *m*-CPP, their psychotic symptoms worsened, although the drug has no effect on normal individuals (Krystal et al., 1993). Since both clozapine and the $5\text{-}HT_2$ receptor antagonist ritanserin reversed the symptoms, their use for treatment-resistant psychosis is suggested.

Clozapine. Clozapine is the best-known atypical antipsychotic. Preclinical animal testing shows that it blocks apomorphine or amphetamine-induced hyperactivity, but does not produce catalepsy except at high doses. Chronic treatment with clozapine does not increase D_2 re-

Clozapine
(Clozaril)

ceptors, but, like sulpiride, it increases D_1 receptors. Clinical trials demonstrated that the antipsychotic effect of clozapine was usually equal to or greater than that of the more conventional neuroleptics such as chlorpromazine and haloperidol. It is the first antipsychotic that demonstrated a significant effect on negative symptoms, as well as reducing anxiety and tension (Meltzer, 1994; Tamminga and Gerlach, 1987). Unfortunately, the effect on negative symptoms is not very great, and this effect has not been consistently reported. Meltzer (1994) has also found improvements in scores on the Quality of Life Scale, which means that patients significantly improve their function in important components of daily living. Cognitive function also improves, as shown on tests of verbal fluency, immediate and delayed recall, and some frontal lobe functions. Among all available neuroleptics, clozapine is considered to be the least likely to induce TD, and it additionally suppresses some kinds of tremors, such as parkinsonian tremors (Pakkenberg and Pakkenberg, 1986). For this reason some clinicians recommend a treatment combination of clozapine and haloperidol. Although clozapine is no more effective than standard neuroleptics in treating the positive symptoms of schizophrenia, it is often effective in those patients who do not respond to classical antipsychotic treatment. Clozapine produces significant improvement in 60% of patients who do not respond to typical neuroleptics. However, response to clozapine may not be evident until after 6 months of treatment, although 30% will respond by 6 weeks (Meltzer, 1995). Why there is such a long delay in effectiveness is not known.

Clozapine is not without side effects. Some of these stem from its affinity for α-adrenergic and cholinergic receptors, which when blocked may lead to cardiovascular irregularities such as orthostatic hypotension and tachycardia. Clozapine also decreases the seizure threshold and produces hypersalivation and weight gain. A more serious side effect is the high incidence of bone marrow toxicity and agranulocytosis (AGC), a serious blood abnormality. By more careful monitoring of blood cell count, restricted use of the drug, and use of granulocyte colony–stimulating factor drugs which reduce recovery time, the incidence of AGC decreased from 0.38% to 0.06% of clozapine-treated patients, and the mortality rate in AGC patients decreased from 42% to 19%. This improvement brings the incidence of AGC into line with more conventional neuroleptics (Tamminga and Gerlach, 1987). However, because of the profile of clozapine's side effects, the risk/benefit assessment used by most clinicians precludes the use of the drug as a first line of treatment (Meltzer, 1994). Rather it is used for treatment-resistant patients or those who cannot tolerate conventional neuroleptics and are noncompliant because of it. However, because of the limited market and the cost of frequent blood screening, clozapine is significantly more expensive than conventional antipsychotic drugs.

Risperidone.   The development of risperidone has been particularly exciting because initial clinical trials suggest that it possesses many of the benefits of clozapine without the risk of blood disorders. Risperidone is chemically unrelated to any other antipsychotic and is a potent 5-HT_{2A}, 5-HT_7, α_1- and α_2-adrenergic, and histamine H_1 receptor antagonist (see Figure 18.8). It is also a D_2 recep-

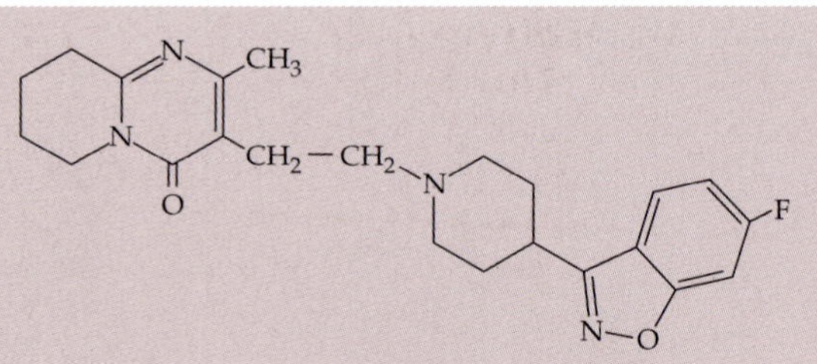

**Risperidone
(Risperdal)**

tor antagonist comparable to haloperidol, though it is a relatively weak antagonist at D_1 and D_4 receptors (see Meltzer, 1995). Preclinical testing shows that risperidone blocks apomorphine-induced hyperactivity at a dose that produces only mild catalepsy, so its profile suggests antipsychotic effectiveness with low extrapyramidal symptoms.

Marder (1994) summarizes four well-designed, double-blind studies that compared risperidone and haloperidol, two of which also utilized a placebo condition. Overall, risperidone and haloperidol were significantly more effective than the placebo in reducing symptoms, using a positive and negative syndrome scale, and risperidone, at most doses, was significantly more effective than haloperidol. Figure 18.9 represents data compiled from several trials of multiple doses of risperidone compared with haloperidol (20 mg) and placebo (Lindenmayer, 1994). Clearly, administration of placebo produced only minimal changes in the scores for the three categories: positive symptoms, negative symptoms, and general psychopathology. Haloperidol clearly improved the positive symptoms but had little effect on the other two measures. Risperidone (6 mg) improved all 7 items on the positive scale, all 7 on the negative scale, and 13 out of 16 items on the psychopathology scale. Risperidone (16 mg) did slightly less well overall, and 10 mg risperidone produced the least improvement, although still better than those produced by haloperidol. Apparently 6 mg risperidone is the most effective dose, although why 10 mg did not produce better results is a matter of concern and certainly will be addressed in future clinical trials.

The same series of trials (Marder, 1994) showed that patients on risperidone required one-tenth the medication for treating extrapyramidal symptoms that patients on haloperidol did, demonstrating low incidence of motor side effects with the drug. Several studies showed that there was no significant difference between risperi-

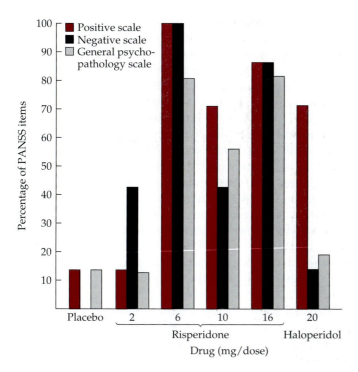

18.9 PERCENTAGE OF POSITIVE AND NEGATIVE SYNDROME SCALE (PANSS) ITEMS significantly improved from baseline values after administration of risperidone and haloperidol. Risperidone improved scores on both the positive and negative scales, while haloperidol improved positive scale scores only. The 6-mg doses of risperidone were most effective in improving scores. The data are compiled from four studies constituting the North American Fixed-Dose Trial. (After Lindenmayer, 1994.)

great potential in treating many conditions for which typical neuroleptic drugs have been used in the past, such as manic–depressive illness, psychotic depression, childhood psychosis, and so forth (Meltzer, 1995).

Neurochemical Hypotheses of Schizophrenia

In order to identify the neurochemical basis for any mental disorder, three general approaches can be taken. First, neurochemical correlates of animal and human models of the disorder are studied. This productive line of research, however, is dependent on the characteristics of the model chosen, in terms of homology to the disorder, validity, reliability, and so forth (see Chapter 2, Part II). Second, neuropharmacologists attempt to elucidate the neuronal mechanisms of the action of drugs that are effective in alleviating symptoms. This must be done with the realization that pharmacological manipulations may produce changes that compensate for the disease without acting at the locus of the disorder. Third, the functioning of neurotransmitter systems in patient populations is assessed. In the past, the methods included examining biological fluids (blood, CSF, urine) as well as postmortem brain tissue for evidence of changes in neurotransmitter turnover. More recently, brain imaging techniques have provided a window into the functioning CNS of the patient population. Using these three approaches, evidence strongly suggests that although several neurotransmitters may play a role in schizophrenic symptoms, malfunction of DA transmission is extremely important.

The Dopamine Hypothesis

The finding that the sympathomimetic drug amphetamine can produce a psychotic reaction that can be reversed by a DA receptor blocking antipsychotic drug, initially prompted the hypothesis of a catecholamine mechanism in schizophrenia. Amphetamine and cocaine, which enhances DA transmission by blocking reuptake, and the DA receptor agonist apomorphine can exacerbate psychotic symptoms in schizophrenics and produce symptoms of psychosis in a healthy individual. Thus, the DA-induced psychotomimetic effects of these drugs suggests that excessive DA neurotransmission is responsible for at least some schizophrenic symptoms. Both amphetamine-induced toxic psychosis in humans and amphetamine- (or apomorphine-) induced stereotyped behavior in rats were described above.

It is well known that amphetamine potentiates the activity of the catecholamines at the synapse by causing release of catecholamines and preventing reuptake into the presynaptic terminal. The relative importance of NE and DA to the various pharmacological effects of amphetamine is clear. Garver and colleagues (1975) found that blocking DA receptors with pimozide or haloperidol before administering amphetamine prevented the appear-

done at low doses (6 mg) and placebo on their assessment for extrapyramidal symptoms (Abnormal Involuntary Movement Scale), although increasing doses did produce more classic extrapyramidal signs. One study suggested that risperidone can partially mask TD symptoms (Chouinard et al., 1993), but data on the incidence of TD following long-term drug use is not yet available. At least one of the studies showed a significant onset of effectiveness for risperidone within the first week of treatment. Although some of the patients in the clinical trials may have been treatment-resistant, there have not been double-blind tests of efficacy comparing risperidone with clozapine, so it is not clear whether risperidone is effective in that population (Meltzer, 1995). The drug additionally needs to be examined for effects on cognitive function.

The most common side effects with risperidone are insomnia, anxiety, agitation, sedation, dizziness, hypotension, weight gain, and menstrual disturbances (Borison et al., 1992). Since blood abnormalities are not part of its clinical picture, weekly monitoring is unnecessary. The overall clinical picture is a bright one at present. Risperidone has the potential to be useful as a first choice antipsychotic agent and is also considered to have

ance of stereotypy and hyperactivity, suggesting that DA is likely to be the significant neurotransmitter in these behaviors. Support for this conclusion comes from lesion experiments in which destruction of the DA-containing pathways reduces or abolishes amphetamine-induced stereotypy (Creese and Iversen, 1974). In addition, stereotyped behavior can be elicited by intracerebral injection of amphetamine into forebrain DA areas, including the striatum and globus pallidus (Costall, Naylor, and Olley, 1972). This effect can be blocked by systemic (Costall, Naylor, and Olley, 1972) or intracerebral (Pijnenburg, Honig, and van Rossum, 1975a) administration of DA blockers, such as haloperidol.

Elucidation of the neurochemical mechanism responsible for the effectiveness of antipsychotic drugs, as described above, also suggests DA as a significant factor in schizophrenia. The correlation between D_2 (and in some cases D_4) receptor binding and clinical efficacy is well documented, as are the PET studies showing the degree of D_2 receptor occupancy produced by neuroleptic drugs. The time-dependent development of depolarization blockade following chronic neuroleptic treatment also argues for the importance of dopaminergic function in the disorder. Finally, the drug-induced changes in DA turnover as determined by plasma HVA levels further enhances the DA hypothesis of schizophrenia.

Since models of schizophrenia and the mechanism of action of neuroleptics both point to a pivotal role for DA in at least some of the symptoms of schizophrenia, DA function in the clinical population needs to be evaluated. To do that, many experiments have attempted to measure plasma or CSF DA metabolites, turnover of DA, DA receptor characteristics in the brains of schizophrenics postmortem or in vivo using PET technology, or indirect indices of DA transmission, such as neuroendocrine function. Each of these topics will be described briefly in subsequent sections. For an excellent and more complete review, see Meltzer (1987).

Plasma measurements of HVA in schizophrenics have proven to be a useful tool to evaluate DA turnover when experimental parameters are carefully controlled. Variables relevant to these measurements include diet, activity, stress, age, sex, weight, circadian and seasonal variation, and neuroleptic treatment (Kendler, Mohs, and Davis, 1983), in addition to factors such as diagnostic subclass, duration of illness, and so forth. An additional concern is that regional differences in dopaminergic cell activity, even if very large, would be diluted out by whole-brain contributions to the total metabolite measured. Also, most plasma HVA comes from several sources, and the majority does not originate in brain or even from cells where DA acts as a neurotransmitter (Friedhoff and Silva, 1995). However, although the exact contribution from each source is not known, plasma HVA is generally accepted as a reasonable measure of brain DA turnover. Validity of the HVA measure is demonstrated by DA agonist- and antagonist-induced changes in the concentration of the metabolite. One explanation may be that neuroleptics produce a correlated effect on the diverse pools of HVA, so even though only a small portion reflects DA neuron activity, HVA levels are predictive of DA cell function.

Unfortunately steady state plasma HVA levels (as well as CSF levels) are not consistently different between schizophrenic and control subjects, nor are HVA levels correlated with symptom type or severity. However, most investigators have found that chronic antipsychotic treatment significantly reduces plasma HVA over several weeks of treatment and that the reduction predicts favorable treatment outcome. Davila, Manero, and Zumarraga (1988) and others have shown that neuroleptics produce an initial increase in HVA during the first 4 days of treatment, followed by a subsequent decrease, and that both the increase and decrease signal a good treatment outcome. Patients displaying predominantly negative symptoms show neither the increase nor the decrease in HVA.

Although steady state DA neuron activity, as reflected by levels of the HVA metabolite, is not significantly different in unmedicated schizophrenics, evaluation of receptor number or sensitivity of coupling mechanisms subsequent to receptor binding may identify a postsynaptic dopaminergic defect. In fact, several studies have found increased D_2 receptors in the basal ganglia, nucleus accumbens, and substantia nigra of postmortem schizophrenic brains (Owen et al., 1984; Mackay et al., 1982; Seeman et al., 1984). In contrast, D_1 receptors do not seem to be different (Pimoule et al., 1985). PET scan quantification of DA receptors in the striatum of living schizophrenics has found slight increases in D_2 receptors (Crawley et al., 1986; Sedvall et al., 1986), although these results are not found consistently (Martinot et al., 1990). Some of the disparities may be due to the radioligand chosen to label the receptor, or to other methodological differences. When increased D_2 receptors are found, they most often occur in patients with positive symptoms. Also the more acutely ill patients have higher D_2 striatal receptors than the chronically ill or than controls (see Kahn and Davis, 1995).

Evaluation of receptor binding studies is done cautiously because contamination of results by prior antipsychotic drug treatment is possible. Chronic administration of typical antipsychotics increases D_2 but not D_1 receptor density in the brain (Porceddu et al., 1986). However, a number of studies reported D_2 increases using drug-naive schizophrenics (see Kahn and Davis, 1995; Wong, 1986). In addition, without a measure of DA turnover it is not possible to rule out a presynaptic *deficit* in DA synthesis or release as a mechanism to induce receptor supersensitivity. One study of schizophrenic patients (Bjerkenstedt et al., 1985) found elevated plasma and CSF levels of six amino acids that compete with tyrosine for transport into the brain. The authors argue that by limiting tyrosine transport, synthesis of DA may be reduced in schizophrenics, leading to subsequent increases in D_2 receptors. Additionally, differences in reported results may be due to changes in the psychiatric state of the schizophrenic patient, for instance, during the acute phase, chronic stage, or remission.

Since prolactin release from the anterior pituitary is controlled by a tonic inhibitory effect of DA neurotransmission, the secretion of the hormone is frequently used as an index of DA activity and effectiveness of neuroleptic drugs. If schizophrenia is due to excessive DA neurotransmission, then reduced levels of prolactin should be found in schizophrenic individuals. In general, no differences have been reported in circulating prolactin levels in unmedicated patients in comparison with controls. However, several studies have found a relationship between specific symptoms and prolactin secretion (Rubin, 1987).

Much of the evidence provided thus far has been synthesized into a DA imbalance hypothesis described by Davis and colleagues (Kahn and Davis, 1995; Davis et al., 1991). They suggest that schizophrenia can be characterized by hypodopaminergia in mesocortical neurons along with hyperdopaminergia in mesolimbic DA neurons. They propose that the negative symptoms and cognitive defects are related to impaired prefrontal cortex function, which may be explained by impoverished mesocortical DA cell function. In contrast, the therapeutic effects of neuroleptics (particularly on positive symptoms) are related to reducing DA function in mesolimbic neurons. The functional relationship between these two effects is discussed in the neurodevelopmental model of schizophrenia (see below).

Despite the array of evidence that DA is important to the etiology of schizophrenia, it is unlikely that a single neurotransmitter or locus of pathology will explain the diverse constellation of behaviors called schizophrenia. Certainly it is possible that while some schizophrenics may experience either excessive or reduced DA transmission as the basis for particular symptoms of the disorder, other symptoms may not be directly related to that amine. Other forms of schizophrenia may also have distinct etiologies, or they may demonstrate altered DA function at a discrete time in the life history of the disorder. Altered DA function may also be subsequent to other factors occurring earlier in the disease process, factors such as viral infection, morphological changes, cellular toxicity, or autoimmune disorders.

It is highly likely that neurotransmitters other than DA are significant to the disorder, despite the fact that antipsychotics seem to owe their effectiveness to reducing DA neurotransmission. Since CNS processing involves integration of excitatory and inhibitory signals from numerous sources mediated via several neurotransmitters, schizophrenia may well be due to excessive non-

dopaminergic inhibitory inputs that can be countered by reducing DA-mediated inhibition. Alternatively, schizophrenia could be due to a reduction in excitatory neurotransmission that can be balanced by a reduction in DA-induced inhibition. Several research groups have suggested that 5-HT cells that interact both anatomically and functionally with DA cells almost certainly play a modulatory role in the disorder (see Roth and Meltzer, 1995). In addition, dopaminergic and glutamatergic interactions also have significant ramifications regarding mental disorders (see Bunney, Bunney, and Carlsson, 1995). Some of the concerns raised are addressed in subsequent sections of this chapter dealing with alternative hypotheses of neurochemical etiology. Others will be left for future investigation.

The Neurodevelopmental Model

Although the DA hypothesis of schizophrenia has received the most attention, it is very likely that the pathogenesis of schizophrenia is far more complex. For example, Weinberger (1987, 1995) has developed a model that attempts to unify the data regarding symptom subsets with the evidence for neurochemical and neurodegenerative changes in schizophrenia. He argues for a neurodevelopmental model in which an initial brain abnormality interacts with a normal maturational sequence such that pathological behavior patterns occur much later in development. His model attempts to address specifically three separate issues regarding schizophrenia: (1) the classic onset during late adolescence or early adulthood, (2) the significance of stress in both onset and relapse, and (3) the apparent selective efficacy of antipsychotic drugs for reducing the positive symptoms of the disorder.

Previously in this chapter, evidence was presented showing that anatomical pathology exists in various limbic and diencephalic structures and in the prefrontal cortex of schizophrenic brains postmortem. Several CT and MRI studies in living patients found enlarged ventricles and wide cortical sulci indicative of tissue loss, as well as reduced tissue mass in the temporal lobe and prefrontal cortex (reviewed by Gur and Pearlson, 1993). Many of the differences were not very large in magnitude, and they did not always present a consistent locus of pathology; nevertheless, any lesion in these brain areas would be expected to have widespread effects because of the many interconnections among the brain structures. Although most studies indicate that the tissue loss in a particular area is not active and progressing at the time symptoms develop, it is clear from developmental studies that the effects of a lesion may not manifest themselves until the brain system matures. For example, in the case of the dorsolateral prefrontal cortex (DLPFC), development and myelination are delayed until after puberty, a characteristic time for the onset of symptoms of schizophrenia. In addition to the observed cell pathology in this region, schizophrenics frequently show reduced cerebral blood flow in the dorsolateral prefrontal cortex during a mentally challenging task.

Several pieces of evidence hint at the idea that negative symptoms of schizophrenia (flat affect, social withdrawal, lack of motivation, poor insight, and intellectual impairment) are associated with reduced frontal lobe function. First, the negative symptoms closely resemble those found in patients with lesions of the frontal lobe. The magnitude of negative symptoms is associated with prefrontal hypometabolism, such as low glucose utilization and reduced blood flow (Wolkin et al., 1992). Second, animal studies show that DLPFC damage produces deficits in behaviors requiring insight and strategy. Neuropsychological testing in humans has also shown a relationship between poor test performance in tasks requiring frontal lobe function and decreased DA function as determined by lowered CSF HVA concentrations (see Kahn and Davis, 1995). Daniel and colleagues (1991) additionally showed that increasing cerebral blood flow to the frontal cortex with amphetamine was correlated with improved test scores on frontal lobe function.

The importance of DA to the complex cognitive functioning regulated by the DLPFC has been further revealed in monkeys with DA mesocortical neuronal lesions. Such damage results in a failure in delayed response tasks. Other animal research shows that DA agonists enhance physiological activity in the DLPFC as measured by prefrontal glucose utilization. Additionally, mesocortical DA neurons respond to stress with increased DA turnover. In fact, mesocortical cells are responsive not only to acute stress but also to learned stress, for instance, when an animal is returned to a previously stressful environment, as during the learned helplessness procedure. Based on the assumption that negative symptoms are associated with low DA function, several attempts have been made to reverse the symptoms with DA agonists. Although most have not been successful, one study using a DA reuptake inhibitor, mazindol, showed a significant improvement in negative symptoms compared with controls (see Kahn and Davis, 1995).

In sum, these results may be interpreted to suggest that the onset of negative symptoms of schizophrenia is due to the occurrence of early mesocortical damage that is expressed as aberrant behavior only at a time of normal functional maturity of the system. Thus, complex cognitive functions, including insightful behavior and the ability to respond to the social stresses prevalent at adolescence, might be expected to be compromised, although some of the symptoms, such as social awkwardness and excessive shyness, may manifest themselves as a portion of early premorbid history. In fact, many of the negative symptoms resemble signs of Parkinson's disease, which are known to be due to DA cell loss. If the symptoms are caused by DA cell loss, the neuroleptic-induced blockade of DA receptors is not likely to be an effective treatment. However, environmental stress management techniques and social skills training, which reduce the demand on the prefrontal system, predictably lessen the frequency of relapse.

Lesioning of prefrontal DA neurons produces chronic subcortical DA hyperactivity, manifested by increased DA turnover, upregulation of postsynaptic D_2 receptors, and increased striatal responsiveness to amphetamine and apomorphine, expressed in behavior (see Kahn and Davis, 1995). In addition, when DA agonists such as apomorphine are injected into the prefrontal cortex, DA metabolites are reduced in the striatum. Thus, an inhibitory role for cortical–limbic feedback is proposed. Similar neurochemical DA overactivity is reported in some studies of schizophrenic patients. Furthermore, studies of epileptic patients suggest that psychotic experiences, hallucinations, unexplainable experiences, perceptual distortions, and irrational fears are associated with electrical discharge in limbic areas, particularly in the temporal lobe, amygdala, and hippocampus. Thus, Weinberger (1995) suggests that excessive mesolimbic DA activity following mesocortical cell loss could explain the more florid positive symptoms of schizophrenia, those most readily reversed by neuroleptic-induced DA receptor blockade.

The neurodevelopmental model shown in Figure 18.10 makes no attempt to identify the etiology of the postulated early mesocortical deficit (indicated with an X) which could be due to one of many things, including maternal nutrition, obstetrical complications, viral infection, and other possibilities discussed above. However, Weinberger argues that such a lesion produces few symptoms early in life, but reveals itself later at a time when social stresses demand maximum prefrontal cognitive function. The loss of the DA input prevents the individual from making appropriate responses and instead leads to confused thinking, perseverance of inappropriate behavior, and social withdrawal. The loss of inhibitory cortical feedback onto subcortical neurons (shaded-color lines) plus the stress-induced increase in mesolimbic cell function (heavy line) leads to agitation, fearfulness, and hallucinations.

The appeal of this model of schizophrenia is in its ability to incorporate many distinct pieces of the puzzle and in providing several testable hypotheses. However, at this time, empirical support is lacking for many of the central assumptions. Further evaluation using techniques in neurochemistry, neuroanatomy, and psychopharmacology is required.

The Role of Norepinephrine

Several lines of evidence suggest that norepinephrine may play a role in psychosis. Several studies have reported elevations in NE concentration in the blood or CSF of schizophrenics (see Meltzer, 1987), which may reflect general arousal or response to stress. Dajas and

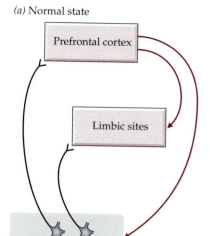

(a) Normal state

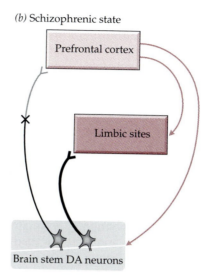

(b) Schizophrenic state

18.10 SCHEMATIC REPRESENTATION OF THE NEURODEVELOPMENTAL MODEL. *(a)* The normal state, in which the mesocortical pathway and prefrontal areas provide inhibitory feedback onto limbic areas and the mesolimbic neurons. *(b)* An early defect in schizophrenia (x) reduces mesocortical function, causing negative symptoms, and subsequently removes inhibitory control of limbic structures, producing the positive symptoms associated with excess subcortical DA activity. (After Weinberger, 1987.)

coworkers (1983) found a correlation between elevated plasma NE, positive symptoms, overall psychopathology, and paranoid symptoms. Kemali and colleagues (1985) reported a relationship between CNS NE concentration, psychosis ratings, and EEG measures.

Since presynaptic α_2-receptor sites normally exert an inhibitory effect on neurotransmitter release, one possible cause of the elevated NE levels could be a reduced number or diminished affinity of α_2-receptors. At least one group has demonstrated a significant decrease in number of α_2 binding sites for [^{3}H]clonidine and [^{3}H]yohimbine in schizophrenics after a 2-week drug-free period (Rosen et al., 1985). Follow-up studies showed a correlation between reduced binding and severity of negative symptoms as well as resistance to antipsychotic treatment. This might suggest a possible therapeutic role for α_2-receptor agonists. β-adrenergic blocking drugs, such as propranolol, have also been found useful in some cases, perhaps due to postsynaptic noradrenergic blockade (Eccleston et al., 1985).

The Serotonin Hypothesis

The importance of 5-HT in the symptoms and treatment of schizophrenia has been reviewed by Roth and Meltzer (1995) and will be only briefly summarized here. The basis for the serotonin hypothesis is the knowledge that functional alterations in the 5-HT system, which have been documented in schizophrenics, have effects on other neurotransmitter systems, such as glutamate, NE, ACh, and DA. Further, manipulation of the 5-HT system can modify symptoms of schizophrenia, as well as modulate side effects. The clinical effectiveness of clozapine lends substantial support to the hypothesis because it has high affinity for several subtypes of 5-HT receptors. Also, in some cases, serotonergic agonists exacerbate schizophrenic symptoms and further impair performance on neuropsychological tests.

Unfortunately neuroendocrine challenge studies in schizophrenics have not provided consistent results, and Roth and Meltzer (1995) suggest a complex serotonergic abnormality in the disorder. Most studies show reduced neuroendocrine responses (e.g., plasma prolactin or cortisol levels) to indirect serotonergic agonists (such as fenfluramine or tryptophan) in the patient population. These studies have been limited due to the lack of specific challenge agonists and antagonists for the many recently discovered 5-HT receptor subtypes. However, clozapine very effectively antagonizes the neuroendocrine responses to 5-HT agonists while conventional antipsychotics do not.

The evaluation of 5-HIAA in CSF of schizophrenics has provided no clear conclusion, although several results are encouraging. For example, Csernansky and coworkers (1990) found a correlation between CSF 5-HIAA and negative symptom rating, which would suggest increased 5-HT function associated with the deficit symptoms. Weinberger, Berman, and Illowsky (1988) also found that CSF levels of 5-HIAA were related to frontal lobe function testing (Wisconsin card sort) and prefrontal regional blood flow. Others (Lewine et al., 1991) found that while neither CSF 5-HIAA nor HVA levels were indicative of ventricular enlargement, the ratio of HVA to 5-HIAA was negatively correlated with ventricular size. This type of data reflects the intimate but complex relationship that exists between the two neurotransmitter systems. Serotonin, acting via several distinct receptor subtypes, has both inhibitory and excitatory actions on DA cell function. For a more complete discussion of the potential role of 5-HT in the etiology of schizophrenia, see Roth and Meltzer (1995).

Other Neurotransmitter Systems

Because ACh, GABA, and endorphins modulate or interact with DA transmission, each has been investigated regarding its potential role in the development of schizophrenia or in a particular pattern of symptoms presented. No consistent differences in the levels, turnover, or receptors of these neurotransmitters have been found in schizophrenics, although there are many provocative results requiring further investigation. A review by Meltzer (1987) briefly summarizes the current status of research in this area.

Pharmacologically modifying the CNS cholinergic function apparently has no effect on the psychotic symptoms of schizophrenia or the course of the disease. Although GABA interacts in a complex manner with DA and is generally believed to have a regulatory effect on cognitive and affective behaviors, GABA mimetics do not have any consistent action on psychosis (Tamminga and Gerlach, 1987). The potential role of endogenous opiates in schizophrenia is described further in Chapter 12, and the interaction between DA and endorphins can be found in Schmauss and Emrich (1985).

The Supersensitivity–Subsensitivity Hypothesis

In an attempt to explain the therapeutic latency of antipsychotic drugs, Freed (1988) suggested that the rapid DA receptor blockade may be secondary in importance to the drugs' slower action on the excitatory glutamate synapses formed by the corticostriatal pathway. His argument, presented in Figure 18.11, is based on the idea that chronic antipsychotic treatment not only increases

DA receptors (thus restoring some of the normal inhibitory effect on the follower cell), but also decreases the receptors for the excitatory glutamatergic input to the same cells. Thus striatal cells normally receive both excitatory input from the glutamate corticostriatal cells and inhibitory input from the DA nigrostriatal cells (Figure 18.11a). When neuroleptics are administered, the balance is altered by the blockade of the inhibitory input (Figure 18.11b). With chronic neuroleptic treatment, the striatal cells respond by increasing the number of inhibitory DA receptors and reducing the excitatory glutamate receptors (Figure 18.11c). In support of the hypothesis, Freed provides some evidence from lesion experiments, which show that neurotoxic lesions of the nigrostriatal DA pathway not only produce supersensitivity of DA receptors on the follower cells, but also result in a 40% decrease in striatal [^{3}H]glutamate binding (Roberts et al., 1982). Further, chronic neuroleptic administration decreased the behavioral response of mice to the glutamate agonist quisqualic acid. An alternative explanation for the reduced glutamate binding is the presence of glutamate receptors on the DA cells themselves.

Conversely, the same group and others (see Freed, 1988) found that cortical lesions that reduce glutamatergic input to the striatum not only lead to increases in striatal glutamate receptors but also to decreases in DA receptors. While these results are cited in support of the

(a) Glutamate (+) and dopamine (–) in balance.

(b) Acute neuroleptic blockade; excess glutamate excitation.

(c) Chronic neuroleptic blockade; decrease in glutamate and increase in dopamine restores balance.

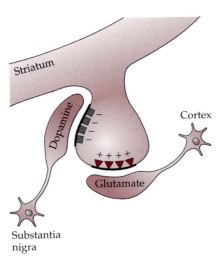
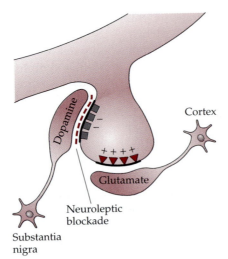
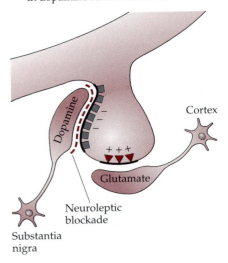
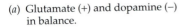

18.11 THE SUPERSENSITIVITY–SUBSENSITIVITY HYPOTHESIS proposed by Freed (1988). The underlying assumption is that excitatory (glutamate) and inhibitory (dopamine) influences on striatal cells are normally in balance (a). Acute neuroleptic DA blockade produces excess glutamate-mediated excitation (b). Striatal cells respond during chronic neuroleptic-induced DA blockade by both decreasing excitatory glutamate input and increasing inhibitory dopamine receptors to restore the neuronal balance (c). (After Freed, 1988.)

supersensitivity–subsensitivity hypothesis, once again, an alternative explanation may be the localization of DA receptors on the glutamate-containing neurons.

The supersensitivity–subsensitivity hypothesis is a novel approach in examining the underlying etiology of schizophrenia. The notion of both increasing and decreasing receptor sensitivities following a selective neurotoxic lesion in order to maintain a physiological balance is appealing. It provides ample opportunities for further testing using biochemical, electrophysiological, and behavioral measures. As with the previously discussed models, this hypothesis does not attempt to pinpoint the site of the disorder, but provides a testable model to uncover one link in a series of neuronal events that leads to schizophrenic behavior.

A second model that emphasizes glutamatergic input to the striatum has been proposed by Grace (1992), who summarizes a large amount of data. This model is based on the evidence for presynaptic glutamate modulation of DA function. Stimulation of corticostriatal fibers or the application of glutamate to DA terminals increases DA levels in the striatum without increasing DA cell firing. In addition, stress also increases DA metabolites without increasing DA cell firing, and its effect can be antagonized by glutamate receptor (NMDA) blockers. This glutamate-induced increase in DA release may be counterbalanced in vivo by glutamate-induced activation of GABA cell firing, which subsequently inhibits DA cell function. These DA modulatory actions by glutamate and GABA may provide a tonic DA cell function that can be altered by DA axon discharge that releases synaptic DA (phasic response), ultimately eliciting a behavioral response. The tonic DA cell function can also modify the phasic response of the DA cell because the low-level tonic DA release can act on autoreceptors to reduce the amount of DA released by subsequent action potentials. Thus, one would anticipate that cortical glutamate-induced tonic DA levels should normally modulate (by reducing) DA cell firing, producing less phasic DA release. Thus, if schizophrenics showed low glutamate activity, one would anticipate an abnormally large action potential–induced DA release and subsequent elevation in HVA. These neurochemical changes have been suggested as the basis for the positive symptoms of schizophrenia.

The relationship of this model to schizophrenia is based on the existing evidence of low glutamate activity in those with the disorder. Since cortical cells that project to subcortical centers are heavily glutamatergic, the hypofrontality of many schizophrenics may reflect low glutamate function. Furthermore, some direct evidence for low CSF glutamate levels in schizophrenics has been found, although not universally. An increase in glutamate binding in the postmortem striatum suggests an up-regulation of its receptors in response to reduced glutamate function (Kornhuber et al., 1989). In addition,

synaptosomes prepared from postmortem schizophrenic brains show reduced depolarization-induced efflux of glutamate (Sherman et al., 1991).

Changes in glutamate receptors in numerous brain areas of schizophrenics have been described (Ulas and Cotman, 1993), with some variability that is attributed to long postmortem intervals, varying drug histories, various stages of the disorder, and so forth. Of particular interest is the discovery that many of the classic neuroleptics interact with the NMDA receptor–ion channel complex. For instance, in at least one report, chronic haloperidol up-regulated the PCP binding site within the NMDA receptor–ion channel (see Ulas and Cotman, 1993). Furthermore, clozapine also modifies glutamatergic function. Clozapine inhibits binding to the PCP site and increases glutamate levels in the rat medial prefrontal cortex. The interaction of neuroleptic drugs with the glutamate neurons suggests that the glutamate NMDA receptor–ion channel complex may be a novel target for new antipsychotic drugs. One method involves facilitating glutamate transmission by activating the NMDA receptor–ion channel complex with glycine. Early studies using this amino acid have provided mixed results (see Ulas and Cotman, 1993; Bunney, Bunney, and Carlsson, 1995); however, this and other techniques for potentiating glutamate function remain to be evaluated more fully. For a detailed discussion of the interaction of glutamate and DA in the production of schizophrenic symptoms, as well as an analysis of the neuronal circuitry and receptor types involved, see Bunney, Bunney, and Carlsson (1995).

Summary

The positive symptoms of schizophrenia are significantly reduced by the classic and the atypical antipsychotic drugs in a majority of schizophrenic patients. Evidence suggests a central role for DA receptor blockade in the mechanism of action of the effective drugs, particularly in limbic and cortical areas of the brain. Further chemical refinements that improve the drugs' specificities for receptor subtypes may enhance their safety, selectivity, and effectiveness. Thus the nature and function of the DA systems have been extensively evaluated (see Chapter 8), as well as their integration with other neurotransmitter systems.

A significant amount of evidence also points to a role for DA in the etiology of schizophrenia. However, abnormalities in DA transmission do not account for all aspects of the disorder, nor is the DA hypothesis free from contradictions. In considering the biological defects in schizophrenia, we must recall not only the intricate interaction among the neural circuits underlying complex human behaviors, but also the role of genetics in the disorder, involvement of neurodevelopmental insults, and the evidence for structural CNS differences. Several neurochemical hypotheses, which are not necessarily mutually exclusive, have been briefly described. It is helpful to recall that, superimposed on the complexity of neural function, we must also evaluate the contribution of unique social and psychological factors that impinge on the individual to produce a distinctive constellation of symptoms.

Great strides have been made in understanding the complex function of various neurotransmitter systems. With the continued development and refinement of neurobiological techniques, greater precision in the measurement and regulation of brain function is inevitable. Unfortunately, application of these techniques in diagnoses and treatment of human psychopathology lags behind the advances in basic research because of the complexities of human behavior.

Chapter 19

Affective Disorders

Part I
Affective Disorders and Antidepressant Drugs

Clinical Profile

The second major class of psychoses comprises the affective disorders, which are characterized by extreme and inappropriate exaggerations of mood without the severely disturbed thought processes that are characteristic of schizophrenia. The disturbances in thinking and motor behavior that do occur are consistent with the exaggerated mood, although the mood does not reflect a realistic appraisal of the environment at the time.

The affective disorders are often considered less devastating than schizophrenia because most individuals have extended periods of normalcy between their episodes of affective disorder, during which time they are capable of normal social or occupational functioning. For example, even without treatment, 40% of patients hospitalized with depression recover within a year. Although some individuals may suffer only a single episode, for most, depressive periods are recurrent.

In comparison to schizophrenia, affective disorders are much more prevalent. Estimates of their incidence suggest that 10% to 20% of the U.S. population will experience a significant episode of affective disorder at some time in their lives, and perhaps 4% of the world's population suffers from severe depression at any one time. Approximately 1 out of 50 cases of affective disorder is sufficiently severe to require hospitalization.

Description

The DSM-IV describes two principal types of affective disorder: major depression and bipolar disorder. **Depression** refers to the affective state of sadness that occurs in response to a variety of human situations such as loss of a loved one, failure to achieve goals, or disappointment in love. Pathological depression differs only in intensity and duration or quality of the emotional state. The dysphoric mood is characterized by loss of interest in almost everything and the inability to experience pleasure in anything (anhedonia). Most depressed patients express feelings of hopelessness, worthlessness, sadness, guilt, and desperation. Frequently patients exhibit loss of appetite, insomnia, crying, diminished sexual desire, loss of ambition, fatigue, and motor retardation or agitation. Physical symptoms may include localized pain, severe digestive disturbances, and difficulty breathing. Severe depression can be extremely debilitating. Individuals may stop eating or caring for themselves physically, sometimes remaining in bed for prolonged periods. Self-devaluation and loss of self-esteem are very common and are combined with a complete sense of hopelessness about the future, which may end in suicide. One estimate of suicide rates suggests that 7% to 15% of depressed individuals commit suicide, in contrast to the total population rate of 1% to 1.5%. Untreated episodes of depression usually last from 7–14 months and recur throughout life, often increasing in frequency in later life. Later episodes tend to occur more abruptly and are less likely to be preceded by increased psychosocial stress (see Gold, Goodwin, and Chrousos, 1988a).

Because the symptoms and consequences of depression are so severe, depression is the subject of much clinical and pharmacological research. The patterns of symptoms vary significantly from individual to individual. This heterogeneity in the population of depressed patients adds to the variability of results in experiments attempting to correlate mental state with changes in neurochemistry. Numerous attempts have been made to identify subgroups of depressed individuals, and they have been classified on the basis of several factors, including age (senile–involutional), motor activity (agitated–retarded depression), stimulus preceding onset (endogenous–exogenous or reactive), or clinical features (neurotic–psychotic). DSM-IV recognizes one subtype of depression that may have an endogenous basis: depression with melancholia. Patients of this subtype display many vegetative symptoms, including reduced appetite, decreased sex drive, disturbed sleep with early morning awakening, and autonomic signs of stress. The patients are characterized by intense arousal centered on feelings of personal inadequacy and inevitable loss. Although such classification has not been extremely useful for identifying a therapeutic protocol, it has been of some value in biological studies that assume multiple etiologies for the subtypes.

Mania involves symptoms that are almost the exact opposite of those of depression; elation is the primary symptom. Manic individuals feel faultless, full of fun, bursting with energy. Their need for sleep is significantly reduced. They tend to be more talkative than usual and subjectively experience racing thoughts and ideas. They tend to make impulsive decisions of the grandiose sort and have unlimited confidence in themselves. The manic individual becomes involved in activities that have a high potential for negative consequences that goes unrecognized, such as foolish business investments, reckless driving, buying sprees, or sexual indiscretions. Some manic individuals, however, are capable of highly productive efforts when channeled appropriately. In some individuals, the predominant mood is irritability, belligerence, and impatience. Those individuals who alternate between periods of mania and depression are manic–depressive, and are suffering from **bipolar disorder**, while recurring episodes of major depression constitute **unipolar depression**.

Demography

Major depression can be found worldwide, although there may be culturally determined symptoms. The prevalence of depressive symptoms ranges from 13% to 20% of the population. The risk factors associated with the disorder are being a woman, particularly between the ages of 35 and 45, having a family history of depression or alcoholism, experiencing parental death before the age of 11, childhood exposure to a disruptive, hostile, and negative family environment, having had recent negative life events preceding the depressive episode, and being divorced or separated (Weissman and Boyd, 1984). In general, females are two to three times as likely to develop major depression as males. Whites are slightly more likely to develop the disorder than blacks; no socioeconomic differences are apparent. The first episode of depression can occur at any age, although the median age is about 40 years. Although their symptoms may differ from those in adults, children and adolescents can develop depression. In contrast to depression, bipolar disorder affects men and women equally (0.65% versus 0.88%), and the average age of onset is in the late 20s or early 30s.

Relationship to Stress

Despite existing research on the subject, the significance of stress in the development of affective disorders is unclear. Although psychosocial factors in some cases may precipitate major depression, many episodes of depression are unrelated to real-life problems and stresses. One possible explanation is that stress-induced episodes may be more prevalent early in the course of the disorder, while in later life the same individual may experience episodes independent of life stresses (Gold, Goodwin, and Chrousos, 1988). A second consideration is that, although for the average individual stress does not necessarily lead to mental disorders, stress in the susceptible individual may precipitate a variety of emotional and cognitive difficulties. Although depressed individuals tend to report more stressful events in their lives, it is seldom clear whether the stress preceded the depression or whether the depression preceded the stress. Clearly, depression leads to occupational stress following poor performance, social stresses, and isolation from friends, as well as marital problems. Since depression is not more frequent among the poor, we might conclude that socioeconomic stress is unrelated to the disorder. Furthermore, major depression is relatively resistant to psychotherapy or positive environmental change (without adjunctive pharmacotherapy), contrary to what one might expect if it were merely a product of stressful life situations.

Genetics

Research into the heritability of affective disorders leads one to conclude that a genetic propensity to develop the disorders plays some role in their etiology. Genetic studies of affective illness are important because they provide direction for clinical research into the origin, progression, and definition of the disease. In addition, such research can be used to identify other disorders that may be cotransmitted genetically with the affective disorders. This type of research may also identify etiological markers, that is, unusual physical or biochemical parameters that cotransmit with the disorder and have the potential to aid in early diagnosis. Ultimately, precise localization and modification of the genes that play a significant part in these and other disorders may be possible. Excellent summaries of the issues regarding the genetics of affective illness are found in reviews by Gershon and colleagues (1987) and Mackinnon and Mitchell (1994).

Many epidemiological studies report several times higher rates of affective illness in first-degree relatives (parents, siblings, and offspring) of individuals with an affective disorder than in the general population. Differences in the estimates from various studies are likely due to differences in methods and criteria for diagnosis and in population sampling. A cultural difference has been reported that demonstrates a higher lifetime prevalence of affective illness in individuals born after 1940. The basis for this difference is unknown, but it contributes to the disparities in epidemiological results.

One further well-documented finding shows that there is a significant amount of unipolar depression in relatives of bipolar patients, although bipolar depression does not occur more frequently in family members of patients with major depression. These results suggest a partial genetic overlap of the two disorders (Gershon et al., 1987). These authors have also reported an association between bipolar illness and schizoaffective disorder and cyclothymic personality, which are related but diagnostically discrete syndromes (see DSM-IV). Furthermore, anorexia and bulimia have a familial association with affective disorders. Familial studies also suggest that unipolar depression may consist of several subgroups, one of which may be cotransmitted with alcoholism. More recent results have found that among children or adolescents hospitalized for severe depression, higher rates of affective disorders and alcoholism exist among their adult relatives.

The best evidence for a heritable component to affective illness comes from twin studies, which show a difference between monozygotic and dizygotic twins in their rate of concordance for affective illness. One report using the Danish Twin Register evaluated 110 same-sex twin pairs born between 1870 and 1920 (Bertelsen, Havvald, and Hauge, 1977). Concordance for unipolar depression in monozygotic twins was 54%, while dyzygotic twins had a concordance of 19%. The difference in concordance for bipolar illness was even greater (79% in monozygotic vs. 24% in dizygotic twins), suggesting a stronger heritable component for manic–depressive disorder.

Examination of the biological and foster families of adopted children who developed affective disorders showed a high incidence (31%) of affective disorder in the biologic parents of 29 bipolar adoptees compared

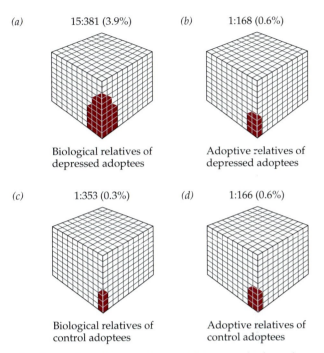

19.1 THE OCCURRENCE OF SUICIDES among biological (*a*) and adoptive (*b*) relatives of adopted bipolar patients, as well as suicide rate of biological (*c*) and adoptive (*d*) relatives of mentally healthy adopted individuals. The ratios of the number of relatives who commit suicide to total number of relatives shows a sixfold increase in suicide among biological relatives of depressed adoptees. (After Kety, 1979.)

with the biological (2%) or adoptive (9%) parents of normal adoptees (Mendlewicz and Rainer, 1977). Furthermore, biological relatives of 71 adoptees with affective disorders included significantly more suicides (3.9%) than adoptive relatives of those individuals (0.6%) or biological (0.3%) or adoptive (0.6%) relatives of control adoptees (Kety, 1979). Figure 19.1 shows the ratios of suicides to total family members for both depressed adoptees and control adoptees.

These earlier heritability studies demonstrate that prenatal or perinatal events predispose some individuals to affective disorders. They do not, however, rule out environmental factors, such as stress, in determining onset or symptomatology. At this time, the heritability of the major affective disorders is apparent, although much work remains to elucidate the type of genetic transmission and to identify the specific genetic defect.

Physiological Correlates of Depression

The heterogeneous diagnosis of depression is made up of at least several subtypes that have not been effectively identified through clinical evaluation or treatment response variables. Although several physiological measures have yielded interesting differences among patients, the results have not produced a definitive delineation of subtypes. Since many of the vegetative symptoms of the disorders reflect potential changes in the hypothalamic regulation of feeding, libido, sleep, and circadian hormone release, it is not surprising that research on depression has focused on these functions.

Biological Rhythms: Cortisol Secretion

Excessive secretion of adrenal cortisol in response to a higher than normal release of adrenocorticotropin (ACTH) from the pituitary is the most consistent neuroendocrine abnormality identified in depressed individuals (Kandel, 1991c). Approximately 50% of depressed patients show this elevation, which is characterized by blunted circadian rhythms. The patients' elevated cortisol levels persist during the afternoon and evening, at which time normal individuals show much lower concentrations than their peak levels in the morning (Figure 19.2).

The ACTH-induced release of adrenal cortisol is normally regulated by hypothalamic secretion of corticotropin-releasing factor (CRF). CRF is in turn regulated by hypothalamic neurotransmitters, including norepinephrine, acetylcholine, and GABA. Gold, Goodwin, and Chrousos (1988b) provide several pieces of evidence to suggest that the abnormal cortisol levels found in some depressed individuals are due to a defect in the brain at or above the level of the hypothalamus (i.e., neurotransmitter regulation of CRF secretion). Animal studies have shown that intracerebroventricular administration of CRF elicits responses similar to those found in some depressed individuals and which reflect a state of anxiety: sympathetic arousal, increased adrenal response, anorexia, and decreased libido.

Under normal circumstances, adrenal steroids are beneficial in preparing the organism for stress and maintaining stability within the CNS, but when corticosteroid levels are persistently elevated, several systems begin to show pathological changes. Among the potentially damaging effects are neuronal atrophy in the hippocampus, leading to cognitive impairment, imbalances in the 5-HT system correlated with anxiety, and elevated insulin and corticosteroids associated with depression (see McEwen et al., 1994).

Dexamethasone suppression test.   Since approximately 50% of depressed patients demonstrate hypercortisolism, clinical research has focused on methods to evaluate hypothalamic–pituitary–adrenal axis function. The most commonly used research tool is the dexamethasone suppression test (DST). Dexamethasone is a synthetic glucocorticoid that suppresses ACTH production, which results in a decrease in cortisol levels. Those individuals who do not suppress cortisol levels are considered to be abnormal responders.

Since many depressed patients have elevated cortisol levels, it is not surprising that some individuals with major depression are dexamethasone nonresponders. It had been hoped that the nonresponders represent a therapeutically distinct population; one for which successful neurochemical treatments might be predicted by their evidence of hormonal imbalance. Although some evidence suggests that 90% of nonresponders have an excellent recovery following treatment with tricyclic antidepressants (Georgotas, 1985), most studies do not seem to provide evidence for a consistent difference in antidepressant effectiveness between normal and abnormal responders.

Reviewing the literature in which dexamethasone suppression was evaluated along with clinical improvement following antidepressant treatment, Arana and Baldessarini (1987) found a small but statistically significant difference in response rate to antidepressant drugs. Nonsuppressors (abnormal) improved at a rate of 81.6% while suppressors improved at a 73.5% rate. A summary of nine well-controlled studies also examined the minimal difference in the rate of successful drug treatment for responders versus nonresponders (Kathol and Carter, 1990). The average success rate in these studies was 76% in the normal response group versus 69% in the abnormal response group, indicating only a marginal difference in response rate between the two groups). It seems quite evident that lacking an abnormal cortisol response does not indicate ineffectiveness of pharmacotherapy, nor does the test suggest that distinct antidepressant treatment is required.

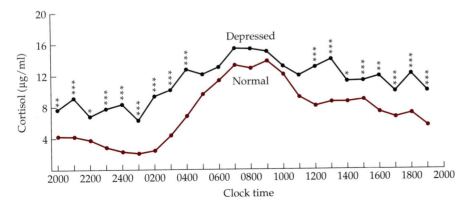

19.2 AVERAGE PLASMA CORTISOL CONCENTRATIONS measured every hour in 7 unipolar depressed patients and 54 control subjects. The normal reduction in plasma cortisol occurring in the early morning and in the evening is significantly blunted in depressed patients. (*$p < 0.05$; **$p < 0.01$; ***$p < 0.001$) (After Kandel, 1991c.)

Despite the lack of predictive value of DST regarding treatment effectiveness, one potential value of DST testing is predicting early relapse after terminating successful treatment with antidepressants. Several studies suggest that there is significantly greater probability of relapse in those patients who remain dexamethasone nonresponders as compared with those who show normal cortisol suppression following successful treatment (Kathol and Carter, 1990).

Biological Rhythms: Sleep and REM

Sleep disturbances of various types are among the most common symptoms of major depressive disorders. Because this symptom occurs in the vast majority of depressed individuals, it has generated significant research interest. The normal sleep cycle is quite regular, with four stages of non-REM sleep, lasting 90–120 minutes, followed by a 10–15 minute period of rapid eye movement (REM) sleep, during which dreaming occurs. For healthy adults the cycle is repeated regularly throughout the night, but for individuals suffering from depression, a variety of irregularities occur (James and Amsterdam, 1990).

Among the sleep abnormalities in depressed individuals is a decrease in time spent in slow-wave or deep sleep (stages 3 and 4), leading to repeated awakenings and more frequent changes between sleep stages than usual. In addition, an altered distribution of REM episodes throughout the night has been well documented. The most reliable finding is that the onset of REM occurs earlier after the onset of sleep. Although decreased REM latency may be correlated with severity of symptoms, it may also be a stable trait marker or a vulnerability factor for depression. Giles and colleagues (Giles et al., 1987) found that those depressed patients undergoing treatment who show a reduced REM latency during an episode of depression have a greater probability of relapse and a decreased time for depression to recur. They suggest that those patients with stable reduced REM latency may have associated physiological abnormalities that are slow to change in response to therapy. Therefore, if the abnormalities persist, it suggests that the individual may be biologically vulnerable to relapse.

In addition to reduced latency of REM onset, REM is also significantly increased during the first one-third of the night in depressed individuals, while nondepressed individuals have proportionately more REM in the final one-third of sleep. Also, while normal REM periods tend to increase in duration during the night, unipolar depressed patients do not show such a pattern. When ocular movement is measured, depressed individuals show more frequent eye movements during REM, which suggests more intense dreaming (see James and Amsterdam, 1990).

Although these rather consistent sleep irregularities in depressed individuals are intriguing, other patients with clinical conditions such as alcoholism, schizophrenia, and anorexia also show similar REM variations. Sleep abnormalities may also occur in narcolepsy, in those with sleep apnea, and following sleep deprivation in healthy individuals (James and Amsterdam, 1990). Perhaps the most important result of the REM sleep findings is that it has led to the investigation of circadian rhythms and the potentially useful therapeutic approach, sleep deprivation.

Chronobiological research evaluates the role of altered circadian rhythms in depression. Although humans are adjusted to the 24-hour day because of external environmental signals, under free-run conditions when no external cues are available, the endogenous circadian period is closer to 25 hours. Body functions that operate on circadian rhythms, such as body temperature, hormone secretion, and sleep–waking, are under the control of several distinct oscillators, which may desynchronize and fail to maintain the same rhythm especially when no external cues are available. For that reason, some individuals may become desynchronized according to external cues and may fail to coordinate individual circadian body functions.

The abnormalities in sleep patterns found in depressed individuals resemble the sleep patterns of normal individuals who must alter their time of sleep by a 12-hour period. Other indicators of biological rhythms, such as body temperature and hormonal secretion (e.g., cortisol), are also altered in some depressed patients. Given the nature of these physiological changes, the possibility of a "phase advance" in biological rhythms must be considered. Alternatively, a desynchronization (mismatching) of the timing oscillators that regulate REM sleep and the sleep–waking cycle may exist. Further discussion of these hypotheses, along with current references and their implications for therapy, can be found in the reviews by James and Amsterdam (1990), Gold, Goodwin, and Chrousos (1988b), and Wirz-Justice (1995).

Sleep deprivation treatment. The chronobiological hypotheses have led to treatment of depressive disorders, particularly of the endogenous type, with manipulations of the sleep–waking cycle (Wehr, 1990; Wu and Bunney, 1990). According to a summary of results compiled from 61 studies completed over 20 years, involving over 1,700 individuals, total sleep deprivation significantly reduced depressive symptoms in 59% of the patients (Wu and Bunney, 1990). Figure 19.3 shows a typical profile of symptoms before and after sleep deprivation in a group of unipolar depressed patients. Unfortunately, efficacy of this therapy is usually lost after the first night of sleep following deprivation. Although improvement was not related to age, sex, or length of illness, Nasrallah and Coryell (1982) found that sleep deprivation transiently alleviated depression most effectively in those individuals who were dexamethasone nonsuppressors. Of the non-

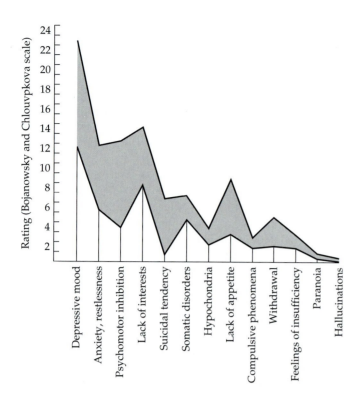

19.3 THE EFFECT OF SLEEP DEPRIVATION ON A PROFILE OF SYMPTOMS IN PATIENTS WITH UNIPOLAR DEPRESSION. The shaded area represents the difference in rating score before and after sleep deprivation therapy. (After Pflug, 1988.)

those given antidepressant medication relapsed after sleeping.

Partial sleep deprivation, especially during the second half of the night, also seems to be effective in reducing symptoms, particularly in conjunction with antidepressant medication. Many of the clinical trials utilized classic antidepressant medication along with total or partial sleep deprivation, and reported that the depressed patients improve more quickly with combined sleep deprivation therapy than with antidepressants alone. Van Bemmel and Van den Hoofdakker (1981) found that clomipramine plus a four-night schedule of partial sleep deprivation was significantly more effective than either clomipramine alone or four nights of sleep deprivation alone. Following one night of total deprivation, subsequent sleep was limited to 2 or 5 hours a night as a maintenance therapy.

Based on the chronobiological hypothesis that the onset of REM is abnormally early relative to sleep onset, attempts have been made to correct the relationship by moving bedtime to earlier in the evening. Such a phase-advance technique has met with some apparent success without the need for deprivation of sleep (Sack et al., 1985). A review by Berger and Riemann (1993) considers the use of phase-advance techniques, partial sleep deprivation, and napping variables (such as duration, timing, and REM architecture) to enhance the antidepressant effects of total sleep deprivation.

In an attempt to unify the existing data, Wu and Bunney (1990) have modified earlier models of sleep biochemistry and developed a theory of the depression-

suppressors, 57% showed some improvement, compared with only 7% of normal dexamethasone suppressors. The therapeutic effect of sleep deprivation in neurotic depression tends to be less pronounced than for endogenous depression. In addition, the neurotic depression group is atypical in that their response tends to appear on the second day after sleep deprivation (Pflug, 1988).

The timing of the antidepressant effect of sleep deprivation has been examined in several studies, and their combined results are shown in Figure 19.4. Depression ratings from eight studies (34 patients responding and 6 nonresponding to sleep deprivation therapy) were transformed to scores on a visual analog scale (Wu and Bunney, 1990). The mean scores are shown before, during, and after sleep deprivation and after the first night of recovery sleep. The average depression scores for the responders showed a gradual decrease during the day before sleep deprivation, reflecting the diurnal decrease in symptoms after waking that is typical in endogenously depressed individuals. That decrease in symptoms continues during the hours of sleep deprivation and into the next day. Following a single night of sleep, however, symptoms returned in these individuals. In other experiments examining relapse (17 studies with 158 subjects), 83% of the patients not receiving medication relapsed after one night's sleep, while only 59% of

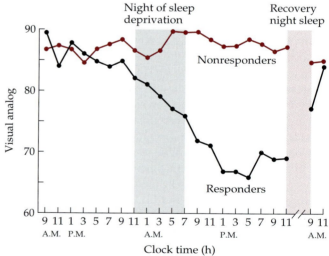

19.4 EFFECTS OF SLEEP DEPRIVATION ON MOOD RATING for depressed patients after one night of total sleep deprivation and after one recovery night of sleep. The data, taken from eight separate experiments, have been transformed to an analog scale that represents the extremes from high depression to no depression. The two curves represent those patients who responded to sleep deprivation treatment and those who were nonresponders. (After Wu and Bunney, 1990.)

inducing effects of sleep and the antidepressant action of wakefulness. They suggest that during sleep, a depression-inducing substance is released that may be a natural sleep-satiety factor. This factor would then be metabolized or eliminated during periods of wakefulness. If depressed individuals either release excessive depression-inducing substance or fail to metabolize the substance adequately, the sleep-satiety factor would be elevated, producing early morning waking or other sleep irregularities associated with depression. This hypothesis could explain why sleep deprivation (i.e., preventing release of the factor) alleviates depression for many and why napping (i.e., inducing release of the factor), even for as short a period as several minutes, exacerbates depressive symptoms for some patients. This theory also explains the frequent occurrence of diurnal mood swings, with worsening of symptoms early in the day followed by gradual improvement.

Despite the appeal of such a model, no unique depression-inducing substance released during sleep has been identified or isolated. The authors have suggested several candidates: (1) growth hormone, which is a sleep-released substance in humans, (2) cortisol, which shows abnormal rhythms in depressed individuals, or (3) neurochemical events related to REM episodes, such as increased cholinergic cell firing and reduced NE and 5-HT activity. Much more investigation is required before pharmacological intervention can be developed to mimic the therapeutic effects of sleep cycle regulation.

Whether sleep deprivation and phase-shift techniques are effective because of biological clock alterations or are due to REM deprivation is not clear. Unfortunately, many of the studies reporting success with sleep or REM deprivation are either case studies with a single subject or uncontrolled studies on a small scale, rather than the placebo-controlled, double-blind procedures optimally employed in clinical research. However, the fact that most of the classical antidepressant drugs reduce REM sleep contributes to the argument that REM sleep may be critical to mood changes in depressed patients. Of course, since sleep and REM are regulated by synergistic actions of several neurotransmitter systems, the sleep therapies and antidepressant drug therapies may have identical neurochemical bases.

Seasonal Affective Disorder (SAD)

Scheduling sleep earlier in the evening may have a transient antidepressant effect because it restores the phase relationship between sleep and other endogenous circadian rhythms. An alternative mode of phase shifting is by exposure to bright artificial light, which shifts circadian rhythms in humans much the way day length regulates seasonal rhythms in animals. Apparently, a subset of depressed individuals exists who experience recurring bouts of depression that begin with the onset of shorter days and longer nights in the fall and show remission in

the spring as the daylight hours increase. These individuals are described as having seasonal affective disorder (SAD). In contrast to the early waking characteristic of endogenous depression, these individuals tend to sleep longer in the morning, suggesting a circadian shift in the opposite direction. Moreover, shifts in the pattern of melatonin production (a pineal gland hormone regulated by light exposure) are another characteristic of a subset of depressed patients with this unique circadian phase change. Lewy and Sack (1990) present evidence of significant antidepressant effects (assessed with the Hamilton Depression Rating Scale) after 1 week of exposure to bright artificial light from 6:00–8:00 A.M. compared to evening light exposure (8:00–10:00 P.M.) or to baseline measures in the same individuals. The efficacy of light treatment for depressed patients other than those suffering from SAD is controversial. However, research into hormonal and physiological differences in the seasonally depressed patient, as well as experimental results from several laboratories, provides intriguing possibilities (Skewer et al., 1988; Terman et al., 1989). A recent review (Wirz-Justice, 1995) summarizes various circardian hypotheses and provides a discussion of the conceptual approach to examining the complex circadian rhythms as well as their neuropharmacological regulation.

Biogenic Amine Hypothesis

The discovery of a genetic link in the incidence of affective disorders prompted the search for a psychobiological explanation for these behaviors. The characteristic somatic symptoms that accompany these disorders, (e.g., the sleep disturbances and loss of appetite), the circadian cycle of depression, and the high incidence of associated endocrine and metabolic disorders further implicate altered biogenic amine function and neuroendocrine regulation as underlying mechanisms in affective disorders.

In addition, during the 1950s several drugs that altered mood and behavior were clinically tested and evaluated for their neurochemical mechanisms of action. For instance, reserpine, which is an effective agent in treating hypertension because it reduces sympathetic (adrenergic) constriction of blood vessels, was found to induce depression in a significant number of patients. The prolonged central depressant properties of reserpine are assumed to be due to the drug-induced inhibition of vesicular storage of several neurotransmitters, which are subsequently metabolized intraneuronally by MAO. The depression in mood that follows reserpine administration is considered by clinicians to be indistinguishable from naturally occurring depression. It became evident that a number of drugs that reduce the biogenic amine levels precipitate depression. In addition, effective antidepressant drugs of several different classes can at least acutely increase intracellular monoamine levels and also reverse reserpine-induced depression. From these early observations, the monoamine hypothesis of depression was formulated. It suggests that depression is related to a deficit of monoamines (particularly NE or 5-HT) at critical synapses, whereas mania is associated with an excess of monoamines at critical synapses (Schildkraut, 1965).

Because reserpine depletes stores of several monoamines, including DA, NE, and 5-HT, and the early antidepressant drugs had relatively nonselective effects on the same amines, the importance of a particular neurotransmitter to the development of depression was not immediately clear. Historically, in the United States, the catecholamines have been the focus of attention, whereas in Europe, serotonin has generated the most research interest. While understanding drug mechanisms has provided many valuable clues regarding the etiology of affective disorders, we must be fully aware of the potential fallacy in assuming that a given drug specifically restores a neurochemical error underlying the pathological condition. It is equally reasonable to assume that the drug works at a distance from a principal disease locus and that it restores a balance among a constellation of neurons, leading ultimately to a change in behavior. No longer are neurotransmitter systems considered in isolation, but rather as a part of a complex network of interacting systems.

It is now quite evident that the biogenic amine hypothesis as originally stated is too simplistic to account for the complex syndrome of affective disorders, which includes changes in mood, sleep, sexual activity, appetite, body temperature, motor activity, cognitive function, and so forth. Nor can the original hypothesis explain the fact that the antidepressant drugs rapidly alter amine concentrations, whereas their therapeutic effects are typically delayed by several weeks. In addition, there is no apparent direct relationship between the potency of the antidepressant effects in vitro on amines and the effective therapeutic dosage. For example, those tricyclic antidepressants that effectively elevate amine levels in vitro at low doses are not necessarily more potent clinically. Further, measurements of amine or metabolite concentrations in various fluids (e.g., blood, urine, CSF) taken from untreated depressed individuals have not consistently supported the original amine hypothesis. Also, many of the newest "second generation" antidepressants do not share similar neurochemical actions with the classic drugs upon which the amine hypothesis was based. A modified hypothesis must also take into account the significant neuroendocrine feedback regulation of behavior. Perhaps most significant is the consideration of the dynamic functioning of neurons in response to neurochemical changes induced acutely by drugs or environmental factors and those induced chronically by pathology underlying the disease.

The remainder of this chapter will consider the effectiveness of antidepressant drugs and their mode of action, experiments on animal behavior, and measurements of altered biogenic amines in human biological fluids.

Antidepressant Screening with Animal Models

Animal models are used to study the neurobiology of depression, to elucidate the mechanism of action of antidepressant drugs, and to screen new compounds for antidepressant action. As is true for most human behavioral disorders, the development of an appropriate animal model for major depression is difficult. The manifestations of depression are described in uniquely human terms, and inferences about the subjective state of an animal can be misleading. Also, drugs in this class, when administered acutely, rarely have much effect on normal animal behavior and in general do not produce significant increases in motor activity. In this respect, the lack of drug effects in animals resembles that found in healthy humans, in whom antidepressants do not cause euphoria or arousal, but may be dysphoric and unpleasant.

As is true for other measures of behavioral pharmacology (see Chapter 2, Part II), all models of depression or tests for antidepressant action should be evaluated for simplicity, cost, speed of performance, and reliability. In addition, any method ideally should have high validity. That means it should be sensitive enough to identify all known antidepressant agents, yet be selective enough to differentiate these drugs from other classes that do not have clinically useful antidepressant action.

Reserpine-Induced Sedation

One screening method used to identify clinically useful antidepressants is the antagonism or reversal of reserpine-induced effects. The rationale for this animal model is the high incidence of reserpine-induced depression in individuals treated for cardiovascular disorders, such as hypertension. The validity of the animal model has been demonstrated by the almost universal ability of clinically significant antidepressant agents to antagonize reserpine's sedative effect, although some new atypical antidepressants do not consistently produce the expected antagonism (Porsolt, Lenegre, and McArthur, 1991). It is important to keep in mind that although reversing reserpine-induced sedation indicates antidepressant action, drug-induced states of hyperactivity in animals do not. For instance, amphetamine, which can produce increased motor activity, is not generally considered an effective antidepressant. Thus, the predictive value of animal tests must be evaluated cautiously.

Reserpine-induced sedation is one of the oldest methods used in drug screening because in terms of face validity, it seems to be most analogous to human depression. However, other reserpine-induced effects provide an equally appropriate measure of drug-induced antagonism. Symptoms of the autonomic syndrome, including ptosis, miosis, prolapse of nictitating membrane, and hypersecretion of tears and saliva, also provide a ready measure and are frequently used in animal research, as is reserpine-induced hypothermia. In most cases, the novel antidepressant is compared with the effectiveness of a classic antidepressant, such as imipramine, in reversing reserpine's effects.

Behavioral Despair Syndrome

More complex measures of antidepressant activity involve use of behavioral models. One such model, developed by Porsolt and coworkers (1978), is the behavioral despair syndrome in rodents. In this task the animals are forced to swim in a water-filled container with no possible escape. After early unsuccessful attempts to escape, the animals assume an immobile posture except for the minimal movements needed to keep their heads above water. Effective antidepressants reduce the time spent in this "freezing" phase of immobility that occurs in untreated animals. The drugs also provide significant protection against water-immersion stress-induced ulcers and immobilization-induced ulcers. A modification of the method that is somewhat less stressful to the animals is the evaluation of immobility induced by suspending a rodent by the tail (Steru et al., 1985). A wide variety of antidepressants are effective in modifying this immobilization response, including a large number of atypical antidepressants that are inactive in other tests. Unfortunately, many other compounds not identified as antidepressants also reduce immobility under test conditions. Among these are some GABA agonists, calcium antagonists, atypical antipsychotics, and other drugs. Despite this difficulty, the test is widely used and is simple to perform and easily automated (Porsolt, Lenegre, and McArthur, 1991).

Learned Helplessness

A second classical behavioral model is that of learned helplessness, originally developed by Seligman (1975). In this paradigm, the subjects are initially exposed to aversive events (e.g., repetitive foot shock) over which they have no control. When the same subjects are placed in a new situation in which a response would alter an aversive event, they fail to make the appropriate response. Although the animals show signs of anxiety, their earlier experience in which their behavior had no effect on their environment, apparently reduces future attempts to cope. Since depressed humans frequently fail to respond to environmental changes and express feelings of hopelessness and the belief that nothing they do has an effect, the theoretical framework for learned helplessness as a model for depression is clear (Hamilton and Timmons, 1990; Willner, 1994).

Klein and Seligman (1976) demonstrated the learned helplessness phenomenon in humans using noxious noise as the uncontrollable aversive stimulus. These subjects showed clear cognitive deficiencies in later testing.

They were not only significantly less successful in complex problem solving, but also less persistent. Furthermore, the subjects were less likely to recognize a consistent rule that provided the solutions. The isomorphism of this behavioral model with human depression is further enhanced by neurochemical similarities that will be described in later sections of this chapter (see below).

While providing an appealing model for depression, the learned helplessness procedure is fairly time-consuming and therefore is not used as a rapid screening device for antidepressant drugs. However, it is sensitive to a large number of antidepressant agents, including some from the newer atypical class, when treatment follows the exposure to unavoidable noxious stimuli and occurs during the learning in stage 2. It is of particular interest that antianxiety drugs are not effective when administered in the same way, but can prevent learned helplessness if they are administered during exposure to the uncontrolled shocks (Porsolt, Lenegre, and McArthur, 1991; also see Feldman, 1962; 1968).

Olfactory Bulbectomy Model

The olfactory bulbectomy model in rodents has received considerable attention in the literature and provides a sensitive procedure for the screening of antidepressant drugs. The procedure involves the surgical removal of the olfactory bulbs followed by a recovery period and testing in any one of several designs, most often passive avoidance acquisition (see Chapter 2). The theoretical framework for such a model reflects the importance of limbic system modulation of emotion and memory for appropriate survival behavior (Richardson, 1991). Under normal circumstances, feeling good or bad following particular activities either reinforces or discourages our repetition of those actions. Accordingly, pathological emotional states, which reflect abnormalities in biological function, are responsible for the loss of normal reinforcement contingencies, thus depriving the individual of the survival value of emotions. The advantages of the model, as summarized by Richardson (1991), include several neurochemical and behavioral parallels between the olfactory bulbectomized rat and the patient with major depression (Table 19.1). The test is sensitive to a wide range of clinically active antidepressants, including both the classical tricyclics some atypical antidepressants. Additionally, the bulbectomy-induced deficits in behaviors similar to human symptoms of depression are modified only by chronic administration of effective antidepressant drugs and not by acute administration.

Other promising models include intracranial self-stimulation, chronic stress, social separation in primates, and many others. Willner (1994), Porsolt, Lenegre, and McArthur (1991), and Geyer and Markou (1995), provide excellent discussions of both behavioral models and pharmacological interaction models of depression in terms of predictive value, validity, and reliability. Discussion of

Table 19.1 Similarities between Humans with Major Depressive Disorder and Olfactory Bulbectomized Rats

Characteristic	Depressed patient	Olfactory bulbectomized rat
Neurotransmitter systems	Probable abnormalities in NE, 5-HT, ACh, GABA, and other neurotransmitters	Demonstrated abnormalities in NE, 5-HT, ACh, GABA, and other neurostransmitters
Neuroanatomical substrate	Probable dysregulation of the limbic–hypothalamic axis	Demonstrated dysregulation of the limbic–hypothalamic axis
Endocrine system	Elevated plasma corticosteroids (cortisol)	Elevated plasma corticosteroids (corticosterone)
Mood	Depressed mood, sadness, hopelessness	Not testable
Activity and sleep	Agitation, sleep disorder	Hyperactivity, abnormal sleep pattern
Motivation	No interest in food, weight loss, no interest in sex	Abnormal daily eating pattern, reduced weight gain, abnormal lordosis and other sexual behaviors
Aggression	Hyperirritability	Hyperreactity, increased aggression
Learning and cognition	Insensitivity to positive and negative reinforcement	Deficits in learning tasks involving positive or negative reinforcement
	Cognitive disorder; verbalization of persistent inappropriate ideas	Performance of perseverative maladaptive behavior
Response to drug therapy	Characteristic response to chronic but not acute antidepressants (MAOIs effective in atypical depression)	Characteristic response to chronic but not acute antidepressants except for MAOIs

Source: After Richardson, 1991.

clinical measures of depression, such as the Hamilton Depression Rating Scale, is provided by Kellner (1994).

Effectiveness of Pharmacotherapy

Pharmacological treatment of depressive disorders includes the three major classes of antidepressants: monoamine oxidase inhibitors, tricyclic antidepressants, and the second-generation antidepressants, which include the selective serotonin uptake blockers. In addition, there are several types of atypical antidepressants as well as electroconvulsive therapy (ECT). Lithium therapy will be considered separately because of its primary importance in treating bipolar disorder. Evidence compiled over the years from double-blind, placebo-controlled trials of antidepressant drugs from all classes have shown them to be effective in alleviating symptoms in approximately 65% to 75% of patients with major depression. In contrast, placebo response rate averages 35% after one month of treatment (Burke and Preskorn, 1995). Furthermore, there is no evidence that efficacy of a specific drug or specific antidepressant class is superior. In those instances in which high doses are used, success rate may increase to 85%.

The effectiveness of the antidepressants includes reduction of virtually all of the symptoms of major depression described in the DSM-IV, although the vegetative symptoms (e.g., sleep disturbances, changes in appetite, etc.) are often the most rapidly improved. Immediate improvement of symptoms occurs in only a very small number of cases. Significant changes in symptoms usually require 1–3 weeks of drug treatment, while maximum effectiveness may not be achieved until after 4–6 weeks of therapy. The slow onset of effectiveness is characteristic for all types of antidepressants, including electroconvulsive therapy.

The modest 65% to 75% rate of effectiveness of these drugs compared with placebo may in part be explained by the difficulties confronted in controlled clinical testing, not the least of which is the high rate of spontaneous recovery and a contribution by the placebo effect. In addition, many studies are short in duration (4 weeks or less), providing insufficient time for drug effectiveness to be revealed. Moreover, it is difficult to estimate the optimum dosage for a given patient since most clinical trials until recently did not monitor plasma levels of the drugs. It is apparent that steady state plasma levels vary widely (up to 40-fold) for the same dose administered to different individuals. The factor most responsible for this difference in blood drug levels is genetic variation in the ability to metabolize the drugs, although diet, smoking, and use of other medications may also play a role (Simpson and Singh, 1990). Further, steady state levels, that is, when the amount of drug eliminated daily equals the amount absorbed, are achieved only after about 5–7 days of consistent antidepressant treatment. For these reasons dosage requirements must be individualized.

Furthermore, while some classic antidepressants, such as imipramine, have a linear relationship between plasma level and therapeutic response, others, such as nortriptyline, have a curvilinear relationship, requiring plasma levels to fall within a relatively narrow "therapeutic window." Data regarding the relationship between plasma level and therapeutic response is not available for many conventionally used antidepressants. Evidence suggests that at least half of the nonresponding individuals may show significant improvement at increased dosages (Quitkin, 1985).

Finally, the initial selection of subjects, the method of diagnosis, and the characteristics of subjects completing the study may jeopardize an unbiased evaluation of the results of a clinical trial. Because ethical concerns are raised in treating a seriously ill and potentially suicidal individual with a placebo, most studies use mild or moderately depressed outpatients for subjects rather than more seriously ill hospitalized individuals. Such patient selection may help to explain the disparity between results reported in the psychiatric literature and those that an individual clinician observes. Alternatively, when using severely depressed patients in a study, an experimental antidepressant may be compared with an antidepressant known to be effective as the control condition. Additionally, the use of outpatients makes compliance with the drug administration schedule a significant variable. Patients unaware of the slow onset of effectiveness may lose hope and terminate drug taking if no effect occurs within the first few weeks. Others who experience relief may terminate drug taking early, being unaware of the high probability of relapse. Still others may fail to follow the prescribed drug regimen or be dropped from the study due to undesirable side effects. Since statistical evaluation usually includes only those patients who continue the full course of treatment, unbiased evaluation of drug effectiveness may be compromised by the dropout rate.

Selection of patients based on DSM-IV criteria greatly improves the probability of homogeneous subtypes of depression, although different symptoms may be emphasized in selecting them for various studies. Comparisons between studies are improved by the frequent use of the Hamilton rating scale for depression as the dependent variable. A 50% reduction in the Hamilton score is the usual operational definition of "improvement." However, 50% improvement may still leave the patient with significant symptoms. Hence, the study may indicate successful treatment while the pa-

tient may report relative failure. An excellent discussion of the methodological issues relevant to the evaluation of antidepressant medication within depressive subtypes can be found in Brotman, Falk, and Gelenberg (1987).

Depression Subtypes

Despite the development of new antidepressant drugs, no single class of antidepressants is clearly more effective than another. Nevertheless, recent approaches to therapeutics have attempted to identify subtypes of depression that will predict differential responsiveness to the antidepressant compounds on the whole.

Brotman and colleagues (1987) have identified six general subtypes of depression that may aid in predicting antidepressant efficacy: major depression with melancholia or endogenous features, major depression without melancholia (atypical), major depression with psychotic features (delusional), bipolar depression, dysthymic disorder, and "treatment resistant" depression. The majority of depressed patients exhibit symptoms of major depression with melancholia and are those who show the most favorable response to antidepressants, especially the tricyclic antidepressants (TCAs) (Burke and Preskorn, 1995). Clusters of symptoms for individuals within this group may further predict effectiveness. Among those positive predictors are psychomotor retardation, anhedonia (loss of enjoyment in usually pleasurable activities), emotional withdrawal, early morning waking, and a diurnal mood swing that is worse in the morning. A family history of major depression and good response to previous antidepressant therapy also predict a positive response to pharmacotherapy. Poor prognosis may be related to the presence of agitation, delusions, neurotic or hypochondriacal symptoms, and hysterical personality traits. Oddly, the duration of the illness, the number of prior episodes, and the age of the patient all show no clear relationship to favorable or unfavorable response to antidepressants (Simpson and Singh, 1990; Brotman, Falk, and Gelenberg, 1987), although a general belief among psychiatrists is that TCAs are the most effective treatment for the most severely melancholic depressed patients (Burke and Preskorn, 1995).

Antidepressant medication is less effective in treating depression with psychotic features (delusional depression) unless the thought disorder is concomitantly treated with antipsychotic drugs. One double-blind study (Spiker et al., 1985) reported clinical effectiveness in 78% of patients treated with amitriptyline (Elavil), a tricyclic antidepressant, plus perphenazine, an antipsychotic drug, compared with 41% effectiveness for amitriptyline alone and 19% improvement with perphenazine alone. Clearly, the combination treatment greatly improves the probability of recovery in these patients. Others have advocated the augmentation of antidepressant treatment with lithium carbonate (Rybakowski, 1990) or electroconvulsive therapy.

The use of antidepressants alone in treating the depressive phase of bipolar depression has generated contradictory points of view. While some report that antidepressants may precipitate mania in the individual despite his or her depressed state, others find little support for the finding (Brotman, Falk, and Gelenberg, 1987). Bipolar depression is often treated with a combination of lithium carbonate to control the mania and an antidepressant drug that alleviates the depression. Further discussion of treatment for bipolar disorder is found in the section below on lithium carbonate.

Individuals with dysthymic disorder (depressive neurosis) are those who have experienced several years of a persistent depressed mood and associated symptoms. Such "minor" depression may precede an episode of major depression by several years or may accompany it, producing "double depression." Coexistence of dysthymic disorder correlates with a poorer prognosis for recovery from major depression and a greater likelihood of relapse once the episode of major depression is alleviated. Treatment of the premorbid neurotic depressive traits must be monitored, and they are treated most effectively with TCAs after recovery from the episode of major depression (Keller et al., 1983). Long-term antidepressant treatment in combination with psychotherapy that emphasizes the interpersonal aspect of the depression rather than intrapsychic conflicts has been found to reduce the residual dysthymic symptoms (Weissman et al., 1981).

For some years clinical impressions have maintained that endogenous depression responded better to TCAs, while monoamine oxidase inhibitors (MAOIs) were more effective in treating atypical depression. Evaluating their relative effectiveness has been difficult because the definition of "atypical" is not uniform. While some investigators emphasize opposite vegetative symptoms (e.g., increased sleep and overeating), others emphasize anxiety and panic attacks, or the presence of histrionic personality and rejection sensitivity. Several reviews (Brotman, Falk, and Gelenberg, 1987; Murphy et al., 1987; Simpson and Singh, 1990) have cited evidence collected in a number of large double-blind studies, which conclude that TCAs and MAOIs are equally effective in reducing symptoms of atypical depression. However, others (see Burke and Preskorn, 1995) report that some clinical features predict a preferential response to MAOIs. Among these features are irritability, hypersensitivity, hypersomnia, overeating, and psychomotor agitation. In addition, MAOIs may be significantly more effective than other antidepressants for nonendogenously depressed patients with prominent anxiety symptoms, panic attacks, or hysteroid dysphoria (Brotman, Falk, and Gelenberg, 1987; Sitsen and Montgomery, 1994).

For those individuals who are not responsive to antidepressant trials, the combination of an MAOI and a TCA may provide relief. However, many consider the combination to be particularly dangerous unless drug dosages, diet restrictions, and use of other medications are strictly monitored. Other therapeutic combinations that may be effective include a TCA or MAOI in combination with lithium, thyroid hormone, stimulants, L-tryptophan, neuroleptics, or ECT. For further discussion of both short- and long-term pharmacotherapy of depression as well as the diagnostic characteristics of "treatment resistant" individuals, refer to Burke and Preskorn (1995), Gerner and Rosenlicht (1990), Prien and Kocsis (1995), Sitsen and Montgomery (1994), or the monograph edited by Roose and Glassman (1990).

Monoamine Oxidase Inhibitors

The first discovery of true antidepressant action was based on serendipitous clinical observations. Used in the early 1950s to treat tuberculosis, iproniazid had a significant mood-elevating effect that was unrelated to its effects on tuberculosis. Such observations prompted clini-

Iproniazid

cal trials of iproniazid as an antidepressant drug. It was only after the discovery of its antidepressant action that the drug's ability to inhibit MAO was discovered. Although iproniazid has been withdrawn from the U.S. market because of hepatotoxicity (that is, impaired liver function), other MAOIs have been developed and are effective in a variety of depressed patients.

The history of the clinical use of MAOIs has been rather cyclic in this country. Although met with enthusiasm following their introduction in the 1950s, the MAOIs fell into disfavor because of their reputation for having severe and dangerous side effects, unlike the later TCAs. More recently, it has become apparent that when used carefully with appropriate dietary restrictions, MAOIs are as safe as TCAs and may have a special place in therapeutic strategies for treating affective disorders. Although they are no more effective than other antidepressants overall, the MAOIs can work in patients who respond poorly to the TCAs and some of the newer second-generation antidepressants. In addition to the treatment of affective disorders, MAOIs also have been used in the treatment of several anxiety states, such as phobic disorders, panic attacks, posttraumatic stress disorder, and obsessive–compulsive disorder, with some reported success. The drugs also may be effective agents in the treatment of bulimia, in prophylaxis of migraine headaches, in reducing narcoleptic attacks, and in potentiating the effects of L-DOPA in the treatment of Parkinson's disease (see Andrews and Nemeroff, 1994; McDaniel, 1986).

Structure and Pharmacokinetics

The chemical classification of the MAOIs comprises two groups: the hydrazines, such as phenelzine (Nardil) and isocarboxazid (Marplan), and the nonhydrazines, including tranylcypromine (Parnate) and pargyline (Table

$$\text{—CH}_2\text{—CH}_2\text{—NH—NH}_2$$

Phenelzine

19.2). The selective MAOIs, which are primarily experimental in nature, are divided into groups based on their ability to inhibit the A or B form of MAO (see below). All of the drugs are administered orally because they are readily absorbed from the GI tract and reach peak blood levels 2 to 4 hours after ingestion. Metabolism occurs in the liver, either through acetylation of the hydrazine group or oxidative degradation of other groups. Several of the MAOIs (e.g., phenelzine and tranylcypromine) are structurally related to amphetamine. Metabolism of tranylcypromine produces measurable levels of the sympathomimetic agent in plasma following drug overdose. Deprenyl is almost totally metabolized to methamphetamine and amphetamine. Significant levels of the metabolites are found in the urine of individuals receiving deprenyl for 3 days (Reynolds et al., 1978; see McDaniel, 1986, for a more detailed discussion).

Interaction with Monoamine Oxidase

The enzyme MAO is located intracellularly and is associated with the outer mitochondrial membrane in most mammalian tissues. The normal intraneuronal function of MAO is to oxidatively deaminate a variety of monoamines that have neurotransmitter function and also some amines found in the diet, such as tyramine and β-phenylethylamine. The inhibition of MAO deamination of neurotransmitters not contained in protective synaptic vesicles acutely increases the amount of neurotransmitter available for release. A single dose of MAOI increases norepinephrine, epinephrine, dopamine, and serotonin in brain, heart, intestine, and blood, and thus presumably prolongs and increases the action of the transmitters at their receptors. However, some compensatory decrease in the rate of synthesis occurs due to end-product inhibition of tyrosine hydroxylase. While amine levels increase within hours, several weeks of administration are usually required to produce effective antidepressant action clinically. Thus, the dynamic feedback regulation of neurons must play a significant part in modulating the mechanism of action of MAOIs.

Selective MAO-A and MAO-B inhibition.   Isoenzymes of brain MAO (MAO-A and MAO-B) have been identified on the basis of pH optima, thermostability, substrate preference, and pharmacological inhibition. Although their specificities are far from absolute, MAO-A acts more efficiently to deaminate 5-HT, NE, epinephrine, normetanephrine, octopamine, and DA, and is inhibited by clorgyline. MAO-B deaminates DA, tyramine, phenylethylamine, and *N*-methylhistamine, and is antagonized by deprenyl. At high concentrations, the selectivity is lost, and all the amines may be deaminated by either enzyme. Since human brain contains more MAO-

Table 19.2	**Chemical Classification and Reversibility of MAO Inhibitors**		
Type	**Chemical classification**	**Drug**	**Reversibility**
Nonselective	Hydrazines	Iproniazid	–
		Isocarboxazid	–
		Phenelzine[a]	–
		Nialamide	–
	Nonhydrazines	Pargyline	–
		Tranylcypromine[a]	–
Selective[b]	MAO-A inhibitors	Clorgyline	–
		Cimoxatone	+
		Amiflamine	+
		Moclobemide	+
	MAO-B inhibitors	Deprenyl	–
		Caroxazone	+

[a]Most commonly prescribed in the United States.
[b]Primarily investigational.

B than MAO-A, DA is metabolized primarily by MAO-B. In contrast, in rat brain DA is primarily deaminated by MAO-A (McDaniel, 1986). Such species differences require consideration when evaluating in vitro studies of these agents.

Intravenous injection of clorgyline inhibits MAO-A in brain (and elsewhere) and increases endogenous levels of 5-HT and NE (Yang and Neff, 1974). In contrast, deprenyl significantly raises the levels of exogenously administered phenylethylamine (PEA), but not NE or 5-HT. The multiple forms of MAO provide therapeutic potential to selectively increase the availability of a particular biogenic amine in a specific area of the brain in order to modify a disease state, while simultaneously maintaining the levels of other amines that may be responsible for side effects. It is generally assumed that inhibition of MAO-A is responsible for the antidepressant action of MAOIs, while MAO-B inhibition is related to at least some of the side effects. Although they are still in the investigative stage, clinical trials show that selective MAOIs seem to be more readily accepted by patients because of reduced intensity of side effects. In addition, they have a greater margin of safety. However, their overall effectiveness is apparently not dramatically different from conventional MAOIs. Further research is required before the drugs will be readily available clinically. Table 19.2 lists some of the selective MAOIs.

Mechanism of Antidepressant Effects

The classic MAOIs act on the MAO enzymes in an irreversible manner, preventing the enzymatic deamination of monoamines for as long as several weeks. The inhibitory effect is apparently a two-step interaction between drug and enzyme. The first step forms a reversible bond that is sensitive to competitive inhibition. The second step involves formation of a covalent bond between the drug and a portion of the enzyme. Termination of drug inhibition necessitates the removal of the drug-bound MAO from the mitochondrial membrane and resynthesis of the enzyme. Because of this process, the drugs have a long duration of action despite their relatively short plasma half-life. Two weeks may be required to restore the enzyme after drug termination.

Although the drugs' interaction with the MAO enzymes have been studied in detail, the importance of MAO inhibition specific to therapeutic efficacy is not known. Acute treatment with an MAOI increases levels of NE, 5-HT, DA, and other endogenous amines in rat brain. Left unresolved is whether elevation of these amines is important to the antidepressant actions of the drug, as originally proposed by the biogenic amine hypothesis of affective disorders, or whether the initial effects on transmitter availability induce time-dependent alterations in receptors or changes in second messenger function further downstream. The possibility of a single amine being pivotal in the etiology of each disorder sub-

type is unlikely, and investigations of the potential involvement of several neurotransmitters have produced a proliferation of research.

Historically, the amines NE and 5-HT were the first to be investigated, but evidence on the relative importance of each has been inconsistent. Spector, Shore, and Brodie (1960) showed that in a species (rabbits) in which both catecholamines and 5-HT are increased by MAO inhibition, increases in motor activity were best correlated with increased levels of NE. In a different species (cats) in which MAO inhibition produces an increase in 5-HT without changing NE levels, no behavioral excitation was observed. On the other hand, at least one study demonstrated that the antidepressant effect of tranylcypromine was reversed by depletion of 5-HT with the synthesis inhibitor p-chlorophenylalanine (Shopsin, Friedman, and Gershon, 1976), and several studies have shown a therapeutic effect of the 5-HT precursor 5-hydroxytryptophan and a potentiation of MAOI antidepressant action by L-tryptophan.

The more recent research into the behavioral effects of the specific MAO-A and MAO-B inhibitors has provided some evidence regarding neurotransmitter specificity. For example, low doses of deprenyl that selectively inhibit MAO-B do not produce antidepressant effects, while higher doses of deprenyl that act on both isoenzymes do reduce depression. This distinction suggests that antidepressant action following MAO inhibition is related to NE and 5-HT, while changes in DA are less significant (see Sitsen and Montgomery, 1994). However, despite improved techniques that give neuropharmacologists a window into the intricate changes occurring following MAOI treatment, the question of the relative importance of NE and 5-HT to the therapeutic efficacy of MAOIs has not been fully resolved. Evidence discussed in more detail below suggests an interdependent nature for the two amines, which may additionally be related to drug-induced changes in coupling mechanisms between the receptors and second messenger systems. Summaries of the effects of MAOIs on various amines are available (Charney et al., 1990; Murphy et al., 1987). Further discussion of neuropharmacological effects of chronic MAOIs follows in the section on mechanism of action of antidepressants.

Side Effects

MAO inhibitors (like all other therapeutic agents) have multiple effects that are not restricted to amines in the brain but occur at peripheral sites as well, producing side effects. For example, MAOIs generally cause dry mouth and orthostatic hypotension (a drop in blood pressure when the individual stands up due to blunted cardiovascular reflexes). Sleep disturbances, including insomnia, frequent awakenings, and reduced sleep time are common side effects and are often the reason cited for discontinuing treatment. However, the drug-induced reduction in REM sleep may be related to efficacy (see previous section on sleep). A rebound increase in REM following abrupt withdrawal of MAOIs is a well-documented phenomenon. Other side effects include overeating (particularly of carbohydrates), which may lead to excessive weight gain, impaired sexual responses, such as impotence in men and inorgasmia in women, and fluid retention in the lower extremities.

The drugs in this class have very little effect on animal behavior. Although these drugs given alone do not increase motor activity, pretreatment with an MAOI does prevent reserpine-induced depression. It is interesting to note that these drugs are not self-administered by animals and do not have a euphoric or stimulating effect on normal human subjects; instead they may induce dysphoria and unpleasant side effects, and are rarely abused.

Because MAOIs are not specific for MAO, they have the potential to cause adverse effects unrelated to MAO function. They generally inhibit the class of enzymes called the mixed-function oxidase system (for example, cytochrome P_{450}), which degrades many other drugs as well as several naturally occurring biogenic amines. For this reason the potential for complex actions and significant drug interactions is great. For instance, since they alter an organism's ability to metabolize barbiturates, alcohol, opiates, aspirin, procaine, atropine, cocaine, and others, the effects of these drugs can be prolonged and intensified in the presence of MAOIs. In addition, MAOIs potentiate the action of sympathomimetics, particularly those that indirectly increase adrenergic function, such as amphetamine and tyramine. Such potentiation may result in massive sympathetic overactivity leading to hypertension, throbbing headache, sweating, tachycardia, and hyperpyrexia. The most extreme case is the tyramine-induced hypertensive crisis.

Although rare, the most serious toxic effect of MAOIs is the hypertensive crisis that occurs following ingestion of tyramine. Tyramine is a naturally occurring amine formed as a by-product of fermentation in many foods, including cheeses, certain meats, pickled products, and others. Tyramine is normally oxidatively deaminated by MAO in the liver, but when the enzyme is inhibited, high levels of circulating tyramine release supranormal stores of NE at nerve endings, producing dramatic increases in blood pressure. Such a drug-induced hypertensive crisis is also known as the "tyramine-cheese reaction." Dietary restrictions reduce the threat of such a side effect occurring.

Tricyclic and Second-Generation Antidepressants

Tricyclic antidepressants are the drugs most often chosen first to treat depression. Their name is derived from their characteristic three-ring structure, which is similar to the phenothiazine nucleus found in classic antipsychotic drugs. In fact, the prototypical tricyclic compound, imipramine (Tofranil), was originally tested for antipsychotic activity because of its similarity in structure to the phenothiazines. Contrary to all expectations, clinical trials showed that imipramine was ineffective in quieting agitated psychotic patients. However, the drug did appear to elevate the mood of some depressed patients. Thus, further trials for its use as an antidepressant followed. Table 19.3 provides a list of several of the often prescribed classic tricyclic antidepressants along with the newer and more experimental second-generation antidepressants, which fall into three categories: modified tricyclic compounds, the specific 5-HT uptake blockers, and the atypical antidepressants.

The antidepressant effects of the commonly used tricyclic compounds are essentially the same; they differ primarily in their relative potencies. Several newer antidepressant drugs, such as fluoxetine (Prozac), mianserin (Tolvon), nomifensine (Merital), and bupropion (Wellbutrin) have been developed to modify neurotransmitter function more selectively, with the hope of targeting specific symptoms with more rapid action and fewer side

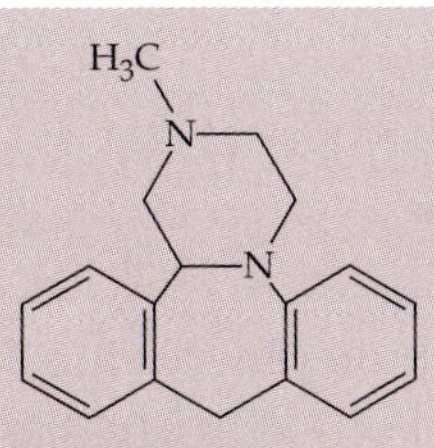

Mianserin 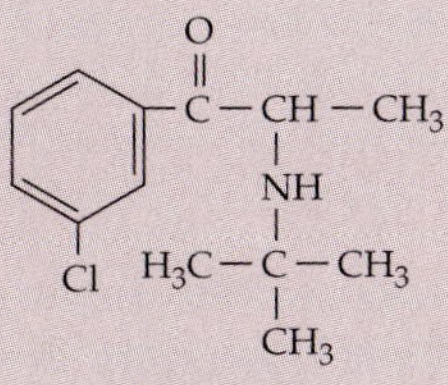   Bupropion

effects. The second-generation antidepressants will be described following a general discussion of the tricyclics.

Tricyclic antidepressant action is generally attributed to inhibition of the neuronal uptake mechanism that normally terminates the action of the neurotransmitter. By inhibiting reuptake, the duration of transmitter action at the synapse is prolonged. The tricyclics do not inhibit the uptake of amines into storage granules, but inhibit only the uptake from the extraneuronal space into the axon terminal. For example, following intracisternal administration of [^{3}H]norepinephrine, treatment with TCAs inhibits the uptake of labeled NE and increases the concentration of O-methylated metabolites without changing the amount of deaminated metabolites. The increase in O-methylated metabolites is a consequence of reuptake inhibition and the subsequent exposure to extraneuronal metabolism by COMT. Uptake inhibition by the tricyclic compounds also occurs for 5-HT.

In general, the tertiary amine tricyclic compounds, such as imipramine and amitriptyline, show little specificity for uptake inhibition of NE or 5-HT. Figure 19.5 provides a visual representation of the relative NE and 5-HT blocking potencies of several TCAs and some atypical antidepressants. The figure is based on experiments

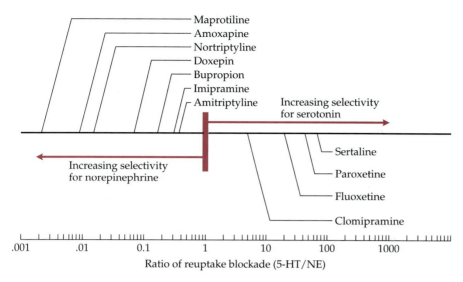

19.5 SELECTIVITY OF ANTIDEPRESSANTS IN INHIBITING REUPTAKE OF [³H]NE AND [³H]5-HT INTO RAT BRAIN SYNAPTOSOMES. A ratio of 1 (midline) indicates that a drug is equally potent in blocking NE and 5-HT reuptake; the greater the difference from 1, the more selective the drug. Drugs with more potent 5-HT uptake inhibition have values greater than 1; those with more potent NE uptake inhibition have values less than 1. Although based on potency of reuptake inhibition, the figure represents selectivity: it shows that sertraline is more selective for 5-HT than is paroxetine, but does not show that paroxetine is four times more potent than sertraline at 5-HT blockade. Likewise, bupropion is a weak uptake blocker that is more selective for NE than for 5-HT, but it blocks DA more potently than it blocks either NE or 5-HT. (After Richelson, 1993.)

Amitriptyline

that measured the amount of [³H]norepinephrine and [³H]5-HT taken up in vitro into synaptosomes prepared from rat brain in the presence of the antidepressant. Although there is general agreement on the effectiveness of antidepressant reuptake inhibition relative to neurotransmitter, some differences in reported results exist depending upon the experimental procedures used to evaluate reuptake. It is also important to note that the potency of an antidepressant in inhibiting amine uptake in vitro may be different from its potency in reuptake blockade in vivo. In addition, there is no apparent relationship between potency for uptake inhibition and potency for clinical effectiveness. Furthermore, relatively specific 5-HT uptake blockers such as zimelidine often modify other aspects of neurotransmitter function. For instance, chronic zimelidine reduces the number of β-adrenergic receptors and reduces the sensitivity of the cAMP generating system to NE as well as reducing the formation of the NE metabolite MHPG.

Although their antidepressant action is often attributed to amine uptake inhibition, many of the TCAs have significant direct effects on receptors. Imipramine, for

Table 19.3 Tricyclic and Second Generation Antidepressants	
Class	**Antidepressant**
Classic tricyclics	Imipramine (Tofranil), amitriptyline (Elavil), desipramine (Norpramine), nortriptyline (Aventyl)
Modified tricyclics	Iprindole (Tertran), doxepine (Sinequan), amoxapine (Asendin), trimipramine (Surmontil), protriptyline (Vivactyl)
5-HT uptake blockers	Fluoxetine (Prozac), clomipramine (Anafranil), citalopram (Cipramil), fluvoxamine (Luvox), sertraline (Zoloft), venlafaxine (Effexor), paroxetine (Paxil)
Atypical antidepressants	Maprotiline (Ludiomil), nomifensine (Merital), mianserin (Tolvon), bupropion (Wellbutrin), trazodone (Desyrel), nefazodone (Serzone)

example, has an IC_{50} value of less than 200 nM for histamine (H_1), muscarinic cholinergic, and adrenergic (α_1) receptors. This potent block of receptors may be responsible for the drowsiness and sedation, the anticholinergic side effects, and the orthostatic hypotension, respectively, that are commonly observed. The newer antidepressant mianserin binds effectively to H_1, α_1, α_2, muscarinic, and $5-HT_2$ receptors. Thus, although mianserin is a relatively weak in vivo blocker of NE uptake, it may increase NE transmission by releasing NE subsequent to blockade of presynaptic α_2-receptors. These plus several other examples of antidepressants with high affinities for multiple receptors are listed in Table 19.4. It should be noted that for many of the newer specific 5-HT uptake blockers, such as fluoxetine, no significant receptor binding occurs, perhaps explaining their distinct constellation of side effects. Since the antidepressant actions of the available drugs are very similar, a particular antidepressant is chosen on the basis of the side effects it produces in relationship to the needs of the individual and its duration of action (see Andrews and Nemeroff, 1994; Potter, Rudorfer, and Manji, 1991).

Pharmacodynamics

The tricyclic compounds are administered orally and are readily absorbed from the GI tract. Plasma levels of drug vary significantly (20–40-fold) from individual to individual despite administration of the same dosage. The variable plasma levels are apparently genetically determined since identical twins show identical plasma concentrations. Differences in the rate of metabolism are the most likely basis for this variability. Although for some tricyclic drugs, a therapeutic window of effectiveness has been identified, in some instances there appears to be little correlation between plasma drug levels and clinical response (Davis, Comaty, and Janicak, 1988).

Metabolism involves several steps, including demethylation and oxidation, which produce active metabolites (e.g., the conversion of imipramine to desipramine). The active metabolites are readily bound to plasma protein and so remain in the body longer, prolonging the drug half-life. The accumulation of active metabolites contributes to the incidence of side effects and toxicity. The final steps in metabolism include hydroxylation and conjugation with glucuronic acid, producing inactive products that are excreted in the urine.

Pharmacological Side Effects

As is true for their structural relatives, the phenothiazines, some of the most frequent side effects of TCAs involve their anticholinergic actions, including dry mouth, constipation, dizziness, tachycardia, palpitations, blurred vision, and urinary retention. Sedation, weakness, and fatigue are frequent side effects that limit the drugs' usefulness for some individuals. Headache is common, as is the occurrence of a fine, persistent tremor.

Sleep rhythms are altered by increasing slow-wave or deep sleep, so fewer nighttime awakenings occur. The total amount of REM sleep is reduced. Effects on the cardiovascular system occur in many cases and are likely to be due to the block of NE uptake in neurons innervating the heart tissue. Tachycardia, development of cardiac arrhythmias, and the dulling of cardiovascular reflexes that adjust for changes in posture (which leads to orthostatic hypotension) are serious side effects, particularly for individuals with known cardiac disorders.

Acute overdosage is characterized by hyperpyrexia, hypertension, seizures, and coma. Cardiac depression and arrest become life threatening. Treatment includes gastric lavage and the maintenance of vital functions with resuscitative equipment. Convulsions may be controlled with intravenous diazepam and hypertension may be treated with short acting α-adrenergic blockers. Physostigmine may be useful in reversing the anticholinergic CNS effects. The significant potential for life-threatening consequences following overdose (5–10 times normal dose) means that caution must be applied when prescribing TCAs to suicidal depressed patients.

Effects on Behavior

The tricyclic compounds, like the MAO inhibitors, are dysphoric for normal individuals. When tricyclic compounds are given to normal individuals, they feel sleepy and tend to be quieter, light-headed, and ataxic. These effects, in combination with a variety of somatic side effects (e.g., dry mouth and blurred vision) make the use

Table 19.4   In Vitro Acute Receptor Affinity of Selected Antidepressant Drugs

Drug	α_1	α_2	H_1	M^b
	Receptor affinity[a]			
Amitriptyline	+++	±	++++	++++
Nortriptyline	+	0	+	++
Imipramine	++	0	+	++
Desipramine	+	0	0	+
Maprotiline	+	0	++	+
Amoxapine	++	0	+	+
Fluoxetine	0	0	—	0
Trazodone	++	±	±	0
Bupropion	0	0	—	0
Nomifensine	0	0	—	+
Iprindole	0	—	0	0
Mianserin	++	+++	+++	+
Alprazolam	0	0	0	0

[a] + to +++ = low to high affinity; ± = weak affinity; 0 = lacking affinity.
[b] M = muscarinic ACh receptor.
Source: After Rudorfer and Potter, 1989.

of these drugs unpleasant and anxiety-provoking for most people. For this reason, drugs in this class have little behavioral reinforcement value and hence, low abuse potential. In contrast, when given to a depressed patient over a 2- to 3-week period, a definite elevation in mood occurs.

Animals respond to TCAs in a manner similar to humans. When given to rats, imipramine depresses spontaneous activity, causes ataxia, and prolongs hexobarbital induced sleeping time. However, if given before reserpine, imipramine induces excitation and exploratory behavior that is presumed to result from the spillover of free catecholamines onto receptors. If imipramine is given after the effects of reserpine have developed or if catecholamine stores are first depleted by administration of α-methyltyrosine, only partial reversal occurs. These data suggest that imipramine's acute behavioral effects are produced by increasing the action of catecholamines. For the same reason, imipramine potentiates the actions of amphetamine, a sympathomimetic that releases catecholamines from the presynaptic terminal. Reuptake blockade by TCAs enhances amphetamine-induced hyperactivity. Also, although tricyclic compounds given alone reduce the rate of electrical self-stimulation in normally positive hypothalamic stimulation sites, imipramine and amphetamine administered together produce self-stimulation at a rate much higher than amphetamine alone (Stein and Seifter, 1961). In a similar manner, imipramine intensifies and increases the duration of amphetamine-induced hyperthermia, although alone, imipramine does not increase body temperature and may in some cases lower it (Jori and Garattini, 1965).

Newer Antidepressant Drugs

Recently new compounds with a wide variety of chemical structures have been developed in an attempt to produce a more effective and safer antidepressant that might have a more rapid onset of action. The earliest of these were modifications of the tricyclic nucleus, such as iprindole (Prondol), doxepine (Sinequan), and amoxapine (Asendin). In an attempt to develop a drug with fewer side effects, two bicyclic compounds were developed in the mid-1970s that prevented the uptake of 5-HT without affecting NE or DA. Fluoxetine and zimelidine are the prototypes for the serotonin-specific reuptake inhibitors (SSRIs). Newer SSRIs include sertraline (Zoloft), paroxetine (Paxil), clomipramine (Anafranil), and fluvoxamine (Luvox). Another SSRI that is presently available in Europe is citalopram (Cipramil). Still other new drugs have a selective action on catecholamine uptake without affecting 5-HT (e.g., maprotiline [Ludiomil] and nomifensine [Merital]), block both 5-HT and NE uptake, such as venlafaxine (Effexor), block 5-HT uptake and also 5-HT receptors (e.g., trazodone [Desyrel] and nefazodone [Serzone]), or have no effect on uptake at all, but

Doxepin

act on a subclass of receptors (e.g., mianserin [Tolvon]). A summary of major characteristics of selected newer antidepressant drugs appears in Table 19.5.*

In general, all of the newer drugs in use are found to be more effective than placebo, and are approximately equal to the earlier TCAs in relieving symptoms associated with moderately severe, unipolar, major depressive disorders. None of the newer compounds clearly stand out as superior to the others, and none has yet been found to work in a selective fashion on a given subtype of depression. All of them produce significant undesirable side effects. The most significant difference is in the nature of side effects, which is related to their neurochemical mechanisms of action. However, many of the newer drugs are considered safer if taken as an overdose than either the TCAs or the MAOIs. However, some, such as bupropion, can cause toxic effects, such as grand mal seizures, at five times the normal therapeutic dose (Burke and Preskorn, 1995).

While both types of newer antidepressants have fewer anticholinergic side effects and autonomic nervous system effects than the classic TCAs, the second-generation antidepressants can be divided into two groups based on their ability to produce either stimulation and agitation or sedation and drowsiness. Those drugs with a stimulant profile, including the selective 5-HT uptake inhibitors, seem to have several qualities distinct from those drugs with a sedative profile. The sedative group in general has the advantage of a longer half-life, which means that these drugs require only a single administration daily; hence greatly increasing the likelihood of compliance and subsequent effectiveness. In addition, their sedative nature is useful in alleviating insomnia. However, most of the antidepressants with a sedative profile, with the exception of mianserin, demonstrate some cardiotoxicity, making them less useful for geriatric patients who have diagnosed cardiac problems. Moreover, the sedative antidepressants also produce weight gain, an undesirable side effect for some individuals. Reviews of the clinical neuropharmacology of fluoxetine and other 5-HT uptake blockers are provided by Kilts (1994) and Montgomery (1995).

---

*Discussion of relative merits of the various atypical antidepressants is beyond the scope of this chapter, but can be found in reviews by Andrews and Nemeroff (1994), Potter, Rudorfer, and Manji (1991), and Sitsen and Montgomery (1994).

Table 19.5   Significant Characteristics of Second Generation Antidepressants

Drug	Mechanism	Clinical profile	Side effects	Half-life (hr)
Amoxapine	NE uptake inhibitor; mixed receptor action	Sedating, useful in psychotic depression	Lower cardiotoxicity; some anticholinergic effects; increased seizures and potential for parkinsonian symptoms	8
Bupropion	DA uptake inhibitor	Stimulant, slower onset of action, three doses per day	Few anticholinergic effects and low cardiotoxicity; causes agitation, anxiety, GI upset, weight loss, headache and insomnia; possible seizures; aggravates schizophrenia	14
Fluoxetine	5-HT uptake inhibitor	Stimulant, slow onset, one dose per day	No anticholinergic effects and no cardiotoxicity; causes insomnia, headache, nausea, anxiety, and sexual dysfunction; pharmacokinetic interactions with TCAs and benzodiazepines	60
Maprotiline	NE uptake inhibitor	Sedating	Some anticholinergic effects; increased seizures and skin rashes	43
Mianserin	Mixed receptor binding, no uptake inhibition	Strong sedative, one dose per day, possible relapse in long-term use	No anticholinergic effects and low cardiotoxicity; increased seizures; possible bone marrow depression and allergic reactions	27
Nomifensine	NE and DA uptake inhibition, mixed receptor activity	Stimulant, two doses per day, withdrawn from market	Less anticholinergic and not cardiotoxic; produces insomnia, allergic reactions, orofacial dyskinesia	3
Trazodone	Weak 5-HT uptake inhibitor, mixed receptor activity, chemically unique	Strong sedative, short onset, questionable efficacy in severe depression, less potent than tricyclics	Low anticholinergic effects and low seizure incidence; increased drowsiness and cognitive changes; may cause cardiac arrhythmias and priapism	9

Fluoxetine may deserve special mention because it has met wide acceptance as an antidepressant of first choice and also has been used to treat several distinct disorders: panic and anxiety disorders, obsessive–compulsive disorder, as an appetite suppressant in obesity, and as a means to control alcohol consumption in alcoholics. Its prestigious position in the pharmacological arsenal seems to be based on its reputation for minimal serious side effects related to cardiovascular toxicity and anticholinergic effects. Instead, it causes a new constellation of potentially hazardous side effects, including nervousness and anxiety, sexual dysfunction, motor restlessness, extrapyramidal movement disorders, muscle rigidity, nausea, headache, and insomnia. Some recent claims of previously unknown side effects, such as violent and suicidal behavior, need to be evaluated further. Fluoxetine's long half-life is an additional advantage, although onset of clinical effectiveness is no better than conventional antidepressants.

Modifications of drug molecules produce new antidepressants with different effects. For example, sertraline has the advantage of slow and steady absorption from the GI tract and enhanced bioavailability in the presence of food. The drug venlafaxine produces an earlier onset of action for some patients (Potter and Manji, 1994b). Other experimental compounds from novel chemical classes are being evaluated for specific antidepressant action (Ferris et al., 1995). Furthermore, 5-HT receptor agonists may have potential as antidepressant agents. In particular, the drugs buspirone and gepirone, which act selectively on 5-HT$_{1A}$ receptors, demonstrate potential antidepressant effects in animal models (see Deakin, 1994). Clinical trials of the 5-HT$_{1A}$ agonists (Robinson et al., 1990) show small but significant improvements in depressed patients based on changes in the Hamilton Depression Rating Scale, which suggests genuine antidepressant effects rather than reduction of anxiety in a depressive illness. Since these drugs are best known for their antianxiety effects, the reader is directed to Chapter 16 for detail.

Part I Summary

The MAOIs, tricyclics, and second-generation antidepressants provide significant relief for a majority of individuals suffering from affective disorders. Current interest is focused on identifying novel antidepressant therapy with more rapid onset of effectiveness and reduced side effects. To achieve that goal, neuropharmacology research emphasizes selective modification of brain chemistry. In addition, research on physiological correlates of depression and the development of animal models are allowing researchers to identify depression subtypes that may differentially respond to antidepressant treatment in a predictable fashion.

Part II
Neurochemistry of Depression and Antidepressant Action

The time course of the effectiveness of MAOIs and tricyclic and second-generation antidepressants has suggested to many that the acute changes in neurochemistry induced by these therapeutic antidepressants are alone not enough to provide relief, but must be followed by adaptational changes in neuronal function. For instance, acute increases in the neurotransmitters NE, DA, and 5-HT occur following a single administration of antidepressant. This acute increase in neurotransmitter levels is accompanied temporally by a slowing of neuronal firing in the raphe nuclei and locus coeruleus, suggesting a negative feedback on cell firing rate mediated by somatodendritic autoreceptors. There is also a reduced rate of neurotransmitter synthesis, which reflects an additional autoreceptor effect. However, with prolonged administration of antidepressant, cell firing and neurotransmitter synthesis rates adjust and transmitter levels return to normal. Since clinical effectiveness of antidepressants requires several weeks of administration, it is clear that clinical efficacy cannot be related to amine levels, but must be due to subsequent neuronal adaptations, such as alterations in receptor number or affinity, or changes in response of second messenger systems.

The general pattern of down-regulation of postsynaptic receptors following chronic antidepressant treatment fits our present understanding of neurotransmitter function. That is, we expect that any chronic increase above normal in neuronal function will lead to a subsequent reduction in receptor number or affinity. With refinements in radioligand receptor binding, families of receptor subtypes have been identified and localized, and the research literature on this subject has expanded exponentially. A comprehensive picture of the mechanism of therapeutic efficacy must consider not only the specific drug, but also the receptor subtype examined, its localization within the CNS, the interaction among receptors, and the time course for the drug-induced changes on individual receptor types. For example, down-regulation of postsynaptic receptors dampens the system while down-regulation of presynaptic receptors may enhance neuronal function. Also the rate and/or extent of down-regulation for pre- and postsynaptic receptors may vary.

In addition to drug-induced changes in receptor number or ligand affinity for the receptor, many questions are being raised regarding the biochemical consequences subsequent to ligand binding. For instance, a well-documented finding is that chronic antidepressants reduce the ability of NE to increase cAMP, a result interpreted as a down-regulation of β-receptors. However, antidepressant effects on the catalytic unit of adenylyl cyclase itself and on G protein coupling between receptor and catalytic unit are also being evaluated. In addition, single-unit electrophysiological recordings provide unique information regarding the effect of chronic drug treatment on ion conductance and gating in neuronal membranes subsequent to the initial receptor binding.

Somewhat further removed from receptor binding is the measurement of behaviors known to be mediated by a particular neurotransmitter or mediated by a particular subtype of receptor. Effects of chronic treatment on the animal's response to a specific agonist tells indirectly about underlying neurochemical changes. The behavioral endpoints utilized vary widely and include such things as hypothalamic self-stimulation, clonidine-induced hypotension, amphetamine-induced locomotor activity, 5-HT-agonist–induced sedation, and many others.

Yet another way to investigate the neurochemical changes and behavior is to consider neurotransmitter turnover in patients treated with antidepressant drugs. Most often neurotransmitter metabolites in the body fluids of patients are measured at several time points in an attempt to correlate neurotransmitter utilization and clinical condition (see Murphy et al., 1987). However, this technique has many technical difficulties relating to disease state, diagnostic uncertainty, and estimation of CNS function based on peripheral measures.

Each of these techniques makes a significant contribution to an integrated evaluation of antidepressant drug effects on CNS function and psychopathology. To summarize the vast literature regarding each of these areas is beyond the scope of this chapter. Instead, selected studies will be summarized and citations will direct the reader to current review articles.

Norepinephrine

The importance of norepinephrine to the etiology of depression is suggested by its role in neuroendocrine function, reward mechanisms, attention and arousal, and response to stress, each of which may contribute to the symptomatology of the affective disorders. While clinical studies of NE utilization in depression are far from unanimous, it is clear that regulation of the adrenergic system is altered in depressed individuals as reflected in their differences in metabolites, in receptor sensitivity to agonist challenge, and in altered endocrine response to adrenergic stimulation. Several reviews provide details regarding altered NE function in individuals suffering from affective disorders (Brown, Steinberg, and van Praag, 1994; Caldecott-Hazard et al., 1991; Charney et al., 1994; Schatzberg and Schildkraut, 1995; Siever, 1987). The importance of NE to the effectiveness of the antidepressant treatments currently available has been extensively investigated. Our discussion will focus on drug-induced changes in NE turnover, pre- and postsynaptic responses, and NE regulation of cAMP formation. (For a review of catecholamine regulation, see Chapter 8.)

Effects of antidepressants on α_2-autoreceptors. As shown in Figure 19.6, multiple adrenergic receptors have a potential role in antidepressant effects. For example, neuropharmacological research has examined long-term effects of the drugs on the α_2-autoreceptors, which provide feedback regulation of adrenergic cell function. The α_2-receptors located at the nerve terminal respond to elevated extracellular concentrations of NE by reducing the amount of NE released by subsequent action potentials. The α_2-receptors located on NE cell bodies (somatodendritic receptors) in the locus coeruleus inhibit the firing of NE cells. Since α_2-receptors acutely reduce NE cell function by decreasing the rate of firing and reducing NE release, α_2-receptor subsensitivity would be expected to increase both of those cell functions. One way to determine potential changes in α_2-receptor–mediated function is to measure specific responses following the administration of clonidine, a relatively specific α_2-receptor agonist. Among the responses measured in animal studies are changes in cell firing rate, depression of NE turnover, and hypothermia and sedation. In humans, the hypotensive effect and clonidine-induced changes in plasma MHPG, growth hormone, cortisol, blood pressure, heart rate, and sedation are assessed following acute and chronic antidepressant treatment.

Using physiological measures of α_2-receptor function, the majority of experiments show that chronic, but not acute, antidepressant treatment produces a reduction in autoreceptor responsiveness (Murphy et al., 1987). Chronic desipramine, amitriptyline, and the MAO-A inhibitor clorgyline reduce clonidine-induced changes in plasma MHPG, blood pressure, and sedation. Electroconvulsive therapy and sleep deprivation therapy also reduce α_2 response in some cases. However, not all antidepressants reduce α_2 sensitivity. For example, chlorimipramine and trazodone do not reliably reduce α_2-receptor sensitivity, and chronic mianserin treatment seems to increase α_2 sensitivity in both animal and human studies. In addition, the growth hormone response to clonidine, which is a postsynaptic α_2-receptor function, does not seem to change in response to prolonged antidepressant treatment (see Charney et al., 1990).

Studies of α_2-receptor binding have produced conflicting results of decreases, increases, and no change reported following prolonged antidepressant treatment. In addition, receptor number does not consistently parallel receptor response. For example, Garcia-Sevilla (1990) reported that the elevated binding of [³H]clonidine to platelets in depressed individuals before treatment was reduced following chronic treatment with antidepressants, such as amitriptyline or ECT. However, this effect has not been universally reported, and physiological responses such as the clonidine-induced inhibition of prostaglandin E₁–stimulated cAMP do not show a parallel change in sensitivity. Additionally, the animal studies that showed reduced [³H]clonidine binding to tissue prepared from discrete brain areas after antidepressant treatment have not provided results consistent with physiological measures. We might conclude that results from ligand binding studies in peripheral tissues, such as platelets, or from discrete brain areas may not reflect CNS changes in distinct physiologically responsive re-

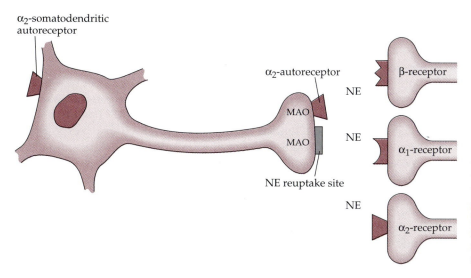

19.6 POTENTIAL MULTIPLE SITES OF ANTIDEPRESSANT ACTION ON NE NEUROTRANSMISSION. Increased synaptic NE following MAO inhibition or NE reuptake blockade can act on β-receptors, α_1-receptors, postsynaptic α_2-receptors, or α_2-autoreceptors on the terminal, soma, and dendrites.

ceptor systems. In addition, correlations between in vitro binding and physiological response do not necessarily exist even in the same tissue. Despite affinity between ligand and membrane protein, the membrane protein cannot be considered a functional receptor unless a relationship between occupancy and biological response is shown (see Leonard, 1994). Further, drug-induced changes in physiological response may more closely coincide with postreceptor cellular changes.

In order to test a possible depression-associated defect in signal transduction, Karege and coworkers (Karege et al., 1996) measured platelet phosphoinositide hydrolysis in drug-free depressed patients and control subjects. They found that α_2-receptor and thrombin receptor–mediated increases in [^{3}H]PIP$_2$ metabolites were potentiated in the depressed patients. In contrast, NaF-induced increase in [^{3}H]PIP$_2$ turnover, which acts by directly stimulating the G protein without receptor interaction, was not different in the two groups. In this experiment it was not directly determined whether the elevated α_2-receptor function was due to increased receptor number or increased coupling to the transducer. However, the parallel change in thrombin-mediated PIP$_2$ turnover suggests a defect in heterologous receptor–G protein interaction in depressed patients. The effects of chronic antidepressants on this second messenger system were not determined.

If we assume that chronic antidepressant treatment does indeed reduce the effectiveness of the presynaptic α_2-receptors, we would expect to find a gradual increase in NE cell firing and turnover. Such a result coincides to some extent with experimental evidence on NE turnover.

Effects on NE turnover.   In contrast with the acutely induced reduction in cell firing in the locus coeruleus and reduced rate of NE synthesis following antidepressant treatment, chronic treatment leads to a gradual increase in locus coeruleus firing, although the rates never return to the levels of untreated animals (McMillen, German, and Shore, 1980). Although NE synthesis also increases, it also may not be restored to predrug levels. Thus, the subsensitivity of the α_2-receptors that we assume are responsible for these physiological effects is apparently not complete, although an alternative explantion is that a second competing mechanism may contribute to the changes in NE function. The picture is complicated by the fact that not all antidepressants acutely reduce locus coeruleus firing and decrease synthesis. Some (e.g., amitriptyline and chlorimipramine) have a dual action at higher doses that may have opposing actions on NE cell function: uptake inhibition plus antagonist action on α_2-receptors. Thus, one might not expect to see α_2 desensitization, or a change in turnover with chronic use of these drugs. Willner (1985b) summarizes the effects on NE turnover, in animals. In general, an increase in NE

turnover occurs following desmethylimipramine, protriptyline, imipramine, ECT, and selected atypical antidepressants, while no significant change occurs following chronic amitriptyline, chlorimipramine, MAOIs, and several atypical antidepressants such as iprindole and maprotiline.

Measurement of NE turnover in patient populations is complicated by the interaction of drug effects with pre-existing disease factors and current clinical state. Demographic variables such as gender, age, diet, caffeine intake, tobacco, time of day, state of activity, and medication status also must be controlled for. In addition, those experiments measuring metabolites in plasma or urine must make the assumption that changes in peripheral NE function parallel changes in CNS NE function. Assuming peripheral measures to be an accurate reflection of CNS activity is not clearly warranted. However, measuring MHPG is more indicative of CNS function than measuring other metabolites such as normetanephrine, which is formed preferentially in peripheral NE neurons.

Despite the initial reduction in noradrenergic cell firing and NE synthesis, MHPG in biological fluids of humans undergoing treatment is usually found to be elevated, suggesting an increase in turnover with chronic antidepressant use. Increased MHPG in light of reduced firing may explain the reports of reduced levels of brain NE. Reports on firing rate, NE synthesis, and MHPG levels, each a measure of NE turnover, unfortunately vary among studies using different antidepressants. The disparity may represent differences in methodologies of measurement, selection of treatment duration, or differences in basal turnover rate in patients preceding pharmacological intervention. A unified pharmacological explanation seems unlikely given the broad chemical spectrum of antidepressant agents.

How the drug-induced changes in MHPG interact with existing biochemical parameters in depressed patients is not clear. As is usually the case, the variability in a given group of depressed patients is much greater than that for controls or for patients with bipolar disorder. Such variability may mean that within the depressed group, two subsets of individuals exist who have significantly high and low levels of MHPG. Schatzberg and Schildkraut (1995) summarize evidence suggesting that 24-hour urinary MHPG levels may predict response to particular antidepressant drugs. In general, patients with a low urinary excretion of MHPG prior to treatment tended to show a better clinical response to imipramine, desmethylimipramine, nortriptyline, and maprotiline than patients with high basal MHPG excretion. Furthermore, some evidence suggests that the low values of urinary MHPG in acutely depressed individuals increase toward control levels following successful drug therapy. Early research found that high urinary MHPG patients have low CSF 5-HIAA, and hence respond better to amitriptyline and 5-HT uptake blockers.

For instance, Beckman and Goodwin (1975) measured urinary MHPG in unipolar depressed patients who were subsequently treated for 4 weeks with either imipramine or amitriptyline. In the imipramine group, the responders had significantly lower pretreatment MHPG levels than those who showed no clinical improvement. In contrast, those responders in the amitriptyline group showed higher pretreatment MHPG levels than those who did not respond to treatment. Although such results are intriguing, they are not yet consistent enough to provide a laboratory method to predict clinical efficacy of a specific drug in a particular patient.

In summary, it can be said that complex relationships exist between NE and its urinary and CSF metabolites relative to diagnostic categories. Although some variation can be explained on the basis of severity of illness, circadian and diurnal changes may also contribute significantly. The phase-shift found in the timing of fluctuations in MHPG (Wehr, Muscettola, and Goodwin, 1980) could explain why MHPG levels in patients and controls is inconsistent, particularly when measured in single–time point studies. Detailed discussion of clinical correlates evaluating adrenergic mechanisms in depression are provided by Caldecott-Hazard and colleagues (1991), Schatzberg and Schildkraut (1995), and Siever (1987).

Postsynaptic α_1-Receptors

The chronic administration of various antidepressant treatments including ECT have not produced consistent changes in α_1-receptor binding using dihydroergocryptine, WB4101, or prazosin as labeled ligands (Charney et al., 1990). However, while Menkes, Aghajanian, and Galleger (1983) found no increase in labeled prazosin binding to spinal cord, thalamus, or cortex following chronic desmethylimipramine, amitriptyline, or iprindol treatment, they did report an increase in the ability of the α_1-agonist phenylephrine to displace bound α_1-antagonist prozosin. This suggests that the antidepressant treatment may increase sensitivity to α_1-agonists without changing the binding characteristics of the labeled α_1-antagonist, perhaps by converting the receptor to an agonist-preferring state.

The enhancement of the agonist binding suggested by Menkes, Aghajanian, and Galleger (1983) may explain the increased α_1-receptor sensitivity demonstrated in electrophysiological and other functional studies. Chronic imipramine, desmethylimipramine, amitriptyline, chlorimipramine, and iprindol enhance the postsynaptic electrophysiological effects of iontophoretically applied NE in selected areas of the brain. Alpha$_1$-mediated responses in the lateral geniculate nucleus of the thalamus were enhanced by chronic treatment, and both α_1 and 5-HT responses were increased in the facial motor nucleus and the amygdala (Menkes and Aghajanian, 1981). Neither fluoxetine nor chlorpromazine had the same effects.

Behavioral models thought to reflect the sensitivity of α_1-receptors may provide information regarding the effects of antidepressants on overall integrated functioning. Chronic treatment with both classic and second-generation antidepressants apparently potentiates clonidine- and apomorphine-induced aggression in mice in a manner antagonized by α_1-receptor blockers. In the same experimental designs, the 5-HT uptake inhibitors, citalopram and fluoxetine were ineffective (Maj et al., 1982). In depressed patients, phenylephrine-induced dilation of the iris, which is mediated by α_1-receptors, has been shown to increase following chronic MAOIs, but the corticosteroid response to amphetamine, although low in depressed patients, does not change following TCA or ECT administration (see Heninger and Charney, 1987). It would appear from these results that consistent changes in α_1 receptor number or function do not occur for antidepressants from several classes.

Changes in β-Receptors and cAMP

The earliest evidence for altered postsynaptic sensitivity involved antidepressant-induced changes in the NE-stimulated formation of cAMP by adenylyl cyclase, an effect antagonized by β-receptor blockers such as propranolol. Classic studies showed that reserpine and other treatments, such as 6-OHDA, that reduce NE synaptic activity produce both sedation in animals and a supersensitivity of the cAMP generating system (Williams and Pirch, 1974). Altered second-messenger function occurs presumably because the postsynaptic β-receptor, which is coupled to adenylyl cyclase, responds to a reduction in impulse traffic with an increased sensitivity to exogenously applied neurotransmitter. In an analogous fashion, an increase in synaptic activity might be expected to reduce postsynaptic responses. In fact, chronic administration of imipramine or related tricyclics for 3–6 weeks produces a subsensitivity to NE in brain slices (Vetulani, Stawarz, and Sulser, 1976). That is, the formation of cAMP after the addition of NE to rat cortex slices is significantly less in animals pretreated for several weeks with imipramine or another tricyclic antidepressant than in nontreated animals or in those receiving only an acute injection of the drug. Similar results occurred with chronic TCAs, MAOIs, ECT, and lithium, as well as following chronic treatment with the atypical antidepressants iprindole and mianserin, and the 5-HT uptake inhibitor zimelidine (Sulser, 1983). Of the antidepressants evaluated, only fluoxetine, citalopram, and bupropion do not seem to alter sensitivity of the β-receptor–linked cAMP generating system. The time course of β-receptor sensitivity is dose dependent, but in general, coincides with the onset of clinical effectiveness, which takes between 1 and 3 weeks (see Caldecott-Hazard et al., 1991; Willner, 1985).

Changes in second messenger response to NE can most easily be explained by a modification of β-receptors. Long-term, but not short-term, antidepressant treatment has been shown to reduce the number of β-adrenergic receptors in rat cortex and limbic forebrain without altering the affinity of the receptor for transmitter (Peroutka and Snyder, 1980). Enhancement of NE function by administration of an α_2-antagonist (yohimbine) in combination with desmethylimipramine (DMI) led to down-regulation of β-receptors in rat brain in a shorter treatment time than DMI alone (Ursillo et al., 1980). Unfortunately, a clinical trial of DMI and yohimbine did not prove to be more effective than desmethylimipramine alone (Heninger and Charney, 1987). Further refinement of the binding assay has led to the conclusion that β_1-receptors, but not β_2-receptors, are modified by antidepressant drugs (Minneman, Wolfe, and Molinoff, 1982). Discrete localization of the receptor subtypes may explain some of the disparities in reported experimental results and also the regional specificity of changes in reported binding following drug treatment. The antidepressants tested in these early experiments included several tricyclics, the modified tricyclic iprindole, and the MAO inhibitor pargyline. Since then, the down-regulation of β-receptors has been confirmed for many other antidepressants, including many of the second-generation antidepressants, ECT, lithium under some conditions, and possibly REM sleep deprivation. In those cases in which antidepressants, such as mianserin, zimelidine, and nisoxetine, reduce the cAMP response to exogenous NE, but not the number of β-receptors, a modification of G protein coupling or the catalytic function of adenylyl cyclase has been proposed.

Also, although chronic treatment with the atypical antidepressant mianserin does not affect β-receptor density, Pilc and Enna (1987) showed that mianserin prevents or reverses the supersensitivity of cortical β-receptors caused by 6-OHDA or by reserpine. These findings suggest that some antidepressant-induced changes in β-receptors may depend on receptor sensitivity at the time of antidepressant treatment (see Leonard, 1994) and may restore elevated receptor levels to control conditions but not reduce receptor number to below normal concentrations.

Animal studies show that other β-receptor–mediated behaviors are also reduced by most antidepressant treatments (see Heninger and Charney, 1987). Included among these are salbutamol-induced inhibition of exploratory behavior and isoproterenol-induced drinking. In contrast, human clinical studies of melatonin secretion, which is under β-receptor control, show a net increase rather than the anticipated decrease in secretion after chronic antidepressants. However, since nocturnal melatonin secretion is low in depressed individuals and shows a blunted circadian rhythm, a further subsensitivity may not be measurable (see Charney et al., 1990; Charney et al., 1994).

Because down-regulation of β-receptors and β-receptor function was found after chronic treatment with

most of the effective antidepressants, a revised model of antidepressant action was proposed (Sulser, Vetulani, and Mobley, 1978). It suggests that depression may be a state characterized by hypersensitive catecholamine receptors and that effective antidepressant treatment desensitizes the receptor mechanism. Some support for this model comes from several studies that examined β-receptor density in the postmortem brains of depressed individuals and individuals committing suicide. Although some reported no significant difference in binding, others that used drug-free individuals and evaluated regional distribution found increased β-receptor density in the frontal cortex of individuals who committed violent suicides (Arango, Ernsberger, and Marzuk,1990; see also Caldecott-Hazzard et al., 1991; Charney et al., 1994).

Although the model utilizes the most consistent neurochemical data and emphasizes long-term changes that temporally coincide with clinical efficacy, several criticisms have been leveled at it. First, chlorpromazine, an antipsychotic agent structurally similar to imipramine but having little antidepressant action, also produces subsensitivity to NE (Schultz, 1976), as does the sympathomimetic amphetamine. Thus, it is possible that the change in receptor function may be unrelated to therapeutic action. Second, several studies that examined the relative potencies for clinical effectiveness and ability to desensitize β-receptors showed a negative correlation between the two effects. In these studies, the most effective antidepressants had the least effect on down-regulation of receptors. Third, despite the down-regulation of β-receptors, there is little evidence to support the idea that NE function is thereby reduced beyond basal levels. The possibility that down-regulation restores NE function only to preantidepressant levels must be considered. In such a case, the receptor change is only compensating for the drug-induced neurochemical change, not the neurochemical abnormalities underlying the disorder. In addition, treatments, such as triiodothyronine (T_3), that tend to enhance therapeutic effects of antidepressants might be expected to also enhance down-regulation of β-receptors. However, T_3 increases β-receptor density and reduces TCA-induced down-regulation. Finally, since the role of β-receptors in regulating human behaviors is not known, further research is needed to develop a probe into the neurochemistry of depressed patients.

Serotonin

There is considerable evidence (see Chapter 9) suggesting that 5-HT has significant influence on sensitivity to pain, emotionality, and response to negative consequences as well as to reward. The effects of 5-HT on sleep, eating, and thermoregulation are likewise well documented. Rats with depleted stores of 5-HT are irritable and aggressive, likely to perform behaviors despite threat of punishment, appear oversensitive to pain, and show altered patterns of eating and satiety. Parallels in humans suffering from major affective disorders can be readily drawn; they frequently report increased pain sensitivity, disturbed sleep, changes in appetite, and loss of sexual interest, along with characteristic mood changes.

Function in depressed individuals. The most common method of determining the level of 5-HT function in patient populations is by measuring the principal 5-HT metabolite, 5-HIAA. Over many years, reduced 5-HIAA in CSF has been reported for subsets of depressed individuals compared with healthy controls. Unfortunately other studies failed to replicate these results. Some of the difficulty in replication includes the fact that 50% of the lumbar CSF 5-HIAA is supplied by peripheral sources, which may or may not change in parallel with brain 5-HIAA. Other factors contributing to experimental disparities include stress-related effects on 5-HIAA, circadian and diurnal influences, gender differences, diet, sleep disturbances, presence of psychoses, and other factors. Also, evidence suggests that low 5-HIAA may be more specifically a marker for suicidal tendencies (Golden et al., 1991; see also Chapter 8) rather than for major affective disorder in general. Therefore, patient populations that vary in the percentage of suicidal subgroups may report variable results. In addition, low CSF 5-HIAA has been associated with aggressive, hostile, anxious, and impulsive behavior, as in the case of violent suicide attempts, impulsive murder, or other types of antisocial behavior (Brown and Linnoila, 1990; see Golden et al., 1991). Unfortunately, there is no consensus on whether high or low 5-HIAA is correlated with depressive symptoms other than suicide, nor is there agreement regarding the relationship between pretreatment 5-HIAA levels and antidepressant treatment outcome. Also, in some cases, TCAs and MAOIs have been found to further reduce the already low levels of CSF 5-HIAA in depressed individuals.

The availability of tryptophan, the 5-HT precursor, is one measure of 5-HT function that frequently appears abnormal in depressed patients. The conversion of tryptophan to 5-hydroxytryptophan by tryptophan hydroxylase is the rate-limiting step in the synthesis of 5-HT. Because the normal concentration of tryptophan does not saturate the enzyme, the amount of available tryptophan can regulate synthesis. Numerous studies report significantly lower levels of plasma free (unbound) tryptophan in depressed patients, although such differences are not found universally (Moller et al., 1983). Lower tryptophan in depressed patients is supported by other reports of an inverse relationship between depression scores in unipolar patients and the ratio of plasma tryptophan to neutral amino acids. The use of the ratio is significant because neutral amino acids compete with tryptophan for transport via a specialized carrier across the blood–brain barrier. Further, citalopram increased the plasma tryptophan/neutral amino acid ratio in clinical trials (see Maes and Meltzer, 1995).

In one double-blind, placebo-controlled study, Delgado and coworkers (1990) rapidly depleted tryptophan in patients who had experienced an antidepressant-induced remission of symptoms. Total and free tryptophan levels were reduced by 87% and 91%, respectively, following the ingestion of a tryptophan-free 16–amino acid drink. Depression scores showed that 14 out of 21 patients experienced a recurrence of symptoms following the drink, despite continued antidepressant medication. The depression scores were negatively correlated with free plasma tryptophan levels. In another placebo-controlled, double-blind crossover study (Lam et al., 1996), patients with seasonal affective disorder in clinical remission after light therapy underwent rapid tryptophan depletion. Six out of ten patients had a clinically significant relapse of depressive symptoms when tryptophan was reduced to 20% of normal. Although tryptophan has little therapeutic effect on depression, it is of interest to note that several studies have demonstrated an enhancement of antidepressant action by the addition of 5-HTP to classic antidepressants that are known to potentiate 5-HT function.

Another method of evaluating 5-HT function in depressed individuals is to measure 5-HT uptake by blood platelets. Platelets have a serotonin transport mechanism that is very similar, if not identical, to the transporter found in the brain. Platelets serve as an accessible model for 5-HT uptake into CNS neurons. In addition to directly measuring 5-HT uptake, the number of transporter sites and their affinity can also be measured, using [^{3}H]imipramine binding. Because imipramine inhibits reuptake in 5-HT neurons by competing with 5-HT, the drug becomes a useful tool to evaluate transporter protein function (Meltzer and Arora, 1991). Most, but not all, studies using platelets from depressed patients have found a reduced uptake of 5-HT, along with a decrease in the number of uptake sites, without a difference in affinity for 5-HT (Poirier et al., 1986; see Maes and Meltzer, 1995). Others find decreased uptake only in selected subtypes of depression, for instance, unipolar depression or nondelusional depression. Furthermore, while some report a normalization of 5-HT uptake in patients responding to antidepressants (see Caldecott-Hazard et al., 1991), others find that TCAs, zimelidine, and lithium cause a further decrease in platelet uptake after several weeks of treatment (see Brown, Steinberg, and van Praag, 1994). There is no evidence that reduced pretreatment 5-HT uptake predicts successful treatment outcome. Whether reduced uptake enhances 5-HT utilization by prolonging synaptic action or reduces 5-HT function by increasing the 5-HT that acts on autoreceptors is not known. How uptake-inhibiting antidepressant drugs further modify this function also is unclear. The possibility that the change in 5-HT uptake reflects an adaptive response to low 5-HT function in depressed individuals is one explanation.

Effects of antidepressant drugs.   As was true for the evaluation of antidepressant effects on NE function, the action of chronic drug treatment must take into account the many regulatory steps that constitute neurotransmitter function. Included are drug effects on neurotransmitter synthesis, release, and reuptake, MAO activity, autoreceptor-mediated modification of release, autoreceptor regulation of firing rate, postsynaptic receptor effects, and second messenger activity. Temporal changes in each aspect of function during chronic drug administration may not occur in synchrony. Furthermore, changes that occur may be either in concert or antagonistic. In addition, acute changes are less significant to therapeutic efficacy than those structural or genomic changes that occur with chronic treatment.

The acute effects of antidepressants on 5-HT closely resemble those modifying NE function. While most antidepressants, including the tricyclics, the specific 5-HT uptake inhibitors, ECT, and MAOIs, increase available 5-HT, the negative feedback mediated by 5-HT autoreceptors slows the firing rate of cells in the raphe nuclei and reduces 5-HT synthesis. The subsequent reduction in turnover is most evident for the most effective 5-HT uptake inhibitors, while imipramine and amitriptyline give variable results, and desmethylimipramine, iprindol, and mianserin produce no reported change in 5-HT turnover following acute treatment (see Willner, 1985a). Reductions in CSF levels of 5-HIAA are recorded in depressed patients following 5-HT uptake blockers as well, although it is difficult to do repeated samplings under those circumstances. However, there seems to be little correlation between 5-HIAA levels and therapeutic effectiveness with either tricyclics or specific 5-HT uptake blockers (see Maes and Meltzer, 1995; Meltzer and Lowy, 1987).

MAOIs also reduce CSF and urinary concentrations of 5-HIAA in depressed patients. This decrease in 5-HIAA is apparently greater for the clinically effective MAO-A inhibitor clorgyline than for the less effective MAO-B inhibitor deprenyl. Once again, the changes in 5-HIAA do not seem to be correlated with patient improvement (Murphy et al., 1987).

The slow onset of efficacy of antidepressants makes long-term neurochemical changes most important to investigate. The 5-HT uptake inhibition that occurs with some of these drugs does not undergo significant tolerance or desensitization. Autoreceptor-mediated suppression of serotonergic neuron activity *does,* however, desensitize following chronic antidepressant treatment (see Artigas et al., 1996). Consequently, 5-HT uptake inhibitors produce only modest increases in synaptic 5-HT concentrations when first administered, but later cause much greater neurotransmitter elevations. These findings have led Blier, de Montigny, and their colleagues to hypothesize that the therapeutic lag associated with the selective serotonin reuptake inhibitors (SSRIs) is related to the time required for 5-HT autoreceptor desensitization (Artigas et al., 1996; Blier and de Montigny, 1994). The investigators further predicted that concomitant administration of an autoreceptor blocker with the antidepressant should hasten the therapeutic response by precluding the acute autoreceptor-mediated dampening of serotonergic transmission. Preliminary data involving treatment of patients with the SSRI paroxetine, along with the somatodendritic autoreceptor antagonist pindolol, appear to support this prediction (Artigas et al., 1996). Perhaps at least some of the other classes of antidepressants act through a similar desensitization of presynaptic α_2-receptors, as described earlier.

Postsynaptic effects.   Most studies report that chronic treatment with ECT, tricyclics, or atypical antidepressants has little effect on the number or affinity of 5-HT$_1$ receptor sites in rat brain, although several MAOIs have been shown to reduce binding to those sites. In contrast, a significant decrease in 5-HT$_2$ receptors, labeled with [^{3}H]spiroperidol, occurs following chronic use of antidepressants. This down-regulation is one of the most consistent effects of chronic antidepressant treatment. Table 19.6 provides a summary of the variety of antidepressant agents that, in general, reduce binding to 5-HT$_2$ sites. The information in the table has been compiled from a large number of studies utilizing a variety of treatment schedules, brain areas, and tissue preparations; discrepancies in results have been found that are not reflected in this table. The down-regulation of receptors is evidently not confined to traditional tricyclic compounds, but also results from treatment with many of the atypical antidepressants as well as the MAOIs, while the clinically less effective MAO-B inhibitor deprenyl has no apparent effect on 5-HT$_2$ receptors. Unfortunately, the clinically effective use of chronic ECT not only does not reduce 5-HT$_2$ receptors, but may actually increase binding to these sites (see Caldecott-Hazard et al., 1991).

Oddly, the postsynaptic electrophysiological response to either direct iontophoretic application of agonist or electrical stimulation of ascending neurons is enhanced by long-term antidepressant treatment. In a series of studies, DeMontigny (1981) examined the electrophysiological responses of single cells in rat forebrain to microiontophoretic application of 5-HT. This study found that following 2 days of antidepressant treatment, the sensitivity of the neurons to 5-HT was not changed. After 4–7 days of pretreatment, the response of the cells to exogenously applied 5-HT was moderately increased, and, following 15 days of antidepressant administration, there was a large increase in sensitivity to 5-HT. The time course of this physiological change is related to the clinical antidepressant effects; that is, the antidepressant action generally requires 2 weeks or more of drug administration. In addition, the study found that several drugs with a similar structure (FG-4963 and chlorpromazine), but without antidepres-

Table 19.6 Effects of Treatment with Chronic Antidepressants or Electroconvulsive Therapy (ECT) on [³H]Spiroperidol Binding to 5-HT₂ Sites and Electrophysiological Response to Exogenous 5-HT

Antidepressant treatment	Effect on binding[a]	Response to 5-HT[a]
Tricyclics		
Amitriptyline	↓ or =	↑
Chlorimipramine	↓	↑
Desmethylimipramine	most ↓	↑
Imipramine	↓ or =	↑
Atypical antidepressants		
Fluoxetine	↓ or =	=
Zimelidine	↓	=
Citalopram	=	?
Iprindole	↓	↑
Mianserin	↓	↑
Trazodone	↓	↑
MAOIs		
Tranylcypromine	↓	↓
Clorgyline	↓	↓
Deprenyl	=	=
ECT	= or ↑	↑

[a] ↑, enhancement; =, no change; ↓, reduction; ?, unknown.
Source: After Willner, 1985a.

sant activity, did not increase sensitivity of the cells to 5-HT. Furthermore, iprindole, which is clinically effective but does not work by amine uptake blockade, significantly increased 5-HT sensitivity in forebrain cells. Others have reported enhanced response following a variety of antidepressants, including tricyclics, mianserin, and ECT, in several brain areas (see Table 19.6). Among the exceptions are several highly effective drugs (e.g., clorgyline and fluoxetine) that do not lead to enhanced responsiveness. Clorgyline decreases rather than increases the response of cortical cells to 5-HT. Worthy of mention is the finding that those antidepressants that induce supersensitivity do not necessarily do so in all brain areas that have 5-HT receptors. In several cases, such as for chlorimipramine and desmethylimipramine, the supersensitivity that develops is limited to subcortical serotonergic areas and may reflect differential responses based on distinct receptor subtypes. Unfortunately, no attempts have been made to correlate the electrophysiological response with changes in receptor number in the same brain areas of antidepressant-treated animals. Although the argument for enhanced sensitivity of 5-HT neurons in response to antidepressants in general is among the most consistent, the fact that the enhanced physiological response occurs in brain areas where 5-HT₂ receptors are reduced is difficult to reconcile (see Caldecott-Hazard et al., 1991).

The complexities involved in the physiological evaluation of drugs that possess potent presynaptic as well as postsynaptic effects is demonstrated by the effects of zimelidine. During chronic treatment with zimelidine, postsynaptic electrophysiological measures show a developing supersensitivity to electrical stimulation of ascending 5-HT pathways, but not to directly applied agonist. Such an apparent anomaly may be explained by the action of the drug to increase the amount of neurotransmitter released with each action potential rather than to change postsynaptic mechanisms. Despite apparent discrepancies, an overall increase in 5-HT-mediated neurotransmission has been suggested as a common mechanism of action of antidepressant drugs (Blier, DeMontigny, and Chaput, 1990; DeMontigny, Blier, and Chaput, 1984).

At least some experiments using behavioral probes in animals are in agreement with the electrophysiological data showing enhanced 5-HT response. Among the behaviors that are enhanced are agonist-induced hyperactivity, 5-HTP-induced head twitches, and 5-HT-mediated hyperthermia. Surprisingly, divergent results occur with the most powerful 5-HT uptake inhibitors (zimelidine, fluoxetine, and chlorimipramine), which decrease the response to 5-HT agonists. It is noteworthy that neither fluoxetine nor zimelidine enhanced the electrophysiological response to 5-HT (see Table 19.6), while chlorimipramine did. The behavioral studies are sometimes difficult to interpret because the responses usually require high concentrations of agonist stimulation. High drug concentrations preclude receptor subtype specificity, and action on supersensitive receptors may produce signs of toxicity. Also, when using behavioral probes, interactions of pre- and postsynaptic receptors are difficult to tease apart.

Probes in human studies tend to rely on neuroendocrine responses (see Brown, Steinberg, and van Praag, 1994; Meltzer and Lowy, 1987) such as L-tryptophan-induced elevations of prolactin, a response that tends to be reduced in depressed individuals. This prolactin response to exogenous tryptophan is restored in depressed patients following chronic administration of certain antidepressants, such as tranylcypromine, desipramine, and amitriptyline, but not others, such as zimelidine. Perhaps serotonin contributes differentially to the symptoms associated with subtypes of depression. One large-scale study (Price et al., 1991) found that prolactin responses to intravenous tryptophan were blunted in nonmelancholic patients compared with melancholic and psychotic depressed individuals. Differential growth hormone responses also were reported. Unfortunately no comparisons of pre- and postdrug hormone levels were made, so we have no indication as to how antidepressant treatment altered the hormonal responses in these groups. However, results did show that nondepressed control subjects experienced a decrease in positive feelings in response to tryptophan (i.e., feeling talkative, happy, and energetic), while depressed patients reported a decrease in fearfulness and enhancement of calmness.

Abnormal function of the hypothalamic–pituitary–adrenal (HPA) axis is a consistent finding among depressed individuals, as demonstrated by excess cortisol secretion and failure to respond to dexamethasone (see discussion above). Several pieces of evidence summarized by Maes and Meltzer (1995) show a significant relationship between HPA axis function and CNS 5-HT. For example, hippocampal 5-HT receptors are a significant locus of control of the HPA axis. Decreased hippocampal regulation may elevate HPA axis activity by modifying hormonal feedback mechanisms. In turn, glucocorticoids have been reported to increase 5-HT synthesis and turnover in several areas of the rat brain (Chaouloff, 1993) and increase 5-HT$_2$ receptor density in prefrontal cortex (Kuroda et al., 1992). Further research in this area is warranted, since disorders in both peripheral and central 5-HT receptors and their relationship to abnormal HPA axis function may be interrelated and significant to the psychopathology of depression. Holsboer (1995) reviews current issues in the neuroendocrinology of mood disorders.

NE–5-HT Interactions

Countless experiments over years of research have shown multiple abnormalities in both 5-HT and NE function in depressed individuals. Neurochemical changes produced by chronic antidepressants also involve both systems. Among the most consistent neurochemical changes are down-regulation of β-receptors and 5-HT$_2$ receptors and an enhanced physiological response to 5-HT.

The inability to identify a single neurotransmitter responsible for antidepressant action may reflect the important interactions among several systems in CNS functioning. Decades ago, Brodie and Shore (1957) suggested a synergistic action of NE and 5-HT. They hypothesized that serotonin is a transmitter in the "trophotropic" system, which is involved with normal conservation and relaxation and which functions much like the parasympathetic division of the autonomic nervous system. Norepinephrine was proposed to act in the "ergotropic" system, which functions during times of stress, aggression, and adaptation to environmental change and which is similar to the sympathetic division of the autonomic nervous system. Thus, depression may be related to a reduced adrenergic function in combination with an increase in 5-HT sensitivity. More recent research also suggests complex interactions between NE and 5-HT to explain antidepressant efficacy.

Caldecott-Hazard and coworkers (1991) have suggested that antidepressant action on both NE and 5-HT systems can involve either parallel or serial interactions. Parallel mechanisms mean that antidepressants act on NE and 5-HT systems independently, but simultaneously. Serial mechanisms imply that antidepressants act on either NE or 5-HT initially, and that the two neuronal systems subsequently interact anatomically and neurochemically. Evidence exists to support each of these mechanisms and, in addition, some antidepressants may be clinically effective despite having effects on only a single neurotransmitter system.

An obvious example of drugs that work by parallel mechanisms is the MAOIs, which increase neuronal content of both NE and 5-HT by inhibiting the enzyme that metabolizes each of them. Second, several TCAs, such as amitriptyline, imipramine, nortriptyline, and amoxepine, block the reuptake of both NE and 5-HT and ultimately lead to subsequent receptor changes. Differences in relative affinities of the TCAs for NE and 5-HT reuptake transporter proteins (discussed previously) explain why some TCA actions may be parallel, but not necessarily equivalent in intensity. Third, many antidepressants bind to receptors in both transmitter systems, although the relationship between receptor binding and clinical efficacy is not clear. For example, doxepin blocks both 5-HT$_2$ and α_1-receptors while mianserin acts on α_2- and 5-HT$_2$ receptors. Evidence for a series mechanism comes from the neurochemical changes induced by the specific 5-HT uptake inhibitors, such as sertraline and fluvoxamine. Although their ability to specifically block 5-HT reuptake is clear, these drugs also down-regulate β-receptors and desensitize β-receptor–coupled adenylyl cyclase (Sulser, 1989). Since these drugs do not directly modify NE action, it is assumed that their adrenergic effects are indirect via a series mechanism. In a similar manner, β-receptor agonists, such as salbutamol, increase serotonin-mediated function, such as 5-HTP-induced behaviors.

Other evidence for a series mechanism is controversial. Numerous experiments have shown that by destroying 5-HT terminals with the neurotoxin 5,6-dihydroxytryptamine, the down-regulation of β-receptors following chronic desmethylimipramine or ECT is prevented (Sulser and Sanders-Bush, 1987). The data have been interpreted by some as a demonstration that intact 5-HT cells are necessary for β-receptor down-regulation, in support of a serial mechanism of action. Sulser (1989) proposes a "serotonin–norepinephrine" hypothesis in which adrenergic information flow involves multiple feedback loops that utilize a variety of neurotransmitters, including 5-HT. NE function has an oscillator role that determines adaptation or amplification of important functions. Disturbances in any one of the systems that modulate NE can lead to psychopathology, including depressive disorders.

An alternative interpretation concludes that serotonergic neurons are unnecessary for desmethylimipramine- or ECT-induced β-receptor down-regulation because the antidepressants down-regulate only those β-receptors that are in a high-affinity state. Conversely, lesioning 5-HT neurons increases the number of β-receptors in the low-affinity state. Therefore, when both conditions (antidepressant treatment and 5-HT neuron lesions) exist, the total number of receptors appears to be unchanged, despite a down-regulation of β-receptors with high affinity and an increase in low-affinity β-receptors. Whether one or both of these interpretations is correct may depend on further investigations into regional brain differences and molecular studies of gene expression and protein synthesis (see Caldecott-Hazard et al., 1991).

Regardless of interpretation of the down-regulation data, the existence of anatomical connections between NE and 5-HT systems is well documented. Furthermore, neurochemical interactions involving NE influence on 5-HT cells and 5-HT influence on NE cells is clear (see Brown, Steinberg, and van Praag, 1994). Lastly, the contribution of each of the neurotransmitters to portions of the whole depression syndrome means that complex neurochemical interactions are a certainty.

In attempts to clarify the interactive nature of neurotransmitter systems, research emphasis has shifted. Current attention is being focused beyond changes in pre- and postsynaptic receptors and neurotransmitter release and metabolism, toward disturbances in postreceptor signal transduction. Postreceptor transduction is where the integration of multiple incoming signals utilizing distinct neurotransmitters occurs. Refinements in our understanding of neurotransmitter regulation of second messenger systems provides a focus for investigations into the pathophysiology of depression and potential target sites for psychotherapeutic agents. Current research emphasizes the role of neurotransmitter receptor–G protein coupling, components of the cAMP second messenger system such as protein kinase and phosphorylated proteins, and receptor-mediated changes in the phosphatidylinositol (PI) cycle, as well as modifications in conductance of calcium in its role as an intracellular mediator. A detailed review of some of these changes in CNS signal transduction in affective disorders and treatment is provided by Hudson and colleagues (Hudson et al., 1993). Specific issues of interest include investigations into the importance of cAMP-dependent protein kinase as a potential target for antidepressant drug action (Perez et al., 1994). Also, diagnosis and treatment strategies may be aided by research into altered platelet α_2-receptor–mediated changes in the PI cycle (Karege et al., 1996). Similarly, the correlation between β-receptor–coupled stimulatory G protein function and the severity of depression (Avissar et al., 1996) provides one more area of research that may clarify previous contradictory evidence.

Other Neurotransmitters

Acetylcholine. Evidence for cholinergic modification of mood has been summarized by Janowsky and Overstreet (1995). Cholinergic supersensitivity is observed in many depressed individuals. Cholinomimetics induce components of a "model depression" such as flattened affect, psychomotor depression, anhedonia, and apathy, as well as elevated levels of ACTH and cortisol and changes in sleep architecture.

Acetylcholine is implicated in the altered sleep patterns described in depressed patients, which include earlier onset of REM sleep and increased total REM sleep time, particularly in the first half of the sleep period. Cholinergic stimulation with physostigmine or the muscarinic agonist arecoline can mimic the sleep changes seen in depression. Further indication that ACh function may be altered in depressed individuals comes from neuroendocrine evidence showing that cholinergic cells are involved in circadian changes in pituitary–adrenal function, as well as in stress-induced ACTH release. The fact that drugs that increase ACh function exacerbate depressive symptoms in depressed individuals is of further interest. Unfortunately, evaluation of anticholinergics as antidepressive agents produced mixed reports (see Janowsky and Risch, 1984)

Blockade of muscarinic receptors by the tricyclic antidepressants is responsible for many of the autonomic side effects, such as dry mouth, that are seen with TCA treatment. However, neither the MAOIs nor ECT share this property, nor do most of the atypical antidepressants designed to diminish the incidence of autonomic side effects. Furthermore, tolerance to the anticholinergic effects of the tricyclics occurs in most patients within a short time after drug exposure. Thus, while most evidence suggests that anticholinergic action is not a significant therapeutic basis for the clinically useful antidepressants, ACh interaction with NE, DA, and 5-HT systems may nevertheless play a role in mood modification, particularly regarding responses to stress. For more information regarding cholinergic effects on appetitive behaviors, sleep and arousal, HPA axis function, and stress, see Caldecott-Hazard and colleagues (1991) and Janowsky and Overstreet (1995).

Histamine.   Antidepressants also act at histamine receptors of the H_1 type (Peroutka and Snyder, 1980). This action, however, does not seem to correlate with clinical effectiveness, but is likely to be related to side effects, such as sedation. Kanof and Greengard (1978) and Green and Maayani (1977) have found that the drugs are very effective competitive inhibitors of histamine-stimulated adenylyl cyclase in the hippocampus and neocortex. In these brain areas, the histamine receptor complex that is coupled to adenylyl cyclase is of the H_2 type. All the antidepressants tested were capable of shifting the dose–response curve for histamine-induced cAMP production to the right, indicating that more histamine was required to produce a given amount of cAMP in the presence of these drugs. The low concentration of antidepressant required for this effect suggests that the histamine-sensitive adenylyl cyclase may be antagonized in vivo at pharmacologically effective doses.

Although the physiological function of histamine neurons in the brain is not known, acute blockade of histamine receptors may reduce cAMP in postsynaptic cells and hence modify the function of other neural networks. With prolonged drug administration, protein synthesis may be affected in these cells and subsequently modify the function of various neurotransmitters, ultimately modifying behavior.

Dopamine.   Interest in dopamine and its relationship to depression stems initially from knowledge of the role of DA in the initiation and modulation of movement, motivation, and reinforcement, and in hypothalamic–pituitary function. Current emphasis on the mesolimbic DA pathway as the neural locus of reward and dependence for a variety of psychoactive drugs (Koob, 1992) implicates DA dysfunction in the anhedonic quality of depression and concomitant loss of motivation. Further, the increased incidence of depression in Parkinson's disease patients (see Chapter 20) and the depressant effects of dopamine-depleting drugs or DA antagonists support the idea that DA has a role in depression.

Animal models of depression further implicate DA in depressive states. Animals with "learned helplessness" exhibit behaviors similar to depressed individuals (see Chapter 2). The syndrome is accompanied by DA depletion in both the caudate and nucleus accumbens.

DA antagonists not only exacerbate the behavioral effects of learned helplessness, but they also prevent antidepressant-induced improvement of the condition (Muscat, Sampson, and Willner, 1990).

In humans suffering from major affective disorder, levels of CSF HVA, dopamine's major metabolite, tend to be reduced, although substantial variability has been reported. In general, antidepressant treatment fails to alter HVA levels in patients experiencing drug-induced reduction of symptoms. MAOIs reduce CSF HVA, although the effect is much less than that reported for MHPG or 5-HIAA levels in the CSF. Furthermore, deprenyl, the less effective antidepressant that inhibits MAO-B, was at least as effective as clorgyline, the MAO-A inhibitor, in reducing the DA metabolite (Murphy et al., 1987). Finally, HVA levels are not predictive of clinical response to classical antidepressants. Interpretation of the data on HVA concentration is not clear-cut. Many results suggest that CSF HVA is correlated with motor activity rather than mood (Willner, 1995). Also, CSF HVA comes predominantly from the basal ganglia because of the dense dopamine terminals located there, and because of close proximity to the ventricles. Mesolimbic and mesocortical DA fibers contribute much less to CSF HVA. Thus, CSF measures of the metabolite do not reflect neural activity in those DA neurons that are most meaningful to the depressive disorder.

Numerous studies have shown that chronic, but not acute, treatment with tricyclics, selected atypical antidepressants, ECT, and REM sleep deprivation enhance apomorphine- and amphetamine-induced motor activity in rats. Several studies also have shown supersensitivity in the nigrostriatal system by examining apomorphine-induced circling in unilaterally lesioned animals or by measuring sterotyped behavior following amphetamine treatment. Others have shown potentiation of DA-mediated behaviors following antidepressant treatment that suggests increased sensitivity of mesolimbic D_2 receptors (Serra et al., 1990). However, the neurochemical basis for this enhanced sensitivity to DA is unclear since no change in D_2 receptor number occurs following chronic antidepressant treatment. Furthermore, electrophysiological, neurochemical, and behavioral approaches in animal studies have failed to find changes in DA autoreceptors following chronic antidepressant treatment, despite several early reports of autoreceptor subsensitivity. In addition, chronic treatment does not consistently alter dopamine turnover. Whether the increased sensitivity to DA is due to changes in second messenger systems or interactions with other subtypes of DA receptors is still unknown (see Kapur and Mann, 1992).

In humans, neuroendocrine methods are the only way of examining DA receptor function. DA in the tuberoinfundibular pathway apparently has excitatory control over growth hormone release and inhibitory control over prolactin. Clinical studies of prolactin and growth hormone regulation in depressed patients have not demonstrated consistent evidence of altered dopamine sensitivity. However, in challenge studies, approximately two-thirds of the researchers have reported antidepressant-induced increases in apomorphine- and DOPA-induced prolactin inhibition, indicative of DA supersensitivity. Why results in these and in animal studies of neuroendocrine function are not more consistent is not clear. Although it seems unlikely at this time that the receptor changes are related to clinical efficacy, they may be responsible for the initiation of mania by antidepressants administered to bipolar patients. Several reviews of the potential role of dopamine mechanisms in affective disorders are available (Kapur and Mann, 1992; Jimerson, 1987; Willner, 1995).

Part II Summary

In summary, we have provided evidence to suggest that the original biogenic amine hypothesis is too simplistic to account for all available data. Certainly, insufficient NE and 5-HT alone cannot be the pathological condition underlying depressive disorders. Subsequent attempts to reconcile some of the discrepancies in the earlier hypotheses have emphasized long-term changes in receptor function or second messenger activity. These hypotheses argue for chronic antidepressant-induced changes in α_2-adrenergic, α_1-adrenergic, β-adrenergic, or 5-HT$_2$ receptors. Changes in receptor signal transduction mechanisms may also be important.

Although the early emphasis was on catecholamine systems, subsequent studies of 5-HIAA levels, plasma tryptophan, and neuroendocrine responses to serotonergic drugs suggest that altered 5-HT function is a likely factor in depression. Nevertheless, there does not seem to be a uniform explanation regarding the effects of antidepressant treatments on serotonergic function, particularly because of difficulties in separating the pre- and postsynaptic actions of these drugs. Thus, while chronic antidepressant administration tends to down-regulate 5-HT$_2$ receptors, 5-HT-mediated physiological and behavioral responses are often increased. One area of current interest is the apparent desensitization of 5-HT autoreceptors to repeated antidepressant treatments. This phenomenon has been hypothesized to account for the therapeutic lag associated with SSRI therapy. A similar process may occur for α_2 autoreceptors and other classes of antidepressants.

Antidepressant drugs clearly have significant effects not only on NE and 5-HT, but also on ACh, DA, histamine, and both opioid (see Chapter 12) and nonopioid peptides (see Plotsky, Owens, and Nemeroff, 1995). The interactions of these neurotransmitter systems are evident on many levels—neuroanatomical, neurochemical, and behavioral. The importance of such interactions to a coherent theory of depression and effective treatment cannot be overemphasized, although we cannot provide more than a cursory overview within the limitations of a single chapter.

An underlying assumption of much depression research is that all antidepressants operate through a common mechanism of action. This assumption may not be correct, however. Consideration of individual symptoms or symptom clusters and their relationship to transmitter function may provide a more productive approach. Alternatively, one might consider the interactive effects of several transmitter systems that ultimately sum to provide clinical efficacy. Siever and Davis (1985) have emphasized the importance of abnormalities in regulation of neurotransmitter function, rather than simple increases or decreases in individual components. Persistent impairment in homeostatic regulatory mechanisms might make an individual vulnerable to sudden changes in neurotransmitter output, as might occur during changing environmental events. It is clear that much more research is needed before a unified theory is developed.

Part III
Other Therapies for Affective Disorders

Electroconvulsive Therapy

In the early 1900s a Hungarian psychiatrist noted that several of his patients showed improvement in their psychiatric state after having spontaneous seizures. This observation prompted others to produce convulsions in psychiatric patients by administering either camphor and oil, or, more recently, a synthetic camphor derivative, pentylenetetrazol (Metrazol), or insulin. Such treatment was the predecessor of electroconvulsive therapy (ECT), which was introduced in 1938 and is used today to treat affective disorders. Although ECT has been used for about 60 years, we do not yet understand the neurochemical basis for its effectiveness. Clinical evaluations have shown ECT to be as good as or better than antidepressant drugs in treating depression in certain types of patients. Although ECT produces no pain or awareness of the seizure and has a relatively low incidence of side effects, a great deal of controversy exists over its use, and public concern has limited its use over the last few years. However, one can view seizure therapy as a complex process to elicit persistent biochemical changes in the brain similar to those produced by the antidepressant drugs. Recent reviews of the technique, utilization, and adverse effects can be found in Weiner and Krystal (1994) and Khan and colleagues (Khan et al., 1993).

Effectiveness. Although used originally for major depressive disorder and melancholia, the effective use of ECT has been expanded to the treatment of delusional depression, schizoaffective disorders, schiophrenia, and mania. Generally, ECT is used on the depressed patient who is unresponsive to pharmacotherapy. Its efficacy, 80% to 90%, is higher than that of more conventional forms of treatment. However, since its administration is technically difficult and expensive, its use is limited to the most resistant cases. In the case of delusional depression, which has reported improvement rates of 30% for tricyclic drugs, 50% for antipsychotic drugs, and 65% to 70% for their combined pharmacotherapy, ECT treatment frequently shows 85% to 90% improvement (see Fink, 1987). Therefore, ECT may be the first course of treatment for delusional depression, particularly in middle-aged or elderly patients, who respond most favorably. Highly suicidal patients also are good candidates for ECT treatment. There is unfortunately no good predictor of efficacy of ECT in a given patient. However, patients with high scores on the Hamilton Depression Scale, those who display prominent vegetative features, such as eating and sleeping disorders, and those who display agitation, cognitive impairment, or withdrawal tend to be helped by ECT treatment. As is true for the antidepressant drugs, ECT treatments must be administered several times a week for several weeks in order to be effective (e.g., 3 times a week for 3 weeks).

Weiner and Krystal (1994) and Fink (1987) describe the characteristics of ECT that enhance its effectiveness and safety. ECT is performed on patients anesthetized with an ultrashort-acting barbiturate. A muscle relaxant, such as succinylcholine, and continuous oxygenation are also usually administered. The mood changes following ECT are due to the cerebral seizure and not to convulsions, hypoxia, or other peripheral events. Curare or succinylcholine (which block cholinergic action at the muscles) prevent convulsions (i.e., the motor effect at muscles), but not the brain seizure, and do not reduce the clinical effectiveness of the therapy. Hyperoxygenation also has no effect on the effectiveness of ECT. The physiological manifestation best correlated with the antidepressant action of ECT is the appearance of a seizure activity pattern followed by a postseizure period of electrical silence. Within the last few years, seizure activity has been monitored by EEG to determine seizure duration, since muscle relaxation prevents direct observation of the behavioral correlate of seizure activity. Alternatively, seizure-induced tachycardia or observation of convulsive movements in one limb blocked from the muscle relaxing effects of succinylcholine by a blood pressure cuff, are used to monitor seizure duration.

The method of producing the seizure, by either electricity or various drugs (e.g., pentylenetetrazol or flurothyl) does not alter the effectiveness of the treatment. Electroshock is most often used because it does not produce the fear reaction that pentylenetetrazol frequently does, and ECT produces seizure more reliably than flurothyl. Furthermore, ECT is easier and safer to administer and apparently produces the least discomfort and side effects to the patient. For some patients, such as those with cardiovascular disorders, the elderly, medically ill, or pregnant individuals, ECT is significantly safer than drug therapies (Fink, 1987).

Improvements in sleep, appetite, menstrual cycle, and sex drive are correlated with the therapeutic effects on mood. These vegetative functions, normally considered to be under hypothalamic control, may be important to the therapeutic process. Fink (1984) suggests that antidepressant activity produced by ECT may be due to the stimulation of the hypothalamic–pituitary axis, leading to the release of peptides into the blood.

Side effects.   With the routine use of anesthesia, muscle relaxation, and oxygenation, side effects of ECT have been minimized (Khan et al., 1993; Weiner and Krystal, 1994). The most significant side effect is cognitive impairment, taking the form of confusion and memory loss. In particular, ECT disrupts the ability to retain information over a delay producing anterograde amnesia. The anterograde amnesia rarely lasts longer than a few weeks after ECT termination. Some patients, however, demonstrate significant retrograde amnesia for events preceding the treatment. Patients may have difficulty remembering events that occurred during the series of ECT treatments and several months or even years prior to the treatment. Apparently, both the amount and type of current and the placement of electrodes alters the effectiveness of treatment as well as the side effects. Although bilateral placement of electrodes tends to be more effective in alleviating depression than unilateral placement, cognitive impairment tends to be less with unilateral placement. In a similar fashion, sine wave current is more effective than brief pulses, but is more likely to produce cognitive impairment. We can conclude that technical factors in treatment administration strongly determine the magnitude of the antidepressant effects and the side effects resulting from ECT. However, it has been suggested that ECT effectiveness and side effects are independent of one another, implying that they are produced by distinct neurochemical mechanisms (Sackeim, 1994). ECT enhances activity in a number of transmitter systems in the brain (see below), which may be related to its effectiveness in the treatment of depression. In contrast, ECT-induced reduction in cholinergic transmission has been associated with its effects on memory and cognition, as well as depression (Mann and Kapur, 1994).

Drug interactions.   Classic antidepressant drugs are rarely used in patients treated with ECT since little evidence of improved effectiveness for dual treatment exists. However, the ECT sequence of treatment must often be started while plasma levels of antidepressants are still fairly high. Although cardiovascular side effects were once considered a danger associated with the antidepressant–ECT combination, newer ECT techniques minimize these side effects. The use of lithium and ECT tends to be avoided because their combination may lead to severe cognitive impairment. In contrast, combinations of antipsychotic drugs and ECT increases effectiveness for some patients, especially for those with mania and schizophrenia (Khan et al., 1993).

Mechanism of Action

The massive discharges of electrical activity that are induced by ECT produce widespread changes in body homeostasis affecting the central nervous system, the autonomic nervous system, the endocrine system, and whole body musculature. Because of these widespread effects, it is easy to find biochemical changes following ECT, but more difficult to correlate those changes with efficacy. Even though ECT effects may initially appear to be generalized to all CNS function, increasing evidence suggests that ECT has considerable pharmacological specificity. Current research emphasizes changes resulting from chronic ECT, since a single seizure does not produce clinical antidepressant effects. In addition, important controls are used to confirm that the changes detected are induced by ECT rather than anoxia, muscle convulsions, or coincidental drug treatment.

It has proven difficult to summarize the neurochemical changes in animals after electroshock because the many parameters of ECT administration vary from laboratory to laboratory. These factors include differences in stimulating electrode properties, placement of electrodes on the skull, direction and amount of current passed through the tissue, the nature of the seizure discharge following ECT, and the acute or chronic nature of the treatment. Despite the many experimental variables, there have been a large number of reports of ECT effects on brain chemistry (Fochtmann, 1994; Sackheim, Devanand, and Nobler, 1995). A correlation between some of these biochemical changes and antidepressant action may soon be identified.

Among the possibly significant effects of ECT is a change in electrolyte concentration. Most often Na^+, K^+, and Ca^{2+} have been studied because changes in the concentration of these ions across cell membranes link the electrical excitation of a cell with intracellular metabolic events. A significant decrease occurs in the level of Ca^{2+} in the CSF, blood, and urine following a series of seizures. The ECT-induced change in Ca^{2+} appears around the time when antidepressant effects are beginning (Fink, 1984). However, subsequent studies showed no change in Ca^{2+} channels using either the L-type channel antagonist [^{3}H]nitrendipine or a probe that labels N-type Ca^{2+} channels in any brain area examined (Gleiter and Nutt, 1989).

In an attempt to find a common link with antidepressant drug treatment, research has been focused on changes in neurotransmitter turnover, receptor binding,

and metabolism in both animal (Fochtmann, 1994; Gleiter and Nutt, 1989) and human studies (Mann and Kapur, 1994). In general, a variety of studies suggest that chronic ECT enhances the function of several neurotransmitter systems, including NE, 5-HT, DA, and GABA. These changes are likely to be the basis for the antidepressant effects of ECT. In contrast, ECT seems to dampen cholinergic function. Since ACh is strongly implicated in learning and memory (see Chapter 7), reduced cholinergic activity may be the basis for the cognitive side effects.

One of the earliest and most consistent findings of receptor change is the down-regulation of β_1-, but not β_2-receptors in the cerebral cortex and hippocampus following chronic treatment with ECT and other antidepressant treatments (see Caldecott-Hazard et al., 1991). The time course of receptor change correlates with the onset of clinical effectiveness, that is, after six electroshock treatments over a two-week period. Down-regulation of receptor number coincides with the reduced sensitivity of limbic forebrain adenylyl cyclase to stimulation by NE after chronic ECT (Vetulani, et al., 1976). Similar subsensitivity of the enzyme does not occur acutely, suggesting that chronic overexposure to NE is responsible for the change in enzyme sensitivity. Microdialysis and other studies demonstrate significant acute increases in brain NE levels and tyrosine hydroxylase activity (Sackheim, Devanand, and Nobler, 1995). ECT also prevents the development of hypersensitivity of the limbic forebrain NE system after reserpine administration. Thus, the therapeutic effects of ECT may be related to the development of subsensitivity of the postsynaptic adenylyl cyclase that is responsive to NE (Sulser, 1987).

In addition, binding to α_2-receptors also decreases following repeated ECT (Stanford and Nutt, 1982). This down-regulation may explain the behavioral evidence showing reduced responses (e.g., sedation and hypothermia) to clonidine following chronic ECT. Once again, brain microdialysis measures of extracellular NE suggest that both β-receptor and α_2-receptor down-regulation represent adaptive responses to the increase in synaptic NE (see Gleiter and Nutt, 1989).

In contrast to the down-regulation of 5-HT$_2$ receptors found following chronic antidepressant treatment, chronic ECT produces an increase in those receptors (see Kapur and Mann, 1993; Nutt and Glue, 1993). The increase in receptors may explain the enhancement of some 5-HT$_2$-mediated behaviors, such as hyperactivity and electrophysiological response, found by several investigators. An inhibition of K^+-evoked release of endogenous 5-HT from rat cortical slices has been found, and may be responsible for the 5-HT$_2$ receptor up-regulation (Green, Heal, and Vincent, 1987).

In contrast to the increase in 5-HT$_2$ receptors, behavioral and biochemical evidence demonstrates a down-regulation of 5-HT$_{1A}$ serotonin receptors. The 5-HT$_{1A}$ serotonin receptor agonist 8-OH-DPAT causes symptoms of the serotonin syndrome (which in rats includes hindlimb abduction, forepaw treading, lateral head-weaving, resting tremor, and hindlimb rigidity) as well as increased eating and hyperreactivity (see Lucki and Wieland, 1990). Following chronic ECT, profound and long-lasting subsensitivity to 8-OH-DPAT occurs for the behaviors that constitute the serotonin syndrome. The behavioral subsensitivity to the 5-HT$_{1A}$ agonist is apparent immediately following a series of electroshock treatments and persists for at least 10 days following the last treatment (Goodwin, DeSouza, and Green, 1987). The reduced sensitivity to 8-OH-DPAT after ECT is particularly interesting given that antidepressant drugs tend to increase behavioral responses mediated by 5-HT and have been implicated in the appearance of the serotonin syndrome in patients taking various combinations of medications, for example, fluoxetine and tryptophan or sertraline and an MAOI (see Bodner et al., 1995). In humans the syndrome is characterized by disorientation and restlessness, rigidity and hyperreflexia, especially in the legs, and autonomic instability, which includes nausea, shivering, flushing, tachycardia, and blood pressure changes (also see Chapter 9).

Other laboratories have investigated the effect of ECT on dopamine systems. Among the most consistent findings is the increased behavioral response to DA agonists following acute and chronic ECT treatment (see Sackheim, Devanand, and Nobler, 1995). For example, chronic electroshock treatments in animals enhance hyperactivity following methamphetamine and apomorphine administration. Since D$_1$ receptor agonists appear to be more effective than D$_2$ agonists, a selective modification of DA receptors is suggested. Selective D$_1$ receptor binding in rat substantia nigra is significantly increased by chronic ECT treatment (Fochtmann et al., 1989). However, it is not clear how this receptor change is related to the significant increase in DA and DA metabolite concentration following ECT, as reported in several microdialysis studies (see Nutt and Glue, 1993).

The ECT-induced effects on DA are further complicated by the clinical evidence that ECT has the unusual characteristic of producing antipsychotic effects and also anti-parkinsonian effects. Clearly a complex pattern of changes in DA function (along with other neurotransmitters) must be responsible for this distinct profile of clinical effects. Some researchers have advocated the use of ECT in combination with antipsychotic drugs in the treatment of schizophrenia to reduce extrapyramidal side effects (see Sackheim, Devanad, and Nobler, 1995).

ECT also produces changes in acetylcholine and in adenosine receptors. Chronic ECT-induced decreases in muscarinic cholinergic receptors in rat cerebral cortex, hippocampus, and striatum are reported by several groups. In addition, atropine-induced increases in muscarinic receptors can be prevented by concurrent ECT. Given that anticholinergic drugs impair certain types of memory in animals and humans, it is not surprising that the ECT-induced side effects of memory loss and confusion are attributed to the ECT-induced down-regulation of cholinergic receptors (see Mann and Kapur, 1994). An up-regulation of adenosine receptors following ECT begins after 3 daily electroshock treatments, increases to a maximum after 6 treatments, and persists for at least 14 days after 10 daily treatments (Gleiter et al., 1989). The authors suggest that the change in adenosine receptors represents another adaptive phenomenon because electrical seizure threshold rises during the course of ECT. Furthermore, over the same period, the electrically induced seizure duration decreases. The importance of adenosine to this change is demonstrated with the adenosine antagonist caffeine, which increases seizure duration.

Lithium Carbonate

The second major class of affective disorders is bipolar disorder (manic–depressive syndrome), which is characterized by extreme mood swings varying from mania to severe depression. Manic episodes may be characterized by euphoria, extreme hyperactivity, increased sexual activity, extreme financial irresponsibility, hostility, and violence.

For the majority of patients with bipolar disorder, lithium carbonate (Carbolith, Lithane) is the most effective medication and is the usual drug of choice. It is clearly superior to placebo in the treatment of acute mania after 2 weeks of treatment, although extending treatment for 5 weeks is necessary in some patients to achieve significant effects. One possible explanation is that despite significant plasma levels of lithium, uptake into cells is less for some individuals (Dunner and Clayton, 1987). For that reason, uptake into erythrocytes, which indicates intracellular levels, is compared with plasma levels in nonresponsive patients. For those with a low erythrocyte level, the dose of lithium can be raised, leading to increased cell uptake and subsequent symptom reduction.

Not only does lithium have acute antimanic effects, but it is also useful for reducing the frequency and severity of recurrent episodes of mania and depression. Lithium prevented relapses in 64% of manic–depressive patients compared with 21% of placebo-treated patients who did not relapse (Davis, 1976). Some evidence exists to suggest that lithium is less effective in preventing recurrence of depression than mania (Bunney and Garland-Bunney, 1987). Since 20% to 40% of patients with acute mania also experience psychotic symptoms, a combination of neuroleptics and lithium may be used, although some evidence of increased toxicity has been suggested with this dual treatment.

While lithium carbonate is widely recognized as the drug of choice for bipolar disorder, its use as an adjunct to antidepressant treatment for unipolar depression, delusional type, and treatment-resistant depression has also been suggested (Jefferson and Greist, 1990). The neurochemical basis for its potentiation of antidepressant action is unknown, but the enhancement of serotonergic systems has generated the greatest experimental support. Detailed discussion is provided by Bunney and Garland-Bunney (1987) and Rybakowski (1990).

Pharmacokinetics

Lithium is a member of the alkali metal family, which also includes sodium, potassium, rubidium, cesium, and francium. With an atomic number of 3 and an atomic weight of about 7, it is the smallest member of the family. It is prepared in the United States for therapeutics as lithium carbonate. The drug is readily absorbed from the GI tract and reaches peak blood levels within 30 minutes to 3 hours. Depot binding to protein is minimal, and the drug is not metabolized, but is excreted by the kidney in its intact form.

The effective therapeutic range of lithium concentration in blood is 0.7–1.2 mM, although no tests are available to determine the effective therapeutic blood drug level for a given individual. Side effects may include impaired concentration and memory, tremor, weight gain, and impaired renal function. Since toxic effects occur at blood levels of 2.0 mM, the therapeutic index is quite low, and a patient's blood level of lithium must be monitored closely. Acute toxic effects include vomiting, diarrhea, polydipsia, ataxia, tremor, fatigue, irritability, seizures, and coma (Jefferson and Greist, 1990). The low therapeutic index also means that in animal experiments, it is difficult to determine whether the effects of lithium on neurochemistry or neurophysiology are related to the therapeutic or the toxic effects of the drug. For a review of therapeutic effects and side effects as well as pharmacokinetics, see Calabrese, Bowden, and Woyshville (1995).

Biological Effects of Lithium

Electrolytes. Electrolytes are essential for neuronal function, for carrying electrical current, and also for the maintenance of neurotransmitter and its release. Because lithium belongs to the same group of elements as sodium and potassium and has a monovalent charge when ionized, it is reasonable to suspect that lithium, which has no known biological function, may exert its therapeutic effect by modifying neuronal ionic mechanisms. Lithium also has an ionic radius similar to those of magnesium and calcium; thus its action may also be related to interaction with these divalent cations. In some biological systems (e.g., isolated nerve preparation), lithium can partially substitute for sodium in carrying the current. However, the substitution is not complete because lithium is not extruded by the active, energy-requiring sodium pump (Peach, 1975). Hence, its antimanic action may be related to its ability to alter membrane excitability.

Several investigators have found that in red blood cells the ratio of intracellular to extracellular lithium ion (Li^+) is higher in bipolar patients than in normal controls when both have been administered lithium (Ramsey, 1981). Li^+ is moved across the membrane by an Li^+–Na^+ countertransport system that does not require energy but is driven by the electrochemical gradient for Na^+ across the membrane. Because the system appears to be under genetic control and is associated with increased vulnerability to bipolar disorder (Dorus et al., 1983), it is possible that the altered Li^+ concentration in red blood cells of manic–depressive individuals represents a genetic deficiency in their cell membrane transport. Although the blood cell transport may not be directly related to the psychotropic action of Li^+, it acts as a model and suggests an important potential site for the drug action within the CNS. However, on the whole, results of studies that examined Li^+ interactions with or substitution for K^+, Na^+, and Mg^{2+} have been quite inconsistent. A relationship between lithium's therapeutic effect in the treatment of mania and its effects on these ions has not been found (Ramsey, 1981).

The best evidence for an ionic mechanism of action for Li^+ involves Ca^{2+}. By competing for Ca^{2+} binding sites, lithium could affect Ca^{2+}-dependent release of neurotransmitter, alter Ca^{2+}-dependent cAMP production, or modify Ca^{2+}-mediated second messenger function. Abnormal Ca^{2+} metabolism is known to frequently produce emotional symptoms that disappear when normal function is restored. Carman and coworkers (1979) found a correlation between CSF levels of Ca^{2+} and the severity of depression. They also reported a change in plasma Ca^{2+} with the onset of mania. Finally, they showed consistent decreases in total Ca^{2+} in CSF and serum following successful electroconvulsive shock treatment. The decrease does not occur initially but develops after 3 or 4 treatments, in close relation with clinical improvement. Unfortunately, although Li^+ administration has been found to antagonize Ca^{2+} actions in some patients, these results, once again, are not consistent. Furthermore, administration of parathyroid hormone (which acutely increases serum Ca^{2+} levels) to manic–depressive individuals has not been found to alter their mood (Gerner et al., 1977).

In addition to acting on neuronal ionic mechanisms, lithium has a wide range of biological effects on a variety of systems, such as carbohydrate, fatty acid, and prostaglandin metabolism, antidiuretic hormone secretion, thyroid function, and the immune system (see Bach and Gallicchio, 1990). Furthermore, Li^+ has significant actions on biogenic amine metabolism.

Effects on serotonin. It should come as no surprise that the effects of lithium on 5-HT have been investigated extensively. In vitro studies on animal cells indicate that lithium enhances 5-HT actions, and this effect tends to persist during chronic treatment. Lithium is known to elevate brain tryptophan, 5-HT, and 5-HIAA. These as well as other indications of increased 5-HT turnover are described by Price and coworkers (Price et al., 1990).

Lithium also enhances 5-HT function by increasing release of 5-HT from brain slices (Friedman and Wang, 1988). Chronic, but not acute, lithium treatment elicits an increase in depolarization-induced efflux of [^{3}H]5-HT from superfused slices of parietal cortex, hippocampus, and hypothalamus. The fact that chronic treatment is necessary suggests that the change in 5-HT release may be due to an adaptive response of the cells, for instance, a change in autoreceptor regulation. Indirect evidence for desensitization of either autoreceptors or transduction mechanisms comes from testing the effects of 5-HT agonists and antagonists. Following chronic lithium treatment, the 5-HT agonist 5-methoxytryptamine is significantly less effective in reducing [^{3}H]5-HT release, while the 5-HT antagonist methiothepin less effectively enhances release of [^{3}H]5-HT.

Hotta and Yamawaki (1988) further demonstrated a distinct effect of lithium on release and receptor response in discrete brain areas. They found that short-term (3 days) lithium treatment enhanced K$^+$-evoked release from rat hippocampal slices, but not from frontal cortex. In hippocampal slices, the inhibitory effect of 5-HT on the release of [^{3}H]5-HT was significantly attenuated, but autoreceptor function was unchanged in cortical slices. The authors suggest that the acute effect of lithium on the autoreceptors may lead to the development of down-regulation of 5-HT$_1$ receptors, which occurs in the hippocampus but not in the cortex. Previously, others reported that Li$^+$ treatment did indeed reduce 5-HT receptors in the hippocampus and striatum, but not in the hypothalamus or cortex (Maggi and Enna, 1980). A preliminary examination of receptor subtypes showed reduced 5-HT$_2$ receptors in the frontal cortex and 5-HT$_1$ receptors in the hippocampus.

Whether lithium's long-term effects are mediated by altered 5-HT function, or whether they are due to an ionic effect on receptor interconversion between high and low affinity states, is not known. For instance, Battaglia, Shannon, and Titeler (1983) found Li$^+$ to be 5 times more potent than Na$^+$ or K$^+$ in decreasing 5-HT affinity for the 5-HT$_2$ receptor.

Clinically, evidence also favors a lithium-induced augmentation of 5-HT function, although results are less consistent. Despite the inconsistencies, large clinical studies tend to support the idea that lithium therapy increases CSF levels of 5-HIAA in patients with affective disorder, although these increases were not always statistically significant. Platelet uptake of 5-HT may be acutely depressed following lithium treatment (Poirier et al., 1988), but in general seems to be significantly elevated after long-term treatment (see Price et al., 1990). Studies examining the challenge effects of 5-HT agonists on neuroendocrine function in patients with affective disorder also produce complex results. Several reports show an enhanced cortisol response to fenfluramine (a 5-HT releaser) in patients treated with lithium or an increased prolactin release following intravenous tryptophan (see Price et al., 1990). However, others (Manji et al., 1991) report no statistically significant effects of lithium on prolactin, corticotropin, or cortisol responses to clomipramine challenge.

Effects on norepinephrine. The ability of lithium to decrease catecholamine activity has been cited in support of the catecholamine hypothesis of affective disorders. Lithium apparently enhances the uptake of NE and 5-HT into both synaptosomes and brain slices. Increasing monoamine uptake effectively reduces the action of the neurotransmitters at the synapse. Neurochemical changes such as these may suggest a basis for the acute antimanic effects as well as the prophylactic effects of lithium.

Lithium also reduces the release of [^{3}H]NE from electrically stimulated brain slices but does not change the spontaneous release of the amine. It is likely that this action of lithium is related to its competitive interference with the role of calcium in the excitation–secretion coupling mechanism (Katz and Kopin, 1969). The inhibition of release by lithium can be reversed by adding excess calcium.

The effect of lithium on NE turnover is not so clear. Corrodi and coworkers (1967) found that acute administration of LiCl increased the rate of disappearance of NE after treatment with the synthesis inhibitor α-methyltyrosine. Schildkraut, Schanberg, and Kopin (1966) found a similar decrease in [^{3}H]NE after intracisternal injection of the labeled amine. An increase in tritiated deaminated metabolite and a decrease in [^{3}H]normetanephrine suggests that lithium increases intracellular deamination by MAO, a result in accord with the enhanced neurotransmitter uptake by lithium. In another report, low dosages of lithium administration produced significantly reduced NE content in rat brain stem, hypothalamus, and midbrain, and elevated levels in cortical areas without corresponding changes in the NE metabolite MHPG (Ahluwalia and Singhal, 1980). Others have reported, however, that prolonged lithium administration produces no change in NE or DA turnover (Bliss and Ailion, 1970). Thus, a clear relationship between long-term clinical efficacy of lithium and its ability to alter NE turnover is not immediately apparent.

Our modified hypothesis of mania and depression might lead us to speculate that increased synaptic activity during mania induces a state of receptor down-regulation. Evidence seems to suggest, however, that lithium is unable to block the development of β-receptor subsensitivity induced by experimental manipulation, for example, following chronic imipramine treatment in rats (Rosenblatt et al., 1979). In fact, reports suggest that lithium alone either decreases β-receptors in rat cortex (Trieser and Kellar, 1979) or produces no significant change in β-receptor binding (Gross, Dodt, and Hanft, 1988). Further, Treiser and Kellar (1979) and others have shown that lithium is capable of reversing reserpine-induced β-receptor supersensitivity in rat cerebral cortex, while not affecting the increase in α-receptors. It would seem that lithium's effect on NE receptors does not fit our revised model. Although lithium-induced modification of β-receptors may be a significant factor in drug action, it is difficult at this point to imagine how changes in receptor binding can explain the unique characteristics of lithium's antimania and antidepressant actions as well as prophylaxis for the cycling disorder.

Effects on Second Messenger Systems

cAMP. While the effects of lithium on neurotransmitter receptors are varied and at times contradictory, consideration of the drug's effects on second messengers may help to reconcile some of the disparities. It is apparent that lithium alters the transduction of the neurotransmitter-initiated signal by modifying the function of second messengers such as adenylyl cyclase and phosphoinositide cycling or receptor–effector coupling via G proteins.

Lithium inhibits the synthesis of cAMP by adenylyl cyclase in many brain regions, including the cerebral cortex, caudate, and hippocampus, but not in the brain stem or cerebellum. In addition, lithium, at clinically relevant doses, reduces the ability of NE to stimulate adenylyl cyclase activity above basal levels in human postmortem brain tissue (Newman et al., 1983), as well as in animals (Ebstein, Hermoni, and Belmaker, 1980). Such results suggest that lithium reduces the postsynaptic action of NE on second messenger systems. Furthermore, lithium pretreatment prevents reserpine-induced increases in NE-induced cAMP formation in rat cerebral cortex at a dose that does not directly inhibit NE-sensitive adenylyl cyclase. This neurochemical effect may be indicative of the prophylactic effect of lithium (Ebstein, Hermoni, and Belmaker, 1980).

The inhibitory action of lithium on NE-sensitive adenylyl cyclase is a consistent finding, but lithium clearly has distinctive effects on the adenylyl cyclase that is coupled to receptors other than NE. For example, instead of inhibition, lithium seems to have a stimulatory effect on DA-sensitive adenylyl cyclase (Reches, Ebstein, and Belmaker, 1978) or no effect at all in ex vivo studies (Newman and Belmaker, 1987). Serotonin-stimulated adenylyl cyclase activity is apparently increased in rat hippocampus after 3 weeks, but not after 5 days, of Li$^+$ treatment, despite a reduction in density of 5-HT$_1$ receptors (Hotta and Yamawaki, 1986). Also, at higher concentrations, lithium modifies hormone-sensitive adenylyl cyclase in kidney, thyroid, and platelets as well as in brain (see Bunney and Garland-Bunney, 1987). The

drug's ability to act on these second messenger systems normally regulated by antidiuretic hormone, thyroid-stimulating hormone, and prostaglandins may explain some of its therapeutic as well as toxic effects, such as induced diabetes insipidus or hypothyroidism.

More detailed examination of the adenylyl cyclase transduction mechanism has led many investigators to evaluate the effects of chronic lithium on postreceptor function (see Jope and Williams, 1994). Several in vitro studies in rat brain have shown that lithium inhibits GTP-, Gpp(NH)p-, fluoride-, forskolin-, and Ca^{2+}-camodulin-stimulated adenylyl cyclase activity, all of which normally activate adenylyl cyclase at points beyond the membrane receptor (Mork and Geisler, 1989b; Newman and Belmaker, 1987). Sodium fluoride, GTP, and GTP analogs increase cAMP synthesis via G protein activation, while Ca^{2+}-dependent calmodulin activation of adenylyl cyclase may work by a direct effect on the catalytic subunit. Forskolin, once believed to act solely on the catalytic unit, has been found to bind to a high-affinity site on the G$_s$ protein as well as to a low-affinity site on the catalytic unit. Nevertheless, in all of these cases, adenylyl cyclase activation occurs at a point beyond the neurotransmitter receptor; hence, the inhibition of their actions by lithium suggests an action beyond the receptor stage.

Mork and Geisler (1989a) went on to demonstrate that long-term (4 week) pretreatment of rats with lithium produced a reduction in isoprenaline-induced increases in cAMP production in cortical membranes. This ex vivo effect of lithium could be overcome by elevating GTP concentrations. Thus, the results suggest that lithium may reduce NE-induced adenylyl cyclase activation by altering the normal agonist/receptor enhancement of GTP stimulation. The same researchers have shown that not only short-term but also long-term pretreatment of rats with lithium also reduces Gpp(NH)p- and forskolin-stimulated adenylyl cyclase, suggesting a postreceptor action.

Belmaker and coworkers (Belmaker et al., 1990) more directly examined the effect of lithium on the β-receptor agonist-induced increase in GTP binding to G protein. They found that lithium at therapeutic concentrations (0.4–1.2 mM) blocked the usual increase in cerebral cortex GTP binding to G$_s$ following isoproterenol stimulation. The pretreatment had no effect on basal GTP binding. Experiments in which rats were treated with lithium carbonate for 21 days before measuring GTP binding to G proteins produced similar results. On the basis of this information, they propose that the effects of Li$^+$ on G protein–GTP binding following adrenergic agonist stimulation have essentially the same net effect on catecholamine neural transmission that long-term antidepressants have. Lithium and antidepressant actions differ, however, in that the latter work via down-regulation of receptors, while lithium acts distal to the receptor. The similarity of effects, however, does not necessarily correlate with antidepressant action, nor does it explain the antimanic or prophylactic effects of lithium.

Once again, the results in humans are less consistent. Ebstein and coworkers found that euthymic patients show reduced basal adenylyl cyclase activity, as well as inhibition of forskolin- and sodium fluoride–stimulated activity in platelets after lithium treatment (Ebstein et al., 1988). It is believed that the inhibition may be due to lithium's ability to compete with the essential Mg^{2+} cation for a regulatory site on the enzyme (Mork and Geisler, 1989b). Such an effect is not likely to explain the therapeutic effects of the drug, since Ebstein and his group showed that 3 weeks of treatment in 10 manic patients significantly reduced the affinity of lithium for adenylyl cyclase (Ebstein et al., 1987). Furthermore, the effects of long-term lithium treatment in rats could not be reversed by increasing Mg^{2+}, suggesting that the long-term inhibition must be due to a mechanism other than competition with Mg^{2+}. The finding that lithium's long-term effects could be reversed by increasing GTP concentrations suggests that an important action of lithium may be on the G proteins in human as well as in animal tissues (Mork and Geisler, 1989a). Some evidence for altered G protein subunits ($G_{s\alpha}$) in the pathogenesis of bipolar disorder exists (Young, Porrino, and Iadarola, 1991). Lithium may have several inhibitory sites: competing for the Mg^{2+} site acutely (demonstrated only in vitro) and an inhibitory action on GTP activation, which has been seen ex vivo.

In contrast to Ebstein's findings, Risby and colleagues (1991) found elevated basal and Gpp(NH)p-stimulated adenylyl cyclase in platelets from normal human volunteers treated for 2 weeks with lithium carbonate. Interestingly, such an increase was not found in the lymphocytes from the same subjects. What they did find was that lithium induced an increase in the ratio of low- to high-affinity dissociation constants for β-receptor binding in the lymphocytes, suggesting an altered coupling between β-receptors and stimulatory G proteins. Whether the differences between studies have to do with subject variations (patients or healthy volunteers) or differences in methodologies has not been resolved. Risby and colleagues (1991) provide an excellent discussion of the issues, develop a model for the lithium-adenylyl cyclase interaction, and provide a brief but excellent review of G protein mediation of receptor-regulated adenylyl cyclase.

In addition to its effects on brain NE and NE-sensitive adenylyl cyclase, lithium also alters the metabolism of other neurotransmitters, including 5-HT, ACh, and GABA. However, the results of experiments investigating their role in lithium's therapeutic action have not produced a cohesive model of drug action.

Effects on the phosphoinositide (PI) cycle. Neurotransmitter regulation of the PI second messenger system is also altered by lithium at concentrations considered therapeutically relevant (Sherman et al., 1986). Since PI regulates a wide variety of cell functions that are mediated by intracellular Ca^{2+} mobilization and protein kinase C activity, lithium-induced modification of the PI cycle can have many effects.

Although the PI cycle is complex, there are some basic features generally agreed upon. Agonist–receptor binding via a G protein mediator triggers the phosphodiesteratic cleavage of phosphatidylinositol-4,5-bisphosphate (PIP_2) by phospholipase C. PIP_2 cleavage produces two products: inositol trisphosphate (IP_3) and diacylglycerol (DAG). IP_3 is responsible for the mobilization of intracellular Ca^{2+}, while DAG activates protein kinase C by enhancing its affinity for calcium. IP_3 can then undergo dephosphorylation by phosphatase enzymes to yield free inositol, which is recycled into PIP_2. IP_3 can also be phosphorylated to form IP_4, a precursor to IP_5. A schematic diagram of a portion of the PI cycle is in Figure 19.7. Chapter 6 provides further background material on the PI second messenger system.

One particularly significant action of lithium on the PI cycle is the inhibition of the phosphatase that converts inositol monophosphate (IP_1) into inositol. Early experiments showed that acute systemic administration of lithium at therapeutic concentrations could reduce inositol levels in rat cerebral cortex, while producing a parallel increase in IP_1 and to a lesser extent IP_3 and IP_4. The inositol/inositol monophosphate effect was found in several brain regions, such as the hypothalamus, hippocampus, and caudate, but not in the cerebellum or corpus callosum. It is conceivable that low levels of inositol may compromise the resynthesis of phosphoinositides, thereby reducing the subsequent receptor response to stimulation. The importance of the phospholipid metabolism effect of lithium has been proposed as a potential explanation for its mood-stablizing effect. Lithium's effects on the PI cycle have generated a good deal of excitement: because the phospholipid second messenger is coupled to both excitatory and inhibitory neurotransmitter receptors, lithium can have an antimanic and/or an antidepressant effect.

There is some indirect evidence for altered PI metabolism in manic–depressive individuals. For example, these individuals show increases in sensitivity to agonist-stimulated accumulation of inositol phosphates, activity of protein kinase C, and intracellular Ca^{2+} responses, along with elevated resting levels of intracellular Ca^{2+} (see Atack, Broughton, and Pollack, 1995a). Each of these are assumed to reflect altered PI function in these patients. In addition, platelet membrane PIP_2 levels are elevated during the manic phase of the disorder (Brown, Mallinger, and Renbaum, 1993), while CSF inositol tends to be low. How these clinical findings relate to PI signal transduction is not clear.

Unfortunately, most knowledge about PI metabolism comes from studies using tissue other than CNS.

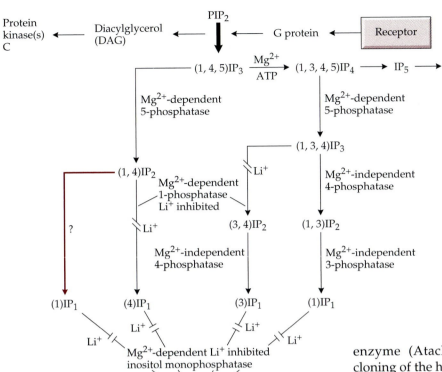

19.7 THE PHOSPHOINOSITIDE CYCLE INCLUDING THE SYNTHESIS AND METABOLISM OF MULTIPLE SECOND MESSENGERS. Not shown is the reincorporation of inositol into the membrane-bound phosphoinositides. Note that Li^+ can inhibit several of the phosphatases, although it is most potent on the monophosphatases, resulting in an increase in levels of inositol monophosphate and a decrease in inositol levels. (After Nahorski, 1988.)

Thus, a general model of PI regulation should not be assumed. For instance, in brain, despite lithium-induced depression of inositol formation, the levels of PIP_2 remain relatively unchanged unless pilocarpine, a cholinergic agonist that increases PI turnover, is administered to lithium-treated animals. Under such challenging conditions, a significant decrease in rat cerebral cortex phosphoinositides occurs (Atack, Broughton, and Pollack, 1995a; Ragan, 1990). Nevertheless, several investigators have found that lithium seems to reduce the effects of neurotransmitters on the PI cycle in cortical slices prepared from lithium-treated animals (Kendall and Nahorski, 1987; Ragan, 1990). In rat brain slices, Li^+ reduces agonist-induced increases in IP_3 and IP_4, and subsequently reduces the mobilization of intracellular Ca^{2+}. These effects can be reversed by the addition of exogenous inositol (administered as myo-inositol), but not by an inactive analog of inositol (scyllo-inositol). Results such as these demonstrate the importance of lithium-induced depletion of inositol in the drug's biochemical effects.

The importance of inositol monophosphatase inhibition to the intracellular effects of lithium can be demonstrated using several newly synthesized inhibitors of the enzyme. For example, one phosphatase antagonist, L690488, reduces agonist-stimulated increases in IP_3 and IP_4, as well as several other measures of PI signaling, just as we have seen with lithium. The potential therapeutic usefulness of phosphatase inhibition has led to detailed biochemical, kinetic, and structural evaluation of the

enzyme (Atack, Broughton, and Pollack, 1995b). The cloning of the human and rat enzymes, X-ray crystallography showing the three-dimensional structure, and determination of the amino acid sequences constituting the active sites for substrate and metal binding have paved the way for development of novel inhibitors of the enzyme, which may have significant clinical utility.

Inhibition of inositol monophosphatases is only one of the potential sites proposed for lithium action on second messenger systems. As was true for lithium effects on adenylyl cyclase, lithium appears to differentially alter the PI cycle regulated by ACh, NE and 5-HT in various brain areas. For example, Casebolt and Jope (1989) examined receptor-coupled inositol phospholipid hydrolysis in brain slices from rats treated with lithium for 30 days. Lithium significantly reduced NE-stimulated PI hydrolysis in the cortex, hippocampus, and striatum, while the effects of 5-HT were attenuated in hippocampal and striatal slices, but not in the cortex. In contrast, although carbachol induced a concentration-dependent, fivefold maximal increase in hydrolysis in cortical slices from control animals, lithium pretreatment had only a small inhibitory effect. In addition, lithium apparently had no effect on the PI response to carbachol in hippocampus, but had a significant inhibitory effect in striatal slices. The finding that lithium pretreatment did not alter NaF-induced PI hydrolysis in the cortex may mean that lithium alters receptor function in that region rather than acting further downstream in the second messenger sequence. NaF is believed to directly activate the G protein coupled to phospholipase C, which cleaves the inositol phospholipids. Rather than G protein–enzyme uncoupling, lithium may uncouple the receptor from the G protein, as has been described in an earlier section regarding receptor-coupled adenylyl cyclase (see Atack, Broughton, and Pollack, 1995a).

Avissar, Schreiber, and Danon (1988) suggested G proteins as the common site for antimanic and antidepressant effects, perhaps by competition between Li$^+$ and Mg^{2+} ions, which are known to be essential for GTP binding to G proteins. They showed that lithium inhibited the isoprenaline- and carbachol-induced increase in [^{3}H]GTP binding to cortical membranes both in vitro and ex vivo. In addition, lithium pretreatment inhibited the ability of Gpp(NH)p to modulate muscarinic agonist binding.

Whether lithium works via monophosphatase inhibition or receptor–G protein uncoupling, its inhibition of the receptor-mediated stimulation of phosphoinositide turnover alters synaptic transmission. Worley and coworkers have shown that lithium antagonizes receptor-mediated electrophysiological effects on postsynaptic responses in hippocampal cells (Worley, Heller, and Snyder, 1988). The dampening of phosphoinositide-mediated signal transduction in both inhibitory and excitatory neurons may explain the antimanic as well as antidepressant effects of lithium. A model of such action, originally proposed by Berridge, Downes, and Hanley (1982), is discussed by Atack, Broughton, and Pollack, (1995a). A detailed discussion of the biochemical effects of lithium on the PI cycle is available in a review by Jope and Williams (1994).

Lithium Effects on Gene Expression

It is clear that G protein function is an integral part of both the cAMP and PI second messenger systems. Since lithium must be chronically administered to be effective, and many patients are maintained on the drug for extended periods, it is not surprising that lithium has effects on gene expression. Lithium alters the protein and mRNA levels of several components of the second messenger systems described. Lithium's effects on gene expression and protein phosphorylation are summarized by Jope and Williams (1994). In general, chronic lithium reduces mRNA levels for several of the G protein subunits (e.g., $G_{s\alpha}$, $G_{i1\alpha}$, $G_{i2\alpha}$) in rat cerebral cortex, though reductions in the corresponding proteins are not always reported. In contrast, chronic lithium increases adenylyl cyclase mRNA levels and the corresponding protein. Further, chronic lithium enhances pilocarpine- or carbachol-induced increases in c-fos mRNA. The transcription factor c-fos regulates the expression of other genes and is induced by stimuli that activate protein kinase C (among other mechanisms). The fact that lithium can modify c-fos expression means that the drug can affect the expression of other genes, resulting in widespread actions on cell function. Li$^+$ also changes mRNA levels of numerous proteins, including peptides (such as prodynorphin and neuropeptide Y), enzymes (such as tyrosine hydroxylase), and the glucocorticoid receptor. Recent evidence suggests that chronic lithium produces transcriptional

and posttranscriptional effects via protein kinase C–induced alterations in transcription regulatory factors (Manji and Lenox, 1994).

Alternative Drug Therapies for Bipolar Disorder

Alternative therapies to lithium in treating bipolar disorder have been developed because lithium has potentially toxic side effects and, in combination with neuroleptics, poses particular difficulties for some patients. Furthermore, some patients, such as the rapid-cycling bipolar patients (i.e., those having more than 4 cyclic episodes in a year), are resistant to the therapeutic effects of lithium. Of these alternative treatments, the anticonvulsant drug carbamazepine (Tegretol) is most frequently used. Carbamazepine is a structurally atypical anticonvulsant drug because it resembles the tricyclic antidepressants. Its use as an anticonvulsant derives, in part, from the knowledge that it is effective in inhibiting limbic afterdischarges and the seizures that follow repeated limbic stimulation. Its use as an antimanic agent was suggested by the proposal that repeated stress and episodes of affective illness might sensitize limbic structures, such as occurs in electrophysiological stimulation-induced kindling (Post et al., 1984). Since patients treated with car-

Carbamazepine

bamazepine for temporal lobe epilepsy also show improvements in mood and cognition (Dalby, 1975), its trial use in affective illness seemed warranted.

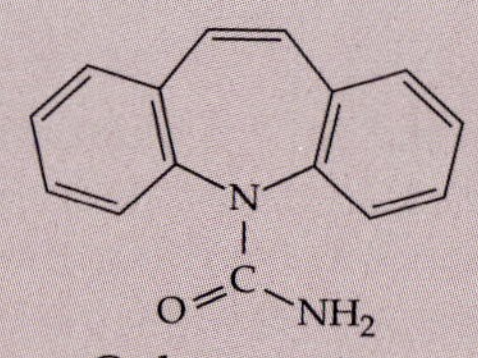

A series of clinical trials that compared the effectiveness of carbamazepine with that of lithium is summarized by Post and colleagues (1984). In these trials, patients with DSM-III-diagnosed affective illness were studied in a double-blind, placebo-controlled, off-on-off-on design. Comparative results are shown in Figure 19.8. It is apparent that the extent of effectiveness and the time course of efficacy in reducing manic symptoms is virtually identical for the two agents. Carbamazepine was also reported to be effective in the attenuation of symptoms during the depressive phase of the illness, although the results were less dramatic than they were during treatment of the manic phase. Furthermore, of seven patients who were unresponsive to lithium treatment, six of them showed a good overall prophylactic response to carbamazepine in terms of reduced frequency and severity of episodes. These results support the use of carbamazepine in patients unresponsive to lithium (Post, Weiss, and Chuang, 1992).

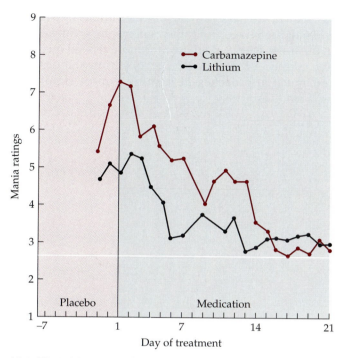

19.8 TIME COURSE AND EXTENT OF EFFECTIVENESS OF CAR-BAMAZEPINE AND LITHIUM IN REDUCING MANIC SYMP-TOMS in patients with bipolar disorder. (After Post et al., 1984.)

The most common side effects of carbamazepine include a mild sedation and ataxia, appearance of an itchy rash, nausea, tremors, weight gain, and cognitive changes. Reduced white blood cell count also occurs. Many of the side effects can be controlled by modifying the dose. Calabrese, Bowden, and Woyshville (1995) provide a more complete discussion.

Another anticonvulsive drug that has demonstrated effectiveness as a "mood stabilizer" in bipolar disorder is valproate (Depakene), a simple branched-chain fatty acid. Its effectiveness for acute mania seems to be unrelated to the patient's response to other therapies, such as lithium and carbamazepine, and so it can be used for patients who are refractory to the usual treatments. It is also used for patients with rapid-cycling bipolar disorder and for bipolar disorder with some organic component, such as head trauma preceding the onset of illness. Serious side effects are rare, although liver function may be compromised in some individuals, particularly in children treated with multiple drugs. Other side effects include GI upset, sedation, hand tremor, and loss of hair. Guay (1995) provides a recent review of effectiveness, adverse effects, and potential for drug interaction with this treatment.

Other treatments receiving some consideration as antimanic agents include clonidine, lorazepam, clonazepam, verapamil (McElroy et al., 1992), and electroconvulsive therapy. A brief summary of their effective-

ness is provided by Dunner and Clayton (1987) and by Mauri and colleagues (1990).

Part III Summary

Despite some controversy surrounding its use, electroconvulsive therapy (ECT) is another valuable treatment for depression, particularly for patients who are resistant to standard antidepressant drugs. The therapeutic efficacy of ECT depends on the induction of cerebral seizures and, presumably, secondary changes in neurotransmitter systems and signal transduction mechanisms. Repeated ECT treatments lead to down-regulation of β_1- and α_2-adrenergic receptors, NE-sensitive adenylyl cyclase activity, and 5-HT$_1$ receptors, but they lead to an increased density of 5-HT$_2$ receptors. It is not yet clear which of these effects are responsible for the antidepressant action of ECT.

Bipolar disorder is most commonly treated with lithium carbonate instead of antidepressant drugs or ECT. The neurochemical effects of acute and chronic lithium administration are very complex, and include altered electrolyte balance, enhanced serotonergic function, reduced activity of NE-sensitive adenylyl cyclase, and blockade of inositol monophosphatase, an important enzyme in the phosphoinositide second messenger system. Lithium should be thought of as a "mood stabilizer" rather than a stimulant or depressant, and thus it is likely to have some actions (but not others) in common with antidepressant medications. Other mood stabilizers introduced more recently include the anticonvulsant compounds carbamazepine and valproate.

From the preceding discussion of drug treatment for affective disorders, it should be clear that the mechanism of action of the most effective agents is not always known. Clinically, the course of therapy for individual patients is most often empirically derived. However, ultimately subpopulations of patients responding to a particular pharmacological treatment will be identified, and this information will provide an essential step in the understanding of pharmacological treatment, CNS biochemistry, and its relationship to the affective disorders.

This chapter has discussed the most recent hypotheses regarding the neurochemical bases for the affective disorders, as well as the neurochemical rationale for treatment as it is currently understood. The biogenic amine hypothesis of affective disorders and its modifications continue to provide a driving force for neuropharmacological research. Although the therapeutic effectiveness of the conventional antidepressant treatments lends support to the importance of the amine neurotransmitters, there is still much to be learned about the drugs' mechanisms of action. The development of novel antidepressants with more specific neurochemical loci, including direct modification of second messenger systems, promises to elucidate the neurochemistry of psychotherapeutics and provide more effective treatment in the future.

Quite clearly, the research described has produced as many questions as answers. We hope that the critical assessment we have provided of the various hypotheses will not discourage, but rather will inspire greater efforts in the neuroscience field, toward more refined quantitative methods, better-controlled experimental designs, and novel approaches in treating a most significant problem.

Chapter 20

Parkinson's Disease and Alzheimer's Disease

Neurodegenerative disorders are of interest to neuropharmacologists for several reasons. First, the behavioral deficits that occur when particular chemically coded neuronal populations are damaged can provide critical insights into the functions of these systems. For example, the discovery of a profound depletion of striatal dopamine (DA) in patients with Parkinson's disease triggered a massive amount of research on the role of this transmitter in movement control. Second, pharmacological manipulation of neurotransmitter activity is one of the major therapeutic strategies used in the treatment of neurodegenerative disorders. This final chapter will therefore present current information and theories concerning two prominent neurodegenerative disorders of aging: Parkinson's disease and Alzheimer's disease.

Part I
Parkinson's Disease

The history of Parkinson's disease (PD) has recently been summarized by Kopin (1993a). It is difficult to determine whether PD has been present throughout human history. Because it is primarily a disease of aging, there may have been few PD cases when the average human life span was decades less than it is now. According to Kolb and Whishaw (1990), many of the individual symptoms of PD were observed by physicians as far back as the second century Greek physician Galen. However, it wasn't until the early 19th century that London physician James Parkinson first recognized the disorder as a distinct clinical entity. In 1817, Parkinson published an account of six patients suffering from a movement disorder characterized by tremor, a bent posture, and, as the disorder progressed, increasing difficulty in initiating voluntary movement. The disease was initially called "shaking palsy" or "paralysis agitans," but was later named Parkinson's disease by the French neurologist Charcot.

When we refer to PD in this chapter, we are specifically referring to idiopathic ("of spontaneous origin; without known cause") parkinsonism. However, parkinsonian symptoms may occur under a wide variety of conditions (Gybels, 1994). Some of these conditions are disease-related, as in postencephalitic parkinsonism. Certain drugs can also produce parkinsonian symptoms, such as the DA receptor-blocking agents used in the treatment of schizophrenia (see Chapter 18).

Any disorder can be characterized by a prevalence ratio, which refers to the proportion of a population that suffers from the disorder at a particular point in time. Because PD is primarily a disease of aging, its prevalence ratio increases dramatically as older cohorts are examined (Schoenberg, 1987; Figure 20.1). Furthermore, epidemiological studies have found PD in all countries that have been studied to date (Zhang and Roman, 1993). However, it is important to determine whether prevalence ratios vary across different geographic areas and/or ethnic groups to identify possible causes of or risk fac-

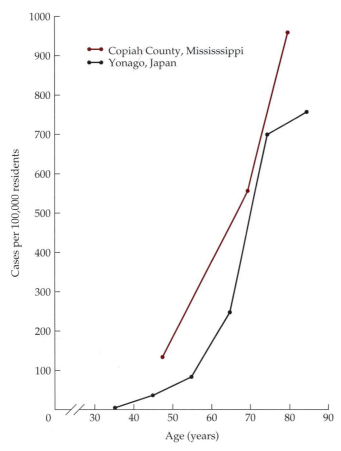

20.1 AGE-SPECIFIC PREVALENCE RATIOS OF PARKINSON'S DISEASE in Copiah County, Mississippi and Iyonago, Japan. (After Schoenberg, 1987.)

sent. Because PD is a progressive degenerative disorder, the kinds of symptoms present and their severity depend significantly on the length of time since onset, the rapidity of functional decline, and whether or not the patient has been receiving medication.

Motor Disturbances

The movement disturbances of PD can be separated into positive symptoms (behaviors rarely, if ever, seen in healthy individuals) and negative symptoms (deficit in or loss of a normal behavioral capacity) (Kolb and Whishaw, 1990).

Positive motor symptoms.   The positive symptoms of PD are (1) tremor, (2) muscular rigidity, and (3) involuntary movements. PD patients typically exhibit a 4–6-Hz resting tremor that is particularly prominent in the distal extremities and that disappears during sleep (Struppler, Erbel, and Velho, 1978). Tremor of the hands is often called a "pill rolling" tremor because it resembles the movements involved in rolling a pill between the thumb and forefinger. Also common in PD is a postural tremor that occurs when antigravity muscles are stimulated in the course of postural maintenance. This type of tremor may be manifested as a shaking of the limbs (when held against gravity) or as a generalized shaking of the trunk. The second symptom, muscle rigidity (i.e., tonically increased muscle tone), occurs in both extensor and flexor muscles. The nature of this rigidity can be seen most clearly when a limb is moved passively around a joint. In such cases, the force is initially resisted, but eventually a short movement occurs. The force is then resisted again and the process is repeated, resulting in an eventual extension or flexion of the limb, but in a series of jerky steps. As the limb movement resembles the action of a cog, this condition has been termed "cogwheel rigidity." The third positive symptom, involuntary movements, is also called akathesia. Such movements consist mainly of constant shifts in posture, which may sometimes be used to relieve tremor or stiffness (Kolb and Whishaw, 1990).

Negative motor symptoms.   The two major types of negative symptoms in parkinsonian patients are (1) bradykinesia (poverty or slowing of movement) and (2) postural disturbances. Bradykinesia may be manifested by difficulty in walking, absence of facial expression ("masked facies"), poverty of blinking, and a lack of spontaneous speech. Patients have problems both in initiating walking and in maintaining a normal gait, and consequently they typically shuffle their feet in short steps. Unfortunately, the difficulties associated with bradykinesia are exacerbated by the postural disturbances of PD, which include a difficulty in maintaining normal position of body parts (e.g., a drooping head) and impaired righting (standing up from a supine position). In the most extreme cases, patients may suffer from periods during which they cannot move at all (akinesia). Nonetheless,

tors for PD. In this case, prevalence ratios must be age-adjusted because age profiles (i.e., percentage of the population between 40 and 50, between 50 and 60, and so forth) vary among different countries and ethnic groups. PD prevalence ratios are usually age-adjusted to the age profile of the United States in 1960, 1970, or some other specified year. Most studies of PD across various countries have found age-adjusted prevalence ratios ranging from approximately 60 cases/100,000 individuals to approximately 180/100,000, although a few groups, such as the inhabitants of rural areas of China, reportedly exhibit lower prevalence ratios (Schoenberg, 1987; Zhang and Roman, 1993). It is presently unclear whether this range of variation is due to differential exposure to environmental risk factors (see below), genetic differences in vulnerability, or interstudy variability in diagnostic criteria, survey techniques, or other key methodological factors.

Behavioral and Psychological Characteristics of Parkinson's Disease

PD is usually thought of as a motor disorder, although we shall see that other types of symptoms are also pre-patients can sometimes briefly overcome even severe bradykinesia or akinesia by extreme effort or when aroused by a sudden strong stimulus (Selby, 1990). This is termed "paradoxical kinesia."

Motor symptom progression. As described by Kolb and Whishaw (1990), the motor symptoms of PD typically begin with a minor tremor in one hand and perhaps a slight muscular stiffness in the limbs. As the disease progresses, the tremor worsens, movements are slowed, blinking is lost, and the masklike facial appearance is observed. The patient subsequently adopts a stooped posture and a shuffling gait (Figure 20.2). Speech becomes laborious, and there are also problems with chewing and swallowing. One approach to classifying the severity of clinical disability in PD is the following staging system developed by Hoehn and Yahr (1967):

> *Stage I.* Unilateral involvement only, usually with minimal or no functional impairment. *Stage II.* Bilateral or midline involvement, with no impairment of balance. *Stage III.* First sign of impaired righting reflexes. Functionally the patient is somewhat restricted in his activities but may have some work potential depending upon the type of employment. Patients are physically capable of leading independent lives, and their disability is mild to moderate. *Stage IV.* Fully developed, severely disabling disease; the patient is still able to walk and stand unassisted but is markedly incapacitated. *Stage V.* Confinement to bed or wheelchair unless aided. (p. 433, italics added)

The Hoehn and Yahr staging system came out of a classic study of the onset and progression of PD in 802 patients seen at Columbia–Presbyterian Medical Center in New York City between 1949 and 1964. In about two-thirds of the cases, symptom onset began between the ages of 50 and 69. Within 5 years of symptom onset, approximately 20% of the patients were severely disabled or dead. The percentage rose to over 80% by 10 to 14 years following symptom onset, although a small subgroup of atypical patients exhibited an extremely slow disease progression in which severe disability had still not occurred after 20 years (Hoehn and Yahr, 1967). It is important to note that these data were obtained well before the advent of current pharmacotherapies that provide substantial symptomatic relief for many patients and, in some cases, may even slow the course of disease progression (see below).

Cognitive Dysfunction

As mentioned earlier, PD is not just a motor disorder. For example, many patients exhibit varying degrees of cognitive dysfunction. In the most extreme cases, the individual may suffer from **dementia**, which refers to a severe impairment of memory, abstract thinking, language, and other cognitive processes. Dementia that is associ-

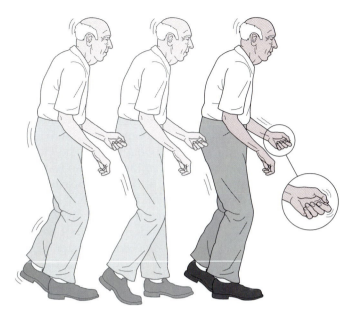

20.2 CLASSIC SYMPTOMS OF LATE-STAGE PARKINSON'S DISEASE, including a stooped and rigid posture, shuffling gait, tremor, a masklike facial appearance, and "pill rolling" (*inset*). (After Markey, 1986.)

ated with PD or other disorders that involve mostly subcortical pathology (see below) is sometimes called "subcortical dementia" to differentiate it from the dementia of Alzheimer's disease (see Part II). Unfortunately, however, the distinction between subcortical and cortical dementia is not clear-cut, either in terms of symptomatology or underlying neuropathology (Brown and Marsden, 1988).

Even nondemented PD patients may show some deficits in concept formation, linguistic function, memory, sequence planning, habit learning, temporal ordering, or visuospatial ability (Growdon, Corkin, and Rosen, 1990; Knowlton, Mangle, and Squire, 1996). Certain of these deficits resemble the abnormalities found in cases of frontal lobe damage (Brown and Marsden, 1990). Anatomical pathways linking the basal ganglia and frontal lobes may thus be critically involved in some of the cognitive aspects of PD (see later discussion). However, other deficits are not attributable to the frontal lobes and may therefore represent more global problems with cortical functioning (Growdon, Corkin, and Rosen, 1990).

Depression

Another relatively common finding in PD is depression. Significant depressive symptomatology has been found in approximately 40% of PD patients (Cummings, 1992). In severe cases, the symptoms meet the criteria for a diagnosis of major depression. It is reasonable to inquire whether depression is a primary feature of PD (i.e., linked to some aspect of PD neuropathology) or a secondary consequence of the progressive and disabling features of the disorder (i.e., some patients become depressed from the realization of what the disease is doing or will do to them). In this regard, Cummings (1992) has summarized evidence demonstrating a higher incidence of depression in PD patients than in patients with other disorders who were matched for degree of functional impairment. Considering PD patients alone, there is no correlation between the degree of depression and Hoehn and Yahr staging scores; however, there is a modest relationship between depression and other measures of functional loss. Together, these findings seem to indicate that depression is a primary feature of PD, at least for some patients. On the other hand, it would not be surprising if the severity of depressive symptomatology increases as motor (and perhaps cognitive) functioning continues to deteriorate over time.

Neuropathological Characteristics of Parkinson's Disease

Histopathological Findings

The first histopathological studies of the brains of PD patients were conducted in the early 1900s. In 1919, Treti-

akoff discovered a striking loss of pigmented cells from the substantia nigra in PD (see Kopin, 1993a). These are DA neurons, mainly in the substantia nigra pars compacta (SNC; A9 cell group), that appear dark even when unstained due to the presence of the neuronal pigment **neuromelanin**. Substantial loss of these cells occurs in the course of normal aging (McGeer, McGeer, and Suzuki, 1977); however, the extent of degeneration is even greater in PD.

In addition to the SNC, there is also significant degeneration within the midbrain A8 and A10 dopaminergic cell groups (Jellinger, 1987, 1990; Figure 20.3). Because of the topographic projections of the A8, A9, and A10 groups, the dopaminergic pathway to the putamen is more heavily damaged than the corresponding pathway to the caudate nucleus. Interestingly, Hirsch, Graybiel, and Agid (1988) found that for the midbrain DA cell groups, there is a strong relationship between the proportion of cells possessing neuromelanin and the percentage lost in PD (Figure 20.4). Further analysis showed that in every cell group, there was relatively greater death of pigmented compared with nonpigmented neurons. Although the reason for this selective vulnerability is not yet clear, some of the recent theories of PD etiology have attempted to explain the relationship between melanization and dopaminergic cell damage (see below).

Dopamine systems in other parts of the nervous system are likewise altered in PD. Within the hypothalamus, there is a diminution of tyrosine hydroxylase–immunoreactive (THI) fibers as well as a decrease in DA concentration (Agid, Javoy-Agid, and Ruberg, 1987; Jellinger, 1990), although the intrinsic hypothalamic neurons (e.g., in the arcuate nucleus) seem to be spared (Matzuk and Saper, 1985). More recently, a Canadian research group reported decreased DA concentrations and TH-immunoreactivity in retinas from PD patients (Nguyen-Legros et al., 1993). There were also some signs of histopathology in relation to

Normal brain

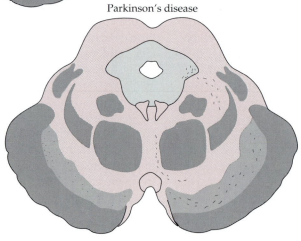

Parkinson's disease

20.3 LOSS OF MIDBRAIN DOPAMINE NEURONS AND FIBERS IN PARKINSON'S DISEASE. Drawings of midbrain sections stained with an antibody to tyrosine hydroxylase from normal (*top*) and parkinsonian (*bottom*) brains reveal fewer dopaminergic cell bodies (left half of each section) and fibers (right half of each section) in the parkinsonian brain. (After Jellinger, 1987.)

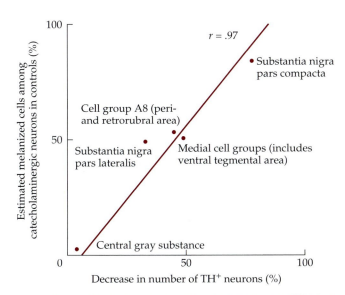

20.4 PROPORTION OF MELANIZED NEURONS IN DIFFERENT DOPAMINE CELL GROUPS AND THEIR VULNERABILITY TO LOSS IN PARKINSON'S DISEASE. (After Graybiel, Hirsch, and Agid, 1990.)

the retinal DA neurons; however, there was little evidence for actual death of these cells.

PD is often thought of as a DA-specific disorder. However, numerous histological studies have demonstrated loss of cells in a number of nondopaminergic cell populations, including noradrenergic neurons of the locus coeruleus (LC) and dorsal vagal nucleus, serotonergic neurons of the dorsal raphe, and cholinergic neurons within the substantia innominata (particularly in the nucleus basalis of Meynert) and in the pedunculopontine nucleus (Jellinger, 1987, 1990). Damage to these important neuronal systems may play a significant role in some of the non-movement-related aspects of PD (see below).

Besides cell loss, the other major histopathological feature of PD was first reported in 1913 by the German neurologist Frederick Lewy, who described the presence of abnormal cytoplasmic inclusions in degenerating brain stem neurons (Kopin, 1993a). These **Lewy bodies**, as they are now called, are spherical, eosinophilic (having an affinity for the acidic dye eosin) structures ranging in size from 5 to 25 μm. Lewy bodies in neurons of the SNC, LC, and other subcortical structures contain a characteristic dense core and peripheral halo. These organelles are also found in cerebral cortical neurons, where they have a somewhat different appearance. Lewy bodies are immunoreactive for a number of different proteins, including neurofilament proteins, tubulin, certain microtubule-associated polypeptides, and ubiquitin (Jellinger, 1990). The expression of ubiquitin, which is a protein that targets other proteins for degradation (Jennissen, 1995), is generally elevated in dying cells. The presence of Lewy bodies in brain stem neurons is often

considered to be a neuropathological hallmark of PD, although some patients who are diagnosed as having PD on the basis of clinical symptomatology and drug responsiveness do not exhibit brain stem Lewy bodies upon postmortem examination (Brooks, 1995). Moreover, Lewy bodies are also found in a number of other neurodegenerative disorders.

Little attention has been paid to the possibility of striatal pathology in PD. However, McNeill and coworkers (1988) reported measurable reductions in dendritic length, dendritic arborization, and spine density in medium spiny neurons in the striatum of advanced PD brains. These intriguing findings suggest that the long-term loss of DA input to these cells may cause atrophication, a process that could be partly responsible for the reduced efficacy of DA replacement therapy over time (see below).

Abnormalities in Neurotransmitter Systems

Dopamine. It was not until the late 1950s that DA was shown to be present in the brain and concentrated in the corpus striatum (caudate and putamen). Beginning in the early 1960s, studies by Oleh Hornykiewicz and other investigators found that postmortem brain tissues from PD patients exhibited a profound depletion of DA in the striatum, globus pallidus, and substantia nigra (reviewed by Agid, Javoy-Agid, and Ruberg, 1987; Hornykiewicz, 1973). Within the striatum, the putamen was found to be more severely affected than the caudate nucleus. Also significantly reduced were the DA metabolite homovanillic acid (HVA) and activities of the DA synthesizing enzymes TH and aromatic L–amino acid decarboxylase. Moreover, there was a significant correlation between the degree of cell loss in the substantia nigra and the reduction in striatal DA.

Subsequent research showed that DA depletion also occurs in limbic system structures, the neocortex, and the hypothalamus of PD patients, although the dopaminergic pathways innervating these areas are not affected as severely as the nigrostriatal pathway (Agid, Javoy-Agid, and Ruberg, 1987). Moreover, available data indicate that the descending dopaminergic system that innervates the spinal cord may be spared in PD. On the other hand, given the previously cited work showing some loss of DA even in the retina of PD patients, it is probably premature to assume that any DA neurons are completely unaffected in this disorder.

Besides DA and its metabolites, another useful presynaptic dopaminergic marker is the DA plasma membrane transporter (uptake site), which can be labeled with several radioligands. Membrane binding and autoradiographic studies on postmortem brain samples have found large decreases in DA transporter binding in the caudate, putamen, and nucleus accumbens (Chinaglia et al., 1992; Niznik et al., 1991). As in the case of

DA itself, loss of transporters was significantly greater in the putamen than in the caudate nucleus (Niznik et al., 1991).

It is interesting to note that PD symptoms generally do not begin to appear until striatal DA levels decline by at least 70% to 80% (Agid, Javoy-Agid, and Ruberg, 1987). The nigrostriatal system presumably has considerable reserve capacity to endure deficits of over 50% without symptomatic manifestation. On the other hand, **compensatory responses** by the surviving dopaminergic neurons and also by the postsynaptic cells in the striatum help mitigate the progressive loss of DA innervation. One type of compensatory response is indicated by the observation that levels of HVA do not decline as much as the DA concentration, leading to an increased HVA/DA ratio in the striatum, substantia nigra, and to a lesser extent in other brain areas (Agid, Javoy-Agid, and Ruberg, 1987; Zigmond et al., 1990; Figure 20.5). This finding, which is consistent with results from animal models involving partial lesions of the nigrostriatal DA system (see below), indicates an increased metabolic turnover and hence heightened activity of the remaining dopaminergic cells. Such increased activity can apparently compensate functionally for nigrostriatal cell loss until the degree of damage reaches the 70% to 80% level.

A second type of compensatory reaction involves changes in the density and/or sensitivity of DA receptors. Although the results are not entirely consistent, evidence from postmortem brain studies generally indicates modest but significant increases in D_1 and D_2 receptor binding in the putamen of PD patients (Agid, Javoy-Agid, and Ruberg, 1987). Based on numerous animal studies, such changes are presumed to be a type of denervation supersensitivity. The apparent increase in D_2 receptor density is particularly intriguing, since this receptor subtype is thought to be present not only postsynaptically but also on presynaptic nigrostriatal nerve terminals, where it functions as a DA autoreceptor (see Chapter 8). Hence, given the massive degeneration of the putamenal DA innervation in PD and a presumed loss of presynaptic DA receptors, it may be the case that the postsynaptic D_2 receptors in this region are more markedly up-regulated than is apparent from the existing data.

Because of their ability to assess neurochemical functioning in living patients, imaging methods such as positron emission tomography (PET) and single photon emission computed tomography (SPECT) are playing an increasingly important role in PD research. For example, a number of studies have found that PD patients exhibit reduced striatal uptake of the DA precursor dihydroxyphenylalanine ([18F]DOPA) and of DA transporter ligands such as [11C]nomifensine (reviewed by Brooks, 1993). The loss of uptake of these compounds was greatest in the putamen and was correlated with the degree of motor dysfunction. Early in the course of the disorder,

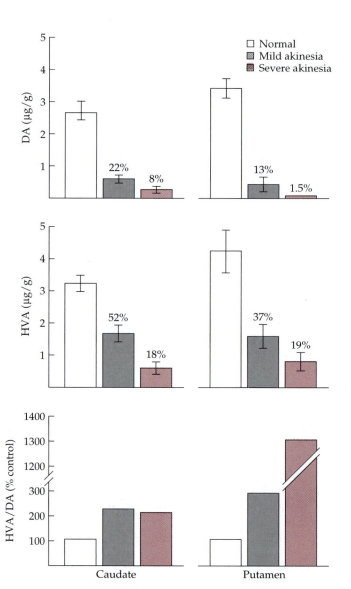

20.5 CHANGES IN DOPAMINE AND HOMOVANILLIC ACID CONCENTRATIONS IN THE CAUDATE AND PUTAMEN OF PARKINSON'S DISEASE PATIENTS. Dopamine (DA) and homovanillic acid (HVA) levels were determined by postmortem analyses of tissue from PD patients who had been classified as either mildly or severely akinesic at the time of death. Severely akinesic patients showed a large increase in the ratio of HVA to DA (an index of DA turnover) in the putamen, which indicates heightened activity in the small number of surviving dopaminergic nerve terminals in this region. (After Zigmond et al., 1990; original data from Bernheimer et al., 1973.)

PD patients often exhibit symptoms on only one side of the body (called hemiparkinsonism). Under these conditions, putamen [18F]DOPA uptake was most altered on the side contralateral to the affected limbs; however, the ipsilateral putamen (i.e., the clinically silent side) also showed a measurable loss of uptake (Garnett, Nahmias, and Firnau, 1984; Nahmias et al., 1985). This was the first demonstration of dopaminergic pathology prior to the appearance of clinical symptomatology. More recently, Frost and colleagues (1993) used [11C]WIN 35,428, a potent cocaine analog (see Chapter 13), to image the DA transporter in relatively early PD patients (Hoehn–Yahr stage II). The researchers found marked decreases in binding in the midbrain and putamen, and a smaller reduction in the caudate nucleus. Together with the [18F]DOPA results, these findings suggest that sensitive imaging methods might be useful in the diagnosis of PD or even for detecting the disorder in at-risk subjects prior to the appearance of clinical symptoms (Madras, 1994; Sawle, 1993).

Imaging of the D_2 receptor in PD has yielded results that are reasonably consistent with the postmortem findings mentioned above. That is, D_2 receptor binding tends to be elevated in the putamen; however, there is little or no effect in the caudate nucleus (Brooks, 1993). On the other hand, more work needs to be performed before any conclusions can be drawn concerning the status of D_1 receptors in vivo in PD.

Norepinephrine. As mentioned earlier, PD involves destruction not only of DA neurons, but also of many noradrenergic cells in the LC. It is not surprising, therefore, that biochemical analyses of PD brains have found 40% to 80% reductions in NE in a variety of brain areas innervated by the LC, including the cerebral cortex, hippocampus, amygdala, thalamus, hypothalamus, nucleus accumbens, and substantia nigra (Agid, Javoy-Agid, and Ruberg, 1987; Gerlach, Jellinger, and Riederer, 1994). There is also a large decline in spinal cord NE, which raises the possibility of damage to the descending noradrenergic pathway that originates in the lateral tegmental cell system (see Chapter 8).

Along with the changes in NE concentration, certain adrenergic receptors may also be altered in PD. Cash and coworkers (1984) reported an increase in frontal cortical β_1-adrenoceptors, a decrease in α_2-receptors, and no change in β_2 or α_1 sites. As discussed earlier for DA receptors, the elevation of β_1-receptors is presumably a response to denervation. The reduction in α_2-receptors probably reflects their partial presynaptic localization and role as adrenergic autoreceptors (Chapter 8).

Serotonin. Serotonergic target structures are not uniformly affected in PD. Various studies have generally reported significant (approximately 50%) reductions in serotonin (5-HT) concentrations in the basal ganglia, cerebral cortex, hippocampus, spinal cord, and possibly the hypothalamus (Agid, Javoy-Agid, and Ruberg, 1987). In contrast, the serotonergic innervation of the amygdala and nucleus accumbens seems to be relatively spared. Little change in 5-HT receptor density has been reported in PD.

Acetylcholine. Changes in cholinergic activity in PD have been examined mainly by measuring the activity of choline acetyltransferase (ChAT). This enzyme is respon-

sible for synthesizing acetylcholine (ACh) and is a specific marker for cholinergic neurons and nerve terminals (see Chapter 7). In PD patients, ChAT activity is significantly reduced in various areas of the cerebral cortex as well as in the hippocampus (Agid, Javoy-Agid, and Ruberg, 1987). These observations are consistent with damage to cholinergic neurons in the basal forebrain (which project to the cortex) and in the septal area (which innervate the hippocampus). In contrast, ChAT activity within the caudate nucleus is normal, which fits with histological findings that indicate no loss of striatal cholinergic interneurons. Moreover, muscarinic receptor binding is significantly elevated in the cortex, but not in the caudate.

Neuropeptides. Regional deficits in various neuropeptides have been found in PD. These effects include decreases in substance P and Met-enkephalin in the SNC and pallidum, and a loss of somatostatin in the frontal cortex and hippocampus (Agid, Javoy-Agid, and Ruberg, 1987). Somatostatin is a peptide that was first discovered as a potent hypothalamic factor that inhibits the release of growth hormone. It was later found in the gastrointestinal tract, the pancreas, and many areas of the CNS, including the cerebral cortex, where it is synthesized by a population of intrinsic cortical neurons. Somatostatin is of particular interest because it was found to be deficient only in PD patients who were demented (Epelbaum et al., 1983). Damage to or destruction of cortical somatostatin-containing cells may therefore be one of the factors contributing to PD dementia (see also next section).

Relationships between Symptomatology and Specific Neurotransmitter Systems

Motor deficits. There is overwhelming evidence that the motor deficits seen in PD (bradykinesia, tremor, and rigidity) stem from the massive loss of DA innervation of the striatum. This notion is supported by several findings:

1. There is a correlation between the degree of DA depletion and the severity of motor symptoms such as bradykinesia (Agid, Javoy-Agid, and Ruberg, 1987).
2. Destruction of the nigrostriatal DA pathway or blockade of striatal DA receptors in either experimental animals or humans causes motor deficits similar to those seen in PD (see below).
3. Pharmacotherapies aimed at increasing DA availability or stimulating DA receptors reduce symptomatology in PD patients (see below).

To understand how a DA deficiency in the striatum can lead to motor deficits, it is necessary to review the anatomy, physiology, and neurochemistry of the basal ganglia, and their afferent and efferent connections with other parts of the brain.

The term "basal ganglia" refers to a collection of subcortical structures, the composition of which varies with different authors. Here we will consider the basal ganglia to include the caudate nucleus, putamen, pallidum, subthalamic nucleus, and substantia nigra pars reticulata (SNR). The caudate and putamen together are referred to as the neostriatum, dorsal striatum, or sometimes just "striatum." The pallidum consists of external and internal segments in primates; in rodents, the homologous structures are the globus pallidus and entopeduncular nucleus.

Intensive study of the basal ganglia has revealed a complex role for this system in cognition and motivation. However, the clearest and best understood function of the basal ganglia involves their participation in motor control. The major anatomical features of basal ganglia circuitry were previously presented in Figure 4.16. The neostriatum receives a massive input from the neocortex via the corticostriatal pathway. Other input comes from the cerebellum by way of the intralaminar nuclei of the thalamus (e.g., the centromedian nucleus), from the SNC, and from the raphe nuclei (not shown). Processing of information within the basal ganglia involves pathways from the striatum to the pallidum and SNR, as well as circuits connecting the pallidum with the subthalamic nucleus. The internal segment of the pallidum and the SNR constitute the output nuclei of the basal ganglia. These structures project to the supplementary motor area and other regions of the frontal cortex by way of the ventral anterior and ventral lateral thalamic nuclei. Other projections terminate in two brain stem target areas: the superior colliculus and the pedunculopontine nucleus (pathways not shown).

Based on the circuitry shown in Figure 4.16, we can see that a loop exists between the cortex and the basal ganglia. Because the cortical inputs to the striatum are so extensive compared with the striatal efferents, anatomists once thought that cortical information was "funneled" into the striatum, thus implying a loss of topographic detail. However, more recent work has given rise to the notion of parallel, rather than converging, circuits that enter the striatum and remain largely segregated through processing in the basal ganglia and eventual output to the frontal cortex (Alexander and Crutcher, 1990). There are roughly five such circuits, based on their target zones within the frontal cortex: (1) a "motor" circuit that projects to the precentral motor fields, (2) an "oculomotor" circuit that projects to the frontal and supplementary eye fields, "prefrontal" circuits projecting to the (3) dorsolateral prefrontal and (4) lateral orbitofrontal cortical areas, and (5) a "limbic" circuit that projects to the anterior cingulate and medial orbitofrontal cortex. These latter pathways to the pre-

frontal and limbic cortices underscore the involvement of the basal ganglia in cognitive and emotional aspects of behavioral regulation. Even within an individual circuit such as the motor circuit, there is evidence for an underlying somatotopic organization (Alexander and Crutcher, 1990). For example, the regions of the primary motor cortex and supplementary motor area that control movement of the right arm project to specific parts of the striatum (mainly the putamen in primates) that represent that limb, and this topographic organization appears to be maintained in the pallidum and substantia nigra.

Now that we have reviewed the anatomy of the basal ganglia and its major input and output pathways, it is necessary to consider the neurotransmitters and neuropeptides that function in these pathways. A simplified diagram illustrating some of the critical transmitters and peptides is presented in Figure 20.6. Beginning with the cerebral cortex, it can be seen that the corticostriatal pathway is excitatory and is thought to use the amino acid transmitter glutamate. The corticostriatal fibers terminate on medium spiny neurons, which constitute the output cells of the striatum. As discussed previously in Chapter 8, the medium spiny neurons fall into two general classes, those that project directly to the output nuclei of the basal ganglia (i.e., the internal pallidal segment [GPi] and the SNR), and those that project to the output nuclei through an indirect route that includes the external pallidal segment (GPe) and the subthalamic nucleus (STN). All of the medium spiny neurons form inhibitory synapses that release γ-aminobutyric acid (GABA). They also contain several neuropeptides, such as substance P, enkephalin, and dynorphin. Peptide expression is regulated by the DA input to the striatum; however, the role of these substances in overall basal ganglia function has not yet been clarified (Gerfen, 1992; Graybiel, 1990). Hence, the remaining discussion will focus on glutamate, GABA, DA from the SNC, and ACh from large cholinergic interneurons in the striatum, which are not illustrated in the figure.

Electrophysiological studies have shown that when an animal is not moving, most striatal neurons are silent, whereas neurons in the GPi and SNR are highly active (Chevalier and Deniau, 1990). When the pallidal and nigral neurons are firing, release of GABA from their terminals produces a powerful inhibition of target cells in the ventral thalamic nuclei, superior colliculi, and pedunculopontine nucleus. When movement is initiated, however, activity in the corticostriatal pathway excites the medium spiny striatal neurons, which leads to a rapid silencing of the inhibitory GPi and SNR neurons through the direct synaptic pathway shown in Figure 20.6. The thalamic, collicular, and pedunculopontine neurons then exhibit a transient burst of activity upon being released from their previous constraint (Figure 20.7). In this way, the basal ganglia do not initiate motor

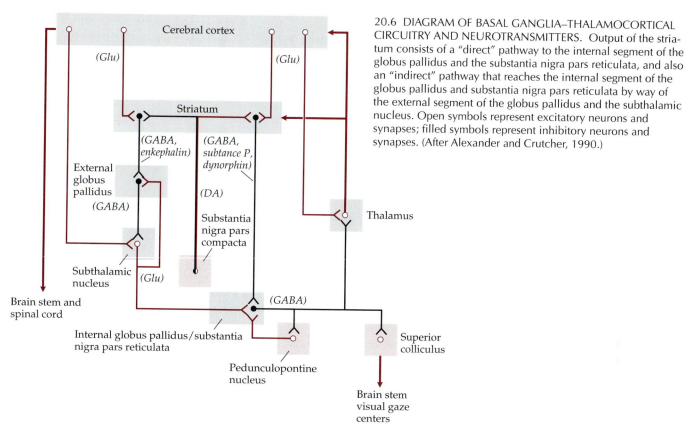

20.6 DIAGRAM OF BASAL GANGLIA–THALAMOCORTICAL CIRCUITRY AND NEUROTRANSMITTERS. Output of the striatum consists of a "direct" pathway to the internal segment of the globus pallidus and the substantia nigra pars reticulata, and also an "indirect" pathway that reaches the internal segment of the globus pallidus and substantia nigra pars reticulata by way of the external segment of the globus pallidus and the subthalamic nucleus. Open symbols represent excitatory neurons and synapses; filled symbols represent inhibitory neurons and synapses. (After Alexander and Crutcher, 1990.)

commands, but rather play a critical role in facilitating or gating such commands by causing synchronized increases in excitability of thalamic and brain stem motor centers (Chevalier and Deniau, 1990).

It is interesting to note that the indirect synaptic pathway from the striatum to the GPi and SNR tends to oppose the action of the direct pathway. That is, the striatum suppresses activity of neurons in the GPe, which releases the STN from prior inhibition by GPe and ultimately causes an excitation of neurons in the GPi and SNR (Figure 20.6). It is not yet clear whether inputs from the direct and indirect pathways project to different neu-

20.7 ELECTROPHYSIOLOGICAL RELATIONSHIPS WITHIN THE DIRECT OUTPUT PATHWAY OF THE STRIATUM. In the absence of movement, most striatal output neurons are silent. Stimulation of these cells by striatal glutamate injection (50 nl of a 30-μM solution) causes a powerful inhibition of tonically active neurons in the substantia nigra pars reticulata and a simultaneous activation of neurons in the superior colliculus and the ventromedial nucleus of the thalamus. The arrow in each histogram denotes the time of glutamate application to the striatum. (After Chevalier and Deniau, 1990.)

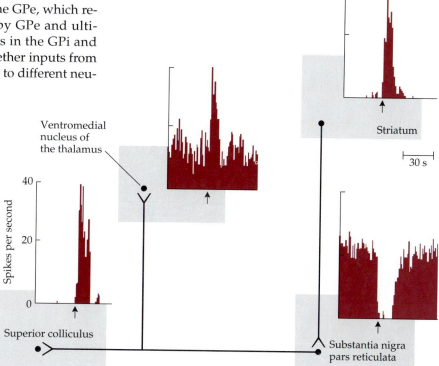

rons within the GPi and SNR, or whether these inputs converge on the same cells. In the latter case, it might be possible that the effect of the indirect pathway on GPi and SNR neurons (which, of course, would tend to *inhibit* thalamic, collicular, and pedunculopontine output) serves a "smoothing" or "braking" function on the motor excitation produced by the direct striatopallidal and striatonigral pathways (Alexander and Crutcher, 1990).

Where does DA fit into this complex picture? As illustrated in Figure 20.6, current evidence suggests that DA exerts a net excitatory influence on striatal output neurons of the direct pathway, but a net inhibitory influence on neurons giving rise to the indirect pathway (Albin, Young, and Penney, 1989; Alexander and Crutcher, 1990). The excitatory effect is thought to be mediated largely by D_1 receptors on the GABA/substance P neurons, whereas the inhibitory effect has been attributed to D_2 receptors on the GABA/enkephalin neurons (Gerfen, 1992; also see Chapter 8). Consistent with their expression of DA receptors, the medium spiny neurons of the striatum do receive a direct dopaminergic input targeted mainly to dendritic spines and shafts (Kötter, 1994; Smith and Bolam, 1990). Of particular interest is the observation that the DA-containing terminals only seem to innervate spines that receive some other, nondopaminergic input (Freund, Powell, and Smith, 1984). As shown in Figure 20.8, these other inputs are frequently terminals of the corticostriatal pathway. Consequently, dopaminergic fibers are well situated anatomically to modulate (i.e., either facilitate or dampen) the excitatory responses elicited by the glutamatergic corticostriatal synapses, and such modulation has indeed been found in studies of striatal slices (Cepeda, Buchwald, and Levine, 1993).

A second important dopaminergic innervation of the striatum is thought to involve axoaxonal synapses directly on the corticostriatal terminals. There is anatomical evidence for axoaxonal contacts between DA and corticostriatal nerve endings in the striatum (Bouyer et al., 1984). Furthermore, pharmacological studies have found that D_2 receptor agonists inhibit glutamate release from corticostriatal terminals (Maura, Giardia, and Raiteri, 1988; Yamamoto and Davy, 1992). This represents another potential mechanism by which DA inhibits the activity of striatal output neurons. However, attempts to demonstrate the actual presence of D_2 receptors on terminals of the corticostriatal pathway have yielded equivocal results

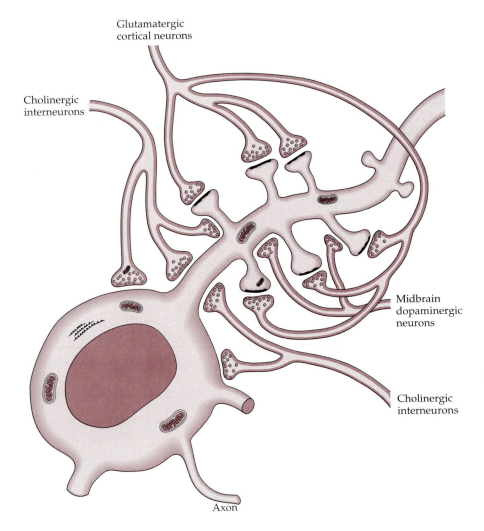

Glutamatergic cortical neurons

Cholinergic interneurons

Midbrain dopaminergic neurons

Cholinergic interneurons

Axon

20.8 TOPOGRAPHICAL ARRANGEMENT OF SYNAPTIC INPUTS TO STRIATAL MEDIUM SPINY NEURONS. Glutamatergic corticostriatal fibers terminate mainly on the heads of distal dendritic spines, whereas many midbrain dopaminergic fibers appear to terminate on the necks of these spines and on the dendritic shafts. Inputs from cholinergic interneurons are found more proximal to the cell soma. (After Smith and Bolam, 1990.)

(see Calabresi et al., 1996). Indeed, recent work by Hersch and coworkers. (1995) using a D_2 receptor–specific antibody found no immunostaining of putative corticostriatal nerve endings. Although somewhat troubling, this finding does not necessarily invalidate the pharmacological results because the presynaptic DA receptors in this system might be of the D_3 or D_4 subtype (both of which are recognized by typical D_2 receptor drugs).

Having considered the characteristics of the dopaminergic innervation of the striatum, we can now see how the loss of this innervation can lead to the symptoms of PD (particularly bradykinesia). Loss of DA inputs will tend to decrease activity of the direct pathway neurons and increase activity of the indirect pathway cells. Both effects should result in enhanced firing of the inhibitory GPi and SNR neurons, thereby shutting down the thalamic and brain stem motor circuits. Loss of activity in these circuits is presumably the major cause of PD-related bradykinesia and also contributes to rigidity. The production of parkinsonian tremor is still not well understood, but it is believed to originate from oscillatory activity within the basal ganglia–thalamic–cortical loop described above (Lee, 1987).

Another transmitter that may be involved in the motor symptoms of PD is ACh. Animal studies have shown that the striatal cholinergic interneurons become hyperactive following loss of DA input (Stoof et al., 1992). As these cells exert an excitatory influence on the medium spiny neurons, they may contribute to the abnormal output of the basal ganglia. There is a long-standing theory that the motor deficits of PD result from an abnormal cholinergic/dopaminergic balance within the striatum, although this view has been superseded by the model presented above, in which direct glutamate–DA interactions are thought to be of prime importance. Nevertheless, we shall see later that cholinergic antagonism has been one of the important therapeutic approaches in PD, particularly before the advent of DA replacement therapies.

Cognitive deficits. Several hypotheses have been advanced to account for the cognitive deficits found in a proportion of PD patients. We mentioned earlier that some of these deficits resemble abnormalities associated with frontal lobe damage. Because the prefrontal cortex is one of the major targets of basal ganglia output, it is possible that striatal DA depletion is important in the cognitive as well as motor symptoms of PD (Brown and Marsden, 1990). Likewise, partial loss of the direct dopaminergic innervation of the frontal cortex from the midbrain (although not as severe as the damage to the nigrostriatal tract) could provide another contributory role for DA. However, DA is unlikely to be the sole source of cognitive dysfunction in PD, as replacement therapy with L-dihydroxyphenylalanine (L-DOPA) at best improves some cognitive functions, but not others (see Growdon, Corkin, and Rosen, 1990).

ACh has also been implicated in PD-related cognitive disorders. As we shall see in Part II of this chapter, degeneration of the cholinergic pathways from the basal forebrain to the cortex and hippocampus is thought to underlie many of the severe cognitive symptoms of Alzheimer's disease. Partial damage to these same pathways could provoke milder cognitive deficits in some PD patients (Agid, Javoy-Agid, and Ruberg, 1987).

Finally, current evidence suggests that dementia in PD may occur through several different mechanisms (Jellinger, 1987). In some cases, postmortem examination of the brains of demented patients found a pathology resembling Alzheimer's disease, including significant cortical atrophy and the presence of senile plaques and tangles (see Part II). In other cases, such pathology was mostly lacking; however, there was particularly severe damage to the ascending cholinergic system.

Depression. Relatively little is known about the source of depression in PD. Based on the major theories of depression (Chapter 19), it is reasonable to conclude that depletion of NE and/or 5-HT may play an important role in the depressive symptomatology displayed by some PD patients (Gerlach, Jellinger, and Riederer, 1994; Mayeux, 1990). DA could also be involved, based on its putative role in brain reward mechanisms, affect, and motivation (Cummings, 1992; see also Chapter 8).

Models of Parkinson's Disease

Experimental models of PD serve at least two important functions. First, they are essential in the development and testing of new therapeutic strategies, whether pharmacological or otherwise. Second, some models may also provide insights into the possible causative mechanisms of the disease. In this section, we will present and evaluate several different models of PD, and this information will then be used to discuss recent hypotheses concerning the etiology of PD.

Early Animal Models

Pharmacological dopamine depletion models. Heikkila, Sonsalla, and Duvoisin (1989) have reviewed various animal models of PD. Because the motor symptoms of PD are due to deficits in striatal DA, such symptoms can be reproduced with some degree of fidelity by pharmacological manipulations that cause DA depletion. The two most commonly used drugs for this purpose are reserpine and α-methyl-*p*-tyrosine (AMPT). As discussed previously in Chapter 8, reserpine produces a long-lasting inhibition of the vesicular monoamine transporter, thereby causing a depletion of vesicular stores of DA, NE, and 5-HT. Overdose of humans with reserpine or treatment of laboratory animals (i.e., rats or mice) with this compound can lead to motor symptoms closely resembling those of PD (Heikilla, Sonsalla, and Duvoisin,

1989). Moreover, administration of L-DOPA produces a temporary reversal of these symptoms.

Although reserpinization was the first model of PD to be developed, it is a poor model for several reasons. The first problem is the lack of selectivity of the drug for the DA system. Even though PD itself exhibits some degree of noradrenergic and serotonergic involvement, the damage to these systems is considerably less than the damage to the nigrostriatal DA pathway. Consequently, a compound that depletes all three monoamines by over 90% is too nonselective. The second problem is that reserpinized animals respond not only to L-DOPA but also to amphetamine. Unfortunately, amphetamine has little therapeutic value for PD patients, indicating that reserpinization cannot reliably be used to screen for new parkinsonian medications. Finally, the effects of reserpine are transient because the drug does not produce any degenerative changes in the brain. This lack of parallelism is important because the striatum may undergo different compensatory reactions to dopaminergic denervation than to pharmacological depletion.

Some of these same problems are associated with the AMPT model of PD. AMPT depletes both DA and NE by blocking TH, the first enzyme in the catecholamine biosynthetic pathway. AMPT-treated animals again show parkinsonian-like bradykinesia, but as in the case of reserpine, the motor deficits are temporary because no neural damage has occurred.

The 6-OHDA lesion model.   A major advance in modelling PD came with the introduction of the catecholamine neurotoxin 6-hydroxydopamine (6-OHDA) (Heikkila, Sonsalla, and Duvoisin, 1989). This substance is transported into the cell bodies and fibers of both dopaminergic and noradrenergic neurons. It causes massive degeneration of nerve terminals and can also affect cell bodies, particularly when administered to the cell body regions. Reasonable selectivity for DA can be produced by pretreating the subjects with desipramine, an NE transporter blocker that inhibits 6-OHDA uptake into the noradrenergic neurons. Further selectivity for the nigrostriatal tract can be achieved by injecting the toxin directly into the striatum, substantia nigra, or medial forebrain bundle (which contains the axons of the nigrostriatal tract).

The most widely used 6-OHDA model for studying PD utilizes animals with unilateral lesions of the nigrostriatal pathway (Heikkila, Sonsalla, and Duvoisin, 1989). These animals are easy to maintain in the laboratory because they show few, if any, behavioral deficits upon gross examination. However, they exhibit predictable behavioral responses to dopaminergic drugs. As described previously in Chapter 8, indirectly acting DA agonists like amphetamine elicit rotational behavior ipsilateral to the side of the lesion. In contrast, direct DA agonists like apomorphine or L-DOPA lead to contralateral rotation.

Hence, drugs that act like apomorphine or L-DOPA in this system are potential candidate therapeutic agents for PD.

It is, of course, also possible to lesion the nigrostriatal DA pathway bilaterally with 6-OHDA. This produces a syndrome of severe bradykinesia that more closely resembles the actual symptoms of PD. As expected, L-DOPA and other agents used in the treatment of PD cause enhanced motor function. Nevertheless, the bilateral lesion model is used much less frequently than the unilateral lesion model. This is probably because the more severely damaged animals have great difficulty in eating and drinking, particularly during the early postsurgical period, and thus are difficult to maintain.

Zigmond and his colleagues (1990) have extensively studied the compensatory neurochemical processes that occur in the 6-OHDA-lesioned rat. These investigators have shown, for example, that extracellular DA levels in the striatum (determined by microdialysis) do not decrease until tissue DA depletion exceeds 80% (Figure 20.9). Likewise, significant behavioral impairment occurred only with severe (bilateral) damage to the nigrostriatal system. Several compensatory mechanisms may underlie the disparity between total tissue DA and extracellular DA levels in incompletely lesioned animals, including increased firing by the remaining dopaminergic neurons and a possible increase in the amount of DA released per action potential. Finally, DA receptor up-regulation occurs in the denervated striatum, but only when the DA depletion exceeds 90%. These findings show striking parallels to the situation believed to occur in PD, in which clinical symptoms do not occur until striatal DA loss reaches about 80%, remaining nigral cells show increased firing and DA turnover (see Figure 20.5), and striatal D_2 receptors may not up-regulate until the dopaminergic denervation is fairly severe. On this basis, therefore, the 6-OHDA-lesioned rat models not only some of the behavioral properties of PD, but also the adaptive neural responses characteristic of loss of DA input to the striatum.

The MPTP Model

The PD model currently favored by most researchers is the syndrome produced by the novel DA neurotoxin 1-methyl-4-phenyl-1,2,3,6-tetrahydropyridine (**MPTP**). MPTP-induced parkinsonism not only mimics the basic

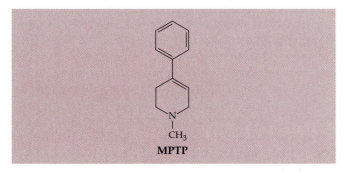

MPTP

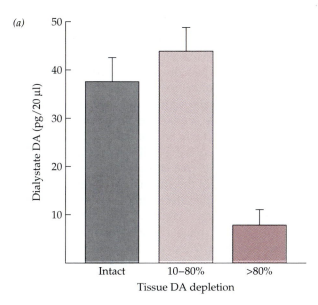

(a)

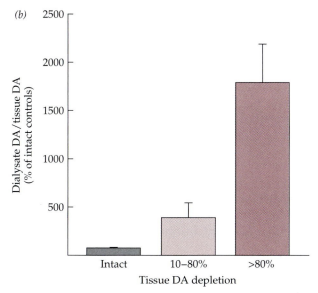

(b)

20.9 EFFECT OF 6-HYDROXYDOPAMINE LESIONS ON STRI-ATAL DOPAMINE OVERFLOW AND TISSUE DOPAMINE CONTENT IN RATS. Rats were given 6-OHDA lesions to deplete striatal DA. Striatal DA overflow was measured by microdialysis, after which tissues were obtained and total DA content was measured. DA overflow did not decline compared with intact control animals until the depletion of striatal DA content exceeded 80% (a). Consequently, a large increase in the ratio of dialysate DA to tissue DA was found in the highly depleted subgroup (b). These findings suggest a compensatory increase in the activity of the surviving dopaminergic nerve terminals, which was also shown for PD patients in Figure 20.5. (After Zigmond et al., 1990.)

land. Kidston had studied chemistry and was using a home laboratory to synthesize various drugs for his own recreational use. At that time, he became interested in synthesizing 1-methyl-4-phenyl-propionoxypiperidine (MPPP), which was originally developed in 1947 by Albert Ziering at the Hoffman–LaRoche Institute. MPPP is a potent analog of the analgesic meperidine (Demerol), and of course Kidston was interested in this "designer" drug for its "high" rather than for its effect on pain sensitivity.

For several months, Kidston synthesized this compound and injected it intravenously without incident. On one occasion, however, he was in a hurry and took some shortcuts in the chemical procedure. When he injected the resulting product, it produced a powerful burning sensation that had not occurred previously. More importantly, within 3 days he was exhibiting such severe bradykinesia that he was unable to speak or move. Initially diagnosed as a catatonic schizophrenic, Kidston was treated with haloperidol (exactly the wrong choice, as things turned out). When haloperidol treatment and a subsequent regimen of electroconvulsive therapy failed to improve his condition, Kidston was seen by a neurologist, who recognized the symptoms as classical parkinsonism. Although PD is extremely rare in patients so young, the neurologist treated Kidston with L-DOPA, which caused a dramatic return of motor function.

Because of the unusual nature of the case, Kidston was subsequently referred to Irwin Kopin and his research team at the nearby National Institute of Mental Health (NIMH). Fortunately, a small amount of Kidston's toxic drug product was still clinging to his glassware at home. When this was analyzed by NIMH chemist Sanford Markey, it was found to contain trace amounts of MPTP, which was an unanticipated by-product of Kidston's procedural shortcuts. Markey tested the influence of MPPP alone (which is not neurotoxic) and mixtures of MPPP and MPTP on rats to see if these substances had any damaging effects. Although the subjects exhibited initial bradykinesia and rigidity in response to the drugs, the effect always wore off within a few hours. We now know that the choice of rats as subjects was unlucky, since this species happens to show resistance to MPTP's neurotoxic action.

symptoms of the idiopathic disorder, but has also opened up a whole new area of research concerning possible etiologic mechanisms. Moreover, as we shall see, several humans have had the misfortune to ingest this compound at neurotoxic doses, thereby providing researchers with an extensive opportunity to study a chemically induced human parkinsonian syndrome.

Discovery of MPTP neurotoxicity. The story of how MPTP neurotoxicity was discovered reads like a detective novel.* The tale begins in 1976 with a student named Barry Kidston, who was then living in Bethesda, Mary-

---

*Readers interested in a complete account of this story are referred to *The Case of the Frozen Addicts* by Langston (one of the major scientific participants) and Palfreman (1995). Most of the present account is based on this source.

Despite his mishap, Kidston continued to abuse drugs (including the L-DOPA with which he was being treated!) until he became depressed in late 1978 and died of a cocaine overdose. When his brain was examined histologically at autopsy, it showed the massive degeneration of pigmented nigral neurons that is a hallmark of PD. Kidston's case study was published the following year by Kopin's group (Davis et al., 1979), even though they could not confirm that MPTP or any other specific substance had caused the neural degeneration.

This report received little attention at the time of its publication and for the next several years. However, in the summer of 1982, six young to middle-aged men and women in northern California suddenly manifested severe parkinsonian symptoms much like those of Barry Kidston. Eventually, all six cases came to the attention of J. William Langston, chief neurologist at the Santa Clara Valley Medical Center and also on the staff at Stanford University Medical School. All patients responded positively to L-DOPA therapy and were considered to be suffering from a parkinsonian-like disorder. However, as in Kidston's case, the patients were too young, and their symptoms emerged much too rapidly, for this to be typical PD. It was quickly determined that all six patients were heroin users who had tried a new batch of drug prior to the onset of their symptoms. Further investigation revealed that this material was obtained from a local "drug designer" who had, like Kidston before him, attempted to synthesize MPPP and had inadvertently produced MPTP again. These findings were published by Langston and his colleagues in a *Science* article in which they hypothesized a relationship between MPTP and the production of parkinsonian symptoms in their patients

(Langston et al., 1983). Indeed, these investigators later became aware of several professional chemists who had worked with MPTP years earlier, before its toxicity was suspected, and who had developed parkinsonism. Yet direct proof of a causal connection was still lacking.

The critical breakthrough came when Burns, Kopin, and their colleagues were able to induce a striking parkinsonian syndrome in rhesus monkeys by repeated intravenous injection of MPTP (Burns et al., 1983). Daily doses of the drug for 5 to 8 days led to progressive loss of motor function until the subjects demonstrated virtually all of the characteristic features of PD, including bradykinesia or akinesia, rigidity, tremor, hunched posture, eyelid closure, masked facies, difficulty in swallowing, and drooling. These symptoms were reversed by L-DOPA treatment (Figure 20.10). Postmortem examination of the brains of several MPTP-treated animals revealed extreme loss of dopaminergic cells in the SNC and a corresponding depletion of striatal DA. Thus, researchers finally had a model that not only mimicked the neurochemical aspects of PD but was also degenerative and progressive. Although progressivity was quite rapid in the intravenously injected animals and drug addicts, it seemed to be slower in the affected chemists, presumably because they ingested much smaller doses over a period of time through accidental skin exposure and/or inhalation.

Characteristics of MPTP neurotoxicity. It is necessary to compare the neurochemical and histopathological features of MPTP-induced parkinsonism with the features of PD itself to determine how well this experimental syndrome models the idiopathic disorder. Burns and

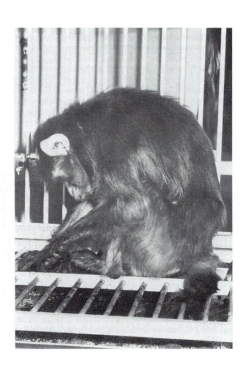
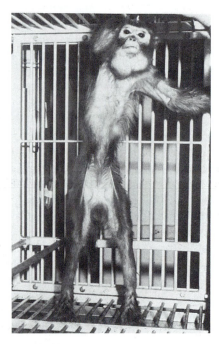

20.10 PARKINSONIAN BEHAVIOR OF A MPTP-TREATED MONKEY AND REVERSAL BY L-DOPA TREATMENT. An adult rhesus monkey was given four daily doses of 0.3 mg/kg of MPTP intravenously followed by three daily doses of 0.38 mg/kg for a cumulative dose of 17.1 mg over 7 days. The animal was subsequently treated for a 2-month period with oral Sinemet (100 mg of L-DOPA plus 10 mg of the peripheral decarboxylase inhibitor carbidopa) five times daily at 4-hour intervals. When treatment was withheld for 16 hours, the animal showed symptoms of akinesia and hunched posture (*left*). Thirty minutes after the first photograph was taken, the animal was given a dose of Sinemet and a second photograph was taken 90 minutes later (*right*). L-DOPA treatment reversed the MPTP-induced behavioral abnormalities. (From Burns et al., 1983.)

coworkers (1985) studied eight patients with PD, six patients with MPTP parkinsonism (four of the California drug addicts and two MPTP-exposed chemists), and six normal control subjects with respect to monoamine metabolite concentrations in their cerebrospinal fluid (CSF). Both the MPTP and PD groups exhibited varying degrees of motor dysfunction (e.g., the PD patients ranged from stage II to stage IV on the Hoehn and Yahr scale). Both the MPTP and PD subjects exhibited dramatic decreases in CSF levels of the DA metabolite HVA (Figure 20.11). In contrast, plasma-adjusted levels of the NE metabolite 3-methoxy-4-hydroxyphenylethylene glycol (MHPG) were unexpectedly higher in the MPTP than in the PD group. There were no significant group differences in CSF concentrations of the 5-HT metabolite 5-hydroxyindoleacetic acid (5-HIAA), although 5-HIAA levels in PD patients tended to be lower than those in controls. These data suggest that the noradrenergic and serotonergic systems may be less severely damaged (or not damaged at all) in MPTP-induced parkinsonism than in idiopathic PD.

The most complete characterization of MPTP neurotoxicity has been carried out in nonhuman primates, particularly rhesus, vervet (African green), and squirrel monkeys. In the original rhesus monkey study of MPTP, Burns and colleagues (1983) found reduced CSF levels of HVA, MHPG, and 5-HIAA during the course of drug treatment, although only HVA remained markedly lower in one subject sampled 3 months later. Several MPTP-treated monkeys were sacrificed at various time points following drug administration, and their brains were removed for neurochemical and histopathological examination. Short-term studies (sacrificing the animals at 1–5 days posttreatment) were consistent with the CSF measurements in showing reduced HVA, MHPG, and 5-HIAA in most brain areas examined. In several other

subjects studied at about 1 or 2 months posttreatment, the investigators found a marked loss of dopaminergic neurons in the substantia nigra, signs of degenerating DA fibers in the putamen, and a massive depletion of DA in the caudate nucleus and especially the putamen. In contrast, the locus coeruleus, nucleus accumbens, and olfactory tubercle appeared histologically normal.

Subsequent research on primates treated with MPTP led to great variability in outcome, which was due to experimental differences in dosing regimens and species differences in vulnerability. In some cases, animals exhibited long-term parkinsonian symptoms, whereas in other cases the subjects recovered after showing initial motor deficits. Neurochemical differences were also found between MPTP-induced parkinsonism and PD. For example, investigators reported approximately equal losses of DA in the caudate and putamen of MPTP-treated animals (Burns et al., 1983; Elsworth et al., 1987), which differs from PD, in which the putamen is more severely affected. Furthermore, early studies seemed to indicate that MPTP selectively targets the nigrostriatal DA pathway while sparing other DA systems and other monoamine transmitters known to be affected in PD (Burns et al., 1983; Langston et al., 1984).

More recent work, however, has demonstrated that appropriate drug treatment regimens can bring about neurochemical effects closely resembling those of PD. For example, Moratalla and coworkers (1992) were able to induce a pattern of nigrostriatal degeneration in which the putamen was more severely affected than the caudate nucleus in squirrel monkeys. Other studies carried out on several different primate species have shown that MPTP is capable of producing damage to the mesolimbic and mesocortical DA pathways as well as to the noradrenergic system (Elsworth et al., 1990; Forno et al., 1986; Mitchell et al., 1985). In fact, Hornykiewicz and

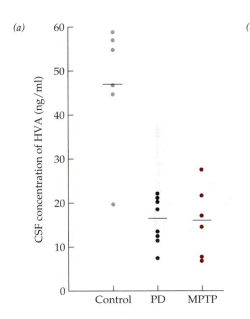

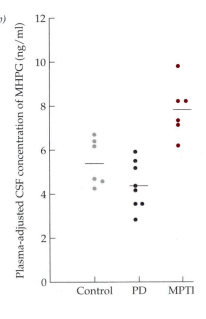

20.11 CSF HVA AND MHPG CONCENTRATIONS IN PARKINSON'S DISEASE AND MPTP-INDUCED PARKINSONISM. The symbols depict individual patient data points and the horizontal bars depict group means. Because plasma free (unconjugated) MHPG crosses the blood–brain barrier and influences CSF MHPG levels (Kopin et al., 1983), the CSF MHPG data were adjusted by subtracting 0.9 times the plasma free MHPG level. (After Burns et al., 1985.)

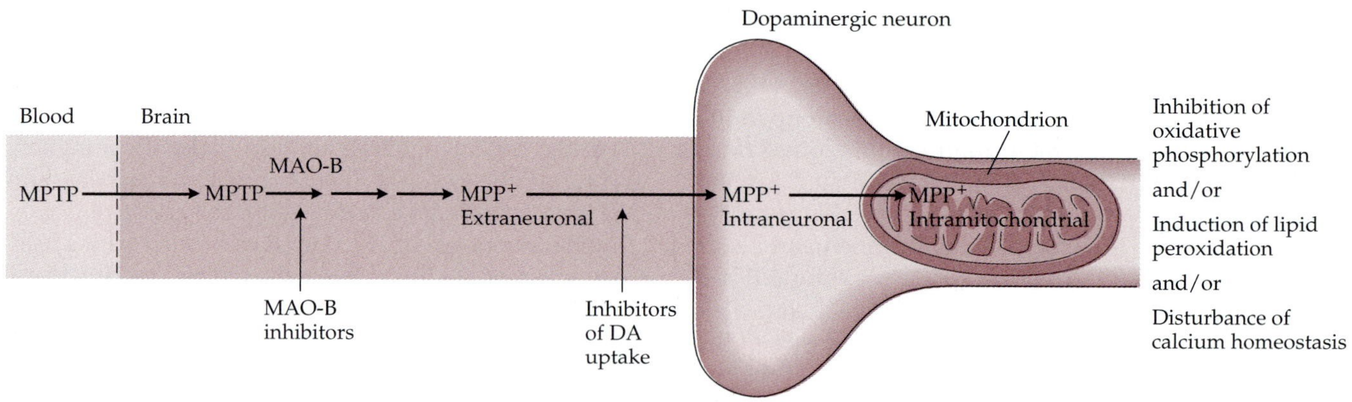

Dopaminergic neuron

20.12 BIOCHEMICAL MECHANISMS THOUGHT TO UNDERLIE MPTP TOXICITY IN DOPAMINERGIC NEURONS. MPTP crosses the blood–brain barrier and is converted by MAO-B to the toxic metabolite MPP^+. MPP^+ is transported into dopaminergic neurons by the plasma membrane DA transporter and then enters mitochondria, where it inhibits oxidative phosphorylation and produces other damaging effects. (After Gerlach et al., 1991.)

Pifl (1994) have developed a rhesus monkey MPTP model that exhibits cortical and subcortical monoamine changes closely resembling those found in PD. Moreover, careful examination of the brains of several monkeys treated with MPTP has even revealed the presence of eosinophilic inclusions resembling the Lewy bodies of PD (Forno et al., 1986; 1988). Taken together, these findings provide strong support for MPTP-induced neurotoxicity in primates as a useful model of PD.

Mechanisms of MPTP action.   The principal theory of the mechanism of MPTP neurotoxicity is presented in Figure 20.12 (see reviews by Gerlach et al., 1991; Tipton and Singer, 1993). MPTP is known to reach the brain from the peripheral circulation and therefore must be able to cross the blood–brain barrier. However, this compound itself is not the neurotoxic agent. Rather, MPTP is first oxidized by the enzyme monoamine oxidase (MAO) to the intermediate product 1-methyl-4-phenyl-1,2-dihydropyridinium ion ($MPDP^+$), which is then further oxidized to the toxic agent 1-methyl-4-phenylpyridinium ion (MPP^+) (Figure 20.13). MAO-B is mainly responsible for MPP^+ formation, as MPTP-induced damage can be prevented by pretreating subjects with an MAO-B inhibitor, but not with an MAO-A inhibitor (Cohen et al., 1984; Heikkila et al., 1984). Further evidence comes from studies of neuronal cell cultures, in which cultures that express only MAO-A are insensitive to MPTP but are destroyed by MPP^+, whereas cultures expressing MAO-B are vulnerable to MPTP toxicity (Buckman, 1991).

Where does MPTP oxidation to MPP^+ occur in the brain? There appears to be little or no MAO-B in dopaminergic neurons (Westlund et al., 1985; also see Chapter 8). However, astrocytes do possess this MAO

isozyme and readily produce MPP^+ from MPTP (Di Monte et al., 1992; Marini et al., 1992). Researchers therefore assume that in the striatum (and presumably in other affected areas), MPP^+ is formed in astrocytes and then taken up by nerve terminals. With respect to the DA system, several lines of evidence demonstrate that the plasma membrane DA transporter mediates MPP^+ uptake and, in fact, confers sensitivity to MPTP. First, MPP^+, but not MPTP, is a good substrate for the DA transporter (Javitch et al., 1985). Second, blockade of the DA transporter in vivo by administration of a DA uptake inhibitor prevents MPTP toxicity (Javitch et al., 1985; Schultz et al., 1986). Finally, nonneuronal cells became vulnerable to MPP^+-induced damage when transfected with the DA transporter (Kitayama, Shimada, and Uhl, 1992; Pifl, Giros, and Caron, 1993).

There is evidence that MPP^+ binds to neuromelanin within dopaminergic neurons (D'Amato, Lipman, and Snyder, 1986), which may cause it to accumulate within these cells and to persist for an extended period of time. However, the site of action of MPP^+ toxicity is thought to be the mitochondria (see Figure 20.12). Of particular importance is the demonstration that MPP^+ inhibits oxidative phosphorylation by blocking the activity of complex I of the mitochondrial respiratory chain (see Gerlach et al., 1991; Tipton and Singer, 1993). This results in a rapid reduction in ATP synthesis, leading to cell damage or death. Other theories advanced to explain MPP^+ toxicity

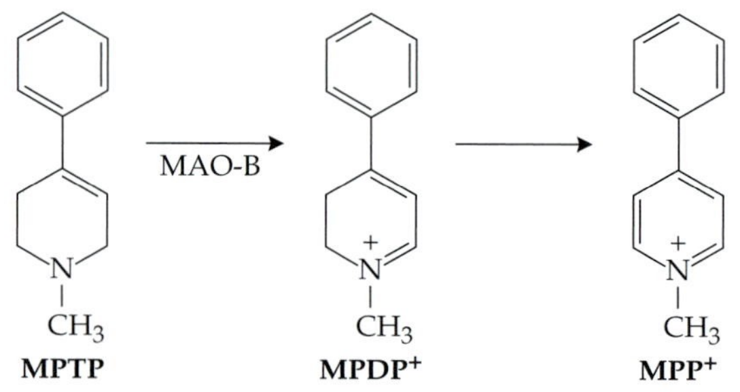

20.13 MPTP METABOLISM.

include oxidative stress (see below) and/or disruption of cellular Ca^{2+} regulation. Energy depletion following inhibition of mitochondrial respiration appears to be an adequate explanation of MPP^+ toxicity, although the other factors mentioned could contribute to the damaging effects of this compound.

Species differences in MPTP sensitivity. Researchers have discovered dramatic species differences in sensitivity to the neurotoxic and behavioral effects of MPTP treatment. As mentioned earlier, primates (both human and nonhuman) are quite vulnerable to this toxin. In contrast, rats exhibit transient behavioral deficits after acute MPTP administration, but they are relatively resistant to the toxic effects of repeated drug treatment (see Heikkila, Sonsalla, and Duvoisin, 1989). MPTP's effects on mice occupy an intermediate position between those seen in primates and in rats. Mice are less sensitive to MPTP than primates; however, a definite parkinsonian syndrome can be produced in some strains of mice (e.g., C57BL/6) using appropriate treatment regimens (Heikkila, Sonsalla, and Duvoisin, 1989; Sundström et al., 1994).

Several factors may account for these species differences, including differences in MPP^+ pharmacokinetics, capillary MAO-B activity, and substantia nigra neuromelanin content. First, primates may be more sensitive to MPTP toxicity in part because MPP^+ is cleared from their brain much more slowly than it is from the brains of mice or rats (Johannessen et al., 1985; Langston and Irwin, 1986). Second, Kalaria, Mitchell, and Harik (1987) proposed that species differences in MPTP sensitivity are related to the activity of MAO-B in brain capillaries. That is, high levels of MAO-B (such as are found in rats) were hypothesized to convert most of the MPTP to MPP^+ within the capillary endothelium. Due to its ionization, MPP^+ is presumably unable to cross the endothelial cell membrane and gain access to nerve cells. Third, the substantia nigra of primates has a high neuromelanin content compared with that of rodents, which may contribute to differences in MPTP toxicity between these orders (D'Amato, Lipman, and Snyder, 1986). These hypotheses are not mutually exclusive, and it is certainly possible (if not likely) that multiple factors are involved in determining species-specific sensitivity to MPTP.

Pathogenesis of Parkinson's Disease

The Oxidative Stress Hypothesis

Research on the pathogenesis of PD has focused on the nigrostriatal dopaminergic system, as this system is most strongly affected and is principally responsible for parkinsonian motor deficits. Investigators do not yet have a clear understanding of how the dopaminergic neurons in the SNC come to be destroyed in PD; how-

$$O_2 \xrightarrow{+1e^-} \cdot O_2^- \xrightarrow[+2H^+]{+1e^-} H_2O_2 \xrightarrow[+1H^+]{+1e^-} \cdot OH + H_2O$$

| Superoxide radical | Hydrogen peroxide | Hydroxyl radical |

20.14 FORMATION OF HYDROGEN PEROXIDE AND OXY-RADICALS FROM MOLECULAR OXYGEN BY ONE-ELECTRON TRANSFER REACTIONS. (After Fahn and Cohen, 1992.)

ever, current theories focus on the idea that this process occurs largely through a mechanism of oxidative stress. As shown in Figure 20.14, electron transfer reactions can convert molecular oxygen (O_2) to hydrogen peroxide and the free radicals superoxide radical and hydroxyl radical (which together are called **oxyradicals**). A free radical is any molecular species with an unpaired electron. Such species are extremely reactive with other compounds and therefore have a short lifetime after they are formed. The oxyradicals under discussion here are powerful oxidizing agents that can cause extensive injury and even cell death through multiple mechanisms, including damage to nucleic acids, oxidation of proteins, and lipid peroxidation (see Fahn and Cohen, 1992). The latter process refers to the oxidation of polyunsaturated fatty acids in membrane phospholipids, which leads to disturbed membrane function. One reason why free radicals are so dangerous is that reaction of a free radical with a nonradical compound can lead to the formation of other free radicals, thus establishing a chain reaction.

Oxyradicals and hydrogen peroxide are created in the normal course of cell metabolism as by-products of certain enzymatic and nonenzymatic reactions and of electron transfer reactions within mitochondria. However, these substances are usually maintained at low levels through the actions of two types of protective mechanisms: (1) cellular antioxidants such as tocopherol (vitamin E) and ascorbate (vitamin C), which can react with free radicals and stop the chain reaction, and (2) enzymes such as superoxide dismutase, glutathione peroxidase, and catalase, which catalyze the removal of reactive species. Superoxide dismutase converts superoxide radicals to hydrogen peroxide, and hydrogen peroxide is metabolized to water by either catalase or glutathione peroxidase (Figure 20.15). In the latter reaction, reduced glutathione (GSH) is converted to its oxidized form (GSSG), which can then be returned to the reduced state by glutathione reductase. It is interesting to note that the hydroxyl radical is so reactive that there is no enzyme to remove it. Therefore, protection against this species requires that its formation be minimized (e.g., by rapidly eliminating hydrogen peroxide). Under normal conditions, a balance is maintained between the formation and removal of oxyradicals and hydrogen peroxide so that cells are protected from the damaging effects of these substances. However, if this balance is altered by increased production of oxidizing species and/or re-

$$2 \cdot O_2^- + 2H^+ \xrightarrow[\text{Superoxide dismutase}]{} H_2O_2 + O_2$$

$$2GSH + H_2O_2 \xrightarrow[\text{Glutathione peroxidase}]{} GSSG + 2H_2O$$

$$GSSG + NADPH + H^+ \xrightarrow[\text{Glutathione reductase}]{} 2GSH + NADP^+$$

$$2H_2O_2 \xrightarrow[\text{Catalase}]{} O_2 + 2H_2O$$

20.15 ENZYMATIC METABOLISM OF SUPEROXIDE RADICAL AND HYDROGEN PEROXIDE.

duced activity of the removal mechanisms, then the affected cells are considered to be under oxidative stress. The presence of oxidative stress may be indicated by (1) loss of reducing substances such as tocopherol, ascorbate, or glutathione, (2) decreased activity of protective enzymes such as superoxide dismutase, (3) altered "redox status" of cells, as suggested by an increased ratio of the oxidized compared with the reduced form of glutathione, and (4) appearance of molecular damage, including peroxidized lipids, oxidized proteins, or damaged DNA (Fahn and Cohen, 1992). In the sections that follow, we will consider possible sources of oxidative stress in the dopaminergic system and then review evidence that this process may be responsible for the cell death that occurs in PD.

Possible sources.   Oxidative stress could be produced by several processes that take place in dopaminergic neurons as well as in some other monoaminergic cells. First, hydrogen peroxide is one of the products of MAO deamination (see Chapter 8). Thus, every molecule of DA catabolized within the cell gives rise to a molecule of hydrogen peroxide (which, as we have seen, can be converted to the even more dangerous hydroxyl radical). Cohen (1983) first proposed that the MAO reaction may be a source of oxidative stress in PD, and this remains an important hypothesis.

Second, catecholamines can undergo nonenzymatic auto-oxidation in the presence of molecular oxygen. This process gives rise to toxic quinones as well as hydrogen peroxide and oxyradicals as by-products (Graham, 1978). Moreover, DA auto-oxidation is considered to be the mechanism of neuromelanin formation. Hence, auto-oxidation may play a role in the particularly severe loss of melanized neurons in PD.

Finally, there is much interest in the possible role of iron in generating hydroxyl radicals. The formation of hydroxyl radicals from hydrogen peroxide can be catalyzed nonenzymatically by ferrous ions in a so-called Fenton-type reaction. A by-product of this reaction is the oxidation of ferrous (Fe^{2+}) to ferric (Fe^{3+}) ions. The

potential damaging effect of iron was shown by Triggs and Willmore (1984), who demonstrated increased lipid peroxidation in rats administered Fe^{2+} intracerebrally. The substantia nigra contains a high concentration of iron, and neuromelanin appears to be capable of reducing Fe^{3+} to Fe^{2+}, thereby driving the Fenton-type reaction (Youdim et al., 1990). Figure 20.16 illustrates the hypothesis that MAO, iron, and neuromelanin in DA neurons may function together to cause the formation of hydroxyl radicals with resulting lipid peroxidation and other types of cell damage. This hypothesis is supported by reports that intranigral injection of iron induces degeneration of nigrostriatal neurons, striatal DA depletion, and motor deficits in rats (Ben-Shachar et al., 1992; Sengstock et al., 1992, 1993).

Evidence.   There are several lines of evidence suggesting that nigral neurons are under oxidative stress in PD. First, increased lipid peroxidation has been observed in nigral tissue obtained from postmortem PD patients compared with tissue from age-matched controls (Jenner et al., 1992). Second, iron levels in the nigra are also elevated in PD (Gerlach et al., 1994). This increase in iron could stimulate Fenton-type reactions, thereby creating hydroxyl radicals and causing the lipid peroxidation found in other studies. Third, substantia nigra from PD patients showed considerable reductions in both total and reduced glutathione concentrations (Jenner et al., 1992). This indicates an abnormality in the glutathione pathway, which serves an important protective function in detoxifying hydrogen peroxide.

These findings provide substantial evidence that DA neurons in the substantia nigra are under oxidative stress in PD. However, a number of questions remain unanswered at this time. What is the source of this stress? Is oxidative stress a sufficient explanation to account for dopaminergic cell loss in PD? And finally, is oxidative stress also present in the nondopaminergic cell populations that are damaged in PD? In the remaining parts of this section, we will consider other factors that may also play an important role in the pathogenesis of PD.

Mitochondrial Dysfunction

Considering that inhibition of mitochondrial respiration (specifically at complex I) is thought to be the principal mechanism of MPP^+ neurotoxicity, several investigators have looked for evidence of mitochondrial dysfunction in PD. Although some inconsistent findings have been reported from different laboratories (see DiMauro, 1993), Schapira and coworkers (Schapira, Cooper et al., 1990; Schapira, Mann et al., 1990) have performed several studies demonstrating a deficiency in mitochondrial complex I specific to the substantia nigra in PD. This is an interesting and potentially important parallel to the complex I inhibition that occurs following MPTP administration.

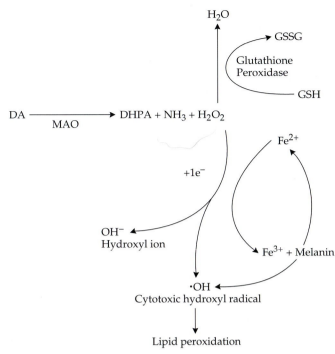

20.16 BIOCHEMICAL REACTIONS LEADING TO OXIDATIVE STRESS AND LIPID PEROXIDATION IN DOPAMINERGIC NEURONS. Deamination of DA to DHPA (3,4,-dihydroxyphenylacetaldehyde) by MAO leads to the formation of a molecule of H_2O_2. Although H_2O_2 can be inactivated by glutathione peroxidase, it can also be converted to a hydroxyl radical by the action of Fe^{2+} ions (Fenton-type reaction). Melanin present inside the cell is thought to help reduce Fe^{3+} back to Fe^{2+}, thereby driving the formation of hydroxyl radicals and eventual lipid peroxidation. (After Youdim et al., 1990.)

The Environmental Toxin Hypothesis

The discovery that a toxic chemical (i.e., MPTP) can reproduce so many of the neuropathological, neurochemical, and behavioral characteristics of PD naturally raises the question of whether PD itself might be caused by exposure to toxins in the environment (reviewed by Tanner, 1989; Tanner and Langston, 1990). Most individuals presumably would not ingest a high dose of the toxin acutely (as was the case for the MPTP-exposed drug addicts), but rather, would experience gradual exposure over long periods of time. Since PD was first identified as a distinct clinical entity in early nineteenth-century England, it is tempting to suggest that the culprit is a chemical or chemicals associated with the advent of industrialism in Europe and elsewhere. This hypothesis leads to two predictions: (1) that the prevalence of PD in industrialized countries has been rising since the beginning of the industrial revolution, and (2) that its prevalence is greater in highly industrialized than in developing countries. It is difficult to address the first prediction since prevalence data have been available only since the mid-1950s. In Rochester, Minnesota, where thorough records are available, there was no change in the incidence of PD from 1955 to 1979 (Tanner, 1989). With regard to differences between countries, there is a trend for PD prevalence to be greater in long-industrialized countries than in countries that began industrialization more recently (Tanner, 1989; Tanner and Langston, 1990). These intriguing findings, which are based on door-to-door community surveys followed by neurological verification, are consistent with the environmental toxin hypothesis. Nevertheless, this hypothesis remains speculative at the present time, since no environmental chemical has yet been linked to substantia nigra damage and PD.

Conclusions

We conclude this discussion by considering four general models of PD etiology, taking into account the gradual decline in striatal DA levels with "normal" aging and the finding that DA must be depleted by at least 80% before clinical symptomatology is manifested (see Figure 20.17). The first model proposes that PD patients are born with an abnormally low number of substantia nigra neurons and hence a low level of striatal DA. This idea is not supported by any available data, although it must be noted that the nature of the model makes it extremely difficult to test in practice. The second model proposes an abrupt decline in striatal DA as a consequence of acute damage from some environmental insult. This is one version of the environmental toxin hypothesis described in the pre-

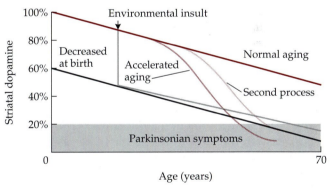

20.17 THEORETICAL POSSIBILITIES CONCERNING THE LOSS OF STRIATAL DOPAMINE IN PARKINSON'S DISEASE. Current evidence suggests that striatal DA concentrations slowly decline as a function of normal aging, and that a reduction of approximately 80% in striatal DA levels is necessary for parkinsonian symptoms to appear (shaded area). According to different theoretical possibilities, reaching this 80% reduction could occur if (1) some genetic or prenatal event causes a large decrease in dopaminergic neurons and striatal DA levels at birth, which is then followed by the normal age-related rate of decline; (2) an environmental insult (e.g., neurotoxin exposure) causes a relatively abrupt reduction in DA levels, followed by a further decline to levels at which symptoms appear; (3) some unknown factor causes an acceleration of the process underlying the normal age-related decline in DA levels; or (4) a second process, different from that involved in normal aging, causes an accelerated loss of DA. (After Langston, 1990a.)

vious section. A third possibility is that some process (e.g., exposure to a toxin) causes an acceleration of the age-related reduction in DA, thereby causing the individual to develop PD. If oxidative stress is responsible for the usual loss of dopaminergic neurons over time, then one can see how a gradual acceleration of this process would eventually lead to parkinsonism. Finally, PD could be caused by a pathological mechanism that differs from the processes involved in normal aging.

We do not know which of these models (if any) is correct, although the second and third seem best at bringing together the current evidence for oxidative stress and mitochondrial dysfunction in PD, along with the possibility of a toxic factor. Any model, however, should take into consideration changes in vulnerability that occur in the course of aging. That is, the amount of oxidative stress and cell damage produced in the nigrostriatal system by MPTP is substantially greater in old animals than in young ones (Ali et al., 1994; Ricaurte et al., 1987). If antioxidants or other protective mechanisms become less effective over time, then the nigrostriatal system could be more vulnerable to insult and could perhaps undergo the accelerated aging shown in Figure 20.17.

Treatment of Parkinson's Disease

Pharmacotherapies

Drugs administered in the early stages. Over 125 years ago, Ordenstein administered belladonna alkaloids (which possess anticholinergic activity; see Chapter 7) to PD patients in order to manage their severe drooling behavior (cited in Kopin, 1993a). This treatment unexpectedly also led to some improvement in the patients' motor deficits and formed the basis of PD pharmacotherapy for many years. Improvement in anticholinergic treatment occurred with the later introduction of synthetic compounds such as benztropine mesylate (Cogentin; as discussed in Chapter 8, this drug is also a DA uptake inhibitor) and trihexyphenidyl (Artane) (Corbin, 1949; Dorshay and Constable, 1949). These compounds are still widely prescribed today, particularly in the early stages of PD. It is still somewhat unclear why anticholinergic (more specifically, antimuscarinic) drugs are efficacious

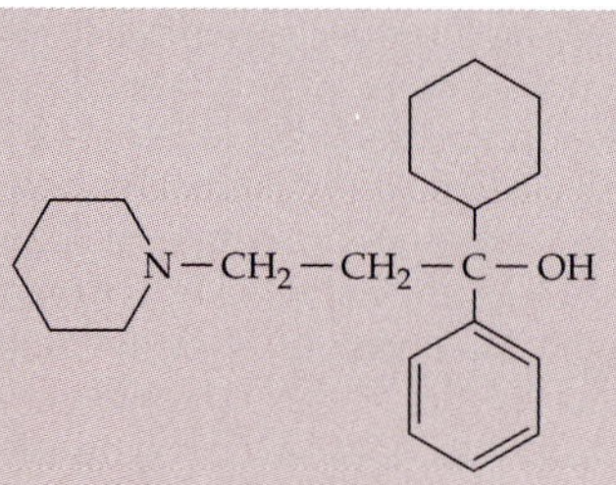

Trihexyphenidyl

in treating PD. However, the prevailing theory is that DA regulates striatal ACh such that in the absence of nigrostriatal input, excessive cholinergic activity is partially responsible for the abnormalities in striatal outflow.

Amantadine (Symmetrel) is another compound that is commonly prescribed in the early stages of PD. The mechanism underlying amantadine's therapeutic benefit is not fully understood; however, the drug has been found to stimulate DA synthesis and release (Leonard, 1992).

Levodopa therapy. Early studies by Bertler and Rosengren (1959) and by Carlsson and his colleagues (1958) set the stage for the development of the first rational phar-

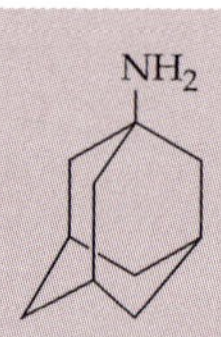

Amantadine

macotherapy for PD. These investigators demonstrated the presence of high levels of DA in the striatum and further showed that the DA precursor L-3,4-dihydroxyphenylalanine (L-DOPA; also called **levodopa**) reversed the tranquilization and parkinsonian-like motor impairment induced by reserpine treatment. When, a few years later, PD patients were found to be suffering from a massive depletion of DA in the striatum, there was immediate interest in testing whether DA replacement using levodopa might reverse the symptoms of the disorder. However, initial attempts at levodopa therapy had disappointing results due to severe side effects, including nausea and vomiting (see Kopin, 1993a). Nevertheless, these problems were subsequently overcome by Cotzias and coworkers (1967, 1969), who minimized adverse reactions by gradually increasing the dose of levodopa until a sufficiently high, therapeutically efficacious regimen was attained.

Levodopa is converted to DA in the brain by the enzyme aromatic L–amino acid decarboxylase (AADC; see Chapter 8). However, this enzyme is also found in many peripheral organs such as the intestine, liver, and kidneys, as well as in the brain capillary endothelial cells. Peripheral decarboxylation therefore results in only a very small percentage of orally administered levodopa reaching dopaminergic neurons in the brain. This problem led to the introduction of two compounds, carbidopa and benserazide, that block AADC peripherally but do not cross the blood–brain barrier (Chapter 8; Papavasiliou et al., 1972; Pletscher, 1973). Coadministration of peripheral decarboxylase inhibitors with levodopa dramatically increases the availability of levodopa to the brain by reducing its extracerebral metabolism. Consequently, the standard DA replacement therapy for PD involves the administration of levodopa combined with either carbidopa (trade name Sinemet) or benserazide (trade name Madopar).

The therapeutic action of levodopa in PD clearly stems from its ability to raise DA levels in the striatum (Hornykiewicz, 1974). However, the conversion of exogenously administered levodopa to DA does not seem to mimic the normal process of DA synthesis in several ways. For example, various studies suggest that most of the DA formed from levodopa remains in the cytoplasm and is not stored in vesicles (Melamed, 1992). If true, this would imply that DA may either passively leak out of the surviving dopaminergic nerve terminals or be transported in the reverse direction by the plasma membrane DA transporter. In either case, release would not be under the stimulus-dependent control that governs release of DA located in the vesicular compartment of the terminals. Likewise, the normal negative feedback mechanisms regulating DA synthesis and release appear to be absent in the case of levodopa-derived DA (Melamed, 1992; Ponzio et al., 1983). Finally, there is good evidence that levodopa can be decarboxylated to DA in serotonergic as well as in dopaminergic neurons (Arai et al., 1994). This DA causes 5-HT release, probably by displacing 5-HT from intracellular storage sites (Ng et al., 1970). Whether levodopa decarboxylation in nondopaminergic cells plays any role in its therapeutic effects is not known at this time.

Problems associated with levodopa therapy. Levodopa therapy typically remains effective for several years after the beginning of treatment. However, within 3 to 5 years, many patients begin to experience response fluctuations despite maintaining the same treatment regimen (Chase et al., 1990; Rinne, 1983). Initial response fluctuations are temporally related to drug ingestion. That is, the patient experiences a "wearing off" of the levodopa-induced motor facilitation before the next dose is due. Later, the patient may begin to show "on–off" effects in which sudden periods of tremors, freezing, or rigidity alternate with periods of mobility in an unpredictable pattern that is unrelated to drug dosing. Other complications arising from long-term levodopa treatment include the development of dyskinesias (abnormal involuntary movements) and, in advanced cases, dopaminergic psychoses (Fischer et al., 1990; Rinne, 1983).

Clinicians have been most concerned with the motor problems (particularly the "on–off" effects and dyskinesias) associated with levodopa because these problems may become so severe as to render the patient functionally disabled. Although the mechanisms underlying these response fluctuations are not yet known, various investigators have hypothesized that such fluctuations may stem from long-term changes in drug pharmacokinetics, alterations in receptor sensitivity, or continuing progression of the disease process (i.e., further loss of

dopaminergic nerve terminals in the striatum). If levodopa decarboxylation to DA eventually occurs mainly in nondopaminergic cells, then the release of this DA would not be under normal physiological control and might shift abruptly to produce sudden alterations in motor function. Exposure of postsynaptic receptors to extreme variations in DA concentrations might additionally cause abnormalities in receptor expression and/or signal transduction (Chase et al., 1990).

The eventual development of response fluctuations and dyskinesias has led some clinicians to argue that the initiation of levodopa therapy should be put off as long as possible, particularly in the case of younger patients (see Quinn, 1994). In contrast, other clinicians find no harm in early levodopa administration (Caraceni, 1994). Although this issue remains unresolved, other pharmacotherapies are now available that may delay disease progression and thus permit a delay in beginning levodopa treatment without compromising the patient's quality of life (see section below on deprenyl).

Approaches to improving levodopa therapy. Since levodopa is inevitably prescribed for most, if not all, PD patients, researchers have shown great interest in developing ways to enhance levodopa efficacy and reduce troublesome response fluctuations. One strategy, which is dietary, is based on the fact that levodopa is transported across the blood–brain barrier by the large neutral amino acid carrier. The amino acids transported by this carrier compete with levodopa as well as with each other for access to the transport sites. As consumption of protein increases the circulating concentrations of these amino acids, levodopa access to the brain will be inhibited. Consequently, research has shown that restricting dietary protein intake improves the efficacy of levodopa treatment and reduces the dose requirement (Pincus and Barry, 1987). Some clinicians are now recommending that PD patients eat meals containing a 7:1 ratio of carbohydrate to protein in order to minimize motor response fluctuations.

Over 10 years ago, researchers found that "off" periods could be significantly reduced by continuous dopaminergic stimulation through intravenous or intraduodenal infusion of levodopa (reviewed by Hutton and Morris, 1994; Schelosky and Poewe, 1993). These findings support the hypothesis that response fluctuations are at least partially related to erratic delivery of levodopa-derived DA to striatal neurons. However, continuous drug infusions are not practical for outpatient therapy. This problem has led to the development of several sustained-release levodopa preparations: Sinemet CR, Madopar CR, and Madopar HBS. Although these preparations use different delivery systems to control drug release rate, they all yield sustained elevations in plasma levodopa concentrations compared with the standard formulations (Figure 20.18). Sustained-release prepara-

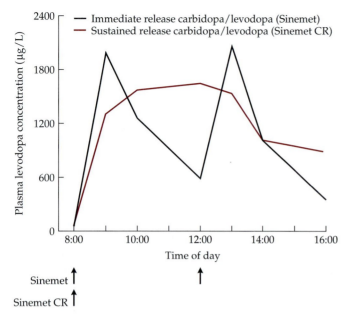

20.18 COMPARISON OF PLASMA LEVODOPA CONCENTRA-TIONS PRODUCED BY IMMEDIATE-RELEASE AND SUSTAINED-RELEASE SINEMET. Fourteen PD patients received two doses of immediate-release Sinemet (100 mg levodopa plus 25 mg carbidopa) or one dose of sustained-release Sinemet CR (200 mg levodopa plus 50 mg carbidopa) at the times indicated by the arrows. (After Hutton and Morris, 1994; original data from Goetz et al., 1988.)

When peripheral decarboxylation is prevented (as with the use of carbidopa or benserazide), *O*-methylation becomes another important metabolic pathway by which levodopa is inactivated peripherally. It should be possible, therefore, to enhance levodopa efficacy by combining COMT inhibition with a peripheral decarboxylase inhibitor. COMT inhibitors, including several compounds mentioned in Chapter 8, are thus under development as potential adjuncts to levodopa therapy (Kopin, 1993b).

A fourth approach, which has been in use for many years, involves the administration of DA receptor agonists either alone or as supplements to levodopa treatment (Montastruc, Rascol, and Senard, 1993). Among the major agonists used in treating PD are the ergot derivatives bromocriptine, lisuride, and pergolide, all of which exert greater potency at D_2 than at D_1 receptors (see Chapter 8). The nonselective DA agonist apomorphine is also useful in some patients, although it must be given subcutaneously or by another nonoral route because of nausea and vomiting that occur following oral administration (Montastruc, Rascol, and Senard, 1993). Unlike levodopa, direct receptor agonists do not depend on the presence of intact dopaminergic terminals for conversion to an active agent. Hence these compounds are helpful in smoothing out response fluctuations when given as adjuncts to levodopa therapy. Some investigators have proposed that long-term treatment with levodopa but not DA receptor agonists may hasten the loss of residual dopaminergic neurons in PD (see Ogawa, 1994). The combination of such concerns with the well-documented decrease in levodopa efficacy over time has led to a strong interest in developing new therapeutic approaches. Indeed, a number of selective D_1 and D_2 agonists are currently being tested for efficacy in animal models of PD (e.g., Belluzi et al., 1994; Gnanalingham et al., 1995; Vermeulen et al., 1994).

Deprenyl. Nonselective MAO inhibitors were considered as potential therapeutic agents for PD many years

tions have been found more beneficial to patients with predictable "wearing-off" effects than to more advanced patients with severe "on–off" effects (Hutton and Morris, 1994; Schelosky and Poewe, 1993).

Yet another strategy to improve levodopa efficacy is to inhibit its conversion to metabolites other than DA. As shown in Figure 20.19, levodopa is a substrate not only for AADC (which converts it to DA), but also for the enzyme catechol-*O*-methyltransferase (COMT). The resulting intermediate, 3-*O*-methyldopa, is then oxidatively deaminated to 3-methoxy-4-hydroxyphenyllactic acid.

20.19 ALTERNATIVE PATHWAY OF LEVODOPA METABOLISM.

ago. Yet they were of little use initially because they had poor efficacy when administered alone and produced potentially dangerous hypertensive reactions when given with levodopa (Kopin, 1993). The development of the selective MAO-B inhibitor (–)deprenyl (also known as selegiline) (see Chapter 8) addressed this problem, however, because it could be administered safely with levodopa without producing hypertension. Initial studies showed that combined levodopa and deprenyl therapy was useful in prolonging the effects of levodopa and in reducing "on–off" effects (Birkmayer et al., 1975). But a major breakthrough occurred 10 years later when Birkmayer and coworkers (1985) reported an increased life expectancy in patients given deprenyl along with levodopa. Coming in the wake of the discovery of MPTP neurotoxicity and the emerging oxidative stress hypothesis of PD, this finding generated considerable interest in the possibility that treatment with deprenyl or antioxidant compounds might actually be able to retard the progress of PD, instead of just ameliorating the symptoms (as is thought to be the case with levodopa).

To determine the effectiveness of deprenyl in treating early PD, two separate double-blind, placebo-controlled clinical studies were begun in 1986 and 1987. One study of 54 patients, which was conducted by Langston's group, tested the effects of daily treatment with 10 mg deprenyl compared with placebo. This dose of deprenyl produces a 90% inhibition of MAO-B in the human brain (Riederer and Youdim, 1986). The second study, which was organized by Ira Shoulson and Stanley Fahn at the University of Rochester, involved 800 patients spread over 28 clinical centers (23 American and 5 Canadian). This study was designed to test the efficacy of both deprenyl and α-tocopherol, which is the active ingredient of vitamin E and which acts as an antioxidant and free radical scavenger. The subjects were divided into four groups: (1) deprenyl (10 mg daily) only, (2) tocopherol (2,000 IU daily) only, (3) both deprenyl and tocopherol, and (4) placebo. Because of its design, the large study was called the DATATOP (Deprenyl and Tocopherol Antioxidant Therapy of Parkinsonism) project.

The subjects in both studies were in the early stages of PD and were either previously untreated (Langston) or were required to forgo other medications during the course of the study (DATATOP). Both studies utilized the same subject end point, namely, a clinical determination that the patient's condition had deteriorated sufficiently to warrant the initiation of levodopa therapy. Cumulative probability of reaching the end point was calculated according to the method of Kaplan and Meier (1958). In addition, subjects in both studies were evaluated with respect to symptom severity a few weeks following the beginning of treatment (wash-in evaluation), at specified intervals during the treatment phase, and after discontinuation of treatment but prior to the initiation of levodopa therapy (wash-out evaluation). The wash-in and wash-out assessments in both studies were important tests of whether deprenyl (and/or tocopherol, in the DATATOP project) produced *symptomatic* improvement in the subjects rather than (or in addition to) retarding the progression of the disorder. If so, then the patients were expected to show significant symptom improvement during the wash-in period as well as significant symptom worsening during wash-out.

Initial data analysis in the DATATOP project was carried out by comparing the combined deprenyl alone and deprenyl + tocopherol groups with the combined tocopherol alone and placebo groups. The results of this analysis, as well as those from the Langston study, showed that daily deprenyl treatment caused a striking decrease in the probability of reaching the clinical end point over the first 600 days (Tetrud and Langston, 1989; The Parkinson Study Group, 1989; Figure 20.20). A later report following completion of the DATATOP project confirmed these initial results, provided additional information concerning the effects of deprenyl treatment, and showed that tocopherol did not influence the progression of PD (The Parkinson Study Group, 1993).

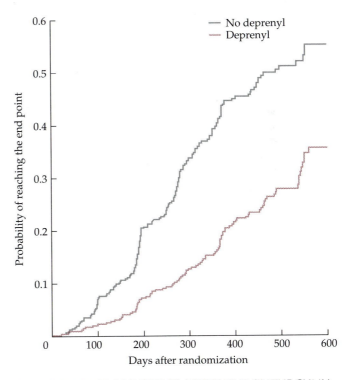

20.20 INFLUENCE OF DEPRENYL TREATMENT ON THE CUMULATIVE PROBABILITY OF REACHING THE STUDY END POINT DURING THE FIRST 600 DAYS OF THE DATATOP STUDY. PD patients treated with deprenyl (with or without tocopherol), had a much lower cumulative probability of reaching the study end point (defined as the need to begin levodopa therapy) than patients not given deprenyl. Cumulative probabilities were determined according to the method of Kaplan and Meier (1958). The group difference was highly significant statistically. (After The Parkinson Study Group, 1989.)

Based on these and other findings, deprenyl should now be considered one of the drugs of choice for the initial treatment of PD (Myllylä et al., 1992; The Parkinson Study Group, 1993). Furthermore, even when the point is reached that levodopa administration must be started, continuation of deprenyl as an adjunct therapy appears to reduce the levodopa dose requirement (Myllylä et al., 1995). Despite these clinical considerations, however, controversy remains as to what kind of action is being exerted by deprenyl (Langston, 1990b). Some investigators (e.g., Ward, 1994) have argued that the results of the DATATOP project can be explained entirely by a direct treatment effect, and therefore that the study provided no evidence for neuroprotection. The DATATOP researchers state that the results of the wash-in and wash-out evaluations indicated significant improvement in PD symptomatology; however, they argue for the presence of an additional protective effect. This possibility is supported by preliminary postmortem findings of reduced loss of nigral neurons in deprenyl-treated patients (Rinne et al., 1991).

Recent animal studies have even shown that deprenyl can mediate neuronal "rescue" in addition to neuronal protection (Tatton, 1993). In these experiments, C57BL mice were given five consecutive daily treatments of 30 mg/kg MPTP, which usually causes a 35% to 40% loss of nigral neurons in this strain. When deprenyl treatment (every second day) was begun 72 hours *after* the last dose of MPTP, however, the cell loss averaged only 12% to 18%. This effect could be produced by a deprenyl dose as low as 0.01 mg/kg, which produces little or no inhibition of MAO-B activity. These results suggest that deprenyl saved damaged neurons that would otherwise have died in the absence of the delayed treatment.

A number of possible mechanisms may underlie the therapeutic actions of deprenyl in PD. As space limitations do not permit a full account of these mechanisms, interested readers are referred to recent reviews by Berry, Juorio, and Paterson (1994b) and Gerlach, Youdim, and Riederer (1994). It is also worth noting that amphetamine and methamphetamine are among the major metabolites of deprenyl. These compounds probably have little effect on the motor symptoms of PD, but they could produce mood elevation in treated patients.

Pallidotomy

Despite the advances in PD pharmacotherapy discussed above, many patients still reach a stage at which drug treatments begin to lose their efficacy. This has prompted a continuing search for other therapeutic approaches, including some that involve surgery. As discussed in Wichmann, Vitek, and DeLong (1995), stereotaxic lesioning of the GPi (known as pallidotomy) has been used to treat PD patients since the 1930s. Although early results were not promising, subsequent changes in the target area within the GPi coupled with the development of more re-

fined electrode placement techniques have led to recent successes with this approach. Because of the permanent nature of brain lesions, however, this treatment remains the last recourse after pharmacotherapy has failed.

Tissue Grafting

Perhaps the most intriguing approach to the treatment of PD is the attempt to restore dopaminergic function by means of intracerebral tissue grafts. This is the only method currently available that could, in principle, *reverse* the course of the illness rather than simply retard its progression or alleviate its symptoms. Readers may be surprised to learn that intracerebral tissue grafting dates back at least to 1890 (see review by Fisher and Gage, 1993). The modern era of research and clinical application of grafting, however, did not begin until the 1970s. In this section, we will consider the current status of tissue grafting in the treatment of PD.

Adrenal medullary grafts.　One approach developed to restore DA to the striatum is the implantation of adrenal medullary tissue either into a lateral ventricle or into the striatum itself (reviewed by Freed, Poltorak, and Becker, 1990). Although adrenal medullary chromaffin cells normally secrete mainly epinephrine and norepinephrine, they were found to contain substantial amounts of DA (and were presumed to secrete some of this transmitter) when removed from their normal neural and hormonal control mechanisms. One important consideration in performing adrenal medullary grafts is that the patient can donate his or her own tissue (autologous transplantation),* which avoids the ethical problems associated with obtaining human fetal tissue (see below) and also precludes the need for immunosuppression to prevent a heterologous transplant (a transplant from a different individual) from being rejected by the host.

The first experimental study of adrenal medulla grafts was carried out by Freed and colleagues (1981), who showed that such grafts decreased apomorphine-induced rotational behavior in rats with unilateral 6-OHDA lesions of the substantia nigra. Within a few years, the technique was modified for application to humans, and since the mid-1980s, hundreds of PD patients around the world have received adrenal medullary transplants. Unfortunately, only a few studies have been carried out to ascertain the safety and efficacy of this procedure. Some positive effects have been reported, particularly when grafts are placed into the cerebral ventricle rather than in the striatum (Fisher and Gage, 1993; Freed, Poltorak, and Becker, 1990). On the other hand, the studies have been plagued by numerous problems, including either the death of grafted tissue or its failure

---

*Only one adrenal medulla is needed to maintain adequate epinephrine secretion in the patient.

to express tyrosine hydroxylase (TH), an unacceptable incidence of adverse side effects and patient mortality, and various methodological flaws. One problem inherent in this type of work is the lack of control groups (e.g., matched subjects receiving sham surgery or grafts of nondopamine-secreting tissue) because of ethical considerations. Despite these concerns, adrenal medullary grafts could eventually become a valuable treatment if graft survival and DA secretion were improved.

Nigral tissue grafts. The major alternative to adrenal medullary grafts is the grafting of fetal substantia nigra (SN) tissue. As before, animal studies initially demonstrated that this procedure alleviated many of the behavioral deficits produced by 6-OHDA lesions (Fisher and Gage, 1993), thereby paving the way for subsequent application of the technique to PD. Human fetal SN grafts were first carried out in 1987 in Sweden and Mexico (Lindvall et al., 1989; Madrazo et al., 1988), and according to Zabek and coworkers (1994), over 100 patients worldwide have now received such grafts. Although some of these surgical procedures have been carried out in the United States, fetal tissue grafting has been politically controversial here because of the need for abortuses as tissue donors.

Several studies have been published concerning the outcome of human SN grafting. As summarized in the recent review by Olanow, Kordower, and Freeman (1996), the results have generally shown increased striatal [18F]DOPA uptake (as indicated by PET scanning)

and mild to moderate improvement in motor symptoms (although not enough improvement to warrant cessation of levodopa therapy). Despite this modest therapeutic benefit, much has been learned from these initial clinical trials. It is now clear that clinical outcome depends on several methodological variables, including the number of tissue donors (due to cell loss, six or more fetal donors may be required for one effective graft), the age of the donors (between 5.5 and 9 weeks postconception seems to be optimal), proper tissue storage, and implant site (Olanow, Kordower, and Freeman, 1996). Careful attention to these and other important variables should increase the therapeutic benefit derived from fetal SN grafts.

One might assume that fetal SN tissue implanted into a host with nigrostriatal pathway damage (either experimentally induced or PD-related) restores behavioral function simply by providing a reinnervation of the denervated striatum. Evidence that such reinnervation can occur is presented in Figure 20.21, which shows TH-immunoreactive cells and fibers in both a rat and a human nigral graft. Reinnervation, however, is but one possible mechanism underlying the therapeutic efficacy of tissue grafts. Other possibilities include (1) passive diffusion of neurotransmitter molecules to target sites in the host brain (this may be important, for example, if reinnervation occurs only within a limited area around the graft), (2) surgical disruption of the blood–brain barrier, thus allowing increased entry of blood-borne neurotransmitter molecules or drugs (e.g., levodopa) into the

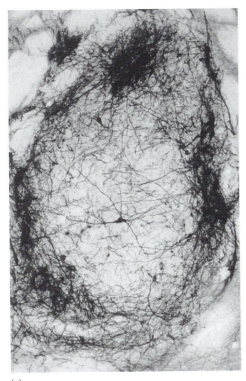

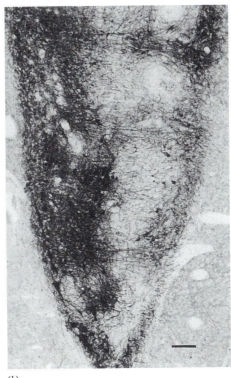

(a)　　　　　　(b)

20.21 TYROSINE HYDROXYLASE–IMMUNOREACTIVE CELLS AND FIBERS IN HUMAN FETAL GRAFTS implanted into an immunosuppressed rat (a) and a Parkinson's disease patient (b). Scale bar = 100 μm. (From Olanow, Kordower, and Freeman, 1996. Fetal nigral transplantation as a therapy for Parkinson's disease. *Trends in Neuroscience.* 19:102–109.)

area of the graft, and (3) graft-induced stimulation of trophic activity and axonal sprouting in the host brain (Dunnett and Björklund, 1994). Several of these mechanisms could be operative with regard to fetal SN or adrenal medullary grafts in PD patients.

Future directions in brain grafting.   Because of the limited availability of healthy human fetal tissues and the moral issues surrounding elective abortion, there is an urgent need to develop methods that do not require human fetal material. One such approach currently being investigated is the grafting of genetically engineered cells. Fibroblasts (immature connective tissue cells) have been genetically modified to express TH (and hence synthesize DOPA) or to express brain-derived neurotrophic factor (BDNF), a trophic factor previously found to enhance the survival of cultured dopaminergic neurons. Implantation of TH-containing fibroblasts in rats reduced the rotational asymmetry caused by a unilateral 6-OHDA lesion (Wolff et al., 1989), whereas fibroblasts that expressed BDNF partially protected nigral DA neurons from the toxic effects of MPTP (Frim et al., 1994).

A second novel approach involves the use of xenografts, that is, tissue grafts obtained from a donor of another species. The first reported xenografts for the treatment of PD were carried out in 1995 and involved the transplantation of fetal pig cells into several patients (see Travis, 1995). No outcome results from these clinical studies have yet been published at the time of this writing. Nevertheless, genetically engineered cells or xenografts may eventually provide ready sources of tissue for the treatment of PD or other degenerative disorders such as Alzheimer's disease.

Part I Summary

Parkinson's disease is a neurodegenerative disorder of aging. The classic symptoms of PD involve the motor system and include resting tremor, bradykinesia (or akinesia), rigidity, and postural disturbances. Some PD patients also show symptoms of dementia or depression.

Histological studies of PD brains have revealed a massive loss of neurons in the substantia nigra pars compacta and several other dopaminergic cell groups, along with a less pronounced reduction in noradrenergic, serotonergic, and cholinergic neurons. Melanized (pigmented) catecholaminergic neurons seem to be particularly likely to die in PD. Cell loss is manifested by depletions of DA, NE, and 5-HT in various terminal areas of these neurotransmitters.

PD-related motor deficits can be attributed mainly to damage to the DA innervation of the neostriatum (caudate nucleus and putamen). The neostriatum is part of a complex loop between the basal ganglia and the neocortex. Other important parts of this circuit are the pallidum, the subthalamic nucleus, the substantia nigra pars reticulata, and the ventral anterior and ventral lateral nuclei of the thalamus. DA is thought to modulate the excitatory action of the glutamatergic corticostriatal inputs to the medium spiny striatal neurons in such a way as to facilitate the activity of thalamic and brain stem motor centers that are under striatal regulation. Destruction of the nigrostriatal pathway in PD presumably causes inhibition of these centers, thus leading to bradykinesia and rigidity.

Two pharmacological treatments provide reasonable experimental models of PD in laboratory animals. The first is unilateral lesioning of the nigrostriatal pathway with the catecholamine neurotoxin 6-hydroxydopamine. This procedure produces a rotational asymmetry that can be used to screen potential therapeutic treatments for PD. The other important model is produced by administration of the neurotoxin 1-methyl-4-phenyl-1,2,3,6-tetrahydropyridine (MPTP). Appropriate MPTP regimens in nonhuman primates can reproduce most of the behavioral and neurochemical deficits found in PD. The mechanism of MPTP toxicity has been widely studied. Systemically administered MPTP crosses the blood–brain barrier and enters astrocytes, where it is oxidized by MAO-B to the toxic metabolite 1-methyl-4-phenylpyridinium ion (MPP^+). MPP^+ is taken up by dopaminergic neurons via the plasma membrane DA transporter, after which it blocks mitochondrial oxidative phosphorylation and exerts other deleterious effects on cell functioning. These biochemical reactions eventually result in the death of the cell.

The cause of idiopathic PD is still unknown, but most current theories emphasize a possible role for free radicals and oxidative stress. Formation of free radicals (particularly oxyradicals) in dopaminergic neurons can stem from DA metabolism by MAO, nonenzymatic autooxidation of DA, and Fenton reactions catalyzed by Fe^{2+} ions. Abnormally high levels of oxyradicals can lead to lipid peroxidation, formation of oxidized proteins, and DNA damage, all of which may contribute to cell damage and death. There is evidence for oxidative damage to nigral DA neurons in PD, although the cause of such damage is presently unknown.

Several therapeutic approaches are used in the treatment of PD. Anticholinergic drugs are widely prescribed, as is the DA-releasing compound amantadine. But the most important therapeutic agent is the DA precursor levodopa, which is typically combined with a peripheral decarboxylase inhibitor to reduce extracerebral metabolism of the drug. Unfortunately, over time, the efficacy of levodopa gradually declines, and patients begin to suffer response fluctuations ("wearing-off" effects, "on–off" effects, and dyskinesias). Such fluctuations can be reduced somewhat by reducing dietary protein intake and by taking a sustained-release levodopa preparation. There is also recent interest in the

MAO-B inhibitor deprenyl as a therapeutic agent in PD. Two large clinical trials indicate that treatment with deprenyl during the early stages of PD retards the progress of the disease so that the beginning of levodopa therapy can be delayed.

Despite the findings with deprenyl, current pharmacotherapies for PD are unable to reverse or even halt the disease progression. This problem has led to the development of a different therapeutic approach that involves the grafting of either adrenal medullary or fetal nigral tissue into the host brain. This technique was first developed in laboratory animals, where it was shown to alleviate many of the behavioral symptoms of experimental parkinsonism. Patients who have received brain grafts have sometimes shown clinical improvement, although the benefits are not yet sufficient to justify the use of this procedure on a routine basis.

Part II
Alzheimer's Disease

Introduction

One of the most feared aspects of aging is the deterioration of memory and cognitive function (dementia) that occurs among the elderly with increasing frequency with advancing years. There are, however, notable examples of extraordinary creative work among people in their 70s and 80s. For example, Haydn composed such masterworks as *The Creation* when he was in his late 70s, and Verdi completed his operatic masterpieces *Othello* and *Falstaff* when he was 74 and 80, respectively. These examples merely highlight the fact that many elderly people are mentally alert and productive in their 7th, 8th, and even 9th decade of life. Nevertheless, a significant proportion of otherwise healthy elderly persons show a significant decline in mental function in later life. It has been estimated that 10% of the population over 65 years old suffers from mild to moderate dementia, and 4% to 5% suffer from severe dementia. The incidence of severe dementia rises from less than 1% at ages 65 to 70 to over 15% by age 85 (Terry and Katzman, 1983). In the United States alone, senile dementia afflicts several million people, and with the increasing longevity of the population, the number of such patients requiring complete and continuous institutional care will rise to epidemic proportions. Among the elderly in nursing homes, 60% to 80% are there because of mental infirmity. Considering Alzheimer's disease (AD) alone, which is the major cause of senile dementia, the total cost of patient care has recently been estimated at nearly $600 billion (see Gualtieri et al., 1995). The scope of age-related dementia has spurred a significant increase in research as to its causes and possible prevention or re-

versal by pharmaceutical agents. Indeed, sales of Alzheimer's disease–related drugs may reach $3 billion in the United States by the year 2000 (Gualtieri et al., 1995).

The onset of senile dementia is characterized by increasing impairment of memory of recent events such as what a patient had for breakfast an hour earlier, though detailed recall of the distant past may be essentially intact. Inevitably the patients lose their cognitive abilities, that is, their abilities to read, write, calculate, and use language appropriately; they cannot feed or dress themselves, they do not recognize their own families, they get lost when only a short distance from home, and ultimately do not even know their own names. For many years, these symptoms were thought to be the normal consequences of aging. Later medical advances showed that some cases of dementia are caused by cerebrovascular accidents (strokes), viral and bacterial infections, alcoholism, and arteriosclerosis with resulting deficiencies in the blood supply to the brain, leading to cell death and marked brain shrinkage. The most common cause of senile dementia, however, is AD.

Alzheimer's disease takes its name from a German neurologist named Alois Alzheimer. In 1907, Alzheimer published a landmark case study describing a set of previously unidentified histopathological features in the brain of a 51-year-old woman who had been demented at the time of her death. Although many years passed before this disorder was studied in detail, by the mid-1960s the neuropathology was more clearly delineated by examination of postmortem tissue samples and, in some cases, of brain tissues taken during diagnostic biopsies of AD patients.

Dementia attributable to AD usually occurs in the later stages of aging (i.e., after the age of 65), in which case it has sometimes been called senile dementia of the Alzheimer's type (SDAT). The corresponding terminology used for dementia occurring before the age of 65 is presenile dementia. However, there is no convincing evidence for a difference in the type of neuropathology seen in presenile dementia compared with SDAT, so we will use AD to refer to Alzheimer's-type dementia regardless of the age of onset. On the other hand, AD is occasionally inherited within families, in which case it is called **familial AD**. It is appropriate to distinguish familial from nonfamilial (i.e., sporadic) AD because familial AD can be traced to several identified genetic mutations, whereas genetic variation accounts only for differences in susceptibility to sporadic AD (discussed further below). Familial AD usually, though not always, has an early onset. Moreover, brain pathology and dementia are generally more severe in early-onset AD cases, and the course of the disease from onset to death is shorter (Raskind, Carta, and Bravi, 1995). But even sporadic AD is associated with a reduced life span, making AD one of the leading causes of death among the elderly.

Behavioral and Psychological Characteristics

Dementia

Hasegawa and Aoba (1994) proposed three stages of increasing intellectual impairment in AD. Stage 1 (termed the "amnesia stage") corresponds to the early clinical symptoms, which are typically manifested as short-term memory deficits, dyscalculia (impairment in using mathematics), constructional apraxia (impairment in basic visual–motor integrative ability), and loss of spontaneity. Examples of short-term memory problems might include repeatedly asking the same question every few minutes, or forgetting a telephone number during the act of dialing. This stage may last for 2–4 years before progressing to the next stage.

In stage 2 (the "confusional stage"), there is a continuing decline in cognitive functioning. The patient exhibits dysphasia (impairment in speaking and writing), agnosia (inability to comprehend sensory stimuli; for example, failure to identify common objects, familiar individuals, or sounds), disorientation in time and place, severe mental confusion, personality changes, behavioral disturbances such as extreme aggressiveness or wandering, and even sometimes psychotic episodes. Stage 3 (the "dementia stage") involves complete dementia, in which the patient is withdrawn and unresponsive, bedridden, incontinent, and unable to care for himself. At this point, the individual typically must be maintained in a nursing facility. Ultimately the patient is likely to die from a secondary illness or problem such as bronchopneumonia, urinary infection, or aspiration.

Other Behavioral and Psychiatric Symptoms

Although the core symptoms of AD involve cognitive deficits and eventual dementia, other behavioral and psychiatric problems can also occur in AD patients. Even Alzheimer's original patient suffered not only from cognitive decline but also from paranoid delusions. According to Lawlor (1994), major depression occurs in 5% to 15% of AD patients and may cause a worsening of cognitive function. Even more prevalent are delusions or hallucinations, which have been reported in approximately 20% to 40% of cases (see Lawlor, 1994). Certain kinds of delusional thinking (for example, that caregivers are stealing the patient's money or other belongings) can lead to combativeness and even violent behavior.

Neuropathology

Gross postmortem examination of the brains of AD patients reveals a marked atrophy of the cortical gyri (Figure 20.22). As we shall see below, this tissue loss results from a combination of cell death and the loss of neuronal fibers and synapses.

Histological Features

Plaques and tangles. As first described by Alzheimer, the classic neurohistopathological signs of AD are the presence of abnormal structures called **senile plaques** and **neurofibrillary tangles** (NFTs) (Color Plate 6). These structures are seen in most areas of the neocortex as well as in the hippocampus, amygdala, some thalamic and hypothala-

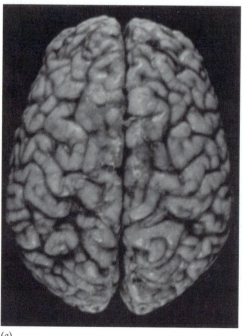
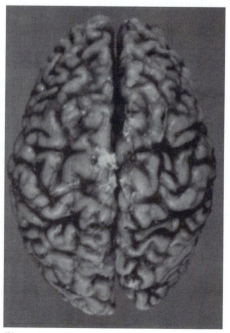

(a)   (b)

20.22 CEREBRAL CORTICAL ATROPHY IN ALZHEIMER'S DISEASE. (a) Normal brain; and (b) AD brain. (From Terry, Masliah, and Hansen, 1994; courtesy of Robert D. Terry.)

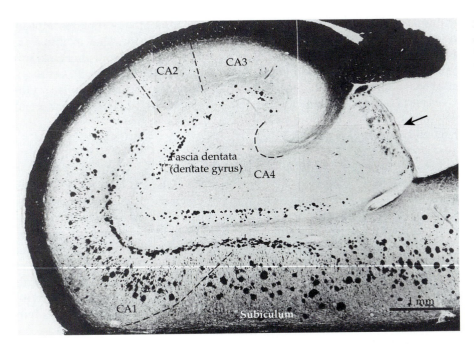

20.23 PATTERN OF AMYLOID PLAQUES AND OTHER DEPOSITS IN THE HIPPOCAMPAL FORMATION OF AN ALZHEIMER'S PATIENT. Many large β-amyloid-containing plaques are present in the hippocampal CA1 area and the subiculum. Smaller deposits can also be seen, such as in the molecular layer of the dentate gyrus (fascia dentata). The arrow denotes fluffy reactive material at the surface of the dentate gyrus. The dashed lines indicate approximate boundaries between the labeled anatomical regions. The tissue, which was silver-stained, was obtained from an 80-year-old demented woman with late-stage AD. (From Braak and Braak, 1991, *Acta Neuropathol.*, Springer-Verlag. Courtesy of Heiko Braak and Eva Braak.)

mic nuclei, locus coeruleus, dorsal raphe nucleus, and nuclei of the basal forebrain cholinergic system (Hardy et al., 1985; Pearson and Powell, 1989). Brain regions associated with the medial temporal lobe (i.e., entorhinal cortex, uncal cortex, parahippocampal gyrus, hippocampus, and corticomedial amygdala) generally exhibit the most severe histopathology in AD (Figure 20.23), whereas the primary sensory and motor cortices show somewhat less pathology (particularly with respect to the density of NFTs). There is evidence that AD histopathology begins in the medial temporal lobe and then spreads to other areas via cortico–cortical and cortico–subcortical connections (see below and also De Lacoste and White, 1993). A corollary of this hypothesis is that disconnection between the hippocampus and neocortex plays a major role in the clinical symptomatology of AD.

Alzheimer (1907) wrote that NFTs appeared to represent an abnormality in the fibrous structure of the neuron. Subsequent electron microscopic studies demonstrated that these elements are composed mainly of pairs of filaments wound around each other in a helical arrangement, thus giving rise to the term **paired helical filaments** (PHFs) (Terry, Masliah, and Hansen, 1994). The classic method for visualizing NFTs is based on their affinity for certain silver-based stains. NFTs are sometimes seen in small amounts in the neuronal cytoplasm, or they may completely occupy the cell body, replacing the normal cellular organelles and extending into the dendrites. Masses of NFTs are sometimes observed extraneuronally in the entorhinal cortex and hippocampus, presumably as a residue ("tombstone") of cells that have died. As we shall see later, PHFs (and hence NFTs) are composed mainly of an abnormal form of tau, an axonal microtubule-associated protein (see Chapter 3). How-

ever, immunohistochemical staining studies have found that NFTs are also immunoreactive for a number of other substances, including (but not limited to) neurofilament proteins, several protein kinases, and a protein called **β-amyloid** that is believed to play an important role in AD histopathology (see later discussion of AD pathogenesis) (Yen et al., 1995).

Several different types of senile plaques have been found in the brains of AD patients (Terry, Masliah, and Hansen, 1994). Some are called **neuritic plaques** because they possess dystrophic and degenerating neurites (neuronal processes) along with reactive microglia and astrocytes. These neurites may appear as large, bulbous structures containing many subcellular organelles, or they may contain large numbers of PHFs. Neuritic plaques also contain β-amyloid filaments and, in many cases, a dense extracellular core made up largely of an insoluble amyloid deposit (such plaques are sometimes termed "mature plaques").* In mature plaques, the dystrophic neurites are seen to surround the β-amyloid core (see Color Plate 6). Yet other plaques, called **diffuse plaques**, contain β-amyloid protein fibers and some unstructured amyloid, but no neurites. These may represent the earliest stage of plaque formation. Finally, **burned-out plaques** possess a dense amyloid core with reactive astrocytes, but no neurites. These are regarded as the end stage of plaque formation, after the dystrophic neurites have degenerated and presumably been phagocytized. Like NFTs, senile plaques can be impregnated by silver stains. Other important methods for visualizing plaques

---

*Although the assumption is often made that senile plaques always possess an amyloid core, this is not necessarily the case (see Roses, 1994).

involve staining with the fluorescent dye thioflavin S or with Congo red, which gives the plaques a birefringent appearance when viewed under polarized light.

It is interesting to note that AD patients usually show signs of β-amyloid deposition in at least some small to medium-sized cerebral blood vessels (Terry, Masliah, and Hansen, 1994). Such amyloid angiopathy occurs within the brain, but even more severely in the vessels of the meninges. On the other hand, the degree of vascular amyloid deposition does not seem to correlate with the incidence of plaques or tangles, and there is no current evidence suggesting a contribution of this process to AD-related dementia.

Although the presence of large numbers of plaques and tangles at postmortem examination is an important criterion for confirming a diagnosis of AD, neither of these structures is unique to AD. Varying concentrations of senile plaques (particularly of the diffuse type) along with occasional NFTs can be found in the brains of non-demented aged individuals. Moreover, substantial numbers of NFTs occur in the substantia nigra in postencephalitic Parkinson's disease (PD) and in the neocortex in dementia pugilistica (boxing dementia; also known colloquially as being "punch drunk") (Terry, Masliah, and Hansen, 1994).

Other histological features. Several other histopathological structures occur in AD, including **neuropil threads**, **Hirano bodies**, and **granulovacuolar bodies** (Terry, Masliah, and Hansen, 1994). Neuropil threads are fine fibrils typically found within dendrites. Like the NFTs, they possess tau protein–containing PHFs (Braak et al., 1986).

Hirano bodies are rodlike filamentous structures appearing within or near pyramidal neurons. They exhibit actin immunoreactivity and thus may represent abnormal microfilaments (Goldman, 1983; see Chapter 3). Granulovacuolar bodies are granule-containing vacuoles (cytoplasmic inclusions) that are particularly apparent in hippocampal pyramidal cells.

Neuron and Synapse Loss in the Cortex and Hippocampus

As reviewed by Terry, Masliah, and Hansen (1994), AD is characterized by an extensive loss of neurons in the neocortex and hippocampus. Recent work indicates that the neuronal loss found in AD is not simply an exaggeration of the normal aging process, but is distinct from the pattern of loss seen in non-AD aged brains (West et al., 1994). Neuron death in the cortex is associated with reactive gliosis, as shown by increased immunoreactivity to the astrocytic protein glial fibrillary acidic protein (GFAP; Schechter, Yen, and Terry, 1981).

As discussed below, AD also involves significant damage to several important subcortical nuclei with major projections to the cerebral cortex. Damage to the efferent fibers from these nuclei as well as to intrinsic cortical neurons should have a deleterious effect on synaptic interactions within the cortex. It is therefore not surprising that a number of recent studies have found marked reductions in cortical synaptic density in AD (Terry, Masliah, and Hansen, 1994; Figure 20.24). Loss of synaptic connectivity could be an important mediating factor in Alzheimer's dementia and probably also contributes to the gross brain atrophy seen in Figure 20.22.

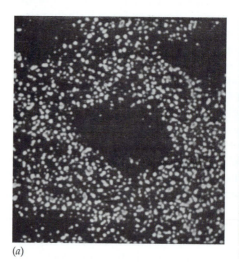 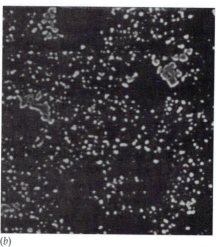 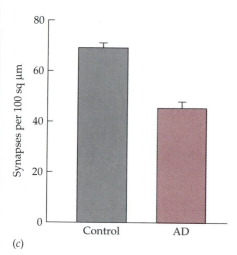

(a)   (b)   (c)

20.24 LOSS OF SYNAPSES IN ALZHEIMER'S DISEASE. Nerve terminals were labeled by immunohistochemistry for the synaptic vesicle protein synaptophysin, imaged by laser scanning confocal microscopy, and counted. For measurement purposes, each terminal was assumed to make one synaptic contact. The photomicrographs illustrate the appearance of nerve terminals in the frontal cortex of a normal aged subject (a) and an AD patient (b). The density of synaptophysin-labeled terminals was significantly decreased in AD (c). (From Terry, Masliah, and Hansen, 1994; photomicrographs courtesy of Robert D. Terry.)

Abnormalities in Neurotransmitter Systems

Acetylcholine. Although the existence of neuritic plaques and NFTs was described by Alzheimer himself, neurotransmitter-related abnormalities were not discovered until the advent of biochemical and histochemical techniques for studying transmitters and their synthetic and catabolic enzymes in brain tissue. The initial findings were reported by Bowen et al. (1976) and several other research teams, who found a marked loss of basal forebrain cholinergic neurons (particularly in the nucleus basalis of Meynert, NBM), and also large reductions in cholinergic markers such as ChAT, acetylcholinesterase (AChE), and synaptosomal choline uptake in cholinergic target areas such as the cortex, hippocampus, and amygdala (reviewed by Bartus et al., 1985; Coyle, Price, and DeLong, 1983; Geula and Mesulam, 1994). Neurochemical indices of cholinergic damage were supported by diagnostic biopsies of the frontal and temporal lobes of AD patients showing that the biochemical deficits are related to degeneration of the presynaptic terminals of axons emanating from the NBM and projecting directly to the cortex (Sims et al., 1983). All areas of the cortex are not uniformly affected, however. The temporal lobe shows the greatest loss of cholinergic enzyme activity, whereas the cingulate cortex and primary visual cortex are among the least affected areas (Geula and Mesulam, 1994).

A comparison of the number of cells in the basal forebrain cholinergic system between the brains of age-related normals and Alzheimer's patients showed that in normals the cell population may drop from a high of 400,000 to 475,000 in the young to less than half (approximately 140,000) in the elderly, whereas in Alzheimer's patients the cell population dropped to as low as 45,000 to 100,000 cells, and even as low as 5% of normal subjects (Price et al., 1982). Thus, it was estimated that the reserve capacity of normal functioning of this system was lost when the cholinergic cell count fell below 140,000 cells (McGeer, 1984). Interestingly, it appears that AD does not affect the large populations of cholinergic neurons in the basal ganglia, the nuclei of the cranial and spinal motor nerves, or the cholinergic cells of the pre- and postganglionic neurons of the autonomic nervous system.

Some, but not all, cholinergic receptor subtypes are altered in AD. The densities of cortical and hippocampal muscarinic M2 and nicotinic receptors are reduced in the brains of AD patients (Flynn et al., 1995; Quirion et al., 1989; Whitehouse et al., 1986), whereas muscarinic M1 receptors are relatively unaffected. One possible reason for this difference is that at least some M2 and nicotinic receptors are believed to be located presynaptically, where they function as autoreceptors or heteroreceptors modulating the release of other transmitters. Damage to cholinergic or other cortical afferents along with a relative sparing of postsynaptic cells could therefore lead to a differential loss of these receptor subtypes. Despite the preservation of M1 receptors in AD, however, Mash and her colleagues have presented evidence for abnormal functioning of this receptor subtype (see Flynn et al., 1995). More specifically, the receptors show a reduced ability to couple normally to G proteins and to activate phospholipase C (see Chapter 7). These findings indicate a major deficit in postsynaptic cholinergic functioning in AD, even though most of the M1 receptors are still present.

Other neurotransmitters. There are indications that other neurotransmitter systems may also be compromised in AD. For example, neuronal cell loss, decreased synthesizing enzyme activity, and NFTs have been observed in the locus coeruleus (Geula and Mesulam, 1994). Noradrenergic deficits were also found in the cortex (particularly in the cingulate cortex, where the concentrations of NE and its metabolites are highest) and in the hypothalamus (Rossor and Iversen, 1986). These deficits are presumed to be the result of damage to the axonal projections from the locus coeruleus. In contrast, there is no consistent evidence for a reduction in cortical adrenergic receptors in AD (Court and Perry, 1991).

The serotonergic system is likewise compromised in AD. The presence of NFTs and a modest loss of neurons have been found in the dorsal raphe nucleus (Geula and Mesulam, 1994). In the cortex, there is some loss of both presynaptic (5-HT concentrations and 5-HT uptake sites) and postsynaptic (5-HT_1 and 5-HT_2 receptors) serotonergic markers (Court and Perry, 1991).

Several investigators have reported significant losses of cortical somatostatin neurons and receptors in AD (Geula and Mesulam, 1994; Rossor and Iversen, 1986). Cholinergic fibers innervate cortical somatostatin neurons and stimulate somatostatin release. This relationship raises the intriguing possibility that somatostatin neurons may be damaged, at least in part, due to the loss of their cholinergic innervation.

Relationships between Alzheimer's Neuropathology and Symptomatology

Many attempts have been made to correlate either the severity of histopathology (i.e., density of plaques or tangles) or the reduction in neurochemical (generally cholinergic) markers with the degree of dementia exhibited by patients at the time of their death. In general, researchers have not found reliable correlations between plaques, tangles, or other pathological structures and symptom severity in AD patients. On the other hand, a few studies have suggested that the degree of synapse loss might be a better indicator of symptom severity (see Terry, Masliah, and Hansen, 1994), which also fits well from a functional perspective. Also correlated with the degree of dementia is the loss of cortical ChAT activity (reviewed by Geula and Mesulam, 1994). Nevertheless, we saw in Chapter 7 that the relationship between the cholinergic system and cognitive processes (particularly learning and memory) is still uncertain, and Geula and Mesulam (1994) have argued that the cholinergic deficits in AD cannot be held completely responsible for the devastating progression of functional loss in this disorder.

Deficits in other neurotransmitter systems have been linked mainly with noncognitive aspects of AD symptomatology. This is particularly true for the noradrenergic system, dysfunction of which may be involved in the depressive symptomatology observed in some AD patients (Court and Perry, 1991; Lawlor, 1994).

Diagnosis of Alzheimer's Disease

As discussed in Berg and Morris (1994), the clinical diagnosis of AD is fraught with difficulties. The principal reason for this problem is that the presence of dementia is not specific to AD, since severe loss of cognitive function can arise from a variety of factors (Haase, 1977). Consequently, a firm diagnosis of AD is generally not possible until the patient's brain is examined histologically at autopsy and the density of senile plaques is ascertained (Khachaturian, 1985). Nevertheless, an assessment of the patient's clinical symptomatology may permit a diagnosis of *probable AD*, which can then be used as a guideline for patient care and treatment. One set of diagnostic criteria for probable AD is found in the *Diagnostic and Statistical Manual of Mental Disorders* (DSM-IV) of the American Psychiatric Association (APA). Another set of criteria was developed in 1984 by a joint work group of the National Institute of Neurological and Communicative Disorders and Stroke (NINCDS) and the Alzheimer's Disease and Related Disorders Association (ADRDA) (McKhann et al., 1984). Some of these criteria are presented in Table 20.1.

If therapeutic approaches can eventually be developed to retard or halt the course of AD progression, then additional screening procedures based on AD-related neural deficits would be useful in confirming the clinical diagnosis of probable AD, thereby identifying patients who would benefit from such therapies. Early screening for AD (i.e., before cognitive decline even begins) could also prove valuable, particularly in individuals who are at increased risk for developing the disorder. One possible approach is to use PET and SPECT imaging, which have already shown large AD-related reductions in blood flow and glucose utilization in the temporal, parietal, and frontal cortices (Rapoport, 1991; Waldemar, 1995). Smaller but still significant metabolic deficits were also observed in the sensorimotor cortex, occipital cortex, basal ganglia, and thalamus. In a recent application of this approach, Reiman et al. (1996) used PET to study cognitively normal individuals 50 to 65 years old (mean age 55 years) who are at high risk for developing late-

onset AD because they are homozygous for the *E4* allele of the apolipoprotein E gene (see below). Compared with age-matched controls, the at-risk group showed deficits in glucose utilization in the parietal, temporal, prefrontal, and posterior cingulate cortex, which corresponds closely to the areas of greatest metabolic abnormality in patients with a clinical diagnosis of probable AD. Thus, it may be possible to identify individuals with incipient AD and to make use of appropriate therapeutic interventions, once such interventions become available.

Pathogenesis of Alzheimer's Disease

Despite a considerable amount of research, the exact mechanisms responsible for AD have yet to be determined. Many investigators, however, believe that abnormalities in β-amyloid protein play a key role in AD pathogenesis. As we shall see, this hypothesis is particularly well supported in cases of familial (i.e., inherited) AD, but may also be valid in the nonfamilial form of the disorder. Because of this emphasis on β-amyloid, we will begin with a discussion of the structure and origin of this protein.

β-Amyloid Protein

β-amyloid precursor protein.   Recent biochemical and molecular biological studies have shed new light on the structure and synthesis of amyloid protein. The β-amyloid protein (abbreviated Aβ) was first purified independently by two research groups (Glenner and Wong, 1984; Masters et al., 1985) and found to be a peptide made up of varying numbers of amino acids (usually 40 to 42), with a molecular weight of about 4 kDa.

The Aβ peptide is synthesized as part of a much larger protein called β-amyloid precursor protein (APP) (reviewed by Gandy and Greengard, 1994). Cloning studies by several laboratories have shown that APP is derived from a single gene (Goldgaber et al., 1987; Robakis et al., 1987; Tanzi et al., 1987). However, alternative splicing of the primary gene transcript gives rise to a family of proteins containing either 695, 751, or 770 amino acids. Following RNA splicing and translation, newly synthesized APP molecules are inserted into the cell membrane such that there is one transmembrane domain that contains part of the Aβ segment (Figure 20.25). The remainder of the molecule includes a short segment in the cytoplasm and an extensive extracellular region. APP molecules are subjected to considerable posttranslational modification, including glycosylation and sulfation of the extracellular region, and potential phosphorylation of several sites within the cytoplasmic domain.

The alternatively spliced forms of APP differ with respect to the presence or absence of two domains in the extracellular part of the protein. One of these domains is designated KPI, because it is homologous to a Kunitz-

Table 20.1 Major NINCDS/ADRDA Criteria for the Diagnosis of Probable Alzheimer's Disease

I. The criteria for the clinical diagnosis of "probable Alzheimer's disease" include:

Dementia established by clinical examination and documented by the Mini-Mental test (Folstein, Folstein, and McHugh, 1975), Blessed Dementia Scale (Blessed, Tomlinson, and Roth, 1968), or some similar examination, and confirmed by neuropsychological tests;

Deficits in two or more areas of cognition;

Progressive worsening of memory and other cognitive functions;

Onset between ages 40 and 90, most often after age 65; and

Absence of systemic disorders or other brain diseases that in and of themselves could account for the progressive deficits in memory and cognition.

II. The diagnosis of "probable Alzheimer's disease" is supported by:

Progressive deterioration of specific cognitive functions such as language (aphasia), motor skills (apraxia), and perception (agnosia);

Impaired activities of daily living and altered patterns of behavior;

Family history of similar disorders, particularly if confirmed neuropathologically;

Laboratory results of:

normal lumbar puncture as evaluated by standard techniques,

normal pattern or nonspecific changes in EEG, such as increased slow-wave activity, or

evidence of cerebral atrophy on CT with progression documented by serial observation.

Source: After McKhann et al., 1984.

type protease inhibitor (Figure 20.25). Proteases are enzymes that degrade proteins, hence protease inhibitors protect potential substrate proteins from such degradation. The second domain, which is designated OX-2, shows some homology to a rat thymocyte antigen. The KPI-containing isoforms of APP (APP$_{751}$ and APP$_{770}$) are found in many types of cells, whereas APP$_{695}$ (which lacks the KPI domain) is found only in neurons and is the major APP isoform in these cells (Cordell, 1994).

APP processing. As we shall see below, mutations in the APP gene can produce inherited (familial) forms of AD. However, these instances represent only a small percentage of AD cases. Attention therefore has turned to the possible role of abnormal APP processing in AD pathogenesis. APP in cell membranes is processed by proteolytic breakdown that gives rise to various fragments of the original molecule. Whether or not the damaging Aβ peptide is produced depends on the sites of

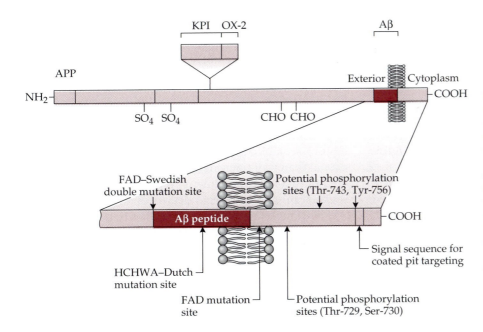

20.25 STRUCTURE OF THE AMYLOID PRECURSOR PROTEIN (APP). APP is a membrane protein that exists in three isoforms, which vary with respect to the presence or absence of a Kunitz-type, protease inhibitor-like domain (KPI) and a domain that is homologous to a rat thymocyte antigen (OX-2). Also illustrated are known APP mutation sites, potential phosphorylation sites within the cytoplasmic domain, glycosylation (CHO) and sulfation (SO$_4$) sites within the extracellular domain, and a signal sequence that targets the protein for coated pit–mediated endocytosis. Amino acid numbering is based on the APP$_{770}$ sequence. (After Gandy and Greengard, 1994.)

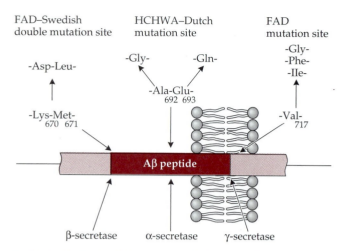

FAD–Swedish
double mutation site

HCHWA–Dutch
mutation site

FAD
mutation site

-Asp-Leu-

-Gly-   -Gln-

-Gly-
-Phe-
-Ile-

-Lys-Met-
670 671

-Ala-Glu-
692 693

-Val-
717

Aβ peptide

β-secretase   α-secretase   γ-secretase

20.26 SITES OF APP PROCESSING AND AMYLOIDOGENIC MUTATIONS. APP is subject to proteolytic cleavage at the three sites designated α-, β-, and γ-secretase. Cleavage by α-secretase releases most of the extracellular region of the molecule, which is harmless. Joint action by β- and γ-secretase, however, releases the amyloidogenic peptide Aβ into the extracellular fluid. The illustrated missense mutations have been found in kindreds with autosomal dominant inheritance of either FAD or a related disorder called hereditary cerebral hemorrhage with amyloidosis (HCHWA). (After Schellenberg, 1995.)

protein cleavage. Current evidence indicates that initial cleavage of APP usually occurs by an as yet unidentified protease that has been termed α-secretase (reviewed by Checler, 1995). The site of α-secretase action is located *within* the Aβ domain of APP (Figure 20.26). This results in the release of most of the extracellular region of the molecule (known as soluble APP, or s-APP) into the extracellular fluid. It is interesting to note that s-APP secretion is enhanced by protein kinase C activation, possibly through stimulation of α-secretase activity (Checler, 1995). Further proteolytic processing of the remainder of the APP molecule is carried out by a different protease that has been called γ-secretase. This reaction yields two small harmless fragments that are eventually catabolized. We can see that the action of α-secretase precludes amyloidogenesis, because amyloid deposits are formed only from the complete Aβ peptide.

In the hypothesized processing pathway necessary for amyloid deposition, a different protease termed β-secretase cleaves APP at the N-terminus of Aβ (Figure 20.26). This causes the secretion of a truncated form of s-APP. More importantly, however, subsequent action of γ-secretase liberates the Aβ peptide. When Aβ is secreted from cells, it is initially in a soluble form; over time, however, it adopts an insoluble β-pleated sheet conformation, which is found in AD senile plaques.

Recent studies have unexpectedly shown that Aβ is released by normal neuronal and glial cells in culture (Checler, 1995) and is also detectable in the cerebrospinal fluid (CSF) and plasma of healthy humans (Seubert et

al., 1992). These findings suggest that some β-secretase activity may be present even in non-AD brain tissue. One hypothesis that needs to be tested is that AD amyloidogenesis might be related either to increased β-secretase activity or to decreased clearance of Aβ from the extracellular space.

The cellular sites of APP processing are not yet clear. The available evidence indicates that some APP molecules are targeted to the cell surface, which is likely to be a major site of s-APP liberation and may also be important for Aβ production and release. On the other hand, some APP appears to be internalized by coated pits and to undergo proteolytic processing within the lysosomal compartment (Checler, 1995; Selkoe, 1994).

Normal functions of APP. The presence of the KPI domain in s-APP suggests that one function of APP may be to inhibit proteolytic activity under certain conditions (Gandy and Greengard, 1994; Selkoe, 1994). This hypothesis is supported by the finding that a previously discovered protease inhibitor called protease nexin II, which is produced by blood platelets, is actually s-APP released by the action of α-secretase on APP_{751} in the platelet membrane. Protease nexin II is thought to play an important role in the mechanisms of coagulation and wound repair (see Mattson et al., 1993). Other research on APP has led to a variety of additional proposed functions, including modulation of cell growth and development as well as cell adhesion (Selkoe, 1994). As more information becomes available concerning the normal roles of APP and its breakdown products, it may eventually become possible to target various steps in APP processing in an attempt to slow down or halt the amyloidogenic process (Cordell, 1994).

Tau Protein

We mentioned earlier that the major component of NFTs is a protein called tau. The characteristics of this protein and its role in the formation of NFTs is reviewed in Goedert (1993) and in Kosik and Greenberg (1994). Tau refers to a group of proteins (six isoforms in human brain, which are generated by alternative mRNA splicing) with molecular weights ranging from 50 to 64 kDa. Tau is a microtubule-associated protein believed to serve an important function in tubulin polymerization and microtubule stabilization. Tau is generally restricted to the axonal region of neurons, and it can therefore be considered the axonal complement to MAP2, a microtubule-associated protein specific to dendrites.

Although tau contains a number of potential phosphorylation sites, in the normal adult brain only two or three of these sites are phosphorylated. In PHFs from AD brain, however, tau was found to be phosphorylated at six to eight sites. This could occur because of overactivity of the kinases responsible for tau phosphorylation and/or underactivity of phosphoprotein phosphatases that normally dephosphorylate tau. Tau hyperphosphorylation is thought to somehow promote disassociation of the protein from microtubules and self-aggregation into the PHFs found in NFTs. It is also important to note that these changes in tau structure alter its subcellular distribution such that PHFs are found throughout affected neurons, not just within the axon. Several antibodies (e.g., Alz50) are available that are relatively selective for hyperphosphorylated tau protein and are therefore useful for staining NFTs and other sites where abnormal tau is present.

Genetics of Alzheimer's Disease

Recent work has shown that AD is a genetically heterogeneous disorder. We will begin our review of AD genetics by demonstrating its relationship to Down syndrome, a well-known congenital disorder. This is followed by a consideration of familial AD (FAD), a general type of AD in which the disease is inherited as an autosomal dominant trait. Finally, we will discuss recent findings concerning the role of genetics in sporadic AD.

Alzheimer's disease and Down syndrome.

Early in the search for genetic mechanisms in AD pathogenesis, researchers made the important discovery that patients suffering from a form of mental retardation known as Down syndrome (DS) exhibit a brain pathology virtually identical to that found in AD (Coyle et al., 1988). The cause of DS is nondisjunction of chromosome 21 during meiosis, thus causing the resulting gamete (ovum or sperm) to have 24 chromosomes instead of the normal 23. When such a gamete is fertilized, the resulting zygote contains three copies of chromosome 21 rather than the usual pair. This condition is therefore known as trisomy 21, which is one of a number of abnormal chromosome duplications that cause serious fetal defects. All cell divisions thereafter will retain the three copies of chromosome 21, and the resulting offspring will have Down syndrome, which includes not only mental retardation but also cardiac, gastrointestinal, and facial anomalies.

Before the advent of modern medical techniques, DS patients usually had a rather short life span. With current standards of treatment and care, however, these individuals may live to the age of 50 or more. As the life span of DS patients increased, it was found that many of them became demented by as early as 30–40 years of age. In the course of this process, the individual regressed from the limited intelligence of a child to a person who was disoriented, unable to speak or comprehend language, and incontinent. These are, of course, symptoms like those of AD. Moreover, postmortem examination of the brains of DS patients showed that AD-type neuropathology (i.e., plaques and tangles) was present in all individuals age 40 or older (Wisniewski, Wisniewski, and Wen, 1985). These findings were the first to suggest that some gene or genes on chromosome 21 might be involved in the genesis of AD, and they eventually led to a genetic analysis of this disorder.

Familial Alzheimer's disease: APP gene mutations.

Important progress in the study of FAD genetics occurred when the cloning and mapping of the *APP* gene demonstrated its presence on chromosome 21 (St George-Hyslop et al., 1987). Subsequent research has shown that missense mutations (i.e., mutations involving alteration of a single nucleotide codon, which results in a change in amino acid) at several positions of this gene lead either to early-onset FAD or to AD-related disorders (reviewed by Schellenberg, 1995; Van Broeckhoven, 1995; see Figure 20.26).

The first mutation to be identified in the *APP* gene involves the substitution of a glutamine (Gln) residue for glutamate (Glu) at position 693. This particular mutation does not cause AD, but rather a disorder called hereditary cerebral hemorrhage with amyloidosis, Dutch type (HCHWA-D). HCHWA-D is characterized by the onset of strokes after the age of 25, cerebral amyloid angiopathy (i.e., deposition of amyloid Aβ deposits in cerebral blood vessels), and a life span usually not exceeding 60 years. Although few AD-type amyloid plaques or NFTs have been found in the brains of HCHWA-D patients, the presence of cerebral amyloid angiopathy (which also occurs to some extent in AD) provides a significant linkage to AD. Moreover, another Dutch kindred (family) has been identified that exhibits a mutation at position 692 instead of 693. In this case, a glycine (Gly) residue is substituted for alanine (Ala), thereby producing a mixture of HCHWA-D and AD (i.e., cerebral hemorrhage and presenile dementia).

Perhaps the most important kindreds are those that exhibit the standard AD neuropathology and that also show an autosomal dominant inheritance of the disorder. Several such kindreds have now been shown to express *APP* gene mutations at different loci than those described above and to suffer from a severe, early-onset form of AD (family age-of-onset means in these kindreds generally range from 45 to 60 years: Schellenberg, 1995). At least 11 different families have been found in which the valine (Val) at position 717 in the APP molecule is altered either to isoleucine (Ile; the most common mutation at this position), phenylalanine (Phe), or glycine (Gly) (Van Broeckhoven, 1995; Figure 20.26). It is interesting to note that this position is within the APP transmembrane domain, but *outside* of the Aβ peptide sequence. Cells transfected with the *APP* gene containing either the Ile-717 or Phe-717 mutation did not exhibit abnormal amounts of Aβ secretion; however, they secreted an increased ratio of the *long* form of the peptide (Aβ$_{1-42}$) compared with the *short* form (Aβ$_{1-40}$) (Suzuki et al., 1994). Since Aβ$_{1-42}$ forms aggregates in vitro more readily than Aβ$_{1-40}$, it is thought to be more pathogenic.

A single Swedish kindred has been identified with a double mutation of APP in which lysine- (Lys-) 670 and methionine- (Met-) 671 are replaced by aspartate- (Asp-) 670 and leucine- (Leu-) 671. The amino acids at positions 670 and 671 are immediately adjacent to the beginning of the Aβ sequence, which of course is at the putative β-secretase cleavage site (Figure 20.26). Cells transfected with the APP gene bearing this double mutation showed a much greater secretion of Aβ than cells transfected with the wild-type gene (Cai, Golde, and Younkin, 1993; Citron et al., 1992). More importantly, Citron and colleagues (1994) recently found increased Aβ secretion in cultured fibroblasts from Swedish kindred members with AD symptomatology as well as in cells from several younger family members who were still asymptomatic. These findings support the hypothesized role of aberrant APP processing in AD pathogenesis within this kindred.

Familial Alzheimer's disease: other gene mutations.   Researchers have found that only a very small percentage of FAD cases can be accounted for by the above-mentioned mutations in the APP gene (Wasco, Peppercorn, and Tanzi, 1993). This has led to an ongoing search for other genetic loci responsible for the remaining 97% to 98% of cases. One such locus has been found on chromosome 14 and designated *AD3* (*AD1* refers to the chromosome 21 locus associated with APP mutations, whereas *AD2* is a genetic locus on chromosome 19 that influences vulnerability to sporadic AD; see below) (Schellenberg, 1995; Van Broeckhoven, 1995). *AD3* kindreds suffer from an extremely severe form of AD that shows onset as early as 30 years of age.

Sherrington and colleagues (1995) recently identified a gene within the *AD3* locus which, when mutated, appears to be responsible for many instances of early-onset FAD. This gene was initially termed *S182* and subsequently given the name *presenilin-1* (*PS-1*). The function of the PS-1 protein is still unknown; however, its putative structure suggests that it is probably an integral membrane protein and therefore could serve as some kind of novel receptor, channel, or structural membrane protein. Interestingly, immunoreactivity for PS-1 was observed in senile plaques of brains obtained not only from *AD3*-linked AD patients but also from patients suffering from sporadic AD, HCHWA-D, Down syndrome, and other disorders involving cerebral amyloidosis (Wisniewski et al., 1995). Further evidence for a relationship between the *AD3* locus and amyloid comes from the recent finding of increased APP mRNA transcription in cultured fibroblasts from a Canadian kindred that exhibits *AD3*-linked AD (Querfurth et al., 1995). Finally, allelic variation in *PS-1* was recently reported to affect the risk for late-onset sporadic AD, suggesting a more general role for the PS-1 protein in AD pathogenesis (Wragg et al., 1996).

There are other FAD kindreds that do not exhibit mutations in either the *APP* or *PS-1* genes. Among these are the Volga German kindreds, which represent a subset of German families that emigrated to the Volga River region of Russia in the 1760s, and then emigrated again to the United States in the early 1900s (Schellenberg, 1995). The mutation responsible for FAD in the Volga German kindreds was recently mapped to chromosome 1, and a candidate gene was identified and variously named *STM2*, *E5-1*, or *presenilin-2* (*PS-2*; Levy-Lahad et al., 1995; Rogaev et al., 1995). The PS-2 protein shows significant sequence homology to PS-1, indicating that they both may be members of a family of proteins involved in AD pathogenesis.

Late-onset Alzheimer's disease and apolipoprotein E.   As mentioned earlier, most instances of AD do not show a simple pattern of inheritance. For this reason, researchers long believed that there was no genetic component at all to late-onset (especially sporadic) AD. However, this view was shattered several years ago when a locus on chromosome 19 (i.e., the *AD2* locus) was found to be associated with differential risk for late-onset familial and sporadic AD (Schellenberg, 1995; Van Broeckhoven, 1995). Subsequent work showed that the critical gene within this locus is the gene for **apolipoprotein E** (apoE; Corder et al., 1993; Saunders et al., 1993).

There are three major alleles of the *apoE* gene, designated *apoE2*, *apoE3*, and *apoE4*. The most common allele in the U.S. population is *apoE3*, whereas the least common is *apoE2*. Because each individual possesses two doses of the *apoE* gene, and the gene alleles may be either the same or different, we can see that six genotypes are possible (i.e., *E2/E2*, *E2/E3*, *E2/E4*, *E3/E3*, etc.). Table 20.2 shows the proportion of each of these genotypes in the U.S. population and the typical age of onset of AD associated with that genotype. Figure 20.27 further illustrates the relationship between genotype and age of onset of AD. It is clear from these data that compared with allele *E3*, allele *E4* heightens the risk for late-onset AD, whereas allele *E2* exerts somewhat of a protective effect (i.e., the individual is likely to develop the disease later in life). In addition, the *apoE* genotype seems to be related not only to the risk for AD, but also the severity of the disease. Soininen and Riekkinen (1996) recently summarized evidence that AD patients homozygous for the *E4* allele (i.e., possessing an *E4/E4* genotype) exhibited lower hippocampal volume, greater loss of hippocampal and frontal cortical ChAT activity, and more impairment of delayed memory than did *E3* homozygotes.

What is the function of apoE, and how might it participate in AD pathogenesis? As summarized in several recent reviews, (Rubinsztein, 1995; Strittmatter and Roses, 1995), apoE is a 34-kDa glycoprotein containing 299 amino acids. Outside of the nervous system, this

Table 20.2   Prevalence of *apoE* Genotypes in the U.S. Population and Age of Onset of Alzheimer's Disease

apoE genotype	Prevalence in U.S. population (%)	Typical age of onset of Alzheimer's Disease (years)
E2/E2	<1	?[a]
E2/E3	11	>90
E2/E4	5	80–90
E3/E3	60	80–90
E3/E4	21	70–80
E4/E4	2	<70

[a]The typical age of onset of AD in individuals with the *E2/E2* genotype has not been determined because of the low prevalence of this genotype in the population.
Source: After Roses, 1995.

protein is an important constituent of circulating lipoprotein complexes that are involved in the blood transport of cholesterol and triglycerides and their uptake by adipose cells. Within the nervous system, apoE is mainly synthesized by nonmyelinating glia (i.e., satellite

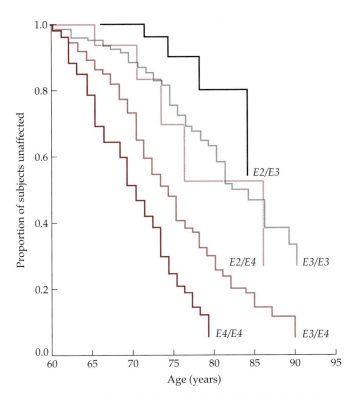

20.27 ALZHEIMER'S DISEASE AGE-OF-ONSET CURVES IN RELATION TO *aPOE* GENOTYPE. The subject population consisted of 72 late-onset AD families (containing a total of 158 AD-diagnosed and 220 unaffected individuals) along with 103 autopsy-confirmed cases of sporadic AD and 198 aged controls. The mean age of onset for AD was estimated to be more than 90 years for subjects with the *E2/E3* genotype, compared with approximately 68 years for *E4* homozygous subjects. It can also be seen that virtually all members of the latter group who lived to the age of 80 or older developed AD. (After Roses, 1994.)

Schwann cells) in the PNS and by astrocytes in the CNS. On the other hand, apoE immunoreactivity was recently demonstrated in the cytoplasm of neurons, suggesting either that these cells possess a low level of apoE synthetic activity or that they take up the protein from the extracellular fluid (Han et al., 1994). Synthesis of apoE rises dramatically following injury to either the PNS or CNS, which suggests a role for this protein in the salvage and reutilization of membrane lipids liberated by tissue damage.

There are several lines of evidence suggesting an involvement of apoE in AD histopathology. Diedrich and coworkers (1991) reported increased astrocytic apoE mRNA in the brains of AD patients. ApoE immunoreactivity has been found in both NFTs and amyloid plaques in AD, Down syndrome, and several other amyloidogenic disorders (Kida et al., 1994; Namba et al., 1991; Wisniewski and Frangione, 1992). Deposition of apoE appears very early in plaque formation and may even precede Aβ deposition (Yamaguchi et al., 1994). Moreover, homozygous *apoE4* patients exhibited much greater plaque formation than age-matched patients who were homozygous for the *E3* allele (Schmechel et al., 1993). This effect could be related to the observation that the apoE3 and apoE4 proteins differentially modulate the formation of Aβ fibrils in vitro (Evans et al., 1995). Both isoforms act as inhibitors of amyloid fibril formation; however, apoE3, but not apoE4, can dimerize, and the resulting apoE3 dimer is a much more potent inhibitor than either the apoE3 or the apoE4 monomer. Consequently, amyloid deposition in vivo may occur more rapidly in the presence of apoE4 than in the presence of apoE3, which could also be related to the increased symptom severity observed in *apoE4* homozygotes that was mentioned earlier.

Summary of Alzheimer's disease genetics.   As we have seen, AD is an unexpectedly heterogeneous disorder genetically (Table 20.3). Early-onset forms of FAD that

Table 20.3   Genetic Factors in Alzheimer's Disease

Type	Chromosome	Gene	Genetic effect	Typical age of onset (years)	Incidence among all AD cases
I. Early-onset familial	21	APP	Direct linkage	50s	<20 known families worldwide
II. Early-onset familial	14	PS-1	Direct linkage	40s	<2%
III. Early-onset familial	1	PS-2	Direct linkage	50s	Volga–German kindreds
IV. Late-onset familial and sporadic	19	ApoE	Risk factor	Allele-dependent	>95%

Source: After Roses, 1995b.

show a pattern of simple autosomal dominance inheritance have been linked to mutations in three different genes, namely *APP*, *PS-1*, and *PS-2*. These mutations are thought to directly (in the case of *APP*) or indirectly (in the cases of *PS-1* and *PS-2*) affect APP processing, Aβ deposition, and amyloid plaque formation. Variation in a fourth gene, which codes for apoE, has been shown to influence the risk for and severity of late-onset familial and sporadic AD. The *E4* allele (particularly when present in two doses) enhances the likelihood of developing AD and also increases the severity of neuropathology and behavioral symptomatology compared with the *E3* or *E2* alleles (the latter of which seems to exert somewhat of a protective effect). There is evidence for involvement of apoE in amyloid deposition and Aβ fibril formation, but as we shall see below, some investigators have hypothesized that other actions of apoE may be even more important in AD pathogenesis.

Theories of Alzheimer's Disease Pathogenesis

There is no question about the fact that the brains of AD patients are characterized by the presence of senile plaques, NFTs, and loss of nerve cells and synapses. There is, however, much disagreement about the mechanisms underlying AD neuropathology and the sequence of events that occurs over the course of the disease. In this section, we briefly consider some of the major theories that have been proposed to account for AD pathogenesis.

The amyloid cascade hypothesis.   Probably the most influential theory of AD pathogenesis has been the "amyloid cascade hypothesis" (Hardy and Allsop, 1991; Hardy and Higgins, 1992; Selkoe, 1991). According to this hypothesis, APP synthesis and/or processing may become abnormal due to the influence of various genetic or environmental factors (Figure 20.28). This change causes enhanced secretion and/or reduced clearance of Aβ, formation of Aβ-containing senile plaques, and the appearance of vascular amyloid. Amyloid deposits subsequently exert a toxic effect on neurons (see Kosik and Coleman, 1992), leading to intraneuronal changes including the development of NFTs and neuropil threads. Finally, the accumulated histological damage causes neuronal death, neurotransmitter deficits, and dementia. The process of amyloid deposition and plaque formation is presumed to begin in temporal lobe limbic system structures and then to spread over neuronal pathways by some unknown mechanism (Hardy, 1992). It would be foolhardy to suggest that Aβ is *directly* responsible for all of the cellular and behavioral effects of AD, because numerous events are interposed between the initial biochemical abnormality and the ultimate clinical disorder. As stated by Selkoe, the central idea of the amyloid cas-

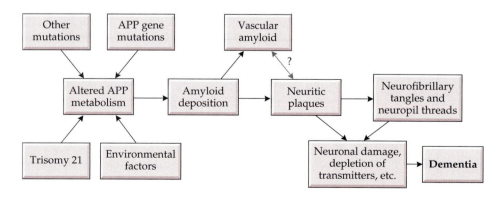

20.28 THE AMYLOID CASCADE HYPOTHESIS OF ALZHEIMER'S DISEASE. (After Hardy and Allsop, 1991.)

cade hypothesis is that "Aβ deposition is a necessary but not sufficient factor for the pathogenesis of AD" (Selkoe, 1994, p. 438).

The amyloid cascade hypothesis is supported by many clinical and experimental findings. First and foremost, AD brains always exhibit cerebral amyloid deposition and the formation of amyloid-containing plaques. Of course, this is a tautological statement because AD is histologically *defined*, at least in part, by the presence of a minimum age-adjusted density of amyloid plaques. A better way of thinking about this issue, therefore, is to note that amyloid plaques represent a major feature of a recognizable constellation of behavioral symptoms and histopathological markers that is medically diagnosed as AD. In both Down syndrome and AD, amyloid deposition (in the form of diffuse plaques) is the first observable histopathological event and should therefore be considered of primary importance according to the amyloid cascade hypothesis (Hardy and Allsop, 1991).

Another line of reasoning is that the formation of senile plaques, NFTs, and other histopathological markers of AD can be caused by genetic anomalies such as trisomy 21 and missense mutations of the *APP* gene that give rise to abnormal APP processing and enhanced Aβ secretion. Individuals suffering from such anomalies invariably develop an Alzheimer's-type dementia as they age. As discussed earlier, FAD is more commonly caused by other genetic defects; however, these may indirectly affect APP metabolism and the rate of Aβ formation.

One of the most recent approaches to assessing the amyloid cascade hypothesis is the creation of transgenic mice engineered to express either wild-type or mutant human APP. Several of these transgenic strains have shown little or no neuropathology (see review by Higgins and Cordell, 1995). On the other hand, Higgins, Cordell, and their colleagues at the Scios Nova company found diffuse amyloid deposits and staining for hyperphosphorylated tau (Alz50 antibody) in mice engineered for excessive neuronal expression of wild-type APP_{751} (L. S. Higgins et al., 1994; 1995). In young mice (2–3 months of age), the histopathology was mild and thus similar to that seen in early AD. Old (22 months of age) subjects, however, showed a substantially greater density of histopathological structures, suggesting the presence of an ongoing degenerative process. Another research group created mice expressing one of the rare FAD-related APP mutations (Val → Phe at position 717). As these animals matured and then aged, they exhibited striking Alzheimer's-type neuropathology, including a high density of amyloid deposits, amyloid fibril formation, gliosis, and formation of dystrophic neurites (Games et al., 1995). Interestingly, however, there was no evidence for abnormal tau staining in this transgenic model.

In evaluating the current status of APP transgenic mouse research, two important points should be made. First, no one has yet succeeded in creating a model that reproduces *all* of the crucial neuropathological features of AD, including mature neuritic plaques *and* NFTs, as well as cortical and subcortical cell loss. Second, although not all of the transgenic strains have been examined behaviorally, those that have been tested generally show no more than moderate behavioral deficits. Therefore, the severe cognitive disturbances characteristic of AD dementia likewise have yet to be produced in an APP transgenic animal model.

Are neurofibrillary changes primary events? Although the amyloid cascade hypothesis has dominated the field of AD research since its inception, it has been criticized on several grounds. First, even though diffuse amyloid deposits may be present very early in AD, they are also found in nondemented aged individuals with no other signs of AD histopathology (see Davies, 1994). We do not know whether these individuals might have eventually developed AD had they lived long enough. Nevertheless, it is possible that diffuse amyloid plaques are a common feature of normal aging, not the harbinger of AD as postulated by the amyloid cascade hypothesis.

A second issue is that if β-amyloid deposition somehow leads to neuronal pathology and NFT formation, then there should be a reasonably similar spatial pattern of plaques and tangles in the brains of AD patients. Yet, these structures do not develop in the same regional pattern as the disease progresses (Braak and Braak, 1991), nor are they closely aligned with each other within a given brain area (Armstrong, Myers, and Smith, 1993). A possible counterargument to this objection is that plaques and tangles do not correlate spatially because tangles are present mainly in the cell body and proximal dendrites, whereas plaques may be formed at the nerve terminals which could be many millimeters away for some neurons.

Perhaps a more important dissociation between β-amyloid and NFTs is the observation that some individuals exhibit plaques but few or no tangles at postmortem examination, whereas others have been found with low to intermediate levels of neurofibrillary structures (i.e., NFTs and neuropil threads) but no amyloid deposits (Braak and Braak, 1991). These findings raise the possibility that senile plaques and neurofibrillary structures are formed independently of one another. In that case, understanding one pathogenic process (e.g., the mechanism by which plaques are formed) is not necessarily helpful in understanding other aspects of AD pathogenesis.

On the other hand, it is possible that the neurofibrillary changes occur first, leading eventually to neuronal damage and the release of intracellular factors (including PHF–tau) that enhance amyloid aggregation and fibril formation (Figure 20.29). There are several problems with this hypothesis, including how it can account for the onset of neurofibrillary abnormalities in patients

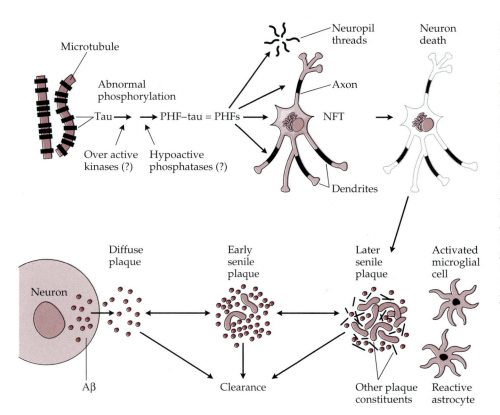

20.29 HYPOTHETICAL RELATIONSHIP BETWEEN NEUROFIBRILLARY TANGLES, NEURON DEATH, AND AMYLOID PLAQUE FORMATION. Aβ may normally be present in the extracellular space (either in a soluble form or as diffuse amyloid deposits) at a level that is regulated by the relative rates of secretion and clearance. One alternative to the amyloid cascade hypothesis proposes that the primary pathology in AD involves the tau hyperphosphorylation–NFT cascade, which results in neuron death and the subsequent release of PHF–tau and other intracellular proteins that somehow promote Aβ aggregation/fibrillogenesis and senile plaque formation. Factors released from nearby activated microglia and reactive astrocytes may also contribute to this process. (After Trojanowski et al., 1995.)

with *APP* gene mutations. Nevertheless, the hypothesis is supported by the extensive neuropathological staging work of Braak and Braak (1991). These investigators found that the distribution pattern of amyloid deposits was too variable to be used for developing a reliable staging system of AD neuropathology. In contrast, NFTs and neuropil threads were usually first observed in a very specific cell population of the temporal lobe, namely, the transentorhinal Pre-α cells, which are important projection neurons connecting the cortex to the hippocampus. There are typically few or no silver-stainable amyloid deposits in the transentorhinal region at this time, and this disparity may persist even in later neuropathological stages. Braak and Braak (1991, 1995) hypothesize that AD neurofibrillary pathology begins in the transentorhinal and entorhinal regions (stages I and II), radiates out to the hippocampus, amygdala, and other parts of the limbic system (stages III and IV), and finally shows a massive involvement of the neocortex (stages V and VI). The early stages of neurofibrillary pathology are shown in Figures 20.30 and 20.31. The pathogenic process is proposed to take up to 50 years from initiation to end-stage disease (Braak and Braak, 1995). Most importantly, since AD is generally believed to originate in temporal lobe structures, this hypothesis implicates neurofibrillary changes as primary events in AD pathogenesis.

What is the role of apoE?   Although researchers have clearly established that the *apoE4* allele is an important risk factor for late-onset AD, the role of the apoE protein in AD pathogenesis has not yet been elucidated. One hypothesis is that apoE acts as a "pathological chaperone" protein that binds to Aβ and promotes the formation of amyloid fibrils and eventually plaques (Wisniewski and Frangione, 1992). However, an alternative viewpoint has been advanced by Strittmatter, Roses, and their colleagues (Strittmatter et al., 1994). These investigators acknowledge that the rate of plaque formation is dependent on *apoE* genotype, but they argue that this effect is not a critical feature of AD pathogenesis. Rather, this research group has found evidence that apoE3, but not apoE4, binds to unphosphorylated tau and retards its phosphorylation. Based on these results, it is hypothesized that the presence of apoE3 (and presumably also apoE2), but not apoE4, in neurons slows the rate of tau phosphorylation, thereby impeding the generation of PHFs and the development of NFTs. Over a life span of 60 years or more, even a small difference in the rate at which tangles form and neurons are lost could have a marked effect on the incidence of AD. This hypothesis is still quite preliminary (see Gearing et al., 1994; Selkoe, 1994), but it is nevertheless an intriguing notion that fits well with the idea presented in the previous section that neurofibrillary abnormalities are a primary feature of AD pathogenesis.

Other factors.   Yet other factors have been hypothesized to participate in the destructive process that occurs in AD. For example, there is substantial evidence that a

(a) Stage I

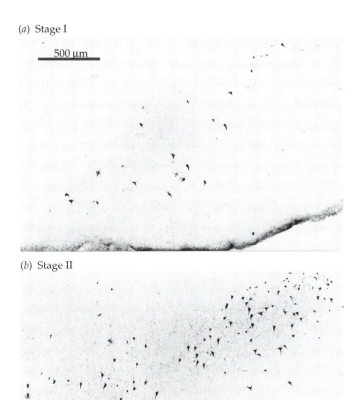

(b) Stage II

(c) Stage IV

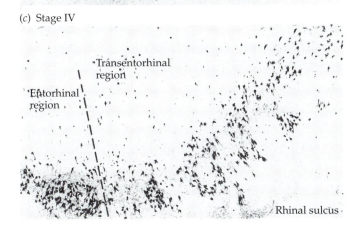

20.30 STAGING OF NEUROFIBRILLARY PATHOLOGY IN THE TRANSENTORHINAL REGION. (a) In stage I, only a few scattered NFT-containing cells are visible. (b) In stage II, the density of NFTs is increased (particularly within the band of Pre-α cells descending from right to left in the photomicrograph), and neuropil threads (thin stained fibrils) are visible. (c) In stage IV, there is a dense accumulation of NFTs and neuropil threads in both the transentorhinal and entorhinal regions (demarcated by the dashed line). Tissue samples were obtained from a 67-year-old nondemented man (a), a 65-year-old nondemented man (b), and a 64-year-old demented man (c). All sections were silver-stained. (From Braak and Braak, 1991, *Acta Neuropathol.*, Springer-Verlag. Courtesy of Heiko Braak and Eva Braak.)

inflammatory processes accelerate the process of neural degeneration that is initiated by the mechanisms described earlier (McGeer and McGeer, 1995).

One of the most recent hypotheses of AD pathogenesis concerns a possible role of free radicals and oxidative stress (see review by Smith et al., 1995). In the earlier section on PD, we saw that the hypothesized mechanisms of free radical formation in that disorder depend partly on the distinctive characteristics of the midbrain dopaminergic neurons. Different mechanisms might be involved in AD, however, since the DA system is relatively spared in this case. Recent findings have generated considerable interest in nitric oxide (NO) as a potential source of free radicals in AD. This gaseous messenger substance (see Chapter 6) can give rise to highly reactive free radicals and has been previously implicated in certain types of neurotoxicity. Benzing and Mufson (1995) reported an increased density of neurons staining for nicotinamide adenine dinucleotide phosphate–diaphorase (NADPH–d) in the substantia innominata (an important site of basal forebrain cholinergic neurons) of postmortem AD brains. As NADPH–d is a recognized histochemical marker for NO synthesis, this finding raises the possibility that cholinergic cell loss in AD could result from NO-dependent free radical formation. NO could also arise from microglia, as these cells can be stimulated to release NO by combined exposure to Aβ and the cytokine interferon-γ (Goodwin, Uemura, and Cunnick, 1995), and such stimulation can lead to cholinergic neuron loss in mixed neuronal/glial cultures (McMillian et al., 1995). The free radical hypothesis of neuron death in AD is a novel idea, but one that clearly deserves further consideration.

Treatment of Alzheimer's Disease

Since there is at present no cure for AD (nor is one yet on the horizon), current treatment strategies must be palliative in nature (i.e., aimed at alleviating symptoms without curing the disorder). Of course, we previously encountered a similar situation with respect to PD. Palliative therapy of AD attempts to improve memory and other cognitive functions, consequently enhancing the patient's daily living skills, easing the burden placed on

chronic inflammatory process is present in the AD brain (reviewed by Aisen and Davis, 1994; McGeer and McGeer, 1995). One type of evidence is that acute phase proteins such as α₁-antichymotrypsin, α₂-macroglobulin, and C-reactive protein, which are synthesized in response to inflammation, are found in senile plaques. Other signs of an inflammatory reaction in AD include stimulation of inflammatory cytokines like interleukin-(IL) 1 and IL-6, activation of the complement system (which serves to promote cell destruction and phagocytosis), and the presence of activated microglia. As pointed out by Aisen and Davis (1994, p. 1108), "inflammatory cells and mediators may be 'innocent bystanders,' reacting to tissue destruction without contributing to it." On the other hand, it is also possible that

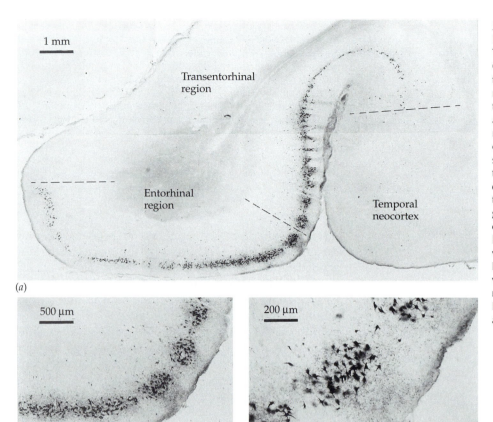

20.31 STAGE III NEUROFIBRILLARY PATHOLOGY IN THE TRANSENTORHINAL AND ENTORHINAL REGIONS. (*a*) A frontal section showing that in stage III of Braak and Braak, neurofibrillary pathology is restricted to the Pre-α layer of the transentorhinal and entorhinal regions. No NFTs or neuropil threads are visible in the adjacent temporal neocortex. (*b*) and (*c*) show progressively higher magnifications of the Pre-α layer around the middle dashed line in (*a*), which separates the transentorhinal and entorhinal regions. Note that the affected cells are organized into clusters (also called islands) in the transentorhinal region, which are also visible to some extent in Figure 20.29*c*. The silver-stained tissue was obtained from an 82-year-old demented woman. (From Braak and Braak, 1995; courtesy of Heiko Braak and Eva Braak.)

caregivers by the patient, and slowing the onset of dependence and disability. As reviewed by Lamy (1994), a number of measurement instruments have been devised to assess how well these treatment goals are met. Such instruments include comprehensive assessments of dementia (such as the Blessed Dementia Scale and the Mini-Mental test, which are mentioned in Table 20.1), noncognitive behavioral assessment measures, neuropsychological tests, scales that evaluate daily living activities or caregiver burden, and global staging and quality-of-life scales. Nevertheless, many clinical studies of AD treatment have primarily focused on memory tests or dementia ratings, with much less emphasis on other aspects of treatment outcome.

Early Treatment Concepts

Early attempts at AD therapy were based on the hypothesis that age-related cognitive deficits are the result of impaired cerebral blood flow. Consequently, vasodilators and anticoagulants were administered, which resulted in subjective reports of improvement in some patients. More objective assessment by psychological testing, however, failed to find significant treatment-related changes. Tests of stimulant drugs such as methylphenidate and pentylenetetrazol (see Chapters 8 and 10) showed limited usefulness in reversing cognitive deficits, although methylphenidate was of some value in al-

leviating fatigue, motor retardation, and depressed mood (Crook, 1985).

Nootropics

Nootropics (from Gk. *noos* = "mind," and *tropein* = "toward"; see Giurgea, 1980), which are also called **cognitive enhancers**, represent a structurally diverse group of drugs thought to enhance various processes of attention, learning, or memory. According to Schindler (1994), for a drug to be considered a nootropic, it should exert the greatest cognition-enhancing effects under conditions of neural impairment, and it should generally not produce the kinds of behavioral effects associated with classic psychotropic agents (e.g., psychomotor stimulants, antidepressants, neuroleptics, sedative–hypnotics, anxiolytics, opiates, or cannabinoids). The possible utility of nootropics is based mainly on their efficacy in animal models used to screen potential therapeutic agents in treating Alzheimer's dementia (Porsolt, Roux, and Wettstein, 1995).

The pyrrolidone derivative piracetam is the prototypical nootropic and was used as the basis for developing a family of analogs such as aniracetam, oxiracetam, and pramiracetam. These drugs have repeatedly proved effective in enhancing performance in various learning and memory tasks in rodents, including tasks involving amnesia induced by the general muscarinic antagonist

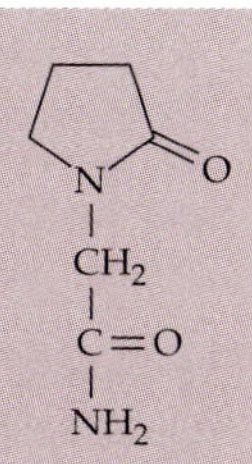

Piracetam

scopolamine (Schindler, 1994). Unfortunately, however, clinical trials suggest that only a small subset of patients (perhaps 10% to 30%) responds positively to nootropics, whereas the majority show little or no effect (Mondadori, 1993; Schindler, 1994). The reason for this response heterogeneity is not clear, but it could reflect variation in the amount or location of neural damage already sustained by different patients. A number of nootropics have already been licensed for use in Europe and Japan, but not in the United States where there seems to be less enthusiasm for these compounds.

The mechanism of action of piracetam-derived nootropics is unclear despite considerable study. Various findings suggest mediation by the cholinergic system, excitatory amino acid receptors, and even adrenal steroid hormones (Mondadori, 1993). Other types of nootropics that differ structurally from piracetam are thought to function by altering different neurotransmitter systems, blocking certain ion channels, or enhancing cerebral blood flow and oxygenation (Sarter, 1991).

Pharmacological Treatment of Cholinergic Deficits

Up to now, most treatment strategies have been based on the "cholinergic hypothesis" of cognitive dysfunction in AD (see Bartus et al., 1982). Consequently, the remainder of this chapter is devoted to ACh-oriented therapies. Although we shall see that some success has been attained in this area, a recent review acknowledges that "despite generally encouraging results [with cholinergic drugs] no agent to date has proved to be dramatically effective [in alleviating AD symptomatology]" (Gualtieri et al., 1995; p. 500).

One obvious limitation of cholinergic therapies is the possibility discussed earlier that AD-associated cognitive deficits are related more closely to cell loss and synaptic damage in the cortex and hippocampus than to decreased functioning of the basal forebrain cholinergic system. In the coming years, we may see the development of pharmacological agents that can selectively target aspects of APP processing and Aβ secretion, tau phosphorylation, or apoE metabolism, depending on which of these processes (if any) proves to be critical to AD pathogenesis. Until that time, however, treatments based on ACh or other potentially relevant neurotransmitters (e.g., glutamate) are likely to remain at the forefront of AD therapy.

Acetylcholine replacement. The idea that cholinergic deficits might play a significant role in AD dementia was a welcome event for those seeking pharmacological approaches to AD therapy. This led to a major effort to develop a neurotransmitter replacement therapy for AD, hopefully emulating the success story enjoyed by PD researchers with levodopa. As described earlier, postsynaptic muscarinic receptors are still present in AD, raising the possibility that supplying ACh precursors or agonists would relieve behavioral symptoms, and possibly even halt progression of the disease.

The first and safest approach was to enhance the patients' diet with large supplements of the ACh precursor choline or of lecithin (phosphatidylcholine, from which choline is liberated by hydrolysis). Increasing plasma choline levels was thought to possibly elevate brain concentrations of ACh, thereby leading to symptom amelioration. The results of this approach, however, were disappointing. A review of 17 clinical trials involving choline or lecithin treatment in AD showed little or no cognitive improvement in almost all cases (Bartus et al., 1982). One limitation of this strategy is that only about 1% of plasma choline is incorporated into ACh, with the remainder entering alternative metabolic pathways (McGeer, 1984).

Acetylcholinesterase inhibition. Early studies revealed that ACh action can be prolonged with AChE inhibitors such as physostigmine and tetrahydroaminoacridine (THA). Physostigmine produced mild improvement in some AD patients, especially when supplemented with dietary lecithin, but unfortunately its effects were short-acting (Crook, 1985; McGeer, 1984). A modest benefit was also found with THA (tacrine), and this compound was approved for use in AD treatment in 1993 under the trade name Cognex.

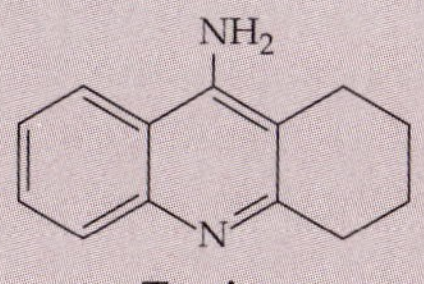

Tacrine

Figure 20.32 illustrates the design and results of a large multicenter study of tacrine efficacy in AD (Davis et al., 1992). The investigators initially enrolled 632 male and female subjects at least 50 years old and with a diagnosis of probable AD. During the first phase of the study (dose titration), the subjects were rotated on a double-blind basis between placebo, 40 mg/day tacrine (given as four equal doses), and 80 mg/day tacrine over a 6-week period (Figure 20.32a). Over the next 2 weeks (placebo baseline), all subjects received placebo to establish baseline data for the subsequent study phases. During this time, the researchers analyzed data from the

(a)

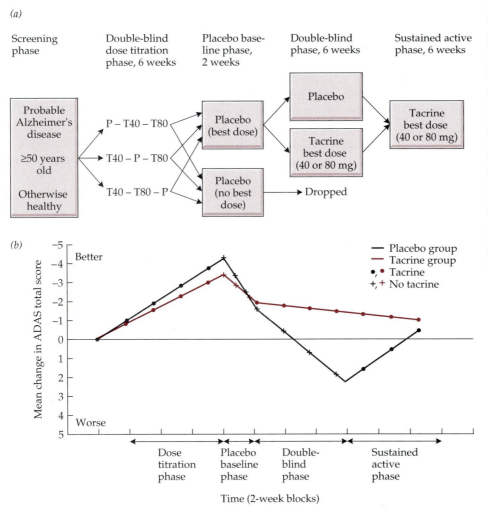

(b)

20.32 EFFICACY OF TACRINE IN TREATING ALZHEIMER'S DISEASE. (a) Study design. P = placebo; T40 and T80 = 40 and 80 mg/day of tacrine, respectively. Each treatment condition lasted 2 weeks. (b) Mean change in ADAS (Alzheimer's Disease Assessment Scale) total score as a function of study phase. All subjects received tacrine during the dose titration and sustained active phases, whereas all were given placebo during the placebo baseline phase. Some subjects were dropped after this phase, but remaining subjects received either tacrine or placebo during the double-blind phase as shown. Note that data are presented *only* from subjects who responded positively to tacrine during the first phase. (After Davis et al., 1992.)

dose titration phase to determine which subjects met the study criterion for a significant response to tacrine (the criterion was set at a 4-point improvement in total score on the Alzheimer's Disease Assessment Scale, ADAS). Adequate data for evaluation were obtained on 563 subjects, of which 231 (41%) met the criterion and were permitted to continue in the study (215 actually entered the next phase) while the remaining subjects were dropped. In the third phase (double-blind), subjects were divided into two groups, tacrine ($n = 103$) versus placebo ($n = 112$). Each tacrine subject received his or her "best dose," that is, the dose (40 or 80 mg/day) that yielded the greatest improvement during the dose titration phase. The last phase of the study (sustained active) was an open phase in which all subjects received their best dose of tacrine.

ADAS results from the tacrine responders are shown in Figure 20.32b. Mean ADAS scores consistently increased (i.e., symptoms worsened) when the patients were receiving the placebo, whereas the scores tended to decrease when tacrine therapy was initiated (note both groups in the double-blind phase and the placebo group in the sustained active phase) and remained relatively stable over the course of continuous treatment (tacrine group during the double-blind and sustained active phases). These results demonstrate a significant effect of tacrine on AD symptomatology (particularly cognitive function, since the cognitive subscale constitutes about 85% of the ADAS). On the other hand, the total ADAS score for both groups during the placebo baseline phase was approximately 35, indicating that a treatment-induced change of a few points was quite small, even though it may have reached statistical significance. Indeed, tacrine administration failed to significantly alter patient scores on the Mini-Mental State Examination or on the Clinical Global Impression of Change scale, further demonstrating the limited efficacy of this compound in AD.

The therapeutic effects of tacrine do not correlate closely with its anti-AChE activity, and therefore other neurochemical actions of the drug may contribute to its behavioral activity (Freeman and Dawson, 1991; Lamy,

1994). Furthermore, tacrine produces problematic side effects in many patients, including hepatotoxicity in some cases (Watkins et al., 1994). Because of tacrine's limited clinical value and potential side effects, pharmaceutical companies have been developing new AChE inhibitors such as galanthamine, huperzine, metrifonate, SM-10888, and velnacrine (Gualtieri et al., 1995; Lamy, 1994). Furthermore, systemic side effects of cholinesterase inhibition could be ameliorated in the future by the advent of brain-selective AChE inhibitors (see Enz et al., 1993). Nevertheless, continuing deterioration of the cholinergic system means that anti-AChE treatment for AD is likely to show reduced efficacy over time, as has been found for levodopa therapy for PD.

Current interest in ACh-based therapy is particularly focused on the possible use of drugs that target either muscarinic or nicotinic receptors (Gualtieri et al., 1995). M1-selective agonists might lead to clinical improvement by directly activating postsynaptic muscarinic receptors (which, as discussed earlier, are largely intact), whereas M2-selective *antagonists* might be effective by blocking presynaptic autoreceptors and thereby enhancing ACh release (Doods et al., 1993). Nicotinic cholinergic agonists could also be of value, particularly as researchers develop new compounds with selectivity for central nicotinic receptors (Holladay, Lebold, and Lin, 1995). Wilson et al. (1995) recently reported the results of a pilot study of nicotine patch therapy in AD patients. A double-blind, placebo-controlled trial was carried out on six patients with probable AD. All subjects were tested in three sequential phases: 7 days of placebo, 8 days of nicotine treatment, and then 7 days of placebo again (drug wash-out phase). The investigators found improved learning during the treatment phase that persisted somewhat during washout. On the other hand, memory, global cognition, and other behavioral measures were not significantly affected. Nicotine administration caused mild side effects and also a decrease in nighttime sleep, which is a potentially serious complication because it significantly increases the burden on patient caregivers.

Neurotrophic Therapy

The pharmacotherapies described above can produce symptom relief, but cannot prevent or halt the course of AD. A better therapeutic approach, therefore, would be to attempt to rescue the cholinergic neurons (or other cell populations) that are under attack. Appel (1981) hypothesized that neurodegenerative disorders might result from deficits in neurotrophic factors, proteins that have been found to promote neuronal survival, growth, or differentiation. Even if this hypothesis is not correct, supplementation with appropriate factors could potentially retard, halt, or even reverse the process of neural degeneration. In the case of AD, particular attention has been directed toward a neurotrophic factor known as nerve growth factor (NGF).

NGF is the prototypic neurotrophic factor, having been identified and characterized in early studies by the Nobel Laureate Rita Levi-Montalcini and her colleagues (see Levi-Montalcini, 1987). Her work showed that in the peripheral nervous system, the presence of NGF is essential to the survival and growth of developing sympathetic and sensory neurons. NGF is synthesized and secreted by tissues that are innervated by these neuronal populations. Following its release, NGF is internalized by sympathetic and sensory nerve terminals, after which it is retrogradely transported to the cell body, where it exerts its trophic effects. Within its cells of origin, NGF is believed to exist as a 140-kDa, 5-subunit complex containing two α-, one β-, and two γ- subunits. However, the subunits dissociate prior to secretion and only the β-subunit (known as β-NGF) is released. This peptide, which is a 13-kDa homodimer, is thus responsible for NGF's neurotrophic activity (Maness et al., 1994).

Studies by a number of laboratories have shown that NGF belongs to a class of neurotrophic factors termed **neurotrophins**. Other members of this group are brain-derived neurotrophic factor (BDNF), neurotrophin-3 (NT-3), and NT-4/5 (Lindsay et al., 1994; Maness et al., 1994). These substances are all found within the brain, although they differ significantly in their regional distribution and may act on different cell populations.

Two distinct receptors for NGF have been identified. One is a low-affinity receptor that was previously mentioned in Chapter 7. In humans, this receptor has a molecular weight of approximately 75 kDa and has therefore been designated p75[NGFR] (Maness et al., 1994; Meakin and Shooter, 1992). Investigators have also found a separate group of neurotrophin receptors possessing tyrosine kinase activity (see Chapter 6). One of these tyrosine receptor kinases (trk's), known as p140[trkA] or simply trk A, is a 140-kDa high-affinity receptor for NGF. Although this issue is still controversial, there is a possibility that the two types of receptors interact to mediate the effects of NGF on its cellular targets.

Whereas NGF in the peripheral nervous system exerts trophic activity on noradrenergic (sympathetic) neurons, this is not the case for central noradrenergic neurons. Instead, there is considerable evidence that NGF in the brain is a trophic factor for cholinergic neurons, particularly basal forebrain neurons that innervate the cerebral cortex and hippocampus. This view is based on the following findings (see Maness et al., 1994; Tuszynski and Gage, 1994):

1. Levels of NGF protein and mRNA expression are highest in the hippocampus and cortex.
2. NGF receptors are found in the medial septal/diagonal band cholinergic complex (which projects to the hippocampus) and in the nucleus basalis (which innervates the cortex).
3. When NGF is injected into the hippocampus and cortex, it is taken up by nerve terminals and transported back to the cholinergic cell bodies.

4. The cholinergic neurons respond to NGF by increasing their ChAT activity.

5. Treatment with anti-NGF antiserum during prenatal development reduces the population of cholinergic neurons in vivo and in cell culture.

6. In adult animals, damaging the ascending cholinergic pathways, either by lesioning the target area (e.g., the neocortex) or by cutting the axons (e.g., the fimbria–fornix, which contains the fibers of the septo–hippocampal pathway), leads to degeneration and death of many of the cholinergic cell bodies. These cells can be rescued, however, by treatment with NGF.

7. NGF treatment has been found to improve learning and memory both in aged animals and in animals with lesion-induced cholinergic degeneration.

The above findings strongly suggest that NGF is synthesized and released by cortical and hippocampal neurons that receive a cholinergic innervation, is taken up by basal forebrain cholinergic cells, and exerts a trophic influence on these cells. As the basal forebrain cholinergic neurons and their targets are among the cell populations most heavily damaged in AD, Hefti and his colleagues suggested that NGF might be an appropriate therapeutic agent for treating AD (Hefti, Hartikka, and Knüsel, 1989; Hefti and Weiner, 1986). In considering this proposal, it is important to determine whether the levels of NGF or its receptors are altered in AD. Several studies have found reduced NGF receptor density in AD (Maness et al., 1994), which is not surprising since the cholinergic neurons that express these receptors are already damaged. The status of NGF synthesis in AD is less clear, although recent studies by Crutcher, Scott, and their coworkers (Crutcher et al., 1993; Scott et al., 1995) may help clarify the situation. Using an enzyme-linked immunosorbent assay (ELISA), these investigators compared the brains of AD patients and control subjects with respect to NGF-like immunoreactivity in the neocortex, hippocampus, amygdala, putamen, cerebellum, and nucleus basalis. NGF levels were unexpectedly found to be elevated in the cortex, hippocampus, and putamen of the AD brains; however, the levels were significantly lower in the nucleus basalis (Figure 20.33). The finding of increased NGF in cholinergic projection areas, but a decrease in a region of cholinergic cell bodies, could be due to several factors, including increased NGF synthesis by target neurons in response to cholinergic denervation, decreased release and hence increased accumulation of NGF by the synthesizing cells, or impaired uptake or retrograde transport of NGF by the cholinergic neurons. A separate experiment demonstrated that many nucleus basalis neurons that were immunoreactive for p75[NGFR] (the low-affinity NGF receptor), and therefore should have contained NGF, exhibited little or no NGF immunoreactivity. Thus, deficient uptake or retrograde transport may be among the factors responsible for the low levels of nucleus basalis NGF found in AD.

Tuszynski and Gage (1994) discuss several important issues related to the therapeutic use of NGF in AD. The first issue concerns the source of the peptide. Human recombinant β-NGF would be an ideal source, but it is not yet available in large enough amounts for broad clinical use. A second issue involves the route of administration. Because NGF is too large to cross the blood–brain barrier, it would have to be administered directly into the brain. Third, treatment with NGF could

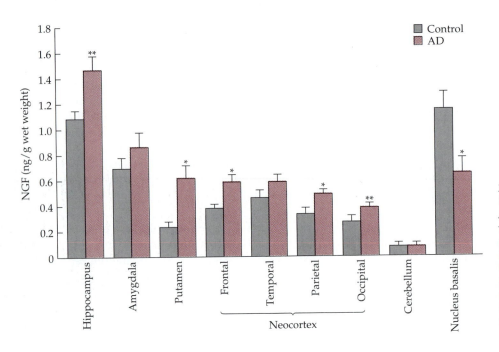

20.33 ALTERATION IN REGIONAL NGF-LIKE IMMUNOREACTIVITY IN ALZHEIMER'S DISEASE. Compared with control brains, brains from AD patients showed significant increases in NGF-like immunoreactivity in the hippocampus, putamen, and all regions of the neocortex, but a significant decrease in the nucleus basalis. (*$p < 0.05$; **$p < 0.01$) (After Scott et al., 1995.)

cause adverse systemic effects or unwanted sprouting of sympathetic fibers, as found in some animal studies. Fourth, NGF therapy should begin as early as possible in the disorder (which would require widespread screening and reliable methods for early diagnosis), and the treatment might have to be continued for the remainder of the patient's lifetime. Finally, some investigators believe that it is still too early to begin trials with NGF, whereas others argue that the potential benefits mitigate in favor of initiating small-scale clinical testing.

At the time of this writing, we know of a single case study in Sweden in which NGF treatment was administered to a 69-year-old patient diagnosed with probable AD and having moderate cognitive deficits (Seiger et al., 1993). In this instance, 75 µg/day of purified mouse β-NGF was infused intracerebroventricularly over a period of 3 months. No adverse effects of the treatment were observed. PET scans performed before, at the completion of, and 3 months after the termination of NGF infusion found treatment-related increases in both cerebral blood flow and nicotinic receptor binding, although only the blood flow change persisted after the treatment had ended. There was also a persistent reduction in the incidence of abnormal slow-wave cortical EEG activity and a transient improvement in one measure of cognitive performance (delayed word recognition), but not in other cognitive measures.

These findings point to the feasibility and apparent safety of chronic NGF administration to AD patients, and further indicate that some neurological and behavioral improvement can be produced by this treatment. In the future, therapy with NGF or other neurotrophins that could also be efficacious may be accomplished by cerebral implantation of NGF-secreting cells, thereby eliminating the problem of continuous peptide infusion (see, for example, Emerich et al., 1994; Martinez-Serrano, Fischer, and Björklund, 1995).

Tissue Grafting

The final therapeutic approach to be discussed involves the technique of tissue grafting to replace the cholinergic neurons that degenerate in AD. This is similar to the use of mesencephalic tissue grafts as described in the section on PD. At the time of this writing, however, it appears that no AD patient has yet received any graft. The present discussion will therefore summarize work using animal models, with the understanding that this methodology is under development for future clinical application.

Research on cholinergic cell grafting has been reviewed by Fisher and Gage (1993), Kimble (1990), and Sinden, Gray, and Hodges (1994). In most cases, assessment of cholinergic cell grafts has been carried out in animals (usually rats) with prior damage to the cholinergic system. Such damage may be produced by performing lesions of the nucleus basalis by infusion of either an excitotoxin (see Chapter 7 for a discussion of methodologi-

cal problems concerning this approach) or the partially selective cholinergic toxin ethylcholine mustard aziridinium ion (AF-64A). Alternatively, the medial septal nucleus or the fimbria–fornix are given electrolytic or radiofrequency lesions. (Excitotoxic lesions have been used much less frequently with the septum than with the nucleus basalis.)

The grafted tissue is generally taken from the basal forebrain region of fetal rats at 14–17 days of embryonic development (rats have a gestation period of 22–23 days). Differentiated cholinergic neurons are present by this time, but neurite outgrowth from the cells is minimal. The tissue is usually mechanically and enzymatically dissociated prior to grafting, and the resulting cell suspension is implanted directly into the cholinergic denervated area (i.e., into the neocortex in the case of a nucleus basalis lesion, or into the hippocampus in the case of a medial septal or fimbria–fornix lesion). The rationale for positioning the graft in an abnormal location is that the graft cell axons typically do not reach their intended target area when placed at a distance from that area.

Numerous studies have demonstrated that cholinergic grafts carried out under these conditions result in good graft viability. There is also an extensive literature showing some improvement in lesion-induced behavioral deficits following grafting, but not all deficits are ameliorated (Sinden, Gray, and Hodges, 1994). Functional recovery has also been observed in monkeys with fimbria–fornix lesions after intrahippocampal grafting of cholinergic-rich tissue (Ridley and Baker, 1991). Compared with rats, nonhuman primates have more sophisticated cognitive abilities and a CNS organization closer to that of humans. Thus, more primate work needs to be performed to determine the potential utility of the cholinergic graft approach. Ultimately, however, the best grafts might be those that provide trophic support to the AD brain rather than mere neurotransmitter replacement.

Part II Summary

Alzheimer's disease is a disorder of aging that is characterized by progressive loss of cognitive functioning, eventually culminating in complete dementia. Some patients also suffer from depression, paranoid delusions, or hallucinations. Several types of neuropathology are found in the brains of AD patients, most notably senile plaques and neurofibrillary tangles. The plaques typically possess a β-amyloid core surrounded by dystrophic neurites and reactive glial cells. NFTs are composed mainly of hyperphosphorylated tau, which is a microtubule-associated protein. The most severe histopathology occurs in limbic brain areas such as the hippocampus and amygdala, as well as in cortical association areas within the frontal, temporal, and parietal lobes. AD patients also show a marked loss of neurons in the cerebral cortex and hippocampus and a reduction in cortical synapse density.

AD histopathology is generally thought to begin in temporal lobe structures and to spread outward to other cortical and subcortical areas. This has been shown most dramatically in the case of neurofibrillary pathology, which appears to originate specifically in the Pre-α cells of the transentorhinal and entorhinal regions. At autopsy, the most severe histopathology is seen in limbic brain areas such as the hippocampus and amygdala, as well as in cortical association areas within the frontal, temporal, and parietal lobes.

Several neurotransmitter systems are affected in AD, particularly the ascending cholinergic system that originates in the basal forebrain. This is shown by a massive loss of cholinergic neurons in the nucleus basalis and other basal forebrain areas, as well as reductions in cholinergic nerve terminals in the cortex and hippocampus. On the other hand, postsynaptic cholinergic receptors seem to be largely intact. There is also some damage to neurons that use NE, 5-HT, or the neuropeptide somatostatin as their transmitter.

There has been considerable controversy concerning the relationship between loss of cognitive function and AD neuropathology. Various investigators have hypothesized that cognitive deficits correlate best with plaque density, NFT density, severity of synapse loss, or severity of cholinergic damage. It is important for this issue to be resolved, since it has significant implications for the targeting of therapeutic interventions. Less attention has been paid to other symptoms of AD, although noradrenergic dysfunction is thought to play a central role in AD-related depression.

Because dementia can occur from a variety of causes, living patients can be diagnosed only as suffering from probable AD. Confirmation of the diagnosis may be accomplished at autopsy by measuring the density of senile plaques in the brain (as plaques and NFTs are also not unique to AD, one must be able to exclude other possible sources of histopathology). Recent work suggests that imaging techniques such as PET and SPECT may be helpful in identifying patients with incipient AD, even before clinical symptoms are apparent.

Studies on the pathogenesis of AD have focused on the Aβ peptide, which is the form of amyloid present in senile plaques, and the processing of its precursor, APP. APP is a transmembrane protein that is a normal constituent of neurons as well as many other cell types throughout the body. Alternative splicing of the APP transcript gives rise to three isoforms, of which the shortest (APP$_{695}$) is found only in nerve cells. APP can be cleaved at several different sites within its extracellular and transmembrane domains, thereby releasing peptides of varying sizes into the extracellular fluid. The action of two unidentified proteases called β- and γ-secretase liberates the amyloidogenic peptide Aβ, whereas a different protease (α-secretase) yields harmless breakdown products. Therefore, many researchers believe that changes in APP processing or other mechanisms involved in Aβ release or extracellular clearance may be critical to AD pathogenesis by altering the availability of Aβ for plaque formation.

The role of Aβ in AD pathogenesis is clearest in cases of early-onset familial Alzheimer's disease (FAD), which is inherited in an autosomal dominant pattern, or in related disorders. Several missense mutations of the *APP* gene have been linked to severe early-onset FAD or other disorders involving amyloid deposition. Moreover, the *APP* gene is located on chromosome 21, and Down syndrome patients (who possess an extra copy of the same chromosome) exhibit AD-like histopathology and become demented as early as 40 years of age. FAD can also be caused by mutations in other genes (*PS-1* and *PS-2*), and the relationship between these mutations and Aβ disposition remains to be determined.

Early-onset FAD represents only a small fraction of all AD cases. Most cases are sporadic and occur later in life (i.e., after the age of 65). Recent studies have shown that the risk for late-onset sporadic or familial AD is strongly associated with allelic variation in the *apoE* gene. This gene codes for apolipoprotein E, a protein that serves an important lipid transport function in the bloodstream and which is also found in the nervous system. Possession of the *E4* allele of *apoE* (especially two doses) enhances the likelihood of developing AD and also increases the severity of neuropathology and behavioral symptomatology compared with the *E3* and *E2* alleles. In fact, the latter seems to exert somewhat of a protective effect with regard to delaying the onset of AD.

The view that extracellular β-amyloid deposition and senile plaque formation are primary to AD pathogenesis has been termed the amyloid cascade hypothesis. There are alternative hypotheses, however, based on the notion that intracellular abnormalities leading to neurofibrillary pathology (e.g., formation of NFTs) and eventual cell death occur first and are most central to AD pathogenesis. This controversy should eventually be resolved as the molecular features of AD continue to be unraveled. The presumptive role of apoE must also be considered: Different investigators have reported evidence that apoE can bind to both Aβ and tau protein, and could therefore be involved in the development of plaques or tangles. Finally, other hypotheses of AD pathogenesis have been proposed involving inflammatory processes and free radical–mediated neuronal death.

At present, AD pharmacotherapy is not nearly as well developed as in the case of PD. One general approach involves the use of nootropics, or cognitive enhancers, which may act by a variety of neurochemical mechanisms. Several nootropics based on the prototypical compound piracetam have been licensed in Europe and Japan, but are not currently available in the United States. Another major avenue of drug development and testing is aimed at restoring cholinergic activity, even though the relationship between cholinergic deficits and cognitive decline has been debated. The earliest approach, which was to provide dietary supplementation with the ACh precursor choline or with the choline-containing lipid lecithin, proved ineffectual. Slightly more promising is AChE inhibition, such as with the drug tacrine, which is currently in clinical use. A third approach is to manipulate the cholinergic system using postsynaptic receptor agonists or autoreceptor antagonists. It will be interesting to see whether such agents show greater efficacy in treating AD symptomatology than the drugs currently in use.

As we saw earlier for PD, pharmacotherapies eventually lose efficacy, in part because of the continuing degenerative process, which is not ameliorated by currently available treatment. This raises the question of whether other methods could be devised to halt or even reverse the course of the disorder. With regard to the cholinergic system in AD, this aim is being investigated using two approaches: treatment with NGF (which has trophic effects on central cholinergic neurons), and grafting of fetal cholinergic-rich tissue. Both approaches are still under development; however, they both have a theoretical advantage over simple pharmacotherapies because they are aimed at increasing the number of viable cholinergic neurons in the patient's brain.

Nevertheless, it seems likely that preventing the cognitive deterioration associated with AD will require much more than saving the ACh system. Therapeutic interventions must be found to inhibit the mechanisms that engender plaque and tangle formation, cell death, and synapse loss in both cortical and subcortical areas.

References

Aaronson, B., and Hoffer, A. (1970). *Psychedelics*. Anchor/Doubleday, Garden City, New York.

Abel, E. L. (1985). Late sequelae of fetal alcohol syndrome. In *Alcohol and the Developing Brain* (U. Rydberg, C. Alling, and J. Engel, Eds.), pp. 125–133. Raven Press, New York.

Abel, E. L., and Sokol, R. J. (1991). A revised conservative estimate of the incidence of FAS and its economic impact. *Alcohol. Clin. Exp. Res.*, 15, 514–524.

Abood, M. E., and Martin, B. R. (1992). Neurobiology of marijuana abuse. *Trends Pharmacol. Sci.*, 13, 201–206.

Abraham, W. C., Dragunow, M., and Tate, W. P. (1991). The role of immediate early genes in the stabilization of long-term potentiation. *Mol. Neurobiol.*, 5, 297–314.

Aceto, M. D., Scates, S. M., Lowe, J. A., and Martin, B. R. (1995). Cannabinoid-precipitated withdrawal by a selective antagonist: SR 141716A. *Eur. J. Pharmacol.*, 282, R1–R2.

Adam, K. (1984). Are poor sleepers changed into good sleepers by hypnotic drugs? In *Sleep, Benzodiazepines and Performance* (I. Hindmarch, H. Ott and T. Roth, Eds.), pp. 44–55. Springer-Verlag, New York.

Adams, R. N. (1990). In vivo electrochemical measurements in the CNS. *Prog. Neurobiol.*, 35, 297–311.

Adham, N., et al. (1993). Cloning of another human serotonin (5-H$_{1F}$): A fifth 5-HT$_1$ subtype coupled to the inhibition of adenylate cyclase. *Proc. Natl. Acad. Sci. U.S.A.*, 90, 408–412.

Aggleton, P. J. (1993). Behavioural tests for the recognition of non-spatial information by rats. In *Behavioural Neuroscience: A Practical Approach*, Vol. 1 (A. Sahgal, Ed.), pp. 81–93. Oxford University Press, New York.

Aghajanian, G. K. (1981). The modulatory role of serotonin at multiple receptors in brain. In *Serotonin Neurotransmission and Behavior* (B. L. Jacobs and A. Gelperin, Eds.), pp. 156–185. MIT Press, Cambridge, MA.

Aghajanian, G. K., and Bunney, B. S. (1977). Dopamine "autoreceptors": Pharmacological characterization by microiontophoretic single cell recording studies. *Arch. Pharmacol.*, 297, 1–7.

Aghajanian, G. K., Cederbaum, J. M., and Wang, R. Y. (1977). Evidence for norepinephrine-mediated collateral inhibition of locus coeruleus neurons. *Brain Res.*, 136, 570–577.

Aghajanian, G. K., and Haigler, H. J. (1974). Mode of action of LSD on serotonergic neurons. *Adv. Biochem. Psychopharmacol.*, 10, 167–178.

Aghajanian, G. K., Haigler, H. J., and Bennett, J. L. (1975). Amine receptors in CNS. III. 5-Hydroxytryptamine in brain. In *Handbook of Psychopharmacology*, Vol. 6 (L. L. Iversen, S. D. Iversen, and S. H. Snyder, Eds.), pp. 63–96. Plenum Press, New York.

Aghajanian, G. K., and Lakoski, J. M. (1984). Hyperpolarization of serotonergic neurons by serotonin and LSD: Studies in brain slices showing increased K$^+$ conductance. *Brain Res.*, 305, 181–185.

Aghajanian, G. K., Sprouse, J. S., and Rasmussen, K. (1987). Physiology of the midbrain serotonin system. In *Psychopharmacology: The Third Generation of Progress* (H. Y. Meltzer, Ed.), pp. 141–149. Raven Press, New York.

Aghajanian, G. K., and van der Maelen, C. P. (1982). Alpha-2 adrenoceptor-mediated hyperpolarization of locus coeruleus neurons: Intracellular studies in vivo. *Science*, 215, 1394–1396.

Aghajanian, G. K., and Wang, Y. Y. (1987). Common alpha-2 and opiate effector mechanisms in the locus coeruleus: Intracellular studies in brain slices. *Neuropharmacology*, 26, 789–800.

Agid, Y., Javoy-Agid, F., and Ruberg, M. (1987). Biochemistry of neurotransmitters in Parkinson's disease. *Mov. Disord.*, 2 , 166–230.

Agnati, L. F., Zoli, M., Pich, E. M., Benfenati, F., and Fuxe, K. (1990). Aspects of neural plasticity in the central nervous system. VII. Theoretical aspects of brain communication and computation. *Neurochem. Int.*, 16, 479–500.

Aguayo, L. G., and Albuquerque, E. X. (1987). Phencyclidine blocks two potassium currents in spinal neurons in cell culture. *Brain Res.*, 436, 9–17.

Agurell, S., Halldin, M., Lindgren, J.-E., Ohlsson, A., Widman, M., Gillespie, H., and Hollister, L. (1986). Pharmacokinetics and metabolism of Δ^1-tetrahydrocannabinol and other cannabinoids with emphasis on man. *Pharmacol. Rev.*, 38, 21–43.

Ahlquist, R. P. (1948). A study of adrenotropic receptors. *Am. J. Physiol.*, 153, 586–600.

Ahlquist, R. P. (1979). Adrenoreceptors. *Trends Pharmacol. Sci.*, 1, 16–17.

Ahluwali, P., and Singhal, R. L. (1980). Effect of low-dose lithium administration and subsequent withdrawal on biogenic amines in rat brain. *Br. J. Pharmacol.*, 71, 601–607.

Aichner, F., and Willeit, J. (1986). Magnetic resonance imaging of the central nervous system. In *PET and NMR: New Perspectives in Neuroimaging and in Clinical Neurochemistry* (L. Battistin and F. Gerstenbrand, Eds.), pp. 381–405. Alan R. Liss, New York.

Aimone, L. D., and Yaksh, T. L. (1989). Opioid modulation of capsaicin-evoked release of substance P from spinal cord in vivo. *Peptides*, 10, 1127–1131.

Airaksinen, M. S., Paetau, A., Paljärvi, L., Reinikainen, K., Riekkinen, P., Suomalainen, R., and Panula, P. (1991). Histamine neurons in human hypothalamus: Anatomy in normal and Alzheimer diseased brains. *Neuroscience*, 44, 465–481.

Aisen, P. S., and Davis, K. L. (1994). Inflammatory mechanisms in Alzheimer's disease: Implications for therapy. *Am. J. Psychiatry*, 151, 1105–1113.

Akaike, A., Ohno, Y., Sasa, M., and Takaori, S. (1987). Excitatory and inhibitory effects of dopamine on neuronal activity of the caudate nucleus neurons in vitro. *Brain Res.*, 418, 262–272.

Akert, K., Moore, K., Pfenninger, K., and Sandri, C. (1969). Contributions of new impregnation methods and freeze etching to the problems of synaptic fine structure. *Prog. Brain Res.*, 31, 223–240.

Akert, K., Peper, K., and Sandri, C. (1975). Structural organization of motor end plate and central synapses. In *Cholinergic Mechanisms* (P. G. Waser, Ed.), pp. 43–57. Raven Press, New York.

Akesson, T. R., and Micevych, P. E. (1988). Estrogen concentration by substance P-immunoreactive neurons in the medial basal hypothalamus of the female rat. *J. Neurosci. Res.*, 19, 412–419.

Akil, H., Bronstein, D., and Mansour, A., (1988). Overview of the endogenous opioid systems: Anatomical, biochemical and functional issues. In *Endorphins, Opiates and Behavioural Processes* (R. J. Rodgers and S. J. Cooper, Eds.), pp. 1–23.Wiley, New York.

Akil, H., and Liebeskind, J. C. (1975). Monoaminergic mechanisms of stimulation-produced analgesia. *Brain Res.*, 94, 279–296.

Akil, H., Mayer, D. J., and Liebeskind, J. C. (1976). Antagonism of stimulation-produced analgesia by naloxone, a narcotic antagonist. *Science*, 191, 961–962.

Akil, H., Richardson, D. E., Barchas, J. D., and Li, C. H. (1978). Appearance of beta-endorphin-like immunoreactivity in human ventricular cerebrospinal fluid upon analgesic electrical stimulation. *Proc. Natl. Acad. Sci. U.S.A.*, 75, 5170–5172.

Akil, H., Richardson, D. E., Hughes, J., and Barchas, J. D. (1978). Enkephalin-like material elevated in ventricular cerebrospinal fluid of pain patients after analgesic focal stimulation. *Science*, 201, 463–465.

Akil, H., Watson, S., Young, E., Lewis, M. E., Khachaturian, H., and Walker, J. W. (1984). Endogenous opioids: Biology and function. *Annu. Rev. Neurosci., 7*, 223–255.

Akunne, H. C., Johannessen, J. N., de Costa, B. R., Rice, K. C., and Rothman, R. B. (1992). MPTP lesions of the nigrostriatal dopaminergic projection decreases [3H]1-[1-(2-thienyl)cyclohexyl]-piperidine binding to PCP site 2: Further evidence that PCP site 2 is associated with the biogenic amine reuptake complex. *Neurochem. Res., 17*, 261–264.

Akunne, H. C., Reid, A. A., Thurkauf, A., Jacobson, A. E., De Costa, B. R., Rice, K. C., Heyes, M. P., and Rothman, R. B. (1991). [3H]1-[2-(2-thienyl)cyclohexyl]piperidine labels two high-affinity binding sites in human cortex: Further evidence for phencyclidine binding sites associated with the biogenic amine reuptake complex. *Synapse, 8*, 289–300.

Alavi, A., and Reivich, M. (1986). Determination of regional function with 18-F-flurodeoxyglucose: Comparison with nuclear magnetic resonance imaging. In *PET and NMR: New Perspectives in Neuroimaging and in Clinical Neurochemistry* (L. Battistin and F. Gerstenbrand, Eds.), pp. 355–380. Alan R. Liss, New York.

Albers, R. W., Siegel, G. J., and Stahl, W. L. (1989). Membrane transport. In *Basic Neurochemistry: Molecular, Cellular, and Medical Aspects* (4th ed.) (G. J. Siegel, B. W. Agranoff, R. W. Albers, and P. B. Molinoff, Eds.), pp. 49–70. Raven Press, New York.

Albert, P. R. (1992). Molecular biology of the 5-HT$_{1A}$ receptor: Low-stringency cloning and eukaryotic expression. *J. Chem. Neuroanat., 5*, 283–288.

Alberts, P. (1993). Subtype classification of presynaptic α_2-adrenoceptors. *Gen. Pharmacol., 24*, 1–8.

Albin, M. S., Bunegin, L., and Garcia, C. (1990). Ketamine and postanesthetic emergence reactions. In *Status of Ketamine in Anesthesiology* (E. F. Domino, Ed.), pp. 17–25. NPP Books, Ann Arbor.

Albin, R. L., Young, A. B., and Penney, J. B. (1989). The functional anatomy of basal ganglia disorders. *Trends Neurosci., 12*, 366–375.

Albuquerque, E. X., Aguayo, L. G., Warnick, J. E., Ickowicz, R. K., and Blaustein, M. P. (1983). Interactions of phencyclidine with ion channels of nerve and muscle: Behavioral implications. *Fed. Proc., 42*, 2584–2589.

Alcoholics Anonymous (1955). *The Story of How Thousands of Men and Women Have Recovered from Alcoholism.* AA World Services, New York.

Alexander, G. E., and Crutcher, M. D. (1990). Functional architecture of basal ganglia circuits: Neural substrates of parallel processing. *Trends Neurosci., 13*, 266–271.

Alford, S., and Grillner, S. (1991). The involvement of GABA$_B$ receptors and coupled G-proteins in spinal GABAergic presynaptic inhibition. *J. Neurosci., 11*, 3718–3726.

Ali, S. F., David, S. N., Newport, G. D., Cadet, J. L., and Slikker, W. Jr. (1994). MPTP-induced oxidative stress and neurotoxicity are age-dependent: Evidence from measures of reactive oxygen species and striatal dopamine levels. *Synapse, 18*, 27–34.

Allaoua, H., and Chicheportiche, R. (1989). Anaesthetic properties of phencyclidine (PCP) and analogues may be related to their interaction with Na$^+$ channels. *Eur. J. Pharmacol., 163*, 327–335.

Allen, R. M., and Young, S. J. (1978). Phencyclidine-induced psychosis. *Am. J. Psychiatry, 135*, 1081–1084.

Allen, T. O., Adler, N. T., Greenberg, J. H., and Reivich, M. (1981). Vaginocervical stimulation selectively increases metabolic activity in the rat brain. *Science, 211*, 1070–1072.

Alling, C. (1985). Biochemical maturation of the brain and the concept of vulnerable periods. In *Alcohol and the Developing Brain* (U. Rydberg, C. Alling, and J. Engel, Eds.), pp. 5–10. Raven Press, New York.

Almay, B. G. L., Johansson, F., Von Knorring, L., Sakurada, T., and Terenius, L. (1985). Long-term high frequency transcutaneous electrical nerve stimulation (hi-TNS) in chronic pain. Clinical response and effects on CSF-endorphins, monoamine metabolites, substance P-like immunoreactivity (SPLI) and pain measures. *J. Psychosom. Res., 29*, 247–257.

Alreja, M., and Aghajanian, G. K. (1993). Opiates suppress a resting sodium-dependent inward current in addition to activating an outward potassium current in locus coeruleus neurons. *J. Neurochem., 13*, 3525–3532.

Alzheimer, A. (1907). Uber eine eigenartige Erkrankung der Hirnrinde (On a peculiar disease of the cerebral cortex). *Allge. Z. Psychiatr., 64*, 146–148.

Amano, K., et al. (1982). Endorphins and pain relief. Further observations on electrical stimulation of the lateral part of the periaqueductal gray mattter during rostral mesencephalic reticulotomy for pain relief. *J. Appl. Neurophysiol., 45*, 123–135.

Amara, S. G., and Kuhar, M. J. (1993). Neurotransmitter transporters: Recent progress. *Annu. Rev. Neurosci., 16*, 73–93.

American Psychiatric Association. (1987). *Diagnostic and Statistical Manual of Mental Disorders* (3rd ed., revised). American Psychiatric Association, Washington, D.C.

American Psychiatric Association. (1994). *Diagnostic and Statistical Manual of Mental Disorders* (4th ed.). American Psychiatric Association, Washington, D.C.

Andén, N. E., Fuxe, K., Hamberger, B., and Hökfelt, T. (1966). A quantitative study of the nigro-neostriatal dopamine neuron system in the rat. *Acta Physiol. Scand., 67*, 306–312.

Andersen, P. H. (1989). The dopamine uptake inhibitor GBR 12909: Selectivity and molecular mechanism of action. *Eur. J. Pharmacol., 166*, 493–504.

Andersen, P. H., Gingrich, J. A., Bates, M. D., Dearry, A., Falardeau, P., Senogles, S. E., and Caron, M. G. (1990). Dopamine receptor subtypes: Beyond the D$_1$/D$_2$ classification. *Trends Pharmacol. Sci., 11*, 231–236.

Andersen, P. H., Grønvald, F. C., Hohlweg, R., Hansen, L. B., Guddal, E., Braestrup, C., and Nielsen, E. B. (1992). NNC-112, NNC-687 and NNC-756, new selective and highly potent dopamine D$_1$ receptor antagonists. *Eur. J. Pharmacol., 219*, 45–52.

Andersen, P. H., and Jansen, J. A. (1990). Dopamine receptor agonists: Selectivity and dopamine D$_1$ receptor efficacy. *Eur. J. Pharmacol., 188*, 335–347.

Anderson, E. J., McFarland, D., and Kimelberg, H. K. (1992). Serotonin uptake by astrocytes in situ. *Glia, 6*, 154–158.

Andersson, K. (1975). Effects of cigarette smoking on learning and retention. *Psychopharmacologia, 41*, 1–5.

Andersson, K. K., Cox, D. D., Que, L. Jr., Flatmark, T., and Haavik, J. (1988). Resonance Raman studies on the blue-green-colored bovine adrenal tyrosine 3-monooxygenase (tyrosine hydroxylase). *J. Biol. Chem., 263*, 18621–18626.

Andrade, R. (1992). Electrophysiology of 5-HT$_{1A}$ receptors in the rat hippocampus and cortex. *Drug Dev. Res., 26*, 275–286.

Andrade, R., and Chaput, Y. (1991). The electrophysiology of serotonin receptor subtypes. In *Serotonin Receptor Subtypes: Basic and Clinical Aspects* (S. J. Peroutka, Ed.), pp. 103–124. Wiley-Liss, New York.

Andreasen, N. C. (1987). The diagnosis of schizophrenia. *Schizophr. Bull., 13*, 25–38.

Andreasen, N. C. (1990). Positive and negative symptoms: Historical and conceptual aspects. In *Modern Problems of Pharmacopsychiatry* (T. A. Ban, A. M. Freedman, C. G. Gottfries, R. Levy, P. Pinchot, and W. Poldinger, Eds.), pp. 1–42. S. Karger, Basel.

Andreasen, N. C., Arndt, S., Alliger, R., Miller, D., and Flaum M. (1995). Symptoms of schizophrenia: Methods, meanings, and mechanisms. *Arch. Gen. Psychiatry, 15*, 341–351.

Andreasen, N. C., Arndt, S., O'Leary, D., Flaum, M., and Nopoulos, P. (1995). Clinical presentation and cognitive disfunction in schizophrenia. In *Critical Issues in the Treatment of Schizophrenia* (N. Brunello, G. Racagni, S. Z. Langer, and J. Mendlewicz, Eds.), pp. 1–8. Karger, Basel.

Andreasen, N. C., Flashman, L., Flaum, M., Arndt, S., Swayze, V., O'Leary, D. S., Ehrhardt, I. C., and Yuh, W. T. (1994). Regional brain abnormalities in schizophrenia measured with magnetic resonance imaging. *JAMA, 272*, 1763–1769.

Andreasen, N., Nasrallah, H. A., Dunn, V., Olson, S. C., Grove, W. M., Ehrhardt, J. C., Coffman, J. A., and Crossett, J. H. W. (1986). Structural abnormalities in the frontal system in schizophrenia. *Arch. Gen. Psychiatry, 43*, 136–144.

Andrews, J. M., and Nemeroff, C. B. (1994). Contemporary management of depression. *Am. J. Med., 97*(6A), 24s–32s.

Andrews, J. S., and Broekkamp, C. L. E. (1993). Procedures to identify anxiolytic or anxiogenic agents. In *Behavioural Neuroscience: A Practical Approach*, Vol. 2 (A. Sahgal, Ed.), pp. 37–54. Oxford University Press, New York.

Angeletti, P. U. (1971). Chemical sympathectomy in newborn animals. *Neuropharmacology, 10*, 55–59.

Angulo, J. A., and McEwen, B. S. (1994). Molecular aspects of neuropeptide regulation and function in the corpus striatum and nucleus accumbens. *Brain Res. Rev., 19*, 1–28.

Angus, J. A., Dyke, A. C., and Korner, P. I. (1990). Estimation of the role of presynaptic α_2-adrenoceptors in the circulation: Influence of neuronal uptake. *Ann. N.Y. Acad. Sci., 604*, 55–68.

Anholt, R. R. H. (1986). Mitochondrial benzodiazepine receptors as potential modulators of intermediary metabolism. *Trends Pharmacol. Sci.*, 7, 506–511.

Anis, N. A., Berry, S. C., Burton, N. R., and Lodge, D. (1983). The dissociative anesthetics, ketamine and phencyclidine, selectively reduce excitation of central mammalian neurones by N-methyl-aspartate. *Br. J. Pharmacol.*, 79, 565–575.

Antin, J., Gibbs, J., Holt, J., Young, R. C., and Smith, G. P. (1975). Cholecystokinin elicits the complete behavioral sequence of satiety in rats. *J. Comp. Physiol. Psychol.*, 89, 784–790.

Aoki, C., Joh, T. H., and Pickel, V. M. (1987). Ultrastructural localization of β-adrenergic receptor-like immunoreactivity in the cortex and neostriatum of rat brain. *Brain Res.*, 437, 264–282.

Appel, J. B., and Freedman, D. X. (1968). Tolerance and cross tolerance among psychotomimetic drugs. *Psychopharmacologia*, 13, 267–274.

Appel, J. B., and Rosecrans, J. A. (1984). Behavioral pharmacology of hallucinogens in animals: Conditioning studies. In *Hallucinogens: Neurochemical, Behavioral, and Clinical Perspectives* (B. L. Jacobs, Ed.), pp. 77–94. Raven Press, New York.

Appel, S. H. (1981). A unifying hypothesis for the cause of amyotrophic lateral sclerosis, Parkinsonism, and Alzheimer disease. *Ann. Neurol.*, 10, 499–505.

Appleyard, M. E. (1992). Secreted acetylcholinesterase: Non-classical aspects of a classical enzyme. *Trends Neurosci.*, 15, 485–490.

Aprison, M. H., and Daly, E. C. (1978). Biochemical aspects of transmission at inhibitory synapses: The role of glycine. In *Advances in Neurochemistry*, Vol. 3 (B. W. Agranoff and M. H. Aprison, Eds.), pp. 203–294. Plenum Press, New York.

Aprison, M. H., and Werman, R. (1965). The distribution of glycine in cat spinal cord and roots. *Life Sci.*, 4, 2075–2083.

Apter, A., van Praag, H. M., Plutchik, R., Sevy, S., Korn, M., and Brown, S.-L. (1990). Interrelationships among anxiety, aggression, impulsivity, and mood: A serotonergically linked cluster? *Psychiatry Res.*, 32, 191–199.

Arai, R., Karasawa, N., Geffard, M., Nagatsu, T., and Nagatsu, I. (1994). Immunohistochemical evidence that central serotonin neurons produce dopamine from exogenous l-DOPA in the rat, with reference to the involvement of aromatic L-amino acid decarboxylase. *Brain Res.*, 667, 295–299.

Arana, G. W., and Baldessarini, R. J. (1987). Clinical use of the dexamethasone suppression test in psychiatry. In *Psychopharmacology: The Third Generation of Progress* (H. Y. Meltzer, Ed.), pp. 609–618. Raven Press, New York.

Arango, V., Ernsberger, P., and Marzuk, P. M. (1990). Autoradiographic demonstration of increased serotonin 5-HT$_2$ and β-adrenergic receptor binding sites in the brain of suicide victims. *Arch. Gen. Psychiatry*, 47, 1038–1045.

Arbuthnott, G. W., Fairbrother, I. S., and Butcher, S. P. (1990). Dopamine release and metabolism in the rat striatum: An analysis by in vivo brain microdialysis. *Pharmacol. Ther.*, 48, 281–293.

Arch, J. R. S., Ainsworth, A. T., Cawthorne, M. A., Piercy, V., Sennitt, M. V., Thody, V. E., Wilson, C., and Wilson, S. (1984). Atypical β-adrenoceptor on brown adipocytes as target for anti-obesity drugs. *Nature*, 309, 163–165.

Argiolas, A., and Gessa, G. L. (1991). Central functions of oxytocin. *Neurosci. Biobehav. Rev.*, 15, 217–231.

Ariano, M. A., and Sibley, D. R. (1994). Dopamine receptor distribution in the rat CNS: Elucidation using anti-peptide antisera directed against D$_{1A}$ and D$_3$ subtypes. *Brain Res.*, 649, 95–110.

Arluison, M., Agid, Y., and Javoy, F. (1978). Dopaminergic nerve endings in the neostriatum of the rat. 1. Identification by intracerebral injections of 5-hydroxydopamine. *Neuroscience*, 3, 657–673.

Armstrong, C. M., and Hille, B. (1972). The inner *quaternary* ammonium ion receptor in potassium channels of the node of Ranvier. *J. Gen. Physiol.*, 59, 388–400.

Armstrong, R. A., Myers, D., and Smith, C. U. M. (1993). The spatial patterns of plaques and tangles in Alzheimer's disease do not support the "cascade hypothesis." *Dementia*, 4, 16–20.

Armstrong, R. C., and Montminy, M. R. (1993). Transsynaptic control of gene expression. *Annu. Rev. Neurosci.*, 16, 17–29.

Arnaud, N. J. (1993). Metabolism of caffeine and other components of coffee. In *Caffeine, Coffee, and Health* (S. Garattini, Ed.), pp. 43–95. Raven Press, New York.

Arnhoff, F. N. (1975). Social consequences of policy toward mental illness. *Science*, 188, 1277–1281.

Arnold, A. P. (1985). Gonadal steroid-induced organization and reorganization of neural circuits involved in bird song. In *Synaptic Plasticity* (C. W. Cotman, Ed.), pp. 263–285. Guilford Press, New York.

Arnold, A. P., Bottjer, S. W., Nordeen, E. S., Nordeen, K. W., and Sengelaub, D. R. (1987). Hormones and critical periods in behavioral and neural development. In *Imprinting and Cortical Plasticity* (J. P. Rauschecker and P. Marler, Eds.), pp. 55–97. John Wiley, New York.

Arnold, E. B., Molinoff, P. B., and Rutledge, C. O. (1977). The release of endogenous norepinephrine and dopamine from cerebral cortex by amphetamine. *J. Pharmacol. Exp. Ther.*, 202, 544–557.

Arnt, J., Hyttel, J., and Sánchez, C. (1992). Partial and full dopamine D$_1$ receptor agonists in mice and rats: Relation between behavioural effects and stimulation of adenylate cyclase in vitro. *Eur. J. Pharmacol.*, 213, 259–267.

Aronson, M., and Olegård, R. (1985). Fetal alcohol effects in pediatrics and child psychology. In *Alcohol and the Developing Brain* (U. Rydberg, C. Alling, and J. Engel, Eds.), pp. 135–145. Raven Press, New York.

Aronson, S. C., Black, J. E., McDougle, C. J., Scanley, B. E., Jatlow, P., Kosten, T. R., Heninger, G. R., and Price, L. H. (1995). Serotonergic mechanisms of cocaine effects in humans. *Psychopharmacology*, 119, 179–185.

Arrang, J.-M., Garbarg, M., Lancelot, J.-C., Lecomte, J.-M., Pollard, H., Robba, M., Schunack, W., and Schwartz, J.-C. (1987). Highly potent and selective ligands for histamine H$_3$-receptors. *Nature*, 327, 117–123.

Arrang, J.-M., Garbarg, M., and Schwartz, J.-C. (1983). Auto-inhibition of brain histamine release mediated by a novel classs (H$_3$) of histamine receptor. *Nature*, 302, 832–837.

Arrang, J.-M., Garbarg, M., and Schwartz, J.-C. (1987). Autoinhibition of histamine synthesis mediated by presynaptic H$_3$-receptors. *Neuroscience*, 23, 149–157.

Artigas, F., Romero, L., de Montigny, C., and Blier, P. (1996). Acceleration of the effect of selected antidepressant drugs in major depression by 5-HT$_{1A}$ antagonists. *Trends Neurosci.*, 19, 378–383.

Artola, A., and Singer, W. (1993). Long-term depression of excitatory synaptic transmission and its relationship to long-term potentiation. *Trends Neurosci.*, 16, 480–487.

Arvanitaki, A., and Chalazonitis, N. (1961). Excitatory and inhibitory processes. In *Nervous Inhibition* (E. Fleury, Ed.), pp. 194–231. Pergamon Press, London.

Åsberg, M., Schalling, D., Träskman-Bendz, L., and Wägner, A. (1987). Psychobiology of suicide, impulsivity, and related phenomena. In *Psychopharmacology: The Third Generation of Progress* (H. Y. Meltzer, Ed.), pp. 655–668. Raven Press, New York.

Åsberg, M., Träskman, L., and Thorén, P. (1976). 5-HIAA in the cerebrospinal fluid: A biochemical suicide predictor? *Arch. Gen. Psychiatry*, 33, 1193–1197.

Ascher, P., and Nowak, L. (1988). The role of divalent cations in the N-methyl-D-aspartate responses of mouse central neurons in culture. *J. Physiol. (Lond.)*, 399, 247–266.

Ash, A. S. F., and Schild, H. O. (1966). Receptors mediating some actions of histamine. *Br. J. Pharmacol. Chemother.*, 27, 427–439.

Ashman, D. F., Lipton, R., Melicow, M. M., and Price, T. D. (1963). Isolation of adenosine 3',5'-monophosphate and guanosine 3',5'-monophosphate from rat urine. *Biochem. Biophys. Res. Commun.*, 11, 330–334.

Asin, K. E., Bednarz, L., Nikkel, A. L., Gore, P. A. Jr., and Nadzan, A. M. (1992). A-71623, a selective CCK-A receptor agonist, suppresses food intake in the mouse, dog, and monkey. *Pharmacol. Biochem. Behav.*, 42, 699–704.

Aston-Jones, G. (1985). Behavioral functions of locus coeruleus derived from cellular attributes. *Physiol. Psychol.*, 13, 118–126.

Aston-Jones, G., and Bloom, F. E. (1981a). Activity of norepinephrine-containing locus coeruleus neurons in behaving rats anticipates fluctuations in the sleep–waking cycle. *J. Neurosci.*, 1, 876–886.

Aston-Jones, G., and Bloom, F. E. (1981b). Norepinephrine-containing locus coeruleus neurons in behaving rats exhibit pronounced responses to non-noxious environmental stimuli. *J. Neurosci.*, 1, 887–900.

Aston-Jones, G., Ennis, M., Pieribone, V. A., Nickell, W. T., and Shipley, M. T. (1986). The brain nucleus locus coeruleus: Restricted afferent control of a broad efferent network. *Science*, 234, 734–737.

Aston-Jones, G., Rajkowski, J., Kubiak, P., and Alexinsky, T. (1994). Locus coeruleus neurons in monkey are selectively activated by attended cues in a vigilance task. *J. Neurosci.*, 14, 4467–4480.

Atack, J. R., Broughton, H. B., and Pollack, S. J. (1995a). Inositol monophosphatase—a putative target for lithium in the treatment of bipolar disorder. *Trends Neurosci.*, 18, 343–349.

Atack, J. R., Broughton, H. B., and Pollack, S. J. (1995b). Structure and mechanism of inositol monophosphatase. *FEBS Lett.*, 361, 1–7.

Atkinson, J., Richtand, N., Schworer, C., Kuczenski, R., and Soderling, T. (1987). Phosphorylation of purified rat striatal tyrosine hydroxylase by Ca^{2+}/calmodulin-dependent protein kinase II: Effect of an activator protein. *J. Neurochem.*, 49, 1241–1249.

Auerbach, S. B., Minzenberg, M. J., and Wilkinson, L. O. (1989). Extracellular serotonin and 5-hydroxyindoleacetic acid in hypothalamus of the unanesthetized rat measured by in vivo dialysis coupled to high-performance liquid chromatography with electrochemical detection: Dialysate serotonin reflects neuronal release. *Brain Res.*, 499, 281–290.

Avissar, S., Barki-Harrington, L, Nechamkin, Y., Roitman, G, and Schreiber, G. (1996). Reduced β-adrenergic receptor-coupled G_s protein function and G_{sa} immunoreactivity in mononuclear leukocytes of patients with depression. *Biol. Psychiatry*, 39, 755–760.

Avissar, S., Schreiber, G., and Danon, A. (1988). Lithium inhibits adrenergic and cholinergic increases in GTP binding in rat cortex. *Nature*, 331,440–442.

Awapara, J., Landua, A. J., Fuerst, R., and Seale, B. (1950). Free γ-aminobutyric acid in brain. *J. Biol. Chem.*, 187, 35–39.

Awouters, F. (1985). The pharmacology of ketanserin, the first selective serotonin S_2-antagonist. *Drug Dev. Res.*, 6, 263–300.

Axelrod, J. (1971). Noradrenaline: Fate and control of its biosynthesis. *Science,* 173, 598–606.

Axt, K. J., Mamounas, L. A., and Molliver, M. E. (1994). Structural features of amphetamine neurotoxicity in the brain. In *Amphetamine and its Analogs* (A. K. Cho, Ed.), pp. 315–367. Academic Press, San Diego.

Azami, J., Llewelyn, M. D., and Roberts, M. H. T. (1982). The contribution of nucleus reticularis paragigantocellularis and nucleus raphe magnus to the analgesia produced by systemically administered morphine, investigated with the microinjection technique. *Pain*, 12, 229–246.

Azari, N. P., Pietrini, P., Horwitz, B., Pettigrew, K. D., Leonard, H. L., Rapoport, J. L., Schapiro, M. B., and Swedo, S. E. (1993). Individual differences in cerebral metabolic patterns during pharmacotherapy in obsessive–compulsive disorder: A multiple regression/discriminant analysis of positron emission tomographic data. *Biol. Psychiatry*, 34, 798–809.

Azmitia, E. C. (1978). The serotonin-producing neurons of the midbrain median and dorsal nuclei. In *Handbook of Psychopharmacology*, Vol. 9 (L. L. Iversen, S. D. Iversen, and S. H. Snyder, Eds.), pp. 233–314. Plenum Press, New York.

Azorlosa, J. L., Greenwald, M. K., and Stitzer, M. L. (1995). Marijuana smoking: Effects of varying puff volume and breathhold duration. *J. Pharmacol. Exp. Ther.*, 272, 560–569.

Azrin, N. H. (1976). Improvements in the community reinforcement approach to alcoholism. *Behav. Res. Ther.*, 14, 339–348.

Azuma, S. D., and Chasnoff, I. J. (1993). Outcome of children prenatally exposed to co-

caine or other drugs: A path analysis of three-year data. *Pediatrics*, 92, 396–402.

Azzaro, A. J., Amedro, J. B., Brown, L. M., Smith, D. J., and Williams, G. M. (1988). The effect of selective Type A or Type B monoamine oxidase inhibition on the intrasynaptosomal deamination of [³H]serotonin in rat spinal cord tissue. *Naunyn Schmiedebergs Arch. Pharmacol.*, 338, 9–13.

Azzaro, A. J., Ziance, R. J., and Rutledge, C. O. (1974). The importance of neuronal uptake of amines for amphetamine-induced release of ³H-norepinephrine from isolated brain tissue. *J. Pharmacol. Exp. Ther.*, 189, 110–118.

Baber, N. S., Dourish, C. T., and Hill, D. R. (1989). The role of CCK, caerulein, and CCK antagonists in nociception. *Pain*, 39, 307–328.

Babu, Y. S., Sack, J. S., Greenhough, T. J., Bugg, C. E., Means, A. R., and Cook, W. J. (1985). Three-dimensional structure of calmodulin. *Nature*, 315, 37–40.

Bach, A. W. J., Lan, N. C., Johnson, D. L., Abell, C. W., Bembenek, M. E., Kwan, S.-W., Seeburg, P. H., and Shih, J. C. (1988). cDNA cloning of human liver monoamine oxidase A and B: Molecular basis of differences in enzymatic properties. *Proc. Natl. Acad. Sci. U.S.A.*, 85, 4934–4938.

Bach, R. O., and Gallicchio, V. S. (Eds.), (1990). *Lithium and Cell Physiology*. Springer-Verlag, New York.

Backover, A. (1991). Native Americans: Alcoholism, FAS put a race at risk. *Guidepost* (Am. Assoc. Counsel. Dev.), May 9, 1–8.

Bagetta, G., Nisticò, G., and Bowery, N. B. (1991). Characteristics of tetanus toxin and its exploitation in neurodegenerative studies. *Trends Pharmacol. Sci.*, 12, 285–289.

Bailey, C. H., and Chen, M. (1983). Morphological basis of long-term habituation and sensitization in *Aplysia. Science,* 220, 91–93.

Baimbridge, K. G., Celio, M. R., and Rogers, J. H. (1992). Calcium-binding proteins in the nervous system. *Trends Neurosci.*, 15, 303–308.

Baker, L. E., Riddle, E. E., Saunders, R. B., and Appel, J. B. (1993). The role of monoamine uptake in the discriminative stimulus effects of cocaine and related compounds. *Behav. Pharmacol.*, 4, 69–79.

Bakker, C. B., and Amini, F. B. (1961). Observations on the psychotomimetic effects of Sernyl. *Compr. Psychiatry*, 2, 269–280.

Balazs, R., Machiyama, Y., Hammond, B. J., Julian, T., and Richter, D. (1970). The operation of γ-aminobutyrate bypath of the tricarboxylic acid cycle in brain tissue in vitro. *Biochem. J.*, 116, 445–461.

Baldessarini, R. J. (1985). Drugs and the treatment of psychiatric disorders. In *The Pharmacological Basis of Therapeutics* (A. G. Gilman, L. S. Goodman, T. W. Rall and F. Murad, Eds.), pp. 387–445. Macmillan, New York.

Balfour, D. J. K. (1990). Nicotine as the basis for the smoking habit. In *Psychotropic Drugs of Abuse. International Encyclopedia of Pharmacology and Therapeutics*, Section 130 (D. J. K. Balfour, Ed.) pp. 453–481. Pergamon Press, New York.

Ball, J. C., and Corty, E. (1988). Basic issues pertaining to the effectiveness of methadone

maintenance treatment. *NIDA Res. Monogr.*, 86, 178–191.

Ballarín, M., Fredholm, B. B., Ambrosio, S., and Mahy, N. (1991). Extracellular levels of adenosine and its metabolites in the striatum of awake rats: Inhibition of uptake and metabolism. *Acta Physiol. Scand.*, 142, 97–103.

Ballenger, J., Goodwin, F., Major, L., and Brown, G. (1979). Alcohol and central serotonin metabolism in man. *Arch. Gen. Psychiatry*, 36, 324–327.

Bals-Kubik, R., Shippenberg, T. S., and Herz, A. (1990). Involvement of mu- and delta-receptors in mediating the reinforcing effects of beta-endorphin in the rat. *Eur. J. Pharmacol.*, 175, 63–69.

Balster, R. L. (1986). Clinical implications of behavioral pharmacology research on phencyclidine. *NIDA Res. Monogr.*, 64, 148–162.

Balster, R. L., and Chait, L. D. (1976). The behavioral pharmacology of phencyclidine. *Clin. Toxicol.*, 9, 513–528.

Balster, R. L., and Prescott, W. R. (1992). Δ^9-Tetrahydrocannabinol discrimination in rats as a model for cannabis intoxication. *Neurosci. Biobehav. Rev.*, 16, 55–62.

Balster, R. L., and Woolverton, W. L. (1980). Continuous-access phencyclidine self-administration by rhesus monkeys leading to physical dependence. *Psychopharmacology*, 70, 5–10.

Balster, R. L., and Woolverton, W. L. (1981). Tolerance and dependence to phencyclidine. In *PCP (Phencyclidine): Historical and Current Perspectives* (E. F. Domino, Ed.), pp. 293–306. NPP Books, Ann Arbor.

Bandura, A., O'Leary, A., Taylor, C. B., Gauthier, J., and Gossard, D. (1987). Perceived self-efficacy and pain control: Opioid and non-opioid mechanisms. *J. Personality Soc. Psychol.*, 53, 563–571.

Barasch, J. M., Tamir, H., Nunez, E. A., and Gershon, M. D. (1987). Serotonin-storing secretory granules from thyroid parafollicular cells. *J. Neurosci.*, 7, 4017–4033.

Barbeau, A., Rondeau, D. B., and Jolicoeur, F. B. (1980). Behavioral effects of substance P in rats. *Int. J. Neurol.*, 14, 239–252.

Barber, R. P., Vaughn, J. E., Saito, K., McLaughlin, B. J., and Roberts, E. (1978). GABAergic terminals are presynaptic to primary afferent terminals in the substantia gelatinosa of the rat spinal cord. *Brain Res.*, 141, 35–55.

Bard, J. A., Zgombick, J., Adham, N., Vaysse, P., Branchek, T. A., and Weinshank, R. L. (1993). Cloning of a novel human serotonin receptor (5-HT$_7$) positively linked to adenylate cyclase. *J. Biol. Chem.*, 268, 23422–23426.

Bargar, T. M., Broersma, R. J., Creemer, L. C., McCarthy, J. R., Hornsperger, J.-M., Palfreyman, M. G., Wagner, J., and Jung, M. J. (1986). Unsaturated heterocyclic amines as potent time-dependent inhibitors of dopamine β-hydroxylase. *J. Med. Chem.*, 29, 315–317.

Bargmann, W., and Scharrer, E. (1951). The site of origin of the hormones of the posterior pituitary. *Am. Sci.*, 39, 255–259.

Baribeau, J., and Laurent, J. P. (1991). Longitudinal studies of clinical and ERP correlates of thought disorder and positive/negative symptoms in schizophrenia. In *Biological Basis of Schizophrenic Disorders* (T. Nakazawa, Ed.), pp. 19–30. Karger, New York.

Barinaga, M. (1992). How scary things get that way. *Science*, 258, 887–888.

Barinaga, M. (1993). Secrets of secretion revealed. *Science*, 260, 487–489.

Barker, E. L., Westphal, R. S., Schmidt, D., and Sanders-Bush, E. (1994). Constitutively active 5-hydroxytryptamine$_{2C}$ receptors reveal novel inverse agonist activity of receptor ligands. *J. Biol. Chem.*, 269, 11687–11690.

Barker, J. C., Gratz, E., Owen, D. G., and Study, R. E. (1984). Pharmacological effects of clinically important drugs on the excitability of cultured mouse spinal neurons. In *Actions and Interactions of GABA and Benzodiazepines* (N. G. Bowery, Ed.), pp. 203–216. Raven Press, New York.

Barker, J. L., and Gainer, H. (1973). Pentobarbital: Selective depression of excitatory postsynaptic potentials. *Science*, 182, 720–722.

Barnard, E. A. (1995). The molecular biology of GABA$_A$ receptors and their structural determinants. In *GABA$_A$ Receptors and Anxiety: From Neurobiology to Treatment* (G. Biggio, E. Sanna, and E. Costa, Eds.), pp. 1–16. Raven Press, New York.

Barnes, D. E., Hanauer, S. A., Slade, J., Bero, L. A., Glantz, S. A. (1995). Environmental tobacco smoke: The Brown and Williamson Documents. *JAMA*, 248–253.

Barnes, J. M., Barnes, N. M., and Cooper, S. J. (1992). Behavioural pharmacology of 5-HT$_3$ receptor ligands. *Neurosci. Biobehav. Rev.*, 16, 107–113.

Barnett, G., Licko, V., and Thompson, T. (1985). Behavioral pharmacokinetics of marijuana. *Psychopharmacology*, 85, 51–56.

Barnett, J. V., and Kuczenski, R. (1986). Desensitization of rat striatal dopamine-stimulated adenylate cyclase after acute amphetamine administration. *J. Pharmacol. Exp. Ther.*, 237, 820–825.

Baron, J. C., and Maziere, B. (1986). Positron emission tomography studies of central receptors in humans. In *PET and NMR: New Perspectives in Neuroimaging and in Clinical Neurochemistry* (L. Battistin and F. Gerstenbrand, Eds.), pp. 83–99. Alan R. Liss, New York.

Baron, M. (1995). Genes and psychosis: Old wine in new bottles? *Acta Psychiatr. Scand.*, 92, 81–86.

Barr, G. A., Paredes, W., and Bridger, W. H. (1985). Place conditioning with morphine and phencyclidine: Dose dependent effects. *Life Sci.*, 36, 363–368.

Barraco, R. A., Martens, K. A., Parizon, M., and Normile, H. J. (1993). Adenosine A$_{2a}$ receptors in the nucleus accumbens mediate locomotor depression. *Brain Res. Bull.*, 31, 397–404.

Barrett, J. E., and Gleeson, S. (1991). Anxiolytic effects of 5-H^{1A} agonists, 5-HT$_3$ antagonists and benzodiazepines: Conflict and drug discrimination studies. In *5-HT$_{1A}$ Agonists, 5-HT$_3$ Antagonists and Benzodiazepines: Their Comparative Behavioral Pharmacology* (R. J. Rogers and J. Gleeson, Eds.), pp. 59–105. Wiley, New York.

Barrett, J. E., and Vanover, K. E. (1993). 5-HT receptors as targets for the development of novel anxiolytic drugs: Models, mechanisms and future directions. *Psychopharmacology*, 112, 1–12.

Barrett, R. L., and Appel, J. B. (1989). Effects of stimulation and blockade of dopamine receptor subtypes on the discriminative stimulus properties of cocaine. *Psychopharmacology*, 99, 13–16.

Barron, J., and Sandman, C. A. (1983). Relationship of sedative-hypnotic response to self-injurious behavior and stereotypy by mentally retarded clients. *Am. J. Ment. Retard.*, 88, 177–186.

Bartecchi, C. E., MacKenzie, T. D., and Schrier, R. W. (1994). The human costs of tobacco use. *N. Engl. J. Med.*, 330, 907–912.

Bartfai, T., Iverfeldt, K., Brodin, E., and Ögren, S.-O. (1986). Functional consequences of coexistence of classical and peptide neurotransmitters. *Prog. Brain Res.*, 68, 321–330.

Bartfai, T., Iverfeldt, K., Fisone, G., and Serfözö, P. (1988). Regulation of the release of coexisting neurotransmitters. *Annu. Rev. Pharmacol. Toxicol.*, 28, 285–310.

Barthó, L., and Holzer, P. (1985). Search for a physiological role of substance P in gastrointestinal motility. *Neuroscience*, 16, 1–32.

Bartus, R. T., Dean, R. L. III, Beer, B., and Lippa, A. S. (1982). The cholinergic hypothesis of geriatric memory dysfunction. *Science*, 217, 408–417.

Bartus, R. T., Dean, R. L., Pontecorvo, M. J., and Flicker, C. (1985). The cholinergic hypothesis: A historical overview, current perspective, and future directions. *Ann. N.Y. Acad. Sci.*, 444, 332–358.

Bassuk, E. L., and Gerson, S. (1978). Deinstitutionalization and mental health services. *Sci. Am.*, 238 (2), 46–53.

Battaglia, G., Shannon, M., Borgundvaag, B., and Titeler, M. (1983). Properties of ^{3}H-prazosin labeled α$_1$-adrenergic receptors in rat brain and porcine neurointermediate lobe tissue. *J. Neurochem.*, 41, 538–542.

Battaglia, G. Shannon, M., and Titeler, M. (1983). Modulation of brain S$_2$ serotonin receptors by lithium, sodium, and potassium chloride. *Life Sci.*, 32, 2597–2601.

Bättig, K., and Welzl, H. (1993). Psychopharmacological profile of caffeine. In *Caffeine, Coffee, and Health* (S. Garattini, Ed.), pp. 213–253. Raven Press, New York.

Baulieu, E. E. (1981). Steroid hormones in the brain: Several mechanisms? In *Steroid Hormone Regulation of the Brain* (K. Fuxe, J. A. Gustafsson, and L. Wetterberg, Eds.), pp. 3–14. Pergamon Press, Oxford.

Baumgarten, H. G., Björklund, A., Lachenmayer, L., Rensch, A., and Rosengren, E. (1974). De- and regeneration of the bulbospinal serotonin neurons in the rat following 5,6- or 5,7-dihydroxytryptamine treatment. *Cell Tissue Res.*, 152, 271–281.

Baumgarten, H. G., Björklund, A., Nobin, A., and Stenevi, U. (1971). Long-lasting selective depletion of brain serotonin by 5,6-dihydroxytryptamine. *Acta Physiol. Scand. Suppl.*, 373, 1–15.

Baumgarten, H. G., Jenner, S., Björklund, A., Klemm, H. P., and Schlossberger, H. G. (1982). Serotonin neurotoxins. In *Biology of Serotonergic Transmission* (N. N. Osborne, Ed.), pp. 249–277. Wiley, Chichester.

Baumgarten, H. G., Klemm, H. P., Lachenmayer, L., Björklund, A., Lovenberg, W., and Schlossberger, H. G. (1978). Mode and mechanism of action of neurotoxic indoleamines: A review and a progress report. *Ann. N.Y. Acad. Sci.*, 305, 3–24.

Baumgold, J. (1992). Muscarinic receptor-mediated stimulation of adenylyl cyclase. *Trends Pharmacol. Sci.*, 13, 339–340.

Baxter, C. F. (1976). Some recent advances in studies of GABA metabolism and compartmentation. In *GABA in Nervous System Function* (E. Roberts, T. N. Chase, and D. B. Tower, Eds.), pp. 61–87. Raven Press, New York.

Baxter, G. S., Boyland, P., Gaster, L. M., and King, F. D. (1993). Quaternized renzapride as a potent and selective 5-HT$_4$ receptor agonist. *Bioorg. Med. Chem. Lett.*, 3, 633–634.

Baxter, G., Kennett, G., Blaney, F., and Blackburn, T. (1995). 5-HT$_2$ receptor subtypes: A family re-united? *Trends Pharmacol. Sci.*, 16, 105–110.

Baxter, M. G., Bucci, D. J., Gorman, L. K., Wiley, R. G., and Gallagher, M. (1995). Selective immunotoxic lesions of basal forebrain cholinergic cells: Effects on learning and memory in rats. *Behav. Neurosci.*, 109, 714–722.

Bean, A. J., During, M. J., and Roth, R. H. (1990). Effects of dopamine autoreceptor stimulation on the release of colocalized transmitters: In vivo release of dopamine and neurotensin from rat prefrontal cortex. *Neurosci. Lett.*, 108, 143–148.

Bean, A. J., and Roth, R. H. (1991). Extracellular dopamine and neurotensin in rat prefrontal cortex in vivo: Effects of median forebrain bundle stimulation frequency, stimulation pattern, and dopamine autoreceptors. *J. Neurosci.*, 11, 2694–2702.

Beardsley, P. M., Balster, R. L., and Harris, L. S. (1986). Dependence on tetrahydrocannabinol in rhesus monkeys. *J. Pharmacol. Exp. Ther.*, 239, 311–319.

Bearsdley, P. M., Hayes, B. A., and Balster, R. L. (1990). The self-administration of MK-801 can depend upon drug-reinforcement history, and its discriminative stimulus properties are phencyclidine-like in rhesus monkeys. *J. Pharmacol. Exp. Ther.*, 252, 953–959.

Beavo, J. A., and Reifsnyder, D. H. (1990). Primary sequence of cyclic nucleotide phosphodiesterase isozymes and the design of selective inhibitors. *Trends Pharmacol. Sci.*, 11, 150–155.

Becker, C.-M. (1995). Glycine receptors: Molecular heterogeneity and implications for disease. *The Neuroscientist*, 1, 130–141.

Beckmann, H., and Goodwin, F. K. (1975). Antidepressant response to tricyclics and urinary MHPG in unipolar patients: Clinical response to imipramine and amitriptyline. *Arch. Gen. Psychiatry*, 32, 17–21.

Beckwith, B. E., Petros, T. V., Couk, D. I., and Tinius, T. P. (1990). The effects of vasopressin on memory in healthy adult volunteers: Theoretical and methodological issues. *Ann. N.Y. Acad. Sci.*, 579, 215–226.

Becquet, D., Faudon, M., and Hery, F. (1990). The role of serotonin release and autoreceptors in the dorsalis raphe nucleus in the control of serotonin release in the cat caudate nucleus. *Neuroscience*, 39, 639–647.

Beecher, H. K. (1957). The measurement of pain. *Pharmacol. Rev.*, 9, 59–209.

Beitner-Johnson, D., Guitart, X., and Nestler, E. J. (1991). Dopaminergic brain reward regions of Lewis and Fischer rats display different levels of tyrosine hydroxylase and other morphine- and cocaine-regulated phosphoproteins. *Brain Res.*, 561, 146–149.

Bekkers, J. M. (1993). Enhancement by histamine of NMDA-mediated synaptic transmission in the hippocampus. *Science*, 261, 104–106.

Bekkers, J. M., and Stevens, C. F. (1990). Presynaptic mechanism for long-term potentiation in the hippocampus. *Nature, 346*, 724–729.

Belin, M. F., Nanopoulos, D., Didier, M., Aguera, M., Steinbusch, H., Verhofstad, A., Maitre, M., and Pujol, J. F. (1983). Immunohistochemical evidence for the presence of γ-aminobutyric acid and serotonin in one nerve cell: A study on the raphe nuclei of the rat using antibodies to glutamate decarboxylase and serotonin. *Brain Res., 275*, 329–339.

Bell, C. (1989). Peripheral dopaminergic nerves. *Pharmacol. Ther., 44*, 157–179.

Bell, R., and Hobson, H. (1994). 5-HT$_{1A}$ receptor influences on rodent social and agonistic behavior: A review and empirical study. *Neurosci. Biobehav. Rev., 18*, 325–338.

Belluzi, J. D., Domino, E. F., May, J. M., Bankiewicz, K. S., and McAfee, D. A. (1994). N-0923, a selective dopamine D$_2$ receptor agonist, is efficacious in rat and monkey models of Parkinson's disease. *Mov. Disord., 9*, 147–154.

Belmaker, R. H. (1984). The lessons of platelet monoamine oxidase. *Psychol. Med., 14*, 249–253.

Belmaker, R. H., Schreiber-Avissar, S., Schreiber, G., Kaplan, Z., Givant, Y., Lichtenberg, P., and Zohar, J. (1990). Does the effect of lithium on G-proteins have behavioral correlates? In *Lithium and Cell Physiology* (R. O. Bach and V. S. Gallicchio, Eds.), pp. 94–101. Springer-Verlag, New York.

Ben-Ari, Y., and Aniksztejn, L. (1995). Role of glutamate metabotropic receptors in long-term potentiation in the hippocampus. *Semin. Neurosci., 7*, 127–135.

Ben-Shachar, D., Eshel, G., Riederer, P., and Youdim, M. B. H. (1992). Role of iron and iron chelation in dopaminergic-induced neurodegeneration: Implication for Parkinson's disease. *Ann. Neurol., 32*, S105–S110.

Benes, F. M., Davidson, J., and Bird, E. D. (1986). Quantitative cytoarchitectural studies of the cerebral cortex of schizophrenics. *Arch. Gen. Psychiatry, 43*, 31–35.

Benfenati, F., and Valtorta, F. (1993). Protein phosphorylation in the nerve terminal. *Neurochem. Int., 23*, 27–34.

Benjamin, A. M., and Quastel, J. H. (1981). Acetylcholine synthesis in synaptosomes: Mode of transfer of mitochondrial acetyl coenzyme A. *Science, 213*, 1495–1497.

Bennett, B. A., Hyde, C. E., Pecora, J. R., and Clodfelter, J. E. (1993). Differing neurotoxic potencies of methamphetamine, mazindol, and cocaine in mesencephalic cultures. *J. Neurochem., 60*, 1444–1452.

Bennett, G. W., Marsden, C. A., Fone, K. C. F., Johnson, J. V., and Heal, D. J. (1989). TRH–catecholamine interactions in brain and spinal cord. *Ann. N.Y. Acad. Sci., 553*, 106–120.

Bennett, J. P., and Snyder, S. H. (1975). Stereospecific binding of *d*-lysergic acid diethylamide (LSD) to brain membranes: Relationship to serotonin receptors. *Brain Res., 94*, 523–544.

Bennett, J. P. Jr., and Yamamura, H. I. (1985). Neurotransmitter, hormone, or drug receptor binding methods. In *Neurotransmitter Receptor Binding* (2nd ed.) (H. I. Yamamura, S. J. Enna, and M. J. Kuhar, Eds.), pp. 61–89. Raven Press, New York.

Benovic, J. L., Shorr, R. G. L., Caron, M. G., and Lefkowitz, R. J. (1984). The mammalian β$_2$-adrenergic receptor: Purification and characterization. *Biochemistry, 23*, 4510–4518.

Benowitz, N. L. (1988). Pharmacologic aspects of cigarette smoking, and nicotine addiction. *N. Engl. J. Med., 319*, 1318–1330.

Benowitz, N. L. (1990a). Clinical pharmacology of caffeine. *Annu. Rev. Med., 41*, 227–288.

Benowitz, N. L. (1990b). Clinical pharmacology of inhaled drugs of abuse: Implication in understanding nicotine dependence. *NIDA Res. Monogr., 99*, 12–29.

Benowitz, N. L., Hall, S. M., Herning, R. I., et al. (1983). Smokers of low yield cigarettes do not consume less nicotine. *N. Engl. J. Med., 309*, 139–142.

Bensimon, G., Lacomblez, L., Meininger, V., and the ALS/Riluzole Study Group. (1994). A controlled trial of riluzole in amyotrophic lateral sclerosis. *N. Engl. J. Med., 330*, 585–591.

Bentley, P. J. (1981). *Elements of Pharmacology.* Cambridge University Press, New York.

Benton, D., and Brain, P. F. (1988). The role of opioid mechanisms in social interaction and attachment. In *Endorphins, Opiates and Behavioural Processes* (R. J. Rodgers and S. J. Cooper, Eds.), pp. 217–235. John Wiley and Sons, Ltd., New York.

Benveniste, H., and Huttemeier, P. C. (1990). Microdialysis: Theory and application. *Prog. Neurobiol., 35*, 195–215.

Benyhe, S. (1994). Morphine: New aspects in the study of an ancient compound. *Life Sci., 55*, 969–979.

Benzing, W. C., and Mufson, E. J. (1995). Increased number of NADPH-d-positive neurons within the substantia innominata in Alzheimer's disease. *Brain Res., 670*, 351–355.

Berendsen, H. H. B., Jenck, F., and Broekkamp, C. L. E. (1990). Involvement of 5-HT$_{1C}$-receptors in drug induced penile erections in rats. *Psychopharmacology, 101*, 57–61.

Berg, L., and Morris, J. C. (1994). Diagnosis. In *Alzheimer Disease* (R. D. Terry, R. Katzman, and K. L. Bick, Eds.), pp. 9–25. Raven Press, New York.

Berger, B., Gaspar, P., and Verney, C. (1991). Dopaminergic innervation of the cerebral cortex: Unexpected differences between rodents and primates. *Trends Neurosci., 14*, 21–27.

Berger, F. M., and Ludwig, B. J. (1964). Meprobamate and related compounds. In *Medicinal Chemistry*, Vol. 1, *Psychopharmacological Agents* (M. Gordon, Ed.), pp. 103–135. Academic Press, New York.

Berger, M. and Riemann, D. (1993). REM sleep in depression—an overview. *J. Sleep Res., 2*, 211–223.

Berger, P. A., and Nemeroff, C. B. (1987). Opioid peptides in affective disorders. In *Psychopharmacology: The Third Generation of Progress* (H. Y. Meltzer, Ed.), pp. 637–646. Raven Press, New York.

Berger-Sweeney, J., Heckers, S., Mesulam, M.-M., Wiley, R. G., Lappi, D. A., and Sharma, M. (1994). Differential effects on spatial navigation of immunotoxin-induced cholinergic lesions of the medial septal area and nucleus basalis magnocellularis. *J. Neurosci., 14*, 4507–4519.

Bergman, H., Borg, S., Hindmarsh, T., Indestrom, C-M., and Mutzell, S. (1980). Computed tomography of the brain and neuropsychological assessment of male alcoholic patients and a random sample from the general male population. *Acta Psychiatr. Scand. Suppl., 286*, 77–88.

Bergman, J., Madras, B. K., Johnson, S. E., and Spealman, R. D. (1989). Effects of cocaine and related drugs in nonhuman primates. III. Self-administration by squirrel monkeys. *J. Pharmacol. Exp. Ther., 251*, 150–155.

Berkenbosch, F., DeVente, J., Schipper, J., and Steinbusch, H. W. M. (1987). Quantitative immunocytochemistry of monoamines, neuropeptides and second messengers in nonbiological and biological models. In *Monoaminergic Neurons: Light Microscopy and Ultrascructure* (H. W. M. Steinbusch, Ed.), pp. 167–177. Wiley, New York.

Bernheimer, H., Birkmayer, W., Hornykiewicz, O., Jellinger, K., and Seitelberger, F. (1973). Brain dopamine and the syndromes of Parkinson and Huntington—Clinical, morphological and neurochemical correlations. *J. Neurol. Sci., 20*, 415–455.

Bero, L. A., Barnes, D. E., Hanauer, S. A., Slade, J., Glantz, S. A. (1995). Lawyer control of the tobacco industry's external research program: The Brown and Williamson Documents. *JAMA, 241*–247.

Berridge, C. W., Arnsten, A. F. T., and Foote, S. L. (1993). Noradrenergic modulation of cognitive function: Clinical implications of anatomical, electrophysiological and behavioural studies in animal models. *Psychol. Med., 23*, 557–564.

Berridge, C. W., and Foote, S. L. (1991). Effects of locus coeruleus activation on electroencephalographic activity in neocortex and hippocampus. *J. Neurosci., 11*, 3135–3145.

Berridge, M. J. (1993). Inositol trisphosphate and calcium signalling. *Nature, 361*, 315–325.

Berridge, M. J., Downes, C. P., and Hanley, M. R. (1982). Lithium amplifies agonist-dependent phosphatidylinositol responses in brain and salivary glands. *Biochem. J., 206*, 587–595.

Berry, J., van Gorp, W. G., Herzberg, D. S., Hinkin, C., Boone, K., Steinman, L., and Wilkins, J. N. (1993). Neuropsychological deficits in abstinent cocaine abusers: Preliminary findings after two weeks of abstinence. *Drug Alcohol Depend., 32*, 231–237.

Berry, M. D., Juorio, A. V., and Paterson, I. A. (1994a). The functional role of monoamine oxidases A and B in the mammalian central nervous system. *Prog. Neurobiol., 42*, 375–391.

Berry, M. D., Juorio, A. V., and Paterson, I. A. (1994b). Possible mechanisms of action of (-)deprenyl and other MAO-B inhibitors in some neurologic and psychiatric disorders. *Prog. Neurobiol., 44*, 141–161.

Bertelsen, A., Harvald, B., and Hauge, M. (1977). A Danish twin study of manic-depressive disorders. *Br. J. Psychiatry, 130*, 330–351.

Berthold, C. W. III, Gonzales, R. A., and Moerschbaecher, J. M. (1992). Prazosin attenuates the effects of cocaine on motor activity but not on schedule-controlled behavior in the rat. *Pharmacol. Biochem. Behav., 43*, 111–115.

Bertler, A., and Rosengren, E. (1959). Occurrence and distribution of catecholamines in brain. *Acta Physiol. Scand.*, 47, 350–361.

Bett, W. R. (1946). Benzedrine sulphate in clinical medicine: A survey of the literature. *Postgrad. Med. J.*, 22, 205–218.

Bettler, B., and Mulle, C. (1995). Review: Neurotransmitter receptors II. AMPA and kainate receptors. *Neuropharmacology*, 34, 123–139.

Betz, H. (1991). Glycine receptors: Heterogeneous and widespread in the mammalian brain. *Trends Neurosci.*, 14, 458–461.

Betz, H., and Becker, C.-M. (1988). The mammalian glycine receptor: Biology and structure of a neuronal chloride channel protein. *Neurochem. Int.*, 13, 137–146.

Betz, W. J., and Bewick, G. S. (1992). Optical analysis of synaptic vesicle recycling at the frog neuromuscular junction. *Science*, 255, 200–203.

Beutler, E. (1993). Modern diagnosis and treatment of Gaucher's disease. *Am. J. Dis. Child.*, 11, 1175–1183.

Biaggioni, I., Paul, S., Puckett, A., and Arzubiaga, C. (1991). Caffeine and theophylline as adenosine receptor antagonists in humans. *J. Pharmacol. Exp. Ther.*, 258, 588–593.

Bianchine, J. R. (1985). Drugs for Parkinson's disease, spasticity, and acute muscle spasms. In *The Pharmacological Basis of Therapeutics* (A. G. Gilman, L. S. Goodman, T. W. Rall, and F. Murad, Eds.), pp. 473–490. Macmillan, New York.

Bibliography on Smoking and Health. (1985). Smoking cessation methods. pp. 329–333, Technical Information Center, Office on Smoking and Health, Park Bldg., Room 116, 5600 Fishers Lane, Rockville, Maryland, 20857.

Bickel, W. K., DeGrandpre, R. J., Higgins, S. T., and Hughes, J. R. (1990). Behavioral economics of drug self-administration. I. Functional equivalence of response requirement and drug dose. *Life Sci.*, 47, 1501–1510.

Bickford, P. C., Palmer, M. R., Rice, K. C., Hoffer, B. J., and Freedman, R. (1981). Electrophysiological effects of phencyclidine on rat hippocampal pyramidal neurons. *Neuropharmacology*, 20, 733–742.

Bidaut-Russell, M., Devane, W. A., and Howlett, A. C. (1990). Cannabinoid receptors and modulation of cyclic AMP accumulation in the rat brain. *J. Neurochem.*, 55, 21–26.

Biel, J. H., and Bopp, B. A. (1978). Amphetamines: Structure–activity relationships. In *Handbook of Psychopharmacology*. Vol. 11, *Stimulants* (L. L. Iversen, S. D. Iversen, and S. H. Snyder, Eds.), pp. 1–39. Plenum Press, New York.

Biggio, G., Casu, M., Klimek, V., and Gessa, G. L. (1980). Dopamine synthesis: Tolerance to haloperidol and supersensitivity to apomorphine depend on pre-synaptic receptors. *Adv. Biochem. Psychopharmacol.*, 24, 18–22.

Biguet, N. F., Buda, M., Lamouroux, A., Samolyk, D., and Mallet, J. (1986). Time course of the changes in TH mRNA in rat brain and adrenal medulla after a single injection of reserpine. *EMBO J.*, 5, 287–291.

Billingsley, M. L., Galloway, M. P., and Roth, R. H. (1984). Possible role of protein carboxymethylation in the autoreceptor-mediated regulation of dopamine neurons. In *Neurology and Neurobiology*, Vol. 8B, *Catecholamines* (E. Usdin, A. Carlsson, A. Dahlstrom, and J. Engel, Eds.), pp. 37–41. Alan R. Liss, New York.

Billington, C. J., Levine, A. S., and Morley, J. E. (1983). Are peptides truly satiety agents? A method of testing for neurohumoral satiety effects. *Am. J. Physiol.*, 245, R920–R926.

Birkmayer, W., Knoll, J., Riederer, P., Youdim, M. B. H., Hars, V., and Marton, J. (1985). Increased life expectancy resulting from addition of L-deprenyl to Madopar treatment in Parkinson's disease: A longterm study. *J. Neural Transm.*, 64, 113–127.

Birkmayer, W., Riederer, P., Youdim, M. B. H., and Linauer, W. (1975). The potentiation of the anti-akinetic effect after L-dopa treatment by an inhibitor of MAO-B, deprenyl. *J. Neural Transm.*, 36, 303–326.

Birks, R., and MacIntosh, F. C. (1961). Actylcholine metabolism of a sympathetic ganglion. *Can. J. Biochem. Physiol.*, 39, 787–827.

Birnbaumer, L. (1990). G proteins in signal transduction. *Annu. Rev. Pharmacol. Toxicol.*, 30, 675–705.

Birnbaumer, L., Abramowitz, J., and Brown, A. M. (1990). Receptor–effector coupling by G proteins. *Biochim. Biophys. Acta,* 1031, 163–224.

Birnbaumer, M., Seibold, A., Gilbert, S., Ishido, M., Barberis, C., Antaramian, A., Brabet, P., and Rosenthal, W. (1992). Molecular cloning of the receptor for human antidiuretic hormone. *Nature*, 357, 333–335.

Bischoff, S., Baumann, P., Krauss, J., Maître, L., Vassout, A., Storni, A., and Chouinard, G. (1994). CGP 25454A, a novel and selective presynaptic dopamine autoreceptor antagonist. *Naunyn Schmiedebergs Arch. Pharmacol.*, 350, 230–238.

Bischoff, S., Heinrich, M., Sonntag, J. M., and Krauss, J. (1986). The D-1 dopamine receptor antagonist SCH 23390 also interacts potently with brain serotonin (5-HT$_2$) receptors. *Eur. J. Pharmacol.*, 129, 367–370.

Bishop, M.L., Duben-Engelkirk, S.L., and Fody, E.P. (1996). *Clinical Chemistry: Principles, Procedures, Correlations* (3rd ed.), Lippincott, New York.

Bittiger, H., Froestl, W., Mickel, S. J., and Olpe, H.-R. (1993). GABA$_B$ receptor antagonists: From synthesis to therapeutic applications. *Trends Pharmacol. Sci.*, 14, 391–394.

Bjerkenstedt, L., Edman, G., Hagenfeldt, L., Sedvall, G., and Wiesel, F-A. (1985). Plasma amino acids in relation to cerebrospinal fluid monoamine metabolites in schizophrenic patients and healthy controls. *Br. J. Psychiatry*, 147, 276–282.

Björklund, A., Baumgarten, H. B., and Rensch, A. (1975). 5,7-dhydroxytryptamine: Improvement of its selectivity for serotonin neurons in the CNS by pretreatment with desipramine. *J. Neurochem.*, 24, 833–835.

Black, I. B., Adler, J. E., Dreyfus, C. F., Friedman, W. F., LaGamma, E. F., and Roach, A. H. (1987). Biochemistry of information storage in the nervous system. *Science*, 236, 1263–1268.

Black, I. B., Chikaraishi, D. M., and Lewis, E. J. (1985). Trans-synaptic increase in RNA coding for tyrosine hydroxylase in a rat sympathetic ganglion. *Brain Res.*, 339, 151–153.

Black, J. W., Duncan, W. A. M., Durant, C. J., Ganellin, C. R., and Parsons, M. E. (1972). Definition and antagonism of histamine H$_2$-receptors. *Nature*, 236, 385–390.

Blackburn, J. R., Pfaus, J. G., and Phillips, A. G. (1992). Dopamine functions in appetitive and defensive behaviours. *Prog. Neurobiol.*, 39, 247–279.

Blackwell, B. (1973). Psychotropic drugs in use today. The role of diazepam in medical practice. *JAMA*, 225, 1637–1641.

Blaha, C. D., and Lane, R. F. (1987). Chronic treatment with classical and atypical antipsychotic drugs differentially decreases dopamine release in striatum and nucleus accumbens in vivo. *Neurosci. Lett.*, 78, 199–204.

Blair, L. A. C., Levitan, E. S., Marshall, J., Dionne, V. E., and Barnard, E. A. (1988). Single subunits of the GABA$_A$ receptor form ion channels with properties of the native receptor. *Science*, 242, 577–579.

Blakely, R. D., Berson, H. E., Fremeau, R. T. Jr., Caron, M. G., Peek, M. M., Prince, H. K., and Bradley, C. C. (1991). Cloning and expression of a functional serotonin transporter from rat brain. *Nature*, 354, 66–70.

Blaschko, H. (1939). The specific action of L-dopa decarboxylase. *J. Physiol.*, 96, 50P–51P.

Blasi, J., Chapman, E. R., Link, E., Binz, T., Yamasaki, S., De Camilli, P., Südhof, T. C., Niemann, H., and Jahn, R. (1993). Botulinum neurotoxin A selectively cleaves the synaptic protein SNAP-25. *Nature,* 365, 160–163.

Blass, E. M., Fitzgerald, E., and Kehoe, P. (1987). Interactions between sucrose, pain and isolation distress. *Pharmacol. Biochem. Behav.* 26, 483–489.

Bleuler, E. P. (1950). *Dementia Praecox or the Group of Schizophrenias* (J. Zinkin, trans.). International Universities Press, New York.

Blier, P., and de Montigny, C. (1994). Current advances and trends in the treatment of depression. *Trends Pharmacol. Sci.*, 15, 220–226.

Blier, P., de Montigny, C., and Chaput, Y. (1990). A role for the serotonin system in the mechanism of action of antidepressant treatments: Preclinical evidence. *J. Clin. Psychiatry*, 51 (Suppl. 4), 14–20.

Bliss, E. L., and Ailion, J. (1970). The effect of lithium upon brain neuroamines. *Brain Res.*, 24, 305–310.

Bliss, T. V. P., and Collingridge, G. L. (1993). A synaptic model of memory: Long-term potentation in the hippocampus. *Nature*, 361, 31–39.

Bliss, T. V. P., and Lømo, T. (1973). Long-lasting potentiation of synaptic transmission in the dentate area of the anaesthetized rabbit following stimulation of the perforant path. *J. Physiol.* (Lond.), 232, 331–356.

Blobel, G., Walter, P., Chang, G. N., Goldman, B. M., Erickson, A. H., and Lingappa, V. R. (1979). Translocation of proteins across membranes: The signal hypothesis and beyond. *Symp. Soc. Exp. Biol.*, 33, 9–36.

Block, R. I., Farinpour, R., and Braverman, K. (1992). Acute effects of marijuana on cognition: Relationships to chronic effects and smoking techniques. *Pharmacol. Biochem. Behav.*, 43, 907–917.

Block, R. I., Farinpour, R., and Schlechte, J. A. (1991). Effects of chronic marijuana use on testosterone, luteinizing hormone, follicle stimulating hormone, prolactin and cortisol in men and women. *Drug Alcohol Depend.*, 28, 121–128.

Block, R. I., and Ghoneim, M. M. (1993). Effects of chronic marijuana use on human cognition. *Psychopharmacology*, 110, 219–228.

Block, R. I., and Wittenborn, J. R. (1986). Marijuana effects on the speed of memory retrieval in the letter-matching task. *Int. J. Addictions*, 21, 281–285.

Blombery, P. A., Kopin, I. J., Gordon, E. K., Markey, S. P., and Ebert, M. H. (1980). Conversion of MHPG to vanillylmandelic acid: Implications for the importance of urinary MHPG. *Arch. Gen. Psychiatry*, 37, 1095–1098.

Bloom, F. E. (1985a). Neurohumoral transmission in the central nervous system. In *The Pharmacological Basis of Therapeutics* (A. G. Gilman, L. S. Goodman, T. W. Rall and F. Murad, Eds.), pp. 236–259. Macmillan, New York.

Bloom, F. E. (1985b). Neuropeptides and other mediators in the central nervous system. *J. Immunol.*, 135, 743s–754s.

Bloom, F. E., Algeri, S., Groppetti, A., Revuelta, A., and Costa, E. (1969). Lesions of central norepinephrine terminals with 6-OH-dopamine: Biochemistry and fine structure. *Science*, 166, 1284–1286.

Bloom, F. E., and Fawcett, D. W. (1986). *A Textbook of Histology*. Saunders, Philadelphia.

Bloom, F. E., Segal, D., Ling, N., and Guillemin, R (1976). Endorphins: Profound behavorial effects in rats suggest new etiological factors in mental illness. *Science*, 194, 630–632.

Blum, K., Noble, E. P., Sheridan, P. J. et al. (1990). Allelic association of human dopamine D_2 receptor gene in alcoholism. *JAMA*, 263, 2055–2060.

Blum, R. H., et al. (1969). *Society and Drugs*, Vol. 1, *Drugs*. Jossey-Bass, San Francisco.

Blumstein, L. K., and Crawley, J. N. (1983). Further characterization of a simple, automated exploratory model for the anxiolytic effects of benzodiazepines. *Pharmacol. Biochem. Behav.*, 18, 37–40.

Blundell, J. E. (1991). Pharmacological approaches to appetite suppression. *Trends Pharmacol. Sci.*, 12, 147–157.

Blundell, J. E., and Hill, A. J. (1989). Do serotoninergic drugs decrease energy intake by reducing fat or carbohydrate intake? Effect of *d*-fenfluramine with supplemented weight-increasing diets. *Pharmacol. Biochem. Behav.*, 31, 773–778.

Blundell, J. E., and Hill, A. J. (1991). Appetite control by dexfenfluramine in the treatment of obesity. *Rev. Contemp. Pharmacother.*, 2, 79–92.

Blusztajn, J. K., Liscovitch, M., Mauron, C., Richardson, U. I., and Wurtman, R. J. (1987). Phosphatidylcholine as a precursor of choline for acetylcholine synthesis. *J. Neural Transm.*, 24 (Suppl.), 247–259.

Boadle-Biber, M. C. (1993). Regulation of serotonin synthesis. *Prog. Biophys. Mol. Biol.*, 60, 1–15.

Boadle-Biber, M. C., Johannessen, J. N., Narasimhachari, N., and Phan, T.-H. (1986). Tryptophan hydroxylase: Increase in activity by electrical stimulation of serotonergic neurons. *Neurochem. Int.*, 8, 83–92.

Boadle-Biber, M. C., and Phan, T.-H. (1987). Involvement of calmodulin-dependent phosphorylation in the activation of brainstem tryptophan hydroxylase induced by depolarization of slices or other treatments that

raise intracellular free calcium levels. *Biochem. Pharmacol.*, 36, 1174–1176.

Bobker, D. H., and Williams, J. T. (1990). Ion conductances affected by 5-HT receptor subtypes in mammalian neurons. *Trends Neurosci.*, 13, 169–173.

Bochet, P., Audinat, E., Lambolez, B., Crépel, F., Rossier, J., Iino, M., Tsuzuki, K., and Ozawa, S. (1994). Subunit composition at the single-cell level explains functional properties of a glutamate-gated channel. *Neuron*, 12, 383–388.

Bockaert, J., Fozard, J. R., Dumuis, A., and Clarke, D. E. (1992). The 5-HT$_4$ receptor: A place in the sun. *Trends Pharmacol. Sci.*, 13, 141–145.

Bockaert, J., Pin, J., and Fagni, L. (1993). Metabotropic glutamate receptors: An original family of G protein-coupled receptors. *Fundam. Clin. Pharmacol.*, 7, 473–485.

Bodian, D. (1962). The generalized vertebrate neuron. *Science*, 137, 323–326.

Bodner, R. A., Lynch, T., Lewis, L., and Kahn, D. (1995). Serotonin syndrome. *Neurology*, 45, 219–223.

Bogerts, B., Meertz, E., and Schonfeldt-Bausch, R. (1985). Basal ganglia and limbic system pathology in schizophrenia: A morphometric study of brain volume and shrinkage. *Arch. Gen. Psychiatry*, 42, 784–791.

Bohn, M. C., Cupit, L., Marciano, F., and Gash, D. M. (1987). Adrenal medulla grafts enhance recovery of striatal dopaminergic fibers. *Science*, 237, 913–916.

Boja, J. W., Mitchell, W. M., Patel, A., Kopajtic, T. A., Carroll, F. I., Lewin, A. H., Abraham, P., and Kuhar, M. J. (1992). High-affinity binding of [^{125}I]RTI-55 to dopamine and serotonin transporters in rat brain. *Synapse*, 12, 27–36.

Boksa, P., and Quirion, R. (1987). ^{3}H-Methylcarbachol, a new radioligand for nicotinic cholinergic receptors in brain. *Eur. J. Pharmacol.*, 139, 323–333.

Bolam, J. P., and Smith, Y. (1990). The GABA and substance P input to dopaminergic neurones in the substantia nigra of the rat. *Brain Res.*, 529, 57–78.

Bolch, B. (1990). Detection of messenger RNAs by in situ hybridization with nonradioactive probes. In *In Situ Hybridization Histochemistry* (M.F. Chesselet, Ed.), pp.23–38. CRC Press, Boston.

Bondy, C. A., Whitnall, M. H., Brady, L. S., and Gainer, H. (1989). Coexisting peptides in hypothalamic neuroendocrine systems: Some functional implications. *Cell. Mol. Neurobiol.*, 9, 427–446.

Bönisch, H. (1984). The transport of (–)-amphetamine by the neuronal noradrenaline carrier. *Naunyn Schmiedebergs Arch. Pharmacol.*, 327, 267–272.

Bonner, T. I. (1989). The molecular basis of muscarinic receptor diversity. *Trends Neurosci.*, 12, 148–151.

Bonnet, J.-J., Lemasson, M.-H., and Costentin, J. (1984). Simultaneous evaluation by a double labelling method of drug-induced uptake inhibition and release of dopamine in synaptosomal preparation of rat striatum. *Biochem. Pharmacol.*, 33, 2129–2135.

Bonnie, R. J., and Whitebread, C. H. II (1974). *The Marijuana Conviction. A History of Marijuana Prohibition in the United States*. University Press of Virginia, Charlottesville.

Book, A. A., Wiley, R. G., and Schweitzer, J. B. (1992). Specificity of 192 IgG-saporin for NGF-positive cholinergic basal forebrain neurons in the rat. *Brain Res.*, 590, 350–355.

Bordi, F., and Meller, E. (1989). Enhanced behavioral stereotypies elicited by intrastriatal injection of D_1 and D_2 dopamine agonists in intact rats. *Brain Res.*, 504, 276–283.

Borgers, D., and Menzel, R. (1984). Who smokes the most? An analysis of cigarette consumption in W. Germany by occupations: Implications for prevention strategies. *Berl Munch Tierarztl Wochenschr*, 126, 1092–1096.

Borison, R. L., Pathiraja, A. P., Diamond, B. I., and Meibach, R. C. (1992). Risperidone: Clinical safety and efficacy in schizophrenia. *Psychopharmacol. Bull.*, 28, 213–218.

Bormann, J. (1988). Electrophysiology of GABA$_A$ and GABA$_B$ receptor subtypes. *Trends Neurosci.*, 11, 112–116.

Bormann, J., and Feigenspan, A. (1995). GABA$_C$ receptors. *Trends Neurosci.*, 18, 515–519.

Bormann, J., Hamill, O. P., and Sakmann, B. (1987). Mechanism of anion permeation through channels gated by glycine and γ-aminobutyric acid in mouse cultured spinal neurones. *J. Physiol.*, 385, 243–286.

Borowsky, B., Mezey, E., and Hoffman, B. J. (1993). Two glycine transporter variants with distinct localization in the CNS and peripheral tissues are encoded by a common gene. *Neuron*, 10, 851–863.

Boulanger, J. P., Uhde, T. W., Wolff, E. A. III, and Post, R. M. (1984). Increased sensitivity to caffeine in patients with panic disorders. *Arch. Gen. Psychiatry*, 41, 1067–1071.

Boulenguez, P., Segu, L., Chauveau, J., Morel, A., Lanoir, J., and Delaage, M. (1992). Biochemical and pharmacological characterization of serotonin-O-carboxymethylglycyl[^{125}I]iodotyrosinamide, a new radioiodinated probe for 5-HT$_{1B}$ and 5-HT$_{1D}$ binding sites. *J. Neurochem.*, 58, 951–959.

Boulter, J., Hollmann, M., O'Shea-Greenfield, A., Hartley, M., Deneris, E., Maron, C., and Heinemann, S. (1990). Molecular cloning and functional expression of glutamate receptor subunit genes. *Science*, 249, 1033–1037.

Bouthenet, M. L., Ruat, M., Sales, N., Garbarg, M., and Schwartz, J.-C. (1988). Detailed mapping of histamine H$_1$–receptors in guinea-pig central nervous system established by autoradiography with [^{125}I]iodobolpyramine. *Neuroscience*, 26, 553–600.

Bouyer, J. J., Park, D. H., Joh, T. H., and Pickel, V. M. (1984). Chemical and structural analysis of the relation between cortical inputs and tyrosine hydroxylase-containing terminals in rat neostriatum. *Brain Res.*, 302, 267–275.

Bovet, D., and Staub, A. M. (1937). Action protectrice des éthers phénoliques au cours de l'intoxication histaminique. *C. R. Seances Soc. Biol. Fil.*, 124, 547–549.

Bovetto, S., and Richard, D. (1995). Functional assessment of the 5-HT 1A-, 1B-, 2A/2C- and 3-receptor subtypes on food intake and metabolic rate in rats. *Am. J. Physiol.*, 268, R14–R20.

Bowden, C. L. (1990). Clinical management of anxiety. *Hosp. Pract.*, 25 (Suppl. 2), 31–42.

Bowen, D. M., Smith, C. B., White, P., and Davison, A. N. (1976). Neurotransmitter-related enzymes and indices of hypoxia in senile dementia and other abiotrophies. *Brain*, 99, 459–496.

Bowers, M.B. (1987). The role of drugs in production of schizophreniform psychoses and related disorders. In *Psychopharmacology: The Third Generation of Progress* (H.Y. Meltzer, Ed.), pp. 819–823. Raven Press, New York.

Bowery, N. (1989). GABA_B receptors and their significance in mammalian pharmacology. *Trends Pharmacol. Sci.*, 10, 401–407.

Bowyer, J. F., Spuhler, K. P., and Weiner, N. (1984). Effects of phencyclidine, amphetamine and related compounds on dopamine release from and uptake into striatal synaptosomes. *J. Pharmacol. Exp. Ther.*, 229, 671–680.

Boyce, S., Rupniak, N. M. J., Steventon, M., and Iversen, S. D. (1990). CCK-8S inhibits L-dopa-induced dyskinesias in parkinsonian squirrel monkeys. *Neurology*, 40, 717–718.

Boyce, S., Rupniak, N. M. J., Tye, S., Steventon, M. J., and Iversen, S. D. (1990). Modulatory role for CCK-B antagonists in Parkinson's disease. *Clin. Neuropharmacol.*, 13, 339–347.

Boyson, S. J., McGonigle, P., and Molinoff, P. B. (1986). Quantitative autoradiographic localization of the D_1 and D_2 subtypes of dopamine receptors in rat brain. *J. Neurosci.*, 6, 3177–3188.

Bozarth, M. (1987). Intracranial self-administration procedures for the assessment of drug reinforcement. In *Methods of Assessing the Reinforcing Properties of Abused Drugs* (M. Bozarth, Ed.), pp. 173–188. Springer, New York.

Bozarth, M. A. (1989). New perspectives on cocaine addiction: Recent findings from animal research. *Can. J. Physiol. Pharmacol.*, 67, 1158–1167.

Bozarth, M. A., and Wise, R. A. (1984). Anatomically distinct opiate receptor fields mediate reward and physical dependence. *Science*, 224, 516–518.

Bozarth, M. A., and Wise, R. A. (1985). Toxicity associated with long-term intravenous heroin and cocaine self-administration in the rat. *JAMA*, 254, 81–83.

Braak, H., and Braak, E. (1991). Neuropathological stageing of Alzheimer-related changes. *Acta Neuropathol.*, 82, 239–259.

Braak, H., and Braak, E. (1995). Staging of Alzheimer's disease-related neurofibrillary changes. *Neurobiol. Aging*, 16, 271–284.

Braak, H., Braak, E., Grundke-Iqbal, I., and Iqbal, K. (1986). Occurrence of neuropil threads in the senile human brain and in Alzheimer's disease: A third location of paired helical filaments outside of neurofibrillary tangles and neuritic plaques. *Neurosci. Lett.*, 65, 351–355.

Bradberry, C. W., and Roth, R. H. (1989). Cocaine increases extracellular dopamine in rat nucleus accumbens and ventral tegmental area as shown by *in vivo* microdialysis. *Neurosci. Lett.*, 103, 97–102.

Bradford, H. F. (1986). *Chemical Neurobiology: An Introduction to Neurochemistry*. W. H. Freeman, New York.

Bradley, P. B., Engel, G., Feniuk, W., Fozard, J. R., Humphrey, P. P. A., Middlemiss, D. N., Mylecharane, E. J., Richardson, B. P., and Saxena, P. R. (1986). Proposals for the classification and nomenclature of functional receptors for 5-hydroxytryptamine. *Neuropharmacology*, 25, 563–576.

Brady, J. V., and Lukas, S. E. (Eds.) (1984). Testing drugs for physical dependence potential and abuse liability. *NIDA Res. Monogr.*, 52.

Brady, K. T., Lydiard, R. B., Malcolm, R., and Ballenger, J. C. (1991). Cocaine-induced psychosis. *J. Clin. Psychiatry*, 52, 509–512.

Brady, R. O. (1975). Lipidoses. In *The Nervous System*, Vol. 2, *The Clinical Neurosciences* (D. B. Tower, Ed.), pp. 219–217. Raven Press, New York.

Braestrup, C., Albrechtsen, R., and Squires, R. F. (1977). High densities of benzodiazepine receptors in human cortical areas. *Nature*, 269, 702–704.

Braestrup, C., Honoré, T., Nielsen, M., Petersen, E. N., and Jensen, L. H. (1984). Ligands for benzodiazepine receptors with positive and negative efficacy. *Biochem. Pharmacol.*, 33, 859–862.

Braestrup, C., and Squires, R. F. (1977). Specific benzodiazepine receptors in rat brain characterized by high-affinity [³H]diazepam binding. *Proc. Natl. Acad. Sci. U.S.A.*, 74, 3805–3809.

Brain, P. F. (1981). Differentiating types of attack and defense in rodents. In *Multidisciplinary Approaches to Aggression Research* (P. F. Brain and D. Benton, Eds.), pp. 53–77. Elsevier/North Holland, Amsterdam.

Brammer, G. L., Raleigh, M. J., Ritvo, E. R., Geller, E., McGuire, M. T., and Yuwiler, A. (1991). Fenfluramine effects on serotonergic measures in vervet monkeys. *Pharmacol. Biochem. Behav.*, 40, 267–271.

Branch, C. A., and Knuepfer, M. M. (1992). Adrenergic mechanisms underlying cardiac and vascular responses to cocaine in conscious rats. *J. Pharmacol. Exp. Ther.*, 263, 742–751.

Brandsma, J. M., Maultsby, M. C., and Welsh, R. J. (1981). *The Outpatient Treatment of Alcoholism: A Review and Comparative Study*. University Park Press, Baltimore.

Brann, M. R., Buckley, N. J., and Bonner, T. I. (1988). The striatum and cerebral cortex express different muscarinic receptor mRNAs. *FEBS Lett.*, 230, 90–94.

Brant-Zawadzki, M. (1987). Magnetic resonance imaging principles: The bare necessities. In *Magnetic Resonance Imaging of the Central Nervous System* (M. Brant-Zawadzki and D. Norman, Eds.), pp. 1–12. Raven Press, New York.

Braude, M. C., and Ludford, J. P. (1984). Marijuana effects on the endocrine and reproductive systems. *NIDA Res. Monogr.*, 44.

Brazelton, T. B. (1984). *Neonatal Behavioral Assessment Scale* (2nd ed.). J. B. Lippincott, Philadelphia.

Brazier, M. A. B. (1961). *A History of the Electrical Activity of the Brain*. Pitman Medical, London.

Brenner, H. R. (1991). How the motoneuron regulates acetylcholine receptor channel function in muscle. *News Physiol. Sci.*, 6, 281–286.

Brenowitz, E. A. (1991). Altered perception of species-specific song by female birds after lesions of a forebrain nucleus. *Science*, 251, 303–305.

Brewster, W. K., Nichols, D. E., Riggs, R. M., Mottola, D. M., Lovenberg, T. W., Lewis, M. H., and Mailman, R. B. (1990). *trans*-10,11-dihydroxy-5,6,6a,7,8,12b-hexahydrobenzo[a]phenanthridine: A highly potent selective dopamine D_1 full agonist. *J. Med. Chem.*, 33, 1756–1764.

Brill, L., and Lieberman, L. (1969). *Authority and Addiction*. Little, Brown, Boston.

Brinkman, C. (1984). Supplementory motor area of the monkey's cerebral cortex: Short- and long-term deficits after unilateral ablation and the effects of subsequent callosal section. *J. Neurosci.*, 4, 918–929.

Brinley, F. J. (1974). Excitation and conduction in nerve fibers. In *Medical Physiology*, Vol. I (V. B. Mountcastle, Ed.), pp. 34–76. Mosby, St. Louis.

Britton, D. R., Curzon, P., MacKenzie, R. G., Kebabian, J. W., Williams, J. E. G., and Kerkman, D. (1991). Evidence for involvement of both D1 and D2 receptors in maintaining cocaine self-administration. *Pharmacol. Biochem. Behav.*, 39, 911–915.

Britton, K. T., Ehlers, C. L., and Koob, G. F. (1988). Is ethanol antagonist Ro15–4513 selective for ethanol? *Science*, 239, 648–649.

Broadhurst, A. M., and Briley, M. (1988). Catecholamine and 5-H synthesis ex vivo as an index of in vivo neuronal activity and regulation. *Trends Pharmacol. Sci.*, 9, 349–351.

Brobeck, J. R., Tepperman, J., and Long, C. N. H. (1943). Experimental hypothalamic hyperphagia in the albino rat. *Yale J. Biol. Med.*, 15, 831–853.

Brodmann, K. (1909). *Vergleichende localizationlehr der Grosshirnrinde in ihren Prinzipien dargestellt auf Grund des Zellenbaues*. J. A. Barth, Leipzig.

Broman, J., Anderson, S., and Ottersen, O. P. (1993). Enrichment of glutamate-like immunoreactivity in primary afferent terminals throughout the spinal cord dorsal horn. *Eur. J. Neurosci.*, 5, 1050–1061.

Bronstein, D. M., Przewlocki, R., and Akil, H. (1990). Effects of morphine treatment on proopiomelanocortin systems in rat brain. *Brain Res.*, 519, 102–111.

Brooks, D. J. (1993). Functional imaging in relation to parkinsonian syndromes. *J. Neurol. Sci.*, 115, 1–17.

Brooks, D. J. (1995). Parkinson's disease < a single clinical entity? *Q. J. Med.*, 88, 81–91.

Brotman, A. W., Falk, W. E., and Gelenberg, A. J. (1987). Pharmacologic treatment of acute depressive subtypes. In *Psychopharmacology: The Third Generation of Progress* (H. Y. Meltzer, Ed.), pp. 1031–1040.

Brown, A. M., and Birnbaumer, L. (1990). Ionic channels and their regulation by G protein subunits. *Annu. Rev. Physiol.*, 52, 197–213.

Brown, A. S., Mallinger, A. G., and Renbaum, L. C. (1993). Elevated platelet membrane phosphatidylinositol-4,5-bisphosphate in bipolar mania. *Am. J. Psychiatry*, 150, 1252–1254.

Brown, C. S., and Cooke, S. C. (1994). Attention deficit hyperactivity disorder. Clinical features and treatment options. *CNS Drugs*, 1: 95–106.

Brown, E. E., Damsma, G., Cumming, P., and Fibiger, H. C. (1991). Interstitial 3-methoxytyramine reflects striatal dopamine release: An in vivo microdialysis study. *J. Neurochem.*, 57, 701–707.

Brown, E., Prager, J., Lee, H.-Y., and Ramsey, R. G. (1992). CNS complications of cocaine abuse: Prevalence, pathophysiology, and neuroradiology. *Am. J. Radiol.*, 159, 137–147.

Brown, G. L., Ebert, M. H., Goyer, P. F., Jimerson, D. C., Klein, W. J., Bunney, W. E., and Goodwin, F. K. (1982). Aggression, suicide, and serotonin: Relationships to CSF amine metabolites. *Am. J. Psychiatry,* 139, 741–746.

Brown, G. L., Goodwin, F. K., Bellenger, J. C., and Goyer, P. F. (1981). Cerebrospinal fluid amine metabolites and cyclic nucleotides in human aggression. *Psychopharmacol. Bull.,* 17, 63–65.

Brown, G. L., and Linnoila, M. (1990). CSF serotonin metabolite (5-HIAA) studies in depression, impulsivity, and violence. *J. Clin. Psychiatry,* 51 (4, Suppl.), 31–41.

Brown, R. G., and Marsden, C. D. (1988). "Subcortical dementia": The neuropsychological evidence. *Neuroscience,* 25, 363–387.

Brown, R. G., and Marsden, C. D. (1990). Cognitive function in Parkinson's disease: From description to theory. *Trends Neurosci.,* 13, 21–29.

Brown, R., Colter, N., Corsellia, J. A. N., Crow, T. J., Frith, C. D., Jagoe, R., Johnstone, E. C., and Marsh, L. (1986). Postmortem evidence of structural brain changes in schizophrenia. Differences in brain weight, temporal horn area, and parahippocampal gyrus compared with affective disorder. *Arch. Gen. Psychiatry,* 43, 36–42.

Brown, R. T., and Braden, N. J. (1987). Hallucinogens. *Pediatr. Clin. North Am.,* 34 (2), 341–347.

Brown, S.-L., Steinberg, R. L., and van Praag, H. M. (1994). The pathogenesis of depression: Reconsideration of neurotransmitter data. In *Handbook of Depression and Anxiety* (J. A. den Boer and J. M. Ad Sitsen, Eds.), pp. 317–347. Marcel Dekker, New York.

Browne, R. G. (1982). Discriminative stimulus properties of phencyclidine. In *Drug Discrimination: Applications in CNS Pharmacology* (F. C. Colpaert and J. L. Slangen, Eds.), pp. 109–122. Elsevier Biomedical Press, New York.

Browne, R. G. (1986). Discriminative stimulus properties of PCP mimetics. *NIDA Res. Monogr.,* 64, 134–147.

Brücke, T., Kornhuber, J., Angelberger, P., Asenbaum, S., Frassine, H., and Podreka, I. (1993). SPECT imaging of dopamine and serotonin transporters with [^{123}I]β-CIT. Binding kinetics in the human brain. *J. Neural Transm.,* 94, 137–146.

Bruinvels, A. T., Palacios, J. M., and Hoyer, D. (1993). Autoradiographic characterisation and localisation of 5-HT$_{1D}$ compared to 5-HT$_{1B}$ binding sites in rat brain. *Naunyn Schmiedebergs Arch. Pharmacol.,* 347, 569–582.

Brunner, H. G., Nelen, M., Breakefield, X. O., Ropers, H. H., and van Oost, B. A. (1993). Abnormal behavior associated with a point mutation in the structural gene for monoamine oxidase A. *Science,* 262, 578–580.

Brunner, H. G., Nelen, M. R., van Zandvoort, P., Abeling, N. G. G. M., van Gennip, A. H., Wolters, E. C., Kuiper, M. A., Ropers, H. H., and van Oost, B. A. (1993). X-linked borderline mental retardation with prominent behavioral disturbance: Phenotype, genetic localization, and evidence for disturbed monoamine metabolism. *Am. J. Hum. Genet.,* 52, 1032–1039.

Bruns, R. F., Lu, G. H., and Pugsley, T. A. (1987). Adenosine receptor subtypes. In *Topics and Perspectives in Adenosine Research*

(E. Gerlach and B. F. Becker, Eds.), pp. 59–73. Springer-Verlag, Berlin.

Bu, D.-F., Erlander, M. G., Hitz, B. C., Tillakaratne, N. J. K., Kaufman, D. L., Wagner-McPherson, C. B., Evans, G. A., and Tobin, A. J. (1992). Two human glutamate decarboxylases, 65-kDa GAD and 67-kDa GAD, are each encoded by a single gene. *Proc. Natl. Acad. Sci. U.S.A.,* 89, 2115–2119.

Buccafusco, J. J. (1992). Neuropharmacologic and behavioral actions of clonidine: Interactions with central transmitters. *Int. Rev. Neurobiol.,* 33, 55–107.

Buchsbaum, M. S. (1990). The frontal lobes, basal ganglia, and temporal lobes as sites for schizophrenia. *Schizophr. Bull.,* 16, 379–390.

Buchsbaum, M. S., and Haier, R. J. (1987). Functional and anatomical brain imaging: Impact on schizophrenia research. *Schizophr. Bull.,* 13, 129–146.

Buchsbaum, M. S., Wu, J., DeLisi, L. E., Holcomb, H. Kessler, R., Johnson, J., King, A. C., Hazlett, E., Langston, K., and Post, R. M. (1986). Frontal cortex and basal ganglia metabolic rates assessed by positron emission tomography with (^{18}F) 2-deoxyglucose in affective illness. *J. Affect. Disord.,* 10, 137–152.

Buck, K. J., and Harris, R. A. (1991). Neuroadaptive responses to chronic alcohol. *Alcohol. Clin. Exp. Res.,* 15, 460–470.

Buckett, K. J., and Saint, D. A. (1989). Cholecystokinin modulates voltage dependent K$^+$ currents in cultured rat hippocampal neurones. *Neurosci. Lett.,* 107, 162–166.

Buckholtz, N. S., Zhou, D., Freedman, D. X., and Potter, W. Z. (1990). Lysergic acid diethylamide (LSD) administration selectively down-regulates serotonin receptors in rat brain. *Neuropsychopharmacology,* 3 (2), 137–148.

Buckley, N. J. (1990). Molecular pharmacology of cloned muscarinic receptors. In *Transmembrane Signalling, Intracellular Messengers and Implications for Drug Development* (S. R. Nahorski, Ed.), pp. 11–30. Wiley, London.

Buckley, N. J., Bonner, T. I., and Brann, M. R. (1988). Localization of a family of muscarinic receptor mRNAs in rat brain. *J. Neurosci.,* 8, 4646–4652.

Buckman, T. D. (1991). Toxicity of MPTP and structural analogs in clonal cell lines of neuronal origin expressing B type monoamine oxidase activity. *Mol. Chem. Neuropathol.,* 15, 87–102.

Buijs, R. M. (1990). Vasopressin and oxytocin localization and putative functions in the brain. *Acta Neurochir. Suppl.,* 47, 86–89.

Buller, A. L., Larson, H. C., Schneider, B. E., Beaton, J. A., Morrisett, R. A., and Monaghan, D. T. (1994). The molecular basis of NMDA receptor subtypes: Native receptor diversity is predicted by subunit composition. *J. Neurosci.,* 14, 5471–5484.

Bunge, R. P., Bunge, M. B., and Bates, M. (1989). Movement of the Schwann cell process during myelination. *J. Cell Biol.,* 109, 273–284.

Bunney, B. G., Bunney, W. E., and Carlsson, A. (1995). Schizophrenia and glutamate. In *Psychopharmacology: The Fourth Generation of Progress* (F. E. Bloom and D. J. Kupfer, Eds.), pp. 1205–1214. Raven Press, New York.

Bunney, B. S. (1992). Clozapine: A hypothesized mechanism for its unique clinical profile. *Br. J. Psychiatr.,* 160 (Suppl. 17), 17–21.

Bunney, B. S., and Aghajanian, G. K. (1975a). Antipsychotic drugs and central dopaminergic neurons: A model for predicting therapeutic efficacy and incidence of extrapyramidal side effects. In *Predictability in Psychopharmacology: Preclinical and Clinical Correlations* (A. Sudilovsky, S. Gershon and B. Beer, Eds.), pp. 225–245. Raven Press, New York.

Bunney, B. S., and Aghajanian, G. K. (1975b). Evidence for drug action on both pre- and postsynaptic catecholamine receptors in the CNS. In *Pre- and Postsynaptic Receptors* (E. Usdin and W. E. Bunney, Eds.), pp. 89–122. Marcel Dekker, New York.

Bunney, B. S., and Aghajanian, G. K. (1978a). d-Amphetamine-induced depression of central dopamine neurons: Evidence for mediation by both autoreceptors and a striatonigral feedback pathway. *Naunyn Schmiedebergs Arch. Pharmacol.,* 304, 255–261.

Bunney, B. S., and Aghajanian, G. K. (1978b). Mesolimbic and mesocortical dopaminergic systems: Physiology and pharmacology. In *Psychopharmacology: A Generation of Progress* (M. A. Lipton, A. DiMascio, and K. F. Killam, Eds.), pp. 159–169. Raven Press, New York.

Bunney, B. S., Walters, J. R., Roth, R. H., and Aghajanian, G. K. (1973). Dopaminergic neurons: Effect of antipsychotic drugs and amphetamine on single cell activity. *J. Pharmacol. Exp. Ther.,* 185, 560–571.

Bunney, W. E., and Garland-Bunney, B. L. (1987). Mechanism of action of lithium in affective illness: Basic and clinical applications. In *Psychopharmacology: The Third Generation of Progress* (H. Y. Meltzer, Ed.), pp. 553–565. Raven Press, New York.

Bunzow, J. R., Van Tol, H. H. M., Grandy, D. K., Albert, P., Salon, J., Christie, M., Machida, C. A., Neve, K. A., and Civelli, O. (1988). Cloning and expression of a rat D$_2$ dopamine receptor cDNA. *Nature,* 336, 783–787.

Burger, P. M., Hell, J., Mehl, E., Krasel, C., Lottspeich, F., and Jahn, R. (1991). GABA and glycine in synaptic vesicles: Storage and transport characteristics. *Neuron,* 7, 287–293.

Burke, M. J., and Preskorn, S. H. (1995). Short-term treatment of mood disorders with standard antidepressants. In *Psychopharmacology: The Fourth Generation of Progress* (F. E. Bloom and D. J. Kupfer, Eds.), pp. 1053–1066. Raven Press, New York.

Burn, J. H., and Dale, H. H. (1915). The action of certain quaternary ammonium bases. *J. Pharmacol. Exp. Ther.,* 6, 417–438.

Burnham, W. M. (1989). The GABA hypothesis of kindling: Recent assay studies. *Neurosci. Biobehav. Rev.,* 13, 281–288.

Burns, R. S., Chiueh, C. C., Markey, S. P., Ebert, M. H., Jacobowitz, D. M., and Kopin, I. J. (1983). A primate model of parkinsonism: Selective destruction of dopaminergic neurons in the pars compacta of the substantia nigra by N-methyl-4-phenyl- 1,2,3,6-tetrahydropyridine. *Proc. Natl. Acad. Sci. U.S.A.,* 80, 4546–4550.

Burns, R. S., and Lerner, S. E. (1976). Perspectives: Acute phencyclidine intoxication. *Clin. Toxicol.,* 9, 477–501.

Burns, R. S., LeWitt, P. A., Ebert, M. H., Pakkenberg, H., and Kopin, I. J. (1985). The clinical syndrome of striatal dopamine deficiency. Parkinsonism induced by 1-methyl-

4-phenyl-1,2,3,6-tetrahydropyridine (MPTP). *N. Engl. J. Med.*, 312, 1418–1421.

Burnstock, G. (1970). Structure of smooth muscle and its innervation. In *Smooth Muscle* (E. Bulbring, A. F. Beading, A. W. Jones and T. Tomita, Eds.), pp. 1–69. Edward Arnold, London.

Burnstock, G. (1983). Recent concepts of chemical communication between excitable cells. In *Dale's Principle and Communication Between Neurones* (N. N. Osborne, Ed.), pp. 7–35. Pergamon Press, Oxford,

Burnstock, G. (1990a). Noradrenaline and ATP as cotransmitters in sympathetic nerves. *Neurochem. Int.*, 17, 357–368.

Burnstock, G. (1990b). Purinergic mechanisms. *Ann. N.Y. Acad. Sci.*, 603, 1–17.

Burt, D. R., Creese, I., and Snyder, S. H. (1977). Antischizophrenic drugs: Chronic treatment elevates dopamine receptor binding in brain. *Science*, 196, 326–328.

Butcher, S. P., Fairbrother, I. S., Kelly, J. S., and Arbuthnott, G. W. (1988). Amphetamine-induced dopamine release in the rat striatum: An in vivo microdialysis study. *J. Neurochem.*, 50, 346–355.

Butcher, S. P., Fairbrother, I. S., Kelly, J. S., and Arbuthnott, G. W. (1990). Effects of selective monoamine oxidase inhibitors on the in vivo release and metabolism of dopamine in the rat striatum. *J. Neurochem.*, 55, 981–998.

Buterbaugh, G. G., and Michaelson, H. B. (1986). Anticonvulsant properties of phencyclidine and ketamine. *NIDA Res. Monogr.*, 64, 67–79.

Butler, P. D., Weiss, J. M., Stout, J. C., and Nemeroff, C. B. (1990). Corticotropin-releasing factor produces fear-enhancing and behavioral activating effects following infusion into the locus coeruleus. *J. Neurosci.*, 10, 176–183.

Bylund, D. B., Eikenberg, D. C., Hieble, J. P., Langer, S. Z., Lefkowitz, R. J., Minneman, K. P., Molinoff, P. B., Ruffolo, R. R. Jr., and Trendelenburg, U. (1994). IV. International Union of Pharmacology Nomenclature of Adrenoceptors. *Pharmacol. Rev.*, 46, 121–136.

Bzdega, T., Chin, H., Kim, H., HoJung, H., Kozak, C. A., and Klee, W. A. (1993). Regional expression and chromosomal localization of the "delta" opiate receptor gene. *Proc. Natl. Acad. Sci. U.S.A.*, 90, 9305–9399.

Cadet, J. L., Sheng, P., Ali, S., Rothman, R., Carlson, E., and Epstein, C. J. (1994). Attenuation of methamphetamine-induced neurotoxicity in copper/zinc superoxide dismutase transgenic mice. *J. Neurochem.*, 62, 380–383.

Cai, X., Golde, T. E., and Younkin, S. G. (1993). Release of excess amyloid-β protein from a mutant amyloid-β protein precursor. *Science*, 259, 514–516.

Caine, S. B., and Koob, G. F. (1993). Modulation of cocaine self-administration in the rat through D-3 dopamine receptors. *Science*, 260, 1814–1816.

Caine, S. B., and Koob, G. F. (1994). Effects of dopamine D-1 and D-2 antagonists on cocaine self-administration under different schedules of reinforcement in the rat. *J. Pharmacol. Exp. Ther.*, 270, 209–218.

Caine, S. B., Lintz, R., and Koob, G. F. (1993). Intravenous drug self-administration technique in animals. In *Behavioural Neuroscience: A Practical Approach*, Vol. 2 (A. Sahgal, Ed.), pp. 117–144. Oxford University Press, New York.

Calabrese, J. R., Bowden, C, and Woyshville, M. J. (1995). Lithium and the anticonvulsants in the treatment of bipolar disorder. In *Psychopharmacology: The Fourth Generation of Progress* (F. E. Bloom and D. J. Kupfer, Eds.), pp. 1099–1112. Raven Press, New York.

Calabresi, P., Pisani, A., Mercuri, N. B., and Bernardi, G. (1996). The corticostriatal projection from synaptic plasticity to dysfunctions of the basal ganglia. *Trends Neurosci.*, 19, 19–24.

Caldecott-Hazard, S., Morgan, D. G., DeLeon-Jones, F., Overstreet, D. H., and Janowsky, D. (1991). Clinical and biochemical aspects of depressive disorders: II. Transmitter/receptor theories. *Synapse*, 9, 251–301.

Caldwell, A. E. (1970). History of psychopharmacology. In *Principles of Psychopharmacology* (W. G. Clark and J. del Giudice, Eds.), pp. 9–30. Academic Press, New York.

Caldwell, J., Dring, L. G., and Williams, R. T. (1972). Metabolism of [¹⁴C]methamphetamine in man, the guinea pig and the rat. *Biochem. J.*, 129, 11–22.

Callahan, C. M., Grant, T. M., Phipps, P., Clark, G., Novack, A. H., Streissguth, A. P., and Raisys, V. A. (1992). Measurement of gestational cocaine exposure: Sensitivity of infants' hair, meconium, and urine. *J. Pediatr.*, 120, 763–768.

Callahan, P. M., Appel, J. B., and Cunningham, K. A. (1991). Dopamine D_1 and D_2 mediation of the discriminative stimulus properties of *d*-amphetamine and cocaine. *Psychopharmacology*, 103, 50–55.

Callahan, P. M., and Cunningham, K. A. (1993). Discriminative stimulus properties of cocaine in relation to dopamine D_2 receptor function in rats. *J. Pharmacol. Exp. Ther.*, 266, 585–592.

Callahan, P. M., De La Garza, R. II, and Cunningham, K. A. (1994). Discriminative stimulus properties of cocaine: Modulation by dopamine D_1 receptors in the nucleus accumbens. *Psychopharmacology*, 115, 110–114.

Callaway, C. W., Kuczenski, R., and Segal, D. S. (1989). Reserpine enhances amphetamine stereotypies without increasing amphetamine-induced changes in striatal dialysate dopamine. *Brain Res.*, 505, 83–90.

Cameron, O. G., Modell, J. G., and Hariharan, M. (1990). Caffeine and human cerebral blood flow: A positron emission tomography study. *Life Sci.*, 47, 1141–1146.

Campbell, I. (1976). The amotivational syndrome and cannabis use with emphasis on the Canadian scene. *Ann. N.Y. Acad. Sci.*, 282, 33–36.

Camps, M., Kelly, P. H., and Palacios, J. M. (1990). Autoradiographic localization of dopamine D_1 and D_2 receptors in the brain of several mammalian species. *J. Neural Transm.*, 80, 105–127.

Cannon, W. B., and Uridil, J. E. (1921). Studies on the conditions of activity in endocrine glands. VIII. Some effects on the denervated heart of stimulating the nerves of the liver. *Am. J. Physiol.*, 58, 353–354.

Caporael, L. R. (1976). Ergotism: The satan loosed in Salem? *Science*, 192, 21–26.

Cappendijk, S. L. T., and Dzolijc, M. R. (1993). Inhibitory effects of ibogaine on cocaine self-administration in rats. *Eur. J. Pharmacol.*, 241, 261–265.

Caraceni, T. (1994). A case for early levodopa treatment of Parkinson's disease. *Clin. Neuropharmacol.*, 17 (Suppl. 3), S38–S42.

Carboni, E., Cadoni, C., Tanda, G. L., and Di Chiara, G. (1989). Calcium-dependent, tetrodotoxin-sensitive stimulation of cortical serotonin release after a tryptophan load. *J. Neurochem.*, 53, 976–978.

Carboni, E., and Di Chiara, G. (1989). Serotonin release estimated by transcortical dialysis in freely moving rats. *Neuroscience*, 32, 637–645.

Carboni, E., Imperato, A., Perezzani, L., and Di Chiara, G. (1989). Amphetamine, cocaine, phencyclidine and nomifensine increase extracellular dopamine concentrations preferentially in the nucleus accumbens of freely moving rats. *Neuroscience*, 28, 653–661.

Cardno, A. G., and Farmer, A. E. (1995). The case for or against heterogenity in the etiology of schizophrenia: The genetic evidence. *Schizophr. Res.*, 17, 153–159.

Cardno, A. G., and McGuffin, P. (1994). The molecular genetics of schizophrenia. *Neuropathol. Applied Neurobiol.*, 20, 344–349.

Carlberg, M., Gundlach, A. L., Mercer, L. D., and Beart, P. M. (1992). Autoradiographic localization of cholecystokinin A and B receptors in rat brain using [¹²⁵I]D-Tyr²⁵-(Nle²⁸,³¹)-CCK 25–33S. *Eur. J. Neurosci.*, 4, 563–573.

Carlen, P. L., Wortzman, G., Holgate, R. C., Wilkinson, D. A., and Rankin, J. G. (1978). Reversible cerebral atrophy in recently abstinent chronic alcoholics measured by computed tomography scans. *Science*, 200, 1076–1078.

Carlson, J. H., Bergstrom, D., and Walters, J. R. (1987). Stimulation of both D_1 and D_2 receptors appears necessary for full expression of postsynaptic effects of dopamine agonists: A neurophysiological study. *Brain Res.*, 400, 205–218.

Carlson, N. R. (1991). *Physiology of Behavior* (4th ed.). Allyn and Bacon, Boston.

Carlson, A. (1959). The occurrence, distribution and physiological role of catecholamines in the nervous system. *Pharmacol. Rev.*, 11, 490–493.

Carlsson, A. (1975a). Dopaminergic autoreceptors. In *Chemical Tools in Catecholamine Research*, Vol. 2 (O. Almgren, A. Carlsson, and J. Engel, Eds.), pp. 219–225. Amsterdam: North Holland.

Carlsson, A. (1975b). Receptor mediated control of dopamine metabolism. In *Pre- and Postsynaptic Receptors* (E. Usdin and W. E. Bunney, Eds.), pp. 49–63. Marcel Dekker, New York.

Carlsson, A. (1987a). Monoamines of the central nervous system. In *Psychopharmacology: The Third Generation of Progress* (H. Y. Meltzer, Ed.), pp. 39–48, Raven Press, New York.

Carlsson, A. (1987b). Perspectives on the discovery of central monoaminergic neurotransmission. *Annu. Rev. Neurosci.*, 10, 19–40

Carlsson, A., Davis, J. N., Kehr, W., Lindqvist, M., and Atack, C. V. (1972). Simultaneous measurement of tyrosine and tryptophan hydroxylase activities in brain in vivo using an inhibitor of the aromatic amino acid decarboxylase. *Naunyn Schmiedebergs Arch. Pharmacol., 275,* 153–168.

Carlsson, A., and Lindqvist, M. (1963). Effect of chlorpromazine or haloperidol on the formation of 3-methoxytyramine and normetanephrine in mouse brain. *Acta Pharmacol. Toxicol., 20,* 140–144.

Carlsson, A., and Lindqvist, M. (1978). Dependence of 5-HT and catecholamine synthesis on concentrations of precursor amino-acids in rat brain. *Naunyn Schmiedebergs Arch. Pharmacol., 303,* 157–164.

Carlsson, A., Lindqvist, M., and Magnusson, T. (1957). 3,5-dihydroxyphenylalanine and 5-hydroxytryptophan as reserpine antagonists. *Nature, 180,* 1200–1202.

Carlsson, A., Lindquist, M., Magnusson, T., and Waldeck, B. (1958). On the presence of 3-hydroxytyramine in brain. *Science, 127,* 471–472.

Carlton, P. (1983). *A Primer of Behavioral Pharmacology.* W. H. Freeman, New York.

Carman, J. S., Post, R. M., Runkle, D. C., Bunney, W. E., and Wyatt, R. J. (1979). Increased serum calcium and phosphorous states. *Br. J. Psychiatry, 135,* 55–61.

Carmichael, W. W., Biggs, D. F., and Gorham, P. R. (1975). Toxicology and pharmacological action of *Anabaena flos-aquae* toxin. *Science, 187,* 542–544.

Carney, J. M., Uwaydah, I. M., and Balster, R. L. (1977). Evaluation of a suspension system for intravenous self-administration studies of water-insoluble compounds in the rhesus monkey. *Pharmacol. Biochem. Behav., 7,* 357–364.

Caroff, S. N., and Mann, S. C. (1988). Neuroleptic malignant syndrome. *Psychopharmacol. Bull., 24,* 25–29.

Carpenter, W. T., Jr. (1987). Approaches to knowledge and understanding of schizophrenia. *Schizophr. Bull., 13,* 17–24.

Carr, G. D., Fibinger, H. C., and Phillips, A. G. (1989). Conditioned place preference as a measure of drug reward. In *The Neurophamacological Basis of Reward* (J. M. Lieberman and S.J Cooper, Eds.), pp. 264–280. Clarendon, Oxford.

Carr, G. D., and White, N. M. (1986). Anatomical dissociation of amphetamine's rewarding and aversive effects: An intracranial microinjection study. *Psychopharmacology, 89,* 340–346.

Carroll, M. E. (1987). A quantitative assessment of phencyclidine dependence produced by oral self-administration in rhesus monkeys. *J. Pharmacol. Exp. Ther., 242,* 405–412.

Carroll, M. E. (1990). PCP and hallucinogens. *Adv. Alcohol. Subst. Abuse, 9,* 167–190.

Carroll, M. E. (1993). The economic context of drug and non-drug reinforcers affects acquisition and maintenance of drug-reinforced behavior and withdrawal effects. *Drug Alcohol Depend., 33,* 201–210.

Carroll, M. E., and Carmona, G. (1991). Effects of food FR and food deprivation on disruptions in food-maintained performance of monkeys during phencyclidine withdrawal. *Psychopharmacology, 104,* 143–149.

Carroll, M. E., France, C. P., and Meisch, R. A. (1981). Intravenous self-administration of etonitazene, cocaine and phencyclidine in rats during food deprivation and satiation. *J. Pharmacol. Exp. Ther., 217,* 241–247.

Carroll, M. E., Krattiger, K. L., Gieske, D., and Sadoff, D. A. (1990). Cocaine-base smoking in rhesus monkeys: Reinforcing and physiological effects. *Psychopharmacology, 102,* 443–450.

Carroll, M. E., Lac, S. T., Asencio, M., and Kragh, R. (1990a). Fluoxetine reduces intravenous cocaine self-administration in rats. *Pharmacol. Biochem. Behav., 35,* 237–244.

Carroll, M. E., Lac, S. T., Asencio, M., and Kragh, R. (1990b). Intravenous cocaine self-administration in rats is reduced by dietary L-tryptophan. *Psychopharmacology, 100,* 293–300.

Carskadon, M., and Dement, W. (1981). Cumulative effects of sleep restriction on daytime sleepiness. *Psychophysiology, 18,* 107–113.

Carter, C. S. (1992). Oxytocin and sexual behavior. *Neurosci. Biobehav. Rev., 16,* 131–144.

Carter, R. B. (1991). Topical capsaicin in the treatment of cutaneous disorders. *Drug Dev. Res., 22,* 109–123.

Carter, W. E. (Ed.) (1980). *Cannabis in Costa Rica.* Institute for the Study of Human Issues, Philadelphia.

Casebolt, T. L., and Jope, R. S. (1989). Long term lithium treatment selectively reduces receptor-soupled inositol phopholipid hydrolysis in rat brain. *Biol. Psychiatry, 25,* 329–340.

Cases, O., et al. (1995). Aggressive behavior and altered amounts of brain serotonin and norepinephrine in mice lacking MAOA. *Science, 268,* 1763–1766.

Casey, D. E. (1985). In *Dyskinesia: Research and Treatment* (D. E. Casey, A. V. Christensen and J. Gerlach, Eds.), pp. 88–96. Springer, Berlin.

Casey, D. E. (1987). Tardive diskinesia. In *Psychopharmacology: The Third Generation of Progress* (H. Y. Meltzer, Ed.), pp. 1411–1419. Raven Press, New York.

Casey, D. E. (1992). What makes a neuroleptic atypical? In *Novel Antipsychotic Drugs* (H. Y. Meltzer, Ed.), pp. 241–251. Raven Press, New York.

Cash, R., Ruberg, M., Raisman, R., and Agid, Y. (1984). Adrenergic receptors in Parkinson's disease. *Brain Res., 322,* 269–275.

Castle, N. A., Haylett, D. G., and Jenkinson, D. H. (1989). Toxins in the characteriztion of potassium channels. *Trends Neurosci., 12,* 59–65.

Catterall, W. A. (1988). Structure and function of voltage-sensitive ion channels. *Science, 242,* 50–61.

Catterall, W. A. (1993a). Structure and function of voltage-gated ion channels. *Trends Neurosci., 16,* 500–506.

Catterall, W. A. (1993b). Structure and modulation of Na^+ and Ca^{2+} channels. *Ann. N.Y. Acad. Sci., 707,* 1–19.

Cawthorne, M. A. (1981). Is tolerance to anorectic drugs a real phenomenon or an experimental artifact? In *Anorectic Agents: Mechanisms of Action and Tolerance* (S. Garattini and R. Samanin, Eds.), pp. 1–17. Raven Press, New York.

Ceccarelli, B., and Hurlbut, W. P. (1975). The effects of prolonged repetitive stimulation in hemicholinium on the frog neuromuscular junction. *J. Physiol.* (Lond.), 247, 163–188.

Ceccarelli, B., Hurlbut, W. P., and Mauro, A. (1972). Depletion of vesicles from frog neuromuscular junctions by prolonged tetanic stimulation. *J. Cell Biol., 54,* 30–38.

Cederbaum, J. M and Aghajanian, G. K. (1977). Catecholamine receptors on locus coeruleus neurons: Pharmacological characterization. *Eur. J. Pharmacol., 44,* 375–385.

Cella, S. G., Locatelli, V., and Muller, E. E. (1993). Opioid peptides in the regulation of anterior pituitary hormones. In *Opioids II,* Handbook of Experimental Pharmacology, Vol. 104 (A. Herz, Ed.), pp. 473–496. Springer-Verlag, New York.

Cenci, M. A., Campbell, K., Wictorin, K., and Björklund, A. (1992). Striatal c-*fos* induction by cocaine or apomorphine occurs preferentially in output neurons projecting to the substantia nigra in the rat. *Eur. J. Neurosci., 4,* 376–380.

Cepeda, C., Buchwald, N. A., and Levine, M. S. (1993). Neuromodulatory actions of dopamine in the neostriatum are dependent upon the excitatory amino acid receptor subtypes activated. *Proc. Natl. Acad. Sci. U.S.A., 90,* 9576–9580.

Cepeda-Benito, A. A. (1993). A meta-analytical review of the efficacy of nicotine chewing gum. *J. Consult. Clin. Psychol., 61,* 822–830.

Cepeda-Benito, A., and Tiffany, S. T. (1992). Effect of number of conditioning trials on the development of associative tolerance to morphine. *Psychopharmacology, 109,* 172–176.

Chait, L. D., and Burke, K. A. (1994). Preference for high- versus low-potency marijuana. *Pharmacol. Biochem. Behav., 49,* 643–647.

Chait, L. D., Evans, S. M., Grant, K. A., Kamien, J. B., Johanson, C. E., and Shuster, C. R. (1988). Discriminative stimulus and subjective effects of smoked marijuana in humans. *Psychopharmacology, 94,* 206–212.

Chait, L. D., Uhlenhuth, E. H., and Johanson, C. E. (1984). An experimental paradigm for studying the discriminative stimulus properties of drugs in humans. *Psychopharmacology, 82,* 272–274.

Chait, L. D., Uhlenhuth, E. H., and Johanson, C. E. (1986). The discriminative stimulus and subjective effects of *d*-amphetamine, phenmetrazine, and fenfluramine in humans. *Psychopharmacology, 89,* 301–306.

Chalmers, D. T., Lovenberg, T. W., Grigoriadis, D. E., Behan, D. P., and De Souza, E. B. (1996). Corticotrophin-releasing factor receptors: From molecular biology to drug design. *Trends Pharmacol. Sci., 17,* 166–172.

Chan, P., Di Monte, D. A., Luo, J.-J., DeLanney, L. E., Irwin, I., and Langston, J. W. (1994). Rapid ATP loss caused by methamphetamine in the mouse striatum: Relationship between energy impairment and dopaminergic neurotoxicity. *J. Neurochem., 62,* 2484–2487.

Chan-Palay, V., and Palay, S. L. (1977). Immunocytochemical identification of substance P cells and their processes in rat sensory ganglia and their terminals in the spinal cord: Light microscopic studies. *Proc. Natl. Acad. Sci. U.S.A.,* 74, 3597–3601.

Chang, H. T. (1988). Substance P–dopamine relationship in the rat substantia nigra: A light and electron microscopy study of double immunocytochemically labeled materials. *Brain Res.,* 448, 391–396.

Chang, J. K., Fong, B. T. W., Pert, C. B., and Pert, A. (1976). Opiate receptor affinities and behavioral effects of enkephalin: Structure-activity relationship of ten synthetic peptide analogues. *Life Sci., 18,* 1473–1482.

Chang, K-J., and Cuatrecasas, P. (1979). Multiple opiate receptors. *J. Biol. Chem.,* 254, 2610–2618.

Chang, M. M., and Leeman, S. E. (1970). Isolation of a sialogogic peptide from bovine hypothalamic tissue and its characterization as substance P. *J. Biol. Chem.,* 245, 4784–4790.

Chang, R. S. L., Chen, T. B., Bock, M. G., Freidinger, R. M., Chen, R., Rosegay, A., and Lotti, V. J. (1989). Characterization of the binding of [³H]L-365,260: A new potent and selective brain cholecystokinin (CCK-B) and gastrin receptor antagonist radioligand. *Mol. Pharmacol.,* 35, 803–808.

Changeux, J.-P. (1990). The nicotinic acetylcholine receptor: An allosteric protein prototype of ligand-gated ion channels. *Trends Pharmacol. Sci.,* 11, 485–492.

Changeux, J.-P. (1993). Chemical signalling in the brain. *Sci. Am.,* November, 269:58–62.

Changeux, J.-P., Devillers-Thiéry, A., and Chemouilli, P. (1984). Acetylcholine receptor: An allosteric protein. *Science,* 225, 1335–1345.

Chaouloff, F. (1993). Physiopharmacological interactions between stress hormones and central serotonergic systems. *Brain Res. Rev.,* 18, 1–32.

Chaput, Y., de Montigny, C., and Blier, P. (1986). Effects of a selective 5-HT reuptake blocker, citalopram, on the sensitivity of 5-HT autoreceptors: Electrophysiological studies in the rat brain. *Naunyn Schmiedebergs Arch. Pharmacol.,* 333, 342–348.

Charness, M. E., Simon, R. P., and Greenberg, D. A. (1989). Ethanol and the nervous system. *N. Engl. J. Med.,* 321, 442–454.

Charney, D. S., Heninger, G. R., and Jatlow, P. I. (1985). Increased anxiogenic effects of caffeine in panic disorders. *Arch. Gen. Psychiatry,* 42, 233–243.

Charney, D. S., Krystal, J. H., Southwick, S. M., and Delgado, P. L. (1994). The role of noradrenergic function in human anxiety and depression. In *Handbook of Depression and Anxiety* (J. A. den Boer and J. M. A. Sitsen, Eds.), pp. 473–496. Marcel Dekker, New York.

Charney, D. S., Southwick, S. M., Delgado, P. L., and Krystal, J. H. (1990). Current status of the receptor sensitivity hypothesis of antidepressant action: Implications for the treatment of severe depression. In *Pharmacotherapy of Depression: Applications for the Outpatient Practitioner* (J. D. Amsterdam, Ed.), pp. 13–34. Marcel Dekker, New York.

Charuchinda, C., Supavilai, P., Karobath, M., and Palacios, J. M. (1987). Dopamine D₂ receptors in the rat brain: Autoradiographic visualization using a high-affinity selective agonist ligand. *J. Neurosci.,* 7, 1352–1360.

Chase, T. N., Fabbrini, G., Juncos, J. L., and Mouradian, M. M. (1990). Motor response complications with chronic levodopa therapy. *Adv. Neurol.,* 53, 377–381.

Checler, F. (1995). Processing of the β-amyloid precursor protein and its regulation in Alzheimer's disease. *J. Neurochem.,* 65, 1431–1444.

Chen, G., and Bohner, B. (1961). Anticonvulsant properties of 1-(-phenylcyclohexyl) piperidine HCl and certain other drugs. *Proc. Soc. Exp. Biol. Med.,* 106, 632–635.

Chen, G., Ensor, C. R., Russell, D., and Bohner, B. (1959). The pharmacology of 1-(1-phenylcyclohexyl) piperidine HCl. *J. Pharmacol. Exp. Ther.,* 127, 241–250.

Chen, G. G., Chalazonitis, A., Shen, K. F., and Crain, S. M. (1988). Inhibitor of cyclic AMP-dependent protein kinase blocks opioid-induced prolongation of the action potential of mouse sensory ganglion neurons in dissociated cell cultures. *Brain Res.,* 462, 372–377.

Chen, J., Paredes, W., Li, J., Lowinson, J., and Gardner, E. L. (1990). Δ⁹-tetrahydrocannabinol produces naloxone-blockable enhancement of presynaptic basal dopamine efflux in nucleus accumbens of conscious, freely-moving rats as measured by intracerebral microdialysis. *Psychopharmacology,* 102, 156–162.

Chen, J., Paredes, W., Lowinson, J. H., and Gardner, E. L. (1990). Δ⁹-tetrahydrocannabinol enhances presynaptic dopamine efflux in medial prefrontal cortex. *Eur. J. Pharmacol.,* 190, 259–262.

Chen, K., Wu, H.-F., and Shih, J. C. (1993). The deduced amino acid sequences of human platelet frontal cortex monoamine oxidase B are identical. *J. Neurochem.,* 61, 187–190.

Chen, Y., Mestek, A., Liu, J., Hurley, J. A., and Yu, L. (1993). Molecular cloning and functional expression of a "mu"-opioid receptor from rat brain. *Mol. Pharmacol.,* 44, 8–12.

Cheramy, A., Leviel, V., and Glowinski, J. (1981). Dendritic release of dopamine in substantia nigra. *Nature,* 289, 537–542.

Cherkas, M. S. (1965). Synanon Foundation: A radical approach to the problem of addiction. *Am. J. Psychiatry,* 121, 1065–1068.

Chesselet, M.-F. (1990). *In Situ Hybridization Histochemistry.* CRC Press, Boca Raton.

Chevalier, G., and Deniau, J. M. (1990). Disinhibition as a basic process in the expression of striatal functions. *Trends Neurosci.,* 13, 277–280.

Chiang, C. N., and Barnett, G. (1989). Marijuana pharmacokinetics and pharmacodynamics. In *Cocaine, Marijuana, Designer Drugs: Chemistry, Pharmacology, and Behavior* (K. K. Redda, C. A. Walker, and G. Barnett, Eds.), pp. 113–125. CRC Press, Boca Raton.

Chiang, C.-W. N., and Barnett, G. (1984). Marijuana effect and delta-9-tetrahydrocannabinol plasma level. *Clin. Pharmacol. Ther.,* 36: 234–238.

Chiang, P. K., Butler, D. L., and Brown, N. D. (1991). Nicotinic action of anatoxin-a on guinea pig ileum antagonized by thymopentin. *Life Sci.,* 49, PL13–PL19.

Chiappinelli, V. A. (1989). Toxins affecting cholinergic neurons. In *Neuromethods,* Vol. 12, *Drugs as Tools in Neurotransmitter Research* (A. B. Boulton, G. B. Baker, and A. V. Juorio, Eds.), pp. 103–159. Humana Press, Clifton, NJ.

Childers, S. R. (1993). Opioid receptor-coupled second messenger systems. In *Opioids I,* Handbook of Experimental Pharmacology, Vol. 104 (A. Herz, Ed.), pp. 189–216. Springer-Verlag, New York.

Childers, S. R., Fleming, L., Konkoy, C., Marckel, D., Pacheco, M., Sexton, T., and Ward, S. (1992). Opioid and cannabinoid receptor inhibition of adenylyl cyclase in brain. *Ann. N.Y. Acad. Sci.,* 654, 33–51.

Childress, A. R., Hole, A. V., Ehrman, R. N., Robbins, S. J., McLellan, A. T., and O'Brien, C. P. (1993). Cue reactivity and cue reactivity interventions in drug dependence. *NIDA Res. Monogr.,* 137, 73–95.

Childress, A. R., McLellan, T., and O'Brien, C. P. (1986). Abstinent opiate abusers exhibit conditioned craving, conditioned withdrawal and reductions in both through extinction. *Br. J. Addiction,* 81, 655–660.

Chin, J. H. (1989). Adenosine receptors in brain: Neuromodulation and role in epilepsy. *Ann. Neurol.,* 26, 695–698.

Chinaglia, G., Alvarez, F. J., Probst, A., and Palacios, J. M. (1992). Mesostriatal and mesolimbic dopamine uptake binding sites are reduced in Parkinson's disease and progressive supranuclear palsy: A quantitative autoradiographic study using [³H]mazindol. *Neuroscience,* 49, 317–327.

Chio, C. L., Lajiness, M. E., and Huff, R. M. (1994). Activation of heterologously expressed D₃ dopamine receptors: Comparison with D₂ dopamine receptors. *Mol. Pharmacol.,* 45, 51–60.

Chiodo, L. A. (1988). Dopamine-containing neurons in the mammalian central nervous system: Electrophysiology and pharmacology. *Neurosci. Biobehav. Rev.,* 12, 49–91.

Chiodo, L. A. (1992). Dopamine autoreceptor signal transduction in the DA cell body: A "current view." *Neurochem. Int.,* 20 (Suppl.), 81S–84S.

Chiodo, L. A., and Berger, T. W. (1986). Interactions between dopamine and amino acid-induced excitation and inhibition in the striatum. *Brain Res.,* 375, 198–203.

Chiodo, L. A., and Bunney, B. S. (1983). Typical and atypical neuroleptics: Differential effects of chronic administration on the activity of A₉ and A₁₀ midbrain dopamine neurons. *J. Neurosci.,* 3, 1607–1619.

Chipkin, R. E., Iorio, L. C., Coffin, V. L., McQuade, R. D., Berger, J. G., and Barnett, A. (1988). Pharmacological profile of SCH39166: A dopamine D₁ selective benzonaphthazepine with potential antipsychotic activity. *J. Pharmacol. Exp. Ther.,* 247, 1093–1102.

Chiueh, C. C., and Moore, K. E. (1975). Blockade by reserpine of methylphenidate-induced release of brain dopamine. *J. Pharmacol. Exp. Ther.,* 193, 559–563.

Cho, A. K. (1990). Ice: A new dosage form of an old drug. *Science,* 249, 631–634.

Choi, D. W. (1992). Excitotoxic cell death. *J. Neurobiol.,* 23, 1261–1276.

Choi, D. W., Farb, D. H., and Fischbach, G. D. (1977). Chlordiazepoxide selectively augments GABA action in spinal cord cultures. *Nature,* 269, 342–344.

Chopin, P., Moret, C., and Briley, M. (1994). Neuropharmacology of 5-hydroxytryptamine₁B/D receptor ligands. *Pharmacol. Ther.,* 62, 385–405.

Chouinard, G., Jones, B., Remington, G., Bloom, D., Addington, D., MacEwan, G. W., Labelle, A., Beauclair, L., and Arnott, W. (1993). A Canadian multicenter placebo-controlled study of fixed doses of risperidone and haloperidol in the treatment of chronic schizophrenic patients. *J. Clin. Psychopharmacol.,* 13, 25–40.

Christensen, E., Moller, J. E., and Faurbye, A. (1970). Neuropathological investigation of 28 brains from patients with dyskinesia. *Acta Psychiatr. Scand.,* 46, 14.

Christie, B. R., Kerr, D. S., and Abraham, W. C. (1994). Flip side of synaptic plasticity:

Long-term depression mechanisms in the hippocampus. *Hippocampus,* 4, 127–135.

Chu, D. C. M., Albin, R. L., Young, A. B., and Penney, J. B. (1990). Distribution and kinetics of $GABA_B$ binding sites in rat central nervous system: A quantitative autoradiographic study. *Neuroscience,* 34, 341–357.

Chuang, D.-M., and Costa, E. (1974). Biosynthesis of tyrosine hydroxylase in rat adrenal medulla after exposure to cold. *Proc. Natl. Acad. Sci. U.S.A.,* 71, 4570–4574.

Chudomelka, P. J., and Murrin, L. C. (1989). Histamine synthesis in rat hypothalamus is not acutely regulated via histidine decarboxylase. *Neurosci. Lett.,* 107, 216–220.

Ciaranello, R. D. (1978). Regulation of phenylethanolamine *N*-methyltransferase synthesis and degradation. I. Regulation by rat adrenal glucocorticoids. *Mol. Pharmacol.,* 14, 478–489.

Ciaranello, R. D., Wooten, G. F., and Axelrod, J. (1975). Regulation of dopamine β-hydroxylase in rat adrenal glands. *J. Biol. Chem.,* 250, 3204–3211.

Citron, M., Oltersdorf, T., Haass, C., McConlogue, L., Hung, A. Y., Seubert, P., Vigo-Pelfrey, C., Lieberburg, I., and Selkoe, D. J. (1992). Mutation of the β-amyloid precursor protein in familial Alzheimer's disease increases β-protein production. *Nature,* 360, 672–674.

Citron, M., Vigo-Pelfrey, C., Teplow, D. B., Miller, C., Schenk, D., Johnston, J., Winblad, B., Venizelos, N., Lannfelt, L., and Selkoe, D. J. (1994). Excessive production of amyloid β-protein by peripheral cells of symptomatic and presymptomatic patients carrying the Swedish familial Alzheimer disease mutation. *Proc. Natl. Acad. Sci. U.S.A.,* 91, 11993–11997.

Civelli, O., Bunzow, J. R., and Grandy, D. K. (1993). Molecular diversity of the dopamine receptors. *Annu. Rev. Pharmacol. Toxicol.,* 32, 281–307.

Clapham, D. E. (1994). Direct G protein activation of ion channels? *Annu. Rev. Neurosci.,* 17, 441–464.

Clapham, D. E., and Neer, E. J. (1993). New roles for G-protein βγ-dimers in transmembrane signalling. *Nature,* 365, 403–406.

Clark, A. J. (1933). *The Mode of Action of Drugs on Cells.* Arnold, London.

Clark, A. W., Hurlbut, W. P., and Mauro, A. (1972). Changes in the fine structure of the neuromuscular functioning of the frog caused by black widow spider venom. *J. Cell Biol.,* 42, 1–14.

Clark, D., and White, F. J. (1987). Review: D_1 dopamine receptor—The search for a function: A critical evaluation of the D_1/D_2 dopamine receptor classification and its functional implications. *Synapse,* 1, 347–388.

Clark, F. C., and Steele, B. J. (1966). Effects of *d*-amphetamine on performance under a multiple schedule in the rat. *Psychopharmacologia,* 9, 157–169.

Clark, J. A., Deutch, A. Y., Gallipoli, P. Z., and Amara, S. G. 1992. Functional expression and CNS distribution of a β-alanine-sensitive neuronal GABA transporter. *Neuron,* 9, 337–348.

Clarke, P. B. S. (1990). Dopaminergic mechanisms in the locomotor stimulus effects of nicotine. *Biochem. Pharmacol.,* 40, 1427–1432.

Clarke, P. B. S. (1993). Nicotinic receptors in mammalian brain: Localization and relation to cholinergic innervation. *Prog. Brain Res.,* 98, 77–83.

Clarke, P. B. S., and Pert, A. (1985). Autoradiographic evidence for nicotine receptors on nigrostriatal and mesolimbic dopaminergic neurons. *Brain Res.,* 355–358.

Clarke, R. L., Daum, S. J., Gambino, A. J., Aceto, M. D., Pearl, J., Levitt, M., Cumiskey, W. R., and Bogado, E. J. (1973). Compounds affecting the central nervous system. 4. 3β-phenyltropane-2-carboxylic esters and analogs. *J. Med. Chem.,* 16, 1260–1267.

Clarren, S. K. (1990). Fetal alcohol syndrome: Diagnosis, treatment, and mechanisms of teratogenesis. In *Transplacental Disorders: Perinatal Detection, Treatment, and Management (Including Pediatric AIDS),* pp. 37–55. Alan R. Liss, New York.

Clarren, S. K., and Smith, D. W. (1973). The fetal alcohol syndrome. *N. Engl. J. Med.,* 298, 1063–1067.

Clement-Cormier, Y. C., Kebabian, J. W., Petzold, G. L., and Greengard, P. (1974). Dopamine-sensitive adenylate cyclase in mammalian brain: A possible site of action of antipsychotic drugs. *Proc. Natl. Acad. Sci. U.S.A.,* 71, 1113–1117.

Cliffe, I. A., Brightwell, C. I., Fletcher, A., Forster, E. A., Mansell, H. L., Reilly, Y., Routledge, C., and White, A. C. (1993). (S)-N-tert-butyl-3-(4-(2-methoxyphenyl)piperazin-1-yl)-2-phenylpropanamide [(S)-WAY-100135]: A selective antagonist at presynaptic and postsynaptic $5\text{-}HT_{1A}$ receptors. *J. Med. Chem.,* 36, 1509–1510.

Cline, E. J., Scheffel, U., Boja, J. W., Mitchell, W. M., Carroll, F. I., Abraham, P., Lewin, A. H., and Kuhar, M. J. (1992). In vivo binding of [^{125}I]RTI-55 to dopamine transporters: Pharmacology and regional distribution with autoradiography. *Synapse,* 12, 37–46.

Cline, E. J., Terry, P., Carroll, F. I., Kuhar, M. J., and Katz, J. L. (1992). Stimulus generalization from cocaine to analogs with high *in vitro* affinity for dopamine uptake sites. *Behav. Pharmacol.,* 3, 113–116.

Cloninger, C. R. (1987a). Neurogenetic adaptive mechanisms in alcoholism. *Science,* 236, 410–416.

Cloninger, C. R. (1987b). Recent advances in the genetics of anxiety and somatoform disorders. In *Psychopharmacology: The Third Generation of Progress* (H. Y. Meltzer, Ed.), pp. 955–965. Raven Press, New York.

Cloninger, C. R. 1991. D_2 dopamine receptor gene is associated but not linked with alcoholism. *JAMA,* 266:1833–1834.

Cloninger, C. R., Sigvardsson, S., Gilligan, S. R., von Knorring, A. L., Reich, T., and Bohman, M. (1988). Genetic heterogeneity and the classification of alcoholism. *Adv. Alcohol Subst. Abuse,* 7, 3–16.

Coccaro, E. F. (1992). Impulsive aggression and central serotonergic system function in humans: An example of a dimensional brain–behavior relationship. *Int. Clin. Psychopharmacol.,* 7, 3–12.

Coccaro, E. F., Siever, L. J., Klar, H. M., Maurer, G., Cochrane, K., Cooper, T. B., Mohs, R. C., and Davis, K. L. (1989). Serotonergic studies in patients with affective and personality disorders: Correlates with suicidal and aggressive behavior. *Arch. Gen. Psychiatry,* 46, 587–599.

Coggins, P. J., and Zwiers, H. (1991). B-50 (GAP-43): Biochemistry and functional neurochemistry of a neuron-specific protein. *J. Neurochem.,* 56, 1095–1106.

Cohen, A. I., Todd, R. D., Harmon, S., and O'-Malley, K. L. (1992). Photoreceptors of mouse retinas possess D_4 receptors coupled to adenylate cyclase. *Proc. Natl. Acad. Sci. U.S.A.,* 89, 12093–12097.

Cohen, B. D., Rosenbaum, G., Luby, E. D., and Gottlieb, J. S. (1962). Comparison of phencyclidine hydrochloride (Sernyl) with other drugs. *Arch. Gen. Psychiatry,* 6, 395–401.

Cohen, G. (1983). The pathobiology of Parkinson's disease: Biochemical aspects of dopamine neuron senescence. *J. Neural Transm.,* 19 (Suppl.), 89–103.

Cohen, G., Pasik, P., Cohen, B., Leist, A., Mytilineou, C., and Yahr, M. D. (1984). Pargyline and deprenyl prevent the neurotoxicity of 1-methyl-4-phenyl-1,2,3,6-tetrahydropyridine (MPTP) in monkeys. *Eur. J. Pharmacol.,* 106, 209–210.

Cohen, J. B., and Changeux, J.-P. (1975). The cholinergic receptor protein in its membrane environment. *Annu. Rev. Pharmacol.,* 15, 83–103.

Cohen, M. J., and Rickles, W. H. Jr. (1974). Performance on a verbal learning task by subjects of heavy past marijuana usage. *Psychopharmacologia,* 37, 323–330.

Cohen, S. (1969). In *Hearings before the Subcommittee to Investigate Juvenile Delinquency of the Committee on the Judiciary, U.S. Senate, 91st Congress, 1st Session, September 17, 1969,* p. 293. U.S. Government Printing Office. Washington, D.C.

Cohen, S. (1970). The hallucinogens. In *Principles of Psychopharmacology* (W. G. Clarke and J. del Guidice, Eds.), pp. 489–503. Academic Press, New York.

Cohen, S. (1985a). *Reinforcement and Rapid Delivery Systems: Understanding Adverse Consequences of Cocaine. NIDA Res. Monogr.,* 61.

Cohen, S. (1985b). The varieties of psychotic experience. *Psychoactive Drugs,* 17, 291–296.

Cole, S. O. (1978). Brain mechanisms of amphetamine-induced anorexia, locomotion, and stereotypy: A review. *Neurosci. Biobehav. Rev.,* 2, 89–100.

Collier, H. O. J. (1984). Cellular aspects of opioid tolerance and dependence. In *Opioids, Past, Present and Future* (J. Hughes, H.O.J. Collier, M.J. Rance and M.B. Tyers, Eds.), pp. 109–125. Taylor and Frances, London.

Collier, H. O. J., Cuthbert, N. J. and Francis, D. L. (1981). Character and meaning of quasi-morphine withdrawal phenomena elicited by methylxanthines. *Fed. Proc.,* 40, 1513–1518.

Collier, H. O. J., and Roy, A. C. (1974). Morphine-like drugs inhibit the stimulation by E prostaglandins of cyclic AMP formation by rat brain homogenate. *Nature,* 248, 24–27.

Collin, E., Mauborgne, A., Bourgoin, S., Mantelet, S., Ferhat, L., Hamon, M., and Cesselin, F. (1992). Kappa-/mu-receptor interactions in the opioid control of the in vivo release of substance P-like material from the rat spinal cord. *Neuroscience,* 51, 347–355.

Collingridge, G. L., and Bliss, T. V. P. (1987). NMDA receptors: Their role in long-term potentiation. *Trends Neurosci.,* 10, 288–293.

Collingridge, G. L., and Davies, J. (1982). Actions of substance P and opiates in the rat substantia nigra. *Neuropharmacology,* 21, 715–719.

Collins, S. (1993). Recent perspectives on the molecular structure and regulation of the β_2-adrenoceptor. *Life Sci., 52,* 2083–2091.

Collins, S., Altschmied, J., Herbsman, O., Caron, M. G., Mellon, P. L., and Lefkowitz, R. J. (1990). A cAMP response element in the β_2-adrenergic receptor gene confers transcriptional autoregulation by cAMP. *J. Biol. Chem., 265,* 19330–19335.

Collins, S., Caron, M. G., and Lefkowitz, R. J. (1991). Regulation of adrenergic receptor responsiveness through modulation of receptor gene expression. *Annu. Rev. Physiol., 53,* 497–508.

Collins, V. J., Gorospe, C. A., and Rovenstine, E. A. (1960). Intravenous nonbarbiturate, nonnarcotic analgesics: Preliminary studies. I. cyclohexylamines. *Anesth. Analg., 39,* 302–306.

Collis, M. G., and Hourani, S. M. O. (1993). Adenosine receptor subtypes. *Trends Pharmacol. Sci., 14,* 360–366.

Colpaert, F. C., Niemegeers, C. J. E., and Janssen, P. A. J. (1976). Cocaine cue in rats as it relates to subjective drug effects: A preliminary report. *Eur. J. Pharmacol., 40,* 195–199.

Comb, J., Seeburg, P. H., Adelman, J., Eiden, L. and Herbert, E. (1982). Primary structure of the human Met- and Leu-enkephalin precursor and its mRNA. *Nature, 295,* 663–667.

Commissiong, J. W. (1985). Monoamine metabolites: Their relationship and lack of relationship to monoaminergic neuronal activity. *Biochem. Pharmacol., 34,* 1127–1131.

Compton, D. R., Dewey, W. L., and Martin, B. R. (1990). Cannabis dependence and tolerance production. *Adv. Alcohol Subst. Abuse, 9,* 129–147.

Compton, D. R., Rice, K. C., De Costa, B. R., Razdan, R. K., Melvin, L. S., Johnson, M. R., and Martin, B. R. (1993). Cannabinoid structure-activity relationships: Correlation of receptor binding and *in vivo* activities. *J. Pharmacol. Exp. Ther., 265,* 218–226.

Compton, R. P., Contreras, P. C., O'Donohue, T. L., and Monahan, J. B. (1987). The N-methyl-D-aspartate antagonist, 2-amino-7-phosphonoheptanoate, produces phencyclidine-like behavioral effects in rats. *Eur. J. Pharmacol., 136,* 133–134.

Cone, E. J., Johnson, R. E., Moore, J. D., and Roache, J. D. (1986). Acute effects of smoking marijuana on hormones, subjective effects and performance in male human subjects. *Pharmacol. Biochem. Behav., 24,* 1749–1754.

Connell, P. H. (1958). *Amphetamine Psychosis,* Maudsley Monographs No. 5. Oxford, London.

Connor, C. E., and Kuczenski, R. (1986). Evidence that amphetamine and Na^+ gradient reversal increase striatal synaptosomal dopamine synthesis through carrier-mediated efflux of dopamine. *Biochem. Pharmacol., 35,* 3123–3130.

Conquet, F., et al. (1994). Motor deficit and impairment of synaptic plasticity in mice lacking mGluR1. *Nature, 372,* 237–243.

Conry, J. (1990). Neuropsychological deficits in fetal alcohol syndrome and fetal alcohol effects. *Alcohol. Clin. Exp. Res., 14,* 650–655.

Consolazione, A., and Cuello, A. C. (1982). CNS serotonin pathways. In *Biology of Serotonergic Transmission* (N. N. Osborne, Ed.), pp. 29–61. Wiley, Chichester.

Contestabile, A., Migani, P., Poli, A., and Villani, L. (1984). Recent advances in the use of selective neuron-destroying agents for neurobiological research. *Experientia, 40,* 524–534.

Conti, F., Rustioni, A., Petrusz, P., and Towle, A. C. (1987). Glutamate-positive neurons in the somatic sensory cortex of rats and monkeys. *J. Neurosci., 7,* 1887–1901.

Conti, L. H., and Musty, R. E. (1984). The effects of delta-9-tetrahydrocannabinol injections to the nucleus accumbens on the locomotor activity of rats. In *The Cannabinoids: Chemical, Pharmacologic, and Therapeutic Aspects* (S. Agurell, S. L. Dewey, and R. E. Willette, Eds.), pp. 649–655. Academic Press, Orlando.

Conti-Tronconi, B. M., Gotti, C. M., Hunkapiller, M. W., and Raftery, M. A. (1982). Mammalian muscle acetylcholine receptor: a supramolecular structure formed by four related proteins. *Science, 218,* 1227–1229.

Contreras, P. C., Gray, N. M., DiMaggio, D. A., Bremer, M. E., and Bussom, J. A. (1993). Isolation and characterization of an endogenous ligand for the PCP and s receptors from porcine, rat, and human tissue. *NIDA Res. Monogr., 133,* 207–222.

Contreras, P. C., Johnson, S., Freedman, R., Hoffer, B., Olsen, K., Rafferty, M. F., Lessor, R. A., Rice, K. C., Jacobson, A. E., and O'-Donohue, T. L. (1986). Metaphit, an acylating ligand for phencyclidine receptors: Characterization of *in vivo* actions in the rat. *J. Pharmacol. Exp. Ther., 238,* 1101–1107.

Cook, C. E. (1991). Pyrolytic characteristics, pharmacokinetics, and bioavailability of smoked heroin, cocaine, phencyclidine, and methamphetamine. *NIDA Res. Monogr., 115,* 6–23.

Cook, C. E., Brine, D. R., Jeffcoat, A. R., Hill, J. M., Wall, M. E., Perez-Reyes, M., and Di Guiseppi, S. R. (1982). Phencyclidine disposition after intravenous and oral doses. *Clin. Pharmacol. Ther., 31,* 625–634.

Cook, C. E., and Jeffcoat, A. R. (1990). Pyrolytic degradation of heroin, phencyclidine, and cocaine: Identification of products and some observations on their metabolism. *NIDA Res. Monogr., 99,* 97–120.

Cook, E. H. Jr., Fletcher, K. E., Wainwright, M., Marks, N., Yan, S.-Y., and Leventhal, B. L. (1994). Primary structure of the human platelet serotonin 5-HT$_{2A}$ receptor: Identity with frontal cortex serotonin 5-HT$_{2A}$ receptor. *J. Neurochem., 63,* 465–469.

Cook, L., and Davidson, A. B. (1973). Effects of behaviorally active drugs in a conflict-punishment procedure in rats. In *The Benzodiazepines* (S. Garattini, E. Mussini, and L. O. Randall, Eds.), pp. 327–345, Raven Press, New York.

Cook, L., and Sepinwall, J. (1975). Behavorial analysis of the effects and mechanisms of action of benzodiazepines. *Adv. Biochem. Psychopharmacol., 14,* 1–28.

Cooper, J. R., Bloom, F. E., and Roth, R. H. (1991). *The Biochemical Basis of Neuropharmacology* (6th ed.). Oxford University Press, New York.

Cooper, S. J., and Dourish, C. T. (1990). Multiple cholecystokinin (CCK) receptors and CCK-monoamine interactions are instrumental in the control of feeding. *Physiol. Behav., 48,* 849–857.

Cooper, S. J., Dourish, C. T., and Clifton, P. G. (1992). CCK antagonists and CCK–monoamine interactions in the control of satiety. *Am. J. Clin. Nutr., 55,* 291S–295S.

Cooper, S. J., and Kirkham, T. C. (1990). Basic mechanisms of opioids' effects on eating and drinking. In *Opioids, Bulimia, and Alcohol Abuse and Alcoholism* (L. D. Reid, Ed.), pp. 91–110. Springer, New York.

Cooper, S. J., and Kirkham, T. C. (1993). Opioid mechanisms in the control of food consumption and taste preferences. In *Opioids II,* Handbook of Experimental Pharmacology, Vol. 104 (A. Herz, Ed.), pp. 239–262. Springer-Verlag, New York.

Corbin, K. B. (1949). Trihexyphenyl: Evaluation of a new agent in the treatment of Parkinson's disease. *JAMA, 141,* 373–381.

Corcoran, J. J., Wilson, S. P., and Kirshner, N. (1984). Flux of catecholamines through chromaffin vesicles in cultured bovine adrenal medullary cells. *J. Biol. Chem., 259,* 6208–6214.

Cordell, B. (1994). β-Amyloid formation as a potential therapeutic target for Alzheimer's disease. *Annu. Rev. Pharmacol. Toxicol., 34,* 69–89.

Corder, E. H., Saunders, A. M., Strittmatter, W. J., Schmechel, D. E., Gaskell, P. C., Small, G. W., Roses, A. D., Haines, J. L., and Pericak-Vance, M. A. (1993). Gene dose of apolipoprotein E type 4 allele and the risk of Alzheimer's disease in late onset families. *Science, 261,* 921–923.

Cormack, M.-A., Owens, R. G., and Dewey, M. E. (Eds.) (1989). *Reducing Benzodiazepine Consumption.* Springer-Verlag, New York.

Cornfield, L. J., and Nelson, D. L. (1991). Biochemistry of 5-Hydroxytryptamine receptor subtypes: Coupling to second messenger systems. In *Serotonin Receptor Subtypes: Basic and Clinical Aspects* (S. J. Peroutka, Ed.), pp. 81–102. Wiley-Liss, New York.

Correa, N., Opler, L. A. Kay, S. R., and Birmaker, B. (1987). Amantadine in the treatment of neuroendocrine side effects of neuroleptics. *J. Clin. Psychopharmacol., 7,* 91–95.

Corrigall, W. A., and Coen, K. M. (1989). Nicotine maintains robust self-administration in rats on a limited-access schedule. *Psychopharmacology, 99,* 473–478.

Corrigall, W. A., and Coen, K. M. (1991). Selective dopamine antagonists reduce nicotine self-administration. *Psychopharmacology, 104,* 171–176.

Corrigall, W. A., Coen, K. M., and Adamson, K. L. (1994). Self-administered nicotine activates the mesolimbic dopamine system through the ventral tegmental area. *Brain Res., 653,* 278–284.

Corrodi, H., Fuxe, K., and Hokfelt, T. (1967). The effect of some psychoactive drugs on central monoamine neurons. *Psychopharmacologia, 11,* 363–368.

Corrodi, H., Fuxe, K., Hokfelt, T., and Schou, M. (1967). The effect of lithium on cerebral monoamine neurons. *Psychopharmacologia, 11,* 345–353.

Corsellis, J. A. N., and Bruton, C. J. (1983). Neuropathology of status epilepticus in humans. *Adv. Neurol., 34,* 129–139.

Corssen, G., and Domino, E. F. (1966). Dissociative anesthesia: Further pharmacologic studies and first clinical experience with the phencyclidine derivative CI-581. *Anesth. Analg., 45,* 29–40.

Cortés, R., Probst, A., Tobler, H.-J., and Palacios, J. M. (1986). Muscarinic cholinergic receptor subtypes in the human brain. II. Quantitative autoradiographic studies. *Brain Res., 362,* 239–253.

Corwin, R. L., Gibbs, J., and Smith, G. P. (1991). Increased food intake after type A but not type B cholecystokinin receptor blockade. *Physiol. Behav., 50,* 255–258.

Cosgrove, J., and Newell, T. G. (1991). Recovery of neuropsychological functions during reduction in use of phencyclidine. *J. Clin. Psychol., 47,* 159–169.

Costa, E., Groppetti, A., and Naimzada, M. K. (1972). Effects of amphetamine on the turnover rate of brain catecholamines and motor activity. *Br. J. Pharmacol., 44,* 742–751.

Costa, E., Guidotti, A., and Mao, C. C. (1975). Evidence for involvement of GABA in the action of benzodiazepines: Studies on rat cerebellum. *Adv. Biochem. Psychopharmacol., 14,* 113–130.

Costa, M., Furness, J. B., Llewellyn-Smith, I. J., Murphy, R., Bornstein, J. C., and Keast, J. R. (1985). Functional roles for substance P-containing neurones in the gastrointestinal tract. In *Substance P: Metabolism and Biological Actions* (C. C. Jordan and P. Oehme, Eds.), pp. 99–119. Taylor and Francis, London.

Costall, B. (1993). The breadth of action of the 5-HT$_3$ receptor antagonists. *Int. Clin. Psychopharmacol., 8* (Suppl. 2), 3–9.

Costall, B., and Naylor, R. J. (1991). Anxiolytic effects of 5-H$_3$ antagonists in animals. In *5-HT$_{1A}$ Agonists, 5-HT$_3$ Antagonists and Benzodiazepines: Their Comparative Behavioral Pharmacology* (R. J. Rodgers and S. J. Cooper, Eds.), pp. 133–157 Wiley, New York.

Costall, B., and Naylor, R. J. (1993). The pharmacology of the 5-HT$_4$ receptor. *Int. Clin. Psychopharmacol., 8* (Suppl. 2), 11–18.

Costall, B., Naylor, R. J., and Olley, J. E. (1972). Stereotypic and anti-cataleptic activities of amphetamine after intracerebral injections. *Eur. J. Pharmacol., 18,* 83–94.

Côté, L., and Crutcher, M. D. (1991). The basal ganglia. In *Principles of Neural Science* (3rd ed.) (E. R. Kandel, J. H. Schwartz, and T. M. Jessell, Eds.), pp. 647–659. Elsevier, New York.

Cotman, C. W. (Ed.). (1985). *Synaptic Plasticity.* Guilford Press, New York.

Cotman, C. W., and McGaugh, J. L. (1980). *Behavioral Neuroscience.* Academic Press, New York.

Cotman, C. W., and Nieto-Sampedro, M. (1984). Cell biology of synaptic plasticity. *Science, 225,* 1287–1294.

Cotzias, G. C., Papavasiliou, P. S., and Gellene, R. (1969). Modification of parkinsonism—chronic treatment with L-dopa. *N. Engl. J. Med., 280,* 337–343.

Cotzias, G. C., Van Woert, M. H., and Schiffer, L. M. (1967). Aromatic amino acids and modification of parkinsonism. *N. Engl. J. Med., 276,* 374–378.

Coull, J. T. (1994). Pharmacological manipulations of the α$_2$-noradrenergic system. *Drugs Aging, 5,* 116–126.

Court, J. A., and Perry, E. K. (1991). Dementia: The neurochemical basis of putative transmitter orientated therapy. *Pharmacol. Ther., 52,* 423–443.

Cowley, G., Springen, K., Iarovici, D. and Hager, M. (1991). Sweet dreams or nightmare? *Newsweek,* August 19, 1991, pp. 44–51.

Cox, B. M. (1993). Opioid receptor-G protein interactions: Acute and chronic effects of opioids. In *Opioids I,* Handbook of Experimental Pharmacology, Vol. 104 (A. Herz, Ed.), pp. 145–188. Springer-Verlag, New York.

Coyle, J. T. (1983). Neurotoxic action of kainic acid. *J. Neurochem., 41,* 1–11.

Coyle, J. T., Murphy, T. H., Puttfarcken, P. S., Lyons, E. W., and Vornov, J. J. (1991). The non-excitatory mechanisms of glutamate-induced neurotoxicity. *Epilepsy Res., 10,* 41–48.

Coyle, J. T., Oster-Granite, M. L., Reeves, R. H., and Gearhart, J. D. (1988). Down syndrome, Alzheimer's disease and the trisomy 16 mouse. *Trends Neurosci., 11,* 390–394.

Coyle, J. T. and Pert, C. B. (1976). Ontogenetic development of 3H-naloxone binding in rat brain. *Neuropharmacology, 15,* 555–560.

Coyle, J. T., Price, D. L., and DeLong, M. R. (1983). Alzheimer's disease: A disorder of cortical cholinergic innervation. *Science, 219,* 1184–1189.

Coyle, J. T., and Puttfarcken, P. (1993). Oxidative stress, glutamate, and neurodegenerative disorders. *Science, 262,* 689–695.

Coyle, J. T., and Schwarcz, R. (1976). Model for Huntington's chorea: Lesions of striatal neurons with kainic acid. *Nature, 263,* 244–246.

Coyle, S., Napier, T. C., and Breese, G. R. (1985). Ontogeny of tolerance to haloperidol: Behavioral and biochemical measures. *Dev. Brain Res., 23,* 27–38.

Crawley, J. C. W., et al. (1986). Dopamine receptors in schizophrenia studied in vivo. *Lancet, II,* 224–225.

Crawley, J. N. (1985a). Clarification of the behavioral functions of peripheral and central cholecystokinin: Two separate peptide pools. *Peptides, 6* (Suppl. 2), 129–136.

Crawley, J. N. (1985b). Comparative distribution of cholecystokinin and other neuropeptides: Why is this peptide different from all other peptides? *Ann. N.Y. Acad. Sci., 448,* 1–8.

Crawley, J. N. (1988). Behavioral analysis of antagonists of the peripheral and central effects of cholecystokinin. In *Cholecystokinin Antagonists* (R. Y. Wang and R. Schoenfeld, Eds.), pp. 243–262. Alan R. Liss, New York.

Crawley, J. N. (1991). Cholecystokinin–dopamine interactions. *Trends Pharmacol. Sci., 12,* 232–236.

Crawley, J. N. (1992). Subtype-selective cholecystokinin receptor antagonists block cholecystokinin modulation of dopamine-mediated behaviors in the rat mesolimbic pathway. *J. Neurosci., 12,* 3380–3391.

Crawley, J. N., Corwin, R. L., Robinson, J. K., Felder, C. C., Devane, W. A., and Axelrod, J. (1993). Anandamide, an endogenous ligand of the cannabinoid receptor, induces hypomotility and hypothermia in vivo in rodents. *Pharmacol. Biochem. Behav., 46,* 967–972.

Crawley, J. N., Fiske, S. M., Durieux, C., Derrien, M., and Roques, B. P. (1991). Centrally administered cholecystokinin suppresses feeding through a peripheral-type receptor mechanism. *J. Pharmacol. Exp. Ther., 257,* 1076–1080.

Creasey, W. A. (1979). *Drug Disposition in Humans.* Oxford University Press, New York.

Creese, I. (1985). Receptor binding as a primary drug screen. In *Neurotransmitter Receptor Binding* (2nd ed.) (H. Yamamura, S. Enna, and M. Kuhar, Eds.), pp. 189–233. Raven Press, New York.

Creese, I., Burt, D. R., and Snyder, S. (1976). Dopamine receptor binding predicts clinical and pharmacological potencies of antischizophrenic drugs. *Science, 194,* 481–483.

Creese, I., Burt, D. R., and Snyder, S. H. (1977). Dopamine receptor binding enhancement accompanies lesion-induced behavioral supersensitivity. *Science, 197,* 596–598.

Creese, I., and Iversen, S. D. (1974). The role of forebrain dopamine systems in amphetamine induced stereotyped behavior in the rat. *Psychopharmacologia, 39,* 345–357.

Criswell, H. E., Simson, P. E., Duncan, G. E., McCown, T. J., Herbert, J. S., Morrow, A. L., and Breese, G. R. (1993). Molecular basis for regionally specific action of ethanol on γ-aminobutyric acid$_A$ receptors: Generalization to other ligand-gated ion channels. *J. Pharmacol. Exp. Ther., 267,* 522–1993.

Crook, T. (1985). Clinical drug trials in Alzheimer's disease. *Ann. N.Y. Acad. Sci., 444,* 428–436.

Crow, T. J. (1980). Molecular pathology of schizophrenia: More than one disease process? *Br. Med. J., 280,* 66–68.

Crow, T. J., Ball, J., and Bloom, S. R. (1989). Schizophrenia as an anomaly of development of cerebral asymmetry: A postmortem study and a proposal concerning the genetic basis of the disease. *Arch. Gen. Psychiatry, 46,* 1145–1150.

Crow, T. J., Cross, A. J., Johnstone, E. C., Owen, F. Owens, D. G. C., and Waddington, J. L. (1982). Abnormal involuntary movements in schizophrenia: Are they related to the disease process or its treatment? *J. Clin. Psychopharmacol., 2,* 336–340.

Crow, T. J., Johnston, E. C., Longden, A., and Owen, F. (1978). Dopamine and schizophrenia. *Adv. Biochem. Psychopharmacol., 19,* 301–309.

Crutcher, K. A., Scott, S. A., Liang, S., Everson, W. V., and Weingartner, J. (1993). Detection of NGF-like activity in human brain tissue: Increased levels in Alzheimer's disease. *J. Neurosci., 13,* 2540–2550.

Csernansky, J. G., King, R. J., Faustman, W. O., Moses, J. A., Poscher, M. E., and Faull, K. F. (1990). 5-HIAA in cerebrospinal fluid and deficit schizophrenic characteristics. *Br. J. Psychiatry, 156,* 501–507.

Cubells, J. F., Rayport, S., Rajendran, G., and Sulzer, D. (1994). Methamphetamine neurotoxicity involves vacuolation of endocytotic organelles and dopamine-dependent intracellular oxidative stress. *J. Neurosci., 14,* 2260–2271.

Cuello, A. C., Milstein, C., Couture, R., Wright, B., Priestley, J. V., and Jarvis, J. (1984). Characterization and immunocytochemical applications of monoclonal antibodies against enkephalins. *J. Histochem. Cytochem., 32,* 947–957.

Cuello, A. C., Priestley, J. V., and Milstein, C. (1982). Immunocytochemistry with internally labeled monoclonal antibodies. *Proc. Natl. Acad. Sci. U.S.A., 79,* 665–669.

Cuello, A. C., Ribeiro-da-Silva, A., Ma, W., De Koninck, Y., and Henry, J. L. (1993). Organization of substance P primary sensory neurons: Ultrastructural and physiological correlates. *Regul. Pept., 46,* 155–164.

Cumming, P., Damsma, G., Fibiger, H. C., and Vincent, S. R. (1991). Characterization of extracellular histamine in the striatum and bed nucleus of the stria terminalis of the rat: An in vivo microdialysis study. *J. Neurochem.*, 56, 1797–1803.

Cummings, J. L. (1992). Depression and Parkinson's disease: A review. *Am. J. Psychiatry*, 149, 443–454.

Cunningham, K. A., and Callahan, P. M. (1991). Monoamine reuptake inhibitors enhance the discriminative state induced by cocaine in the rat. *Psychopharmacology*, 104, 177–180.

Cunningham, K. A., and Lakoski, J. M. (1990). The interaction of cocaine with serotonin dorsal raphe neurons. Single-unit extracellular recording studies. *Neuropsychopharmacology*, 3, 41–50.

Cunningham, M. D., Ferkany, J. W., and Enna, S. J. (1993). Excitatory amino acid receptors: A gallery of new targets for pharmacological intervention. *Life Sci.*, 54, 135–148.

Curtis, D. R., and Eccles, R. M. (1958). The excitation of Renshaw cells by pharmacological agents applied electrophoretically. *J. Physiol.* (Lond.), 141, 435–445.

Curtis, D. R., and Koizumi, K. (1961). Chemical transmitter substances in brain stem of cat. *J. Neurophysiol.*, 24, 80–90.

Curtis, D. R., Phillis, J. W., and Watkins, J. C. (1960). The chemical excitation of spinal neurones by certain acidic amino acids. *J. Physiol.*, 150, 656–682.

Curzon, G. (1981). The turnover of 5-hydroxytryptamine. In *Central Neurotransmitter Turnover* (C. J. Pycock and P. V. Taberner, Eds.), pp. 59–80. Croom Helm, London.

Curzon, G., and Kennett, G. A. (1990). *m*-CPP: A tool for studying behavioural responses associated with 5-HT$_{1C}$ receptors. *Trends Pharmacol. Sci.*, 11, 181–182.

Czajkowski, C., Kaufmann, C., and Karlin, A. (1993). Negatively charged amino acid residues in the nicotinic receptor δ subunit that contribute to the binding of acetylcholine. *Proc. Natl. Acad. Sci. U.S.A.*, 90, 6285–6289.

Dabadie, H., Mons, N., and Geffard, M. (1990). Simultaneous detection of tryptamine and dopamine in rat substantia nigra and raphe nuclei using specific antibodies. *Brain Res.*, 512, 138–142.

Dackis, C. A., and Gold, M. S. (1985). New concepts in cocaine addiction: The dopamine depletion hypothesis. *Neurosci. Biobehav. Rev.*, 9, 469–477.

Dafters, R., and Anderson, G. (1982). Conditioned tolerance to the tachycardia effect of ethanol in humans. *Psychopharmacology*, 78, 365–367.

Dahlström, A., and Fuxe, K. (1964). Evidence for the existence of monoamine-containing neurons in the central nervous system. I. Demonstration of monoamines in the cell bodies of brainstem neurons. *Acta Physiol. Scand.*, 62 (Suppl. 232), 1–55.

Dahlström, A., and Fuxe, K. (1965). Evidence for the existence of monoamine neurons in the central nervous system. II. Experimentally induced changes in the intraneuronal levels of bulbospinal neuron system. *Acta Physiol. Scand.*, 64 (Suppl. 247), 7–36.

Dajas, F., Barbeito, L., Martinez-Pesquera, G., Lista, A., Puppo, D., and Puppo-Touriz, H. (1983). Plasma noradrenalin and clinical psychopathology in schizophrenia. *Neuropsychobiology*, 10, 70–74.

Dalby, M. A. (1975). Behavioral effects of carbamazepine. Complex partial siezures and their treatment. *Adv. Neurol.*, 11, 331–343.

Dale, H. H. (1914). The action of certain esters and ethers of choline and their relation to muscarine. *J. Pharmacol.*, 6, 147–190.

Dale, H. H. (1935). Pharmacology and nerve-endings. Walter Ernest Dixon Memorial Lecture for 1934. *Proc. R. Soc. Med., Ther. Sect.*, 28, 319–332.

Dale, H. H., Feldberg, W., and Vogt, M. (1936). Release of acetylcholine at voluntary motor nerve endings. *J. Physiol.* (Lond.), 86, 353–380.

Dale, N., Schacher, S., and Kandel, E. R. (1988). Long-term facilitation in *Aplysia* involves imcrease in transmitter release. *Science*, 239, 282–285.

Dal Toso, R., Sommer, B., Ewert, M., Herb, A., Pritchett, D. B., Bach, A., Shivers, B. D., and Seeburg, P. H. (1989). The dopamine D$_2$ receptor: Two molecular forms generated by alternative splicing. *EMBO J.*, 8, 4025–4034.

Daly, J. W. (1993). Mechanism of action of caffeine. In *Caffeine, Coffee, and Health* (S. Garattini, Ed.), pp. 97–150. Raven Press, New York.

Daly, S. A., and Waddington, J. L. (1992). New classes of selective D-1 dopamine receptor antagonist provide further evidence for two directions of D-1:D-2 interaction. *Neurochem. Int.*, 20 (Suppl.), 135S–139S.

Daly, S. A., and Waddington, J. L. (1993). Behavioural effects of the putative D-3 dopamine receptor agonist 7-OH-DPAT in relation to other "D-2-like" agonists. *Neuropharmacology*, 32, 509–510.

D'Amato, R. J., Lipman, Z., and Snyder, S. H. (1986). Selectivity of the Parkinsonian neurotoxin MPTP: Toxic metabolite MPP$^+$ binds to neuromelanin. *Science*, 231, 987–989.

D'Amour, F. E., and Smith, D. L. (1941). A method for determining loss of pain sensation. *J. Pharmacol., Exp. Ther.*, 72, 74–79.

Danbolt, N. C., Storm-Mathisen, J., and Kanner, B. I. (1992). An [Na$^+$–K$^+$] coupled L-glutamate transporter purified from rat brain is located in glial cell processes. *Neuroscience*, 51, 295–310.

Daniel, D. G., et al. (1991). The effect of amphetamine on regional cerebral blood flow during cognitive activation in schizophrenia. *J. Neurosci.*, 11, 1907–1917.

Daniel, P. M., Love, E. R., Moorhouse, S. R., and Pratt, O. E. (1981). The effect of insulin upon the influx of tryptophan into the brain of the rabbit. *J. Physiol.* (Lond.), 312, 551–562.

Da Prada, M., Cesura, A. M., Launay, J. M., and Richards, J. G. (1988). Platelets as a model for neurones? *Experientia*, 44, 115–126.

Darley, C. F., Tinklenberg, J. R., Roth, W. T., Vernon, S., and Kopell, B. S. (1977). Marijuana effects on long-term memory assessment and retrieval. *Psychopharmacology*, 52, 239–241.

Darmon, M. C., Guibert, B., Leviel, V., Ehret, M., Maitre, M., and Mallet, J. (1988). Sequence of two mRNAs encoding active rat tryptophan hydroxylase. *J. Neurochem.*, 51, 312–316.

Das, G., and Laddu, A. (1993). Cocaine: Friend or foe? (Part 1). *Int. J. Clin. Pharmacol. Ther. Toxicol.*, 31, 449–455.

Daubner, S. C., Lauriano, C., Haycock, J. W., and Fitzpatrick, P. F. (1992). Site-directed mutagenesis of serine 40 of rat tyrosine hydroxylase: Effects of dopamine and cAMP-dependent phosphorylation on enzyme activity. *J. Biol. Chem.*, 267, 12639–12646.

Daugé, V., Steimes, P., Derrien, M., Beau, N., Roques, B. P., and Féger, J. (1989). CCK8 effects on motivational and emotional states of rats involve CCKA receptors of the postero-median part of the nucleus accumbens. *Pharmacol. Biochem. Behav.*, 34, 157–163.

Davidson, N. (1976). *Neurotransmitter Amino Acids.* Academic Press, London.

Davies, B. M., and Beech, H. R. (1960). The effect of 1-arylcyclohexylamine (Sernyl) on twelve normal volunteers. *J. Ment. Sci.*, 106, 912–924.

Davies, P. (1994). Neuronal abnormalities, not amyloid, are the cause of dementia in Alzheimer disease. In *Alzheimer Disease* (R. D. Terry, R. Katzman, and K. L. Bick, Eds.), pp. 327–33. Raven Press, New York.

Davies, R. F., Rossi, J. III, Panksepp, J., Bean, N. J., and Zolovick, A. J. (1983). Fenfluramine anorexia: A peripheral locus of action. *Physiol. Behav.*, 30, 723–730.

Davila, R., Manero, E., and Zumarraga, M. (1988). Plasma homovanillic acid as a predictor of response to neuroleptics. *Arch. Gen. Psychiatry*, 45, 564–567.

Davis, G. C., William, A. C., Markey, S. P., Ebert, M. H., Caine, E. D., Reichert, C. M., and Kopin, I. J. (1979). Chronic Parkinsonism secondary to intravenous injection of meperidine analogues. *Psychiatry Res.*, 1, 249–254.

Davis, J. M. (1976). Maintenance therapy in psychiatry 1. Affective disorders. *Am. J. Psychiatry*, 133, 1–13.

Davis, J. M., Comaty, J. E., and Janicak, P. G. (1988). Clinical applicability of antidepressant plasma levels. In *Affective Disorders* (No. 3) (F. Flach, Ed.), pp. 140–150. W. W. Norton & Co., New York.

Davis, K. L., Kahn, R. S., Ko, G., and Davidson, M. (1991). Dopamine in schizophrenia: A review and reconceptualization. *Am. J. Psychiatry*, 148, 1474–1486.

Davis, K. L., et al. (1992). A double-blind, place-controlled multicenter study of tacrine for Alzheimer's disease. *N. Engl. J. Med.*, 327, 1253–1259.

Davis, M. (1979). Diazepam and flurazepam: Effects on conditioned fear as measured with the potentiated startle paradigm. *Psychopharmacology*, 62, 1–7.

Davis, M., Kehne, J. H., Commissaris, J., and Geyer, M. A. (1984). Effects of hallucinogens on unconditioned behaviors in animals. In *Hallucinogens: Neurochemical, Behavioral, and Clinical Perspectives* (B. L. Jacobs, Ed.), pp. 35–75. Raven Press, New York.

Davis, R., et al. (1993). Subtype selective muscarinic agonists: Potential therapeutic agents for Alzheimer's disease. *Prog. Brain Res.*, 98, 439–445.

Davis, S., Butcher, S. P., and Morris, R. G. M. (1992). The NMDA receptor antagonist D-2-amino-5-phosphopentanoate (D-AP5) impairs spatial learning and LTP in vivo at intracerebral concentrations comparable to those that block LTP in vitro. *J. Neurosci.,* 12, 21–34.

Davis, V. E., and Walsh, M. S. (1970a). Alcohol, amines and alkaloids: A possible biochemical basis for alcohol addiction. *Science,* 167, 105–107.

Davis, V. E., and Walsh, M. S. (1970b). Rebuttal. *Science,* 169, 1105–1106.

Davis, V. E., and Walsh, M. S. (1970c). Rebuttal. *Science,* 170, 1114–1115.

Dawson, G. R., Heyes, C. M., and Iversen, S. D. (1992). Pharmacological mechanisms and animal models of cognition. *Behav. Pharmacol.,* 3, 285–297.

Dawson, T. M., Gehlert, D. R., McCabe, R. T., Barnett, A., and Wamsley, J. K. (1986). D-1 dopamine receptors in the rat brain: A quantitative autoradiographic analysis. *J. Neurosci.,* 6, 2352–2365.

Day, N. L., and Richardson, G. A. (1993). Cocaine use and crack babies: Science, the media, and miscommunication. *Neurotoxicol. Teratol.,* 15, 293–294.

Day, R., Trujillo, K. A., and Akil, H. (1993). Prodynorphin biosynthesis and posttranslational processing. In *Opioids I,* Handbook of Experimental Pharmacology, Vol. 104 (A. Herz, Ed.), pp. 449–470. Springer-Verlag, New York.

Deadwyler, S. A., Heyser, C. J., Michaelis, R. C., and Hampson, R. E. (1990). The effects of delta-9-tHC on mechanisms of learning and memory. *NIDA Res. Monogr.* 97, 79–93.

Deakin, J. F. W. (1994). The clinical anxiolytic and antidepressant efficacy of drugs with actions on serotonin systems. In *Handbook of Depression and Anxiety* (J. A. den Boer and J. M. Ad Sitsen, Eds.), pp. 447–472. Marcel Dekker, Inc., New York.

Dearry, A., Gingrich, J. A., Falardeau, P., Fremeau, R. T. Jr., Bates, M. D., and Caron, M. G. (1990). Molecular cloning and expression of the gene for a human D_1 dopamine receptor. *Nature,* 347, 72–76.

De Biasi, S., and Rustioni, A. (1988). Glutamate and substance P coexist in primary afferent terminals in the superficial laminae of spinal cord. *Proc. Natl. Acad. Sci. U.S.A.,* 85, 7820–7824.

de Blas, A. (1988). Endogenous benzodiazepines in brain. *Trends Neurosci.,* 11, 489–490.

De Blas, A. L., Park, D., and Friedrich, P. (1987). Endogenous benzodiazepine-like molecules in the human, rat and bovine brains studied with monoclonal antibody to benzodiazepines. *Brain Res.,* 413, 275–284.

De Blas, A. L., and Sotelo, C. (1987). Localization of benzodiazepine-like molecules in the rat brain. A light and electron microscopy immunocytochemistry study with an anti-benzodiazepine monoclonal antibody. *Brain Res.,* 413, 285–296.

Decavel, C., Lescaudron, L., Mons, N., and Calas, A. (1987). First visualization of dopaminergic neurons with a monoclonal antibody to dopamine: A light and electron microscopic study. *J. Histochem. Cytochem.,* 35, 1245–1251.

Decker, M. W., Brioni, J. D., Bannon, A. W., and Arneric, S. P. (1995). Diversity of neuronal nicotinic acetylcholine receptors: Lessons from behavior and implications for CNS therapeutics. *Life Sci.,* 56, 545–570.

Decker, M. W., and McGaugh, J. L. (1991). The role of interactions between the cholinergic

system and other neuromodulatory systems in learning and memory. *Synapse,* 7, 151–168.

Deckert, J., Morgan, P. F., and Marangos, P. J. (1988). Adenosine uptake site heterogeneity in the mammalian CNS? Uptake inhibitors as probes and potential neuropharmaceuticals. *Life Sci.,* 42, 1331–1345.

De Clerck, F., and de Chaffoy de Courcelles, D. (1990). Serotonergic amplification in platelet function: Mechanisms and in vivo relevance. *Prog. Pharmacol. Clin. Pharmacol.,* 7, 51–59.

DeFeudis, F. V. (1974). *Central Cholinergic Systems and Behavior.* Academic Press, New York.

Deitrich, R. A., Dunwiddie, T. V., Harris, R. A., and Erwin, V. G. (1989). Mechanism of action of ethanol: Initial central nervous system actions. *Pharmacol. Rev.,* 41, 489–537.

Deitrich, R. A., and Erwin, V. G. (1975). Involvement of biogenic amine metabolism in ethanol addiction. *Fed. Proc.,* 34, 1962–1968.

De Keyser, J. (1993). Subtypes and localization of dopamine receptors in human brain. *Neurochem. Int.,* 22, 83–93.

Dekker, A. J. A. M., Connor, D. J., and Thal, L. J. (1991). The role of cholinergic projections from the nucleus basalis in memory. *Neurosci. Biobehav. Rev.,* 15, 299–317.

De Lacoste, M.-C., and White, C. L. III (1993). The role of cortical connectivity in Alzheimer's disease pathogenesis: A review and model system. *Neurobiol. Aging,* 14, 1–16.

Delarue, C., Becquet, D., Idres, S., Hery, F., and Vaudry, H. (1992). Serotonin synthesis in adrenochromaffin cells. *Neuroscience,* 46, 495–500.

Delarue, C., Lefebvre, H., Idres, S., Leboulenger, F., HomoDelarche, F., Lihrmann, I., Feuilloley, M., and Vaudry, H. (1988). Sertonin stimulates corticosteroid secretion by frog adrenocortical tissue in vitro. *J. Steroid Biochem.,* 29, 519–525.

Delfs, J. M., Schreiber, L., and Kelley, A. E. (1990). Microinjection of cocaine into the nucleus accumbens elicits locomotor activation in the rat. *J. Neurosci.,* 10, 303–310.

Delgado, P. L., Charney, D. S., Price, L. H., Aghajanian, G. K., Landis, H., and Heninger, G. R. (1990). Serotonin function and the mechanism of antidepressant action. *Arch. Gen. Psychiatry,* 47, 411–418.

DeLisi, L. E., Hoff, A. L., Schwartz, J. E., Shields, G. W., Halthore, S. N. Gupta, S. M., Henn, F. A., and Anand, A. K. (1991). Brain morphology in first-episode schizophrenic-like psychotic patients: A quantitative magnetic resonance imaging study. *Biol. Psychiatry,* 29, 159–175.

Della-Fera, M. A., Baile, C. A., Schneider, B. S., and Grinker, J. A. (1981). Cholecystokinin antibody injected in cerebral ventricles stimulates feeding in sheep. *Science,* 212, 687–689.

Della-Fera, M. A., Coleman, B. D., and Baile, C. A. (1990). CNS injection of CCK in rats: Effects on real and sham feeding and gastric emptying. *Am. J. Physiol.,* 258, R1165–R1169.

Demellweek, C., and Goudie, A. J. (1983). Behavioural tolerance to amphetamine and other psychostimulants: The case for considering behavioural mechanisms. *Psychopharmacology,* 80, 287–307.

Dement, W., Seidel, W., and Carskadon, M. (1984). Issues in the diagnosis and treat-

ment of insomnia. In *Sleep, Benzodiazepines and Performance: Experimental Methodologies and Research Prospects* (I. Hindmarch, H. Ott, and T. Roth, Eds.), pp. 11–43. Springer-Verlag, New York.

Demet, E. M., and Halaris, A. E. (1979). Origin and distribution of 3-methoxy-4-hydroxyphenylglycol in body fluids. *Biochem. Pharmacol.,* 28, 3043–3050.

de Montigny, C. (1981). Enhancement of the 5-HT neurotransmission by antidepressant treatments. *J. Physiol.,* 77, 455–461.

de Montigny, C., and Blier, P. (1992). Electrophysiological evidence for the distinct properties of presynaptic and postsynaptic 5-HT_{1A} receptors: Possible clinical relevance. In *Serotonin Receptor Subtypes: Pharmacological Significance and Clinical Implications* (S. Z. Langer, N. Brunello, G. Racagni, and J. Mendlewicz, Eds.), pp. 80–88. Karger, Basel.

de Montigny, C., Blier, P., and Chaput, Y. (1984). Electrophysiologically-identified serotonin receptors in the rat CNS. *Neuropharmacology,* 23, 1511–1520.

Denizeau, F., and Sourkes, T. L. (1978). Regional transport of tryptophan in rat brain. *J. Neurochem.,* 28, 951–959.

De Robertis, E. (1967). Ultrastructure and cytochemistry of the synaptic region. *Science,* 156, 907–914.

De Robertis, E., and Bennett, H. S. (1954). Submicroscopic vesicular component in the synapse. *Fed. Proc.,* 13, 53.

De Robertis, E. D. P., and Bennett, H. S. (1955). Some features of the submicroscopic morphology of synapses in frog and earthworm. *J. Biophys. Biochem. Cytol.,* 1, 47–58.

De Robertis, E., Rodrigues de Lores Arnaiz, G., and Pallegrino de Iraldi, A. (1962). Isolation of synaptic vesicles from nerve endings of rat brain. *Nature,* 194, 794–795.

Descarries, L., Bosler, O., Berthelet, F., and Des Rossiers, M. H. (1980). Dopaminergic nerve endings visualized by high resolution autoradiography in adult rat neostriatum. *Nature,* 284, 620–622.

Descarries, L., Séguéla, P., and Watkins, K. C. (1991). Nonjunctional relationships of monoamine axon terminals in the cerebral cortex of adult rat. In *Volume Transmission in the Brain: Novel Mechanisms for Neural Transmission* (K. Fuxe and L. F. Agnati, Eds.), pp. 53–62. Raven Press, New York.

De Souza, E. B., Battaglia, G., and Insel, T. R. (1990). Neurotoxic effects of MDMA on brain serotonin neurons: Evidence from neurochemical and radioligand binding studies. *Ann. N.Y. Acad. Sci.,* 600, 682–698.

Deutch, A. Y., and Zahm, D. S. (1992). The current status of neurotensin–dopamine interactions: Issues and speculations. *Ann. N.Y. Acad. Sci.,* 668, 232–252.

Deutsch, D. G., and Chin, S. A. (1993). Enzymatic synthesis and degradation of anandamide, a cannabinoid receptor agonist. *Biochem. Pharmacol.,* 46, 791–796.

Deutsch, J. A. (1983a). The cholinergic synapse and the site of memory, In *The Physiological Basis of Memory* (2nd ed.). (J. A. Deutsch, Ed.), pp. 367–386, Academic Press, New York.

Deutsch, J. A. (1983b). Dietary control and the stomach. *Prog. Neurobiol.,* 20, 313–332.

Deutsch, J. A., and Hardy, W. T. (1977). Cholecystokinin produces bait shyness in rats. *Nature,* 266, 196.

Devane, W. A., and Axelrod, J. (1994). Enzymatic synthesis of anandamide, an endogenous ligand for the cannabinoid receptor, by brain membranes. *Proc. Natl. Acad. Sci. U.S.A.*, 91, 6698–6701.

Devane, W. A., Dysarz, F. A. III, Johnson, M. R., Melvin, L. S., and Howlett, A. C. (1988). Determination and characterization of a cannabinoid receptor in rat brain. *Mol. Pharmacol.*, 34, 605–613.

Devane, W. A., et al.(1992). Isolation and structure of a brain constituent that binds to the cannabinoid receptor. *Science*, 258, 1946–1949.

Devine, D. P., Leone, P., Pocock, D., and Wise, R. A. (1993). Differential involvement of ventral tegmental mu, delta and kappa opioid receptors in modulation of basal mesolimbic dopamine release: in vivo microdialysis studies. *J. Pharmacol. Exp. Ther.*, 266, 1236–1246.

Dewey, W. L. (1986). Cannabinoid pharmacology. *Pharmacol. Rev.*, 38, 151–178.

De Wit, H., and Wise, R. A. (1977). Blockade of cocaine reinforcement in rats with the dopamine receptor blocker pimozide, but not with the noradrenergic blockers phentolamine or phenoxybenzamine. *Canad. J. Psychol.*, 31, 195–203.

Dews, P. B. (1955). Studies on behavior. I. Differential sensitivity to pentobarbital of pecking performance in pigeons depending on the schedule of reward. *J. Pharmacol. Exp. Ther.*, 113, 393–401.

Dews, P. B. (1958). Studies on behavior. IV. Stimulant actions of methamphetamine. *J. Pharmacol. Exp. Ther.*, 122, 137–147.

Dews, P. B., and Wenger, G. R. (1977). Rate-dependency of the behavioral effects of amphetamine. In *Advances in Behavioral Pharmacology, Volume 1* (T. Thompson and P. B. Dews, Eds.), pp. 167–227. Academic Press, New York.

Diamandis, E. P. (1990). Analytical methodology for immunoassays and DNA hybridization assays: Current status and selected systems: Critical review. *Clin. Chim. Acta*, 194, 19–50.

Diana, M., Pistis, M., Carboni, S., Gessa, G. L., and Rossetti, Z. L. (1993). Profound decrement of mesolimbic dopaminergic neuronal activity during ethanol withdrawal syndrome in rats: Electrophysiological and biochemical evidence. *Proc. Natl. Acad. Sci. U.S.A.*, 90, 7966–7969.

Diana, M., Pistis, M., Muntoni, A., and Gessa, G. (1995). Profound decrease of mesolimbic dopaminergic neuronal activity in morphine withdrawn rats. *J. Pharmacol. Exp. Ther.*, 272, 781–785.

Di Chiara, G., and Imperato, A. (1985). Alcohol preferentially stimulates dopamine release from the nucleus accumbens in freely moving rats. *Eur. J. Pharmacol.*, 115, 131–132.

Di Chiara, G., and Imperato, A. (1986). Preferential stimulation of dopamine release in the nucleus accumbens by opiates, alcohol and barbiturates: Studies by transcerebral dialysis in freely moving rats. *Ann. N.Y. Acad. Sci.*, 473, 367–381.

Di Chiara, G., and Imperato, A. (1988). Drugs abused by humans preferentially increase synaptic dopamine concentrations in the mesolimbic system of freely moving rats. *Proc. Natl. Acad. Sci. U.S.A.*, 85, 5274–5278.

Di Chiara, G., and North, R. A. (1992). Neurobiology of opiate abuse. *Trends Pharmacol. Sci.*, 13, 185–193.

Di Chiara, G., Tanda, G. L., Frau, R., and Carboni, E. (1992). Heterologous monoamine reuptake: Lack of transmitter specificity of neuron-specific carriers. *Neurochem. Int.*, 20 (Suppl.), 231S–235S.

Dichter, M. A. (1988). Modulation of inhibition and the transition to seizures. In *Mechanisms of Epileptogenesis: The Transition to Seizure* (M. A. Dichter, Ed.), pp. 169–181. Plenum Press, New York.

Diedrich, J. F., Minnigan, H., Carp, R. I., Whitaker, J. N., Race, R., Frey, W. II, and Haase, A. T. (1991). Neuropathological changes in scrapie and Alzheimer's disease are associated with increased expression of apolipoprotein E and cathepsin D in astrocytes. *J. Virol.*, 65, 4759–4768.

DiFiglia, M. (1990). Excitotoxic injury of the neostriatum: A model for Huntington's disease. *Trends Neurosci.*, 13, 286–289.

DiFranza, J. R., Richards, J. W. Jr., Paulman, P. M., Wolf-Gillespie, N., Fletcher, C., Jaffe, R. D., and Murray, D. (1991). RJR Nabisco's cartoon camel promotes Camel cigarettes to children. *JAMA*, 266, 3149–3153.

Diksic, M. (1992). Alpha-methyl tryptophan as a tracer for in vivo studies of brain serotonin system, from autoradiography to positron emission tomography. *J. Chem. Neuroanat.*, 5, 349–354.

Diksic, M., Nagahiro, S., Chaly, T., Sourkes, T. L., Yamamoto, Y. L., and Feindel, W. (1991). Serotonin synthesis rate measured in living dog brain by positron emission tomography. *J. Neurochem.*, 56, 153–162.

Diksic, M., Nagahiro, S., Sourkes, T. L., and Yamamoto, Y. L. (1990). A new method to measure brain serotonin synthesis in vivo. I. Theory and basic data for a biological model. *J. Cereb. Blood Flow Metab.*, 10, 1–12.

Diliberto, E. J. Jr., Daniels, A. J., and Viveros, O. H. (1991). Multicompartmental secretion of ascorbate and its dual role in dopamine β-hydroxylation. *Am. J. Clin. Nutr.*, 54, 1163S–1172S.

DiMauro, S. (1993). Mitochondrial involvement in Parkinson's disease: The controversy continues. *Neurology*, 43, 2170–2172.

Di Monte, D. A., Wu, E. Y., Irwin, I., DeLanney, L. E., and Langston, J. W. (1992). Production and disposition of 1-methyl-4-phenylpyridinium in primary cultures of mouse astrocytes. *Glia*, 5, 48–55.

Dingledine, R., McBain, C. J., and McNamara, J. O. (1990). Excitatory amino acid receptors in epilepsy. *Trends Pharmacol. Sci.*, 11, 334–338.

Dirksen, R. (1990). Opioid receptors and pain. *Pharmacol Weekbl*[*Sci*]., 12, 41–45.

Dixon, R. A. F., et al. (1986). Cloning of the gene and cDNA for mammalian β-adrenergic receptor and homology with rhodopsin. *Nature*, 321, 75–79.

Dixon, W. E. (1906). Vagus inhibition. *Br. Med. J.*, ii, 1807.

Djamgoz, M. B. A., and Wagner, H.-J. (1992). Localization and function of dopamine in the adult vertebrate retinal. *Neurochem. Int.*, 20, 139–191.

Doble, A., and Martin, I. L. (1992). Multiple benzodiazepine receptors: No reason for anxiety. *Trends Pharmacol. Sci.*, 13, 76–81.

Dodd, J., and Castellucci, V. F. (1991). Smell and taste. In *Principles of Neural Science*, (3rd ed.) (E. R. Kandel, J. H. Schwartz and T. M. Jessell, Eds.), pp. 512–529. Elsevier, New York.

Doenicke, A. (1984). Modern trends in the investigation of new hypnotics in anesthesia. In *Sleep, Benzodiazepines and Performance: Experimental Methodologies and Research Prospects* (I. Hindmarch, H. Ott, and T. Roth, Eds.), pp. 119–132. Springer-Verlag, New York

Dole, V. P. (1988). Implications of methadone maintenance for theories of narcotic addiction. *JAMA*, 260, 3025–3029.

Dole, V. P., and Nyswander, M. E. (1965). A medical treatment for diacetylmorphine (heroin) addiction. *JAMA*, 193, 646–650.

Doll, R. and Hill, A. B. (1964). *Br. Med. J.*, 1, 1399–1410.

Donnerer, J., Oka, K., Brossi, A., Rice, K. C., and Spector, S. (1986). Presence and formation of codeine and morphine in the rat. *Proc. Nat. Acad. Sci. U.S.A.*, 83, 4566–4567.

Doods, H. N., et al. (1993). Therapeutic potential of CNS-active M2 antagonists: Novel structures and pharmacology. *Life Sci.*, 52, 497–503.

Dores, R. and Akil, H. (1987). Species specific processing of pro-dynorphin in the posterior pituitary of mammals. *Endocrinology*, 120, 230–238.

Dores, R., Jain, M. and Akil, H. (1986). Characterization of the forms of beta-endorphin and alpha-MSH in the caudal medulla of the rat and guinea pig. *Brain Res.*, 377, 251–260.

Dori, I., Dinopoulos, A., Cavanagh, M. E., and Parnavelas, J. G. (1992). Proportion of glutamate- and aspartate-immunoreactive neurons in the efferent pathways of the rat visual cortex varies according to the target. *J. Comp. Neurol.*, 319, 191–204.

Dori, I., Petrou, M., and Parnavelas, J. G. (1989). Excitatory transmitter amino acid-containing neurons in the rat visual cortex: A light and electron microscopic immunocytochemical study. *J. Comp. Neurol.*, 290, 169–184.

Dornan, W. A., Akesson, T. R., and Micevych, P. E. (1990). A substance P projection from the VMH to the dorsal midbrain central gray: Implication for lordosis. *Brain Res. Bull.*, 25, 791–796.

Dornan, W. A., Malsbury, C. W., and Penney, R. B. (1987). Facilitation of lordosis by injection of substance P into the midbrain central gray. *Neuroendocrinology*, 45, 498–506.

Dorshay, L. J., and Constable, K. (1949). Active therapy for parkinsonism. *JAMA*, 140, 1317.

Dorus, E., Cox, N. J., Gibbons, R. D., Shaughnessy, R., Pandey, G. N., and Cloninger, R. (1983). Lithium ion transport and affective disorders within families of bipolar patients. *Arch. Gen. Psychiatry*, 40, 545–552.

Dougherty, G. G. Jr. and Ellinwood, E. H. Jr. (1981). Chronic *d*-amphetamine in nucleus accumbens: Lack of tolerance or reverse tolerance of locomotor activity. *Life Sci.*, 28, 2295–2298.

Douglas, W. W. (1985). Histamine and 5-hydroxytryptamine (serotonin) and their anyagonists. In *Goodman and Gilman's Pharmacological Basis of Therapeutics* (7th ed.). (A. G. Gilman, L. S. Goodman, T. W. Rall and F. Murad, Eds.), pp. 605–638, Macmillan, New York.

Dourish, C. T., Hutson, P. H., Kennett, G. H., and Curzon, G. (1986). 8-OH-DPAT-induced hyperphagia: Its neural basis and possible therapeutic relevance. *Appetite*, 7 (Suppl.), 127–140.

Dourish, C. T., Rycroft, W., and Iversen, S. D. (1989). Postponement of satiety by blockade of brain cholecystokinin (CCK-B) receptors. *Science,* 245, 1509–1511.

Dowd, D. J., Edwards, C., Englert, D., Mazurkiewicz, J. E., and Ye, H. Z. (1983). Immunofluorescent evidence for exocytosis and internalization of secretory granule membrane in isolated chromaffin cells. *Neuroscience,* 10, 1025–1033.

Drachman, D. B. (1987). Myasthenia gravis: A model disorder of acetylcholine receptors. In *Molecular Neurobiology in Neurology and Psychiatry* (E. R. Kandel, Ed.), pp. 65–82. Raven Press, New York.

Dragunow, M. (1988). Purinergic mechanisms in epilepsy. *Prog. Neurobiol.,* 31, 85–108.

Dragunow, M., Robertson, G. S., Faull, R. L. M., Robertson, H. A., and Jansen, K. (1990). D_2 dopamine receptor antagonists induce Fos and related proteins in rat striatal neurons. *Neuroscience,* 37, 287–294.

Dray, A. (1992). Mechanism of action of capsaicin-like molecules on sensory neurons. *Life Sci.,* 51, 1759–1765.

Drew, W. G., and Miller, L. L. (1974). Cannabis: Neural mechanisms and behavior—a theoretical review. *Pharmacology,* 11, 12–32.

Dring, L. G., Smith, R. L., and Williams, R. T. (1970). The metabolic fate of amphetamine in man and other species. *Biochem. J.,* 116, 425–435.

Dropp, J. J. (1976). Mast cells in mammalian brain. I. Distribution. *Acta Anat.,* 94, 1–21.

Drukarch, B., and Stoof, J. C. (1990). D-2 dopamine autoreceptor selective drugs: Do they really exist? *Life Sci.,* 47, 361–376.

Drummond, A. H. (1987). Lithium and inositol lipid-linked signalling mechanisms. *Trends Pharmacol. Sci.,* 8, 129–133.

Drummond, D. C. (1991). Comprehensive strategies for the therapy of alcoholism: Where have we gone wrong? *Alcohol Acohol.* Suppl. 1, 49–56.

Dua, A. K., Pinsky, C, and LaBella, F. S. (1985). Peptidases that terminate the action of enkephalins. Consideration of physiological importance for amino-, carboxy-, endo-, and pseudoenkephalinase. *Life Sci.,* 37, 985–992.

Du Bois-Raymond, E. (1877). Gesammelte Abhandl. d. allgem *Muskel-und Nervenphysik,* 2, 700.

Duda, N. J., and Moore, K. E. (1985). Simultaneous determination of 5-hydroxytryptophan and 3,4-dihydroxyphenylalanine in rat brain by HPLC with electrochemical detection following electrical stimulation of the dorsal raphe nucleus. *J. Neurochem.,* 44, 128–133.

Dudley, M. W., Howard, B. D., and Cho, A. K. (1990). The interaction of the beta-haloethyl benzylamines, xylamine, and DSP-4 with catecholaminergic neurons. *Annu. Rev. Pharmacol. Toxicol.,* 30, 387–403.

Duggan, A. W., and Fleetwood-Walker, S. M. (1993). Opioids and sensory processing in the central nervous system. In *Opioids I,* Handbook of Experimental Pharmacology, Vol. 104 (A. Herz, Ed.), pp. 731–771. Springer-Verlag, New York.

Duggan, A. W., Hall, J. G., and Headly P. M. (1976). Morphine, enkephalin and the substantia gelatinosa. *Nature,* 264, 456–458.

Duggan, A. W., Morton, C. R., Zhao, Z. Q., and Hendry, I. A. (1987). Noxious heating of the skin releases immunoreactive substance P in the substantia gelatinosa of the cat: A study with antibody microprobes. *Brain Res.,* 403, 345–349.

Dumuis, A., Bouhelal, R., Sebben, M., and Bockaert, J. (1988). A 5-HT receptor in the central nervous system, positively coupled with adenylate cyclase, is antagonized by ICS205–930. *Eur. J. Pharmacol.,* 146, 187–188.

Dunant, Y. (1986). On the mechanism of acetylcholine release. *Prog. Neurobiol.,* 26, 55–92.

Dunant, Y., and Israël, M. (1993). Ultrastructure and biophysics of acetylcholine release: Central role of the mediatophore. *J. Physiol.* (Paris), 87, 179–192.

Duncan, G. E., and Stumpf, W. E. (1991). Brain activity patterns: Assessment by high resolution audioradiographic imaging of radiolabeled 2-deoxyglucose and glucose uptake. *Prog. Neurobiol.,* 37, 365–382.

Dunlap, K., Luebke, J. I., and Turner, T. J. (1995). Exocytotic Ca^{2+} channels in mammalian central neurons. *Trends Neurosci.,* 18, 89–98.

Dunn, A. J., and Berridge, C. W. (1987). Corticotropin-releasing factor administration elicits a stress-like activation of cerebral catecholaminergic systems. *Pharmacol. Biochem. Behav.,* 27, 685–691.

Dunn, A. J., and Berridge, C. W. (1990). Physiological and behavioral responses to corticotropin-releasing factor administration: Is CRF a mediator of anxiety or stress responses? *Brain Res. Rev.,* 15, 71–100.

Dunner, D. L., and Clayton, P. J. (1987). Drug treatment of bipolar disorder. In *Psychopharmacology: The Third Generation of Progress* (H. Y. Meltzer, Ed.), pp. 1077–1083. Raven Press, New York.

Dunnett, S. B. (1985). Comparative effects of cholinergic drugs and lesions of the nucleus basalis or fimbria-fornix on delayed matching in rats. *Psychopharmacology,* 87, 357–363.

Dunnett, S. B., and Björklund, A. (1994). Mechanisms of function of neural grafts in the injured brain. In *Functional Neural Transplantation* (S. B. Dunnett and A. Björklund, Eds.), pp. 531–567. Raven Press, New York.

Dunnett, S. B., Everitt, B. J., and Robbins, T. W. (1991). The basal forebrain–cortical cholinergic system: Interpreting the functional consequences of excitotoxic lesions. *Trends Neurosci.,* 14, 494–501.

Dunnett, S. B., Whishaw, I. Q., Jones, G. H., and Bunch, S. T. (1987). Behavioural, biochemical and histochemical effects of different neurotoxic amino acids injected into nucleus basalis magnocellularis of rats. *Neuroscience,* 20, 653–669.

Durazzo, T. C., Gauvin, D. V., Goulden, K. L., Briscoe, R. J., and Holloway, F. A. (1994). Cocaine-induced conditioned place approach in rats: The role of dose and route of administration. *Pharmacol. Biochem. Behav.,* 49, 1001–1005.

Durcan, M. J., and Morgan, P. F. (1989). Evidence for adenosine A_2 receptor involvement in the hypomobility effects of adenosine analogues in mice. *Eur. J. Pharmacol.,* 168, 285–290.

Dworkin, S. I., Gleeson, S., Meloni, D., Koves, T. R., and Martin, T. J. (1995). Effects of ibogaine on responding maintained by food, cocaine and heroin reinforcement in rats. *Psychopharmacology,* 117, 257–261.

Dyck, L. E. (1989). Release of some endogenous trace amines from rat striatal slices in the presence and absence of a monoamine oxidase inhibitor. *Life Sci.,* 44, 1149–1156.

Eberwine, J.H., Valentino, K.L. and Barchas, J.D. (1994). *In Situ Hybridization in Neurobiology,* Oxford University Press, New York.

Ebstein, R. P., Hermoni, M., and Belmaker, R. H. (1980). The effect of lithium on noradrenaline-induced cyclic AMP accumulation in rat brain: Inhibition after chronic treatment and absence of supersensitivity. *J. Pharmacol. Exp. Ther.,* 213, 161–167.

Ebstein, R. P., Lever, B., Bennett, E. R., Dayek, D. B., Newman, M. E., Shapira, B., and Kindler, S. (1988). Lithium modulation of second messenger signal amplification in man: Inhibition of phosphatidylinositol-specific phopholipase C and adenylate cyclase activity. *Psychiatry Res.,* 24, 45–52.

Ebstein, R. P., Moscovich, D., Zeevi, S., Amiri, Z., and Lerer, B. (1987). Effect of lithium in vitro and after chronic treatment on human platelet adenylate cyclase activity: Postreceptor modification of second messenger signal amplification. *Psychiatry Res.,* 21, 221–228.

Eccles, J. C. (1957). *The Physiology of Nerve Cells.* Johns Hopkins Press, Baltimore.

Eccles, J. C. (1964a). Ionic mechanisms of postsynaptic inhibition. *Science,* 145, 1140–1147.

Eccles, J. C. (1964b). *The Physiology of Synapses.* Academic Press, New York.

Eccles, J. C. (1967). Postsynaptic inhibition in the central nervous system. In *The Neurosciences, A Study Program* (G. C. Quarton, T. Melnechuk, and F. O. Schmitt, Eds.), pp. 408–426. The Rockefeller University Press, New York.

Eccles, J. C., Fatt, P., and Koketsu, K. (1954). Cholinergic and inhibitory synapses in a pathway from motor-axon collaterals to motoneurones. *J. Physiol.* (Lond.), 126, 524–562.

Eccleston, D., Fairbairn, A. F., Hassanyeh, F., McClelland, H. A., and Stephens, D. A. (1985). The effect of propranalol and thioridazine on positive and negative symptoms of schizophrenia. *Br. J. Psychiatry,* 147, 623–630.

Eccleston, D., Loose, R., Pullar, I. A., and Sugden, R. F. (1970). Exercise and urinary excretion of cyclic AMP. *Lancet,* 2, 612–613.

Edelman, A. M., Raese, J. D., Lazar, M. A., and Barchas, J. D. (1978). In vitro phosphorylation of a purified preparation of bovine corpus striatal tyrosine hydroxylase. *Commun. Psychopharmacol.,* 2, 461–465.

Egeland, J. A., et al. (1987). Bipolar affective disorders linked to DNA markers on chromosome 11. *Nature,* 325, 783–787.

Ehrenkranz, J. R. L., and Hembree, W. C. (1986). Effects of marijuana on male reproductive function. *Psychiatric Ann.,* 16, 243–248.

Ehrman, R. N., Robbins, S. J., Childress, A. R., and O'Brien, C. P. (1992). Conditioned responses to cocaine-related stimuli in cocaine abuse patients. *Psychopharmacology,* 107, 523–529.

Eide, F. F., Lowenstein, D. H., and Reichardt, L. F. (1993). Neurotrophins and their receptors: Current concepts and implications for neurologic disease. *Exp. Neurol.,* 121, 200–214.

Eilam, D., Talangbayan, H., Canaran, G., and Szechtman, H. (1992). Dopaminergic control of locomotion, mouthing, snout contact, and grooming: Opposing roles of D_1 and D_2 receptors. *Psychopharmacology, 106,* 447–454.

Einhorn, L. C., Johansen, P. A., and White, F. J. (1988). Electrophysiological effects of cocaine in the mesoaccumbens dopamine system: Studies in the ventral tegmental area. *J. Neurosci., 8,* 100–112.

Eipper, B.A. and Mains, R.E. (1981). Further analysis of posttranslational processing of β-endorphin in rat intermediate pituitary. J. Biol. Chem., 256, 5689–5695.

Eisner, B. (1989). *Ecstasy: The MDMA Story.* Ronin Publishing Company, Berkeley.

Elam, M., Yao, T., Svensson, T. H., and Thorén, P. (1984). Regulation of locus coeruleus neurons and splanchnic, sympathetic nerves by cardiovascular afferents. *Brain Res., 290,* 281–287.

Elbert, T., Pantev, C., Weinbruch, C., Rockstraw, B., and Taub, E. (1995). Increased cortical representation of the fingers of the left hand in string players. *Science, 270,* 305–307.

Elchisak, M. A., Maas, J. W., and Roth, R. H. (1977). Dihydroxyphenylacetic acid conjugate: Natural occurrence and demonstration of probenecid-induced accumulation in rat striatum, olfactory tubercles and frontal cortex. *Eur. J. Pharmacol., 41,* 369–378.

Elde, R., and Hokfelt, T. (1993). Coexistence of opioid peptides with other neurotransmitters. In *Opioids I,* Handbook of Experimental Pharmacology, Vol. 104 (A. Herz, Ed.), pp. 585–624. Springer-Verlag, New York.

Elfvin, L.-G., Lindh, B., and Hökfelt, T. (1993). The chemical neuroanatomy of sympathetic ganglia. *Annu. Rev. Neurosci., 16,* 471–507.

Elkawad, A. O., and Woodruff, G. N. (1976). Studies on the behavioural pharmacology of a cyclic analogue of dopamine following its injection into the brains of conscious rats. *Brit. J. Pharmacol., 54,* 107–114.

Ellinwood, E. H. Jr. (1967). Amphetamine psychosis: I. Description of the individuals and process. *J. Nerv. Ment. Dis., 144,* 273–283.

Ellinwood, E. H. Jr., and Nikaido, A. M. (1987). Perceptual neuro-motor pharmacodynamics of psychotropic drugs. In *Psychopharmacology: The Third Generation of Progress* (H. Y. Meltzer, Ed.), pp. 1457–1466. Raven Press, New York.

Ellinwood, E. H. Jr., Sudilovsky, A., and Nelson, L. M. (1973). Evolving behavior in the clinical and experimental amphetamine (model) psychosis. *Am. J. Psychiatry, 130,* 1088–1093.

Elliott, P. J., and Iversen, S. D. (1986). Behavioural effects of tachykinins and related peptides. *Brain Res., 381,* 68–76.

Elliott, T. R. (1904). On the action of adrenalin. *J. Physiol. (Lond.), 31,* XX–XXI.

Elliott, T. R. (1905). The action of adrenaline. *J. Physiol.* (Lond.), 32, 401–467.

Ellisman, M. H. (1981). Topographic organization of the elements of the cytoskeleton. *Neurosci. Res. Prog. Bull., 20,* 79–91.

Ellison, G.D. (1991). Animal models of hallucinations. Continuous stimulants. In *Neuromethods, Vol. 18: Animal Models in Psychiatry I* (A. Boulton, G. Baker, and M. Martin-Iverson, Eds.), pp. 151–195. Humana Press, Clifton, NJ.

Ellison, G. (1992). Continuous amphetamine and cocaine have similar neurotoxic effects in lateral habenular nucleus and fasciculus retroflexus. *Brain Res., 598,* 353–356.

Ellison, G. (1995). The N-methyl-D-aspartate antagonists phencyclidine, ketamine and dizocilpine as both behavioral and anatomical models of the dementias. *Brain Res. Rev., 20,* 250–267.

Ellison, G., Eison, M. S., Huberman, H. S., and Daniel, F. (1978). Long-term changes in dopaminergic innervation of caudate nucleus after continuous amphetamine administration. *Science, 201,* 276–278.

Elsmore, T. F., and Fletcher, G. V. (1972). Δ⁹-tetrahydrocannabinol: Aversive effects in rat at high doses. *Science, 175,* 911–912.

Elsworth, J. D., Deutch, A. Y., Redmond, D. E. Jr., Sladek, J. R. Jr., and Roth, R. H. (1987). Effects of 1-methyl-4-phenyl- 1,2,3,6-tetrahydropyridine (MPTP) on catecholamines and metabolites in primate brain and CSF. *Brain Res., 415,* 293–299.

Elsworth, J. D., Deutch, A. Y., Redmond, D. E. Jr., Sladek, J. R. Jr., and Roth, R. H. (1990). MPTP reduces dopamine and norepinephrine concentrations in the supplementary motor area and cingulate cortex of the primate. *Neurosci. Lett., 114,* 316–322.

Elsworth, J. D., Roth, R. H., and Redmond, D. E. Jr. (1983). Relative importance of 3-methoxy-4-hydroxyphenylglycol and 3,4-dhydroxyphenylglycol as norepinephrine metabolites in rat, monkey, and humans. *J. Neurochem., 41,* 786–793.

Elverfors, A., and Nissbrandt, H. (1992). Effects of *d*-amphetamine on dopaminergic neurotransmission; a comparison between the substantia nigra and the striatum. *Neuropharmacology, 31,* 661–670.

Emerich, D. F., Winn, S. R., Harper, J., Hammang, J. P., Baetge, E. E., and Kordower, J. H. (1994). Implants of polymer-encapsulated human NGF-secreting cells in the nonhuman primate: Rescue and sprouting of degenerating cholinergic basal forebrain neurons. *J. Comp. Neurol., 349,* 148–164.

Emmett-Oglesby, M. W., Peltier, R. L., Depoortere, R. Y., Pickering, C. L., Hooper, M. L., Gong, Y. H., and Lane, J. D. (1993). Tolerance to self-administration of cocaine in rats: Time course and dose-response determination using a multi-dose method. *Drug Alcohol Depend.* 32, 247–256.

Emorine, L., Blin, N., and Strosberg, A. D. (1994). The human β₃-adrenoceptor: The search for a physiological function. *Trends Pharmacol. Sci., 15,* 3–7.

Emoto, H., Tanaka, M., Koga, C., Yokoo, H., Tsuda, A., and Yoshida, M. (1993). Corticotropin-releasing factor activates the noradrenergic neuron system in the rat brain. *Pharmacol. Biochem. Behav., 45,* 419–422.

Engberg, G., and Svensson, T. H. (1979). Amphetamine-induced inhibition of central noradrenergic neurons: A pharmacological analysis. *Life Sci., 24,* 2245–2254.

Engel, G. L. (1980). The clinical application of the biopsychosocial model. *Am. J. Psychiatry, 137,* 535–544.

Enna, S. J., Wood, J. H., and Snyder, S. H. (1977). γ-Aminobutyric acid (GABA) in human cerebrospinal fluid: Radioreceptor assay. *J. Neurochem.,* 28, 1121–1124.

Enz, A., Amstutz, R., Boddeke, H., Gmelin, G., and Malanowski, J. (1993). Brain selective inhibition of acetylcholinesterase: A novel approach to therapy for Alzheimer's disease. *Prog. Brain Res.,* 98, 431–438.

Epelbaum, J., Ruberg, M., Moyse, E., Javoy-Agid, F., Dubois, B., and Agid, Y. (1983). Somatostatin and dementia in Parkinson's disease. *Brain Res., 278,* 376–379.

Eränkö, O. (1955). Histochemistry of noradrenaline in the adrenal medulla of rats and mice. *Endocrinology, 57,* 363–367.

Eränkö, O. (Ed.) (1976). *Structure and Function of the Small Intensely Fluorescent Sympathetic Cells.* Fogarty International Center Proceedings, No. 30. DHEW Publication No. (NIH) 76–942. Superintendent of Documents, Washington, D.C.

Erard, R., Luisada, P. V., and Peele, R. (1980). The PCP psychosis: Prolonged intoxication or drug-precipitated functional illness? *Psychedel. Drugs, 12,* 235–245.

Erdö, S. L. (1991). Excitatory amino acid receptors in the mammalian periphery. *Trends Pharmacol. Sci., 12,* 426–429.

Erecińska, M. (1987). The neurotransmitter amino acid transport systems: A fresh outlook on an old problem. *Biochem. Pharmacol., 36,* 3547–3555.

Erickson, J. D., and Eiden, L. E. (1993). Functional identification and molecular cloning of a human brain vesicle monoamine transporter. *J. Neurochem., 61,* 2314–2317.

Erickson, J. D., Eiden, L. E., and Hoffman, B. J. (1992). Expression cloning of a reserpine-sensitive vesicular monoamine transporter. *Proc. Natl. Acad. Sci. U.S.A., 89,* 10993–10997.

Erlander, M. G., Tillakaratne, N. J. K., Feldblum, S., Patel, N., and Tobin, A. J. (1991). Two genes encode distinct glutamate decarboxylases. *Neuron, 7,* 91–100.

Erspamer, V. (1940). Pharmacology of enteramine. I. Action of acetone extract of rabbit stomach mucosa on blood pressure and on surviving isolated organs. *Naunyn Schmiedebergs Arch. Exp. Path. Pharmakol., 196,* 343–365.

Erspamer, V., and Asero, B. (1952). Identification of enteramine, the specific hormone of the enterochromaffin cell system, as 5-Hdroxytrypamine. *Nature,* 169, 800–801.

Esplin, D. W., and Zablocka, B. (1965). Central nervous system stimulants. In *The Pharmacological Basis of Therapeutics* (L. S. Goodman and A. Gilman, Eds.), pp. 345–353. Macmillan, New York.

Esposito, R. U., Porrino, L. J., and Seeger, T. F. (1989). Brain stimulation reward measurement and mapping by psychophysical techniques and quantitative 2-(¹⁴C)deoxyglucose autoradiography. In *Methods of Assessing the Reinforcing Properties of Abused Drugs* (M. A. Bozarth, Ed.), pp. 421–447. Springer, New York.

Essig, C. (1970). Barbiturate dependence. In *Drug Dependence* (R. T. Harris, W. M. McIsaac, and C. R. Schuster, Eds.), pp. 219–140. University of Texas Press, Austin.

Essman, W. B. (1978). Serotonin distribution in tissues and fluids. In *Serotonin in Health and Disease,* Vol. I. *Availability, Localization and Disposition* (W. B. Essman, Ed.), pp. 15–169. Spectrum, New York.

Ettenberg, A., and Geist, T. D. (1991). Animal model for investigating the anxiogenic effects of self-administered cocaine. *Psychopharmacology, 103,* 455–461.

Ettenberg, A., Pettit, H. O., Bloom, F. E., and Koob, G. F. (1982). Heroin and cocaine intravenous self-administration in rats: Mediation by separate neural systems. *Psychopharmacology*, 78, 204–209.

Ettenberg, A., van der Kooy, D., Le Moal, M., Koob, G. F., and Bloom, F. E. (1983). Can aversive properties of (peripherally-injected) vasopressin account for its putative role in memory? *Behav. Brain Res.*, 7, 331–350.

Evans, C. J., Keith, D. E., Jr., Morrison, H., Magendzo, K., and Edwards, R. H. (1992). Cloning of a delta opioid receptor by functional expression. *Science*, 258, 1952–1955.

Evans, K. C., Berger, E. P., Cho, C.-G., Weisgraber, K. H., and Lansbury, P. T. Jr. (1995). Apolipoprotein E is a kinetic but not a thermodynamic inhibitor of amyloid formation: Implications for the pathogenesis and treatment of Alzheimer disease. *Proc. Natl. Acad. Sci. U.S.A.*, 92, 763–767.

Evans, K. R., and Vaccarino, F. J. (1990). Amphetamine- and morphine-induced feeding: Evidence for involvement of reward mechanisms. *Neurosci. Biobehav. Rev.*, 14, 9–22.

Evans, R. I., Henderson, A., Hill, P., and Raines, B. (1979). Smoking in children and adolescents: Psychosocial determinants and prevention strategies. In *The Behavioral Aspects of Smoking* (N. A.. Krasnegor, Ed.), pp. 69–96, NIDA Res. Mongr. 26, Natl. Inst. on Drug Abuse, Rockville, MD.

Evans, S. M., Critchfield, T. S., and Griffiths, R. R. (1994). Caffeine reinforcement demonstrated in a majority of moderate caffeine users. *Behav. Pharmacol.*, 5, 231–238.

Evans, W. O. (1961). A new technique for the investigation of some analgesic drugs on a reflexive behavior in the rat. *Psychopharmacologia*, 2, 318–325.

Evarts, E. V., Kimura, M., Wurtz, R. H., and Hikosaka, O. (1984). Behavioral correlates of activity in basal ganglia neurons. *Trends Neurosci.*, 7, 447–453.

Evenden, J. L., and Ryan, C. N. (1990). Behavioral responses to psychomotor stimulant drugs: Localization in the central nervous system. In *Psychotropic Drugs of Abuse* (D. J. K. Balfour, Ed.), pp. 1–21. Pergamon Press, New York.

Evinger, E. J., Ernsberger, P., Regunathan, S., Joh, T. J., and Reis, D. J. (1994). A single transmitter regulates gene expression through two separate mechanisms: Cholinergic regulation of phenylethanolamine *N*-methyltransferase mRNA via nicotinic and muscarinic pathways. *J. Neurosci.*, 14, 2106–2116.

Evinger, M. J., Towle, A. C., Park, D. H., Lee, P., and Joh, T. H. (1992). Glucocorticoids stimulate transcription of the rat phenylethanolamine *N*-methyltransferase (PNMT) gene in vivo and in vitro. *Cell. Mol. Neurobiol.*, 12, 193–215.

Ewing, A. G., Bigelow, J. C., and Wightman, R. M. (1983). Direct in vivo monitoring of dopamine released from two striatal compartments in the rat. *Science*, 221, 169–171.

Faden, A. I. (1993). Role of endogenous opioids in central cardiovascular regulation and dysregulation. In *Opioids II*, Handbook of Experimental Pharmacology, Vol. 104 (A. Herz, Ed.), pp. 191–204. Springer-Verlag, New York.

Fagerström, K. O. (1978). Measuring degree of physical dependence to tobacco smoking with reference to individuation of treatment. *Addict. Behav.*, 3, 235–241.

Fagerström, K. O., Schneider, N. G., and Lunell, E. (1993). Effectiveness of nicotine patch and nicotine gum as individual versus combined treatments for tobacco withdrawal symptoms. *Psychopharmacology*, 111, 271–277.

Fagervall, I., and Ross, S. B. (1986). A and B forms of monoamine oxidase within the monoaminergic neurons of the rat brain. *J. Neurochem.*, 47, 569–576.

Faglia, G., and Persani, L. (1991). Thyrotropin-releasing hormone: Basic and clinical aspects. In *Brain Endocrinology* (2nd ed.) (M. Motta, Ed.), pp. 315–350. Raven Press, New York.

Fahn, S., and Cohen, G. (1992). The oxidant stress hypothesis in Parkinson's disease: Evidence supporting it. *Ann. Neurol.*, 32, 804–812.

Falck, B., Hillarp, N. A., Thieme, G., and Torp, A. (1962). Fluorescence of catecholamines and related compounds with formaldehyde. *J. Histochem. Cytochem.*, 10, 348–354.

Falkson, G., and van Zyl, A. (1989). A phase I study of a new 5-H_3-receptor antagonist, BRL43694A, an agent for the prevention of chemotherapy-induced nausea and vomiting. *Cancer Chemother. Pharmacol.*, 24, 193–196.

Fallon, J. H., and Seroogy, K. B. (1985). The distribution and some connections of cholecystokinin neurons in the rat brain. *Ann. N.Y. Acad. Sci.*, 448, 121–132.

Farde, L., Halldin, C., Müller, L., Suhara, T., Karlsson, P., and Hall, H. (1994). PET study of [^{11}C]β-CIT binding to monoamine transporters in the monkey and human brain. *Synapse*, 16, 93–103.

Farde, L., Nordstrom, A-L., Wiesel, F-A., Pauli, S., Halldin, C., Sedvall, G. (1992). Positron emission tomographic analysis of central D_1 and D_2 dopamine receptor occupancy in patients treated with classical neuroleptics and clozapine. *Arch. Gen. Psychiatry*, 49, 538–544.

Farnebo, L.-O., and Hamberger, B. (1971). Drug-induced changes in the release of [^{3}H]-noradrenaline from field stimulated rat iris. *Br. J. Pharmacol.*, 43, 97–106.

Farrant, M., Gibbs, T. T., and Farb, D. H. (1990). Molecular and cellular mechanisms of GABA/benzodiazepine-receptor regulation: Electrophysiological and biochemical studies. *Neurochem. Res.*, 15, 175–191.

Fatt, P., and Katz, B. (1952). Spontaneous subthreshold activity of motor nerve endings. *J. Physiol.* (Lond.), 117, 109–128.

Fawcett, D. W. (1986). *A Textbook of Histology*. Saunders, Philadelphia.

Feinberg, A. P., and Snyder, S. H. (1975). Phenothiazine drugs: Structure-activity relationships explained by a conformation that mimics dopamine. *Proc. Natl. Acad. Sci. U.S.A.*, 72, 1899–1903.

Feinberg, I. (1982). Schizophrenia: Caused by a fault in programmed synaptic elimination during adolescence? *J. Psychiatr. Res.*, 17, 319–334.

Felder, C. C., Briley, E. M., Axelrod, J., Simpson, J. T., Mackie, K., and Devane, W. A. (1993). Anandamide, an endogenous cannabimimetic eicosanoid, binds to the cloned human cannabinoid receptor and stimulates receptor-mediated signal transduction. *Proc. Natl. Acad. Sci. U.S.A.*, 90, 7656–7660.

Feldman, H. W. (1980). *Angel dust in four American cities: an ethnographic study of PCP users*. United States Department of Health and Human Services (DHHS publication no. ADM 81–1039), Rockville, MD.

Feldman, R. S., and Lewis, E. (1962). Response differences of psychotropic drugs in rats during chronic anxiety states. *J. Neuropsychiat.*, 3 (Suppl. 1), S27–S41.

Feldman, R. S., and Quenzer, L. F. (1984). *Fundamentals of Neuropsychopharmacology*. Sinauer Associates, Sunderland, MA.

Ferno, O., Lichmeckert, S. J. A., and Lundgren, C. E. G. (1973). A substitute for tobacco smoking. *Psychopharmacologia*, 31, 201–204.

Fernstrom, J. D. (1988a). Carbohydrate ingestion and brain serotonin synthesis: Relevance to a putative control loop for regulating carbohydrate ingestion, and effects of aspartame consumption. *Appetite*, 11 (Suppl.), 35–41.

Fernstrom, J. D. (1988b). Tryptophan, serotonin and carbohydrate appetite: Will the real carbohydrate craver please stand up! *J. Nutr.*, 118, 1417–1419.

Fernstrom, J. D. (1990). Aromatic amino acids and monoamine synthesis in the central nervous system: Influence of the diet. *J. Nutr. Biochem.*, 1, 508–517.

Fernstrom, J. D., and Fernstrom, M. H. (1994). Dietary effects on tyrosine availability and catecholamine synthesis in the central nervous system: Possible relevance to the control of protein intake. *Proc. Nutr. Soc.*, 53, 419–429.

Fernstrom, J. D., and Wurtman, R. J. (1971). Brain serotonin content: Physiological dependence on plasma tryptophan levels. *Science*, 173, 149–152.

Fernstrom, J. D., and Wurtman, R. J. (1972a). Brain serotonin content: Physiological regulation by plasma neutral amino acids. *Science*, 178, 414–416.

Fernstrom, J. D., and Wurtman, R. J. (1972b). Elevation of plasma tryptophan by insulin in rat. *Metabolism*, 21, 337–342.

Fernstrom, J. D., and Wurtman, R. J. (1974). Nutrition and the brain. *Sci. Am.*, 230, 84–91.

Fernstrom, M. H., and Fernstrom, J. D. (1995). Brain tryptophan concentrations and serotonin synthesis remain responsive to food consumption after the ingestion of sequential meals. *Am. J. Clin. Nutr.*, 61, 312–319.

Fernstrom, M. H., Massoudi, M. S., and Fernstrom, J. D. (1990). Effect of 8-hydroxy-2-(Di-*n*-propylamino)-tetralin on the tryptophan-induced increase in 5-hydroxytryptophan accumulation in rat brain. *Life Sci.*, 47, 283–289.

Ferrari, C. M., O'Connor, D. A., and Riley, A. L. (1991). Cocaine-induced taste aversions: Effect of route of administration. *Pharmacol. Biochem. Behav.*, 38, 267–271.

Ferraro, D. P. (1980). Acute effects of marijuana on human memory and cognition. In *Marijuana Research Findings: 1980. NIDA Res. Monogr. 31* (R. C. Petersen, Ed.), pp. 98–119. U.S. Government Printing Office, Washington, D.C.

Ferré, S., O'Connor, W. T., Fuxe, K., and Ungerstedt, U. (1993). The striopallidal neuron: A main locus for adenosine-dopamine interactions in the brain. *J. Neurosci.*, 13, 5402–5406.

Ferré, S., Rubio, A., and Fuxe, K. (1991). Stimulation of adenosine A_2 receptors induces catalepsy. *Neurosci. Lett.*, 130, 162–164.

Ferré, S., von Euler, G., Johansson, B., Fredholm, B. B., and Fuxe, K. (1991). Stimulation of high-affinity adenosine A_2 receptors decreases the affinity of dopamine D_2 receptors in rat striatal membranes. *Proc. Natl. Acad. Sci. U.S.A.*, 88, 7238–7241.

Ferris, R. M., Brieaddy, L., Mehta, N., Hollingsworth, E., Rigdon, G., Wang, C., Soroko, F., Wastila, W., and Cooper, B. (1995). Pharmacological properties of 403U76, a new chemical class of 5-hydroxytryptamine- and noradrenalin-reuptake inhibitor. *J. Pharm. Pharmacol.*, 47, 775–781.

Ferris, R. M., and Tang, F. L. M. (1979). Comparison of the effects of the isomers of amphetamine, methylphenidate and deoxypipradol on the uptake of L-[^{3}H]norepinephrine and [^{3}H]dopamine by synaptic vesicles from rat whole brain, striatum and hypothalamus. *J. Pharmacol. Exp. Ther.*, 210, 422–428.

Ferris, R. M., Tang, F. L. M., and Maxwell, R. A. (1972). A comparison of the capacities of isomers of amphetamine, deoxypipradol and methylphenidate to inhibit the uptake of tritiated catecholamines into rat cerebral cortex slices, synaptosomal preparations of rat cerebral cortex, hypothalamus and striatum and into adrenergic nerves of rabbit aorta. *J. Pharmacol. Exp. Ther.*, 181, 407–416.

Fertuck, H. C., and Salpeter, M. M. (1974). Localization of acetylcholine receptor by ^{125}I-labeled alpha-bungarotoxin binding at mouse motor endplates. *Proc. Natl. Acad. Sci. U.S.A.*, 71, 1376–1378.

ffrench-Mullen, J. M. H., and Rogawski, M. A. (1989). Interactions of phencyclidine with voltage-dependent potassium channels in cultured rat hippocampal neurons: Comparison with block of the NMDA receptor-ionophore complex. *J. Neurosci.*, 9, 4051–4061.

Fialkov, M. J. (1985). Biologic and psychosocial determinants in the etiology of alcoholism: Chronic effects. In *Alcohol and the Brain* (R. E. Tarter and D. H. Van Thiel, Eds.), pp. 245–263. Plenum Press, New York.

Fibiger, H. C. (1991). Cholinergic mechanisms in learning, memory and dementia: A review of recent evidence. *Trends Neurosci.*, 14, 220–223.

Fielding, S., and Szewczak, M. R. (1984). Pharmacology of nomifensine: A review of animal studies. *J. Clin. Psychiatry*, 45 (section 2), 12–20.

Fields, H. L. (1987). *Pain*. McGraw-Hill, New York.

Fields, H. L. (1993). Brainstem mechanisms of pain modulation. In *Opioids II*, Handbook of Experimental Pharmacology, Vol. 104 (A. Herz, Ed.), pp. 3–20. Springer-Verlag, New York.

Fields, H. L., Heinricher, M. M. and Mason, P. M. (1991). Neurotransmitters in nociceptive modulatory circuits. *Ann. Rev. Neurosci.*, 14, 219–245.

File, S. E. (1980). The use of social interactions as a method for detecting anxiolytic activity of chlordiazepoxide-like drugs. *J. Neurosci. Methods*, 2, 219–238.

File, S. E., Baldwin, H. A., Johnston, A. L., and Wilks, L. J. (1988). Behavioral effects of acute and chronic administration of caffeine in the rat. *Pharmacol. Biochem. Behav.*, 30, 809–815.

Fineberg, N. A., Bullock, T., Montgomery, D. B., and Montgomery, S. A. (1992). Serotonin reuptake inhibitors are the treatment of choice in obsessive compulsive disorder. *Int. Clin. Psychopharmacol.*, 7 (Suppl. 1), 43–47.

Fink, J. S., and Smith, G. P. (1980). Relationships between selective denervation of dopamine terminal fields in the anterior forebrain and behavioral responses to amphetamine and apomorphine. *Brain Res.*, 201, 107–127.

Fink, J. S., Weaver, D. R., Rivkees, S. A., Peterfreund, R. A., Pollack, A. E., Adler, E. M., and Reppert, S. M. (1992). Molecular cloning of the rat A_2 adenosine receptor: Selective co-expression with D_2 dopamine receptors in rat striatum. *Mol. Brain Res.*, 14, 186–195.

Fink, M. (1984). Theories of the antidepressant efficacy of convulsive therapy (ECT). In *Neurobiology of Mood Disorders* (R. M. Post and J. C. Ballenger, Eds.), pp. 721–730. Williams and Wilkins, Baltimore.

Fink, M. (1987). Convulsive therapy in affective disorders: A decade of understanding and acceptance. In *Psychopharmacology: The Third Generation of Progress* (H. Y. Meltzer, Ed.), pp. 1077–1083. Raven Press, New York.

Finn, I. B., and Holtzman, S. G. (1986). Tolerance to caffeine-induced stimulation of locomotor activity in rats. *J. Pharmacol. Exp. Ther.*, 238, 542–546.

Fiorino, D. F., Coury, A., Fibiger, H. C., and Phillips, A. G. (1993). Electrical stimulation of reward sites in the ventral tegmental area increases dopamine transmission in the nucleus accumbens of the rat. *Behav. Brain Res.*, 55, 131–141.

Fischer, J. F., and Cho, A. K. (1979). Chemical release of dopamine from striatal homogenates: Evidence for an exchange diffusion model. *J. Pharmacol. Exp. Ther.*, 208, 203–209.

Fischer, P., Danielczyk, W., Simanyi, M., and Streifler, B. (1990). Dopaminergic psychoses in advanced Parkinson's disease. *Adv. Neurol.*, 53, 391–397.

Fischer, P. M., Schwartz, M. P., Richards, J. W. Jr., Goldstein, A. O., and Rojas, T. H. (1991). Brand logo recognition by children aged from 3 to 6 years. Mickey Mouse and Old Joe the camel. *JAMA*, 266, 3145–3148.

Fischman, M. W. (1987). Cocaine and the amphetamines. In *Psychopharmacology: The Third Generation of Progress* (H. Y. Meltzer, Ed.), pp. 1543–1553. Raven Press, New York.

Fischman, M. W., and Schuster, C. R. (1977). Long-term behavioral changes in the rhesus monkey after multiple daily injections of *d*-methylamphetamine. *J. Pharmacol. Exp. Ther.*, 201, 593–605.

Fischman, M. W., and Schuster, C. R. (1980). Cocaine effects in sleep-deprived humans. *Psychopharmacology*, 72, 1–8.

Fischman, M. W., Schuster, C. R., Javaid, J., Hatano, Y., and Davis, J. (1985). Acute tolerance development to the cardiovascular and subjective effects of cocaine. *J. Pharmacol. Exp. Ther.*, 235, 677–682.

Fisher, L. A. (1989). Corticotropin-releasing factor: Endocrine and autonomic integration of responses to stress. *Trends Pharmacol. Sci.*, 10, 189–193.

Fisher, L. A. (1993). Central actions of corticotropin-releasing factor on autonomic nervous activity and cardiovascular functioning. *Ciba Found. Symp.*, 172, 243–257.

Fisher, L. J., and Gage, F. H. (1993). Grafting in the mammalian central nervous system. *Physiol. Rev.*, 73, 583–616.

Fisher, R. S. (1993). Emerging antiepileptic drugs. *Neurology*, 43 (Suppl. 5), S12–S20.

Fisher, S. K., Heacock, A. M., and Agranoff, B. W. (1992). Inositol lipids and signal transduction in the nervous system: An update. *J. Neurochem.*, 58, 18–38.

Flaum, M., and Andreasen, N. (1995). The reliability of distinguishing primary versus secondary negative symptoms. *Compr. Psychiatry*, 36, 421–427.

Flaum, M., Swayze, V. W., O'Leary, D. S., Yuh, W. T. C., Ehrhardt, J. C., Arndt, S. V., and Andreasen, N. C. (1995). Effects of diagnosis, laterality and gender on brain morphology in schizophrenia. *Am. J. Psychiatry* 152, 704–714.

Fleck, M. W., Henze, D. A., Barrionuevo, G., and Palmer, A. M. (1993). Aspartate and glutamate mediate excitatory synaptic transmission in area CA1 of the hippocampus. *J. Neurosci.*, 13, 3944–3955.

Fleetwood-Walker, S. M., Hope, P. J., Mitchell, R., El-Yassir, N., and Molony, V. (1988). The influence of opioid receptor subtypes on the processing of nociceptive inputs in the spinal dorsal horn of the cat. *Brain Res.*, 451, 213–226.

Fletcher, G. H., and Starr, M. S. (1988). Intracerebral SCH 23390 and catalepsy in the rat. *Eur. J. Pharmacol.*, 149, 175–178.

Fletcher, P. J., Currie, P. J., Chambers, J. W., and Coscina, D. V. (1993). Radiofrequency lesions of the PVN fail to modify the effects of serotonergic drugs on food intake. *Brain Res.*, 630, 1–9.

Fletcher, P. J., Ming, Z. H., Zack, M. H., and Coscina, D. V. (1992). A comparison of the effects of 5-HT$_1$ agonists TFMPP and RU 24969 on feeding following peripheral or medial hypothalamic injection. *Brain Res.*, 580, 265–272.

Fleurel-Balter, C., Beange, F., Nordmann, J., and Nordmann, R. (1983). Brain membrane disordering by administration of a single ethanol dose. *Pharmacol. Biochem. Behav.*, 18 (Suppl. 1), 25–29.

Flood, J. F., Silver, A. J., and Morley, J. E. (1990). Do peptide-induced changes in feeding occur because of changes in motivation to eat? *Peptides*, 11, 265–270.

Floor, E., Leventhal, P. S., Wang, Y., Meng, L., and Chen, W. (1995). Dynamic storage of dopamine in rat brain synaptic vesicles in vitro. *J. Neurochem.*, 64, 689–699.

Florez, J., and Hurle, M. A. (1993). Opioids in respiration and vomiting. In *Opioids II*, Handbook of Experimental Pharmacology, Vol. 104 (A. Herz, Ed.), pp. 263–292. Springer-Verlag, New York.

Fluharty, S. J., Snyder, G. L., Stricker, E. M., and Zigmond, M. J. (1983). Short- and long-term changes in adrenal tyrosine hydroxylase activity during insulin-induced hypoglycemia and cold stress. *Brain Res.*, 267, 384–387.

Flynn, D. D., Ferrari-DiLeo, G., Levey, A. I., and Mash, D. C. (1995). Differential alterations in muscarinic receptor subtypes in

Alzheimer's disease: Implications for cholinergic-based therapies. *Life Sci.*, 56, 869–876.

Fochtmann, L. J. (1994). Animal studies of electroconvulsive therapy: Foundations for future research. *Psychopharmacol. Bull.*, 30, 321–444.

Fochtmann, L. J., Cruciani, R., Aiso, M., and Potter, W. Z. (1989). Chronic electroconvulsive shock increases D-1 receptor binding in rat substantia nigra. *Eur. J. Pharmacol.*, 167, 305–306.

Foley, K. M. (1993). Opioid analgesics in clinical pain management. In *Opioids II*, Handbook of Experimental Pharmacology, Vol. 104 (A. Herz, Ed.), pp. 687–744. Springer-Verlag, New York.

Foltin, R. W., and Fischman, M. W. (1994). Effects of buprenorphine on the self-administration of cocaine by humans. *Behav. Pharmacol.*, 5, 79–89.

Foltin, R. W., Fischman, M. W., and Levin, F. R. (1995). Cardiovascular effects of cocaine in humans: Laboratory studies. *Drug Alcohol Depend.*, 37, 193–210.

Fonnum, F. (1984). Glutamate: A neurotransmitter in mammalian brain. *J. Neurochem.*, 42, 1–11.

Fonnum, F. (1987). Biochemistry, anatomy, and pharmacology of GABA neurons. In *Psychopharmacology: The Third Generation of Progress* (H. Y. Meltzer, ed.), pp. 173–182. Raven Press, New York.

Ford, A. P. D., and Clarke, D. E. (1993). The 5-HT$_4$ receptor. *Med. Res. Rev.*, 13, 633–662.

Forney, R. B., and Harger, R. N. (1971). The alcohols. In *Drill's Pharmacology of Medicine* (4th ed.) (J. R. DiPalma, Ed.), 275–302. McGraw-Hill, New York.

Forney, R. B., Hughes, F. W., Harger, R. N., and Richards, A. B. (1964). Alcohol distribution in the vascular system. *Q. J. Stud. Alcohol*, 25, 205–217.

Forno, L. S., Langston, J. W., Delanney, L. E., and Irwin, I. (1988). An electron microscopic study of MPTP-induced inclusion bodies in an old monkey. *Brain Res.*, 488, 150–157.

Forno, L. S., Langston, J. W., Delanney, L. E., Irwin, I., and Ricaurte, G. A. (1986). Locus coeruleus lesions and eosinophilic inclusions in MPTP-treated monkeys. *Ann. Neurol.*, 20, 449–455.

Fort, J. (1970). A world view of drugs. In *Society and Drugs* (R. H. Blum et al., Eds.), pp. 229–243. Jossey-Bass, San Francisco.

Fortier, I., Marcoux, S., and Beaulac-Baillargeon, L. (1993). Relation of caffeine intake during pregnancy to intrauterine growth retardation and preterm birth. *Am. J. Epidemiol.*, 137, 931–940.

Fossom, L. H., Carlson, C. D., and Tank, A. W. (1991). Stimulation of tyrosine hydroxylase gene transcription rate by nicotine in rat adrenal medulla. *Mol. Pharmacol.*, 40, 193–202.

Fossom, L. H., Sterling, C., and Tank, A. W. (1991). Activation of tyrosine hydroxylase by nicotine in rat adrenal gland. *J. Neurochem.*, 57, 2070–2077.

Foster, T. C., and McNaughton, B. L. (1991). Long-term synaptic enhancement in hippocampal field CA1 is due to increased quantal size, not quantal content. *Hippocampus*, 1, 79–91.

Fouriezos, G., and Wise, R. A. (1976). Pimozide-induced extinction of intracranial self-stimulation: Response patterns rule out motor or performance deficits. *Brain Res.*, 103, 377–380.

Fowler, C. J., and Ross, S. B. (1984). Selective inhibitors of monoamine oxidase A and B: Biochemical, pharmacological, and clinical properties. *Med. Res. Rev.*, 4, 323–358.

Fox, C. F. (1972). The structure of cell membranes. *Sci. Am.*, 226 (2), 30–38.

France, C. P., Woods, J. H., and Ornstein, P. (1989). The competitive N-methyl-D-aspartate (NMDA) antagonist CGS 19755 attenuates the rate-decreasing effects of NMDA in monkeys without producing ketamine-like discriminative stimulus effects. *Eur. J. Pharmacol.*, 159, 133–139.

Francis, S. H., and Corbin, J. D. (1994). Progress in understanding the mechanism and function of cyclic GMP-dependent protein kinase. *Adv. Pharmacol.*, 26, 115–170.

Frank, D. A., Bresnahan, K., and Zuckerman, B. S. (1993). Maternal cocaine use: Impact on child health and development. *Adv. Pediat.*, 40, 65–99.

Frank, D. A., et al. (1988). Cocaine use during pregnancy: Prevalence and correlates. *Pediatrics*, 82, 888–895.

Frankel, D., Khana, J. M., and LeBlanc, A. E. (1978). Effect of *p*-chlorophenylalanine on the loss and maintenance of tolerance to ethanol. *Psychopharmacology*, 56, 139–143.

Frankel, D., Khana, J. M., LeBlanc, A. E., and Kalant, H. (1975). Effect of *p*-chlorophenylalanine on the acquisition of tolerance to ethanol and pentobarbital. *Psychopharmacologia*, 44, 247–252.

Fraser, H. F., Wikler, A., Essig, C., and Isbell, H. (1958). Degree of physical dependence induced by secobarbital or pentobarbital. *JAMA*, 166, 126–129.

Fraser, K. A., and Davison, J. S. (1992). Cholecystokinin-induced *c-fos* expression in the rat brain stem is influenced by vagal nerve integrity. *Exp. Physiol.*, 77, 225–228.

Frazer, A., Maayani, S., and Wolfe, B. B. (1990). Subtypes of receptors for serotonin. *Annu. Rev. Pharmacol. Toxicol.*, 30, 307–348.

Fredericks, A. B., and Benowitz, N. L. (1980). An abstinence syndrome following chronic administration of delta-9-tetrahydrocannabinol in rhesus monkeys. *Psychopharmacology*, 71, 201–202.

Frederickson, R. C. A., and Norris, F. H. (1976). Enkephalin-induced depression of single neurons in brain areas with opiate receptors: Antagonism by naloxone. *Science*, 194, 440–442.

Frederking, W. (1955). Intoxicant drugs (mescaline and Lysergic acid diethylamide) in Psychotherapy. *J. Nerv. Ment. Dis.*, 1, 241–243.

Fredholm, B. B., and Dunwiddie, T. V. (1988). How does adenosine inhibit transmitter release? *Trends Pharmacol. Sci.*, 9, 130–134.

Freed, W. J. (1988). The therapeutic latency of neuroleptic drugs and nonspecific postjunctional supersensitivity. *Schizophr. Bull.*, 14, 269–277.

Freed, W. J., Morihisa, J. M., Spoor, E., Hoffer, B. J., Olson, L., Seiger, Å., and Wyatt, R. J. (1981). Transplanted adrenal chromaffin cells in rat brain reduce lesion-induced rotational behaviour. *Nature*, 292, 351–352.

Freed, W. J., Poltorak, M., and Becker, J. B. (1990). Intracerebral adrenal medulla grafts: A review. *Exp. Neurol.*, 110, 139–166.

Freedman, J. E., and Weight, F. F. (1988). Single K$^+$ channels activated by D$_2$ dopamine receptors in acutely dissociated neurons from rat corpus striatum. *Proc. Natl. Acad. Sci. U.S.A.*, 85, 3618–3622.

Freeman, A. S., and Bunney, B. S. (1984). The effects of phencyclidine and N-allylnormetazocine on midbrain dopamine neuronal activity. *Eur. J. Pharmacol.*, 104, 287–293.

Freeman, A. S., Meltzer, L. T., and Bunney, B. S. (1985). Firing properties of substantia nigra neurons in freely moving rats. *Life Sci.*, 36, 1983–1994.

Freeman, S. E., and Dawson, R. M. (1991). Tacrine: A pharmacological review. *Prog. Neurobiol.*, 36, 257–277.

French, E. D. (1994). Phencyclidine and the midbrain dopamine system: Electrophysiology and behavior. *Neurotoxicol. Teratol.*, 16, 355–362.

French, E. D., and Ceci, A. (1990). Non-competitive N-methyl-D-aspartate antagonists are potent activators of ventral tegmental A$_{10}$ dopamine neurons. *Neurosci. Lett.*, 119, 159–162.

French, E. D., and Vantini, G. (1984). Phencyclidine-induced locomotor activity in the rat is blocked by 6-hydroxydopamine lesion of the nucleus accumbens: Comparisons to other psychomotor stimulants. *Psychopharmacology*, 82, 83–88.

French, E. D., Mura, A., and Wang, T. (1993). MK-801, phencyclidine (PCP), and PCP-like drugs increase burst firing in rat A10 dopamine neurons: Comparison to competitive NMDA antagonists. *Synapse*, 13, 108–116.

French, E. D., Pilapil, C., and Quirion, R. (1985). Phencyclidine binding sites in the nucleus accumbens and phencyclidine-induced hyperactivity are decreased following lesions of the mesolimbic dopamine system. *Eur. J. Pharmacol.*, 116, 1–9.

Freud, S. (1936). *The Problem of Anxiety*. Norton, New York.

Freund, T. F., Powell, J. F., and Smith, A. D. (1984). Tyrosine hydroxylase-immunoreactive boutons in synaptic contact with identified striatonigral neurons, with particular reference to dendritic spines. *Neuroscience*, 13, 1189–1215.

Freygang, W., and Sokoloff, L. (1958). Quantitative measurement of regional circulation in the central nervous system by use of radioactive inert gas. *Adv. Biol. Med. Phys.*, 6, 263–279.

Frezza, M., Di Padova, C., Pozzato, G., Terpin, M., Barona, E., and Lieber, C. S. (1990). High blood levels of alcohol in women: The role of decreased alcohol dehydrogenase activity and first-pass metabolism. *N. Engl. J. Med.*, 322, 95–99.

Fride, E., and Mechoulam, R. (1993). Pharmacological activity of the cannabinoid receptor agonist, anandamide, a brain constituent. *Eur. J. Pharmacol.*, 231, 313–314.

Friedhoff, A. J., and Silva, R. R. (1995). The effects of neuroleptics on plasma homovanillic acid. In *Psychopharmacology: The Fourth Generation of Progress* (F. E. Bloom and D. J. Kupfer, Eds.), pp. 1229–1234. Raven Press, New York.

Friedman, E., and Wang, H-Y. (1988). Effect of chronic lithium threatment on 5-hydroxytryptamine autoreceptors and release of 5-[^{3}H]hydroxytryptamine from rat brain cortical, hippocampal and hypothalamic slices. *J. Neurochem.*, 50, 195–201.

Frielle, T., Collins, S., Daniel, K. W., Caron, M. G., Lefkowitz, R. J., and Kobilka, B. K. (1987). Cloning of the cDNA for the human β_1-adrenergic receptor. *Proc. Natl. Acad. Sci. U.S.A.*, 84, 7920–7924.

Frielle, T., Kobilka, B., Lefkowitz, R. J., and Caron, M. G. (1988). Human β_1- and β_2-adrenergic receptors: Structurally and functionally related receptors derived from distinct genes. *Trends Neurosci.*, 11, 321–324.

Frim, D. M., Uhler, T. A., Galpern, W. R., Beal, M. F., Breakefield, X. O., and Isacson, O. (1994). Implanted fibroblasts genetically engineered to produce brain-derived neurotrophic factor prevent 1-methyl-4-phenyl-pyridinium toxicity to dopaminergic neurons in the rat. *Proc. Natl. Acad. Sci. U.S.A.*, 91, 5104–5108.

Fritsch, G., and Hitzig, E. (1870). Ueber die elektrische Erregbarkeit des Grosshirns. In *Some Papers on the Cerebral Cortex* (G. von Bonin, Trans.), 1960. pp. 73–96, Thomas, Springfield, IL.

Froehlich, J. C., Harts, J., Lumeng, L., and Li, T. K. (1990). Naloxone attenuates voluntary ethanol intake in rats selectively bred for high ethanol preference. *Pharmacol. Biochem. Behav.*, 35, 385–390.

Froehlich, J. C., Zweifel, M., Harts, J., Lumens, L., and Li, T.-K. (1991). Importance of delta opioid receptors in maintaining high alcohol drinking. *Psychopharmacology*, 103, 467–472.

Frohman, L. A. (1980). Neurotransmitters as regulators of endocrine function. In *Neuroendocrinology* (D. T. Krieger and J. C. Hughes, Eds.), pp. 44–57. Sinauer Associates, Sunderland, MA.

Frost, J. J., Rosier, A. J., Reich, S. G., Smith, J. S., Ehlers, M. D., Snyder, S. H., Ravert, H. T., and Dannals, R. F. (1993). Positron emission tomographic imaging of the dopamine transporter with ^{11}C-WIN 35,428 reveals marked declines in mild Parkinson's disease. *Ann. Neurol.*, 34, 423–431.

Fukunaga, K., Stoppini, L., Miyamoto, E., and Muller, D. (1993). Long-term potentiation is associated with increased activity of Ca^{++}/calmodulin-dependent protein kinase II. *J. Biol. Chem.*, 268, 7863–7867.

Fuller, R. W. (1992). Effects of *p*-chloroamphetamine on brain serotonin neurons. *Neurochem. Res.*, 17, 449–456.

Fuller, R. W. (1994). Uptake inhibitors increase extracellular serotonin concentrations measured by brain microdialysis. *Life Sci.*, 55, 163–167.

Fuller, R. W., and Clemens, J. A. (1991). Pergolide: A dopamine agonist at both D_1 and D_2 receptors. *Life Sci.*, 49, 925–930.

Fuller, R. W., and Hemrick-Luecke, S. (1980). Long-lasting depletion of striatal dopamine by a single injection of amphetamine in iprindole-treated rats. *Science*, 209, 305–307.

Fuller, R. W., and Wong, D. T. (1989). Fluoxetine: A serotonergic appetite suppressant drug. *Drug Dev. Res.*, 17, 1–15.

Fuller, R. W., and Wong, D. T. (1990). Serotonin uptake and serotonin uptake inhibition. *Ann. N.Y. Acad. Sci.*, 600, 68–80.

Fuller, R. W., Wong, D. T., and Robertson, D. W. (1991). Fluoxetine, a selective inhibitor of serotonin uptake. *Med. Res. Rev.*, 11, 17–34.

Furchgott, R. F. (1984). The role of endothelium in the responses of vascular smooth muscle to drugs. *Annu. Rev. Pharmacol. Toxicol.*, 24, 175–197.

Furchgott, R. F., and Zawadzki, J. V. (1980). The obligatory role of endothelial cells in the relaxation of arterial smooth muscle by acetylcholine. *Nature*, 288, 373–376.

Furness, J. B., Morris, J. L., Gibbins, I. L., and Costa, M. (1989). Chemical coding of neurons and plurichemical transmission. *Annu. Rev. Pharmacol. Toxicol.*, 29, 289–306.

Furshpan, E. J., and Potter, D. D. (1959). Transmission at the giant motor synapses of the crayfish. *J. Physiol.* 145, 289–325.

Furuichi, T., and Mikoshiba, K. (1995). Inositol 1,4,5-trisphosphate receptor-mediated Ca^{2+} signaling in the brain. *J. Neurochem.*, 64, 953–960.

Fuxe, K. (1965). Evidence for the existence of monoamine neurons in the central nervous system. IV. Distribution of monoamine nerve terminals in the central nervous system. *Acta Physiol. Scand.*, 64 (Suppl. 247), 37–85.

Fuxe, K., Agnati, L. F., Kalia, M., Goldstein, M., Andersson, K., and Härfstrand, A. (1985). Dopaminergic systems in the brain and pituitary. In *Basic and Clinical Aspects of Neuroscience: The Dopaminergic System* (E. Flückiger, E. E. Müller, and M. O. Thorner, Eds.), pp. 11–25. Springer-Verlag, Berlin.

Fyer, A. J., Liebowitz, M. R., Gorman, J. M., Compeas, R., Levin, A., Davies, S. O., Goetz, D., and Klein, D. F. (1987). Discontinuation of alprazolam treatment in panic patients. *Am. J. Psychiatry*, 144, 303–308.

Gaddum, J. H. (1953). Antagonism between lysergic acid diethylamide and 5-hydroxytryptamine. *J. Physiol.* (Lond.), 121, 15P.

Gaddum, J. H., and Picarelli, Z. P. (1957). Two kinds of tryptamine receptor. *Br. J. Pharmacol. Chemother.*, 12, 323–328.

Gainer, H., Russell, J. T., and Loh, Y. P. (1985). The enzymology and intracellular organization of peptide precursor processing: The secretory vesicle hypothesis. *Neuroendocrinology*, 40, 171–184.

Gale, K. (1992). GABA and epilepsy: Basic concepts from preclinical research. *Epilepsia*, 33 (Suppl. 5), S3–S12.

Gall, C., Lauterborn, J., Isackson, P., and White, J. (1990). Seizures, neuropeptide regulation and mRNA expression in the hippocampus. *Prog. Brain Res.* 83, 371–390.

Gallager, D. W., and Tallman, J. F. (1990). Relationship of $GABA_a$ receptor heterogeneity to regional differences in drug response. *Neurochem. Res.*, 15, 113–118.

Gallistel, C. R. (1983). Self-stimulation. In *The Physiological Basis of Memory* (J. A. Deutsch, Ed.), pp. 269–349. Academic Press, New York.

Galloway, M. P. (1990). Regulation of dopamine and serotonin synthesis by acute administration of cocaine. *Synapse*, 6, 63–72.

Games, D., et al. (1995). Alzheimer-type neuropathology in transgenic mice overexpressing V717F β-amyloid precursor protein. *Nature*, 373, 523–527,

Gandy, S., and Greengard, P. (1994). Processing of Alzheimer Aβ-amyloid precursor protein: Cell biology, regulation, and role in Alzheimer disease. *Int. Rev. Neurobiol.*, 36, 29–50.

Ganellin, C. R. (1982). Chemistry amd structure–activity relationship of drugs acting at histamine receptors. In *Pharmacology of Histamine Receptors* (C. R. Ganellin and M. E. Parsons, Eds.), pp. 10–102. Wright PSG, Bristol.

Gantz, I., Munzert, G., Tashiro, T., Schäffer, M., Wang, L., DelValle, J., and Yamada, T. (1991). Molecular cloning of the human histamine H_2 receptor. *Biochem. Biophys. Res. Commun.*, 178, 1386–1392.

Gantz, I., Schäffer, M., DelValle, J., Logsdon, C., Campbell, V., Uhler, M., and Yamada, T. (1991). Molecular cloning of a gene encoding the histamine H_2 receptor. *Proc. Natl. Acad. Sci. U.S.A.*, 88, 429–433.

Gao, Y., Baldessarini, R. J., Kula, N. S., and Neumeyer, J. L. (1990). Synthesis and dopamine receptor affinities of enantiomers of 2-substituted apomorphines and their *N*-*n*-propyl analogues. *J. Med. Chem.*, 33, 1800–1805.

Gaoni, Y., and Mechoulam, R. (1964). Isolation, structure and partial synthesis of of an active component of hashish. *J. Am. Chem. Soc.*, 86, 1646–1647.

Garau, L., Govoni, S., Stefanini, E., Trabucchi, M., and Spano, P. F. (1978). Dopamine receptors: Pharmacological and anatomical evidences indicate that two distinct dopamine receptor populations are present in rat striatum. *Life Sci.*, 23, 1745–1750.

Garcia-Sevilla, J. A. (1990). Platelet alpha 2 adrenoceptor function in depression and response to drug treatment. In *Antidepressants: Thirty Years On* (B. E. Leonard and P. S. J. Spencer, Eds.), pp. 163–169. Clinical Neuroscience Publishers, London.

Gardner, C. R. (1985). Inhibition of ultrasonic distress vocalizations in rat pups by chlordiazepoxide and diazepam. *Drug Dev. Res.*, 5, 185–193.

Gardner, C. R. (1986). Recent developments in 5-HT-related pharmacology of animal models of anxiety. *Pharmacol. Biochem. Behav.*, 24, 1479–1485.

Gardner, E. L., and Lowinson, J. H. (1991). Marijuana's interaction with brain reward systems: Update 1991. *Pharmacol. Biochem. Behav.*, 40, 571–580.

Garey, R. E., and Heath, R. G. (1976). The effects of phencyclidine on the uptake of ^{3}H-catecholamines by rat striatal and hypothalamic synaptosomes. *Life Sci.*, 18, 1105–1110.

Garnett, E. S., Nahmias, C., and Firnau, G. (1984). Central dopaminergic pathways in hemiparkinsonism examined by positron emission tomography. *Can. J. Neurol. Sci.*, 11, 174–179.

Garrett, B. E., and Holtzman, S. G. (1994). D_1 and D_2 receptor antagonists block caffeine-induced stimulation of locomotor activity in rats. *Pharmacol. Biochem. Behav.*, 47, 89–94.

Garris, P. A., Ciolkowski, E. L., Pastore, P., and Wightman, M. (1994). Efflux of dopamine from the synaptic cleft in the nucleus accumbens of the rat brain. *J. Neurosci.*, 14, 6084–6093.

Garthwaite, J. (1991). Glutamate, nitric oxide and cell–cell signalling in the nervous system. *Trends Neurosci.*, 14, 60–67.

Garver, D. L., Schlemmer, R. F., Maas, J. W., and Davis, J. M. (1975). A schizophreniform behavioral psychosis mediated by dopamine. *Am. J. Psychiatry*, 132, 33–38.

Gasic, G. P., and Hollmann, M. (1992). Molecular neurobiology of glutamate receptors. *Annu. Rev. Physiol.,* 54, 507–536.

Gastaut, H., Naquet, R., Poire, R., and Tassinari, C. A. (1965). Treatment of status epilepticus with diazepam (Valium). *Epilepsia,* 6, 167–182.

Gately, P. F., Segal, D. S., and Geyer, M. A. (1986). The behavioral effects of depletions of brain serotonin induced by 5,7-dihydroxytryptamine vary with time after administration. *Behav. Neural Biol.,* 45, 31–42.

Gavish, M., Katz, Y., Bar-Ami, S., and Weizman, R. (1992). Biochemical, physiological, and pathological aspects of the peripheral benzodiazepine receptor. *J. Neurochem.,* 58, 1589–1601.

Gawin, F. H. (1991). Cocaine addiction: Psychology and neurophysiology. *Science,* 251, 1580–1586.

Gawin, F. H., and Ellinwood, E. H. Jr. (1988). Cocaine and other stimulants. Actions, abuse, and treatment. *N. Engl. J. Med.,* 318, 1173–1182.

Gawin, F. H., and Kleber, H. D. (1986). Abstinence symptomatology and psychiatric diagnosis in cocaine abusers. Clinical observations. *Arch. Gen. Psychiatry,* 43, 107–113.

Gawin, F. H., and Kleber, H. D. (1988). Evolving conceptualizations of cocaine dependence. *Yale J. Biol. Med.,* 61, 123–136.

Gearing, M., Rebeck, G. W., Hyman, B. T., Tigges, J., and Mirra, S. S. (1994). Neuropathology and apolipoprotein E profile of aged chimpanzees: Implications for Alzheimer disease. *Proc. Natl. Acad. Sci. U.S.A.,* 91, 9382–9386.

Geddes, J. W., Chang-Chui, H., Cooper, S. M., Lott, I. T., and Cotman, C. W. (1986). Density and distribution of NMDA receptors in the human hippocampus in Alzheimer's disease. *Brain Res.,* 399, 156–161.

Geffard, M., Buijs, R. M., Sequela, P., Pool, C. W., and LeMoal, M. (1984). First demonstration of highly specific and sensitive antibodies against dopamine. *Brain Res.,* 294, 161–165.

Gehlert, D. R., and Wamsley, J. K. (1985). Dopamine receptors in the rat brain: Quantitative autoradiographic localization using [³H]sulpiride. *Neurochem. Int.,* 7, 717–723.

Gehlert, D. R., Yamamura, H. I., and Wamsley, J. K. (1985). γ-aminobutyric acid$_B$ receptors in the rat brain: Quantitative autoradiographic localization using [³H](-)baclofen. *Neurosci. Lett.,* 56, 183–188.

Geiger, J. D., and Nagy, J. I. (1990). Adenosine deaminase and [³H]nitrobenzylthioinosine as markers of adenosine metabolism and transport in central purinergic systems. In *Adenosine and Adenosine Receptors* (M. Williams, Ed.), pp. 225–288. Humana Press, Clifton, N. J.

Geller, I. (1962). Use of approach avoidance behavior (conflict) for evaluating depressant drugs. In *Psychosomatic Medicine* (J. H. Nodine and J. H. Moyer, Eds.), pp. 267–274. Lea and Febiger, Philadelphia.

Geller, I., Hartmann, R. J., Croy, D. J., and Haber, B. (1974). Attenuation of conflict behavior with cinanserin, a serotonin antagonist: Reversal of the effect with 5-hydroxytryptophan and α-methyl tryptamine. *Res. Commun. Clin. Pathol. Pharmacol.,* 7, 165–174.

Geller, I., and Seifter, J. (1960). The effects of meprobamate, barbiturates, *d*-amphetamine and promazine on experimentally-induced conflict in the rat. *Psychopharmacologia,* 1, 482–492.

Georgotas, A. (1985). Affective disorders: Pharmacotherapy. In *Comprehensive Textbook of Psychiatry/IV* (H. I. Kaplan and B. J. Sadock, Eds.), pp. 821–833. Williams and Wilkins, Baltimore.

Gerard, N. P., Bao, L., Xiao-Ping, H., and Gerard, C. (1993). Molecular aspects of the tachykinin receptors. *Regul. Pept.,* 43, 21–35.

Gerfen, C. R. (1992). The neostriatal mosaic: Multiple levels of compartmental organization in the basal ganglia. *Annu. Rev. Neurosci.,* 15, 285–320.

Gerfen, C. R., Engber, T. M., Mahan, L. C., Susel, Z., Chase, T. N., Monsma, F. J. Jr., and Sibley, D. R. (1990). D₁ and D₂ dopamine receptor-regulated gene expression of striatonigral and striatopallidal neurons. *Science,* 250, 1429–1432.

Gerfen, C. R., and Young, W. S. III. (1988). Distribution of striatonigral and striatopallidal peptidergic neurons in both patch and matrix compartments: An in situ hybridization histochemistry and fluorescent retrograde tracing study. *Brain Res.,* 460, 161–167.

Gerlach, M. Ben-Schachar, D., Riederer, P., and Youdim, M. B. H. (1994). Altered brain metabolism of iron as a cause of neurodegenerative diseases? *J. Neurochem.,* 63, 793–807.

Gerlach, J. (1991). New antipsychotics: Classification, efficacy, and adverse effects. *Schizophr. Bull.,* 17, 289–309.

Gerlach, J., Casey, D. E., and Korsgaard, S. (1986). In *Movement Disorders* (N. S. Shah and A. G. Donald, Eds.), pp. 119–147. Plenum Press, New York.

Gerlach, M., Jellinger, K., and Riederer, P. (1994). The possible role of noradrenergic deficits in selected signs of Parkinson's disease. In *Noradrenergic Mechanisms in Parkinson's Disease* (M. Briley and M. Marien, Eds.), pp. 59–71. CRC Press, Boca Raton.

Gerlach, M., Riederer, P., Przuntek, H., and Youdim, M. B. H. (1991). MPTP mechanisms of neurotoxicity and their implications for Parkinson's disease. *Eur. J. Pharmacol. Mol. Pharmacol. Sect.,* 208, 273–286.

Gerlach, M., Youdim, M. B. H., and Riederer, P. (1994). Is selegiline neuroprotective in Parkinson's disease? *J. Neural Trans.,* 41 (Suppl.), 177–188.

German, D. C., and Manaye, K. F. (1993). Midbrain dopaminergic neurons (nuclei A8, A9, and A10): Three-dimensional reconstruction in the rat. *J. Comp. Neurol.,* 331, 297–309.

Gerner, R. H., Post, R. M., Spiegel, A. M., and Murphy, D. L. (1977). Effects of parathormone and lithium treatment on calcium and mood in depressed patients. *Biol. Psychiatry,* 12, 145–151.

Gershon, E. S., Berrettini, W., Nurnberger, J., and Goldin, L. R. (1987). Genetics of affective illness. In *Psychopharmacology: The Third Generation of Progress* (H. Y. Meltzer, Ed.), pp. 481–491. Raven Press, New York.

Gershon, M. D. (1982). Enteric serotonergic neurones. In *Biology of Serotonergic Transmission* (N. N. Osborne, Ed.), pp. 363–399. Wiley, Chichester.

Geula, C., and Mesulam, M.-M. (1994). Cholinergic systems and related neuropathological predilection patterns in Alzheimer disease. In *Alzheimer Disease* (R. D. Terry, R.

Katzman, and K. L. Bick, Eds.), pp. 263–291. Raven Press, New York.

Geyer, M. A., and Markou, A. (1995). Animal models of psychiatric disorders. In *Psychopharmacology: The Fourth Generation of Progress* (F. E. Bloom and D. J. Kupfer, Eds.), pp. 787–798. Raven Press, New York.

Ghez, C. (1991). The cerebellum. In *Principles of Neural Science* (3rd ed.) (E. R. Kandel, J. H. Schwartz, and T. M. Jessell, Eds.), pp. 626–646. Elsevier, New York.

Ghosh, A., and Greenberg, M. E. (1995). Calcium signaling in neurons: Molecular mechanisms and cellular consequences. *Science,* 268, 239–247.

Giannini, A. J. (1989). Phencyclidine. In *Drugs of Abuse* (A. J. Giannini and A. E. Slaby, Eds.), pp. 145–159. Medical Economics Books, Oradell.

Gianoulakis, C., Angelogianni, P., Meany, M., Thavundayil, J., and Twar, V. (1990). Endorphins in individuals with high and low risk for development of alcoholism. In *Opioids, Bulimia, and Alcohol Abuse and Alcoholism* (L. D. Reid, Ed.), pp 229–246, Springer-Verlag, New York.

Gibb, J. W., Johnson, M., Stone, D., and Hanson, G. R. (1990). MDMA: Historical perspectives. *Ann. N.Y. Acad. Sci.,* 600, 601–612.

Gibb, J. W., Stone, D. M., Johnson, M., and Hanson, G. R. (1989). Role of dopamine in the neurotoxicity induced by amphetamine and related designer drugs. *NIDA Res. Monogr.,* 94, 161–178.

Gibbins, R. J., Kalant, H., and Le Blanc, A. E. (1968). A technique for accurate measurement of moderate degrees of alcoholic intoxication in small animals. *J. Pharmacol. Exp. Ther.,* 159, 236–242.

Gibbs, D. M. (1986). Vasopressin and oxytocin: Hypothalamic modulators of the stress response: A review. *Psychoneuroendocrinology,* 11, 131–140.

Gibbs, J., Young, R. C., and Smith, G. P. (1973). Cholecystokinin decreases food intake in rats. *J. Comp. Physiol. Psychol.,* 84, 488–495.

Gieringer, D. H. (1988). Marijuana, driving, and accident safety. *J. Psychoactive Drugs,* 20, 93–101.

Giesler, G. J., Katter, J. T., and Dado, R. J. (1994). Direct spinal pathways to the limbic system for nociceptive information. *Trends Neurosci.,* 17, 244–250.

Gil-Ad, I., Dickerman, Z., Amdursky, S., and Laron, A. (1986). Diurnal rhythm of plasma beta-endorphin, cortisol and growth hormone in schizophrenics as compared to control subjects. *Psychopharmacology,* 88, 496–499.

Gilbert, R. F. T., Emson, P. C., Hunt, S. P., Bennett, G. W., Marsden, C. A., Sandberg, B. E. B., Steinbusch, H. W. M., and Verhofstad, A. A. J. (1982). The effects of monoamine neurotoxins on peptides in the rat spinal cord. *Neuroscience,* 7, 60–87.

Giles, D. E., Jarrett, R. B., Roffwarg, H. P., and Rush, A. J. (1987). Reduced rapid eye movement latency: A prediction of recurrence in depression. *Neuropsychopharmacology,* 1, 33–39.

Giles, H. G., Corrigall, W. A., Khouw, V., and Sellers, E. M. (1982). Plasma protein binding of phencyclidine. *Clin. Pharmacol. Ther.,* 31, 77–82.

Gill, E. W., Paton, W. D. M., and Pertwee, R. G. (1970). Preliminary experiments on the chemistry and pharmacology of cannabis. *Nature*, 228, 134–136.

Gillberg, C., Terenius, L. and Lonnerholm, G. (1985). Endorphin activity in childhood psychosis. *Arch. Gen. Psychiatry*, 42, 780–783.

Gillin, J. C., Salin-Pascual, R., Velazquez-Moctezuma, J., Shiromani, P., and Zoltoski, R. (1993). Cholinergic receptor subtypes and REM sleep in animals and normal controls. *Prog. Brain Res.*, 98, 379–387.

Gillin, J. C., Stoff, D. M., and Wyatt, R. J. (1978). Transmethylation hypothesis: A review. In *Psychopharmacology: A Generation of Progress* (M. A. Lipton, A. DiMascio, and K. F. Killam, Eds.), pp. 1097–1112. Raven Press, New York.

Gilman, A.G., Goodman, L.S., Rall T.W. and Murad, F. (Eds.) (1985). *The Pharmacological Basis of Therapeutics* (7th ed.), Macmillan, New York.

Gillman, P. K., Bartlett, J. R., Bridges, P. K., Hunt, A., Patel, A. J., Kantamaneni, B. D., and Curzon, G. (1981). Indolic substances in plasma, cerebrospinal fluid, and frontal cortex of human subjects infused with saline or tryptophan. *J. Neurochem.*, 37, 410–417.

Giros, B., and Caron, M. (1993). Molecular characterization of the dopamine transporter. *Trends Pharmacol. Sci.*, 14, 43–49.

Giros, B., Jaber, M., Jones, S. R., Wightman, R. M., and Caron, M. G. (1996). Hyperlocomotion and indifferences to cocaine and amphetamine in mice lacking the dopamine transporter. *Nature*, 379, 606–612.

Giros, B., Sokoloff, P., Martres, M.-P., Riou, J.-F., Emorine, L. J., and Schwartz, J.-C. (1989). Alternative splicing directs the expression of two D_2 receptor isoforms. *Nature*, 342, 923–926.

Gittleman-Klein, R., Mannuzza, S., Shenker, R., and Bonagura, N. (1985). Hyperactive boys almost grown up: I. Psychiatric status. *Arch. Gen. Psychiatry*, 42, 937–947.

Giurgea, C. E. (1980). *Fundamentals to a Pharmacology of the Mind*. Thomas, Springfield, Illinois.

Glantz, S. A., Barnes, D. E., Bero, L., Hanauer, P., and Slade, J. (1995). Looking through a keyhole at the tobacco industry: The Brown and Williamson Documents. *JAMA*, 219–224.

Glaser, S. B. (1980). Anybody got a match? Treatment research and the matching hypothesis. In *Alcholism Treatment in Transition* (G. Edwards and M. Grant, Eds.), pp. 178–196. Croom Helm, London.

Gleeson, S., and Barrett, J. E. (1990). 5-HT_{1A} agonist effects on punished responding of squirrel monkeys. *Pharmacol. Biochem. Behav.*, 37, 335–337.

Gleiter, C. H., Deckert, J., Nutt, D. J., and Marangos, P. J. (1989). Electroconvulsive shock (ECS) and the adenosine neuromodulatory system: Effect single and repeated ECS on the adenosine A_1 and A_2 receptors, adenylate cyclase, and the adenosine uptake site. *J. Neurochem.*, 52, 641–646.

Gleiter, C. H., and Nutt, D. J. (1989). Chronic electroconvulsive shock and neurotransmitter receptors. *Life Sci.*, 44, 985–1006.

Glenner, G. G., and Wong, C. W. (1984). Alzheimer's disease: Initial report of the purification and characterization of a novel cerebrovascular amyloid protein. *Biochem. Biophys. Res. Commun.*, 120, 885–890.

Glennon, R. (1990a). Do classical hallucinogens act as 5-HT_2 agonists or antagonists? *Neuropsychopharmacology*, 3, 509–517.

Glennon, R. (1990b). Serotonin receptors: Clinical implications. *Neurosci. Biobehav. Rev.*, 14, 35–47.

Glennon, R. A., Darmani, N. A., and Martin, B. R. (1991). Multiple populations of serotonin receptors may modulate the behavioral effects of serotonergic agents. *Life Sci.*, 48, 2493–2498.

Glennon, R. A., Hong, S.-S., Dukat, M., Teitler, M., and Davis, K. (1994). 5-(Nonyloxy)tryptamine: A novel high-affinity 5-HT1Db serotonin receptor agonist. *J. Med. Chem.*, 37, 2828–2830.

Glennon, R. A., Naiman, N. A., Pierson, M. E., Titeler, M., Lyon, R. A., Herndon, J. L., and Misenheimer, B, (1989). Stimulus properties of arylpiperazines: NAN-190, a potential 5-HT_{1A} serotonin antagonist. *Drug. Dev. Res.*, 16, 335–343.

Glennon, R. A., Titeler, M., and McKenny, J. D. (1984). Evidence for 5-HT_2 involvement in the mechanism of action of hallucinogenic agents. *Life Sci.*, 35, 2505–2511.

Glick, S. D. (1976). Screening and therapeutics: Animal models and human problems. In *Behavioral Pharmacology* (S. D. Glick and J. Goldfarb, Eds.), pp. 339–361. Mosby, St. Louis.

Glick, S. D., Kuehne, M. E., Raucci, J., Wilson, T. E., Larson, D., and Keller, R. W. Jr., and Carlson, J. N. (1994). Effects of *iboga* alkaloids on morphine and cocaine self-administration in rats: Relationship to tremorigenic effects and to effects on dopamine release in nucleus accumbens and striatum. *Brain Res.*, 657, 14–22.

Glowa, J. R., Bacher, J. D., Herkenham, M., and Gold, P. W. (1991). Selective anorexigenic effects of corticotropin releasing hormone in the rhesus monkey. *Prog. Neuropsychopharmacol. Biol. Psychiatry*, 15, 379–391.

Gmerek, D.E., Kykstra, L.A. and Woods, J.H. (1987). Kappa opioids in rhesus monkeys: III Dependence associated with chronic administration. *J. Pharmacol. Exp. Ther.*, 242, 429–436.

Gnanalingham, K. K., Hunter, A. J., Jenner, P., and Marsden, C. D. (1995). The differential behavioural effects of benzazepine D_1 dopamine agonists with varying efficacies, co-administered with quinpirole in primate and rodent models of Parkinson's disease. *Psychopharmacology*, 117, 287–297.

Gnegy, M. E. (1993). Calmodulin in neurotransmitter and hormone action. *Annu. Rev. Pharmacol. Toxicol.*, 32, 45–70.

Goddard, G. V., McIntyre, D. C., and Leech, C. K. (1969). A permanent change in brain function resulting from daily electrical stimulation. *Exp. Neurol.*, 25, 295–330.

Goeders, N. E., Dworkin, S. I., and Smith, J. E. (1986). Neuropharmacological assessment of cocaine self-administration into the medial prefrontal cortex. *Pharmacol. Biochem. Behav.*, 24, 1429–1440.

Goeders, N. E., and Smith, J. E. (1983). Cortical dopaminergic involvement in cocaine reinforcement. *Science*, 221, 773–775.

Goeders, N. E., and Smith, J. E. (1993). Intracranial cocaine self-administration into the medial prefrontal cortex increases dopamine turnover in the nucleus accumbens. *J. Pharmacol. Exp. Ther.*, 265, 592–600.

Goedert, M. (1993). Tau protein and the neurofibrillary pathology of Alzheimer's disease. *Trends Neurosci.*, 16, 460–465.

Goetz, C. G., Tanner, C. M., Shannon, K. M., Carroll, V. S., Klawans, H. L., Carvey, P. M., and Gilley, D. (1988). Controlled-release carbidopa/levodopa (CR4–Sinemet) in Parkinson's disease patients with and without motor fluctuations. *Neurology*, 38, 1143–1146.

Gold, L. H., Balster, R. L., Barrett, R. L., Britt, D. T., and Martin, B. R. (1992). A comparison of the discriminative stimulus properties of Δ^9-tetrahydrocannabinol and CP 55,940 in rats and rhesus monkeys. *J. Pharmacol. Exp. Ther.*, 262, 479–486.

Gold, M. S. (1989). Opiates. In *Drugs of Abuse* (A. J. Giannini and A. E. Slaby, Eds.), pp. 127–145. Medical Economics Books, Oradell, New Jersey.

Gold, P. W., Goodwin, F. K., and Chrousos, G. P. (1988a) Clinical and biochemical manifestations of depression, part 1. *N. Engl. J. Med.*, 319, 348–353.

Gold, P. W., Goodwin, F. K., and Chrousos, G. P. (1988b) Clinical and biochemical manifestations of depression, part 2. *N. Engl. J. Med.*, 319, 413–420.

Gold, R. M. (1973). Hypothalamic obesity: The myth of the ventromedial nucleus. *Science*, 182, 488–490.

Gold, R. M., Jones, A. P., Sawchenko, P. E., and Kapatos, G. (1977). Paraventricular area: Critical focus of a longitudinal neurocircuitry mediating food intake. *Physiol. Behav.*, 118, 1111–1119.

Goldberg, H. L., and Finnerty, R. J. (1979). The comparative efficacy of buspirone and diazepam in the treatment of anxiety. *Am. J. Psychiatry*, 136, 1184–1187.

Goldberg, L. (1943). Quantitative studies on alcohol tolerance in man. *Acta Physiol. Scand.*, 5 (Suppl. 16), 1–128.

Goldberg, M. E., Eggers, H. M., and Gowras, P. (1991). The ocular motor system. In *Principles of Neural Science* (3rd ed.) (E. R. Kandel, J. H. Schwartz, and T. M. Jessell, Eds.), pp. 660–678. Elsevier, New York.

Goldberg, M. E., Satama, A. I., and Blum, S. W. (1971). Inhibition of choline acetyltransferase and hexobarbitone-metabolizing enzymes by naphthyl vinylpyridine and analogues. *J. Pharm. Pharmacol.*, 23, 384–385.

Goldberg, S. R., and Schuster, C. R. (1967). Conditioned suppression by a stimulus associated with nalorphin in morphine-dependent monkeys. *J. Exp. Anal. Behav.*, 10, 235–242.

Goldberg, T. E., and Weinberger, D. R. (1995). A case against subtyping in schizophrenia. *Schizophr. Res.*, 17, 147–152.

Golden, R. N., Gilmore, J. H.,, Corrigan, M., Ekstrom, R. D., Knight, B. T., and Garbutt, J. C. (1991). Serotonin, suicide and aggression: Clinical studies. *J. Clin. Psychiatry*, 52:12 (Suppl.), 61–69.

Goldgaber, D., Lerman, M. I., McBride, O. W., Saffiotti, U., and Gajdusek, D. C. (1987). Characterization and chromosomal localization of a cDNA encoding brain amyloid of Alzheimer's disease. *Science*, 235, 877–880.

Goldman, J. E. (1983). The association of actin with Hirano bodies. *J. Neuropathol. Exp. Neurol.*, 42, 146–152.

Goldstein, A. (1994). *Addiction: From Biology to Drug Policy*. Freeman, New York.

Goldstein, D. B. (1983). *Pharmacology of Alcohol.* Oxford University Press, New York.

Goldstein, D. B., and Chin, J. H. (1981). Interaction of ethanol with biological membranes. *Fed. Proc.,* 40, 2073–2076.

Goldstein, M. (1987). Psychosocial issues. *Schizophr. Bull.,* 13, 171–186.

Goldstein, M., Freedman, L. S., Ebstein, R. P., Park, D. H., and Kashimoto, T. (1974). Human serum dopamine-β-hydroxylase: Relationship to sympathetic activity in physiological and pathological states. *Adv. Biochem. Psychopharmacol,* 12, 105–119.

Goldstein, M. J. (1995). Psychoeducation and relapse prevention. An update. In *Critical Issues in the Treatment of Schizophrenia* (N. Brunello, G. Racagni, S. Z. Langer and J. Mendlewicz, Eds.), pp. 134–141. Karger, New York.

Golub, A., and Johnson, B. D. (1994). The shifting importance of alcohol and marijuana as gateway substances among serious drug abusers. *J. Stud. Alcohol,* 55, 607–614.

Gonon, F. G., Suaud-Chagny, M. F., Mermet, C. C., and Buda, M. (1991). Relation between impulse flow and extracellular catecholamine levels as studied by in vivo electrochemistry in CNS. In *Volume Transmission in the Brain: Novel Mechanisms for Neural Transmission* (K. Fuxe and L. F. Agnati, Eds.), pp. 337–350. Raven Press, New York.

Goodman, J. H., and Sloviter, R. S. (1993). Cocaine neurotoxicity and altered neuropeptide Y immunoreactivity in the rat hippocampus; a silver degeneration and immunocytochemical study. *Brain Res.,* 616, 263–272.

Goodman, L. S., and Gilman, A. (Eds.) (1980). *The Pharmacological Basis of Therapeutics.* Macmillan, New York.

Goodman, R.R. and Pasternak, G.W. (1985). Visualization of mu$_1$ opiate receptors in rat brain by using a computerized autoradiographic subtraction technique. *Proc. Natl. Acad. Sci. U.S.A.,* 82, 6667–6671.

Goodman, W. K., Price, L. H., Delgado, P. L., Palumbo, J., Krystal, J. H., Nagy, L. M., Rasmussen, S. A., Heninger, G. R., and Charney, D. S. (1990). Specificity of serotonin reuptake inhibitors in the treatment of obsessive–compulsive disorder. *Arch. Gen. Psychiatry,* 47, 577–585.

Goodwin, D. W. (1979). Alcoholism and heredity: A review and hypothesis. *Arch. Gen. Psychiatry,* 36, 57–61.

Goodwin, D. W. (1991). The genetics of alcoholism. In *Genes, Brain and Behavior* (P. R. McHugh and V. A. McKusick, Eds.), pp. 219–226. Raven Press, New York.

Goodwin, G. M., DeSouza, R. J., and Green, A. R. (1987). Attenuation by electroconvulsive shock and antidepressant drugs of the 5-HT$_{1A}$ receptor-mediated hypothermia and serotonin syndrome produced by 8-OH-DPAT in the rat. *Psychopharmacology,* 91, 500–505.

Goodwin, J. L., Uemura, E., and Cunnick, J. E. (1995). Microglial release of nitric oxide by the synergistic action of β-amyloid and IFN-g. *Brain Res.,* 692, 207–214.

Gordon, E. R. (1966). Effect of aeration on the consumption of ethanol by the isolated perfused rat liver. *Nature,* 209, 1028–1029.

Gordon, E. R. (1968). The utilization of ethanol by the isolated perfused rat liver. *Can. J. Physiol. Pharmacol.,* 46, 609–616.

Gorman, J. M., Fyer, M. R., Liebowitz, M. R., and Klein, D. F. (1987). Pharmacologic provocation of panic attacks. In *Psychopharmacology: The Third Generation of Progress* (H. Y. Meltzer, Ed.), pp. 985–993, Raven Press, New York.

Goshima, Y., Kubo, T., and Misu, Y. (1988). Transmitter-like release of endogenous 3,4-dihydroxyphenylalanine from rat striatal slices. *J. Neurochem.,* 50, 1725–1730.

Gosnell, B. A., Krahn, D. D., and Majchrzak, M. J. (1990). The effects of morphine on diet selection are dependent upon baseline diet preferences. *Pharmacol. Biochem. Behav.,* 37, 207–212.

Goth, A. (1984). *Medical Pharmacology* (11th ed.). Mosby, St. Louis.

Göthert, M. (1980). Serotonin-receptor-mediated modulation of Ca^{2+}-dependent 5-hydroxytryptamine release from neurones of the rat brain cortex. *Naunyn Schmiedebergs Arch. Pharmacol.,* 314, 223–230.

Göthert, M. (1990). Presynaptic serotonin receptors in the central nervous system. *Ann. N.Y. Acad. Sci.,* 604, 102–112.

Gottesfeld, A., Kelly, J. S., and Renaud, L. P. (1972). The in vivo neuropharmacology of amino-oxyacetic acid in the cerebral cortex of the cat. *Brain Res.,* 42, 319–335.

Gottesman, I.I (1991). *Schizophrenia Genesis.* W. H. Freeman, New York.

Gouarderes, C., Cros, J., and Quirion, R. (1985). Autoradiogrphic localization of mu, delta and kappa opioid receptor binding sites in rat and guinea pig spinal cord. *Neuropeptides,* 6, 331–342.

Goudie, A. J., and Leathley, M. J. (1993). Drug discrimination assays. In *Behavioural Neuroscience: A Practical Approach,* Vol. 2 (A. Sahgal, Ed.), pp. 145–168. Oxford University Press, New York.

Gough, A. L., and Olley, J. E. (1978). Catalepsy induced by intrastriatal injections of Δ^9-tHC and 11-OH-Δ^9-tHC in the rat. *Neuropharmacology,* 17, 137–144.

Goyal, R. K. (1989). Muscarinic receptor subtypes: Physiology and clinical implications. *N. Engl. J. Med.,* 321, 1022–1029.

Grabowski, J., and Hall, S. M. (Eds.), (1985a). Pharmacological Adjuncts in Smoking Cessation. *NIDA Res. Monogr.,* 53.

Grabowski, J., and Hall, S. M. (1985b). Tobacco use, treatment strategies, and pharmacological adjuncts: An overview. *NIDA Res. Monogr.,* 53, 1–13.

Grabowski, J., Rhoades, H., Elk, R., Schmitz, J., Davis, C., Creson, D., and Kirby, K. (1995). Fluoxetine is ineffective for treatment of cocaine dependence or concurrent opiate and cocaine dependence: Two placebo-controlled, double-blind studies. *J. Clin. Psychopharmacol.,* 15, 163–174.

Grace, A. A. (1992). The depolarization block hypothesis of neuroleptic action: Implications for the etiology and treatment of schizophrenia. *J. Neural. Transm.,* 36 (Suppl.), 91–131.

Grace, A. A., and Bunney, B. S. (1985). Dopamine. In *Neurotransmitter Actions in the Vertebrate Nervous System* (M. A. Rogawski and J. L. Barker, Eds.), pp. 285–319. Plenum Press, New York.

Grace, A. A., and Bunney, B. S. (1995). Electrophysiological properties of midbrain dopamine neurons. In *Psychopharmacology: The Fourth Generation of Progress* (F. E. Bloom and D. J. Kupfer, Eds.), pp. 163–177. Raven Press, New York.

Graeff, F. G., and Schoenfeld, R. I. (1970). Tryptaminergic mechanisms in punished and nonpunished behavior. *J. Pharmacol. Exp. Ther.,* 173, 277–283.

Grafstein, B., and Foreman, D. S. (1980). Intracellular transport in neurons. *Physiol. Rev.,* 60, 1168–1282.

Graham, A. W., and Aghajanian, G. K. (1971). Effects of amphetamine on single cell activity in a catecholamine nucleus, the locus coeruleus. *Nature,* 234, 100–102.

Graham, D. C. (1978). Oxidative pathways for catecholamines in the genesis of neuromelanin and cytotoxic quinones. *Mol. Pharmacol.,* 14, 633–643.

Graham, D., Esnaud, H., Habert, E., and Langer, S. Z. (1989). A common binding site for tricyclic and nontricyclic 5-hydroxytryptamine uptake inhibitors at the substrate recognition site of the neuronal sodium-dependent 5-hydroxytryptamine transporter. *Biochem. Pharmacol.,* 38, 3819–3826.

Graham, D., and Langer, S. Z. (1992). Advances in sodium-ion coupled biogenic amine transporters. *Life Sci.,* 51, 631–645.

Gram, L., Sabers, A., and Dulae, O. (1992). Treatment of pediatric epilepsies with γ-vinyl GABA (vigabatrin). *Epilepsia,* 33 (Suppl. 5), S26–S29.

Gray, E. G. (1959). Axo-somatic and axo-dendritic synapses of the cerebral cortex: An electron microscopic study. *J. Anat.,* 93, 420–423.

Graybiel, A. M. (1990). Neurotransmitters and neuromodulators in the basal ganglia. *Trends Neurosci.,* 13, 244–254.

Graybiel, A. M., Hirsch, E. C., and Agid, Y. (1990). The nigrostriatal system in Parkinson's disease. *Adv. Neurol.,* 53, 17–29.

Graybiel, A. M., Moratalla, R., and Robertson, H. A. (1990). Amphetamine and cocaine induce drug-specific activation of the *c-fos* gene in striosome-matrix compartments and limbic subdivisions of the striatum. *Proc. Natl. Acad. Sci. U.S.A.,* 87, 6912–6916.

Green, A. R., Heal, D. J., and Vincent, N. D. (1987). The effects of single and repeated electroconvulsive shock administration on the release of 5-hydroxytryptamine and noradrenaline from cortical slices of rat brain. *Br. J. Pharmacol.,* 92, 25–30.

Green, J. P., and Maayani, S. (1977). Tricyclic antidepressant drugs block histamine H$_2$ receptors in brain. *Nature,* 269, 163–165.

Green, S. (1991). Benzodiazepines, putative anxiolytics and animal models of anxiety. *Trends Neurosci.,* 14, 101–104.

Greenblatt, D. J. (1990). Pharmacokinetics and pharmacodynamics. *Hosp. Pract.,* 25 (Suppl. 2), 9–18.

Greenblatt, D. J., and Shader, R. I. (1987). Pharmacokinetics of antianxiety agents. In *Psychopharmacology: The Third Generation of Progress* (H. Y. Meltzer, Ed.), pp. 1377–1386. Raven Press, New York.

Greene, R. W., and Haas, H. L. (1991). The electrophysiology of adenosine in the mammalian central nervous system. *Prog. Neurobiol.,* 36, 329–341.

Greenfield, S. A. (1991). A noncholinergic action of acetylcholinesterase (AChE) in the brain: From neuronal secretion to the generation of movement. *Cell. Mol. Neurobiol.,* 11, 55–77.

Greengard, P., Valtorta, F., Czernik, A. J., and Benfenati, F. (1993). Synaptic vesicle phosphoproteins and regulation of synaptic function. *Science*, 259, 780–785.

Greenough, W. T., Juraska, J. M., and Volkmar, F. R. (1979). Maze training effects on dendritic branching in occipital cortex of adult rats. *Behav. Neural Biol.*, 26, 287–297.

Greenshaw, A. J. (1993). Behavioural pharmacology of 5-HT$_3$ receptor antagonists: A critical update on therapeutic potential. *Trends Pharmacol. Sci.*, 14, 265–270.

Greifenstein, F. E., Yoshitake, J., DeVault, M., and Gajewski, J. E. (1958). A study of 1-aryl cyclo hexyl amine for anesthesia. *Anesth. Analg.*, 37, 283–294.

Griffiths, R. R., and Ator, N. A. (1980). Benzodiazepine self-administration in animals and humans: A comprehensive literature review. *NIDA Res. Monogr.*, 33, 22–36.

Griffiths, R. R., Bigelow, G. E., and Liebson, I. A. (1986). Human coffee drinking: Reinforcing and physical dependence producing effects of caffeine. *J. Pharmacol. Exp. Ther.*, 239, 416–425.

Griffiths, R. R., Evans, S. M., Heishman, S. J., Preston, K. L., Sannerud, C. A., Wolf, B., and Woodson, P. P. (1990a). Low-dose caffeine discrimination in humans. *J. Pharmacol. Exp. Ther.*, 252, 970–978.

Griffiths, R. R., Evans, S. M., Heishman, S. J., Preston, K. L., Sannerud, C. A., Wolf, B., and Woodson, P. P. (1990b). Low-dose caffeine physical dependence in humans. *J. Pharmacol. Exp. Ther.*, 255, 1123–1132.

Griffiths, R. R., and Sannerud, C. A. (1987). Abuse of and dependence on benzodiazepines and other anxiolytic/sedative drugs. In *Psychopharmacology: The Third Generation of Progress* (H. Y. Meltzer, Ed.), pp. 1535–1541. Raven Press, New York.

Grigoriadis, D. E., Heroux, J. A., and De Souza, E. B. (1993). Characterization and regulation of corticotropin-releasing factor receptors in the central nervous, endocrine and immune systems. *Ciba Found. Symp.*, 172, 85–107.

Grimm, U., Moser, U., Mutschler, E., and Lambrecht, G. (1994). Muscarinic receptors: Focus on presynaptic mechanisms and recently developed novel agonists and antagonists. *Pharmazie*, 49, 711–726.

Grinker, R. R., and Spiegel, J. P. (1945). *Men Under Stress*. Blakiston, Philadelphia.

Grinspoon, L. (1977). *Marijuana Reconsidered* (2nd ed.). Harvard University Press, Cambridge, MA.

Grinspoon, L., and Bakalar, J. B. (1979). The amphetamines: Medical uses and health hazards. In *Amphetamine Use, Misuse, and Abuse* (D. E. Smith, et al., Eds.), pp. 3–10. Hall, Boston.

Grinspoon, L., and Bakalar, J. B. (1985). *Cocaine. A Drug and its Social Evolution* (Rev. ed.). Basic Books, New York.

Grinspoon, L., and Hedblom, P. (1975). *The Speed Culture: Amphetamine Use and Abuse in America*. Harvard University Press, Cambridge, MA.

Gritz, E. R., and Jarvik, M. E. (1978). Nicotine and smoking. In *Handbook of Psychopharmacology*, Vol. 11 (L. L. Iversen, S. D. Iversen, and S. H. Snyder, Eds.), pp. 425–464. Plenum Press, New York.

Grob, C. S., Bravo, G. L., Walsh, R. N., and Liester, M. B. (1992). The MDMA-neurotoxicity controversy: Implications for clinical research with novel psychoactive agents. *J. Nerv. Ment. Dis.*, 180, 355–356.

Gross, G., Dodt, C., and Hanft, G. (1988). Effect of chronic lithium administration on adrenoceptor binding and adrenoceptor regulation in rat cerebral cortex. *Naunyn Schmiedebergs Arch. Pharmacol.*, 337, 267–272.

Grossman, C. J., Kilpatrick, G. J., and Bunce, K. T. (1993). Development of a radioligand binding assay for 5-HT$_4$ receptors in guinea-pig and rat brain. *Br. J. Pharmacol.*, 109, 618–624.

Groves, P. M., Ryan, L. J., Diana, M., Young, S. J., and Fisher, L. J. (1989). Neuronal actions of amphetamine in the rat brain. *NIDA Res. Monogr.*, 94, 127–145.

Growdon, J. H., Corkin, S., and Rosen, T. J. (1990). Distinctive aspects of cognitive dysfunction in Parkinson's disease. *Adv. Neurol.*, 53, 365–376.

Grucker, D., Mauss, Y., Armspach, J. P., Dumitresco, B., Gounot, D., and Chambron, J. (1986). In vivo state and distribution of water in the brain as studied by NMR proton relaxation. In *PET and NMR: New Perspectives in Neuroimaging and in Clinical Neurochemistry* (L. Battistin and F. Gerstenbrand, Eds.), pp. 303–314. Alan R. Liss, New York.

Grunfeld, Y., and Edery, H. (1969). Psychopharmacological activity of the active constituents of hashish and some related cannabinoids. *Psychopharmacologia*, 14, 200–210.

Gu, X. F., and Azmitia, E. C. (1993). Integrative transporter-mediated release from cytoplasmic and vesicular 5-hydroxytryptamine stores in cultured neurons. *Eur. J. Pharmacol.*, 235, 51–57.

Gualtieri, C. T., Ondrusek, M. G., and Finley, C. (1985). Attention deficit disorders in adults. *Clin. Neuropharmacol.*, 8, 343–356.

Gualtieri, F., Dei, S., Manetti, D., Romanelli, M. N., Scapecchi, S., and Teodori, E. (1995). The medicinal chemistry of Alzheimer's and Alzheimer-like diseases with emphasis on the cholinergic hypothesis. *Farmaco*, 50, 489–503.

Guastella, J., Brecha, N., Weigmann, C., Lester, H., and Davidson, N. (1992). Cloning, expression, and localization of a rat brain high-affinity glycine transporter. *Proc. Natl. Acad. Sci. U.S.A.*, 89, 7189–7193.

Guastella, J., Nelson, N., Nelson, H., Czyzyk, L., Keynan, S., Miedel, M. C., Davidson, N., Lester, H. A., and Kanner, B. I. (1990). Cloning and expression of a rat brain GABA transporter. *Science*, 249, 1303–1306.

Guay, D. R. (1995). The emerging role of valproate in bipolar disorder and other psychiatric disorders. *Pharmacotherapy*, 15, 631–647.

Guidotti, A. (1978). Synaptic mechanisms in the action of benzodiazepines. In *Psychopharmacology: A Generation of Progress* (M. A. Lipton, A. DiMascio, and K. F. Killam, Eds.), pp. 1349–1357. Raven Press, New York.

Guidotti, A., Corda, M. G., and Costa, E. (1983). Strategies for the isolation and characterization of an endogenous effector of the benzodiazepine recognition sites. *Adv. Biochem. Psychopharmacol.*, 38, 95–103.

Guidotti, A., and Costa, E. (1973). Involvement of adenosine 3',5'-monophosphate in the activation of tyrosine hydroxylase elicited by drugs. *Science*, 179, 902–904.

Guidotti, A., and Costa, E. (1974). A role for nicotinic receptors in the regulation of the adenylate cyclase of adrenal medulla. *J. Pharmacol. Exp. Ther.*, 189, 665–675.

Guidotti, A., and Costa, E. (1977). Trans-synaptic regulation of tyrosine 3-mono-oxygenase biosynthesis in rat adrenal medulla. *Biochem. Pharmacol.*, 26, 817–823.

Guidotti, A., Ferrero, P., Fujimoto, M., Santi, R. M., and Costa, E. (1986). Studies on the endogenous ligands (endocoids) for the benzodiazepine β-carboline binding sites. *Adv. Biochem. Psychopharmacol.*, 137–148.

Guitart, X., Thompson, M. A., Mirante, C. K., Greenberg, M. E., and Nestler, E. J. (1992). Regulation of CREB phosphorylation by acute and chronic morphine in the rat locus coeruleus. *J. Neurochem.*, 58, 1168–1171.

Gunne, L. M., Änggård, E., and Jönsson, L. E. (1972). Clinical trials with amphetamine-blocking drugs. *Psychiatry Neurol. Neurochir. (Amst.)*, 75, 225–226.

Gunne, L. M., Lindstrom, L., and Terenius, J. (1977). Naloxone-induced reversal of schizophrenic hallucinations. *J. Neural Transm.*, 40, 13–20.

Gur, R. E. (1995). Functional brain-imaging studies in schizophrenia. In *Psychopharmacology: The Fourth Generation of Progress* (F. E. Bloom and D. J. Kupfer, Eds.), pp. 1185–1192. Raven Press, New York.

Gur, R. E., and Pearlson, G. D. (1993). Neuroimaging in schizophrenia research. *Schizophr. Bull.*, 19, 337–353.

Gurwitz, D., and Sokolovsky, M. (1980). Induced interconversion of agonist affinity states in muscarinic receptor from mouse brain: Effects of temperature and sugars. *Biochem. Biophys. Res. Commun.*, 94, 493–500.

Guttman, N., and Kalish, H. I. (1956). Discriminability and stimulus generalization. *J. Exp. Psychol.*, 51, 79–88.

Guyenet, P. G., and Cabot, J. B. (1981). Inhibition of sympathetic preganglionic neurons by catecholamines and clonidine: Mediation by an α-adrenergic receptor. *J. Neurosci.*, 1, 908–917.

Gybels, J. M. (1994). Defining idiopathic Parkinson's disease. In *Noradrenergic Mechanisms in Parkinson's Disease* (M. Briley and M. Marien, Eds.), pp. 1–9. CRC Press, Boca Raton.

Haas, H. L. (1985). Histamine. In *Neurotransmitter Actions in the Vertebrate Nervous System* (M. A. Rogawski and J. L. Barker, Eds.), pp. 321–337. Plenum Press, New York.

Haase, G. R. (1977). Diseases presenting as dementia. In *Dementia* (2nd ed.). (C. E. Wells, Ed.), pp. 27–67. F. A. Davis Co., Philadelphia.

Haavik, J., Martinez, A., and Flatmark, T. (1990). pH-dependent release of catecholamines from tyrosine hydroxylase and the effect of phosphorylation of Ser-40. *FEBS Lett.*, 262, 363–365.

Hadfield, H. G., Crane, P., King, M. E., Nugent, E. A., Milio, C., and Narasimhachari, N. (1985). Determination of 13 catecholamines, indoleamines, metabolites and precursors in less than 20 minutes during a single HPLC run. *J. Liquid Chromotogr.*, 8, 2689–2697.

Haefely, W. E. (1977). Synaptic pharmacology of barbiturates and benzodiazepines. *Agents Actions,* 7/3, 353–359.

Haefely, W. E. (1978). Behavioral and neuropharmacological aspects of drugs used in anxiety and related states. In *Psychopharmacology: A Generation of Progress* (M. A. Lipton, A. DiMascio, and K. F. Killem, Eds.), pp. 1359–1374. Raven Press, New York.

Haefely, W. E. (1983). Antagonists of benzodiazepines: Functional aspects. *Adv. Biochem. Psychopharmacol.,* 38, 73–93.

Haefely, W. E. (1989). Pharmacology of the benzodiazepine receptor. *Eur. Arch. Psychiatry Neurol. Sci.,* 238, 294–301.

Haefely, W., Kulcsár, A., Möhler, H., Pieri, L., Polc, P., and Schaffner, R. (1975). Possible involvement of GABA in the central actions of benzodiazepines. *Adv. Biochem. Psychopharmacol.,* 14, 131–151.

Hagan, J. J., and Morris, R. J. M. (1987). The cholinergic hypothesis of memory: A review of animal experiments. In *The Handbook of Psychopharmacology,* Vol. 6 (S. Snyder, L. L. Iversen, and S. D. Iversen, Eds.), pp. 237–323. Plenum Press, New York.

Hagberg, H., Andersson, P., Lacerwicz, J., Jacobsen, I., Butcher, S., and Sandberg, M. (1987). Extracellular adenosine, inosine, hypoxanthine, and xanthine in relation to tissue nucleotides and purines in rat striatum during transient ischemia. *J. Neurochem.,* 49, 227–231.

Hahn, M., Hahn, S. L., Stone, D. M., and Joh, T. H. (1992). Cloning of the rat gene encoding choline acetyltransferase, a cholinergic neuron-specific marker. *Proc. Natl. Acad. Sci. U.S.A.,* 89, 4387–4391.

Haier, R. (1980). The diagnosis of schizophrenia: A review of recent developments. *Schizophr. Bull.,* 6, 417–428.

Hall, J. (1988). Fluoxetine: Efficacy against placebo and by dose: An overview. *Br. J. Psychiatry,* 153 (Suppl. 3), 59–63.

Hall, Z. W. (1992). The nerve terminal. In *An Introduction to Molecular Neurobiology* (Z. W. Hall, Ed.), pp. 148–178. Sinauer Associates, Sunderland, MA.

Halldin, M. M., Widman, M., Agurell, S., Hollister, L. E., and Kanter, S. L. (1984). Acidic metabolites of delta-1-tetrahydrocannabinol excreted in the urine of man. In *The Cannabinoids: Chemical, Pharmacologic, and Therapeutic Aspects* (S. Agurell, W. L. Dewey, and R. E. Willette, Eds.), pp. 211–218. Academic Press, New York.

Hallman, H., Sundström, E., and Jonsson, G. (1984). Effects of the noradrenaline neurotoxin DSP 4 on monoamine neurons and their transmitter turnover in rat CNS. *J. Neural Transm.,* 60, 89–102.

Halperin, R., Guerin, J. Jr., and Davis, K. L. (1989). Regional differences in the induction of behavioral supersensitivity by prolonged treatment with atypical neuroleptics. *Psychopharmacology,* 98, 386–391.

Hamberger, A., Chiang, G. H., Nylén, E. S., Scheff, S. W., and Cotman, C. W. (1979). Glutamate as a CNS transmitter. I. Evaluation of glucose and glutamine as precursors for the synthesis of preferentially released glutamate. *Brain Res.,* 168, 513–530.

Hamberger, A., Nyström, B., and Silfvenius, H. (1992). Extracellular and intracellular amino acids in the CNS of patients with epilepsy and other neurological disorders. *Epilepsy Res.* (Suppl. 8), 375–381.

Hamblin, M. W., McGuffin, R. W., Metcalf, M. A., Dorsa, D. M., and Merchant, K. M. (1992). Distinct 5-HT$_{1B}$ and 5-HT$_{1D}$ serotonin receptors in rat: Structural and pharmacological comparison of the two cloned receptors. *Mol. Cell. Neurosci.,* 3, 578–587.

Hamill, O. P., Marty, A., Neher, E., Sakmann, B., and Sigworth, F. J. (1981). Improved patch-clamp techniques for high rresolution current recording from cells and cell-free membrane patches. *Pflügers Arch.,* 391, 85–100

Hamilton, L. W., and Timmons, C. R. (1990). *Principles of Behavioral Pharmacology: A Biopsychological Perspective.* Prentice-Hall, Englewood, N. J.

Hammer, R., Berrie, C. P., Birdsall, N. J. M., Burgen, A. S. V., and Hulme, E. C. (1980). Pirenzepine distinguishes between different subclasses of muscarinic receptors. *Nature,* 283, 90–92.

Hammer, R. P., and Hauser, K. F. (1992). Consequences of early exposure to opioids on cell proliferation and neuronal morphogenesis. In *Development of the Central Nervous System: Effects of Alcohol and Opiates,* pp. 319–339. Wiley-Liss, Inc, New York.

Hamon, M., Gozlan, H., El Mestikawy, S., Emerit, M. B., Bolaños, F., and Schechter, L. (1990). The central 5-HT$_{1A}$ receptors: Pharmacological, biochemical, functional, and regulatory properties. *Ann. N.Y. Acad. Sci.,* 600, 114–131.

Hampson, R. E., Foster, T. C., and Deadwyler, S. A. (1989). Effects of Δ-9-tetrahydrocannabinol on sensory evoked hippocampal activity in the rat: Principal components analysis and sequential dependency. *J. Pharmacol. Exp. Ther.,* 251, 870–877.

Han, J. S. (1993). Acupuncture and stimulation produced analgesia. In *Opioids II,* Handbook of Experimental Pharmacology, Vol. 104 (A. Herz, Ed.), pp. 105–125. Springer-Verlag, New York.

Han, J. S., Chen, X. H., Sun, S. L., Xu, X. J., Yuan, Y., Uan, S. C., Hao, J. X., and Terenius, L. (1991). Effect of low- and high-frequency TENS on met-enkephalin-Arg-Phe and dynorphin A immunoreactivity in human lumbar CSF. *Pain,* 47, 295–298.

Han, S. H., Einstein, G., Weisgraber, K. H., Strittmatter, W. J., Saunders, A. M., Pericak-Vance, M., Roses, A. D., and Schmechel, D. E. (1994). Apolipoprotein E is localized to the cytoplasm of human cortical neurons: A light and electron microscopic study. *J. Neuropathol. Exp. Neurol.,* 53, 535–544.

Hanauer, S. A., Slade, J., Barnes, D. E., Bero, L. A., and Glantz, S. A. (1995). Lawyer control of internal scientific research to protect against product liability lawsuits: The Brown and Williamson Documents. *JAMA,* 274, 234–240.

Handelmann, G. E., Contreras, P. C., and O'Donohue, T. L. (1987). Selective memory impairment by phencyclidine in rats. *Eur. J. Pharmacol.,* 140, 69–73.

Handley, S. (1994). Future prospects for the pharmacological treatment of anxiety. *CNS Drugs,* 2, (5) 397–414.2

Hanse, E., and Gustafsson, B. (1994). Onset and stabilization of NMDA receptor-dependent hippocampal long-term potentiation. *Neurosci. Res.,* 20, 15–25.

Hanson, M. D. (1984). Smokeless tobacco and oral carcinoma: A review of the literature. *Va. Dent. J.,* 61, 30–32.

Hanuš, L., Gopher, A., Almog, S., and Mechoulam, R. (1993). Two new unsaturated fatty acid ethanolamides in brain that bind to the cannabinoid receptor. *J. Med. Chem.,* 36, 3032–3034.

Haracz, J. L., Tschanz, J. T., Wang, Z., White, I. M., and Rebec, G. V. (1993). Striatal single-unit responses to amphetamine and neuroleptics in freely moving rats. *Neurosci. Biobehav. Rev.,* 17, 1–12.

Harbuz, M. S., and Lightman, S. L. (1989). Responses of hypothalamic and pituitary mRNA to physical and psychological stress in the rat. *J. Endocrinol.,* 122, 705–711.

Hardy, J. (1992). An 'anatomical cascade hypothesis' for Alzheimer's disease. *Trends Neurosci.,* 15, 200–201.

Hardy, J., Adolfsson, R., Alafuzoff, I., Bucht, G., Marcusson, J., Nyberg, P., Perdahl, E., Wester, P., and Windblad, B. (1985). Transmitter deficits in Alzheimer's disease. *Neurochem. Int.,* 4, 545–563.

Hardy, J., and Allsop, D. (1991). Amyloid deposition as the central event in the aetiology of Alzheimer's disease. *Trends Pharmacol. Sci.,* 12, 383–388.

Hardy, J. A., and Higgins, G. A. (1992). Alzheimer's disease: The amyloid cascade hypothesis. *Science,* 256, 184–185.

Harger, R. N., Hulpieu, H. R., and Lamb, E. B. (1937). The speed with which various parts of the body reach equilibrium in the storage of ethyl alcohol. *J. Biol. Chem.,* 120, 689–704.

Harper, C. G., and Kril, J. J. (1990). Neuropathology of alcoholism. *Alcohol Alcohol.,* 25, 207–216.

Harris, G. C., and Aston-Jones, G. (1994). Involvement of D2 dopamine receptors in the nucleus accumbens in the opiate withdrawal syndrome. *Nature,* 371, 155–157.

Harris, G. W. (1948). Neural control of the pituitary gland. *Physiol. Rev.,* 28, 139–179.

Harris, G. W. (1955). *Neural Control of the Pituitary Gland.* Edward Arnold, London.

Harris, J. E., and Baldessarini, R. J. (1973). Uptake of [^{3}H]-catecholamines by homogenates of rat corpus striatum and cerebral cortex: Effects of amphetamine analogues. *Neuropharmacology,* 12, 669–679.

Harris, R. A., and Allan, A. M. (1985). Functional coupling of γ-aminobutyric acid receptors to chloride channels in brain membranes. *Science,* 228, 1108–1110.

Harris, R. T., Waters, W., and McLendon, D. (1974). Evaluation of reinforcing capability of delta-9-tetrahydrocannabinol in rhesus monkeys. *Psychopharmacologia,* 37, 23–29.

Harro, J., Vasar, E., and Bradwejn, J. (1993). CCK in animal and human research on anxiety. *Trends Pharmacol. Sci.,* 14, 244–249.

Hartig, P. R., Branchek, T. A., and Weinshank, R. L. (1992). A subfamily of 5-HT$_{1D}$ receptor genes. *Trends Pharmacol. Sci.,* 13, 152–159.

Hartig, P. R., Hoffman, B. J., Kaufman, M. J., and Hirata, F. (1990). The 5-HT$_{1C}$ receptor. *Ann. N.Y. Acad. Sci.,* 600, 149–167.

Hartig, P. R., and Lever, J. (1990). Serotonin receptors. In *Quantitative Imaging: Neuroreceptors, Neurotransmitters, and Enzymes* (J. J. Frost and H. N. Wagner Jr., Eds.), pp. 153–165. Raven Press, New York.

Harvey, J. A. (1978). Neurotoxic actions of halogenated amphetamines. *Ann. N.Y. Acad. Sci.,* 305, 289–304.

Harvey, S. C. (1985). Hypnotics and sedatives. In *The Pharmacological Basis of Therapeutics* (A. Gilman, L. S. Goodman, T. W. Rall, and

F. Murad, Eds.), pp. 339–371. Macmillan, New York.

Hasegawa, K., and Aoba, A. (1994). Symptoms, diagnosis and epidemiology of dementia. In *Anti-Dementia Agents*, pp. 13–31. Academic Press Ltd.

Hatsukami, D., Hughes, J., and Pickens, R. (1984). Tobacco withdrawal symptoms. *Psychopharmacology*, 84, 231–236.

Hatton, G. I. (1990). Emerging concepts of structure–function dynamics in adult brain: The hypothalamo-neurohypophysial system. *Prog. Neurobiol.*, 34, 437–504.

Haubrich, D. R., and Wang, P. F. L. (1976). Inhibition of acetylcholine synthesis by juglone and 4-(1=naphthylvinyl)pyridine. *Biochem. Pharmacol.*, 25, 669–672.

Hausdorff, W. P., Caron, M. G., and Lefkowitz, R. J. (1990). Turning off the signal: Desensitization of β-adrenergic receptor function. *FASEB J.*, 4, 2881–2889.

Hawkins, J. D., Catalano, R. F., and Miller, J. Y. (1992). Risk and protective factors for alcohol and other drug problems in adolescence and early adulthood: Implications for substance abuse prevention. *Psychol. Bull.*, 112, 64–105.

Haxby, J. V., Duara, R., Grady, C. L., Cutler, N. R., and Rapoport, S. I. (1985). Relations between neuropsychology and cerebral metabolic asymmetries in early Alzheimer's disease. *J. Cereb. Blood Flow Metab.*, 5, 193–200.

Hayashi, T. (1954). Effects of sodium glutamate on the nervous system. *Keio J. Med.*, 3, 183–192.

Haycock, J. W. (1990). Phosphorylation of tyrosine hydroxylase in situ at serine 8, 19, 31, and 40. *J. Biol. Chem.*, 265, 11682–11691.

Haycock, J. W. (1993). Multiple signaling pathways in bovine chromaffin cells regulate tyrosine hydroxylase phosphorylation at Ser[19], Ser[31], and Ser[40]. *Neurochem. Res.*, 18, 15–26.

Haycock, J. W., Ahn, N. B., Cobb, M. H., and Krebs, E. G. (1992). ERK1 and ERK2, two microtubule-associated protein kinases, mediate the phosphorylation of tyrosine hydroxylase at serine 31 in situ. *Proc. Natl. Acad. Sci. U.S.A.*, 84, 1677–1681.

Haycock, J. W., and Haycock, D. A. (1991). Tyrosine hydroxylase in rat brain dopaminergic nerve terminals: Multiple-site phosphorylation in vivo and in synaptosomes. *J. Biol. Chem.*, 266, 5650–5657.

Heather, N. (1990). Treatment of alcohol problems, with special reference to the behavioral approach. In *Psychotropic Drugs of Abuse* (D. J. K. Balfour, Ed.), pp. 283–312. Pergamon Press, New York.

Heather, N., and Robertson I. (1983). *Controlled Drinking*. Methuen, London.

Hebb, D. O. (1949). *The Organization of Behavior*. Wiley, New York.

Hechtman, P., and Kaplan, F. (1993). Tay-Sachs disease screening and diagnosis: Evolving technologies. *DNA Cell Biol.*, 8, 651–665.

Heffner, T. G., Drawbaugh, R. B., and Zigmond, M. J. (1974). Amphetamine and operant behavior in rats: Relationship between drug effect and control response rate. *J. Comp. Physiol. Psychol.*, 8, 1031–1043.

Hefti, F., Hartikka, J., and Knüsel, B. (1989). Function of neurotrophic factors in the adult and aging brain and their possible use in the treatment of neurodegenerative diseases. *Neurobiol. Aging*, 10, 515–533.

Hefti, F., and Weiner, W. J. (1986). Nerve growth factor and Alzheimer's disease. *Ann. Neurol.*, 20, 275–281.

Heijna, M. H., Padt, M., Hogenboom, F., Schoffelmeer, A. N. M., and Mulder, A. H. (1991). Opioid receptor-mediated inhibition of ^{3}H-dopamine but not ^{3}H-noradrenaline release from rat mediobasal hypothalamus slices. *Neuroendocrinology*, 54, 118–126.

Heikkila, R. E., Cabbat, F. S., and Mytilineou, C. (1977). Studies on the capacity of mazindol and dita to act as uptake inhibitors or releasing agents for ^{3}H-biogenic amines in rat brain tissue slices. *Eur. J. Pharmacol.*, 45, 329–333.

Heikkila, R. E., Manzino, L., Cabbat, F. S., and Duvoisin, R. C. (1984). Protection against the dopaminergic neurotoxicity of 1-methyl-4-phenyl-1,2,5,6-tetrahydropyridine by monoanime oxidase inhibitors. *Nature*, 11, 467–469.

Heikkila, R. E., Orlansky, H., and Cohen, G. (1975). Studies on the distinction between uptake inhibition and release of [^{3}H]dopamine in rat brain tissue slices. *Biochem. Pharmacol.*, 24, 847–852.

Heikkila, R. E., Sonsalla, P. K., and Duvoisin, R. C. (1989). Biochemical models of Parkinson's disease. In *Neuromethods*, Vol. 12, *Drugs as Tools in Neuroscience Research* (A. B. Boulton, G. B. Baker, and A. V. Juorio, Eds.), pp. 351–384. Humana Press, Clifton, N. J.

Heilig, M., Engel, J. A., and Söderpalm, B. (1993). C-fos antisense in the nucleus accumbens blocks the locomotor stimulant action of cocaine. *Eur. J. Pharmacol.*, 236, 339–340.

Heineman, W. R., Halsall, H. B., Wehmeyer, K. R., Doyle, M. J., and Wright, D. S. (1987). Immunoassay with electrochemical detection. In *Methods of Biochemical Analysis*, Vol. 32 (David Glick, Ed.), pp. 345–393. Wiley, New York.

Heinrichs, R. W. (1993). Schizophrenia and the brain: Conditions for a neuropsychology of madness. *Am. Psychol.*, 48, 221–233.

Heise, G. A. (1987). Facilitation of memory and cognition by drugs. *Trends Pharmacol. Sci.*, 8, 65–68.

Heishman, S. J., and Henningfield, J. E. (1992). Stimulus functions of caffeine in humans: Relation to dependence potential. *Neurosci. Biobehav. Rev.*, 16, 273–287.

Heishman, S. J., and Taylor, R,C., and Henningfield, J. E. (1994). Nicotine and smoking: A review of effects on human performance. *Exp. Clin. Psychopharmacol.*, 345–395.

Helke, C. J., Krause, J. E., Mantyh, P. W., Couture, R., and Bannon, M. J. (1990). Diversity in mammalian tachykinin peptidergic neurons: Multiple peptides, receptors, and regulatory mechanisms. *FASEB J.*, 4, 1606–1615.

Helm, C. A., and Israelachvili, J. N. (1993). Forces between phospholipid bilayers and relationship to membrane fusion. *Methods Enzymol.*, 220, 130–143.

Hemby, S. E., Martin, T. J., Co, C., Dworkin, S. I., and Smith, J. E. (1995). The effects of intravenous heroin administration on extracellular nucleus accumbens dopamine concentrations as determined by *in vivo* microdialysis. *J. Pharmacol. Exp. Ther.*, 273, 591–598.

Hemmings, H. C. Jr., Walaas, S. I., Ouimet, C. C., and Greengard, P. (1987). Dopaminergic regulation of protein phosphorylation in the striatum: DARPP-32. *Trends Neurosci.*, 10, 377–383.

Hen, R. (1992). Of mice and flies: Commonalities among 5-HT receptors. *Trends Pharmacol. Sci.*, 13, 160–165.

Henderson, R. L., Tennant, F. S., and Guerney, R. (1972). Respiratory manifestations of hashish smoking. *Arch. Otolaryngol.*, 95, 248–251.

Hendin, H., Pollinger, A., Ulman, R., and Carr, A. C. (1981). *Adolescent Marijuana Abusers and Their Families*. NIDA Res. Monogr., 40.

Heninger, G. R., and Charney, D. S. (1987). Mechanism of action of antidepressant treatments: Implications for the etiology and treatment of depressive disorders. In *Psychopharmacology: The Third Generation of Progress* (H. Y. Meltzer, Ed.), pp. 535–544. Raven Press, New York.

Henley, J. M. (1994). Kainate-binding proteins: Phylogeny, structures and possible functions. *Trends Pharmacol. Sci.*, 15, 182–190.

Henningfield, J. E. (1992). Nicotine: an old fashioned addiction. In *The Encyclopedia of Psychoactive Drugs* (S. H. Snyder, Ed.). Chelsea House, New York.

Henry, J.-P., and Scherman, D. (1989). Radioligands of the vesicular monoamine transporter and their use as markers of monoamine storage vesicles. *Biochem. Pharmacol.*, 38, 2395–2404.

Herkenham, M. (1987). Mismatches between neurotransmitter and receptor localizations in brain: Observations and implications. *Neuroscience*, 243, 1–38.

Herkenham, M. (1991). Mismatches between neurotransmitter and receptor localizations in brain: Implications for endocrine functions in brain. In *Volume Transmission in the Brain: Novel Mechanisms for Neural Transmission* (K. Fuxe and L. F. Agnati, Eds.), pp. 63–87. Raven Press, New York.

Herkenham, M., Lynn, A. B., de Costa, B. R., and Richfield, E. K. (1991). Neuronal localization of cannabinoid receptors in the basal ganglia of the rat. *Brain Res.*, 547, 267–274.

Herkenham, M., Lynn, A. B., Johnson, M. R., Melvin, L. S., de Costa, B. R., and Rice, K. C. (1991). Characterization and localization of cannabinoid receptors in rat brain: A quantitative *in vitro* autoradiographic study. *J. Neurosci.*, 11, 563–583.

Herkenham, M., Lynn, A. B., Little, M. D., Johnson, M. R., Melvin, L. S., de Costa, B. R., and Rice, K. R. (1990). Cannabinoid receptor localization in brain. *Proc. Natl. Acad. Sci. U.S.A.*, 87, 1932–1936.

Herkenham, M., and McLean, S. (1986). Mismatches between receptor and transmitter localizations in the brain. In *Quantitative Receptor Autoradiography* (C. A. Boast, E. W. Snowhill, and C. A. Altar, Eds.), pp. 131–171. Alan R. Liss, New York.

Herman, B. H., Hammock, M. K., Egan, J., Arthur-Smith, A., Chatoor, I., and Werner, A. (1989). Role for opioid peptides in self-injurious behavior: Dissociation from autonomic nervous system functioning. *Dev. Pharmacol. Ther.*, 12, 81–89.

Hernandez, L., Auerbach, S., and Hoebel, B. G. (1988). Phencyclidine (PCP) injected in the nucleus accumbens increases extracellular dopamine and serotonin as measured by microdialysis. *Life Sci.*, 42, 1713–1723.

Herrick, C. L. (1893). Report upon the pathology of a case of general paralysis. *J. Comp. Neurol.*, 3, 141–162.

Herrick, C. L., and Tight, W. G. (1890). The central nervous system of rodents: Preliminary report. *Bull. Sci. Lab. Denison Univ.*, 5, 35–95.

Hersch, S. M., et al. (1995). Electron microscopic analysis of D1 and D2 dopamine receptor proteins in the dorsal striatum and their synaptic relationships with motor corticostriatal afferents. *J. Neurosci.*, 15, 5222–5237.

Hersch, S. M., Gutenkunst, C.-A., Rees, H. D., Heilman, C. J., and Levey, A. I. (1994). Distribution of m1–m4 muscarinic receptor proteins in the rat striatum: Light and electron microscopic immunocytochemistry using subtype-specific antibodies. *J. Neurosci.*, 14, 3351–3363.

Hess, W. R. (1954). Diencephalon. Autonomic and Extrapyramidal Functions. *Monogr. Biol. Med.* Vol. 3.

Hetherington, A. W., and Ranson, S. W. (1940). Hypothalamic lesions and adiposity in the rat. *Anat. Rec.*, 78, 149–172.

Heuser, J. E. (1976). Morphology of synaptic vesicle discharge and reformation at the frog neuromuscular junction. In *Motor Innervation of Muscle* (S. Thesleff, Ed.), pp. 51–115. Academic Press, London.

Heuser, J. E. (1977). Synaptic vesicle exocytosis revealed in quick-frozen frog neuromuscular junctions treated with 4-aminopyridine and given a single electrical shock. In *Society for Neuroscience Symposia*, Vol. 2 (W. M. Cowan and J. A. Ferrendelli, Eds.), pp. 215–239. Society for Neuroscience, Bethesda, MD.

Heuser, J. E., and Reese, T. S. (1973). Evidence for recycling of synaptic vesicle membrane at the frog neuromuscular junction. *J. Cell Biol.*, 57, 315–344.

Heuser, J. E., and Reese, T. S. (1977). Structure of the synapse. In *Handbook of Physiology, The Nervous System*, Vol. 1 (J. M. Brookhart and V. B. Mountcastle, Eds.), pp. 261–294. American Physiological Society, Washington, D.C.

Heuser, J. E., Reese, T. S., and Landis, D. M. D. (1974). Functional changes in frog neuromuscular junction studied with freeze-fracture. *J. Neurocytol.*, 3, 109–131.

Hewlett, W. A., Vinogradov, S., Martin, K., Berman, S., and Csernansky, J. G. (1992). Fenfluramine stimulation of prolactin in obsessive–compulsive disorder. *Psychiatry Res.*, 42, 81–92.

Hewson, G., Leighton, G. E., Hill, R. G., and Hughes, J. (1988). The cholecystokinin receptor antagonist L364,718 increases food intake in the rat by attenuation of the action of endogenous cholecystokinin. *Br. J. Pharmacol.*, 93, 79–84.

Heym, J., and Jacobs, B. L. (1987). Serotonergic mechanisms of hallucinogenic drug effects. *Monogr. Neural Sci.*,13, 55–81.

Heym, J., Rasmussen, K., and Jacobs, B. L. (1984). Some behavioral effects of hallucinogens are mediated by a postsynaptic serotonergic action: Evidence from single unit studies in freely moving cats. 101, 57–68.

Heyser, C. J., Chen, W.-J., Miller, J., Spear, N. E., and Spear, L. P. (1990). Prenatal cocaine exposure induces deficits in Pavlovian conditioning and sensory preconditioning among infant rat pups. *Behav. Neurosci.*, 104, 955–963.

Heyser, C. J., Spear, N. E., and Spear, L. P. (1992). Effects of prenatal exposure to cocaine on conditional discrimination learning in adult rats. *Behav. Neurosci.*, 106, 837–845.

Hieble, J. P., et al. (1995). International Union of Pharmacology X. Recommendation for nomenclature of α_1-adrenoceptors: Consensus update. *Pharmacol. Rev.*, 47, 267–270.

Hieble, J. P., and Ruffolo, R. R. Jr. (1991a). Functions mediated by β-adrenoceptor activation. In *Progress in Basic and Clinical Pharmacology*, Vol. 7, *β-Adrenoceptors: Molecular Biology, Biochemistry and Pharmacology* (R. R. Ruffolo Jr., Ed.), pp. 173–209. Karger, Basel.

Hieble, J. P., and Ruffolo, R. R. Jr. (1991b). Subclassification of β-adrenoceptors. In *Progress in Basic and Clinical Pharmacology*, Vol. 7. *β-Adrenoceptors: Molecular Biology, Biochemistry and Pharmacology* (R. R. Ruffolo Jr., Ed.), pp. 1–25. Karger, Basel.

Higgins, C. W., Whitley, K. N., and Dunn, J. D. (1984). A comparison between smoking related attitudes and behaviors among Kentucky public school children whose families are or are not involved in tobacco production. *J. Sch. Health*, 54, 185–187.

Higgins, L. S., and Cordell, B. (1995). Genetically engineered animal models of human neurodegenerative disorders. *Neurodegeneration*, 4, 117–129.

Higgins, L. S., Holtzman, D. M., Rabin, J., Mobley, W. C., and Cordell, B. (1994). Transgenic mouse brain histopathology resembles early Alzheimer's disease. *Ann. Neurol.*, 35, 598–607.

Higgins, L. S., Rodems, J. M., Catalano, R., Quon, D., and Cordell, B. (1995). Early Alzheimer disease-like histopathology increases in frequency with age in mice transgenic for β-APP751. *Proc. Natl. Acad. Sci. U.S.A.*, 92, 4402–4406.

Higgins, S. T., Bickel, W. K., and Hughes, J. R. (1994). Influence of an alternative reinforcer on human cocaine self-administration. *Life Sci.*, 55, 179–187.

Higgins, S. T., Bickel, W. K., Hughes, J. R., Lynn, M., Capeless, M. A., and Fenwick, J. W. (1990). Effects of intranasal cocaine on human learning, performance and physiology. *Psychopharmacology*, 102, 451–458.

Higgins, S. T., Budney, A. J., and Bickel, W. K. (1994). Applying behavioral concepts and principles to the treatment of cocaine dependence. *Drug Alcohol Depend.*, 34, 87–97.

Higgins, S. T., Budney, A. J., Bickel, W. K., Badger, G. J., Foerg, F. E., and Ogden, D. (1995). Outpatient behavioral treatment for cocaine dependence: One-year outcome. *Exp. Clin. Psychopharmacol.*, 3, 205–212.

Higgins, S. T., Budney, A. J., Bickel, W. K., Hughes, J. R., Foerg, F., and Badger, G. (1993). Achieving cocaine abstinence with a behavioral approach. *Am. J. Psychiatry*, 150, 763–769.

Higley, J. D., Mehlman, P. T., Taub, D. M., Higley, S. B., Suomi, S. J., Vickers, J. H., and Linnoila, M. (1992). Cerebrospinal fluid monoamine and adrenal correlates of aggression in free-ranging rhesus monkeys. *Arch. Gen. Psychiatry*, 49, 436–441.

Hilakivi, L. A., Hilakivi, I., and Kiianmaa, K. (1987). Neonatal antidepressant administration suppresses concurrent active (REM) sleep and increases adult alcohol consumption in rats. *Alcohol Alcohol.* (Suppl. 1), 339–343.

Hildebrand, J., Bourgeois, F., Buyse, M., Przedborski, S., and Goldman, S. (1990). Reproducibility of monoamine metabolite measurements in human cerebrospinal fluid. *Acta Neurol. Scand.*, 81, 427–430.

Hill, D. R., and Bowery, N. G. (1981). ^{3}H-baclofen and ^{3}H-GABA bind to bicuculline-insensitive $GABA_B$ sites in rat brain. *Nature*, 290, 149–152.

Hill, S. J. (1987). Histamine receptors in the mammalian nervous system: Biochemical studies. *Prog. Med. Chem.*, 24, 29–84.

Hille, B. (1970). Ionic channels in nerve membranes. *Prog. Biophys. Mol. Biol.*, 21, 1–32.

Hille, B. (1992). *Ionic Channels of Excitable Membranes* (2nd ed.). Sinauer Associates, Sunderland, MA.

Hille, B. (1994). Modulation of ion-channel function by G protein-coupled receptors. *Trends Neurosci.*, 17, 531–536.

Hille, B., and Catterall, W. A. (1989). Electrical excitability and ionic channels. In *Basic Neurochemistry* (G. J. Siegel, B. W. Agranoff, R. W. Albers, and P. B. Molinoff, Eds.), pp. 71–90. Raven Press, New York.

Himmelsbach, C. K. (1943). Can the euphoric analgetic and physical dependence effects of drugs be separated? With reference to physical dependence. *Fed. Proc.*, 2, 201–203.

Hindmarch, I. (1984). Psychological performance models as indicators of the effects of hypnotic drugs on sleep. In *Sleep, Benzodiazepines and Performance: Experimental Methodologies and Research Prospects* (I. Hindmarch, H. Ott, and T. Roth, Eds.), pp. 58–68. Springer-Verlag, New York

Hindmarch, I., and Ott, H. (1984). Sleep, benzodiazepines and performance: Issues and comments. In *Sleep, Benzodiazepines and Performance: Experimental Methodologies and Research Prospects* (I. Hindmarch, H. Ott, and T. Roth, Eds.), pp. 194–202. Springer-Verlag, New York.

Hiroi, N., and White, N. M. (1990). The reserpine-sensitive dopamine pool mediates (–)-amphetamine-conditioned reward in the place preference paradigm. *Brain Res.*, 510, 33–42.

Hiroi, N., and White, N. M. (1991). The amphetamine conditioned place preference: Differential involvement of dopamine receptor subtypes and two dopaminergic terminal areas. *Brain Res.*, 552, 141–152.

Hirota, N., Kuraishi, Y., Hino, Y., Sato, Y., Satoh, M., and Takagi, H. (1985). Met-enkephalin and morphine but not dynorphin inhibit noxious stimuli-induced release of substance P from rabbit dorsal horn in situ. *Neuropharmacology*, 24, 567–570.

Hirsch, E., Graybiel, A. M., and Agid, Y. A. (1988). Melanized dopaminergic neurons are differentially susceptible to degeneration in Parkinson's disease. *Nature*, 334, 345–348.

Hjorth, S. (1993). Serotonin 5-HT$_{1A}$ autoreceptor blockade potentiates the ability of the 5-HT reuptake inhibitor citalopram to increase nerve terminal output of 5-HT in vivo: A microdialysis study. *J. Neurochem.*, 60, 776–779.

Hjorth, S., and Tao, R. (1991). The putative 5-HT$_{1B}$ receptor agonist CP-93,129 suppresses rat hippocampal 5-HT release in vivo: Comparison with RU 24969. *Eur. J. Pharmacol.*, 209, 249–252.

Hobson, J. A., Lydic, R., and Baghdoyan, H. A. (1986). Evolving concepts of sleep cycle generation: From brain centers to neuronal populations. *Behav. Brain Sci.*, 9, 371–448.

Hodgkin, A. L. (1964a). *The Conduction of the Nervous Impulse.* Liverpool University Press, Liverpool.

Hodgkin, A. L. (1964b). The ionic basis of nervous conduction. *Science,* 145, 1148–1153.

Hodgkin, A. L., and Huxley, A. F. (1952). A quantitative description of membrane current and its application to conduction and excitation in nerve. *J. Physiol.* (Lond.), 117: 500–544.

Hoebel, B. G., Monaco, A. P., Hernandez, L., Aulisi, E. F., Stanley, B. G., and Lenard, L. (1983). Self-injection of amphetamine directly into the brain. *Psychopharmacology,* 81, 158–163.

Hoehn, M. M., and Yahr, M. D. (1967). Parkinsonism: Onset, progression, and mortality. *Neurology,* 17, 427–442.

Hoffer, A. (1970). Treatment of alcoholism with psychedelic therapy. In *Psychedelics.* (B. Aronson and A. Hoffer, Eds.) pp. 357–366. Anchor/Doubleday, Garden City, New York.

Hoffer, A., and Osmond, H. (1959). The adrenochrome model and schizophrenia. *J. Nerv. Ment. Dis.,* 128, 18–35.

Hoffman, B. J., Mezey, E., and Brownstein, M. J. (1991). Cloning of a serotonin transporter affected by antidepressants. *Science,* 254, 579–580.

Hoffman, D. C. (1989). The use of place conditioning in studying the neuropharmacology of drug reinforcement. *Brain Res. Bull.,* 23, 373–387.

Hoffman, P. L., and Tabakoff, B. (1990). Ethanol and guanine nucleotide binding proteins: A selective interaction. *FASEB J.,* 4, 2612–2622,

Hofmann, A. (1970). The discovery of LSD and subsequent investigations on natural occurring hallucinogens. In *Discoveries in Biological Psychiatry* (F. J. Ayd and B. Blackwell, Eds.), pp. 93–106. Lippincott, Philadelphia.

Hofmann, F. G. (1983). *A Handbook on Drug and Alcohol Abuse,* (2nd ed.). Oxford University Press, New York.

Hogarty, G. E., Goldberg, S. C., and the Collaborative Study Group. (1974). Drug and sociotherapy in the aftercare of schizophrenic patients: One year relapse rates. *Arch. Gen. Psychiatry,* 28, 54–64.

Hökfelt, T. (1991). Neuropeptides in perspective: The last ten years. *Neuron,* 7, 867–879.

Hökfelt, T., Johansson, O., and Goldstein, M. (1984a). Central catecholamine neurons as revealed by immunohistochemistry with special reference to adrenaline neurons. In *Handbook of Chemical Neuroanatomy,* Vol. 2, *Classical Transmitters in the CNS,* Part I (A. Björklund and T. Hökfelt, Eds.), pp. 157–276. Elsevier, Amsterdam.

Hökfelt, T., Johansson, O., and Goldstein, M. (1984b). Chemical anatomy of the brain. *Science,* 225:1326–1334.

Hökfelt, T., Johansson, O., Ljungdahl, Å., Lundberg, J. M., and Schultzberg, M. (1980). Peptidergic neurons. *Nature,* 284, 515–521.

Hökfelt, T., Kellerth, J. O., Nilsson, G., and Pernow, B. (1975a). Experimental immunohistochemical studies on the localization and distribution of substance P in cat primary sensory neurons. *Brain Res.,* 100, 234–252.

Hökfelt, T., Kellerth, J. O., Nilsson, G., and Pernow, B. (1975b). Substance P: Localization

in the central nervous system and in some primary sensory neurons. *Science,* 190, 889–890.

Hökfelt, T., Ljungdahl, A., Fuxe, K., and Johansson, O. (1974c). Dopamine nerve terminals in the rat limbic cortex: Aspects of the dopamine hypothesis of schizophrenia. *Science,* 184, 177–179.

Hökfelt, T., Ljungdahl, A., Terenius, L., Elde, R., and Nilsson, G. (1977). Immunohistochemical analysis of peptide pathways possibly related to pain and analgesia: Enkephalin and substance P. *Proc. Natl. Acad. Sci. U.S.A.,* 74, 3081–3085.

Hökfelt, T., et al. (1985). Distribution of cholecystokinin-like immunoreactivity in the nervous system. Co-existence with classical neurotransmitters and other neuropeptides. *Ann. N.Y. Acad. Sci.,* 448, 255–274.

Hökfelt, T., et al. (1987). Coexistence of peptides with classical neurotransmitters. *Experientia,* 43, 768–780.

Hökfelt, T., et al. (1989). Distribution of TRH-like immunoreactivity with special reference to coexistence with other neuroactive compounds. *Ann. N.Y. Acad. Sci.,* 553, 76–105.

Hokin, M. R., and Hokin, L. E. (1953). Enzyme secretion and the incorporation of P^{32} into phospholipides of pancreas slices. *J. Biol. Chem.,* 203, 967–977.

Holden, C. (1989). Flipping the main switch in the central reward system. *Science,* 246, 1378–179.

Holden, C. (1991). Probing the complex genetics of alcoholism. *Science,* 251, 163–164.

Holladay, M. W., Lebold, S. A., and Lin, N.-H. (1995). Structure-activity relationships of nicotinic acetylcholine receptor agonists as potential treatments for dementia. *Drug Dev. Res.,* 35, 191–213.

Hollander, E., DeCaria, C. M., Nitescu, A., Gully, R., Suckow, R. F., Cooper, T. B., Gorman, J. M., Klein, D. F., and Liebowitz, M. R. (1992). Serotonergic function in obsessive–compulsive disorder: Behavioral and neuroendocrine responses to oral *m*-chlorophenylpiperazine and fenfluramine in patients and healthy volunteers. *Arch. Gen. Psychiatry,* 49, 21–28.

Hollister, L. E. (1974). Structure-activity relationships in man of cannabis constituents, and homologs and metabolites of Δ^9-tetrahydrocanabinol. *Pharmacology,* 11, 3–11.

Hollister, L. E. (1978). Psychotomimetic drugs in man. In *Handbook of Psychopharmacology,* Vol. 11 (L. L. Iversen, S. D. Iversen, and S. H. Snyder, Eds.), pp. 389–424. Plenum Press, New York.

Hollister, L. E. (1986). Health aspects of cannabis. *Pharmacol. Rev.,* 38, 1–20.

Hollmann, M., Hartley, M., and Heinemann, S. (1991). Ca^{2+} permeability of KA-AMPA-gated glutamate receptor channels depends on subunit composition. *Science,* 252, 851–853.

Hollmann, M., and Heinemann, S. (1994). Cloned glutamate receptors. *Annu. Rev. Neurosci.,* 17, 31–108.

Hollmann, M., Maron, C., and Heinemann, S. (1994). N-Glycosylation site tagging suggests a three transmembrane domain topology for the glutamate receptor GluR1. *Neuron,* 13, 1331–1343.

Hollt, V. (1993). Regulation of opioid peptide gene expression. In *Opioids I,* Handbook of

Experimental Pharmacology, Vol. 104 (A. Herz, Ed.), pp. 307–346. Springer-Verlag, New York.

Holmsen, H. (1985). Platelet activation and serotonin. In *Serotonin and the Cardiovascular System* (P. M. Vanhoutte, Ed.), pp. 75–86. Raven Press, New York.

Holsboer, F. (1995). Neuroendocrinology of mood disorders. In *Psychopharmacology: The Fourth Generation of Progress* (F. E. Bloom and D. J. Kupfer, Eds.), pp. 957–970. Raven Press, New York.

Holt, J., Antin, J., Gibbs, J., Young, R. C., and Smith, G. P. (1974). Cholecystokinin does not produce bait shyness in rats. *Physiol. Behav.,* 12, 497–498.

Holtz, P. (1950). Ueber die sympathicomimetische Wirksamkeit von Gehirnextrackten. *Acta Physiol. Scand.,* 20, 354–362.

Holtzman, E. J., Haris, H. W. Jr., Kolakowski, L. F. Jr., Guay-Woodford, L. M., Botelho, B., and Ausiello, D. A. (1993). A molecular defect in the vasopressin V2-receptor gene causing nephrogenic diabetes insipidus. *N. Engl. J. Med.,* 328, 1534–1537.

Holtzman, S. G., Mante, S., and Minneman, K. P. (1991). Role of adenosine receptors in caffeine tolerance. *J. Pharmacol. Exp. Ther.,* 256, 62–68.

Holzer, P. (1988). Local effector functions of capsaicin-sensitive sensory nerve endings: Involvement of tachykinins, calcitonin gene-related peptide and other neuropeptides. *Neuroscience,* 24, 739–768.

Holzer, P. (1991). Capsaicin: Cellular targets, mechanisms of action, and selectivity for thin sensory neurons. *Pharmacol. Rev.,* 43, 143–201.

Holzman, P. S. (1987). Recent studies of psychophysiology in schizophrenia. *Schizophr. Bull.,* 13, 65–92.

Holzwarth, M. A., and Brownfield, M. S. (1985). Serotonin coexists with epinephrine in rat adrenal medullary cells. *Neuroendocrinology,* 41, 230–236.

Hommer, D. W., Skolnick, P., and Paul, S. M. (1987). The benzodiazepine/GABA receptor complex and anxiety. In *Psychopharmacology: The Third Generation of Progress* (H. Y. Meltzer, Ed.), pp. 977–983. Raven Press, New York.

Hong, M., Jenner, P., and Marsden, C. D. (1987). Comparison of the acute actions of amine-depleting drugs and dopamine receptor antagonists on dopamine function in the brain in rats. *Neuropharmacology,* 26, 237–245.

Hooker, W. D., and Jones, J. T. (1987). Increased susceptibility to memory intrusions and the Stroop interference effect during acute marijuana intoxication. *Psychopharmacology,* 91, 20–24.

Horger, B. A., Shelton, K., and Schenk, S. (1990). Preexposure sensitizes rats to the rewarding effects of cocaine. *Pharmacol. Biochem. Behav.,* 37, 707–711.

Horn, A. S. (1990). Dopamine uptake: A review of progress in the last decade. *Prog. Neurobiol.,* 34, 387–400.

Horn, J. P. (1992). The heroic age of neurophysiology. *Hosp. Pract.,* July, 65–74.

Hornykiewicz, O. (1973). Metabolism of dopamine and L-DOPA in human brain. In *Frontiers in Catecholamine Research* (E. Usdin and S. H. Snyder, Eds.), pp. 1101–1107. Pergamon Press, New York.

Hornykiewicz, O. (1974). The mechanisms of action of L-dopamine in Parkinson's disease. *Life Sci.*, 15, 1249–1259.

Hornykiewicz, O., and Pifl, C. (1994). The validity of the MPTP primate model for the neurochemical pathology of idiopathic Parkinson's disease. In *Noradrenergic Mechanisms in Parkinson's Disease* (M. Briley and M. Marien, Eds.), pp. 11–23. CRC Press, Boca Raton.

Horwitz, B., Soncrant, T., and Rapoport, S. (1986). New approach to the examination of data derived with PET. In *PET and NMR: New Perspectives in Neuroimaging and in Clinical Neurochemistry* (L. Battistin and F. Gerstenbrand, Eds.), pp. 151–171. Alan R. Liss, New York.

Hosey, M. M. (1992). Diversity of structure, signaling and regulation within the family of muscarinic cholinergic receptors. *FASEB J.*, 6, 845–852.

Hotchkiss, A. J., and Gibb, J. W. (1980). Long-term effects of multiple doses of methamphetamine on tryptophan hydroxylase and tyrosine hydroxylase activity in rat brain. *J. Pharmacol. Exp. Ther.*, 214, 257–262.

Hotchkiss, A. J., Morgan, M. E., and Gibb, J. W. (1979). The long-term effects of multiple doses of methamphetamine on neostriatal tryptophan hydroxylase, tyrosine hydroxylase, choline acetyltransferase and glutamate decarboxylase activities. *Life Sci.*, 25, 1373–1378.

Hotta, I., and Yamawaki, S. (1986). Lithium decreases 5-HT$_1$ receptors but increases 5-HT-sensitive adenylate cyclase activity in rat hippocampus. *Biol. Psychiatry*, 21, 1382–1390.

Hotta, I., and Yamawaki, S. (1988). Possible involvement of presynaptic 5-HT autoreceptors in effect of lithium on 5-HT release in hippocampus of rat. *Neuropharmacology*, 27, 987–992.

Hough, L. B. (1988). Cellular localization and possible functions for brain histamine: Recent progress. *Prog. Neurobiol.*, 30, 469–505.

Hourani, S. M. O., and Cusack, N. J. (1991). Pharmacological receptors on blood platelets. *Pharmacol. Rev.*, 43, 243–298.

Houser, C. R. (1991). GABA neurons in seizure disorders: A review of immunocytochemical studies. *Neurochem. Res.*, 16, 295–308.

Howard, J. L., and Pollard, G. T. (1990). Effects of buspirone in the Geller–Seifter conflict test with incremental shock. *Drug Dev. Res.*, 19, 37–49.

Howell, L. L., and Byrd, L. D. (1991). Characterization of the effects of cocaine and GBR 12909, a dopamine uptake inhibitor, on behavior in the squirrel monkey. *J. Pharmacol. Exp. Ther.*, 258, 178–185.

Howlett, A. C. (1995). Pharmacology of cannabinoid receptors. *Annu. Rev. Pharmacol. Toxicol.*, 35, 607–634.

Howlett, A. C., Bidaut-Russell, M., Devane, W. A., Melvin, L. S., Johnson, M. R., and Herkenham, M. (1990). The cannabinoid receptor: Biochemical, anatomical and behavioral characterization. *Trends Neurosci.*, 13, 420–423.

Hoyer, D. (1990). Serotonin 5-HT$_3$, 5-HT$_4$, and 5-HT-M receptors. *Neuropsychopharmacology*, 3, 371–383.

Hoyer, D., Clarke, D. E., Fozard, J. R., Hartig, P. R., Martin, G. R., Mylecharane, E. J., Saxena, P. R., and Humphrey, P. P. A. (1994). VII. International Union of Pharmacology classification of receptors for 5-hydroxytryptamine (serotonin). *Pharmacol. Rev.*, 46, 157–203.

Hoyer, D., and Schoeffter, P. (1991). 5-HT receptors: Subtypes and second messengers. *J. Recept. Res.*, 11, 197–214.

Hrdina, P. D. (1986). Binding sites for antidepressants. In *Neuromethods,* Vol. 4. *Receptor Binding* (A. A. Boulton, G. B. Baker, and P. D. Hrdina, Eds.), pp. 455–498. Humana Press, Clifton, NJ.

Hu, X.-T., and Wang, R. Y. (1988). Comparison of effects of D-1 and D-2 dopamine receptor agonists on neurons in the rat caudate putamen: An electrophysiological study. *J. Neurosci.*, 8, 4340–4348.

Hu, X-T., and Wang, R. Y. (1989). Haloperidol and clozapine: Differential effects on the sensitivity of caudate-putamen neurons to dopamine agonists and cholecystokinin following one-month continuous treatment. *Brain Res.*, 486, 325–333.

Huang, J.-T., and Ho, B. T. (1974). Discriminative stimulus properties of d-amphetamine and related compounds in rats. *Pharmacol. Biochem. Behav.*, 2, 669–673.

Huang, K.-P., and Huang, F. L. (1993). How is protein kinase C activated in CNS? *Neurochem. Int.*, 22, 417–433.

Hubner, C. B., and Koob, G. F. (1987). Ventral pallidal lesions produce decreases in cocaine and heroin self-administration in the rat. *Proc. Soc. Neurosci.*, 13, 1717.

Hubner, C. B., and Moreton, J. E. (1991). Effects of selective D1 and D2 dopamine antagonists on cocaine self-administration in the rat. *Psychopharmacology*, 105, 151–156.

Hudson, C. J., Young, L. T., Li, P. P., and Warsh, J. J. (1993). CNS signal transduction in the pathophysiology and pharmacotherapy of affective disorders and schizophrenia. *Synapse*, 13, 278–293.

Hughes, J. (1975). Search for the endogenous ligand of the opiate receptor. *Neurosci. Res. Prog. Bull.*, 13, 55–58.

Hughes, J., Boden, P., Costall, B., Domeney, A., Kelly, E., Horwell, D. C., Hunter, J. C., Pinnock, R. D., and Woodruff, G. N. (1990). Development of a class of selective cholecystokinin type B receptor antagonists having potent anxiolytic activity. *Proc. Natl. Acad. Sci. U.S.A.*, 87, 6728–6732.

Hughes, J., Smith, T. W., Kosterlitz, H. W., Fothergill, L. A., Morgan, B. A., and Morris, H. R. (1975). Identification of two related pentapeptides from the brain with potent opiate agonist activity. *Nature*, 258, 577–579.

Hughes, J., Smith, T., Morgan, B., and Fothergill, L. (1975). Purification and properties of enkephalin: The possible endogenous ligand for the morphine receptor. *Life Sci.*, 16, 1753–1758.

Hughes, J. R., Gust, S. W., Skog, K., and Fenwick, J. W. (1991). Symptoms of tobacco withdrawal. *Arch. Gen. Psychiary*, 48, 52–59.

Hughes, J. R., Hatsukami, D. K., Pickens, R. W., Krahn, D., Malin, S., and Luknic, A. (1984). Effect of nicotine on tobacco withdrawal syndrome. *Psychopharmacology*, 83, 82–87.

Hughes, J. R., Higgins, S. T., Bickel, W. K., Hunt, W. K., Fenwick, J. W., Gulliver, S. B., and Mireault, G. C. (1991). Caffeine self-administration, withdrawal, and adverse effects among coffee drinkers. *Arch. Gen. Psychiatry*, 48, 611–617.

Hulme, E. C., Birdsall, N. J. M., and Buckley, N. J. (1990). Muscarinic receptor subtypes. *Annu. Rev. Pharmacol. Toxicol.*, 30, 633–673.

Hume, R. I., Dingledine, R., and Heinemann, S. F. (1991). Identification of a site in glutamate receptor subunits that controls calcium permeability. *Science*, 253, 1028–1031.

Humphrey, P. P. A., and Feniuk, W. (1991). Mode of action of the anti-migraine drug sumatriptan. *Trends Pharmacol. Sci.*, 12, 444–446.

Humphrey, P. P. A., Hartig, P., and Hoyer, D. (1993). A proposed new nomenclature for 5-HT receptors. *Trends Pharmacol. Sci.*, 14, 233–236.

Hunt, G. M., and Azrin, N. H. (1973). A community-reinforcement approach to alcoholism. *Behav. Res. Ther.*, 11, 91–104.

Hunter, A. E., et al. (1991). Granisetron, a selective 5-H$_3$ receptor antagonist, for the prevention of radiation induced emesis during total body irradiation. *Bone Marrow Transpl.*, 7, 439–441.

Hunter, W. S. (1913). The delayed reaction in animals and children. *Behav. Monogr.*, 2, 1–86.

Hurd, Y. L., and Herkenham, M. (1992). Influence of a single injection of cocaine, amphetamine or GBR 12909 on mRNA expression of striatal neuropeptides. *Mol. Brain Res.*, 16, 97–104.

Hurd, Y. L., and Herkenham, M. (1993). Molecular alterations in the neostriatum of human cocaine addicts. *Synapse*, 13, 357–369.

Hurd, Y. L., Kehr, J., and Ungerstedt, U. (1988). In vivo microdialysis as a technique to monitor drug transport: Correlation of extracellular cocaine levels and dopamine overflow in the rat brain. *J. Neurochem.*, 51, 1314–1316.

Huszti, Z. (1990). Histamine inactivation in the brain: Aspects of N-methylation. *J. Neural. Transm.*, 29 (Suppl.), 107–118.

Hutchings, D. E. (1993). The puzzle of cocaine's effects following maternal use during pregnancy: Are there reconcilable differences? *Neurotoxicol. Teratol.*, 15, 281–286.

Hutson, P. H., Donohoe, T. P., and Curzon, G. (1988). Infusion of the 5-hydroxytryptamine agonists RU24969 and TFMPP into the paraventricular nucleus of the hypothalamus causes hypophagia. *Psychopharmacology*, 95, 550–552.

Huttner, W. B. (1993). Snappy exocytoxins. *Nature*, 365, 104–105.

Hutton, J. T., and Morris, J. L. (1994). Therapeutic advantages of sustained release levodopa formulations in Parkinson's disease. *CNS Drugs*, 2, 110–119.

Hyman, S. E., and Nestler, E. J. (1993). *The Molecular Foundations of Psychiatry*. American Psychiatric Press, Washington, D.C.

Hyttel, J. (1983). SCH 23390: The first selective dopamine D-1 antagonist. *Eur. J. Pharmacol.*, 91, 153–154.

Icard-Liepkalns, C., Biguet, N. F., Vyas, S., Robert, J. J., Sassone-Corsi, P., and Mallet, J. (1992). AP-1 complex and c-*fos* transcription are involved in TPA provoked and transsynaptic inductions of the tyrosine hydroxylase gene: Insights into long-term regulatory mechanisms. *J. Neurosci. Res.*, 32, 290–298.

Ichimura, T., Isobe, T., Okuyama, T., Yamauchi, T., and Fujisawa, H. (1987). Brain 14–3–3 protein is an activator protein that activates tryptophan 5-monooxygenase and tyrosine 3-monooxygenase in the presence of Ca^{2+} calmodulin-dependent protein kinase II. *FEBS Lett.*, 219, 79–82.

Illes, P. (1989). Modulation of transmitter and hormone release by multiple neuronal opioid receptors. *Rev. Physiol. Biochem. Pharmacol.*, 112, 139–233.

Imeri, L., Bianchi, S., Angeli, P., and Mancia, M. (1994). Selective blockade of different brain stem muscarinic receptor subtypes: Effects on the sleep–wake cycle. *Brain Res.*, 636, 68–72.

Imperato, A., Honoré, T., and Jensen, L. H. (1990). Dopamine release in the nucleus caudatus and in the nucleus accumbens is under glutamatergic control through non-NMDA receptors: A study in freely-moving rats. *Brain Res.*, 530, 223–228.

Inada, T., Polk, K., Purser, C., Hume, A., Hoskins, B., Ho, I. K., and Rockhold, R. W. (1992). Behavioral and neurochemical effects of continuous infusion of cocaine in rats. *Neuropharmacology*, 31, 701–708.

Ingram, S. M., Krause, R. G. II, Baldino, F. Jr., Skeen, L. C., and Lewis, M. E. (1989). Neuronal localization of cholecystokinin mRNA in the rat brain by using in situ hybridization histochemistry. *J. Comp. Neurol.*, 287, 260–272.

Innis, R. B., Andrade, R., and Aghajanian, G. K. (1985). Substance K excites dopaminergic and non-dopaminergic neurons in rat substantia nigra. *Brain Res.*, 335, 381–383.

Innis, R. B., and Snyder, S. H. (1980). Distinct cholecystokinin receptors in brain and pancreas. *Proc. Natl. Acad. Sci. U.S.A.*, 77, 6917–6921.

Insel, T. R. (1988). Obsessive–compulsive disorder: A neuroethological perspective. *Psychopharmacol. Bull.*, 24, 365–369.

Insel, T. R. (1990). Oxytocin and maternal behavior. In *Mammalian Parenting: Biochemical, Neurobiological, and Behavioral Determinants* (N. A. Krasnegor and R. S. Bridges, Eds.), pp. 260–280. Oxford University Press, New York.

Insel, T. R. (1992a). Neurobiology of obsessive compulsive disorder: A review. *Int. Clin. Psychopharmacol.*, 7 (Suppl. 1), 31–33.

Insel, T. R. (1992b). Oxytocin: A neuropeptide for affiliation: Evidence from behavioral, receptor autoradiographic, and comparative studies. *Psychoneuroendocrinology*, 17, 3–35.

Insel, T. R., Battaglia, G., Johannessen, J. N., Marra, S., and De Souza, E. B. (1989). 3,4-methylenedioxymethamphetamine ("Ecstasy") selectively destroys brain serotonin terminals in rhesus monkeys. *J. Pharmacol. Exp. Ther.*, 249, 713–720.

Insel, T. R., Hill, J. L., and Mayor, R. B. (1986). Rat pup ultrasonic isolation calls: Possible mediation by the benzodiazepine receptor complex. *Pharmacol. Biochem. Behav.*, 24, 1263–1267.

Insel, T. R., Ninan, P. T., Aloi, J., Jimerson, D. C., Skolnick, P., and Paul, S. M. (1984). A benzodiazepine receptor-mediated model of anxiety. *Arch. Gen. Psychiatry*, 41, 741–750.

Insel, T. R., and Shapiro, L. E. (1992). Oxytocin receptor distribution reflects social organization in monogamous and polygamous voles. *Proc. Natl. Acad. Sci. U.S.A.*, 89, 5981–5985.

Insel, T. R., Wang, Z.-X., and Ferris, C. F. (1994). Patterns of brain vasopressin receptor distribution associated with social organization in microtine rodents. *J. Neurosci.*, 14, 5381–5392.

Invernizzi, R., Carli, M., Clemente, A. D., and Samanin, R. (1991). Administration of 8-hydroxy-2-(Di-*n*-propylamino)tetralin in raphe nuclei dorsalis and medianus reduces serotonin synthesis in the rat brain: Differences in potency and regional sensitivity. *J. Neurochem.*, 56, 243–247.

Irwin, M., Vale, W., and Rivier, C. (1990). Central corticotropin-releasing factor mediates the suppressive effect of stress on natural killer cytotoxicity. *Endocrinology*, 126, 2837–2844.

Isbell, H. (1950). Addiction to barbiturates and barbiturate abstinence syndrome. *Ann. Intern. Med.*, 33, 108–121.

Isbell, H., Altschul, S., Kornetsky, C. H., Eisenman, A. J., Flanary, H. G., and Fraser, H. F. (1950). Chronic barbiturate intoxication. *Arch. Neurol. Psychiatry*, 64, 1–28.

Isbell, H., Gorodetzsky, C. W., Jasinski, D., Claussen, U., v. Spulak, F., and Korte, F. (1967). Effects of (-)Δ⁹-trans-tetrahydrocannabinol in man. *Psychopharmacologia*, 11, 184–188.

Isbell, H., Miner, E. J., and Logan, C. R. (1959). Cross tolerance between *d*-2 brom-lysergic acid diethylamide (BOL-148) and *d*-diethylamide of lysergic acid (LSD-25). *Psychopharmacologia*, 1, 109–116.

Isbell, H., Wolbach, A. B., and Miner, E. J. (1961). Cross tolerance between LSD and psilocybin. *Psychopharmacologia*, 2, 147–159.

Isbell, H., Wolbach, A., and Rosenberg, D. (1962). Observations on direct and cross tolerance with LSD and dextroamphetamine in man. *Fed. Proc.*, 2, 416.

Isenschmid, D. S., Fischman, M. W., Foltin, R. W., and Caplan, Y. H. (1992). Concentration of cocaine and metabolites in plasma of humans following intravenous administration and smoking of cocaine. *J. Anal. Toxicol.*, 16, 311–314.

Israel, Y., and Mardones, J. (1971). *Biological Basis of Alcoholism*. Wiley, New York.

Itoh, S., and Lal, H. (1990). Influences of cholecystokinin and analogues on memory processes. *Drug Dev. Res.*, 21, 257–276.

Itoh, Y., Oishi, R., Nishibori, M., and Saeki, K. (1991). Characterization of histamine release from the rat hypothalamus as measured by in vivo microdialysis. *J. Neurochem.*, 56, 769–774.

Iversen, L. L. (1974). Uptake mechanisms for neurotransmitter amines. *Biochem. Pharmacol.*, 23, 1927–1935.

Iversen, L. L. (1975a). Dopamine receptors in the brain. *Science*, 188, 1084–1089.

Iversen, L. L. (1975b). Uptake processes for biogenic amines. In *Handbook of Psychopharmacology*, Vol. 3 (L. L. Iversen, S. D. Iversen, and S. H. Snyder, Eds.), pp. 381–442. Plenum Press, New York.

Iversen, L. L. (1979). The chemistry of the brain. *Sci. Am.*, 241 (3), 134–149.

Ivy, A. C., and Oldberg, E. A. (1928). A hormone mechanism for gallbladder contraction and evacuation. *Am. J. Physiol.*, 86, 599–613.

Ivy, M. T., and Carroll, P. T. (1988). Evidence to suggest that the spontaneous release of acetylcholine from rat hippocampal tissue is carrier-mediated. *Neurochem. Res.*, 13, 325–328.

Iyengar, R. (1993). Molecular and functional diversity of mammalian G_s-stimulated adenylyl cyclases. *FASEB J.*, 7, 768–775.

Izquierdo, I., and Medina, J. H. (1991). GABA$_A$ receptor modulation of memory: The role of endogenous benzodiazepines. *Trends Pharmacol. Sci.*, 12, 260–263.

Izzo, J. L. Jr., Horwitz, D., and Keiser, H. R. (1979). Reduction in human urinary MHPG excretion by guanethidine: Urinary MHPG as index of sympathetic nervous activity. *Life Sci.*, 24, 1403–1406.

Jackson, A., and Sanger, D. J. (1988). Is the discriminative stimulus produced by phencyclidine due to an interaction with N-methyl-D-aspartate receptors? *Psychopharmacology*, 96, 87–92.

Jackson, D. M., and Westlind-Danielsson, A. (1994). Dopamine receptors: Molecular biology, biochemistry and behavioural aspects. *Pharmacol. Ther.*, 64, 291–369.

Jacobs, B. L. (1976). An animal behavior model for studying central serotonergic synapses. *Life Sci.*, 19, 777–786.

Jacobs, B. L. (1987). How hallucinogenic drugs work. *Am. Sci.*, 75, 386–392.

Jacobs, B. L., and Azmitia, E. C. (1992). Structure and function of the brain serotonin system. *Physiol. Rev.*, 72, 165–229.

Jacobs, B. L., and Fornal, C. A. (1993). 5-HT and motor control: A hypothesis. *Trends Neurosci.*, 16, 346–352.

Jacobs, B. L., Wilkinson, L. O., and Fornal, C. A. (1990). The role of brain serotonin: A neurophysiologic perspective. *Neuropsychopharmacology*, 3, 473–479.

Jacobs, S., and Cuatrecasas, P. (1983). Insulin receptors. *Annu. Rev. Pharmacol. Toxicol.*, 23, 461–479.

Jacobson, R. (1986). The contribution of sex and drinking history to CT scan changes in alcoholics. *Psychol. Med.*, 16, 547–599.

Jacobson, S. (1972). Neurocytology. In *An Introduction to the Neurosciences* (B. A. Curtis, S. Jacobson, and E. M. Marcus, Eds.), pp. 36–71. Saunders, Philadelphia.

Jacquet, Y. F., and Marks, N. (1976). The C-fragment of β-lipotropin: An endogenous neuroleptic or antipsychotogen? *Science*, 194, 632–635.

Jacquet, Y. F., Marks, N., and Li, C. H. (1976). Behavioral and biochemical properties of "opioid" peptides. In *Opiates and Endogenous Opiate Peptides* (H. Kosterlitz, Ed.), pp. 411–414. Elsevier/North-Holland, Amsterdam.

Jaeger, C. B., Ruggiero, D. A., Albert, V. R., Joh, T. H., and Reis, D. J. (1984). Immunocytochemical localization of aromatic-L-amino acid decarboxylase. In *Handbook of Chemical Neuroanatomy*, Vol. 2 (A. Björklund and T. Hökfelt, Eds.), pp. 387–408. Elsevier, Amsterdam.

Jaeger, C. B., Ruggiero, D. A., Albert, V. R., Park, D. H., Joh, T. H., and Reis, D. J. (1984). Aromatic L-amino acid decarboxylase in the rat brain: Immunocytochemical localization in neurons of the brain stem. *Neuroscience*, 11, 691–713.

Jaffe, J. H. (1975). Drug addiction and drug abuse. In *The Pharmacological Basis of Therapeutics* (5th ed.) (L. S. Goodman and A. Gilman, Eds.), pp. 284–324. Macmillan, New York.

Jaffe, J. H. (1985). Drug addiction and drug abuse. In *The Pharmacological Basis of Thera-*

peutics (A. G. Gilman, L. S. Goodman, T. W. Rall and F. Murad, Eds.), pp. 532–581, Macmillan, New York.

Jaffe, J. H. (1987). Pharmacologic agents in treatment of drug dependence. In *Psychopharmacology: The Third Generation of Progress* (H. Y. Meltzer, Ed.), pp. 1605–1616, Raven Press, New York.

Jaffe, J. H., and Jarvik, M. E. (1978). Tobacco use and tobacco use disorder. In *Psychopharmacology: A Generation of Progress* (M. A.Lipton, A. DiMascio, and K. F. Killam, Eds.), pp. 1665–1676. Raven Press, New York.

Jaim-Etcheverry, G., and Zieher, L. M. (1980). DSP 4: A novel compound with neurotoxic effects on noradrenergic neurons of adult and developing rats. *Brain Res.*, 188, 513–523.

JAMA Editorial: (1995). The Brown and Williamson Documents: Where do we go from here? *JAMA*, 274, 3, 256–258.

James, J. E. (1994a). Chronic effects of habitual caffeine consumption on laboratory and ambulatory blood pressure levels. *J. Cardiovasc. Risk*, 1, 159–164.

James, J. E. (1994b). Does caffeine enhance or merely restore degraded psychomotor performance? *Neuropsychobiology*, 30, 124–125.

James, S. P., and Amsterdam, J. D. (1990). Sleep and affective disorders. In *Pharmacotherapy of Depression* (J. D. Amsterdam, Ed.), pp. 427–440. Marcel Dekker, New York.

Jan, L. Y., and Jan, Y. N. (1994). Potassium channels and their evolving gates. *Nature*, 371, 119–122.

Jan, Y. N., and Jan, L. Y. (1983). A LHRH-like peptidergic neurotransmitter capable of "action at a distance" in autonomic ganglia. *Trends Neurosci.*, 6, 320–325.

Janowsky, D. S., and Davis, J. M. (1976). Methylphenidate, dextroamphetamine, levoamphetamine effects on schizophrenic symptoms. *Arch. Gen. Psychiatry*, 33, 304–308.

Janowsky, D. S., Khaled, M. K., and Davis, J. M. (1974). Acetylcholine and depression. *Psychosomatic Med.*, 36, 248–257.

Janowsky, D. S., and Overstreet, D. H. (1995). The role of acetylcholine mechanisms in mood disorders. In *Psychopharmacology: The Fourth Generation of Progress* (F. E. Bloom and D. J. Kupfer, Eds.), pp. 945–956. Raven Press, New York.

Janowsky, D. S., and Risch, S. C. (1984). Cholinomimetic and anticholinergic drugs used to investigate an acetylcholine hypothesis of affective disorders and stress. *Drug Dev. Res.*, 4, 125–142.

Jarvik, M. E. (1970). Drugs used in the treatment of psychiatric disorders. In *The Pharmacological Basis of Therapeutics* (L. S. Goodman and A. Gilman, Eds.), pp. 151–203. Macmillan, New York.

Jarvik, M. E. (1979). Biological influences on cigarette smoking. *NIDA Res. Monogr.*, 26, 7–46.

Jarvis, M. F., Murphy, D. E., and Williams, M. (1987). Quantitative autoradiographic localization of NMDA receptors in rat brain using [³H]CPP: Comparison with [³H]TCP binding sites. *Eur. J. Pharmacol.*, 141, 149–152.

Jarvis, M. F., and Williams, M. (1989). Direct autoradiographic localization of adenosine A_2 receptors in the rat brain using the A_2-selective agonist, [³H]CGS 21680. *Eur. J. Pharmacol.*, 168, 243–246.

Jarvis, M. J. (1993). Does caffeine intake enhance absolute levels of cognitive performance? *Psychopharmacology*, 110, 45–52.

Jasper, H. H., Proctor, L. D., Knighton, R. S., Noshay, W. C., and Costello, R. T. (Eds.). (1958). *Reticular Formation of the Brain*. Little, Brown, Boston.

Jatlow, P. (1988). Cocaine: Analysis, pharmacokinetics, and metabolic disposition. *Yale J. Biol. Med.*, 61, 105–113.

Javitch, J. A., D'Amato, R. J., Strittmatter, S. M., and Snyder, S. H. (1985). Parkinsonism-inducing neurotoxin, *N*-methyl-4-phenyl-1,2,3,6-tetrahydropyridine: Uptake of the metabolite *N*-methyl-4-phenylpyridine by dopamine neurons explains selective toxicity. *Proc. Natl. Acad. Sci. U.S.A.*, 82, 2173–2177.

Javitt, D. C., and Zukin, S. R. (1991). Recent advances in the phencyclidine model of schizophrenia. *Am. J. Psychiatry*, 148, 1301–1308.

Javoy, F., and Glowinski, J. (1971). Dynamic characteristics of the "functional compartment" of dopamine in dopaminergic terminals of the rat striatum. *J. Neurochem.*, 18, 1305–1311.

Jefferson, J. W., and Greist, J. H. (1990). The clinical application of lithium. In *Pharmacotherapy of Depression* (J. D. Amsterdam, Ed.), pp. 111–127. Marcel Dekker, New York.

Jellinek, E.M. (1960). *The Disease Concept of Alcoholism*. Hillhouse Press, New York

Jellinger, K. (1987). The pathology of parkinsonism. In *Movement Disorders 2* (C. D. Marsden and S. Fahn, Eds.), pp. 124–165. Butterworths, London.

Jellinger, K. (1990). New developments in the pathology of Parkinson's disease. *Adv. Neurol.*, 53, 1–16.

Jenck, F., Quirion, R., and Wise, R. A. (1987). Opioid receptor subtypes associated with ventral tegmental facilitation and periaqueductal gray inhibition of feeding. *Brain Res.*, 423, 39–44.

Jenner, P., Dexter, D. T., Sian, J., Schapira, A. H. V., and Marsden, C. D. (1992). Oxidative stress as a cause of nigral cell death in Parkinson's disease and incidental Lewy body disease. *Ann. Neurol.*, 32, S82–S87.

Jenner, P., Rupniak, N. M. J., and Marsden, D. C. (1985). In *Dyskinesias: Research and Treatment* (D.E Casey, T. N. Chase, A. V. Christensen, and J. Gerlach, Eds.), pp. 174–181. Springer-Verlag, New york.

Jennissen, H. P. (1995). Ubiquitin and the enigma of intracellular protein degradation. *Eur. J. Biochem.*, 231, 1–30.

Jensen, T. S., and Yaksh, T. L. (1986). Examination of spinal monoamine receptors through which brainstem opiate-sensitive systems act in the rat. *Brain Res.*, 363, 114–127.

Jessell, T. M. (1991). Cell migration and axon guidance. In *Principles of Neural Science* (3rd ed.) (E. R. Kandel, J. H. Schwartz, and T. M. Jessell, Eds.), pp. 908–928. Elsevier, New York.

Jessell, T. M., and Iversen, L. L. (1977). Opiate analgesics inhibit substance P release from rat trigeminal nucleus. *Nature*, 268, 549–551.

Jessell, T. M., and Kelly, D. D. (1991). Pain and analgesia. In *Principles of Neural Science* (3rd ed.) (E. R. Kandel, J. H. Schwartz and T. M. Jessell, Eds.), pp. 385–399. Elsevier, New York.

Jeste, D. V., and Wyatt, R. J. (1982). Therapeutic strategies against tardive dyskinesia. *Arch. Gen. Psychiatry*, 39, 803–816.

Jiang, Q., Mosberg, H. I., and Porreca, F. (1990). Selective modulation of morphine antinociceptive potency, but not development of tolerance, by delta agonists in the mouse. *J. Pharmacol. Exp. Ther.*, 254, 683–689.

Jimerson, D. C. (1987). Role of dopamine mechanisms in the affective disorders. In *Psychopharmacology: The Third Generation of Progress* (H. Y. Meltzer, Ed.), pp. 505–511. Raven Press, New York.

Joh, T. H., Geghman, C., and Reis, D. (1973). Immunochemical demonstration of increased accumulation of tyrosine hydroxylase protein in sympathetic ganglia and adrenal medulla elicited by reserpine. *Proc. Natl. Acad. Sci. U.S.A.*, 70, 2767–2771.

Joh, T. H., Park, D. H., and Reis, D. J. (1978). Direct phosphorylation of brain tyrosine hydroxylase by cyclic AMP-dependent protein kinase: Mechanism of enzyme activation. *Proc. Natl. Acad. Sci. U.S.A.*, 75, 4744–4748.

Johannessen, J. N., Chiueh, C. C., Burns, R. S., and Markey, S. P. (1985). Differences in the metabolism of MPTP in the rodent and primate parallel differences in sensitivity to its neurotoxic effect. *Life Sci.*, 36, 219–224.

Johanning, H., Plenge, P., and Mellerup, E. (1992). Serotonin receptors in the brain of rats treated chronically with imipramine or RU24969: Support for the 5-HT$_{1B}$ receptor being a 5-HT autoreceptor. *Pharmacol. Toxicol.*, 70, 131–134.

Johannson, O., and Lundberg, J. M. (1982). Ultrastructural localization of vasoactive intestinal polypeptide-like immunoreactivity in large dense-core vesicles of "cholinergic type" nerve terminals in cat exocrine glands. *Neuroscience*, 6, 847.

Johansen, P. A., Hu, X.-T., and White, F. J. (1991). Relationship between D_1 dopamine receptors, adenylate cyclase, and the electrophysiological responses of rat accumbens neurons. *J. Neural Transm.*, 86, 97–113.

Johanson, C. E., Balster, R. L., and Bonese, K. (1976). Self-administration of psychomotor stimulant drugs: The effects of unlimited access. *Pharmacol. Biochem. Behav.*, 4, 45–51.

Johanson, C. E., and Fischman, M. W. (1989). The pharmacology of cocaine related to its abuse. *Pharmacol. Rev.*, 41, 3–52.

Johanson, C. E., and Uhlenhuth, E. H. (1980). Drug preference and mood in humans: *d*-amphetamine. *Psychopharmacology*, 71, 275–279.

Johanson, C. E., Woolverton, W. L., and Schuster, C. R. (1987). Evaluating laboratory models of drug dependence. In *Psychopharmacology: The Third Generation of Progress* (H. Y. Meltzer, Ed.), pp. 1617–1625. Raven Press, New York.

Johansson, B., Ahlberg, S., van der Ploeg, I., Brené, S., Lindefors, N., Persson, H., and Fredholm, B. B. (1993). Effect of long term caffeine treatment on A_1 and A_2 adenosine receptor binding and on mRNA levels in rat brain. *Naunyn Schmiedebergs Arch. Pharmacol.*, 347, 407–414.

Johansson, E. K., Tucker, S. M., Ginn, H. B., Martin, B. R., and Aceto, M. D. (1992). Functional and dispositional tolerance develops during continuous cocaine exposure. *Eur. J. Drug Metab. Pharmacokinet.*, 17, 155–162.

Johansson, O., Hökfelt, T., Pernow, P., Jeffcoate, S. L., White, N., Steinbusch, H. W. M., Verhofstad, A. A. J., Emson, P. C., and Spindel, E. (1981). Immunohistochemical support for three putative transmitters in one neuron: Coexistence of 5-hydroxytryptamine, substance P- and thyrotropin releasing hormone-like immunoreactivity in medullary neurons projecting to the spinal cord. *Neuroscience, 6*, 1857–1881.

Johnson, D. A., Lee, N. M., Cook, R., and Loh, M. H. (1979). Ethanol-induced fluidization of lipid bilayers: Required presence of cholesterol in membranes for the expression of tolerance. *Mol. Pharmacol., 15*, 739–746.

Johnson, E. W., Wolfe, B. B., and Molinoff, P. B. (1989). Regulation of subtypes of β-adrenergic receptors in rat brain following treatment with 6-hydroxydopamine. *J. Neurosci., 9*, 2297–2305.

Johnson, J. W., and Ascher, P. (1987). Glycine potentiates the NMDA response in cultured mouse brain neurons. *Nature, 325*, 529–531.

Johnson, K. M. (1982a). Acute and chronic phencyclidine administration: Effects on the conversion of ^{3}H-tryptophan to ^{3}H-serotonin in rat forebrain. *J. Neural Transm., 53*, 179–186.

Johnson, K. M. (1982b). Phencyclidine: Behavioral and biochemical evidence against the anticholinergic hypothesis. *Pharmacol. Biochem. Behav., 17*, 53–57.

Johnson, K. M. (1983). Phencyclidine: Behavioral and biochemical evidence supporting a role for dopamine. *Fed. Proc., 42*, 2579–2583.

Johnson, K. M., and Hillman, G. R. (1982). Comparisons between phencyclidine, its monohydroxylated metabolites, and the stereoisomers of N-allyl-N-normetazocine (SKF 10047) as inhibitors of the muscarinic receptor and acetylcholinesterase. *J. Pharmacol., 34*, 462–464.

Johnson, K. M., and Jeng, Y.-J. (1991). Pharmacological evidence for N-methyl-Dp-aspartate receptors on nigrostriatal dopaminergic nerve terminals. *Can. J. Pysiol. Pharmacol., 69*, 1416–1421.

Johnson, K. M., and Jones, S. M. (1990). Neuropharmacology of phencyclidine: Basic mechanisms and therapeutic potential. *Annu. Rev. Pharmacol. Toxicol., 30*, 707–750.

Johnson, K. M., Snell, L. D., Sacaan, A. I., and Jones, S. M. (1989). Pharmacological regulation of the phencyclidine-binding site associated with the N-methyl-D-aspartate receptor-operated ion channel. *Drug Dev. Res., 17*, 281–287.

Johnson, K. M., Snell, L. D., Sacaan, A. I., and Jones, S. M. (1993). Pharmacologic regulation of the NMDA receptor-ionophore complex. *NIDA Res. Monogr., 133*, 13–39.

Johnson, M. R., and Melvin, L. S. (1986). The discovery of nonclassical cannabinoid analgetics. In *Cannabinoids as Therapeutic Agents* (R. Mechoulam, Ed.), pp. 121–145. CRC Press, Boca Raton.

Johnson, R. G. Jr. (1987). Proton pumps and chemiosmotic coupling as a generalized mechanism for neurotransmitter and hormone transport. *Ann. N.Y. Acad. Sci., 493*, 162–177.

Johnson, R. L., and Koerner, J. F. (1988). Excitatory amino acid neurotransmission. *J. Med. Chem., 31*, 2057–2066.

Johnston, A. L., and File, S. E. (1986). 5-HT and anxiety: Promises and pitfalls. *Pharmacol. Biochem. Behav., 24*, 1467–1470.

Johnston, G. A. R. (1995). GABA$_C$ receptors. *Prog. Brain Res., 100*, 61–65.

Johnston, J. (1991). Panic researchers find therapies but not causes. *J. NIH Res., 3*, 11, 30–32.

Johnstone, M., Evans, V., and Baigel, S. (1959). Sernyl (CI-395) in clinical anesthesia. *Br. J. Anaesth, 31*, 433–439.

Jonakait, G. M., Tamir, H., Gintzler, A. R., and Gershon, M. D. (1979). Release of [^{3}H]serotonin and its binding protein from enteric neurons. *Brain Res., 174*, 55–69.

Jones, B. E. (1990). Influence of the brainstem reticular formation, including intrinsic monoaminergic and cholinergic neurons, on forebrain mechanisms of sleep and waking. In *The Diencephalon and Sleep* (M. Mancia and G. Marini, Eds.), pp. 31–48. Raven Press, New York.

Jones, B. J., Paterson, I. A., and Roberts, M. H. T. (1986). Microinjections of methyl-β-carboline-carboxylate into the dorsal raphe nucleus: Behavioral consequences. *Pharmacol. Biochem. Behav., 24*, 1487–1489.

Jones, D. T., and Reed, R. R. (1989). G$_{olf}$: An olfactory neuron-specific G protein involved in odorant signal transduction. *Science, 244*, 790–795.

Jones, E. G.. (Ed.) (1983). *The Structural Basis of Neurobiology*. Elsevier, New York

Jones, E. G., and Cowan, W. M. (1983). The nervous tissue. In *The Structural Basis of Neurobiology* (E. G. Jones, Ed.), 282–370. Elsevier, New York.

Jones, K. L., Smith, D. W., Ulleland, C. N., and Streissguth, A. P. (1973). Pattern of malformation in offspring of chronic alcoholic mothers. *Lancet, 1*, 1267–1271.

Jones, R. T. (1987a). Drug of abuse profile: Cannabis. *Clin. Chem., 33*, 72B-81B.

Jones, R. T. (1987b). Tobacco dependence. In *Psychopharmacology: The Third Generation of Progress* (H. Y. Meltzer, Ed.), pp. 1589–1595. Raven Press, New York.

Jones, R. T. (1990). The pharmacology of cocaine smoking in humans. *NIDA Res. Monogr., 99*, 30–41.

Jones, R. T. (1992). What have we learned from nicotine, cocaine, and marijuana about addiction? In *Addictive States* (C. P. O'Brien and J. H. Jaffe, Eds.), pp. 109–122. Raven Press, New York.

Jones, R. T., Benowitz, N., and Bachman, J. (1976). Clinical studies of cannabis tolerance and dependence. *Ann. N.Y. Acad. Sci., 282*, 221–239.

Jones, S. M., Snell, L. D., and Johnson, K. M. (1987). Phencyclidine selectively inhibits N-methyl-D-asparate-induced hippocampal [^{3}H]norepinephrine release. *J. Pharmacol. Exp. Ther., 240*, 492–497.

Jones, S. V. P. (1993). Muscarinic receptor subtypes: Modulation of ion channels. *Life Sci., 52*, 457–464.

Jonsson, G., Hallman, H., Ponzio, F., and Ross, S. (1981). DSP 4—(N-(2-chloroethyl-)N-ethyl-2-bromobenzylamine)—a useful denervation tool for central and peripheral noradrenaline neurons. *Eur. J. Pharmacol., 72*, 173–188.

Jope, R. S., and Williams, M. B. (1994). Lithium and brain signal transduction systems. *Biochem. Pharmacol., 47*, 429–441.

Jorenby, D. E., Keehn, D. S., and Flore, M. C. (1995). Comparative efficacy and tolerability of nicotine replacement therapies. *CNS Drugs, 3* (3), 227–236.

Jori, A., and Garattini, S. (1965). Interaction between imipramine-like agents and catecholamine-induced hyperthermia. *J. Pharmacol., 17*, 480–488.

Josselyn, S. A., and Beninger, R. J. (1991). Behavioral effects of intrastriatal caffeine mediated by adenosinergic modulation of dopamine. *Pharmacol. Biochem. Behav., 39*, 97–103.

Jouvet, M. (1969). Biogenic amines and the states of sleep. *Science, 163*, 32–41.

Joyce, E. M., and Iversen, S. D. (1984). Dissociable effects of 6-OHDA-induced lesions of neostriatum on anorexia, locomotor activity and stereotypy: The role of behavioural competition. *Psychopharmacology, 83*, 363–366.

Julien, R. M. (1985). A *Primer of Drug Action* (4th ed.). W. H. Freeman, San Francisco.

Justice, J. B. Jr., Nicolaysen, L. C., and Michael, A. C. (1988). Modeling the dopaminergic nerve terminal. *J. Neurosci. Methods, 22*, 239–252.

Kaddis, F. G., Wallace, L. J., and Uretsky, N. J. (1993). AMPA/kainate antagonists in the nucleus accumbens inhibit locomotor stimulatory response to cocaine and dopamine agonists. *Pharmacol. Biochem. Behav., 46*, 703–708.

Kahn, R. S., and Davis, K. L. (1995). New developments in dopamine and schizophrenia. In *Psychopharmacology: The Fourth Generation of Progress* (F. E. Bloom and D. J. Kupfer, Eds.), pp. 1193–1204. Raven Press, New York.

Kaila, K. (1994). Ionic basis of GABA$_A$ receptor channel function in the nervous system. *Prog. Neurobiol., 42*, 489–537.

Kakidani, H., Furutani, Y., Takehashi, H., Noda, M., Morimoto, Y., Hirone, T., Asai, M., Inayama, S., Nakanishi, S., and Numa, S. (1982). Cloning and sequence analysis of cDNA for porcine beta-neo-endorphin, dynorphin precursor. *Nature, 298*, 245–249.

Kalant, H., Khana, J. M., Lin, G. Y., and Chung, S. (1976). Ethanol: A direct inducer of drug metabolism. *Biochem. Pharmacol., 25*, 337–342.

Kalant, H., Le Blanc, A. E., Guttman, M., and Khana, J. M. (1972). Metabolic and pharmacologic interaction of ethanol and etronidazole in the rat. *Can. J. Physiol. Pharmacol., 50*, 476–484.

Kalaria, R. N., Mitchell, M. J., and Harik, S. I. (1987). Correlation of 1-methyl-4-phenyl-1,2,3,6-tetrahydropyridine neurotoxicity with blood-brain barrier monoamine oxidase activity. *Proc. Natl. Acad. Sci. U.S.A., 84*, 3521–3535.

Kales, A., Scharf, M. B., and Kales, J. D. (1978). Rebound insomnia: A new clinical syndrome. *Science, 201*, 1039–1041.

Kales, A., Soldatos, C. R., Bixler, E. O., and Kales, J. D. (1983). Early morning insomnia with rapidly eliminated benzodiazepines. *Science, 220*, 95–97.

Kalia, M. (1991). Reversible, short-lasting, and dose-dependent effect of (–)-fenfluramine on neocortical serotonergic axons. *Brain Res., 548*, 111–125.

Kalivas, P. W. (1995). Interactions between dopamine and excitatory amino acids in behavioral sensitization to psychostimulants. *Drug Alcohol Dep.,* 37, 95–100.

Kalivas, P. W., Sorg, B. A., and Hooks, M. S. (1993). The pharmacology and neural circuitry of sensitization to psychostimulants. *Behav. Pharmacol.,* 4, 315–334.

Kalivas, P. W., and Weber, B. (1988). Amphetamine injection into the A10 dopamine region sensitizes rats to peripheral amphetamine and cocaine. *J. Pharmacol. Exp. Ther.,* 245, 1095–1102.

Kalsner, S. (1990). Heteroreceptors, autoreceptors, and other terminal sites. *Ann. N.Y. Acad. Sci.,* 604, 1–6.

Kalsner, S., and Westfall, T. C. (Eds.) (1990). Presynaptic receptors and the question of autoregulation of neurotransmitter release. *Ann. N.Y. Acad. Sci.,* 604, 1–652.

Kanai, Y., Smith, C. P., and Hediger, M. A. (1993). The elusive transporters with a high affinity for glutamate. *Trends Neurosci.,* 16, 365–370.

Kandel, D. B., and Davies, M. (1992). Progression to regular marijuana involvement: Phenomenology and risk factors for near-daily use. In *Vulnerability to Drug Abuse* (M. Glantz and R. Pickens, Eds.), pp. 211–253. American Psychological Association, Washington, D.C.

Kandel, D. B., and Faust, R. (1975). Sequence and stages in patterns of adolescent drug use. *Arch. Gen Psychiatry,* 32, 923–932.

Kandel, D. B., and Logan, J. A. (1984). Patterns of drug use from adolescence to young adulthood: I. Periods of risk for initiation, continued use, and discontinuation. *Am. J. Pub. Health,* 74, 660–666.

Kandel, D. B., Yamaguchi, K., and Chen, K. (1992). Stages of progression in drug involvement from adolescence to adulthood: Further evidence for the gateway theory. *J. Stud. Alcohol,* 53, 447–457.

Kandel, E. R. (1976). *Cellular Basis of Behavior: An Introduction to Behavioral Neurobiology.* W. H. Freeman, San Francisco.

Kandel, E. R. (1979). *Behavioral Biology of Aplysia.* New York.

Kandel, E. R. (1991a). Brain and behavior. In *Principles of Neural Science* (3rd ed.) (E. R. Kandel, J. H. Schwartz and T. M. Jessell, Eds.), pp. 5–17. Elsevier, New York.

Kandel, E. R. (1991b). Cellular mechanisms of learning and the biological basis of individuality. In *Principles of Neural Science* (3rd ed.) (E. R. Kandel, J. H. Schwartz, and T. M. Jessell, Eds.), pp. 1009–1031. Elsevier, New York.

Kandel, E. R. (1991c). Disorders of mood: Depression, mania, and anxiety disorders. In *Principles of Neural Science* (3rd ed.) (E. R. Kandel, J. H. Schwartz, and T. M. Jessell, Eds.), pp. 869–883. Elsevier, New York.

Kandel, E. R. (1991d). Disorders of thought: Schizophrenia. In *Principles of Neural Science* (3rd ed.) (E. R. Kandel, J. H. Schwartz, and T. M. Jessell, Eds.), pp. 853–868. Elsevier, New York.

Kandel, E. R. (1991e). Nerve cells and behavior. In *Principles of Neural Science* (3rd ed.) (E. R. Kandel, J. H. Schwartz, and T. M. Jessell, Eds.), pp. 18–32. Elsevier, New York.

Kandel, E. R. (1991f). Perception of motion, depth, and form. In *Principles of Neural Science* (3rd ed.) (E. R. Kandel, J. H. Schwartz, and T. M. Jessell, Eds.), pp. 440–456. Elsevier, New York.

Kandel, E. R., Castelucci, V. F., Goelet, P., and Schacher, S. (1987). Cell-biological interrelationships between short-term and long-term memory. In *Molecular Neurobiology in Neurology and Psychiatry* (E. R. Kandel, Ed.), pp. 111–132. Raven Press, New York.

Kandel, E. R., and Jessell, T. M. (1991). Touch. In *Principles of Neural Science* (3rd ed.) (E. R. Kandel, J. H. Schwartz, and T. M. Jessell, Eds.), pp. 367–384. Elsevier, New York.

Kandel, E. R., and Schwartz, J. H. (1982). Molecular biology of learning: Modulation of transmitter release. *Science,* 218, 433–443.

Kandel, E. R., and Schwartz, J. H. (1991). Directly gated transmission at central synapses. In *Principles of Neural Science* (3rd ed.) (E. R. Kandel, J. H. Schwartz, and T. M. Jessell, Eds.), pp. 153–172. Elsevier, New York.

Kandel, E. R., Siegelbaum, S. A., and Schwartz, J. H. (1991). Synaptic transmission. In *Principles of Neural Science* (3rd ed.) (E. R. Kandel, J. H. Schwartz, and T. M. Jessell, Eds.), pp. 123–134. Elsevier, New York.

Kane, J. M. (1987). Treatment of schizophrenia. *Schizophr. Bull.,* 13, 147–170.

Kane, J. M. (1995). Tardive dyskinesia: Epidemiological and clinical presentation. In *Psychopharmacology: The Fourth Generation of Progress* (F. E. Bloom and D. J. Kupfer, Eds.), pp. 1485–1495. Raven Press, New York.

Kane, J. M., Honigfeld, G., Singer, J., and Meltzer, H. (1988). Clozapine in treatment-resistant schizophrenics. *Psychopharmacol. Bull.,* 24, 62–67.

Kane, J. M., and Lieberman, J. A. (1987). Maintenance pharmacotherapy in schizophrenia. In *Psychopharmacology: The Third Generation of Progress* (H. Y. Meltzer, Ed.), pp. 1103–1109. Raven Press, New York.

Kaneyuki, H., Yokoo, H., Tsuda, A. et al. (1991). Psychological stress increases dopamine tunover selectively in mesoprefrontal dopamine neurons of rats: Reversal by diazepine. *Brain Res.,* 557, 154–161.

Kanner, B. I. (1983). Bioenergetics of neurotransmitter transport. *Biochim. Biophys. Acta,* 726, 293–316.

Kanof, P. D., and Greengard, P. (1978). Brain histamine receptors as targets for antidepressant drugs. *Nature,* 272, 329–333.

Kantorovich, N. (1930). An attempt at associative-reflex therapy in alcoholism. *Psychol. Abstracts,* 4, 493.

Kao, I., Drachman, D. B., and Price, D. L. (1976). Botulinum toxin: Mechanism of presynaptic blockade. *Science,* 193, 1256–1258.

Kaplan, A., Szabo, L. L., and Opheim, K. E. (1988). Chapter 2. In *Clinical Chemistry: Interpretation and Techniques* (3rd ed.), pp. 5–85. Lea & Febiger, Philadelphia.

Kaplan, C. D., Bieleman, B., and TenHouten, W. D. (1992). Are there 'casual users' of cocaine? *Ciba Found. Symp.,*166, 57–80.

Kaplan, E. L., and Meier, P. (1958). Nonparametric estimation from incomplete observations. *J. Am. Stat. Assoc.,* 53, 457–481.

Kaplan, G. P., Hartman, B. K., and Creveling, C. R. (1979). Immunohistochemical demonstration of catechol-O-methyltransferase in mammalian brain. *Brain Res.,* 167, 241–250.

Kapur, S., and Mann, J. J. (1992). Role of the dopaminergic system in depression. *Biol. Psychiatry,* 32, 1–17.

Kapur, S., and Mann, J. J. (1993). Antidepressant action and the neurobiologic effects of ECT: Human studies. In *The Clinical Science*
of Electroconvulsive Therapy (C. E. Coffey, Ed.), pp. 235–250. American Psychiatric Press, Washington, D.C.

Karch, S. B. (1993). *The Pathology of Drug Abuse.* CRC Press, Boca Raton.

Karczmar, A. G. (1993). Brief presentation of the story and present status of studies of the vertebrate cholinergic system. *Neuropsychopharmacology,* 9, 181–199.

Karege, F., Bovier, P., Rudolph, W., and Gaillard, J. M. (1996). Platelet phosphoinositide signaling system: An overstimulated pathway in depression. *Biol. Psychiatry,* 39, 697–702.

Karler, R., and Calder, L. D. (1992). Excitatory amino acids and the actions of cocaine. *Brain Res.,* 582, 143–146.

Karler, R., Calder, L. D., Chaudhry, I. A., and Turkanis, S. A. (1989). Blockade of 'reverse tolerance' to cocaine and amphetamine by MK-801. *Life Sci.,* 45, 599–606.

Karler, R., Calder, L. D., and Turkanis, S. A. (1991). DNQX blockade of amphetamine behavioral sensitization. *Brain Res.,* 552, 295–300.

Karler, R., Finnegan, K. T., and Calder, L. D. (1993). Blockade of behavioral sensitization to cocaine and amphetamine by inhibitors of protein synthesis. *Brain Res.,* 603, 19–24.

Karobath, M., and Leitich, H. (1974). Antipsychotic drugs and dopamine-stimulated adenylate cyclase prepared from corpus striatum of rat brain. *Proc. Natl. Acad. Sci. U.S.A.,* 71, 2915–2918.

Karobath, M., and Sperk, G. (1979). Stimulation of benzodiazepine receptor binding by g-aminobutyric acid. *Proc. Natl. Acad. Sci. U.S.A.,* 76, 1004–1006.

Kathol, R. G., and Carter, J. L. (1990). Use of hypothalamic-pituitary-adrenal axis tests in patients with major depression. In *Pharmacotherapy of Depression* (J. D. Amsterdam, Ed.), pp. 57–74. Marcel Dekker, New York.

Kato, T., Dong, B., Ishii, K., and Kinemuchi, H. (1986). Brain dialysis: In vivo metabolism of dopamine and serotonin by monoamine oxidase A but not B in the striatum of unrestrained rats. *J. Neurochem.,* 46, 1277–1282.

Katz, B. (1966). *Nerve, Muscle and Synapse.* McGraw-Hill, New York.

Katz, B., and Thesleff, S. (1957). A study of the "desensitization" produced by acetylcholine at the motor end-plate. *J. Physiol.* (Lond.), 138, 63–80.

Katz, J. L., Winger, G. D., and Woods, J. H. (1991). Abuse liability of benzodiazepines and 5-HT$_{1A}$ agonists. In *5-HT$_{1A}$ Agonists, 5-HT$_3$ Antagonists and Benzodiazepines: Their Comparative Behavioral Pharmacology* (R. J. Rodgers and S. J. Cooper, Eds.), pp. 317–341. Wiley, New York.

Katz, R. I., and Kopin, I. J. (1969). Release of norepinephrine^{+3}H evoked from brain slices by electrical-field stimulation-calcium dependency and the effects of lithium, ouabain, and tetrodotoxin. *Biochem. Pharmacol.,* 18, 1935–1939.

Kaufman, C. A., and Wyatt, R. J. (1987). Neuroleptic malignant syndrome. In *Psychopharmacology: The Third Generation of Progress* (H. Y. Meltzer, Ed.), pp. 1421–1430. Raven Press, New York.

Kaufman, D. L., and Tobin, A. J. (1993). Glutamate decarboxylases and autoimmunity in insulin-dependent diabetes. *Trends Pharmacol. Sci.,* 14, 107–109.

Kaufman, M. J., Spealman, R. D., and Madras, B. K. (1991). Distribution of cocaine recognition sites in monkey brain: I. In vitro autoradiography with [³H]CFT. *Synapse*, 9, 177–187.

Kaufman, S. (1973). Cofactors of tyrosine hydroxylase. In *Frontiers in Catecholamine Research* (E. Usdin and S. H. Snyder, Eds.), pp. 53–60. Pergamon Press, New York.

Kaufman, S. (1977). Mixed function oxygenases: General considerations. In *Structure and Function of Monoamine Enzymes* (E. Usdin, N. Weiner, and M. B. H. Youdim, Eds.), pp. 3–22. Marcel Dekker, New York.

Kaymakçalan, S. (1972). Physiological and psychological dependence on THC in rhesus monkeys. In *Cannabis and its Derivatives* (W. D. M. Paton and J. Crown, Eds.), pp. 142–149. Oxford, London.

Kaymakçalan, S. (1981). The addictive potential of cannabis. *Bull. Narc.*, 31, 21–31.

Kebabian, J. W., and Calne, D. B. (1979). Multiple receptors for dopamine. *Nature*, 277, 93–96.

Kebabian, J. W., Petzold, G. L., and Greengard, P. (1972). Dopamine-sensitive adenylate cyclase in caudate nucleus of rat brain, and its similarity to the "dopamine receptor." *Proc. Natl. Acad. Sci. U.S.A.*, 69, 2145–2149.

Kehoe, P. (1988). Opioids, behavior and learning. In *The Handbook of Behavioral Neurobiology: Developmental Psychobiology and Behavioral Ecology* (E. M. Blass, Ed.), pp. 309–340. Plenum Press, New York.

Kehoe, P., and Blass, E. M. (1986). Behaviorally functional opioid system in infant rats II. Evidence for pharmacological, physiological and psychological mediation of pain and stress. *Behav. Neurosci.*, 5, 624–630.

Kehoe, P., and Boylan, B. (1994). Behavioral effects of kappa opioid receptor stimulation on neonatal rats. *Behav. Neurosci.*, 108, 418–423.

Keinänen, K., Wisden, W., Sommer, B., Werner, P., Herb, A., Verdoorn, T. A., Sakmann, B., and Seeburg, P. H. (1990). A family of AMPA-selective glutamate receptors. *Science*, 249, 556–560.

Kelleher, R. T., and W. H. Morse. (1964). Escape behavior and punished behavior. *Fed. Proc.*, 23, 808–817.

Keller, M. B., Labori, B. W., Endicott, J., Coryell, W., Klerman, G. L., et al. (1983). Double depression: Two-year follow up. *Am. J. Psychiatry*, 140, 689–694.

Kelley, A. E. (1993). Locomotor activity and exploration. In *Behavioural Neuroscience: A Practical Approach*, Vol. 2 (A. Sahgal, Ed.), pp. 1–21. Oxford University Press, New York.

Kelley, A. E., Lang, C. G., and Gauthier, A. M. (1988). Induction of oral stereotypy following amphetamine microinjection into a discrete subregion of the striatum. *Psychopharmacology*, 95, 556–559.

Kellner, R. (1994). The measurement of depression and anxiety. In *Handbook of Depression and Anxiety* (J. A. den Boer and J. M. Ad Sitsen, Eds.), pp. 133–158. Marcel Dekker, New York.

Kelly, D. D. (1991a). Disorders of sleep and consciousness. In *Principles of Neural Science* (3rd ed.) (E. R. Kandel, J. H. Schwartz, and T. M. Jessell, Eds.), pp. 805–819. Elsevier, New York.

Kelly, D. D. (1991b). Sleep, and dreaming. In *Principles of Neural Science* (3rd ed.) (E. R.

Kandel, J. H. Schwartz, and T. M. Jessell, Eds.), pp. 792–804. Elsevier, New York.

Kelly, J. P. (1991a). Hearing. In *Principles of Neural Science* (3rd ed.) (E. R. Kandel, J. H. Schwartz, and T. M. Jessell, Eds.), pp. 481–499. Elsevier, New York.

Kelly, J. P. (1991b). The neural basis of perception and movement. In *Principles of Neural Science* (3rd ed.) (E. R. Kandel, J. H. Schwartz, and T. M. Jessell, Eds.), pp. 283–295. Elsevier, New York.

Kelly, J. P., and Dodd, J. (1991). Anatomical organization of the nervous system. In *Principles of Neural Science* (3rd ed.) (E. R. Kandel, J. H. Schwartz, and T. M. Jessell, Eds.), pp. 273–282. Elsevier, New York.

Kelly, P. H., and Iversen, S. D. (1976). Selective 6-OHDA induced destruction of mesolimbic dopamine neurons: Abolition of psychostimulant-induced locomotor activity in rats. *Eur. J. Pharmacol.*, 40, 45–56.

Kelly, P. H., Seviour, P. W., and Iversen, S. D. (1975). Amphetamine and apomorphine responses in the rat following 6-ODA lesions of the nucleus accumbens septi and corpus striatum. *Brain Res.*, 94, 507–522.

Kemali, D., Maj, M., Iorio, G., Marciano, F., Nolfe, G., Galderisi, S., and Salvati, A. (1985). Relationship between CSF noradrenaline levels, C-EEG indicators of activation and psychosis ratings in drug-free schizophrenic patients. *Acta Psychiatr. Scand.*, 71, 19–24.

Kemp, J. A., and Leeson, P. D. (1993). The glycine site of the NMDA receptor: Five years on. *Trends Pharmacol. Sci.*, 14, 20–25.

Kemper, T. D. (1978). *A Social Interactional Theory of Emotions*. Wiley-Interscience, New York.

Kendall, D. A., and Nahorski, S. R. (1987). Acute and chronic lithium treatments influence agonist and depolarization-stimulated inositol phopholipid hydrolysis in rat cerebral cortex. *J. Pharmacol. Exp. Ther.*, 241, 1023–1027.

Kendler, K. S., Mohs, R. C., and Davis, K. L. (1983). The effects of diet and physical activity on plasma homovanillic acid in normal human subjects. *Psychiatry Res.*, 8, 215–223.

Kendrick, K. M., Keverne, E. B., Hinton, M. R., and Goode, J. A. (1992). Oxytocin, amino acid and monoamine release in the region of the medial preoptic area and bed nucleus of the stria terminalis of the sheep during parturition and suckling. *Brain Res.*, 569, 199–209.

Kennedy, M. B. (1992). Second messengers and neuronal function. In *An Introduction to Molecular Neurobiology* (Z. W. Hall, ed.), pp. 207–246. Sinauer Associates, Sunderland, MA.

Kennett, G. A., Dourish, C. T., and Curzon, G. (1987). 5-HT₁ᵦ agonists induce anorexia at a postsynaptic site. *Eur. J. Pharmacol.*, 141, 429–435.

Kent, C., and Coupland, R. E. (1984). On uptake and storage of 5-hydroxytryptamine, 5-hydroxytryptophan and catecholamines by adrenal chromaffin cells and nerve endings. *Cell Tissue Res.*, 236, 189–195.

Keshavan, M. S., Anderson, S., and Pettegrew, J. W. (1994). Is schizophrenia due to excessive synaptic pruning in the prefrontal cortex? The Feinberg hypothesis revisited. *J. Psychiatr. Res.*, 28, 239–265.

Kesner, R. P., Dakis, M., and Bolland, B. L. (1993). Phencyclidine disrupts long- but not short-term memory within a spatial learning task. *Psychopharmacology*, 111, 85–90.

Kesner, R. P., Hardy, J. D., and Novak, J. M. (1983). Phencyclidine and behavior: II. Active avoidance learning and radial arm maze performance. *Pharmacol. Biochem. Behav.*, 18, 351–356.

Kety, S. S. (1979). Disorders of the human brain. *Sci. Am.*, 241, 202–214.

Keverne, E. B., and Kendrick, K. M. (1990). Neurochemical changes accompanying parturition and their significance for maternal behavior. In *Mammalian Parenting: Biochemical, Neurobiological, and Behavioral Determinants* (N. A. Krasnegor and R. S. Bridges, Eds.), pp. 281–304. Oxford University Press, New York.

Khachaturian, Z. S. (1985). Diagnosis of Alzheimer's disease. *Arch. Neurol.*, 42, 1097–1105.

Khachaturian, H., Schaefer, M. K. H., and Lewis, M. E. (1993). Anatomy and function of the endogenous opioid systems. In *Opioids I*, Handbook of Experimental Pharmacology, Vol. 104 (A. Herz, Ed.), pp. 471–497. Springer-Verlag, New York.

Khan, A., Mirolo, H. H., Hughes, D., and Bierut, L. (1993). Electroconvulsive therapy. *Psychiatr. Clin. North Am.*, 16, 497–513.

Kiba, H., and Jayaraman, A. (1994). Nicotine induced *c-fos* expression in the striatum is mediated mostly by dopamine D₁ receptor and is dependent on NMDA stimulation. *Mol. Brain Res.*, 23, 1–13.

Kida, E., Golabek, A. A., Wisniewski, T., and Wisniewski, K. E. (1994). Regional differences in apolipoprotein E immunoreactivity in diffuse plaques in Alzheimer's disease brain. *Neurosci. Lett.*, 167, 73–76.

Kieffer, B. L., Befort, K, Gaveriaux-Ruff, C., and Hirth, C. G. (1992). The "mu"-opioid receptor: Isolation of a cDNA by expression cloning and pharmacological characterization. *Proc. Natl. Acad. Sci. U.S.A.*, 89, 12048–12052.

Kilbey, M. M., and Ellinwood, E. H. Jr. (1977). Reverse tolerance to stimulant-induced abnormal behavior. *Life Sci.*, 20, 1063–1076.

Kilbinger, H., Dietrich, C., and von Bardeleben, R. S. (1992). Functional relevance of presynaptic muscarinic autoreceptors. *J. Physiol. (Paris)*, 86, 77–81.

Kilbourn, M. R., DaSilva, J. N., Frey, K. A., Koeppe, R. A., and Kuhl, D. E. (1993). In vivo imaging of vesicular monoamine transporters in human brain using [¹¹C]-tetrabenazine and positron emission tomography. *J. Neurochem.*, 60, 2315–2318.

Kilpatrick, G. J., Bunce, K. T., and Tyers, M. B. (1990). 5-H₃ receptors. *Med. Res. Rev.*, 10, 441–475.

Kilpatrick, G. J., Jones, B. J., and Tyers, M. B. (1987). Identification and distribution of 5-HT₃ receptors in rat brain using radioligand binding. *Nature*, 330, 746–748.

Kilts, C. D. (1994). Recent pharmacologic advances in antidepresant therapy. *Am. J. Med.*, 97, 3s-12s.

Kim, K.-S., Lee, M. K., Carroll, J., and Joh, T. H. (1993). Both the basal and inducible transcription of the tyrosine hydroxylase gene are dependent upon a cAMP response element. *J. Biol. Chem.*, 268, 15689–15695.

Kim, K.-S., Park, D. H., Wessel, T. C., Song, B., Wagner, J. A., and Joh, T. H. (1993). A dual role for the cAMP-dependent protein kinase in tyrosine hydroxylase gene expression. *Proc. Natl. Acad. Sci. U.S.A.*, 90, 3471–3475.

Kim, K.-S., Wessel, T. C., Stone, D. M., Carver, C. H., Joh, T. H., and Park, D. H. (1991). Molecular cloning and characterization of cDNA encoding tryptophan hydroxylase from rat central serotonergic neurons. *Mol. Brain Res.*, 9, 277–283.

Kim, K.-T., Park, D. H., and Joh, T. H. (1993). Parallel up-regulation of catecholamine biosynthetic enzymes by dexamethasone in PC12 cells. *J. Neurochem.*, 60, 946–951.

Kimble, D. P. (1990). Functional effects of neural grafting in the mammalian central nervous system. *Psychol. Bull.*, 108, 462–479.

Kimelberg, H. K. (1986). Occurrence and functional significance of serotonin and catecholamine uptake by astrocytes. *Biochem. Pharmacol.*, 35, 2273–2281.

Kiritsy-Roy, J. A., Halter, J. B., Gordon, S. M., Smith, M. J., and Terry, L. C. (1990). Role of the central nervous system in hemodynamic and sympathoadrenal responses to cocaine in rats. *J. Pharmacol. Exp. Ther.*, 255, 154–160.

Kirkham, T. C., and Cooper, S. J. (1991). Opioid peptides in relation to the treatment of obesity and bulimia. In *Peptides: A Target for New Drug Development* (S. R. Bloom and G. Burnstock, Eds.), pp. 28–44, IBC Technical Services, London.

Kish, P. E., Fisher-Bovenkerk, C., and Ueda, T. (1989). Active transport of γ-aminobutyric acid and glycine into synaptic vesicles. *Proc. Natl. Acad. Sci. U.S.A.*, 86, 3877–3881.

Kitahama, K., Arai, R., Maeda, T., and Jouvet, M. (1986). Demonstration of monoamine oxidase type B in serotonergic and type A in noradrenergic neurons in the cat dorsal pontine tegmentum by an improved histochemical technique. *Neurosci. Lett.*, 71, 19–24.

Kitahama, K., Geffard, M., Okamura, H., Nagatsu, I., Mons, N., and Jouvet, M. (1990). Dopamine- and DOPA-immunoreactive neurons in the cat forebrain with reference to tyrosine hydroxylase-immunohistochemistry. *Brain Res.*, 518, 83–94.

Kitayama, S., Shimada, S., and Uhl, G. R. (1992). Parkinsonism-inducing neurotoxin MPP$^+$: Uptake and toxicity in nonneuronal COS cells expressing the dopamine transporter cDNA. *Ann. Neurol.*, 32, 109–111.

Kito, S., and Miyoshi, R. (1985). Autoradiographic studies of neurotransmitter receptors. In *Recent Research on Neurotransmitter Receptors* (H. Yoshida, Ed.), pp. 82–92. Excerpta Medica, Amsterdam.

Klaassen, C. D. (1985). Nonmetallic environmental toxicants: Air pollutants, solvents and vapors, and pesticides. In *The Pharmacological Basis of Therapeutics* (A. G. Gilman, A. S. Goodman, T. W. Rall, and F. Murad, Eds.), pp. 1628–1650. Macmillan, New York.

Klann, E., Chen, S.-J., and Sweatt, J. D. (1993). Mechanism of protein kinase C activation during the induction and maintenance of long-term potentiation probed using a selective peptide substrate. *Proc. Natl. Acad. Sci. U.S.A.*, 90, 8337–8341.

Kleber, H. D. (1995). Pharcotherapy, current and potential, for the treatment of cocaine dependence. *Clin. Neuropharmacol.*, 18 (Suppl. 1), S96–S109.

Kleiman, M. A. R. (1989). *Marijuana: Costs of Abuse, Costs of Control.* Greenwood Press, New York.

Klein, D. C., and Seligman, M. E. P. (1976). Reversal of performance deficits and perceptual deficits in learned helplessness and depression. *J. Abnorm. Psychol.*, 85, 11–26.

Kleinman, K. M., Vaughn, R. L., and Christ, T. S. (1973). Effects of cigarette smoking and smoking deprivation on paired-associate learning of high and low meaningful nonsense syllables. *Psychol. Rep.*, 32, 963–966.

Kleinman, P. H., Miller, A. B., Millman, R. B., Woody, G. E., Todd, T., Kemp, J., and Lipton, D. S. (1990). Psychopathology among cocaine abusers entering treatment. *J. Nerv. Ment. Dis.*, 178, 442–447.

Klemm, W. R., and Foster, D. M. (1986). Alcohol, in a single pharmacological dose, decreases brain gangliosides. *Life Sci.*, 39, 897–902.

Klerman, G. L. (1984). Ideology and science in the individual psychotherapy of schizophrenia. *Schizophr. Bull.*, 10, 608–612.

Kleven, M. S., Anthony, E. W., and Woolverton, W. L. (1990). Pharmacological characterization of the discriminative stimulus effects of cocaine in rhesus monkeys. *J. Pharmacol. Exp. Ther.*, 254, 312–317.

Kleven, M. S., Woolverton, W. L., and Seiden, L. S. (1988). Lack of long-term monoamine depletions following repeated or continuous exposure to cocaine. *Brain Res. Bull.*, 21, 233–237.

Kley, N., and Loeffler, J. P. (1993). Molecular mechanisms in proenkephalin gene regulation. In *Opioids I*, Handbook of Experimental Pharmacology, Vol. 104 (A. Herz, Ed.), pp. 379–392. Springer-Verlag, New York.

Klonoff, H. (1974). Marijuana and driving in real-life situations. *Science*, 186, 317–324.

Kloog, Y., Rehavi, M., Maayani, S., and Sokolovsky, M. (1977). Anticholinesterase and antiacetylcholine activity of 1-phenylcyclohexylamine derivatives. *Eur. J. Pharmacol.*, 45, 221–227.

Klopfer, P. H. (1971). Mother love: What turns it on? *Am. Sci.*, 59, 404–407.

Klotz, I. M. (1983). Ligand–receptor interactions: What we can and cannot learn from binding measurements. *Trends Pharmacol. Sci.*, 4, 253–255.

Klüver, H., and Bucy, P. C. (1939). Preliminary analysis of the functions of the temporal lobes in monkeys. *Arch. Neurol. Psychiatry*, 42, 979–1000.

Knapp, R. J., Vaughn, L. K., Fang, S.-N., Bogert, C. L., Yamamura, M. S., Hruby, V. J., and Yamamura, H. I. (1990). A new, highly selective CCK-B receptor radioligand ([^{3}H]-[N-methyl-Nle^{28,31}]CCK$_{26+33}$): Evidence for CCK-B heterogeneity. *J. Pharmacol. Exp. Ther.*, 255, 1278–1286.

Knepper, S. M., Grunewald, G. L., and Rutledge, C. O. (1988). Inhibition of norepinephrine transport into synaptic vesicles by amphetamine analogs. *J. Pharmacol. Exp. Ther.*, 247, 487–494.

Knoblich, G., Curtis, D., Faustman, W. O., Zarcone, V., Stewart, S. Mefford, I., and King, R. (1992). Increased CSF HVA with craving in long-term abstinent cocaine abusers. *Biol. Psychiatry*, 32, 96–100.

Knowlton, B. J., Mangels, J. A., and Squire, L. R. (1996). A neostriatal habit learning system in humans. *Science*, 273, 1399–1402.

Kobilka, B. (1992). Adrenergic receptors as models for G protein-coupled receptors. *Annu. Rev. Neurosci.*, 15, 87–114.

Kobilka, B., et al. (1987). cDNA for the human β$_2$-adrenergic receptor: A protein with multiple membrane-spanning domains and encoded by a gene whose chromosal location is shared with that of the receptor for platelet-derived growth factor. *Proc. Natl. Acad. Sci. U.S.A.*, 84, 46–50.

Koda, L. Y., and Gibb, J. W. (1973). Adrenal and striatal tyrosine hydroxylase activity after methamphetamine. *J. Pharmacol. Exp. Ther.*, 185, 42–48.

Koe, B. K., Nielsen, J. A., Macor, J. E., and Heym, J. (1992). Biochemical and behavioral studies of the 5-HT$_{1B}$ receptor agonist, CP-94,253. *Drug Dev. Res.*, 26, 241–250.

Koe, B. K., and Weissman, A. (1966). Parachlorophenylalanine: A specific depletor of brain serotonin. *J. Pharmacol. Exp. Ther.*, 154, 499–516.

Koek, W., Colpaert, F. C., Woods, J. H., and Kamenka, J.-M. (1989). The phencyclidine (PCP) analog N-[1-(2-benzo(b)thiophenyl)-cyclohexyl)piperidine shares cocaine-like but not other characteristic behavioral effects with PCP, ketamine, and MK-801. *J. Pharmacol. Exp. Ther.*, 250, 1019–1027.

Koek, W., Jackson, A., and Colpaert, F. C. (1992). Behavioral pharmacology of antagonists at 5-HT$_2$/5-HT$_{1C}$ receptors. *Neurosci. Biobehav. Rev.*, 16, 95–105.

Koek, W., Woods, J. H., and Colpaert, F. C. (1990). N-Methyl-D-aspartate antagonism and phencyclidine-like activity: A drug discrimination analysis. *J. Pharmacol. Exp. Ther.*, 253, 1017–1025.

Koek, W., Woods, J. H., Jacobson, A. E., and Rice, K. C. (1987). Phencyclidine (PCP)-like discriminative stimulus effects of metaphit and of 2-amino-5-phosphonovalerate in pigeons: Generality across different training doses of PCP. *Psychopharmacology*, 93, 437–442.

Koek, W., Woods, J. H., and Ornstein, P. (1987). A simple and rapid method for assessing similarities among directly observable behavioral effects of drugs: PCP-like effects of 2-amino-5-phosphonovalerate in rats. *Psychopharmacology*, 91, 297–304.

Koek, W., Woods, J. H., and Winger, G. D. (1988). MK-801, a proposed noncompetitive antagonist of excitatory amino acid neurotransmission, produces phencyclidine-like behavioral effects in pigeons, rats and rhesus monkeys. *J. Pharmacol. Exp. Ther.*, 245, 969–974.

Koelle, G. B. (1975a). Anticholinesterase agents. In *The Pharmacological Basis of Therapeutics* (5th ed.) (L. S. Goodman and A. Gilman, Eds.), pp. 445–466. Macmillan, New York.

Koelle, G. B. (1975b). Neuromuscular blocking agents. In *The Pharmacological Basis of Therapeutics* (5th ed.) (L. S. Goodman and A. Gilman, Eds.), pp. 575–588. Macmillan, New York.

Koelle, G. B. (1975c). Parasympathomimetic agents. In *The Pharmacological Basis of Therapeutics* (5th ed.) (L. S. Goodman and A. Gilman, Eds.), pp. 467–476. Macmillan, New York.

Koelle, G. B. (1990). Early evidence of presynaptic receptors. *Ann. N.Y. Acad. Sci.*, 604, 488–491.

Koenig, J. H., Kosaka, T., and Ikeda, K. (1989). The relationship between the number of synaptic vesicles and the amount of transmitter released. *J. Neurosci.,* 9, 1937–1942.

Koester, J. (1991a). Membrane potential. In *Principles of Neural Science* (3rd ed.) (E. R. Kandel, J. H. Schwartz, and T. M. Jessell, Eds.), pp. 81–94. Elsevier, New York.

Koester, J. (1991b). Passive membrane properties of the neuron. In *Principles of Neural Science* (3rd ed.) (E. R. Kandel, J. H. Schwartz, and T. M. Jessell, Eds.), pp. 95–103. Elsevier, New York.

Koester, J. (1991c). Voltage-gated ion channels and the generation of the action potential. In *Principles of Neural Science* (3rd ed.) (E. R. Kandel, J. H. Schwartz, and T. M. Jessell, Eds.), pp. 104–119. Elsevier, New York.

Kohler, G., and Milstein, C. (1975). Continuous cultures of fused cells secreting antibody of predefined specificity. *Nature,* 256, 495–497.

Kolata, G. B. (1981a) Clues to the cause of senile dementia. *Science,* 211, 1032–1033.

Kolata, G. B. (1981b). Drug found to help heart attack survivors. *Science,* 214, 774–775.

Kolb, B., and Whishaw, I. Q. (1990). *Fundamentals of Neuropsychology* (3rd ed.). Freeman, New York.

Kolbe, L. J., and Newman, I. M. (1984). The role of school health education in preventing heart, lung and blood diseases. *J. Sch. Health,* 54, 15–26.

Kollonitsch, J., Patchell, A. A., Marburg, S., Maycock, A. L., Perkins, L. M., Doldouras, G. A., Duggan, D. E., and Aster, S. D. (1978). Selective inhibitors of biosynthesis of aminergic neurotransmitters. *Nature,* 274, 906–908.

Komori, K., Fujii, T., and Nagatsu, I. (1991). Do some tyrosine hydroxylase-immunoreactive neurons in the human ventrolateral arcuate nucleus and globus pallidus produce only L-DOPA? *Neurosci. Lett.,* 133, 203–206.

Konkoy, C. S., and Childers, S. R. (1989). Dynorphin-selective inhibition of adenylyl cyclase in guinea pig cerebellum membranes. *Mol. Pharmacol.,* 36, 627–633.

Konradi, C., Cole, R. L., Heckers, S., and Hyman, S. E. (1994). Amphetamine regulates gene expression in rat striatum via transcription factor CREB. *J. Neurosci.,* 14, 5623–5634.

Konradi, C., Svoma, E., Jellinger, K., Riederer, P., Denney, R., and Thibault, J. (1988). Topographic immunocytochemical mapping of monoamine oxidase-A, monoamine oxidase-B and tyrosine hydroxylase in human post mortem brain stem. *Neuroscience,* 26, 791–802.

Koob, G. F. (1992). Drugs of abuse: Anatomy, pharmacology and function of reward pathways. *Trends Pharmacol. Sci.,* 13, 177–184.

Koob, G. F., and Bloom, F. E. (1988). Cellular and molecular mechanisms of drug dependence. *Science,* 242, 715–723.

Koob, G. F., and Goeders, N. E. (1989). Neuroanatomical substrates of drug self-administration. In *The Neuropharmacological Basis of Reward* (S. J. Cooper and J. M. Lieberman, Eds.), pp. 214–263. Clarendon, Oxford.

Koob, G. F., Heinrichs, S. C., Pich, E. M., Menzaghi, F., Baldwin, H., Miczek, K., and Britton, K. T. (1993). The role of corticotropin-releasing factor in behavioural responses to stress. *Ciba Found. Symp.,* 172, 277–295.

Koob, G. F., Maldonado, R., and Stinus, L. (1992). Neural substrates of opiate withdrawal. *Trends Neurosci.,* 15, 186–191.

Koolhaas, J. M., and Bohus, B. (1991). Animal models of human aggression. In *Neuromethods,* Vol. 19. *Animal Models in Psychiatry,* II (A. A. Boulton, G. B. Baker, and M. T. Martin-Iverson, Eds.), pp. 249–271. Humana Press, Clifton, NJ.

Koop, C. E. (1989). *Reducing the Health Consequences of Smoking: 25 Years of Progress.* U.S. Government Printing Office, Washington, D.C.

Kopin, I. J. (1985). Catecholamine metabolism: Basic aspects and clinical significance. *Pharmacol. Rev.,* 37, 333–364.

Kopin, I. J. (1987). Neurotoxins affecting biogenic aminergic neurons. In *Psychopharmacology: The Third Generation of Progress* (H. Y. Meltzer, Ed.), pp. 351–358. Raven Press, New York.

Kopin, I. J. (1993a). Parkinson's disease: Past, present, and future. *Neuropsychopharmacology,* 9, 1–12.

Kopin, I. J. (1993b). The pharmacology of Parkinson's disease therapy. An update. *Annu. Rev. Pharmacol.,* 32, 467–495.

Korn, H., Sur, C., Charpier, S., Legendre, P., and Faber, D. S. (1994). The one-vesicle hypothesis and multivesicular release. In *Molecular and Cellular Mechanisms of Neurotransmitter Release* (L. Stjärne, P. Greengard, S. Grillner, T. Hökfelt, and D. Ottoson, Eds.), pp. 301–322. Raven Press, New York.

Kornblum, H. I., Hurlbut, D. E., and Leslie, F. M. (1987). Postnatal development of multiple opioid receptors in rat brain. *Dev. Brain Res.,* 37, 21–41.

Kornhuber, J., Mack-Burkhardt, F., Riederer, P., Hebenstreit, G. F., Reynolds, G. P., Andrews, H. B., and Beckmann, H. (1989). [³H]MK-801 binding sites in postmortem brain regions of schizophrenic patients. *J. Neural Transm.,* 77, 231–236.

Kosik, K. S., and Coleman, P. D. (1992). Is β-amyloid neurotoxic? *Neurobiol. Aging,* 13, 535–630.

Kosik, K. S., and Greenberg, S. M. (1994). Tau protein and Alzheimer disease. In *Alzheimer Disease* (R. D. Terry, R. Katzman, and K. L. Bick, Eds.), pp. 335–344. Raven Press, New York.

Kosofsky, B. E., and Molliver, M. E. (1987). The serotoninergic innervation of cerebral cortex: Different classes of axon terminals arise from dorsal and median raphe nuclei. *Synapse,* 1, 153–168.

Kosten, T. R., Rosen, M. I., Schottenfeld, R., and Ziedonis, D. (1992). Buprenorphine for cocaine and opiate dependence. *Psychopharmacol. Bull.,* 28, 15–19.

Kosterlitz, H. W., and Hughes, J. (1975). Some thoughts on the significance of enkephalin, the endogenous ligand. *Life Sci.,* 17, 91–96.

Kosterlitz, H. W., Lydon, R. J., and Watt, A. J. (1970). The effects of adrenaline, noradrenaline and isoprenaline on inhibitory α- and β-adrenoceptors in the longitudinal muscle of the guinea-pig ileum. *Br. J. Pharmacol.,* 39, 398–413.

Kosterlitz, H. W., and Waterfield, A. A. (1975). In vitro models in the study of structure-activity relationships of narcotic analgesics. *Annu. Rev. Pharmacol.,* 15, 29–47.

Kötter, R. (1994). Postsynaptic integration of glutamatergic and dopaminergic signals in the striatum. *Prog. Neurobiol.,* 44, 163–196.

Kovács, G. L., and De Wied, D. (1994). Peptidergic modulation of learning and memory processes. *Pharmacol. Rev.,* 46, 269–291.

Kovelman, J. A., and Scheibel, A. B. (1984). A neurohistological correlate of schizophrenia. *Biol. Psychiatry,* 19, 1601–1621.

Kovner, R., and Stamm, J. S. (1972). Disruption of short-term visual memory by electrical stimulation of inferotemporal cortex in the monkey. *J. Comp. Physiol. Psychol.,* 81, 163–172.

Kow, L.-M., and Pfaff, D. W. (1988). Neuromodulatory actions of peptides. *Annu. Rev. Pharmacol. Toxicol.,* 28, 163–188.

Kozlowski, G. P., Nilaver, G., and Zimmerman, E. A. (1983). Distribution of neurohypophysial hormones in the brain. *Pharmacol. Ther.,* 21, 325–349.

Kozlowski, L. T. (1984). Pharmacological approaches to smoking modification. In *Behavioral Health: A Handbook of Health Enhancement and Disease Prevention* (J. D. Matarazzo, A. J. Herd, N. E. Miller, and S. M. Weiss, Eds.), pp. 713–728. Wiley, New York.

Kraepelin, E. (1913). *Textbook of Psychiatry* (R. M. Barclay, trans.). Livingston, Edinburgh.

Kramer, J. C., Fischman, V. S., and Littlefield, D. C. (1967). Amphetamine abuse: Pattern and effects of high doses taken intravenously. *JAMA,* 201, 89–93.

Krasnegor, N. A. (Ed.) (1978). Behavioral Tolerance: Research and Treatment Implications. *NIDA Res. Monogr.,* 18.

Kravitz, E. A., Kuffler, S. W., and Potter, D. D. (1963). Gamma-aminobutyric acid and other blocking compounds in Crustacea. III. Their relative concentrations in separated motor and inhibitory axons. *J. Neurophysiol.,* 26, 739–751.

Kreek, M. J. (1987). Multiple drug abuse patterns and medical consequences. In *Psychopharmacology: The Third Generation of Progress* (H. Y. Meltzer, Ed.), pp. 1597–1604. Raven Press, New York.

Kreek, M. J. (1991). Using methadone effectively: Achieving goals by application of laboratory, clinical and evaluation research and by development of innovative programs. *NIDA Res. Monogr.,* 106, 245–266.

Kreutz, M. R., Acworth, I. N., Lehnert, H., and Wurtman, R. J. (1990). Systemic administration of thyrotropin-releasing hormone enhances striatal dopamine release in vivo. *Brain Res.,* 536, 347–352.

Krevsky, B., Cowan, A., Maurer, A. H., Butt, W., and Fisher, R. S. (1991). Effects of selective opioid agonists on feline colonic transit. *Life Sci.,* 48, 1597–1602.

Krisanda, T. J. (1993). Flumazenil: An antidote for benzodiazepine toxicity. *Am. Fam. Physician,* 47, 891–895.

Krishek, B. J., Xie, X., Blackstone, C., Huganir, R. L., Moss, S. J., and Smart, T. G. (1994). Regulation of GABA_A receptor function by protein kinase C phosphorylation. *Neuron,* 12, 1081–1095.

Krnjević, K. (1993). Central cholinergic mechanisms and function. *Prog. Brain Res.,* 98, 285–292.

Kromer, W. (1993). Gastrointestinal effects of opioids. In *Opioids II,* Handbook of Experimental Pharmacology, Vol. 104 (A. Herz, Ed.), pp. 163–190. Springer-Verlag, New York.

Krueger, B. K. (1990). Kinetics and block of dopamine uptake in synaptosomes from rat caudate nucleus. *J. Neurochem.*, 55, 260–267.

Kruesi, M. J. P. (1989). Cruelty to animals and CSF 5-HIAA. *Psychiatry Res.*, 28, 115–116.

Kruesi, M. J. P., Rapoport, J. L., Hamburger, S., Hibbs, E., Potter, W. Z., Lenane, M., and Brown, G. L. (1990). Cerebrospinal fluid monoamine metabolites, aggression, and disruptive behavior disorders of children and adolescents. *Arch. Gen. Psychiatry*, 47, 419–426.

Kruk, M. R. (1991). Ethology and pharmacology of hypothalamic aggression in the rat. *Neurosci. Biobehav. Rev.*, 15, 527–538.

Krystal, J. H., Seibyl, J. P., Price, L. H., Woods, S. W., Heninger, G. R., Aghajanian, G. K., and Charney, D. S. (1993). m-Chlorophenylpiperazine effects in neuroleptic-free schizophrenic patients: Evidence implicating serotonergic systems in the positive symptoms of schizophrenia. *Arch. Gen. Psychiatry*, 50, 624–635.

Kubo, T., Fukuda, K., et al. (1986). Cloning, sequencing and expression of complementary DNA encoding the muscarinic acetylcholine receptor. *Nature*, 323, 411–416.

Kubo, T., Maeda, A., et al. (1986). Primary structure of porcine cardiac muscarinic acetylcholine receptor deduced from the cDNA sequence. *FEBS Lett.*, 209, 367–372.

Kubota, Y., Inagaki, S., and Kito, S. (1986). Innervation of substance P neurons by catecholaminergic terminals in the neostriatum. *Brain Res.*, 375, 163–167.

Kuczenski, R. (1983). Biochemical actions of amphetamine and other stimulants. In *Stimulants: Neurochemical, Behavioral, and Clinical Perspectives* (I. Creese, Ed.), pp. 31–61. Raven Press, New York.

Kuczenski, R., and Segal, D. S. (1992a). Differential effects of amphetamine and dopamine uptake blockers (cocaine, nomifensine) on caudate and accumbens dialysate dopamine and 3-methoxytyramine. *J. Pharmacol. Exp. Ther.*, 262, 1085–1094.

Kuczenski, R., and Segal, D. S. (1992b). Regional norepinephrine response to amphetamine using dialysis: Comparison to caudate dopamine. *Synapse*, 11, 164–169.

Kuczenski, R., and Segal, D. S. (1994). Neurochemistry of amphetamine. In *Amphetamine and its Analogs* (A. K. Cho, Ed.), pp. 81–113. Academic Press, San Diego.

Kuczenski, R., Segal, D. S., and Aizenstein, M. L. (1991). Amphetamine, cocaine, and fencamfamine: Relationship between locomotor and stereotypy response profiles and caudate and accumbens dopamine dynamics. *J. Neurosci.*, 11, 2703–2712.

Kuhar, M. J. (1982). Localization of drug and neurotransmitter receptors in brain by light microscopic autoradiography. In *Handbook of Psychopharmacology*, Vol. 15 (L. Iversen, S. Iversen, and S. Snyder, Eds.), pp. 299–320. Plenum Press, New York.

Kuhar, M. J. (1985). The mismatch problem in receptor mapping studies. *Trends Neurosci.*, 8, 190–191.

Kuhar, M. J., Boja, J. W., and Cone, E. J. (1990). Phencyclidine binding to striatal cocaine receptors. *Neuropharmacology*, 29, 295–297.

Kuhar, M. J., Murrin, L. C., Maloup, A. T., and Klemm, N. (1978). Dopamine receptor binding in vivo: The feasibility of autoradiographic studies. *Life Sci.*, 22, 203–210.

Kuhar, M. J., Roth, R. H., and Aghajanian, G. K. (1972). Synaptosomes from forebrain of rats

with midbrain raphe lesions: Selective reduction of serotonin uptake. *J. Pharmacol. Exp. Ther.*, 181, 36–45.

Kuhl, D. E., Markham, C. H., Metter, E. J., Riege, W. H., Phelps, M. E., and Mazziotta, J. C. (1985). Local cerebral glucose utilization in symptomatic and presymptomatic Huntington's disease. In *Brain Imaging and Brain Function* (L. Sokoloff, Ed.), pp. 199–209. Raven Press, New York.

Kuhl, D. E., Metter, E. J., and Riege, W. H. (1985). Patterns of cerebral glucose utilization in depression, multiple infarct dementia, and Alzheimer's disease. In *Brain Imaging and Brain Function* (L. Sokoloff, Ed.). pp. 211–226. Raven Press, New York.

Kuhn, C. M., and Schanberg, S. M. (1978). Metabolism of amphetamine after acute and chronic administration to the rat. *J. Pharmacol. Exp. Ther.*, 207, 544–554.

Kuhn, D. M., Appel, J. B., and Greenburg, I. (1974). An analysis of some discriminative properties of *d*-amphetamine. *Psychopharmacologia*, 39, 57–66.

Kuhn, D. M., and Lovenberg, W. (1982). Role of calmodulin in the activation of tryptophan hydroxylase. *Fed. Proc.*, 41, 2258–2264.

Kühn, D. M., and Lovenberg, W. (1983). Hydroxylases. In *Handbook of Neurochemistry* (2nd ed.), Vol. 4. *Enzymes in the Nervous System* (A. Lajtha, Ed.), pp. 133–150. Plenum Press, New York.

Kühn, D. M., Wolf, W. A., and Youdim, M. B. H. (1985). 5-Hydroxytryptamine release in vivo from a cytoplasmic pool: Studies on the 5-HT behavioural syndrome in reserpinized rats. *Br. J. Pharmacol.*, 84, 121–129.

Kühn, D. M., Wolf, W. A., and Youdim, M. B. H. (1986). Serotonin neurochemistry revisited: A new look at some old axioms. *Neurochem. Int.*, 8, 141–154.

Kuhn, H., and Wilden, U. (1987). Light-dependent activation and ATP-dependent deactivation of cGMP-phosphodiesterase in rod outer segments: Interactions between proteins involved. In *Discussions in Neurosciences*, Vol. 4, No. 3, *Sensory Transduction* (A. J. Hudspeth, P. R. MacLeish, F. L. Margolis, and T. N. Wiesel, Eds.), pp. 75–79. Fondation pour l'Etude du Système Nerveux, Geneva.

Kupfermann, I. (1991a). Genetic determinants of behavior. In *Principles of Neural Science* (3rd ed.) (E. R. Kandel, J. H. Schwartz, and T. M. Jessell, Eds.), pp. 987–996. Elsevier, New York.

Kupfermann, I. (1991b). Hypothalamus and limbic system: Motivation. In *Principles of Neural Science* (3rd ed.) (E. R. Kandel, J. H. Schwartz, and T. M. Jessell, Eds.), pp. 750–760. Elsevier, New York.

Kupfermann, I. (1991c). Hypothalamus and limbic system: Peptidergic neurons, homeostasis, and emotional behavior. In *Principles of Neural Science* (3rd ed.) (E. R. Kandel, J. H. Schwartz, and T. M. Jessell, Eds.), pp. 735–749. Elsevier, New York.

Kupfermann, I. (1991d). Localization of higher cognitive and affective functions: The association cortices. In *Principles of Neural Science* (3rd ed.) (E. R. Kandel, J. H. Schwartz, and T. M. Jessell, Eds.), pp. 823–838. Elsevier, New York.

Kuroda, Y., Mikuni, M., Ogawa, T., and Takahashi, K. (1992). Effect of ACTH, adrenalectomy and the combination treatment on the density of 5-HT2 receptor binding sites in

neocortex of rat forebrain and 5-HT2 receptor-mediated wet-dog shake behaviors. *Psychopharmacology*, 108, 27–32.

Kursar, J. D., Nelson, D. L., Wainscott, D. B., and Baez, M. (1994). Molecular cloning, functional expression, and mRNA tissue distribution of the human 5-hydroxytryptamine$_{2B}$ receptor. *Mol. Pharmacol.*, 46, 227–234.

Kurz, E. M., Sengelaub, D. R., and Arnold, A. P. (1986). Androgens regulate the dendritic length of mammalian motoneurons in adulthood. *Science*, 232, 395–398.

Kushner, L., Lerma, J., Zukin, R. S., and Bennett, M. V. L. (1988). Coexpression of N-methyl-D-aspartate and phencyclidine receptors in *Xenopus* oocytes injected with rat brain mRNA. *Proc. Natl. Acad. Sci. U.S.A.*, 85, 3250–3254.

Kushner, M. G., Sher, K. J., and Beitman, B. D. (1990). The relation between alcohol problems and the anxiety disorders. *Am. J. Psychiatry*, 147, 685–695.

Kvetňansky, R., Weise, V. K., and Kopin, I. J. (1970). Elevation of adrenal tyrosine hydroxylase and phenylethanolamine-N-methyl transferase by repeated immobilization of rats. *Endocrinology*, 87, 744–749.

Lacey, M. G., Mercuri, N. B., and North, R. A. (1987). Dopamine acts on D$_2$ receptor to increase potassium conductance in neurones of the rat substantia nigra pars compacta. *J. Physiol.* (Lond.), 392, 397–416.

Lacey, M. G., Mercuri, N. B., and North, R. A. (1990). Actions of cocaine on rat dopaminergic neurones *in vitro*. *Br. J. Pharmacol.*, 99, 731–735.

Lacomblez, L., Bensimon, G., Leigh, P. N., Guillet, P., and Meininger, V., for the Amyotrophic Lateral Sclerosis/Riluzole Study Group II. (1996). Dose-ranging study of riluzole in amyotrophic lateral sclerosis. *Lancet*, 347, 1425–1431.

Lader, M. (1991). Can buspirone induce rebound, dependence or abuse? *Br. J. Psychiatry*, 159 (Suppl. 12), 45–51.

Laduron, P. M., and Leysen, J. E. (1979). Domperidone, a specific in vitro dopamine antagonist, devoid of in vivo central dopaminergic activity. *Biochem. Pharmacol.*, 28, 2161–2165.

Laferrere, B., Nguyen, M., Bonhomme, G., Legall, A., Basdevant, A., and Guy-Grand, B. (1991). Effect of BIM-18216, a novel cholecystokinin receptor antagonist, on food intake reduction induced by cholecystokinin. *Behav. Neurosci.*, 105, 705–709.

LaHoste, G. J., and Marshall, J. F. (1989). Nonadditivity of D$_2$ receptor proliferation induced by dopamine denervation and chronic selective antagonist administration: Evidence from quantitative autoradiography indicates a single mechanism of action. *Brain Res.*, 502, 223–232.

LaHoste, G. J., and Marshall, J. F. (1992). Dopamine supersensitivity and D$_1$/D$_2$ synergism are unrelated to changes in striatal receptor density. *Synapse*, 12, 14–26.

Lahti, A. C., Koffel, B., LaPorte, D., and Tamminga, C. A. (1995). Subanesthetic doses of ketamine stimulate psychosis in schizophrenia. *Neuropsychopharmacology*, 13, 9–19.

Lal, H. (1977). *Discriminative Stimulus Properties of Drugs*. Plenum Press, New York.

Lal, H., Gianutsos, G., and Miksic, S. (1977). Discriminable stimuli produced by narcotic analgesics. In *Discriminative Stimulus Properties of Drugs* (H. Lal, Ed.), pp. 23–47. Plenum Press, New York.

Lam, R. W., Zis, A. P., Grewal, A., Delgado, P. L. Charney, D. S., and Krystal, J. H. (1996). Effects of rapid tryptophan depletion in patients with seasonal affective disorder in remission after light therapy. *Arch. Gen. Psychiatry, 53*, 41–44.

Lam, W., Sze, P. C., Sacks, H. S. et al., (1987). Meta-analysis of randomized controlled trials of nicotine chewing gum. *Lancet, 2*, 27–30

Lamb, R. J., and Griffiths, R. R. (1987). Self-injection of *d,l*-3,4-methylenedioxymethamphetamine (MDMA) in the baboon. *Psychopharmacology, 91*, 268–272.

Lambert, J. J., Belelli, D., Hill-Venning, C., and Peters, J. A. (1995). Neurosteroids and GABA$_A$ receptor function. *Trends Pharmacol. Sci., 16*, 295–303.

Lambrecht, G., Moser, U., Grimm, U., Pfaff, O., Hermanni, U., Hildebrandt, C., Waelbroeck, M., Christophe, J., and Mutschler, E. (1993). New functionally selective muscarinic agonists. *Life Sci., 52*, 481–488.

Lamy, P. P. (1994). The role of cholinesterase inhibitors in Alzheimer's disease. *CNS Drugs, 1*, 146–165.

Landfield, P. W., Cadwallader, L. B., and Vinsant, S. (1988). Quantitative changes in hippocampal structure following long-term exposure to Δ^9-tetrahydrocannabinol: Possible mediation by glucocorticoid systems. *Brain Res., 443*, 47–62.

Landis, S. C. (1990). Target regulation of neurotransmitter phenotype. *Trends Neurosci., 13*, 344–350.

Landmann, R. (1992). Beta-adrenergic receptors in human leukocyte subpopulations. *Eur. J. Clin. Invest., 22* (Suppl. 1), 30–36.

Lands, A. M., Arnold, A., McAuliff, J. P., Luduena, F. P., and Brown, T. G. Jr. (1967). Differentiation of receptor systems activated by sympathomimetic amines. *Nature, 214*, 597–598.

Lang, J., and Costa, T. (1989). Chronic exposure of NG 108–15 cells to opiate agonists does not alter the amount of the guanine nucleotide-binding proteins G$_i$ and G$_o$. *J. Neurochem., 53*, 1500–1506.

Lange, W., and Krueger, G. von. (1932). Über Ester der Monoflurophosphosäure. *Berl. Dtsch. Chem. Ges., 65*, 1598–1601.

Langer, S. Z. (1974). Presynaptic regulation of catecholamine release. *Biochem. Pharmacol.,* 1793–1800.

Langer, S. Z. (1987). Presynaptic regulation of monoaminergic neurons. In *Psychopharmacology: The Third Generation of Progress* (H. Y. Meltzer, Ed.), pp. 151–158, Raven Press, New York.

Langer, S. Z., Adler, E., Enero, M. A., and Stefano, F. J. E. (1971). The role of the alpha receptor in regulating noradrenaline overflow by nerve stimulation. Proceedings of the 25th International Congress of the International of Physiological Science, Munich, 335.

Langer, S. Z., and Arbilla, S. (1984). The amphetamine paradox in dopaminergic neurotransmission. *Trends Biochem. Sci., 9*, 387–390.

Langer, S. Z., and Arbilla, S. (1990). Presynaptic receptors on peripheral noradrenergic neurons. *Ann. N.Y. Acad. Sci., 604*, 7–16.

Langley, J. N. (1906). On nerve endings and on special excitable substances in cells. *Proc. R. Soc. Lond. B, 78*, 170–194.

Langley, J. N. (1921). *The Autonomic Nervous System.* Cambridge University Press, London.

Langrod, J., Brill, L., Lowinson, J., and Joseph, H. (1972). Methadone maintenance from research to treatment. In *Major Modalities in the Treatment of Drug Abuse* (L. Brill and L. Lieberman, Eds.), pp. 107–141. Behavioral Publications, New York.

Langston, J. W. (1990a). Predicting Parkinson's disease. *Neurology, 40* (Suppl. 3), 70–74.

Langston, J. W. (1990b). Selegiline as neuroprotective therapy in Parkinson's disease: Concepts and controversies. *Neurology, 40* (Suppl. 3), 61–66.

Langston, J. W., Ballard, P., Tetrud, J. W., and Irwin, I. (1983). Chronic parkinsonism in humans due to a product of meperidine-analog synthesis. *Science, 219*, 979–980.

Langston, J. W., Forno, L. S., Rebert, C. S., and Irwin, I. (1984). Selective nigral toxicity after systemic administration of 1-methyl-4-phenyl-1,2,5,6-tetrahydropyridine (MPTP) in the squirrel monkey. *Brain Res., 292*, 390–394.

Langston, J. W., and Irwin, I. (1986). MPTP: Current concepts and controversies. *Clin. Neuropharmacol., 9*, 485–507.

Langston, J. W., and Palfreman, J. (1995). *The Case of the Frozen Addicts.* Pantheon Books, New York.

Largent, B. L., Gundlach, A. L., and Snyder, S. H. (1986). Pharmacological and autoradiographic discrimination of *sigma* and phencyclidine receptor binding sites in brain with (–)-[^{3}H]SKF 10,047, (–)-[^{3}H]-3-[3-hydroxyphenyl]-N-(1-propyl)piperidine and [^{3}H]-1-[1-(2-thienyl)cyclohexyl]piperidine. *J. Pharmacol. Exp. Ther., 238*, 739–748.

Largis, E. E., Burns, M. G., Muenkel, H. A., Dolan, J. A., and Claus, T. H. (1994). Antidiabetic and antiobesity effects of a highly selective β$_3$-adrenocepter agonist (CL 316,-243). *Drug Dev. Res., 32*, 69–76.

Lasagna, L., Mosteller, F., von Felsinger, J. M., and Beecher, H. K. (1954). A study of the placebo response. *Am. J. Med., 16*, 770–779.

Lasek, R. J. (1980). *Trends Neurosci., 3*, 87.

Lasek, R. J., Gainer, H., and Barker, J. L. (1977). Cell-to-cell transfer of glial proteins to the squid giant axon. *J. Cell Biol., 74*, 501–523.

Lashley, K. S. (1950). In search of the engram. *Symp. Soc. Exp. Biol., 4*, 454–482.

László, F. A., László, F. A. Jr., and De Wied, D. (1991). Pharmacology and clinical perspectives of vasopressin antagonists. *Pharmacol. Rev., 43*, 73–108.

Laties, V. G., and Weiss, B. (1981). The amphetamine margin in sports. *Fed. Proc., 40*, 2689–2692.

Law, P. Y., Wu, J., Koehler, J. E., and Loh, H. H. (1981). Demonstration and characterization of opiate inhibition of the striatal adenylate cyclase. *J. Neurochem., 36*, 1834–1846.

Lawlor, B. A. (1994). Non-cognitive disturbances in Alzheimer's disease. *Hum. Psychopharmacol., 9*, 393–396.

Lawton, C. L., and Blundell, J. E. (1992). The effect of *d*-fenfluramine on intake of carbohydrate supplements is influenced by the hydration of the test diets. *Behav. Pharmacol., 3*, 517–523.

Lazareno, S., Buckley, N. J., and Roberts, F. F. (1990). Characterization of muscarinic M4

binding sites in rabbit lung, chicken heart, and NG108–15 cells. *Mol. Pharmacol., 38*, 805–815.

Le, A. D., Khana, J. M., Kalant, H., and Leblanc, A. E. (1981a). The effect of lesions in the dorsal, median and magnus raphe nuclei on the development of tolerance to ethanol. *J. Pharmacol. Exp. Ther., 218*, 525–529.

Le, A. D., Khana, J. M., Kalant, H., and Leblanc, A. E. (1981b). Effect of modification of brain serotonin (5-HT), norepinephrine (NE) and dopamine (DA) on ethanol tolerance. *Psychopharmacology, 75*, 231–235.

Leander, J. D., Rathbun, R. C., and Zimmerman, D. M. (1988). Anticonvulsant effects of phencyclidine-like drugs: Relation to N-methyl-D-aspartic acid antagonism. *Brain. Res., 454*, 368–372.

Leander, J. D., Zerbe, R. L., and Hart, J. C. (1985). Diuresis and suppression of vasopressin by kappa opioids: Comparison with mu and delta opioids and clonidine. *J. Pharmacol. Exper. Ther., 234*, 463–469.

Leanza, G., Nilsson, O. G., Wiley, R. G., and Björklund, A. (1995). Selective lesioning of the basal forebrain cholinergic system by intraventricular 192 IgG-saporin: Behavioural, biochemical and stereological studies in the rat. *Eur. J. Neurosci., 7*, 329–343.

Lear, J. (1986). Principles of single and multiple radionuclide autoradiography. In *Positron Emission Tomography and Autoradiography: Principles and Applications for the Brain and Heart* (M. Phelps, J. Mazziotta, and H. Schelbert, Eds.), pp. 197–235. Raven Press, New York.

Leathwood, P. D. (1987). Tryptophan availability and serotonin synthesis. *Proc. Nutr. Soc., 46*, 143–156.

Lebel, L. A., and Koe, B. K. (1992). Binding studies with the 5-H$_{1B}$ receptor agonist [^{3}H]CP-96,501 in brain tissues. *Drug Dev. Res., 27*, 253–264.

Le Blanc, A. E., Lalant, H., and Gibbins, R. J. (1975). Acute tolerance to ethanol in the rat. *Psychopharmacologia, 41*, 43–46.

Leccese, A. P., and Lyness, W. H. (1984). The effects of putative 5-hydroxytryptamine receptor active agents on D-amphetamine self-administration in controls and rats with 5,7-dihydroxytryptamine median forebrain bundle lesions. *Brain Res., 303*, 153–162.

Lechan, R. M., and Segerson, T. P. (1989). Pro-TRH gene expression and precursor peptides in rat brain: Observations by hybridization analysis and immunocytochemistry. *Ann. N.Y. Acad. Sci., 553*, 29–59.

LeDoux, J. E. (1993). Emotional memory systems in the brain. *Behav. Brain Res., 58*, 69–79.

Lee, C. Y. (1972). Chemistry and pharmacology of polypeptide toxins in snake venoms. *Annu. Rev. Pharmacol., 12*, 265–286.

Lee, C. Y., Tseng, L. F., and Chiu, T. H. (1967). Influence of denervation on localization of neurotoxins from clopid venoms in rat diaphragm. *Nature, 215*, 1177–1178.

Lee, R. G. (1987). The pathophysiology of essential tremor. In *Movement Disorders 2* (C. D. Marsden and S. Fahn, Eds.), pp. 423–437. Butterworths, London.

Lee, S. L., Sevarino, K., Roos, B. A., and Goodman, R. H. (1989). Characterization and expression of the gene encoding rat thyrotropin-releasing hormone (TRH). *Ann. N.Y. Acad. Sci.*, 553, 14–28.

Lee, T. P., Kuo, J. F., and Greengard, P. (1972). Role of muscarinic cholinergic receptors in regulation of guanosine 3′,5′-cyclic monophosphate content in mammalian brain, heart muscle, and intestinal smooth muscle. *Proc. Natl. Acad. Sci. U.S.A.*, 69, 3287–3291.

Leeb-Lundberg, F., Snowman, A., and Olsen, R. W. (1980). Barbiturate receptor sites are coupled to benzodiazepine receptors. *Proc. Natl. Acad. Sci. U.S.A.*, 77, 7468–7472.

Lefebvre, D. L., Giaid, A., Bennett, H., Larivière, R., and Zingg, H. H. (1992). Oxytocin gene expression in rat uterus. *Science*, 256, 1553–1555.

Lefkowitz, R. J., Hausdorff, W. P., and Caron, M. G. (1990). Role of phosphorylation in desensitization of the β-adrenoceptor. *Trends Pharmacol. Sci.*, 11, 190–194.

Leibowitz, S. F. (1974a). Adrenergic receptor mechanisms in eating and drinking. In *The Neurosciences: Third Study Program* (F. O. Schmitt and F. G. Worden, Eds.), pp. 713–719. MIT Press, Cambridge, MA.

Leibowitz, S. F. (1974b). Norepinephrine-elicited eating: Involvement of neuroendocrine systems of the paraventricular nucleus. *Soc. Neurosci. Abstr.*, 301.

Leibowitz, S. F. (1978). Paraventricular nucleus: A primary site mediating adrenergic stimulation of feeding and drinking. *Pharmacol. Biochem. Behav.*, 8, 163–175.

Leibowitz, S. F. (1986). Brain monoamines and peptides: Role in the control of eating behavior. *Fed. Proc.*, 45, 1396–1403.

Leibowitz, S. F. (1992). Neurochemical–neuroendocrine systems in the brain controlling macronutrient intake and metabolism. *Trends Neurosci.*, 15, 491–497.

Leibowitz, S. F., and Shor-Posner, G. (1986). Brain serotonin and eating behavior. *Appetite*, 7 (Suppl.), 1–14.

Leibowitz, S. F., Weiss, G. F., and Suh, J. S. (1990). Medial hypothalamic nuclei mediate serotonin's inhibitory effect on feeding behavior. *Pharmacol. Biochem. Behav.*, 37, 735–742.

Leichter, J. (1989). Growth of fetuses of rats exposed to ethanol and cigarette smoke during gestation. *Growth Dev. Aging*, 129–134.

Lejoyeux, M., Adès, J., and Rouillon, F. (1994). Serotonin syndrome: Incidence, symptoms and treatment. *CNS Drugs*, 2, 132–143.

Lembeck, F. (1953). Zur Frage der zentralen Übertragung afferenter Impulse. III. Mitteilung. Das Vorkommen und die Bedeutung der Substanz P in den dorsalen Wurzeln des Rückenmarks. *Arch. Exp. Pathol. Pharmakol.*, 219, 197–213.

Lemberger, L. (1980). Potential therapeutic usefulness of marijuana. *Annu. Rev. Pharmacol. Toxicol.*, 20, 151–172.

Lemberger, L., Fuller, R. W., and Zerbe, R. L. (1985). Use of specific serotonin uptake inhibitors as antidepressants. *Clin. Neuropharmacol.*, 8, 299–317.

Lemke, G. (1992a). Gene regulation in the nervous system. In *An Introduction to Molecular Neurobiology* (Z. W. Hall, Ed.), pp. 313–354. Sinauer Associates, Sunderland, MA.

Lemke, G. (1992b). Myelin and myelination. In *An Introduction to Molecular Neurobiology* (Z. W. Hall, Ed.), pp. 281–309. Sinauer Associates, Sunderland, MA.

Léna, C., and Changeux, J.-P. (1993). Allosteric modulations of the nicotinic acetylcholine receptor. *Trends Neurosci.*, 16, 181–186.

Lennard, H. L., Epstein, L. J., and Rosenthal, M. S. (1972). The methadone illusion. *Science*, 176, 881–884.

Leonard, B. E. (1992). *Fundamentals of Psychopharmacology*. Wiley, New York.

Leonard, B. E. (1994). Effects of antidepressants on specific neurotransmitters: Are such effects relevant to the therapeutic action? In *Handbook of Depression and Anxiety* (J. A. den Boer and J. M. Ad Sitsen, Eds.), pp. 379–404. Marcel Dekker, New York.

Lesch, K.-P., Wolozin, B. L., Estler, H. C., Murphy, D. L., and Riederer, P. (1993). Isolation of a cDNA encoding the human brain serotonin transporter. *J. Neural Transm. Gen. Sect.*, 91, 67–72.

Lesch, K.-P., Wolozin, B. L., Murphy, D. L., and Riederer, P. (1993). Primary structure of the human platelet serotonin uptake site: Identity with the brain serotonin transporter. *J. Neurochem.*, 60, 2319–2322.

Lester, B. M., Corwin, M. J., Sepkoski, C., Seifer, R., Peucker, M., McLaughlin, S., and Golub, H. L. (1991). Neurobehavioral syndromes in cocaine-exposed newborn infants. *Child Dev.*, 62, 694–705.

Levenson, T. (1995). Accounting for taste. *The Sciences*, January/February, 13–15.

Lévesque, D., et al. (1992). Identification, characterization, and localization of the dopamine D_3 receptor in rat brain using 7-[H]-hydroxy-N,N,-di-n-propyl-2-aminotetralin. *Proc. Natl. Acad. Sci. U.S.A.*, 89, 8155–8159.

Levey, A. I., Kitt, C. A., Simonds, W. F., Price, D. L., and Brann, M. R. (1991). Identification and localization of muscarinic acetylcholine receptor proteins in brain with subtype-specific antibodies. *J. Neurosci.*, 11, 3218–3226.

Levi, G., and Raiteri, M. (1993). Carrier-mediated release of neurotransmitters. *Trends Neurosci.*, 16, 415–419.

Levi-Montalcini, R. (1987). The nerve growth factor 35 years later. *Science*, 237, 1154–1162.

Leviel, V., Gobert, A., and Guibert, B. (1989). Direct observation of dopamine compartmentation in striatal nerve terminal by "in vivo" measurement of the specific activity of released dopamine. *Brain Res.*, 499, 205–213.

Leviel, V., Gobert, A., and Guibert, B. (1990). The glutamate-mediated release of dopamine in the rat striatum: Further characterization of the dual excitatory-inhibitory function. *Neuroscience*, 39, 305–312.

Levin, E. D. (1992). Nicotinic systems and cognitive function. *Psychopharmacology*, 108, 417–431.

Levin, F. R., and Lehman, A. F. (1991). Meta-analysis of desipramine as an adjunct in the treatment of cocaine addiction. *J. Clin. Psychopharmacol.*, 11, 374–378.

Levine, R. R. (1983). *Pharmacology: Drug Actions and Reactions* (3rd ed.). Little, Brown, Boston.

Levitan, I. B. (1994). Modulation of ion channels by protein phosphorylation and dephosphorylation. *Annu. Rev. Physiol.*, 56, 193–212.

Levitt, P., Pintar, J. E., and Breakefield, X. O. (1982). Immunocytochemical demonstration of monoamine oxidase B in brain astro-

cytes and serotonergic neurons. *Proc. Natl. Acad. Sci. U.S.A.*, 79, 6385–6389.

Levitzki, A. (1988). From epinephrine to cyclic AMP. *Science*, 241, 800–806.

Levy-Lahad, E., et al. (1995). Candidate gene for the chromosome 1 familial Alzheimer's disease locus. *Science*, 269, 973–977.

Lewander, T. (1971). A mechanism for the development of tolerance in rats. *Psychopharmacologia*, 21, 17–31.

Lewander, T. (1994). Overcoming the neuroleptic-induced deficit syndrome: Clinical observations with remoxipride. *Acta Psychiatrica Scand.*, 380 (Suppl.), 64–67.

Lewine, R. R., Risch, S. C., Risby, E., Stipetic, M., Jewart, R. D., Eccard, M., Caudle, J., and Pollard, W. (1991). Lateral ventricle-brain ratio and balance between CSF HVA and 5-HIAA in schizophrenia. *Am. J. Psychiatry*, 148, 1189–1194.

Lewis, E. J., and Asnani, L. P. (1992). Soluble and membrane-bound forms of dopamine β-hydroxylase are encoded by the same mRNA. *J. Biol. Chem.*, 267, 494–500.

Lewis, E. J., Tank, A. W., Weiner, N., and Chikaraishi, D. M. (1983). Regulation of tyrosine hydroxylase mRNA by glucocorticoid and cyclic AMP in a rat pheochromocytoma cell line. *J. Biol. Chem.*, 258, 14632–14637.

Lewis, M. J., and June, H. L. (1990). Neurobehavioral studies of ethanol reward and activation. *Alcohol*, 7, 213–219.

Lewis, P. R., and Shute, C. C. D. (1978). Cholinergic pathways in CNS. In *Handbook of Psychopharmacology*, Vol. 9 (L. L. Iversen, S. D. Iversen, and S. D. Snyder, Eds.), pp. 315–355. Plenum Press, New York.

Lewy, A. J., and Sack, R. L. (1990). The use of light therapy in the treatment of depression. In *Pharmacotherapy of Depression* (J. D. Amsterdam, Ed.), pp. 185–199. Marcel Dekker, New York.

Leysen, J. E. (1990). Gaps and peculiarities in 5-HT_2 receptor studies. *Neuropsychopharmacology*, 3, 361–369.

Li, C. H., and Chung, D. (1976). Isolation and structure of an untriakontapeptide with opiate activity from camel pituitary glands. *Proc. Natl. Acad. Sci. U.S.A.*, 73, 1145–1148.

Li, H. (1975). The origin and use of cannabis in eastern Asia. In *Cannabis and Culture* (V. Rubin, Ed.), pp. 51–62. Mouton, The Hague.

Li, M., Yasuda, R. P., Wall, S. J., Wellstein, A., and Wolfe, B. B. (1991). Distribution of m2 muscarinic receptors in rat brain using antisera selective for m2 receptors. *Mol. Pharmacol.*, 40, 28–35.

Li, P. P., Warsh, J. J., and Godse, D. D. (1983). Rat brain norepinephrine metabolism: Substantial clearance through 3,4-dhydroxyphenylethyleneglycol formation. *J. Neurochem.*, 41, 1065–1071.

Li, T. K. (1986). Animal studies in the genetics of alcoholism. *Alcohol. Clin. Exp. Res.*, 9, 475–492.

Liang, N. Y., and Rutledge, C. O. (1982). Comparison of the release of [^{3}H]dopamine from isolated corpus striatum by amphetamine, fenfluramine and unlabelled dopamine. *Biochem. Pharmacol.*, 31, 983–992.

Liao, D., Hessler, N. A., and Malinow, R. (1995). Activation of postsynaptically silent synapses during pairing-induced LTP in CA1 region of hippocampal slice. *Nature*, 375, 400–404.

Liao, D., Jones, A., and Malinow, R. (1992). Direct measurement of quantal changes underlying long-term potentiation in CA1 hippocampus. *Neuron*, 9, 1089–1097.

Libet, B. (1992). Introduction to slow synaptic potentials and their neuromodulation by dopamine. *Can. J. Physiol. Pharmacol.*, 70, S3–S11.

Licata, A., Taylor, S., Berman, M., and Cranston, J. (1993). Effects of cocaine on human aggression. *Pharmacol. Biochem. Behav.*, 45, 549–552.

Lidberg, L., Tuck, J. R., Åsberg, M., Scalia-Tomba, G. P., and Bertilsson, L. (1985). *Acta Psychiatr. Scand.*, 71, 230–236.

Liddle, R. A. (1994). Cholecystokinin. In *Gut Peptides: Biochemistry and Physiology* (J. H. Walsh and G. J. Dockray, Eds.), pp. 175–216. Raven Press, New York.

Lidsky, T. I. (1995). Reevaluation of the mesolimbic hypothesis of antipsychotic drug action. *Schizophr. Bull.*, 21, 67–74.

Lieberman, J. A. (1994). Clinical biological studies of atypical antipsychotics: Focus on the serotonin/dopamine systems. *J. Clin. Psychiatry*, 12, 24–28.

Lieberman, L., and Brill, L. (1972). Rational authority. In *Major Modalities in the Treatment of Drug Abuse* (L. Brill and L. Lieberman, Eds.), pp. 67–84. Behavioral Publications, New York.

Liester, M. B., Grob, C. S., Bravo, G. L., and Walsh, R. N. (1992). Phenomenology and sequelae of 3,4-methylenedioxymethamphetamine use. *J. Nerv. Ment. Dis.*, 180, 345–352.

Lightman, S. L., and Young, W. S. III (1987). Vasopressin, oxytocin, dynorphin, enkephalin and corticotrophin-releasing factor mRNA stimulation in the rat. *J. Physiol.* (Lond.), 394, 23–39.

Limbird, L. E. (1986). *Cell Surface Receptors: A Short Course on Theory and Methods.* Martinus Nijhoff Publishing, Boston.

Lin, J.-S., Fort, P., Kitahama, K., Panula, P., Denney, R. M., and Jouvet, M. (1991). Immunochemical evidence for the presence of type B monoamine oxidase in histamine-containing neurons in the posterior hypothalamus of cats. *Neurosci. Lett.*, 128, 61–65.

Lin, J.-S., Sakai, K., and Jouvet, M. (1988). Evidence for histaminergic arousal mechanisms in the hypothalamus of cat. *Neuropharmacology*, 27, 111–122.

Lin, J.-S., Sakai, K., Vanni-Mercier, G., Arrang, J.-M., Garbarg, M., Schwartz, J.-C., and Jouvet, M. (1990). Involvement of histaminergic neurons in arousal mechanisms demonstrated with H3–receptor ligands in the cat. *Brain Res.*, 523, 325–330.

Lincoln, T. M., and Cornwell, T. L. (1993). Intracellular cyclic GMP receptor proteins. *FASEB J.*, 7, 328–338.

Lindberg, I. (1991). The new eukaryotic precursor processing proteinases. *Mol. Endocrinol.*, 5, 1361–1365.

Linden, D. J. (1994). Long-term synaptic depression in the mammalian brain. *Neuron*, 12, 457–472.

Linden, J. (1994). Cloned adenosine A3 receptors: Pharmacological properties, species differences and receptor functions. *Trends Pharmacol. Sci.*, 15, 298–306.

Lindenmayer, J-P. (1994). Risperidone: Efficacy and side effects. *J.Clin. Psychiatry*, 12, 53–58.

Linder, R. L., Lerner, S. E., and Burns, R. S. (1981). *PCP: The Devil's Dust.* Wadsworth Publishing Co., Belmont, CA.

Lindsay, R. M., Wiegand, S. J., Altar, C. A., and DiStefano, P. S. (1994). Neurotrophic factors: From molecule to man. *Trends Neurosci.*, 17, 182–190.

Lindvall, O., and Björklund, A. (1974a). The glyoxylic acid fluorescence method: A detailed account of the methodology for the visualization of central catecholamine neurons. *Histochemistry*, 39, 97–127.

Lindvall, O., and Björklund, A. (1974b). The organization of the ascending catecholamine neuron systems in the rat brain as revealed by the glyoxylic acid fluorescence method. *Acta Physiol. Scand. Suppl.*, 412, 1–48.

Lindvall, O., and Björklund, A. (1983). Dopamine and norepinephrine containing neuron systems: Their anatomy in the rat brain. In *Chemical Neuroanatomy* (P. C. Emson, Ed.), pp. 229–255. Raven Press, New York.

Lindvall, O., and Bjorklund, A. (1987). Localization of monoamines by aldehyde-induced fluorescence in the central nervous system. In *Monoaminergic Neurons: Light Microscopy and Ultrastructure* (H. W. M. Steinbusch, Ed.), pp. 27–78. Wiley, New York.

Lindvall, O., et al. (1989). Human fetal dopamine neurons grafted into the striatum in two patients with severe Parkinson's disease. A detailed account of methodology and a 6-month follow-up. *Arch. Neurol.*, 46, 615–631.

Ling, G. S. F., MacLeod, J. M., Lee, S., Lockhart, S. H., and Pasternak, G. W. (1984). Separation of morphine analgesia from physical dependence. *Science*, 226, 462–464.

Lingjærde, O. (1990). Blood platelets as a model system for studying serotonergic dysfunction and effects of antidepressants. *Pharmacol. Toxicol.*, 66 (Suppl. 3), 61–68.

Linnoila, M., Virkkunen, M., George, T., and Higley, D. (1993). Impulse control disorders. *Int. Clin. Psychopharmacol.*, 8 (Suppl. 1), 53–56.

Lippa, A. S., Meyerson, L. R., and Beer, B. (1982). Molecular substrates of anxiety: Clues from the heterogeneity of benzodiazepine receptors. *Life Sci.*, 31, 1409–1417.

Lipper, S., and Kornetsky, C. (1971). Effect of chlorpromazine on conditional avoidance as a function of CS-US interval length. *Psychopharmacologia*, 22, 144–150.

Lipton, S. A., and Rosenberg, P. A. (1994). Excitatory amino acids as a final common pathway for neurologic disorders. *N. Engl. J. Med.*, 330, 613–622.

Liska, K. (1986). *Drugs and the Human Body.* Macmillan, New York.

Littleton, J. T., and Bellen, H. J. (1995). Synaptotagmin controls and modulates synaptic-vesicle fusion in a Ca^{2+}-dependent manner. *Trends Neurosci.*, 18, 177–183.

Liu, J., Nickolenko, J., and Sharp, F. R. (1994). Morphine induces *c-fos* and *junB* in striatum and nucleus accumbens via D1 and N-methyl-D-aspartate receptors. *Proc. Natl. Acad. Sci. U.S.A.*, 91, 8537–8541.

Liu, Q.-R., López-Corcuera, B., Mandiyan, S., Nelson, H., and Nelson, N. (1993). Cloning and expression of a spinal cord- and brain-specific glycine transporter with novel structural features. *J. Biol. Chem.*, 268, 22802–22808.

Liu, Y., Peter, D., Roghani, A., Schuldiner, S., Prive, G. G., Eisenberg, D., Brecha, N., and Edwards, R. H. (1992). A cDNA that suppresses MPP+ toxicity encodes a vesicular amine transporter. *Cell*, 70, 539–551.

Ljungberg, T., Apicella, P., and Schultz, W. (1992). Responses of monkey dopamine neurons during learning of behavioral reactions. *J. Neurophysiol.*, 67, 145–163.

Llinás, R. R. (1977). Calcium and transmitter release in squid synapse. In *Society for Neuroscience Symposia*, Vol. 2. *Approaches to the Cell Biology of Neurons* (W. M. Cowan and J. A. Ferrendelli, Eds.), pp. 139–160. Society for Neuroscience, Bethesda, MD.

Llinás, R., Sugimori, M., and Silver, R. B. (1992). Microdomains of high calcium concentration in a presynaptic terminal. *Science*, 256, 677–679.

Lloyd, K. G., Bossi, L., Morselli, P. L., Munari, C., Rougier, M., and Loiseau, H. (1986). Alterations of GABA-mediated synaptic transmission in human epilepsy. *Adv. Neurol.*, 44, 1033–1044.

Lloyd, K. G., and Morselli, P. L. (1987). Psychopharmacology of GABAergic drugs. In *Psychopharmacology: The Third Generation of Progress* (H. Y. Meltzer, Ed.), pp. 183–195. Raven Press, New York.

Lodge, D., and Anis, N. A. (1982). Effects of phencyclidine on excitatory amino acid activation of spinal interneurones in the cat. *Eur. J. Pharmacol.*, 77, 203–204.

Lodge, D., and Johnston, G. A. R. (1985). Effect of ketamine on amino acid-evoked release of acetylcholine from rat cerebral cortex in vitro. *Neurosci. Lett.*, 56, 371–375.

Loewenstein, W. R. (1981). Junctional intercellular communication: The cell to cell membrane channel. *Physiol. Rev.*, 61, 829–913.

Loewi, O. (1921). Ueber humorale Uebertragbarkeit der Herznervenwirkung. *Pflügers Arch.*, 189, 239–242.

Löffelholz, K., Klein, J., and Köppen, A. (1993). Choline, a precursor of acetylcholine and phospholipids in the brain. *Prog. Brain Res.*, 98, 197–200.

Lolait, S. J., O'Carroll, A.-M., McBride, O. W., Konig, M., Morel, A., and Brownstein, M. J. (1992). Cloning and characterization of a vasopressin V2 receptor and possible link to nephrogenic diabetes insipidus. *Nature*, 357, 336–339.

London, E. D. (1993). Studies of σ receptors and metabolic responses to σ ligands in the brain. *NIDA Res. Monogr.*, 133, 55–68.

Longoni, R., Spina, L., Mulas, A., Carboni, E., Garau, L., Melchiorri, P., and Di Chiara, G. (1991). (D-Ala2)deltorphin II: D1-dependent stereotypies and stimulation of dopamine release in the nucleus accumbens. *J. Neurosci.* 11: 1565–1576.

Lookingland, K. J., Shannon, N. J., Chapin, D. S., and Moore, K. E. (1986). Exogenous tryptophan increases synthesis, storage, and intraneuronal metabolism of 5-hydroxytryptamine in the rat hypothalamus. *J. Neurochem.*, 47, 205–212.

Loosen, P. T. (1988). TRH: Behavioral and endocrine effects in man. *Prog. Neuropsychopharmacol. Biol. Psychiatry*, 12, S87–S117.

Lorenz, K. (1966). *On Aggression.* Harcourt Brace Jovanovich, New York.

Löscher, W., and Hönack, D. (1992). The behavioural effects of MK-801 in rats: Involvement of dopaminergic, serotonergic and noradrenergic systems. *Eur. J. Pharmacol.*, 215, 199–208.

Lotsof, H. (1986). Rapid Method for Interrupting the Cocaine and Amphetamine Abuse

Syndrome. Patent No. 4,587,243, U.S. Patent Office.

Loughlin, S. E., Massamiri, T. R., Kornblum, H. I., and Leslie, F. M. (1985). Postnatal development of opioid systems in rat brain. *Neuropeptides,* 5, 469–472.

Louie, A. K., Law, P.-Y., and Loh, H. H. (1985). Molecular mechanisms of opiate tolerance and dependence in a clonal cell line. *NIDA Res. Monogr.,* 62, 117–128.

Lovenberg, T. W., Erlander, M. G., Baron, B. M., Racke, M., Slone, A. L., Siegel, B. W., Craft, C. M., Burns, J. E., Danielson, P. E., and Sutcliffe, J. G. (1993). Molecular cloning and functional expression of 5-HT$_{1E}$-like rat and human 5-hydroxytryptamine receptor genes. *Proc. Natl. Acad. Sci. U.S.A.,* 90, 2184–2188.

Lovenberg, W., Bruckwick, E. A., Alexander, R. W., Horwitz, D., and Keiser, H. R. (1974). Evaluation of serum dopamine-β-hydroxylase activity as an index of sympathetic nervous activity in man. *Adv. Biochem. Psychopharmacol.,* 12, 121–128.

Luby, E. D., Cohen, B. D., Rosenbaum, G., Gottlieb, J. S., and Kelley, R. (1959). Study of a new schizophrenomimetic drug—Sernyl. *Arch. Neurol. Psychiatry,* 81, 363–369.

Lucas, D. R., and Newhouse, J. P. (1957). The toxic effect of sodium L-glutamate on the inner layers of the retina. *Arch. Ophthalmol.,* 58, 193–201.

Lucas, S. E., and Griffiths, R. R. (1982). Precipitated withdrawal by a benzodiazepine antagonist (Ro 15 1788) after 7 days of diazepam. *Science,* 217, 1161–1163.

Lucki, I. (1992). 5-HT$_1$ receptors and behavior. *Neurosci. Biobehav. Rev.,* 16, 83–93.

Lucki, I., and Frazer, A. (1981). Prevention of the serotonin syndrome by repeated administration of monoamine oxidase inhibitors but not tricyclic antidepressants. *Psychopharmacology,* 205, 205–211.

Lucki, I., and Harvey, J. A. (1979). Increased sensitivity to *d*- and *l*-amphetamine action after midbrain raphe lesions as measured by locomotor activity. *Neuropharmacology,* 18, 243–249.

Lucki, I., and Wieland, S. (1990). 5-hydroxytryptamine$_{1A}$ receptors and behavioral responses. *Neuropsychopharmacology,* 3, 481–493.

Luckman, S. M., Antonijevic, I., Leng, G., Dye, S., Douglas, A. J., Russell, J. A., and Bicknell, R. J. (1993). The maintenance of normal parturition in the rat requires neurohypophysial oxytocin. *J. Neuroendocrinol.,* 5, 7–12.

Lüddens, H., Korpi, E. R., and Seeburg, P. H. (1995). GABA$_A$/benzodiazepine receptor heterogeneity: Neurophysiological implications. *Neuropharmacology,* 34, 245–254.

Lüddens, H., Pritchett, D. B., Köhler, M., Killisch, I., Keinänen, K., Monyer, H., Sprengel, R., and Seeburg, P. H. (1990). Cerebellar GABA$_A$ receptor selective for a behavioural alcohol antagonist. *Nature,* 346, 648–651.

Ludwig, B. J., and Piech, E. C. (1951). Some anticonvulsant agents derived from 1, 3 propanediols. *J. Am. Chem. Soc.,* 73, 5779–5781.

Luetje, C. W., Patrick, J., and Séguéla, P. (1990). Nicotine receptors in the mammalian brain. *FASEB J.,* 4, 2753–2760.

Luisada, P. V. (1978). The phencyclidine psychosis: Phenomenology and treatment. *NIDA Res. Monogr.,* 21, 241–253.

Lukas, S. E., Griffiths, R. R., Brady, J. V., and Wurster, R. M. (1984). Phencyclidine-analogue self-injection by the baboon. *Psychopharmacology,* 83, 316–320.

Lundberg, J. M., and Hökfelt, T. (1983). Coexistence of peptides and classical neurotransmitters. *Trends Neurosci.,* 6, 325–333.

Lundeen, J. E., and Gordon, J. H. (1986). Computer analysis of binding data. In *Receptor Binding in Drug Research* (R. A. O'Brien, Ed.), pp. 31–49. Marcel Dekker, New York.

Lundquist, F. (1971). The metabolism of alcohol. In *Biological Basis of Alcoholism* (Y. Israel and J. Mardones, Eds.), pp. 1–52. Wiley, New York.

Luo, S., and Li, E. T. S. (1992). Effect of 5-HT agonists on rats fed single diets with varying proportions of carbohydrate and protein. *Psychopharmacology,* 109, 212–216.

Luque, J. M., Nelson, N., and Richards, J. G. (1995). Cellular expression of glycine transporter 2 messenger RNA exclusively in rat hindbrain and spinal cord. *Neuroscience,* 64, 525–535.

Lyon, M., and Robbins, T. W. (1975). The action of central nervous system stimulant drugs: A general theory concerning amphetamine effects. In *Current Developments in Psychopharmacology,* Volume 2 (W. Essman and L. Valzelli, Eds.), pp. 79–163. Spectrum Publications, New York.

MacCrae, J. R., Scoles, M. T., and Siegel, S. (1987). The contribution of Pavlovian conditioning to drug tolerance and dependence. *Br. J. Addict.,* 82, 371–380.

Macdonald, R., and Barker, J. L. (1978a). Benzodiazepines specifically modulate GABA-mediated postsynaptic inhibition in cultured mammalian neurones. *Nature,* 271, 563–564.

MacDonald, R. L., and Barker, J. L. (1978b). Specific antagonism of GABA-mediated post-synaptic inhibition in cultured mammalian spinal cord neurons: A common mode of convulsant action. *Neurology,* 28, 325–330.

Macdonald, R. L., and Kelly, K. M. (1994). Mechanisms of action of currently prescribed and newly developed antiepileptic drugs. *Epilepsia,* 35 (Suppl. 4), S41–S50.

Macdonald, R. L., and Olsen, R. W. (1994). GABA$_A$ receptor channels. *Annu. Rev. Neurosci.,* 17, 569–602.

Macdonald, R. L., Twyman, R. E., Rogers, C. J., and Weddle, M. G. (1988). Pentobarbital regulation of the kinetic properties of GABA receptor chloride channels. In *Chloride Channels and Their Modulation by Neurotransmitters and Drugs* (G. Biggio and E. Costa, Eds.), pp. 61–71. Raven Press, New York.

Machida, C. A., Bunzow, J. R., Searles, R. P., Van Tol, H., Tester, B., Neve, K. A., Teal, P., Nipper, V., and Civelli, O. (1990). Molecular cloning and expression of the rat β$_1$-adrenergic receptor gene. *J. Biol. Chem.,* 265, 12960–12965.

Maciewicz, R., Phipps, B. S., Grenier, J., and Poletti, C. E. (1984). Edinger-Westphal nucleus: Cholecystokinin immunocytochemistry and projections to spinal cord and trigeminal nucleus in the cat. *Brain Res.,* 299, 139–145.

MacIntosh, F. C. (1941). Distribution of acetylcholine in peripheral and central nervous system. *J. Physiol.* (Lond.), 99, 436–442.

MacIntosh, F. C., and Oborin, P. E. (1953). Release of acetylcholine from intact cerebral cortex. *Abstr. 19th Int. Physiol. Congr.,* 580–581.

Mack, F., and Bönisch, H. (1979). Dissociation constants and lipophilicity of catecholamines and related compounds. *Naunyn Schmiedebergs Arch. Pharmacol.,* 310, 1–9.

Mackay, A. V. P., Iversen, L. L., Lassor, M., Spokes, E., Bird, E., Arregui, A., Creese, I., and Snyder, S. (1982). Increased brain dopamine and dopamine receptors in schizophrenia. *Arch. Gen. Psychiatry,* 39, 991–997.

Mackay, C. J., Cox, T., Burrows, G., and Lazzerini, T. (1978). An inventory for the measurement of self-reported stress and arousal. *Br. J. Clin. Psychol.,* 17, 283–284.

Mackie, K., and Hille, B. (1992). Cannabinoids inhibit N-type calcium channels in neuroblastoma-glioma cells. *Proc. Natl. Acad. Sci. U.S.A.,* 89, 3825–3829.

Mackinnon, A., and Mitchell, P. B. (1994). The genetics of anxiety and depression. In *Handbook of Depression and Anxiety* (J. A. den Boer and J. M. Ad Sitsen, Eds.), pp. 71–118. Marcel Dekker, New York.

MacKinnon, R. (1995). Pore loops: An emerging theme in ion channel structure. *Neuron,* 14, 889–892.

Macmillan, F. M., and Cuello, A. C. (1986). Monoclonal antibodies in neurochemistry: The state of the art. In *Neurochemistry: Modern Methods and Applications* (P. Panula, H. Paivarinta, and S. Soinila, Eds.), pp. 49–74. Alan R. Liss, New York.

Macor, J. E., et al. (1990). 3-(1,2,5,6-tetrahydropyrid-4-yl)pyrrolo[3,2,-b]pyrid-5-one: A potent and selective serotonin (5-HT$_{1B}$) agonist and rotationally restricted phenolic analogue of 5-methoxy-3-(1,2,5,6-tetrahydropyrid-4-yl)indole. *J. Med. Chem.,* 33, 2087–2093.

Maddox, V. H. (1981). The historical development of phencyclidine. In *PCP (Phencyclidine): Historical and Current Perspectives* (E. F. Domino, Ed.), pp. 1–8. NPP Books, Ann Arbor.

Maddrell, S. H. P., and Nordmann, J. J. (1979). *Neurosecretion.* Wiley, New York.

Madras, B. K. (1994). ^{11}C-WIN 35,428 for detecting dopamine depletion in mild Parkinson's disease. *Ann. Neurol.,* 35, 376–377.

Madras, B. K., Spealman, R. D., Fahey, M. A., Neumeyer, J. L., Saha, J. K., and Milius, R. A. (1989). Cocaine receptors labeled by [^{3}H]2β-carbomethoxy-3β-(4-fluorophenyl)-tropane. *Mol. Pharmacol.,* 36, 518–524.

Madrazo, I., et al. (1988). Transplantation of fetal substantia nigra and adrenal medulla to the caudate nucleus in two patients with Parkinson's disease. *N. Engl. J. Med.,* 318, 51.

Maes, M., and Meltzer, H. Y. (1995). The serotonin hypothesis of major depression. In *Psychopharmacology: The Fourth Generation of Progress* (F. E. Bloom and D. J. Kupfer, Eds.), pp. 933–944. Raven Press, New York.

Maggi, A., and Enna, S. J. (1980). Regional alterations in rat brain neurotransmitter systems following chronic lithium treatment. *J. Neurochem.,* 34, 888–894.

Maggio, J. E. (1988). Tachykinins. *Annu. Rev. Neurosci.,* 11, 13–28.

Mahan, L. C., Burch, R. M., Monsma, F. J. Jr., and Sibley, D. R. (1990). Expression of striatal D$_1$ dopamine receptors coupled to inositol phosphate production and Ca^{2+} mobilization in *Xenopus* oocytes. *Proc. Natl. Acad. Sci. U.S.A.,* 87, 2196–2200.

Maier, N. R. F. (1949). *Frustration*. McGraw-Hill, New York.

Mailleux, P., and Vanderhaeghen, J.-J. (1992). Distribution of neuronal cannabinoid receptor in the adult rat brain: A comparative receptor binding radioautography and *in situ* hybridization histochemistry. *Neuroscience*, 48, 655–668.

Mailleux, P., and Vanderhaeghen, J.-J. (1993). Dopaminergic regulation of cannabinoid receptor mRNA levels in the rat caudate-putamen: An in situ hybridization study. *J. Neurochem.*, 61, 1705–1712.

Mailleux, P., Verslype, M., Preud'homme, X., and Vanderhaeghen, J.-J. (1994). Activation of multiple transcription factor genes by tetrahydrocannabinol in rat forebrain. *Neuroreport*, 5, 1265–1268.

Maj, J. Rogoz, Z., Skuza, G., and Sowinska, H. (1982). Effects of chronic treatment with antidepressants on aggressiveness induced by clonidine in mice. *J. Neural Trans.*, 55, 19–25.

Majorossy, K., Rethelyi, M., and Szentagothai, J. (1965). The large glomerular synapse of the pulvinar. *J. Hirnforsch.*, 7, 415–432.

Makita, Y., Okuno, S., and Fujisawa, H. (1990). Involvement of activator protein in the activation of tryptophan hydroxylase by cAMP-dependent protein kinase. *FEBS Lett.*, 268, 185–188.

Makriyannis, A., and Rapaka, R. S. (1990). The molecular basis of cannabinoid activity. *Life Sci.*, 47, 2173–2184.

Maldonado, R., Robledo, P., Chover, A. J., Caine, S. B., and Koob, G. F. (1993). D_1 dopamine receptors in the nucleus accumbens modulate cocaine self-administration in the rat. *Pharmacol. Biochem. Behav.*, 45, 239–242.

Maldonado, R., Stinus, L., Gold, L. H., and Koob, G. F. (1992). Role of different brain structures in the expression of the physical morphine withdrawal syndrome. *J. Pharmacol. Exp. Ther.*, 261,669–677.

Malenka, R. C. (1991). Postsynaptic factors control the duration of synaptic enhancement in area CA1 of the hippocampus. *Neuron*, 6, 53–60.

Malenka, R. C. (1995). LTP and LTD: Dynamic and interactive processes of synaptic plasticity. *The Neuroscientist*, 1, 35–42.

Malenka, R. C., Kauer, J. A., Perkel, D. J., Mauk, M. D., Kelly, P. T., Nicoll, R. A., and Waxham, M. N. (1989). An essential role for postsynaptic calmodulin and protein kinase activity in long-term potentiation. *Nature*, 340, 554–557.

Malenka, R. C., and Nicoll, R. A. (1993). NMDA-receptor-dependent synaptic plasticity: Multiple forms and mechanisms. *Trends Neurosci.*, 16, 521–527.

Maley, B. E., Engle, M. G., Humphreys, S., Vascik, D. A., Howes, K. A., Newton, B. W., and Elde, R. P. (1990). Monoamine synaptic structure and localization in the central nervous system. *J. Electron Microsc. Tech.*, 15, 20–33.

Malgouris, C., Flamand, F., and Doble, A. (1993). Autoradiographic studies of RP 62203, a potent 5-HT$_2$ receptor antagonist: Pharmacological characterization of [^{3}H]RP 62203 binding in the rat brain. *Eur. J. Pharmacol.*, 233, 37–45.

Malinow, R. (1994). LTP: Desperately seeking resolution. *Science,* 266, 1195–1196.

Malinow, R., Schulman, H., and Tsien, R. W. (1989). Inhibition of postsynaptic PKC or CaMKII blocks induction but not expression of LTP. *Science*, 245, 862–866.

Malosio, M.-L., Marquèze-Pouey, B., Kuhse, J., and Betz, H. (1991). Widespread expression of glycine receptor subunit mRNAs in the adult and developing rat brain. *EMBO J.*, 10, 2401–2409.

Manabe, T., and Nicoll, R. A. (1994). Long-term potentiation: Evidence against an increase in transmitter release probability in the CA1 region of the hippocampus. *Science,* 265, 1888–1892.

Manabe, T., Renner, P., and Nicoll, R. A. (1992). Postsynaptic contribution to long-term potentiation revealed by the analysis of miniature synaptic currents. *Nature,* 355, 50–55.

Mandel, R. J., Hartgraves, S. L., Severson, J. A., Woodward, J. J., Wilcox, R. E., and Randall, P. K. (1993). A quantitative estimate of the role of striatal D-2 receptor proliferation in dopaminergic supersensitivity: The contribution of mesolimbic dopamine to the magnitude of 6-OHDA lesion-induced agonist sensitivity in the rat. *Behav. Brain Res.,* 59, 53–64.

Mandell, A. J., and Knapp, S. (1977). Regulation of serotonin biosynthesis in brain: Role of the high affinity uptake of tryptophan into serotonergic neurons. *Fed. Proc.,* 36, 2142–2148.

Maness, L. M., Kastin, A. J., Weber, J. T., Banks, W. A., Beckman, B. S., and Zadina, J. E. (1994). The neurotrophins and their receptors: Structure, function, and neuropathology. *Neurosci. Biobehav. Rev.,* 18, 143–159.

Manji, H. K. (1992). G proteins: Implications for psychiatry. *Am. J. Psychiatry,* 149, 746–760.

Manji, H. K., Hsiao, J., Risby, E., Oliver, J., Rudorfer, M. V., and Potter, W. (1991). The mechanisms of action of lithium-effects on serotonergic and noradrenergic systems in normal subjects. *Arch. Gen. Psychiatry,* 48, 505–512.

Manji, H. K., and Lenox, R. H. (1994). Long-term action of lithium: A role for transcriptional and posttranscriptional factors regulated by protein kinase C. *Synapse,* 16, 11–28.

Mann, J. J., and Kapur, S. (1994). Elucidation of biochemical basis of the antidepressant action of electroconvulsive therapy by human studies. *Psychopharmacol. Bull.,* 30, 445–453.

Mann, P. J. G., and Quastel, J. H. (1940). Benzedrine (β-phenylisopropylamine) and brain metabolism. *Biochem. J.,* 34, 414–431.

Manning, C., and Gengo, F. M. (1993). Effects of drugs on human functioning: Antihistamines. In *Progress in Basic and Clinical Pharmacology,* Vol. 9, *Effects of Drugs on Human Functioning* (S. Streufert and F. M. Gengo, Eds.), pp. 52–69. Karger, Basel.

Manning, M., and Sawyer, W. H. (1989). Discovery, development, and some uses of vasopressin and oxytocin antagonists. *J. Lab. Clin. Med.,* 114, 617–632.

Männistö, P. T. (1994). Clinical potential of catechol-O-methyltransferase (COMT) inhibitors as adjuvants in Parkinson's disease. *CNS Drugs,* 1, 172–179.

Männistö, P. T., Kaakkola, S., Nissinen, E., Linden, I.-B., and Pohto, P. (1988). Properties of novel effective and highly selective inhibitors of catechol-O-methyltransferase. *Life Sci.,* 43, 1465–1471.

Manno, J. E., Manno, B. R., Kiplinger, G. F., and Forney, R. B. (1974). Motor and mental performance with marijuana: Relationship to administered dose of Δ^9-tetrahydrocannabinol and its interaction with alcohol. In *Marijuana: Effects on Human Behavior* (L. L. Miller, Ed.), pp. 45–72. Academic Press, New York.

Mansbach, R. S., and Balster, R. L. (1991). Pharmacological specificity of the phencyclidine discriminative stimulus in rats. *Pharmacol. Biochem. Behav.,* 39, 971–975.

Mansbach, R. S., Nicholson, K. L., Martin, B. R., and Balster, R. L. (1994). Failure of Δ^9-tetrahydrocannabinol and CP 55,940 to maintain intravenous self-administration under a fixed-interval schedule in rhesus monkeys. *Behav. Pharmacol.,* 5, 219–225.

Manschreck, T. C., Laughery, J. A., Weisstein, C. C., Allen, D., Humblestone, B., Neville, M., Podlewski, H., and Mitra, N. (1988). Characteristics of freebase cocaine psychosis. *Yale J. Biol. Med.,* 61, 115–122.

Mansour, A., Fox, C. A., Akil, H., and Watson, S. J. (1995). Opioid-receptor mRNA expression in the rat CNS: Anatomical and functional implications. *Trends Neurosci.,* 18, 22–29.

Mansour, A., Khachaturian, H., Lewis, M. E., Akil, H., and Watson, S. J. (1987). Autoradiographic differentiation of mu, delta, kappa opioid receptors in the rat forebrain and midbrain. *J. Neurosci.,* 7, 2445–2464.

Mansour, A., Khachaturian, H., Lewis, M. E., Akil, H., and Watson, S. J. (1988). Anatomy of CNS opioid receptors. *Trends Neurosci.,* 11, 308–314.

Mansour, A., and Watson, S. J. (1993). Anatomical distribution of opioid receptors in mammalians: An overview. In *Opioids I,* Handbook of Experimental Pharmacology, Vol. 104 (A. Herz, Ed.), pp. 79–106. Springer-Verlag, New York.

Mantle, T. J., Tipton, K. F., and Garrett, N. J. (1976). Inhibition of monoamine oxidase by amphetamine and related compounds. *Biochem. Pharmacol.,* 25, 2073–2077.

Manyam, B. V. (1987). Influence of precursors on brain GABA level. *Clin. Neuropharmacol.,* 10, 38–46.

Manyam, N. V. B., Katz, L., Hare, T. A., Gerber, J. C. III, and Grossman, M. H. (1980). Levels of γ-aminobutyric acid in cerebrospinal fluid in various neurologic disorders. *Arch. Neurol.,* 37, 352–355.

Maragos, W. F., Penney, J. B., and Young, A. B. (1988). Anatomic corelation of NMDA and ^{3}H-TCP-labeled receptors in rat brain. *J. Neurosci.,* 8, 493–501.

Marchbanks, R. M. (1975). Biochemistry of cholinergic neurons. In *Handbook of Psychopharmacology,* Vol. 3 (L. L. Iversen, S. D. Iversen and S. H. Snyder, Eds.), pp. 247–326. Plenum Press, New York.

Marcus, R., and Coulston, A. M. (1985a). The vitamins. In *The Pharmacological Basis of Therapeutics* (A. G. Gilman, L. S. Goodman, T. W. Rall, and F. Murad, Eds.), pp. 1544–1572. Macmillan, New York.

Marcus, R., and Coulston, A. M. (1985b). Water-soluble vitamins. In *The Pharmacological Basis of Therapeutics* (A. G. Gilman, L. S. Goodman, T. W. Rall and F. Murad, Eds.), pp. 372–386. Macmillan, New York.

Marcusson, J. O., and Ross, S. B. (1990). Binding of some antidepressants to the 5-hydroxytryptamine transporter in brain and platelets. *Psychopharmacology,* 102, 145–155.

Marder, S. R. (1994). Risperidone: Efficacy. *J. Clin. Psychiatry,* 12, 49–52.

Mårdh, G., Sjöquist, B., and Änggård, E. (1981). Norepinephrine metabolism in man using deuterium labelling: The conversion of 4-hydroxy-3-methoxyphenylglycol to 4-hydroxy-3-methoxymandelic acid. *J. Neurochem.,* 36, 1181–1185.

Maren, S., and Baudry, M. (1995). Properties and mechanisms of long-term synaptic plasticity in the mammalian brain: Relationships to learning and memory. *Neurobiol. Learn. Memory,* 63, 1–18.

Maren, S., Tocco, G., Standley, S., Baudry, M., and Thompson, R. F. (1993). Postsynaptic factors in the expression of long-term potentiation (LTP): Increased glutamate receptor binding following LTP induction in vivo. *Proc. Natl. Acad. Sci. U.S.A.,* 90, 9654–9658.

Marglin, S. H., Milano, W. C., Mattie, M. E., and Reid, L. D. (1989). PCP and conditioned place preferences. *Pharmacol. Biochem. Behav.,* 33, 281–283.

Margules, D. L., and Stein, L. (1967). Neuroleptics vs. tranquilizers: Evidence from animal behavior studies of mode and site of action. In *Neuropsychopharmacology* (H. Brill, J. O. Cole, P. Denicker, H. Hippius, and P. B. Bradley, Eds.), pp. 108–120. Excerpta Medica Foundation, New York.

Margules, D. L., and Stein, L. (1968). Increase of "antianxiety" activity and tolerance of behavioral depressions during chronic administration of oxazepam. *Psychopharmacologia,* 13, 74–80.

Marini, A. M., Lipsky, R. H., Schwartz, J. P., and Kopin, I. J. (1992). Accumulation of 1-methyl-4-phenyl-1,2,3,6-tetrahydropyridine in cultured cerebellar astrocytes. *J. Neurochem.,* 58, 1250–1258.

Markey, S. P. (1986). MPTP: A new tool to understand Parkinson's Disease. *Discussions in Neurosciences, Vol. III, No. 4.* Fondation pour l'Etude du Système Nerveux Central et Périphérique, Geneva.

Marlatt, G. A., and George, W. H. (1984). Relapse prevention: Introduction and overview of the model. *Br. J. Addict.,* 79, 261–274.

Marquis, K. L., and Moreton, J. E. (1987). Animal models of intravenous phencyclinoid self-administration. *Pharmacol. Biochem. Behav.,* 27, 385–389.

Marsden, C. A., Bennett, G. W., Fone, K. C. F., and Johnson, J. V. (1989). Functional interactions between TRH and 5-hydroxytryptamine (5-HT) and proctolin in rat brain and spinal cord. *Ann. N.Y. Acad. Sci.,* 553, 121–134.

Marsden, C. A., Joseph, M. H., Kruk, Z. L., Maidment, N. T., O'Neill, R. D., Schenk, J. O., and Stamford, J. A. (1988). In vivo voltammetry: Present electrodes and methods. *Neuroscience,* 25, 389–400.

Marshall, B. E., and Wollman, H. 1985. General anesthetics. In *The Pharmacological Basis of Therapeutics* (A. G. Gilman, L. S. Goodman, T. W. Rall, and F. Murad, Eds.), pp. 276–301. Macmillan, New York.

Marshall, C. R. (1913). Studies on the pharmaceutical action of tera-alkyl-ammonium compounds. *Trans. R. Soc. Edinburgh,* 17–40

Marshall, E. F., Stirling, G. S., Tait, A. C., and Todrick, A. (1960). The effect of irproniazid and imipramine on the blood platelet 5-hydroxytryptamine level in man. *Br. J. Pharmacol.,* 15, 35–41.

Marshall, F. H., Barnes, S., Hughes, J., Woodruff, G. N., and Hunter, J. C. (1991). Cholecystokinin modulates the release of dopamine from the anterior and posterior nucleus accumbens by two different mechanisms. *J. Neurochem.,* 56, 917–922.

Marshall, I. G., and Parsons, S. M. (1987). The vesicular acetylcholine transport system. *Trends Neurosci.,* 10, 174–177.

Marshall, J. F., O'Dell, S. J., and Weihmuller, F. B. (1993). Dopamine-glutamate interactions in methamphetamine-induced neurotoxicity. *J. Neural. Transm. (Gen. Sect.),* 91, 241–254.

Marshall, J. F., Richardson, J. S., and Teitelbaum, P. (1974). Nigrostriatal bundle damage and the lateral hypothalamic syndrome. *J. Comp. Physiol. Psychol.,* 87, 808–830.

Marshall, J. M. (1974). Vertebrate smooth muscle. In *Medical Physiology* Vol. 1 (V. B. Mountcastle, Ed.), pp. 121–148. Mosby, St. Louis.

Martin, B. R. (1982). Long-term disposition of phencyclidine in mice. *Drug Metab. Dis.,* 10, 189–195.

Martin, B. R. (1986). Cellular effects of cannabinoids. *Pharmacol. Rev.,* 38, 45–74.

Martin, B. R., and Boni, J. (1990). Pyrolysis and inhalation studies with phencyclidine and cocaine. *NIDA Res. Monogr.,* 99, 141–158.

Martin, D. L. (1987). Regulatory properties of brain glutamate decarboxylase. *Cell. Mol. Neurobiol.,* 7, 237–253.

Martin, D. L., and Rimvall, K. (1993). Regulation of γ-aminobutyric acid synthesis in the brain. *J. Neurochem.,* 60, 395–407.

Martin, J. H. (1991a). Coding and processing of sensory information. In *Principles of Neural Science* (3rd ed.) (E. R. Kandel, J. H. Schwartz, and T. M. Jessell, Eds.), pp. 329–340. Elsevier, New York.

Martin, J. H. (1991b). The collective electrical behavior of cortical neurons: The electroencephalogram of the mechanism of epilepsy. In *Principles of Neural Science* (3rd ed.) (E. R. Kandel, J. H. Schwartz, and T. M. Jessell, Eds.), pp. 770–791. Elsevier, New York.

Martin, J. H., Brust, J. C. M., and Hilal, S. (1991). Imaging the living brain. In *Principles of Neural Science* (3rd ed.) (E. R. Kandel, J. H. Schwartz, and T. M. Jessell, Eds.), pp. 309–324. Elsevier, New York.

Martin, L. J., Blackstone, C. D., Huganir, R. L., and Price, D. L. (1992). Cellular localization of a metabotropic glutamate receptor in rat brain. *Neuron,* 9, 259–270.

Martin, S. D., Yeragani, V. K., Lodhi, R., and Galloway, M. P. (1989). Clinical ratings and plasma HVA during cocaine abstinence. *Biol. Psychiatry,* 26, 356–362.

Martin, T. R., and Bracken, M. B. (1987). The association between low birth weight and caffeine consumption during pregnancy. *Am. J. Epidemiol.,* 126, 813–821.

Martin, W. R., Eades, C. G., Thompson, J. A., Huppler, R. E., and Gilbert, P. E. (1976). The effects of morphine- and nalorphine- like drugs in the nondependent and morphine-dependent chronic spinal dog. *J. Pharmacol. Exp. Ther.,* 197, 517–532.

Martin, W. R., Sloan, J. W., Sapira, J. D., and Jasinski, D. R. (1971). Physiologic, subjective, and behavioral effects of amphetamine, methamphetamine, ephedrine, phen-

metrazine, and methylphenidate in man. *Clin. Pharmacol. Ther.,* 12, 245–258.

Martinez, J. L. Jr., Schulteis, G., and Weinberger, S. B. (1991). How to increase and decrease the strength of memory traces: The effects of drugs and hormones. In *Learning and Memory* (2nd ed.), pp. 149–198. Academic Press, New York.

Martinez-Serrano, A., Fischer, W., and Björklund, A. (1995). Reversal of age-dependent cognitive impairments and cholinergic neuron atrophy by NGF-secreting neural progenitors grafted to the basal forebrain. *Neuron,* 15, 473–484.

Martinot, J-L., et al. (1990). Striatal D_2 dopaminergic receptors assessed with positron emission tomography and [^{76}Br]bromospiperone in untreated schizophrenic patients. *Am. J. Psychiatry,* 147, 44–50.

Martres, M. P., Sokoloff, P., Giros, B., and Schwartz, J.-C. (1992). Effects of dopaminergic transmission interruption on the D_2 isoforms in various cerebral tissues. *J. Neurochem.,* 58, 673–679.

Marwaha, J., Palmer, M. R., Woodward, D. J., Hoffer, B. J., and Freedman, R. (1980). Electrophysiological evidence for presynaptic actions of phencyclidine on noradrenergic transmission in rat cerebellum. *J. Pharmacol. Exp. Ther.,* 215, 606–613.

Marx, J. L. (1980). Calmodulin: A protein for all seasons. *Science,* 208, 274–276.

Mash, D. C., and Potter, L. T. (1986). Autoradiographic localization of M1 and M2 muscarine receptors in the rat brain. *Neuroscience,* 19, 551–564.

Mason, S. T. (1984). *Catecholamines and Behaviour.* Cambridge University Press, Cambridge.

Masserano, J. M., Vuilliet, P. R., Tank, A. W., and Weiner, N. (1989). The role of tyrosine hydroxylase in the regulation of catecholamine synthesis. In *Handbook of Experimental Pharmacology,* Vol. 90/II (U. Trendelenburg and N. Weiner, Eds.), pp. 427–469. Springer-Verlag, Berlin.

Massoulié, J., Pezzementi, L., Bon, S., Krejci, E., and Vallette, F.-M. (1993). Molecular and cellular biology of cholinesterases. *Prog. Neurobiol.,* 41, 31–91.

Masters, C. L., Multhaup, G., Simms, G., Pottgiesser, J., Martins, R. N., and Beyreuther, K. (1985). Neuronal origin of a cerebral amyloid: Neurofibrillary tangles of Alzheimer's disease contain the same protein as the amyloid of plaque cores and blood vessels. *EMBO J.,* 4, 2757–2763.

Masters, R. E., and Houston, J. (1970). Toward an individual psychedelic psychotherapy. In *Psychedelics.* (B. Aaronson and H. Osmond, (Eds.), Anchor/Doubleday, Garden City, New York.

Matera, C., Warren, W. B., Moomjy, M., Fink, D. J., and Fox, H. E. (1990). Prevalence of use of cocaine and other substances in an obstetric population. *Am. J. Obstet. Gynecol.,* 163, 797–801.

Mathers, D. A. (1987). The $GABA_A$ receptor: New insights from single-channel recording. *Synapse,* 1, 96–101.

Matsubara, S., Arora, R. C., and Meltzer, H. Y. (1991). Serotonergic measures in suicide brain: $5-HT_{1A}$ binding sites in frontal cortex of suicide victims. *J. Neural Transm. Gen. Sect.,* 85, 181–194.

Matsuda, L. A., Bonner, T. I., and Lolait, S. J. (1993). Localization of cannabinoid receptor mRNA in rat brain. *J. Comp. Neurol.*, 327, 535–550.

Matsuda, L. A., Lolait, S. J., Brownstein, M. J., Young, A. C., and Bonner, T. I. (1990). Structure of a cannabinoid receptor and functional expression of the cloned cDNA. *Nature*, 346, 561–564.

Matsumoto, R. R. (1989). GABA receptors: Are cellular differences reflected in function? *Brain Res. Rev.*, 14, 203–225.

Matsushima, E. (1991). Schizophrenia and eye movements. In *Biological Basis of Schizophrenic Disorders* (T. Nakazawa, Ed.) pp. 31–42. Japan Scientific Societies Press, Karger, New York.

Matteoli, M., Reetz, A. T., and De Camilli, P. (1991). Small synaptic vesicles and large dense-core vesicles: Secretory organelles involved in two modes of neuronal signaling. In *Volume Transmission in the Brain: Novel Mechanisms for Neural Transmission* (K. Fuxe and L. F. Agnati, Eds.), pp. 181–193. Raven Press, New York.

Mattes, R. D., Shaw, L. M., Owens-Edling, J., Engelman, K., and Elsohly, M. A. (1993). Bypassing the first-pass effect for the therapeutic use of cannabinoids. *Pharmacol. Biochem. Behav.*, 44, 745–747.

Matthews, J. C., and Collins, A. (1983). Interactions of cocaine and cocaine congeners with sodium channels. *Biochem. Pharmacol.*, 32, 455–460.

Mattson, M. P., Barger, S. W., Lieberburg, I., Smith-Swintosky, V. L., and Rydel, R. E. (1993). β-Amyloid precursor protein metabolites and loss of neuronal Ca^{2+} homeostasis in Alzheimer's disease. *Trends Neurosci.*, 16, 409–414.

Matzuk, M. M., and Saper, C. B. (1985). Preservation of hypothalamic dopaminergic neurons in Parkinson's disease. *Ann. Neurol.*, 18, 552–555.

Mauborgne, A., Javoy-Agid, F., Legrand, J. C., Agid, Y., and Cesselin, F. (1983). Decrease of substance P-like immunoreactivity in the substantia nigra and pallidum of parkinsonian brains. *Brain Res.*, 268, 167–170.

Maura, G., Giardi, A., and Raiteri, M. (1988). Release-regulating D-2 dopamine receptors are located on striatal glutamatergic nerve terminals. *J. Pharmacol. Exp. Ther.*, 247, 680–684.

Mauri, M. C., Percudani, M., Regazzetti, M. G., and Ahamura, A. C. (1990). Alternative prophylactic treatment to lithium in bipolar disorder. *Clin. Neuropharmacol.*, 13, Suppl. 1, S90–S96.

Maurice, T., Vignon, J., Kamenka, J.-M., and Chicheportiche, R. (1991). Differential interaction of phencyclidine-like drugs with the dopamine uptake complex in vivo. *J. Neurochem.*, 56, 553–559.

Maxwell, D. S. (1984). Developmental effects of alcohol. In *Alcoholism* (I. J. West, Moderator). *Ann. Intern. Med.*, 100, 406–407.

Mayberg, H. S., and Frost, J. J. (1990). Opiate receptors. In *Quantitative Imaging: Neuroreceptors, Neurotransmitters, and Enzymes* (J. J. Frost and H. N. Wagner, Jr., Eds.), pp. 81–95. Raven Press, Ltd., New York.

Maycox, P. R., Hell, J. W., and Jahn, R. (1990). Amino acid neurotransmission: Spotlight on synaptic vesicles. *Trends Neurosci.*, 13, 83–87.

Mayer, D. J., and Hayes, R. L. (1975). Stimulation-produced analgesia: Development of

tolerance and cross-tolerance to morphine. *Science*, 188, 941–943.

Mayer, D. J., and Liebeskind, J. C. (1974). Pain reduction by focal electrical stimulation of the brain: An anatomical and behavioral analysis. *Brain Res.*, 68, 73–93.

Mayer, D. J., Price, D. D.. amd Rafi, A. (1975). Antagonism of acupuncture analgesia in man by narcotic antagonist anloxone. *Brain Res.*, 121, 368–372.

Mayer, L. A., and Parker, L. A. (1993). Rewarding anad aversive properties of IP and SC cocaine: Assessment by place and taste conditioning. *Psychopharmacology*, 112, 189–194.

Mayer, M. L., Vyklicky, L. Jr., and Sernagor, E. (1989). A physiologist's view of the N-methyl-D-aspartate receptor: An allosteric ion channel with multiple regulatory sites. *Drug Dev. Res.*, 17, 263–280.

Mayeux, R. (1990). The "serotonin hypothesis" for depression in Parkinson's disease. *Adv. Neurol.*, 53, pp. 163–166.

Mayeux, R., and Kandel, E. R. (1991). Disorders of language: The aphasias. In *Principles of Neural Science* (3rd ed.) (E. R. Kandel, J. H. Schwartz, and T. M. Jessell, Eds.), pp. 839–851. Elsevier, New York.

Maynert, E. W., and Klingman, G. I. (1960). Acute tolerance to intravenous anesthetics in dogs. *J. Pharmacol. Exp. Ther.*, 128, 192–200.

Mazziotta, J. C., and Phelps, M. E. (1985). Human neuropsychological imaging studies of local brain metabolism: Strategies and results. In *Brain Imaging and Brain Function* (L. Sokoloff, Ed.), pp. 121–137. Raven Press, New York.

Mazziotta, J. C., and Phelps, M. E. (1986). Positron emission tomography studies of the brain. In *Positron Emission Tomography and Autoradiography: Principles and Applications for the Brain and Heart* (M. Phelps, J. Mazziotta, and H. Schelbert, Eds.), pp. 493–579. Raven Press, New York.

McBain, C. J., and Mayer, M. L. (1994). N-Methyl-D-aspartic acid receptor structure and function. *Physiol. Rev.*, 74, 723–760.

McBride, P., DeMeo, M. D., Sweeney, J. A., Halper, J., Mann, J. J., and Shear, M. K. (1992). Neuroendocrine and behavioral responses to challenge with the indirect serotonin agonist *dl*-fenfluramine in adults with obsessive–compulsive disorder. *Biol. Psychiatry*, 31, 19–34.

McCann, U., Hatzidimitriou, G., Ridenour, A., Fischer, C., Yuan, J., Katz, J., and Ricaurte, G. (1994). Dexfenfluramine and serotonin neurotoxicity: Further preclinical evidence that clinical caution is indicated. *J. Pharmacol. Exp. Ther.*, 269, 792–798.

McCann, U., Ridenour, A., Shaham, Y., and Ricaurte, G. A. (1994). Serotonin neurotoxicity after (±)3,4-methylenedioxymethamphetamine (MDMA; "Ecstasy"): A controlled study in humans. *Neuropsychopharmacology*, 10, 129–138.

McCarron, M. M., Schulze, B. W., Thompson, G. A., Conder, M. C., and Goetz, W. A. (1981). Acute phencyclidine intoxication: Clinical patterns, complications, and treatment. *Ann. Emerg. Med.*, 10, 290–297.

McClearn, G.E. (1988) Animal models in alcohol research. *Alcohol. Clin. Exp. Res.*,12, 573–576

McCormick, D. A. (1989). GABA as an inhibitory neurotransmitter in human cerebral cortex. *J. Neurophysiol.*, 62, 1018–1027.

McCormick, D. A. (1991). Electrophysiological consequences of activation of adrenoceptors in the CNS. In *Adrenoceptors: Structure, Mechanisms, Function. Advances in Pharmacological Sciences*, pp. 159–169. Birkhäuser, Basel.

McCormick, D. A. (1992). Neurotransmitter actions in the thalamus and cerebral cortex and their role in neuromodulation of thalamocortical activity. *Prog. Neurobiol.*, 39, 337–388.

McCormick, D. A., and Prince, D. A. (1988). Noradrenergic modulation of firing pattern in guinea pig and cat thalamic neurons, in vitro. *J. Neurophysiol.*, 59, 978–996.

McCormick, D. A., and Williamson, A. (1989). Convergence and divergence of neurotransmitter action in human cerebral cortex. *Proc. Natl. Acad. Sci. U.S.A.*, 86, 8098–8102.

McCulloch, J. (1982). Mapping functional alterations in the CNS with $[^{14}C]$deoxyglucose. In *Handbook of Psychopharmacology*, Vol. 15 (L. Iversen, S. Iversen, and S. Snyder, Eds.), pp. 321–410. Plenum Press, New York.

McCullough, L. D., and Salamone, J. D. (1992). Increases in extracellular dopamine levels and locomotor activity after direct infusion of phencyclidine into the nucleus accumbens. *Brain Res.*, 577, 1–9.

McDaniel, K. D. (1986). Clinical pharmacology of monoamine oxidase inhibitors. *Clin. Neuropharmacol.*, 9, 207–234.

McDowell, J., and Kitchen, I. (1987). Development of opioid systems: Peptides, receptors and pharmacology. *Brain Res. Rev.*, 12, 397–421.

McElroy, J., Zeller, K., Amy, K., Ward, K., Cawley, J., Mazzola, A., Keim, W., and Rohrbach, K. (1993). In vivo agonist properties of 7-hydroxy-N,N-di-N-propyl-2-aminotetralin, a dopamine D_3-selective receptor ligand. *Drug Dev. Res.*, 30, 257–259.

McElroy, S., Keck, P. E., Pope, H. G., and Hudson, J. I. (1992). Valproate in the treatment of bipolar disorder: Literature review and clinical guidelines. *J. Clin. Psychopharmacol.*, 12 (Suppl. 1), 42s–52s.

McEwen, B. S. (1980). The brain as a target organ of endocrine hormones. In *Neuroendocrinology* (D. T. Krieger and J. C. Hughes, Eds.), pp. 33–43. Sinauer Associates, Sunderland, MA.

McEwen, B. S., Davis, P. G., Parsons, B., and Pfaff, D. W. (1979). The brain as a target for steroid hormone action. *Annu. Rev. Neurosci.*, 2, 65–112.

McEwen, B. S., Frankfurt, M., Kuroda, Y., Magarinos, A. M., McKittrick, C., and Watanabe, Y. (1994). Dysregulation of the hypothalamo-pituitary-adrenal axis in depressive illness: Interactions between antidepressants, glucocorticoids, serotonin and excitatory amino acids. In *Critical Issues in the Treatment of Affective Disorders* (S. Z. Langer, N. Bunello, G. Racagni, and J. Mendlewicz, Eds.), pp. 75–81. Karger, Basel.

McGaugh, J. L., Introini-Collison, I. B., and Castellano, C. (1993). Involvement of opioid peptides in learning and memory. In *Opioids II,*, Handbook of Experimental

Pharmacology, Vol. 104 (A. Herz, Ed.), pp. 429–448. Springer-Verlag, New York.

McGeer, P. L. (1984). Aging, Alzheimer's disease, and the cholinergic system. Can. J. Physiol. Pharmacol., 62, 741–754.

McGeer, P. L., Eccles, J. C., and McGeer, E. G. (1978). Molecular Neurobiology of the Mammalian Brain. Plenum Press, New York.

McGeer, P. L., Hattori, T., and McGeer, E. G. (1975). Chemical and autoradiographic analysis of γ-aminobutyric acid transport in Purkinje cells of the cerebellum. Exp. Neurol., 47, 26–41.

McGeer, P. L., and McGeer, E. G. (1989). Amino acid neurotransmitters. In Basic Neurochemistry (G. Siegel, B. Agranoff, R. W. Albers, and P. Molinoff, Eds.), pp. 311–332. Raven Press, New York.

McGeer, P. L., and McGeer, E. G. (1995). The inflammatory response system of brain: Implications for therapy of Alzheimer and other neurodegenerative disorders. Brain Res. Rev., 21, 195–218.

McGeer, P. L., McGeer, E. G., and Suzuki, J. S. (1977). Aging and extrapyramidal function. Arch. Neurol., 34, 33–35.

McGehee, D. S., Heath, M. J. S., Gelber, S., DeVay, P., and Role, L. W. (1995). Nicotine enhancement of fast excitatory synaptic transmission in CNS by presynaptic receptors. Science, 269, 1692–1696.

McGlade-McCulloh, E., Yamamoto, H., Tan, S.-E., Brickey, D. A., and Soderling, T. R. (1993). Phosphorylation and regulation of glutamate receptors by calcium/calmodulin-dependent protein kinase II. Nature, 362, 640–642.

McGlothlin, W. H., and Arnold, D. (1971). LSD revisited, a ten year follow-up of medical LSD use. Arch. Gen. Psychiatry, 24, 35–49.

McGlothlin, W. H., and West, L. J. (1968). The marihuana problem: An overview. Am. J. Psychiatry, 125, 370–378.

McGregor, A., Lacosta, S., and Roberts, D. C. S. (1993). L-tryptophan decreases the breaking point under a progressive ratio schedule of intravenous cocaine reinforcement in the rat. Pharmacol. Biochem. Behav., 44, 651–655.

McGregor, A., and Roberts, D. C. S. (1994). Mechanisms of abuse. In Amphetamine and its Analogs (A. K. Cho, Ed.), pp. 243–266. Academic Press, San Diego.

McGregor, I. S., Atrens, D. M., and Jackson, D. M. (1992). Cocaine facilitation of prefrontal cortex self-stimulation: A microstructural and pharmacological analysis. Psychopharmacology, 106, 239–247.

McKay, J. R., Rutherford, M. J., Alterman, A. I., Cacciola, J. S., and Kaplan, M. R. (1995). An examination of the cocaine relapse process. Drug Alcohol Depend., 38, 35–43.

McKelvy, J. F., and Blumberg, S. (1986). Inactivation and metabolism of neuropeptides. Annu. Rev. Neurosci., 9, 415–434.

McKernan, R. M., and Whiting, P. J. (1996). Which GABA$_A$-receptor subtypes really occur in the brain? Trends Neurosci., 19, 139–143.

McKhann, G., Drachman, D., Folstein, M., Katzman, R., Price, D., and Stadlan, E. M. (1984). Clinical diagnosis of Alzheimer's disease: Report of the NINCDS-ADRDA Work Group under the auspices of the Department of Health and Human Services Task Force on Alzheimer's Disease. Neurology, 34, 939–944.

McKinney, M. (1993). Muscarinic receptor subtype-specific coupling to second messengers in neuronal systems. Prog. Brain Res., 98, 333–340.

McKinney, M., Miller, J. H., and Aagaard, P. J. (1993). Pharmacological characterization of the rat hippocampal muscarinic autoreceptor. J. Pharmacol. Exp. Ther., 264, 74–78.

McKinney, M., and Richelson, E. (1989). Muscarinic receptor regulation of cyclic GMP and eicosanoid production. In The Muscarinic Receptors (J. H. Brown, Ed.), pp. 309–339. Humana Press, Clifton, NJ.

McLaughlin, B. J., Wood, J. G., Saito, K., Barber, R., Vaughn, J. E., Roberts, E., and Yu, J.-Y. (1974). The fine structural localization of glutamate decarboxylase in synaptic terminals of rodent cerebellum. Brain Res., 76, 377–391.

McLean, S., Rothman, R., and Herkenham, M. (1986). Autoradiographic localiztion of mu- and delta-opiate receptors in the forebrain of the rat. Brain Res., 378, 49–60.

McLellan, A. T., and Alterman, A. I. (1991). Patient treatment matching: A conceptual and methodological review with suggestions for future research. NIDA Res. Monogr., 106, 114–135.

McLellan, A. T., and Childress, A. R. (1985). Aversive therapies for substance abuse: Do they work? J. Subst. Abuse Treatment, 2, 187–191.

McLennan, H. (1970). Synaptic Transmission (2nd ed.). Saunders, Philadelphia.

McMahon, A., and Sabban, E. L. (1992). Regulation of expression of dopamine β-hydroxylase in PC12 cells by glucocorticoids and cyclic AMP analogues. J. Neurochem., 59, 2040–2047.

McMillan, D. E., Dewey, W. L., and Harris, L. S. (1971). Characteristics of tetrahydrocannabinol tolerance. Ann. N.Y. Acad. Sci., 191, 83–99.

McMillen, B. A. (1983). CNS stimulants: Two distinct mechanisms of action for amphetamine-like drugs. Trends Pharmacol. Sci., 4, 429–432.

McMillen, B. A., German, D. C., and Shore, P. A. (1980). Functional and pharmacological significance of brain dopamine and norepinephrine storage pools. Biochem. Pharmacol., 29, 3045–3050.

McMillian, M., Kong, L.-Y., Sawin, S. M., Wilson, B., Das, K., Hudson, P., Hong, J.-S., and Bing, G. (1995). Selective killing of cholinergic neurons by microglial activation in basal forebrain mixed neuronal/glial culture. Biochem. Biophys. Res. Commun., 215, 572–577.

McNamara, J. O. (1994). Cellular and molecular basis of epilepsy. J. Neurosci., 14, 3413–3425.

McNamara, J. O., Bonhaus, D. W., and Shin, C. (1993). The kindling model of epilepsy. In Concepts and Models in Epilepsy Research (P. Schwartzkroin, Ed.), pp. 27–47. Cambridge University Press, New York.

McNamara, R. K., and Skelton, R. W. (1993). The neuropharmacological and neurochemical basis of place learning in the Morris water maze. Brain Res. Rev., 18, 33–49.

McNaughton, P. A. (1990). Light response of vertebrate photoreceptors. Physiol. Rev., 70, 847–883.

McNeill, T. H., Brown, S. A., Rafols, J. A., and Shoulson, I. (1988). Atrophy of medium spiny I striatal dendrites in advanced

Parkinson's disease. Brain Res., 455, 148–152.

McNeilly, A. S., Robinson, I. C. A. F., Houston, M. J., and Howie, P. W. (1983). Release of oxytocin and prolactin in response to suckling. Br. Med. J., 286, 257–259.

Meador-Woodruff, J. H., Damask, S. P., and Watson, S. J. Jr. (1994). Differential expression of autoreceptors in the ascending dopamine systems of the human brain. Proc. Natl. Acad. Sci. U.S.A., 91, 8297–8301.

Meador-Woodruff, J. H., Haskett, R. F., Grunhaus, L., Akil, H., Watson, S. J., and Greden, J. F. (1987). Postdexamethasone plasma cortisol and B-endorphin levels in depression: Relationship to severity of illness. Biol. Psychiatry, 22, 1137–1150.

Meador-Woodruff, J. H., Mansour, A., Grandy, D. K., Damask, S. P., Civelli, O., and Watson, S. J. Jr. (1992). Distribution of D$_5$ dopamine receptor mRNA in rat brain. Neurosci. Lett., 145, 209–212.

Meakin, S. O., and Shooter, E. M. (1992). The nerve growth family of receptors. Trends Neurosci., 15, 323–331,

Mechoulam, R. (1986). The pharmacohistory of Cannabis sativa. In Cannabinoids as Therapeutic Agents (R. Mechoulam, Ed.), pp. 1–19. CRC Press, Boca Raton.

Mechoulam, R., and Feigenbaum, J. J. (1987). Towards cannabinoid drugs. Prog. Med. Chem., 24, 159–207.

Mechoulam, R., Hanus, L., and Martin, B. R. (1994). Search for endogenous ligands of the cannabinoid receptor. Biochem. Pharmacol., 48, 1537–1544.

Mechoulam, R., Vogel, Z., and Barg, J. (1994). CNS cannabinoid receptors. Role and therapeutic implications for CNS disorders. CNS Drugs, 2, 255–260.

Medina, J. H., Pena, C., Piva, M., Paladini, A. C., and De Robertis, E. (1988). Biochem. Biophys. Res. Commun., 152, 534–539.

Meek, J. L., and Neff, N. H. (1972). Tryptophan 5-hydroxylase: Approximation of half-life and rate of axonal transport. J. Neurochem., 19, 1519–1525.

Meek, J. L., and Neff, N. H. (1973). The rate of formation of 3-methoxy-4-hydroxyphenylethyleneglycol sulfate in brain as an estimate of the rate of formation of norepinephrine. J. Pharmacol. Exp. Ther., 184, 570–575.

Mefford, I. N., Baker, T. L., Boehme, R., Foutz, A. S., Ciaranello, R. D., Barchas, J. D., and Dement, W. C. (1983). Narcolepsy: Biogenic amine deficits in an animal model. Science, 220, 629–632.

Meghji, P., and Newby, A. C. (1990). Sites of adenosine formation, action and inactivation in the brain. Neurochem. Int., 16, 227–232.

Mehlman, P. T., Higley, J. D., Faucher, I., Lilly, A. A., Taub, D. M., Vickers, J., Suomi, S. J., and Linnoila, M. (1994). Low CSF 5-HIAA concentrations and severe aggression and impaired impulse control in nonhuman primates. Am. J. Psychiatry, 151, 1485–1491.

Mehta, A. K., and Ticku, M. K. (1988). Ethanol potentiation of GABAergic transmission in cultured spinal cord neurons involves γ-aminobutyric acid$_A$-gated chloride channels. J. Pharmacol. Exp. Ther., 246, 558–564.

Meisch, R. A., and George, F. R. (1988). Influence of genetic factors on drug-reinforced behavior in animals. NIDA Res. Monogr., 89, 9–24.

Meister, B., Hökfelt, T., Steinbusch, H. W. M., Skagerberg, G., Lindvall, O., Geffard, M., Joh, T. H., Cuello, A. C., and Goldstein, M. (1988). Do tyrosine hydroxylase-immuno-reactive neurons in the ventrolateral arcuate nucleus produce dopamine or only L-DOPA? *J. Chem. Neuroanat.*, 1, 59–64.

Meites, J. (1977). The 1977 Nobel prize in physiology or medicine. *Science*, 198, 594–596.

Melamed, E. (1992). Biochemical and functional differences between dopamine formed from endogenous tyrosine and exogenous L-DOPA in nigrostriatal dopaminergic neurons. *Neurochem. Int.*, 20 (Suppl.), 115S-117S.

Meldrum, B. (1991). Excitotoxicity and epileptic brain damage. *Epilepsy Res.*, 10, 55–61.

Melia, K. R., and Duman, R. S. (1991). Involvement of corticotropin-releasing factor in chronic stress regulation of the brain noradrenergic system. *Proc. Natl. Acad. Sci. U.S.A.*, 88, 8382–8386.

Meliska, C. J., Landrum, R. E., and Landrum, T. A. (1990). Tolerance and sensitization to chronic and subchronic oral caffeine: Effects on wheel-running in rats. *Pharmacol. Biochem. Behav.*, 35, 477–479.

Meliska, C. J., Landrum, R. E., and Loke, W. H. (1985). Caffeine effects: Interaction of drug and wheel-running experience. *Pharmacol. Biochem. Behav.*, 23, 633–635.

Mellanby, J., and Green, J. (1981). How does tetanus toxin act? *Neuroscience*, 6, 281–300.

Meller, E., Bohmaker, K., Goldstein, M., and Basham, D. A. (1993). Evidence that striatal synthesis-inhibiting autoreceptors are dopamine D$_3$ receptors. *Eur. J. Pharmacol.*, 249, R5–R6.

Mellinger, G. D., Somers, R. H., Davidson, S. T., and Manheimer, D. I. (1976). The amotivational syndrome and the college student. *Ann. N.Y. Acad. Sci.*, 282, 37–55.

Mello, N. K. (1987). Alcohol abuse and alcoholism. In *Psychopharmacology: The Third Generation of Progress* (H. Y. Meltzer, Ed.), pp. 1515–1520. Raven Press, New York.

Mello, N. K., Mendelson, J. H., Bree, M. P., and Lukas, S. E. (1989). Buprenorphine suppresses cocaine self-administration by rhesus monkeys. *Science*, 245, 859–862.

Meltzer, H. Y. (1987). Biological studies in schizophrenia. *Schiz Bull.*, 13, 93–128.

Meltzer, H. Y. (1994). Clozapine and other atypical neuroleptics: Efficacy, side effects, optimal utilization. *J.Clin.Psychiat.*, 12, 38–42.

Meltzer, H. Y. (1995). Atypical antipsychotic drugs. In *Psychopharmacology: The Fourth Generation of Progress* (F. E. Bloom and D. J. Kupfer, Eds.), pp. 1277–1286. Raven Press, New York.

Meltzer, H. Y., and Arora, R. C. (1991). Platelet serotonin studies in affective disorders: Evidence for a serotonergic abnormality. In *5-hydroxytryptamine in Psychiatry: A Spectrum of Ideas* (M. Sandler, A. Coppen, and S. Harnett, Eds.), pp. 50–89. Oxford University Press, New York.

Meltzer, H. Y., and Lowy, M. T. (1987). The serotonin hypothesis of depression. In *Psychopharmacology: The Third Generation of Progress* (H. Y. Meltzer, Ed.), pp. 513–526. Raven Press, New York.

Meltzer, H. Y., Matsubara, S., and Lee, J.-C. (1989). Classification of typical and atypical antipsychotic drugs on the basis of dopa-mine D-1, D-2 and serotonin$_2$ pK_i values. *J. Pharmacol. Exp. Ther.*, 251, 238–246.

Melville, L. D., Smith, G. P., and Gibbs, J. (1992). Devazepide antagonizes the inhibitory effect of cholecystokinin on intake in sham-feeding rats. *Pharmacol. Biochem. Behav.*, 43, 975–977.

Mendelson, J. H. (1968). Ethanol-C^{14} metabolism in alcoholics and nonalcoholics. *Science*, 159, 319–320.

Mendelson, J. H. (1987). Marijuana. In *Psychopharmacology: The Third Generation of Progress* (H. Y. Meltzer, Ed.), pp. 1565–1571. Raven Press, New York.

Mendlewicz, J., and Rainer, J. D. (1977). Adoption study supporting genetic transmission in manic-depressive illness. *Nature*, 268, 327–329.

Meng, G., Xie, G-X., Thompson, R. C., Mansour, A., Goldstein, A., Watson, S. J., and Akil, H. (1993). Cloning and pharmacological characterization of a rat "kappa" opioid receptor. *Proc. Natl. Acad. Sci. U.S.A.*, 90, 9954–9958.

Mengod, G., et al. (1992). Visualization of dopamine D$_1$, D$_2$, and D$_3$ receptor mRNAs in human and rat brain. *Neurochem. Int.*, 20 (Suppl.), 33S–43S.

Menkel, M., Terry, P., Pontecorvo, M., Katz, J. L., and Witkin, J. M. (1991). Selective σ ligands block stimulant effects of cocaine. *Eur. J. Pharmacol.*, 201, 251–252.

Menkes, D. B., and Aghajanian, G. K. (1981). Alpha$_1$-adrenoreceptor-mediated responses in the lateral geniculate are enhanced by chronic antidepressant treatment. *Eur. J. Pharmacol.*, 74, 27–35.

Menkes, D. B., Aghajanian, G. K., and Galleger, D. W. (1983). Chronic antidepressant treatment enhances agonist affinity of brain alpha$_1$-adrenoreceptors. *Eur. J. Pharmacol.*, 87, 35–41.

Mercuri, N. B., Calabresi, P., and Bernardi, G. (1992). The electrophysiological actions of dopamine and dopaminergic drugs on neurons of the substantia nigra pars compacta and ventral tegmental area. *Life Sci.*, 51, 711–718.

Meselson, M., and Robinson, J. P. (1980). Chemical warfare and chemical disarmament. *Sci. Am.*, 242 (4), 38–47.

Meyer, J. S., Mirochnick, M., Frank, D. A., and Zuckerman, B. S. (1996). Adversity in the newborn infant: psychological and physiological effects of prenatal cocaine exposure. In *The Psychology of Adversity* (R. S. Feldman, Ed.), pp. 3–22. University of Massachusetts Press, Amherst.

Meyer, J. S., Robinson, P., and Todtenkopf, M. S. (1994). Prenatal cocaine reduces haloperidol-induced catalepsy on postnatal day 10. *Neurotoxicol. Teratol.*, 16, 193–194.

Meyer, J. S., Shearman, L. P., Collins, L. M., and Maguire, R. L. (1993). Cocaine binding sites in fetal rat brain: Implications for prenatal cocaine action. *Psychopharmacology*, 112, 445–451.

Meyer, M. B., and Tonascia, J. A. (1977). Maternal smoking, pregnancy complications and perinatal mortality. *Am. J. Obstet. Gynecol.*, 128, 494–502.

Meyer, M. E., Van Hartesveldt, C., and Potter, T. J. (1993). Locomotor activity following intra-accumbens microinjections of dopamine D$_1$ agonist SK&F 38393 in rats. *Synapse*, 13, 310–314.

Meyer, R. E. (1972). *Guide to Drug Rehabilitation*. Beacon Press, Boston.

Michaelis, E. K. (1990). Fetal alcohol exposure: Cellular toxicity and molecular events involved in toxicity. *Alcohol. Clin. Exp. Res.*, 14, 819–826.

Mickel, E. J. (1969). *The Artificial Paradises in French Literature*. University of North Carolina Press, Chapel Hill.

Miczek, K. A., DeBold, J. F., and Thompson, M. (1984). Pharmacological, hormonal, and behavioral manipulations in the analysis of aggressive behavior. In *Ethopharmacological Aggression Research* (K. A. Miczek, M. R. Kruk, and B. Olivier, Eds.), pp. 1–26. Alan R. Liss, New York.

Miczek, K. A., Mos, J., and Olivier, B. (1989). Serotonin, aggression and self-destructive behavior. *Psychopharmacol. Bull.*, 25, 399–403.

Middlebrooks, J. C., Clock, A. E., Xu, L., and Green, D. M. (1994). A panoramic code for sound location by cortical neurons. *Science*, 264, 842–844.

Middlemiss, D. N., and Tricklebank, M. D. (1992). Centrally active 5-HT receptor agonists and antagonists. *Neurosci. Biobehav. Rev.*, 16, 75–82.

Mileson, B. E., Lewis, M. H., and Mailman, R. B. (1991). Dopamine receptor "supersensitivity" occurring without receptor up-regulation. *Brain Res.*, 561, 1–10.

Millan, M. J. (1990). K-Opioid receptors and analgesia. *Trends Pharmacol. Sci.*, 11, 70–76.

Millan, M. J., Audinot, V., Rivet, J.-M., Gobert, A., Vian, J., Prost, J.-F., Spedding, M., and Peglion, J.-L. (1994). S 14297, a novel selective ligand at cloned human dopamine D$_3$ receptors, blocks 7-OH-DPAT-induced hypothermia in rats. *Eur. J. Pharmacol.*, 260, R3–R5.

Miller, B. A. (1990). The interrelationships between alcohol and drugs and family violence. *NIDA Res. Monogr.*,103, 177–207.

Miller, H. H., Shore, P. A., and Clarke, D. E. (1980). *In vivo* monoamine oxidase inhibition by *d*-amphetamine. *Biochem. Pharmacol.*, 29, 1347–1354.

Miller, L. L., and Branconnier, R. J. (1983). Cannabis: Effects on memory and the cholinergic limbic system. *Psychol. Bull.*, 93, 441–456.

Miller, N. S., and Gold, M. S. (1989). The diagnosis of marijuana (*Cannabis*) dependence. *J. Subst. Abuse Treatment*, 6, 183–192.

Miller, N. S., Gold, M. S., and Pottash, A. C. (1989). A 12-step treatment approach for marijuana (*Cannabis*) dependence. *J. Subst. Abuse Treatment*, 6, 241–250.

Miller, R. J., Wickens, J. R., and Beninger, R. J. (1990). Dopamine D-1 and D-2 receptors in relation to reward and performance: A case for the D-1 receptor as a primary site of therapeutic action of neuroleptic drugs. *Prog. Neurobiol.*, 34, 143–183.

Milligan, G. (1993). Agonist regulation of cellular G protein levels and distribution: Mechanisms and functional implications. *Trends Pharmacol. Sci.*, 14, 413–418.

Milligan, G., Bond, R. A., and Lee, M. (1995). Inverse agonism: Pharmacological curiosity or potential therapeutic strategy? *Trends Pharmacol. Sci.*, 16, 10–13.

Mills, P. J., and Dimsdale, J. E. (1993). The promise of adrenergic receptor studies in psychophysiologic research. II. Applications, limitations, and progress. *Psychosom. Med.,* 55, 448–457.

Milner, J. D., and Wurtman, J. (1986). Catecholamine synthesis: Physiological coupling to precursor supply. *Biochem. Pharmacol.,* 35, 875–881.

Milner, R. J., and Sutcliffe, J. G. (1988). Molecular neurobiological strategies applied to the nervous system. In *Discussions in Neurosciences,* Vol. V, No. 2. Fondation pour l'Etude du système Nerveux Central et Périphérique, Geneva.

Minneman, K. P., and Esbenshade, T. A. (1994). α_1-adrenergic receptor subtypes. *Annu. Rev. Pharmacol. Toxicol.,* 34, 117–133.

Minneman, K. P., Wolfe, B. B., and Molinoff, P. B. (1982). Selective changes in the density of beta$_1$-adrenergic receptors in rat striatum following chronic drug treatment and adrenalectomy. *Brain Res.,* 252, 309–314.

Minz, B. (1955). *The Role of Humoral Agents in Nervous Activity.* Thomas, Springfield, IL.

Mirsky, I. E., Piker, P., Rosenbaum, M., and Lederer, H. (1941). "Adaptation" of the central nervous system to various concentrations of alcohol in the blood. *Q. J. Stud. Alcohol,* 2, 35–45.

Misu, Y., and Goshima, Y. (1993). Is L-DOPA an endogenous neurotransmitter? *Trends Pharmacol. Sci.,* 14, 119–123.

Mitchell, I. J., Cross, A. J., Sambrook, M. A., and Crossman, A. R. (1985). Sites of the neurotoxic action of 1-methyl-4-phenyl-1,2,3,6-tetrahydropyridine in the macaque monkey include the ventral tegmental area and the locus coeruleus. *Neurosci. Lett.,* 61, 195–200.

Mitchell, K., Oke, A. F., and Adams, R. N. (1994). In vivo dynamics of norepinephrine release–reuptake in multiple terminal field regions of rat brain. *J. Neurochem.,* 63, 917–926.

Mitler, M. (1982). The multiple sleep latency test as an evaluation for excessive somnolence. In *Sleeping and Waking Disorders: Indications and Techniques* (C. Guilleminault, Ed.). Addison Wesley, Palo Alto.

Miyasaka, K., Kanai, S., Ohta, M., Kawanami, T., Kono, A., and Funakoshi, A. (1994). Lack of satiety effect of cholecystokinin (CCK) in a new rat model not expressing the CCK-A receptor gene. *Neurosci. Lett.,* 180, 143–146.

Mochizuki, T., Yamatodani, A., Okakura, K., Horii, A., Inagaki, N., and Wada, H. (1992). Circadian rhythm of histamine release from the hypothalamus of freely moving rats. *Physiol. Behav.,* 51, 391–394.

Mody, I., and MacDonald, J. F. (1995). NMDA receptor-dependent excitotoxicity: The role of intracellular Ca^{2+} release. *Trends Pharmacol. Sci.,* 16, 356–359.

Mogenson, G. J., Jones, D. L., and Yim, C. Y. (1980). From motivation to action: Functional interface between the limbic system and the motor system. *Prog. Neurobiol.,* 14, 69–97.

Moghaddam, B., and Gruen, R. J. (1991). Do endogenous excitatory amino acids influence striatal dopamine release? *Brain Res.,* 544, 329–330.

Möhler, H., and Okada, T. (1977a). Benzodiazepine receptor: Demonstration in the central nervous system. *Science,* 198, 849–851.

Möhler, H., and Okada, T. (1977b). Properties of [^{3}H] diazepam binding to benzodiazepine receptors in rat cerebral cortex. *Life Sci.,* 20, 2101–2110.

Möhler, H., Richards, J. G., and Wu, J. Y. (1981). Autoradiographic localization of benzodiazepine receptors in immunocytochemically identified gamma-aminobutyrergic synapses. *Proc. Natl. Acad. Sci. U.S.A.,* 78, 1935–1938.

Moller, S. E., Kirk, L., Brandrup, E., Hollnagel, M., Kaldan, B., and Odum, K. (1983). Tryptophan availability in endogenous depression–Relation to efficacy of L-tryptophan treatment. *Adv. Biol. Psychiatry,* 10, 30–46.

Molliver, M. E. (1987). Serotonergic neuronal systems: What their anatomic organization tells us about function. *J. Clin. Psychopharmacol.,* 7, (Suppl. 6), 3S–23S.

Molliver, M. E., Berger, U. V., Mamounas, L. A., Molliver, D. C., O'Hearn, E., and Wilson, M. A. (1990). Neurotoxicity of MDMA and related compounds: Anatomic studies. *Ann. N.Y. Acad. Sci.,* 600, 640–664.

Molloy, A. G., O'Boyle, K. M., Pugh, M. T., and Waddington, J. L. (1986). Locomotor behaviors in response to new selective D-2 and D-2 dopamine receptor agonists, and the influence of selective antagonists. *Pharmacol. Biochem. Behav.,* 25, 249–253.

Molloy, A. G., and Waddington, J. L. (1984). Dopaminergic behaviour stereospecifically promoted by the D$_1$ agonist *R*-SK&F 38393 and selectively blocked by the D$_1$ antagonist SCH 23390. *Psychopharmacology,* 82, 409–410.

Monaghan, D. T., Bridges, R. J., and Cotman, C. W. (1989). The excitatory amino acid receptors: Their classes, pharmacology, and distinct properties in the function of the central nervous system. *Annu. Rev. Pharmacol. Toxicol.,* 29, 365–402.

Monaghan, D. T., and Cotman, C. W. (1985). Distribution of N-methyl-D-aspartate-sensitive L-[^{3}H]glutamate-binding sites in rat brain. *J. Neurosci.,* 5, 2909–2919.

Moncada, S., Palmer, R. M. J., and Higgs, E. A. (1991). Nitric oxide: Physiology, pathophysiology, and pharmacology. *Pharmacol. Rev.,* 43, 109–142.

Monck, J. R., and Fernandez, J. M. (1994). The exocytotic fusion pore and neurotransmitter release. *Neuron,* 12, 707–716.

Mondadori, C. (1993). The pharmacology of the nootropics; new insights and new questions. *Behav. Brain Res.,* 59, 1–9.

Monsma, F. J. Jr., McVittie, L. D., Gerfen, C. R., Mahan, L. C., and Sibley, D. R. (1989). Multiple D$_2$ dopamine receptors produced by alternative RNA splicing. *Nature,* 342, 926–929.

Montastruc, J. L., Rascol, O., and Senard, J. M. (1993). Current status of dopamine agonists in Parkinson's disease management. *Drugs,* 46, 384–393.

Montgomery, S. A. (1995). Selective serotonin reuptake inhibitors in the acute treatment of depression. In *Psychopharmacology: The Fourth Generation of Progress* (F. E. Bloom and D. J. Kupfer, Eds.), pp. 1043–1052. Raven Press, New York.

Monti, J. M. (1993). Involvement of histamine in the control of the waking state. *Life Sci.,* 53, 1331–1338.

Monyer, H., Seeburg, P. H., and Wisden, W. (1991). Glutamate-operated channels: Developmentally early and mature forms arise by alternative splicing. *Neuron,* 6, 799–810.

Moody, C. A., Frambes, N. A., and Spear, L. P. (1992). Psychopharmacological responsiveness to the dopamine agonist quinpirole in normal weanlings and in weanling offspring exposed gestationally to cocaine. *Psychopharmacology,* 108, 256–262.

Moore, K. E., and Demarest, K. T. (1984). Regulation of tuberoinfundibular dopaminergic neurons: The role of prolactin. In *Catecholamines,* Part B. *Neuropharmacology and Central Nervous System: Theoretical Aspects* (E. Usdin, A. Carlsson, A. Dahlström, and J. Engel, Eds.), pp. 451–462. Alan R. Liss, New York.

Moore, K. E., and Dominic, J. A. (1971). Tyrosine hydroxylase inhibitors. *Fed. Proc.,* 30, 859–870.

Moore, R. Y., and Bloom, F. E. (1979). Central catecholamine neuron systems: Anatomy and physiology of the norepinephrine and epinephrine systems. *Annu. Rev. Neurosci.,* 2, 113–168.

Moran, T. H., Robinson, P. H., Goldrich, M. S., and McHugh, P. R. (1986). Two brain cholecystokinin receptors: Implications for behavioral actions. *Brain Res.,* 362, 175–179.

Moratalla, R., Quinn, B., DeLanney, L. E., Irwin, I., Langston, J. W., and Graybiel, A. M. (1992). Differential vulnerability of primate caudate-putamen and striosome-matrix dopamine systems to the neurotoxic effects of 1-methyl-4-phenyl-1,2,3,6-tetrahydropyridine. *Proc. Natl. Acad. Sci. U.S.A.,* 89, 3859–3863.

Moreines, R. (1989). The psychedelics. In *Drugs of Abuse* (A. J. Giannini and A. E. Slaby, Eds.), pp. 207–241. Medical Economics Books, Oradell.

Morel, A., O'Carroll, A.-M., Brownstein, M. J., and Lolait, S. J. (1992). Molecular cloning and expression of a rat V1a arginine vasopressin receptor. *Nature,* 356, 523–526.

Morell, P. (Ed.) (1978). *Myelin.* Plenum Press, New York.

Morell, P. (Ed.) (1984). *Myelin* (2nd ed.). Plenum Press, New York.

Morell, P., and Norton, W. T. (1980). Myelin. *Sci. Am.,* 242 (5), 88–118.

Morelli, M., Mennini, T., and Di Chiara, G. (1988). Nigral dopamine autoreceptors are exclusively of the D$_2$ type: Quantitative autoradiography of [^{125}I]iodosulpride and [^{125}I]SCH 23982 in adjacent brain sections. *Neuroscience,* 27, 865–870.

Moret, C., and Briley, M. (1990). Serotonin autoreceptor subsensitivity and antidepressant activity. *Eur. J. Pharmacol.,* 180, 351–356.

Morgan, D. G., and May, P. C. (1990). Age-related changes in synaptic neurochemistry. In *Handbook of the Biology of Aging* (3rd ed.) (L. T. Landmesser, Ed.), pp. 219–253. Academic Press, San Diego.

Morgan, I. G., and Chubb, I. W. (1991). How peptidergic neurons cope with variation in physiological stimulation. *Neurochem. Res.,* 16, 705–714.

Morgan, J. I., and Curran, T. (1989a). Role of the immediate-early genes, *c-fos* and *c-jun*, in stimulus-transcription coupling in the mammalian central nervous system. In *The Assembly of the Nervous System,* pp. 235–246. Alan R. Liss, New York.

Morgan, J. I., and Curran, T. (1989b) Stimulus-transcription coupling in neurons: Role of cellular immediate-early genes. *Trends Neurosci.,* 12, 459–462.

Morgan, J. I., and Curran, T. (1991). Stimulus-transcription coupling in the nervous sytem. *Annu. Rev. Neurosci., 14,* 421–452.

Morgan, J. P. (1979). The clinical pharmacology of amphetamine. In *Amphetamine Use, Misuse, and Abuse* (D. E. Smith, D. R. Wesson, M. E. Buxton, R. B. Seymour, J. T. Ungerleider, J. P. Morgan, A. J. Mandell, and G. Jara, Eds.), pp. 3–10. Hall, Boston.

Morgan, K. (1984). Effects of two benzodiazepines on the speed and accuracy of perceptual–motor performance in the elderly. In *Sleep, Benzodiazepines and Performance: Experimental Methodologies and Research Prospects* (I. Hindmarch, H. Ott, and T. Roth, Eds.), pp. 79–83. Springer-Verlag, New York.

Morgan, M. E., and Gibb, J. W. (1980). Short-term and long-term effects of methamphetamine on biogenic amine metabolism in extra-striatal dopaminergic nuclei. *Neuropharmacology, 19,* 989–995.

Morgenroth, V. H. III, Boadle-Biber, M., and Roth, R. H. (1974). Tyrosine hydroxylase: Activation by nerve stimulation. *Proc. Natl. Acad. Sci. U.S.A., 71,* 4283–4287.

Morimoto, K. (1989). Seizure-triggering mechanisms in the kindling model of epilepsy: Collapse of GABA-mediated inhibition and activation of NMDA receptors. *Neurosci. Biobehav. Rev., 13,* 253–260.

Morimoto, K., and Goddard, G. V. (1986). Kindling induced changes in EEG recorded during stimulation from the site of stimulation: Collapse of GABA-mediated inhibition and onset of rhythmic synchronous burst. *Exp. Neurol., 94,* 571–584.

Mork, A., and Geisler, A. (1989a). Effects of GTP on hormone-stimulated adenylate cyclase activity in cerebral cortex, striatum, and hippocampus from rats treated chronically with lithium. *Biol. Psychiatry, 26,* 279–288.

Mork, A., and Geisler, A. (1989b). The effects of lithium in vitro and ex vivo on adenylate cyclase in brain are exerted by distinct mechanisms. *Neuropharmacology, 28,* 307–311.

Morley, J. E. (1990). Appetite regulation by gut peptides. *Annu. Rev. Nutr., 10,* 383–395.

Morley, J. E., Levine, A. S., Bartness, T. J., Nizielski, S. E., Shaw, M. J., and Hughes, J. J. (1985). Species differences in the response to cholecystokinin. *Ann. N.Y. Acad. Sci., 448,* 413–416.

Moroni, F., and Pepeu, G. (1984). The cortical cup technique. In *Measurement of Neurotransmitter Release In Vivo* (C. A. Marsden, Ed.), pp. 63–80. Wiley & Sons, New York.

Morot-Gaudry, Y., Bourgoin, S., and Hamon, M. (1981). Kinetic characteristics of newly synthesized ^{3}H-5-HT in the brain of control and reserpinized mice: Evidence for the heterogeneous distribution of 5-HT in serotoninergic neurons. *Naunyn Schmiedebergs Arch. Pharmacol., 316,* 311–316.

Morris, B. J., and Johnston, H. M. (1995). A role for hippocampal opioids in long-term functional plasticity. *Trends Neurosci., 18,* 350–355.

Morris, J. F., and Pow, D. V. (1991). Widespread release of peptides in the central nervous system: Quantitation of tannic acid-captured exocytoses. *Anat. Rec., 231,* 437–445.

Morris, J. L., and Gibbins, I. L. (1989). Co-localization and plasticity of transmitters in peripheral, autonomic and sensory neurons. *Int. J. Dev. Neurosci., 7,* 521–531.

Morris, R. G. M. (1984). Development of a water-maze procedure for studying spatial learning in the rat. *J. Neurosci. Methods, 11,* 47–60.

Morris, R. G. M. (1989). Synaptic plasticity and learning: Selective impairment of learning in rats and blockade of long-term potentiation in vivo by the N-methyl-D-aspartate receptor antagonist AP5. *J. Neurosci., 9,* 3040–3057.

Morris, R. G. M., Anderson, E., Lynch, G. S., and Baudry, M. (1986). Selective impairment of learning and blockage of long-term potentiation by an N-methyl-D-aspartate receptor antagonist, AP5. *Nature, 319,* 774–776.

Morrison, J. H., Foote, S. L., Molliver, M. E., Bloom, F. E., and Lidov, H. G. W. (1982). Noradrenergic and serotonergic fibers innervate complementary layers in monkey primary visual cortex: An immunohistochemical study. *Proc. Natl. Acad. Sci. U.S.A., 79,* 2401–2405.

Morrison, J. H., Grzanna, R., Molliver, M. E., and Coyle, J. T. (1978). The distribution and orientation of noradrenergic fibers in neocortex of the rat: An immunofluorescence study. *J. Comp. Neurol., 181,* 17–40.

Morrow, A. L., and Creese, I. (1986). Characterization of α_1-adrenergic receptor subtypes in rat brain: A reevaluation of [^{3}H]WB4101 and [^{3}H]prazosin binding. *Mol. Pharmacol., 29,* 321–330.

Mos, J., Olivier, B., and Tulp, M. T. M. (1992). Ethopharmacological studies differentiate the effects of various serotonergic compounds on aggression in rats. *Drug Dev. Res., 26,* 343–360.

Moseley, I. (1986). *Diagnostic Imaging in Neurological Disease*, Churchill Livingstone, New York.

Moskowitz, A. S., and Goodman, R. R. (1985). Autoradiographic distribution of mu$_1$ and mu$_2$ opioid binding in mouse central nervous sytem. *Brain Res., 360,* 117–129.

Moskowitz, M. A. (1992). Neurogenic versus vascular mechanisms of sumatriptan and ergot alkaloids in migraine. *Trends Pharmacol. Sci., 13,* 307–311.

Moss, S. J., Smart, T. G., Blackstone, C. D., and Huganir, R. L. (1992). Functional modulation of GABA$_A$ receptors by cAMP-dependent protein phosphorylation. *Science, 257,* 661–665.

Motulsky, H. J., and Insel, P. A. (1987). In vitro methods for studying human adrenergic receptors: Methods and applications. In *Adrenergic Receptors in Man*, Vol. 8 (P. Insel, Ed.), pp. 139–161. Marcel Dekker, New York.

Mount, H., Boksa, P., Chaudieu, I., and Quirion, R. (1990). Phencyclidine and related compounds evoke [^{3}H]dopamine release from rat mesencephalic cell cultures by a mechanism independent of the phencyclidine receptor, sigma binding site, or dopamine uptake site. *Can. J. Physiol. Pharmacol., 68,* 1200–1206.

Mountcastle, V. B., and Baldessarini, R. J. (1974). Synaptic transmission. In *Medical Physiology*, Vol. 1 (V. B. Mountcastle, Ed.), pp. 182–223. Mosby, St. Louis.

Moussa, B. H., Youdim, M. H., and Bourgoin, S. (1974). Purification of pig brainstem tryptophan hydroxylase and some of its properties. *Adv. Biochem. Psychopharmacol., 11,* 13–17.

Moyer, K. E. (1968). Kinds of aggression and their physiological basis. *Commun. Behav. Biol. A, 2,* 65–87.

Mudge, A. W., Leeman, S. E., and Fishbach, G. D. (1979). Enkephalin inhibits release of substance P from sensory neurons in culture and decreases action potential duration. *Proc. Natl. Acad. Sci. U.S.A., 76,* 526–530.

Mudgett-Hunter, M. (1986). Monoclonal antibodies. In *The Heart and Cardiovascular System* (H. Fozzard, E. Haber, R. Jennings, A. Katz, and H. Morgan, Eds.), pp. 189–201. Raven Press, New York.

Mueller, R. A., Thoenen, H., and Axelrod, J. (1969). Inhibition of trans-synaptically increased tyrosine hydroxylase activity by cycloheximide and actinomycin D. *Mol. Pharmacol., 5,* 463–469.

Mugnaini, E., and Oertel, W. H. (1985). An atlas of the distribution of GABAergic neurons and terminals in the rat CNS as revealed by GAD immunohistochemistry. In *Handbook of Chemical Neuroanatomy*, Vol. 4. *GABA and Neuropeptides in the CNS*, Part I (A. Björklund and T. Hökfelt, Eds.), pp. 436–608. Elsevier, Amsterdam.

Muir, J. L., Page, K. J., Sirinathsinghji, D. J. S., Robbins, T. W., and Everitt, B. J. (1993). Excitotoxic lesions of basal forebrain cholinergic neurons: Effects on learning, memory and attention. *Behav. Brain Res., 57,* 123–131.

Mulder, A. H., Frankhuysen, A. L., Stoof, J. C., Wemer, J., and Schoffelmeer, A. N. M. (1984). Catecholamine receptors, opiate receptors, and presynaptic modulation of neurotransmitter release in the brain. In *Neurology and Neurobiology*, Vol. 8B: *Catecholamines* (E. Usdin, A. Carlsson, A. Dahlstrom, and J. Engel, Eds.), pp. 47–58. Alan R. Liss, New York.

Mulder, A. H., and Schoffelmeer, A. N. M. (1993). Multiple opioid receptors and presynaptic modulation of neurotransmitter release in the brain. In *Opioids I*, Handbook of Experimental Pharmacology, Vol. 104 (A. Herz, Ed.), pp. 125–144. Springer-Verlag, New York.

Müller, O. A., and von Werder, K. (1991). Corticotropin-releasing hormone. In *Brain Endocrinology* (2nd ed.) (M. Motta, Ed.), pp. 351–375. Raven Press, New York.

Mulligan, K. A., and Törk, I. (1988). Serotoninergic innervation of the cat cerebral cortex. *J. Comp. Neurol., 270,* 86–110.

Mumford, J. P., and Cannon, D. J. (1994). Vigabatrin. *Epilepsia, 35* (Suppl. 5), S25–S28.

Munck, A., Guyre, P. M., and Holbrook, N. J. (1984). Physiological functions of glucocorticoids in stress and their relation to pharmacological actions. *Endocrinol. Rev., 5,* 25–44.

Munro, S., Thomas, K. L., and Abu-Shaar, M. (1993). Molecular characterization of a peripheral receptor for cannabinoids. *Nature, 365,* 61–65.

Murase, S., Nisell, M., Grenhoff, J., and Svensson, T. H. (1992). Decreased sensory responsiveness of noradrenergic neurons in the rat locus coeruleus following phencyclidine or dizocilpine (MK-801): Role of NMDA antagonism. *Psychopharmacology, 109,* 271–276.

Murphy, D. L., Aulakh, C. S., Garrick, N. A., and Sunderland, T. (1987). Monoamine oxidase inhibitors as antidepressants: Implications for the mechanism of action of antidepressants and the psychobiology of the affective disorders and some related disorders. In *Psychopharmacology: The Third Generation of Progress* (H. Y. Meltzer, Ed.), pp. 545–552. Raven Press, New York.

Murphy, D. L., Mitchell, P. B., and Potter, W. Z. (1995). Novel pharmacological approaches to the treatment of depression. In *Psychopharmacology: The Fourth Generation of Progress* (F. E. Bloom and D. J. Kupfer, Eds.), pp. 1143–1154. Raven Press, New York.

Murphy, D. L., Pigott, T. A., and Insel, T. R. (1990). Obsessive–compulsive disorder and anxiety. In *Handbook of Anxiety*, Vol. 3., *The Neurobiology of Anxiety* (G. D. Burrows, M. Roth, and R. Noyes Jr., Eds.), pp. 269–287. Elsevier, Amsterdam.

Murphy, D. L., and Wyatt, R. J. (1972). Reduced platelet monoamine oxidase activity in chronic schizophrenia. *Nature*, 238, 225–226.

Murphy, D. L., Zohar, J., Benkelfat, C., Pato, M. T., Pigott, T. A., and Insel, T. R. (1989). Obsessive–compulsive disorder as a 5-HT subsystem-related behavioural disorder. *Br. J. Psychiatry*, 155 (Suppl. 8), 15–24.

Murphy, R. B., Schneider, L. H., and Smith, G. P. (1988). Peripheral loci for the mediation of cholecystokinin-induced satiety. In *Cholecystokinin Antagonists* (R. Y. Wang and R. Schoenfeld, Eds.), pp. 73–91. Alan R. Liss, New York.

Murrin, L. C., Morgenroth, V. H. III, and Roth, R. H. (1976). Dopaminergic neurons: Effects of electrical stimulation on tyrosine hydroxylase. *Mol. Pharmacol.*, 12, 1070–1081.

Muscat, R., Sampson, D., and Willner, P. (1990). Dopaminergic mechanism of imipramine action in an animal model of depression. *Biol. Psychiatry*, 28, 223–230.

Mussap, C. J., Geraghty, D. P., and Burcher, E. (1993). Tachykinin receptors: A radioligand binding perspective. *J. Neurochem.*, 60, 1987–2009.

Musto, D. F. (1991). Opium, cocaine and marijuana in American history. *Sci. Am.*, 265, 40–47.

Mutt, V., and Jorpes, J. E. (1971). Hormonal polypeptides of the upper intestine. *Biochem. J.*, 125, 57P–58P.

Myerson, A. (1936). Effect of benzedrine sulfate on mood and fatigue in normal and in neurotic persons. *Arch. Neurol. Psychiatry*, 36, 816–822.

Myllylä, V. V., Heinonen, E. H., Vuorinen, J. A., Kilkku, O. I., and Sotaniemi, K. A. (1995). Early selegiline therapy reduces levodopa dose requirement in Parkinson's disease. *Acta Neurol. Scand.*, 91, 177–182.

Myllylä, V. V., Sotaniemi, K. A., Vuorinen, J. A., and Heinonen, E. H. (1992). Selegiline as initial treatment in de novo parkinsonian patients. *Neurology*, 42, 339–343.

Myrsten, A. L., Post, B., Frankenhaeuser, M., and Elgerot, A. (1975). Immediate effects of cigarette smoking as related to different smoking habits. *Percept. Mot. Skills*, 40, 515–523.

Naber, D. (1993). Opioids in the etiology and treatment of psychiatric disorders. In *Opioids II,*, Handbook of Experimental Pharmacology, Vol. 104 (A. Herz, Ed.), pp. 781–801. Springer-Verlag, New York.

Nabeshima, T., Yamaguchi, K., Ishikawa, K., Furukawa, H., and Kameyama, T. (1987). Potentiation in phencyclidine-induced serotonin-mediated behaviors after intracerebroventricular administration of 5,7-dihydroxytryptamine in rats. *J. Pharmacol. Exp. Ther.*, 243, 1139–1146.

Nader, M. A., Hedeker, D., and Woolverton, W. L. (1993). Behavioral economics and drug choice: effects of unit price on cocaine self-administration by monkeys. *Drug Alcohol Depend.*, 33, 193–199.

Nader, M. A. and Woolverton, W. L. (1992). Effects of increasing response requirement on choice between cocaine and food in rhesus monkeys. *Psychopharmacology*, 108, 295–300.

Nagahiro, S., Takada, A., Diksic, M., Sourkes, T.L., Missala, K., and Yamamoto, Y.L. (1990). A new method to measure brain serotonin synthesis in vivo. II. A practical autoradiographic method tested in normal and lithium-treated rats. *J. Cereb. Blood Flow Metab.*, 10, 13–21.

Nagai, T., McGeer, P. L., Araki, M. and McGeer, E. G. (1984). GABA-T-intensive neurons in the rat brain. In *Classical Transmitters and Transmitter Receptors in the CNS, Part II. Handbook of Chemical Neuroanatomy*, Vol. 3 (A. Björklund, T. Hökfelt and M. J. Kuhar, Eds.), pp. 247–272. Elsevier, Amsterdam.

Nagatsu, T. (1991). Genes for human catecholamine-synthesizing enzymes. *Neurosci. Res.*, 12, 315–345.

Nagatsu, T., Hidaka, H., Kuzuya, H., and Takeya, K. (1970). Inhibition of dopamine β-hydroxylase by fusaric acid (5-butylpicolinic acid) in vitro and in vivo. *Biochem. Pharmacol.*, 19, 35–44.

Nagatsu, T., and Ichinose, H. (1991). Comparative studies on the structure of human tyrosine hydroxylase with those of the enzyme of various mammals. *Comp. Biochem. Physiol.*, 98C, 203–210.

Nagatsu, T., Levitt, M., and Udenfriend, S. (1964). Tyrosine hydroxylase: The initial step in norepinephrine biosynthesis. *J. Biol. Chem.*, 238, 2910–2917.

Nagy, J. I., Geiger, J. D., and Staines, W. A. (1990). Adenosine deaminase and purinergic regulation. *Neurochem. Int.*, 16, 211–221.

Nahas, G. G. (1975). *Marijuana—Deceptive Weed*. Raven Press, New York.

Nahmias, C., Garnett, E. S., Firnau, G., and Lang, A. (1985). Striatal dopamine distribution in Parkinsonian patients during life. *J. Neurol. Sci.*, 69, 223–230.

Nahorski, S. R. (1988). Inositol polyphosphates and neuronal calcium homeostasis. *Trends Neurosci.*, 11, 444–448.

Naito, S. and Ueda, T. (1985). Characterization of glutamate uptake into synaptic vesicles. *J. Neurochem.*, 44, 99–109.

Nakajima, S. (1989). Subtypes of dopamine receptors involved in the mechanism of reinforcement. *Neurosci. Biobehav. Rev.*, 13, 123–128.

Nakajima, S., Daval, J.-C., Morgan, P. F., Post, R. M., and Marangos, P. J. (1989). Adenosinergic modulation of caffeine-induced c-fos mRNA expression in mouse brain. *Brain Res.*, 501, 307–314.

Nakajima, S., Liu, X., and Lau, C. L. (1993). Synergistic interaction of D_1 and D_2 dopamine receptors in the modulation of the reinforcing effect of brain stimulation. *Behav. Neurosci.*, 107, 161–165.

Nakanishi, S., Inoue, A., Kita, T., Nakamura, M., Chung, A.C.Y., Cohen, S.N. and Numa, S. (1979). Nucleotide sequence of cloned cDNA for bovine corticotropin-beta-lipotropin precursor. *Nature*, 278, 423–427.

Namba, Y., Tomonaga, M., Kawasaki, H., Otomo, E., and Ikeda, K. (1991). Apolipoprotein E immunoreactivity in cerebral amyloid deposits and neurofibrillary tangles in Alzheimer's disease and kuru plaque amyloid in Creutzfeldt-Jakob disease. *Brain Res.*, 541, 163–166.

Nanson, J. L., and Hiscock, M. (1990). Attention deficits in children exposed to alcohol prenatally. *Alcohol. Clin. Exp. Res.*, 14, 656–661.

Narahashi, T., Moore, J. W., and Scott, W. R. (1964). Tetrodotoxin blockage of sodium conductance increase in lobster giant axons. *J. Gen. Physiol.*, 47, 965–974.

Naranjo, C. A., Sellers, E. M., and Larwin, M. O. (1986). Modulation of ETOH intake by 5-HT uptake inhibitors. *J. Neuropsychiatry Clin. Neurosci.*, 47 (Suppl.), 16–22.

Naranjo, C. A., Sellers, E. M., Roach, C. A., Woodley, D. V., Sanchez-Craig, M., et al. (1984). Zimelidine-induced variations in alcohol intake by non-depressed heavy drinkers. *Clin. Pharmacol. Ther.*, 35, 374–381.

Naranjo, C., Sellers, E., and Wu, P. (1985). Moderation of ethanol drinking; Role of enhanced serotonergic neurotransmission. In *Research Advances in New Psychopharmacological Treatments for Alcoholism* (C. Naranjo and E. Sellers, Eds.), pp 171–186, Excerpta Medica, New York.

Nasrallah, H. A. (1993). Neurodevelopmental pathogenesis of schizophrenia. *Psychiatr. Clin. North Am.*, 16, 269–280.

Nasrallah, H. B., and Coryel, W. H. (1982). Dexamethasone nonsuppression predicts the antidepressant effects of sleep deprivation. *Psychiatry Res.*, 68, 61–64.

Nastuk, M. A., and Fallon, J. R. (1993). Agrin and the molecular choreography of synapse formation. *Trends Neurosci.*, 16, 72–76.

Nastuk, W. L. (1974). Neuromuscular transmission. In *Medical Physiology*, Vol. 1 (V. B. Mountcastle, Ed.), pp. 151–181. Mosby, St. Louis.

Nathan, C. and Rolland, Y. (1987). Pharmacological treatments that affect CNS activity: serotonin. *Ann. N. Y. Acad. Sci.*, 499, 277–296.

Nathan, P. E. (1990). Residual effects of alcohol. *NIDA Res. Monogr.*, 101,112–123.

Nathanson, M. H. (1937). The central action of beta-aminopropylbenzene (benzedrine). Clinical observations. *JAMA*, 108, 528–531.

National Institute on Drug Abuse. (1991). *National Household Survey on Drug Abuse. Population Estimates, 1990*. U.S. Dept. of Health and Human Services, Rockville, Maryland.

Nayeem, N., Green, T. P., Martin, I. L., and Barnard, E. A. (1994). Quaternary structure of the native $GABA_A$ receptor determined by electron microscope image analysis. *J. Neurochem.*, 62, 815–818.

Negin, E. (1985). Just a pinch between your cheek and gum. *Public Citizen*, Spring, 28–32.

Neisewander, J. L., O'Dell, L. E., and Redmond, J. C. (1995). Localization of dopamine receptor subtypes occupied that reverse cocaine-induced locomotion. *Brain Res.*, 671, 201–212.

Nemeroff, C. B., Kalivas, P. W., Golden, R. N., and Prange, A. J., Jr. (1984). Behavioral effects of hypothalamic hypophysiotropic hormones, neurotensin, substance P and other neuropeptides. *Pharmacol. Ther., 24,* 1–56.

Nemeroff, C. B., Berger, P. A. and Bissette, G. (1987). Peptides in schizophrenia. In *Psychopharmacology: The Third Generation of Progress* (H.Y. Meltzer, Ed.), pp. 727–743. Raven Press, New York.

Nestler, E. J. (1992). Molecular mechanisms of drug addiction. *J. Neurosci., 12,* 2439–2450.

Nestler, E. J., Alreja, M., and Aghajanian, G. K. (1994). Molecular and cellular mechanisms of opiate action: studies in the rat locus coeruleus. *Brain Res. Bull., 35,* 521–528.

Nestoros, J. N. (1980). Ethanol specifically potentiates GABA-mediated neurotransmission in feline cerebral cortex. *Science, 209,* 708–710.

Netter, F. H. (1983). *The Ciba Collection of Medical Illustrations.* Vol. 1, *Nervous System,* Part 1, *Anatomy and Physiology.* Ciba Pharmaceutical Company, West Caldwell, NJ.

Neuman, R. S. and Zebrowska, G. (1992). Serotonin (5-HT$_2$) receptor mediated enhancement of cortical unit activity. *J. Physiol. Pharmacol.,70,* 1604–1609.

Neuspiel, D. R. and Hamel, S. C. (1991). Cocaine and infant behavior. *Dev. Behav. Pediat.,* 12, 55-64.

Newby, A. C. (1984). The solubilization of membrane proteins. In *Brain Receptor Methodologies* (P. J. Marangos, I. C. Campbell, and R. M. Cohen, Eds.), pp. 76–93. Academic Press, New York.

Newman, H. W., and Lehman, A. J. (1938). Nature of acquired tolerance to alcohol. *J. Pharmacol. Exp. Ther., 62,* 301–306.

Newman, M. E., and Belmaker, R. H. (1987). Effects of lithium in vitro and ex vivo on components of the adenylate cyclase system in membranes from the cerebral cortex of the rat. *Neuropharmacology, 26,* 211–217.

Newman, M. E., Klein, E., Birmaker, B., Feinsod, M., and Belmaker, R. H. (1983). Lithium at therapeutic concentrations inhibits human brain noradrenaline-sensitive cyclic AMP accumulation. *Brain Res., 278,* 380–381.

Newmeyer, J. A. (1979). The epidemiology of amphetamine use. In *Amphetamine Use, Misuse, and Abuse* (D. E. Smith, D. R. Wesson, M. E. Buxton, R. B. Seymour, J. T. Ungerleider, J. P. Morgan, A. J. Mandell, and G. Jara, Eds.), pp. 55–72. Hall, Boston.

Ng, L. K. Y., Chase, T. N., Colburn, R. W., and Kopin, I. J. (1970). L-dopa-induced release of cerebral monoamines. *Science, 170,* 76–77.

Nguyen-Legros, J., Harnois, C., Di Paolo, T., and Simon, A. (1993). The retinal dopamine system in Parkinson's disease. *Clin. Vision Sci.,* 8, 1–12.

Nicholas, A. P., Pieribone, V. A., and Hökfelt, T. (1993). Cellular localization of messenger RNA for beta-1 and beta-2 adrenergic receptors in rat brain: An in situ hybridization study. *Neuroscience, 56,* 1023–1039.

Nicholas, A. P., Pieribone, V., and Hökfelt, T. (1993b). Distributions of mRNAs for alpha-2 adrenergic receptor subtypes in rat brain: an in situ hybridization study. *J. Comp. Neurol.,328,* 575–594.

Nicholls, D. and Attwell, D. (1990). The release and uptake of excitatory amino acids. *Trends Pharmacol. Sci.,11,* 462–468.

Nicholls, D. G. (1989). Release of glutamate, aspartate, and γ-aminobutyric acid from isolated nerve terminals. *J. Neurochem., 52,* 331–341.

Nicholls, D. G. (1994). *Proteins, Transmitters and Synapses.* Blackwell Scientific Publications, Oxford.

Nicholls, J. G., Martin, A. R., and Wallace, B. G. (1992). *From Neuron to Brain* (3rd ed.). Sinauer Associates, Sunderland, MA.

Nicklas, W. J., Zeevalk, G. and Hyndman, A. (1987). Interactions between neurons and glia in glutamate/glutamine compartmentation. *Biochem. Soc. Trans., 15,* 208–213.

Nicolaysen, L. C. and Justice, J. B. Jr. (1988). Effects of cocaine on release and uptake of dopamine in vivo: differentiation by mathematical modeling. *Pharmacol. Biochem. Behav.,* 31, 327–335.

Nicolaysen, L. C., Pan, H.-T., and Justice, J. B. Jr. (1988). Extracellular cocaine and dopamine concentrations are linearly related in rat striatum. *Brain Res., 456,* 317–323.

Nicoll, R. A. (1978a). Pentobarbital: Differential postsynaptic action on sympathetic ganglion cells. *Science, 199,* 451–452.

Nicoll, R. A. (1978b). Selective actions of barbiturates on synaptic transmission. In *Psychopharmacology: A Generation of Progress* (M. A. Lipton, A. DiMascio, and K. F. Killam, Eds.), pp. 1337–1348. Raven Press, New York.

Nicoll, R. A. (1988). The coupling of neurotransmitter receptors to ion channels in the brain. *Science, 241,* 545–551.

Nicoll, R. A. and Alger, B. E. (1979). Presynaptic inhibition: transmitter and ionic mechanisms. *Int. Rev. Neurobiol., 21,* 217–258.

Nicoll, R. A., and Iwamoto, E. T. (1978). Action of pentobarbital on sympathetic ganglion cells. *J. Neurophysiol., 41,* 4:977–986.

Nicoll, R. A., Kauer, J. A., and Malenka, R. C. (1988). The current excitement in long-term potentiation. *Neuron,1,* 97–103.

Nicoll, R. A., Malenka, R. C., and Kauer, J. A. (1990). Functional comparison of neurotransmitter receptor subtypes in mammalian central nervous system. *Physiol. Rev.,70,* 513–565.

Nielsen, E. B. and Jepsen, S. (1985). Antagonism of the amphetamine cue by both classical and atypical antipsychotic drugs. *Eur. J. Pharmacol.,11,* 167–176.

Nielsen, E. B. and Scheel-Krüger, J. (1986). Cueing effects of amphetamine and LSD: Elicitation by direct microinjection of the drugs into the nucleus accumbens. *Eur. J. Pharmacol.,125,* 85–92.

Nielsen, J. A., Chapin, D. S., and Moore, K. E. (1983). Differential effects of d-amphetamine, β-phenylethylamine, cocaine and methylphenidate on the rate of dopamine synthesis in terminals of nigrostriatal and mesolimbic neurons and on the efflux of dopamine metabolites into cerebroventricular perfusates of rats. *Life Sci., 33,* 1899–1907.

Nielsen, K. H. and Blaustein, J. D. (1990). Many progestin receptor-containing neurons in the guinea pig ventrolateral hypothalamus contain substance P: Immunocytochemical evidence. *Brain Res., 517,* 175–181.

Nieuwenhuys, R. (1985). *Chemoarchitecture of the Brain.* Springer-Verlag, Berlin.

Nikodijević, O., Daly, J. W., and Jacobson, K. A. (1990). Characterization of the locomotor depression produced by an A$_2$-selective adenosine agonist. *FEBS Lett., 261,* 67–70.

Nilsson, O. G., Leanza, G., Rosenblad, C., Lappi, D. A., Wiley, R. G., and Bjorklund, A. (1992). Spatial learning impairments in rats with selective immunolesion of the forebrain cholinergic system. *Neuroreport,3,* 1005–1008.

Ninan, P. T., Insel, T. M., Cohen, R. M., Cook, J. M., Skolnick, P., and Paul, S. M. (1982). Benzodiazepine receptor-mediated experimental "anxiety" in primates. *Science, 218,* 1332–1334.

Nisell, M., Nomikos, G. G., and Svensson, T. H. (1994). Systemic nicotine-induced dopamine release in the rat nucleus accumbens is regulated in the ventral tegmental area. *Synapse,16,* 36–44.

Nishikawa, T., Umino, A., Tanii, U. Y., Hashimoto, A., Nata, N. Takashima, M., Takahashi, K., and Toru, M. (1991). Dysfunction of excitatory amino acidergic systems and schizophrenic disorders. In *Biological Basis of Schizophrenic Disorders* (T. Nakazawa, Ed.) pp. 65–76. Japan Scientific Societies Press, Karger, New York.

Nissen, M. J., Knopman, D. S., and Schachter, D. L. (1987). Neurochemical dissociation of memory systems. *Neurology, 37,* 789–794.

Nissinen, E., Lindén, I.-B., Schultz, E., Kaakkola, S., Männistö, P. T., and Pohto, P. (1988). Inhibition of catechol-O-methyltransferase activity by two novel disubstituted catechols in the rat. *Eur. J. Pharmacol., 153,* 263–269.

Niznik, H. B., Fogel, E. F., Fassos, F. F., and Seeman, P. (1991). The dopamine transporter is absent in Parkinsonian putamen and reduced in the caudate nucleus. *J. Neurochem., 56,* 192–198.

Noback, C. R. (1967). *The Human Nervous System.* McGraw-Hill, New York

Noback, C. R., and Demarest, R. J. (1977). *The Nervous System.* McGraw-Hill, New York.

Noble, E. P. (1984). The biochemistry and pathophysiology of alcoholism. *Ann. Intern. Med., 100,* 405–416.

Noble, E. P., Blum, K., Ritchie, T., Montgomery, A., and Sheridan, P. J. (1991). Allelic association of the D$_2$ dopamine receptor gene with receptor-binding characteristics in alcoholism. *Arch. Gen. Psychiatry, 48,* 648–654.

Noda, M., Furutani, Y., et al. (1983). Cloning and sequence analysis of calf cDNA and human genomic DNA encoding alpha-subunit precursor of muscle acetylcholine receptor. *Nature, 305,* 818–823.

Noda, M., Shimizu, S., et al. (1986). Primary structure of Electrophorus electricus sodium channel deduced from cDNA sequence. *Nature, 312,* 121–127.

Noguchi, K., Morita, Y., Kiyama, H., Ono, K., and Tohyama, M. (1988). A noxious stimulus induces the preprotachykinin-A gene expression in the rat dorsal root ganglion: a quantitative study using in situ hybridization histochemistry. *Mol. Brain Res., 4,* 31–35.

Nomikos, G. G. and Spyraki, C. (1988). Cocaine-induced place conditioning: Importance of route of administration and other procedural variables. *Psychopharmacology, 94,* 167–173.

Nomikos, G. G., Damsma, G., Wenkstern, D., and Fibiger, H. C. (1990). In vivo characterization of locally applied dopamine uptake inhibitors by striatal microdialysis. *Synapse, 6,* 106–112.

Nordmann, J. J., and Artault, J.-C. (1992). Membrane retrieval following exocytosis in isolated neurosecretory nerve endings. *Neuroscience, 49*, 201–207.

Nordstrom, A-L., Farde, L., and Halldin, C. (1992). Time course of D_2-dopamine receptor occupancy examined by PET after single oral doses of haloperidol. *Psychopharmacology, 106*, 433–438.

Nordstrom, A-L., Farde, L., and Halldin, C. (1993). High 5-HT_2 receptor occupancy in clozapine treated patients demonstrated by PET. *Psychopharmacology, 110*, 365–367.

Nordström, P. and Åsberg, M. (1992). Suicide risk and serotonin. *Int. Clin. Psychopharmacol., 6* (Suppl. 6), 12–21.

Norenberg, M. D. (1979). The distribution of glutamine synthetase in the rat central nervous system. *J. Histochem. Cytochem., 27*, 756–762.

North, R. A. (1989). Drug receptors and the inhibition of nerve cells. *Br. J. Pharmacol., 98*, 13–28.

North, R.A. (1993). Opioid actions on membrane ion channels. In *Opioids I*, Handbook of Experimental Pharmacology, Vol. 104 (A. Herz, Ed.), pp. 773–797. Springer-Verlag, New York.

North, R.A. and Williams, J.T. (1976). Enkephalin inhibits firing of myenteric neurons. *Nature, 264*, 460–461.

North, R. A., Williams, J. T., Surprenant, A., and Christie, M. J. (1987). 1 and δ receptors belong to a family of receptors that are coupled to potassium channels. *Proc. Natl. Acad. Sci. U.S.A., 84*, 5487–5491.

Norton, W. T. (1976). Formation, structure, and biochemistry of myelin. In *Basic Neurochemistry* (G. J. Sieger, R. W. Albers, R. Katzman and B. W. Agranoff, Eds.), pp. 74–99. Little Brown, Boston.

Nottebohm, F. (1979). Origins and mechanisms in the establishment of cerebral dominance. In *Handbook of Behavioral Neurobiology*, Vol. 2, *Neuropsychology*. (M. S. Gazzaniga, Ed.), pp. 295–344. Plenum Press, New York.

Novick, D.M., Pascarelli, E.F., Joseph, H., Salsitz, E.A., Richman, B.L., DesJarlais, D.C., Anderson, M., Dole, V.P. and Nyswander, M.E. (1988). Methadone maintenance. *JAMA, 259*, 3299–3302.

Nuechterlein, K. H., and Dawson, M. E. (1995). Neurophysiological and psychophysiological approaches to schizophrenia. In *Psychopharmacology: The Fourth Generation of Progress* (F. E. Bloom and D. J. Kupfer, Eds.), pp. 1235–1244. Raven Press, New York.

Nulman, I., Rovet, J., Altmann, D., Bradley, C., Einarson, T., and Koren, G. (1994). Neurodevelopment of adopted children exposed in utero to cocaine. *Can. Med. Assoc. J., 151*, 1591–1597.

Nusser, Z., Mulvihill, E., Streit, P., and Somogyi, P. (1994). Subsynaptic segregation of metabotropic and ionotropic glutamate receptors as revealed by immunogold localization. *Neuroscience, 61*, 421–427.

Nutt, D. J., and Glue, P. (1993). The neurobiology of ECT: Animal studies. In *The Clinical Science of Electroconvulsive Therapy* (C. E. Coffey, Ed.), pp. 235–250. American Psychiatric Press, Washington, D.C.

Nyberg. F. (1993). CSF opioids in pathophysiology. In *Opioids II*, Handbook of Behavioral Neurology, Vol. 104 (A. Herz, Ed.), pp. 653–671. Springer-Verlag, New York.

Nyberg, F. and Terenius, L. (1988). Neurochemical methods in the study of the role of endorphins in psychiatric disorders. In *Endorphins, Opiates and Behavioural Processes* (R.J. Rodgers and S.J. Cooper, Eds.) John Wiley and Sons, Ltd., New York.

Oades, R. D. (1987). Attention deficit disorder with hyperactivity (ADDH): The contribution of catecholaminergic activity. *Prog. Neurobiol., 29*, 365–391.

Obata, K., Ito, M., Ochi, R., and Sato, N. (1967). Pharmacological properties of the postsynaptic inhibition by Purkinje cell axons and the action of γ-aminobutyric acid on Deiter's neurones. *Exp. Brain Res., 4*, 43–57.

Obata, K., and Takeda, K. (1969). Release of γ-aminobutyric acid into the fourth ventricle induced by stimulation of the cat's cerebellum. *J. Neurochem., 16*, 1043–1047.

O'Brien, C. P. (1993). Opioid addiction. In *Opioids II*, Handbook of Behavioral Neurology, Vol. 104 (A. Herz, Ed.), pp. 803–824. Springer-Verlag, New York.

O'Brien, C. P. (1994). Treatment of alcoholism as a chronic disorder. In *Toward a Molecular Basis of Alcohol Use and Abuse* (B. Jansson, H. Jörnvall, U. Rydberg, L. Terenius and B. L. Vallee, Eds.). pp. 349–359, Birkhäuser Verlag, Basel, Switzerland.

O'Brien, C. P., Childress, A. R., McLellan, A. T., and Ehrman, R. (1993). Developing treatments that address classical conditioning. *NIDA Res. Monogr., 135*, 71–91.

Ochoa, E. L. M. (1994). Nicotine-related brain disorders: The neurobiological basis of nicotine dependence. *Cell. Mol. Neurobiol., 14*, 195–225.

Ochoa, E. L. M., Chattopadhyay, A., and McNamee, M. G. (1989). Desensitization of the nicotinic acetylcholine receptor: Molecular mechanisms and effect of modulators. *Cell. Mol. Neurobiol., 9*, 141–178.

Ochs, S. (1972). Fast transport of materials in mammalian nerve fibers. *Science, 176*, 252–260.

Ochs, S. (1975). Axoplasmic transport. In *The Nervous System*, Vol. 1 (D. B. Tower, Ed.), pp. 137–146. Raven Press, New York.

Ochs, S. (1981). Axoplasmic transport. In *Basic Neurochemistry* (3rd ed.) (C. J. Siegel, R. W. Albers, B. W. Agranoff and R. Katzman, Eds.), pp. 425–442. Little, Brown, Boston.

O'Dell, S. J., Weihmuller, F. B., and Marshall, J. F. (1991). Multiple methamphetamine injections induce marked increases in extracellular striatal dopamine which correlate with subsequent neurotoxicity. *Brain Res., 564*, 256–260.

O'Dell, S. J., Weihmuller, F. B., and Marshall, J. F. (1993). Methamphetamine-induced dopamine overflow and injury to striatal dopamine terminals: Attenuation by dopamine D_1 or D_2 antagonists. *J. Neurochem., 60*, 1792–1799.

O'Donohue, T. L., Millington, W. R., Handelmann, G. E., Contreras, P. C., and Chronwall, B. M. (1985). On the 50th anniversary of Dale's law: Multiple neurotransmitter neurons. *Trends Pharmacol. Sci., 6*, 305–308.

O'Dowd, B. F. (1993). Structures of dopamine receptors. *J. Neurochem., 60*, 804–816.

Oechsli, F. W. and Seltzer, C. C. (1984). Teenage smoking and antecedent parental characteristics: A prospective study. *Pub. Health, 98*, 103–108.

Offermanns, S., and Schultz, G. (1994). Complex information processing by the transmembrane signaling system involving G proteins. *Naunyn Schmiedebergs Arch. Pharmacol., 350*, 329–338.

Ogawa, N. (1994). Levodopa and dopamine agonists in the treatment of Parkinson's disease: Advantages and disadvantages. *Eur. Neurol., 34* (Suppl. 3), 20–28.

Ogborne, A. C., and Glaser, F. B. (1981). Characteristics of affiliates of Alcoholics Anonymous: A review of the literature. *J. Stud. Alcohol, 42*, 661–675.

Ohisalo, J. J. (1987). Regulatory functions of adenosine. *Med. Biol., 65*, 181–191.

Ojesjo, L. (1981). Long-term outcome in alcohol abuse and alcoholism among males in the Lundby general population, Sweden. *Br. J. Addict., 76*, 391–400.

Okamoto, M. (1984). Barbiturate tolerance and physical dependence: Contribution of pharmacological factors. *NIDA Res. Monogr., 54*, 333–347.

Oksenberg, D., Marsters, S. A., O'Dowd, B. F., Jin, H., Havlik, S., Peroutka, S. J., and Ashkenazi, A. (1992). A single amino-acid difference confers major pharmacological variation between human and rodent 5-HT_{1B} receptors. *Nature, 360*, 161–163.

Okuno, S., and Fujisawa, H. (1985). A new mechanism for regulation of tyrosine 3-monooxygenase by end product and cyclic AMP-dependent protein kinase. *J. Biol. Chem., 260*, 2633–2635.

Olanow, C. W., Kordower, J. H., and Freeman, T. B. (1996). Fetal nigral transplantation as a therapy for Parkinson's disease. *Trends Neurosci., 19*, 102–109.

Olasmaa, M., Guidotti, A., Grayson, D., and Costa, E. (1991). Regulation of medullary tyrosine hydroxylase (TH) expression by nicotinic and VIP receptor activation. *J. Neurochem., 56* (Suppl.), S20.

Oldendorf, W. H. (1975). Permeability of the blood-brain barrier. In *The Nervous System*, Vol. 1 (D. B. Tower, Ed.), pp. 279–289. Raven Press, New York.

Oldendorf, W. H. (1980). *The Quest for an Image of Brain: Computerized Tomography in the Perspective of Past and Future Imaging Methods*. Raven Press, New York.

Oldendorf, W. H. (1985). Principles of imaging structure by NMR. In *Brain Imaging and Brain Function* (L. Sokoloff, Ed.), pp. 245–257. Raven Press, New York.

Oldendorf, W. H. (1992). Some relationships between addiction and drug delivery to the brain. *NIDA Res. Monogr. 120*, 13–25.

Olds, J., and Milner, P. (1954). Positive reinforcement produced by electrical stimulation of septal area and other regions of the rat brain. *J. Comp. Physiol. Psychol., 47*, 419–427.

Olenick, N. L., and Chalmers, D. K. (1991). Gender-specific drinking styles in alcoholics and nonalcoholics. *J. Stud. Alcohol, 52*, 325–330.

Olivier, B., and Mos, J. (1992). Rodent models of aggressive behavior and serotonergic drugs. *Prog. Neuropsychopharmacol. Biol. Psychiatry, 16*, 847–870.

Olivier, B., Tulp, M. T. M., and Mos, J. (1991). Serotonergic receptors in anxiety and aggression: Evidence from animal pharmacology. *Hum. Psychopharmacol., 6*, S73–S78.

Ollat, H., Parvez, H., and Parvez, S. (1988). Alcohol and central neurotransmission. *Neurochem. Int.* 13, 275–300.

Olney, J. W. (1969). Brain lesions, obesity, and other disturbances in mice treated with monosodium glutamate. *Science,* 164, 719–721.

Olney, J. W. (1989). Excitatory amino acids and neuropsychiatric disorders. *Biol. Psychiatry,* 26, 505–525.

Olney, J. W., Ho, O. L., and Rhee, V. (1971). Cytotoxic effects of acidic and sulphur containing amino acids on the infant mouse central nervous system. *Exp. Brain Res.,* 14, 61–76.

Olney, J. W., Labruyere, J., and Price, M. T. (1989). Pathological changes induced in cerebrocortical neurons by phencyclidine and related drugs. *Science,* 244, 1360–1362.

Olney, J. W., Labruyere, J., Wang, G., Wozniak, D. F., Price, M. T., and Sesma, M. A. (1991). NMDA antagonist neurotoxicity: Mechanism and prevention. *Science,* 254, 1515–1518.

Olney, J. W., Rhee, V., and Ho, O. L. (1974). Kainic acid: A powerful neurotoxic analogue of glutamate. *Brain Res.,* 77, 507–512.

Olpe, H.-R., Karlsson, G., Pozza, M. F., Brugger, F., Steinmann, M., Van Riezen, H., Fagg, G., Hall, R. G., Froestl, W., and Bittiger, H. (1990). CGP 35348: A centrally active blocker of GABA$_B$ receptors. *Eur. J. Pharmacol.,* 187, 27–38.

Olsen, R. W. (1987). The gamma-butyric acid/benzodiazepine/barbiturate receptor chloride ion channel complex of mammalian brain. In *Synaptic Function* (W. E. Gall and W. M. Cowan, Eds.), pp. 257–271. Wiley, New York.

Olsen, R. W., Sapp, D. M., Bureau, M. H., Turner, D. M., and Kokka, N. (1991). Allosteric actions of central nervous system depressants including anesthetics on subtypes of the inhibitory γ-aminobutyric acid$_A$ receptor–chloride channel complex. *Ann. N.Y. Acad. Sci.,* 625, 145–154.

Olson, G. A., Olson, R. D., and Kastin, A. J. (1989). Endogenous opiates. *Peptides,* 11, 1277–1304.

Olton, D. S. (1985). Strategies for the development of animal models of human memory impairments. *Ann. N.Y. Acad. Sci.,* 444, 113–121.

Olton, D. S., Collison, C., and Werz, M. A. (1977). Spatial memory and radial arm maze performance in rats. *Learn. Motiv.,* 8, 289–314.

O'Malley, K. L., Harmon, S., Tang, L., and Todd, R. D. (1992). The rat dopamine D$_4$ receptor: Sequence, gene structure, and demonstration of expression in the cardiovascular system. *New Biol.,* 4, 137–146.

O'Malley, S. S., Jaffe, A. J., Chang, G., Schattenfeld, R. S., Meyer, R. E., and Rounseville, B. (1992). Naltrexone and coping skills therapy for alcohol dependence. *Arch. Gen. Psychiatry,* 49, 881–887.

Onali, P., Mosca, E., and Olianas, M. C. (1992). Presynaptic dopamine autoreceptors and second messengers controlling tyrosine hydroxylase activity in rat brain. *Neurochem. Int.,* 20 (Suppl.), 89S–93S.

Onken, L. S., Blaine, J. D., and Boren, J. J., Eds. (1993). Behavioral treatments for drug abuse and dependence. *NIDA Res. Monogr.,* 137.

Onodera, K., Yamatodani, A., Watanabe, T., and Wada, H. (1994). Neuropharmacology of the histaminergic neuron system in the brain and its relationship with behavioral disorders. *Prog. Neurobiol.,* 42, 685–702.

Oorshot, D. E., and Jones, D. G. (1987). The vesicle hypothesis and its alternatives: A critical assessment. *Curr. Top. Res. Synapses,* 4, 85–153.

Ornstein, P. L., Arnold, M. B., Augenstein, N. K., Lodge, D., Leander, J. D., and Schoepp, D. D. (1993). (3SR,4aRS,6RS,8aRS)-6-[2-(1H-tetrazol-5-yl)ethyl]decahydroisoquinoline-3-carboxylic acid: A structurally novel, systemically active, competitive AMPA receptor antagonist. *J. Med. Chem.,* 36, 2046–2048.

Orrego, F., and Villanueva, S. (1993). The chemical nature of the main central excitatory transmitter: A critical appraisal based upon release studies and synaptic vesicle localization. *Neuroscience,* 56, 539–555.

Osborne, N. N. (1982). Evidence for serotonin being a neurotransmitter in the retina. In *Biology of Serotonergic Transmission* (N. N. Osborne, Ed.), pp. 401–430. Wiley, Chichester.

O'Shea, K. S., and Kaufman, M. H. (1979). The teratogenic effect of acetaldehyde: Implications for the study of the fetal alcohol syndrome. *J. Anat.,* 128, 65–76.

Osmond, H. (1957). A review of the clinical effects of psychotomimetic agents. *Ann. N.Y. Acad. Sci.,* 66, 418–434.

Ostrowski, J., Kjelsberg, M. A., Caron, M. G., and Lefkowitz, R. J. (1992). Mutagenesis of the β$_2$-adrenergic receptor: How structure elucidates function. *Annu. Rev. Pharmacol. Toxicol.,* 32, 167–183.

Oswald, R., and Changeux, J. P. (1981). Ultraviolet light-induced labeling by noncompetitive blockers of the acetylcholine receptor from *Torpedo marmorata. Proc. Natl. Acad. Sci. U.S.A.,* 78, 3925–3929.

Otsuka, M., Iversen, L. L., Hall, Z. W., and Kravitz, E. A. (1966). Release of gamma-aminobutyric acid from inhibitory nerves of lobster. *Proc. Natl. Acad. Sci. U.S.A.,* 56, 1110–1115.

Otsuka, M., and Yanagisawa, M. (1987). Does substance P act as a pain transmitter? *Trends Pharmacol. Sci.,* 8, 506–510.

Otsuka, M., and Yoshioka, K. (1993). Neurotransmitter functions of mammalian tachykinins. *Physiol. Rev.,* 73, 229–308.

Ottersen, O. P., Storm-Mathisen, J., and Somogyi, P. (1988). Colocalization of glycine-like and GABA-like immunoreactivities in Golgi cell terminals in the rat cerebellum: A postembedding light and electron microscopic study. *Brain Res.,* 450, 342–353.

Overton, D. A. (1984). State dependent learning and drug discriminations. In *Handbook of Psychopharmacology,* Vol. 18 (L. L. Iversen, S. D. Iversen, and S. H. Snyder, Eds.), pp. 59–112. Plenum Press, New York.

Overton, D. A. (1987). Drugs as discriminative stimuli. In *Methods of Assessing the Reinforcing Properties of Abused Drugs* (M. A. Bozarth, Ed.), pp. 291–340. Springer, New York.

Oviedo, A., Glowa, J., and Herkenham, M. (1993). Chronic cannabinoid administration alters cannabinoid receptor binding in rat brain: A quantitative autoradiographic study. *Brain Res.,* 616, 293–302.

Owen, R., Owen, F., Poulter, M., and Crow, T. J. (1984). Dopamine D$_2$ receptors in substantia nigra in schizophrenia. *Brain Res.,* 299, 152–154.

Owens, M. J., and Nemeroff, C. B. (1991). Physiology and pharmacology of corticotropin-releasing factor. *Pharmacol. Rev.,* 43, 425–473.

Padua, R., Geiger, J. D., Dambock, S., and Nagy, J. I. (1990). 2'-Deoxycoformycin inhibition of adenosine deaminase in rat brain: In vivo and in vitro analysis of specificity, potency, and enzyme recovery. *J. Neurochem.,* 54, 1169–1178.

Pakkenberg, H., and Packkenberg, B. (1986). Clozapine in the treatment of tremor. *Acta Neurol. Scand.,* 73, 295–297.

Palacios, J. M., Boddeke, H. W. G. M., and Pombo-Villar, E. (1991). Cholinergic neuropharmacology: An update. *Acta Psychiatr. Scand.,* 366 (Suppl.), 27–33.

Palacios, J. M., and Kuhar, M. J. (1980). Beta-adrenergic receptor localization by light microscopic autoradiography. *Science,* 208, 1378–1380.

Palacios, J. M., and Kuhar, M. J. (1983). Beta-adrenergic receptor localization in rat brain by light microscopic autoradiography. *Neurochem. Int.,* 4, 473–490.

Palacios, J. M., Waeber, C., Bruinvels, A. T., and Hoyer, D. (1992). Direct visualization of serotonin$_{1D}$ receptors in the human brain using a new iodinated radioligand. *Mol. Brain Res.,* 13, 175–179.

Palacios, J. M., Wamsley, J. K., and Kuhar, M. J. (1981). The distribution of histamine H$_1$ receptors in the rat brain: An autoradiographic study. *Neuroscience,* 6, 15–38.

Palade, G. E. (1954). Electron microscope observations of interneuronal and neuromuscular synapses. *Anat. Rec.,* 118, 335–336.

Palay, S. L. (1956). Synapses in the central nervous system. *J. Biophys. Biochem. Cytol.,* 2 (Suppl.), 193–202.

Pallanti, S., and Mazzi, D. (1992). MDMA (Ecstasy) precipitation of panic disorder. *Biol. Psychiatry,* 32, 91–95.

Palmer, E., Monaghan, D. T., and Cotman, C. (1989). *Trans*-APCD, a selective agonist of the phosphoinositide-coupled excitatory amino acid receptor. *Eur. J. Pharmacol.,* 166, 585–587.

Palmer, M. R., and Hoffer, B. J. (1990). GABAergic mechanisms in the electrophysiological actions of ethanol on cerebellar neurons. *Neurochem. Res.,* 15, 145–151.

Panicker, M. M., Parker, I., and Miledi, R. (1991). Receptors of the serotonin 1C subtype expressed from cloned DNA mediate the closing of K$^+$ membrane channels encoded by brain mRNA. *Proc. Natl. Acad. Sci. U.S.A.,* 88, 2560–2562.

Panksepp, J., Siviy, S. M., and Normansell, L. A. (1985). Brain opioids and social emotions. In *Biology of Social Attachments* (M. Reite and T. Fields, Eds.). Academic Press, New York.

Panula, P., Airaksinen, M. S., Pirvola, U., and Kotilainen, E. (1990). A histamine-containing neuronal system in human brain. *Neuroscience,* 34, 127–132.

Panula, P., Yang, H.-Y. T., and Costa, E. (1984). Histamine-containing neurons in the rat hypothalamus. *Proc. Natl. Acad. Sci. U.S.A.,* 81, 2572–2576.

Papadopoulos, V. (1993). Peripheral-type benzodiazepine/diazepam binding inhibitor receptor: Biological role in steroidogenic cell function. *Endocrinol. Rev.*, 14, 222–240.

Papavasiliou, P. S., Cotzias, G. C., Duby, S. E., Steck, A. J., Fehling, C., and Bell, M. A. (1972). Levodopa in parkinsonism: Potentiation of central effects with a peripheral inhibitor. *New Engl. J. Med.*, 286, 8–14.

Papazian, D. M., Schwartz, T. L., Tempel, B. L., Jan, Y. N., and Jan, L. Y. (1987). Cloning of genomic and complementary DNA from *Shaker*, a putative potassium channel gene from *Drosophila*. *Science*, 237, 749–753.

Pappas, G. D. (1975). Ultrastructural basis of synaptic transmission. In *The Nervous System*, Vol. 1 (D. B. Tower, Ed.), pp. 19–30. Raven Press, New York.

Pardridge, W. M. (1984). Transport of nutrients and hormones through the blood–brain barrier. *Fed. Proc.*, 43, 201–204.

Paredes, R. G., and Ågmo, A. (1992). GABA and behavior: The role of receptor subtypes. *Neurosci. Biobehav. Rev.*, 16, 145–170.

Parker, E. M., and Cubeddu, L. X. (1986a). Effects of d-amphetamine and dopamine synthesis inhibitors on dopamine and acetylcholine neurotransmission in the striatum. I. Release in the absence of vesicular transmitter stores. *J. Pharmacol. Exp. Ther.*, 237, 179–192.

Parker, E. M., and Cubeddu, L. X. (1986b). Effects of d-amphetamine and dopamine synthesis inhibitors on dopamine and acetylcholine neurotransmission in the striatum. II. Release in the presence of vesicular transmitter stores. *J. Pharmacol. Exp. Ther.*, 237, 193–203.

Parker, E. M., and Cubeddu, L. X. (1988). Comparative effects of amphetamine, phenylethylamine and related drugs on dopamine efflux, dopamine uptake and mazindol binding. *J. Pharmacol. Exp. Ther.*, 245, 199–210.

Parker, E. M., Grisel, D. A., Iben, L. G., and Shapiro, R. A. (1993). A single amino acid difference accounts for the pharmacological distinctions between the rat and human 5-hydroxytryptamine$_{1B}$ receptors. *J. Neurochem.*, 60, 380–383.

Parker, L. A., and Gillies, T. (1995). THC-induced place and taste aversions in Lewis and Sprague-Dawley rats. *Behav. Neurosci.*, 109, 71–78.

Parkinson, J. (1817). *An Essay on the Shaking Palsy*. Sherwood, Neely, and Jones, London.

The Parkinson Study Group. (1989). Effect of deprenyl on the progression of disability in early Parkinson's disease. *N. Engl. J. Med.*, 321, 1364–1371.

The Parkinson Study Group. (1993). Effects of tocopherol and deprenyl on the progression of disability in early Parkinson's disease. *N. Engl. J. Med.*, 328, 176–183.

Parnavelas, J. G., and Papadopoulos, G. C. (1989). The monoaminergic innervation of the cerebral cortex is not diffuse and nonspecific. *Trends Neurosci.*, 12, 315–319.

Parola, A. L., Yamamura, H. I., and Laird, H. E. II (1993). Peripheral-type benzodiazepine receptors. *Life Sci.*, 52, 1329–1342.

Parrott, A. C. (1994). Acute pharmacodynamic tolerance to the subjective effects of cigarette smoking. *Psychopharmacology*, 116, 93–97.

Pasinetti, G. M., Morgan, D. G., Johnson, S. A., Millar, S. L., and Finch, C. E. (1990). Tyrosine hydroxylase mRNA concentration in midbrain dopaminergic neurons is differentially regulated by reserpine. *J. Neurochem.*, 55, 1793–1799.

Pasternak, G. W. (1987). Opioid receptors. In *Psychopharmacology: The Third Generation of Progress* (H. Y. Meltzer, Ed.), pp. 281–288. Raven Press, New York.

Pasternak, G. W. (1993). Pharmacological mechanisms of opioid analgesics. *Clin. Neuropharmacol.*, 16, 1–18.

Pasternak, G. W., Goodman, R., and Snyder, S. H. (1975). An endogenous morphine-like factor in mammalian brain. *Life Sci.*, 16, 1765–1769.

Paterson, I. A., Juorio, A. V., and Boulton, A. A. (1990). 2-penylethylamine: A modulator of catecholamine transmission in the mammalian central nervous system? *J. Neurochem.*, 55, 1827–1837.

Paton, W. (1969). A pharmacologic approach to drug dependence and drug tolerance. In *Scientific Basis of Drug Dependence* (H. Steinberg, Ed.), pp. 31–47. J. A. Churchill, London.

Patrick, J., Séquéla, P., Vernino, S., Amador, M., Luetje, C., and Dani, J. A. (1993). Functional diversity of neuronal nicotinic acetylcholine receptors. *Prog. Brain Res.*, 98, 113–120.

Patrick, S. L., Thompson, T. L., Walker, J. M., and Patrick, R. L. (1991). Concomitant sensitization of amphetamine-induced behavioral stimulation and in vivo dopamine release from rat caudate nucleus. *Brain Res.*, 538, 343–346.

Patthy, L., and Nikolics, K. (1993). Functions of agrin and agrin-related proteins. *Trends Neurosci.*, 16, 76–81.

Paul, S. M., and Purdy, R. H. (1992). Neuroactive steroids. *FASEB J.*, 6, 2311–2322.

Pavlov, I. (1928). *Lectures on Conditioned Reflexes* (W. H. Gantt, trans.). International, New York.

Pazos, A., Cortés, R., and Palacios, J. M. (1985). Quantitative autoradiographic mapping of serotonin receptors in the rat brain. II. Serotonin-2 receptors. *Brain Res.*, 346, 231–249.

Peach, M. J. (1975). Cations: Calcium, magnesium, barium, lithium, and ammonium. In *The Pharmacological Basis of Therapeutics* (5th ed.) (L. S. Goodman and A. Gilman, Eds.), pp. 782–797. Macmillan, New York.

Pearson, R. C. A., and Powell, T. P. S. (1989). The neuroanatomy of Alzheimer's disease. *Rev. Neurosci.*, 2, 101–122.

Pedersen, C. A., Ascher, J. A., Monroe, Y. L., and Prange, A. J. Jr. (1982). Oxytocin induces maternal behavior in virgin female rats. *Science*, 216, 648–650.

Pedersen, C. A., Caldwell, J. D., Jirikowski, G. F., and Insel, T. R. (Eds.) (1992). Oxytocin in maternal, sexual, and social behaviors. *Ann. N.Y. Acad. Sci.*, 652.

Pedersen, C. A., Caldwell, J. D., Walker, C., Ayers, G., and Mason, G. A. (1994). Oxytocin activates the postpartum onset of rat maternal behavior in the ventral tegmental and medial preoptic areas. *Behav. Neurosci.*, 108, 1163–1171.

Pedersen, C. A., and Prange, A. J. Jr. (1985). Oxytocin and mothering behavior in the rat. *Pharmacol. Ther.*, 28, 287–302.

Pedersen, U. B., Norby, B., Jensen, A. A., Schiødt, M., Hansen, A., Suhr-Jessen, P., Scheideler, M., Thastrup, O., and Andersen, P. H. (1994). Characteristics of stably expressed human dopamine D_{1a} and D_{1b} receptors: Atypical behavior of the dopamine D_{1b} receptor. *Eur. J. Pharmacol.*, 267, 85–93.

Peele, S. (1991). What we now know about treating alcoholism and other addictions. *Harvard Health Lett.*, 8 (6), 5–7.

Pelletier, G., Steinbusch, H. W. M., and Verhofstad, A. A. J. (1981). Immunoreactive substance P and serotonin present in the same dense-core vesicles. *Nature*, 293, 71–72.

Pellow, S., Chopin, P., File, S. E., and Briley, M. (1985). Validation of open:closed arm entries in an elevated plus-maze as a measure of anxiety in the rat. *J. Neurosci. Methods* 14, 149–167.

Pellow, S., and File, S. E. (1986). Anxiolytic and anxiogenic drug effects on exploratory activity in the elevated plus-maze: A novel test of anxiety in the rat. *Pharmacol. Biochem. Behav.*, 24, 525–529.

Penfield, W. G., and Jasper, H. H. (1954). *Epilepsy and the Functional Anatomy of the Human Brain*. Little, Brown, Boston.

Penfield, W. G., and Rasmussen, T. (1950). *The Cerebral Cortex of Man*. Macmillan, New York.

Penfield, W. G., and Roberts, L. (1959). *Speech and Brain Mechanisms*. Princeton University Press, Princeton, NJ.

Peng, L., Hertz, L., Huang, R., Sonnewald, U., Petersen, S. B., Westergaard, N., Larsson, O., and Schousboe, A. (1993). Utilization of glutamine and of TCA cycle constituents as precursors for transmitter glutamate and GABA. *Dev. Neurosci.*, 15, 367–377.

Peoples, S. A., and Guttmann, E. (1936). Hypertension produced with benzedrine. Its psychological accompaniments. *Lancet*, I, 1107–1109.

Peralta, V., deLeon, J., and Cuestra, M. J. (1992). Are there more than two syndromes in schizophrenia? A critique of the positive-negative dichotomy. *Br. J. Psychiatry*, 161, 335–343.

Perez, J., Mori, S., Brunello, N., and Racagni, G. (1994). Cyclic AMP protein kinase as an intracellular target for the action of antidepressant drugs. In *Critical Issues in the Treatment of Affective Disorders* (S. Z. Langer, N. Bunello, G. Racagni, and J. Mendlewicz, Eds.), pp. 110–117. Karger, Basel.

Perez-Reyes, M. (1990). Marijuana smoking: Factors that influence the bioavailability of tetrahydrocannabinol. *NIDA Res. Monogr.*, 99, 42–62.

Perez-Reyes, M., White, W. R., McDonald, S. A., Hicks, R. E., Jeffcoat, A. R., Hill, J. M., and Cook, C. E. (1991). Clinical effects of daily methamphetamine administration. *Clin. Neuropharmacol.*, 14, 352–358.

Peris, J., Boyson, S. J., Cass, W. A., Curella, P., Dwoskin, L. P., Larson, G., Lin, L.-H., Yasuda, R. P., and Zahniser, N. R. (1990). Persistence of neurochemical changes in dopamine systems after repeated cocaine administration. *J. Pharmacol. Exp. Ther.*, 253, 38–44.

Perl, T. M., Bédard, L., Kosatsky, T., Hockin, J. C., Todd, E. C. D., and Remis, R. S. (1990). An outbreak of toxic encephalopathy caused by eating mussels contaminated with domoic acid. *N. Engl. J. Med.*, 322, 1775–1780.

Peroutka, S. J., and Snyder, S. H. (1979). Multiple serotonin receptors: Differential binding of [^{3}H]5-hydroxytryptamine, [^{3}H]lysergic acid diethylamide and [^{3}H]spiroperidol. *Mol. Pharmacol.*, 16, 687–699.

Peroutka, S. J., and Snyder, S. H. (1980). Long-term antidepressant treatment decreases spiroperidol-labeled serotonin receptor binding. *Science,* 210, 88–90.

Peroutka, S. J., and Snyder, S. H. (1982). Radioactive ligand binding studies: Identification of multiple serotonin receptors. In *Biology of Serotonergic Transmission* (N. N. Osborne, Ed.), pp. 279–298. Wiley, Chichester.

Persohn, E., Malherbe, P., and Richards, J. G. (1992). Comparative molecular neuroanatomy of cloned GABA$_A$ receptor subunits in the rat CNS. *J. Comp. Neurol.,* 326, 193–216.

Pert, C. B., and Snyder, S. H. (1973). Properties of opiate receptor binding in rat brain. *Proc. Natl. Acad. Sci. U.S.A.,* 70, 2243–2247.

Pert, C. B., and Snyder, S. H. (1974). Opiate receptor binding of agonists and antagonists affected differentially by sodium. *Mol. Pharmacol.,* 10, 868–879.

Pertwee, R. G. (1972). The ring test: A quantitative method for assessing the 'cataleptic' effect of cannabis in mice. *Br. J. Pharmacol.,* 46, 753–763.

Pertwee, R. G. (1990). The central neuropharmacology of psychotropic cannabinoids. In *Psychotropic Drugs of Abuse* (D. J. K. Balfour, Ed.), pp. 355–429. Pergamon Press, Elmsford.

Pertwee, R., Griffin, G., Fernando, S., Li, X., Hill, A., and Makriyannis, A. (1995). AM630, a competitive cannabinoid receptor antagonist. *Life Sci.,* 56, 1949–1955.

Peters, A., Palay, S. L., and Webster, H. deF. (1991). *The Fine Structure of the Nervous System: Neurons and their Supporting Cells* (3rd ed.). Oxford University Press, New York.

Peters, J. A., Malone, H. M., and Lambert, J. J. (1992). Recent advances in the electrophysiological characterization of 5-HT$_3$ receptors. *Trends Pharmacol. Sci.,* 13, 391–397.

Petersen, E. N., and Buss Lassen, J. (1981). A water lick paradigm using drug-experienced rats. *Psychopharmacology,* 75, 236–239.

Petersen, R. C. (1977). Cocaine: An overview. *NIDA Res. Monogr.,* 13, 17–34.

Petersen, S. E., Fox, P. T., Posner, M. I., Minton, M., and Raichli, M. E. (1988). Positron emission tomographic studies of the cortical anatomy of single word processing. *Nature,* 331, 585–589.

Peto, R. (1986). Influence of dose and duration of smoking on lung cancer rates. In *Tobacco: A Major International Health Hazard* (D. Zaridze and R. Peto, Eds.), International Agency for Research on Cancer, TARC Scientific Publications No. 74, Lyons, France.

Petralia, R. S., Wang, Y.-X., and Wenthold, R. J. (1994a). Histological and ultrastructural localization of the kainate receptor subunits, KA2 and GluR6/7, in the rat nervous system using selective antipeptide antibodies. *J. Comp. Neurol.,* 349, 85–110.

Petralia, R. S., Wang, Y.-X., and Wenthold, R. J. (1994b). The NMDA receptor subunits NR2A and NR2B show histological and ultrastructural localization patterns similar to those of NR1. *J. Neurosci.,* 14, 6102–6120.

Petralia, R. S., and Wenthold, R. J. (1992). Light and electron immunocytochemical localization of AMPA-selective glutamate receptors in the rat brain. *J. Comp. Neurol.,* 318, 329–354.

Petralia, R. S., Yokotani, N., and Wenthold, R. J. (1994). Light and electron microscope distribution of the NMDA receptor subunit NMDAR1 in the rat nervous system using a selective anti-peptide antibody. *J. Neurosci.,* 14, 667–696.

Petrusz, P., Merchenthaler, I., Maderdrut, J. L., and Heitz, P. U. (1985). Central and peripheral distribution of corticotropin-releasing factor. *Fed. Proc.,* 44, 229–235.

Petry, N., Furmidge, L., Tong, Z.-Y., Martin, C., and Clark, D. (1993). Time sampling observation procedure for studying drug effects: Interaction between *d*-amphetamine and selective dopamine receptor antagonists in the rat. *Pharmacol. Biochem. Behav.,* 44, 167–180.

Pettit, H. O., Ettenberg, A., Bloom, F. E., and Koob, G. F. (1984). Destruction of dopamine in the nucleus accumbens selectively attenuates cocaine but not heroin self-administration in rats. *Psychopharmacology,* 84, 167–173.

Pettit, H. O., and Justice, J. B. Jr. (1991). Effect of dose on cocaine self-administration behavior and dopamine levels in the nucleus accumbens. *Brain Res.,* 539, 94–102.

Pettit, H. O., Pan, H.-T., Parsons, L. H., and Justice, J. B. Jr. (1990). Extracellular concentrations of cocaine and dopamine are enhanced during chronic cocaine administration. *J. Neurochem.,* 55, 798–804.

Pfefferbaum, A., Lim, K., Rosenbloom, M., and Zipursky, R. B. (1990). Brain magetic resonance imaging: Approaches for investigating schizophrenia. *Schizophr. Bull.,*16, 452–476.

Pflug, B. (1988). Sleep deprivation in treatment of depression. In *Affective Disorders—Directions in Psychiatry* (Monogr. series, No. 3), pp. 175–185. W. W. Norton, New York.

Philippu, A. (1984). Use of push–pull cannulae to determine the release of endogenous neurotransmitters in distinct brain areas of anaesthetized and freely moving animals. In *Measurement of Neurotransmitter Release In Vivo* (C. A. Marsden, Ed.), pp. 3–38. Wiley, New York.

Philippu, A., and Beyer, J. (1973). Dopamine and noradrenaline transport into subcellular vesicles of the striatum. *Naunyn Schmiedebergs Arch. Pharmacol.,* 278, 387–402.

Phipps, B. S., Maciewicz, R., Sandrew, B. B., Poletti, C. E., and Foote, W. E. (1983). Edinger-Westphal neurons that project to spinal cord contain substance P. *Neurosci. Lett.,* 36, 125–131.

Pi, F., and García-Sevilla, J. A. (1992). α$_2$-autoreceptor-mediated modulation of tyrosine hydroxylase activity in noradrenergic regions of the rat brain in vivo. *Naunyn Schmiedebergs Arch. Pharmacol.,* 345, 653–660.

Piazza, P. V., Deminière, J.-M., Le Moal, M., and Simon, H. (1989). Factors that predict individual vulnerability to amphetamine self-administration. *Science,* 245, 1511–1513.

Pickel, V. M., and Teitelman, G. (1987). Immunocytochemistry of single and multiple antigens with special reference to the enzymes of catecholamine neurons. In *Monoaminergic Neurons: Light Microscopy and Ultrastructure* (H. W. M. Steinbusch, Ed.), pp. 79–109. Wiley, New York.

Pickens, R. W., Miesch, R. A., and Thompson, T. (1978). Drug self-administration: An analysis of the reinforcing effects of drugs. In *Handbook of Psychopharmacology.* Volume 12, *Drugs of Abuse* (L. L. Iversen, S. D. Iversen, and S. H. Snyder, Eds.), pp. 1–37. Plenum Press, New York.

Pickens, R. W., Svikis, D. S., McGue, M., Lykken, D. T., Heston, L. L., and Clayton, P. J. (1991). Heterogeneity in the inheritance of alcoholism: A study of male and female twins. *Arch. Gen. Psychiatry,* 48, 19–28.

Pierce, J. P., Gilpin, E., Burns, D. M., Whalen, E. Posbrook. B., Shopland, D., and Johnson, M. (1991). Does tobacco advertising target young people to start smoking? Evidence from California. *JAMA* 266, 3154–3158.

Piercey, M. F., Moon, M. W., and Blinn, J. R. (1985). The role of substance P as a central nervous system neurotransmitter. In *Substance P: Metabolism and Biological Actions* (C. C. Jordan and P. Oehme, Eds.), pp. 165–176. Taylor and Francis, London.

Pifl, C., Giros, B., and Caron, M. G. (1993). Dopamine transporter expression confers cytotoxicity to low doses of the Parkinsonism-inducing neurotoxin 1-methyl-4-phenylpyridinium. *J. Neurosci.,* 13, 4246–4253.

Pijnenburg, A. J. J., Honig, W. M. M., Van der Heyden, J. A. M., and Van Rossum, J. M. (1976). Effects of chemical stimulation of the mesolimbic dopamine system upon locomotor activity. *Eur. J. Pharmacol.,* 35, 45–58.

Pijnenburg, A. J. J., Honig, W. M. M., and van Rossum, J. M. (1975a). Antagonism of apomorphine- and d-amphetamine-induced stereotyped behaviour by injection of low doses of haloperidol into the caudate nucleus and the nucleus accumbens. *Psychopharmacologia,* 45, 65–71.

Pijnenburg, A. J. J., Honig, W. M. M., and Van Rossum, J. M. (1975b). Effects of antagonists upon locomotor stimulation induced by injection of dopamine and noradrenaline into the nucleus accumbens of nialamide-pretreated rats. *Psychopharmacologia,* 41, 175–180.

Pilc, A., and Enna, S. J. (1987). Supersensitive β-adrenergic receptors are down regulated in rat brain by mianserin administration. *J. Neural Trans.,* 70, 71–76.

Pilowsky, P. M., Suzuki, S., and Minson, J. B. (1994). Antisense oligonucleotides: A new tool in neuroscience. *Clin. Exp. Pharmacol. Physiol.,* 21, 935–944.

Pimoule, C., Schoemaker, H., Reynolds, G. P., and Langer, S. Z. (1985). [^{3}H]SCH-23390 labeled D$_1$ dopamine receptors are unchanged in schizophrenia and Parkinson's disease. *Eur. J. Pharmacol.,* 114, 235–237.

Pincus, J. H., and Barry, K. (1987). Influence of dietary protein on motor fluctuations in Parkinson's disease. *Arch. Neurol.,* 44, 270–272.

Pinder, R. M., and Wieringa, J. H. (1993). Third-generation antidepressants. *Med. Res. Rev.,* 13, 259–325.

Pintar, J. E., and Scott, R. E. M. (1993). Ontogeny of mammalian opioid systems. In *Opioids I,* Handbook of Experimental Pharmacology, Vol. 104 (A. Herz, Ed.), pp. 711–730. Springer-Verlag, New York.

Piomelli, D., Pilon, C., Giros, B., Sokoloff, P., Martres, M.-P., and Schwartz, J.-C. (1991). Dopamine activation of the arachidonic acid cascade as a basis for D$_1$/D$_2$ synergism. *Nature,* 353, 164–166.

Pisegna, J. R., De Weerth, A., Huppi, K., and Wank, S. A. (1992). Molecular cloning of the human brain and gastric cholecystokinin receptor: Structure, functional expression and chromosomal localization. *Biochem. Biophys. Res. Commun.,* 189, 296–303.

Pitts, D. K., and Marwah, J. (1987). Electrophysiological actions of cocaine on noradrenergic neurons in rat locus ceruleus. *J. Pharmacol. Exp. Ther.,* 240, 345–351.

Pitts, D. K., and Marwah, J. (1989). Autonomic actions of cocaine. *Can. J. Physiol. Pharmacol.,* 67, 1168–1176.

Pizzi, M., Da Prada, M., Valerio, A., Memo, M., Spano, P. F., and Haefely, W. E. (1988). Dopamine D_2 receptor stimulation inhibits inositol phosphate generating system in rat striatal slices. *Brain Res.,* 456, 235–240.

Plessinger, M. A., and Woods, J. R. J. (1991). The cardiovascular effects of cocaine use in pregnancy. *Reprod. Toxicol.,* 5, 99–113.

Pletscher, A. (1973). Effect of inhibitors of extracerebral decarboxylase on levodopa metabolism. *Adv. Neurol.,* 3, 49–58.

Pletscher, A. (1988). Platelets as models: Use and limitations. *Experientia,* 44, 152–155.

Pletscher, A., Shore, P. A., and Brodie, B. B. (1955). Serotonin release as a possible mechanism of reserpine action. *Science,* 122, 374–375.

Plotsky, P. M., Owens, M. J., and Nemeroff, C. B. (1995). Neuropeptide alterations in mood disorders. In *Psychopharmacology: The Fourth Generation of Progress* (F. E. Bloom and D. J. Kupfer, Eds.), pp. 971–982. Raven Press, New York.

Plutchik, R., and van Praag, H. (1989). The measurement of suicidality, aggressivity and impulsivity. *Prog. Neuropsychopharmacol. Biol. Psychiatry,* 13, S23–S34.

Pohl, M., Mauborgne, A., Bourgoin, S., Benoliel, J. J., Hamon, M., and Cesselin, F. (1989). Neonatal capsaicin treatment abolishes the modulations by opioids of substance P release from rat spinal cord slices. *Neurosci. Lett.,* 96, 102–107.

Pohorecky, L. A., and Brick, J. (1990). Pharmacology of ethanol. In *Psychotropic Drugs of Abuse* (D. J. K. Balfour, Ed.), pp. 189–281. Pergamon Press, New York.

Poirier, M. F., Benkelfat, C., Loo, H., Sechter, D., Zarifian, E., Galzin, A. M., and Langer, S. Z. (1986). Reduced Bmax of tritiated-imipramine binding to platelets of depressed patients free of previous medication with 5HT uptake inhibitors. *Psychopharmacology,* 89, 456–461.

Poirier, M. F., Galzin, A. M., Pimoule, C., Schoemaker, H., LeQuanBui, K. H., Meyer, P., Gay, C., Loo, H., and Langer, S. Z. (1988). Short-term lithium administration to healthy volunteers produces long-lasting pronounced changes in platelet serotonin uptake but not imipramine binding. *Psychopharmacology,* 94, 521–526.

Polak, J. M., and McGee, J.O'D. (1990). *In Situ Hybridization: Principles and Practice.* Oxford University Press, New York.

Polc, P., Mohler, H., and Haefely, W. (1974). The effect of diazepam on spinal cord activities: Possible sites and mechanisms of action. *Naunyn Schmiedebergs Arch. Pharmacol.,* 284, 319–337.

Pollard, H., Moreau, J., Arrang, J. M., and Schwartz, J.-C. (1993). A detailed autoradiographic mapping of histamine H_3 receptors in rat brain areas. *Neuroscience,* 52, 169–189.

Pollard, M., Bouthenet, M. L., Moreau, J., Souil, E., Verroust, P., Ronco, P., and Schwartz, J.-C. (1989). Detailed immunoautoradiographic mapping system comparison with enkephalins and SP. *Neuroscience,* 30, 339–376.

Polster, M. R. (1993). Drug-induced amnesia: Implications for cognitive neuropsychological investigations of memory. *Psychol. Bull.,* 114, 477–493.

Pomerleau, C. S., and Pomerleau, O. F. (1992). Euphoriant effects of nicotine in smokers. *Psychopharmacology,* 108, 460–465.

Pomerleau, O. F. (1992). Nicotine and the central nervous system: Behavioral effects of cigarette smoking. *Am. J. Med.,* 93 (Suppl. 1A), 1A2S–1A7S.

Poncelet, M., Chermat, R., Soubrie, P., and Simon, P. (1983). The progressive ratio schedule as a model for studying the psychomotor stimulant activity of drugs in the rat. *Psychopharmacology,* 80, 184–189.

Ponzio, F., Achilli, G., Perego, C., Rinaldi, G., and Algeri, S. (1983). Does acute L-DOPA increase active release of dopamine from dopaminergic neurons? *Brain Res.,* 273, 45–51.

Pope, H. G. Jr., Gruber, A. J., and Yurgelun-Todd, D. (1995). The residual neuropsychological effects of cannabis: The current status of research. *Drug Alcohol Depend.,* 38, 25–34.

Popik, P., Layer, R. T., and Skolnick, P. (1995). 100 years of ibogaine: Neurochemical and pharmacological actions of a putative anti-addictive drug. *Pharmacol. Rev.,* 47, 235–253.

Porceddu, M. L., Origini, E., Mele, S., and Biggio, G. (1986). ^{3}H-SCH-23390 binding sites in the rat substantia nigra: Evidence for a presynaptic localization and innervation by dopamine. *Life Sci.,* 39, 321–328.

Poritsky, R. (1969). Two and three dimensional ultrastructure of boutons and glial cells on the motoneuronal surface in the cat spinal cord. *J. Comp. Neurol.,* 135, 423–452.

Porreca, F., and Burks, T. F. (1993). Supraspinal opioid receptors in antinociception. In *Opioids II,* Handbook of Experimental Pharmacology, Vol. 104 (A. Herz, Ed.), pp. 21–51. Springer-Verlag, New York.

Porrino, L. J., Domer, F. R., Crane, A. M., and Sokoloff, L. (1988). Selective alterations in cerebral metabolism within the mesocorticolimbic dopaminergic system produced by acute cocaine administration in rats. *Neuropsychopharmacology,* 1, 109–118.

Porrino, L. J., and Lucignani, G. (1987). Different patterns of local brain energy metabolism associated with high and low doses of methylphenidate. Relevance to its action in hyperactive children. *Biol. Psychiatry,* 22, 126–138.

Porrino, L. J., Lucignani, G., Dow-Edwards, D., and Sokoloff, L. (1984). Correlation of dose-dependent effects of acute amphetamine administration on behavior and local cerebral metabolism in rats. *Brain Res.,* 307, 311–320.

Porsolt, R. D., Anton, G., Blavet, N., and Jalfre, M. (1978). Behavioral despair in rats: A new model sensitive to antidepressant treatments. *Eur. J. Pharmacol.,* 47, 379–391.

Porsolt, R. D., Lenegre, A., and McArthur, R. A. (1991). Pharmacological models of depression, In *Animal Models in Psychopharmacology, Advances in Pharmacological Sciences,* Birkhauser Verlag, Basel.

Porsolt, R. D., Roux, S., and Wettstein, J. G. (1995). Animal models of dementia. *Drug Dev. Res.,* 35, 214–229.

Portoghese, P. S. (1993). Selective nonpeptide opioid antagonists. In *Opioids I,* Handbook of Experimental Pharmacology, Vol. 104 (A. Herz, Ed.), pp. 279–294. Springer-Verlag, New York.

Post, R. M., Ballenger, J. C., Uhde, T., and Bunney, W. (1984). Efficacy of carbamazepine in manic-depressive illness: Implications for underlying mechanisms. In *Neurobiology of Mood Disorders* (R. M. Post and J. C. Ballenger, Eds.), pp. 777–816. Williams and Wilkins, Baltimore.

Post, R. M., and Contel, N. R. (1983). Human and animal studies of cocaine: Implications for the development of behavioral pathology. In *Stimulants: Neurochemical, Behavioral, and Clinical Perspectives* (I. Creese, Ed.), pp. 169–203. Raven Press, New York.

Post, R. M., and Weiss, S. R. B. (1988). Psychomotor stimulant vs. local anesthetic effects of cocaine: Role of behavioral sensitization and kindling. *NIDA Res. Monogr.,* 88, 217–238.

Post, R. M., Weiss, S. R. B., and Chuang, D-M. (1992). Mechanisms of action of anticonvulsants in affective disorders: Comparison with lithium. *J. Clin. Psychopharmacol.,* 12 (Suppl.), 23s–35s.

Potter, W. Z., and Manji, H. K. (1993). Are monoamine metabolites in cerebrospinal fluid worth measuring? *Arch. Gen. Psychiatry,* 50, 653–656.

Potter, W. Z., and Manji, H. K. (1994a). Catecholamines in depression: An update. *Clin. Chem.,* 40, 279–287.

Potter, W. Z., and Manji, H. K. (1994b). Clinical onset of antidepressant action: Implications for new drug development. In *Critical Issues in the Treatment of Affective Disorders* (S. Z. Langer, N. Bunello, G. Racagni, and J. Mendlewicz, Eds.), pp. 118–126. Karger, Basel.

Potter, W. Z., Rudorfer, M. V., and Manji, H. (1991). The pharmacological treatment of depression. *N. Engl. J. Med.,* 325, 633–642.

Powley, T. L. (1977). The ventromedial hypothalamic syndrome, satiety, and a cephalic phase hypothesis. *Psychol. Rev.,* 84, 89–126.

Prange, A. J. Jr., Wilson, I. C., Knox, A., McClane, T. K., and Lipton, M. A. (1970). Enhancement of imipramine by thyroid stimulating hormone: Clinical and theoretical implications. *Am. J. Psychiatry,* 127, 191–199.

Pranzatelli, M. R., Murthy, J. N., and Tailor, P. T. (1993). Novel regulation of 5-HT_{1C} receptors: Down-regulation induced both by 5-$HT_{1C/2}$ receptor agonists and antagonists. *Eur. J. Pharmacol.,* 244, 1–5.

Pratt, W. B., and Taylor, P. (Eds.). (1990). *Principles of Drug Action.* Churchill Livingstone, New York.

Prensky, A. L. (1975). Metabolic disorders of genetic origin: Disorders of amino, organic, and nucleic acids and carbohydrate metabolism. In *The Nervous System,* Vol. 2 (D. B. Tower, Ed. in Chief), pp. 205–217. Raven Press, New York.

Prescott, C. A., and Gottesman, I. I. (1993). Genetically mediated vulnerability to schizophrenia. *Psychiatr. Clin. North Am.,* 16, 245–268.

Preston, K., and Jasinski, D. R. (1991). Abuse liability studies of opioid agonist-antagonists in humans. *Drug Alcohol Depend.,* 28, 49–82.

Price, D. L., Whitehouse, P. J., Struble, R. G., Clark, A. W., Coyle, J. T., DeLong, M. R., and Hedreen, J. C. (1982). Basal forebrain cholinergic systems in Alzheimer's disease and related dementias. *Neurosci. Comment.*, 1, 84–92.

Price, H. L. (1975). General anesthetics: Intravenous anesthetics. In *The Pharmacological Basis of Therapeutics* (L. S. Goodman and A. Gilman, Eds.), pp. 97–101. Macmillan, New York.

Price, L. H., Charney, D. S., Delgado, P. L., and Heninger, G. R. (1990). Lithium and serotonin function: Implications for the serotonin hypothesis of depression. *Psychopharmacology*, 100, 3–12.

Price, L. H., Charney, D. S., Delgado, P. C., and Heninger, G. R. (1991). Serotonin function and depression: Neuroendocrine and mood responses to intravenous L-tryptophan in depressed patients and healthy comparison subjects. *Am. J. Psychiatry*, 148, 1518–1525.

Price, W. P., Ahier, R. G., Middlemiss, D. N., Singh, L., Trickelbank, M. D., and Wong, E. H. F. (1988). In vivo labeling of the NMDA receptor channel complex by [³H]MK801. *Eur. J. Pharmacol.*, 158, 279–282.

Prien, R. F., and Kocsis, J. H. (1995). Long-term treatment of mood disorders. In *Psychopharmacology: The Fourth Generation of Progress* (F. E. Bloom and D. J. Kupfer, Eds.), pp. 1067–1080. Raven Press, New York.

Prince, D. A., and Stevens, C. F. (1992). Adenosine decreases neurotransmitter release at central synapses. *Proc. Natl. Acad. Sci. U.S.A.*, 89, 8586–8590.

Pritchett, D. B., Sontheimer, H., Gorman, C. M., Kettenmann, H., Seeburg, P. H., and Schofield, P. R. (1988). Transient expression shows ligand gating and allosteric potentation of GABA$_A$ receptor subunits. *Science*, 242, 1306–1308.

Pritchett, D. B., Sontheimer, H., Shivers, B. D., Ymer, S., Kettenmann, H., Schofield, P. R., and Seeburg, P. H. (1989). Importance of a novel GABA$_A$ receptor subunit for benzodiazepine pharmacology. *Nature*, 338, 582–585.

Proudfit, H. K. (1988). Pharmacological evidence for the modulation of nociception by noradrenergic neurons. *Prog. Brain Res.*, 77, 357–370.

Przewlocki, R. (1993). Opioid systems and stress. In *Opioids II*, Handbook of Experimental Pharmacology, Vol. 104 (A. Herz, Ed.), pp. 293–324. Springer-Verlag, New York.

Purdy, R. H., Morrow, A. L., Moore, P. H. Jr., and Paul, S. M. (1991). Stress-induced elevations of γ-aminobutyric acid type A receptor-active steroids in the rat brain. *Proc. Natl. Acad. Sci. U.S.A.*, 88, 4553–4557.

Purpura, D. F. (1974). Dendritic spine "dysgenesis" and mental retardation. *Science*, 186, 1126–1128.

Purves, D., Voyvodic, J. T., and Yawo, H. (1987). Nerve terminal remodeling visualized in living mice by repeated examination of the same neuron. *Science*, 238, 1122–1126.

Quarles, R. H. (1975). Glycoproteins in the nervous system. In *The Nervous System*, Vol. 1 (D. B. Tower, Ed.), pp. 493–501. Raven Press, New York.

Quastel, J. H., Tennenbaum, M., and Wheatley, A. H. M. (1936). Choline ester formation in, and choline esterase activities of, tissues in vitro. *Biochem. J.*, 30, 1668–1681.

Querfurth, H. W., Wijsman, E. M., St George-Hyslop, P. H., and Selkoe, D. J. (1995). bAPP mRNA transcription is increased in cultured fibroblasts from the familial Alzheimer's disease-1 family. *Mol. Brain Res.*, 28, 319–337.

Quinn, N. P. (1994). A case against early levodopa treatment of Parkinson's disease. *Clin. Neuropharmacol.*, 17 (Suppl. 3), S43–S49.

Quirion, R. (1985). Multiple tachykinin receptors. *Trends Neurosci.*, 8, 183–185.

Quirion, R., Aubert, I., Araujo, D. M., Hersi, A., and Gaudreau, P. (1993). Autoradiographic distribution of putative muscarinic receptor sub-types in mammalian brain. *Prog. Brain Res.*, 98, 85–93.

Quirion, R., Aubert, I., Lapchak, P. A., Schaum, R. P., Teolis, S., Gauthier, S., and Araujo, D. M. (1989). Muscarinic receptor subtypes in human neurodegenerative disorders: Focus on Alzheimer's disease. *Trends Pharmacol. Sci.*, 10 (Suppl.), 80–84.

Quirion, R., Bowen, W. D., Itzhak, Y., Junien, J. L., Musacchio, J. M., Rothman, R. B., Su, T.-P., Tam, S. W., and Taylor, D. P. (1992). A proposal for the classification of sigma binding sites. *Trends Pharmacol. Sci.*, 13, 85–86.

Quirion, R., Chicheportiche, R., Contreras, P. C., Johnson, K. M., Lodge, D., Tam, S. W., Woods, J. H., and Zukin, S. R. (1987). Classification and nomenclature of phencyclidine and sigma receptor sites. *Trends Neurosci.*, 10, 444–445.

Quirion, R., and Pilapil, C. (1991). Distribution of multiple opioid receptors in the human brain. In *Receptors in the Human Nervous System* (F. A. O. Mendelsohn, Ed.), pp. 103–121. Academic Press, New York.

Quitkin, F. M. (1985). The importance of dosage in prescribing antidepressants. *Br. J. Psychiatry*, 147, 593–597.

Radian, R., Bendahan, A., and Kanner, B. I. (1986). Purification and identification of the functional sodium- and chloride-coupled γ-aminobutyric acid transport glycoprotein from rat brain. *J. Biol. Chem.*, 261, 15437–15441.

Radian, R., Ottersen, O. P., Storm-Mathisen, J., Castel, M., and Kanner, B. I. (1990). Immunocytochemical localization of the GABA transporter in rat brain. *J. Neurosci.*, 10, 1319–1330.

Rafferty, M. F., Mattson, M., Jacobson, A. E., and Rice, K. C. (1985). A specific acylating agent for the [³H]phencyclidine receptors in rat brain. *FEBS Lett.*, 181, 318–322.

Ragan, C. I. (1990). The effect of lithium on inositol phosphate metabolism. In *Lithium and Cell Physiology* (R. O. Bach and V. S. Gallicchio, Eds.), pp. 102–120. Springer-Verlag, New York.

Rahwan, R. G. (1975). Toxic effects of ethanol: Possible role of acetaldehyde, tetrahydroisoquinolines, and tetrahydro-β-carbolines. *Toxicol. Appl. Pharmacol.*, 34, 3–27.

Rainbow, T. C., Parsons, B., and Wolfe, B. B. (1984). Quantitative autoradiography of β$_1$- and β$_2$-adrenergic receptors in rat brain. *Proc. Natl. Acad. Sci. U.S.A.*, 81, 1585–1589.

Rainey, J. M. Jr. and Crowder, M. K. (1975). Prolonged psychosis attributed to phencyclidine: Report of three cases. *Am. J. Psychiatry*, 132, 1076–1078.

Rainnie, D. G., Grunze, H. C. R., McCarley, R. W., and Greene, R. W. (1994). Adenosine inhibition of mesopontine cholinergic neurons: Implications for EEG arousal. *Science*, 263, 689–692.

Raiteri, M., Angelini, F., and Levi, G. (1974). A simple apparatus for studying the release of neurotransmitters from synaptosomes. *Eur. J. Pharmacol.*, 25, 411–414.

Raiteri, M., Bertollini, A., Angelini, F., and Levi, G. (1975). d-Amphetamine as a releaser or reuptake inhibitor of biogenic amines in synaptosomes. *Eur. J. Pharmacol.*, 34, 189–195.

Raiteri, M., Cerrito, F., Cervoni, A. M., and Levi, G. (1979). Dopamine can be released by two mechanisms differentially affected by the dopamine transport inhibitor nomifensine. *J. Pharmacol. Exp. Ther.*, 208, 195–202.

Raiteri, M., Levi, G., and Federico, R. (1974). d-Amphetamine and the release of ³H-norepinephrine from synaptosomes. *Eur. J. Pharmacol.*, 28, 237–240.

Raiteri, M., Marchi, M., and Paudice, P. (1990). Presynaptic muscarinic receptors in the central nervous system. *Ann. N.Y. Acad. Sci.*, 604, 113–129.

Raiteri, M., Paudice, P., and Vallebuona, F. (1993). Release of cholecystokinin in the central nervous system. *Neurochem. Int.*, 22, 519–527.

Raja, S. N., and Guyenet, P. G. (1980). Effects of phencyclidine on the spontaneous activity of monoaminergic neurons. *Eur. J. Pharmacol.*, 63, 229–233.

Rajendra, S., and Schofield, P. R. (1995). Molecular mechanisms of inherited startle syndromes. *Trends Neurosci.*, 18, 80–82.

Raleigh, M. J., McGuire, M. T., Brammer, G. L., Pollack, D. B., and Yuwiler, A. (1991). Serotonergic mechanisms promote dominance acquisition in adult male vervet monkeys. *Brain Res.*, 559, 181–190.

Raleigh, M. J., McGuire, M. T., Brammer, G. L., and Yuwiler, A. (1984). Social and environmental influences on blood serotonin concentrations in monkeys. *Arch. Gen. Psychiatry*, 41, 405–410.

Rall, T. W., and Schleifer, L. S. (1985). Drugs effective in the therapy of the epilepsies. In *The Pharmacological Basis of Therapeutics* (A. G. Gilman, L. S. Goodman, T. W. Rall, and F. Murad, Eds.), pp. 446–472. Macmillan, New York.

Ramamoorthy, S., Bauman, A. L., Moore, K. R., Han, H., Yang-Feng, T., Chang, A. S., Ganapathy, V., and Blakely, R. D. (1993). Antidepressant- and cocaine-sensitive human serotonin transporter: Molecular cloning, expression, and chromosomal localization. *Proc. Natl. Acad. Sci. U.S.A.*, 9, 2542–2546.

Ramsey, T. A. (1981). Manic-depressive illness and the pharmacology of lithium. In *Neuropharmacology of the CNS and Behavioral Disorders* (G. C. Palmer, Ed.), pp. 111–121. Academic Press, New York.

Rand, M. J. (1989). Neuropharmacological effects in relation to cholinergic mechanisms. *Prog. Brain Res.*, 9, 3–11.

Randall, C. L., Ekblad, U., and Anton, R. F. (1990). Perspectives on the pathophysiology of fetal alcohol syndrome. *Alcohol. Clin. Exp. Res.,* 14, 807–812.

Randall, C. L., and Taylor, W. J. (1979). Prenatal ethanol exposure in mice: Teratogenic effects. *Teratology,* 19, 305–312.

Randall, L. O., Heise, G. A., Schallek, W., Bagdon, R. E., Banziger, R., Boris, A., Moe, R. A., and Abrams, W. B. (1961). Pharmacological and clinical studies on valium, a new psychotherapeutic agent of the benzodiazepine class. *Curr. Ther. Res. Clin. Exp.,* 3, 405–425.

Randall, L. O., and Kapell, B. (1973). Pharmacological activity of some benzodiazepines and their metabolites. In *The Benzodiazepines* (S. Garattini, E. Mussini, and L. O. Randall, Eds.), pp. 27–51. Raven Press, New York.

Randall, L. O., Schallek, W., Heise, G. A., Keith, E. F., and Bagdon, R. E. (1960). The psychosedative properties of methaminodiazepoxide. *J. Pharmacol. Exp. Ther.,* 129, 163–171.

Randrup, A., and Munkvad, I. (1967). Stereotyped activities produced by amphetamine in several animal species and man. *Psychopharmacologia,* 11, 300–310.

Rankin, H., Hodgson, R., and Stockwell, T. (1983). Cue exposure and response prevention with alcoholics: A controlled trial. *Behav. Res. Ther.,* 21, 435–446.

Ransom, R. W., and Deschenes, N. (1990). Polyamines regulate glycine interaction with the N-methyl-D-aspartate receptor. *Synapse,* 5, 294–298.

Rao, T. S., Kim, H. S., Lehmann, J., Martin, L. L., and Wood, P. L. (1990a). Interactions of phencyclidine receptor agonist MK-801 with dopaminergic system: Regional studies in the rat. *J. Neurochem.,* 54, 1157–1162.

Rao, T. S., Kim, H. S., Lehmann, J., Martin, L. L., and Wood, P. J. (1990b). Selective activation of dopaminergic pathways in the mesocortex by compounds that act at the phencyclidine (PCP) binding site: Tentative evidence for PCP recognition sites not coupled to N-methyl-D-aspartate (NMDA) receptors. *Neuropharmacology,* 29, 225–230.

Rapoport, R. M., and Murad, F. (1983). Agonist induced endothelium-dependent relaxation in rat thoracic aorta may be mediated through cyclic GMP. *Circ. Res.,* 52, 352–357.

Rapoport, S. I. (1991). Positron emission tomography in Alzheimer's disease in relation to disease pathogenesis: A critical review. *Cerebrovasc. Brain Metab. Rev.,* 3, 297–335.

Rapp, P. R., and Amaral, D. G. (1992). Individual differences in the cognitive and neurobiological consequences of normal aging. *Trends Neurosci.,* 15, 340–345.

Rapport, M. M., Green, A. A., and Page, I. H. (1948). Crystalline serotonin. *Science,* 108, 329–330.

Rash, J. E., Walrond, J. P., and Morita, M. (1988). Structural and functional correlates of synaptic transmission in the vertebrate neuromuscular junction. *J. Electron Microsc. Tech.,* 10, 153–185.

Raskind, M. A., Carta, A., and Bravi, D. (1995). Is early-onset Alzheimer disease a distinct subgroup within the Alzheimer disease population? *Alzheimer Dis. Assoc. Disord.,* 9 (Suppl. 1), S2–S6.

Rasmussen, K. (1994). CCK, schizophrenia, and anxiety: CCK-B antagonists inhibit the activity of brain dopamine neurons. *Ann. N.Y. Acad. Sci.,* 713, 300–311.

Rasmussen, K., Beitner-Johnson, D. B., Krystal, J. H., Aghajanian, G. K., and Nestler, E. J. (1990). Opiate withdrawal and the rat locus coeruleus: Behavioral, electophysiological, and biochemical correlates. *J. Neurosci.,* 10, 2308–2317.

Rasmusson, D. D. (1993). Cholinergic modulation of sensory inforamtion. *Prog. Brain Res.,* 98, 357–364.

Ravard, S., and Dourish, C. T. (1990). Cholecystokinin and anxiety. *Trends Pharmacol. Sci.,* 11, 271–273.

Rawlin, J. W. (1968). Street level abuse of amphetamines. In *Amphetamine Abuse* (J. R. Russo, Ed.), pp. 51–65. Thomas, Springfield, IL.

Rawlins, J. N. P., and Deacon, R. M. J. (1993). Further developments of maze procedures. In *Behavioural Neuroscience: A Practical Approach,* Vol. 2 (A. Sahgal, Ed.), pp. 95–106. Oxford University Press, New York.

Raz, S., and Raz, N. (1990). Structural brain abnormalities in the major psychoses: A quantitative review of the evidence from computerized imaging. *Psychol. Bull.,* 108, 93–108.

Razdan, R. K. (1986). Structure-activity relationships in cannabinoids. *Pharmacol. Rev.,* 38, 75–149.

Reavill, C., and Stolerman, I. P. (1990). Locomotor activity in rats after administration of nicotine agonists locally. *Br. J. Pharmacol.,* 99, 273–278.

Rebec, G. V., and Bashore, T. R. (1984). Critical issues in assessing the behavioral effects of amphetamine. *Neurosci. Biobehav. Rev.,* 8, 153–159.

Rebec, G. V., Curtis, S. D., and Zimmerman, K. S. (1982). Dorsal raphe neurons: Self-inhibition by an amphetamine-induced release of endogenous serotonin. *Brain Res.,* 251, 374–379.

Reches, A., Ebstein, R. P., and Belmaker, R. H. (1978). The differential effect of lithium on noradrenaline and dopamine-sensitive accumulation of cyclic AMP in guinea pig brain. *Psychopharmacology,* 58, 213–216.

Redmond, D. E. Jr. (1987). Studies of the nucleus coeruleus in monkeys and hypotheses for neuropsychopharmacology. In *Psychopharmacology: The Third Generation of Progress* (H. Y. Meltzer, Ed.), pp. 967–975. Raven Press, New York.

Reeder, L. G. (1977). Sociocultural factors in the etiology of smoking behavior: An assessment. *NIDA Res. Monogr.,* 17, 186–201.

Reetz, A., Solimena, M., Matteoli, M., Folli, F., Takei, K., and De Camilli, P. (1991). GABA and pancreatic b-cells: Colocalization of glutamic acid decarboxylase (GAD) and GABA with synaptic-like microvesicles suggests their role in GABA storage and secretion. *EMBO J.,* 10, 1275–1284.

Regoli, D., Drapeau, G., Dion, S., and Couture, R. (1988). New selective agonists for neurokinin receptors: Pharmacological tools for receptor characterization. *Trends Pharmacol. Sci.,* 9, 290–295.

Rehfeld, J. F. (1980). Cholecystokinin. *Trends Neurosci.,* March, 65–67.

Rehfeld, J. F., Hansen, H. F., Marley, P. D., and Stengaard-Pedersen, K. (1985). Molecular forms of cholecystokinin in the brain and the relationship to neuronal gastrins. *Ann. N.Y. Acad. Sci.,* 448, 11–23.

Reid, M. S., Herrera-Marschitz, M., Hökfelt, T., Lindefors, N., Persson, H., and Ungerstedt, U. (1990). Striatonigral GABA, dynorphin, substance P and neurokinin A modulation of nigrostriatal dopamine release: Evidence for direct regulatory mechanisms. *Exp. Brain Res.,* 82, 293–303.

Reiman, E. M., Caselli, R. J., Yun, L. S., Chen, K., Bandy, D., Minoshima, S., Thibodeau, S. N., and Osborne, D. (1996). Preclinical evidence of Alzheimer's disease in persons homozygous for the *e4* allele for apolipoprotein E. *N. Engl. J. Med.,* 334, 752–758.

Reinis, S., and Goldman, J. M. (1982). *The Chemistry of Behavior.* Plenum Press, New York.

Reis, D. J., Joh, T. H., and Ross, R. A. (1975). Effects of reserpine on activities and amounts of tyrosine hydroxylase and dopamine-β-hydroxylase in catecholamine neuronal systems in rat brain. *J. Pharmacol. Exp. Ther.,* 193, 775–784.

Reith, M. E. A. (1990). 5-HT$_3$ receptor antagonists attenuate cocaine-induced locomotion in mice. *Eur. J. Pharmacol.,* 186, 327–330.

Reith, M. E. A., Benuck, M., and Lajtha, A. (1987). Cocaine disposition in the brain after continuous or intermittent treatment and locomotor stimulation in mice. *J. Pharmacol. Exp. Ther.,* 243, 281–287.

Reivich, M., Alavi, A., Fieschi, C., Greenberg, J., and Gur, R. (1986). Cerebral metabolic and hemodynamic effects of sensory and cognitive stimuli in normal subjects. In *PET and NMR: New Perspectives in Neuroimaging and in Clinical Neurochemistry* (L. Battistin and F. Gerstenbrand, Eds.), pp. 65–81. Alan R. Liss, New York.

Remmer, H. (1962). Drugs as activators of drug enzymes. In *Metabolic Factors Controlling Duration of Drug Action,* Vol. 6 (B. B.Brodie and E. G. Erdos, Eds.), p. 235f. Macmillan, New York.

Reppert, S. M., Artman, H. G., Swaminathan, S., and Fischer, D. A. (1981). Vasopressin exhibits a rhythmic daily pattern in cerebrospinal fluid but not in blood. *Science,* 213, 1256–1257.

Rexed, B. (1954). A cytoarchitectonic atlas of the spinal cord in the cat. *J. Comp. Neurol.,* 100, 297–379.

Reynolds, A. K., and Randall, L. O. (1957). *Morphine and Allied Drugs.* University of Toronto Press, Toronto.

Reynolds, G. P., Elsworth, J. D., Blau, K., Sandler, M., Lees, A. J., and Stern, G. M. (1978). Deprenyl is metabolized to methamphetamine and amphetamine in man. *Br. J. Clin. Pharmacol.,* 6, 542–544.

Reynolds, I. J., Rothermund, K., Rajdev, S., Fauq, A. H., and Kozikowski, A. P. (1992). [^{125}I]Thienylphencyclidine, a novel ligand for the NMDA receptor. *Eur. J. Pharmacol.,* 226, 53–58.

Ribeiro, P., Wang, Y., Citron, B. A., and Kaufman, S. (1992). Regulation of recombinant rat tyrosine hydroxylase by dopamine. *Proc. Natl. Acad. Sci. U.S.A.,* 89, 9593–9597.

Ricaurte, G. A., DeLanney, L. E., Irwin, I., and Langston, J. W. (1987). Older dopaminergic neurons do not recover from the effects of MPTP. *Neuropharmacology,* 26, 97–99.

Ricaurte, G. A., Finnegan, K. T., Irwin, I., and Langston, J. W. (1990). Aminergic metabolites in cerebrospinal fluid of humans previously exposed to MDMA: Preliminary observations. *Ann. N.Y. Acad. Sci.,* 600, 699–710.

Ricaurte, G. A., Forno, L. S., Wilson, M. A., De-Lanney, L. E., Irwin, I., Molliver, M. E., and Langston, J. W. (1988). (±)3,4-mthylenedioxymethamphetamine selectively damages central serotonergic neurons in nonhuman primates. *JAMA*, 260, 51–55.

Ricaurte, G. A., Guillery, R. W., Seiden, L. S., Schuster, C. R., and Moore, R. Y. (1982). Dopamine nerve terminal degeneration produced by high doses of methylamphetamine in the rat brain. *Brain Res.*, 235, 93–103.

Ricaurte, G. A., Martello, A. L., Katz, J. L., and Martello, M. B. (1992). Lasting effects of (±)-3,4-methylenedioxymethamphetamine (MDMA) on central serotonergic neurons in nonhuman primates: Neurochemical observations. *J. Pharmacol. Exp. Ther.*, 261, 616–622.

Ricaurte, G. A., Molliver, M. E., Martello, M. B., Katz, J. L., Wilson, M. A., and Martello, A. L. (1991). Dexfenfluramine neurotoxicity in brains of non-human primates. *Lancet*, 338, 1487–1488.

Ricaurte, G. A., Schuster, C. R., and Seiden, L. S. (1980). Long-term effects of repeated methylamphetamine administration on dopamine and serotonin neurons in the rat brain: A regional study. *Brain Res.*, 193, 153–163.

Ricaurte, G. A., Seiden, L. S., and Schuster, C. R. (1984). Further evidence that amphetamines produce long-lasting dopamine neurochemical deficits by destroying dopamine nerve fibers. *Brain Res.*, 303, 359–364.

Richard, P., Moos, F., and Freund-Mercier, M.-J. (1991). Central effects of oxytocin. *Physiol. Rev.*, 71, 331–370.

Richards, J. G., Schoch, P., and Jenck, F. (1991). Benzodiazepine receptors and their ligands. In *5-HT$_{1A}$ Agonists, 5-HT$_3$ Antagonists and Benzodiazepines: Their Comparative Behavioural Pharmacology* (R. J. Rogers and S. J. Cooper, Eds.), pp. 1–30. Wiley, New York.

Richards, M. H. (1991). Pharmacology and second messenger interactions of cloned muscarinic receptors. *Biochem. Pharmacol.*, 42, 1645–1653.

Richardson, G., Carskadon, M., Flagg, W., van den Hoed, J., Dement, W., and Mitler, M. (1978). Excessive daytime sleepiness in man: Multiple sleep latency measurement in narcoleptic and control subjects. *Electroencephalogr. Clin. Neurophysiol.*, 45, 621–627.

Richardson, J. S. (1991). The olfactory bulbectomized rat as a model of major depressive disorder. *Neuromethods*, 19.

Richardson, J. S., and Zaleski, W. A. (1983). Naloxone and self-mutilation. *Biol. Psychiatry*, 18, 99–101.

Richardson, N. R., and Roberts, D. C. S. (1991). Fluoxetine pretreatment reduces breaking points on a progressive ratio schedule reinforced by intravenous cocaine self-administration in the rat. *Life Sci.*, 49, 833–840.

Richardson, R. T., and DeLong, M. R. (1988). A reappraisal of the functions of the nucleus basalis of Meynert. *Trends Neurosci.*, 11, 264–267.

Richelson, E. (1993). Treatment of acute depression. *Psychiatr. Clin. North Am.*, 16, 461–478.

Richelson, E. (1995). Cholinergic transduction. In *Psychopharmacology: The Fourth Generation of Progress*. (F. E. Bloom and D. J. Kupfer, Eds.), pp. 125–134. Raven Press, New York.

Richelson, E., and Pfenning, M. (1984). Blockade by antidepressants and related compounds of biogenic amine uptake into rat brain synaptosomes: Most antidepressants selectively block norepinephrine uptake. *Eur. J. Pharmacol.*, 104, 277–286.

Richfield, E. K. (1991). Quantitative autoradiography of the dopamine uptake complex in rat brain using [^{3}H]GBR 12935: Binding characteristics. *Brain Res.*, 540, 1–13.

Richter, D. (1988). Molecular events in expression of vasopressin and oxytocin and their cognate receptors. *Am. J. Physiol.*, 255, F207–F219.

Rickels, K. (1980). Benzodiazepines: Clinical use patterns. *NIDA Res. Monogr.*, 33, 43–60.

Rickels, K., and Schweizer, E. E. (1987). Current pharmacotherapy of anxiety and panic. In *Psychopharmacology: The Third Generation of Progress* (H. Y. Meltzer, Ed.), pp. 1193–1203. Raven Press, New York.

Ridley, R. M., and Baker, H. F. (1982). Stereotypy in monkeys and humans. *Psychol. Med.*, 12, 61–72.

Ridley, R. M., and Baker, H. F. (1991). Can fetal neural transplants restore function in monkeys with lesion-induced behavioural deficits? *Trends Neurosci.*, 14, 36–370.

Riederer, P., and Youdim, M. B. H. (1986). Monoamine oxidase activity and monoamine metabolism in brains of parkinsonian patients treated with l-deprenyl. *J. Neurochem.*, 46, 1359–1365.

Rigdon, G. C., and Wang, C. M. (1991). Serotonin uptake blockers inhibit the firing of presumed serotonergic dorsal raphe neurons in vitro. *Drug Dev. Res.*, 22, 135–140.

Rinaldi-Carmona, M., Barth, F., Héaulme, M., Alonso, R., Shire, D., Congy, C., Soubrié, P., Brelière, J.-C., and Le Fur, G. (1995). Biochemical and pharmacological characterisation of SR141716A, the first potent and selective brain cannabinoid receptor antagonist. *Life Sci.*, 56, 1941–1947.

Rinne, J. O., Roytta, M., Paljarvi, L., Rummukainen, J., and Rinne, U. K. (1991). Selegiline (deprenyl) treatment and death of nigral neurons in Parkinson's disease. *Neurology*, 41, 859–861.

Rinne, U. K. (1983). Problems associated with long-term levodopa treatment of Parkinson's disease. *Acta Neurol. Scand.*, 95 (Suppl.), 19–26.

Risby, E. D., Hsiao, J. K., Husseini, K., Manji, M. D., Bitran, M. D., Moses, F., Zhou, D. F., and Potter, W. Z. (1991). The mechanisms of action of lithium, II. Effects on adenylate cyclase activity and β-adrenergic receptor binding in normal subjects. *Arch. Gen. Psychiatry*, 48, 513–524.

Risch, S. C. (1982). Beta-endorphin hypersecretion in depression: Possible cholinergic mechanisms. *Biol. Psychiatry*, 17, 1071–1079.

Risner, M. E. (1982). Intravenous self-administration of phencyclidine and related compounds in the dog. *J. Pharmacol. Exp. Ther.*, 221, 637–644.

Ritchie, J. M. (1985). The aliphatic alcohols. In *The Pharmacological Basis of Therapeutics* (A. G. Gilman, L. S. Goodman, T. W. Rall and F. Murad, Eds.), pp. 372–386. Macmillan, New York.

Ritchie, J. M., and Greene, N. M. (1985). Local anesthetics. In *The Pharmacological Basis of Therapeutics* (A. G. Gilman, L. S. Goodman, T. W. Rall and F. Murad, Eds.), pp. 302–321. Macmillan, New York.

Ritchie, J. M., and Rogart, R. B. (1977). The binding of saxitoxin and tetrodotoxin to excitable tissue. *Rev. Physiol. Biochem. Pharmacol.* 79, 1–50.

Ritter, R. C., Brenner, L. A., and Tamura, C. S. (1994). Endogenous CCK and the peripheral neural substrates of intestinal satiety. *Ann. N.Y. Acad. Sci.*, 713, 255–267.

Ritz, M. C., and Kuhar, M. J. (1989). Relationship between self-administration of amphetamine and monoamine receptors in brain: Comparison with cocaine. *J. Pharmacol. Exp. Ther.*, 248, 1010–1017.

Ritz, M. C., Lamb, R. J., Goldberg, S. R., and Kuhar, M. J. (1987). Cocaine receptors on dopamine transporters are related to self-administration of cocaine. *Science*, 237, 1219–1223.

Rivett, A. J., Francis, A., and Roth, J. A. (1983a). Distinct cellular localization of membrane-bound and soluble forms of catechol-*O*-methyltransferase in brain. *J. Neurochem.*, 40, 215–219.

Rivett, A. J., Francis, A., and Roth, J. A. (1983b). Localization of membrane-bound catechol-*O*-methyltransferase. *J. Neurochem.*, 40, 1494–1496.

Rivier, C., Rivier, J., and Vale, W. (1986). Stress-induced inhibition of reproductive functions: Role of endogenous corticotropin-releasing factor. *Science*, 231, 607–609.

Rivier, C., and Vale, W. (1984a). Corticotropin-releasing factor (CRF) acts centrally to inhibit growth hormone secretion in the rat. *Endocrinology*, 114, 2409–2411.

Rivier, C., and Vale, W. (1984b). Influence of corticotropin-releasing factor on reproductive functions in the rat. *Endocrinology*, 114, 914–921.

Robakis, N. K., Ramakrishna, N., Wolfe, G., and Wisniewski, H. M. (1987). Molecular cloning and characterization of a cDNA encoding the cerebrovascular and neuritic plaque amyloid peptides. *Proc. Natl. Acad. Sci. U.S.A.*, 84, 4190–4194.

Robbins, T. W. (1978). The acquisition of responding with conditioned reinforcement: Effect of pipradrol, methylphenidate, *d*-amphetamine and nomifensine. *Psychopharmacology*, 58, 79–87.

Robbins, T. W., Cador, M., Taylor, R., and Everitt, B. J. (1989). Limbic–striatal interactions in reward-related processes. *Neurosci. Biobehav. Rev.*, 13, 155–162.

Robbins, T. W., Everitt, B. J., Marston, H. M., Wilkinson, J., Jones, G. H., and Page, K. J. (1989). Comparative effects of ibotenic acid- and quisqualic acid-induced lesions of the substantia innominata on attentional function in the rat: Further implications for the role of the cholinergic neurons of the nucleus basalis in cognitive processes. *Behav. Brain Res.*, 35, 221–240.

Robbins, T. W., and Sahakian, B. J. (1983). Behavioral effects of psychomotor stimulant drugs: Clinical and neuropsychological implications. In *Stimulants: Neurochemical, Behavioral, and Clinical Perspectives* (I. Creese, Ed.), pp. 301–338. Raven Press, New York.

Robel, P., and Baulieu, E.-E. (1994). Neurosteroids: Biosynthesis and function. *Trends Endocrinol. Metab.*, 5, 1–8.

Roberts, D. C. S. (1993). Self-administration of GBR 12909 on a fixed ratio and progressive ratio schedule in rats. *Psychopharmacology*, 111, 202–206.

Roberts, D. C. S., Corcoran, M. E., and Fibiger, H. C. (1977). On the role of ascending catecholaminergic systems in intravenous self-administration of cocaine. *Pharmacol. Biochem. Behav.,* 6, 615–620.

Roberts, D. C. S., and Koob, G. F. (1982). Disruption of cocaine self-administration following 6-hydroxydopamine lesions of the ventral tegmental area in rats. *Pharmacol. Biochem. Behav.,* 17, 901–904.

Roberts, D. C. S., and Ranaldi, R. (1995). Effect of dopaminergic drugs on cocaine reinforcement. *Clin. Neuropharmacol.,* 18 (Suppl. 1), S84–S95.

Roberts, E. (1975). GABA in nervous system function—an overview. In *The Nervous System* Vol. 1 (D. B. Tower, Ed.), pp. 541–552. Raven Press, New York.

Roberts, E. (1986). Metabolism and nervous system disease: A challenge for our times. Part II. *Metab. Brain Dis.,* 1, 91–117.

Roberts, E., and Frankel, S. (1950). γ-Aminobutyric acid in brain: Its formation from glutamic acid. *J. Biol. Chem.,* 187, 55–63.

Roberts, J. L., Levin, N., Lorang, D., Lundblad, J. R., Dermer, S., and Blum, M. (1993). Regulation of pituitary proopiomelanocortin gene expression. In *Opioids I,* Handbook of Experimental Pharmacology, Vol. 104 (A. Herz, Ed.), pp. 347–378. Springer-Verlag, New York.

Roberts, P. J., McBean, G. J., Sharif, N. A., and Thomas, E. M. (1982). Striatal glutamatergic function: Modifications following specific lesions. *Brain Res.,* 235, 83–91.

Roberts, S. S. (1990). A marker gene for alcoholism? *J. NIH Res.,* 2 (5), 24–26.

Roberts-Lewis, J. M., Roseboom, P. H., Iwaniec, L. M., and Gnegy, M. E. (1986). Differential down-regulation of D1-stimulated adenylate cyclase activity in rat forebrain after *in vivo* amphetamine treatments. *J. Neurosci.,* 6, 2245–2251.

Robertson, G. S., Damsma, G., and Fibiger, H. C. (1991). Characterization of dopamine release in the substantia nigra by in vivo microdialysis in freely moving rats. *J. Neurosci.,* 11, 2209–2216.

Robertson, R. T., and Yu, J. (1993). Acetylcholinesterase and neural development: New tricks for an old dog? *News Physiol. Sci.,* 8, 266–272.

Robichaud, R. C., and Sledge, K. L. (1969). The effects of *p*-chlorophenylalanine on experimentally induced conflict in the rat. *Life Sci.,* 8, 965–696.

Robinson, B. G., Frim, D. M., Schwartz, W. J., and Majzoub, J. A. (1988). Vasopressin mRNA in the suprachiasmatic nuclei: Daily regulation of polyadenylate tail length. *Science,* 241, 342–344.

Robinson, D. S., Rickels, K., Feighner, J., Fabre, L. F., Gammans, R. E., Shrotriya, R. C., alms, D. R., Andary, J. J., and Messina, M. E. (1990). Clinical effects of the 5-HT$_{1A}$ partial agonists in depression: A composit analysis of buspirone in the treatment of depression. *J. Clin. Psychopharmacol.,* 10, 67s–73s.

Robinson, J. H., and Pritchard, W. S. (1995). Reply to Stolerman and Jarvis. *Psychopharmacology,* 117, 16–17.

Robinson, T. E., and Becker, J. B. (1986). Enduring changes in brain and behavior produced by chronic amphetamine administration: A review and evaluation of animal models of amphetamine psychosis. *Brain Res. Rev.,* 157–198.

Robinson, T. E., and Berridge, K. C. (1993). The neural basis of drug craving: An incentive-sensitization theory of addiction. *Brain Res. Rev.,* 18, 247–291.

Robinson, T. E., and Camp, D. M. (1990). Does amphetamine *preferentially* increase the extracellular concentration of dopamine in the mesolimbic system of freely moving rats? *Neuropsychopharmacology,* 3, 163–173.

Robison, G. A., Butcher, R. W., and Sutherland, E. W. (1971). *Cyclic AMP.* Academic Press, New York.

Robison, G. A., Coppen, A. J., Whybrow, P. C., and Prange, A. J. (1970). Cyclic AMP in affective disorders. *Lancet,* 2, 1028–1029.

Robitaille, N-M., Dagenais, G. R., and Christe (1984). Factors determining tobacco usage in the Quebec region. *Union Medicale du Canada,* 113, 21–23.

Robledo, P., and Koob, G. F. (1993). Two discrete nucleus accumbens projection areas differentially mediate cocaine self-administration in the rat. *Behav. Brain Res.,* 55, 159–166.

Robledo, P., Maldonado-Lopez, R., and Koob, G. F. (1992). Role of dopamine receptors in the nucleus accumbens in the rewarding properties of cocaine. *Ann. N.Y. Acad. Sci.,* 654, 509–512.

Rodríguez de Fonseca, F., Gorriti, M. A., Fernández-Ruiz, J. J., Palomo, T., and Ramos, J. A. (1994). Downregulation of rat brain cannabinoid binding sites after chronic Δ⁹-tetrahydrocannabinol treatment. *Pharmacol. Biochem. Behav.,* 47, 33–40.

Roffman, M., Reddy, C., and Lal, H. (1972). Alleviation of morphine-withdrawal symptoms by conditional stimuli: Possible explanation for "drug hunger" and "relapse." In *Drug Addiction: Experimental Pharmacology* (J. M. Singh, L. Miller, and H. Lal, Eds.), pp. 223–226. Futura, Mt. Kisco, NY.

Roffwarg, H. P. (1979). Diagnostic classification of sleep and arousal disorders (1st ed.). *Sleep,* 2, 1–207.

Rogaev, E. I., et al. (1995). Familial Alzheimer's disease in kindreds with missense mutations in a gene on chromosome 1 related to the Alzheimer's disease type 3 gene. *Nature,* 376, 775–778.

Rogawski, M. A. (1985). Norepinephrine. In *Neurotransmitter Actions in the Vertebrate Nervous System* (M. A. Rogawski and J. L. Barker, Eds.), pp. 241–284. Plenum Press, New York.

Rogawski, M. A. (1993). Therapeutic potential of excitatory amino acid antagonists: Channel blockers and 2,3-benzodiazepines. *Trends Pharmacol. Sci.,* 14, 325–331.

Rogue, P., Hanauer, A., Zwiller, J., Malviya, A. N., and Vincendon, G. (1991). Up-regulation of dopamine D$_2$ receptor mRNA in rat striatum by chronic neuroleptic treatment. *Eur. J. Pharmacol.,* 207, 165–168.

Roland, P. E., Larsen, B., Lassen, N. A., and Skinhöf, E. (1980). Supplementory motor area and other cortical areas in organization of voluntary movements in man. *J. Neurophysiol.,* 43, 118–136.

Role, L. W., and Kelly, J. P. (1991). The brain stem: Cranial nerve nuclei and the monoaminergic systems. In *Principles of Neural Science* (3rd ed.) (E. R. Kandel, J. H. Schwartz, and T. M. Jessel, Eds.), pp. 683–699. Elsevier, New York.

Romano, G. J., Mobbs, C. V., Lauber, A., Howells, R. D., and Pfaff, D. W. (1990). Differen-tial regulation of proenkephalin gene expression by estrogen in the ventromedial hypothalamus of male and remale rats: Implications for the molecular basis of a sexually differentiated behavior. *Brain Res.,* 536, 63–68.

Ronne-Engström, E., Hillered, L., Flink, R., Spännare, B., Ungerstedt, U., and Carlson, H. (1992). Intracerebral microdialysis of extracellular amino acids in the human epileptic focus. *J. Cereb. Blood Flow Metab.,* 12, 873–876.

Ronnett, G. V., and Snyder, S. H. (1992). Molecular messengers of olfaction. *Trends Neurosci.,* 15, 508–513.

Roose, S. P., and Glassman, A. H. (Eds.). (1990). *Treatment Strategies for Refractory Depression.* American Psychiatric Press, Washington, D.C.

Roques, B. P., Beaumont, A., Dauge, V., and Fournie-Zaluski, M. C. (1993). Peptidase inactivation of enkephalins: Design of inhibitors and biochemical, pharmacological, and clinical applications. In *Opioids I,* Handbook of Experimental Pharmacology, Vol. 104 (A. Herz, Ed.), pp. 547–584. Springer-Verlag, New York.

Rorsman, P., Berggren, P.-O., Bokvist, K., Ericson, H., Möhler, H., Östenson, C.-G., and Smith, P. A. (1989). Glucose-inhibition of glucagon secretion involves activation of GABA$_A$-receptor chloride channels. *Nature,* 341, 233–236.

Rosecran, J. S., and Spitz, H. I. (1987). Cocaine reconceptualized: Historical overview. In *Cocaine Abuse* (H. I. Spitz and J. S. Rosecran, Eds.), pp. 5–16. Brunner/Mazel, New York.

Roseman, S. (1974). Complex carbohydrates and intercellular adhesion. In *The Cell Surface in Development* (A. Moscona, Ed.), pp. 255–271. Wiley, New York.

Rosen, J., Silk, K. R., Rice, H. E., and Smith, C. B. (1985). Platelet alpha-2-adrenergic dysfunction in negative symptom schizophrenia: A preliminary study. *Biol. Psychiatry,* 20, 539–545.

Rosenbaum, G., Cohen, B. D., Luby, E. D., Gottlieb, J. S., and Yelen, D. (1959). Comparison of Sernyl with other drugs. *Arch. Gen. Psychiatry,* 1, 651–656.

Rosenbaum, J. F. (1990). Drug treatment of panic disorder. *Hosp. Pract.* (Suppl. 2), 25, 31–42.

Rosenberg, P. A., and Dichter, M. A. (1989). Extracellular cyclic AMP accumulation and degradation in rat cerebral cortex in dissociated cell culture. *J. Neurosci.,* 9, 2654–2663.

Rosenblatt, J. E., Pert, C. B., Tallman, J. F., Pert, A., and Bunney, W. E., Jr. (1979). The effect of imipramine and lithium on α- and β-receptor binding in rat brain. *Brain Res.,* 160, 186–191.

Rosenzweig, M. R., Bennett, E. L., and Diamond, M. C. (1972). Brain changes in response to experience. *Sci. Am.,* 226 (2), 22–29.

Roses, A. D. (1994). Apolipoprotein E affects the rate of Alzheimer disease expression: β-amyloid burden is a secondary consequence dependent on APOE genotype and duration of disease. *J. Neuropathol. Exp. Neurol.,* 53, 429–437.

Rosett, H. L. (1980). A clinical perspective of the fetal alcohol syndrome. *Alcoholism,* 4, 119–122.

Ross, S. B. (1976). Long-term effects of N-2-chloroethyl-N-ethyl-2-bromobenzylamine hydrochloride on noradrenergic neurons in the rat brain and heart. *Br. J. Pharmacol., 58,* 521–527.

Ross, S. B. (1982). The characteristics of serotonin uptake systems. In *Biology of Serotonergic Transmission* (N. N. Osborne, Ed.), pp. 159–195. Wiley, Chichester.

Rossetti, Z. L., Hmaidan, Y., and Gessa, G. L. (1992). Marked inhibition of mesolimbic dopamine release: A common feature of ethanol, morphine, cocaine and amphetamine abstinence in rats. *Eur. J. Pharmacol., 221,* 227–234.

Rossier, J. (1993). Biosynthesis of enkephalins and proenkephalin-derived peptides. In *Opioids I,* Handbook of Experimental Pharmacology, Vol. 104 (A. Herz, Ed.), pp. 423–448. Springer-Verlag, New York.

Rossor, M., and Iversen, L. L. (1986). Noncholinergic neurotransmitters in Alzheimer's disease. *Br. Med. Bull., 42,* 70–74.

Rostène, W., Boja, J. W., Scherman, D., Carroll, F. I., and Kuhar, M. J. (1992). Dopamine transport: Pharmacological distinction between the synaptic membrane and the vesicular transporter in rat striatum. *Eur. J. Pharmacol., 218,* 175–177.

Roszak, T. (1969). *The Making of a Counter Culture.* Doubleday, Garden City, New York.

Roth, B. L., and Meltzer, H. Y. (1995). The role of serotonin in schizophrenia. In *Psychopharmacology: The Fourth Generation of Progress* (F. E. Bloom and D. J. Kupfer, Eds.), pp. 1215–1228. Raven Press, New York.

Roth, N., Lutiger, B., Hasenfratz, M., Bättig, K., and Knye, M. (1992). Smoking deprivation in "early" and "late" smokers and memory functions. *Psychopharmacology, 106,* 253–260.

Roth, R. H. (1984). CNS dopamine autoreceptors: Distribution, pharmacology, and function. *Ann. N.Y. Acad. Sci., 430,* 27–53.

Roth, R. H., Morgenroth, V. H., and Salzman, P. M. (1975). Tyrosine hydroxylase: Allosteric activation induced by stimulation of central noradrenergic neurons. *Naunyn Schmiedebergs Arch. Pharmacol., 289,* 327–343.

Roth, R. H., Tam, S. Y., Ida, Y., Yang, J. X., and Deutch, A. Y. (1988). Stress and the mesocorticolimbic dopamine systems. *Ann. N.Y. Acad. Sci., 537,* 138–147.

Roth, R. H., Wolf, M. E., and Deutsch, A. Y. (1987). Neurochemistry of midbrain dopamine systems. In *Psychopharmacology: The Third Generation of Progress* (H. Y. Meltzer, Ed.), pp. 81–94. Raven Press, New York.

Rothman, J. E. (1981). The Golgi apparatus: Two organelles in tandem. *Science, 213,* 1212–1219.

Rothman, R. B., Holaday, J. W., and Porreca, F. (1993). Allosteric coupling among opioid receptors: Evidence for an opioid receptor complex. In *Opioids I,* Handbook of Experimental Pharmacology, Vol. 104 (A. Herz, Ed.), pp. 217–237. Springer-Verlag, New York.

Rothman, R. B., Long, J. B., Bykov, V., Jacobson, A. E., Rice, K. C., and Holaday, J. W. (1988). Beta-FNA binds irreversibly to the opiate receptor complex: In vivo and in vitro evidence. *J. Pharmacol. Exp. Ther., 247,* 405–416.

Rothman, R. B., Reid, A. A., Monn, J. A., Jacobson, A. E., and Rice, K. C. (1989). The psychotomimetic drug phencyclidine labels two high affinity binding sites in guinea pig brain: Evidence for *N*-methyl-D-aspartate-coupled and dopamine reuptake car-

rier-associated phencyclidine binding sites. *Mol. Pharmacol., 36,* 887–896.

Rothman, S. M., and Olney, J. W. (1987). Excitotoxicity and the NMDA receptor. *Trends Neurosci., 10,* 299–302.

Rothstein, J. D., Jin, L., Dykes-Hoberg, M., and Kuncl, R. W. (1993). Chronic inhibition of glutamate uptake produces a model of slow neurotoxicity. *Proc. Natl. Acad. Sci. U.S.A., 90,* 6591–6595.

Rothstein, J. D., Martin, L. J., and Kuncl, R. W. (1992). Decreased glutamate transport by the brain and spinal cord in amyotrophic lateral sclerosis. *N. Engl. J. Med., 326,* 1464–1468.

Rothstein, J. D., Martin, L., Levey, A. I., Dykes-Hoberg, M., Jin, L., Wu, D., Nash, N., and Kuncl, R. W. (1994). Localization of neuronal and glial glutamate transporters. *Neuron, 13,* 713–725.

Rothstein, J. D., Tsai, G., Kuncl, R. W., Clawson, L., Comblath, D. R., Drachman, D. B., Pestronk, A., Stauch, B. L., and Coyle, J. T. (1990). Abnormal excitatory amino acid metabolism in amyotrophic lateral sclerosis. *Ann. Neurol., 28,* 18–25.

Rothwell, N. J. (1990). Central effects of CRF on metabolism and energy balance. *Neurosci. Biobehav. Rev., 14,* 263–271.

Rothwell, N. J., and Le Feuvre, R. A. (1992). Thermogenesis, brown adipose tissue and dexfenfluramine in animal studies. *Int. J. Obes., 16* (Suppl. 3), S67–S71.

Rottenberg, H., Waring, A., and Rubin, E. (1981). Tolerance and cross-tolerance in chronic alcoholics: Reduced membrane binding of ethanol and other drugs. *Science, 213,* 583–585.

Roueché, B. (1966). Cultural factors and drinking patterns. *Ann. N.Y. Acad. Sci., 133,* 846–855.

Rounsaville, B. J., Anton, S. F., Carroll, K., Budde, D., Prusoff, B. A., and Gawin, F. (1991). Psychiatric diagnoses of treatment-seeking cocaine abusers. *Arch. Gen. Psychiatry, 48,* 43–51.

Rowland, N. E., and Carlton, J. (1986). Neurobiology of an anorectic drug: Fenfluramine. *Prog. Neurobiol., 27,* 13–62.

Rowland, N. E., Kalehua, A. N., Li, B.-H., Semple-Rowland, S. L., and Streit, W. J. (1993). Loss of serotonin uptake sites and immunoreactivity in rat cortex after dexfenfluramine occur without parallel glial reactions. *Brain Res., 624,* 35–43.

Roy, A., Adinoff, B., and Linnoila, M. (1988). Acting out hostility in normal volunteers: Negative correlation with levels of 5HIAA in cerebrospinal fluid. *Psychiatry Res., 24,* 187–194.

Roy, A., and Linnoila, M. (1989). CSF studies on alcoholism and related disorders. *Prog. Neuropsychopharmacol. Biol. Psychiatry, 13,* 505–511.

Ruat, M., Traiffort, E., Arrang, J.-M., Leurs, R., and Schwartz, J.-C. (1991). Cloning and tissue expression of a rat histamine H₂–receptor gene. *Biochem. Biophys. Res. Commun., 179,* 1470–1478.

Ruat, M., Traiffort, E., Arrang, J.-M., Tardivel-Lacombe, J., Diaz, J., Leurs, R., and Schwartz, J.-C. (1993). A novel rat serotonin (5-HT₆) receptor: Molecular cloning, localization and stimulation of cAMP accumulation. *Biochem. Biophys. Res. Commun., 193,* 268–276.

Ruat, M., Traiffort, E., Bouthenet, M. L., Schwartz, J.-C., Hirschfeld, J., Buschauer, A., and Schunack, W. (1990). Reversible and irreversible labeling and autoradiographic localization of the cerebral histamine H₂ receptor using [¹²⁵I]iodinated probes. *Proc. Natl. Acad. Sci. U.S.A., 87,* 1658–1662.

Rubin, P., et al. (1991). Altered modulation of prefrontal and subcortical brain activity in newly diagnosed schizophrenia and schizophreniform disorder: A regional cerebral blood flow study. *Arch. Gen. Psychiatry, 48,* 987–995.

Rubin, R. T. (1987). Prolactin and schizophrenia. In *Psychopharmacology: The Third Generation of Progress* (H. Y. Meltzer, Ed.), pp. 803–808. Raven Press, New York.

Rubin, V., and Comitas, L. (1975). *Ganja in Jamaica.* Mouton, The Hague.

Rubinstein, J. E., and Hitzemann, R. J. (1990). Further evidence against the coupling of dopamine receptors to phosphoinositide hydrolysis in rat striatum. *Biochem. Pharmacol., 39,* 1965–1970.

Rubinsztein, D. C. (1995). Apolipoprotein E: A review of its roles in lipoprotein metabolism, neuronal growth and repair and as a risk factor for Alzheimer's disease. *Psychol. Med., 25,* 223–229.

Rudnick, G., and Wall, S. C. (1992). *p*-Chloroamphetamine induces serotonin release through serotonin transporters. *Biochemistry, 31,* 6710–6718.

Ruffolo, R. R. Jr., Nichols, A. J., Stadel, J. M., and Hieble, J. P. (1991). Structure and function of α-adrenoreceptors. *Pharmacol. Rev., 43,* 475–505.

Ruffolo, R. R. Jr., Nichols, A. J., Stadel, J. M., and Hieble, J. P. (1993). Pharmacologic and therapeutic applications of α₂-adrenoceptor subtypes. *Annu. Rev. Pharmacol. Toxicol., 32,* 243–279.

Ruffolo, R. R. Jr., Stadel, J. M., and Hieble, J. P. (1994). α-Adrenoreceptors: Recent developments. *Med. Res. Rev., 14,* 229–270.

Rupp, A., and Keith, S. J. (1993). The costs of schizophrenia: Assessing the burden. *Psychiatr. Clin. North Am., 16,* 413–444.

Ruskin, D. N., and Marshall, J. F. (1994). Amphetamine- and cocaine-induced Fos in the rat striatum depends on D₂ dopamine receptor activation. *Synapse, 18,* 233–240.

Russell, D., and Kenny, G. N. C. (1992). 5-HT₃ antagonists in postoperative nausea and vomiting. *Br. J. Anaesth., 69* (Suppl. 1), 63S–68S.

Russell, M. A. H. (1977). Smoking problems: An overview. In *Research on Smoking* (Jarvik, M. E., Cullen, J. W., Gritz, E. R., Vogt, T. M., and West, L. J. Eds.) pp. 13–34, U.S. Government Printing Office, Washington, D.C.

Russell, M. A. H., Raw, M., and Jarvis, M. J. (1980). Clinical use of nicotine chewing gum. *Br. Med. J., 1,* 1599–1602.

Russell, W. L., Henry, D. P., Phebus, L. A., and Clemens, J. A. (1990). Release of histamine in rat hypothalamus and corpus striatum in vivo. *Brain Res., 512,* 95–101.

Rusted, J. M., and Warburton, D. M. (1989). Cognitive models and cholinergic drugs. *Neuropsychobiology, 21,* 31–36.

Ryan, L. J., Linder, J. C., Martone, M. E., and Groves, P. M. (1990). Histological and ultrastructural evidence that D-amphetamine causes degeneration in neostriatum and frontal cortex of rats. *Brain Res.*, 518, 67–77.

Ryan, L. J., Martone, M. E., Linder, J. C., and Groves, P. M. (1988). Cocaine, in contrast to d-amphetamine, does not cause axonal terminal degeneration in neostriatum and agranular frontal cortex of Long-Evans rats. *Life Sci.*, 43, 1403–1409.

Ryan, T. A., Reuter, H., Wendland, B., Schweizer, F. E., Tsien, R. W., and Smith, S. J. (1993). The kinetics of synaptic vesicle recycling measured at single presynaptic boutons. *Neuron*, 11, 713–724.

Rybakowski, J. K. (1990). Lithium potentiation of antidepressants. In *Pharmacotherapy of Depression* (J. D. Amsterdam, Ed.), pp. 225–239. Marcel Dekker, New York.

Rylander, G. (1972). Psychoses and the punding and choreiform syndromes in addiction to central stimulant drugs. *Psychiatry, Neurol., Neurochir. (Amst.)*, 75, 203–212.

Rylett, R. J. and Schmidt, B. M. (1993). Regulation of the synthesis of acetylcholine. *Prog. Brain Res.*, 98, 161–166.

Sack, D. A., Nurnberger, J., Rosenthal, N. E., Ashburn, E., and Wehr., T. A. (1985). Potentiation of antidepressant medications by phase advance of the sleep-wake cycle. *Am. J. Psychiatry*, 142, 606–608.

Sackeim, H. A. (1994). Central issues regarding the mechanisms of action of electroconvulsive therapy: Directions for future research. *Psychopharmacol. Bull.*, 30, 281–308.

Sackeim, H. A., Devanand, D. P., and Nobler, M. S. (1995). Electroconvulsive therapy. In *Psychopharmacology: The Fourth Generation of Progress* (F. E. Bloom and D. J. Kupfer, Eds.), pp. 1123–1142. Raven Press, New York.

Sagar, S. M., and Sharp, F. R. (1993). Early response genes as markers of neuronal activity and growth factor action. *Adv. Neurol.*, 59, 273–284.

Sahgal, A. (1984). A critique of the vasopressin–memory hypothesis. *Psychopharmacology*, 83, 215–228.

Sahgal, A. (1993). Passive avoidance procedures. In *Behavioural Neuroscience: A Practical Approach*, Vol. 1 (A. Sahgal, Ed.), pp. 49–56. Oxford University Press, New York.

Sahley, T. L., and Panksepp, J. (1987). Brain opioids and autism: An updated analysis of possible linkages. *J. Autism Devel. Disorders*, 17, 201–216.

Saito, A., Williams, J. A., and Goldfine, I. D. (1981). Alterations in brain cholecystokinin receptors after fasting. *Nature*, 289, 599–600.

Saito, K., Barber, R., Wu, J.-Y., Matsuda, T., Roberts, E., and Vaughn, J. E. (1974). Immunohistochemical localization of glutamate decarboxylase in rat cerebellum. *Proc. Natl. Acad. Sci. U.S.A.*, 71, 269–273.

Sakimura, K., Kutsuwada, T., Ito, I., Manabe, T., Takayama, C., Kushiya, E., Yagi, T., Aizawa, S., Inoue, Y., Sugiyama, H., and Mishina, M. (1995). Reduced hippocampal LTP and spatial learning in mice lacking NMDA receptor ε1 subunit. *Nature*, 373, 151–155.

Sakmann, B. (1992). Elementary steps in synaptic transmission revealed by currents through single ion channels. *Science*, 256, 503–512.

Sakurada, O., Kennedy, C., Jehle, J., Brown, J., Carbin, G., and Sokoloff, L. (1978). Measurement of local cerebral blood flow with iodo[^{14}C]antipyrine. *Am. J. Physiol.*, 234, H59–H66.

Sakurai, Y., Ohta, H., Shimazoe, T., Kataoka, T., Fujiwara, M., and Ueki, S. (1985). Delta-9-tetrahydrocannabinol elicited ipsilateral circling behavior in rats with unilateral nigral lesion. *Life Sci.*, 37, 2181–2185.

Salamone, J. D. (1992). Complex motor and sensorimotor functions of striatal and accumbens dopamine: Involvement in instrumental behavior processes. *Psychopharmacology*, 107, 160–174.

Salm, A. K., and McCarthy, K. D. (1992). The evidence for astrocytes as a target for central noradrenergic activity: Expression of adrenergic receptors. *Brain Res. Bull.*, 29, 265–275.

Salt, T. E., and Hill, R. G. (1983). Neurotransmitter candidates of somatosensory primary afferent fibres. *Neuroscience*, 10, 1083–1103.

Salter, M. W., De Koninck, Y., and Henry, J. L. (1993). Physiological roles for adenosine and ATP in synaptic transmission in the spinal dorsal horn. *Prog. Neurobiol.*, 41, 125–156.

Salvaterra, P. M., and Vaughn, J. E. (1989). Regulation of choline acetyltransferase. *Int. Rev. Neurobiol.*, 31, 81–143.

Sammet, S., and Graefe, K.-H. (1979). Kinetic analysis of the interaction between noradrenaline and Na^+ in neuronal uptake: Kinetic evidence for co-transport. *Naunyn Schmiedebergs Arch. Pharmacol.*, 309, 99–107.

Samson, H. H., and Harris, R. A. (1992). Neurobiology of alcohol abuse. *Trends Pharmacol. Sci.*, 206–211.

Sanberg, P. R. (1980). Haloperidol-induced catalepsy is mediated by postsynaptic dopamine receptors. *Nature*, 284, 472–473.

Sánchez, C., Arnt, J., Hyttel, J., and Moltzen, E. K. (1993). The role of serotonergic mechanisms in inhibition of isolation-induced aggression in male mice. *Psychopharmacology*, 110, 53–59.

Sanders-Bush, E. (1990). Adaptive regulation of central serotonin receptors linked to phosphoinositide hydrolysis. *Neuropsychopharmacology*, 3, 411–415.

Sanders-Bush, E., Gallagher, D. A., and Sulser, F. (1974). On the mechanism of brain 5-hydroxytryptamine depletion by p-chloroamphetamine and related drugs and the specificity of their action. *Adv. Biochem. Psychopharmacol.*, 10, 185–194.

Sanders-Bush, E., and Martin, L. L. (1982). Storage and release of serotonin. In *Biology of Serotonergic Transmission* (N. N. Osborne, Ed.), pp. 95–118. Wiley, Chichester.

Sandman, C. A., Datta, P. C., Barron, J., Hoehler, F. K., Williams, C., and Swanson, J. M. (1983). Naloxone attenuates self-abusive behavior in developmentally disabled clients. *Appl. Res. Mental Retardation*, 4, 5–11.

Sangameswaran, L., Fales, M. M., Friedrich, P., and De Blas, A. L. (1986). Purification of a benzodiazepine from bovine brain and detection of benzodiazepine-like immunoreactivity in human brain. *Proc. Natl. Acad. Sci. U.S.A.*, 83, 9236–9240.

Sanger, D. J., Benavides, J., Perrault, G., Morel, E., Cohen, C., Joly, D., and Zivkovic, B. (1994). Recent developments in the behavioral pharmacology of benzodiazepine (w) receptors: Evidence for the functional significance of receptor subtypes. *Neurosci. Biobehav. Rev.*, 18, 355–372.

Santiago, M., and Westerink, B. H. C. (1991). The regulation of dopamine release from nigrostriatal neurons in conscious rats: The role of somatodendritic autoreceptors. *Eur. J. Pharmacol.*, 204, 79–85.

Santiago, M., and Westerink, B. H. C. (1992). Simultaneous recording of the release of nigral and striatal dopamine in the awake rat. *Neurochem. Int.*, 20 (Suppl.), 107S–110S.

Sargent, P. B. (1992). Electrical signalling. In *An Introduction to Molecular Neurobiology* (Z. W. Hall, Ed.), pp. 33–80. Sinauer Associates, Sunderland, MA.

Sargent, P. B. (1993). The diversity of neuronal nicotinic acetylcholine receptors. *Annu. Rev. Neurosci.*, 16, 403–443.

Sarnyai, Z., Höhn, J., Szabó, G., and Penke, B. (1992). Critical role of endogenous corticotropin-releasing factor (CRF) in the mediation of the behavioral action of cocaine in rats. *Life Sci.*, 51, 2019–2024.

Sarter, M. (1991). Taking stock of cognition enhancers. *Trends Pharmacol. Sci.*, 12, 456–461.

Satel, S. L., Southwick, S. M., and Gawin, F. H. (1991). Clinical features of cocaine-induced paranoia. *Am. J. Psychiatry*, 148, 495–498.

Sato, M., Chen, C.-C., Akiyama, K., and Otsuki, S. (1983). Acute exacerbation of paranoid psychotic state after long-term abstinence in patients with previous methamphetamine psychosis. *Biol. Psychiatry*, 18, 429–440.

Sattin, A., and Rall, T. W. (1970). The effect of adenosine and adenine nucleotides on the cyclic adenosine 3′,5′-phosphate content of guinea pig cerebral cortical slices. *Mol. Pharmacol.*, 6, 13–23.

Saudou, F., Amara, D. A., Dierich, A., LeMeur, M., Ramboz, S., Segu, L., Buhot, M.-C., and Hen, R. (1994). Enhanced aggressive behavior in mice lacking 5-HT$_{1B}$ receptor. *Science*, 265, 1875–1878.

Saunders, A. M., et al. (1993). Association of apolipoprotein E allele *E4* with late-onset familial and sporadic Alzheimer's disease. *Neurology*, 43, 1467–1472.

Saussy, D. L., Goetz, A. S., King, H. K., and True, T. A. (1994). BMY 7378 is a selective antagonist of α_{1D}-adrenoceptors: Further evidence that vascular α_1-adrenoceptors are of the α_{1D}-subtype. *Can. J. Physiol. Pharmacol.*, 72 (Suppl. 1), 323.

Savasta, M., Palacios, J. M., and Mengod, G. (1990). Regional distribution of the messenger RNA coding for the neuropeptide cholecystokinin in the human brain examined by in situ hybridization. *Mol. Brain Res.*, 7, 91–104.

Savio, T., and Schwab, M. E. (1989). Rat CNS white matter, but not gray matter, is nonpermissive for neuronal cell adhesion and fiber outgrowth. *J. Neurosci.*, 9, 1126–1133.

Sawada, M., and Nagatsu, T. (1986). Stimulation of the serotonin autoreceptor prevents the calcium–calmodulin-dependent increase of serotonin biosynthesis in rat raphe slices. *J. Neurochem.*, 46, 963–967.

Sawchenko, P. E., Imaki, T., Potter, E., Kovács, K., Imaki, J., and Vale, W. (1993). The functional neuroanatomy of corticotropin-releasing factor. *Ciba Found. Symp.*, 172, 5–29.

Sawchenko, P. E., and Swanson, L. W. (1989). Organization of CRF immunoreactive cells and fibers in the rat brain: Immunohistochemical studies. In *Corticotropin-Releasing*

Factor: Basic and Clinical Studies of a Neuropeptide (E. B. DeSouza and C. B. Nemeroff, Eds.), pp. 29–51. CRC Press, Boca Raton.

Sawle, G. V. (1993). The detection of preclinical Parkinson's disease: What is the role of positron emission tomography? *Mov. Disord.*, 8, 271–277.

Saykin, A. J., Gur, R. C., Gur, R. E., Mozley, P. D., Mozley, M. S., Resnick, S. M., Kester, B., and Stafiniak, P. (1991). Neuropsychological function in schizophrenia: Selective impairment in memory and learning. *Arch. Gen. Psychiatry*, 48, 618–624.

Scallet, A. C., Uemura, E., Andrews, A., Ali, S. F., McMillan, D. E., Paule, M. G., Brown, R. M., and Slikker, W. Jr. (1987). Morphometric studies of the rat hippocampus following chronic delta-9-tetrahydrocannabinol (THC). *Brain Res.*, 436, 193–198.

Scanzello, C. R., Hatzidimitriou, G., Martello, A. L., Katz, J. L., and Ricaurte, G. A. (1993). Serotonergic recovery after (±)3,4-(methylenedioxy)methamphetamine injury: Observations in rats. *J. Pharmacol. Exp. Ther.*, 264, 1484–1491.

Scatton, B. (1993). The NMDA receptor complex. *Fundam. Clin. Pharmacol.*, 7, 389–400.

Scatton, B. (1994). Excitatory amino acid receptor antagonists: A novel treatment for ischemic cerebrovascular diseases. *Life Sci.*, 55, 2115–2124.

Schaechter, J. D., and Wurtman, R. J. (1989). Tryptophan availability modulates serotonin release from rat hypothalamic slices. *J. Neurochem.*, 53, 1925–1933.

Schapira, A. H. V., Cooper, J. M., Dexter, D., Clark, J. B., Jenner, P., and Marsden, C. D. (1990). Mitochondrial complex I deficiency in Parkinson's disease. *J. Neurochem.*, 54, 823–827.

Schapira, A. H. V., Mann, V. M., Cooper, J. M., Dexter, D., Daniel, S. E., Jenner, P., Clark, J. B., and Marsden, C. D. (1990). Anatomic and disease specificity of NADH CoQ$_1$ reductase (complex I) deficiency in Parkinson's disease. *J. Neurochem.*, 55, 2142–2145.

Schatzberg, A. F., and Schildkraut, J. J. (1995). Recent studies on norepinephrine systems in mood disorders. In *Psychopharmacology: The Fourth Generation of Progress* (F. E. Bloom and D. J. Kupfer, Eds.), pp. 911–920. Raven Press, New York.

Schechter, M. D., and Cook, P. G. (1975). Dopaminergic mediation of the interoceptive cue produced by *d*-amphetamine in rats. *Psychopharmacologia*, 42, 185–193.

Schechter, M. D., and Rosecrans, J. A. (1972). Lysergic acid diethylamide (LSD) as a discriminative cue: Drugs with similar properties. *Psychopharmacologia*, 26, 313–316.

Schechter, M. D. and Rosecrans, J. A. (1973). D-amphetamine as a discriminative cue: drugs with similar stimulus properties. *Eur. J. Pharmacol.*, 21, 212–216.

Schechter, R., Yen, S. H. C., and Terry, R. D. (1981). Fibrous astrocytes in senile dementia of the Alzheimer type. *J. Neuropathol. Exp. Neurol.*, 40, 95–101.

Scheel-Krüger, J. (1986). Dopamine-GABA interactions: Evidence that GABA transmits, modulates, and mediates dopaminergic functions in the basal ganglia and the limbic system. *Acta Neurol. Scand.* (Suppl.), 107, 1–54.

Scheel-Krüger, J., Braestrup, C., Nielson, M., Golembiowska, K., and Mogilnicka, E.

(1977). Cocaine: Discussion on the role of dopamine in the biochemical mechanism of action. In *Cocaine and Other Stimulants* (E. H. Ellinwood Jr. and M. M. Kilbey, Eds.), pp. 373–408. Plenum Press, New York.

Scheffel, U., Dannals, R. F., Cline, E. J., Ricaurte, G. A., Carroll, F. I., Abraham, P., Lewin, A. H., and Kuhar, M. J. (1992). [$^{123/125}$I]RTI-55, an in vivo label for the serotonin transporter. *Synapse*, 11, 134–139.

Scheibel, M. E., and Scheibel, A. B. (1967). Anatomical basis of attention mechanisms in vertebrate brains. In *The Neurosciences, A Study Program* (G. C. Quarton, T. Melnechuk, and F. O. Schmitt, Eds.), pp. 577–602. Rockefeller University Press, New York.

Scheinin, M., Lomasney, J. W., Hayden-Hixson, D. M., Schambra, U. B., Caron, M. G., Lefkowitz, R. J., and Fremeau, R. T. Jr. (1994). Distribution of α_2-adrenergic receptor subtype gene expression in rat brain. *Mol. Brain Res.*, 21, 133–149.

Schellenberg, G. D. (1995). Genetic dissection of Alzheimer disease, a heterogeneous disorder. *Proc. Natl. Acad. Sci. U.S.A.*, 92, 8552–8559.

Scheller, R. H., and Hall, Z. W. (1992). Chemical messengers at synapses. In *An Introduction to Molecular Neurobiology* (Z. W. Hall, Ed.), pp. 119–147. Sinauer Associates, Sunderland, MA.

Schelling, T. C. (1992). Addictive drugs: The cigarette experience.

Schelosky, L., and Poewe, W. (1993). Current strategies in the drug treatment of advanced Parkinson's disease—new modes of dopamine substitution. *Acta Neurol. Scand.*, 87 (Suppl. 146), 46–49.

Schenker, S., Becker, H. C., Randall, C. L., Phillips, D. K., Baskin, G. S., and Henderson, G. I. (1990). Fetal alcohol syndrome: Current status of pathogenesis. *Alcohol. Clin. Exp. Res.*, 14, 635–647.

Schenker, S., Yang, Y., Johnson, R. F., Downing, J. W., Schenken, R. S., Henderson, G. I., and King, T. S. (1993). The transfer of cocaine and its metabolites across the term human placenta. *Clin. Pharmacol. Ther.*, 53, 329–339.

Schiavo, G., Benfenati, F., Poulain, B., Rossetto, O., de Laureto, P. P., DasGupta, B. R., and Montecucco, C. (1992). Tetanus and botulinum-B neurotoxins block neurotransmitter release by proteolytic cleavage of synaptobrevin. *Nature*, 359, 832–834.

Schildkraut, J. J. (1965). The catecholamine hypothesis of affective disorders: A review of supporting evidence. *Am. J. Psychiatry*, 122, 509–522.

Schildkraut, J. J., Schanberg, S. M., and Kopin, I. J. (1966). The effects of lithium ion on [^{3}H]norepinephrine metabolism in brain. *Life Sci.*, 5, 1479–1483.

Schiller, P. W. (1993). Development of receptor-selective opioid peptide analogs as pharmacologic tools and as potential drugs. In *Opioids I*, Handbook of Experimental Pharmacology, Vol. 104 (A. Herz, Ed.), pp. 681–710. Springer-Verlag, New York.

Schindler, U. (1994). The utility of nootropics in primary senile dementia. In *Anti-Dementia Agents*, pp. 167–205. Academic Press Ltd.

Schinelli, S., Paolillo, M., and Corona, G. L. (1994). Opposing actions of D$_1$- and D$_2$-dopamine receptors on arachidonic acid release and cyclic AMP production in striatal neurons. *J. Neurochem.*, 62, 944–949.

Schiørring, E. (1981). Psychopathology induced by "speed drugs." *Pharmacol. Biochem. Behav.*, 14 (Suppl. 1), 109–122.

Schipper, J., and Tilders, F. J. H. (1982). Quantification of formaldehyde induced fluorescence and its application in neurobiology. *Brain Res. Bull.*, 9, 69–80.

Schlessinger, J., and Ullrich, A. (1992). Growth factor signaling by receptor tyrosine kinases. *Neuron*, 9, 383–391.

Schlicker, E., Göthert, M., and Hillenbrand, K. (1985). Cyanopindolol is a highly potent and selective antagonist at the presynaptic serotonin autoreceptor in the rat brain cortex. *Naunyn Schmiedebergs Arch. Pharmacol.*, 331, 398–401.

Schmauss, C., Doherty, C., Yaksh, T. L. (1983). The analgesic effects of intrathecally administered partial agonist nalbuphine hydrochloride. *Eur. J. Pharmacol.*, 86, 1–7.

Schmauss, C., and Emrich, H. M. (1985). Dopamine and the action of opiates: A reevaluation of the dopamine hypothesis of schizophrenia with special consideration of the role of endogenous opioids in the pathogenesis of schizophrenia. *Biol. Psychiatry*, 20, 1211–1231.

Schmauss, C., and Emrich, H. M. (1988). Narcotic antagonist and opioid treatment in psychiatry. In *Endorphins, Opiates and Behavioural Processes* (R. J. Rodgers and S. J. Cooper, Eds.), pp. 327–351. Wiley, New York.

Schmechel, D. E., Saunders, A. M., Stittmatter, W. J., Crain, B. J., Hulette, C. M., Joo, S. H., Pericak-Vance, M. A., Goldgaber, D., and Roses, A. D. (1993). Increased amyloid β-peptide deposition in cerebral cortex as a consequence of apolipoprotein E genotype in late-onset Alzheimer disease. *Proc. Natl. Acad. Sci. U.S.A.*, 90, 9649–9653.

Schneider, N. G., and Jarvik, M. E. (1985). Nicotine gum vs. placebo gum: Comparisons of withdrawal symptoms and success rates. *NIDA Res. Monogr.*, 53, 83–101.

Schneider, S. P., and Fyffe, R. E. W. (1992). Involvement of GABA and glycine in recurrent inhibition of spinal motoneurons. *J. Neurophysiol.*, 68, 397–406.

Schnoll, S. H., and Daghestani, A. N. (1986). Treatment of marijuana abuse. *Psychiatric Ann.*, 16, 249–254.

Schoch, P., Richards, J. G., Häring, P., Takacs, B., Stähli, C., Staehelin, T., Haefely, W., and Möhler, H. (1985). Co-localization of GABA$_A$ receptors and benzodiazepine receptors in the brain shown by monoclonal antibodies. *Nature*, 314, 168–171.

Schoeffter, P., Fozard, J. R., Stoll, A., Siegl, H., Seiler, M. P., and Hoyer, D. (1993). SDZ 216–525, a selective and potent 5-H$_{1A}$ receptor antagonist. *Eur. J. Pharmacol.*, 244, 251–257.

Schoenberg, B. S. (1987). Environmental risk factors for Parkinson's disease: The epidemiologic evidence. *Can. J. Neurol. Sci.*, 14, 407–413.

Schoepfer, R., et al. (1994). Molecular biology of glutamate receptors. *Prog. Neurobiol.*, 42, 353–357.

Schoepp, D. D. (1994). Novel functions for subtypes of metabotropic glutamate receptors. *Neurochem. Int.*, 24, 439–449.

Schoepp, D. D., and Conn, P. J. (1993). Metabotropic glutamate receptors in brain function and pathology. *Trends Pharmacol. Sci.*, 14, 13–20.

Schofield, P. R.,et al. (1987). Sequence and functional expression of the GABA_A receptor shows a ligand-gated receptor super-family. *Nature,* 328, 221–227.

Schofield, P. R., Shivers, B. D., and Seeburg, P. H. (1990). The role of receptor subtype diversity in the CNS. *Trends Neurosci.,* 13, 8–11.

Schooler, N. R., and Hogarty, G. E. (1987). Medication and psychosocial stagies in the treatment of schizophrenia. In *Psychopharmacology: The Third Generation of Progress* (H. Y. Meltzer, Ed.), pp. 1111–1119. Raven Press, New York.

Schuckit, M. A. (1986). Genetic aspects of alcoholism. *Ann. Emerg. Med.,* 15, 991–996.

Schuckit, M. A. (1987). Biology of risk for alcoholism. In *Psychopharmacology: The Third Generation of Progress* (H. Y. Meltzer, Ed.), pp. 1527–1533. Raven Press, New York.

Schuetze, S. (1986). Embryonic and adult acetylcholine receptors: Molecular basis of developmental changes in ion channel properties. *Trends Neurosci.,* 9, 386–388.

Schulman, H., and Hanson, P. I. (1993). Multifunctional Ca²⁺/calmodulin-dependent protein kinase. *Neurochem. Res.,* 18, 65–77.

Schultz, J. (1976). Psychoactive drug effects on a system which generates cyclic AMP in brain. *Nature,* 261, 417–418.

Schultz, W., Scarnati, E., Sundström, E., Tsutsumi, T., and Jonsson, G. (1986). The catecholamine uptake blocker nomifensine protects against MPTP-induced parkinsonism in monkeys. *Exp. Brain Res.,* 63, 216–220.

Schulz, S., Yuen, P. S. T., and Garbers, D. L. (1991). The expanding family of guanylyl cyclases. *Trends Pharmacol. Sci.,* 12, 116–120.

Schulze, G. E., McMillan, D. E., Bailey, J. R., Scallet, A., Ali, S. F., Slikker, W. Jr., and Paule, M. G. (1988). Acute effects of Δ-9-tetrahydrocannabinol in rhesus monkeys as measured by performance in a battery of complex operant tests. *J. Pharmacol. Exp. Ther.,* 245, 178–186.

Schulze, G. E., McMillan, D. E., Bailey, J. R., Scallet, A., Ali, S. F., Slikker, W. Jr., and Paule, M. G. (1989). Acute effects of marijuana smoke on complex operant behavior in rhesus monkeys. *Life Sci.,* 45, 465–475.

Schulze, H. G., and Gorzalka, B. B. (1991). Oxytocin effects on lordosis frequency and lordosis duration following infusion into the medial pre-optic area and ventromedial hypothalamus of female rats. *Neuropeptides,* 18, 99–106.

Schumacher, M., Coirini, H., Johnson, A. E., Flanagan, L. M., Frankfurt, M., Pfaff, D. W., and McEwen, B. S. (1993). The oxytocin receptor: A target for steroid hormones. *Reg. Pept.,* 45, 115–119.

Schuster, C. R., Dockens, W. S., and Woods, J. H. (1966). Behavioral variables affecting the develfopment of amphetamine tolerance. *Psycopharmacologia (Berl.),* 9, 170–182.

Schutz, Y., Munger, R., Dériaz, O., and Jéquier, E. (1992). Effect of dexfenfluramine on energy expenditure in man. *Int. J. Obes.,* 16 (Suppl. 3), S61–S66.

Schwartz, D. H., Hernandez, L., and Hoebel, B. G. (1990a). Serotonin release in lateral and medial hypothalamus during feeding and its anticipation. *Brain Res. Bull.,* 25, 797–802.

Schwartz, D. H., Hernandez, L., and Hoebel, B. G. (1990b). Tryptophan increases extracellular serotonin in the lateral hypothalamus of food-deprived rats. *Brain Res. Bull.,* 25, 803–807.

Schwartz, J.-C. (1983a). Metabolism of enkephalins and the inactivating neuropeptidase concept. *Trends Neurosci.,* 6, 45–48.

Schwartz, J.-C. (1983b). Two distinct classes of dopamine receptor mediating actions of antipsychotics: Binding and behavioral studies. In *Molecular Pharmacology of Neurotransmitter Receptors* (T. Sagawa, H. I. Yamamura and K. Kuriyama, Eds.), pp. 163–173. Raven Press, New York.

Schwartz, J.-C., Arrang, J.-M., and Garbarg, M. (1986). Three classes of histamine receptors in the brain. *Trends Pharmacol. Sci.,* 7, 24–28.

Schwartz, J.-C., Arrang, J. M., Garbarg, M., Pollard, H., and Ruat, M. (1991). Histaminergic transmission in the mammalian brain. *Physiol. Rev.,* 71, 1–52.

Schwartz, J.-C., Bouthenet, M.-L., Giros, B., Gros, C., Llorens-Cortes, C., and Pollard, H. (1991). Neuropeptidases and neuropeptide inactivation in the brain. In *Volume Transmission in the Brain: Novel Mechanisms for Neural Transmission* (K. Fuxe and L. F. Agnati, Eds.), pp. 381–394. Raven Press, New York.

Schwartz, J.-C., Giros, B., Martres, M.-P., and Sokoloff, P. (1993). Multiple dopamine receptors as molecular targets for antipsychotics. In *International Academy of Biomedical Drug Research,* Vol. 4. *New Generation of Antipsychotic Drugs: Novel Mechanisms of Action* (N. Brunello, J. Mendlewicz, and J. Racagni, Eds.), pp. 1–14. Karger, Basel.

Schwartz, J.-C., Lampart, C., and Rose, C. (1972). Histamine formation in rat brain in vivo: Effects of histidine loads. *J. Neurochem.,* 19, 801–810.

Schwartz, J.-C., Pollard, H., and Quach, T. T. (1980). Histamine as a neurotransmitter in mammalian brain: Neurochemical evidence. *J. Neurochem.,* 35, 26–33.

Schwartz, J. H. (1980). The transport of substances in nerve cells. *Sci. Am.,* 242 (4), 152–171.

Schwartz, J. H. (1991a). The cytology of neurons. In *Principles of Neural Science* (3rd ed.) (E. R. Kandel, J. H. Schwartz, and T. M. Jessell, Eds.), pp. 37–48. Elsevier, New York.

Schwartz, J. H. (1991b). Synaptic vesicles. In *Principles of Neural Science* (3rd ed.) (E. R. Kandel, J. H. Schwartz, and T. M. Jessell, Eds.), pp. 225–234. Elsevier, New York.

Schwartz, J. H. (1991c). Synthesis and trafficking of neural proteins. In *Principles of Neural Science* (3rd ed.) (E. R. Kandel, J. H. Schwartz, and T. M. Jessell, Eds.), pp. 49–65. Elsevier, New York.

Schwarz, K. R. (1986). The principles of recptor binding studies. In *The Heart and Cardiovascular System* (H. A. Fozzard, E. Haber, R. Jennings, A. Katz, and H. Morgan, Eds.), pp. 169–188. Raven Press, New York.

Schweizer, E., and Rickels, K. (1986). Failure of buspirone to manage benzodiazepine withdrawal. *Am. J. Psychiatry,* 143, 1590–1592.

Schweizer, E., and Rickels, K. (1991). Serotonergic anxiolytics: A review of their clinical efficacy. In *5-HT_1A Agonists, 5-HT_3 Antagonists and Benzodiazepines: Their Comparative Behavioural Pharmacology* (R. J. Rogers and S. J. Cooper, Eds.), pp. 365–376. Wiley, New York.

Scott, J. D. (1991). Cyclic nucleotide-dependent protein kinases. *Pharmacol. Ther.,* 50, 123–145.

Scott, S. A., Mufson, E. J., Weingartner, J. A., Skau, K. A., and Crutcher, K. A. (1995). Nerve growth factor in Alzheimer's disease: Increased levels throughout the brain coupled with declines in nucleus basalis. *J. Neurosci.,* 15, 6213–6221.

Scuderi, P., Wetchler, B., Sung, Y.-F., Mingus, M., DuPen, S., Claybon, L., Leslie, J., Talke, P., Apfelbaum, J., Sharifi-Azad, S., and Williams, M. F. (1993). Treatment of postoperative nausea and vomiting after outpatient surgery with the 5-HT_3 antagonist ondansetron. *Anesthesiology,* 78, 15–20.

Sedvall, G. (1992). The current status of PET scanning with respect to schizophrenia. *Neuropsychopharmacology,* 7, 41–54.

Sedvall, G. and Farde, L. (1995). Chemical brain anatomy in schizophrenia. *Lancet,* 346, 743–749.

Sedvall, G., Farde, L., Persson, A., and Wiesel, F. A. (1986). Imaging of neurotransmitter receptors in the living human brain. *Arch. Gen. Psychiatry,* 43, 995–1005.

Seeburg, P. H. (1993). The TIPS/TINS Lecture: The molecular biology of mammalian glutamate receptor channels. *Trends Pharmacol. Sci.,* 14, 297–303.

Seeman, P. (1980). Brain dopamine receptors. *Pharmacol. Rev.,* 32, 229–313.

Seeman, P. (1990). Atypical neuroleptics: Role of multiple receptors, endogenous dopamine, and receptor linkage. *Acta Psychiatr. Scand.,* 82 (Suppl. 358), 14–20.

Seeman, P. (1992). Dopamine receptor sequences: Therapeutic levels of neuroleptics occupy D_2 receptors, clozapine occupies D_4. *Neuropsychopharmacology,* 7, 261–284.

Seeman, P. (1995). Dopamine receptors: Clinical correlates. In *Psychopharmacology: The Fourth Generation of Progress* (F. E. Bloom and D. J. Kupfer, Eds.), pp. 295–302. Raven Press, New York.

Seeman, P., and Grigoriadis, D. (1987). Dopamine receptors in brain and periphery. *Neurochem. Int.,* 10, 1–25.

Seeman, P., Ulpian, C., Bergeron, C., Riederer, P., Jellinger, L., Gabriel, E., Reynolds, G. P., and Tourtellotte, W. W. (1984). Bimodal distribution of dopamine receptor densities in brains of schizophrenics, *Science,* 225, 728–731.

Seeman, P., and Van Tol, H. H. M. (1994). Dopamine receptor pharmacology. *Trends Pharmacol. Sci.,* 15, 264–270.

Segal, B. M. (1987). Drinking motivation and the causes of alcoholism: An overview of the problem and a multidisciplinary model. *Alcohol Alcohol.,* 22 (3), 301–311.

Segal, D. S., and Kuczenski, R. (1992). In vivo microdialysis reveals a diminished amphetamine-induced DA response corresponding to behavioral sensitization produced by repeated amphetamine pretreatment. *Brain Res.,* 571, 330–337.

Segal, D. S., and Kuczenski, R. (1994). Behavioral pharmacology of amphetamine. In *Amphetamine and its Analogs* (A. K. Cho, Ed.), pp. 115–150. Academic Press, San Diego.

Segal, M. (1986). Cannabinoids and analgesia. In *Cannabinoids as Therapeutic Agents* (R. Mechoulam, Ed.), pp. 105–120. CRC Press, Boca Raton.

Seidel, W. F., Roth, T., Roehrs, T., Zorick, F., and Dement, W. C. (1984). Treatment of a 12-hour shift of sleep schedule with benzodiazepines. *Science,* 224, 1262–1264.

Seiden, L. S., Fischman, M. W., and Schuster, C. R. (1975/76). Long-term methamphetamine induced changes in brain catecholamines in tolerant rhesus monkeys. *Drug Alcohol Depend.*, 1, 215–219.

Seiden, L. S., and Kleven, M. S. (1989). Methamphetamine and related drugs: Toxicity and resulting behavioral changes in response to pharmacological probes. *NIDA Res. Monogr.*, 94, 146–160.

Seiden, L. S., and Ricaurte, G. A. (1987). Neurotoxicity of methamphetamine and related drugs. In *Psychopharmacology: The Third Generation of Progress* (H. Y. Meltzer, Ed.), pp. 359–366. Raven Press, New York.

Seiden, L. S., Sabol, K. E., and Ricaurte, G. A. (1993). Amphetamine: Effects on catecholamine systems and behavior. *Annu. Rev. Pharmacol. Toxicol.*, 32, 639–677.

Seiger, A., et al. (1993). Intracranial infusion of purified nerve growth factor to an Alzheimer patient: The first attempt of a possible future treatment strategy. *Behav. Brain Res.*, 57, 255–261.

Seiler, N., and Lajtha, A. (1987). Functions of GABA in the vertebrate organism. In *Neurotrophic Activity of GABA During Development*, pp. 1–56. Alan R. Liss, New York.

Selby, G. (1990). Clinical features. In *Parkinson's Disease* (G. M. Stern, Ed.), pp. 333–388. Chapman and Hall, London.

Self, D. W., and Stein, L. (1992). Receptor subtypes in opioid and stimulant reward. *Pharmacol. Toxicol.*, 70, 87–94.

Seligman, M. E. P. (1975). *Helplessness: On Depression, Development and Death*, Freeman, San Francisco.

Selkoe, D. J. (1991). The molecular pathology of Alzheimer's disease. *Neuron*, 6, 487–498.

Selkoe, D. J. (1994). Alzheimer's disease: A central role for amyloid. *J. Neuropathol. Exp. Neurol.*, 53, 438–447.

Selkoe, D. J., Bell, D. S., Podlisny, M. B., Price, D. L., and Cork, L. C. (1987). Conservation of brain amyloid proteins in aged mammals and humans with Alzheimer's disease. *Science*, 235, 873–877.

Sellers, E. M., and Bendayan, R. (1987). Pharmacokinetics of psychotropic drugs in selected patient populations. In *Psychopharmacology: The Third Generation of Progress* (H. Y. Meltzer, Ed.), pp. 1397–1406. Raven Press, New York.

Selye, H. (1950). *Stress: The Physiology and Pathology of Exposure to Systemic Stress*. Acta, Montreal.

Sengstock, G. W., Olanow, C. W., Dunn, A. J., and Arendash, G. W. (1992). Iron induces degeneration of nigrostriatal neurons. *Brain Res. Bull.*, 28, 645–649.

Sengstock, G. W., Olanow, C. W., Menzies, R. A., Dunn, A. J., and Arendash, G. W. (1993). Infusion of iron into the rat substantia nigra: Nigral pathology and dose dependent loss of dopaminergic markers. *J. Neurosci. Res.*, 35, 67–82.

Sepinwall, J., and Cook, L. (1980). Mechanism of action of the benzodiazepines: Behavioral aspect. *Fed. Proc.*, 39, 3024–3031.

Serra, G., Cullu, M., D'Augila, P. S., DeMontis, M. G., and Gessor, G. L. (1990). On the mechanism involved in the behavioral supersensitivity to DA-agonists induced by chronic antidepressants. In *Dopamine in Mental Depression* (G. L. Gessa and G. Serra, Eds.), pp. 121–138. Pergamon Press, Oxford.

Sesack, S. R., and Pickel, V. M. (1992). Prefrontal cortical efferents in the rat synapse on unlabeled neuronal targets of catecholamine terminals in the nucleus accumbens septi and on dopamine neurons in the ventral tegmental area. *J. Comp. Neurol.*, 320, 145–160.

Seubert, P., et al. (1992). Isolation and quantification of soluble Alzheimer's β-peptide from biological fluids. *Nature*, 359, 325–327.

Seutin, V., Verbanck, P., Massotte, L., and Dresse, A. (1991). Acute amphetamine-induced subsensitivity of A_{10} dopamine autoreceptors in vitro. *Brain Res.*, 558, 141–144.

Severson, H. H. (1984). Adolescent social drug use: School prevention program. *Sch. Psychol. Rev.*, 13, 150–161

Shader, R. I., and Greenblatt, D. J. (1977). Clinical implications of benzodiazepines pharmacokinetics. *Am. J. Psychiatry*, 134, 652–656.

Shannon, H. E. (1981). Evaluation of phencyclidine analogs on the basis of their discriminative stimulus properties in the rat. *J. Pharmacol. Exp. Ther.*, 216, 543–551.

Shannon, N. J., Gunnet, J. W., and Moore, K. E. (1986). A comparison of biochemical indices of 5-hydroxytryptaminergic neuronal activity following electrical stimulation of the dorsal raphe nucleus. *J. Neurochem.*, 47, 958–965.

Sharif, N. A. (1989). Quantitative autoradiography of TRH receptors in discrete brain regions of different mammalian species. *Ann. N.Y. Acad. Sci.*, 553, 147–175.

Sharkey, J., Glen, K. A., Wolfe, S., and Kuhar, M. J. (1988). Cocaine binding at sigma receptors. *Eur. J. Pharmacol.*, 149, 171–174.

Sharkey, J., Ritz, M. C., Schenden, J. A., Hanson, R. C., and Kuhar, M. J. (1988). Cocaine inhibits muscarinic cholinergic receptors in heart and brain. *J. Pharmacol. Exp. Ther.*, 246, 1048–1052.

Sharma, S. K., Klee, W. A., and Nirenberg, M. (1975). Dual regulation of adenylate cyclase accounts for narcotic dependence and tolerance. *Proc. Natl. Acad. Sci. U.S.A.*, 72, 3092–3096.

Sharma, S. K., Nirenberg, M., and Klee, W. A. (1975). Morphine receptors as regulators of adenylate cyclase activity. *Proc. Natl. Acad. Sci. U.S.A.*, 72, 590–594.

Sharman, D. F. (1981). The turnover of catecholamines. In *Central Neurotransmitter Turnover* (C. J. Pycock and P. V. Taberner, Eds.), pp. 20–58. Croom Helm, London.

Sharp, T., Bramwell, S. R., Clark, D., and Grahame-Smith, D. G. (1989). In vivo measurement of extracellular 5-hydroxytryptamine in hippocampus of the anaesthetized rat using microdialysis: Changes in relation to 5-hydroxytryptaminergic neuronal activity. *J. Neurochem.*, 53, 234–240.

Sharp, T., Bramwell, S. R., Hjorth, S., and Grahame-Smith, D. G. (1989). Pharmacological characterization of 8-OH-DPAT-induced inhibition of rat hippocampal 5-HT release in vivo as measured by microdialysis. *Br. J. Pharmacol.*, 98, 989–997.

Sharp, T., and Hjorth, S. (1990). Application of brain microdialysis to study the pharmacology of the 5-HT$_{1A}$ autoreceptor. *J. Neurosci. Methods*, 34, 83–90.

Sharp, T., Zetterström, T., Ljungberg, T., and Ungerstedt, U. (1987). A direct comparison of amphetamine-induced behaviours and

regional brain dopamine release in the rat using intracerebral dialysis. *Brain Res.*, 401, 322–330.

Sharpless, S. K. (1970). Hypnotics and sedatives: 1. The barbiturates. In *The Pharmacological Basis of Therapeutics* (L. S. Goodman and A. Gilman, Eds.), pp. 98–120. Macmillan, New York.

Shaw, D. M., Camps, F. E., and Eccleston, E. G. (1967). 5-hydroxytryptamine in the hindbrain of depressive suicides. *Br. J. Psychiatry*, 113, 1407–1411.

Shearman, L. P., Collins, L. M., and Meyer, J. S. (1996). Characterization and localization of [^{125}I]RTI-55–labeled cocaine binding sites in fetal and adult rat brain. *J. Pharmacol. Exp. Ther.*, 277, 1770–1783.

Shen, R.-Y., Asdourian, D., and Chiodo, L. A. (1992). Microiontophoretic studies of the effects of D-1 and D-2 receptor agonists on type I caudate nucleus neurons: Lack of synergistic interaction. *Synapse*, 11, 319–329.

Shen, Y., Monsma, F. J. Jr., Metcalf, M. A., Jose, P. A., Hamblin, M. W., and Sibley, D. R. (1993). Molecular cloning and expression of a 5-hydroxytryptamine$_7$ serotonin receptor subtype. *J. Biol. Chem.*, 268, 18200–18204.

Shepherd, G. M. (1988). *Neurobiology* (2nd ed.). Oxford University Press, New York.

Shepherd, G. M., and Greer, C. A. (1990). Olfactory bulb. In *The Synaptic Organization of the Brain* (3rd ed.) (G. M. Shepherd, Ed.), pp. 133–169. Oxford University Press, New York.

Sherer, M. A. (1988). Intravenous cocaine: Psychiatric effects, biological mechanisms. *Biol. Psychiatry*, 24, 865–885.

Sherer, M. A., Kumor, K. M., and Jaffe, J. H. (1989). Effects of intravenous cocaine are partially attenuated by haloperidol. *Psychiatry Res.*, 27, 117–125.

Sherman, A. D., Davidson, A. T., Baruah, S., Hegwood, T. S., and Waziri, R. (1991). Evidence of glutamatergic deficiency in schizophrenia. *Neurosci. Lett.*, 121, 77–80.

Sherman, W. R., Gish, B. G., Honchar, M. P., and Munsell, L. Y. (1986). Effects of lithium on phosphoinositide metabolism in vivo. *Fed. Proc.*, 45, 2639–2646.

Sherrington, C. S. (1897). The central nervous system. In *A Textbook of Physiology*, Vol. 3 (M. Foster, Ed.), Macmillan, London.

Sherrington, R., et al. (1995). Cloning of a gene bearing missense mutations in early-onset familial Alzheimer's disease. *Nature*, 375, 754–760.

Sherwin, A. L., Quesney, F., Gauthier, S., Olivier, A., Robitaille, Y., McQuaid, P., Harvey, C., and van Gelder, N. (1984). Enzyme changes in actively spiking areas of human epileptic cerebral cortex. *Neurology*, 34, 927–933.

Sherwin, A. L., and van Gelder, N. M. (1986). Amino acid and catecholamine markers of metabolic abnormalities in human focal epilepsy. *Adv. Neurol.*, 44, 1011–1032.

Sherwood, N. (1993). Effects of nicotine on human psychomotor performance. *Hum. Psychopharmacol.*, 8, 155–184.

Shi, D., Nikodijević, O., Jacobson, K. A., and Daly, J. W. (1993). Chronic caffeine alters the density of adenosine, adrenergic, cholinergic, GABA, and serotonin receptors and calcium channels in mouse brain. *Cell. Mol. Neurobiol.*, 13, 247–261.

Shiffman, S. M. (1979). The tobacco withdrawal syndrome. *NIDA Res. Monogr.*, 23, 158–185.

Shimizu, N., Nakane, H., Hori, T., and Hayashi, Y. (1994). CRF receptor antagonist attenuates stress-induced noradrenaline release in the medial prefrontal cortex of rats. *Brain Res.,* 654, 145–148.

Shimizu, T., and Wolfe, L. S. (1990). Arachidonic acid cascade and signal transduction. *J. Neurochem.,* 55, 1–15.

Shiomi, H. Watson, S. J., Kelsey, J. E., and Akil, H. (1986). Pre-translational and post-translational mechanism for regulating beta-endorphin/ACTH cells: Studies in anterior lobe. *Endocrinology,* 119, 1793–1799.

Shippenberg, T. S. (1993). Motivational effects of opioids. In *Opioids II,*, Handbook of Experimental Pharmacology, Vol. 104 (A. Herz, Ed.), pp. 633–650. Springer-Verlag, New York.

Shippenberg, T. S., Herz, A., Spanagel, R., and Bals-Kubik, R. (1991). Neural substrates mediating the motivational effects of opioids. *Biol. Psychiatry,* 2, 33–35.

Shivers, B. D., Killisch, I., Sprengel, R., Sontheimer, H., Köhler, M., Schofield, P. R., and Seeburg, P. H. (1989). Two novel GABA$_A$ receptor subunits exist in distinct neuronal subpopulations. *Neuron,* 3, 327–337.

Shopsin, B., Friedman, E., and Gershon, J. (1976). Parachlorophenylalanine reversal of tranylcypromine effects in depressed patients. *Arch. Gen. Psychiatry,* 33, 811–822.

Shorr, R. G. L., Lefkowitz, R. J., and Caron, M. G. (1981). Purification of the β-adrenergic receptor: Identification of the hormone binding subunit. *J. Biol. Chem.,* 256, 5820–5826.

Shorr, R. G. L., Strohsacker, M. W., Lavin, T. N., Lefkowitz, R. J., and Caron, M. G. (1982). The β$_1$-adrenergic receptor of the turkey erythrocyte: Molecular heterogeneity revealed by purification and photoaffinity labeling. *J. Biol. Chem.,* 257, 12341–12350.

Shulgin, A. T. (1978). Psychotomimetic drugs: Structure activity relationships. In *Handbook of Psychopharmacology,* Vol. 11 (L. L. Iversen, S. D. Iversen, and S. H. Snyder, Eds.), pp. 243–333. Plenum Press, New York.

Shuster, C. R., Lucchesi, B. R., and Emley, G. S. (1979). The effect of d-amphetamine, meprobamate and lobeline on the cigarette smoking of normal human subjects. *NIDA Res. Monogr.,* 23, 91–99.

Shuster, L. (1992). Pharmacokinetics, metabolism, and disposition of cocaine. In *Cocaine: Pharmacology, Physiology, and Clinical Strategies* (J. M. Lakoski, M. P. Galloway, and F. J. White, Eds.), pp. 1–14. CRC Press, Boca Raton.

Sibley, D. R., Nambi, P., and Lefkowitz, R. J. (1985). Molecular mechanisms of hormone receptor desensitization. In *Molecular Mechanisms of Transmembrane Signalling* (Cohen and Houslay, Eds.), pp. 359–374. Elsevier, Amsterdam.

Sidman, M. (1953). Avoidance conditioning with brief shock and no exteroceptive warning stimulus. *Science,* 118, 157–158.

Siegel, G. J., Albers, R. W., Agranoff, B. W., and Katzman, R. (Eds.) (1981). *Basic Neurochemistry,* Little, Brown, Boston.

Siegel, R. K. (1989). *Intoxication.* Pocket Books, New York.

Siegel, S. (1975). Evidence from rats that morphine tolerance is a learned response. *J. Comp. Physiol. Psychol.,* 89, 498–506.

Siegel, S. (1976). Morphine analgesic tolerance: Its situation specificity supports a Pavlovian conditioning model. *Science,* 193, 323–325.

Siegel, S. (1985). Drug-anticipatory responses in animals. In *Placebo: Theory, Research and Mechanisms* (L. White, B. Tursky, and B. Schwartz, Eds.), pp. 288–305. Guilford Press, New York.

Siegel, S. (1989). Pharmacological conditioning and drug effects. In *Psychoactive Drugs: Tolerance and Sensitization.* (A. J. Goudie and M. W. Emmett-Oglesby, Eds.), pp. 115–180. Humana, Clifton, N. J.

Siegel, S., Hinson, R. E., and Krank, M. D. (1981). Morphine-induced attenuation of morphine tolerance. *Science,* 212, 1533–1534.

Siegelbaum, S. A., and Koester, J. (1991). Ion channels. In *Principles of Neural Science* (3rd ed.) (E. R. Kandel, J. H. Schwartz, and T. M. Jessell, Eds.), pp. 66–79. Elsevier, New York.

Sieghart, W. (1995). Structure and pharmacology of γ-aminobutyric acid$_A$ receptor subtypes. *Pharmacol. Rev.,* 181–234.

Siever, L. J. (1987). Role of noradrenergic mechanisms in the etiology of the affective siorders. In *Psychopharmacology: The Third Generation of Progress* (H. Y. Meltzer, Ed.), pp. 493–504. Raven Press, New York.

Siever, L. J., and Davis, K. L. (1985). Overview: Toward a dysregulation hypothesis of depression. *Am. J. Psychiatry,* 142, 1017–1031.

Siever, L. J., Kalus, O. F., and Keefe, R. S. E. (1993). The boundaries of schizophrenia. *Psychiatr. Clin. North Am,* 16, 217–244.

Siggins, G. R., Hoffer, B. J., and Ungerstedt, U. (1974). Electrophysiological evidence for involvement of cyclic adenosine monophosphate in dopamine responses of caudate neurons. *Life Sci.,* 15, 779–792.

Silagy, C., Mant, D., Fowler,G. et al., (1994). A meta-analysis on efficacy of nicotine-replacement therapies in smoking cessation.

Silva, A. J., Paylor, R., Wehner, J. M., and Tonegawa, S. (1992). Impaired spatial learning in α-calcium-calmodulin kinase II mutant mice. *Science,* 257, 206–211.

Silva, A. J., Stevens, C. F., Tonegawa, S., and Wang, Y. (1992). Deficient hippocampal long-term potentiation in α-calcium-calmodulin kinase II mutant mice. *Science,* 257, 201–206.

Silver, A. J., Flood, J. F., Song, A. M., and Morley, J. E. (1989). Evidence for a physiological role for CCK in the regulation of food intake in mice. *Am. J. Physiol.,* 256, R646–R652.

Silver, A. J., and Morley, J. E. (1991). Role of CCK in regulation of food intake. *Prog. Neurobiol.,* 36, 23–34.

Silverman, K., Brooner, R. K., Montoya, I. D., Schuster, C. R., and Preston, K. L. (1995). Differential reinforcement of sustained cocaine abstinence in intravenous polydrug abusers. *NIDA Res. Monogr.,* 153, 212.

Silverman, K., Evans, S. M., Strain, E. C., and Griffiths, R. R. (1992). Withdrawal syndrome after the double-blind cessation of caffeine consumption. *N. Engl. J. Med.,* 327, 1109–1114.

Silverman, K., Mumford, G. K., and Griffiths, R. R. (1994). Enhancing caffeine reinforcement by behavioral requirements following drug ingestion. *Psychopharmacology,* 114, 424–432.

Silverstone, T. (1981). Clinical pharmacology of anorectic drugs. In *Anorectic Agents: Mechanisms of Action and Tolerance* (S. Garattini

and R. Samanin, Eds.), pp. 1–17. Raven Press, New York.

Simantov, R., Kuhar, M. J., Pasternak, G. W., and Snyder, S. H. (1976). The regional distribution of a morphine-like factor enkephalin in monkey brain. *Brain Res.,* 106, 189–197.

Simmonet, G., Taquet, H., Floras, P., Caille, J. M., Legrand, J. C., Vincent, J. D., and Cesselin, F. (1986). Simultaneous determination of radioimmunoassayable methionine-enkephalin and radioreceptor-active pain suffering and non-suffering patients. *Neuropeptides,* 7, 229–240.

Simon, E. J. (1991). Opioid receptors and endogenous opioid peptides. *Med. Res. Rev.,* 11, 357–374.

Simpson, D.D., Joe, G.W. and Bracy, S.A. (1982). Six-year follow-up of opioid addicts after administration to treatment. *Arch. Gen. Psychiatry,* 39, 1318–1326.

Simpson, G. M., and Singh, H. (1990). Tricyclic antidepressants. In *Pharmacotherapy of Depression* (J. D. Amsterdam, Ed.), pp. 75–91. Marcel Dekker, New York.

Sims, K. L., and Bloom, F. E. (1973). Rat brain L-3,4-dihydroxyphenylalanine and L-5-Hdroxytryptophan decarboxylase activities: Differential effect of 6-hydroxy-dopamine. *Brain Res.,* 49, 165–175.

Sims, N. R., Bowen, D. M., Allen, S. J., Smith, C. C. T., Neary, D., Thomas, D. J., and Davison, A. N. (1983). Presynaptic cholinergic dysfunction in patients with dementia. *J. Neurochem.,* 40, 503–509.

Sims, S. M., and Janssen, L. J. (1993). Cholinergic excitation of smooth muscle. *News Physiol. Sci.,* 8, 207–212.

Simson, E. L., Gold, R. M., Standish, L. J., and Pellett, P. L. (1977). Axon-sparing brain lesioning technique: The use of monosodium-L-glutamate and other amino acids. *Science,* 198, 515–517.

Sinden, J. D., Gray, J. A., and Hodges, H. (1994). Cholinergic grafts and cognitive function. In *Functional Neural Transplantation* (S. B. Dunnett and A. Björklund, Eds.), pp. 253–293. Raven Press, New York.

Singh, L., Lewis, A. S., Field, M. J., Hughes, J., and Woodruff, G. N. (1991). Evidence for an involvement of the brain cholecystokinin B receptor in anxiety. *Proc. Natl. Acad. Sci. U.S.A.,* 88, 1130–1133.

Sirinathsinghji, D. J. S., Rees, L. H., Rivier, J., and Vale, W. (1983). Corticotropin-releasing factor is a potent inhibitor of sexual receptivity in the female rat. *Nature,* 305, 232–235.

Sitsen, J. M. A., and Montgomery, S. A. (1994). The pharmacological treatment of depression. In *Handbook of Depression and Anxiety* (J. A. den Boer and J. M. Ad Sitsen, Eds.), pp. 349–377. Marcel Dekker, New York.

Sjolund, B., Terenius, L., and Eriksson, M. (1977). Increased cerebrospinal level of endorphins after electroacupuncture. *Acta Physiol. Scand.,* 100, 382–384.

Skewer, R. G., Jacobsen, F. M., Duncan, C. C., Kelly, K. A., Sack, D. A., Tamarkin, L., Gaist, P. A., Kasper, S., and Rosenthal, N. E. (1988). Neurobiology of seasonal affective disorder and phototherapy. *J. Biol. Rhythms,* 3, 135–154.

Skinner, B. F. (1966). The ontogeny and phylogeny of behavior. *Science,* 153, 1203–1213.

Skinner, B. F. (1981). Selection by consequences. *Science,* 213, 501–504.

Slade, J. (1989). The tobacco epidemic: lessons from history. *J. Psychoactive Drugs*, 21, 281–291.

Slade, J., Bero, L. A., Hanauer, S. A., Barnes, D. E., and Glantz, S. A. (1995). Nicotine and addiction: The Brown and Williamson Documents. *JAMA*, 225–233.

Sladeczek, F., Pin, J.-P., Récasens, M., Bockaert, J., and Weiss, S. (1985). Glutamate stimulates inositol phosphate formation in striatal neurones. *Nature*, 317, 717–719.

Slifer, B. L., Balster, R. L., and Woolverton, W. L. (1984). Behavioral dependence produced by continuous phencyclidine infusion in rhesus monkeys. *J. Pharmacol. Exp. Ther.*, 230, 399–406.

Slopsema, J. S., Van der Gugten, J., and De Bruin, J. P. C. (1982). Regional concentrations of noradrenaline and dopamine in the frontal cortex of the rat: Dopaminegic innervation of the prefrontal subareas and lateralization of prefrontal dopamine. *Brain Res.*, 250, 197–200.

Slotkin, T. A., and Seidler, F. J. (1975). Acute and chronic effects of nicotine on synthesis and storage of catecholamines in the rat adrenal medulla. *Life Sci.*, 16, 1613–1622.

Small, J. G., Milstein, V., Marhenke, J. D., Hall, D. D., and Kellams, J. J. (1987). Treatment outcome with clozapine in tardive dyskinesia, neuroleptic sensitivity, and treatment-resistant psychosis. *J. Clin. Psychiatry*, 48, 263–267.

Smiley, J. F., Levey, A. I., Ciliax, B. J., and Goldman-Rakic, P. S. (1994). D$_1$ dopamine receptor immunoreactivity in human and monkey cerebral cortex: Predominant and extrasynaptic localization in dendritic spines. *Proc. Natl. Acad. Sci. U.S.A.*, 91, p. 5720–5724.

Smith, A. D. (1978). Biochemical studies of the mechanism of release. In *The Release of Catecholamines from Adrenergic Neurons* (D. M. Paton, Ed.), pp. 1–15. Pergamon Press, Oxford.

Smith, A. D., and Bolam, J. P. (1990). The neural network of the basal ganglia as revealed by the study of synaptic connections of identified neurones. *Trends Neurosci.*, 13, 259–265.

Smith, G. B., and Olsen, R. W. (1995). Functional domains of GABA$_A$ receptors. *Trends Pharmacol. Sci.*, 16, 162–168.

Smith, G. P., and Gibbs, J. (1987). The effect of gut peptides on hunger, satiety, and food intake in humans. *Ann. N.Y. Acad. Sci.*, 499, 132–136.

Smith, J. A. M., and Leslie, F. M. (1993). Use of organ systems for opioid bioassay. In *Opioids I*, Handbook of Experimental Pharmacology, Vol. 104 (A. Herz, Ed.), pp. 53–78. Springer-Verlag, New York.

Smith, K. E., Borden, L. A., Hartig, P. R., Branchek, T., and Weinshank, R. L. (1992). Cloning and expression of a glycine transporter reveal colocalization with NMDA receptors. *Neuron*, 8, 927–935.

Smith, M. A., Sayre, L. M., Monnier, V. M., and Perry, G. (1995). Radical AGEing in Alzheimer's disease. *Trends Neurosci.*, 18, 172–176.

Smith, P. B., Compton, D. R., Welch, S. P., Razdan, R. K., Mechoulam, R., and Martin, B. R. (1994). The pharmacological activity of anandamide, a putative endogenous cannabinoid, in mice. *J. Pharmacol. Exp. Ther.*, 270, 219–227.

Smith, R. C., Meltzer, H. Y., Arora, R. C., and Davis, J. M. (1977). Effects of phencyclidine on [^{3}H]catecholamine and [^{3}H]serotonin uptake in synaptosomal preparations from rat brain. *Biochem. Pharmacol.*, 26, 1435–1439.

Smith, R. J. (1979). Study finds sleeping pills overprescribed. *Science*, 204, 287–288.

Smith, S. S., and Augustine, G. J. (1988). Calcium ions, active zones and synaptic transmitter release. *Trends Neurosci.*, 11, 458–464.

Smolen, A. and Beaston-Wimmer, A. (1990). Quantitative analysis of in situ hybridization using image analysis. In *In Situ Hybridization Histochemistry* (M.F. Chesselet, Ed.), p. 175–188. CRC Press, Boston.

Snel, J. (1993). Coffee and caffeine. Sleep and wakefulness. In *Caffeine, Coffee, and Health* (S. Garattini, Ed.), pp. 255–290. Raven Press, New York.

Snell, L. D., and Johnson, K. M. (1985). Antagonism of N-methyl-D-aspartate-induced transmitter release in the rat striatum by phencyclidine-like drugs and its relationship to turning behavior. *J. Pharmacol. Exp. Ther.*, 235, 50–57.

Snell, L. D., and Johnson, K. M. (1986). Characterization of the inhibition of excitatory amino acid-induced neurotransmitter release in the rat striatum by phencyclidine-like drugs. *J. Pharmacol. Exp. Ther.*, 238, 938–946.

Snell, L. D., Mueller, Z. L., Gannon, R. L., Silverman, P. B., and Johnson, K. M. (1984). A comparison between classes of drugs having phencyclidine-like behavioral properties on dopamine efflux *in vitro* and dopamine metabolism *in vivo*. *J. Pharmacol. Exp. Ther.*, 231, 261–269.

Snell, L. D., Yi, S.-J., and Johnson, K. M. (1988). Comparison of the effects of MK-801 and phencyclidine on catecholamine uptake and NMDA-induced norepinephrine release. *Eur. J. Pharmacol.*, 145, 223–226.

Snyder, S. H. (1974a). Catecholamines as mediators of drug effects in schizophrenia. In *The Neurosciences, Third Study Program* (F. O. Schmitt and F. G. Worden, Eds.), pp. 721–232. MIT Press, Cambridge, MA.

Snyder, S. H. (1974b). Psychedelicrazy. In *Madness and the Brain*. McGraw-Hill, New York.

Snyder, S. H. (1985). Adenosine as a neuromodulator. *Annu. Rev. Neurosci.*, 8, 103–124.

Snyder, S. H. (1986). *Drugs and the Brain*. Freeman, New York.

Snyder, S. H., Banerjee, S. P., Yamamura, H., and Greenberg, D. (1974). Drugs, neurotransmitters, and schizophrenia. *Science*, 184, 1243–1253.

Snyder, S. H., Creese, I., and Burt, D. R. (1977). Dopamine receptor binding in the mammalian brain: Revelance to psychiatry. In *Neuroregulators and Psychiatric Disorders* (E. Usdin, D. A. Hamburg and J. Barchas, Eds.), pp. 526–537. Oxford University Press, New York.

Snyder, S. H., Katims, J. J., Annau, Z., Bruns, R. F., and Daly, J. W. (1981). Adenosine receptors and behavioral actions of methylxanthines. *Proc. Natl. Acad. Sci. U.S.A.*, 78, 3260–3264.

Snyder, S. H., Young, A. B., Bennet, J. P., and Mulder, A. H. (1973). Synaptic biochemistry of amino acids. *Fed. Proc.*, 32, 2039–2047.

Sobell, M. B., and Sobell, L. C. (1973). Individualized behavior therapy for alcoholics. *Behav. Res. Ther.*, 4, 49–72.

Sobell, M. B., and Sobell, L. C. (1976). Second-year treatment outcome of alcoholics treated by individualized behavior therapy: Results. *Behav. Res. Ther.*, 14, 195–215.

Sofroniew, M. V. (1983). Vasopressin and oxytocin in the mammalian brain and spinal cord. *Trends Neurosci.*, 6, 467–472.

Soghomonian, J-J. (1990) In situ hybridization histochemistry at the electron microscopic level. In *In Situ Hybridization Histochemistry* (M.F. Chesselet, Ed.), p. 165–174. CRC Press, Boston.

Soininen, H. S., and Riekkinen, P. J. Sr. (1996). Apolipoprotein E, memory and Alzheimer's disease. *Trends Neurosci.*, 19, 224–228.

Sokol, R. J., Miller, S. I., and Reed, G. (1980). Alcohol abuse during pregnancy: An epidemiological study. *Alcohol. Clin. Exp. Res.*, 4, 135–145.

Sokoloff, L. (1984). *Metabolic Probes of Central Nervous System Activity in Experimental Animals and Man*. Sinauer Associates, Sunderland, MA.

Sokoloff, L. (1986). Cerebral circulation, energy metabolism, and protein synthesis: General characteristics and principles of measurement. In *Positron Emission Tomography and Autoradiography: Principles and Application for the Brain and Heart* (M. Phelps, J. Mazziotta, and H. Schelbert, Eds.), pp. 1–71. Raven Press, New York.

Sokoloff, L., Reivich, M., Kennedy, C., DesRosiers, M. H., Patlak, C. S., Pettigrew, K. D., Sakurada, O., and Shinohara, M. (1977). The [^{14}C]-deoxyglucose method for the measurement of local cerebral glucose utilization: Theory, procedure, and normal values in the conscious and anesthetized albino rat. *J. Neurochem.*, 28, 897–916.

Sokoloff, P., Giros, B., Martres, M.-P., and Schwartz, J-C. (1990). Molecular cloning and characterization of a novel dopamine receptor (D$_3$) as a target for neuroleptics. *Nature*, 347, 146–151.

Sokolovsky, M. (1984). Affinity and photoaffinity labeling of receptors. In *Brain Receptor Methodologies* (P. J. Marangos, I. C. Campbell, and R. M. Cohen, Eds.), pp. 153–167. Academic Press, New York.

Soldatos, C. R., Kales, A., and Cadieux, R. (1979). Narcolepsy: Evaluation and treatment. In *Amphetamine Use, Misuse, and Abuse* (D. E. Smith, D. R. Wesson, M. E. Buxton, R. B. Seymour, J. T. Ungerleider, J. P. Morgan, A. J. Mandell, and G. Jara, Eds.), pp. 3–10. Hall, Boston.

Soldo, B. L., Proctor, W. R., and Dunwiddie, T. V. (1994). Ethanol differentially modulates GABA$_A$ receptor-mediated chloride currents in hippocampal, cortical, and septal neurons in rat brain slices. *Synapse*, 18, 94–103.

Solowij, N. (1995). Do cognitive impairments recover following cessation of cannabis use? *Life Sci.*, 56, 2119–2126.

Solowij, N., Michie, P. T., and Fox, A. M. (1991). Effects of long-term cannabis use on selective attention: An event-related potential study. *Pharmacol. Biochem. Behav.*, 40, 683–688.

Solowij, N., Michie, P. T., and Fox, A. M. (1995). Differential impairments of selective attention due to frequency and duration of cannabis use. *Biol. Psychiatry, 37,* 731–739.

Sommer, B., et al. (1990). Flip and flop: A cell-specific functional switch in glutamate-operated channels of the CNS. *Science, 249,* 1580–1585.

Sommer, B., and Seeburg, P. H. (1992). Glutamate receptor channels: Novel properties and new clones. *Trends Pharmacol. Sci., 13,* 291–296.

Sommer, W. (1880). Erkrankung des ammonshornes als aetiologisches moment der epilepsie. *Arch. Psychiatr. Nervenkr., 10,* 631–675.

Soncrant, T. (1986). The use of drugs as probes of cerebral function. In *PET and NMR: New Perspectives in Neuroimaging and in Clinical Neurochemistry* (L. Battistin and F. Gerstenbrand, Eds.), pp. 131–149. Alan R. Liss, New York.

Sonsalla, P. K., Riordan, D. E., and Heikkila, R. E. (1991). Competitive and noncompetitive antagonists at N-methyl-D- aspartate receptors protect against methamphetamine-induced dopaminergic damage in mice. *J. Pharmacol. Exp. Ther., 256,* 506–512.

Sorg, B. A., and Kalivas, P. W. (1991). Behavioral and neurochemical cross-sensitization between footshock stress and cocaine. *Brain Res., 559,* 29–36.

Sotelo, C., Cholley, B., El Mestikawy, S., Gozlan, H., and Hamon, M. (1990). Direct immunohistochemical evidence of the existence of 5-HT$_{1A}$ autoreceptors on serotoninergic neurons in the midbrain raphe nuclei. *Eur. J. Neurosci., 2,* 1144–1154.

Soubrié, P. (1986). Reconciling the role of central serotonin neurons in human and animal behavior. *Behav. Brain Sci., 9,* 319–364.

Spain, J. W., and Klingman, G. I. (1985). Continuous intravenous infusion of phencyclidine in unrestrained rats results in the rapid induction of tolerance and physical dependence. *J. Pharmacol. Exp. Ther., 234,* 415–424.

Spain, J. W., Roth, B. L., and Coscia, C. J. (1985). Differential ontogeny of multiple opioid receptors (mu, delta, and kappa). *J. Neurosci., 5,* 584–588.

Spanagel, R., Herz, A., and Shippenberg, T. S. (1992). Opposing tonically active endogenous opioid systems modulate the mesolimbic dopaminergic pathway. *Proc. Natl. Acad. Sci. U.S.A., 89,* 2046–2050.

Spanos, N. P., and Gottlieb, J. (1976). Ergotism and the Salem village witch trials. *Science, 194,* 1390–1394.

Spealman, R. D. (1993). Modification of behavioral effects of cocaine by selective serotonin and dopamine uptake inhibitors in squirrel monkeys. *Psychopharmacology, 112,* 93–99.

Spealman, R. D., and Bergman, J. (1992). Modulation of the discriminative stimulus effects of cocaine by *mu* and *kappa* opioids. *J. Pharmacol. Exp. Ther., 261,* 607–615.

Spealman, R. D., and Bergman, J. (1994). Opioid modulation of the discriminative stimulus effects of cocaine: Comparison of μ, κ, and δ agonists in squirrel monkeys discriminating low doses of cocaine. *Behav. Pharmacol., 5,* 21–31.

Spector, S., Shore, P. A., and Brodie, B. B. (1960). Biochemical and pharmacological effects of the monoamine oxidase inhibitors, iproniazid, 1-phenyl-2-hydrazinopropane (JB516), and 1-phenyl-3-hydrazinobutane (JB835). *J. Pharmacol. Exp. Ther., 128,* 15–21.

Spencer, D. G. Jr., and Lal, H. (1983). Effects of anticholinergic drugs on learning and memory. *Drug Dev. Res., 3,* 489–502.

Spiker, D. G., et al. (1985). The pharmacological treatment of delusional depression. *Am. J. Psychiatry, 142,* 430–436.

Spilich, G. J., June, L., and Renner, J. (1992). Cigarette smoking and cognitive performance. *J. Addiction, 87,* 1313–1326.

Spoont, M. R. (1992). Modulatory role of serotonin in neural information processing: Implications for human psychopathology. *Psychol. Bull., 112,* 330–350.

Spotts, J. V., and Shontz, F. C. (1980). *Cocaine Users. A Representative Case Approach.* Free Press, New York.

Squire, L. R. (1986). Mechanisms of memory. *Science, 232,* 1612–1619.

Squires, R. F., Benson, D. I., Braestrup, C., Coupet, J., Klepner, C. A., Myers, V., and Beer, B. (1979). Some properties of brain specific benzodiazepine receptors: New evidence for multiple receptors. *Pharmacol. Biochem. Behav., 10,* 825–830.

Squires, R. F., and Braestrup, C. (1977). Benzodiazepine receptors in rat brain. *Nature, 266,* 732–734.

Stabenau, J. R. (1988). Family pedigree studies of biological vulnerability to drug dependence. *NIDA Res. Monogr., 89,* 25–40.

Stacher, G. (1985). Satiety effects of cholecystokinin and ceruletide in lean and obese man. *Ann. N.Y. Acad. Sci., 448,* 431–436.

Stachowiak, M. K., Rigual, R. J., Lee, P. H. K., Viveros, O. H., and Hong, J. S. (1988). Regulation of tyrosine hydroxylase and phenylethanolamine N-methyltransferase mRNA levels in the sympathoadrenal system by the pituitary–adrenocortical axis. *Mol. Brain Res., 3,* 275–286.

Stachowiak, M., Sebbane, R., Stricker, E. M., Zigmond, M. J., and Kaplan, B. B. (1985). Effect of chronic cold exposure on tyrosine hydroxylase mRNA in rat adrenal gland. *Brain Res., 359,* 356–359.

Stachowiak, M., Stricker, E. M., Zigmond, M. J., and Kaplan, B. B. (1988). A cholinergic antagonist blocks cold stress-induced alterations in rat adrenal tyrosine hydroxylase mRNA. *Mol. Brain Res., 3,* 193–195.

Stahl, S. M. (1985). Platelets as pharmacologic models for the receptors and biochemistry of monoaminergic neurons. In *The Platelets: Physiology and Pharmacology* (G. L. Longenecker, Ed.), pp. 307–340. Academic Press, London.

Staines, W. A., Daddona, P. E., and Nagy, J. I. (1987). The organization and hypothalamic projections of the tuberomammillary nucleus in the rat: An immunohistochemical study of adenosine deaminase-positive neurons and fibers. *Neuroscience, 23,* 571–596.

Stanford, C., and Nutt, D. J. (1982). Comparison of the effects of repeated ECS on α$_2$- and β-adrenoreceptors in different regions of rat brain. *Neuroscience, 7,* 1753–1757.

Starke, K. (1971). Influence of α-receptor stimulants on noradrenaline release. *Naturwissenschaften, 58,* 420.

Starke, K., Göthert, M., and Kilbinger, H. (1989). Modulation of neurotransmitter release by presynaptic autoreceptors. *Physiol. Rev., 69,* 864–989.

Staton, D. M., and Solomon, P. R. (1984). Microinjections of d-amphetamine into the nucleus accumbens and caudate-putamen

differentially affect stereotypy and locomotion in the rat. *Physiol. Psychol., 12,* 159–162.

Stäubli, U., Perez, Y., Xu, F., Rogers, G., Ingvar, M., Stone-Elander, S., and Lynch, G. (1994). Centrally active modulators of glutamate receptors facilitate the induction of long-term potentiation in vivo. *Proc. Natl. Acad. Sci. U.S.A., 91,* 11158–11162.

Stäubli, U., Rogers, G., and Lynch, G. (1994). Facilitation of glutamate receptors enhances memory. *Proc. Natl. Acad. Sci. U.S.A., 91,* 777–781.

Stein, L. (1981). Behavioral pharmacology of benzodiazepines. In *Anxiety: New Research and Changing Concepts* (D. F. Klein and J. Rabkin, Eds.), pp. 205–213. Raven Press, New York.

Stein, L., Belluzzi, J. D., Ritter, S., and Wise, C. D. (1974). Self-stimulation reward pathways: Norepinephrine vs. dopamine. *J. Psychiatr. Res., 11,* 115–124.

Stein, L., and Ray, O. (1959). Self-regulation of brain stimulating current intensity in the rat. *Science, 130,* 570–572.

Stein, L., and Seifter, J. (1961). Possible mode of antidepressive action of imipramine. *Science, 134,* 286–287.

Stein, L., Wise, C. D., and Belluzzi, J. D. (1975). Effects of benzodiazepines on central serotonergic mechanisms. In *Mechanisms of Action of Benzodiazepines* (E. Costa and P. Greengard, Eds.), pp. 29–44. Raven Press, New York.

Stein, L., Wise, C. D., and Belluzzi, J. D. (1977). Neuropharmacology of reward and punishment. In *Handbook of Psychopharmacology,* Vol. 8 (L. L. Iversen, S. D. Iversen, and S. H. Snyder, Eds.), pp. 25–53. Plenum Press, New York.

Stein, L., Wise, C. D., and Berger, B. D. (1973). Antianxiety actions of benzodiazepines: Decrease in activity of serotonin neurons in the punishment system. In *The Benzodiazepines* (S. Garattini, E. Mussini, and L. O. Randall, Eds.), pp. 299–326. Raven Press, New York.

Stein, W. D. (1967). *The Movement of Molecules Across Cell Membranes.* Academic Press, New York.

Steinberg, G. K., Saleh, J., and Kunis, D. (1988). Delayed treatment with dextromethorphan and dextrorphan reduces cerebral damage after transient focal ischemica. *Neurosci. Lett., 89,* 193–197.

Steinbusch, H. W. M. (1991). Distribution of histaminergic neurons and fibers in rat brain. *Acta Otolaryngol.* 479 (Suppl.), 12–23.

Steinbusch, H. W. M., DeVente, J., and Schipper, J. (1986). Immunocytochemistry of monoamines in the central nervous system. In *Neurohistochemistry: Modern Methods and Applications* (P. Panula, H. Paivarinta, and S. Soinila, Eds.), pp. 75–105. Alan R. Liss, New York.

Steinbusch, H. W. M., Verhofstad, A. J. J., and Joosten, H. W. M. (1978). Localization of serotonin in central nervous system by immunohistochemistry: Description of a specific and sensitive technique and some applications. *Neuroscience, 3,* 811–819.

Steiner, D. F., and Dyer, E. (1967). The biosynthesis of insulin and a probable precursor of insulin by a human islet cell adenoma. *Proc. Natl. Acad. Sci. U.S.A., 57,* 473–480.

Stellar, E. (1954). The physiology of motivation. *Psychol. Rev., 61,* 5–22.

Stellar, J. R., and Stellar, E. (1985). *The Neurobiology of Motivation and Reward*. Springer-Verlag, New York.

Stenzel-Poore, M. P., Heinrichs, S. C., Rivest, S., Koob, G. F., and Vale, W. W. (1994). Overproduction of corticotropin-releasing factor in transgenic mice: A genetic model of anxiogenic behavior. *J. Neurosci.*, 14, 2579–2584.

Stephens, D. N., Schneider, H. H., Kehr, W., Jensen, L. H., Petersen, E., and Honore, T. (1987). Modulation of anxiety by β-carbolines and other benzodiazepine receptor ligands: Relationship of pharmacological to biochemical measures of efficacy. *Brain Res. Bull.*, 19, 309–318.

Steriade, M., and McCarley, R. W. (1990). *Brainstem Control of Wakefulness and Sleep*. Plenum Press, New York.

Sternbach, L. H. (1973). Chemistry of 1, 4-benzodiazepines and some aspects of the structure-activity relationship. In *The Benzodiazepines* (S. Garattini, E. Mussini, and L. O. Randall, Eds.), pp. 1–26. Raven Press, New York.

Sternberger, L. A. (1986). *Immunocytochemistry*. Wiley, New York.

Sternweis, P. C., and Pang, I.-H. (1990). The G protein–channel connection. *Trends Neurosci.*, 13, 122–126.

Steru, L., Chermat, R., Thierry, B., and Simon, P. (1985). The tail suspension test: A new method for screening antidepressants in mice. *Psychopharmacology*, 85, 367–370.

Stevens, C. F. (1984). Biophysical studies of ion channels. *Science*, 225, 1346–1350.

Stevens, C. F. (1987). An introduction to ion channels. In *Molecular Neurobiology in Neurology and Psychiatry* (E. Kandel, Ed.), pp. 1–6, Raven Press, New York.

Stevens, C. F., and Wang, Y. (1994). Changes in reliability of synaptic function as a mechanism for plasticity. *Nature*, 371, 704–707.

Stewart, C. A., and Morris, R. G. M. (1993). The watermaze. In *Behavioural Neuroscience: A Practical Approach*, Vol. 1 (A. Sahgal, Ed.), pp. 107–122. Oxford University Press, New York.

Stewart, G. R., Zorumski, C. F., Price, M. T., and Olney, J. W. (1990). Domoic acid: A dementia-inducing excitotoxic food poison with kainic acid receptor specificity. *Exp. Neurol.*, 110, 127–138.

Stewart, J., and Druhan, J. P. (1993). The development of both conditioning and sensitization of the behavioral activating effects of amphetamine is blocked by the noncompetitive NMDA receptor antagonist, MK-801. *Psychopharmacology*, 110, 125–132.

Stewart, J., and Vezina, P. (1989). Microinjections of SCH-23390 into the ventral tegmental area and substantia nigra pars reticulata attenuate the development of sensitization to the locomotor activating effects of systemic amphetamine. *Brain Res.*, 495, 401–406.

Stewart, L. C., and Klinman, J. P. (1988). Dopamine beta-hydroxylase of adrenal chromaffin granules: Structure and function. *Annu. Rev. Biochem.*, 57, 551–592.

St. George-Hyslop, et al. (1987). The genetic defect causing Alzheimer's disease maps on chromosome 21. *Science*, 235, 885–890.

Stiglick, A., and Kalant, H. (1982a). Learning impairment in the radial-arm maze following prolonged cannabis treatment in rats. *Psychopharmacology*, 77, 117–123.

Stiglick, A., and Kalant, H. (1982b). Residual effects of prolonged cannabis administration on exploration and DRL performance in rats. *Psychopharmacology*, 77, 124–128.

Stiglick, A., Llewellyn, M. E., and Kalant, H. (1984). Residual effects of prolonged cannabis treatment on shuttle-box avoidance in the rat. *Psychopharmacology*, 84, 476–479.

Stiles, G. L. (1991). Adenosine receptors: Physiological regulation and biochemical mechanisms. *News Physiol. Sci.*, 6, 161–165.

Stolerman, I. (1992). Drugs of abuse: Behavioural principles, methods and terms. *Trends Pharmacol. Sci.*, 13, 170–176.

Stolerman, I. P., and Jarvis, M. J. (1995). The scientific case that nicotine is addictive. *Psychopharmacology*, 117, 2–10.

Stolerman, I. P., and Shoaib, M. (1991). The neurobiology of tobacco addiction. *Trends Parmacol. Sci.*, 12, 467–473.

Stoll, W. A. (1947). Lysergsäure-Diethylamid un phantastikum aus der Mutterkorngruppe. *Schweiz. Arch. Neurol. Psychiat.* 60, 279–323.

Stone, E. A., and Ariano, M. A. (1989). Are glial cells targets of the central noradrenergic system? A review of the evidence. *Brain Res. Rev.*, 14, 297–309.

Stone, E. A., and John, S. M. (1991). Further evidence for a glial localization of rat cortical beta adrenoceptors: Studies of in vivo cyclic AMP responses to catecholamines. *Brain Res.*, 549, 78–82.

Stone, E. A., John, S. M., Bing, G., and Zhang, Y. (1992). Studies on the cellular localization of biochemical responses to catecholamines in the brain. *Brain Res. Bull.*, 29, 285–288.

Stoof, J. C., Drukarch, B., de Boer, P., Westerink, B. H. C., and Groenewegen, H. J. (1992). Regulation of the activity of striatal cholinergic neurons by dopamine. *Neuroscience*, 47, 755–770.

Stoof, J. C., and Kebabian, J. W. (1981). Opposing roles for D-1 and D-2 dopamine receptors in efflux of cyclic AMP from rat neostriatum. *Nature*, 294, 366–368.

Storm-Mathisen, J., and Ottersen, O. P. (1990). Immunocytochemistry of glutamate at the synaptic level. *J. Histochem. Cytochem.*, 38, 1733–1743.

Strain, E. C., Mumford, G. K., Silverman, K., and Griffiths, R. R. (1994). Caffeine dependence syndrome. Evidence from case histories and experimental evaluations. *JAMA*, 272, 1043–1048.

Strait, K. A., and Kuczenski, R. (1986). Dopamine autoreceptor regulation of the kinetic state of striatal tyrosine hydroxylase. *Mol. Pharmacol.*, 29, 561–569.

Strassman, R. J. (1995). Hallucinogenic drugs in psychiatric research and treatment. *J. Nerv. Ment. Dis.*, 183, 3, 127–138.

Streissguth, A. P. (1988). Long term effects of fetal alcohol syndrome. In *Alcohol and Child Family Health*, (G. Robinson, Ed.), p. 135. Vancouver Children's Hopsital, Vancouver.

Streissguth, A. P., Aase, J. M., Clarren, S. K., Randels, S. P., LaDue, R. A., and Smith, D. F. (1991). Fetal alcohol syndrome in adolescents and adults. *JAMA*, 265, 1961–1967.

Streissguth, A. P., Barr, H. M., and Sampson, P. D. (1990). Moderate prenatal alcohol exposure: Effects on child IQ and learning problems at age 7 years. *Alcohol. Clin. Exp. Res.*, 14, 662–669.

Strittmatter, W. J., et al. (1994). Hypothesis: Microtubule instability and paired helical filament formation in the Alzheimer disease brain are related to apolipoprotein E genotype. *Exp. Neurol.*, 125, 163–171.

Strupp, B. J., and Levitsky, D. A. (1985). A mnemonic role for vasopressin: The evidence for and against. *Neurosci. Biobehav. Rev.*, 9, 399–411.

Struppler, A., Erbel, F., and Velho, F. (1978). An overview on the pathophysiology of Parkinsonian and other pathological tremors. *Prog. Clin. Neurophysiol.*, 5, 114–128.

Stryer, L. (1981). *Biochemistry*. W. H. Freeman, San Francisco.

Sturgeon, R. D., Fessler, R. G., and Meltzer, H. Y. (1979). Behavioral rating scales for assessing phencyclidine-induced locomotor activity, stereotyped behavior and ataxia in rats. *Eur. J. Pharmacol.*, 59, 169–179.

Suddath, R. L., Christinson, G. W., Torrey, E. F., Casanova, M. F., and Weinberger, D. R. (1990). Anatomical abnormalities in the brains of monozygotic twins discordant for schizophrenia. *N. Engl. J. Med.*, 322, 789–794.

Südhof, T. C., and Jahn, R. (1991). Proteins of synaptic vesicles involved in exocytosis and membrane recycling. *Neuron*, 6, 665–677.

Sulser, F. (1983). Mode of action of antidepressant drugs. *J. Clin. Psychiatry*, 44, 14–20.

Sulser, F. (1987). Serotonin-norepinephrine receptor interactions in the brain: Implications for the pharmacolgy and pathophysiology of affective disorders. *J. Clin. Psychiatry*, 48 (Suppl.), 12–17.

Sulser, F. (1989). New perspectives on the molecular pharmacology of affective disorders. *Eur. Arch. Psychiatr. Neurol. Sci.*, 238, 231–239.

Sulser, F., and Sanders-Bush, E. (1987). The serotonin-norepinephrine link hypothesis of affective disorders: Receptor-receptor interactions in brain. In *Molecular Basis of Neuronal Responsiveness* (Y. H. Erlich, R. H. Lenox, E. Kornecki, and W. O. Berry, Eds.), pp. 489–502. Plenum Press, New York.

Sulser, F., Vetulani, J., and Mobley, P. L. (1978). Mode of action of antidepressant drugs. *Biochem. Pharmacol.*, 27, 257–261.

Sultatos, L.G. and Soranno, T.M. (1991). Alcohol-induced liver disease. In *Biochemistry and Physiology of Substance Abuse*. (R.R. Watson, Ed.), pp. 71–92, CRC Press, Ann Arbor, MI.

Sulzer, D., Maidment, N. T., and Rayport, S. (1993). Amphetamine and other weak bases act to promote reverse transport of dopamine in ventral midbrain neurons. *J. Neurochem.*, 60, 527–535.

Sulzer, D., and Rayport, S. (1990). Amphetamine and other psychostimulants reduce pH gradients in midbrain dopaminergic neurons and chromaffin granules: A mechanism of action. *Neuron*, 5, 797–808.

The Sumatriptan Auto-Injector Study Group (1991). Self-treatment of acute migraine with subcutaneous sumatriptan using an auto-injector device. *Eur. Neurol.*, 31, 323–331.

Sunahara, R. K., et al. (1990). Human dopamine D_1 gene encoded by an intronless gene on chromosome 5. *Nature*, 347, 146–151.

Sunahara, R. K., et al. (1991). Cloning of the gene for a human dopamine D_5 receptor with higher affinity for dopamine than D_1. *Nature*, 350, 614–619.

Sundström, E., Henriksson, B. G., Mohammed, A. H., and Souverbie, F. (1994). MPTP-treated mice: A useful model for Parkinson's disease? In *Toxin-Induced Models of Neurological Disorders* (M. L. Woodruff and A. J. Nonneman, Eds.), pp. 121–137. Plenum Press, New York.

Surmeier, D. J., Reiner, A., Levine, M. S., and Ariano, M. A. (1993). Are neostriatal dopamine receptors co-localized? *Trends Neurosci.*, 16, 299–305.

Surratt, C. K., Persico, A. M., Yang, X.-D., Edgar, S. R., Bird, G. S., Hawkins, A. L., Griffin, C. A., Li, X., Jabs, E. W., and Uhl, G. R. (1993). A human synaptic vesicle monoamine transporter cDNA predicts posttranslational modifications, reveals chromosome 10 gene localization and identifies *Taq*I RFLPs. *FEBS Lett.*, 318, 325–330.

Sutherland, G., Stapleton, J. A., Russell, M. A., Jarvis, M. J., Hajek, P., Belcher, M., and Feyerabend, C. (1992). Randomised controlled trial of nasal nicotine spray in smoking cessation. *Lancet*, 340, 324–329.

Suwaki, H. (1991). Methamphetamine abuse in Japan. *NIDA Res. Monogr.*, 115, 84–98.

Suzdak, P. D., et al. (1986). A selective imidazobenzodiazepine antagonist of ethanol in the rat. *Science*, 234, 1243–1247.

Suzuki, N., Cheung, T. T., Cai, X.-D., Odaka, A., Otvos, L. Jr., Eckman, C., Golde, T. E., and Younkin, S. G. (1994). An increased percentage of long amyloid β protein secreted by familial amyloid β protein precursor ($bAPP_{717}$) mutants. *Science*, 264, 1336–1340.

Sved, A. F. (1983). Precursor control of the function of monoaminegic neurons. In *Nutrition and the Brain*, Vol. 6, *Physiological and Behavioral Effects of Food Constituents* (R. J. Wurtman and J. J. Wurtman, Eds.), pp. 223–275. Raven Press, New York.

Svensson, K., Carlsson, A., Huff, R. M., Kling-Petersen, T., and Waters, N. (1994). Behavioral and neurochemical data suggest functional differences between dopamine D_2 and D_3 receptors. *Eur. J. Pharmacol.*, 263, 235–243.

Swedberg, M. D. B., Henningfield, J. E., and Goldberg, S. R. (1990). Nicotine dependency: animal studies. In *Nicotine Psychopharmacology: Molecular, Cellular and Behavioural Aspects* (S. Wonnacott, M. A. H. Russell, and I. P. Stolerman, eds.), pp. 38–76. Oxford Science Publications, Oxford.

Swerdlow, N. R., Vaccarino, F. J., Amalric, M., and Koob, G. F. (1986). The neural substrates for the motor-activating properties of psychostimulants: A review of recent findings. *Pharmacol. Biochem. Behav.*, 25, 233–248.

Swerdlow, N. R., van der Kooy, D., Koob, G. F., and Wenger, J. R. (1983). Cholecystokinin produces conditioned place-aversions, not place-preferences, in food-deprived rats: Evidence against involvement in satiety. *Life Sci.*, 32, 2087–2093.

Szatkowski, M., and Attwell, D. (1994). Triggering and execution of neuronal death in brain ischaemia: Two phases of glutamate release by different mechanisms. *Trends Neurosci.*, 17, 359–365.

Szechtman, H., Ornstein, K., Teitelbaum, P., and Golani, I. (1985). The morphogenesis of stereotyped behavior induced by the dopamine receptor agonist apomorphine in the laboratory rat. *Neuroscience*, 14, 783–798.

Szentágothai, J. 1969. Architecture of the cerebral cortex. In *Basic Mechanisms of the Epilepsies* (H. H. Jasper, A. A. Ward, Jr., and A. Pope, Eds.), pp. 13–28. Little, Brown, Boston.

Tabakoff, B., Cornell, N., and Hoffman, P. L. (1986). Alcohol tolerance. *Ann. Emerg. Med.*, 15, 1005–1012.

Tabatabaie, T., Goyal, R. N., Blank, C. L., and Dryhurst, G. (1993). Further insights into the molecular mechanisms of action of the serotonergic neurotoxin 5,7-dihydroxytryptamine. *J. Med. Chem.*, 36, 229–236.

Takagi, H., Morishima, Y., Matsuyama, T., Hayashi, H., Watanabe, T., and Wada, H. (1986). Histaminergic axons in the neostriatum and cerebral cortex of the rat: A correlated light and electron microscopic immunocytochemical study using histidine decarboxylase as a marker. *Brain Res.*, 364, 114–123.

Tallaksen-Greene, S. J., Elde, R., and Wessendorf, M. W. (1993). Regional distribution of serotonin and substance P co-existing in nerve fibers and terminals in the brainstem of the rat. *Neuroscience*, 53, 1127–1142.

Tallan, H. H., Moore, S., and Stein, W. H. (1954). Studies on the free amino acids and related compounds in the tissues of the cat. *J. Biol. Chem.*, 211, 927–939.

Tallman, J. F., Thomas, J. W., and Gallagher, D. W. (1978). GABAergic modulation of benzodiazepine binding site sensitivity. *Nature*, 274, 383–385.

Tam, S. Y., Nobufumi, O., and Roth, R. H. (1987). Precursor control and influence of aspartame on midbrain dopamine neurons. In *Amino Acids in Health and Disease* (S. Kaufman, Ed.), pp. 421–435. Alan R. Liss, New York.

Tam, S. Y., and Roth, R. H. (1985). Selective increase of dopamine metabolism in the prefrontal cortex by the anxiogenic beta carboline FG 7142. *Biochem. Pharmacol.*, 34, 1595–1598.

Tamir, H., and Gershon, M. D. (1990). Serotonin-storing secretory vesicles. *Ann. N.Y. Acad. Sci.*, 600, 53–67.

Tamir, H., Liu, K.-P., Hsiung, S.-C., Adlersberg, M., and Gershon, M. D. (1994). Serotonin binding protein: Synthesis, secretion, and recycling. *J. Neurochem.*, 63, 97–107.

Tamminga, C. A., and Gerlach, J. (1987). New neuroleptics and experimental antipsychotics in schizophrenia. *Psychopharmacology: The Third Generation of Progress* (H. Y. Meltzer, Ed.), pp. 1129–1140. Raven Press, New York.

Tan, S.-E., Wenthold, R. J., and Soderling, T. R. (1994). Phosphorylation of AMPA-type glutamate receptors by calcium/calmodulin-dependent protein kinase II and protein kinase C in cultured hippocampal neurons. *J. Neurosci.*, 14, 1123–1129.

Tanaka, C. (1985). γ-Aminobutyric acid in peripheral tissues. *Life Sci.*, 37, 2221–2235.

Tanaka, C., and Nishizuka, Y. (1994). The protein kinase C family for neuronal signaling. *Annu. Rev. Neurosci.*, 17, 551–567.

Tang, A. H., and Franklin, S. R. (1983). Disruption of brightness discrimination in a shock avoidance task by phencyclidine and its an-tagonism in rats. *J. Pharmacol. Exp. Ther.*, 225, 503–508.

Tang, L., Todd, R. D., and O'Malley, K. L. (1994). Dopamine D_2 and D_3 receptors inhibit dopamine release. *J. Pharmacol. Exp. Ther.*, 270, 475–479.

Tanii, Y., Nishikawa, T., Umino, A., and Takahashi, K. (1990). Phencyclidine increases extracellular dopamine metabolites in rat medial frontal cortex as measured by in vivo dialysis. *Neurosci. Lett.*, 112, 318–323.

Tank, A. W., Curella, P., and Ham, L. (1986). Induction of mRNA for tyrosine hydroxylase by cyclic AMP and glucocorticoids in a rat pheochromocytoma cell line: Evidence for the regulation of tyrosine hydroxylase synthesis by multiple mechanisms in cells exposed to elevated levels of both inducing agents. *Mol. Pharmacol.*, 30, 497–503.

Tank, A. W., Lewis, E. J., Chikaraishi, D. M., and Weiner, N. (1985). Elevation of RNA coding for tyrosine hydroxylase in rat adrenal gland by reserpine treatment and exposure to cold. *J. Neurochem.*, 45, 1030–1033.

Tanner, C. M. (1989). The role of environmental toxins in the etiology of Parkinson's disease. *Trends Neurosci.*, 12, 49–54.

Tanner, C. M., and Langston, J. W. (1990). Do environmental toxins cause Parkinson's disease? A critical review. *Neurology*, 40 (Suppl. 3), 17–30.

Tanouye, M. A., Ferrus, A., and Fujita, S. C. (1981). Abnormal action potentials associated with the Shaker complex locus of *Drosophila*. *Proc. Natl. Acad. Sci. U.S.A.*, 78, 6548–6552.

Tansey, F. A., Farooq, M., and Cammer, W. (1991). Glutamine synthetase in oligodendrocytes and astrocytes: New biochemical and immunocytochemical evidence. *J. Neurochem.*, 56, 266–272.

Tanzi, E. (1893). The facts and the inductions in current histology of the nervous system. *Rev. Sper. Freniat.* 19, 419–472.

Tanzi, R. E., Bird, E. D., Latt, S. A., and Neve, R. l. (1987). The amyloid β-protein gene is not duplicated in brains from patients with Alzheimer's disease. *Science*, 238, 666–669.

Tanzi, R. E., Gusella, J. F., et al. (1987). Amyloid β-protein gene: CDNA, mRNA distribution and genetic linkage near the Alzheimer locus. *Science*, 235, 880–884.

Tart, C. T. (1971). *On Being Stoned. A Psychological Study of Marijuana Intoxication.* Science and Behavior Books, Palo Alto.

Tatton, W. G. (1993). Selegiline can mediate neuronal rescue rather than neuronal protection. *Mov. Disord.*, 8 (Suppl. 1), S20–S30.

Taylor, D., and Ho, B. T. (1978). Comparison of inhibition of monoamine uptake by cocaine, methylphenidate and amphetamine. *Res. Commun. Chem. Pathol. Pharmacol.*, 21, 67–75.

Taylor, D. P., and Schlemmer, R. F. Jr. (1992). Sigma "antagonists." Potential antipsychotics? In *Novel Antipsychotic Drugs* (H. Y. Meltzer, Ed.), pp. 189–201. Raven Press, New York.

Taylor, P. (1985a). Anticholinergic agents. In *The Pharmacological Basis of Therapeutics* (7th ed.) (A. G. Gilman, L. S. Goodman, T. W. Rall, and F. Murad, Eds.), pp. 110–129. Macmillan, New York.

Taylor, P. (1985b). Cholinergic agonists. In *The Pharmacological Basis of Therapeutics* (7th ed.) (A. G. Gilman, L. S. Goodman, T. W. Rall, and F. Murad, Eds.), pp. 100–109. Macmillan, New York.

Taylor, P. (1985c). Ganglionic stimulating and blocking agents. In *The Pharmacological Basis of Therapeutics* (7th ed.) (A. G. Gilman, L. S. Goodman, T. W. Rall, and F. Murad, Eds.), pp. 215–221. Macmillan, New York.

Taylor, P. (1985d). Neuromuscular blocking agents. In *The Pharmacological Basis of Therapeutics* (7th ed.) (A. G. Gilman, L. S. Goodman, T. W. Rall, and F. Murad, Eds.), pp. 222–235. Macmillan, New York.

Taylor, P., and Radić, Z. (1994). The cholinesterases: From genes to proteins. *Annu. Rev. Pharmacol. Toxicol., 34*, 281–320.

Tecott, L.H., Eberwine, J.H., Barchas, J.D. and Valentino, K.L. (1994). Methodological considerations in the utilization of in situ hybridization. In *In Situ Hybridization in Neurobiology* (J.H. Eberwine, K.L. Valentino, and J.D. Barchas, Eds.), pp. 3–23. Oxford University Press, New York.

Tejani-Butt, S. M. (1992). [^{3}H]Nisoxetine: A radioligand for quantitation of norepinephrine uptake sites by autoradiography or by homogenate binding. *J. Pharmacol. Exp. Ther., 260*, 427–436.

Tella, S. R., Schindler, C. W., and Goldberg, S. R. (1992). Cardiovascular effects of cocaine in conscious rats: Relative significance of central sympathetic stimulation and peripheral neuronal monoamine uptake and release mechanisms. *J. Pharmacol. Exp. Ther., 262*, 602–610.

Tella, S. R., Schindler, C. W., and Goldberg, S. R. (1993). Cocaine: Cardiovascular effects in relation to inhibition of peripheral neuronal monoamine uptake and central stimulation of the sympathoadrenal system. *J. Pharmacol. Exp. Ther., 267*, 153–162.

Tempel, A., Kessler, J. A., and Zukin, R. S. (1990). Chronic naltrexone treatment increases expression of preproenkephalin and preprotackykinin mRNA in discrete brain regions. *J. Neurosci., 10*, 741–747.

Tempel, A., and Zukin, R. S. (1987). Neuroanatomical patterns of the mu, delta, and kappa opioid receptors of rat brain as determined by quantitative in vitro autoradiography. *Proc. Natl. Acad. Sci. U.S.A., 84*, 4308–4312.

Tennant, F. S. (1986). The clinical syndrome of marijuana dependence. *Psychiatric Ann., 16*, 225–234.

Tennant, F. S., Jr., Rawson, R. A., and McCann, M. (1981). Withdrawal from chronic phencyclidine (PCP) dependence with desipramine. *Am. J. Psychiatry, 138*, 845–847.

Terakawa, S., Fan, J.-H., Kumakura, K., and Ohara-Imaizumi, M. (1991). Quantitative analysis of exocytosis directly visualized in living chromaffin cells. *Neurosci. Lett., 123*, 82–86.

Terenius, L. (1982). Endorphins and modulation of pain. *Adv. Neurol., 33*, 59–64.

Terenius, L., and Wahlstrom, A. (1974). Inhibitor(s) of narcotic receptor binding in brain extracts and cerebrospinal fluid. *Acta Pharmacol. Toxicol., 35* (Suppl. 1), 87 (Abst.).

Terenius, L., and Wahlstrom, A. (1975). Morphine-like ligand for opiate receptors in human CSF. *Life Sci., 16*, 1759–1764.

Terman, M., Terman, J. S., Quitkin, F. M., McGrath, P. J., Steward, J. W., and Rafferty, B. (1989). Light therapy for seasonal affective disorder: A review of efficacy. *Neuropsychopharmacology, 2*, 1–22.

Terry, R. D., and Katzman, R. (1983). Senile dementia of the Alzheimer type. *Ann. Neurol., 14*, 497–506.

Terry, R. D., Masliah, E., and Hansen, L. A. (1994). Structural basis of the cognitive alterations in Alzheimer disease. In *Alzheimer Disease* (R. D. Terry, R. Katzman, and K. L. Bick, Eds.), pp. 179–196. Raven Press, New York.

Terwilliger, R., Beitner-Johnson, D., Sevarino, K. A., Crain, S. M., Nestler, E. J. (1991). A general model for adaptations in G proteins and the cyclic AMP system in mediating the chronic actions of morphine and cocaine on neuronal function. *Brain Res., 548*, 100–1110.

Teschemacher, H., Opheim, K. E., Cox, B. M., and Goldstein, A. (1975). A peptide-like substance from pituitary that acts like morphine. I. Isolation. *Life Sci., 16*, 1771–1776.

Tessel, R. E. (1990). Noradrenergic processes in the behavioral actions of psychomotor stimulants. *Drug Dev. Res., 20*, 359–368.

Tetrud, J. W., and Langston, J. W. (1989). The effect of deprenyl (selegiline) on the natural history of Parkinson's disease. *Science, 245*, 519–522.

Thaker, G. K., Nguyen, J. A., Strauss, M. E., Jacobson, R., Kaup, B. A., and Tamminga, C. A. (1990). Clonazepam treatment of tardive dyskinesia: A practical GABAmimetic strategy. *Am. J. Psychiatry, 147*, 445–451.

Thaker, G. K., Tamminga, C. A., Alphs, L. D., Lafferman, J., Ferraro, T. N., and Hare, T. A. (1987). Brain gamma-aminobutyric acid abnormality in tardive dyskinesia: Reduction in cerebrospinal fluid GABA levels and therapeutic response to GABA agonist treatment. *Arch. Gen. Psychiatry, 44*, 522–529.

Tharion, W. J., McMenemy, D. J., and Rauch, T. M. (1994). Antihistamine effects on the central nervous system, cognitive performance and subjective states. *Neuropsychobiology, 29*, 97–104.

Theodosis, D. T. 1979. Endocytosis in glial cells (pituicytes) of the rat neurohypophysis demonstrated by the incorporation of horseradish peroxidase. *Neuroscience, 4*, 417–425.

Thesleff, S. (1986). Different kinds of acetylcholine release from the motor nerve. *Int. Rev. Neurobiol., 28*, 59–88.

Thesleff, S., and Sellin, L. C. (1980). Denervation supersensitivity. *Trends Neurosci., 3*, 122–126.

Thiebot, M.-H. (1986). Are serotonergic neurons involved in the control of anxiety and in the anxiolytic activity of the benzodiazepines? *Pharmacol. Biochem. Behav., 24*, 1471–1477.

Thiel, G. (1995). Recent breakthroughs in neurotransmitter release: Paradigm for regulated exocytosis? *News Physiol. Sci., 10*, 42–46.

Thoenen, H. (1970). Induction of tyrosine hydroxylase in peripheral and central adrenergic neurones by cold-exposure of rats. *Nature, 228*, 861–862.

Thoenen, K., and Kreutzberg, G. W. (1981). The role of fast transport in the nervous system. *Neurosci. Res. Progr. Bull., 20*, 1–138.

Thoenen, H., Mueller, R. A., and Axelrod, J. (1969). Trans-synaptic induction of adrenal tyrosine hydroxylase. *J. Pharmacol. Exp. Ther., 169*, 249–254.

Thoenen, H., and Tranzer, J. P. (1968). Chemical sympathectomy by selective destruction of adrenergic nerve endings with 6-hydroxydopamine. *Naunyn Schmiedebergs Arch. Pathol. Exp. Pharmakol., 261*, 271–288.

Thomas, B. L., Book, A. A., and Schweitzer, J. B. (1991). Immunohistochemical detection of a monoclonal antibody directed against the NGF receptor in basal forebrain neurons following intraventricular injection. *J. Neurosci. Methods, 37*, 37–45.

Thomas, H. (1993). Psychiatric symptoms in cannabis users. *Br. J. Psychiatry, 163*, 141–149.

Thomas, J. W., and Tallman, J. F. (1984). Solubilization and characterization of brain benzodiazepine binding sites. In *Brain Receptor Methodologies* (P. J. Marangos, I. C. Campbell, and R. M. Cohen, Eds.), pp. 95–113. Academic Press, New York.

Thomas, J. M., Vagelos, R., and Hoffman, B. B. (1990). Decreased cyclic AMP degradation in NG 108–15 neuroblastoma X glioma hybrid cells and S49 lymphoma cells chronically treated with drugs that inhibit adenylate cyclase. *J. Neurochem., 54*, 402–410.

Thompson, R. C., Mansour, A., Akil, H., and Watson, S. J. (1993). Cloning and pharmacological characterization of a rat "mu" opioid receptor. *Neuron, 11*, 903–913.

Thompson, R. F. (1986). The neurobiology of learning and memory. *Science, 233*, 941–947.

Thompson, T., and Schuster, C. R. (1968). *Behavioral Pharmacology.* Prentice-Hall, Englewood Cliffs, NJ.

Thomson, A. D., Pratt, O. E., Jeyasingham, M., and Shaw, G. K. (1988). Alcohol and brain damage. *Hum. Toxicol., 7*, 455–463.

Thorner, M. W. (1935). The psycho-pharmacology of sodium-amytal. *J. Nerv. Ment. Dis., 81*, 161–167.

Thureson-Klein, Å. (1983). Exocytosis from large and small dense cored vesicles in noradrenergic nerve terminals. *Neuroscience, 10*, 245–252.

Tiberi, M., et al. (1991). Cloning, molecular characterization, and chromosomal assignment of a gene encoding a second D_1 dopamine receptor subtype: Differential expression pattern in rat brain compared with the D_{1A} receptor. *Proc. Natl. Acad. Sci. U.S.A., 88*, 7491–7495.

Tiffany, S. T., Drobes, D. J., and Cepeda-Benito, A. (1992). Contribution of associative and nonassociative processes to the development of morphine tolerance. *Psychopharmacology, 109*, 185–190.

Tims, F. M., and Leukefeld, C. G., (Eds.). (1993a). Cocaine Treatment: Research and Clinical Perspectives. *NIDA Res. Monogr., 135*.

Tims, F. M., and Leukefeld, C. G. (1993b). Treatment of cocaine abusers: Issues and perspectives. *NIDA Res. Monogr., 135*, 1–14.

Tinklenberg, J. R. (1977). Antianxiety medications and the treatment of anxiety. In *Psychopharmacology: From Theory to Practice* (J. D. Barchas, P. A. Berger, R. D. Ciaranello and G. R. Elliott, Eds.), pp. 226–241. Oxford University Press, New York.

Tinklenberg, J. R., and Darley, C. F. (1975). Psychological and cognitive effects of cannabis. In *Cannabis and Man. Psychological and Clinical Aspects and Patterns of Use* (P. H. Connell and N. Dorn, Eds.), pp. 45–65. Churchill Livingstone, Edinburgh.

Tipton, K. F. (1988). Central neurotransmission and alcohol. *Neurochem. Int.*, 13 (3), 301–305.

Tipton, K. F., and Singer, T. P. (1993). Advances in our understanding of the mechanisms of the neurotoxicity of MPTP and related compounds. *J. Neurochem.*, 61, 1191–1206.

Tischler, A. S., Perlman, R. L., Costopoulos, D., and Horwitz, J. (1985). Vasoactive intestinal peptide increases tyrosine hydroxylase activity in normal and neoplastic rat chromaffin cell cultures. *Neurosci. Lett.*, 61, 141–146.

Titeler, M., Weinreich, P., Sinclair, D., and Seeman, P. (1978). Multiple receptors for brain dopamine. *Proc. Natl. Acad. Sci. U.S.A.*, 75, 1153–1156.

Todd, A. J., and Sullivan, A. C. (1990). Light microscopic study of the coexistence of GABA-like and glycine-like immunoreactivities in the spinal cord of the rat. *J. Comp. Neurol.*, 296, 496–505.

Todd, A. R. (1946). Hashish. *Experientia*, II, 55–60.

Tollefson, G. D. (1991). Anxiety and alcoholism: A serotonin link. *Br. J. Psychiatry*, 159 (Suppl. 12), 34–39.

Tomaz, C., Dickinson-Anson, H., McGaugh, J. L., Souza-Silva, M. A., Viana, M. B., and Graeff, F. G. (1993). Localization in the amygdala of the amnesic action of diazepam on emotional memory. *Behav. Brain Res.*, 58, 99–105.

Törk, I. (1990). Anatomy of the serotonergic system. *Ann. N.Y. Acad. Sci.*, 600, 9–35.

Törnwall, M., Kaakkola, S., Tuomainen, P., Kask, A., and Männistö, P. T. (1994). Comparison of two new inhibitors of catechol O-methylation on striatal dopamine metabolism: A microdialysis study in rats. *Br. J. Pharmacol.*, 112, 13–18.

Toth, M., and Shenk, T. (1994). Antagonist-mediated down-regulation of 5-hydroxytryptamine type 2 receptor gene expression: Modulation of transcription. *Mol. Pharmacol.*, 45, 1095–1100.

Towbin, K. E., and Leckman, J. F. (1992). Attention deficit hyperactivity in childhood and adolescence. In *Textbook of Clinical Neuropharmacology and Therapeutics* (2nd ed.). (H. L. Klawans et al., Eds.), pp. 323–333. Raven Press, New York.

Towle, A. C., Breese, G. R., Mueller, R. A., Coyle, S., and Lauder, J. M. (1984). Early postnatal administration of 5,7-DHT: Effects on serotonergic neurons and terminals. *Brain Res.*, 310, 67–75.

Tracey, D. J., De Biasi, S., Phend, K., and Rustioni, A. (1991). Aspartate-like immunoreactivity in primary afferent neurons. *Neuroscience*, 40, 673–686.

Tracqui, P., Morot-Gaudry, Y., Staub, J. F., Brézillon, P., Perault-Staub, A. M., Bougoin, S., and Hamon, M. (1983). Model of brain serotonin metabolism. II. Physiological interpretation. *Am. J. Physiol.*, 244, R206–R215.

Traiffort, E., Arrang, J.-M., Garbarg, M., Ruat, M., Leurs, R., Tardivel-Lacombe, J., Rouleau, A., and Schwartz, J.-C. (1993). Molecular pharmacology of histamine receptors. In *International Academy of Biomedical Drug Research*, Vol. 6., *New Developments in the Therapy of Allergic Disorders and Asthma* (S. Z. Langer, M. K. Church, B. B. Vargaftig, and S. Nicosia, Eds.), pp. 1–9. Karger, Basel.

Traiffort, E., Leurs, R., Arrang, J. M., Tardivel-Lacombe, J., Diaz, J., Schwartz, J.-C., and Ruat, M. (1994). Guinea pig histamine H₁ receptor. I. Gene cloning, characterization, and tissue expression revealed by in situ hybridization. *J. Neurochem.*, 62, 507–518.

Traiffort, E., Pollard, H., Moreau, J., Ruat, M., Schwartz, J.-C., Martinez-Mir, M. I., and Palacios, J. M. (1992). Pharmacological characterization and autoradiographic localization of histamine H₂ receptors in human brain identified with [^{125}I]iodoaminopotentidine. *J. Neurochem.*, 59, 290–299.

Trapp, B. D., Moench, T., Pulley, M. Barbosa, E. et al., (1987). Spatial segregation of mRNA encoding myelin-specific proteins. *Proc. Natl. Acad. Sci. U.S.A.*, 84, 7773–7777.

Travis, J. (1995). Pig cells used for Parkinson's disease. *Sci. News*, 148, 230.

Traynor, J. R., and Elliott, J. (1993). "Delta"-opioid receptor subtypes and cross-talk with "mu"-receptors. *Trends Pharmacol. Sci.*, 14, 84–86.

Treiser, S., and Kellar, K. J. (1979). Lithium effects on adrenergic receptor supersensitivity in rat brain. *Eur. J. Pharmacol.*, 58, 85–86.

Treit, D. (1985). Animal models for the study of anti-anxiety agents: A review. *Neurosci. Biobehav. Rev.*, 9, 203–222.

Treit, D. (1991). Anxiolytic effects of BDZs and 5-HT₁ₐ agonists: Animal models. In *5-H₁ₐ Agonists, 5-HT₃ Antagonists and Benzodiazepines: Their Comparative Behavioural Pharmacology* (R. J. Rogers and S. J. Cooper, Eds.), pp. 107–131. Wiley, New York.

Trendelenburg, U. (1991). Functional aspects of the neuronal uptake of noradrenaline. *Trends Pharmacol. Sci.*, 12, 334–337.

Tricklebank, M. D., Singh, L., Oles, R. J., Preston, C., and Iversen, S. D. (1989). The behavioural effects of MK-801: A comparison with antagonists acting non-competitively and competitively at the NMDA receptor. *Eur. J. Pharmacol.*, 167, 127–135.

Trifaró, J.-M., Vitale, M. L., and Del Castillo, A. R. (1992). Cytoskeleton and molecular mechanisms in neurotransmitter release by neurosecretory cells. *Eur. J. Pharmacol.*, 225, 83–104.

Triggs, W. J., and Willmore, L. J. (1984). *In vivo* lipid peroxidation in rat brain following intracortical Fe²⁺ injection. *J. Neurochem.*, 42, 976–980.

Trojanowski, J. Q., Shin, R.-W., Schmidt, M. L., and Lee, V. M.-Y. (1995). Relationship between plaques, tangles, and dystrophic processes in Alzheimer's disease. *Neurobiol. Aging*, 16, 335–345.

Trujillo, K. A., and Akil, H. (1991). Opiate tolerance and dependence: Recent findings and synthesis. *New Biol.*, 3, 915–923.

Trulson, M. E., Eubanks, E. E., and Jacobs, B. L. (1976). Behavioral evidence for supersensitivity following destruction of central serotonergic nerve terminals by 5,7-dihydroxytryptamine. *J. Pharmacol. Exp. Ther.*, 198, 23–32.

Trulson, M. E., Heym, J., and Jacobs, B. L. (1981). Dissociation between the effects of hallucinogenic drugs and behavior and raphé activity in freely moving cats. *Brain Res.*, 215, 275–293.

Trulson, M. E., and Jacobs, B. L. (1979). Dissociation between the effects of LSD on behavior in raphe unit activity in freely moving cats. *Science*, 205 (3), 515–518.

Tsou, K., Khachaturian, H., Akil, H., and Watson, S. J. (1986). Immunocytochemical localization of proopiomelanocortin-derived peptides in the adult rat spinal cord. *Brain Res.*, 378, 28–37.

Tsou, K., Patrick, S., and Walker, M. J. (1995). Physical withdrawal in rats tolerant to delta-9-tetrahydrocannabinol precipitated by a cannabinoid receptor antagonist. *Eur. J. Pharmacol.*, 280, R13–R15.

Tsuang, M. T., and Farrone, S. V. (1995). The case for heterogeneity in the etiology of schizophrenia. *Schizophr. Res.*, 17, 161–175.

Tsumoto, T. (1992). Long-term potentiation and long-term depression in the neocortex. *Prog. Neurobiol.*, 39, 209–228.

TuFek, S. (1985). Regulation of acetylcholine synthesis in the brain. *J. Neurochem.*, 44, 11–24.

Tulving, E. A. (1987). Multiple memory systems and consciousness. *Hum. Neurobiol.*, 6, 67–80.

Turner, A. J. (1988). Metabolism of neuropeptides. *ISI Atlas Pharmacol.*, 2, 362–366.

Turner, C. E. (1984). Marijuana and cannabis: Research, why the conflict. In *Marijuana '84. Proceedings of the Oxford Symposium on Cannabis* (D. J. Harvey, Ed.), pp. 31–36. IRL Press, Oxford.

Tuszynski, M. H., and Gage, F. H. (1994). Neurotrophic factors and neuronal loss. In *Alzheimer Disease* (R. D. Terry, R. Katzman, and K. L. Bick, Eds.), pp. 405–417. Raven Press, New York.

Twarog, B. M., and Page, I. H. (1953). Serotonin content of some mammalian tissues and urine and a method for its determination. *Am. J. Physiol.*, 175, 157–161.

Tyers, M. B., and Freeman, A. J. (1992). Mechanism of the anti-emetic activity of 5-H₃ receptor antagonists. *Oncology*, 49, 263–268.

Tyler, C. B., and Galloway, M. P. (1992). Acute administration of amphetamine: Differential regulation of dopamine synthesis in dopamine projection fields. *J. Pharmacol. Exp. Ther.*, 261, 567–573.

Tyrer, P. (1992). Anxiolytics not acting at the benzodiazepine receptor: Beta blockers. *Prog. Neuropsychopharmacol. Biol. Psychiatry*, 16, 17–26.

Uchimura, N., and North, R. A. (1990). Actions of cocaine on rat nucleus accumbens neurones *in vitro*. *Br. J. Pharmacol.*, 99, 736–740.

Udenfriend, S., Zaltzman-Nirenberg, P., and Nagatsu, T. (1965). Inhibitors of purified beef adrenal tyrosine hydroxylase. *Biochem. Pharmacol.*, 14, 837–845.

Uhl, G. R. (1992). Neurotransmitter transporters (plus): A promising new gene family. *Trends Neurosci.*, 15, 265–268.

Uhl, G. R., Blum, K., Noble, E., and Smith, S. (1993). Substance abuse vulnerability and D₂ receptor genes. *Trends Neurosci.*, 16, 83–88.

Uhl, G. R., Childers, S., and Pasternak, G. (1994). An opiate-receptor gene family reunion. *Trends Neurosci.*, 17, 89–93.

Uhl, G. R., Ryan, J. P., Schwartz, J. P. (1988). Morphine alters preproenkephalin gene expression. *Mol. Brain Res.*, 391–397.

Ulas, J., and Cotman, C. W. (1993). Excitatory amino acid receptors in schizophrenia. *Schizophr. Bull.*, 19, 105–117.

Ulrich, R. F., and Patten, B. M. (1991). The rise, decline, and fall of LSD. *Perspect. Biol. Med.*, 34, 561–578.

Undie, A. S., and Friedman, E. (1990). Stimulation of a dopamine D₁ receptor enhances inositol phosphates formation in rat brain. *J. Pharmacol. Exp. Ther.*, 253, 987–992.

Ungerstedt, U. (1968). 6-hydroxydopamine induced degeneration of central monoamine neurons. *Eur. J. Pharmacol.*, 5, 107–110.

Ungerstedt, U. (1971a). Adipsia and aphagia after 6-hydroxydopamine induced degeneration of the nigro-striatal dopamine system. *Acta Physiol. Scand.*, 82 (Suppl. 367), 95–122.

Ungerstedt, U. (1971b). Postsynaptic supersensitivity after 6-hydroxydopamine induced degeneration of the nigro-striatal dopamine system. *Acta Physiol. Scand.*, 82 (Suppl. 367), 69–93.

Ungerstedt, U. (1971c). Stereotaxic mapping of the monoamine pathways in the rat brain. *Acta Physiol. Scand.*, 82 (Suppl. 367), 1–48.

Ungerstedt, U. (1971d). Striatal dopamine release after amphetamine or nerve degeneration revealed by rotational behavior. *Acta Physiol. Scand.*, 82 (Suppl. 367), 49–68.

Ungerstedt, U. (1974a). Brain dopamine neurons and behavior. In *The Neurosciences, Third Study Program* (F. O. Schmitt and F. G. Worden, Eds.), pp. 695–703. MIT Press, Cambridge, MA.

Ungerstedt, U. (1974b). Functional dynamics of central monoamine pathways. In *The Neurosciences, Third Study Program* (F. O. Schmitt and F. G. Worden, Eds.), pp. 979–988. MIT Press, Cambridge, MA.

Ungerstedt, U. (1984). Measurement of neurotransmitter release by intracranial dialysis. In *Measurement of Neurotransmitter Release In Vivo* (C. A. Marsden, Ed.), pp. 81–106. Wiley, New York.

United States Department of Health, Education, and Welfare. (1978). *Alcohol and Health: Third Special Report to the U.S. Congress,* U.S.Government Printing Office, Washington, D.C.

United States Department of Health and Human Services. (1988). *The Health Consequences of Smoking: Nicotine Addiction. A Report of the Surgeon General.* U.S. Dept. H.H.S., Rockville, MD.

United States Department of Health and Human Services. (1989). *Reducing the Health Consequences of Smoking: 25 Years of Progress. A Report of the Surgeon General.* U.S. Dept. H.H.S., Rockville, MD.

Unseld, E., and Klotz, U. (1989). Benzodiazepines: Are they of natural origin? *Pharmacol. Res.*, 1, 1–3.

Upton, N. (1994). Mechanisms of action of new antiepileptic drugs: Rational design and serendipitous findings. *Trends Pharmacol. Sci.*, 15, 456–463.

Uranova, N. A., Orlovskaya, D. D., Apel, K. Klintsova, A. J., Haselhorst, U., and Schenk, H. (1991). Morphometric study of synaptic patterns in the rat caudate nucleus and hippocampus under haloperidol treatment. *Synapse*, 7, 253–259.

Uretsky, N. J., Kamal, L., and Snodgrass, S. R. (1979). Effect of divalent cations on the amphetamine-induced stimulation of [³H]catechol synthesis in the striatum. *J. Neurochem.*, 32, 951–960.

Ursillo, R. C., Wiech, N. L., Reisine, T. D., and Yamamura, H. I. (1980). Mechanisms of action of antidepressants. In *Psychopharmacology and biochemistry of Neurotransmitter Receptors* (H. Yamamura, H. Olsen, and E.

Usdin, Eds.), pp. 189–202. Elsevier North Holland, Amsterdam.

Usdin, T. B., Eiden, L. E., Bonner, T. I., and Erickson, J. D. (1995). Molecular biology of the vesicular ACh transporter. *Trends Neurosci.*, 18, 218–224.

Vaillant, G. E. (1983). *The Natural History of Alcoholism.* Harvard University Press, Cambridge, MA.

Vale, R. D., Banker, G., and Hall, Z. W. (1992). The neuronal cytoskeleton. In *An Introduction to Molecular Neurobiology* (Z. W. Hall, Ed.), pp. 247–280. Sinauer Associates, Sunderland, MA.

Vale, W., Spiess, J., Rivier, C., and Rivier, J. (1981). Characterization of a 41–residue ovine hypothalamic peptide that stimulates secretion of corticotropin and β-endorphin. *Science,* 213, 1394–1397.

Valentino, K. L., Tatemoto, K., Hunter, J., and Barchas, J. D. (1986). Distribution of neuropeptide K-immunoreactivity in the rat central nervous system. *Peptides*, 7, 1043–1059.

Valentino, R. J., Page, M., Van Bockstaele, E., and Aston-Jones, G. (1992). Corticotropin-releasing factor innervation of the locus coeruleus region: Distribution of fibers and sources of input. *Neuroscience,* 48, 689–705.

Vallar, L., and Meldolesi, J. (1989). Mechanisms of signal transduction at the dopamine D$_2$ receptor. *Trends Pharmacol. Sci.*, 10, 74–77.

Vallejo, M. (1994). Transcriptional control of gene expression by cAMP-response element binding proteins. *J. Neuroendocrinol.*, 6, 587–596.

Valtin, H. (1982). The discovery of the Brattleboro rat, recommended nomenclature, and the question of proper controls. *Ann. N.Y. Acad. Sci.*, 394, 1–9.

Valtorta, F., Fesce, R., Grohovaz, F., Haimann, C., Hurlbut, W. P., Iezzi, N., Tarelli, F. T., Villa, A., and Ceccarelli, B. (1990). Neurotransmitter release and synaptic vesicle recycling. *Neuroscience,* 35, 477–489.

Van Baar, A. (1990). Development of infants of drug dependent mothers. *J. Child Psychol. Psychiatry,* 31, 911–920.

Van Bemmel, A. L., and Van den Hoofdakker, R. H. (1981). Maintenance of therapeutic effects of total sleep deprivation by limitation of subsequent sleep. *Acta Psychiatr. Scand.*, 63, 453–462.

Van Broeckhoven, C. L. (1995). Molecular genetics of Alzheimer disease: Identification of genes and gene mutations. *Eur. Neurol.*, 35, 8–19.

Vandekamp, J. L., and Collins, A. C. (1994). Prenatal nicotine alters nicotinic receptor development in the mouse brain. *Pharmacol. Biochem. Behav.*, 47, 889–900.

Vanderhaeghen, J. J. (1985). Neuronal cholecystokin. In *Handbook of Chemical Neuroanatomy*, Vol. 4., *GABA and Neuropeptides in the CNS*, Part I (A. Björklund and T. Hökfelt, Eds.), pp. 406–435. Elsevier, Amsterdam.

Vanderhaeghen, J. J., Signeau, J. C., and Gepts, W. (1975). New peptide in the vertebrate CNS reacting with antigastrin antibodies. *Nature,* 257, 604–605.

Van der Kooy, D. (1987). Place conditioning: A simple and effective method for assessing the motivational properties of drugs. In *Methods of Assessing the Reinforcing Proper-*

ties of Abused Drugs (M. A. Bozarth, Ed.), pp. 229–240. Springer-Verlag, New York.

Vandermaelen, C. P. (1985). Serotonin. In *Neurotransmitter Actions* (M. A. Rogawski and J. L. Barker, Eds.), pp. 201–240. Plenum Press, New York.

Vanderwolf, C. H. (1992). The electrocorticogram in relation to physiology and behavior: A new analysis. *Electroencephalogr. Clin. Neurophysiol.*, 82, 165–175.

Van der Zee, P., Koger, H. S., Gootjes, J., and Hespe, W. (1980). Aryl 1,4-dialk(en)ylpiperazines as selective and very potent inhibitors of dopamine uptake. *Eur. J. Med. Chem.*, 15, 363–370.

Van Dyke, C., and Byck, R. (1982). Cocaine. *Sci. Am.*, March, 128–141.

Van Galen, P. J. M., Stiles, G. L., Michaels, G., and Jacobson, K. A. (1992). Adenosine A$_1$ and A$_2$ receptors: Structure-function relationships. *Med. Res. Rev.*, 12, 423–471.

Van Harreveld, A. (1959). Compounds in brain extracts causing spreading depression of cerebral cortical activity and contraction of crustacean muscle. *J. Neurochem.*, 3, 300–315.

Van Harreveld, A., and Fifkova, E. (1975). Swelling of dendritic spines in the facia dentata after stimulation of the perforant fibers as a mechanism of post-tetanic potentiation. *Exp. Neurol.*, 49, 736–749.

Van Putten, T., Marder, S. R., May, P. R., Poland, R. E., and O'Brien, R. (1985). Plasma levels of haloperidol and clinical response. *Psychopharmacol. Bull.*, 21, 69–72.

Van Tol, H. H. M., Bunzow, J. R., Guan, H.-C., Sunahara, R. K., Seeman, P., Niznik, H. B., and Civelli, O. (1991). Cloning of the gene for a human dopamine D$_4$ receptor with high affinity for the antipsychotic clozapine. *Nature,* 350, 610–614.

Van Tol, H. H. M., et al. (1992). Multiple dopamine D$_4$ receptor variants in the human population. *Nature,* 358, 149–152.

Van Wimersma Greidanus, T. B., Burbach, J. P. H., and Veldhuis, H. D. (1986). Vasopressin and oxytocin: Their presence in the central nervous system and their functional significance in brain processes related to behaviour and memory. *Acta Endocrinol.* 276 (Suppl.), 85–94.

Vaught, J. L. (1988). Substance P antagonists and analgesia: A review of the hypothesis. *Life Sci.*, 43, 1419–1431.

Vaught, J. L., Mathiasen, J. H. R., and Raffa, R. B. (1988). Examination of the involvement of supraspinal and spinal mu and delta opioid receptors in analgesia using the mu receptor deficient CXBK mouse. *Pharmcol. Exp. Ther.*, 245, 13–26.

Vautrin, J. (1994). Vesicular or quantal and subquantal transmitter release. *News Physiol. Sci.*, 9, 59–64.

Velazquez-Moctezuma, J., Shiromani, P. J., and Gillin, J. C. (1990). Acetylcholine and acetylcholine receptor subtypes in REM sleep generation. *Prog. Brain Res.* 84, 407–413.

Verdoorn, T. A., Burnashev, N., Monyer, H., Seeburg, P. H., and Sakmann, B. (1991). Structural determinants of ion flow through recombinant glutamate receptor channels. *Science,* 252, 1715–1718.

Vermeulen, R. J., Drukarch, B., Sahadat, M. C. R., Goosen, C., Wolters, E. C., and Stoof, J. C. (1994). The dopamine D$_1$ agonist SKF

81297 and the dopamine D_2 agonist LY 171555 act synergistically to stimulate motor behavior of 1-methyl-4-phenyl-1,2,3,6-ttrahydropyridine-lesioned Parkinsonian rhesus monkeys. *Mov. Disord., 9,* 664–672.

Vernallis, A. B., Conroy, W. G., and Berg, D. W. (1993). Neurons assemble acetylcholine receptors with as many as three kinds of subunits while maintaining segregation among receptor subtypes. *Neuron, 10,* 451–464.

Vescovi, P. P., Pedrazzoni, M., Michelini, M., Maninetti, L., Bernardelli, F., and Passeri, M. (1992). Chronic effects of marihuana smoking on luteinizing hormone, follicle-stimulating hormone and prolactin levels in human males. *Drug Alcohol Depend., 30,* 59–63.

Vetulani, J. Antkiewicz-Michaluk, L., and Rokosz-Pelc, A. (1984). Chronic administration of antidepressant drugs increases the density of cortical ^{3}H-prazosin binding sites in the rat. *Brain Res., 310,* 360–362.

Vetulani, J., Stawarz, R. J., Dingell, J. V., and Sulser, F. (1976). A possible common mechanism of action of antidepressant treatments. *Naunyn Schmiedebergs Arch. Pharmacol., 293,* 109–114.

Vetulani, J., Stawarz, R. J., and Sulser, F. (1976). Adaptive mechanisms of the noradrenergic CAMP generating system in limbic forebrain of the rat: Adaptation to persistent changes in the availability of norepinephrine. *J. Neurochem., 27,* 661–666.

Vezina, P., and Stewart, J. (1989). The effect of dopamine receptor blockade on the development of sensitization to the locomotor activating effects of amphetamine and morphine. *Brain Res., 499,* 108–120.

Vickroy, T. W., and Johnson, K. M. (1982). Similar dopamine-releasing effects of phencyclidine and nonamphetamine stimulants in striatal slices. *J. Pharmacol. Exp. Ther., 223,* 669–674.

Vignon, J., Chicheportiche, R., Chicheportiche, M., Kamenka, J. M., Geneste, P., and Lazdunski, M. (1983). [^{3}H]TCP: A new tool with high affinity for the PCP receptor in rat brain. *Brain Res., 280,* 194–197.

Vignon, J., and Lazdunski, M. (1984). Structure-function relationships in the inhibition of synaptosomal dopamine uptake by phencyclidine and analogues: Potential correlation with binding site identified with [^{3}H]PCP. *Biochem. Pharmacol., 33,* 700–702.

Vignon, J., Pinet, V., Cerruti, C., Kamenka, J.-M., and Chicheportiche, R. (1988). [^{3}H]N-[1-(2-benzo(b)thiophenyl)cyclohexyl]piperidine ([^{3}H]BTCP): A new phencyclidine analog selective for the dopamine uptake complex. *Eur. J. Pharmacol., 148,* 427–436.

Vilaro, M. T., Wiederhold, K.-H., Palacios, J. M., and Mengod, G. (1991). Muscarinic cholinergic receptors in the rat caudate–putamen and olfactory tubercle belong predominantly to the m4 class: In situ hybridization and receptor autoradiography. *Neuroscience, 40,* 159–167.

Vincent, J.-P., Bidard, J.-N., Lazdunski, M., Romey, G., Tourneur, Y., and Vignon, J. (1983). Identification and properties of phencyclidine-binding sites in nervous tissues. *Fed. Proc., 42,* 2570–2573.

Vincent, J.-P., Kartalovski, B., Geneste, P., Kamenka, J. M., and Lazdunski, M. (1979). Interaction of phencyclidine ("angel dust") with a specific receptor in rat brain membranes. *Proc. Natl. Acad. Sci. U.S.A., 76,* 4678–4682.

Vincent, S. R., and Hope, B. T. (1992). Neurons that say NO. *Trends Neurosci., 15,* 108–113.

Virchow, R. (1860). *Cellular Pathology* (F. Chance, trans.) Churchill, London.

Viveros, O. H., and Wilson, S. P. (1983). The adrenal chromaffin cell as a model to study the co-secretion of enkephalins and catecholamines. *J. Auton. Nerv. Syst., 7,* 41–58.

Voegtlin, W. L., and Broz, W. R. (1949). The conditioned reflex treatment of chronic alcoholism. X. An analysis of 3125 admissions over a period of ten and a half years. *Ann. Intern. Med., 30,* 580–597.

Voegtlin, W. L., Lemere, F., Broz, W. R., and O'Hollaran, P. (1941a). Conditioned reflex therapy of chronic alcoholism. IV. A preliminary report on the value of reinforcement. *Q. J. Stud. Alcohol, 2,* 505–511.

Voegtlin, W. L., Lemere, F., Broz, W. R., and O'Hollaran, P. (1941b). Conditioned reflex therapy of chronic alcoholism. V. Follow-up report of 1042 cases. *Am. J. Med. Sci., 203,* 525–528.

Voet, D., and Voet, J. G. (1990). *Biochemistry.* Wiley, New York.

Vogel, G. W. (1984). Sleep laboratory study of lormetazepam in older insomniacs. In *Sleep, Benzodiazepines and Performance: Experimental Methodologies and Research Prospects* (I. Hindmarch, H. Ott, and T. Roth, Eds.), pp. 69–78. Springer-Verlag, New York.

Vogel, J. B., Beer, B., and Clody, D. E. (1971). A simple and reliable conflict procedure for the testing of antianxiety agents. *Psychopharmacology, 2,* 1–7.

Vogel, R. A., Cooper, B. R., Barlow, T. S., Prange, A. J., Mueller, R. A., and Breese, G. R. (1979). Effects of thyrotropin-releasing hormone on locomotor activity, operant performance and ingestive behavior. *J. Pharmacol. Exp. Ther., 208,* 161–168.

Vogel, Z., Barg, J., Levy, R., Saya, D., Heldman, E., and Mechoulam, R. (1993). Anandamide, a brain endogenous compound, interacts specifically with cannabinoid receptors and inhibits adenylate cyclase. *J. Neurochem., 61,* 352–355.

Vogt, M. (1954). The concentration of sympathin in different parts of the central nervous system under normal conditions and after the administration of drugs. *J. Physiol. (Lond.), 123,* 451–481.

Volkmar, F. R., and Greenough, W. T. (1972). Rearing complexity affects branching of dendrites in the visual cortex of the rat. *Science, 176,* 1445–1447.

Volle, R. L., and Koelle, G. B. (1975). Ganglionic stimulating and blocking agents. In *The Pharmacological Basis of Therapeutics* (L. S. Goodman and A. Gilman, Eds.), pp. 565–575. Macmillan, New York.

Volpicelli, J. R., Alterman, A. I., Hayashida, M., and O'Brian, C. P. (1992). Naltrexone in the treatment of alcohol dependence. *Arch. Gen. Psychiatry, 49,* 876–880.

von Euler, U. S. (1946a). The presence of a substance with sympathin properties in spleen extracts. *Acta Physiol. Scand., 11,* 168–186.

von Euler, U. S. (1946b). A specific sympathomimetic ergone in adrenergic nerve fibers (sympathin) and its relations to adrenaline and noradrenaline. *Acta Physiol. Scand., 12,* 73–97.

von Euler, U. S. (1971). Adrenergic neurotransmitter function. *Science, 173,* 202–206.

von Euler, U. S. (1985). The history of substance P. In *Neurotransmitters in Action* (D. Bousfield, Ed.), pp. 143–150. Elsevier, Amsterdam.

von Euler, U. S., and Gaddum, J. H. (1931). An unidentified depressor substance in certain tissue extracts. *J. Physiol. (Lond.), 72,* 74–87.

von Kügelgen, I., and Starke, K. (1991). Noradrenaline–ATP co-transmission in the sympathetic nervous system. *Trends Pharmacol. Sci., 12,* 319–324.

Voytko, M. L., Olton, D. S., Richardson, R. T., Gorman, L. K., Tobin, J. R., and Price, D. L. (1994). Basal forebrain lesions in monkeys disrupt attention but not learning and memory. *J. Neurosci., 14,* 167–186.

Vyas, S., Biguet, N. F., and Mallet, J. (1990). Transcriptional and post-transcriptional regulation of tyrosine hydroxylase gene by protein kinase C. *EMBO J., 9,* 3707–3712.

Wachtel, S. R., Brooderson, R. J., and White, F. J. (1992). Parametric and pharmacological analyses of the enhanced grooming response elicited by the D_1 dopamine receptor agonist SKF 38393 in the rat. *Psychopharmacology, 109,* 41–48.

Wachtel, S. R., Hu, X.-T., Galloway, M. P., and White, F. J. (1989). D_1 dopamine receptor stimulation enables the postsynaptic, but not autoreceptor, effects of D_2 dopamine agonists in nigrostriatal and mesoaccumbens dopamine systems. *Synapse, 4,* 327–346.

Wada, H., Inagaki, N., Yamatodani, A., and Watanabe, T. (1991). Is the histaminergic neuron system a regulatory center for whole-brain activity? *Trends Neurosci., 14,* 415–418.

Waddington, J. L. (1986). Behavioural correlates of the action of selective D-1 dopamine receptor antagonists. Impact of SCH 23390 and SKF 83566, and functionally interactive D-1:D-2 receptor systems. *Biochem. Pharmacol., 35,* 3661–3667.

Waddington, J. L., and Daly, S. A. (1993). Regulation of unconditioned motor behaviour by D_1:D_2 interactions. In D_1:D_2 *Dopamine Receptor Interactions* (J. L. Waddington, Ed.), pp. 51–78. San Diego, Academic Press.

Wade, N. (1978a). Guillemin and Schally: A race spurred by rivalry. *Science, 200,* 510–513.

Wade, N. (1978b). Guillemin and Schally: The three-lap race to Stockholm. *Science, 200,* 411–415.

Wade, N. (1978c). Guillemin and Schally: The years in the wilderness. *Science, 200,* 279–282.

Waeber, C., Sebben, M., Grossman, C., Javoy-Agid, F., Bochaert, J., and Dumuis, A. (1993). [^{3}H]-GR113808 labels 5-HT$_4$ receptors in the human and guinea-pig brain. *Neuroreport, 4,* 1239–1242.

Waelbroeck, M., Tastenoy, M., Camus, J., and Cristophe, J. (1990). Binding of selective antagonists to four muscarinic receptors (M1 to M4) in rat forebrain. *Mol. Pharmacol., 38,* 267–273.

Wafford, K. A., Burnett, D. M., Dunwiddie, T. V., and Harris, R. A. (1990). Genetic differences in the ethanol sensitivity of GABA$_A$ receptors expressed in *Xenopus* oocytes. *Science, 249,* 291–293.

Wafford, K. A., Burnett, D. M., Leidenheimer, N. J., Burt, D. R., Wang, J. B., Kofuji, P., Dunwiddie, T. V., Harris, R. A., and Sikela,

J. M. (1991). Ethanol sensitivity of the GABA$_A$ receptor expressed in *Xenopus* oocytes requires 8 amino acids contained in the g2L subunit. *Neuron,* 7, 27–33.

Wagner, G. C., Ricaurte, G. A., Seiden, L. S., Schuster, C. R., Miller, R. J., and Westley, J. (1980). Long-lasting depletions of striatal dopamine and loss of dopamine uptake sites following repeated administration of methamphetamine. *Brain Res.,* 181, 151–160.

Wainer, B. H., Levey, A. I., Mufson, E. J., and Mesulam, M.-M. (1984). Cholinergic systems in mammalian brain identified with antibodies against choline acetyltransferase. *Neurochem. Int.,* 6, 163–182.

Waksman, G., Hamel, E., Delay-Goyet, P., and Roques, B. P. (1987). Neutral endopeptidase 24.11, mu and delta opioid receptors after selective brain lesions: An autoradiographic study. *Brain. Res.,* 436, 205–216.

Waldemar, G. (1995). Functional brain imaging with SPECT in normal aging and dementia. *Cerebrovasc. Brain Metab. Rev.,* 7, 89–130.

Waldmeier, P. C., and Baumann, P. A. (1990). Presynaptic GABA receptors. *Ann. N.Y. Acad. Sci.,* 604, 136–151.

Waldrop, M. M. (1987). The workings of working memory. *Science,* 237, 1564–1567.

Walker, J. M., Bowen, W. D., Walker, F. O., Matsumoto, R. R., De Costa, B., and Rice, K. C. (1990). Sigma receptors: Biology and function. *Pharmacol. Rev.,* 42, 355–402.

Wall, A.-M., Hinson, R. E., Schmidt, E., Johnston, C., and Streather, A. (1990). Place conditioning with d-amphetamine: The effect of the CS-UCS interval and evidence of a place avoidance. *Anim. Learn. Behav.,* 18, 393–400.

Wall, M. E., Brine, D. R., Jeffcoat, A. R., Cook, C. E., and Perez-Reyes, M. (1981). Phencyclidine metabolism and disposition in man following a 100 1g intravenous dose. *Res. Commun. Subst. Abuse,* 2, 161–172.

Wall, S. J., Yasuda, R. P., Hory, F., Flagg, S., Martin, B. M., Ginns, E. I., and Wolfe, B. B. (1991). Production of antisera selective for m1 muscarinic receptors using fusion proteins: Distribution of m1 receptors in rat brain. *Mol. Pharmacol.,* 39, 643–649.

Wall, S. J., Yasuda, R. P., Li, M., and Wolfe, B. B. (1991). Development of an antiserum against m3 muscarinic receptors: Distribution of m3 receptors in rat tissues and clonal cell lines. *Mol. Pharmacol.,* 40, 783–789.

Wallach, M. B. (1974). Drug-induced stereotyped behavior: Similarities and differences. *Adv. Biochem. Psychopharmacol.,* 12, 241–260.

Waller, M. B., McBride, W. J., Gatto, G. J., Lumeng, L., and Li, T. K. (1984). Intragastric self-infusion of ethanol by ethanol-preferring and -nonpreferring lines of rats. *Science,* 225, 78–80.

Wallis, D. I. (1994). 5-HT receptors involved in initiation or modulation of motor patterns: Opportunities for drug development. *Trends Pharmacol. Sci.,* 15, 288–292.

Walters, J. R., Bergstrom, D. A., Carlson, J. H., Chase, T. N., and Braun, A. R. (1987). D$_1$ dopamine receptor activation required for postsynaptic expression of D$_2$ agonist effects. *Science,* 236, 719–722.

Wamsley, J. K., Alburges, M. E., Hunt, M. A. E., and Bylund, D. B. (1992). Differential local-

ization of a$_2$-adrenergic receptor subtypes in brain. *Pharmacol. Biochem. Behav.,* 41, 267–273.

Wamsley, J. K., Alburges, M. E., McQuade, R. D., and Hunt, M. (1992). CNS distribution of D$_1$ receptors: Use of a new specific D$_1$ receptor antagonist, [^{3}H]SCH 39166. *Neurochem. Int.,* 20 (Suppl.), 123S–128S.

Wamsley, J. K., Gehlert, D. R., and Olsen, R. W. (1986). The benzodiazepine/barbiturate-sensitive convulsant/GABA receptor/chloride ionophore complex: Autoradiographic localization of individual components. In *Benzodiazepine/GABA Receptors and Chloride Channels,* Vol. 5 (R. W. Olsen and J. C. Venter, Eds.), pp. 299–313. Alan R. Liss, New York.

Wang, Z., Ferris, C. F., and De Vries, G. J. (1994). Role of septal vasopressin innervation in paternal behavior in prairie voles (*Microtus ochrogaster*). *Proc. Natl. Acad. Sci. U.S.A.,* 91, 400–404.

Wanibuchi, F., and Usuda, S. (1990). Synergistic effects between D-1 and D-2 dopamine antagonists on catalepsy in rats. *Psychopharmacology,* 102, 339–342.

Wank, S. A., Harkins, R., Jensen, R. T., Shapira, H., De Weerth, A., and Slattery, T. (1992). Purification, molecular cloning, and functional expression of the cholecystokinin receptor from rat pancreas. *Proc. Natl. Acad. Sci. U.S.A.,* 89, 3125–3129.

Wank, S. A., Pisegna, J. R., and De Weerth, A. (1992). Brain and gastrointestinal cholecystokinin receptor family: Structure and functional expression. *Proc. Natl. Acad. Sci. U.S.A.,* 89, 8691–8695.

Ward, C. D. (1994). Does selegiline delay progression of Parkinson's disease? A critical re-evaluation of the DATATOP study. *J. Neurol. Neurosurg. Psychiatry,* 57, 217–220.

Ward, H. K., and Bradford, H. F. (1979). Relative activities of glutamine synthetase and glutaminase in mammalian synaptosomes. *J. Neurochem.,* 33, 339–342.

Warembourg, M. (1985). Steroid receptors in the brain: Topography and some functional implications. *Neurochem. Int.,* 7, 941–952.

Warner, K. E. (1986). *Selling Smoke: Cigarette Advertising and Public Health.* American Public Health Association, Washington, D.C.

Wasco, W., Peppercorn, J., and Tanzi, R. E. (1993). Search for the genes responsible for familial Alzheimer's disease. *Ann. N.Y. Acad. Sci.,* 695, 203–208.

Washton, A. M., Gold, M. S., and Pottash, A. C. (1984). Naltrexone in addicted physicians and business executives. *NIDA Res. Monogr.,* 55, 185–190.

Watanabe, T., Yamatodani, A., Maeyama, K., and Wada, H. (1990). Pharmacology of α-fluoromethylhistidine, a specific inhibitor of histidine decarboxylase. *Trends Pharmacol. Sci.,* 11, 363–367.

Waters, N., Löfberg, L., Haadsma-Svensson, S., Svensson, K., and Carlsson, A. (1994). Differential effects of dopamine D2 and D3 receptor antagonists in regard to dopamine release, in vivo receptor displacement and behaviour. *J. Neural Transm.,* 98, 39–55.

Watkins, J. C. (1984). Excitatory amino acids and central synaptic transmission. *Trends Pharmacol. Sci.,* 5, 373–376.

Watkins, J., and Collingridge, G. (1994). Phenylglycine derivatives as antagonists of metabotropic glutamate receptors. *Trends Pharmacol. Sci.,* 15, 333–342.

Watkins, L. R., and Mayer, D. J. (1982). Organization of endogenous opiate and nonopiate pain control systems. *Science,* 216, 1185–1192.

Watkins, P. B., Zimmerman, H. J., Knapp, M. J., Gracon, S. I., and Lewis, K. W. (1994). Hepatotoxic effects of tacrine administration in patients with Alzheimer's disease. *JAMA,* 271, 992–998.

Watling, K. J. (1992). Nonpeptide antagonists herald new era in tachykinin research. *Trends Pharmacol. Sci.,* 13, 266–269.

Watling, K. J., and Krause, J. E. (1993). The rising sun shines on substance P and related peptides. *Trends Pharmacol. Sci.,* 14, 81–84.

Watson, J. D., Gilman, M., Witkowski, J., and Zoller, M. (1992). *Recombinant DNA* (2nd ed.). W. H. Freeman, New York.

Watson, S. J., Barchas, J. D., and Li, C. H. (1977). P-Lipotropin: Localization of cells and axons in rat brain by immunocytochemistry. *Proc. Natl. Acad. Sci. U.S.A.,* 74, 5155–5158.

Watson, S. J., Trujillo, K. A., Herman, J. P., and Akil, H. (1989). Neuroanatomical and neurochemical substrates of drug-seeking behavior: Overview and future directions. In *Molecular and Cellular Aspects of the Drug Addictions* (A. Goldstein, Ed.), pp.29–87. Springer-Verlag, New York.

Watterson, D. M., and Vincenzi, F. F. (Eds.) (1980). Calmodulin and cell function. *Ann. N.Y. Acad. Sci.,* 356.

Watzman, N., and Barry, H. III. (1968). Drug effects on motor coordination. *Psychopharmacologia,* 12, 414–423.

Way, E. L. (1993). Opioid tolerance and physical dependence and their relationship. In *Opioids II,,* Handbook of Experimental Pharmacology, Vol. 104 (A. Herz, Ed.), pp. 573–596. Springer-Verlag, New York.

Weber, R., Jones, C. R., Palacios, J. M., and Lohse, M. J. (1990). High resolution autoradiography of A$_1$ adenosine receptors with [^{3}H]8–cyclopentyl-1,3-dipropylxanthine ([^{3}H]DPCPX). *J. Neurochem.,* 54, 1344–1353.

Webster, H. H., and Jones, B. E. (1988). Neurotoxic lesions of the dorsolateral pontomesencephalic tegmentum–cholinergic cell area in the cat. II. Effects upon sleep–waking states. *Brain Res.,* 458, 285–302.

Wecker, L. (1990). Choline utilization by central cholinergic neurons. In *Nutrition and the Brain,* Vol. 8 (R. J. Wurtman and J. J. Wurtman, Eds.), pp. 147–162. Raven Press, New York.

Weddington, W. W., Brown, B. S., Haertzen, C. A., Cone, E. J., Dax, E. M., Herning, R. I., and Michaelson, B. S. (1990). Changes in mood, craving, and sleep during short-term abstinence reported by male cocaine addicts. *Arch. Gen. Psychiatry,* 47, 861–868.

Weeks, J. R. (1964). Experimental narcotic addiction. *Sci. Am.,* 210, 46–52.

Wehr, T. A. (1990). Manipulations of sleep and phototherapy: Nonpharmacologic alternatives in the treatment of depression. *Clin. Neuropharmacol.,* 13 (Suppl. 1), S54–S65.

Wehr, T. A., Muscettola, G., and Goodwin, F. K. (1980). Urinary 3-methody-4-hydroxypehnylglycol circadian rhythm. *Arch. Gen. Psychiatry,* 37, 257–263.

Wei, E., and Loh, H. (1976a). Chronic intracerebral infusion of morphine and peptides with osmotic minipumps, and the development of physical dependence. In *Opiates and Endogenous Opioid Peptides* (H. W.

Kosterlitz, Ed.), pp. 303–310. Elsevier/North-Holland, Amsterdam.

Wei, E, and Loh, H. (1976b). Physical dependence on opiate-like peptides. *Science*, 193, 1262–1263.

Weidner, G., and Istvan, J. (1985). Dietary sources of caffeine. *N. Engl. J. Med.*, 313, 1421.

Weil, A. (1972). *The Natural Mind: A New Way of Looking at Drugs and the Higher Consciousness*. Houghton-Mifflin, New York.

Weil, A. T., Zinberg, N. E., and Nelsen, J. M. (1968). Clinical and psychological effects of marihuana in man. *Science*, 162, 1234–1242.

Weinberger, D. R. (1987). Implications of normal brain development for the pathogenesis of schizophrenia. *Arch. Gen Psychiatry*, 44, 660–669.

Weinberger, D. R. (1995). Neurodevelopmental perspecitves on schizophrenia. In *Psychopharmacology: The Fourth Generation of Progress*, (F. E. Bloom and D. J. Kupfer, Eds.), pp. 1171–1183. Raven Press, New York.

Weinberger, D. R., Berman, K. F., and Illowsky, B. P. (1988). Physiological dysfunction of dorsolateral prefrontal cortex in schizophrenia. III. A new cohort and evidence for a monoaminergic mechanism. *Arch. Gen. Psychiatry*, 45, 609–615.

Weinberger, D. R., Berman, K. F., and Zec, R. F. (1986). Physiologic dysfunction of dorsolateral prefrontal cortex in schizophrenia: I. Regional cerebral blood flow evidence. *Arch. Gen. Psychiatry*, 43, 114–124.

Weiner, D. M., Levey, A. I., and Brann, M. R. (1990). Expression of muscarinic acetylcholine and dopamine receptor mRNAs in rat basal ganglia. *Proc. Natl. Acad. Sci. U.S.A.*, 87, 7050–7054.

Weiner, N. (1985a). Atropine, scopolamine, and related muscarinic drugs. In *The Pharmacological Basis of Therapeutics* (7th ed.) (A. G. Gilman, L. S. Goodman, T. W. Rall, and F. Murad, Eds.), pp. 130–144. Macmillan, New York.

Weiner, N. (1985b). Drugs that inhibit adrenergic nerves and block adrenergic receptors. In *The Pharmacological Basis of Therapeutics* (A. G. Gilman, L. S. Goodman, T. W. Rall and F. Murad, Eds.), pp. 181–214. Macmillan, New York.

Weiner, N. (1985c). Norepinephrine, epinephrine, and the sympathomimetic amines. In *The Pharmacological Basis of Therapeutics* (A. G. Gilman, L. S. Goodman, T. W. Rall, and F. Murad, Eds.), pp. 145–180. Macmillan, New York.

Weiner, R. D., and Krystal, A. D. (1994). The present use of electroconvulsive therapy. *Annu. Rev. Med.*, 45, 273–281.

Weinshank, R. L., Adham, N., Macchi, M., Olsen, M. A., Branchek, T. A., and Hartig, P. R. (1991). Molecular cloning and characterization of a high affinity dopamine receptor (D$_{1b}$) and its pseudogene. *J. Biol. Chem.*, 266, 22427–22435.

Weinshank, R. L., Zgombick, J. M., Macchi, M. J., Branchek, T. A., and Hartig, P. R. (1992). Human serotonin 1D receptor is encoded by a subfamily of two distinct genes: 5-HT$_{1Da}$ and 5-HT$_{1Db}$. *Proc. Natl. Acad. Sci. U.S.A.*, 89, 3630–3634.

Weinstein, H., Maayani, S., and Pazhenchevsky, B. (1983). Multiple actions of phencyclidine: Discriminant structure-activity relationships from molecular conforma-

tions and assay conditions. *Fed. Proc.*, 42, 2574–2578.

Weinswig, M. H. (1973). *Use and Misuse of Drugs Subject to Abuse*. Pegasus, New York.

Weintraub, M. (1992a). Long-term weight control: The National Heart, Lung, and Blood Institute funded multimodal intervention study. Introduction. *Clin. Pharmacol. Ther.*, 51, 581–585.

Weintraub, M. (1992b). Long-term weight control study: Conclusions. *Clin. Pharmacol. Ther.*, 51, 642–645.

Weintraub, M., Sundaresan, P. R., Madan, M., Schuster, B., Balder, A., Lasagna, L., and Cox, C. (1992). Long-term weight control study I (weeks 0 to 34). *Clin. Pharmacol. Ther.*, 51, 586–594.

Weiss, B., and Laties, V. G. (1961). Changes in brain tolerance and other behavior produced by salicylates. *J. Pharmacol. Exp. Ther.*, 113, 120–129.

Weiss, B., and Laties, V. G. (1962). Enhancement of human performance by caffeine and the amphetamines. *Pharmacol. Rev.*, 14, 1–36.

Weiss, G. F., Papadakos, P., Knudson, K., and Leibowitz, S. F. (1986). Medial hypothalamic serotonin: Effects on deprivation and norepinephrine-induced eating. *Pharmacol. Biochem. Behav.*, 25, 1223–1230.

Weissman, A., Koe, B. K., and Tenen, S. S. (1966). Antiamphetamine effects following inhibition of tyrosine hydroxylase. *J. Pharmacol. Exp. Ther.*, 151, 339–352.

Weissman, M. M., and Boyd, J. D. (1984). The epidemiology of affective disorders. In *Neurobiology of Mood Disorders* (R. M. Post and J. C. Ballenger, Eds.), pp. 60–75. Williams and Wilkins, Baltimore.

Weissman, M. M., Klerman, G. L., Prusoff, B. A., Sholomskas, D., and Padian, N. (1981). Depressed outpatients: Results one year after treatment with drugs and/or interpersonal psychotherapy. *Arch. Gen. Psychiatry*, 38, 51–55.

Weizman, R., Weizman, A., Kook, K. A., Vocci, F., Deutsch, S. T., and Paul, S. M. (1989). Repeated swim stress alters brain benzodiazepine receptors measured in vivo. *J. Pharmacol. Exp. Ther.*, 249, 701–707.

Weizman, R., Weizman, A., Tyano, S., Szekely, G., Weissman, B. A., and Sarne, Y. (1984). Humoral-endorphin blood levels in autistic schizophrenic and healthy subjects. *Psychopharmacology*, 82, 368–370.

Wellman, P. J., Davies, B. T., Morien, A., and McMahon, L. (1993). Modulation of feeding by hypothalamic paraventricular nucleus α_1- and α_2-adrenergic receptors. *Life Sci.*, 53, 669–679.

Welsh, J. H. (1957). Serotonin as a possible neurohumoral agent. Evidence obtained in lower animals. *Ann. N.Y. Acad. Sci.*, 66, 618–630.

Wender, P. H. (1978). Minimal brain dysfunction: An overview. In *Psychopharmacology: A Generation of Progress* (M. A. Lipton, A. DiMascio and K. F. Killam, Eds.), pp. 1429–1435. Raven Press, New York.

Wenk, G. L. (1993). A primate model of Alzheimer's disease. *Behav. Brain Res.*, 57, 117–122.

Werman, R. (1966). Criteria for identification of a central nervous system transmitter. *Comp. Biochem. Physiol.*, 18, 745–766.

Wernicke, C. (1908). The symptom complex of aphasia. In *Diseases of the Nervous System*

(A. Church, Ed.), 265–324. Appleton, New York.

Wert, R. C., and Raulin, M. L. (1986a). The chronic cerebral effects of cannabis use. I. Methodological issues and neurological findings. *Int. J. Addict.*, 21, 605–628.

Wert, R. C., and Raulin, M. L. (1986b). The chronic cerebral effects of cannabis use. II. Psychological findings and conclusions. *Int. J. Addict.*, 21, 629–642.

Wess, J. (1993a). Molecular basis of muscarinic acetylcholine receptor function. *Trends Pharmacol. Sci.*, 14, 308–313.

Wess, J. (1993b). Mutational analysis of muscarinic acetylcholine receptors: Structural basis of ligand/receptor/G protein interactions. *Life Sci.*, 53, 1447–1463.

Wessel, T. C., and Joh, T. J. (1992). Parallel up-regulation of catecholamine-synthesizing enzymes in rat brain and adrenal gland: Effects of reserpine and correlation with immediate early gene expression. *Mol. Brain Res.*, 15, 349–360.

Wessels-Reiker, M., Haycock, J. W., Howlett, A. C., and Strong, R. (1991). Vasoactive intestinal polypeptide induces tyrosine hydroxylase in PC12 cells. *J. Biol. Chem.*, 266, 9347–9350.

Wessendorf, M. W., and Elde, R. P. (1987). The coexistence of serotonin and substance P-like immunoreactivity in the spinal cord as shown by immunofluorescent double labeling. *J. Neurosci.*, 7, 2352–2363.

Wessinger, W. D., and Owens, M. (1991). Phencyclidine dependence: The relationship of dose and serum concentrations to operant behavioral effects. *J. Pharmacol. Exp. Ther.*, 258, 207–215.

Wessler, I. (1989). Control of transmitter release from the motor nerve by presynaptic nicotinic and muscarinic autoreceptors. *Trends Pharmacol. Sci.*, 10, 110–114.

West, J. R., Goodlett, C. R., Bonthius, D. J., Hamre, K. M., and Marcussen, B. L. (1990). Cell population depletion associated with fetal alcohol brain damage: Mechanisms of BAC-dependent cell loss. *Alcohol. Clin. Exp. Res.*, 14, 813–818.

West, L. J. (Moderator), (1984). Alcoholism. *Ann. Intern. Med.*, 100, 405–416.

West, M. J., Coleman, P. D., Flood, D. G., and Troncoso, J. C. (1994). Differences in the pattern of hippocampal neuronal loss in normal ageing and Alzheimer's disease. *Lancet*, 344, 769–772.

West, R. J., Jarvis, M. J. Russell, M. A. H., Carruthers, M. E., and Feyerabend, C. (1984). Effect of nicotine replacement on the cigarette withdrawal syndrome. *Br. J. Addict.*, 79, 215–219.

West, W. B., Van Groll, B. J., and Appel, J. B. (1995). Stimulus effects of *d*-amphetamine II: DA, NE, and 5-HT mechanisms. *Pharmacol. Biochem. Behav.*, 51, 69–76.

Westerink, B. H. C. (1985). Sequence and significance of dopamine metabolism in the rat brain. *Neurochem. Int.*, 7, 221–227.

Westerink, B. H. C., and De Vries, J. B. (1991). Effect of precursor loading on the synthesis rate and release of dopamine and serotonin in the striatum: A microdialysis study in conscious rats. *J. Neurochem.*, 56, 228–233.

Westerink, B. H. C., Tuntler, J., Damsma, G., Rollema, H., and de Vries, J. B. (1987). The use of tetrodotoxin for the characterization of drug-enhanced dopamine release in conscious rats studied by brain dialysis.

Naunyn Schmiedebergs Arch. Pharmacol., 336, 502–507.

Westerink, B. H. C., and Van Putten, F. M. S. (1987). Simultaneous determination of the rates of synthesis and metabolism of dopamine in various areas of the rat brain: Application to the effects of (–)-amphetamine. *Eur. J. Pharmacol.*, 133, 103–110.

Westlund, K. N., Denney, R. M., Kochersperger, L. M., Rose, R. M., and Abell, C. W. (1985). Distinct monoamine oxidase A and B populations in primate brain. *Science*, 230, 181–183.

Westlund, K. N., Denney, R. M., Rose, R. M., and Abell, C. W. (1988). Localization of distinct monoamine oxidase A and monoamine oxidase B cell populations in human brainstem. *Neuroscience*, 25, 439–456.

Wettstein, J. G., Buéno, L., and Junien, J. L. (1994). CCK antagonists: Pharmacology and therapeutic interest. *Pharmacol. Ther.*, 62, 267–282.

Whishaw, I. Q., and Tomie, J.-A. (1987). Cholinergic receptor blockade produces impairments in a sensorimotor subsystem for place navigation in the rat: Evidence from sensory, motor, and acqusition tests in a swimming pool. *Behav. Neurosci.*, 101, 603–616.

White, F. J., and Wang, R. Y. (1984a). Electrophysiological evidence for A10 dopamine autoreceptor subsensitivity following chronic D-amphetamine treatment. *Brain Res.*, 309, 283–292.

White, F. J., and Wang, R. Y. (1984b). Pharmacological characterization of dopamine autoreceptors in the rat ventral tegmental area: Microiontophoretic studies. *J. Pharmacol. Exp. Ther.*, 231, 275–280.

White, J. D., Stewart, K. D., Krause, J. E., and McKelvy, J. F. (1985). Biochemistry of peptide-secreting neurons. *Physiol. Rev.*, 65, 553–606.

White, J. M., and Rumbold, G. R. (1988). Behavioural effects of histamine and its antagonists: A review. *Psychopharmacology*, 95, 1–14.

White, N. M. (1989). Reward or reinforcement: What's the difference? *Neurosci. Biobehav. Rev.*, 13, 181–186.

White, N. M., Packard, M. G., and Hiroi, N. (1991). Place conditioning with dopamine D_1 and D_2 agonists injected peripherally or into nucleus accumbens. *Psychopharmacology*, 103, 271–276.

White, S. H. (1986). The physical nature of planar bilayer membranes. In *Ion Channel Reconstituition* (C. Miller, Ed.), pp. 3–36. Plenum Press, New York.

White, S. M., Kucharik, R. F., and Moyer, J. A. (1991). Effects of serotonergic agents on isolation-induced aggression. *Pharmacol. Biochem. Behav.*, 39, 729–736.

Whitehouse, P. K., Martino, A. M., Antuono, P. J., Lowenstein, P. R., Coyle, J. T., Price, D. L., and Kellar, K. J. (1986). Nicotinic acetylcholine binding sites in Alzheimer's disease. *Brain Res.*, 371, 146–151.

Whiting, P., McKernan, R. M., and Iversen, L. L. (1990). Another mechanism for creating diversity in γ-aminobutyrate type A receptors: RNA splicing directs expression of two forms of γ2 subunit, one of which contains a protein kinase C phosphorylation site. *Proc. Natl. Acad. Sci. U.S.A.*, 87, 9966–9970.

Whittaker, V. P. (1987). Cholinergic synaptic vesicles from the electromotor nerve terminals of *Torpedo*: Composition and life cycle. *Ann. N.Y. Acad. Sci.*, 493, 77–91.

Wichmann, T., Vitek, J. L., and DeLong, M. R. (1995). Parkinson's disease and the basal ganglia: Lessons from the laboratory and from neurosurgery. *The Neuroscientist*, 1, 236–244.

Widerlöv, E., and Lewander, T. (1978). Inhibition of the in vivo biosynthesis and change of catecholamine levels in rat brain after alpha methyl-*p*-tyrosine: Time and dose–response relationships. *Naunyn Schmiedebergs Arch. Pharmacol.*, 304, 111–123.

Wiemann, J. N., Clifton, D. K., and Steiner, R. A. (1989). Pubertal changes in gonadotropin-releasing hormone and proopiomelanocortin gene expression in the brain of the male rat. *Endocrinology*, 124, 1760–1767.

Wightman, R. M., Amatore, C., Engstrom, R. C., Hale, P. D., Kristensen, E. W., Kuhr, W. G., and May, L. J. (1988). Real-time characterization of DA overflow and uptake in rat striatum. *Neuroscience*, 25, 513–523.

Wightman, R. M., Brown, D. S., Kuhr, W. G., and Wilson, R. L. (1987). Molecular specificity of in vivo electrochemical measurements. In *Voltammetry in the Neurosciences* (J. B. Justice, Ed.), pp. 103–138. Humana Press, Clifton, NJ.

Wikler, A. (1973). Dynamics of drug dependence: Implications of a conditioning theory for research and treatment. *Arch. Gen. Psychiatry*, 28, 611–616.

Wikler, A. (1980). Conditioning processes in dependence and relapse. In *Opioid Dependence: Mechanisms and Treatment*, pp. 167–218. Plenum Press, New York.

Wiklund, L., Toggenburger, G., and Cuénod, M. (1982). Aspartate: Possible neurotransmitter in cerebellar climbing fibers. *Science*, 216, 78–79.

Wildmann, J., Möhler, H., Vetter, W., Ranalder, U., Schmidt, K., and Maurer, R. (1987). Diazepam and N-desmethyldiazepam are found in rat brain and adrenal and may be of plant origin. *J. Neural Transm.*, 70, 383–398.

Wilens, T. E., Biederman, J., Spencer, T. J., and Prince, J. (1995). Pharmacotherapy of adult attention deficit/hyperactivity disorder: A review. *J. Clin. Psychopharmacol.*, 15, 270–279.

Wiley, R. G., Oeltmann, T. N., and Lappi, D. (1991). Immunolesioning: Selective destruction of neurons using immunotoxin to rat NGF receptor. *Brain Res.*, 562, 149–153.

Willetts, J., and Balster, R. L. (1988). The discriminative stimulus effects of N-methyl-D-aspartate antagonists in phencyclidine-trained rats. *Neuropharmacology*, 27, 1249–1256.

Willetts, J., Balster, R. L., and Leander, J. D. (1990). The behavioral pharmacology of NMDA receptor antagonists. *Trends Pharmacol. Sci.*, 11, 423–428.

Williams, B. J., and Pirch, J. H. (1974). Correlation between brain adenyl cyclase activity and spontaneous motor activity in rats after chronic reserpine treatment. *Brain Res.*, 68, 227–234.

Williams, E. F., Rice, K., Mattson, M., Paul, S. M., and Skolnick, P. (1981). In vivo effects of two novel alkylating benzodiazepines,

irazepine and kenazepine. *Pharmacol. Biochem. Behav.*, 14, 487–491.

Williams, J. R., Insel, T. R., Harbaugh, C. R., and Carter, C. S. (1994). Oxytocin administered centrally facilitates formation of a partner preference in female prairie voles (*Microtus ochrogaster*). *J. Neuroendocrinol.*, 6, 247–250.

Willner, P. (1985a). Antidepressants and serotonergic neurotransmission: An integrative review. *Psychopharmacology*, 85, 387–404.

Willner, P. (1985b). *Depression: A Psychobiological Synthesis*. Wiley, New York.

Willner, P. (1994). Animal models of depression. In *Handbook of Depression and Anxiety* (J. A. den Boer and J. M. Ad Sitsen, Eds.), pp. 291–316. Marcel Dekker, New York.

Willner, P. (1995). Dopaminergic mechanisms in depression and mania. In *Psychopharmacology: The Fourth Generation of Progress* (F. E. Bloom and D. J. Kupfer, Eds.), pp. 921–932. Raven Press, New York.

Willoughby, J., Glover, V., and Sandler, M. (1988). Histochemical localisation of monoamine oxidase A and B in rat brain. *J. Neural Transm.*, 74, 29–42.

Willow, M., and Johnston, G. A. R. (1983). Pharmacology of barbiturates: Electrophysiological and neurochemical studies. *Int. Rev. Neurobiol.*, 24, 15–49.

Wilson, A. L., Langley, L. K., Monley, J., Bauer, T., Rottunda, S., McFalls, E., Kovera, C., and McCarten, J. R. (1995). Nicotine patches in Alzheimer's disease: Pilot study on learning, memory, and safety. *Pharmacol. Biochem. Behav.*, 51, 509–514.

Wilson, I. C., Prange, A. J. Jr., McClane, T. K., Rabon, A. M., and Lipton, M. A. (1970). Thyroid hormone enhancement of imipramine in nonretarded depressions. *N. Engl. J. Med.*, 282, 1063–1067.

Wilson, K. M., and Minneman, K. P. (1989). Regional variations in α_1-adrenergic receptor subtypes in rat brain. *J. Neurochem.*, 53, 1782–1786.

Winkler, H., Apps, D. K., and Fischer-Colbrie, R. (1986). The molecular function of adrenal chromaffin granules: Established facts and unresolved topics. *Neuroscience*, 18, 261–290.

Winkler, H., Sietzen, M., and Schober, M. (1987). The life cycle of catecholamine-storing vesicles. *Ann. N.Y. Acad. Sci.*, 493, 3–19.

Winslow, J. T., Hastings, N., Carter, C. S., Harbaugh, C. R., and Insel, T. R. (1993). A role for central vasopressin in pair bonding in monogamous prairie voles. *Nature*, 365, 545–548.

Winslow, J. T., and Insel, T. R. (1991). Infant rat separation is a sensitive test for novel anxiolytics. *Prog. Neuropsychopharmacol. Biol. Psychiatry*, 15, 745–757.

Winslow, J. T., Shapiro, L., Carter, C. S., and Insel, T. R. (1993). Oxytocin and complex social behavior: Species comparisons. *Psychopharmacol. Bull.*, 29, 409–414.

Wirshing, W. C., Marder, S. R., Van Putten, T., and Ames, D. (1995). Acute treatment of schizophrenia. In *Psychopharmacology: The Fourth Generation of Progress*, (F. E. Bloom and D. J. Kupfer, Eds.), pp. 1259–1266. Raven Press, New York.

Wirz-Justice, A. (1988). Platelet research in psychiatry. *Experientia*, 44, 145–152.

Wirz-Justice, A. (1995). Biological rhythms in mood disorders. In *Psychopharmacology: The Fourth Generation of Progress* (F. E. Bloom and D. J. Kupfer, Eds.), pp. 999–1018. Raven Press, New York.

Wisden, W., Laurie, D. J., Monyer, H., and Seeburg, P. H. (1992). The distribution of 13 GABA$_A$ receptor subunit mRNAs in the rat brain. I. Telecephalon, diencephalon, mesencephalon. *J. Neurosci., 12*, 1040–1062.

Wise, C. D., Berger, B. D., and Stein, L. (1973). Evidence of α-noradrenergic reward receptors and serotonergic punishment receptors in the rat brain. *Biol. Psychiatry, 6*, 3–21.

Wise, R. A., Bauco, P., Carlezon, W. A. Jr., and Trojniar, W. (1992). Self-stimulation and drug reward mechanisms. *Ann. N.Y. Acad. Sci., 654*, 192–198.

Wise, R. A., and Bozarth, M. A. (1987). A psychomotor stimulant theory of addiction. *Psychol. Bull., 94*, 469–492.

Wise, R. A., and Rompre, P.-P. (1989). Brain dopamine and reward. *Annu. Rev. Psychol., 40*, 191–225.

Wisniewski, K. E., Wisniewski, H. M., and Wen, G. Y. (1985). Occurrence of neurological changes and dementia of Alzheimer's disease in Down's syndrome. *Ann. Neurol., 17*, 278–282.

Wisniewski, T., and Frangione, B. (1992). Apolipoprotein E: A pathological chaperone protein in patients with cerebral and systemic amyloid. *Neurosci. Lett., 135*, 235–238.

Wisniewski, T., Palha, J., Ghiso, J., and Frangione, B. (1995). S182 protein in Alzheimer's disease neuritic plaques. *Lancet, 346*, 1366.

Witkin, J. M. (1993). Blockade of the locomotor stimulant effects of cocaine and methamphetamine by glutamate antagonists. *Life Sci., 53*, PL 405–410.

Witkin, J. M. (1994). Pharmacotherapy of cocaine abuse: Preclinical development. *Neurosci. Biobehav. Rev., 18*, 121–142.

Witschi, H., Pinkerton, K. E., Coggins, R. E., Penn, A., and Gori, G. B. (1995). Environmenta tobacco smoke: Experimental facts and sociatal issues. *Fundam. Appl. Toxicol., 24*, 3–12.

Witt, D. M., and Insel, T. R. (1991). A selective oxytocin antagonist attenuates progesterone facilitation of female sexual behavior. *Endocrinology, 128*, 3269–3276.

Wojcik, W. J., and Holopainen, I. (1992). Role of central GABA$_B$ receptors in physiology and pathology. *Neuropsychopharmacology, 6*, 201–214.

Wolf, W. A., and Kuhn, D. M. (1990). Modulation of serotonin release: Interactions between the serotonin transporter and autoreceptors. *Ann. N.Y. Acad. Sci., 604*, 505–513.

Wolff, J. A., et al. (1989). Grafting fibroblasts genetically modified to produce L-dopa in a rat model of Parkinson disease. *Proc. Natl. Acad. Sci. U.S.A., 86*, 9011–9014.

Wolff, J. R., Laskawi, R., Spatz, W. B., and Missler, M. (1995). Structural dynamics of synapses and synaptic components. *Behav. Brain Res., 66*, 13–20.

Wolkin, A., Jaeger, J., Brodie, J. D., Wolf, A. P., Fowler, J., Rotrosen, J., Gomez-Mont, F., and Cancro, R. (1985). Persistence of cerebral metabolism abnormalities in chronic schizophrenia as determined by positron emission tomography. *Am. J. Psychiatry, 142*, 564–571.

Wolkin, A., Sanfilipo, M., Wolf, A. P., Angrist, B., Brodle, J. D. Rotrosen, J. (1992). Negative symptoms and hypofrontality in chronic

schizophrenia. *Arch. Gen. Psychiatry, 49*, 959–965.

Wolkowitz, O. M., Gertz, B., Weingartner, H., Beccaria, L., Thompson, K., and Liddle, R. A. (1990). Hunger in humans induced by MK-329, a specific peripheral-type cholecystokinin receptor antagonist. *Biol. Psychiatry, 28*, 169–173.

Wollemann, M., Benyhe, S., and Simon, J. (1993). The kappa-opioid receptor: Evidence for the different subtypes. *Life Sci., 52*, 599–611.

Wong, D. F. (1986). Positron emission tomography reveals elevated D$_2$ dopamine receptors in drug-naive schizophrenics. *Science, 234*, 1558–1561.

Wong, D. L., Zager, E. L., and Ciaranello, R. D. (1982). Effects of hypophysectomy and dexamethasone administration on central and peripheral *S*-adenosylmethionine levels. *J. Neurosci., 2*, 758–764.

Wong, D. T., Threlkeld, P. G., and Robertson, D. W. (1991). Affinities of fluoxetine, its enantiomers, and other inhibitors of serotonin uptake for subtypes of serotonin receptors. *Neuropsychopharmacology, 5*, 43–47.

Wonnacott, S., and Dajas, F. (1994). Neurotoxins: Nature's untapped bounty. *Trends Pharmacol. Sci., 15*, 1–3.

Wonnacott, S., Jackman, S., Swanson, K. L., Rapoport, H., and Albuquerque, E. X. (1991). Nicotinic pharmacology of anatoxin analogs. II. Side chain structure–activity relationships at neuronal nicotinic ligand binding sites. *J. Pharmacol. Exp. Ther., 259*, 387–391.

Wood, A., Tollefson, G. D., and Birkett, M. (1993). Pharmacotherapy of obsessive–compulsive disorder: Experience with fluoxetine. *Int. Clin. Psychopharmacol., 8*, 301–306.

Wood, A. A. (1985). Tobacco advertising's target. (Letter). *Lancet, 1*(8435), 985.

Wood, J., and Garthwaite, J. (1994). Models of the diffusional spread of nitric oxide: Implications for neural nitric oxide signalling and its pharmacological properties. *Neuropharmacology, 33*, 1235–1244.

Wood, J. H., Hare, T. A., Glaeser, B. S., Ballenger, J. C., and Post, R. M. (1979). Low cerebrospinal fluid γ-aminobutyric acid content in seizure patients. *Neurology, 29*, 1203 - 1208.

Wood, P. L., and Altar, C. A. (1988). Dopamine release in vivo from nigrostriatal, mesolimbic, and mesocortical neurons: Utility of 3-methoxytyramine measurements. *Pharmacol. Rev., 40*, 163–187.

Wood, P. L., et al. (1990). A review of the in vitro and in vivo neurochemical characterization of the NMDA/PCP/glycine/ion channel receptor macrocomplex. *Neurochem. Res., 15*, 217–230.

Woodruff, G. N., Hill, D. R., Boden, P., Pinnock, R., Singh, L., and Hughes, J. (1991). Functional role of brain CCK receptors. *Neuropeptides, 19* (Suppl.), 45–56.

Woodruff, G. N., and Hughes, J. (1991). Cholecystokinin antagonists. *Annu. Rev. Pharmacol. Toxicol., 31*, 469–501.

Woods, J. H., France, C. P., Winger, G., Bertalmio, A. J., and Schwarz-Stevens, K. (1993). Opioid abuse liability assessment in rhesus monkeys. In *Opioids II,*, Handbook of Experimental Pharmacology, Vol. 104 (A. Herz, Ed.), pp. 609–632. Springer-Verlag, New York.

Woods, J. H., Katz, J. L., and Winger, G. D. (1992). Benzodiazepines, use, abuse and consequences. *Pharmacological Rev., 44*, 151–347.

Woods, J. H., and Winger, G. (1987). Opioid, receptors, and abuse liability. In *Psychopharmacology: The Third Generation of Progress* (H. Y. Meltzer, Ed.), pp. 1555–1564. Raven Press, New York.

Woods, S. K., and Meyer, J. S. (1991). Exogenous tyrosine potentiates the methylphenidate-induced increase in extracellular dopamine in the nucleus accumbens: A microdialysis study. *Brain Res., 560*, 97–105.

Wooley, D. W., and Shaw, E. N. (1954). Some neurophysiological aspects of serotonin. *Br. Med. J., 2*, 122–125.

Woolf, N. J. (1991). Cholinergic systems in mammalian brain and spinal cord. *Prog. Neurobiol., 37*, 475–524.

Woolfe, G., and MacDonald, A. D. (1944). The evaluation of the analgesic action of pethidine hydrochloride (Demerol). *J. Pharmacol. Exp. Ther., 80*, 300–307.

Woolverton, W. L., and Cervo, L. (1986). Effects of central dopamine depletion on the *d*-amphetamine discriminative stimulus in rats. *Psychopharmacology, 88*, 196–200.

Woolverton, W. L., Goldberg, L. I., and Ginos, J. Z. (1984). Intravenous self-administration of dopamine receptor agonists by rhesus monkeys. *J. Pharmacol. Exp. Ther., 230*, 678–683.

Woolverton, W. L., and Johnson, K. M. (1992). Neurobiology of cocaine abuse. *Trends Pharmacol. Sci., 13*, 193–200.

Worley, P. F., Heller, W. A., and Snyder, S. H. (1988). Lithium blocks a phosphoinositide-mediated cholinergic response in hippocampal slices. *Science, 239*, 1428–1429.

Wragg, M., Hutton, M., Talbot, C., and the Alzheimer's Disease Collaborative Group. (1996). Genetic association between intronic polymorphism in presenilin-1 gene and late-onset Alzheimer's disease. *Lancet, 347*, 509–512.

Wu, D., and Hersh, L. B. (1994). Choline acetyltransferase: Celebrating its fiftieth year. *J. Neurochem., 62*, 1653–1663.

Wu, J. C., Buchsbaum, M. S., and Bunney, W. E. (1991). Positron emission tomography study of phencyclidine users as a possible drug model of schizophrenia. *Jpn. J. Psychopharmacol., 11*, 47–48.

Wu, J. C., and Bunney, W. E. (1990). The biological basis of an antidepressant response to sleep deprivation and relapse: Review and hypothesis. *Am. J. Psychiatry, 147*, 14–21.

Wurtman, J. J. (1990). Carbohydrate craving. Relationships between carbohydrate intake and disorders of mood. *Drugs, 39* (Suppl. 3), 49–52.

Wurtman, J. J., Wurtman, R. J., Berry, E., Gleason, R., Goldberg, H., McDermott, J., Kahne, M., and Tsay, R. (1993). Dexfenfluramine, fluoxetine, and weight loss among female carbohydrate cravers. *Neuropsychopharmacology, 9*, 201–210.

Wurtman, J. J., Wurtman, R. J., Growdon, J. H., Henry, P., Lipscomb, A., and Zeisel, S. H. (1981). Carbohydrate craving in obese people: Suppression by treatments affecting serotoninergic transmission. *Int. J. Eating Dis., 1*, 2–15.

Wurtman, R. J., Larin, F., Mostafapour, S., and Fernstrom, J. D. (1974). Brain catechol synthesis: Control by brain tyrosine concentration. *Science,* 185, 183–184.

Wurtman, R. J., and Wurtman, J. J. (1988). Do carbohydrates affect food intake via neurotransmitter activity? *Appetite,* 11 (Suppl.), 42–47.

Wuster, M., Costa, T., Aktories, K., and Jacobs, K. H. (1984). Sodium regulation of opioid agonist binding is potentiated by pertussis toxin. *Biochem. Biophys. Res. Commun.,* 123, 1107–1115.

Wuster, M., Costa, T., and Gramsch, C. (1983). Uncoupling of receptors is essential for opiate-induced desensitization (tolerance) in neuroblastoma x glioma hybrid cells NG 108–15. *Life Sci.,* 33 (Suppl 1), 341–344.

Wyatt, R. J. (1996). Neurodevelopmental abnormalities and schizophrenia: A family affair. *Arch. Gen. Psychiatry,* 53, 11–15.

Yadin, E., Guarini, V., and Gallistel, C. R. (1983). Unilaterally activated systems in rats self-stimulating at site in the media forebrain bundle, medial prefrontal cortex, or locus coeruleus. *Brain Res.,* 266, 39–50.

Yakeley, J., and Murray, R. M. (1995). Genetic and environmental risk factors for schizophrenia. In *Critical Issues in the Treatment of Schizophrenia* (N. Brunello, G. Racagni, S. Z. Langer, and J. Mendlewicz, Eds.), p. 9–34. Karger, Basel.

Yaksh, T. L. (1993). The spinal actions of opioids. In *Opioids II,,* Handbook of Experimental Pharmacology, Vol. 104 (A. Herz, Ed.), pp. 53–89. Springer-Verlag, New York.

Yaksh, T. L., Jessell, T. M., Gamse, R., Mudge, A. W., and Leeman, S. E. (1980). Intrathecal morphine inhibits substance P release from mammalian spinal cord in vivo. *Nature,* 286, 155–157.

Yalow, R. S. (1978). Radioimmunoassay: A probe for the fine structure of biologic systems. *Science,* 200, 1236–1245.

Yamaguchi, H., Ishiguro, K., Sugihara, S., Nakazato, Y., Kawarabayashi, T., Sun, X., and Hirai, S. (1994). Presence of apolipoprotein E on extracellular neurofibrillary tangles and on meningeal blood vessels precedes the Alzheimer β-amyloid deposition. *Acta Neuropathol.,* 88, 413–419.

Yamamoto, B. K., and Davy, S. (1992). Dopaminergic modulation of glutamate release in striatum measured by microdialysis. *J. Neurochem.,* 58, 1736–1742.

Yamamoto, T., Geiger, J. D., Daddona, P. E., and Nagy, J. I. (1987). Subcellular, regional and immunohistochemical localization of adenosine deaminase in various species. *Brain Res. Bull.,* 19, 473–484.

Yamamura, H. I., and Snyder, S. H. (1973). High affinity transport of choline into synaptosomes of rat brain. *J. Neurochem.,* 21, 1355–1374.

Yamamura, Y., Ogawa, H., Chihara, T., Kondo, K., Onogawa, T., Nakamura, S., Mori, T., Tominaga, M., and Yabuuchi, Y. (1991). OPC-21268, an orally effective, nonpeptide vasopressin V1 receptor antagonist. *Science,* 252, 572–574.

Yamashita, M., Fukui, H., Sugama, K., Horio, Y., Ito, S., Mizuguchi, H., and Wada, H. (1991). Expression cloning of a cDNA encoding the bovine histamine H_1 receptor. *Proc. Natl. Acad. Sci. U.S.A.,* 88, 11515–11519.

Yamatodani, A., Inagaki, N., Panula, P., Itowi, N., Watanabe, T., and Wada, H. (1991). Structure and functions of the histaminergic neurone system. In *Handbook of Experimental Pharmacology,* Vol. 97, *Histamine and Histamine Antagonists* (B. Uvnäs, ed.), pp. 243–283. Springer-Verlag, Berlin.

Yamauchi, T. and Fujisawa, H. (1979). In vitro phosphorylation of bovine adrenal tyrosine hydroxylase by adenosine 3':5'-monophosphate-dependent protein kinase. *J. Biol. Chem.,* 254, 503–507.

Yan, Q., and Johnson, E. M. J. (1989). Immunohistochemical localization and biochemical characterization of nerve growth factor receptor in adult rat brain. *J. Comp. Neurol.,* 290, 585–598.

Yang, H.-Y. T., and Neff, N. H. (1974). The monoamine oxidases of brain: Selective inhibition with drugs and the consequences for the metabolism of biogenic amines. *J. Pharmacol. Exp. Ther.,* 189, 733–740.

Yang, X.-M., and Dunn, A. J. (1990). Central $β_1$-adrenergic receptors are involved in CRF-induced defensive withdrawal. *Pharmacol. Biochem. Behav.,* 36, 847–851.

Yang, X.-M., Gorman, A. L., Dunn, A. J., and Goeders, N. E. (1992). Anxiogenic effects of acute and chronic cocaine administration: Neurochemical and behavioral studies. *Pharmacol. Biochem. Behav.,* 41, 643–650.

Yarden, Y., et al. (1986). The avian β-adrenergic receptor: Primary structure and membrane topology. *Proc. Natl. Acad. Sci. U.S.A.,* 83, 6795–6799.

Yasuda, K., Raynor, K., Kong, H., Breder, C. D., Takeda, J., reisine, T., and Bell, G. I. (1993). Cloning and functional comparison of kappa and delta opioid receptors from mouse brain. *Proc. Natl. Acad. Sci. U.S.A.,* 90, 6736–6740.

Yasuda, N., Greer, M. A., and Aizawa, T. (1982). Corticotropin-releasing factor. *Endocrinol. Rev.,* 3, 123–140.

Yasuda, R. P., Ciesla, W., Flores, L. R., Wall, S. J., Li, M., Satkus, S. A., Weisstein, J. S., Spagnola, B. V., and Wolfe, B. B. (1993). Development of antisera selective for m4 and m5 muscarinic cholinergic receptors: Distribution of m4 and m5 receptors in rat brain. *Mol. Pharmacol.,* 43, 149–157.

Yates, A. J. (1962). *Frustration and Conflict.* Van Nostrand, New York.

Yeh, S. Y., and De Souza, E. B. (1991). Lack of neurochemical evidence for neurotoxic effects of repeated cocaine administration in rats on brain monoamine neurons. *Drug Alcohol Depend.,* 27, 51–61.

Yen, C. I., Stranger, R. L., and Millman, N. (1959). Ataractic suppression of isolation-induced aggressive behavior. *Arch. Int. Pharmacodyn. Ther.,* 123, 179–185.

Yen, S.-H., Liu, W.-K., Hall, F. L., Yan, S.-D., Stern, D., and Dickson, D. W. (1995). Alzheimer neurofibrillary lesions: Molecular nature and potential roles of different compounds. *Neurobiol. Aging,* 16, 381–387.

Ylinen, A. M. A., Miettinen, R., Pitkänen, A., Gulyas, A. I., Freund, T. F., and Riekkinen, P. J. (1991). Enhanced GABAergic inhibition preserves hippocampal structure and function in a model of epilepsy. *Proc. Natl. Acad. Sci. U.S.A.,* 88, 7650–7653.

Yokel, R. A. (1987). Intravenous self-administration: Response rates, the effects of pharmacological challenges, and drug preference. In *Methods of Assessing the Reinforcing Properties of Drugs* (M. A. Bozarth, Ed.), pp. 1–33. Springer-Verlag, New York.

Yokel, R. A., and Wise, R. A. (1975). Increased lever pressing for amphetamine after pimozide in rats: Implications for a dopamine theory of reward. *Science,* 187, 547–549.

Yoshimura, M., and North, R. A. (1983). Substantia gelatinosa neurones in vitro hyperpolarized by enkephalin. *Nature,* 305, 529–530.

Youdim, M. B. H. (1988). Platelet monoamine oxidase B: Use and misuse. *Experientia,* 44, 137–141.

Youdim, M. B. H., Ben-Shachar, D., Yehuda, S., and Riederer, P. (1990). The role of iron in the basal ganglion. *Adv. Neurol.,* 53, 155–162.

Young, A. B. (1984). Glycine receptors in the nervous system. In *Brain Receptor Methodologies,* Vol. 2 (P. J. Marangos, I. Campbell, and R. M. Cohen, Eds.), pp. 37–57. Academic Press, New York.

Young, A. B., Frey, K. A., and Agranoff, B. W. (1986). Receptor assays: In vitro and in vivo. In *Positron Emission Tomography and Autoradiography: Principles and Applications for the Brain and Heart* (M. Phelps, J. Mazziotta, and H. Schelbert, Eds.), pp. 73–111. Raven Press, New York.

Young, A. M., and Herling, S. (1986). In *Behavioral Analysis of Drug Dependence* (S. R. Goldberg and I. P. Stolerman, Eds.), pp 9–67. Academic Press, New York.

Young, A. M., Katz, J. L., and Woods, J. H. (1981). Behavioral effects of levonantradol and nantradol in the rhesus monkey. *J. Clin. Pharmacol.,* 21, 348S–360S.

Young, E., Bronstein, D., and Akil, H. (1993). Proopiomelanocortin biosynthesis, processing and secretion: Functional implications. In *Opioids I,* Handbook of Experimental Pharmacology, Vol. 104 (A. Herz, Ed.), pp. 393–422. Springer-Verlag, New York.

Young, E. A. (1990). Induction of the intermediate lobe POMC system with chronic swim stress and β-adrenergic modulation of this induction. *Neuroendocrinology* 52, 405–411.

Young, J. Z. (1936). Structure of nerve fibers and synapses in some invertebrates. *Cold Spring Harbor Symp. Quant. Biol.,* 4, 1–6.

Young, L. T., Li, P. P., Kish, S. J., Siu, K. P., and Warsh, J. J. (1991). Postmortem cerebral cortex G_{sa}-subunit levels are elevated in bipolar affective disorder. *Brain Res.,* 553, 323–326.

Young, R., and Glennon, R. A. (1986). Discriminative stimulus properties of amphetamine and structurally related phenalkylamines. *Med. Res. Rev.,* 6, 99–130.

Young, R. F. (1989). Brain stimulation. In *Textbook of Pain* (2nd ed.) (P. D. Wall and R. Melzack, Eds.), pp. 925–929. Churchill Livingstone, Edinburgh.

Young, S. T., Porrino, L. J., and Iadarola, M. J. (1991). Cocaine induces striatal c-fos-immunoreactive proteins via dopaminergic D_1 receptors. *Proc. Natl. Acad. Sci. U.S.A.,* 88, 1291–1295.

Young, W. S., and Kuhar, M. J. (1980). Radiohistochemical localization of benzodiazepine receptors in rat brain. *J. Pharmacol. Exp. Ther.,* 212, 337–346.

Yu, D. S. L., Smith, F. L., Smith, D. G., and Lyness, W. H. (1986). Fluoxetine-induced attenuation of amphetamine self-administration in rats. *Life Sci.,* 39, 1383–1388.

Yu, S. S., Lefkowitz, R. J., and Hausdorff, W. P. (1993). β-Adrenergic receptor sequestration: A potential mechanism of receptor resensitization. *J. Biol. Chem.*, 268, 337–341.

Yuen, P. S. T., and Garbers, D. L. (1992). Guanylyl cyclase-linked receptors. *Annu. Rev. Neurosci.*, 15, 193–225.

Zabek, M., Mazurowski, W., Dymecki, J., Stelmachów, J., and Zawada, E. (1994). A long term follow-up of fetal dopaminergic neurons transplantation into the brain of three parkinsonian patients. *Restorative Neurol. Neurosci.*, 6, 97–106.

Zaczek, R., Battaglia, G., Culp, S., Appel, N. M., Contrera, J. F., and De Souza, E. B. (1990). Effects of repeated fenfluramine administration on indices of monoamine function in rat brain: Pharmacokinetic, dose response, regional specificity, and time course data. *J. Pharmacol. Exp. Ther.*, 253, 104–253.

Zaczek, R., Culp, S., and De Souza, E. B. (1991). Interactions of [^{3}H]amphetamine with rat brain synaptosomes. II. Active transport. *J. Pharmacol. Exp. Ther.*, 257, 830–835.

Zager, E. L., and Black, P. McL. (1985). Neuropeptides in human memory and learning processes. *Neurosurgery*, 17, 355–369.

Zagon, I. S., Gibo, D. M., and McLaughlin, P. J. (1992). Ontogeny of zeta, the opioid growth factor receptor, in the rat brain. *Brain Res.*, 596, 149–156.

Zagon, I. S., and McLaughlin, P. J. (1986). Opioid antagonist-induced modulation of cerebral and hippocampal development: Histological and morphometric studies. *Dev. Brain Res.*, 28, 233–246.

Zagon, I. S., and McLaughlin, P. J. (1991). Identification of opioid peptides regulating proliferation of neurons and glia in the developing nervous system. *Brain Res.*, 542, 318–323.

Zahniser, N. R., Cass, W. A., and Fitzpatrick, F. A. (1992). Signal transduction pathways involved in presynaptic receptor-mediated inhibition of dopamine release in rat striatum. *Neurochem. Int.*, 20 (Suppl.), 85S–88S.

Zametkin, A. J., and Rapoport, J. L. (1987). Noradrenergic hypothesis of attention deficit disorder with hyperactivity: A critical review. In *Psychopharmacology: The Third Generation of Progress* (H. Y. Meltzer, Ed.), pp. 837–859. Raven Press, New York.

Zarbin, M. A., Wamsley, J. K., and Kuhar, M. J. (1981). Glycine receptor: Light microscopic autoradiographic localization with [^{3}H]-strychnine. *J. Neurosci.*, 1, 532–547.

Zbinden, G., and Randall, L. O. (1967). Pharmacology of benzodiazepines: Laboratory and clinical correlations. *Adv. Pharmacol.*, 5, 213–291.

Zetterström, T., Vernet, T., Ungerstedt, U., Tossman, U., Jonzon, B., and Fredholm, B. B. (1982). Purine levels in the intact rat brain: Studies with an implanted perfused hollow fibre. *Neurosci. Lett.*, 29, 111–115.

Zezula, J., et al. (1988). Benzodiazepine receptor sites in the human brain: Autoradiographic mapping. *Neuroscience*, 25, 771–795.

Zhang, J., Chiodo, L. A., and Freeman, A. S. (1992). Electrophysiological effects of MK-801 on rat nigrostriatal and mesoaccumbal dopaminergic neurons. *Brain Res.*, 590, 153–163.

Zhang, S.-P., Zhou, L.-W., and Weiss, B. (1994). Oligodeoxynucleotide antisense to the D_1 dopamine receptor mRNA inhibits D_1 receptor-mediated behaviors in normal mice and in mice lesioned with 6-hydroxydopamine. *J. Pharmacol. Exp. Ther.*, 271, 1462–1470.

Zhang, Z.-X., and Roman, G. C. (1993). Worldwide occurrence of Parkinson's disease: An updated review. *Neuroepidemiology*, 12, 195–208.

Zhao, R. R., Fennell, W. H., and Abel, F. L. (1990). Effects of dopamine D_1 and dopamine D_2 receptor agonists on coronary and peripheral hemodynamics. *Eur. J. Pharmacol.*, 190, 193–202.

Zhou, Q.-Y., et al. (1990). Cloning and expression of human and rat D_1 dopamine receptors. *Nature*, 347, 76–80.

Zifa, E., and Fillion, G. (1992). 5-Hydroxytryptamine receptors. *Pharmacol. Rev.*, 44, 401–458.

Zigmond, M. J., Abercrombie, E. D., Berger, T. W., Grace, A. A., and Stricker, E. M. (1990). Compensations after lesions of central dopaminergic neurons: Some clinical and basic implications. *Trends Neurosci.*, 13, 290–296.

Zigmond, R. E. (1985). Biochemical consequences of synaptic stimulation: The regulation of tyrosine hydroxylase by multiple transmitters. *Trends Neurosci.*, 8 (2), 63–69.

Zigmond, R. E., Schon, F., and Iversen, L. L. (1974). Increased tyrosine hydroxylase activity in the locus coeruleus of rat brain stem after reserpine treatment and cold stress. *Brain Res.*, 70, 547–552.

Zigmond, R. E., Schwarzschild, M. A., and Rittenhouse, A. R. (1989). Acute regulation of tyrosine hydroxylase by nerve activity and by neurotransmitters via phosphorylation. *Annu. Rev. Neurosci.*, 12, 415–461.

Zimmermann, H., Volknandt, W., Wittich, B., and Hausinger, A. (1993). Synaptic vesicle life cycle and synaptic turnover. *J. Physiol.* (Paris), 87, 159–170.

Zubieta, J. K., and Frey, K. A. (1993). Autoradiographic mapping of M_3 muscarinic receptors in the rat brain. *J. Pharmacol. Exp. Ther.*, 264, 415–422.

Zuckerman, B., et al. (1989). Effects of maternal marijuana and cocaine use on fetal growth. *N. Engl. J. Med.*, 320, 762–768.

Zukin, R. S., Pellegrini-Giampietro, D. E., Knapp, C. M., and Tempel, A. (1993). Opioid receptor regulation. In *Opioids I*, Handbook of Experimental Pharmacology, Vol. 104 (A. Herz, Ed.), pp. 107–123. Springer-Verlag, New York.

Zukin, S. R., and Zukin, R. S. (1979). Specific [^{3}H]phencyclidine binding in rat central nervous system. *Proc. Natl. Acad. Sci. U.S.A.*, 76, 5372–5376.

Zukin, S. R., Zukin, R. S., Vale, W., Rivier, J., Nichtenhauser, R., Snell, L. D., and Johnson, K. M. (1987). An endogenous ligand of the brain s/PCP receptor antagonizes NMDA-induced neurotransmitter release. *Brain Res.*, 416, 84–89.

Zweben, J. E., and O'Connell, K. (1988). Strategies for breaking marijuana dependence. *J. Psychoactive Drugs*, 20, 121–127.

Illustration Credits

Index

About the book

Editor: Peter Farley
Project Editor: Kerry Falvey
Copy Editors: Norma Roche, Elaine Brown
Production Manager: Christopher Small
Book Production: Janice Holabird
Art: Precision Graphics; Network Graphics; Nancy Haver
Book Design: Bessas & Ackerman
Cover Design: MBDesign
Cover Manufacturer: Henry N. Sawyer Company Inc.
Book Manufacturer: Courier Companies, Inc.